INFECTIOUS DISEASES

For Elsevier

Commissioning Editor: *Sue Hodgson*
Development Editor: *Sven Pinczewski*
Editorial Assistant: *Poppy Garraway*
Project Manager: *Elouise Ball*
Copyeditor: *Isobel Black*
Design: *Charles Gray*
Illustration Manager: *Merlyn Harvey*
Illustrator: *Ethan Danielson*
Marketing Manager(s) (UK/USA): *Clara Toombs/Brenna Christiansen*

INFECTIOUS DISEASES

THIRD EDITION

Edited by

Jonathan Cohen
MB BS FRCP FRCPath FRCPE FMedSci
Professor of Infectious Diseases, and Dean
Brighton and Sussex Medical School
Honorary Consultant Physician, Royal Sussex
County Hospital
Brighton, UK

Steven M Opal
MD
Professor of Medicine Infectious Disease
Division, The Warren Alpert Medical School
of Brown University, Providence, RI, USA

William G Powderly
MD FRCPI
Professor of Medicine and Therapeutics
Head, UCD School of Medicine and
Medical Sciences, Health Sciences Centre
University College Dublin
Dublin, Ireland

Section editors

Thierry Calandra MD PhD
Professor of Medicine
Head, Infectious Diseases
Service, Department
of Internal Medicine
Centre Hospitalier
Universitaire Vaudois
Lausanne, Switzerland

Nathan Clumeck MD PhD
Professor of Infectious Diseases
Head, Department of
Infectious Diseases
St Pierre University Hospital
Brussels, Belgium

Jeremy Farrar FRCP FRCP
(Ed) FMedSci PhD OBE
Director
Oxford University Clinical
Research Unit
The Hospital for Tropical
Diseases
Ho Chi Minh City, Vietnam

Roger G Finch MB BS FRCP
FRCPath FRCPEd FFPM
Professor of Infectious
Diseases
School of Molecular Medical
Science
Division of Microbiology
and Infectious Disease
Nottingham University
Hospitals NHS Trust
Nottingham, UK

Scott M Hammer MD
Professor of Medicine
and Public Health
(Epidemiology)
Columbia University
Presbyterian Hospital
New York, NY, USA

Andy IM Hoepelman
MD PhD
Professor in Medicine,
Infectious Diseases Specialist
Head, Department of Internal
Medicine and Infectious
Diseases
University Medical Center
Utrecht, The Netherlands

Timothy E Kiehn PhD
Chief, Microbiology Service
Memorial Sloan-Kettering
Cancer Center
New York, NY, USA

Kieren A Marr MD
Director, Transplant and
Oncology
John Hopkins University
School of Medicine
Baltimore, MD, USA

Keith P W J McAdam MA
MB BChir FRCP FWACP
Emeritus Professor of Clinical
Tropical Medicine
London School of Hygiene
and Tropical Medicine
London, UK

Didier Raoult MD PhD
Professor, Faculté de
Médecine, Unité des
Rickettsies
WHO Collaborative Center
for Rickettsial Reference and
Research
Marseille, France

Robert T Schooley MD
Professor and Head
Division of Infectious Diseases
Academic Vice Chair
Department of Medicine
University of California
San Diego, La Jolla, CA

Jack D Sobel MD
Professor of Infectious
Diseases
Division Head, Infectious
Diseases
Wayne State University -
Medicine
Detroit, MI, USA

Jos WM van der Meer
MD PhD FRCP
Professor of Medicine
Department of General
Internal Medicine, Nijmegen
Institute for Infection,
Inflammation and Immunity
Radboud University Medical
Centre
Nijmegen, The Netherlands

MOSBY

ELSEVIER

MOSBY is an imprint of Elsevier Limited.
© 2010, Elsevier Limited. All rights reserved.

First published 1999
Second edition 2004
Third edition 2010
Chapters 4, 13, PP37, 120, 121, 126, 182 and 184 are US Government works in the public domain and not subject to copyright.

The right of Jonathan Cohen, Steven M Opal, William G Powderly, Thierry Calandra, Nathan Clumeck, Jeremy Farrar, Roger G Finch, Scott M Hammer, Andy IM Hoepelman, Timothy E Kiehn, Kieren A Marr, Keith PWJ McAdam, Didier Raoult, Robert T Schooley, Jack D Sobel and Jos WM van der Meer to be identified as authors of this work has been asserted by them in accordance with the Copyright, Designs and Patents Act 1988.

ISBN: 978-0-323-04579-7

British Library Cataloguing in Publication Data
Infectious diseases.-3rd ed.
  1. Communicable diseases 2. Communicable diseases - Diagnosis 3. Communicable diseases - Treatment
I. Cohen, J. (Jon), 1949-
616.9
ISBN-13: 9780323045797

Infectious diseases.-3rd ed., Expert consult premium ed.
  1. Communicable diseases 2. Communicable diseases - Diagnosis 3. Communicable diseases - Treatment
I. Cohen, J. (Jon), 1949-
616.9
ISBN-13: 9780723435037

Library of Congress Cataloging in Publication Data
A catalog record for this book is available from the Library of Congress

Notice
Medical knowledge is constantly changing. Standard safety precautions must be followed, but as new research and clinical experience broaden our knowledge, changes in treatment and drug therapy may become necessary or appropriate. Readers are advised to check the most current product information provided by the manufacturer of each drug to be administered to verify the recommended dose, the method and duration of administration, and contraindications. It is the responsibility of the practitioner, relying on experience and knowledge of the patient, to determine dosages and the best treatment for each individual patient. Neither the Publisher nor the author assume any liability for any injury and/or damage to persons or property arising from this publication.

The Publisher

ELSEVIER   your source for books,
             journals and multimedia
             in the health sciences
www.elsevierhealth.com

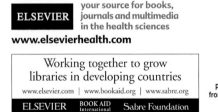

The publisher's policy is to use paper manufactured from sustainable forests

Printed in China
Last digit is the print number: 9 8 7 6 5 4 3 2 1

Contents

Contents

Section 3: Special Problems in Infectious Disease Practice

Jonathan Cohen & Steven M Opal

Contents

Section 4: Infections in the Immunocompromised Host

Thierry Calandra & Kieren A Marr

Volume 2

Section 5: HIV and AIDS

Nathan Clumeck & William G Powderly

PREVENTION

PATHOGENESIS

CLINICAL PRESENTATION

Section 6: International Medicine

Jeremy Farrar & Keith PWJ McAdam

MAJOR TROPICAL SYNDROMES: SKIN AND SOFT TISSUE

MAJOR TROPICAL SYNDROMES: THE CENTRAL NERVOUS SYSTEM

MAJOR TROPICAL SYNDROMES: THE GASTROINTESTINAL TRACT

Contents

Section 8: Clinical Microbiology

Andy IM Hoepelman & Timothy E Kiehn

VIRUSES

BACTERIA

FUNGI

PARASITES

Preface to the Third Edition

These are extraordinary times in the fields of microbiology and infectious diseases. The genomes of essentially all the major bacterial and viral pathogens known to infect humankind have now been sequenced and are available on public databases. The human genome project is now complete and whole genome sequencing of the major malaria parasite *Plasmodium falciparum* and the common fungal pathogen *Candida albicans* are now available on line. We have learned an enormous amount of new information about the molecular mechanisms that underlie microbial pathogenesis and the host response to pathogens since the second edition of this book some five years ago. An expanding number of antiviral and antifungal agents are now available to clinicians, and new generations of vaccine constructs and adjuvants are now entering clinical practice.

Despite these advances, progress has been uneven with very little in the developmental pipeline for novel antibacterial agents, antituberculosis drugs, or chemotherapeutic agents against parasitic infection. We find ourselves increasingly on the defensive against a variety of newly emerging and remerging pathogens. The specter of progressive antimicrobial resistance now threatens the long-term viability of the very foundation of our primary treatment approach against bacterial pathogens, including extensively drug resistant tuberculosis (XDR-TB). Our collective vulnerability to airborne pathogens within our highly mobile and crowded global community has become poignantly evident with the H1N1 swine flu pandemic of 2009 and ongoing threats of human dissemination of H5N1 avian influenza strains. Environmental disruption and global warming largely attributable to our ever expanding human population is likely to have adverse health consequences; among them with be the spread of vector-borne, waterborne and airborne pathogens.

In preparing this third edition we have continued the themes that initially inspired the creation of this textbook of Infectious Diseases. The book maintains its tradition of well illustrated and tightly referenced chapters with an emphasis on clinical practicality along with a detailed review of disease pathogenesis and microbiology. Practice points are found throughout the text that highlight common, and not so common, clinical scenarios that require specific and targeted information to provide informed responses. The interactive website, complete with its frequently updated information sources and a downloadable set of illustrations, will continue to support the print version of the text and now includes a number of innovative new functions. The whole text has been carefully reviewed, many chapters have been totally re-written with new figures added, and new authors and editors have been commissioned to ensure that the material is fresh, up to date and relevant.

We are indebted to the superb group of section editors and the extensive collection of highly skilled, international, contributors for each chapter, without whom the third edition of this book would not have been possible. We would especially like to extend our sincere gratitude to Sue Hodgson, Sven Pinczewski, Poppy Garraway and the staff at Elsevier for their unflappable spirit and their attention to detail throughout this considerable undertaking. Finally, we thank the Section Editors from the second edition who have now stood down: Steven Holland, Dennis Maki, Ragnar Norrby, Allan Ronald, Claus Solberg and Jan Verhoef without whom we would never have been in the position of preparing a third edition. We trust that our readers will find the readily accessible knowledge distilled into these pages to have been well worth the effort in generating the Third Edition of Infectious Diseases.

Jon Cohen
William Powderly
Steven Opal

User Guide

Volumes, sections and color coding
Infectious Diseases is divided into two volumes. The book is divided into eight sections, which are color-coded as follows for reference:

Volume 1

Section 1 – Introduction to infectious diseases

Section 2 – Syndromes by body system

Section 3 – Special problems in infectious disease practice

Section 4 – Infections in the immunocompromised host

Volume 2

Section 5 – HIV and AIDS

Section 6 – International medicine

Section 7 – Anti-infective therapy

Section 8 – Clinical microbiology

Contributors

George J Alangaden MD
Professor of Medicine
Division of Infectious Diseases
Wayne State University School of
Medicine
Detroit, MI, USA

Michael J Aldape PhD
Affiliate Assistant Professor
Department of Microbiology
Molecular Biology and
Biochemistry
University of Idaho at Moscow
Assistant Research Scientist
Infectious Disease Section
Veterans Affairs Medical Center
Boise, ID, USA

**Jérôme Allardet-Servent
MD MSc**
Intensivist
Service de Réanimation
Fondation Hôpital Ambroise Paré
Marseille, France

**Upton D Allen MBBS MS
FAAP FRCPC**
Professor of Paediatrics
Consultant in Infectious Diseases
Division of Infectious Diseases
Hospital for Sick Children
Toronto, Ontario, Canada

Heidi SM Ammerlaan MD
PhD student/Resident in Internal
Medicine
Department of Medical
Microbiology
University Medical Centre
Utrecht, The Netherlands

**Emmanouil Angelakis PhD
MD**
Detection of Molecular
Mechanisms Resulting in Antibiotic
Resistance
Faculté de médecine
Urmite, UMR 6236, CNRS-IRD
Marseille, France

**Andrew Artenstein MD
FACP FIDSA**
Physician-in-Chief
Department of Medicine
Director, Center for Biodefense
and Emerging Pathogens Memorial
Hospital of Rhode Island,
Professor of Medicine and
Community Health
The Warren Alpert Medical School
of Brown University
Providence, RI, USA

**David Asboe MB ChB
Dip GUM FRCP**
Consultant Physician
Department of HIV and
Genitourinary Medicine
Chelsea and Westminster
Hospital Foundation Trust
London, UK

Kingsley B Asiedu MD
Medical Officer
Department of Control of
Neglected Tropical Diseases
World Health Organization
Geneva, Switzerland

John C Atherton MD FRCP
Professor of Gastroenterology;
Director
Nottingham Digestive Diseases
Centre
Biomedical Research Unit
Nottingham Digestive Diseases
Centre
University of Nottingham
Nottingham, UK

**Tar-Ching Aw MBBS PhD
FRCP FRCPC FFOM FFPHM**
Professor and Chair
Department of Community
Medicine
Faculty of Medicine and Health
Sciences
United Arab Emirates University
Al Ain, United Arab Emirates

**Seema Baid-Agrawal MD
FASN**
Attending Nephrologist
Department of Nephrology and
Medical Intensive Care
Campus Virchow-Klinikum
Berlin, Germany

**Robin Bailey BA BM DTMH
PhD FRCP**
Professor of Tropical Medicine
London School of Hygiene and
Tropical Medicine
London, UK

Christopher Bandel MD
Research Fellow
Department of Dermatology
University of Texas Southwestern
Medical School
Dallas, TX, USA

**Philip S Barie MD MBA
FCCM FACS**
Professor of Surgery and Public
Health
Department of Surgery
New York-Presbyterian Hospital
and Weill Medical College P713A
New York, NY, USA

David J Barillo MD FACS
Surgical Intensivist and Chief
Burn Flight Team and Special
Medical Augmentation Response
Team (Burn)
US Army Institute of Surgical
Research
Fort Sam Houston
San Antonio, TX, USA

Pierre-Alexandre Bart MD
Senior Scientist and Clinician
Division of Immunology and Allergy
University Hospital Center
Lausanne, Switzerland

**Roger Bayston MMedSci
PhD MSc FRCPath**
Associate Professor
Surgical Infection
Biomaterials-Related Infection
Group
School of Medical and Surgical
Sciences
University of Nottingham
Nottingham, UK

C. Ben Beard PhD
Chief
Bacterial Diseases Branch
Division of Vector-Borne Infectious
Diseases
US Centers for Disease Control and
Prevention
Fort Collins, CO, USA

**Nick J Beeching MA BM BCh
FRCP (Lond) FRACP FFTM
RCPS (Glasg) DCH DTM&H**
Senior Lecturer in Infectious Diseases
Clinical Group
Liverpool School of Tropical
Medicine
Liverpool, UK

Rodolfo E Bégué MD
Professor of Pediatrics
Chief Infectious Diseases
Department of Pediatrics
Health Sciences Center
Louisiana State University
New Orleans, LA, USA

Yves Benhamou MD PhD
Associate Professor
Service d'Hépato-Gastroentérologie
Hôpital Pitié-Salpêtrière
Paris, France

Constance A Benson MD
Professor of Medicine
Division of Infectious Diseases
University of California, San Diego
San Diego, CA, USA

Elie F Berbari MD
Assistant Professor of Medicine
Division of Infectious Diseases
Section of Orthopedic Infectious
Diseases
Department of Internal Medicine
Mayo Clinic College of Medicine
Rochester, MN, USA

**Anthony R Berendt BM BCh
MRCP(UK)**
Consultant Physician-in-Charge
Bone Infection Unit
Nuffield Orthopaedic Centre
Oxford, UK

Madhav P Bhatta MPH
Doctoral Candidate
Department of Epidemiology
University of Alabama at
Birmingham
Birmingham, AL, USA

Jacques Bille MD
Professor of Medical Microbiology
Institute of Microbiology
University of Lausanne and
University Hospital Centre
Lausanne, Switzerland

Ari Bitnun MD MSc FRCPC
Assistant Professor
University of Toronto
Staff Physician
Division of Infectious Diseases
Hospital for Sick Children
Toronto, Ontario, Canada

**Finn T Black MD DMSc
DTM&H**
Professor of Infectious Diseases and
Tropical Medicine
Department of Infectious Diseases
University Hospital of Aårhus
Aårhus, Denmark

Contributors

Iain Blair MA MB BChir
Associate Professor
Department of Community Medicine
Faculty of Medicine and Health
Sciences
United Arab Emirates University
Al Ain, United Arab Emirates

Stéphane Blanche MD
Professor of Pediatrics
Hôpital Necker Enfant Malades
Paris, France

Thomas P Bleck MD FCCM
Professor of Neurological Sciences
Neurosurgery, Internal Medicine
(Pulmonary/Critical Care Medicine
and Infectious Diseases), and
Anesthesiology;
Assistant Dean, Rush Medical
College; and
Associate Chief Medical Officer
(Critical Care),
Rush University Medical Center
Chicago, IL, USA

**Chantal P Bleeker-Rovers
MD PhD**
Internist specialized in infectious
diseases
Department of Internal Medicine
Division of Infectious Diseases
Radboud University Nijmegen
Medical Center
Nijmegen, The Netherlands

Gijs Bleijenberg PhD
Professor of Clinical Psychology
Expert Centre Chronic Fatigue
University Medical Centre
Nijmegen
Nijmegen, The Netherlands

Karen C Bloch MD MPH
Assistant Professor of Medicine
(Infectious Disease) and Preventive
Medicine
Vanderbilt University Medical
Center
Nashville, TN, USA

Marc JM Bonten MD PhD
Professor of Molecular
Epidemiology of Infectious Diseases
Department of Medical
Microbiology
Julius Centre for Health Sciences
and Primary Care
Utrecht, The Netherlands

**Charles AB Boucher MD
PhD**
Clinical Virologist
Department of Virology
Erasmus Medical Center
Erasmus University
Rotterdam, The Netherlands

Rafik Bourayou MD
Specialist in Pediatrics
Department of Pediatrics
Pediatric Rheumatology and
Pediatric Emergency Medicine
Hôpital de Bicêtre
Le Kremlin-Bicêtre, France

Emilio S Bouza MD PhD
Head
Clinical Microbiology and Infectious
Diseases
Clinical Microbiology and Infectious
Diseases Department
Hospital General Universitario
Gregorio Marañón
Madrid, Spain

**William R Bowie MD
FRCPC**
Professor of Medicine
Division of Infectious Diseases
The University of British Columbia
Vancouver, BC, Canada

Barry D Brause MD
Clinical Professor of Medicine,
Weill-Cornell Medical College
Attending Physician
Hospital for Special Surgery and
New York Presbyterian Hospital
New York, NY, USA

Sylvain Brisse PhD
Researcher
Genotyping of Pathogens and
Public Health Institut Pasteur
Paris, France

**Warwick Britton PhD MB BS
BScMed FRACP FRCP FRCPA
DTM&H**
Bosch Professor of Medicine
and Professor of Immunology,
Centenary Institute and Disciplines
of Medicine
Infectious Diseases and Immunology
University of Sydney
Sydney, NSW, Australia

Itzhak Brook MD MSc
Professor of Pediatric Medicine
Department of Pediatrics
Georgetown University School of
Medicine
Washington, DC, USA

**David WG Brown MBBS
MSc FRCPath FFPH**
Director
Enteric and Respiratory Virus
Laboratory
London, UK

Christian Brun-Buisson MD
Service de Réanimation Médicale
C.H.U. Henri Mondor
University Paris Val-de-Marne
Assistance Publique-Hôpitaux de
Paris
Créteil, France

James CM Brust MD
Assistant Professor of Medicine
Divisions of General Internal
Medicine and Infectious Diseases
Montefiore Medical Center
and Albert Einstein College of
Medicine
Bronx, NY, USA

Amy E Bryant PhD
Affiliate Assistant Professor of
Medicine
University of Washington School of
Medicine
Seattle, WA
Research Scientist
Infectious Disease Section
Veterans Affairs Medical Center
Boise, ID, USA

André Bryskier MD
Consultant in Microbiology and
Infectious Diseases
Romainville
Le Mesnil Le Roi, France

R. Mark L Buller PhD
Professor of Molecular
Microbiology and Immunology
Department of Molecular
Microbiology and Immunology
St Louis University
St Louis, MO, USA

Karen Bush PhD
Adjunct Professor of Biology
Indiana University Bloomington
Bloomington, IN, USA

Thierry Calandra MD PhD
Professor of Medicine
Head, Infectious Diseases Service,
Department of Internal Medicine
Centre Hospitalier
Universitaire Vaudois
Lausanne, Switzerland

**D. William Cameron MD
FRCP FACP**
Professor of Medicine
Divisions of Infectious Diseases and
Respirology
University of Ottawa at The Ottawa
Hospital
Ottawa, ON, Canada

Michel Caraël PhD
Professor Emeritus of Medical
Sociology
Social Sciences Faculty
Free University Brussels
Brussels, Belgium

Michael J Carr BSc PhD
Clinical Scientist
National Virus Reference Laboratory
University College Dublin
Belfield, Dublin
Ireland

Inmaculada Casas PhD
Research Scientist
Alert and Emergency Unit
Virology Service
National Centre of Microbiology
Instituto de Salud Carlos III
Madrid, Spain

**Stephen T Chambers MD
ChB MSc FRACP**
Professor of Pathology,
Christchurch School of Medicine,
University of Otago
Clinical Director of Infectious
Diseases, Christchurch Hospital
Department of Infectious Diseases
Christchurch Hospital
Christchurch, New Zealand

**Katarina G Chiller MD
MPH&TM**
Assistant Clinical Professor of
Dermatology
Emory University School of
Medicine
Atlanta Skin Cancer
Specialists, PC
Atlanta, GA, USA

Tom M Chiller MD MPHTM
Deputy Chief, Mycotic Diseases
Branch
Division of Foodborne, Bacterial
and Mycotic Diseases
National Center for Zoonotic
Vector-Borne and Enteric
Diseases, Centers for Disease
Control and Prevention
Adjunct Assistant Professor of
Infectious Diseases
Emory University school of
Medicine
Atlanta, GA, USA

**Peter L Chiodini BSc MBBS
PhD MRCS FRCP FRCPath**
Consultant Parasitologist
Department of Clinical Parasitology
Hospital for Tropical Diseases
London, UK

**Ian Chopra BA MA PhD DSc
MD(honorary)**
Professor of Microbiology and
Director of the Antimicrobial
Research Centre
Institute of Molecular and Cellular
Biology
University of Leeds
Leeds, UK

Anthony C Chu FRCP
Consultant Dermatologist/Honorary
Senior Lecturer
Head of Dermatology, Unit of
Dermatology
Imperial College School of Medicine
London, UK

Kevin K Chung MD
Medical Intensivist
Medical Director
Burn ICU
US Army Institute of Surgical
Research
San Antonio, TX, USA

Benjamin M Clark MBChB MRCP (UK) DTM&H
Consultant in Infectious Diseases
Department of Infectious Diseases
Fremantle Hospital
Fremantle, WA, Australia

Nathan Clumeck MD PhD
Professor of Infectious Diseases
Head, Department of Infectious Diseases
St Pierre University Hospital
Brussels, Belgium

Clay J Cockerell MD
Professor of Dermatology and Pathology
Departments of Dermatology and Pathology
University of Texas
Dallas, TX, USA

Jonathan Cohen MB BS FRCP FRCPath FRCPE FmedSci
Professor of Infectious Diseases and Dean
Brighton and Sussex Medical School
Honorary Consultant Physician
Royal Sussex County Hospital
Brighton, UK

John Collinge MRCP MD FRCPath
Professor of Neurology
Head of Department
Department of Neurodegenerative Diseases/Director, MRC Prion Unit
Institute of Neurology
University College London
London, UK

Christopher P Conlon MA MD FRCP
Reader in Infectious Diseases and Tropical Medicine
University of Oxford Consultant in Infectious Diseases
Nuffield Department of Medicine
Oxford, UK

G. Ralph Corey MD
Gary Hock Professor of Global Health
Duke University Medical Center
Durham, NC, USA

Alan Cross MD
Professor of Medicine
Center for Vaccine Development and Department of Medicine
University of Maryland School of Medicine
Baltimore, MD, USA

John H Cross PhD
Professor
Tropical Public Health
Department of Preventive Medicine and Biometrics
Uniformed Services University of the Health Sciences
Bethesda, MD, USA

Judith Currier MD
Professor of Medicine
Division of Infectious Diseases
Center for Clinical AIDS Research and Education
David Geffen School of Medicine
University of California
Los Angeles, CA, USA

Carmel M Curtis PhD MRCP
Microbiology Specialist Registrar
Department of Parasitology
The Hospital for Tropical Diseases
London, UK

Gina Dallabetta MD
Director
Technical Support
HIV/AIDS Institute
Family Health International
Arlington, VA, USA

Robert N Davidson MD FRCP DTM&H
Consultant Physician
Hon. Senior Lecturer
Department of Infectious and Tropical Diseases
Northwick Park Hospital
Harrow, Middlesex, UK

Jane Davies MBBS MRCP DTM&H PGCTLCP
Specialist Registrar in Infectious Diseases and Tropical Medicine
Tropical and Infectious Disease Unit, Royal Liverpool University Hospital
Liverpool, UK

Jeremy Day MA MB BChir MRCP(London) DTM&H
Consultant in Infectious Diseases
Wellcome Trust Major Overseas Program
Oxford University Clinical Research Unit
Hospital for Tropical Diseases
Ho Chi Minh City, Vietnam

Nicholas PJ Day DM FRCP FMedSci
Professor of Tropical Medicine
Centre for Tropical Medicine
University of Oxford, UK
Director of the Mahidol Oxford Tropical Medicine Research Unit
Faculty of Tropical Medicine
Mahidol University
Bangkok, Thailand

Cillian F De Gascun MB MRCPI
Senior Registrar in Virology
National Virus Reference Laboratory
University College Dublin
Belfield, Dublin
Ireland

Stéphane de Wit MD PhD
Senior Physician
Division of Infectious Diseases
St Pierre University Hospital
Brussels, Belgium

Jean Delmont MD PhD
Physician, Professor of Infectious Diseases and Tropical Medicine
Infectious Diseases Department
Hôpital Nord, University Hospital of Marseille
Marseille, France

David T Dennis MD MPH DCMT
Medical Epidemiologist
Influenza Coordinator
Vietnam
Division of Influenza
Atlanta, GA, USA

David J Diemert MD FRCP(C) DTM&H
Assistant Professor
Department of Microbiology Immunology and Tropical Medicine
The George Washington School of Medicine
Director of Clinical Trials, Sabin Vaccine Institute
Washington DC, USA

Mehmet Doganay MD
Professor in Infectious Diseases
Department of Infectious Diseases
Faculty of Medicine
Erciyes University
Kayseri, Turkey

Tom Doherty MD FRCP DTM&H
Consultant Physician
Hospital for Tropical Diseases
London, UK

Christiane Dolecek MD
The Hospital for Tropical Diseases
Oxford University Clinical Research Unit
Ho Chi Minh City, Vietnam

Stéphane Y Donati MD
Intensivist
Medico-surgical ICU
Font Pré Hospital
Toulon, France

Arjen M Dondorp MD PhD
Infectious Diseases and Intensive Care Physician
Deputy Director
Mahidol-Oxford Tropical Medicine Research Unit (MORU)
Bangkok, Thailand

Barbara Doudier MD
Physician, Infectious Diseases Fellow
Assistant Professor, Infectious Diseases Department
Hôpital de la Conception
University Hospital of Marseille
Marseille, France

Michel Drancourt MD
Professor of Microbiology, Head of the Clinical Microbiology Laboratory
Unité de Recherche sur les Maladies Infectieuses et Tropicales Emergentes
Medical School, Méditerranée University
Marseille, France

Dimitri M Drekonja MD
Assistant Professor of Medicine
University of Minnesota
Infectious Diseases
VA Medical Center
Minneapolis, MN, USA

Richard H Drew PharmD MS BCPS
Professor, Campbell University College of Pharmacy and Health Sciences
Associate Professor of Medicine (Infectious Diseases)
Duke University School of Medicine
Durham, NC, USA

Jay S Duker MD
Director
New England Eye Center
Professor and Chair of Ophthalmology
Tufts New England Medical Center
Tufts University School of Medicine
Boston, MA, USA

J. Stephen Dummer MD
Professor of Medicine
Division of Infectious Diseases
Vanderbilt University Medical Center
Nashville, TN, USA

Charles N Edwards FRCP FACP FACG
Associate Senior Lecturer
School of Clinical Medicine and Research
University of the West Indies
Barbados

Miquel B Ekkelenkamp MD
Clinical Microbiologist
University Medical Center Utrecht
Utrecht, The Netherlands

Mark C Enright PhD
Professor of Molecular Epidemiology
Department of Infectious Disease Epidemiology
Imperial College London
London, UK

Paul R Epstein MD MPH
Associate Director
Center for Health and the Global Environment
Harvard Medical School
Boston, MA, USA

Veronique Erard MD MSc
Division of Infectious Diseases
Centre Hospitalier University
Vadors Rue du Bugnon
Lausanne, Switzerland

Alice Chijioke Eziefula MBBS MA MRCP MRC Path
Department of Infection
Brighton and Sussex University Hospitals
Brighton, UK

Contributors

Mark B Feinberg MD PhD
Vice President
Policy, Public Health and Medical Affairs
Merck & Co., Inc.
West Point, PA, USA

Florence Fenollar MD PhD
Associate Professor of Clinical Microbiology
Unité des Rickettsies
Faculté de Médecine
Marseille, France

Alan Fenwick OBE
Professor of Tropical Parasitology
Director, Schistosomiasis Control Initiative
Department of Infectious Disease Epidemiology
Imperial College London
London, UK

Luis Fernandez MD FACS
Assistant Professor of Surgery
Department of Surgery
University of Wisconsin School of Medicine and Public Health
Madison, WI, USA

Joshua Fierer MD
Michael and Marci Oxman Professor of Medicine and Pathology
Chief, Infectious Diseases Section
VA San Diego Healthcare System
Director, Microbiology Laboratory
VA San Diego Healthcare System
San Diego, CA, USA

Roger G Finch MB BS FRCP FRCPath FRCPEd FFPM
Professor of Infectious Diseases
School of Molecular Medical Science
Division of Microbiology and Infectious Disease
Nottingham University Hospitals NHS Trust
Nottingham, UK

Charles W Flexner MD
Professor of Medicine
Pharmacology and Molecular Sciences and International Health
Johns Hopkins University
Baltimore, MD, USA

Ad C Fluit PhD
Associate Professor
Department of Medical Microbiology
University Medical Center Utrecht
Utrecht, The Netherlands

Elizabeth Lee Ford-Jones MD FRCPC
Professor of Pediatrics
Division of Infectious Diseases
The Hospital for Sick Children
University of Toronto
Co-editor *Paediatrics and Child Health*
Toronto, ON, Canada

Pierre-Edouard Fournier MD PhD
Associate Professor
Unité des Rickettsies
Faculté dé Medecine, Université de la Méditerranée
Marseille, France

Victoria Fraser MD
J William Campbell Professor of Medicine and Co-Director
Infectious Diseases Division
Washington University School of Medicine
St Louis, MO, USA

Martyn A French MB CRB MD FRCPath FRCP FRACP
Clinical Immunologist and Winthrop Professor of Pathology and Laboratory Medicine
Department of Clinical Immunology
Royal Perth Hospital and School of Pathology and Laboratory Medicine
University of Western Australia
Perth, Australia

Jon S Friedland MA PhD FRCP FRCPE FMedSci
Head, Department of Infectious Diseases and Immunity
Imperial College London
Lead Clinician, Clinical Infection
Imperial College Healthcare
NHS Trust
London, UK

Joseph M Fritz MD
St Lukés Hospital
St Louis, MO, USA

E. Yoko Furuya MD MS
Assistant Professor of Clinical Medicine
Division of Infectious Diseases
Columbia University
New York, NY, USA

Kenneth L Gage PhD
Chief, Flea-borne Disease Activity
Bacterial Diseases Branch
Division of Vector-Borne Infectious Diseases
US Centers for Disease Control and Prevention
Fort Collins, CO, USA

Lynne S Garcia MS FAAM MT(ASCP) CLS(NCA) BLM(AAB)
Director, LSG & Associates
Santa Monica, CA, USA

Arturo S Gastañaduy MD
Associate Professor of Pediatrics
Department of Pediatrics
Louisiana State University Health Sciences Center
New Orleans, LA, USA

Khalil G Ghanem MD PhD
Assistant Professor of Medicine
Division of Infectious Diseases
Johns Hopkins University School of Medicine
Assistant Professor Population Family and Reproductive Health
Johns Hopkins University
Bloomberg School of Public Health
Baltimore, MD, USA

Maddalena Giannella MD
Research Assistant
Clinical Microbiology and Infectious Diseases Department
Hospital General Universitario Gregorio Marañón
Madrid, Spain

Carol A Glaser DVM MD
Chief, Viral and Rickettsial Disease Laboratory Branch
California Department of Public Health
Richmond, CA, USA

Marshall J Glesby MD PhD
Associate Professor of Medicine and Public Health
Division of Infectious Diseases
Department of Medicine
Weill Cornell Medical College
New York, NY, USA

Sarah Glover MBChB MRCP FRCPath
Specialist Registrar in Infectious Diseases and Microbiology
Brighton and Sussex University Hospitals NHS Trust
Brighton, UK

Youri Glupczynski MD
Professor of Microbiology
Laboratoire de Microbiologie
Cliniques universitaires UCL de Mont-Godinne
Yvoir, Belgium

John W Gnann Jr MD
Professor of Medicine,
Pediatrics and Microbiology
Division of Infectious Diseases
University of Alabama at Birmingham and Birmingham Veterans Administration Medical Center
Birmingham, AL, USA

Andrew F Goddard MA MD FRCP
Consultant Gastroenterologist
Digestive Diseases Centre
Derby Hospitals NHS Foundation Trust
Derby, UK

Ellie JC Goldstein MD FIDSA
Director, RM Alden Research Laboratory
Santa Monica, CA
Clinical Professor of Medicine
UCLA School of Medicine
Los Angeles, CA, USA

Iveth J González MD PhD
Scientific Officer
FIND Diagnostics
Geneva, Switzerland

Sherwood L Gorbach MD
Distinguished Professor
Departments of Public Health and Medicine
Tufts University School of Medicine
Boston, MA, USA

Bruno Gottstein PhD AssEVPC CBA
Professor and Director
Institute of Parasitology
Vetsuisse-Faculty and Faculty of Medicine
University of Bern
Bern, Switzerland

Ravi Gowda MBBS MRCP(UK) DTM&H DCH DRCOG MRCGP
Consultant in Infectious Diseases
Department of Infection and Tropical Medicine
University Hospitals Coventry and Warwickshire
Coventry, UK

John D Grabenstein RPh PhD
Senior Medical Director-Adult Vaccines
Merck Vaccines & Infectious Diseases
Merck & Co., Inc.
West Point, PA, USA

John M Grange MBBS MSc MD
Visiting Professor
Centre for Infectious Diseases and International Heatlh
Windeyer Institute for Medical Sciences
London, UK

Michael D Green MD MPH
Professor of Pediatrics and Surgery
University of Pittsburgh School of Medicine
Division of Infectious Diseases
Children's Hospital of Pittsburgh
Pittsburgh, PA, USA

Stephen T Green MD BSc FRCP(Lond, Glas) FFTH DTM&H
Consultant Physician in Infectious Disease and Tropical Medicine
Department of Infection and Tropical Medicine
Royal Hallamshire Hospitals
Sheffield, UK

Danielle T Greenblatt MBChB MRCP
Specialist Registrar
Department of Dermatology
Ealing Hospital NHS Trust
Southall, UK

Brian Greenwood MD
Professor of Tropical Medicine
Department of Infectious and
Tropical Diseases
London School of Hygiene and
Tropical Medicine
London, UK

Aric L Gregson MD
Assistant Clinical Professor of
Medicine
Department of Medicine
Division of Infectious Diseases
University of California
Los Angeles, CA, USA

Andreas H Groll MD
Infectious Disease Research Program
Center for Bone Marrow
Transplantation and Department of
Pediatric Hematology/Oncology
University Children's Hospital
Munster, Germany

**Aditya K Gupta MD PhD
MA(Cantab) CCI CCTI CCRP
DABD FAAD FRCPC**
Professor, Division of Dermatology
Department of Medicine
Sunnybrook and Women's Health
Science Center and the University
of Toronto
London, ON, Canada

**Kok-Ann Gwee MBBS
MMed MRCP FAMS PhD
FRCP**
Consultant Gastroenterologist
Gleneagles Hospital, Singapore
and Adjunct Associate Professor of
Medicine, Yong Loo Lin School of
Medicine
National University of Singapore
Singapore

**William Hall BSc PhD MD
DTMH**
Professor of Medical Microbiology
College of Life Sciences
School of Medicine & Medical
Science
Belfield, Dublin
Ireland

Scott M Hammer MD
Professor of Medicine and Public
Health (Epidemiology)
Columbia University
Presbyterian Hospital
New York, NY, USA

Sajeev Handa MD FMM
Director, Division of Hospital
Medicine
Rhode Island Hospital
Providence, RI, USA

Diane Hanfelt-Goade MD
Assistant Professor
Department of Medicine
The University of New Mexico
School of Medicine
Albuquerque, NM, USA

Alexandre Harari PhD
Project Leader
Service of Immunology and Allergy
Centre Hospitalier Universitaire
Vaudois
Lausanne, Switzerland

Marianne Harris MD CCFPC
Clinical Research Advisor
AIDS Research Program
Providence Health Care
Vancouver, BC, Canada

Barry J Hartman MD
Clinical Professor of Medicine
Department of International
Medicine and Infectious Diseases
Cornell University Medical College
New York
New York, NY, USA

**Roderick J Hay DM FRCP
FRCPath**
Honorary Professor, London School
of Hygiene and Tropical Medicine
Chairman
International Foundation for
Dermatology
London, UK

David K Henderson MD
Deputy Director for Clinical Care
Warren G Magnuson Clinical
Center
National Institutes of Health
Bethesda, MD, USA

Lisa E Hensley MD
Chief of Viral Therapeutics
Department of Viral Therapeutics
Virology Division
Fort Detrick, MD, USA

Luke Herbert FRCOphth
Consultant and Clinical Director
Department of Ophthalmology
The Queen Elizabeth II Hospital
Welwyn Garden City, UK

**David R Hill MD DTM&H
FRCP FFTM**
Honorary Professor, London
School of Hygiene and Tropical
Medicine
Director, National Travel Health
Network and Centre
Hospital for Tropical Diseases
London, UK

**Timothy J Hills
BPharm MRPharmS Dip
Clin Pharm**
Lead Pharmacist Antimicrobials and
Infection Control
Department of Pharmacy
Nottingham University Hospitals
NHS Trust
Nottingham, UK

John David Hinze DO
Pulmonary and Critical Care
Consultants of Austin
Austin, TX, USA

Hans H Hirsch MD MS
Professor of Clinical Virology
Division of Infectious Diseases
University Hospital Basel
Institute for Medical Microbiology
Basel, Switzerland

Bernard Hirschel MD
Division of Infectious Diseases
Unite VIH/SIDA Hôpital Universitaire
de Geneve
Geneva, Switzerland

**Andy IM Hoepelman
MD PhD**
Professor in Medicine, Infectious
Diseases Specialist
Head, Department of
Internal Medicine and Infectious
Diseases
University Medical Center
Utrecht, The Netherlands

Steven M Holland MD
Chief, Laboratory of Clinical
Infectious Diseases
National Institute of Allergy and
Infectious Disease
National Institutes of Health
Bethesda, MD, USA

Mary M Horgan MD FRCPI
Senior Lecturer in Medicine
University College Cork
Consultant in Infectious Diseases
Cork University Hospital
Cork, Ireland

**Robin Howe MA MBBS
FRCPath**
Consultant in Clinical Microbiology
Microbiology Cardiff (Velindre NHS
Trust),
University Hospital of Wales,
Heath Park, Cardiff, UK

James M Hughes MD
Professor of Medicine and Public
Health
Division of Infectious Diseases
Department of Medicine
Emory University School of Medicine
Atlanta, GA, USA

Mark W Hull MD FRCPC
Research Scientist
BC Centre for Excellence in
HIV/AIDS
Vancouver, BC, Canada

Clark B Inderlied PhD
Professor of Clinical Microbiology
Keck School of Medicine
University of Southern California
Los Angeles, CA, USA

Michael G Ison MD MS
Assistant Professor, Divisions of
Infectious Diseases and Organ
Transplantation
Medical Director, Transplant
& Immunocompromised Host
Infectious Diseases Service
Northwestern University Feinberg
School of Medicine
Chicago, IL, USA

**Peter J Jenks PhD MRCP
FRCPath**
Director of Infection Prevention and
Control/Consultant in Microbiology
Department of Microbiology
Plymouth Hospitals NHS Trust
Plymouth, UK

**James R Johnson MD FACP
FIDSA**
Professor of Medicine University of
Minnesota
Infectious Diseases
VA Medical Center
Minneapolis, MN, USA

Theodore Jones MD
Associate Professor
Wayne State University
Detroit, MI, USA

Mettassebia Kanno MD
Assistant Professor of Medicine
Division of Infectious
Diseases
Institute of Human Virology
University of Maryland
Baltimore, MD, USA

Carol Kauffman MD
Professor of Internal Medicine
University of Michigan
Chief, Infectious Diseases Section
VA Ann Arbor Healthcare System
Ann Arbor, MI, UK

Patrick Kelly BVSc PhD
Professor of Small Animal Medicine
Ross University School of Veterinary
Medicine
Basseterre
St Kitts, West Indies

Jason S Kendler MD
Clinical Associate Professor of
Medicine
Weill Cornell Medical College
New York, NY, USA

Yoav Keynan MD
Infectious Disease Fellow
Department of Internal Medicine
Laboratory of Viral Immunology
Department of Medical
Microbiology
Winnipeg, MB, Canada

Ali S Khan MD
Assistant Surgeon General and
Deputy Director
National Center for Zoonotic,
Vector-borne, and Enteric Diseases
Centers for Disease Control and
Prevention
Atlanta, GA, USA

Grace T Kho MD
Department of Dermatology and
Pathology
University of Texas Southwestern
Medical Center
Dallas, TX, USA

**George R Kinghorn MD
FRCP**
Clinical Director, Directorate of
Communicable Diseases
Royal Hallamshire Hospital
Sheffield, UK

Contributors

Paul E Klapper PhD MRCPath
Consultant Clinical Scientist
Honorary Professor of Clinical
Virology,
University of Manchester
Clinical Virology Central
Manchester
University Hospitals
NHS Foundation Trust
Manchester, UK

Jan AJW Kluytmans MD PhD
Professor of Medical Microbiology
and Infection Control
VU University Medical Center
Laboratory for Microbiology and
Infection Control
Amsterdam, The Netherlands

Menno Kok PhD
Senior Staff Member
Medical Faculty
Erasmus MC
Rotterdam, The Netherlands

Isabelle Koné-Paut MD
Professor, Department of Pediatrics
Pediatric Rheumatology and
Pediatric Emergency Medicine
Hôpital de Bicêtre
Le Kremlin-Bicêtre, France

John N Krieger MD
Professor of Urology
Department of Urology
University of Washington and Chief
of Urology
VA Puget Sound Health Care System
Seattle, WA, USA

Aloys CM Kroes MD PhD
Professor of Medical Microbiology
and Clinical Virology
Department of Medical
Microbiology
Leiden University Medical Center
Leiden, The Netherlands

Frank P Kroon MD PhD
Department of Infectious Diseases
C5P
Leiden University Medical Center
Leiden, The Netherlands

Christine J Kubin PharmD BCPS
Clinical Pharmacy Manager
Infectious Diseases
Columbia University College of
Physicians and Surgeons
New York-Presbyterian Hospital
Columbia University Medical Centre
New York, NY, USA

Alberto M La Rosa MD
Director of Clinical Trials Unit
Asociacion Civil Impacta Salud Y
Educacion
Lima, Peru

Tahaniyat Lalani MBBS MHS
Assistant Professor, Division of
Infectious Diseases, Uniformed
Services
University of the Health Sciences
Naval Medical Center Portsmouth
Portsmouth, VA, USA

David G Lalloo MB BS MD FRCP
Professor of Tropical Medicine and
Head, Clinical Research Group
Liverpool School of Tropical Medicine
Liverpool, UK

Harold Lambert MD FRCP FRCPath
Emeritus Professor of Microbial
Diseases
St George's Hospital Medical School
London, UK

Luce Landraud MD PhD
Medical Doctor
Microbiology Department
Archet II-Hospital
Microbial Toxins in Host Pathogen
Interactions
Sophia Antipolis University
Nice, France

Stephen D Lawn BMedSci MBBS MRCP MD DTM&H Dip HIV Med
Reader in Infectious Diseases and
Tropical Medicine
Department of Infectious and
Tropical Diseases
London School of Hygiene and
Tropical Medicine, London, UK
Associate Professor of Infectious
Diseases and HIV Medicine
The Desmond Tutu HIV Centre
Institute for Infectious Disease and
Molecular Medicine
Faculty of Health Sciences
University of Cape Town
Cape Town, South Africa

Phillipe Lehours Pharm PhD
Associate Professor of Bacteriology
Université Victor Segalen
Bordeaux, France

Marc Leone MD PhD
Assistant Professor of Anesthesiology
and Critical Care Medicine
Service d'anesthésie et de
réanimation
Hôpital Nord
Marseille, France

Itzchak Levi MD
Infectious Diseases Unit
Sheba Medical Center
Tel Hashomer
Ramat Gan, Israel

Alexandra M Levitt PhD
Health Scientist
National Center for Preparedness,
Detection, and Control of
Infectious Diseases
Centers for Disease Control and
Prevention
Atlanta, GA, USA

H. D. Alan Lindquist PhD
Microbiologist
Water Infrastructure Protection
Division
National Homeland Security
Research Center
Office of Research and Development
US Environmental Protection Agency
Cincinnati, OH, USA

Graham Lloyd PhD MSc BSc FIBMS CMS
Health Protection Agency
Centre for Applied Microbiology
and Research
Salisbury, UK

David J Looney MD
Associate Professor of Medicine
of Residence
Director, UCSD Center for AIDS
Research Molecular Biology Core
University of California San Diego
San Diego, CA, USA

Franklin D Lowy MD
Professor of Medicine and Pathology
Division of Infectious Diseases
Columbia University
College of Physicians and Surgeons
New York, NY, USA

Benjamin J Luft MD
Edmund D Pellegrino
Professor Chairman,
Department of Medicine
State University of New York
at Stony Brook
Stony Brook, NY, USA

William A Lynn MD FRCP
Medical Director
Consultant in Infectious Diseases
Infection and Immunity Unit
Ealing Hospital
Southall, UK

Mark J Macielag PhD
Senior Research Fellow
Johnson & Johnson Pharmaceutical
Research / Development
Spring House PA, USA

Philip A Mackowiak MD MBA MACP
Director, Medical Care Clinical Center
Professor of Medicine and
Vice-Chairman, VA Maryland
Health Care System
Department of Medicine
University of Maryland School of
Medicine
Baltimore, MD, USA

Paul A MacPherson MD PhD FRCPC
Assistant Professor, University of
Ottawa
Specialist in Infectious Diseases
Ottawa Hospital
Scientist, Ottawa Hospital Research
Institute
Ottawa, ON, Canada

Valérie Maghraoui-Slim MD
Specialist in Pediatrics
Department of Pediatrics
Pediatric Rheumatology and
Pediatric Emergency Medicine
Hôpital de Bicêtre
Le Kremlin-Bicêtre, France

Janice Main FRCP(Ed, Lond)
Reader and Consultant Physician
in Infectious Diseases and General
Medicine
Department of Medicine
Imperial College
London, UK

Vincent Mallet MD PhD
Assistant Professor
Service d'Hepatologie
Université Paris Descartes
Assistance Publique Hôpitaux de
Paris, INSERM U.567
Paris, France

Julie E Mangino MD
Associate Professor of Internal
Medicine
Division of Infectious Diseases
Department of Internal Medicine
OSUMC Medical Director,
Department of Clinical
Epidemiology
The Ohio State University College
of Medicine
Columbus, OH, USA

Oriol Manuel MD
Attending in Transplant Infectious
Diseases
Service of Infectious Diseases
Transplantation Centre
University Hospital of Lausanne
(CHUV)
Lausanne, Switzerland

Oscar Marchetti MD
Privat Docent
Infectious Diseases Service
Department of Medicine
Centre Hospitalier Universitaire
Vaudois and University of Lausanne
Lausanne, Switzerland

Kristen Marks MD MS
Assistant Professor of Medicine
Division of Infectious Diseases
Department of Medicine
Weill Cornell Medical College
New York, NY, USA

Kieren A Marr MD
Director, Transplant and
Oncology
Johns Hopkins University School of
Medicine
Baltimore, MD, USA

Claude Martin MD
Professor of Anesthesiology and
Critical Care Medicine
Service d'anesthésie et de
réanimation
Hôpital Nord
Marseille, France

Pablo Martín-Rabadán MD DTMH
Consultant Physician
Servicio de Microbiologia y
Enjermedades Infecciosas
Hospital General Universitario
Gregorio Maranon
Madrid, Spain

Augusto Julio Martinez MD
(deceased)
Professor of Pathology
Department of Pathology
(Neuropathology)
University of Pittsburg School of
Medicine
Pittsburg, PA, USA

Ellen M Mascini MD PhD
Medical Microbiologist
Laboratory for Medical
Microbiology and Immunology
Alysis Zorggroep Arnhem,
The Netherlands

Kenneth H Mayer MD
Professor of Medicine and
Community Health
Brown University; Director of
Brown University
Infectious Diseases Division
The Miriam Hospital
Providence, RI, USA

Joseph B McCormick MD
Regional Dean and James H Steele
Professor
School of Public Health
University of Texas Houston Health
Science Center
Brownsville, TX, USA

Rose McGready MB BS PhD
Research Clinician
Obstetrics
Shoklo Malaria Research Unit
Tak Province, Thailand

**Michael W McKendrick
MB BS FRCP(Lond)
FRCP(Glasg)**
Lead Consultant Physician
Department of Infection and
Tropical Medicine
South Yorkshire Regional
Department of Infection and
Tropical Medicine
Sheffield, UK

Simon Mead MD
Honorary Consultant Neurologist
and Senior Lecturer
MRC Prion Unit
Institute of Neurology
University College London
London, UK

Francis Mégraud MD
Professor of Bacteriology
Université Victor Segalen
Bordeaux, France

André Z Meheus MD PhD
Professor Emeritus
Department of Epidemiology and
Social Medicine
Campus Drie Eiken
Antwerp, Belgium

**Graeme Meintjes MBChB
MRCP(UK) FCP(SA)
DipHIVMan(SA)**
Honorary Senior Lecturer
Division of Infectious Diseases and
HIV Medicine
Department of Medicine
University of Cape Town
Waterfront, South Africa

**Marian G Michaels
MD MPH**
Professor of Pediatrics and Surgery
University of Pittsburgh School of
Medicine
Division of Pediatric Infectious
Diseases
Pittsburgh, PA, USA

**Michael Miles MSc PhD DSc
FRCPath**
Professor of Medical Protozoology
London School of Hygiene and
Tropical Medicine
London, UK

**Alastair Miller MA FRCP
(Edin) DTM&H**
Consultant Physician
Tropical and Infectious Disease Unit
Royal Liverpool University Hospital
Honorary Fellow
Liverpool School of Tropical Medicine
Liverpool, UK

**Matthew J Mimiaga ScD
MPH**
Research Scientist
The Fenway Institute
Instructor in Psychiatry
Harvard Medical School
Boston, MA, USA

**Marie-Paule Mingeot-
Leclercq MSc PharmD PhD**
Professor of Pharmacology
Biochemistry and Biophysics
Unité de Pharmacologie cellulaire
et moléculaire & Louvain Drug
Research Institute
Université catholique de Louvain
Brussels, Belgium

Thomas G Mitchell PhD
Associate Professor
Department of Molecular Genetics
and Microbiology
Duke University Medical Center
Durham, NC, USA

Pamela A Moise PharmD
Clinical Scientific Director
Cubist Pharmaceuticals, Lexington
MA USA

Julio Montaner MD
Director, Infectious Disease Clinic
St Paul's Hospital
Vancouver, BC, Canada

Caroline B Moore PhD
Principle Clinical Mycologist
Regional Mycology Laboratory
University Hospital of South
Manchester (Wythenshawe
Hospital)
Manchester, UK

Philippe Moreillon MD PhD
Professor
Department of Fundamental
Microbiology
University of Lausanne
Lausanne, Switzerland

**Peter Morgan-Capner BSc
MBBS FRCPath FRCP Hon
FFPHM**
Honorary Professor of Clinical
Virology
Department of Microbiology
Royal Preston Hospital
Preston, UK

**Valentina Montessori MD
FRCPC**
Clinical Assistant Professor
Canadian HIV Trials Network
British Columbia Centre for
Excellence in HIV/AIDS
Division of Infectious Diseases
Vancouver, BC, Canada

Peter Moss MD FRCP DTMH
Consultant in Infectious Diseases
and Honorary Senior Lecturer in
Medicine
Director of Infection Prevention and
Control
Hull and East Yorkshire Hospitals
NHS Trust
East Riding of Yorkshire, UK

Patricia Muñoz MD PhD
Professor of Clinical Microbiology
and Infectious Diseases Department
Hospital General Universitario
Gregorio Marañón
Madrid, Spain

Kurt G Naber MD PhD
Associate Professor of Urology
Technical University Munich
Munich, Germany

Sammy Nakhla MD
State University of
New York at Stony Brook
Stony Brook, NY, USA

Jai P Narain MD
Director
Department of Communicable
Diseases
World Health Organization
New Delhi, India

**Dilip Nathwani MB
FRCP(Lond) FRCP(Edin)
FRCP(Glas) DTM&H**
Consultant Physician and Honorary
Professor of Infection
Infection Unit
Ninewells Hospital and Medical
School
Dundee, UK

Paul Newton MRCP
Reader in Tropical Medicine, Head
of the Laos Collaboration
Group Head/PI and Grant Holding
Senior Scientist
Wellcome Trust-Mahosot Hospital-
Oxford Tropical Medicine Research
Collaboration
Vientiane, Laos

Chinh Nguyen MD
Postdoctoral Fellow
Department of Infectious Diseases
University of Maryland School of
Medicine
Baltimore, MD, USA

**Lindsay E Nicolle BSc
BScMed MD FRCPC**
Professor of Internal Medicine and
Medical Microbiology
University of Manitoba
Winnipeg, MB, Canada

Michael S Niederman MD
Chairman
Department of Medicine
Winthrop-University Hospital
Professor of Medicine
Mineola, NY, USA

**Gary J Noel MD FIDSA
FAAP**
Clinical Professor of Pediatrics
Weill Cornell Medical College
Anti-Infectives Medical Leader
Johnson & Johnson Pharmaceutical
Research and Development
Raritan, NJ, USA

**S. Ragnar Norrby MD PhD
FRCP(Edin)**
Professor and Director General
The Swedish Institute for Infectious
Disease Control
Solna, Sweden

François Nosten MD
Professor
Shoklo Malaria Research Unit
Tak Province, Thailand

**Luigi Daniele Notarangelo
MD**
Professor of Pediatrics and
Pathology, Harvard Medical
School
Director of Research and Molecular
Diagnosis Program on Primary
Immunodeficiencies
Division of Immunology
Children's Hospital
Boston, MA, USA

Paul Nyirjesy MD
Professor
Departments of Obstetrics and
Gynecology and Medicine
Drexel University College of
Medicine
Philadelphia, PA, USA

**P. Ronan O'Connell MD
FRCSI FRCS(Glas)**
Head of Surgery and Surgical
Specialties
UCD School of Medicine and
Medical Fellow, Conway Institute
of Biomolecular and Biomedical
Research University College Dublin
Consultant Surgeon
St Vincent's University Hospital
Dublin, Ireland

Jon S Odorico MD FACS
Associate Professor of Surgery
Director of Pancreas and Islet
Transplantation
Division of Transplantation
University of Wisconsin-Madison
School of Medicine and Public
Health
Madison, WI, USA

Contributors

Edmund LC Ong MBBS FRCP FRCPI MSC DTMH
Consultant Physician and Honorary
Senior Lecturer
Department of Infection and
Tropical Medicine
University of Newcastle Medical
School
Newcastle upon Tyne, UK

Steven M Opal MD
Professor of Medicine,
Infectious Disease Division
The Warren Alpert Medical School
of Brown University
Providence, RI, USA

L. Peter Ormerod BSc MBChB(Hons) MD DSc(Med) FRCP
Professor of Medicine
Chest Clinic
Blackburn Royal Infirmary
Blackburn, UK

Douglas R Osmon MD
Associate Professor of Medicine
Division of Infectious Diseases
Department of Internal Medicine
Mayo Clinic
Rochester, MN, USA

Eric A Ottesen MD
Director, Lymphatic Filariasis
Support Center
Task Force for Global Health
Decatur, GA, USA
Technical Director, Neglected
Tropical Disease Control Program
RTI International
Washington, DC, USA

Gustavo Palacios PhD
Assistant Professor
Center for Infection and Immunity
Mailman School of Public Health
Columbia University
New York, NY, USA

Giuseppe Pantaleo MD
Professor of Medicine
Division of Immunology and Allergy
Department of Medicine
Centre Hospitalier Universitaire
Vaudois (CHUV)
University of Lausanne
Lausanne, Switzerland

Laurent Papazian MD
Intensivist
Service de Réanimation Médicale
Hôpital Sainte Marguerite
Marseille, France

Philippe Parola MD PhD
Associate Professor
Unité de Recherche en Maladies
Infectieuses et Tropicales
Emergentes
Marseille, France

Manuel A Pascual MD
Professor and Chief
Transplantation Center
University of Lausanne
Lausanne, Switzerland

Eleni Patrozou MD
Clinical Instructor in Medicine
Alpert Medical School of Brown
University
Providence, RI, USA
Internist-Infectious Diseases
Consultant, Hygeia Hospital
Athens, Greece Medical Director
The PROLEPSIS Institute
Athens, Greece

Carlos Paya MD PhD
Professor of Medicine, Consultant
Infectious Diseases
Division of Infectious Diseases and
Transplant Center
Mayo Clinic
Rochester, MN, USA

Sharon J Peacock BM MSc FRCP FRCPath PhD
Professor of Clinical Microbiology
Department of Medicine
University of Cambridge
Addenbrooke's Hospital
Cambridge, UK

Jean-Claude Pechère MD
President, International Society of
Chemotherapy
Universities of Geneva and
Marrakech
Geneva, Switzerland

Mark D Perkins MD
Chief Scientific Officer
Foundation for Innovative New
Diagnostics (FIND)
Cointrin, Switzerland

Barry Peters MBBS DFFP MD FRCP
Head of Academic Unit of HIV and
STDs
Department of Infectious Diseases
Kings College London
London, UK

Gaby E Pfyffer PhD FAMH FAAM
Professor of Medical
Microbiology
Head, Department of Medical
Microbiology
Center for Laboratory Medicine
Luzerner Kantonsspital Luzern
Luzern, Switzerland

Paul A Pham PharmD BCPS
Research Associate
Johns Hopkins University School of
Medicine
Division of Infectious Diseases
Baltimore, MD, USA

Peter Piot MD PhD FRCP
Director, Institute for Global Health
at Imperial College
London, UK

Geraldine Placko-Parola MD
Physician, Radiology Fellow
Assistant Professor InfectRadiology
Department Hopital de la
Conception
University Hôspital of Marseille
Marseille, France

Stainslas Pol MD PhD
Liver Unit Hôpital Cochin
Paris, France

Klara M Posfay-Barbe MD MS
Head of Pediatric Infectious
Diseases
Department of Pediatrics
Children's Hospital of Geneva
University Hospitals of Geneva
Geneva, Switzerland

William G Powderly MD FRCPI
Professor of Medicine and
Therapeutics
Head, UCD School of Medicine and
Medical Sciences
Medical Professorial Unit
University College Dublin
Dublin, Ireland

Anton Pozniak MD FRCP
Consultant Physician and Director
of HIV Services
Executive Director of HIV Research
Department of HIV and
Genitourinary Medicine
Chelsea and Westminster
Hospital
London, UK

Guy Prod'hom MD
Head of Bacteriology Unit
Institute of Microbiology
University of Lausanne and
University Hospital Centre
Lausanne, Switzerland

Thomas C Quinn MD MSc
Associate Director for International
Research,
Division of Intramural Research,
National Institute of Allergy and
Infectious Diseases
Bethesda, MD, USA

Daniel W Rahn MD
President and Professor of
Medicine
Medical College of Georgia
Augusta, GA, USA

Aadia I Rana MD
Fellow, Division of Infectious
Diseases
Warren Alpert Medical School of
Brown University
Providence, RI, USA

Didier Raoult MD PhD
Professor, Faculté de Médecine
Unité des Rickettsies
WHO Collaborative Center for
Rickettsial Reference and Research
Marseille, France

Raul Raz MD
Director
Infectious Diseases Unit
Ha'Emek Medical Center
Afula, Israel

Raymund Razonable MD
Consultant, Division of Infectious
Diseases
The William J von Liebig Transplant
Center
Associate Professor of Medicine
Mayo Clinic College of Medicine
Rochester, MN, USA

Robert C Read MD FRCP FIDSA
Professor of Infectious Diseases
University of Sheffield Medical
School
Sheffield, UK

Stephen J Reynolds PhD CIH
Staff Clinician
Division of Intramural Research
National Institute of Allergy and
Infectious Diseases
Bethesda, MD, USA

Malcolm D Richardson PhD FIBiol FRCPath
Director
New England Eye Center
Boston, MA, USA

Christopher C Robinson MD
Director
New England Eye Center
Boston, MA, USA

Suzan HM Rooijakkers PhD
Post-Doctorate
Department of Medical
Microbiology
University Medical Center Utrecht
Utrecht, The Netherlands

Daniel Rosenbluth MD
Professor of Medicine and
Pediatrics
Medical Director, Jacqueline Maritz
Lung Center
Fellowship Director
Division of Pulmonary and Critical
Care Medicine
Washington University School of
Medicine
St Louis, MO, USA

Sergio D Rosenzweig MD
Immunopathogenesis Unit
Clinical Pathophysiology Section
Laboratory of Host Defenses
National Institute of Allergy and
Infectious Diseases
Bethesda, MD, USA

Clarisse Rovery MD
Specialist in Infectious Diseases
Infectious Disease Unit
Hôpital Nord
Marseille, France

Robert H Rubin MD FACP FCCP
Associate Director of Infectious Diseases
Brigham and Women's Hospital
Professor of Medicine, Harvard Medical School
Gordon and Marjorie Osborne Professor of Health Sciences and Technology
Director, Center for Experimental Pharmacology and Therapeutics
Co-Director, The Clinical Investigator Training Program Fellowship
Harvard–MIT Division of Health Sciences and Technology
Massachusetts Institute of Technology
Cambridge, MA, USA

Bina Rubinovitch MD
Sheba Medical Center
Tel Hashomer
Ramat Gan, Israel

Kathleen H Rubins PhD
Principal Investigator/Fellow
Rubins Lab
Whitehead Institute for Biomedical Research
Cambridge, MA, USA

Ethan Rubinstein MD Llb
Sellers Professor and Head
Section of Infectious Diseases
Faculty of Medicine
Winnipeg, Manitoba, Canada

Greg Ryan MB FRCOG FRCSC
Associate Professor
Department of Obstetrics and Gynecology
Division of Fetal and Maternal Medicine
University of Toronto
Toronto, ON, Canada

Stephen Ryder DM FRCP
Consultant Hepatologist
Division of Gastroenterology
Queen's Medical Centre
Nottingham University Hospital
NHS Trust and Biomedical Research Unit
Nottingham, UK

Steven Safren PhD
Director of Behavioral Medicine
The Fenway Institute
Associate Professor in Psychology
Department of Psychiatry
Harvard Medical School
Boston, MA, USA

Vikrant V Sahasrabuddhe MBBS MPH DrPH
Assistant Professor
Department of Pediatrics and Institute for Global Health
Vanderbilt University School of Medicine
Nashville, TN, USA

Pekka AI Saikku MD PhD
Professor of Medical Microbiology
Department of Medical Microbiology
University of Oulu
Oulu, Finland

George Sakoulas MD
Assistant Professor
Department of Pediatrics
University of California
San Diego School of Medicine
La Jolla, CA

Juan Carlos Salazar MD MPH
Associate Professor of Pediatrics
Department of Pediatrics
University of Connecticut Health Center
Director, Division of Infectious Diseases
Connecticut Children's Medical Center
Hartford, CT, USA

Michelle R Salvaggio MD
Instructor of Medicine
Division of Infectious Diseases
University of Alabama at Birmingham and Birmingham Veterans Administration Medical Center
Birmingham, AL, USA

Kirsten Schaffer MD MRCPath
Consultant Microbiologist
Department of Medical Microbiology
St Vincent's University Hospital
Dublin, Ireland

Franz-Josef Schmitz MD PhD
Head, Institute for Laboratory Medicine, Microbiology, Hygiene and Transfusion Medicine Klinikum Minden,
Associate Professor of Medical Microbiology, Institute for Medical Microbiology and Virology
University of Düsseldorf
Düsseldorf, Germany

Robert T Schooley MD
Professor and Head
Division of Infectious Diseases
Academic Vice Chair
Department of Medicine
University of California, San Diego
La Jolla, CA, USA

Richard-Fabian Schumacher MD
Attending Physician, Children's Hospital
Clinica Pediatrica
Universita' degli Studi di Brescia
Brescia, Italy

Euan M Scrimgeour MD FRACP DTM&H FAFPHM
Clinical Associate Professor
Department of Immunology and Microbiology
School of Biomedical, Biomolecular and Clinical Sciences
Perth, Australia

James Seddon MBBS MA MRCPCH DTM&H
London School of Hygiene and Tropical Medicine
London, UK

Harald Seifert MD
Professor of Medical Microbiology and Hygiene
Institute for Medical Microbiology, Immunology and Hygiene
University of Cologne
Cologne, Germany

Graham R Serjeant CMG CD MD FRCP FRCPE
Sickle Cell Trust
Kingston, Jamaica

Beverly E Sha MD
Associate Professor of Medicine
Section of Infectious Diseases
Rush University Medical Center
Chicago, IL, USA

Keerti V Shah MD DrPH
Professor of Molecular Microbiology and Immunology
Johns Hopkins Bloombery School of Public Health
Baltimore, MD, USA

Daniel S Shapiro MD
Director, Clinical Microbiology Laboratory
Lahey Clinic
Burlington, MA
Adjunct Associate Professor of Medicine
Boston University School of Medicine
Boston, MA, USA

Gerard Sheehan MB FRCPI
Senior Lecturer
School of Medicine and Medical Sciences
University College Dublin
Consultant in Infectious Diseases
Mater Misericordiae University Hospital
Dublin, Ireland

Shmuel Shoham MD
Director of Transplant Infectious Diseases
Division of Infectious Diseases
Washington Hospital Center
Washington, DC
Immunocompromised Host Section
Pediatric Oncology Branch
National Cancer Institute
Bethesda, MD, USA

Cameron P Simmons BSc(Hons) PhD
Reader in Tropical Medicine
Oxford University Clinical Research Unit
Hospital for Tropical Diseases
Ho Chi Minh City, Vietnam

Kari A Simonsen MD
Assistant Professor of Pediatrics
Section of Pediatric Infectious Diseases
Nebraska Medical Center
Omaha, NE, USA

Neeraj Singh MBBS
Assistant Professor of Medicine
Division of Nephrology
The Ohio State University Medical Centre
Columbus, OH, USA

Mary PE Slack MAMBBChir FRCPath
Head of Haemophilus Influenzae Reference Unit
Respiratory and Systemic Infection Laboratory
Central Public Health Laboratory
London, UK

Jack D Sobel MD
Professor of Infectious Diseases
Division Head
Infectious Diseases
Wayne State University School of Medicine
Detroit, MI, USA

Madhuri M Sopirala MD MPH
Assistant Professor of Internal Medicine
Division of Infectious Diseases
Department of Internal Medicine
OSUMC
Assistant Medical Director, Clinical Epidemiology
The Ohio State University Medical Center
Columbus, OH, USA

Lisa A Spacek MD PhD
Assistant Professor
Division of Infectious Diseases
Department of Medicine
Johns Hopkins University
Baltimore, MD, USA

Shiranee Sriskandan PhD FRCP MA MBBChir
Professor of Infectious Diseases
Department of Infectious Diseases
Faculty of Medicine
Imperial College School of Medicine
London, UK

Samuel L Stanley Jr MD
President Stony Brook University
Stony Brook, NY, USA

James M Steckelberg MD
Professor of Medicine
Division of Infectious Disease
Department of Internal Medicine
Mayo Clinic
Rochester, MN, USA

Iain Stephenson FRCP MB MA (Cantab)
Senior Lecturer in Infectious Diseases
Infectious Diseases Unit
Leicester Royal Infirmary
Leicester, UK

Dennis L Stevens PhD MD
Professor of Medicine
University of Washington School of Medicine
Chief, Infectious Disease Section
Veterans Affairs Medical Center
Boise, ID, USA

Contributors

Walter L Straus MD MPH
Global Director for Scientific
Affairs-Vaccines
Merck Vaccines and Infectious
Diseases
Merck & Co., Inc.
West Point, PA, USA

Willem Sturm MD PhD
Professor of Medical Microbiology
Department of Medical
Microbiology
Nelson R Madela School of
Medicine
Congella, South Africa

Richard C Summerbell PhD
Senior Researcher
Centraalbureau voor
Schimmelcultures
Royal Netherlands Academy of
Sciences
Utrecht, The Netherlands

Joseph S Susa MD
Clinical Assistant Professor
Dermatology Department
University of Texas Southwestern
Medical Center
Dallas, TX, USA

**Sarah J Tabrizi BSc(Hons)
FRCP PhD**
Reader in Neurology and
Neurogenetics
Department of Neurodegenerative
Diseases/MRC Prion Unit
Institute of Neurology
London, UK

Marc A Tack MD
Infectious Diseases Consultant
Medical Associates of the Hudson
Valley P.C.
Kingston, NY, USA

Randy Taplitz MD
Associate Professor of Clinical
Medicine
Clinical Director
Division of Infectious Diseases
Associate Medical Director of UCSD
Infection Prevention and Clinical
Epidemiology
University of California at San Diego
San Diego, CA, USA

Pablo Tebas MD
Associate Professor of Medicine
Division of Infectious Diseases
University of Pennsylvania
Philadelphia, PA, USA

**Marleen Temmerman MD
MPH PhD**
Professor
Head of Department of Obstetrics
& Gynaecology
International Center for
Reproductive Health
WHO Collaborating Centre
for Research on Sexual and
Reproductive Health
Faculty of Medicine and Health
Sciences
Ghent University
Ghent, Belgium

Steven FT Thijsen MD PhD
Medical Microbiologist
Department of Medical
Microbiology
Diakonessenhuis
Utrecht, The Netherlands

Lora D Thomas MD MPH
Assistant Professor of Medicine
Division of Infectious Diseases
Vanderbilt University Medical Center
Nashville, TN, USA

**Gail Thomson MB ChB
MRCP & DTM&H**
Consultant in Infectious Diseases
North Manchester General Hospital
Manchester, UK

**Guy E Thwaites MA MBBS
MRCP MRCPath PhD**
Wellcome Trust Clinical Research
Fellow
Centre for Molecular Microbiology
and Infection
Imperial College London
London, UK

Umberto Tirelli MD
Director, Division of Medical Oncology
National Cancer Institute
Aviano, Italy

**Nina E Tolkoff-Rubin MD
FACP**
Director of Hemodialysis and CAPD
Units
Medical Director for Renal
Transplantation
Professor of Medicine
Harvard Medical School
Department of Medicine
Massachusetts General Hospital
Boston, MA, USA

Tone Tønjum MD PhD
Professor
Chief Physician
Institute of Microbiology, Centre for
Molecular Biology and Neuroscience
University of Oslo
Rikshospitalet
Oslo, Norway

Francesca J Torriani MD
Professor of Clinical Medicine
Medical Director of UCSD
Infection Prevention and Clinical
Epidemiology
Division of Infectious Diseases
University of California at San Diego
San Diego, CA, USA

Gregory C Townsend MD
Assistant Professor of Medicine
Division of Infectious Diseases
University of Virginia
Charlottesville, VA, USA

Gloria Trallero Masó BSc
Enterovirus Laboratory
Department of Virology
National Center for Microbiology
Instituto de Salud Carlos III
Madrid, Spain

Paul M Tulkens MD PhD
Professor of Pharmacology
Unité de Pharmacologie cellulaire
et moléculaire & Louvain Drug
Research Institute
Université catholique de Louvain
Brussels, Belgium

Allan R Tunkel MD PhD
Professor of Medicine
Drexel University College of Medicine
Chair, Department of Medicine
Monmouth Medical Center
Long Branch, NJ, USA

Emanuela Vaccher MD
Department of Medical Oncology
National Cancer Institute
Aviano, Italy

Anaïs Vallet-Pichard MD
Service d'Hepatologie
Hopital Necker
Paris, France

**Françoise Van Bambeke
PharmD PhD**
Senior Research Associate of
the Belgian Fonds National de la
Recherche Scientifique
Unité de Pharmacologie cellulaire
et moléculaire & Louvain Drug
Research Insitute
Université catholique de Louvain
Brussels, Belgium

**Diederik van de Beek MD
PhD**
Neurologist
Department of Neurology
Center of Infection and Immunity
Amsterdam (CINIMA)
Academic Medical Center
University of Amsterdam
Amsterdam, The Netherlands

**Jos WM van der Meer MD
PhD FRCP**
Professor of Medicine
Department of General Internal
Medicine
Nijmegen Institute for Infection
Inflammation and Immunity
Radboud University Medical Center
Nijmegen, The Netherlands

Anton M van Loon PhD
Director
Department of Virology
University Medical Centre Utrecht
Utrecht, The Netherlands

Jos van Putten MD PhD
Professor of Infection Biology
Infectious Diseases and
Immunology
Utrecht University
Utrecht, The Netherlands

Bernard P Vaudaux MD
Head, Unit of Pediatric Infectious
Diseases and Vaccinology
Department of Pediatrics
Centre Hospitalier Universitaire
Vaudois and Hôpital de l'Enfance
de Lausanne
Lausanne, Switzerland

Sten H Vermund MD PhD
Amos Christie Chair of Global Health
Vanderbilt University School of
Medicine
Nashville, TN, USA

**Hans Verstraelen MD MPH
PhD**
Research Fellow
Department of Obstetrics and
Gynaecology
Ghent University
Ghent, Belgium

Paul Verweij MD PhD
Professor of Medical Microbiology
Department of Medical
Microbiology
Radboud University Nijmegen
Medical Centre
Nijmegen Centre for Molecular Life
Sciences
Nijmegen, The Netherlands

Raphael P Viscidi MD
Professor of Pediatrics
Department of Pediatrics
Johns Hopkins University School of
Medicine
Baltimore, MD, USA

Kumar Visvanathan MD
Director, Innate Immunity
Laboratory and Infectious Diseases
Physician
Centre for Inflammatory Diseases
Department of Medicine (Monash
Medical Centre)
Monash University
Clayton, VIC, Australia

Govinda S Visvesvara PhD
Research Microbiologist
Division of Parasitic Diseases
National Center for Zoonotic,
Vector–Borne and Enteric Diseases
Centers for Disease Control
and Prevention
Atlanta, GA, USA

Lorenz von Seidlein MD PhD
Reader
London School of Hygiene and
Tropical Medicine
London, UK

**Florian ME Wagenlehner
MD PhD**
Consultant Urologist
Clinic for Urology and Pediatric
Urology
Justus-Liebig-University
Giessen, Germany

Victoria Wahl-Jensen MS PhD
Principal Investigator
Virology
United States Army Medical
Research Institute of Infectious
Disease (USAMRIID)
Fort Detrick, MD, USA

Thomas J Walsh MD
Head, Immunocompromised Host
Section
Pediatric Oncology Branch
National Cancer Institute
Bethesda, MD, USA

David C Warhurst BSc PhD DSc FRCPath
Emeritus Professor of Protozoan Chemotherapy
Department of Infections and Tropical Diseases
London School of Hygiene and Tropical Medicine
London, UK

David W Warnock BSc PhD FAAM FRCPath
Director
Division of Foodborne
Bacterial and Mycotic Diseases
National Center for Zoonotic, Vector-borne and Enteric Diseases
Centers for Disease Control and Prevention
Adjunct Professor of Pathology and Laboratory Medicine
Emory University School of Medicine
Atlanta, GA, USA

David A Warrell MA DM DSc FRCP FRCPE HonFCeylonCP FMedSci HonFZS FRGS
Emeritus Professor of Tropical Medicine
Nuffield Department of Clinical Medicine
University of Oxford
Oxford, UK

Mary J Warrell MBBS MRCP FRCPath
Oxford Vaccine Group University of Oxford
Centre for Clinical Vaccinology and Tropical Medicine
Oxford, UK

Adilia Warris MD PhD
Pediatric Infectious Diseases Specialist
Head of the Division of Pediatric Infectious Diseases and Immunology
Department of Pediatrics
Radboud University Nijmegen Medical Center
Nijmegen, The Netherlands

Rainer Weber MD DTMH(Lond)
Head of the Division of Infectious Diseases and Hospital Epidemiology
Division of Infectious Diseases and Hospital Epidemiology
Department of Internal Medicine
University Hospital Zurich
Zurich, Switzerland

Wolfgang Weidner MD
Professor of Urology
Head of Department of Urology
Clinic for Urology, Pediatric Urology and Andrology
Justus-Liebig University
Giessen, Germany

Vivienne C Weston MBBS MSc FRCPath FRCP(UK)
Consultant Medical Microbiologist
Department of Microbiology
Nottingham University Hospitals
NHS Trust
Nottingham, UK

Estella Whimbey MD
Associate Medical Director
University of Washington
Medical Center
Seattle WA, USA

Michael Whitby MD BS DTM&H MPH FRACP FRCPA FRCPath FAFPHM
Director, Infection Management Services
Princess Alexandra Hospital
Brisbane, Australia

Peter J White PhD
Head
Modelling and Economics Unit
Health Protection Agency Centre for Infections, London;
MRC Centre for Outbreak Analysis and Modelling, Department of Infectious Disease Epidemiology
Imperial College London
London, UK

Christopher JM Whitty FRCP DTM&H
Consultant Physician
Hospital for Tropical Diseases
Professor of International Health
London School of Hygiene and Tropical Medicine
London, UK

Rob JL Willems PhD
Associate Professor
Medical Microbiology
University Medical Center Utrecht
Utrecht, The Netherlands

Emrys Williams MBBS MRCP DTM&H FRCPath
Consultant in Medical Microbiology
NPHS Microbiology Bangor
Ysbyty Gwynedd
Bangor, UK

Cara Wilson MD
Associate Professor
Infectious Diseases Division
University of Colorado School of Medicine
Denver, CO, USA

Mary E Wilson MD FACP FIDSA
Associate Clinical Professor of Medicine
Harvard Medical School
Associate Professor of Global Health and Population
Harvard School of Public Health
Washington DC, WA, USA

Richard E Winn MD
Division Director of Pulmonary Medicine and Infectious Diseases,
Scott and White Clinic
Professor of Internal Medicine
Texas A&M College of Medicine
Temple, TX, USA

Kevin L Winthrop MD MPH
Assistant Professor of Infectious Diseases, Ophthalmology, Public Health and Preventive Medicine
Oregon Health and Science University
Portland, OR, USA

Martin J Wiselka MD PhD FRCP
Consultant in Infectious Disease
Leicester Royal Infirmary
Leicester, UK

Hilmar Wisplinghoff MD
Physician
Institute for Medical Microbiology Immunology and Hygiene
University of Cologne
Cologne, Germany

Cameron R Wolfe MD
Fellow
Department of Infectious Diseases and Internal Health
Duke University School of Medicine
Durham, NC, USA

Robin Wood BSc BM MMed DTM&H
Professor of Medicine
The Desmond Tutu HIV Centre
Institute of Infectious Disease and Molecular Medicine
Faculty of Health Sciences
University of Cape Town
Cape Town, South Africa

Natalie Wright BSc
University of Texas Health Science Center
Houston, TX, USA

James R Yankaskas MD MS BS
Professor of Medicine
Cystic Fibrosis/Pulmonary Research and Treatment Center
University of North Carolina
Chapel Hill, NC, USA

Najam A Zaidi MD
Assistant Professor of Medicine (Clinical)
Warren Alpert Medical School of Brown University
Providence, RI, USA

Jonathan M Zenilman MD
Professor of Medicine
Johns Hopkins University School of Medicine
Baltimore, MD, USA

Yaobi Zhang MD PhD
Field Programme Co-ordinator
Schistosomiasis Control Initiative
Department of Infectious Disease Epidemiology
Imperial College London
London, UK

Arie J Zuckerman MD DSc FRCP FRCPath FMedSci
Professor of Medical Microbiology in the University of London
Academic Centre for Travel Medicine and Vaccines
London, UK

Jane Nicola Zuckerman MD FRCP(Edin) FRCPath MRCGP FFPH FFPM FHEA
Senior Lecturer and Honorary Consultant
WHO Centre for Reference, Research and Training in Travel Medicine
Academic Centre for Travel Medicine and Vaccines
University College London Medical School
London, UK

Alimuddin Zumla BSc MBChB MSc PhD FRCP(Lond) FRCP(Edin)
Director, Centre for Infectious Diseases and International Health
Royal Free and University College London Medical School
Consultant Infectious Diseases Physician
University College London NHS Hospitals Trust
London, UK

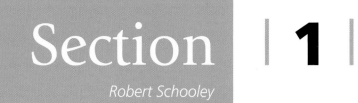

Section | 1 |

Robert Schooley

Introduction to Infectious Diseases

Joshua Fierer
David Looney
Menno Kok
Jean-Claude Pechère

Chapter | **1** |

Nature and pathogenicity of micro-organisms

Human existence would be impossible without the micro-organisms that surround us, as they play critical roles in processes as diverse as photosynthesis, nitrogen fixation, production of vitamins in the human intestine and decomposition of organic matter. They are the sole, true 'recyclers' of our planet. Micro-organisms are also the major driving force behind the evolution of life. They evolved photosynthesis and respiration, which have since been acquired by present-day eukaryotes, and they mediate genome rearrangements in infected host cells.

In a rather simplified view, micro-organisms may be considered to be no more than 'little machines that multiply'. In fact, this is what they do best. We are starting to understand some of the strategies micro-organisms have developed to stay alive, grow and reproduce. The lifestyle of a micro-organism is intimately related to its environment, whether that environment is the human body or a polluted riverbed. Some highly specialized micro-organisms have adapted to the harsh environmental conditions, while others, such as root-colonizing bacteria and our own intestinal flora, have taken advantage of the abundant resources provided by higher organisms.

This chapter focuses on the lifestyle of pathogenic micro-organisms and how they infect us, reproduce and cause disease. We shall use the word 'pathogenicity' to indicate the capacity to cause disease (or damage) in nonimmune individuals. Although the word 'virulence' is often used in the same sense, we mean it to refer to the severity of the illness that is caused. Communicability refers to the transmissibility or infectiousness of micro-organisms.

DEFINITION AND COMPARISON OF INFECTIOUS AGENTS

The definition of an 'infectious agent' was proposed by J Henle in 1840 and put to the test by the German physician Robert Koch. In 1876, Koch reported experiments on mice with *Bacillus anthracis* showing that:
- a single micro-organism could be isolated from all animals suffering from anthrax;
- the disease could be reproduced in an experimental host by infection with a pure culture of this bacterium; and
- the same micro-organism could subsequently be reisolated from the experimental host.

This definition is an oversimplification because many pathogenic microbes have never been cultured (e.g. *Mycobacterium leprae*), others lack a suitable animal host in which the infection can be reproduced (e.g. *Salmonella enterica* serovar Typhi) and some cause disease only under specific conditions.

Infectious agents can be divided into four groups:
- Prions, which consist of only a single protein (PrP). The infectious form (PrP^{TSE})[1] is transmissible as spongiform encephalopathy (see Chapter 22).
- Viruses, which contain proteins and nucleic acids, and virioids which contain only nucleic acid. These characteristically disassemble after cell entry and then assemble their progeny during replication[2] (see Chapters 151 and 152).
- Bacteria, including archaea and eubacteria. Unlike eukaryotes, the DNA genomes of these prokaryotes are not separated from the cell by a membrane. Unlike viruses, they remain enclosed within their own cell envelope throughout their life cycle (see Chapters 165–177).
- Eukaryotes, including fungi (see Chapters 178 and 179), protozoa (see Chapters 180–183) and multicellular parasites (see Chapter 184). These organisms have subcellular compartments, including the nucleus, where DNA transcription occurs.

Table 1.1 compares the properties that define prokaryotes with eukaryotes and Table 1.2 emphasizes the differences between bacteria and fungi, many of which determine the specificity of antimicrobial agents.

GENERAL PROPERTIES AND CLASSIFICATION OF VIRUSES

Taxonomy of viruses

The hierarchical classification system[4] groups viruses in families (-viridae), genera (-virus or -viruses) and species (-virus), emphasizing similarities in the type (DNA or RNA) and nature (single stranded or double stranded, segmented or nonsegmented) of genetic material, and structural features (size, symmetry and presence or absence of a lipid envelope; see Table 1.3). For example, picornaviridae is a family of small, non-enveloped RNA viruses containing the enterovirus genus, which in turn includes poliovirus species of serotypes 1, 2 and 3.[5] The Baltimore classification system[6] emphasizes the relationship of the genetic material of the virus and the viral replication scheme. For example, group IV contains viruses with single-stranded RNA genomes where the mRNA shares the same sense as the viral RNA (+ssRNA), which includes picornaviridae, enterovirus and poliovirus.

Common steps in the replication of viruses

Virus replication involves the following steps.
1. Attachment: Virus particles (virions) must first attach to specific receptor(s) on the surface of a host cell.
2. Penetration: This may proceed via direct fusion with the cell membrane or through endocytosis and pH-mediated fusion.
3. Uncoating: The virion disassembles, freeing nucleic acid and viral proteins needed for replication.

Table 1.1 Comparison of prokaryotes and eukaryotes

Feature	Prokaryotes	Eukaryotes
Chromosome	Single, circular or linear	Yes
Gene organization	Operon-polycistrionic mRNA	Single genes and block of genes
Nucleosomes	No	Yes
Nuclear membrane	No	Yes
Mitosis	No	Yes
Introns in genes	No	Yes
Transcription	Coupled with translation	Separate from translation
mRNA	No terminal polyadenylation (except archaebacteria); polygenic	Terminal polyadenylation; usually monogenic
First amino acid	Unstable formylmethionine (except archaebacteria)	Methionine
Ribosome	70S (30S + 50S)	80S (40S + 60S)
Cell wall	Presence of muramic acid, D-amino acids, peptidoglycan (except archaebacteria and mycoplasma)	No muramic acid, D-amino acids or peptidoglycan
Membrane	No sterols or phosphatidyl-choline (except mycoplasma)	Sterols and phosphatidyl-choline
Endoplasmic reticulum	No	Yes
Mitochondria	No	Yes (*E. histolytica*, *Giardia* and microsporidia have vestigial remnants of mitochondria)
Lysosomes and peroxisomes	No	Yes
Movement	By flagella, composed of a single fiber	Ameboid, by cilia or cilia-like flagella

Table 1.2 Comparison of bacteria and fungi

Characteristics	Bacteria	Fungi
Cell volume (mm³)	0.6–5.0	Yeast: 20–50; molds: greater than yeast
Nucleus	No membrane	Membrane
Mitochondria	No	Yes
Endoplasmic reticulum	No	Yes
Sterol in cytoplasmic membrane	No (except for mycoplasma)	Yes
Cell wall components	Muramic acids and teichoic acids; no chitin, glucans or mannans	Chitin, glucans and mannans; no muramic acids or teichoic acids
Metabolism	Autotropic or heterotropic	Heterotropic
Sensitivity to polyenes	No	Yes

Adapted from Kobayashi.[3]

4. Replication: Viral proteins and messages are expressed. Intermediates such as viral complementary RNA or integrated proviral DNA may be needed.
5. Assembly: New virions containing viral nucleic acid are formed.
6. Release: New virions are released from the cell via lysis of the cell or intra- or extracellular budding.

Structure of viruses

The virion is designed to protect the viral genome and to mediate the migration of the virus and the invasion of the target host cell. Viruses are small, the smallest being ~25–30 nm in diameter, while the largest (mimivirus, an infectious agent of amebae) are 400 nm or more in size.[7] The viral genome is tightly associated with a nucleoprotein in a highly organized core structure, the nucleocapsid. In some virus families, such as (–) strand RNA viruses and retroviruses, the virion contains enzymes required for early stages of virus replication.

The main proteinaceous outer structure of a virus is the capsid or tegument. Clefts or vertices in the assembled capsid, protruding protein spikes or other structures may mediate viral attachment. Alternatively, the capsid is surrounded by an outer lipid membrane (the envelope) derived from membranes of the host cell in a process termed 'budding.' Viral proteins inserted within the envelope then serve as receptors for specific host cell molecules.

The viral genome

Viral genomes consist of DNA or RNA, and range from 1.7 kb to 1.2 Mb in size. There may be only a single gene in the smallest virions, whereas the larger genomes encode hundreds. For example, parvoviridae have only two open reading frames, whereas the vaccinia poxvirus has 263 known genes.

The nucleic acid of all mammalian DNA viruses except the parvoviridae and circoviridae is double stranded (dsDNA, Fig. 1.1). In contrast, the nucleic acid of all mammalian RNA viruses except the reoviruses (e.g. rotavirus, coltivirus) is single stranded (ssRNA). The genome structure may be linear, circular or rod-like, and either non-segmented or segmented. Genome segmentation facilitates genetic exchange between co-infecting virions in a process known as reassortment. Some viral nucleic acid molecules may contain modified nucleotides, which inhibit host cell nucleases and/or mediate recognition by viral polymerase. Linear genomes often contain conserved terminal sequences. When complementary, these allow partial circularization of the genome or formation of panhandle or tube-like structures. Terminal sequences may also allow incomplete replication products to recombine or mediate recognition by proteins that prime transcription or replication. The proviral DNA of retroviruses is flanked by repeat sequences similar to transposable genetic elements.

The genome of ssRNA viruses may have either of two possible polarities. The viral RNA (vRNA) of positive-strand RNA viruses acts directly as mRNA for protein synthesis; they resemble eukaryotic RNAs with a cap at the 5' end and are polyadenylated at the 3' end. In contrast, the RNA-dependent RNA polymerase of (–) ssRNA viruses uses the vRNA as a template for mRNA transcription. Negative-strand RNA genomes have neither cap structures nor poly-A tails, often parasitizing cap structures from cellular pre-mRNA or mRNA. Retroviruses synthesize a dsDNA copy of the positive-strand RNA genome, which integrates into the cellular DNA and then expresses viral messages.

Table 1.3 Classification of viruses

Family name	Example	Genome size (kb) polarity (+ or –) and segments	Morphology	Envelope
DNA viruses				
Single-stranded (Class II)				
Parvoviridae	Human parvovirus B19	5 (±) single	Icosahedral	No
Mixed-stranded (Class VII)				
Hepadnaviridae	Hepatitis B	3 (±) single	Icosahedral	Yes
Double-stranded (Class I)				
Papovaviridae	Wart virus	8 (±) single	Icosahedral	No
Polyomaviridae	JC virus	5 (±) single	Icosahedral	No
Adenoviridae	Adenovirus	36–38 (±) single	Icosahedral	No
Herpesviridae	Herpes simplex	120–220 (±) single	Icosahedral	Yes
Poxviridae	Vaccinia	120–280 (±) single	Complex	Yes
RNA viruses				
Positive-sense (Class IV)				
Picornaviridae	Poliovirus	7.2–8.4 (+) single	Icosahedral	No
Togaviridae	Rubella	12 (+) single	Icosahedral	Yes
Flaviviridae	Yellow fever	10 (+) single	Icosahedral	Yes
Coronaviridae	Infectious bronchitis	16–21 (+) single	Helical	Yes
Negative-sense (Class V)				
Rhabdoviridae	Rabies	13–16 (–) single	Helical	Yes
Paramyxoviridae	Measles	16–20 (–) single	Helical	Yes
Orthomyxoviridae	Influenza	14 (–) 8	Helical	Yes
Bunyaviridae	California encephalitis	13–21 (–) 3	Helical	Yes
Arenaviridae	Lassa fever	10–14 (–) 2	Helical	Yes
Filoviridae	Marburg, Ebola	19 (–) single	Helical	Yes
Reverse (Class VI)				
Retroviridae	HIV-1	3–9 (+) diploid	Icosahedral	Yes
Double-stranded (Class III)				
Reoviridae	Rotavirus	16–27 (±) 10-12	Icosahedral	No

The capsid

The viral genome is protected by one or more protein coats, the nucleocapsid and/or capsid. The capsid is made of structures known as capsomeres, which consist of proteins coded by the viral genome, and accounts for a large portion of the viral mass. Papillomavirus produces only two capsid proteins and poliovirus four, but more complex viruses may encode a much larger variety.

Picornaviruses, adenoviruses and papovaviruses have a nucleocapsid structure with icosahedral symmetry. The capsid consists of 20 triangular facets and 12 corners or apices. Influenza, measles and rabies virus form capsids with helical symmetry. The central core is formed by the nucleic acid genome, around which the nucleocapsid proteins are arranged like the steps of a spiral staircase, forming long cylinders (Fig. 1.2).

More complex virion morphologies also exist. Bacteriophages, which use bacteria as hosts, have additional attachment structures fixed to the capsid. The nucleocapsid of orthopoxviruses, such as variola and vaccinia virus, consists of a network of tubules, sometimes surrounded by an envelope, forming a brick-shaped virion.

The envelope

Enveloped viruses contain nucleocapsids of either icosahedral (e.g. herpesviruses, togavirus) or helical symmetry (e.g. influenza). The outer envelope consists of a lipid bilayer derived from host cell membrane in which the viral glycoproteins are embedded. The viral matrix proteins (M proteins) associate with the envelope, playing an important role in the structural organization of the virion by connecting the capsid to the viral glycoprotein inserted in the lipid bilayer. Besides oligosaccharide residues, the glycoproteins contain a membrane anchor and, in many cases, one or two molecules of fatty acid. Glycoproteins play a key role in the attachment of virions to the cell surface and penetration into the cell.

Some glycoproteins have enzymatic activity, such as the influenza virus neuraminidase, which promotes the release of newly formed viral particles from the host cell membrane. Maturation of protein structures and transcription steps may occur after release from the host cell. For example, the typical conical core of the human immunodeficiency virus retrovirus may be incomplete at release and partial reverse transcription occurs within the virion.[9]

Viral gene expression strategies

In the Baltimore classification, seven major viral replication strategies are distinguished (see Figs 1.1, 1.3 and the following).

In positive-strand RNA viruses (Baltimore Class IV), the viral genome serves immediately as mRNA. The first step in viral infection consists of a complete translation of the genome to produce a polyprotein, which is sequentially processed into smaller polypeptides via enzymatic cleavage which is at least partially autocatalytic. In the early phase, processing of viral structural proteins occurs slowly, due to the low concentrations of mature viral proteases. Viral complementary RNA is synthesized, followed by new viral RNA. As the viral proteases accumulate, core proteins are more efficiently processed, assemble and begin to encapsidate viral RNA. This strategy is used by picornaviruses and flaviviridae, including hepatitis C viruses. In other (+)ssRNA virus families (e.g. togaviridae, coronaviridae, caliciviridae and hepatitis E virus), the viral complementary RNA serves not only for production of

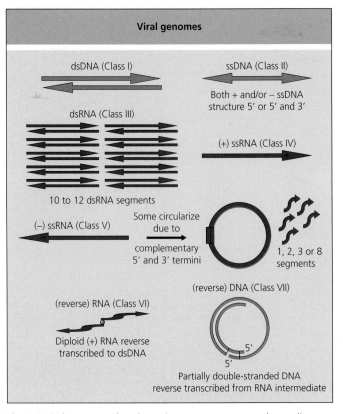

Viral genomes

dsDNA (Class I)

ssDNA (Class II)

Both + and/or – ssDNA
structure 5' or 5' and 3'

dsRNA (Class III)

(+) ssRNA (Class IV)

10 to 12 dsRNA segments

(–) ssRNA (Class V)

Some circularize
due to

complementary
5' and 3' termini

1, 2, 3 or 8
segments

(reverse) DNA (Class VII)

(reverse) RNA (Class VI)

Diploid (+) RNA reverse
transcribed to dsDNA

5'

5'

Partially double-stranded DNA
reverse transcribed from RNA intermediate

Fig. 1.1 Viral genomes. The schematic genomes are grouped according to the Baltimore classification system. DNA is represented by blue shades, RNA in red shades. Arrows indicate direction of DNA/RNA 5' to 3', not necessarily relationship of sense of messenger RNA to that of genome. See Figure 1.2 for a diagram of typical viral structures, Table 1.5 for a list of representative viruses within groups and Figure 1.3 for strategies of viral replication.

full length vRNA, but also subgenomic transcripts encoding structural proteins, allowing regulation of expression.

The RNA-dependent RNA polymerase of (–)ssRNA viruses (Baltimore Class V) must first produce transcripts using the infecting vRNA as a template. Primary transcription may generate a full-length viral complementary RNA (positive-strand) which acts as both mRNA for viral protein synthesis as well as a template for transcription of new viral RNA. This is typical of segmented (–)ssRNA viruses including orthomyxoviridae and most bunyaviridae. Alternatively, the incoming viral RNA may initially be transcribed into mRNA messages for individual genes, which must accumulate before transcription of full-length viral complementary RNA and replication of viral RNA can occur (e.g. paramyxoviridae, rhabdoviridae). The late phases of replication transcription and viral protein synthesis proceed simultaneously.

The arenaviridae and the some bunyaviridae use a somewhat more complicated strategy, termed ambisense. For one or more of the RNA genome segments, both the viral RNA and the viral complementary RNA serve as templates for mRNA transcription by the viral polymerase. This does not result in the formation of complementary double-stranded mRNAs, as different portions of the genome are transcribed from the viral and complementary RNA strands.

Only a few double-stranded RNA viruses (reoviridae, Baltimore Class III) produce human disease. The coltivirus Colorado tick fever virus causes a febrile syndrome with myalgia, headache, rash and occasionally encephalitis. The rotaviruses are important causes of diarrheal illness. Virions have 10–12 dsRNA segments and replication resembles that of (–)ssRNA viruses in that RNA is not infectious, and transcription of segment length mRNAs using the negative strand of the genomic dsRNA must first occur before genome replication. Regulation is accomplished via transcription rate (inverse to segment length) and efficiency of translation (varying up to 100-fold).

In the case of ssDNA viruses (parvoviridae and circoviridae, Baltimore Class II), the incoming genome is first used to express proteins that permit the synthesis of the complementary DNA strand. Double-stranded DNA is a replication intermediate, and DNA replication is dependent on repeats which form DNA structures on one or both ends. These parvoviridae include the B19 erythrovirus that causes erythema infectiosum (fifth disease) in children and exanthem, arthropathy and aplastic crisis in adults. This family also includes the apathogenic adeno-associated dependoviruses (AAV), which serology indicates cause ubiquitous human infection.[10] Parvoviridae have 4.5–5.5 kb ssDNA genomes and only two open reading frames, one of which codes for between two and four nonstructural proteins and the other coats polypeptides. The circoviridae have circular ssDNA genomes. This family includes Torque Teno viruses (TTV, TTMV) which cause widespread human infection without evidence of disease.[11]

Replication of dsDNA viruses (Baltimore Class I) proceeds to lysis or latency depending on cellular conditions. The lytic phase can be subdivided into early and late phases. In the early lytic phase, viral genes alter cellular conditions to allow efficient viral DNA synthesis and transcription, often activating the host cell and inducing cell division. In the late lytic phase, viral proteins accumulate, virions are assembled and released upon death of the cell. In latency, viral gene expression is confined to functions that prevent replication while maintaining the viral genome within the cell, often for the lifetime of the individual. When cellular conditions become favorable, the latent virus can be 'activated' into lytic replication.

There are many dsDNA viruses of medical importance for humans, including:

- herpes simplex viruses (cause of genital and labial herpes, meningitis and encephalitis);
- varicella-zoster virus (the causative agent of chickenpox);
- human cytomegalovirus (frequently causing disease in immunocompromised hosts);
- Epstein–Barr virus (causing infectious mononucleosis);
- adenoviruses (causing respiratory disease and conjunctivitis);

and many others.

In the case of the retroviruses (Baltimore Class VI), the virus enters the cell and uncoats, discharging the preintegration complex, consisting of the polyadenylated, diploid viral RNA genome together with nucleoproteins, the viral reverse transcriptase and the viral integrase. The two RNA genomes are converted to a single, mostly dsDNA copy by reverse transcriptase in a process requiring template switching. The viral integrase then cuts the host genome and inserts the linear viral DNA into the chromosome as a provirus. This process may require cellular activation and/or cell division, though retroviruses can persistent for weeks at stages before integration. Integrated virus may become latent, with limited or no transcription by cellular RNA polymerase II, until conditions allow virus replication.

More complex retroviruses (e.g. spumaviruses, lentiviruses) first transcribe multiply-spliced mRNAs that direct the synthesis of regulatory proteins. As these accumulate, the processing of viral transcripts changes and more singly or unspliced mRNAs coding for viral structural proteins are produced. For example, human immunodeficiency virus (HIV) *Rev* protein, produced from early, multiply-spliced RNA transcripts, prevents splicing and allows nuclear export of singly spliced and unspliced messages.

Hepadnaviruses (Baltimore Class VII), including hepatitis B virus, encode genetic information in DNA but use reverse transcription during infection in the cell to produce the (–) strand of viral DNA, which in turn is used as a template for synthesis of (+) strand viral DNA.

GENERAL PROPERTIES AND CLASSIFICATION OF BACTERIA

Bacteria are small (0.6–4.0 μm) unicellular organisms; 3×10^{12} bacteria weigh in the order of 1 g. Under optimal conditions, a bacterium may divide between two or three times per hour. Theoretically, nearly 300 g of bacterial mass can be produced from a single bacterial cell in

Examples of virions

Adenovirus

HIV-1

Influenza virus

Rabies virus

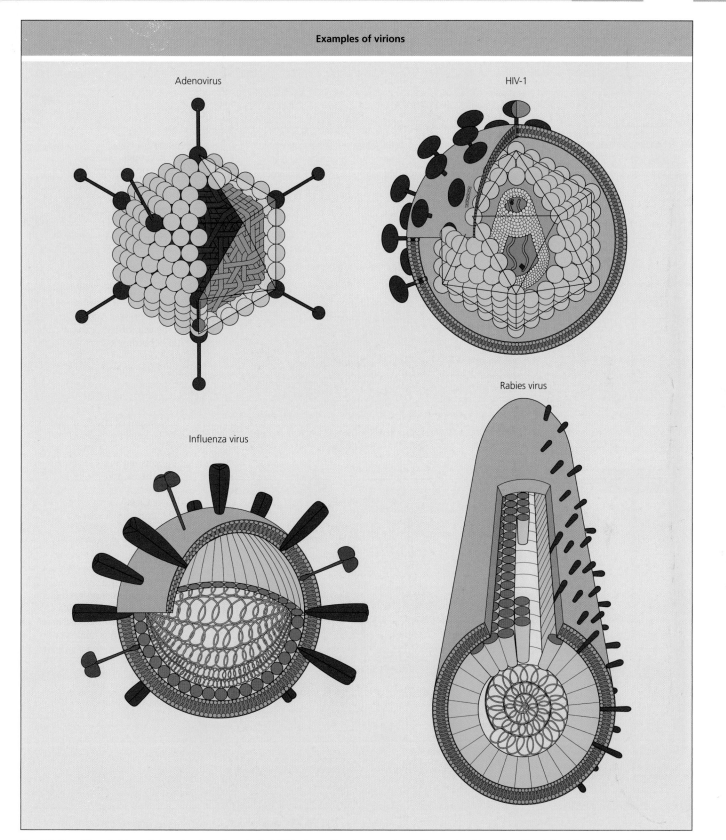

Fig. 1.2 Examples of virions. Adenovirus is an icosahedral DNA virus without an envelope; fibers extend from the 12 points of the icosahedral coat; DNA forms a ribbon-like molecule. Approximate size 8 nm. HIV-1; glycoprotein (GP) molecules protrude through the lipid membrane; the icosahedral capsid encloses a truncated conical nucleocapsid in which the diploid RNA is enclosed. Approximate size 100 nm. Influenza virus is an enveloped RNA virus containing nucleocapsid of helical symmetry; spikes of hemagglutinin and neuraminidase protrude from the lipid bilayer. Approximate size 100–200 nm (variable). Rabies virus is a helical RNA nucleocapsid with a bullet-shaped lipoprotein envelope in which approximately 200 GPs are embedded. Approximate size 150 nm. (The diagram is not to relative scale.) Adapted from Collier and Oxford[8] by permission of Oxford University Press.

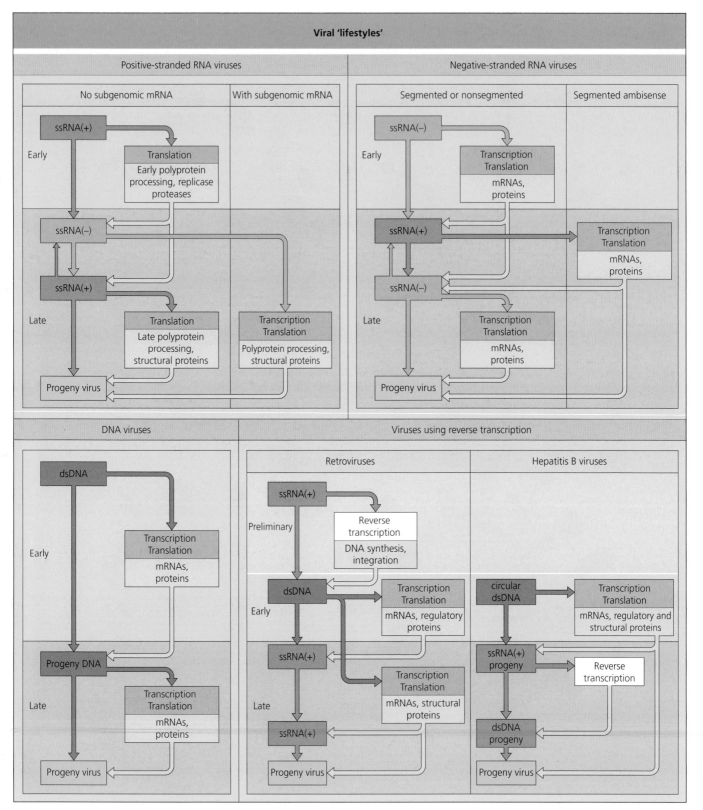

Fig. 1.3 Viral 'lifestyles'. Upper left. Single stranded (+) sense RNA viruses can be subdivided into those which produce subgenomic mRNAs (e.g. togaviridae, coronaviridae, calciviridae), allowing additional regulation of transcription, and those which do not (poliovirus, hepatitis A virus, flaviviridae including hepatitis C virus). Upper right. Negative sense RNA viruses must first transcribe RNA messages from incoming viral RNA (vRNA), as well as making a copy complementary to the viral genomic DNA (vcRNA) to serve as a template for synthesis of new viral RNA. Some (−) ssRNA viruses use both vRNA and vcRNA as templates for transcription of mRNA (arenaviruses, some bunyaviruses). Lower left. Double stranded DNA viruses have early and late lytic phases of replication, and some (e.g. Epstein–Barr herpesvirus) also have latent (usually episomal) phases. Lower right. Viruses using reverse transcription include RNA retroviruses (e.g. HIV), which reverse transcribe a dsDNA copy from diploid (+) ssRNA vRNA, and hepadnaviruses (e.g. HBV) which reverse transcribe the (−) strand of DNA from RNA transcribed from incoming viral DNA. (Courtesy of Menno Kok & Jean-Claude Pechere.)

one day. Such small organisms profit from a favorable cell surface-to-volume ratio, which allows metabolic fluxes largely superior to those attained by the larger eukaryotic cells. Bacteria react very quickly to environmental changes, regulating gene transcription to adapt their physiology.

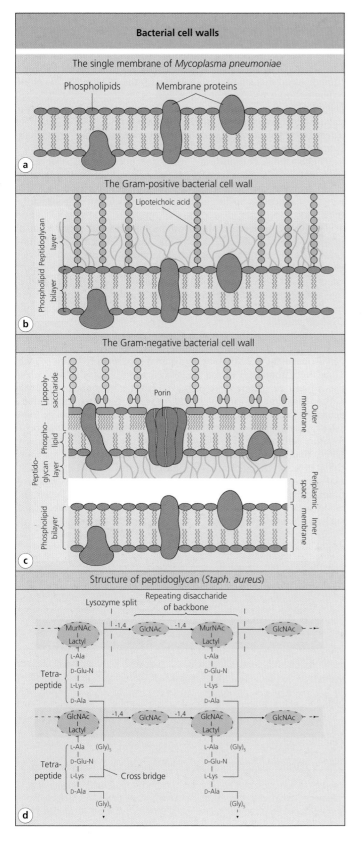

Bacterial cell walls

The single membrane of *Mycoplasma pneumoniae*

Phospholipids   Membrane proteins

a

The Gram-positive bacterial cell wall

Lipoteichoic acid

Peptidoglycan layer

Phospholipid bilayer

b

The Gram-negative bacterial cell wall

Lipopoly-saccharide

Porin

Phospho-lipid

Peptido-glycan layer

Phospholipid bilayer

Outer membrane

Periplasmic space   Inner membrane

c

Structure of peptidoglycan (*Staph. aureus*)

Lysozyme split   Repeating disaccharide of backbone

MurNAc — GlcNAc — MurNAc — GlcNAc
| |
Lactyl   Lactyl
| |
L-Ala   L-Ala
| |
D-Glu-N   D-Glu-N
| |
Tetra-peptide L-Lys   L-Lys
| |
D-Ala   D-Ala

GlcNAc — GlcNAc — GlcNAc — GlcNAc
| |
Lactyl   Lactyl
| |
L-Ala   (Gly)₅   L-Ala   (Gly)₅
| |
D-Glu-N   D-Glu-N
| |
Tetra-peptide L-Lys — Cross bridge — L-Lys
| |
D-Ala   D-Ala
| |
(Gly)₅   (Gly)₅

d

Bacteria were probably the first cells to appear on earth more than 3.5 billion years ago. They have since developed into an overwhelming diversity representing the bulk of the world's biomass today. Although evolution has not led to bacteria associating into multicellular organisms, they are capable of cell-to-cell communication.[12] By using low molecular weight compounds, bacteria have found a way to sense how dense their local population is and decide whether or not to activate developmental programs such as plasmid conjugation, light production (in association with deep-sea fish) or virulence gene expression.

Different cell morphologies can be observed with light microscopy (e.g. spherical cocci, rod-shaped bacilli, curved vibrios, spiral treponemes). Electron microscopy unveils a distinctive cell wall, a simple nuclear body without a nuclear membrane and the presence in the cytoplasm of ribosomes and mesosomes, sometimes granules of reserve material, but no endoplasmic reticulum and no organelles such as mitochondria or chloroplasts. There frequently are appendages such as flagella that are used for motility, pili and fimbriae that may be used for adhesion or for conjugation.

Bacterial dichotomy revealed by a simple staining technique

In 1884, the Danish bacteriologist Hans-Christian Gram developed a simple staining technique that distinguishes two types of bacteria: the Gram-positive and the Gram-negative bacteria. The distinction is based on the ability of one group of bacteria, the Gram-positives, to retain a crystal violet-iodine dye in the presence of an organic solvent such as alcohol or acetone. The solvent dissolves the dye from Gram-negatives and they can be counterstained with other dyes such as safranin. This simple observation reflects distinctive structures. Gram-positive bacteria characteristically have a thick cell wall made up mainly of a vast molecule of peptidoglycan, with protruding chains of teichoic acids. Surrounding the peptidoglycan skeleton in the periplasm of Gram-negative bacteria is an additional asymmetric outer membrane, the outer layer composed of lipopolysaccharide (endotoxin) (Fig. 1.4). *Escherichia coli* is an example of a Gram-negative bacterium; it is rod shaped and growing cells are between 2 μm and 4 μm long.

The rigid cell wall determines the shape of bacteria and allows them to resist the osmotic pressure caused by the large difference in solute concentration between the cytoplasm and the environment. *Mycoplasma* spp. lack peptidoglycan and thus have neither a rigid wall nor a defined shape.

Fig. 1.4 Bacterial cell walls. (a) *Mycoplasma pneumoniae* has a single membrane, made up of phospholipids and membrane proteins. (b) In Gram-positive organisms the cytoplasmic membrane is covered with a thick layer of peptidoglycan; chains of lipoteichoic acid anchored in the cell membrane protrude outside. Negatively charged teichoic acids are covalently attached to the peptidoglycan. Cell wall proteins also are covalently attached to the peptidoglycan. There is no periplasmic space in Gram-positive bacteria. (c) The cell wall of a Gram-negative rod is more complex. The layers are: the cytoplasmic membrane, the periplasmic space, a layer of peptidoglycan which is thinner than that in Gram-positive bacteria and an asymmetric outer membrane. The inner leaflet of the outer membrane is made of phospholipids. The outer leaflet has lipopolysaccharides as its principal lipids; porins, which are channel-forming proteins often organized as trimers, allow the penetration of hydrophilic molecules through the outer membrane. (d) The peptidoglycan of *Staphylococcus aureus* has polysaccharide chains ('backbone') that are alternating residues of *N*-acetylglucosamine (GlcNAc) and *N*-acetylmuramic acid (MurNAc). Tetrapeptides are attached to MurNAc and are linked together by pentaglycines bridging the L-lysine of each tetrapeptide chain to the D-alanine of the neighboring one. (Courtesy of Menno Kok & Jean-Claude Pechere.)

Organization of the bacterial cell

The bacterial cytoplasm does not contain physically separated compartments. DNA replication, transcription, protein synthesis, central metabolism and respiration all take place in the same environment. Complex biochemical processes may nonetheless be spatially organized in the cell. Transcription of DNA into mRNA and translation of the mRNA into protein are coupled processes. This means that polysomes are linked to the DNA, via the enzyme RNA polymerase (Fig. 1.5). The cytoplasmic membrane not only contains numerous metabolite transport systems, but it is the site of intense enzymatic activity as well. Like eukaryotic cells, bacteria possess efflux systems that allow them to expel unwanted substances from the cytoplasm into the environment. Gram-positive bacteria express many important enzymes and ligands in their cell wall. It is estimated that *Listeria monocytogenes* has 42 different cell wall anchored proteins.

The genetic information is usually stored in a single circular chromosome. Bacterial chromosomes vary considerably in size. The *Haemophilus influenzae* chromosome, the first completely sequenced genome of a cellular life form, is 1.83 million base pairs (Mbp) long and encodes 1703 putative proteins.[13] The chromosome of laboratory strains of *E. coli* K12 is approximately 2.5 times bigger (5 Mbp), though still rather small if compared with the 30 Mbp *Bacillus megaterium* genome that is more than 500 times the length of the cell (Fig. 1.6). A few organisms such as *Vibrio cholera* and *Borrelia* spp. have fragmented genomes, and the *Borrelia* genomes are encoded on linear DNA. The advantage to the organisms of such an arrangement is not known.

The bacterial chromosome codes for polypeptides and stable RNA molecules such as transfer RNA and ribosomal RNA molecules. *E. coli* probably contains well over 1500 different polypeptides with a variety of functions, including maintenance of membrane structure; transport; respiration; degradation of nutrients; synthesis of amino acids, sugars, nucleotides, lipids and vitamins; and production of polymers such as DNA, RNA, proteins and polysaccharides. Mobile genetic elements, such as plasmids, bacteriophages and transposable elements, are important sources of genetic variation. They supply genes that are not essential for bacterial growth but may offer a selective advantage under specific conditions. Virulence factors and antibiotic resistance elements are frequently associated with these mobile DNA structures.

Comparison of the genome sequences of the harmless laboratory strains of *E. coli* shows that naturally occurring *E. coli* isolates can differ by up to 1 Mb, ranging from approximately 4.5 to 5.5 Mb. Thus the commensal *E. coli* K12 has a genome of 4.64 Mb, while the human pathogen *E. coli* O157:H7 has a genome of 5.53 Mb. Several uropathogenic *E. coli* (UPEC) have been sequenced and have genomes varying from 4.94 to 5.23 Mb. The differences in genome sizes are largely due to insertions or deletions of large chromosomal regions, referred to as pathogenicity islands. Genomic islands in UPEC that are not found in commensal *E. coli* account for more than 10% of the genome, emphasizing the importance of lateral gene transfer in the evolution of pathogens. The overall gene order, except for the insertions, remains the same in all *E. coli* and is remarkably similar to the gene order in other Enterobacteriaceae such as *Salmonella enterica*.

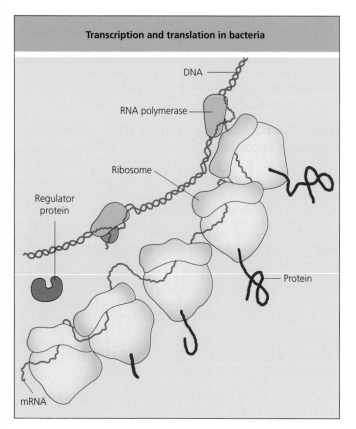

Transcription and translation in bacteria

DNA

RNA polymerase

Ribosome

Regulator protein

Protein

mRNA

Fig. 1.5 Transcription and translation in bacteria (*Escherichia coli*). (Courtesy of Menno Kok & Jean-Claude Pechere.)

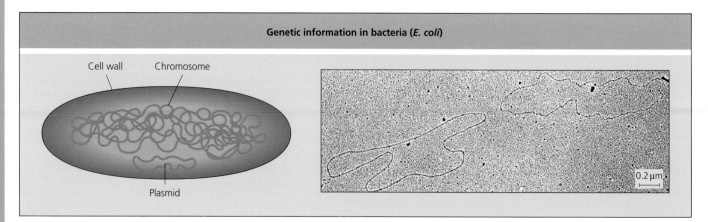

Genetic information in bacteria (*E. coli*)

Cell wall   Chromosome

Plasmid

0.2 μm

Fig. 1.6 Genetic information in bacteria. This example is *Escherichia coli*. Additional genetic information may be supplied by extrachromosomal elements such as plasmids or bacteriophages. Bacteria may carry a variety of these 'mobile genetic elements', which may transfer readily from one cell to another. The electron micrograph shows a 8.65 kb *E. coli* plasmid that confers sulfonamide and streptomycin resistance (left) and a single-stranded derivative of the plasmid (right). (Courtesy of Menno Kok & Jean-Claude Pechere.)

Transcription and translation in bacteria

Gene expression is usually regulated at the level of transcription initiation by regulator proteins and occasionally by small RNA molecules, which interact with the 'promoter DNA' and with the enzyme RNA polymerase (see Fig. 1.5). The promoter is the site where RNA polymerase opens ('melts') the dsDNA to synthesize an RNA copy of one of the two DNA strands. A sigma factor transiently interacts with the polymerase when it binds the promoter DNA and determines the nucleotide sequence specificity of the enzyme. Bacterial cells produce multiple sigma factors, each controlling the expression of a set of genes, and each expressed under different environmental conditions.

Three types of RNA are produced: regulatory RNA, 'stable' RNA and messenger RNA (mRNA). Stable RNAs include the transfer RNA molecules, which position the amino acids on the ribosomes during protein synthesis and are important structural components of the ribosomes. Messenger RNA molecules are generally quite unstable but are protected from premature degradation by ribosomes, the protein synthesis machines.[14] Regulatory RNAs, such as small RNAs (sRNA) in two component systems, may function in a fashion similar to microRNAs in eukaryotes.[15] Transcription and translation are coupled in bacteria; ribosomes bind the mRNA as soon as it 'leaves' RNA polymerase and start protein synthesis by coupling the initiator amino acid (formyl-methionine) to the second amino acid in the coding sequence and uncoupling it from the tRNA molecule. As mRNA elongation proceeds, more ribosomes bind to the mRNA to form a 'polysome'. The polypeptides that are produced by the ribosomes fold either spontaneously or with the help of molecular chaperones into their native structures. Bacterial mRNAs generally encode more than one protein. The bacterial protein synthesis machinery is an important target for antibiotics.

Motility

Many bacterial species can detect very small variations in concentrations of either valuable or harmful substances in the surrounding environment, guiding movement in a process called chemotaxis.[16] Flagella are the effectors of chemotaxis (Fig. 1.7). By changing the direction of flagellar rotation, micro-organisms swim towards sites favorable to survival and growth and away from noxious stimuli. Amino acids and sugars are powerful chemoattractants. Although many pathogenic species are flagellated, a role for motility in virulence has not been established in many cases.

PATHOGENESIS OF INFECTIOUS DISEASE

The key microbial factors involved in the onset and spread of microbial infection can be identified by carefully analyzing the interaction of the micro-organism with its host (Table 1.4). Insight into the intimate relationship between host and pathogen will help us find the answers to the all-important questions: how can we eliminate the cause of disease and how can we reduce its harmful effects on the human body?

One of the major advances in pathogenic microbiology has been the use of molecular techniques to make targeted mutations in organisms. These mutants can then be tested in appropriate animal or tissue culture models to determine if the loss of the gene affects the virulence of the pathogen without affecting its ability to grow *in vitro* in standard media. Genes that are identified as 'virulence' genes are sometimes considered to be 'accessory' genes because they are not required for replication outside the host. A virulence gene can also be cloned into a genetically related nonpathogenic microbe and tested for its ability to confer a new property in that organism such as adhesion or hemolysis.

Virulence factors can be thought of as falling into one of two functional categories, though there can be overlap in the categories. There are purely defensive functions that help the organism to escape the host's innate immune response. Two examples of this are

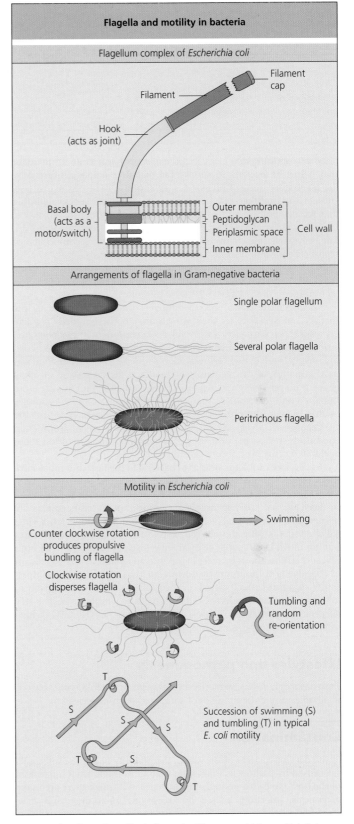

Fig. 1.7 Flagella and motility in bacteria. (Courtesy of Menno Kok & Jean-Claude Pechere.)

the polysaccharide capsule made by *Streptococcus pneumoniae* and the golden pigment made by *Staphylococcus aureus*. The former prevents complement from effectively opsonizing the bacteria for ingestion and destruction by neutrophils, while the carotenoid pigment

Table 1.4 Important steps in microbial pathogenesis

- Encounter
- Attachment to host cells
- Local or general spread in the body (invasion)
- Cell and tissue damage
- Evasion of host defenses
- Shedding from the body

(staphyloxanthin) that gives *Staph. aureus* its name is an antioxidant that helps the bacteria to survive the oxidative damage inflicted by the respiratory burst of phagocytes. In contrast, many exotoxins (e.g. cholera and diphtheria toxins) secreted by the bacteria actively inflict damage on the host and so can be thought of as offensive weapons. Lipopolysaccharides (LPS) serve both functions for the organism. The polysaccharide chains divert the membrane attack component of complement from the inner membrane, making Gram-negative bacilli resistant to the bactericidal action of complement (defensive), while the lipid A end can stimulate exuberant and damaging inflammation by binding to the TLR4/MD-2/CD14 complex.

Because bacteria do not constitutively produce virulence factors that are not necessary for their growth, they transcriptionally regulate expression of virulence genes. Since expression of these regulated virulence genes (or 'accessory genes') may carry a large metabolic cost, organisms regulate their expression in response to environmental signals. Mutation of the regulators often affects the expression of many genes, both positively and negatively, and regulatory mutants are more impaired and less virulent than most single gene mutants. Examples of this include the phoP/Q regulon in *Salmonella enterica* and the agr regulon in *Staph. aureus*. Some regulators sense environmental conditions such as pH or magnesium concentration and others sense bacterial density via quorum sensing.

Viruses face problems similar to bacteria in the host, but must solve them using a limited genetic repertoire. Analogous to bacterial virulence factors, viral genes required for replication and/or pathogenesis in the host that are dispensable for replication in tissue culture are termed accessory genes. For example, simian immunodeficiency virus (SIV) strains lacking the *nef* gene replicate well in certain cell lines but are much less capable of producing disease.[17] Expression of both SIV and HIV *nef* both increases viral infectivity and assists in evasion of adaptive host immunity by downregulation of major histocompatibility complex (MHC) class I, needed for presentation of antigen to allow recognition of infected cells by cytotoxic lymphocytes. The HIV *vif* gene inactivates an innate restrictive factor, APOBEC3G, which otherwise renders progeny virus uninfectious.[18]

Lifestyles and pathogenesis

Each pathogen has its own infection strategy. In the following sections we shall examine the lifestyles of some pathogenic species.

Contamination

In the developed areas of the world, the majority of human infections are caused by pathogens that either belong to the normal microflora of the host (so-called endogenous infections), though there are many exceptions. Infections caused by exogenous micro-organisms have steadily declined over the past century. In contrast, exogenous infections are still prevalent in poorer areas.[19]

Endogenous infections and normal microbial flora of the human host

The fetus in utero is normally sterile but immediately after birth it starts acquiring its indigenous microflora, which will quickly outnumber its own cell content; a normal adult carries more than 10^{14} bacteria, which represents roughly 10 bacteria for each eukaryotic cell. In addition to bacteria, we provide permanent or transient hospitality to an estimated 150 viral species, including numerous remnants of 'endogenous' retroviruses that are inherited in our DNA,[20] to a few fungi, some protozoa and occasionally to worms. The indigenous flora, or 'normal flora' that consists of many species of bacteria and one fungus (*Candida albicans*), is found in any part of the body exposed to the outside environment – the alimentary tract from the mouth to the anus, nose and the oropharynx to the epiglottis, the anterior part of the urethra and the vagina, and the skin (Fig. 1.8). The human microbial population is especially dense in the large intestine; it has been estimated that each gram of stool specimen contains about 10^{12} bacteria. The normal flora is well adapted to its niche and may multiply rapidly under favorable nutritional conditions such as those found in the colon. Although the host's age and physical condition, and especially antibiotic treatment, may induce important variations, the microbial population of the gastrointestinal tract seems to be stable, consisting of more than 99% of obligate anaerobic species. The fecal flora is much more diverse in vegetarians than in omnivores or carnivores, probably reflecting the difficulty of digesting complex carbohydrates found in plants. Facultative anaerobes such as *E. coli*, which are frequently used as markers for environmental pollution with human feces, represent less than 1% of the normal flora.

Transient micro-organisms, ingested with food or water, will normally pass through the proximal small intestine because of the high flow rate and low gastric pH, without being able to penetrate the mucous gel that overlays the intestinal epithelium or to adhere to the epithelial surface. Population levels of the different areas of the gastrointestinal tract are controlled mainly at the level of metabolic competition, the normal flora being well adapted to the low oxidation reduction potentials and tightly adherent to the mucosal epithelium. Pathogens that use the gastrointestinal tract as a portal of entry must find ways of dealing with the fierce microbial competition in the colon, or they target the less densely populated small intestine. Small intestinal pathogens have specific adhesions that allow them to remain attached to epithelial cells or to invade those cells.

The skin is much less densely populated by the indigenous flora. In comparison with the gastrointestinal tract, it supplies a considerably less stable microenvironment and one that is often devoid of water. Nevertheless, there are bacteria within skin appendages in all areas of the skin. Although intact skin is impermeable to bacteria, a number of parasites, among them *Schistosoma mansoni*, which poses a major health threat in developing countries, can penetrate the intact human skin. Skin disruptions due to lacerations or insect bites may allow entry of pathogenic microbes into the body.

The large majority of micro-organisms in the human flora reside on the body surface without creating any damage. This peaceful cohabitation can be called a symbiotic ('both sides win') relationship. Some bacteria find shelter and food in the intestine and, in turn, supply vitamins or digest cellulose. We are just beginning to understand the roles that normal flora play in human nutrition, in maintaining oral tolerance and in developing our innate immune system. If the micro-organisms, rather than the host, derive benefit from the association, those inhabitants of our body are called commensals. True commensals do not invade the host and, therefore, do not elicit an immune response. Parasitism constitutes a third category where the micro-organisms, after invading the host, cause an infection. Some have suggested that chronic infection with highly prevalent viruses, including herpesviruses, may play a protective role against bacterial infection by boosting innate immunity, suggesting a complex, three-way symbiotic relationship.[21]

The separation between parasitism, commensalism and symbiosis is not always clearly defined and the condition of the host may make a big difference. Some micro-organisms, referred to as opportunistic pathogens, are commensals in the majority of people but can cause disease in an immunocompromised host. For instance, *C. albicans* is part of the normal oral flora, but in the absence of adequate numbers of CD4 T cells, as occurs in AIDS, the yeast can proliferate and cause thrush and esophagitis. Similarly, virtually all individuals chronically

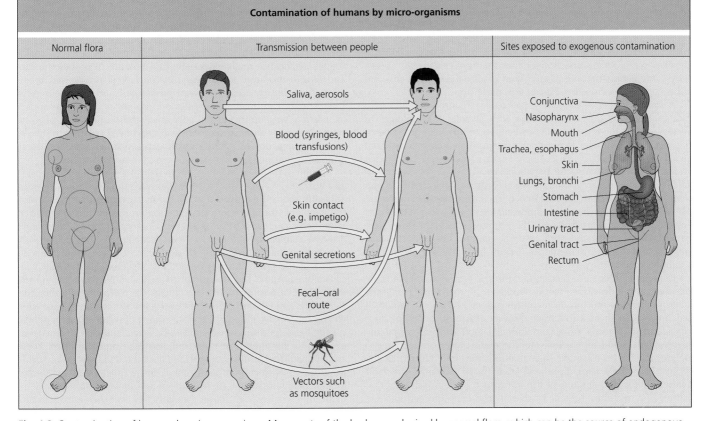

Fig. 1.8 Contamination of humans by micro-organisms. Many parts of the body are colonized by normal flora, which can be the source of endogenous infection. Large numbers of micro-organisms are found in moist areas of the skin (e.g. the groin, between the toes), the upper respiratory tract, the digestive tract (e.g. the mouth, the nasopharynx), the ileum and large intestine, the anterior parts of the urethra, and the vagina. Other routes are interhuman transmission of infections and exposure to exogenous contamination. (Courtesy of Menno Kok & Jean-Claude Pechere.)

infected with human cytomegalovirus (CMV) are asymptomatic, but CMV can cause serious diseases such as colitis and pneumonia when the immune system is suppressed.

The host and its indigenous microflora maintain a delicately balanced relationship that, when disrupted, may lead to the development of infectious disease.

An inevitable consequence of antibiotic treatment is the elimination of susceptible bacteria, which are quickly replaced by antibiotic-resistant species. This phenomenon can cause diseases such as mucosal candidiasis, pseudomembranous colitis or enterococcal superinfection. Even a short course of antibiotics can cause a large change in the composition of the fecal flora.

Probiotics (live micro-organisms) may help to restore the natural flora after antibiotic use, but their usefulness is still not fully established. For example, *Saccharomyces boulardii* may be used to prevent relapses of colitis caused by *Clostridium difficile*, but there are no convincing studies showing efficacy.

Exogenous infections

Exogenous infections occur after direct contamination from microbial populations in the environment.

Humans are continuously in intimate contact with the large exogenous microbial populations in the air, soil and water, which may harbor highly pathogenic bacteria such as *Clostridium tetani* and *Bacillus anthracis*. Important pathogenic species, such as *Salmonella enterica*, *Staph. aureus*, *Clostridium perfringens* and *Clostridium botulinum*, may be present in our food and cause food poisoning or gastroenteritis.

Live animals represent another important source of exogenous micro-organisms. Infectious diseases of animals that may be transmitted to humans (called zoonoses) include cat-scratch fever, brucellosis,

tularemia, toxoplasmosis and rabies. In addition, microbial pathogens can be transmitted from animals to humans by insect vectors such as flies, mosquitoes and ticks. Plague and Lyme disease are examples of vector-borne zoonotic bacterial infection. Many viruses, such as dengue virus, which is transmitted by Aedes mosquitoes, are transmitted by insect vectors. The Sin Nombre hantavirus, which produces hantavirus pulmonary syndrome, is acquired from rodents by aerosolization of their dried, infected urine. Many protozoan pathogens are transmitted by insect bites, malaria being the most important.

The most important sources of exogenous infections are probably humans themselves (see Fig. 1.8). Well-known examples of human-to-human transmission include AIDS and other sexually transmitted diseases, airborne infections such as varicella, rubella, measles and tuberculosis, and fecal–oral infections such as shigellosis and typhoid fever. Vertical transmission of infections to the fetus or newborn is uncommon but they often have devastating effects. They include toxoplasmosis, CMV, rubella, HIV, listeriosis and syphilis. In contrast, vertical transmission of hepatitis B virus (HBV) occurs at or after parturition, and the infants have a high likelihood of becoming asymptomatically but chronically infected. This is common in many populations in South East Asia where HBV is endemic. Cross-infection in hospitals poses enormous problems, especially in intensive care units, but these infections are usually transmitted on fomites or inadvertently on the hands of hospital personnel rather than by direct contact or by droplets.

Several regions of the body may be exposed to exogenous contamination (see Fig. 1.8). Healthy people may be carriers if they harbor and excrete potentially disease-producing micro-organisms. For instance, people recovering from typhoid fever may retain *Salmonella typhi* in the gallbladder and continue to excrete the pathogen in the feces long after recovery from the disease. These people are chronic carriers, even though they have recovered from the illness themselves. Certain bacterial respiratory pathogens have no environmental or animal hosts, and are passed by droplets from person to person. These include *Strep. pyogenes*, *Strep. pneumoniae* and *Neisseria meningitidis*. If newly colonized individuals do not have protective antibodies they are liable to develop symptomatic infections. Other than pre-existing immunity, why some people become ill after they acquire these organisms and others remain asymptomatic is not well understood.

A small number of exogenous pathogens are airborne and establish infection by direct interactions with alveolar macrophages or mucosal dendritic cells. For this to happen the particles must be of a certain size; particles larger than 4 microns in diameter will not reach the terminal airways and very small particles will be trapped in the nasopharynx. Alveolar macrophages are inherently downregulated for inflammatory responses, which is probably necessary to prevent lung damage from the many encounters with particles in the air. However, this makes them ill equipped to kill organisms that they may ingest. *Mycobacterium tuberculosis*, the primary pathogenic fungi such as *Histoplasma capsulatum*, *Paracoccidioides braziliensis* and *Coccidioides immitis*, and the environmental bacterium *Legionella pneumophila* are examples of airborne pathogens.

Exogenous infections, predominant in the past, have dramatically declined in the developed world thanks to improved hygiene, vaccination programs and infection control programs. They are, however, still prevalent in areas with limited resources. Pneumococcal pneumonia, diarrheal diseases from contaminated food and water, malaria, measles, AIDS and tuberculosis are the main causes of mortality in developing countries, other than malnutrition and trauma. In the 1990s there was a large diphtheria epidemic in Russia as the result of the collapse of the public health infrastructure, demonstrating that pathogenic microbes are still in the environment and can become epidemic even in technologically advanced countries if we relax our efforts to contain them.

The infection process

Three stages in the infection process may be functionally distinguished:

- attachment of the micro-organism to the target cell(s) and, for intracellular pathogens, entry into the host cell;
- development of the infection, local multiplication of the pathogen and spread of the micro-organism to distant sites; and
- shedding of the organism and transfer to a new host.

Attachment to host cells

Only a few pathogens have the capacity to penetrate our body directly through the skin. Examples include the cercariae of various schistosome species, which can invade the skin with the help of their glandular secretions. Many other pathogens enter the body after an insect bite (e.g. *Simulium* blackfly bite for *Onchocercus volvulus*, anopheles mosquito bite for malaria) or iatrogenically from intramuscular or intravenous injection of contaminated medications or blood. This can transmit various blood-borne pathogens such as HBV, hepatitis C virus (HCV), HIV, West Nile virus, syphilis and malaria.

Although 'free' micro-organisms exist in the body (for instance, in the lumen of the intestine or in the saliva), most members of the human flora need to be attached to a cellular surface to avoid being swept away by biologic fluxes such as swallowing or the passage of the alimentary bolus. For many microbial and viral pathogens, adherence to the epithelial surface of the respiratory, digestive or reproductive mucosa is a compulsory step in pathogenesis.

Adherence

The approach of micro-organisms to an epithelial surface is guided by a balance between attractive and repulsive forces. Eventually, multiple high-affinity contacts between the microbe or virion and the cellular surface may establish a virtually irreversible association between the two. Even for viruses, attachment may involve multiple different mechanisms. Such contacts may involve nonspecific interactions, such as those between exposed hydrophobic structures on the microbial cell envelope and lipophilic areas on the cell membrane. Glycocalyx, made essentially of a mixture of polysaccharides and 'slime', produced in particular by *Staph. epidermidis*, may mediate nonspecific adherence between prokaryotic and eukaryotic cells. Interestingly, carbohydrate capsules on respiratory pathogens appear to interfere with epithelial cell adherence and bacteria that progress from epithelial colonization to invasion and need capsules to survive after invasion, downregulate capsule expression in order to adhere and invade epithelial cells, the first step in their pathogenesis.

Specific adherence involves microbial adhesins on the one side and host cell receptors on the other. Although the interaction between adhesins and cell receptors may be highly specific, this is not always the case. The specificity can be tested by artificially blocking adherence with an excess of purified adhesin or receptor or with antibodies directed against one of these two. The specificity accounts for the early observation that many pathogens distinctively infect certain areas or organs of the body and not others. For instance, *Strep. pneumoniae* causes pneumonia but not urethritis, whereas *Neisseria gonorrhoeae* exhibits the opposite pattern of specificity. The receptors for poliovirus, rhinovirus and HIV are expressed only by specific cell types, restricting virus infection accordingly. Different strains of influenza virus adhere via the hemagglutinin to different sialic acids, and this largely determines not only their host range but also their organ tropism. These and many other examples support the notion that adhesins determine the tropism of microbial pathogens. On the other hand, cell receptors for many organisms are ubiquitous and these organisms have no tissue or even host restriction, possibly because they encode many adhesins. *Salmonella enterica* serovar Typhimurium encodes 12 different fimbriae, but the binding specificity is known for only two.

Ubiquitous receptors

Fibrinogen, fibronectin, collagen and heparin-related polysaccharides are major components of the extracellular matrix (ECM) that coats the mucosal surface of epithelial cells. Members of the integrin family are involved in the interaction between the ECM and the underlying epithelium. A number of components of the ECM are used as receptors for microbial adhesins and viral receptor proteins. *Staph. aureus* has cell wall proteins that recognize nearly all ECM proteins including fibronectin, elastin, von Willebrand factor, vitronectin and collagen.

Attachment to fibronectin is also required for *Staph. aureus* to invade nonphagocytic cells. Fibronectin specifically binds fibronectin-binding factors on the cell envelopes of other bacteria including *Strep. pyogenes*, *Treponema pallidum*, *Mycobacterium* spp. and *Orientia tsutsugamushi*, the etiologic agent of scrub typhus; fibrinogen binds groups A, C and G streptococci and a member of the integrin family binds the major invasion factor of *Yersinia pseudotuberculosis*. Their abundance and structural conservation among mammalian species make ECM components ideal targets for bacterial adhesins.

Bacterial adhesins

Close contact between micro-organism and host cell represents an essential step in pathogenesis. It optimizes the interaction of microbial virulence factors with the target cell to allow the pathogen to penetrate or cause local cell damage, or both. Other possible functions of adhesins include modulation of the inflammatory response, adhesin-directed degranulation from mast cells and adhesin-mediated bacterial phagocytosis by neutrophils. Bacteria use two general strategies to attach themselves to host cells: fimbrial and afimbrial adhesion (Fig. 1.9).[22]

Pili and fibrillae

Attachment of bacteria to the plasma membrane can be mediated by filamentous structures protruding from the bacterial surface, called

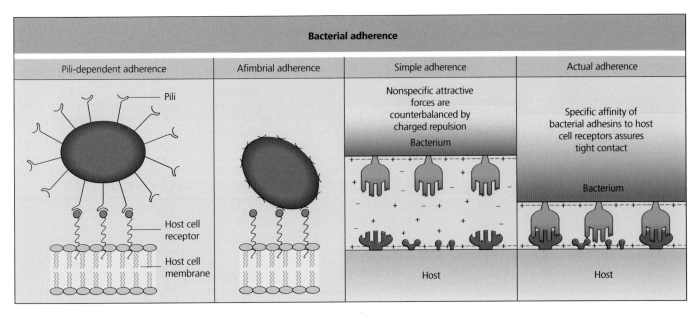

Fig. 1.9 Bacterial adherence. (Courtesy of Menno Kok & Jean-Claude Pechere.)

fimbriae or fibrillae. The classification of these colonization factors is based on morphologic criteria. Fimbriae (or common pili) are rigid hair-like structures with a regular diameter, whereas fibrillae are flexible and have an irregular diameter. These structures are distinct from flagella, which are responsible for bacterial motility (see Fig. 1.7), and sex pili, which are associated with bacterial conjugation.

Twenty different colonization factors have been described for *E. coli*.[23] One of these, the so-called P-pili expressed by uropathogenic *E. coli* strains, mediates adherence of the bacterium to the urinary mucosa to avoid elimination by the urinary flux. P-pili consist of a long and rigid base section attached to an outer membrane scaffold and a short flexible tip (Fig. 1.10).[24] The rigid section is composed of hundreds of pyelonephritis-associated (PapA) pilin subunits arranged in a right-handed helix. The pilus tip is 2 nm in diameter with a 15 nm pitch composed of PapE monomers. The PapG monomer is located at the end of the tip and is the actual adhesin. It recognizes the glycolipid receptor globobiose (α-1–4 linked di-galactose) on the host cell surface.

Afimbrial adhesins

Afimbrial adhesins, such as lectins (carbohydrate-binding proteins), also mediate tight binding between the bacteria and the host cell but, unlike pili, they do not form supramolecular structures. Similar adhesins exist in viruses, fungi and protozoa. Afimbrial binding has been extensively studied in *Strep. pyogenes* (Fig. 1.11). Two surface components are believed to be critical in the colonization of an epithelial surface: lipoteichoic acid and fibronectin-binding protein.

Purified lipoteichoic acid binds to fibronectin and inhibits the binding of *Strep. pyogenes* to oral epithelial cells. The binding properties of *Strep. pyogenes* lipoteichoic acid are confined to the lipid moiety. Similarly, artificially added fibronectin-binding protein inhibits adhesion of *Strep. pyogenes* to epithelial cells even after the streptococci have been depleted of lipoteichoic acid.

The complex surface of this micro-organism also includes the M protein.[26] This protein is a major virulence factor but it does not seem to be involved in adherence to epithelial cells, as was previously assumed. However, the M protein binds fibrinogen in a stoichiometric fashion and exerts an antiphagocytic effect, which may partially explain its role in virulence.

Viral adhesion

Adhesion represents the first in a series of steps that ultimately leads to the delivery of the viral genome to its site of replication. Multiple different viral proteins may be required to mediate attachment, viral fusion and entry into the cell. For example, the HIV gp120 protein first attaches to the CD4 molecule on the cell surface, exposing an area of gp120 that interacts with a seven-loop transmembrane protein co-receptor, finally triggering fusion via a portion of gp41 transmembrane protein. Similarly, different viral proteins in rotavirus interact with membrane carbohydrates, integrins and a heat shock protein to mediate attachment and entry.[27]

For some viruses (typically enveloped viruses, including measles and mumps viruses[28]), attachment proceeds via direct fusion with the cell plasma membrane. These virions have a transmembrane fusion protein that induces contact between the viral and cellular lipid bilayers. Alternatively, attachment may trigger a process of endocytosis, proceeding through clathrin-coated pits, frequently requiring acidification to trigger structural changes in viral proteins that results in escape from the endolysosome into the cytoplasm. This is used by many non-enveloped viruses, including adenovirus, rhinovirus and some other enteroviruses.[29]

Availability of receptors and/or co-receptors on the cell surface determines whether a virus particle will bind. Cell specificity

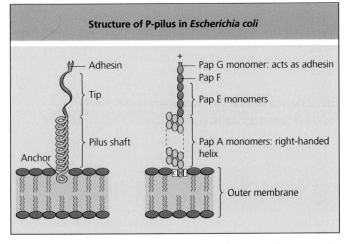

Fig. 1.10 Structure of P-pilus in *Escherichia coli*. (Courtesy of Menno Kok & Jean-Claude Pechere.)

Cell wall of *Streptococcus pyogenes*

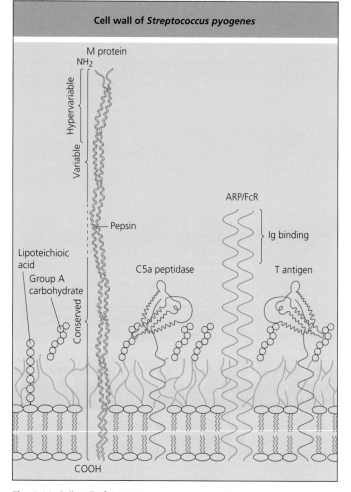

Fig. 1.11 Cell wall of *Streptococcus pyogenes*. The proposed model of the M protein is based on current sequence and structural data. ARP, immunoglobulin A receptor protein; FcR, receptor for the Fc portions of immunoglobulin. Adapted from Kehoe.[25]

('tropism') may be rather relaxed for viruses that use ubiquitous receptors while strongly restricted for viruses requiring two or more cellular receptors. As noted, HIV requires co-expression of CD4 and one of several chemokine receptors for efficient infection, and it principally infects only CD4+ lymphocytes and monocyte/macrophages. In contrast, herpes simplex virus type 1 glycoproteins B and C interact with ubiquitous heparin sulfate present on cell plasma membranes. A second interaction is between glycoprotein D and nectin-1 or herpes virus entry mediator (HVEM) cellular receptors, widely expressed in epithelial cells and some neurons.[30] Herpes simplex virus first infects epithelial cells of the skin and mucosal surfaces, where the initial replication cycles take place, passing into axon termini of neurons. Tropism is not always restricted by surface binding, however. The JC polyoma virus receptor, sialyl ($\alpha2-6$) Gal, has a wide distribution in human tissues, while virus replication is restricted primarily to oligodendrocytes, urothelial cells and perhaps B lymphocytes.[31]

Viral adherence and invasion can be blocked by neutralizing antibodies, which specifically bind the active site(s) of the adhesin(s). However, many viruses have hidden this region in a protein pocket (or 'canyon'), making it physically inaccessible to potentially neutralizing antibodies, thus escaping humoral immunity. In addition, many viruses produce huge amounts of variation due to relative infidelity of viral polymerases, allowing selection and escape of variants during infection.

INVASION

Invasive and noninvasive micro-organisms

Many micro-organisms, including those of the natural flora, remain at the epithelial surface without invading the underlying tissue (Table 1.5). This type of colonization is usually harmless although it may, in some cases, induce damage to adjacent cells through the production of toxins or elicit a local inflammatory or allergic response. Nonpenetrating micro-organisms include *Corynebacterium diphtheriae*, which cause pharyngitis, *Mycoplasma pneumoniae*, which cause pneumonia, and *Trichomonas vaginalis*, a cause of vaginitis.

Other micro-organisms gain access to deeper tissues only after a physical or chemical injury of the epithelial barrier. *Staph. aureus*, a harmless microbe when on the nasal mucosa, may become a dangerous toxin-producing pathogen once it penetrates the body, or can become locally destructive if it can penetrate beneath the stratified epithelium of the epidermis.

Invasive micro-organisms exhibit the capacity to penetrate the target tissue to which they adhere without the need for local disruption of the protective epithelium. Invasive bacteria have developed the capacity to enter host cells that are not naturally phagocytic. Penetration into these 'nonprofessional' phagocytes is achieved by either engulfment or zippering. *Salmonella enterica* and *Shigella* spp. are examples of bacteria that trigger their own engulfment using type III secretion systems to rearrange the host cell cytoskeleton using enzymes that are injected through the host cell membrane resulting in actin rearrangement so that the bacteria are carried into the cell (Fig. 1.12). The bacteria inject additional enzymes that restore the cytoskeleton to its original shape and restore integrity. In contrast, bacteria such as *Listeria monocytogenes* and *Yersinia pseudotuberculosis* use a 'zipper' mechanism to enter cells that starts with binding to integrins on the cell surface, which leads to cytoskeletal rearrangements. *Listeria* uses a second adhesion factor to enter hepatic cells, attaching to the hepatocyte growth factor receptor, which triggers phosphatidylinositol (PI) 3 kinase activation. Surprisingly, *Listeria* enters all cells in a clathrin-dependent, endocytic manner, except that after clathrin and dynamin are recruited there is cytoskeletal rearrangement necessary for the large particle to enter the cell.

In some cases infection remains confined to the epithelial surface (see Table 1.5), but in others the micro-organism may be transported across the superficial epithelium to be released into subepithelial space. This process is called transcytosis and involves the host cell actin network (see below). After transcytosis, the underlying tissues may be invaded and infected and the infection may eventually spread all over the body (e.g. *N. meningitidis* may cross the pharyngeal epithelium and cause meningitis, and *Salmonella enterica* serovar Typhi may cross the intestinal epithelium and infect the reticuloendothelial system causing typhoid fever). Some pathogens such as *Strep. pyogenes* usually cause disease on an epithelial surface, but they are also capable of invading epithelial cells and causing deep tissue infections. For a more detailed analysis of the mechanisms of invasion, we shall use the example of enteroinvasive pathogens.

Enteroinvasive pathogens and the membranous cell gateway

Acute infectious diarrhea may cause the clinical spectrum ranging from watery diarrhea to dysentery (bloody diarrhea). It occurs when the pathogen invades the intestinal mucosa and causes structural damage to the intestine. The immunologic protection of the intestine is performed by the gut-associated lymphoid tissues, which are separated from the intestinal lumen by epithelium. The follicle-associated epithelium is covered by membranous cells (M cells) that play a prominent role because they are specialized in the transport of antigens. Enteroinvasive viruses, protozoa and bacteria exploit the transport facilities provided by M cells to invade the host. Entry into (and passage through) M cells

Table 1.5 Interaction of micro-organisms with epithelial cells

	Order	Micro-organism	Disease
Generally confined to epithelial surfaces	Bacteria	*Bordetella pertussis*	Pertussis
		Chlamydia trachomatis	Trachoma, urethritis
		Corynebacterium diphtheriae	Diphtheria
		Streptococcus pyogenes	Uncomplicated pharyngitis
		Vibrio cholera	Cholera
		E. coli (EPEC)	Diarrhea
	Viruses	Coronaviruses	Common cold
		Rhinoviruses	Common cold
		Rotaviruses	Diarrhea
	Fungi	*Candida albicans*	Thrush
		Trichophyton spp.	Athlete's foot
	Protozoa	*Giardia lamblia*	Diarrhea
		Trichomonas vaginalis	Vaginitis
Enter through the epithelium	Bacteria	*Shigella* spp.	Bacillary dysentery
		Brucella melitensis	Brucellosis
		Neisseria meningitidis	Meningitis
		Salmonella typhi	Typhoid fever
		Treponema pallidum	Syphilis
		Yersinia pestis	Plague
	Viruses	Measles virus	Measles
		Rubella virus	Rubella
		Varicella	Chickenpox
		Poliovirus	Poliomyelitis
	Fungi	*C. albicans*	Disseminated candidiasis
	Protozoa	*Toxoplasma gondii*	Toxoplasmosis
		Entamoeba histolytica	Liver abscess

by these pathogens is preceded by adherence. While its pathogenicity is uncertain, enteric infection by mammalian reovirus type 1 involves initial entry through M cells mediated by the capsid proteins σ1 and μ1.[32] Infection by poliovirus may proceed by a similar route.[33]

Enteroinvasive bacteria such as *Salmonella*, *Shigella* and *Yersinia* spp. appear to distinguish between different subsets of M cells. Membranous cells produce glycocalyx, which contains a distinctive profile of lectin-binding sites. Diversity in lectin-binding sites between different locations of the gut may account for the tropism of enteric pathogens, such as the preferential colonization of colonic mucosa by *Shigella* spp. rather than *Salmonella* spp., which are more commonly found at the end of the ileum. Following adherence, the interactions with the M cells vary according to the pathogen (Fig. 1.13). Enteroadherent *E. coli* are not internalized and hence are not invasive. *Vibrio cholerae* is taken up and transported by the M cells but rapidly killed thereafter. It is considered to be invasive at the cellular level but not at the clinical level.

The *Salmonella* and *Shigella* spp. genes involved in invasion of the eukaryotic host cell are homologous and have been remarkably well conserved with respect to both the individual coding sequences and their genetic organization (Fig. 1.14).[35] Detailed molecular analyses of virulence factors produced by enteroinvasive *Shigella* spp. have revealed that all virulent species harbor a 220 kb plasmid, of which a 31 kb operon, encoding 32 genes, is both necessary and sufficient for invasion of epithelial cells.[36] The *Salmonella* spp. entry functions are clustered in a 35–40 kb pathogenicity island[37] inserted in the chromosome at centisome 63.[38] Using a needle-like complex,[39] the bacteria translocate a number of effector proteins into the cytosol and the plasma membrane of the target cell.[40] Some of these effector proteins specifically modify the activities of cellular GTPases (see Fig. 1.12), inducing the alterations of the cytoskeleton required for bacterial internalization.

An important difference between the pathogenic lifestyles of these two bacterial species involves the intracellular fate of the bacteria. Once internalized, the bacteria are enclosed by a host cell membrane

in an endocytic vesicle, deprived of nutrients. Soon after entry into the epithelial cell, *Shigella* spp. escape from the endosome into the nutritious cytoplasm; however, *Salmonella* spp. have adopted an entirely different strategy. Salmonellae modify the endocytic pathway of the host cell by means of virulence factors encoded largely by pathogenicity islands and, for highly invasive strains, the virulence plasmids, thus avoiding exposure to bactericidal mechanisms of the cell. Although only some of the cellular targets of the translocated bacterial virulence proteins have been identified to date, it is clear that the physiology of the infected cell is profoundly modified to suit bacterial growth and maintenance.

Actin-based intracellular motility of microbial pathogens

Listeria monocytogenes, *Rickettsia* spp., *Shigella* spp. and vaccinia, measles and rabies viruses use active actin modification to move within the cytoplasm of infected cells and to invade neighboring cells. They induce the formation of actin cross-linked filaments, which assemble in characteristic 'comet-like tails' (Fig. 1.15).[41,42] Elongation of the actin filaments generates sufficient force to move the micro-organisms through the cytoplasm at rates of 2–100 mm/min.

The intracellular life cycle of *L. monocytogenes* illustrates this strategy (Fig. 1.16).[43,44] Under natural conditions, *Listeria* first penetrates enterocytes and subsequently spreads through the body to infect a variety of host cells, including endothelial cells, Kupffer cells, hepatocytes, phagocytes and, most importantly, the trophoblasts of the placenta. Entry is facilitated by the products encoded by the internalin (*inl*) family of genes, which seem to confer tropism for different cell types. Once inside the cell, *L. monocytogenes* remains confined to the phagosome for only a short time. Following lysis of the endosomal membrane, it escapes into the cytosol. Membrane lysis is achieved by a production of listeriolysin-O, which attains maximum activity under the acidic conditions of the intravacuolar environment.

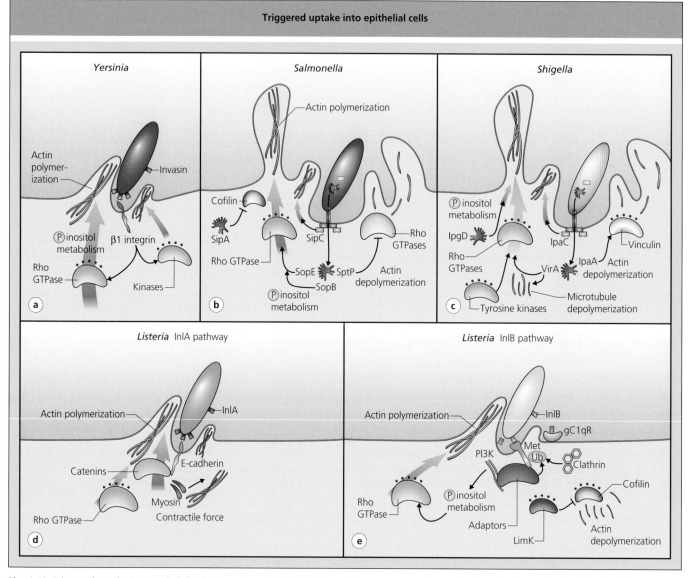

Triggered uptake into epithelial cells

Fig. 1.12 Triggered uptake into epithelial cells. Some invasive bacteria (b and c) express a complex needle-like structure on their cell surface (Type III secretion system) through which they inject proteins that hijack the adjacent cytoskeleton, triggering membrane ruffling that embraces the adjacent bacterium and internalizes it in a vacuole. Others have surface receptors for integrins (a, d and e) which trigger a pinocytic-like response leading to uptake.

Once in the cytosol, the bacteria multiply and migrate towards the plasma membrane by using the actin-based mechanism as described above. Actin polymerization is mediated by the *L. monocytogenes* protein ActA, localized at one end of the bacterium. For spread to neighboring cells, *L. monocytogenes* requires bacterial lecithinase and phospholipase C, which stimulate lysis of the two membranes that separate the bacterium from the cytoplasm of the newly infected cell. Interestingly, most of the virulence genes associated with this process are clustered in a single region of the *L. monocytogenes* chromosome. By spreading in this manner the bacteria are not exposed to human and cellular defenses. However, the intracytoplasmic bacteria stimulate cell innate immune responses via Nod signaling.

Subepithelial invasion and spread through the body

Invasion from the site of infection can only be achieved by microorganisms that effectively resist or subvert the host defense mechanisms in the subepithelial space, most prominently phagocytosis.

Some organisms take advantage of the normal transport of antigens and are carried by dendritic cells to regional lymph nodes. In the lymph nodes, resident macrophages and polymorphonuclear cells actively fight the invaders. As a result, the first line of lymph nodes is often inflamed. If the invading micro-organism is sufficiently virulent or present in sufficiently large numbers, it may pass into efferent lymphatic vessels to be conducted to the bloodstream. The result is primary bacteremia or viremia.

Some microbes can enter directly into the blood vessels via an injury. A typical example is provided by viridians streptococci, which enter the bloodstream during dental extraction, enabling them to infect an abnormal cardiac valve and produce endocarditis. Insect bites (malaria and arthropod-borne viruses) or damage to the blood vessel wall inflicted during infection with hemorrhagic fever viruses are alternative ways to circumvent the body's first line of defense: the mucosal immune system.

Once in the bloodstream, the micro-organisms may circulate as either an extracellular or an intracellular species. Pathogens have been found in polymorphonuclear cells (*Anaplasma*), lymphocytes (HIV), macrophages (*M. tuberculosis*, *Histoplasma capsulatum* and CMV) and

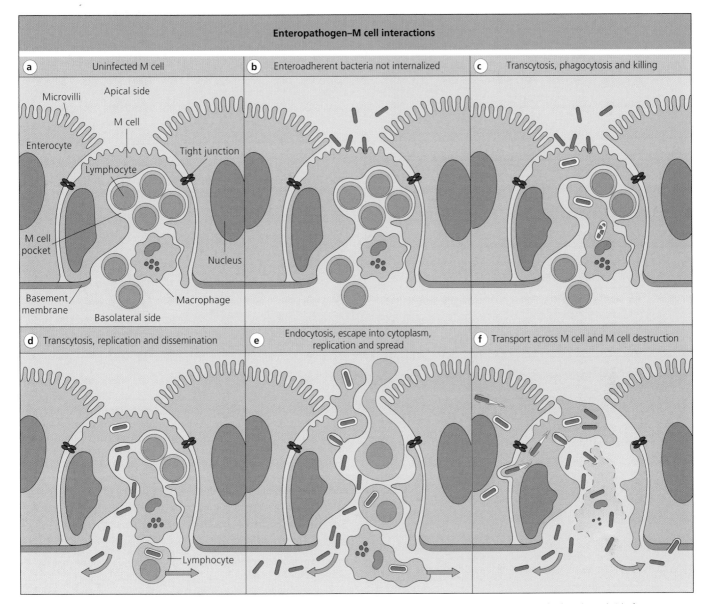

Enteropathogen–M cell interactions

(a) Uninfected M cell

Microvilli   Apical side
Enterocyte
M cell
Lymphocyte
Tight junction
M cell pocket
Nucleus
Basement membrane
Macrophage
Basolateral side

(b) Enteroadherent bacteria not internalized

(c) Transcytosis, phagocytosis and killing

(d) Transcytosis, replication and dissemination

(e) Endocytosis, escape into cytoplasm, replication and spread

(f) Transport across M cell and M cell destruction

Lymphocyte

Fig. 1.13 Enteropathogen–M cell interactions. (a) An uninfected M cell, enclosed between two adjacent enterocytes. The basolateral side forms a pocket where lymphocytes and macrophages are located. (b) Enteroadherent *Escherichia coli* forms microcolonies at the M cell surface, but is not internalized. (c) *Vibrio cholerae* undergoes transcytosis but is efficiently phagocytosed in the submucosa. (d) *Campylobacter jejunii* and *Yersinia* spp. undergo transcytosis, replicate in the submucosa and disseminate. (e) *Salmonella* spp. are transported across M cells, leading to destruction of the M cell. (f) *Shigella flexneri* is endocytosed by M cells, escapes into the cytoplasm, replicates, is propelled by actin tails and spreads to adjacent enterocytes. Adapted from Siebers & Finlay.[34]

even in red blood cells (*Plasmodium* spp., *Bartonella bacilliformis*), which provide protection against potent humoral factors in the serum, such as complement.

Infection of distant target organs

Transported by the bloodstream, the invasive micro-organisms can reach distant target organs and create infective metastases throughout the body. Almost any tissue can be reached, but the organs containing abundant capillary and sinusoid networks (e.g. lungs, liver, kidneys, bone marrow) and macrophages that are exposed directly to circulating blood are especially exposed, because blood flows slowly at these sites and transported micro-organisms get the opportunity to adhere and establish an infection. The epiphyses of long bones in children are an important target for certain pathogens such as *Staph. aureus* and *Haemophilus influenzae*. From the target organs, the invaders may pro-

duce a secondary bacteremia or viremia, in which microbial counts in the blood are generally higher than during primary infections.

The example of measles virus

Inhaled airborne measles virus recognizes membrane co-factor protein (CD46)[45] and/or the signaling lymphocyte activation molecule (SLAM/CD150)[46] as a receptor on the epithelial surface of the respiratory mucosa. Infection in a nonimmune host proceeds with 2–4 days of limited local replication in the lining of the trachea and bronchi. Pulmonary macrophages carry the virus to the regional lymph nodes, where exponential virus replication causes formation of reticuloendothelial giant cells. Progeny virions enter the bloodstream, causing a primary viremia with spread to the spleen, other lymphatic tissue, the lung, nasopharynx, oral mucosa, thymus, liver, skin and the central nervous system over the next 4–5 days, with secondary replication

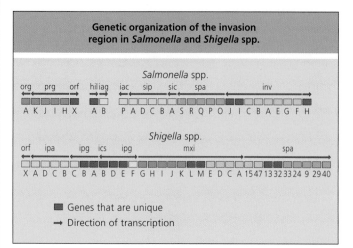

Fig. 1.14 Genetic organization of the invasion region on *Salmonella* and *Shigella* spp. Identical patterns indicate topologically conserved blocks of genes. Each genus has genes that are unique. Despite remarkable genetic similarities, the invasion strategies of the two bacteria are quite different (see Fig. 1.13). Adapted from Galan.[38]

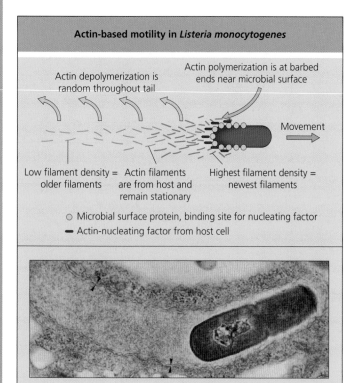

Fig. 1.15 Actin-based motility in *Listeria monocytogenes*. The bacterium moves forwards at the rate of actin-filament growth behind the pathogen. Adapted from Sanders & Theriot.[41] The electron micrograph shows a section of a CaCo-2 cell infected with *Listeria monocytogenes*; the bacterium protrudes into the cytoplasm of an adjacent cell; protrusion is limited by a double membrane (arrowheads).

and increasing viremia. Virus shedding from the nasopharynx begins about 12 days after infection, before symptoms or rash develop, contributing to a secondary attack rate of 80% in susceptible contacts.

These pathogenic steps correspond to different clinical periods. During the 10-day incubation period, infection and primary viremia proceed with no clinical symptoms. Symptoms of fever, malaise, cough and conjunctivitis are concomitant with secondary viremia, followed

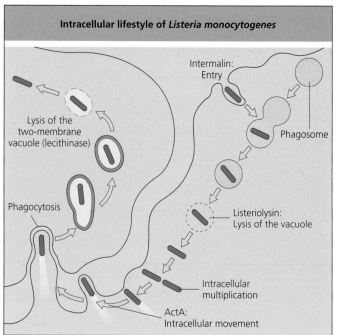

Fig. 1.16 Intracellular life cycle of *Listeria monocytogenes*. (Courtesy of Menno Kok & Jean-Claude Pechere.)

by rash at 12–13 days. The characteristic morbilliform exanthem is associated with a perivascular mononuclear infiltrate, including cytotoxic T cells which migrate to the site of virus infection of dermal endothelial cells and overlying dermis. Virus infection produces epithelial giant cells, but does not directly destroy infected cells in the skin. Leukopenia occurs late in viremia, and immune suppression can be seen from the time of appearance of symptoms until 2–3 weeks after resolution of clinical infection (see Chapter 152).

Serum resistance in *Neisseria gonorrhoeae* and *Salmonella* spp.

Complement is a complex system of circulating proteins that can be activated in three ways:
- by antibodies that interact with C1q;
- by spontaneous hydrolysis of C3 to the enzymatically active C3b that is then stabilized on appropriate surfaces by factors B, D and properdin of the alternative pathway; and
- binding of mannose-binding protein to microbes with subsequent attraction of C1 and mannan-binding lectin-associated serine proteases (MASPs) that proceed to activate C2 and C4.

Complement activation is a major component of the innate immune system, primarily because it can function as an opsonin in people who do not have antibody against the carbohydrates and proteins that form the outer layer of invasive bacteria. Children who are born lacking C3, the central component of all three complement pathways, suffer from repeated bacterial infections and often die in infancy. In contrast, people who are deficient in one of the late complement proteins (C5, 6, 7, 8 or 9) are usually in their teens before they become ill, and the only infections that occur at a higher than expected frequency are disseminated *N. meningitides* and *N. gonorrhoeae*.

In theory, Gram-negative bacteria are susceptible to complement lysis, as the membrane attack unit can insert itself through the outer and inner membranes if C3b binds close enough to the peptidoglycan. However, *Salmonella* and many other Gram-negative bacteria have developed various strategies to prevent complement lysis. These include diverting C3b binding to the ends of the long chain polysaccharide components of LPS that project from the bacterial surface so that the attack component assembles harmlessly at a distance from the inner membrane. Another strategy used by bacteria with short chain polysaccharides is to use outer membrane proteins to bind host regulatory proteins such as factor H and C4 binding protein to their surface.

Most immunocompetent hosts contracting gonorrhea do not develop a systemic disease because complement can kill bacteria that penetrate through the mucosal barrier. However, the clones of *N. gonorrhoeae* that cause disseminated infections in normal hosts are serum resistant, but often lose that property when passed *in vitro*, as they undergo phase variation. A large number of genes in the *N. gonorrhoeae* genome appear to be phase variable, but which of these is responsible for the invasiveness and complement resistance of disseminated gonococcal infection (DGI) strains is not clear. Another strategy used by pathogenic *Neisseria* to escape complement lysis is stimulation of 'blocking antibodies', which are often IgA (noncomplement binding) that recognize outer membrane proteins and prevent the attachment of bactericidal IgG antibodies and complement to the cell surface.

Cell and tissue damage induced by micro-organisms

Infectious disease is often characterized by cell and tissue damage. Paralysis in poliomyelitis, exanthem in varicella, gastroduodenal ulcers in *Helicobacter pylori* infections and bloody diarrhea in shigellosis all result from damage caused directly or indirectly by micro-organisms. Cell damage can be generated by a variety of different mechanisms (Table 1.6).

Bacterial toxins

Bacteria produce a large diversity of toxins, which have been classified according to their mode of action (Table 1.7, Fig. 1.17). Historically, toxins were defined as soluble substances that alter the normal metabolism of the host cells with deleterious effects on the host. However, as we learn more about the mechanisms of action of exotoxins, the distinction between them and secreted enzymes that play a role in pathogenesis is disappearing. The clostridial exotoxins are good examples of proteases that are exotoxins because they have specific cellular targets within nerve cells. These toxins, which are responsible for tetanus and botulism, are zinc metalloproteases that cleave synaptobrevins or a related protein in the same pathway so that docking and fusion of synaptic vesicles are impaired. The substrate specificity of the proteases and the binding affinity of the heavy chain of the toxins are

what determine the different clinical presentations of these diseases. The scalded skin syndrome (SSSS), a blistering skin disorder caused by some strains of *Staph. aureus*, is another example of clinical illness that is the consequence of a secreted protease with a specific target. Cleavage of human desmoglein 1 results in the widespread acantholysis and the flaccid bullous lesions of generalized SSSS.

Cholera toxin ADP ribosylates G_s protein, locking it into the 'on' position, resulting in unregulated activity of adenyl cyclase and high levels of cAMP. The singularity of cholera as an enterotoxin is not due to the specificity of the toxin binding or function but to the location of the pathogen; *V. cholera* is an extracellular mucosal pathogen so only intestinal epithelial cells are exposed to the toxin *in vivo*. Traditionally, exotoxins are said to be excreted toxins. However, some of the so-called exotoxins are actually intracellular and are released into the environment only after cell lysis. The pneumolysin of *Strep. pneumoniae*, for example, is cytoplasmic, the adenylate cyclase of *Bordetella pertussis* is associated with the cytoplasmic membrane and the heat-labile toxin 1 (LT-1) from *E. coli* is periplasmic. The genetic information that encodes bacterial toxins is frequently carried on mobile DNA elements, which may readily pass from one microbial host to another. The toxins associated with diphtheria, cholera, botulism and scarlet fever, as well as Shiga-like toxins in *E. coli*, are encoded by temperate bacteriophages. Genes for LT-1 and methanol-susceptible heat-stable toxin (Sta) of *E. coli* are carried on plasmids.

Toxins deregulate the physiology of the host cell before or during bacterial adhesion and invasion. The bacteria may profit from the induced damage, which compromises the cellular defense against the intruder and release of nutrients from the cytosol. In the case of enteric pathogens, the flux of fluid that characterizes diarrhea makes it more likely that the bacteria will find their way to another host.

The diphtheria toxin as example of an A–B toxin

Diphtheria toxin belongs to the so-called bifunctional A–B toxins (Fig. 1.18). Portion A mediates the enzymatic activity responsible for the toxicity after internalization into the target cell, but cannot penetrate by itself. Portion B is not toxic but binds to a cell receptor localized on the cell surface and mediates the translocation of the A chain into the cytosol. Portion B accounts for the cell specificity of the A–B toxins. The receptor recognized by the B chain of diphtheria toxin is a heparin-binding precursor of epidermal growth factor, an important hormone for growth and differentiation of many different cell types.

Table 1.6 Mechanisms of cell and tissue damage produced by micro-organisms

	Mechanism	Examples
Direct damage by micro-organisms	Production of toxins	See Table 1.7
	Production of enzymes	Proteases, coagulase, DNAses produced by *Staphylococcus aureus*
	Apoptosis	HIV (CD4+ T cells); *Shigella* spp. (macrophages)
	Virus-induced cytopathic effects: Cell enlargement and lysis Formation of syncytium	Cytomegalovirus Respiratory syncytial virus
	Inclusion bodies: Intracytoplasmic Nuclear	Rabies Herpesviruses
	Transformation	Human papillomavirus type 16
Damage via the host immune response	Cytotoxic T cells and natural killer lymphocytes	Production of the measles rash, hepatitis A
	Autoimmunity	Acute rheumatic fever
	Immediate hypersensitivity	Rashes associated with helminthic infections
	Cytotoxic hypersensitivity	Cell necrosis induced by hepatitis B
	Immune complexes	Glomerulonephritis in subacute endocarditis
	Delayed type hypersensitivity	Tuberculous granuloma, caseous necrosis

Table 1.7 Examples of bacterial toxins

Toxin type	Example of sources	Toxin	Targets	Mechanisms	Effects
Endotoxin (LPS, lipid A)	Gram-negative bacteria	Endotoxin	Macrophages, neutrophils, B lymphocytes, endothelial cells, plasma components	Activation of target cells via TLR4, complement activation; release of IL-1, TNF, kinins	Fever, septic shock
Membrane-disrupting toxins	*Staphylococcus aureus*	α-Toxin	Many cell types	Formation of pores	Tissue necrosis
	Listeria monocytogenes	Listeriolysin	Many cell types	Formation of pores at acidic pH	Escape from the phagosome
	Clostridium perfringens	Perfringolysin-O	Many cell types	Phospholipase (removes polar head groups from phospholipids)	Gas gangrene
A–B type toxins	*Clostridium tetani*	Tetanospasmin	Synaptic transmission	Inhibits release of inhibitory neurotransmitters	Spastic paralysis
	Clostridium diphtheriae	Diphtheria toxin	Many cell types	ADP ribosylation of EF-2	Myopathy, polyneuropathy
	Vibrio cholerae	Cholera toxin	Intestinal cells	ADP ribosylation of adenylate cyclase, leading to rise cyclic AMP	Profuse watery diarrhea
Superantigen	*Streptococcus pyogenes*	Streptococcal pyogenic exotoxin	T cells, macrophages	T cell stimulation, release of IL-1, IL-2, TNF; possible enhancement of LPS activities	Fever, rash, toxic shock-like syndrome
	Staphylococcus aureus	Toxic shock toxin	T cells, macrophages	Same as streptococcal pyrogenic toxin	Toxic shock syndrome

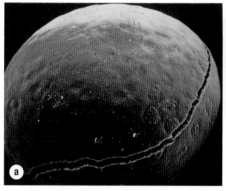
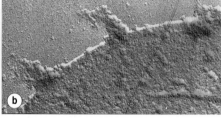

Fig. 1.17 Action of bacterial toxins. (a) *Xenopus* oocyte treated with the cytolytic delta toxin (perfringolysin) of *Clostridium perfringens*. (b) Rabbit erythrocyte exposed to a very small quantity of streptolysin-O, produced by *Streptococcus* A,C,G. Hemoglobin escapes from sites of membrane rupture. (Courtesy of Menno Kok & Jean-Claude Pechere.)

Uptake of diphtheria toxin proceeds via receptor-mediated endocytosis. Acidification of the endocytic vesicle induces a conformational change in the enclosed holotoxin, enabling the A subunit to traverse the membrane and reach its cytoplasmic target. The A subunit of diphtheria toxin catalyzes ADP ribosylation of the elongation factor-2 (EF-2), resulting in its inactivation. The *tox* gene is encoded by a phage and is under the control of the repressor protein DtxR, which forms a complex with iron, DtxR-Fe (Fig. 1.19), binds DNA and represses *tox* expression. Thus diphtheria toxin is only synthesized under low iron conditions, suggesting that it may be produced to stimulate iron release from target cells. Interestingly, the *Pseudomonas aeruginosa* exotoxin A has a very similar structure, but uses a different cell receptor: the α-2 macroglobulin low-density lipoprotein receptor. Like diphtheria toxin, exotoxin enters the cell via receptor-mediated endocytosis but the toxin is released only after passage through the Golgi system.

Hydrolyzing enzymes

Microbial pathogens often secrete hydrolyzing enzymes, such as proteases, hyaluronidases, coagulases and nucleases. As such, these enzymes do not harm the host cells directly and they are therefore not considered to be toxins. However, in the context of an ongoing infection they can facilitate colonization of host tissues by a variety of mechanisms, such as proteolysis of IgA; fluidification of pus; induction of plasma clotting, which may hinder the influx of phagocytes into the focus of infection; and destruction of extracellular DNA nets produced by polymorphonuclear neutrophils (PMNs) as an antimicrobial factor. The release of hydrolytic enzymes by phagocytes damaged by a bacterial toxin may have similar effects.

An example of how one such exoenzyme can nevertheless contribute to the pathogenesis of disease was recently discovered. Host

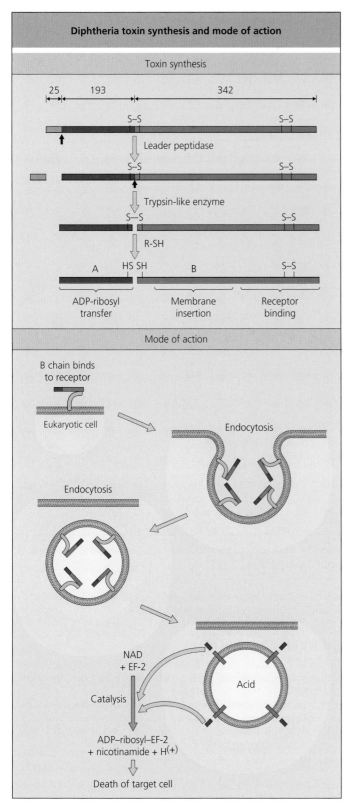

Fig. 1.18 Diphtheria toxin synthesis and mode of action. (Top) The 25-residue leader sequence is cleaved off by the bacterial leader peptidase; the A and B subunits are generated from the precursor protein by a 'trypsin-like enzyme'. Once in the cytoplasm of a targeted eukaryotic cell, the A chain, responsible for ADP-ribosyl transfer, is disconnected from the B chain, responsible for receptor binding and membrane insertion. (Bottom) The B chain binds to a specific receptor on the eukaryotic cell. After endocytosis, acidification in the endosome induces insertion of the B chain into the endosomal membrane and translocation of subunit A into the cytosol, where it catalyzes the ADP ribosylation of EF-2. As a result, protein synthesis is inhibited and the targeted cell dies. (Courtesy of Menno Kok & Jean-Claude Pechere.)

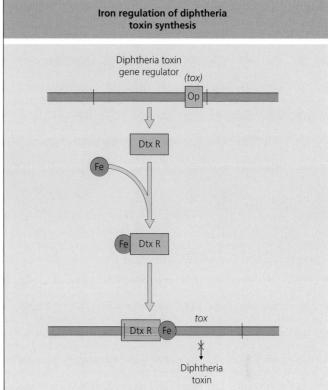

Fig. 1.19 Iron regulation of diphtheria toxin synthesis. High iron concentrations in the environment repress the synthesis of diphtheria toxin. When bound to iron, DtxR-Fe binds to the operator (Op) of the *tox* gene and acts as a transcriptional repressor of the *tox* gene. (Courtesy of Menno Kok & Jean-Claude Pechere.)

proteins that have a sialic acid in a 2,3 linkage to galactose residues at the termini of N- and O-glycan chains are not substrates for the host Ashwell receptor unless the terminal sialic acid is cleaved off. Pathogens such as *Strep. pneumoniae* that secrete a sialidase can remove sialic acids from host platelets that are then cleared from the circulation by the Ashwell receptor. This produces thrombocytopenia but avoids disseminated intravascular coagulation (DIC). Thus, one complication of severe pneumococcal sepsis is due to a secreted enzyme that is not generally considered to be an exotoxin.

Apoptosis

Apoptosis is a process in which the cell activates an intrinsic suicide program. It plays a key role in processes like organ development, tissue repair and maintenance of the dynamic equilibrium of the immune system. These processes critically depend on the generation of self-limiting organized structures through addition of new cells and elimination of 'old' cells. The morphologic changes associated with apoptotic death are a reduction of the volume of the cytosol and nuclear condensation (Fig. 1.20). The genome is fractionated by an endonuclease that cuts the DNA into multiples of 180–200 bp.[47] Finally, the remains of the cell are removed by phagocytosis without triggering an inflammatory response. In necrosis the cell does not participate actively in its own death and the dead cells trigger production of proinflammatory cytokines by macrophages.

Viral infection often triggers apoptosis of infected cells due to interruption of protein synthesis, transcription or signaling. For instance, apoptosis seems to contribute to the depletion of CD4⁺ T cells, both in cell culture and in HIV-infected people.[48] Several different HIV proteins have been noted to both promote and inhibit apoptotic cell death.[49] Similarly, apoptotic cells have also been observed in infections caused by Epstein–Barr virus (EBV) and adenoviruses, though in latency EBV

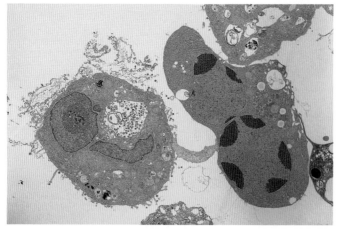

Fig. 1.20 Apoptosis induced by Sendai virus. Morphologic changes in the apoptotic Sendai infected cell (right) include the typical condensation of chromosomal DNA. (Courtesy of Menno Kok & Jean-Claude Pechere.)

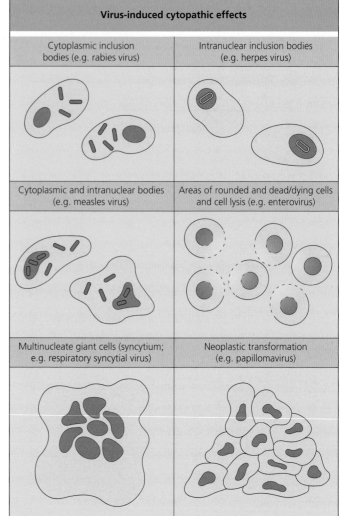

Fig. 1.21 Virus-induced cytopathic effects. (Courtesy of Menno Kok & Jean-Claude Pechere.)

latent membrane protein 1 (LMP-1) inhibits apoptosis.[50] Apoptosis can be seen to be beneficial to the host in that it can eliminate a host cell before it has produced a full complement of progeny virus.

Bacteria can also induce apoptosis. *Bordetella pertussis*, the agent of whooping cough, triggers macrophage apoptosis by interfering with cellular regulation at the level of the cytoplasmic second messenger cyclic AMP (cAMP).[51] The bacterium induces high levels of cytoplasmic cAMP, favoring the induction of apoptosis. *Shigella flexneri*, the etiologic agent of dysentery, can kill macrophages by apoptosis. Cell death is induced by invasion plasmid antigen B (IpaB) encoded by the *Shigella* virulence plasmid (see Fig. 1.14).[52] The *Shigella* IpaB protein binds to the host cytoplasmic enzyme interleukin (IL)-1b converting enzyme (caspase-1) and activates it.[53] Caspase-1 activates the proinflammatory cytokines IL-1 and IL-18 by proteolytic cleavage and initiates one of the proapoptotic pathways. In *Salmonella* infection the IpaB homologue SipB similarly activates caspase-1 to stimulate secretion of the proinflammatory cytokine IL-18 and induce apoptosis.[54] Timely induction of apoptosis in dendritic cells may well allow Salmonellae to exploit the mobility of these host cells to migrate away from the intestinal mucosa and establish systemic infection.

Virus-induced cytopathic effect

Many viruses damage the cells they infect, sometimes inducing visible and distinctive cytopathic effects (Fig. 1.21). Cytopathic effects may be mediated by either the presence of the virus or the host immune response. Poliovirus shuts off host cell protein translation through action of viral protease 2A resulting in cleavage of eIF4G needed for recognition of capped mRNA and cellular protein synthesis[55] and Coxsackie B virus protease 2A cleaves dystrophin in cardiac muscle, contributing to myocarditits.[56] In contrast, infection with hepatitis A and hepatitis C viruses produce very little direct killing of hepatocytes, with most liver damage mediated by the cytotoxic lymphocyte response.

Virus infection may also result in the intracellular accumulation or release of small molecules, such as reactive oxygen or nitric oxide, probably via effects on cellular signaling pathways or induction of innate immune responses. These may play important roles in cell destruction, particularly in macrophages. Rotavirus, CMV and HIV infection produce significant increases in intracellular calcium, a common pathway for the development of irreversible cell injury.

Viral fusion proteins mediate characteristic formation of multinucleated giant cells (syncytia). Examples include respiratory syncytial virus, parainfluenza viruses, measles virus, herpesviruses and some retroviruses. Viral infection can also produce eosinophilic or basophilic inclusion bodies in the cytoplasm or the nucleus. Inclusion bodies represent aggregations of mature virions, sites of viral replication or assembly, or degenerative changes.

Infection and cancer

Infection can favor development of cancer by producing chronic inflammation, impairing immune surveillance and directly altering cell growth and death, for example:

- chronic *H. pylori* infection is associated with gastric adenocarcinoma and mucosa-associated lymphoid tissue (MALT) lymphoma;
- inflammation associated with *M. tuberculosis* infection may lead to adenocarcinoma of the lung; and
- *Schistosoma haematobium* infestation is associated with bladder cancer.

It is possible that different types of infection may act together in promoting neoplasia. For example, human papillomavirus (HPV) has been found to be present in all bladder tumors associated with schistosomiasis but only the minority without parasitic infestation. Expression of some viral genes (oncogenes) can drive cellular proliferation and impair apoptosis, producing disordered growth (transformation) that may lead to cancer. As examples, Burkitt's type lymphomas and craniopharyngioma are associated with EBV, cervical and anogenital carcinomas are associated with HPV, hepatitis B and C infection is associated with hepatocellular carcinoma, Kaposi's sarcoma-associated herpesvirus produces

---

Virus-induced cytopathic effects

Cytoplasmic inclusion bodies (e.g. rabies virus)	Intranuclear inclusion bodies (e.g. herpes virus)
Cytoplasmic and intranuclear bodies (e.g. measles virus)	Areas of rounded and dead/dying cells and cell lysis (e.g. enterovirus)
Multinucleate giant cells (syncytium; e.g. respiratory syncytial virus)	Neoplastic transformation (e.g. papillomavirus)

Kaposi's sarcoma, and adult T-cell leukemia is caused by human T-cell lymphotropic virus type 1.[57]

In the case of HPV, persistent 'high-risk' infections (e.g. HPV16 and 18) may lead to the development of high levels of viral DNA, progressing to invasive carcinoma.[58] The HPV E2 protein regulates expression of E6 and E7 but is disrupted by viral integration, E5 acts as a viral analogue of the platelet-derived growth factor, E6 functions as a ubiquitin ligase to degrade the p53 anti-oncogene, and E7 binds to retinoblastoma protein (Rb) and cyclins A and E, allowing Rb phosphorylation and release of the E-2F, promoting G1 to S cell cycle transition.[59] With further chromosomal destabilization and mutations promoted by enhanced viral expression following DNA integration, the infected cells transform to a malignant phenotype.

Damage resulting from cytotoxic lymphocytes

The most effective host defense mechanism against most viral infections is mediated by the CD8+ cytotoxic T lymphocytes (CTLs). The CTLs recognize, attack and lyse virus-infected cells that present viral antigens on their surface in the context of MHC class I molecules. In addition to CTLs, natural killer lymphocytes can kill virus-infected cells. The cytotoxic reaction contributes to the pathologic and clinical picture of many viral diseases. The characteristic measles rash is produced by infiltration of lymphocytes including CTLs attacking skin cells infected by the measles virus. This explains why children with defects in cell-mediated immunity do not develop a rash during measles infection. In this disease, rash indeed represents a good immune response by the host, whereas its absence may signal uncontrolled viral growth. As previously noted, hepatitis due to hepatitis A and C may be largely or entirely the consequence of immune attack rather than viral cytopathic effects. It is also believed that lymphocyte-induced cytotoxicity contributes to the pathology associated with persistent virus infections such as the subacute sclerosing panencephalitis caused by defective measles virus within the brain.

Harmful immune responses

The destructive potential of the immune system is considerable. It can damage the host in a variety of ways.

Autoimmunity

Autoimmune reactions break the rules of the 'self versus nonself' dichotomy. Autoimmune reactions, directed against 'self-proteins', may result from partial identity of antigenic determinants of the host and an infective agent or from alterations of self-components caused by infection. Acute rheumatic fever occurring after group A streptococcal pharyngitis has been associated with antibodies against antigens found in the cell wall of the streptococcus that also recognize components of the endocardium and the joint synovial membrane molecules and thus induce an autoimmune response. Mycobacterial infection may give rise to antibodies and T cells that are reactive to both the microbial (nonself) and the host (self) heat shock proteins.

Another example of molecular mimicry is the association between production of antiganglioside antibodies, the Miller-Fisher (MFS) variant of the Guillain–Barré syndrome (GBS), and prior *Campylobacter jejunii* infection. This illness is almost certainly due to cross-reacting antibodies against the sialated LPS of *C. jejunii*.

Hypersensitivity reactions

Hypersensitivity reactions occur if the host immune system seemingly overreacts to microbial infection. Hypersensitivity reactions have been classified by Gell and Coombs into four types.

Type I or immediate hypersensitivity

Type I hypersensitivity occurs within minutes of antigen exposure. It results from antigen binding to mast cell-associated IgE. Vasoactive amines are released and anaphylactic reactions may develop. Certain forms of rash after helminth infections seem to be due to this type of hypersensitivity.

Type II or cytotoxic hypersensitivity

Type II hypersensitivity is a consequence of the binding of specific antibodies to cell surface-associated antigens. Antibody binding mediates cytotoxicity via complement activation or natural killer cells. Thus cells bearing microbial antigens may be lysed via an antibody-dependent mechanism. Such a mechanism has been suggested to account for liver cell necrosis during hepatitis B infection.

Type III or immune complex-mediated hypersensitivity

Type III hypersensitivity is induced by classic complement activation, caused by extracellular antibody–antigen complexes. This causes inflammation and changes in vascular permeability and attracts neutrophils to tissues where the immune complexes are deposited, including the kidneys, joints and small vessels of the skin. Glomerulonephritis in malaria and subacute endocarditis are probably due to this mechanism.

Type IV or delayed-type hypersensitivity

Type IV hypersensitivity typically occurs at least 48 hours after exposure to an antigen. It involves activated T cells, which release cytokines, macrophages attracted by these cytokines, and cytotoxic CD8+ T cells. Delayed-type hypersensitivity and granuloma play a major role in tissue damage observed during infections with slow-growing intracellular organisms, such as *M. tuberculosis* (tuberculosis), *M. leprae* (leprosy) and *Histoplasma capsulatum*. Many of the clinical manifestations of chlamydial disease, in particular trachoma, seem to result from a delayed-type hypersensitivity triggered by chlamydial heat shock proteins. In spite of the involvement of bacterial heat shock proteins, this is not an autoimmune phenomenon, because the unique rather than the conserved portions of these proteins seem to be implicated here.

Superantigens and bacterial components associated with toxic and septic shock

Toxic shock and septic shock are exceptionally impressive syndromes associated with a variety of infectious diseases. Severe hypotension, multiple organ failure and intravascular disseminated coagulopathy occur in the most severe cases. Pathogenesis of these syndromes is complex. Various bacterial components, including LPS, peptidoglycans, lipoteichoic acid and (in some cases) exotoxins acting as superantigens (see Table 1.7) trigger an intense, potentially lethal host response. Macrophages, neutrophils and/or T cells play important roles in the cascade of events leading to this condition (see Chapters 9 and 44) by releasing high levels of inflammatory response mediators, notably tumor necrosis factor and IL-1.

How micro-organisms escape host defense

In spite of the efficacy of host defense mechanisms, microbial pathogens can still infect humans and cause disease. This is in part due to the very potent weapons micro-organisms have (a single gram of crystalline botulinum toxin could potentially kill more than 1 million people) but it is also due to the intricate strategies that micro-organisms use to evade host defenses (Table 1.8).

Surviving the phagocyte and complement attack

Immediately after passage through the epithelial surface, the invading micro-organism encounters the most powerful actors of host defense: phagocytes. The two main types of phagocyte are PMNs and macrophages. These 'professional' phagocytes can bind micro-organisms

Table 1.8 Evasion of host defenses

Mechanism	Examples
Surviving the phagocyte and complement attack	
Inhibition of chemotaxis	C5a peptidase by *Streptococcus pyogenes*
Killing the phagocyte before ingestion	α-Toxin and Panton–Valentine leukocidin by *Staphylococcus aureus*
Avoiding ingestion	Bacterial capsules (e.g. *Streptococcus pneumoniae*) K (capsule) and O (LPS) antigens in Gram-negative rods
Avoid complement lysis	Coating with IgA antibodies (*Neisseria meningitidis*) Porin binding factor H and C4 binding protein (*N. gonorrhoeae*) M protein (*Streptococcus pyogenes*)
Surviving within phagocytes	Inhibition of phagolysosome fusion (*Chlamydia trachomatis*) Escape from phagolysosome (*Listeria monocytogenes*) Inhibit NADPH oxidase fusion with phagosome (*Salmonella typhimurium*) Inhibition of acidification of phagosome due to exclusion of the vacuolar H^+-ATPase (*Mycobacterium tuberculosis*)
Antigenic variations	Shift and drift in influenza A virus, pilin variation in *N. gonorrhoeae*
Tolerance	Prenatal infections
Immunosuppression	
Destroying lymphocytes Proteolysis of antibodies	Depletion of $CD4^+$ cells by HIV IgA protease by *Haemophilus influenzae*
Presence in inaccessible sites	Latent infection in dorsal root ganglia (herpes simplex virus)

with a variety of receptors, some of which specifically interact with bacterial surface structure or with antibodies or complement bound to the microbial surface (opsonized micro-organisms). The micro-organisms usually pass into the epithelial cell via phagocytosis or pinocytosis, although some (especially viruses) may enter the cytosol directly.

Bacteria invariably go through an endosomal stage, in which they will be exposed to a multitude of phagocyte defense mechanisms such as acidification, reactive oxygen species, bactericidal peptides, and hydrolytic enzymes released after phagosome–lysosome fusion. In addition, in the endosomal pathway, micro-organisms are deprived of the nutritional wealth of the cytosol. If the pathogens are killed and degraded their microbial antigens may be presented to lymphocytes. However, micro-organisms have developed strategies to avoid, mislead, deregulate or even profit from phagocytes.[60] Organisms like *Salmonella* require acidification of the phagosome and low Ca^{2+}/Mg^{2+} concentrations to trigger the PhoP/PhoQ transcriptional regulatory system that is required for survival inside macrophages. If acidification is prevented, *Salmonella* are killed by macrophages. In contrast, *M. tuberculosis* prevents acidification of the phagosome to varying degrees, and those micro-organisms that reside inside less acidic phagosomes remain metabolically active.

Inhibition of the mobilization of phagocytes

Extracellular micro-organisms can avoid phagocytes by inhibiting chemotaxis or complement activation (see below). A bacterial enzyme that degrades complement protein C5a, a main chemoattractant for phagocytes, has been discovered in *Strep. pyogenes* and *agalactiae*. Pertussis toxin catalyzes ADP ribosylation in neutrophils, which causes a rise in intracellular cAMP levels that ultimately impairs chemotaxis. *Yersinia pestis* employs several secreted enzymes (YOPS) to subvert macrophage phagocytosis and thus remain extracellular.

Killing the phagocytes before being ingested

Many soluble products excreted by bacteria are potentially toxic for phagocytes entering the foci of infection. Streptolysin-O binds to cholesterol in cell membranes, which results in rapid lysis of PMNs. In the process, the lysosomes are also disrupted and release their toxic contents, which may have deleterious effects on the neighboring cells. Other examples of toxins that are directed against phagocytes include the γ toxin of *Clostridium perfringens*, α toxin and Panton–Valentine leukotoxin made by *Staph. aureus*; the latter specifically targets myeloid cells and has species specificity. Many so-called extraintestinal pathogenic *E. coli* are hemolytic because they produce an RTX membrane toxin that damages PMNs, impairing their function in several ways, depending on the local concentration of the toxin. Several toxins from *Clostridium perfringens* produce similar effects. Indeed, pus sampled from gas gangrene may contain numerous Gram-positive rods without any visible PMNs.

'Professional' phagocytes as vectors or refuges

Legionella pneumophila provokes entry in mononuclear phagocytes by accumulating complement factor C3bi on the envelope of the organism. This complement factor is a ligand for the phagocyte receptor CR3, and enhances phagocytosis. Following uptake, *Legionella* remains in the phagosomes, which do not fuse with lysosomes and thus provide protection. Alveolar macrophages are host cells for *M. tuberculosis*.[61] *Salmonella enterica* are ingested by intraepithelial dendritic cells and carried into regional lymph nodes and the systemic circulation by those cells. Many viruses (HIV, dengue virus, measles, etc.) infect and replicate in monocyte macrophages. Infected monocytes may provide HIV with a route through the blood–brain barrier into the CNS[62] and dendritic cells loaded with infectious HIV may activate and infect T cells[63] (see Chapters 120 & 121). *Ehrlichia*, which are small, Gram-negative, obligatory intracellular bacteria, directly infect the cytoplasm of granulocytes or macrophages, depending on the bacterial species. All organisms that have adapted to live inside phagocytic cells have developed mechanisms to escape, disarm or survive the onslaught of antimicrobial factors.

Avoiding ingestion

The surface of numerous pathogenic bacteria is covered with a loose network of polymers, which constitutes the bacterial capsule.[64] Capsular material may be very thin, visible only by electron microscopy, as is the case with the hyaluronate capsule of *Strep. pyogenes*. In some species (*Strep. pneumoniae, Klebsiella pneumoniae*) capsule material is abundant, easily visible with a light microscope and responsible for a mucoid aspect of the bacterial colonies. Most of the capsules are composed of polysaccharides, others are made of proteins or a combination of carbohydrate and protein. Some capsule contents mimic host polysaccharides and are thus recognized as 'self' by the host immune system. Examples are the capsules of *N. meningitidis*, which contain sialic acid, and *Strep. pyogenes*, which contain hyaluronic acid. Proteins that envelop bacteria in S-layers can serve the same function as polysaccharides, as in the cases of *Campylobacter fetus* and *Bacillus anthracis*.

Capsules may protect bacteria from complement activation.[65] As a result, encapsulated bacteria are not immediately recognized as invaders by the phagocytes. Capsulated *Strep. pneumoniae* resist engulfment by macrophages and PMNs and are virulent; however, noncapsulated strains are easily phagocytosed and are avirulent.[66]

Meningococci circulating in the blood are coated with IgA, which is not an activator of the complement cascade. *Schistosoma mansoni* incorporates decay accelerating factors in its membrane; these are host plasma proteins that inhibit deposition of C3 onto host cell membranes. Activation of complement in the blood is thus avoided by the parasite.

Matrix (M) proteins, which form fibrillae (see Fig. 1.11), are considered to be the primary virulence determinants of *Strep. pyogenes*. Matrix protein renders the bacteria resistant to phagocytosis by human neutrophils. Matrix fibrillae are approximately 50–60 nm in length and exhibit a seven-residue periodicity. They exist as stable dimers, arranged in an α-helical, coiled coil configuration, with the carboxyl terminal portion closely associated with the cell wall (see Fig. 1.11). Streptococci that express M proteins on their surface are poorly opsonized by the alternative pathway and resist PMN phagocytosis. In contrast, streptococci that fail to express M protein are readily opsonized and phagocytosed, and are avirulent. Resistance to phagocytosis can be overcome by antibodies directed against type-specific M epitopes.

The mechanism of antiphagocytic activity of M proteins is still unclear. According to one hypothesis, fibrinogen, known to bind to M protein, may hinder access to complement-binding sites on the bacterial surface, disguising the pathogen as 'self'. In another hypothesis, a complement control protein (protein H), which also binds M, may be responsible for the observed complement resistance of virulent *Strep. pyogenes*.

Survival within phagocytes

Once ingested by the phagocyte, the pathogen may survive and grow using a variety of strategies (Fig. 1.22). Some microbes prevent exposure to hydrolytic enzymes by inhibiting fusion of the phagosome and the lysosome, others survive within the phagolysosome because they resist enzymatic degradation or neutralize toxic products to which they are exposed in this compartment. Some bacterial pathogens (such as Salmonellae discussed above) extensively modify endosomes into customized survival vesicles. Certain types of bacteria rapidly escape from the phagolysosome and propagate in the cytoplasm, as described above for *Listeria monocytogenes*. Recent studies suggest that intracellular pathogens, notably *M. tuberculosis*, may inhibit the early host response at the level of host gene expression.

Inhibition of phagolysosomal fusion

Salmonella spp. have developed several strategies to survive and propagate in macrophages; *Salmonella* spp. that lack this capacity to survive in macrophages are avirulent. Several hours after infection *in vitro*, two distinct *Salmonella* populations can be seen in the macrophage. One consists of rapidly dividing bacteria located in large unfused phagosomes. This population may grow rapidly and kill the macrophage, leading to the liberation of intracellular bacteria.[67] *In vivo*, this population may be responsible for the acute stage of salmonellosis.

The second population of *Salmonella* consists of nondividing organisms located in phagolysosomes. This population resists the toxic effect of lysosomal products and is believed to account for the prolonged survival of *Salmonella* spp. in the body. Long-living stromal macrophages of the bone marrow may act as long-term reservoirs and be responsible for the relapses of salmonellosis that are seen in immunosuppressed patients with AIDS. The dormant phase represents a well-regulated physiologic condition associated with nutrient deprivation *in vitro*.

Inactivation of reactive oxygen species

Reactive oxygen species damage DNA and inhibit bacterial oxidative phosphorylation. Bacteria may escape from the damaging effect of

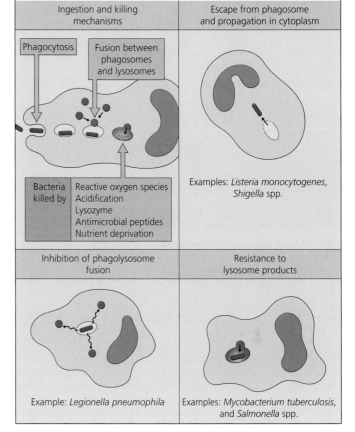

Fig. 1.22 Phagocytosis and bacterial resistance to killing. (Courtesy of Menno Kok & Jean-Claude Pechere.)

reactive oxygen species by rapid detoxification of the bactericidal products and by efficient DNA repair. Several bacterial pathogens produce superoxide dismutase (SOD) and catalase, two enzymes that might eliminate the reactive oxygen species and damage to DNA may be efficiently repaired through a RecA-dependent pathway. In Salmonellae the RecA pathway seems to be more important, as *recA* mutants are avirulent. However, enzymes that inactivate oxygen radicals are also virulence factors.

A SOD encoded by a bacteriophage that is present in many virulent *Salmonella enterica* is expressed under the control of the sigma factor rpoS when the bacteria are inside phagocytes. In contrast, expression of the chromosomally encoded SOD that is in all strains of *Salmonella enterica* is controlled by another sigma factor and expression is repressed in intracellular bacteria. However, the ability of this bacterial species to modify the endocytic pathway of the host cell seems to be the most important mechanism of resistance to reactive oxygen species. In macrophages, virulent Salmonellae localize in phagosomes devoid of NADPH oxidase, the enzyme that drives the respiratory burst.[68]

Resistance to antimicrobial peptides

Several cationic peptides are produced within the lysosomal granules and are believed to kill intracellular pathogens by forming channels in the bacterial cell wall. *Salmonella* spp. resist these antimicrobial peptides by at least two complementary mechanisms, one of which, encoded by the *sap* locus, is characterized in some detail (Fig. 1.23). It seems that the SapA protein forms a complex with the antimicrobial peptides, reducing the deleterious effect on the bacterial membranes.

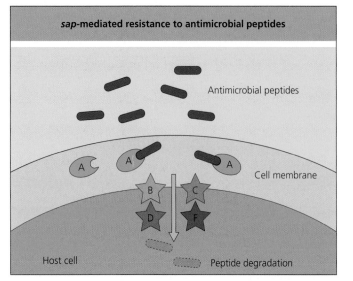

sap-mediated resistance to antimicrobial peptides

Antimicrobial peptides

Cell membrane

A   A   A

B   C

D   F

Host cell   Peptide degradation

Fig. 1.23 Mechanism of resistance to macrophage antimicrobial peptides by *Salmonella* spp. *Salmonella* produces the SapA (A) peptide, which complexes with host cell antimicrobial peptides. Other proteins encoded by the *sap* locus (SapB, SapC and SapD) are required for the transport of the SapA-antimicrobial peptide complex into the cytosol where the antimicrobial peptide is degraded. (Courtesy of Menno Kok & Jean-Claude Pechere.)

Other proteins encoded by the *sap* locus (SapB, SapC and SapD) allow the transport of the SapA–peptide complex into the cytosol. Within the cytosol, peptidases degrade the antimicrobial peptides. Recently it was shown that pili make group B streptococci resistant to Mouse CRAMP and the human homologue LL-37.

Antigenic and phase variations

A powerful survival strategy for a pathogen would be to mislead the specific host immune response by 'changing appearances'. Three examples of molecular mechanisms used to achieve antigenic variation, one each by a bacterium, a virus and a protozoan, are illustrated below (Table 1.9).

Table 1.9 Examples of antigenic variations

Genetic mechanisms	Examples
Recombination between different copies of pilin genes	Pili in *Neisseria gonorrhoeae*
Phase variation – turning expression of an antigen on or off ('flip-flop')	Flagella in *Salmonella*; pili in *N. gonorrhoeae*
Gene reassortment between two strains infecting the same cell	Influenza virus type A
Mutation of surface antigens	Influenza virus type A, B and C; deletion of flagella in *Shigella* spp. (avoids TLR5 signaling)
Gene switch leading to surface glycoprotein changes	*Trypanosoma brucei*
Gene switch leading to production of nonactivating lipopolysaccharides	*Yersinia pestis* growing at 37°C; *Salmonella enterica* growing inside phagosome (PhoP regulated)

Antigenic variation in *Neisseria gonorrhoeae*

Neisseria gonorrhoeae varies the composition of at least three major components of its outer membrane: the pili, which mediate the initial attachment to host cells; the membrane protein P.II, responsible for closer attachment resulting in phagocytosis; and LPS, described earlier.

Antigenic variations in the major pilin subunit are essentially due to recombination between different copies of *pil* genes scattered over the chromosome (Fig. 1.24). Only one or two of these are expressed (*pil*E, where E denotes 'expressed') at any point in time, but an array of antigenically distinct pili may be produced in response to an antibody challenge. In addition to this mechanism, pili are subject to phase variation (i.e. switches between *pil*-positive and *pil*-negative variants). Phase variation is controlled at the transcriptional level.

The P.II protein is similarly subject to genetic variation. As a consequence, the specific immune response never quite catches up with genetic variation in the bacterial population. The combination of this mechanism, LPS sialylation (see above) and IgA protease production, explains the apparent lack of acquired immunity to gonorrhea and makes vaccine development very difficult.

Shift and drift in influenza A viruses

Every year, during seasonal influenza, vaccination programs are confronted with the problem of antigenic variation. Influenza viruses change through drift and shift. Antigenic drift refers to the gradual accumulation of point mutations during annual circulation of influenza as a consequence of the high error rates associated with RNA-dependent RNA polymerase during virus replication. Influenza A virus mutants with antigenic changes tend to have a selective advantage over the nonmutant viral population. The rapidity with which drift can produce change is illustrated by the dramatic increase in amantadine resistance (from 2–12% to >91%) in influenza A/H3N2 strains, associated with a single mutation at position 31 of the M2 protein from 2005 to 2006. As a consequence of antigenic drift, the composition of the influenza vaccine must be evaluated very carefully and updated on an annual basis in order to offer coverage for the strains likely to be circulating at the time.

Antigenic shift refers to the emergence of a novel influenza virus in humans, due to direct introduction of an avian strain or to a new strain produced by recombination and reassortment of two different influenza viruses. Antigenic shift results in dramatic changes in the antigenic composition of the surface hemagglutinin (which binds the host cell receptor) or the neuraminidase (which modifies these receptors) and can cause devastating worldwide epidemics, or pandemics, in the immunologically unprepared population. Recent influenza A pandemics occurred in 1957 (the H2N2 'Asian Flu') and 1968 (the H3N2 'Hong Kong Flu'). An outbreak of avian influenza from exposure to infected poultry in Hong Kong in 1997 caused 18 human deaths. A genetically different strain of A/H5N1 circulated in domestic birds throughout Asia, causing 387 cases and 245 deaths between 2003 and 2008, raising concerns that a new pandemic might arise. Instead, in 2009, an unanticipated, novel H1N1 reassortant influenza A virus with origins in circulating seasonal influenza, avian, and both classic and Eurasian swine strains emerged to cause the latest worldwide influenza A pandemic.[70]

Antigenic variations in *Trypanosoma brucei*

African trypanosomes (*Trypanosoma brucei*) are flagellated protozoa, transmitted to humans by several species of *Glossina* (tsetse). The parasite survives in mammalian body fluids thanks to antigenic variation of the variant surface glycoprotein (VSG), which forms a 15 nm thick monolayer covering most of the parasite surface.[69] Within a single generation, most or all of the 10^7 VSG molecules may be replaced by an unrelated species, stemming from a repertoire of an estimated 1000 genomic copies of the gene. The VSG gene is invariably expressed from a polycistronic transcription unit, in the

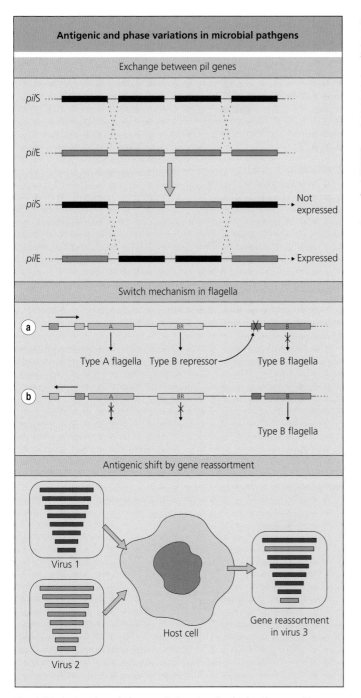

Antigenic and phase variations in microbial pathgens
Exchange between pil genes

pilS

pilE

pilS → Not expressed

pilE → Expressed

Switch mechanism in flagella

(a)

Type A flagella   Type B repressor   Type B flagella

(b)

Type B flagella

Antigenic shift by gene reassortment

Virus 1

Host cell

Gene reassortment in virus 3

Virus 2

Fig. 1.24 Antigenic and phase variations in microbial pathogens. Three mechanisms are shown. (Top) Exchange of DNA between nonexpressed copies of *pil*S and the expressed gene *pil*E in *Neisseria gonorrhoeae* can change the expressed antigen. (Middle) A switch mechanism is responsible for the (mutually exclusive) production of type A and type B flagella in *Salmonella typhimurium*. Phase variation depends on the orientation of a DNA fragment adjacent to the type A flagella gene. When A is expressed (a) from the promoter in the invertable fragment, the repressor for the type B flagella is expressed at the same time. As a consequence the type B flagella gene is repressed. Inversion of the DNA fragment abolishes expression of the A-repressor gene and the B-repressor gene (b). In this situation type B flagella are produced. (Bottom) Antigenic shift by gene reassortment results from infection of a single cell by two different virions. (Courtesy of Menno Kok & Jean-Claude Pechere.)

so-called telomeric expression site adjacent to the telomeric repeats. During chronic infection, patients experience successive episodes of parasitemia, each episode coinciding with the expression of a new VSG on the surface of the parasite. With this strategy, trypanosomes avoid complete eradication by the specific immune response, while maintaining the pathogenic burden at sublethal levels. The closely related *T. brucei brucei*, which causes the bovine disease nagana, does not spread to humans because it is sensitive to high-density lipoprotein in human serum.

IMMUNOSUPPRESSION

The most illustrative example of immunosuppression induced by microbial infection is provided by HIV. Human immunodeficiency virus circulating in the bloodstream readily infects CD4+ lymphocytes, macrophages and dendritic cells. The destruction of CD4+ T-helper cells is particularly detrimental to the host and accounts for the emergence of a variety of opportunistic infections as soon as the T-cell count drops below a critical level. In addition to its general immunosuppressive effects, HIV-1 preferentially infects HIV-1 specific CD4+ T cells, thereby undermining the ability of the host to mount an effective immune response to the virus itself.[71] It has recently been shown that HIV infection rapidly causes a profound depletion of CD4+ T cells in the gut as well as the lymph nodes and peripheral blood. This local immunosuppression may in turn be instrumental in producing continued T-cell activation due to increased bacterial translocation through the damaged mucosal barrier, increasing susceptibility to additional HIV infection.[72]

Other viruses may produce immunosuppression in a more subtle fashion. Measles virus infects macrophages and both B and T lymphocytes, interfering with the immunocompetence of the host for weeks after resolution of clinical disease. As a consequence, in areas with a high prevalence of tuberculosis, measles epidemics may be followed by outbreaks of tuberculosis. Gonococci, meningococci and *Haemophilus influenzae* produce proteases that hydrolyze secretory IgA1 antibodies. Protease-negative mutants of these bacterial strains are less virulent, suggesting a role for mucosal IgA1 antibodies in host defense against these pathogens.

CONCLUSION

Throughout evolution, humans, like all mammalian species, have maintained an intimate relationship with the microbial world. We have survived thanks to the efficient defense mechanisms we have developed against potentially dangerous micro-organisms. Pathogenic micro-organisms are still here because they have found ways of avoiding elimination by their host or by the microbial competition. 'Successful' pathogens have developed strategies to enter the body and reach and colonize their favorite niche, while defying the powerful human immune system.

In this chapter we have looked into microbial survival strategies. Although some of these have been analyzed in 'molecular detail', a lot remains to be discovered. Future remedies for infectious diseases are likely to be aimed at specific molecular interactions between the pathogenic micro-organism and its host.

REFERENCES

References for this chapter can be found online at http://www.expertconsult.com

Host responses to infection

OVERVIEW

The host response to potential microbial pathogens is complex and largely successful in preventing microbial invasion and disease. However, a number of organisms have evolved means of evading host immune mechanisms. This interplay between pathogen and host immune response results in a delicate balance, the weight of which can shift in favor of the pathogen in the setting of acquired immune deficiency states associated with immunosuppressive drugs, human immunodeficiency virus type 1 (HIV-1) infection and pregnancy. This chapter will broadly address the mechanisms that humans have developed to prevent microbial invasion as well as those that aim to rid the body of invading pathogens in order to prevent established infection. Lastly, we will address the consequences to the host of a strong inflammatory response, a form of 'friendly fire' in the body's war against infection.

The immune response can be viewed as consisting of two distinct but interconnecting branches, termed innate and adaptive immunity, that differ in their manner and rapidity of response to pathogens (Fig. 2.1). The innate response, the oldest mechanism of host defense, serves as the first line of response against invading microbes. The innate system is primarily mediated by cells that serve a barrier function, such as intestinal epithelium and skin, and phagocytes

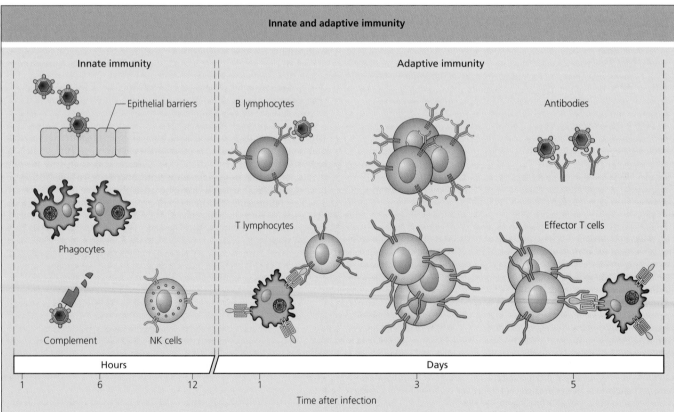

Fig. 2.1 Innate and adaptive immunity. The mechanisms of innate immunity provide the initial defense against infections. Adaptive immune responses develop later and consist of activation of lymphocytes. The kinetics of the innate and adaptive immune responses are approximations and may vary in different infections. From Abbas & Lichtman.[1]

Table 2.1 Innate versus adaptive immunity

	Innate	Adaptive
Components		
Barriers	Mucosal epithelia, skin, antimicrobial peptides	Antibodies secreted at epithelial surfaces, lymphocytes in epithelia
Cells	Phagocytes (neutrophils, macrophages, dendritic cells), natural killer cells	Lymphocytes, antigen-presenting cells (dendritic cells)
Blood proteins	Complement	Antibodies
Antigen receptors	Pattern recognition receptors	T-cell receptors, membrane immunoglobulin
Characteristics		
Specificity	For microbial-associated molecular patterns shared by microbes	For unique linear and conformational determinants (epitopes) of microbial antigens
Diversity	Limited, germline-encoded	Diverse, receptors produced by somatic recombination
Memory	No	Yes

From Abbas & Lichtman.[1] Copyright Elsevier, 2003.

that are recruited early to sites of pathogen invasion. Recognition of pathogens by innate immune cells is mediated by a limited number of germline-encoded pathogen recognition receptors (PRRs) that recognize conserved microbial components called microbial-associated molecular patterns (MAMPs). Conversely, cells of the acquired immune system respond to pathogens at later stages of infection and recognize microbial antigens using highly specific receptors that require gene rearrangement and clonal expansion. Furthermore, acquired immunity is associated with the development of immunologic memory (Table 2.1).

INNATE IMMUNITY

The innate immune response serves several functions in the early response to pathogenic microbes. The first is a barrier function to prevent organisms from invading the body. The second major function is an effector mechanism designed to eliminate microbes that breach the epithelial barriers through recognition, ingestion and killing by phagocytes. A third function is to alert the adaptive immune response to the presence of the pathogen, stimulate the appropriate adaptive effector cells and influence the nature of the adaptive immune response generated based on the nature of the pathogen.

Barrier functions of the innate immune response

Epithelial barriers form the first line of defense against the microbial world surrounding all multicellular organisms. The skin and mucosal surfaces lining the gastrointestinal, respiratory and genitourinary tracts provide both a physical barrier to invasion and also play a critical role in serving as the first geographic location at which interactions between pathogens and host occur.[2] The critical contribution of an

intact skin to the prevention of infection is clearly demonstrated by the direct relationship between percent of body surface area disrupted in burn injuries and mortality associated with the event. Disruption of the integrity of the gastrointestinal tract by cytotoxic chemotherapy compounds the risk of enteric pathogen bacteremia during periods of neutropenia during cancer chemotherapy. In the case of mucosal surfaces, additional physical protection is provided by the secretion of mucus and immunoglobulins in which bacteria and other pathogens are aggregated for clearance by cilia, coughing and/or peristalsis depending on the specific mucosal surface (Fig. 2.2).

In addition to the role played by the skin and mucosal surfaces in providing physical separation and clearance, both organs are heavily fortified with both innate and adaptive effector immune mechanisms. Antimicrobial peptides such as defensins, cathelicidins, lysozyme and lactoferrins provide one of the first lines of immunologic defense and are present at integumentary surfaces on a chronic basis. Immunoglobulins are both secreted into luminal cavities and affixed to the surface of cells lining these surfaces. Finally, cellular defense mechanisms abound in and around integumentary surfaces as locations where antigens are processed and presented to the immune response for amplification and recruitment, where pathogens are physically destroyed by effector cells and where they are actively captured and transported to local lymphoid structures for both secondary processing and destruction. These integrated immunologic functions of cutaneous and mucosal surfaces play critical roles in determining the events that follow any encounter with a potential pathogen.

Recognition and effector functions of the innate immune response

Innate immune recognition by pattern recognition receptors

As noted above, PRRs recognize MAMPs, and many of these microbial-derived products are shared by both commensal organisms as well as pathogens (termed pathogen-associated molecular patterns, PAMPs).[3]

Microbial-associated molecular patterns may be derived from a variety of organisms, including bacteria, fungi, parasites and viruses. These microbial products tend to be highly conserved, are essential to micro-organism survival and may contain carbohydrate, lipid, protein or nucleic acid components. Examples of MAMPs include lipopolysaccharide (LPS) from Gram-negative bacteria, peptidoglycan from Gram-positive bacteria, flagellin from flagellated bacteria, fungal mannans, bacterial CpG DNA, and viral DNA or RNA, to name just a few.

Although PRRs do discriminate between self and nonself, certain PRRs have been reported to recognize host self-antigens, such as heat-shock proteins and fibrinogen.[4,5] Each PRR recognizes a specific MAMP or set of related MAMPs, and their binding results in activation of specific signaling pathways that lead to distinct response patterns. As a result of the conserved nature of MAMPs, a given PRR may recognize multiple organisms that share PAMPs. In turn, a given organism may express multiple MAMPs and thus stimulate multiple PRRs. This specificity, combined with redundancy, ensures an appropriate pathogen-tailored innate, and subsequent adaptive, immune response against microbial invasion. The three major classes of PRRs that will be covered in this chapter include Toll-like receptors (TLRs), Nod-like receptors (NLRs) and C-type lectin receptors (CLRs).

Toll-like receptors

Toll-like receptors, originally identified in the antifungal response of *Drosophila*, are a family of transmembrane PRRs that are evolutionarily conserved from worms to mammals.[6,7] Thirteen mammalian TLR family members, including 10 in humans, have been identified to date, and ligand recognition is mediated by TLR homodimers or, in some cases, heterodimers.[8,9] Toll-like receptors have been further divided into subfamilies based on sequence similarities and recognition of related MAMPs. For instance, TLRs 7, 8 and 9 recognize nucleic

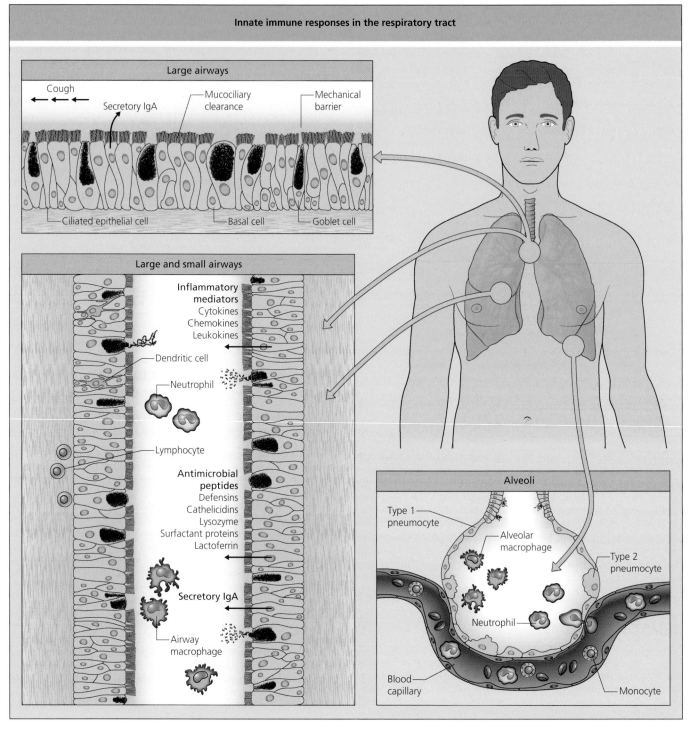

Fig. 2.2 Innate immune responses in the respiratory tract. From Sethi & Murphy.[2] Copyright 2008, Massachusetts Medical Society.

acids, whereas TLRs 1, 2 and 6 recognize lipids. Alternatively, TLR4 recognizes a diverse array of structurally dissimilar ligands.[3]

Toll-like receptors are expressed on both immune and nonimmune cells. On immune cells, TLRs are found on a number of phagocytic and antigen-presenting cells, such as dendritic cells (DCs), macrophages/monocytes and B cells. Toll-like receptors are also reported to be expressed on some subsets of T lymphocytes.[10,11] Among nonimmune cells, TLR expression has been reported on epithelial cells and fibroblasts. Interestingly, TLR expression on intestinal epithelial cells may play an important role in regulating intestinal inflammation.[12] Toll-like receptors may also have differential expression within a cell.

For instance, TLRs 1, 2, 4, 5 and 6 are expressed on the cell surface, whereas TLRs 3, 7, 8 and 9 are expressed intracellularly in compartments such as endosomes. Ligands for intracellular TLRs require internalization before signaling can take place.[3,13]

As noted above, TLRs recognize components of multiple organisms, including Gram-positive and Gram-negative bacteria, mycobacteria, fungi, protozoan parasites and a number of both RNA and DNA viruses (Table 2.2). A number of unique cell wall components of bacteria serve as PAMPs and are recognized by TLRs. Lipopolysaccharide (endotoxin) is a component of enteric Gram-negative bacterial cell walls that binds to CD14, then is able to associate with TLR4 to induce

Table 2.2 Toll-like receptor (TLR) recognition of microbial components

Microbial components	Species	TLR usage
Bacteria		
Lipopolysaccharides	Gram-negative bacteria	TLR4
Diacyl lipopeptides	*Mycoplasma*	TLR6/TLR2
Triacyl lipopeptides	Bacteria and mycobacteria	TLR1/TLR2
Lipotechoic acid	Group B *Streptococcus*	TLR6/TLR2
Peptidoglycans	Gram-positive bacteria	TLR2
Porins	*Neisseria*	TLR2
Lipoarabinomannan	Mycobacteria	TLR2
Flagellin	Flagellated bacteria	TLR5
CpG DNA	Bacteria and mycobacteria	TLR9
Not detected	Uropathogenic bacteria	TLR11
Fungi		
Zymosan	*Saccharomyces cerevisiae*	TLR6/TLR2
Phospholipomannan	*Candida albicans*	TLR2
Mannan	*Candida albicans*	TLR4
Glucuronoxylomannan	*Cryptococcus neoformans*	TLR2 and TLR4
Parasites		
tGPI-mutin	*Trypanosoma*	TLR2
Glycoinositol phospholipids	*Trypanosoma*	TLR4
Hemozoin	*Plasmodium*	TLR9
Profilin-like molecule	*Toxoplasma gondii*	TLR11
Viruses		
DNA	Viruses	TLR9
dsRNA	Viruses	TLR3
ssRNA	RNA viruses	TLR7 and TLR8
Envelope proteins	RSV, MMTV	TLR4
Hemagglutinin protein	Measles virus	TLR2
Not detected	HCMV, HSV1	TLR2
Host		
Heat-shock protein 60, 70		TLR4
Fibrinogen		TLR4

From Akira et al.[3] Copyright Elsevier, 2003.

signaling. Lipopolysaccharide preparations from some nonenteric bacteria have been reported to serve as TLR2 agonists.[14] Components of Gram-positive bacteria, such as lipoteichoic acid (LTA) and peptidoglycan (PG) serve as immune activators primarily by binding to TLR2. Flagellin, the major component of flagella used by many microbes for motility, is a potent activator of TLR5. Flagellins from some pathogenic bacteria have been shown to escape this important host defense mechanism.[15]

Innate recognition of mycobacterial bacteria by TLRs is also an important aspect of the host response to these intracellular organisms. Mycobacterial cell wall products have been shown to stimulate TLR2, TLR4 and TLR2/1 heterodimers.[16,17] In addition to proteins, lipoproteins and lipopolysaccharides, bacterial DNA also may induce an innate immune response. This effect is mediated by binding of unmethylated CpG dinucleotides in genomic bacterial DNA (CpG DNA) to TLR9, a TLR that resides intracellularly in endosomes.

TLRs are also critical components of the host response to fungi, protozoan parasites and viruses. Several cell wall components of fungi are recognized by TLRs 2 and 4, and, interestingly, different morphologic forms of a fungus (e.g. hyphae versus conidia) may preferentially stimulate one TLR over another.[18] As will be further discussed below, TLRs function in collaboration with other PRRs, in particular CLRs, to ward of pathogenic fungal infections. Components of protozoan parasites, including those of *Trypanosoma*, *Plasmodium*, *Toxoplasma* and *Leishmania* spp., have been shown to activate innate immune responses through stimulation of TLR2, TLR4 and TLR9.[19]

Moreover, nucleotide sequences from numerous RNA and DNA viruses are recognized by intracellular TLRs, in particular TLR7/8, TLR9 and TLR3.

- Recognition of viral PAMPs by TLR7/8 appears to play a role in several viral infections. TLR7 and TLR8 show a great deal of sequence homology, are expressed in endosomal membranes and are capable of recognizing viral ssRNA.[20] There is some published evidence to suggest that recognition of HIV-1 RNA sequences by TLR7/8 expressed on APCs such as DCs may be in part responsible for the generalized immune activation that characterizes HIV-1 disease and is associated with disease progression.[21-23]
- TLR9 plays an important role in innate host recognition of DNA viruses such as cytomegalovirus antigen-presenting cells and herpes viruses, as these viruses contain genomes rich in CpG-DNA sequences. TLR9 is expressed on a subpopulation of blood DCs and plasmacytoid DCs (pDCs) that are capable of secreting high levels of type I interferons (IFN, an antiviral cytokine) in response to TLR9 ligation and play a major role in the innate antiviral response to such pathogens.[24]
- TLR3 recognizes dsRNA that can be generated as a replication intermediate or by-product during infections with ssRNA or DNA viruses.[25] TLR3 is expressed in conventional DCs but also in a variety of epithelial cells and in astrocytes in the brain. Despite its wide expression, the role of TLR3 in antiviral immunity remains to be clarified, especially since TLR3 knockout mice do not appear to have increased susceptibility to viral infections.[26]

Finally, envelope proteins from several viruses may bind to and activate extracellular TLRs, such as TLR2 and 4, and this activation generally results in the production of inflammatory cytokines but not antiviral IFNs. This innate cytokine response may be in part responsible for the inflammatory complications associated with certain viral infections.[27]

Upon ligand recognition by TLRs, signaling cascades mediated through intracellular adaptor proteins such as myeloid differentiation factor 88 (MyD88) are induced in a similar manner to that seen with interleukin (IL)-1R signaling. Signaling ultimately results in the activation of transcription factors (such as nuclear factor kappa B, NF-κB), enhanced gene expression and the production of inflammatory cytokines and chemokines.[28] The topic of TLR signaling is too complex to be adequately covered in this chapter and a comprehensive review can be found in West *et al.*[9]

The differences in response patterns mediated by different TLR ligands may be in part explained by differential recruitment of adaptor molecules, although multiple factors are involved, including responder cell type and additional signals received. For instance, distinct adaptor molecules mediate the specific signaling pathways that result in the production of type I IFNs versus inflammatory cytokines (Fig. 2.3). As will be discussed further below, the early innate response

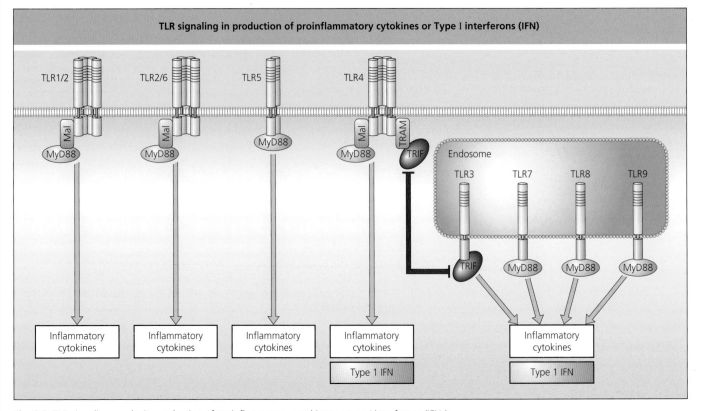

Fig. 2.3 TLR signaling results in production of proinflammatory cytokines or type I interferons (IFNs).

influences the adaptive immune response to a given pathogen that develops later. Thus, the specific early response pattern dictated by the sum of pathogen-specific TLR signals may profoundly influence whether an effective adaptive response is generated.

In addition to the production of cytokines and chemokines, additional programs may be induced upon TLR signaling, depending on the responder cell type. Immature tissue DCs serve as sentinels to sample the environment. Upon appropriate stimulation of DC TLRs by microbial MAMPs, the process of DC maturation is set into motion, ultimately leading to changes in phagocytic/endocytic capacity, secretion of cytokines, enhanced processing and presentation of antigen, upregulation of the major histocompatibility complex (MHC) and co-stimulatory molecules, and migration of DCs to T-cell areas of draining lymph nodes (Fig. 2.4). Mature DCs are then capable of effectively and efficiently presenting antigen to naive T cells. Thus, TLR ligation on DCs serves to link innate and adaptive immunity.[29]

Nod-like receptors

The nucleotide oligomerization domain (Nod) proteins are another more recently described family of germline-encoded PRRs (NLRs) that respond to microbial 'danger signals' in the form of MAMPs.[30,31] Unlike TLRs, NLRs sense MAMPs in the cytoplasm and are felt to be responsible for responding to bacterial and viral pathogens that replicate intracellularly. In some cases, extracellular pathogens can also be sensed by NLRs, especially if a cell contains machinery for transporting virulence factors (such as muropeptides) into the cytoplasm.[32,33] Upon ligand binding, NLRs oligomerize and recruit several adaptor proteins to activate a number of signaling pathways that result in formation of an 'inflammasome' associated with inflammatory cytokine production, production of antimicrobial peptides and, in some cases, rapid cell death.

One difference between pathogenic and nonpathogenic microbes is their ability to escape intracellular compartments and either replicate in the cytosol or inject microbial products into the cytosol for the

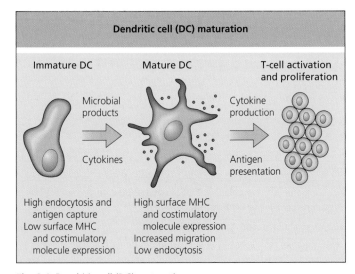

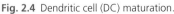

Fig. 2.4 Dendritic cell (DC) maturation.

purpose of manipulating host cellular machinery.[13] Activation of the NLR pathway may then be seen by the host as a sign of extreme danger, requiring a dramatic response with death of the host cell to prevent the microbe from hiding from host defenses within it.[34] Although much remains to be learned about this complex family of PRRs, there is already evidence to suggest that NLRs play an important role in the host response to organisms such as *Listeria monocytogenes*,[35] *Legionella pneumophila*[36] and *Helicobacter pylori*.[33] Like TLRs, NLRs are also likely involved in driving and directing the pathogen-specific adaptive immune response.

C-type lectin receptors

The last group of PRRs that will be reviewed in this chapter are the large family of C-type lectin receptors (CLRs) which are grouped based on organization of their CLR domains and are diverse in function. They are involved in mediating binding, internalization and potentially killing of micro-organisms, especially fungal pathogens.[37] Many of the CLRs recognize carbohydrate MAMPs, such as fungal cell wall mannans. Examples of CLRs include the mannose receptor (MR), dectins 1 and 2, DC-SIGN (dendritic cell-specific ICAM-3-grabbing nonintegrin) and collectins. CLRs are found on a number of phagocytic cells, such as macrophages, DCs and neutrophils. Some of the CLRS such as dectin are able to mediate intracellular signaling,[38] whereas others such as the MR lack classic signaling motifs in their cytoplasmic tail. Despite lack of signaling motifs, several studies have reported NF-κB activation and inflammatory cytokine production following ligation of the MR,[39,40] although the exact role of the MR in phagocytosis and signaling remains controversial.[41]

Dectin-1 binds to β-glucan ligands and has been shown to recognize numerous fungal species, including *Candida*, *Coccidioides*, *Pneumocystis*, *Aspergillus* and *Saccharomyces*. Dectin-mediated signaling results in phagocytosis, respiratory burst, activation of phospholipase and cyclooxygenase, and production in inflammatory cytokines and chemokines that may influence the adaptive immune response.[42] Dectin-2 is a CLR that is upregulated during inflammation and is important for its recognition of fungal hyphae.[43,44]

DC-SIGN is a CLR reported to internalize pathogens as well as to induce signaling, sometimes resulting in production of the immunosuppressive cytokine IL-10.[45] DC-SIGN has been shown to be involved in the innate response against fungal pathogens as well as viruses, such as HIV-1 and hepatitis C virus (HCV).[46-48]

Although CLRs clearly have a role in the innate immune response against microbial pathogens, their actual functions *in vivo* and their relative contribution to the overall innate response require further evaluation.

Collaborative interactions between PRRs

It is clear from the above discussion that multiple PRRs are capable of recognizing potentially pathogenic microbes and the overall innate response to a given pathogen likely utilizes multiple PRRs from several families simultaneously. Much interest has developed over recent years in determining how the different families of PRRs cooperate *in vivo* to induce optimal immune responses. There are a number of ways in which different PRRs might theoretically interact to benefit the host and there is some evidence that these coordinated interactions, or 'collaborations', are in fact necessary for an effective response to a microbe.[49]

Since NLRs recognize microbial ligands in the cytosol, they rely on mechanisms that make those ligands available to them. Herskovits *et al.*[50] reported that phagocytosis and killing of bacteria can generate PAMPs that become available to NLRs. Likewise, CLRs such as dectin may collaborate with TLRs by triggering phagocytosis, phagosome maturation and reactive oxygen production, and enhancing NF-κB activation.[51-53] Thus, it is likely that innate recognition of many microbes involves surface recognition and binding of the organism via CLRs and surface TLRs (e.g. TLR2, 4, 5), followed by internalization and recognition of PAMPs by intracellular PRRs, such as intracellular TLRs (e.g. TLR7/8 or 9) or NLRs, depending on the ability of the organism itself or its products to escape the endosome and reach the cytosol.

Since ligation of many of these PRRs results in induction of signaling cascades, the ultimate response depends on the various signals received. Several studies now suggest that antimicrobial inflammatory responses can be synergistically activated via ligation of multiple PRRs. For instance, concurrent ligation of TLR4 by bacterial LPS and TLR 7, 8 or 9 results in the synergistic production of IL-12 p70, a cytokine that has a significant impact on directing the adaptive immune response.[54-56] Similarly, there is evidence to suggest that

concurrent ligation of TLRs and NLRs results in synergistic production of inflammatory cytokines, such as tumor necrosis factor (TNF) and IL-1β.[57,58]

Additional research is needed to more clearly define these complex receptor networks and the results of such studies could have a major impact on the development of vaccines and vaccine adjuvants.

Phagocytes

Phagocytosis is one of the most basic elements of the immune response with phylogenetic origins in unicellular organisms. Phagocytosis can be undertaken by mononuclear cells, polymorphonuclear cells or natural killer (NK) cells. Although phagocytosis is often thought of as a mechanism by which organisms are merely engulfed and either sequestered or destroyed, the process actually plays the equally important role of providing a mechanism by which organisms are broken down and processed for presentation as antigens to critical elements of the adaptive immune response.[59-63]

Cells of the monocytic lineage are among the most diverse in the immune system and adapt both morphologically and functionally to their geographical location in the body.[64,65] Monocytes originate in the bone marrow and emerge into the peripheral blood as blood monocytes.[62] These cells migrate into tissues and differentiate into cells with a wide variety of morphologies and functions related to host defense (macrophages and dendritic cells), tissue maintenance (glial cells) and structural maintenance (osteoclasts and osteoblasts) (Fig. 2.5).[66-68] Macrophages involved in host defense further differentiate into alveolar macrophages in the lung, Kupffer cells in the liver, Langerhans' cells in the skin and other specialized cells depending on their ultimate

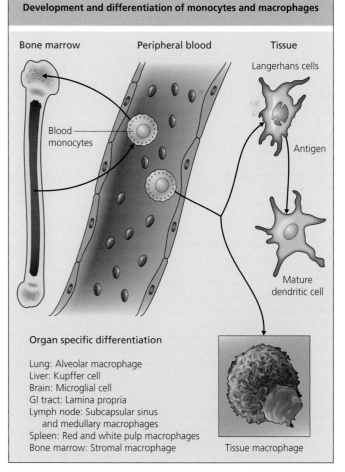

Development and differentiation of monocytes and macrophages

Bone marrow   Peripheral blood   Tissue

Langerhans cells

Blood monocytes

Antigen

Mature dendritic cell

Organ specific differentiation

Lung: Alveolar macrophage
Liver: Kupffer cell
Brain: Microglial cell
GI tract: Lamina propria
Lymph node: Subcapsular sinus and medullary macrophages
Spleen: Red and white pulp macrophages
Bone marrow: Stromal macrophage

Tissue macrophage

Fig. 2.5 Development and differentiation of monocytes and macrophages.

location. In each of these locations, monocytes adapt functions that are particularly suited to their specific locations. In addition to their stereotypical functions related to phagocytosis of foreign organisms, macrophages play important housekeeping roles related to removal of cellular debris, immune complexes and other cellular and subcellular entities requiring recycling.

Mononuclear cells are both resident in tissues on a chronic basis and respond to a number of well-characterized growth factors, chemoattractants and activators that both attract them to sites of inflammation and activate them for more efficient phagocytosis and intracellular killing. Macrophages interact with these stimuli with several families of surface receptors that provide specific instructions to the macrophage depending on the stimulus and the receptor.[69] Macrophages are dependent on growth factors such as granulocyte colony-stimulating factor (G-CSF) and granulocyte-macrophage colony-stimulating factor (GM-CSF) for growth, differentiation and survival. Chemokines, cytokines and microbial products play important roles in directing migration, secretion and activation. Macrophage functions are further directed by interleukins and interferons produced by lymphocytes and NK cells.

Phagocytes can identify pathogens by the presence of PRRs on the cell surface that recognize PAMPs expressed by the target organism.[69,70] Although phagocytes can engulf micro-organisms and other entities through this PRR–PAMP interaction, the process can also be facilitated by the presence of IgG or C3b on the surface of targets. IgG1 and IgG3 bind to the FcγR1 receptor constitutively produced by monocytes and produced after induction on polymorphonuclear cells. These receptors both serve as opsonins to facilitate recognition and tethering of pathogens by the phagocyte and as activators of the phagocyte oxidative burst through several intracellular pathways.[71,72] Binding of any one of several other surface molecules including TLRs, the IL-1 receptor or CD14 can also activate these intracellular pathways. FcR can either activate or downregulate macrophages depending on whether tyrosine-based activation (ITAM) or inhibitory (ITIM) motifs are formed intracellularly. ITIMs and certain other receptors such as signal regulatory proteins (SIRPs) are important in quenching inflammation to prevent excessive tissue damage as the inflammatory process develops momentum. In addition to surface molecules that regulate macrophage activation, a number of intracellular molecules can also mediate these functions. These include nucleotide oligomerization domains (NOD), caspase-associated recruitment domains (CARD) and leucine-rich repeats. The NOD pathway is particularly important in the gastrointestinal tract.

Once activated, macrophages both secrete additional inflammatory and chemotactic molecules and are primed to kill engulfed organisms within the cell. Inflammatory mediators such as IL-6 and IL-1 act remotely to promote the systemic inflammatory (acute phase) response.[73,74] Excessive production of these inflammatory cytokines can be dangerous to the host, contributing to the pathogenesis of septic shock and the systemic inflammatory response syndrome (SIRS). Other macrophage products such as collagenase and elastase may produce local tissue destruction and participate in deleterious processes including arthritis and pulmonary inflammation.

In addition to cells of the macrophage lineage, polymorphonuclear cells are capable of phagocytosis and intracellular killing. These cells are also ubiquitous in the body and are much shorter lived than cells of the mononuclear lineage. Polymorphonuclear cells share many, but not all, of the surface molecules expressed by macrophages. These cells are particularly efficient at intracellular killing, especially after activation, but are less intimately involved in immunoregulation and 'crosstalk' between the innate and adaptive immune systems than monocytes.

Phagocytes kill organisms by a number of means. Activation of the macrophage greatly extends these killing capabilities. Lysozyme which is constitutively produced by macrophages can destroy the integrity of the cell walls of Gram-positive organisms or collaborate with complement to damage Gram-negative organisms. Macrophages and polymorphonuclear cells also produce a number of short peptides termed 'defensins' that can permeabilize the cell walls of ingested bacteria.

The most potent microbicidal functions of phagocytes are mediated by reactive oxygen molecules formed through peroxidase-dependent and -independent pathways and by nitric oxide produced after stimulation by interferon gamma (IFN-γ) or TNF.[75] Genetic or acquired defects in either of these pathways greatly increases susceptibility to pathogens traditionally killed inside the cell such as *Staphylococcus aureus* and *Salmonella*.[76,77]

ADAPTIVE IMMUNITY

As discussed above, whereas innate immunity is an immediate response to conserved microbial products that is limited in scope of recognition by a 'hardwired' set of receptors, the adaptive response is more specific and all-encompassing in its scope of recognition but takes longer to develop. Innate and adaptive responses to a particular microbial pathogen are linked in a complex manner and the inflammatory responses induced by innate activation are often necessary for appropriate activation and direction of the adaptive response.

Adaptive immunity is characterized by several distinctive features that include:[1]

- antigen specificity;
- diversity of responses;
- pathogen-specific memory;
- nonreactivity to self antigens; and
- response self-limitation.

First, the adaptive response is characterized by exquisite specificity for distinct molecules, mediated by a diverse array of surface receptors on B and T lymphocytes. Microbial recognition by the adaptive immune system results in expansion of clones of B and T lymphocytes that express these randomly generated and unique microbe-specific receptors. This specific response is generated upon initial exposure to an infectious pathogen, and the response increases in magnitude and rapidity with each subsequent exposure (termed an 'anamnestic response') to the same pathogen. Thus, the adaptive immune system provides the host with 'memory' for each microbe that is specific, diverse in nature and quick to respond upon reexposure.

Adaptive immunity is comprised of two major types of responses, cell-mediated and humoral immunity (Fig. 2.6). Humoral immunity is mediated by antibodies that are produced by B lymphocytes. Antibodies recognize and bind extracellular microbes and their toxins and neutralize their infectivity. Cell-mediated immunity is primarily mediated by T lymphocytes, with the primary goal of recognizing and fighting intracellular pathogens such as viruses and bacteria that can proliferate inside cells, such as phagocytes. The specific features of both types of response are further described below.

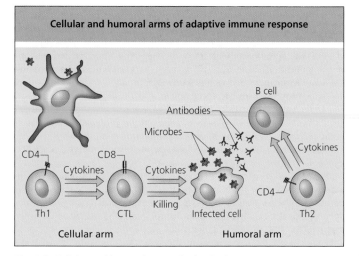

Fig. 2.6 Cellular and humoral arms of adaptive immune response. CTL, cytotoxic T lymphocyte; DC, dendritic cell; Th, T helper cell.

Cellular immune responses

Overview

The components of the cellular immune response include several varieties of T lymphocytes and antigen-presenting cells (APCs), such as DCs and monocyte/macrophages. Antigen-presenting cells capture and process exogenous microbes or process microbes or microbial antigens that are present in the cytoplasm (such as intracellular bacteria or viruses). Processed microbial peptide antigens are expressed in the context of MHC molecules on the surface of APCs and are recognized by surface receptors on T cells (T cell receptors, TCRs).

There are several functionally distinct populations of T cells. Helper T cells express the CD4 molecule, recognize antigen in the context of MHC class II molecules and help to orchestrate the adaptive immune response through the production of cytokines that provide 'help' to B cells and CD8+ T cells. Helper T cells also interact directly with APCs, such as DCs, to enhance their ability to present antigen and stimulate effector CD8 T-cell responses.[78] CD8 T lymphocytes, often called cytotoxic T lymphocytes or CTLs, recognize intracellular antigens presented in the context of widely distributed MHC class I molecules. These effector cells often have cytolytic potential and play an important role in killing infected cells. Another group of T lymphocytes, regulatory T cells, function to inhibit or suppress inflammatory adaptive responses.[79]

The complex interplay between these different cell types is critical to achieve the ultimate goal of cell-mediated immunity, which is to eliminate dangerous microbes without damaging the host through excessive inflammation.

CD4+ T-cell responses

Antigen-specific CD4+ T-cell responses play a central role in the adaptive immune response to microbial pathogens. Naive CD4+ T cells expand in response to antigenic stimulation and differentiate into effector T helper (Th) cells (Fig. 2.7).[80] Two distinct Th cell subsets with differing cytokine profiles and effector functions, Th1 and Th2, were originally described.[81,82]

Th1 cells are involved in mediating inflammatory responses against intracellular pathogens, such as viruses and intracellular bacteria, and produce cytokines such as IFN-γ and IL-2. Activated Th1 cells interact with APCs, such as DCs, to enhance their ability to prime effector CD8+ T cells that recognize intracellular microbial pathogens.[78] They further enhance the expansion of antigen-specific effector CD8+ T cells through the production of IL-2. IFN-γ produced by Th1 cells also serves to activate phagocytic cells, such as macrophages, and enhances their ability to kill ingested organisms. IL-12, a cytokine produced by APCs such as DCs, is important in the development of Th1 cells.[83]

On the other hand, Th2 cells produce IL-4, IL-5, IL-13 and IL-25, and play an important role in the clearance of extracellular pathogens by providing help to B cells, enabling the production of antibodies. Thus, they have a central role in orchestrating the humoral immune response, as will be described in more detail below. Aberrant or uncontrolled Th1 responses may result in inflammatory disorders or autoimmunity, whereas excessive or misdirected Th2 responses may result in atopy and allergy. Thus, a number of immune checks and balances are in place to ensure that activation and expansion of Th cells are tightly regulated. Anti-inflammatory cytokines, such as IL-10[84] and transforming growth factor beta (TGF-β), and regulatory T cells play a role in maintaining a balance between effective antimicrobial activity and excessive inflammation.

More recently, a third subset of T helper cells, Th17 cells, has been described.[85,86] Th17 cells produce several cytokines in the IL-17 family,[87,88] including IL-17A (IL-17), IL-17F and IL-22, have proinflammatory properties and are felt to play a role in clearance of certain extracellular bacterial (e.g. *Klebsiella pneumonia, Mycobacterium tuberculosis*) and fungal (e.g. *Candida*) pathogens.[89–92] The expansion and maintenance of Th17 cells is driven in part by IL-23, a proinflammatory cytokine in the IL-12 family.[85] Th17 cells have been identified in significant numbers in the intestinal mucosae and are postulated to play a key role in intestinal defense against invading microbes.[93–95] Mucosal defense by Th17 cells is likely mediated through a number of mechanisms, including cytokine-enhanced epithelial cell (EC) defensin production and neutrophil recruitment, and by enhancing epithelial integrity by fortifying EC tight junctions.[96,97] In addition to its role in normal host defense, the Th17–IL-23 axis has been implicated in a number of autoimmune diseases as well as in inflammatory bowel disease.[94,95]

CD8+ T-cell responses

CD8+ T cells are considered the primary effector cells responsible for clearance of intracellular pathogens, such as viruses and intracellular bacteria. Naive CD8+ T cells must interact with mature, antigen-loaded DCs in lymphoid tissue in order to differentiate into pathogen-specific effector cells. These activated effector CD8+ T cells are then capable of manifesting both cytolytic and noncytolytic antimicrobial effector functions that include MHC class I-dependent cytolysis of infected target cells and rapid production of β-chemokines and cytokines such as IFN-γ and TNF.[98,99] Cytolytic T lymphocytes (CTLs) proliferate and expand markedly during acute infections, migrate to the sites of infection, then contract into a state of memory. As noted above, CD4 T cells play an important role in the differentiation of CD8+ T cells and perhaps an even more critical role in their memory development.[100] These memory CD8+ T cells form the basis for protective immunity and are capable of rapidly expanding upon future reexposure to the same pathogen.[99]

Although some intracellular pathogens are readily cleared by CTLs, others, such as cytomegalovirus and Epstein–Barr virus, can maintain a state of latency by avoiding such clearance.[101–103] In the case of these chronic infections, ongoing immune surveillance by virus-specific CTLs results in suppression of overt disease, unless the host becomes immunocompromised. In contrast, in the case of pathogens (e.g. HIV-1) with a high mutation rate, escape from detection by CD8+ CTLs is a major mechanism used by the virus to advance its agenda of more active persistence, resulting in chronic progressive disease.[104–106]

Regulatory T-cell responses

Given the inflammatory potential of activated, antigen-specific CD4+ and CD8+ T cells, a number of mechanisms are in place to maintain the balance between the protective and tissue-damaging effects of the adaptive immune response. Regulatory T cells, or T$_{reg}$, are a heterogeneous category of T cells that suppress cytokine secretion and proliferation of effector T cells. This broad category consists of several populations of CD4+ T$_{reg}$, including CD4+CD25^{high} natural T$_{reg}$ cells of thymic origin, peripherally induced, IL-10-producing adaptive type 1

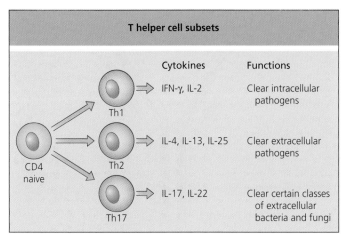

T helper cell subsets

	Cytokines	Functions
Th1	IFN-γ, IL-2	Clear intracellular pathogens
Th2	IL-4, IL-13, IL-25	Clear extracellular pathogens
Th17	IL-17, IL-22	Clear certain classes of extracellular bacteria and fungi

CD4 naive

Fig. 2.7 T helper cell subsets. Adapted from Bettelli *et al.*[79]

regulatory cells (Tr1) and TGF-β-producing T helper type 3 (Th3) cells. In addition, CD8+ and NK regulatory T cells have been described.[107,108]

One challenge in characterizing T_{reg} populations has been the difficulty in finding phenotype markers specific to these cells. The most specific marker to date for characterizing natural T_{reg} cells is the transcription factor forkhead box P3 (Foxp3). Foxp3 has been shown to be critical for the development and suppressive function of CD4+CD25high natural T_{reg} cells by controlling expression of multiple regulatory genes.[109,110] In fact, gene mutations that render Foxp3 dysfunctional result in a severe autoimmune disease in humans.[111,112]

The mechanisms by which regulatory T cells exert their suppressive effects on effector T cells, especially in humans, are not entirely clear, although both indirect mechanisms such as secretion of suppressive cytokines (e.g. IL-10, TGF-β) and direct mechanisms such as blocking T-cell activation or degranulation have been postulated.[107] Also, although antigen-specific T_{reg} cells have been reported in the setting of viral infections such as human papillomavirus,[113] T_{reg} cells may also suppress pathogen-specific CD4+ and CD8+ T cells nonspecifically upon activation. In any event, regulatory T cells are postulated to play a key role in modulating the adaptive immune response in the setting of both acute and chronic infections in order to limit inflammation and prevent tissue damage.

Antigen-presenting cells

Dendritic cells are indispensable in the initiation of the adaptive immune response based on their ability to process exogenous antigens and present them in the context of both MHC class I and II molecules to CD8+ and CD4+ T cells. Dendritic cells are the most potent APCs capable of activating naive, antigen-specific T cells and inducing their proliferation and differentiation into T helper and CTL effector cells. The immunostimulatory capacity of DCs arises in part as a result of high level expression of MHC and co-stimulatory molecules, such as CD40 and CD80. More recently, DCs have also been shown to have a role in stimulating memory T cells.[114]

Dendritic cells exist in an immature state in many tissues, where they serve to sample the environment by internalizing microbes and microbial antigens. In many cases, exposure to such antigens results in DC activation, migration to local lymphoid tissues and subsequent interactions with T cells. As noted above (see Fig. 2.4), the process of DC activation or 'maturation' is a complex one that involves changes in phagocytic capacity, upregulation of MHC and co-stimulatory molecules, changes in chemokine receptor expression that facilitate migration to lymphoid tissue, and production of cytokines and chemokines.[115] These changes are necessary to induce antigen-specific T cells; in fact, exposure of T cells to 'immature' DCs may result in their anergy or tolerance. The innate response of DCs to microbes and their antigens are critical to DC maturation and, in particular, the recognition of MAMPs by the many types of PRR expressed by DCs (such as CLRs and TLRs) regulates each step in the maturation process.[116] As a result, DCs are considered to bridge innate and adaptive immunity.

The type of DC activated, its tissue location and the microbe that is sensed all determine the nature of the innate response. The type of innate response generated, and in particular the cytokine profile of the activated DC, then has a major impact on determining the type of adaptive response that is generated in turn. For instance, an activated DC that produces IL-12 or IL-23 may stimulate inflammatory T cells, whereas activated DCs that produce IL-10 may regulate or suppress T-cell inflammation. Thus, the adaptive immune response cannot be fully understood without an understanding of the upstream, innate signals that influence it.

Humoral immune response

By definition, the humoral immune response consists of immunologic effector molecules that are present in soluble form in plasma and other bodily fluids. The two major components of this response consist of immunoglobulins that are produced by specialized cells of the lymphoid lineage (termed B cells) and a family of complement proteins that are primarily synthesized by liver cells. These proteins are capable of interacting with pathogens alone or in concert to reduce their infectivity or, in some cases, to kill them; however, they are most effective when they contribute to a coordinated immune response that includes both cellular and humoral components.

Antibodies

Immunoglobulins are members of a family of molecules that combine variable regions that provide exquisite specificity for binding to target molecules with constant structural motifs that allow well-defined interactions with other components of the immune response. The variable region of the molecule provides the diversity required to identify and to bind to an essentially limitless range of target molecules while the constant region allows the antibody molecule to channel effector activities of other components of the immune response that lack the ability to specifically identify diverse structural targets.

Antibody structure

Immunoglobulin molecules are composed of four protein chains that are joined by a variable number of disulfide bonds. Each molecule consists to two identical heavy chain proteins and two identical light chain proteins (Fig. 2.8). These proteins are joined in the shape of a 'Y', with the heavy chain proteins providing the base of the 'Y' and part of each of the arms. The base of the 'Y' is termed the constant (Fc) region and serves as the portion of the immunoglobulin molecule that binds to other Fc receptors on the surface of specialized immune cells and that provides a locus for binding the initial protein of the complement cascade. Each light chain pairs with a heavy chain to form one of the two arms of the molecule. These arms are termed the 'antibody binding' (Fab) regions of the molecule. These two arms of the molecule are characterized by major molecular diversity and provide the specificity by which each immunoglobulin molecule defines its optimal binding ligand.

Immunoglobulin classes

Antibodies are subdivided into isotypes (or classes) and are termed IgM, IgG, IgA, IgD and IgE antibodies, based on which of the five different heavy chain molecules are synthesized by the B cell producing the antibody (Fig. 2.9, Table 2.3) Two subclasses of IgA (termed IgA1 and IgA2) and four subclasses of IgG (IgG1, IgG2, IgG3 and IgG4) are

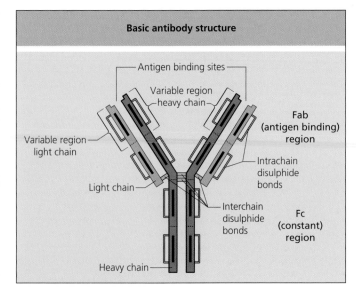

Fig. 2.8 Basic antibody structure.

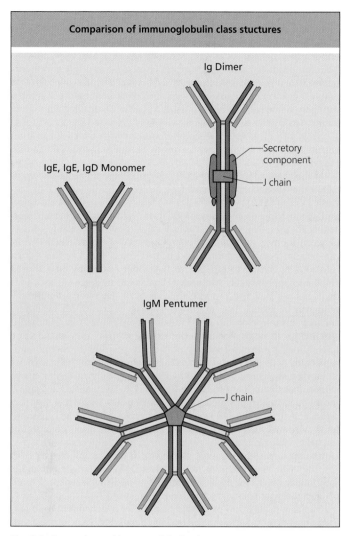

Comparison of immunoglobulin class stuctures

Ig Dimer

IgE, IgE, IgD Monomer

Secretory component

J chain

IgM Pentumer

J chain

Fig. 2.9 Comparison of immunoglobulin class structures.

present in humans. The specific range of functions that can be mediated by an antibody is defined by its subclass. Except for a short period of time in B-cell development when a B cell can produce both IgM and IgD, each B cell can make only one immunoglobulin subclass at any one time. Isotype switching during B-cell development (described in more detail below) is one of the most interesting biologic processes yet defined. In addition to the production of heavy and light chains, B cells producing IgM and IgA can produce a joining (or 'J') protein that results in multimerization of the antibodies produced.

IgM antibodies are the first antibodies produced in response to an antigenic challenge and may appear within the plasma within a week of initially encountering an antigen. IgM antibodies are of relatively low affinity but are produced with a joining piece that results in five molecules possessing 10 binding sites being produced as a molecular unit. This greatly enhanced valency increases the effectiveness of IgM antibodies and partially compensates for the relatively low binding affinity of each Fab unit. Because of the high molecular weight of IgM antibodies, they do not readily leave the vascular space and are usually found in plasma. IgM antibodies primarily function to prevent binding of pathogens to cells or to aggregate pathogens, thereby enhancing physical clearance of the organism.

The four subclasses of IgG antibodies are present in the highest concentration in the plasma because of their long half-lives (~3 weeks) and high production rates. These antibodies, produced in the second wave of response to an antigenic challenge, evolve to much higher affinities than observed in IgM antibodies and diffuse much more widely throughout the body. Approximately 50% of IgG antibody is found outside the vascular space. IgG antibodies are particularly effective in bringing pathogens into contact with effector cells through binding of the Fc portion of the IgG antibody to Fc receptors on these cells.

IgA antibodies, primarily produced as dimers joined by a J piece by B cells residing in submucosal locations, are present in the greatest concentrations on the mucosal surfaces of the respiratory, gastrointestinal and genitourinary tracts. Antibodies of this class are produced in greater quantity than those of all other classes combined. IgA dimers are linked to a secretory component (SC) protein on the internal surface of epithelial membrane cells and then exported into secretions on the apical side of the membrane. Once within secretions most of the SC molecule is cleaved and IgA dimers cross link infectious agents, thereby both blocking adherence of pathogens to mucosal

Table 2.3 Immunoglobulin classes

Antibody class	Subclasses	Heavy chain isotype	Number of units	Molecular weight (kDa)	Complement fixation	FcR binding	Adult serum half-life (days)	Adult serum concentration (μg/ml)
IgM		μ	5	950	Yes	No	10	600–3500
IgG				150			23	6400–13 500
	IgG1	γ1	1		Yes	Yes		
	IgG2	γ2	1		Yes	No		
	IgG3	γ3	1		Yes	Yes		
	IgG4	γ4	1		No	No		
IgA				400			6	700–3100
	IgA1	α1	2		No	Yes		
	IgA2	α2	2		No	Yes		
IgE		ε	1	190	No	Yes	2	0.04
IgD		δ	1	175	No		NA	NA

surfaces and facilitating physical clearance by cilia and other mechanisms. IgM molecules can also be exported through this pathway. Since most IgA antibodies are secreted through mucosal surfaces, serum levels of IgA are much lower than those of IgG. IgA antibodies do not fix complement or bind to Fc receptors, and thus are relatively poor inducers of inflammatory responses. Because of this property, IgA antibodies are thought to be important in binding potential food allergens and facilitating clearance without sensitization.[117] Individuals who lack IgA antibodies have a higher incidence of food allergies than the general population.

IgE antibodies bind tightly and specifically to mast cells where they reside for a prolonged period of time.[118] When IgE antibodies on the surface of mast cells bind an antigen, they trigger the mast cell to release histamine and other inflammatory mediators resulting in an immediate hypersensitivity response. Although the specific role for IgE antibodies in host defense against multicellular parasites has not been fully delineated, these antibodies seem to be integral to the immune response to this group of pathogens.[119]

IgD antibodies are transiently present on the surface of B cells during B-cell development and play a key role in B-cell maturation and selection.

Generation of antibody diversity and isotype switching

The mechanisms by which the immune response selects for high affinity antibodies, regulates production of the appropriate isotypes during induction of the immune response, and by which antibody production is downmodulated following an immunologic challenge, are among the most elegant regulatory mechanisms in nature. This response features a series of DNA rearrangements that result in the creation of massive antibody diversity followed by an efficient mechanism for selecting for B cells producing antibodies of the highest affinity and eliminating those that produce antibodies that bind to antigens of the host.

Antibody diversity is created by a series of rearrangements of DNA as cells mature from pro-B cells to B cells in the bone marrow (Fig. 2.10). These rearrangements result in the joining of four segments of DNA into the necessary components for the heavy chain of an IgM molecule. These components include a constant μ segment as well as three other segments termed V (variable segment), D (diversity segment) and J (joining segment). These latter segments are selected randomly from 130 possible V segments, 27 possible D segments and 6 possible J segments, allowing for over 20 000 possible combinations of V, D and J segments with each μ segment. The splicing mechanisms responsible for this process are themselves 'sloppy' and allow for the insertion and deletion of bases, thereby greatly increasing potential diversity. Once these arrangements have occurred with the heavy chain, the cell is termed a B cell and an analogous process ensues with the light chain to introduce additional diversity as another rearrangement process develops a DNA segment capable of encoding an intact light chain. In the case of the light chain, only the V, J and constant segments are involved. With the light chain, the B cell can choose one of two different possible constant regions termed kappa or lambda for fusion to the V and J segments. Once a DNA sequence capable of encoding a light chain has been assembled, two identical light and two identical heavy chains are synthesized and unite to form a full IgM molecule which is then displayed on the B-cell surface to allow for expansion of those with the appropriate specificity and elimination of any B cells with self-specificity.

B cells first express surface IgM molecules while still in the bone marrow. Since the bone marrow is a reasonably sequestered location, antigens present in the bone marrow are most likely host antigens rather than foreign ones. If a B cell still resident in the marrow encounters an antigen that binds to its surface IgM molecule, it is signaled to either undergo apoptosis or to become anergic and not expand further. Thus, B cells that recognize self-antigens are prevented from further expansion before leaving the marrow.

As B cells leave the marrow, long RNA transcripts are produced that include both the μ and δ segments as well as the previously selected V, D and J segments. Since this messenger RNA can be spliced to produce either a heavy chain for an IgM antibody or one for an IgD antibody, both are produced and B cells express both IgM and IgD simultaneously as they emerge from the marrow. If a B cell expressing both IgM and IgD encounters cognate antigen, it receives what has been termed the 'first signal' and is subsequently capable of proliferating when stimulated by the 'second signal' which is delivered by an activated T cell. If a B cell does not encounter antigen with which it can bind within a week of leaving the marrow, it becomes anergic and can no longer divide.

At this stage of development, B cells express a molecule known as CD40 that is specifically bound by a molecule on the surface of activated T cells (CD40 ligand, or CD154). This results in B-cell activation and stimulation of antibody production. Additional adhesion molecules are then expressed by T and B cells, resulting in stable contact between the two cells and a channel between them by which T cells can secrete specific cytokines and further direct the B cell to switch its antibody isotype to IgG, IgE or IgA. Once bound by an activated T cell and appropriately stimulated, B cells can undergo three or four divisions per day and produce thousands of daughter cells. By this sequence of events, the immune response is capable of randomly creating immunoglobulin molecules of an almost infinite number of specificities through recombination in the marrow but, at the same time, allows for expansion only of those responding to foreign antigens being actively encountered as B cells emerge from the marrow.

Isotype switching is directed by cytokines produced by T cells in close proximity to IgM producing B cells. IL-6, IL-10 and TGF-β signal B cells to switch to production of IgA antibodies, while IL-4 and IL-5 direct a switch to the IgE isotype. Isotype switching to IgG, IgA and IgE is accomplished by another DNA rearrangement with ligation of the heavy chain V, D and J segments to γ, α or ε segments, respectively. Unlike the IgM to IgD isotype switch which is accomplished by RNA splicing, this final isotype switch involves DNA rearrangement and is a permanent event for the B cell. Progeny of an isotype-switched B cell produce only that isotype from that time forward.

Ongoing production of specific antibodies is dependent on ongoing antigenic stimulation in the face of a regulatory bias to cease production of antibodies of a given specificity and ongoing selection of antibodies of even higher specificity. As B cells undergo division, they express increasing amounts of a surface molecule known as Fas and lower levels of Bcl-2. Bcl-2 is required for ongoing division while ligation of Fas results in death by apoptosis. If a B cell encounters an antigen that binds its surface immunoglobulin, it produces higher levels of Bcl-X$_L$ and survives. As B cells divide, the immunoglobulin gene continues to undergo somatic hypermutation. B cells that generate immunoglobulin with a higher affinity for the antigens of interest outcompete other B cells for this antigen and have a selective advantage, thereby further increasing antibody specificity over time. As antigen density decreases with resolution of an infection, for example, B cells cease producing antibodies and cells that survive become memory B cells that are capable of rapid expansion if a related antigen is subsequently encountered.[120]

Antibody functions

Antibodies serve in a number of different roles, both as freestanding molecules and working in concert with other components of the immune response (Table 2.4).

Neutralization

The most straightforward function of antibodies involves direct binding to microbes or toxins to block binding to host cell receptors or to reduce infectivity through a process termed neutralization. Microbial pathogens often gain entrance into target cells by binding with specific ligands on the cell surface. Antibodies that interfere with this interaction reduce the infectivity of organisms by preventing effective

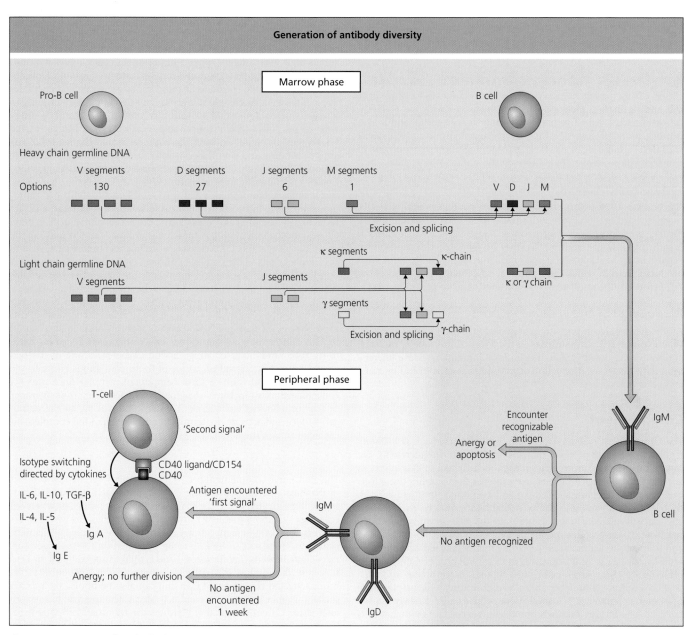

Fig. 2.10 Generation of antibody diversity.

interactions with target cells.[121] Microbial toxins also usually bind to specific molecules on the surface of target cells and interactions with antibodies that interfere with this interaction can markedly reduce the effects of these toxins. Antibodies can also reduce the infectivity of organisms without binding directly to receptor molecules if they interfere with molecular rearrangements involved in infectivity after initial binding has occurred.[122]

Table 2.4 Functions of antibodies

- Cross linking and physical clearance of pathogens
- Neutralization of pathogens
- Initiation and enhancement of complement activity
- Opsonization of pathogens
- Antibody-dependent cellular cytotoxicity
- Modulation of the immune response

Complement activation

Antibodies of the IgM class as well as those of the IgG1, IgG2 and IgG3 subclass can activate complement after binding to the surface of a microbe. IgG1 and IgG3 are usually targeted to protein antigens while antibodies of the IgG2 subclass usually bind to polysaccharide antigens. Individuals with selective IgG2 deficiency exhibit greater susceptibility to encapsulated organisms.[123] As will be described in more detail below, when antibodies activate complement through the classic pathway, the first complement component (C1q) binds to the Fc portions of at least two antibody molecules and sets off a series of molecular interactions with distal components of the complement cascade that culminates in the formation of pores in the wall of the microbe leading to an osmotic death. Complement can also facilitate the formation of large soluble complexes of antibodies and pathogens that can be eliminated from the host. Red blood cells are coated with receptors for complement protein C3b and can transport pathogens coated with this protein to the spleen and liver for ingestion by the reticuloendothelial system.

Opsonization

Antibodies of the IgG1 and IgG3 subclass also target pathogens for ingestion by phagocytic cells of the immune system by binding to the pathogen with the Fab end of the antibody and to a phagocytic cell through Fc receptors on the surface of these cells. In addition to providing a bridging mechanism between the microbe and a phagocytic cell and facilitating phagocytosis, the interaction with the Fc receptor activates the oxidative pathway within the phagocyte and makes it much more effective in killing the pathogen within its phagocytic vacuoles. Pathogens can also be targeted for ingestion by deposition of complement proteins C3b and C4b on the surface of the pathogen.

Antibody-dependent cellular cytotoxicity

Antibodies can also form bridges between pathogens and NK cells, monocytes or granulocytes and activate these cells to secrete microbicidal substances including perforins or granzymes that can kill organisms without requiring that they be ingested. This mechanism is particularly well suited to targets too large for ingestion or for virus producing cells in which these antibodies facilitate destruction of the cell before a full complement of infectious virus can be produced.[124]

Modulation of the immune response

Antibodies are also important for modulation of the immune response. When complexed with antigens in the form of immune complexes, antibodies can downregulate the humoral immune response, thereby modulating ongoing production of antibodies as antigen and immune complexes are cleared.

Complement

The complement system is probably best characterized as a highly regulated series of proteins that play a key role in interfacing the innate and adaptive immune responses.[125,126] The complement system is composed of over 30 interactive proteins that amplify the effects of antibodies, integrate the cellular and humoral responses, assist in the clearance of immune complexes, enhance antigen presentation and can stimulate cellular immunity in the absence of an antibody response. These proteins are highly evolved both in their regulation and in their effector function to provide tightly targeted amplification of the immune response, especially in its earliest phases. Complement proteins are also critical to the cross linking of antibodies and antigens in immune complexes and play a critical role in the clearance of immune complexes.[127] Complement proteins are primarily synthesized by hepatocytes although monocytes and certain epithelial cells can also produce complement components.

Initiation of the complement cascade

The complement cascade can be activated by one of three different types of signal (Fig. 2.11). Once activated by any of these signals, the three signaling pathways converge at an activated protein common to all three pathways, C3b, that then catalyzes the remainder of the cascade to produce a membrane attack complex as well as a family of terminal components with immunoregulatory functions.[126] The classic complement pathway is activated by interactions between pathogens and IgM or IgG.[128,129] The other two pathways do not require antibody for activation and can evolve very early during interactions between pathogen and host. The first of these, termed the 'lectin pathway', is triggered when one or more circulating mannose-binding ligands bind to monosaccharides on the surface of pathogens.[130] The final pathway, termed the 'alternative pathway', is activated when C3b is incorporated into an active complex by a circulating protein known as properdin and stabilized on the surface of a pathogen.[131]

Classic pathway

The classic pathway of complement activation can be triggered when the first component of the complement cascade, C1, interacts with IgM, IgG1, IgG2 or IgG3 molecules that have undergone structural rearrangement following binding to cognate antigen.[128,129] C1 circulates as a huge noncovalently linked polyprotein composed of 22 protein subunits of five different types and is not activated unless it simultaneously encounters Fc regions from at least two immunoglobulin molecules that have bound to an antigenic target. Since IgM circulates as a pentamer, a single IgM molecule can activate C1 after binding to a target antigen. IgG-based activation requires that at least two molecules of antibody bind in close enough proximity to be bridged by the C1 protein. By requiring both the conformational change following antigen binding and simultaneous interaction with more than one Fc region, C1 can freely circulate in its nonactive form and avoid activation by encountering unbound antibody.

Once the C1 molecule is activated by interaction with the appropriate antibody ligands, two of its protein subunits, C1r and C1s, are sequentially activated as proteases. The active C1s serine protease then cleaves another circulating complement protein, C4, to continue the complement cascade. C4 is cleaved into a larger component, C4b, that covalently bonds to the pathogen through either an amide or an ester bond and a smaller soluble component, C4b, that possesses inflammatory activity. When C4b is bound to the membrane of a pathogen, it can, in turn, bind complement protein C2 which then becomes a target for proteolysis by the C1s protease. The larger fragment of this proteolysis, C2a, then gains proteolytic capability and remains bound to C4b and forms a protein dimer that can convert C3 to its active form. C4b binds to circulating C3 and C2a cleaves one of the two chains of the C3 heterodimer. One of these, C3b, binds either to the C4–C2 dimer and forms a three-component complex known as C5 convertase that is capable of cleaving C5 and activating the remainder of the complement cascade, or that can bind directly to the pathogen surface and activate the terminal components of the complement cascade through the alternative pathway.[132]

Alternative pathway

The alternative complement pathway can be activated as a by-product of the classic pathway when the C4–C2 dimer facilitates direct binding of the activated C3 to the pathogen surface as above or when circulating C3 is spontaneously hydrolyzed and acted on by two proteins (factors B and D) to form a free C3 convertase molecule.[131] This molecule can, in turn, activate C3b to be deposited on the pathogen surface where it binds first to factor B and is then trimmed by factor D to form a surface-bound alternative C3b convertase. This molecule forms more activated molecules of C3b and can also be bound by another protein, properdin, and a second activated C3b molecule to form an alternative C5 convertase that activates the terminal components of the complement cascade.

Lectin pathway

Complement can also be deposited on the surface of pathogens displaying certain monosaccharides in a process that is initiated when these polysaccharides bind to one of two multimeric protein complexes composed of either mannose-binding lectin (MBL) or C-reactive protein (CRP).[130,133] In either case, once one of these ligands binds to a monosaccharide on the pathogen surface, proteases analogous to C1r and C1s (MASP1 and MASP2) in the classic pathway are triggered.[134] With MBL the sequence of events is the same as in the classic pathway and results in the deposition of C5 convertase on the surface of the pathogen; with CRP the classic pathway is initiated but the process stops with the formation of C3 convertase, allowing opsonization but not activation of the terminal components of the complement pathway.

Formation of the membrane attack complex

Once the complement cascade has been initiated by one of these three pathways, the process converges on cleavage of C5 into an anaphylotoxin (C5a) and C5b which is bound to the wall of the pathogen by the relevant C5 convertase complex. This process triggers a terminal sequence of binding events for C6 through C9 to form the membrane activation complex.[135] The C9 component of this complex forms

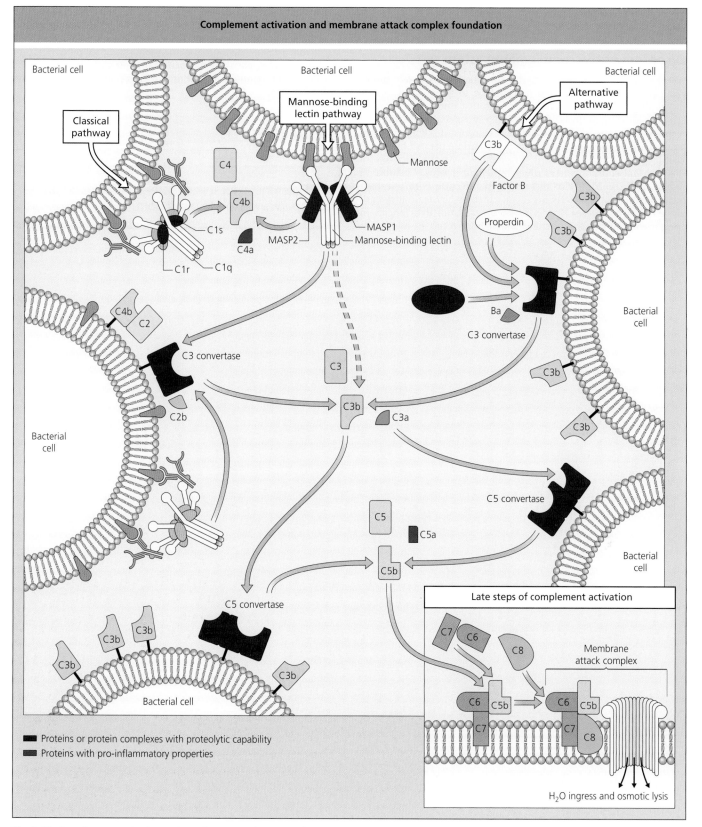

Fig. 2.11 Complement activation and membrane attack complex foundation. Adapted from Walport.[127] Copyright 2001, Massachusetts Medical Society.

a pore in the membrane of the pathogen and allows for the ingress of water, osmotic lysis and death of the target organism.[136]

Disorders of the complement system

As is evident from the above, the complement is a self-amplifying pluripotent system that has evolved to play a central role in amplifying both the innate and adaptive immune responses. From its location in the crossroads of many aspects of the immune response, aberrant or inappropriate activation of complement or an absence of any of several of its key components can have very visible clinical manifestations. Individuals with a deficiency in the terminal components of the complement pathway exhibit an increased susceptibility to disseminated infection with encapsulated organisms, especially organisms such as *Neisseria meningitidis* and *N. gonorrhoeae*.[137-139] On the other hand, deficiencies in components of the complement system that result in inefficient activation of the classic complement pathway may increase the risk for autoimmune diseases such as systemic lupus erythematosus.[140] Disorders in complement proteins responsible for regulation of C3 activation may increase the risk for membranoproliferative glomerulonephritis or paroxysmal nocturnal hemoglobinuria.[126,141] The absence of functional C1 inhibitor is associated with hereditary angioedema.[126]

REFERENCES

References for this chapter can be found online at http://www.expertconsult.com

Chapter | 3 |

John D Grabenstein
Walter L Straus
Mark B Feinberg

Vaccines and vaccination

Before vaccines were developed, children died in large numbers from diphtheria, meningitis and pertussis. From time to time, epidemics of smallpox, measles, poliomyelitis, rubella, and other contagions swept across cities and age groups. Many individuals succumbed to tetanus, hepatitis, rabies and septicemia. Fortunately, scientists and clinicians progressively developed an arsenal of vaccines, increasing both life expectancy and the quality of life. Indeed, the prospects for preventing even more diseases have brightened with the development of new vaccines to prevent severe gastroenteritis, cervical cancer and herpes zoster.

THE VALUE OF VACCINATION

The distinction between vaccines (i.e. the products) and vaccination (i.e. the act of administering vaccines) is important. Edward Jenner's recognition of the value of inoculating cowpox to prevent smallpox in 1796 was nothing less than historic. But smallpox was not contained until wide-scale vaccination programs snuffed out the ability of variola

virus to spread naturally. Indeed, the disease was eventually eradicated in the late 1970s, by means of a global vaccination program.[1,2]

In the last 50 years, vaccines have tended to be used widely more quickly after invention than in Jenner's case. The plummeting rates of *Haemophilus influenzae* type b, pneumococcal disease, meningococcal serogroup C and rotavirus gastroenteritis among children (Figs 3.1–3.4) within a few years after widespread vaccination programs began, clearly show how quickly the benefits of vaccination can be achieved.[3–5]

In notable contrast, pertussis has not yet been controlled, even though adult-formulation acellular pertussis vaccines were introduced in developed countries in recent years. Adolescents and adults provide a large reservoir for this pathogen; uptake of the new vaccines in these cohorts is still insufficient to reduce disease incidence, either among themselves or in younger contacts.[6,7]

As a matter of biologic science and medicine, vaccines are remarkable accomplishments. As a matter of social science, vaccines are similarly impressive. As the number of vaccinated people in a cohort increases, the less likely it is for a contagious person to be able to transmit that infection to others. Above a certain threshold, a condition of 'herd immunity' or 'community immunity' develops.[8–10] At that point,

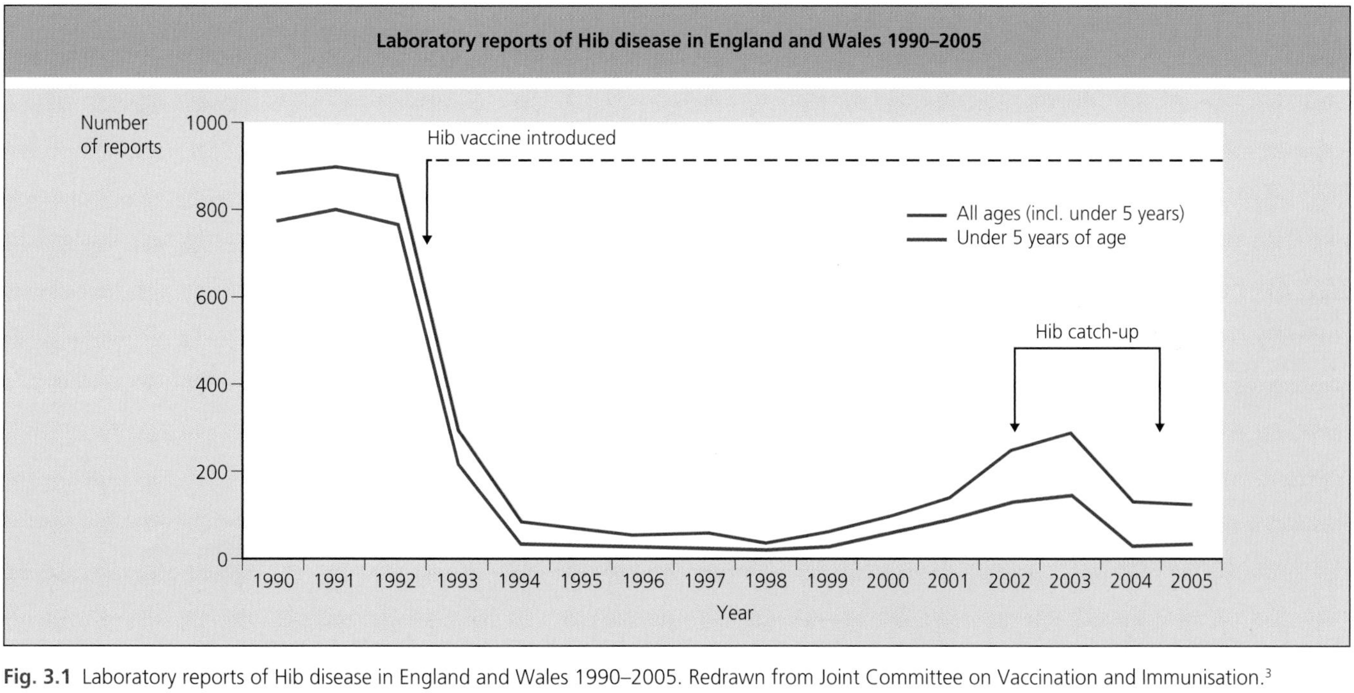

Fig. 3.1 Laboratory reports of Hib disease in England and Wales 1990–2005. Redrawn from Joint Committee on Vaccination and Immunisation.[3]

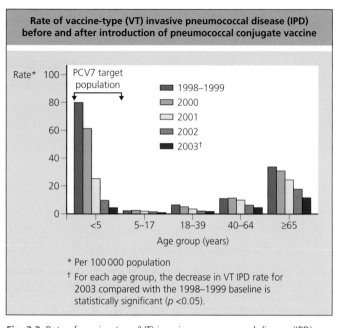

Fig. 3.2 Rate of vaccine-type (VT) invasive pneumococcal disease (IPD) before and after introduction of pneumococcal conjugate vaccine (PCV7), by age group and year. Active Bacterial Core surveillance, United States, 1998–2003. Redrawn from Centers for Disease Control and Prevention.[4]

it is difficult for a chain of transmission to sustain itself, to the advantage of the public's health. In this way, a decision to be vaccinated can offer two distinct forms of benefit:

- the vaccine recipient becomes personally immune to infection; and
- the vaccine recipient helps contribute to the community's collective immunity, making those unable to be vaccinated less vulnerable to infection.

Thus, the vaccine recipient gains personal, direct protection and altruistically helps others at the same time. The threshold to achieve herd or community immunity varies from disease to disease, based on the reproductive and infectious characteristics of the pathogen and the vaccine's efficacy and duration of protection. As two of the most contagious of the childhood diseases, measles and chickenpox require some of the highest proportions of immunity to achieve herd immunity.

In addition to their human benefits through prevention of morbidity and mortality, most vaccination programs are cost-effective. That is, most vaccines either result in net cost savings or correspond to a price per infection or death averted or a quality-adjusted life year gained that is within the range society has been willing to pay for value returned.[11–13] In developed countries, rabies vaccine may be the least cost-effective, at least in some scenarios, with a calculated cost of $2.9 million to $4 billion per life saved.[14]

In stark contrast, preventing 10 diseases among children (i.e. diphtheria, tetanus, pertussis, Hib, poliomyelitis, measles, mumps, rubella, varicella and hepatitis B) averted over 14 million cases of disease and more than 33 500 deaths over the lifetime of the immunized birth cohort of children, saving an estimated $10 billion per year.[15] If indirect economic benefits (e.g. time parents take off from work to care for sick children) are included, the annual savings to society exceed $40 billion. In a ranking of 30 preventive services based on preventable disease burden and cost-effectiveness, childhood vaccination ranked first; the value of increased use of pneumococcal vaccination among those 65 years or older was also noted.[16,17]

With high rates of childhood vaccination in most developed countries, the challenge for contemporary clinical services is to consistently and reliably extend the benefits of vaccination to adolescents and adults. Interest in preventing cervical cancer and genital warts via human papillomavirus (HPV) vaccination or meningitis provides an opportunity to protect against pertussis and other infections as well. Bundling these vaccination efforts for teenagers can provide what is known as the 'adolescent platform' for vaccination.

Efforts to deliver the annual influenza vaccine formulation to the elderly can provide a similar 'adult platform' for assessing vulnerability to pneumococcal disease and herpes zoster ('shingles' or 'zona'). Vaccination assessments before international travel provide an opportunity to assess susceptibilities to both exotic travel-related infections and ubiquitous domestic infections as well. Adults aged from their 30s to their 50s remain perhaps the group least well evaluated for vaccination adequacy, which could often benefit from periodic vaccination check-ups.

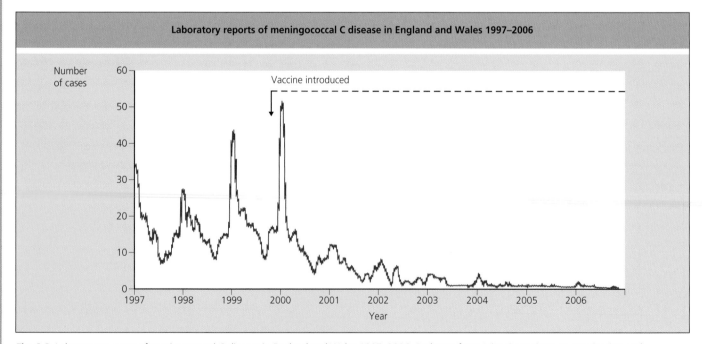

Fig. 3.3 Laboratory reports of meningococcal C disease in England and Wales 1997–2006. Redrawn from Joint Committee on Vaccination and Immunisation.[3]

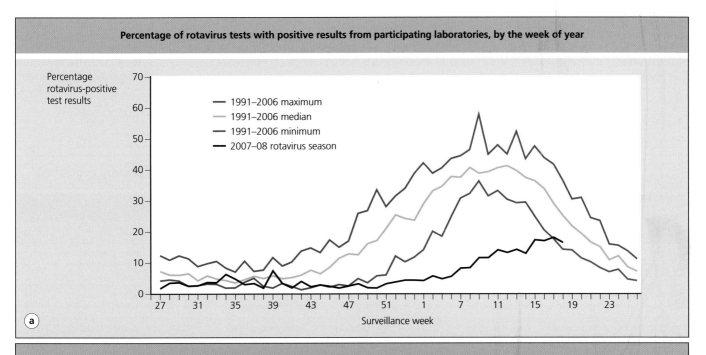

Percentage of rotavirus tests with positive results from participating laboratories, by the week of year

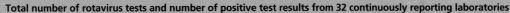

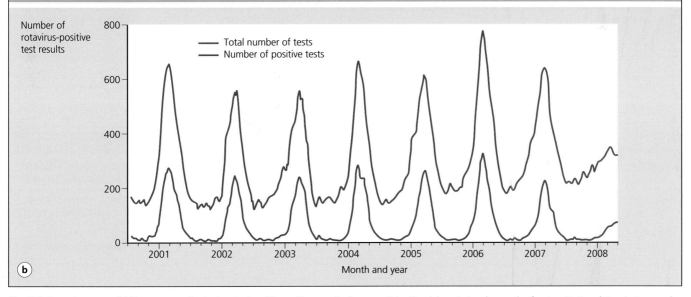

Fig. 3.4 Rotavirus tests. (a) Percentage of rotavirus tests with positive results from participating laboratories, by week of year – National Respiratory and Enteric Virus Surveillance System, United States, 1991–2006 rotavirus seasons and 2007–08 rotavirus season. (b) Total number of rotavirus tests and number of positive test results from 32 continuously reporting laboratories – National Respiratory and Enteric Virus Surveillance System, United States, July 2, 2000–May 3, 2008. Redrawn from Centers for Disease Control and Prevention.[5]

TYPES OF VACCINES, TYPES OF IMMUNITY

A vaccine is a medication used to induce active immunity. Vaccines typically consist of several ingredients, of which antigens (or immunogens) are the principal active ingredients. The specific three-dimensional sites on antigens that bind with antibodies are called epitopes. Vaccines also contain excipients, sometimes called inactive ingredients, necessary to manufacture the vaccine components, stabilize and suspend those components, preserve them against bacterial contamination, or other purposes. Some vaccines contain adjuvants (from the Latin *adjuvare*, to help) or carrier proteins to enhance the immune response to the primary antigens.[18,19]

Vaccines do not protect directly. Rather, they stimulate the immune system to develop a specific state of immunity by means of T lymphocytes, B cells (i.e. plasma cells), antibodies and immunologic mediators (e.g. interferons, interleukins). Vaccines evoke a state of 'active immunity', protection that typically lasts for years or decades. Although their protection tends to be durable, vaccines typically require a period of 10–14 days or more after each dose to elicit an enhanced state of immunity against specific pathogens or diseases.[18]

Most vaccines elicit an immune response similar to what would prevent re-infection in people who survive natural infection. Most pivotal clinical trials of new vaccines evaluate a vaccine's ability to prevent or accelerate clearance of an infection. Once a body of knowledge for a vaccine-disease relationship is established, later vaccines may be evaluated in a simpler manner by comparing antibody responses or serologic or clinical 'correlates of immunity'.

Vaccines can be divided into four major categories, quadrants based on whether the pathogen is a virus or a bacterium and whether the antigen is viable or not (Table 3.1).[18]

Most inactivated whole-microbe vaccines, toxoids and subunit vaccines evoke relatively simple antibody responses, with meager CD8 T-cell responses. In such cases, the humoral (i.e. antibody) response is likely the principal or only protective mechanism. An antibody that neutralizes a circulating toxin is the paragon of this type of vaccine-induced benefit.

Table 3.1 Diseases that can be prevented with vaccines licensed in Europe or the USA, categorized by microbial type and antigenic type*

		'INACTIVATED' VACCINES			
	Live vaccines	**Whole microbe**	**Subunit**	**Other**	**Typical primary populations**
Bacterial diseases					
Anthrax			Cell filtrate		Occupational
Cholera	Live (oral)	Whole			Endemic areas, travelers
Diphtheria				Toxoid	Throughout life
Haemophilus influenzae type b				Protein-conjugated polysaccharide	Infants, children
Meningococcal, some or all of serogroups A, C, Y, and W135			Polysaccharide, polyvalent	Protein-conjugated polysaccharide, polyvalent	Varies by country; children, adolescents, travelers
Pertussis			Multiple acellular components		Throughout life
Pneumococcal			Polysaccharide, polyvalent	Protein-conjugated polysaccharide, polyvalent	Infants, children, elderly, plus underlying chronic diseases
Tetanus				Toxoid	Throughout life
Typhoid	Live (oral)		Vi polysaccharide		Endemic areas, travelers
Tuberculosis (BCG)	Live				Varies by country; children, selected other groups
Viral diseases					
Hepatitis A		Whole			Varies by country; infants, children, adolescents, occupational, travelers
Hepatitis B			Surface antigen		Varies by country; infants, children, adolescents, occupational, travelers
Influenza A and B			Split virus		Elderly, plus other groups, such as children, adolescents, occupational
Japanese encephalitis		Whole			Endemic areas, travelers
Measles	Whole				Infants, children
Mumps	Whole				Infants, children
Papillomavirus, types 6, 11, 16, 18			Virus-like particles		Adolescents, adults
Poliovirus	Whole	Whole			Infants, children
Rabies		Whole			Occupational, postexposure
Rotavirus (mono- or pentavalent)	Whole				Infants
Rubella	Whole				Infants, children
Tick-borne encephalitis		Whole			
Vaccinia (to prevent smallpox)	Whole				Occupational
Varicella	Whole				Infants, children
Yellow fever	Whole				Endemic areas, travelers
Zoster	Whole				Elderly

*Multiple entries within a row indicate availability of more than one type of vaccine for that disease.

In contrast, live-microbe vaccines can induce both humoral and cellular (i.e. specialized lymphocyte) immune responses against the pathogen; however, in most such cases, the actual mechanisms of protection elicited by either natural infection or vaccination are not understood in detail.

In the course of investigating diphtheria and tetanus in 1890, Emil Behring and Shibasaburo Kitasato identified protective substances that they could transfer from one animal to another.[1] These substances were eventually recognized to be IgG antibodies, found in human serum as well as in other animals. Because these antibodies neutralize toxins, they warrant designation as antitoxins or antisera. These pathogen-specific antibodies offer the ability to provide 'passive immunity', the donation of one person's immunity to another person. Such a benefit provides prompt protection. Unfortunately, the protection from these antibodies is relatively short-lived, generally measured in weeks.

In many cases (e.g. diphtheria, tetanus) the quantity of circulating antibody and memory B cells present at the time of infection is very important in predicting protection. In other cases, such as the relatively long incubation period with hepatitis B infection, people who achieve a sufficient level of antibody response, even if their antibody concentration later falls below detectable limits, may remain protected from infection. This strongly indicates a cellular component to their immunity. While some may believe simplistically that vaccines induce 'sterilizing immunity' (i.e. blocking the pathogen from infecting even one cell), this is clearly not the case with several vaccines (e.g. poliovirus, rotavirus, pertussis).

SPECIFIC VACCINE ADVANCES

In 1885, a few years before Behring's achievement, Louis Pasteur did not understand he was attenuating the rabies virus as he dried rabbit tissue and transformed it into the material for a set of vaccinations of increasing potency. But his novel approach was dramatically successful. Although neither Jenner nor Pasteur understood viruses as we understand them today, their preparations contained whole, viable viruses.[1]

Antibodies developed by Behring and his contemporaries (e.g. Paul Ehrlich) relieved suffering and helped reduce case-fatality ratios. But the immunity induced was too short to much affect community transmission of infections. So Gaston Ramon and Alexander Glenny separately developed modified bacterial toxins ('toxoids') in the 1920s that induced active immunization against diphtheria and tetanus.[1]

A few years later, Ramon, Glenny and their respective teams added a variety of compounds to these toxoids, searching for combinations that would make immune responses to vaccination stronger and more durable. Eventually, these researchers focused on aluminum salts, still the most common adjuvant used worldwide. Their adjuvanted products of the 1920s worked quite well. But, as with smallpox vaccine, it was only with vaccination of large segments of populations in the 1950s that diphtheria and tetanus came under control in developed countries.[1] It would take several decades longer for the Expanded Programme on Vaccination to make prevention of diphtheria, tetanus and several other common infections commonplace in developing countries.[20,21]

In this era, most bacteria (unlike viruses) were readily visible via microscopes and thus the main topics of vaccine development. Vaccine researchers like Waldemar Haffkine, Almroth Wright, Wilhelm Kolle and Richard Pfeiffer and their colleagues, between 1890 and 1910, developed the first bacterial vaccines by cultivating the microbes (e.g. those causing plague, cholera, typhoid), inactivating the bacteria with chemicals and/or heat, and then formulating these products into vaccines for administration.[1] These products contained whole bacteria.

Gradually, through the 20th century, additional whole-microbe vaccines were developed and introduced into clinical practice. But slowly subunit vaccines came into being, as Michael Heidelberger and

Oswald Avery identified the capsular antigens of pneumococcal bacteria in the 1920s. Colin MacLeod showed the ability of pneumococcal polysaccharide vaccines to protect against pneumococcal diseases in the 1940s.[1]

Malcolm Artenstein, Irving Goldschneider and Emil Gotschlich developed analogous meningococcal polysaccharide vaccines in the 1960s. Then David Smith and Porter Anderson, Jr, developed the first *Haemophilus influenzae* type b (Hib) polysaccharide vaccine in 1973, subsequently licensed in 1985.[18,22,23]

Unfortunately, polysaccharides do not elicit much of an immune response in young children. John Robbins and Rachel Schneerson solved this problem by developing the technique for conjugating polysaccharides to protein carriers in 1980. This technology was applied first to Hib, then pneumococcal, and finally meningococcal vaccines in succeeding decades.[18,24]

Although whole-cell vaccines were the norm among bacterial vaccines through most of the 20th century, inactivated whole-cell vaccines were entirely replaced by subunit vaccines by 2000 in the USA, and now largely replaced in most developed countries.[18] This transition resulted in fewer injection-site reactions than whole-cell vaccination and more specific immune responses. Whole-inactivated and subunit bacterial vaccines are typically administered with an adjuvant (e.g. an aluminum salt) to enhance a typically modest immunogenicity, relative to live vaccines.

Sometimes research teams approached the goal of vaccine development from very different angles. Perhaps the best-known example was Jonas Salk's injectable, inactivated poliovirus vaccine, developed in 1954, and Albert Sabin's oral, attenuated poliovirus vaccine, developed around 1960.[1,18]

One of the major advances in vaccinology was the discovery by John Enders and his team of how to grow viruses in cell culture in 1954.[1] This breakthrough enabled vaccines against measles, mumps, rubella, varicella and other viruses in the decades that followed. Indeed, most live vaccines in use today were derived by serially propagating initially pathogenic organisms in nonhuman cell culture or at nonphysiologic temperatures for prolonged periods. These conditions allowed evolutionary selection for variants that grow poorly in humans and do not cause clinical symptoms.

Effective vaccines must strike a balance between degree of attenuation and degree of immunogenicity. Modern live vaccines tend to be highly efficacious, with prolonged duration of efficacy. Such vaccines reflect an ability to replicate within vaccinees and expose the immune system to antigens in a manner resembling the nature, anatomic location and effects of natural infection. Because live attenuated vaccines replicate within the vaccinee, they can induce cellular (e.g. CD4, CD8), humoral (B cell) and innate responses and immunologic memory.

In the case of hepatitis B vaccine, the initial vaccines were developed by Maurice Hilleman, Philippe Maupas, and their teams in the mid-1970s.[25,26] These vaccines contained hepatitis B surface antigen (HBsAg) harvested from the serum of chronic carriers. The next step was to harness recombinant DNA technology in the 1980s to develop yeast cells that expressed the same single protein, HBsAg. Such technology is now used to manufacture other vaccines (e.g. human papillomavirus, HPV). HPV vaccines are notable because they consist of virus-like particles (VLPs) that are polymeric spheres built of multiple copies of a single protein.[18]

Most of today's live vaccines are viral vaccines. But there are several remarkable exceptions involving bacteria. In 1921, Albert Calmette and Camille Guérin developed a tuberculosis vaccine, whose common name evokes their memory: bacille Calmette-Guérin (BCG). More recently, live oral vaccines to prevent typhoid or cholera have been licensed (or registered) in various countries.[1,18]

Before closing this section, it is important to note that a vaccination involves far more than the antigen(s) that comprise the active ingredient(s) of a vaccine. The vaccination of one person is the sum of the effects achieved by the antigens, the other components of the vaccine formulation (e.g. adjuvant, carrier proteins), the route of administration, and the number and timing of the vaccine doses. Even then, the product administered is affected by the recipient's genetic characteristics (e.g. major histocompatibility complex polymorphisms) and physiologic condition (e.g. age, nutrition, gender, stress, immune competence). The net effect of all these parameters determines the degree to which a vaccine confers or evokes immunity in that one person. And, as mentioned above, the real societal benefits come when effective vaccines are used on a broad scale.

Considerations in vaccine use

In contrast to drugs, which are typically prescribed to patients to treat existing diseases, vaccines are generally administered to healthy persons with the objective of preventing disease. With the notable exception of communicable diseases, drugs confer benefit only to the patient who is treated. Vaccines benefit both the vaccine recipient as well as society, and are considered one of the major public health resources to improve the health of the general population. These attributes account for several distinct features in vaccine prescribing by health-care practitioners.

While clinical guidelines are relatively recent as a tool in therapeutics, and represent discretionary suggestions, clinical guidelines have long been integral to vaccine use. Examples of common policies for smallpox and diphtheria vaccines date to the early 20th century, although nationwide policies on vaccine use more commonly arose with the introduction of poliovirus and measles vaccines in the 1950s and 1960s.

Typically, vaccine use is guided by recommendations issued by professional bodies or government agencies, which are often coordinated on a national level (Table 3.2). One of the oldest is the Advisory Committee on Immunization Practices (ACIP), which advises the US Centers for Disease Control and Prevention (CDC). Its working structure is analogous to many similar groups around the globe. ACIP interdisciplinary work groups, consisting of technical and program experts drawn from academia, government and professional associations, evaluate the potential population-based value of new vaccines. Their review incorporates evidence derived from preclinical and clinical safety and efficacy data, as well as public health considerations (e.g. disease burden, populations at risk, ease of integration of the vaccine into the health-care system) and a formal health economic analysis. Although ACIP recommendations are nonbinding, they are considered critical peer-reviewed information for professional associations and individual clinicians, as well as governmental and private payers.[27]

ACIP recommendations are summarized in immunization schedules published periodically in the *Morbidity and Mortality Weekly Report* (http://www.cdc.gov/mmwr). The ACIP monitors licensed vaccines throughout their period of availability, which may last for multiple decades, and periodically revises its recommendations as additional information (e.g. safety data, clinical efficacy in populations not studied at licensure, duration of protection) becomes available.

The approach to developing vaccine recommendations in the European Union (EU) is somewhat more complicated, because of the multiple sovereign countries involved. While efforts are underway to coordinate vaccine registration or licensure, there are to date no European regulations to harmonize vaccine policy making. At present, vaccines are evaluated for registration through a centralized procedure by the European Medicines Evaluation Agency (EMEA) and its Committee for Medicinal Products for Human Use (CHMP). Vaccines are reviewed by a country representing the EU as a whole, and ultimately registered through a mutual recognition procedure based upon endorsement by concerned member states, or (occasionally) by individual countries. In contrast, for vaccine policy making, each member country retains its own national advisory committee with responsibility for national recommendations. As a result, there is significant heterogeneity in vaccine recommendations in the EU.[28] With the continuing integration of the EU and increasing ease of travel among populations, the differences in vaccine schedules may create complexity

Table 3.2 Selected national or multinational vaccine policy bodies

Australia	Australian Technical Advisory Group on Immunisation (ATAGI)
Canada	National Advisory Committee on Immunization (NACI); Canadian Immunization Committee (CIC)
European Union	European Technical Advisory Committee of Experts (ETAGE)
France	Conseil supérieur d'hygène publique de France (CSHPF); Comité technique des vaccinations (CTV); Institute de Veille Sanitaire (InVS)
Germany	Ständige Impfkommission (STIKO, Standing Advisory Committee on Vaccinations)
Ireland, Republic of	National Immunisation Advisory Committee (NIAC) of the Royal College of Physicians of Ireland
Korea, Republic of	Korea Advisory Committee on Immunization Practice (KACIP)
Mexico	Consejo Nacional de Vacunación (CONAVA)
Netherlands	National Vaccine Institute (NVI); National Institute for Public Health and the Environment (RNVI)
New Zealand	Immunisation Technical Working Group (ITWG)
Poland	Sera-Vaccine Evaluation Committee
Switzerland	Eidgenössische Kommission für Impffragen (also called Commission fédèrale pour les vaccinations, Commissione federale per le vaccinazioni)
Taiwan	Taiwan Advisory Committee for Immunization Practice (ACIP)
United Kingdom	Joint Committee on Vaccination and Immunisation (JCVI)
United States	Advisory Committee on Immunization Practices (ACIP)
World Health Organization	Strategic Advisory Group of Experts (SAGE)

for practitioners (e.g. providing for infants of immigrants immunized under varying standards) as well as for public health officials. An example of this latter difficulty includes providing for people freely traveling from countries with low hepatitis B endemicity (where hepatitis B vaccination may not be included in the national guidelines) to countries with high hepatitis B endemnicity.

Many developing and mid-income countries lack the regulatory infrastructure and technical expertise to conduct their own formal review of new vaccines. These countries may rely upon assessments made by the World Health Organization (WHO) through its prequalification procedure.[29] The prequalification procedure assesses a candidate vaccine, according to prespecified criteria of quality, safety and efficacy of vaccines, and is often used as a criterion by third-party organizations (e.g. UNICEF) that endorse (and may purchase) vaccines for developing countries. Manufacturers may request review of a vaccine, which involves not only review of safety and efficacy data, but also an inspection by WHO officials of the manufacturing facilities. In addition to the preceding efforts related to product quality, the WHO Strategic Advisory Group of Experts (SAGE) provides vaccine-use recommendations analogous to that of national bodies (see Table 3.2).

Recently, the EMEA recognized an unmet need to evaluate vaccines intended for endemic diseases of the developing world and which may never be licensed (registered) in the EU. A new approach has been introduced, which provides an expert assessment (in contrast to a licensure evaluation) of such vaccines (as well as therapeutic products).[30]

VACCINE SCHEDULES

Vaccination is a cornerstone of care of infants and small children, and is carefully integrated into routine pediatric care. With the introduction of an increasing number of vaccines (usually administered by injection), manufacturers and public health authorities continue to try to simplify the approach to childhood vaccination. The primary approaches involve combination vaccines (i.e. a single dosage form containing components targeted against more than one disease) as well as through administration of multiple vaccines during a minimal number of visits (consistent with safety and efficacy evidence).

To assure safety and efficacy, vaccines are evaluated when given in combination. The timing of pediatric, adolescent and adult vaccinations is typically summarized in composite vaccine schedules, such as those published by the ACIP (Figs 3.5–3.7).[31,32] With the recent introduction of new vaccines (e.g. human papillomavirus, meningococcal conjugate vaccines) and revised recommendations for longstanding vaccines (e.g. pertussis), there is a growing need for a practical approach to vaccinate adolescents and young adults. Because this population receives less routine scheduled clinical care than infants and young children, new approaches are needed to ensure adequate vaccination. This is also true for older adults, for whom coverage with existing vaccines (e.g. influenza, pneumococcal) has long lagged behind that of pediatric coverage with their respective recommended vaccines. Integration of regular reviews of the immune status of adolescents and adults is essential to avoid vaccine-preventable diseases in these cohorts. A variety of approaches are being tested in various countries to enhance vaccination of adolescents and adults. These include alternate delivery sites (e.g. schools, workplaces, pharmacies), more assertive marketing or outreach campaigns, use of standing orders to empower nurses and pharmacists to attend to needed vaccination, and use of electronic health records to help identify those unvaccinated.

Vaccine safety

Because vaccines are usually administered to healthy individuals to prevent disease, both public health authorities and vaccine manufacturers take extraordinary efforts to ensure safety in the development, manufacture and use of vaccines. Because many vaccines include components derived from biologically active material (e.g. pneumococcal vaccine antigens consist of capsular polysaccharides harvested from bacterial culture), there is a necessary emphasis on assuring that vaccines are manufactured in a consistent and defined manner to promote patient safety. Failure to do so could result in tragedy that compromises both patient health and confidence in public health policies.

This situation was exemplified in the so-called Cutter incident of 1955, in which several lots of inactivated poliovirus vaccine (IPV) were inadequately treated, resulting in poliomyelitis in 79 vaccine recipients, as well as 125 family and community contacts.[33,34] Regulators responded to the incident with more intensive requirements for quality control. In following decades, these quality requirements have become more intricate and specific.

Vaccine development follows a parallel pathway to that used for pharmaceutical products. While the details vary for individual vaccines, in general, preclinical research is followed by three phases of human clinical trials. Phase I studies involve safety, immunogenicity and dose ranging in a few dozen healthy volunteers. Phase II studies add safety and immunogenicity information from a few hundred people with the demographic characteristics expected of those intended to receive the final vaccine, as well as an initial assessment of efficacy. Phase III studies are the large-scale efficacy and safety studies in several thousand people that form the pivotal basis for licensure (registration).[18]

Vaccine registration is like that of chemically defined pharmaceuticals in that preclinical and clinical data are submitted to regulators, but the detailed technical specifications describing the process of vaccine manufacture are more extensive than that of pharmaceuticals. To limit the possibility of contamination, vaccine facilities are typically constructed as dedicated plants designated to manufacture a specific vaccine. Following licensure, vaccine manufacture continues to be actively monitored: a sample of each manufactured vaccine lot is

Recommended immunization schedule for persons aged 0–6 years											
Age Vaccine	Birth	1 month	2 months	4 months	6 months	12 months	15 months	18 months	19–23 months	2–3 years	4–6 years
Hepatitis B[1]	HepB	HepB		see footnote 1	HepB						
Rotavirus[2]			RV	RV	*RV*[3]						
Diphtheria, tetanus, pertussis[3]			DTaP	DTaP	DTaP	see footnote 3	DTaP				DTaP
Haemophilus influenzae type b[4]			Hib	Hib	*Hib*[4]	Hib					
Pneumococcal[5]			PCV	PCV	PCV	PCV				PPSV	
Inactivated poliovirus			IPV	IPV		IPV					IPV
Influenza[6]						Influenza (yearly)					
Measles, mumps, rubella[7]						MMR		see footnote 7			MMR
Varicella[8]						Varicella		see footnote 8			Varicella
Hepatitis A[9]						HepA (2 doses)				HepA Series	
Meningococcal[10]										MCV	

Range of recommended ages

Certain high-risk groups

Fig. 3.5 Recommended immunization schedule for persons aged 0–6 years – United States, 2009. Redrawn from Advisory Committee on Immunization Practices.[31] (See reference for detailed footnotes and ancillary information.)

Recommended immunization schedule for persons aged 7–18 years

Vaccine \ Age	7–10 years	11–12 years	13–18 years
Tetanus, diphtheria, pertussis[1]	see footnote 1	Tdap	HepB
Human papillomavirus[2]	see footnote 2	HPV (3 doses)	HPV Series
Meningococcal[3]	MCV	MCV	MCV
Influenza[4]	Influenza (yearly)		
Pneumococcal[5]	PPSV		
Hepatitis A[6]	HepA Series		
Hepatitis A[7]	HepB Series		
Inactivated poliovirus[8]	IPV Series		
Measles, mumps, rubella[9]	MMR Series		
Varicella[10]	Varicella Series		

Range of recommended ages

Catch-up immunization

Certain high-risk groups

Fig. 3.6 Recommended immunization schedule for persons 7–18 years – United States, 2009. Redrawn from Advisory Committee on Immunization Practices.[31] (See reference for detailed footnotes and ancillary information.)

Recommended immunization schedule for adults

Vaccine \ Age	19–26 years	27–49 years	50–59 years	60–64 years	≥65–59 years
Tetanus, diphtheria, pertussis (Td/Tdap)[1,*]	Substitute 1-time dose of Tdap for Td booster; then boost with Td every 10 years				Td booster every 10 years
Human papillomavirus (HPV)[2,*]	3 doses (females)				
Varicella[3,*]	2 doses				
Zoster[4]				1 dose	
Measles, mumps, rubella (MMR)[5,*]	1 or 2 doses		1 dose		
Influenza[6,*]	1 dose annually				
Pneumococcal (polysaccharide)[7,8]	1 or 2 doses				1 dose
Hepatitis A[9,*]	2 doses				
Hepatitis B[10,*]	3 doses				
Meningococcal[11,*]	1 or more doses				

For all persons in this category who meet the age requirements and who lack evidence of immunity (e.g. lack documentation of vaccination or have no evidence of prior infection)

Recommended if some other risk factor is present (e.g. on the basis of medical, occupational, lifestyle or other indications)

No recommendation

Fig. 3.7 Recommended immunization schedule for adults – United States, 2009. Redrawn from Advisory Committee on Immunization Practices.[32] (See reference for detailed footnotes and ancillary information.)

typically provided to the US Food and Drug Administration (FDA) for review. Any change in protocol/manufacture requires formal regulatory review.

Licensed (registered) vaccines undergo extensive safety testing, which may include clinical trials enrolling tens of thousands of individuals. But clinical trials can never be statistically powered to reliably identify extremely rare adverse events. Several post-licensure measures exist to ensure that adverse events associated with vaccine use are identified promptly and completely. Manufacturers are required to promptly communicate to regulators those adverse events reported by providers and consumers, as well those identified in post-marketing studies, along with relevant publications.

In the USA, a spontaneous vaccine adverse event reporting system (VAERS, http://www.vaers.hhs.gov) is administered jointly by the FDA and the CDC. The corresponding system in Canada is called the Canadian Adverse Events Following Immunization Surveillance System (CAEFISS). These surveillance systems and their counterparts worldwide collect vaccine safety information from consumers, providers and manufacturers.

Passive surveillance systems can identify extremely rare events after vaccination (e.g. Guillain-Barré syndrome) and are most appropriately considered a mechanism for signal detection. These systems do not collect information on overall vaccine use and cannot provide quantitative estimates of risk (i.e. strength of association) or of incidence.

Once a potential safety signal is identified, formal epidemiologic studies may be employed to assess strength of association. One mechanism for this type of research is the Vaccine Safety Datalink (VSD) coordinated by the CDC. A network of US managed-care organizations conduct controlled epidemiologic studies to evaluate safety signals. The RotaShield (quadrivalent rhesus-human reassortant rotavirus vaccine) experience provides an example of the manner in which these safety systems operate in a complementary manner. During clinical trials of this vaccine designed to prevent pediatric rotavirus infection, a small but not statistically significant number of cases of intussusception was noted, but considered to occur at background rate. This potential safety concern was noted in the ACIP recommendation. Some months following introduction of RotaShield, the VAERS system became concerned that the number of cases of intussusception occurring in vaccine recipients was larger than expected by background rates and that vaccine use should be temporarily suspended. Several CDC epidemiologic studies then quantified the risk of intussusception in vaccinees, and concluded that it exceeded the expected rate. RotaShield was withdrawn from the market.[35-37] Subsequent rotavirus vaccines were subjected to larger safety studies with special focus on intussusception before they were licensed, with additional post-licensure studies after registration.

Vaccine use in special populations

Pregnancy

Most clinical studies leading to vaccine licensure do not routinely enroll pregnant women; indeed, pregnancy is a common exclusion criterion. As a result, information on vaccine safety in pregnant women is commonly based upon empiric evidence derived from other sources:

- women enrolled in vaccine trials who inadvertently become pregnant during the course of study;
- data made available through passive reporting systems (e.g. VAERS); and
- specific registries (often sponsored by vaccine manufacturers) that collect data prospectively on women seen in clinical practice who happen to become vaccinated while pregnant.[38-41]

Due to concerns regarding teratogenicity, live viral vaccines (e.g. rubella, vaccinia, varicella) are typically contraindicated during pregnancy. There is no convincing evidence of harm resulting from vaccinating pregnant women with inactivated viral or bacterial vaccines, or with toxoids. The risk of hospitalization due to influenza infection is elevated in pregnancy; thus, women pregnant during the influenza

season are recommended for vaccination with inactivated influenza vaccine.[42,43] Because neonatal tetanus is associated with severe infant outcomes, and maternal antibodies to tetanus have been shown to be protective in infants, incompletely vaccinated pregnant women are also recommended for tetanus toxoid vaccination.

Vaccines for international travel

The increasingly globalized society is associated with unprecedented international travel, traveling far from their places of residence, and risking exposure to diseases that are either well controlled or not found in their homeland. In addition, travelers may import infectious diseases back to their homeland. The key principles of vaccination for travel are to ensure that patients are up to date on their routine ('domestic') vaccinations (e.g. tetanus, measles, influenza, and to provide vaccinations against vaccine-preventable diseases in those countries that they will visit. Several websites summarize vaccination recommendations by country (http://www.cdc.gov/travel; http://www.who.int/ith/en). While the decision regarding appropriate vaccination fundamentally belongs to patients and providers, certain vaccines may be required to enter specific countries (e.g. yellow fever) under international health regulations. Evidence of vaccination is provided in standard travel documents recognized by the WHO (International Certificate of Vaccination, http://www.who.int/csr/ihr/icvp/en/print.html).

Immunocompromised populations (see also Chapter 83)

Immunocompromised patients are at increased susceptibility to infection, may not respond to vaccination with adequate immunogenicity, and could face added risk of adverse events after live vaccinations. Increased risk for infection is a sine qua non for immunosuppression. Vaccine recommendations in these populations balance the estimated risk for specific vaccine-preventable infections against known (based usually on empiric data) safety and efficacy information. In general, individuals who will, through medical intervention (e.g. autologous bone marrow transplantation), become immune suppressed, are vaccinated in a timely manner to optimize their vaccine immune response in advance of the period of immune suppression. Live (self-replicating) vaccines may pose a safety concern and are not generally administered to immune-suppressed persons. Killed (or subunit) vaccines are considered safer than live vaccines for these cohorts. Hepatitis B vaccine is of particular interest due to the concern of the risk of infection in a seronegative patient recipient of hepatitis B virus transmitted by solid organ transplant or by transfusion. These patients should be vaccinated well before transplantation to allow induction of immunity. HIV infection is associated with progressive immunodeficiency; recommendations for vaccination are based upon the stage of disease (and by patient age). The reader is referred to specialized texts for detailed information on vaccination in this population.[44-55]

FUTURE PROSPECTS FOR VACCINES

While vaccines provide some of the greatest contributions to improving the health of individuals and populations, tremendous unmet public health opportunities remain. These include both the development of new vaccines for infectious diseases that cannot yet be prevented effectively and programs to meet the needs of cohorts who do not have reliable access to existing vaccines.

Not only will the future bring vaccines to prevent currently uncontrolled diseases, it will likely harness new technologies to do so. Promising new advances may allow DNA or viral-vector vaccines to take their places on shelves next to vaccines consisting of whole microbes, subunits and toxoids. DNA vaccination is accomplished by injecting genetically engineered DNA (in the form of circular plasmids) into the body, where the gene expresses the corresponding immunogenic protein. With viral-vectored vaccines, a suitable virus (e.g. vaccinia, one of the adenoviruses) is genetically engineered to convey genetic material into cells, where it can be expressed. With each of these approaches, intracellular expression can elicit T-cell immunity. Practical challenges to overcome include induction of sufficient immune responses to confer immunity, overcoming pre-existing immunity to the viral vector, and questions about product safety. These approaches are also limited to protein epitopes.

Several resources track the development of new vaccines targeted against outstanding infectious diseases.

The US National Institute of Allergy and Infectious Diseases (http://www3.niaid.nih.gov) publishes *The Jordan Report: Accelerated Development of Vaccines*, to periodically summarize global vaccine development.[56] First issued in 1982, the 2007 edition complements a review of investigational vaccines with a discussion of programmatic issues in vaccine implementation (e.g. development of an approach to vaccinate adolescents).

The World Health Organization also provides a periodic update on the status of vaccines in development, along with its assessment of the outstanding public health need for those vaccines.[57] The American Society for Microbiology does likewise.[58]

In 2000, the Institute of Medicine (IOM, a component of the US National Academy of Sciences) issued a report entitled *Vaccines for the 21st Century: A Tool for Decision Making*.[59] This publication focused upon US public health needs and prioritized 26 candidate vaccine targets (ranked by levels; level I refers to those considered most attractive) based on their public health relevance and the estimated likelihood that they might be licensed within 20 years. In addition, the reviewers included vaccine program implementation considerations, along with a health economic assessment, in their recommendations (Table 3.3).

Notably, the IOM panel did not consider HIV/AIDS, for which a preventive vaccine would be of extraordinary public health value. Efforts to develop a successful HIV vaccine have bedeviled researchers for almost 20 years.[60] The recent failure of an adenovirus vector-based HIV-1 vaccine intended to induce a cell-mediated immunity response, speaks to the scientific uncertainty and technical complexity of successful vaccine development against this pathogen.[61–63] Decisions to develop vaccines are sometimes subject to pressures outside of those considered by expert panels (or by market forces), including specific ethical, legal and regulatory hurdles.[64]

The IOM report also included proposed vaccines for conditions not generally considered infectious (e.g. multiple myeloma), highlighting expectations that future vaccines will expand their scope beyond the traditional limits of infectious diseases. It is worth noting that some current vaccines have public health value beyond the prevention of an infection. Two widely used licensed vaccines help prevent cancer: the hepatitis B vaccines (i.e. to prevent hepatocellular carcinoma) and human papillomavirus vaccines (i.e. to prevent cervical, vaginal and other cancers). Widespread use of hepatitis B vaccine has been associated with a decline in liver cancer deaths.[65,66] In the controlled trials supporting licensure, one of the recently introduced human papillomavirus vaccines has already demonstrated a decrease in the incidence of cervical cancer precursor lesions;[67] however, the long natural history of HPV infection leading to cervical cancer makes it likely that some additional time will be needed for population-based declines in cervical cancer in vaccinated populations to become apparent. Research is underway with therapeutic cancer vaccines, and the reader is referred to specialized texts for additional information.[68]

One of the great and unfortunate paradoxes in public health is that many vaccines have not been readily available or routinely utilized by populations who bear the greatest burden of a disease. While widespread adoption of newly recommended vaccines in industrialized countries usually occurs within a few years, there has historically been a delay in common use in developing countries where vaccine-preventable diseases are often endemic, and where access to therapeutic care is typically hindered by lack of medical resources.

Hepatitis B virus vaccines and *Haemophilus influenzae* type b vaccines, each of which targets important pathogens common in the developing world, only began to be widely introduced there 10–15 years after their licensure in the USA.[69] However, it is possible that global access to new vaccines is beginning to improve.

In affluent countries, rotavirus infection is almost universal, yet mortality is rare.[70,71] In contrast, the WHO estimates that more than 500 000 children die annually due to this infection, with a majority of the deaths concentrated in South and South East Asia.[72] The rotavirus vaccine licensed in the USA in 2006 was associated with a decline in domestic rotavirus cases within just 2 years of widespread use[5] (see Fig. 3.4). Although rotavirus vaccines are not yet widely used in developing countries, clinical trials are presently underway in some developing countries with a high rotavirus burden of illness, and efforts are in place to provide funding and access to this vaccine in a timely fashion.

These programs include networks of organizations, institutions and companies working in vaccine development and use, such as the Global Alliance for Vaccines and Immunization (GAVI), large private foundation contributions (e.g. Bill and Melinda Gates Foundation) and government-supported 'push' mechanisms to encourage development of vaccines specifically for developing world use (e.g. advance market commitments).[73] Initiatives such as these are considered critical to overcome the significant costs (vaccine purchase, delivery and surveillance) that have so far impeded the use of vaccines to reduce the enormous burden of vaccine-preventable diseases in the developing world.[74,75]

Beyond issues of immunology and vaccine technology, those interested in preventing disease through vaccination will need to address society's needs for thorough safety evaluation. The last 20 years have witnessed several concerns about vaccine safety become widely debated (e.g. autism, diabetes, sudden infant death syndrome). Those questions have been answered through epidemiologic and other studies, which

Table 3.3 Priorities for vaccine development, US Institute of Medicine[59]

Level I (highest priority)	Level II	Level III	Level IV
Cytomegalovirus (CMV)	*Chlamydia, Helicobacter pylori*	Parainfluenza	*Borrelia burgdorferi*
Influenza	Hepatitis C virus	Rotavirus	*Coccidioides immitis*
Insulin-dependent diabetes mellitus*	Herpes simplex virus	Group A streptococcus	Enterotoxigenic
Multiple sclerosis*	Human papillomavirus	Group B streptococcus	*Escherichia coli*
Rheumatoid arthritis*	Melanoma*		Epstein–Barr virus
Group B streptococcus	*Mycobacterium tuberculosis*		*Histoplasma capsulatum*
Streptococcus pneumoniae	*Neisseria gonorrhoeae*		*Neisseria meningitidis* type b
Diabetes mellitus	Respiratory syncytial virus		Shigella

Note: HIV/AIDS was omitted from consideration.
*Not usually considered infectious in origin.

now provide a substantial body of scientific evidence. With the success of vaccines in making so many now-preventable diseases recede from public attention, specific efforts are needed to explain what vaccines have accomplished and why continued vaccination is needed to keep these diseases suppressed. Vaccines have improved many millions of lives around the world. Expanded use of existing vaccines and development of new vaccines are likely to add substantially to this remarkable record of achievement.

REFERENCES

References for this chapter can be found online at http://www.expertconsult.com

Chapter | **4** |

Alexandra M Levitt
Ali S Khan
James M Hughes

Emerging and re-emerging pathogens and diseases

INTRODUCTION

Humans and microbes have engaged in an epic struggle for survival since human life began. Rapid microbial evolution and adaptation allow bacteria, viruses and parasites to overcome human defenses (e.g. physiologic mechanisms and manmade drugs) and exploit human behaviors (e.g. sexual practices and methods of food production and preparation). Some zoonotic microbes have 'jumped' from animals to humans to become major human pathogens. The ancestors of smallpox virus and malaria parasites, for example, probably became human pathogens 10 000 years ago when humans began to domesticate animals in settlements that were large enough to sustain human-to-human transmission. In recent times the AIDS virus, one of the most destructive pathogens in human history, evolved from a virus carried by a nonhuman primate.[1]

Human evolution, though far slower and more difficult to observe, has in turn been influenced by microbes. Some pathogens have apparently been sufficiently virulent and widespread over the course of human history to affect the make-up of the human genome. The best evidence for this concerns malaria parasites, which are less likely to kill individuals who have globin gene alleles that make their red blood cells poor hosts for intracellular parasites (e.g. sickle hemoglobin and α- and β-thalassemias).[2] Moreover, most or all components of the human immune system probably evolved to prevent disease agents from co-opting human cellular machinery for microbial gene expression and reproduction. In addition, the human body benefits from the presence of nonpathogenic, symbiotic microbes, such as bacteria in the human gut that synthesize components of the vitamin B complex (folic acid and biotin).

Today, the increasing complexity of human behavior coupled with our ability to change our natural environment has hastened the pace of disease emergence and re-emergence (Fig. 4.1). Many modern human activities facilitate microbial transmission (e.g. air travel and the globalization of the food supply; see Table 4.1),[3-5] while others have decreased it (e.g. improvements in sanitation, antimicrobial drugs, vaccines and disease control and eradication programs). Looking ahead, the most significant risk factor for disease emergence in the 21st century is likely to be population growth and urbanization, leading to the creation of megacities (a city with 10 million inhabitants)[6] throughout the developing world. According to a recent United Nations report (http://www.unfpa.org/swp/2007/english/introduction.html), more than half the world's population will be living in urban areas by the end of 2008, and by 2025 there are likely to be eight new megacities, most of them in the developing world, bringing the total to 28. By 2050, 6.4 billion people will be living in urban areas, out of a total projected population of 9.2 billion. These population increases will be associated with further stresses on resources (e.g. clean air, water and food) and natural habitats (e.g. higher temperatures caused by global warming that allow disease-carrying mosquitoes to move into new areas). Moreover, as human cities expand into forested areas, increased contact between humans and wildlife may lead to human infection with previously unknown animal pathogens that can cause human disease. Intensified livestock production – both traditional and modern – to meet increasing demand may also facilitate the spread of new and re-emerging zoonotic diseases (http://www.ifpri.org/2020/dp/dp28.pdf).

New and re-emerging infectious diseases

Over the past 40 years, more than 40 new human pathogens have been identified and characterized, often by using serologic and molecular methods (Table 4.2). Some of these microbes cause diseases of global importance (e.g. HIV/AIDS, hepatitis C, rotavirus diarrheal disease; and the (H1N1) 2009 influenza pandemic). Others appear to be limited (thus far) to particular countries or continents (e.g. Ebola hemorrhagic fever in central Africa (although simian Ebola has also been identified in the Philippines); Argentinian, Bolivian, Venezuelan and Sabia-associated hemorrhagic fevers in South America; hantavirus pulmonary syndrome in the Americas; and new variant Creutzfeldt–Jakob disease in Europe, Japan, Canada, and Saudi Arabia). A recent example is the 2003 outbreak of severe acute respiratory syndrome (SARS), caused by a novel coronavirus, which spread overnight from Hong Kong to Canada and several other countries by airplane (Fig. 4.2; see also below). In addition to these newly identified diseases, several 'old' threats have re-emerged in new or drug-resistant forms (Table 4.3). These include highly virulent epidemic strains of *Mycobacterium tuberculosis* (see below) and *Clostridium difficile*.[10,11]

Selected examples of major outbreaks since 1993 are listed in Table 4.4.

The essential role of the clinician in disease detection and surveillance

Physicians are in the best possible position to observe and report unusual illnesses, syndromes and disease risk factors. In 1993, for example, an Indian Health Service physician reported a cluster of fatal cases of unexplained respiratory disease in the southwestern United States that proved to be caused by a previously unrecognized hantavirus. In 1999, the first US outbreak of West Nile encephalitis was identified when an infectious disease physician reported unusual neurologic disease in three elderly people who lived in the same area (Fig. 4.3).[12] West Nile encephalitis – whose causative agent is carried by migratory birds in Africa, the Middle East, and Europe and transmitted to humans by mosquito bite – had never before been reported in the Western hemisphere.[13] In 2000, physicians in New York, London and Toronto helped identify an international outbreak

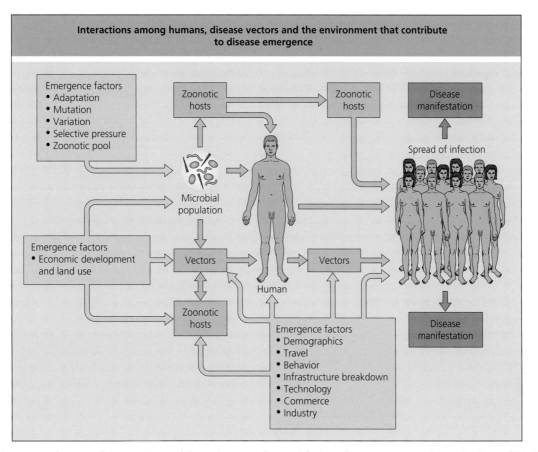

Interactions among humans, disease vectors and the environment that contribute to disease emergence

Fig. 4.1 Interactions among humans, disease vectors and the environment that contribute to disease emergence. *Source*: Institute of Medicine. Emerging infections: microbial threats to health in the United States. Washington, DC: National Academy Press; 1992.[3] (In March 2003, the Institute of Medicine published a reassessment: Microbial threats to health: emergence, detection, and response. Washington DC: National Academy Press; 2003.[4])

of leptospirosis among athletes returning home from a competition in Malaysian Borneo. These physicians reported their findings to Geosentinel, the surveillance network of the International Society of Travel Medicine (http://www.istm.org/geosentinel/main.html),

---

Table 4.1 Factors in the emergence of infectious diseases

Modern demographic, environmental, and behavioral factors that favor the spread of infectious diseases include:

- global travel
- globalization of the food supply and centralized processing of food
- population growth and increased urbanization and crowding
- population movements due to civil wars, famines and other manmade or natural disasters
- irrigation, deforestation and reforestation projects that alter the habitats of disease-carrying insects and animals
- human behaviors, such as intravenous drug use and risky sexual behavior
- increased use of antimicrobial agents and pesticides, hastening the development of resistance
- increased human contact with tropical rainforests and other wilderness habitats that are reservoirs for insects and animals that harbor unknown infectious agents
- deteriorating public health infrastructures in many parts of the world
- changes in climate and weather patterns
- lack of political will to institute disease control measures
- intentional release of pathogenic agents by terrorists.

Adapted from references[3–5].

---

which alerted travel clinics in 11 countries. An astute clinician was also responsible for reporting the first cases of a multistate outbreak of *Cyclospora* infection that was associated with imported raspberries.[14] Later cases were detected in 20 states, the District of Columbia and two Canadian provinces.

The US anthrax attacks in autumn 2001 also highlighted the crucial role of clinicians in monitoring unusual and dangerous diseases. The first case of anthrax (an inhalational case) was recognized in a hospitalized patient by an infectious disease physician in Palm Beach County, Florida, and six of eight anthrax cases detected in New York City (one inhalational and seven cutaneous) were reported to city health authorities by alert physicians. Three were diagnosed by infectious disease physicians (including the inhalational case), one by a dermatologist, one by a public health physician and one by an emergency room physician. Physicians also reported anthrax cases in Washington DC and New Jersey.

As these examples illustrate, the vigilance of physicians and other health-care providers remains the most important factor in infectious disease surveillance and control and in recognition of new and emerging infectious diseases.

Linkages between animal and human disease surveillance

Between 60% and 75% of all emerging and many re-emerging infectious diseases of human health importance are zoonotic.[15] The intimate relationship between animal and human health is illustrated by the emergence of the pandemic (H1N1) 2009 influenza virus, which includes gene segments from humans, birds, and pigs. Other examples include the 1999 outbreak of West Nile encephalitis, which was preceded by die-offs

57

Table 4.2 Newly identified microbial pathogens

	Agent	Type	Disease
1972	Calicivirus (Norwalk agent)	Virus	Acute gastroenteritis
1973	Rotavirus	Virus	Major cause of infantile diarrhea worldwide
1975	Parvovirus B19	Virus	Aplastic crisis in chronic hemolytic anemia
1976	*Cryptosporidium parvum*	Parasite	Acute and chronic diarrhea
1977	Ebola virus	Virus	Ebola hemorrhagic fever
1977	Hantaan virus	Virus	Hemorrhagic fever with renal syndrome (HFRS)
1977	*Legionella pneumophila*	Bacterium	Legionnaires' disease
1977	*Campylobacter jejuni*	Bacterium	Enteric pathogens distributed globally
1980	Human T-lymphotropic virus type 1 (HTLV-1)	Virus	T-cell lymphoma-leukemia
1981	Toxin producing strains of *Staphylococcus aureus*	Bacterium	Toxic shock syndrome
1982	*Escherichia coli* O157:H7	Bacterium	Hemorrhagic colitis; hemolytic uremic syndrome
1982	Human T-lymphotropic virus type 2 (HTLV-2)	Virus	Hairy cell leukemia
1982	*Borrelia burgdorferi*	Bacterium	Lyme disease
1983	Human immunodeficiency virus (HIV)	Virus	Acquired immunodeficiency syndrome (AIDS)
1985	*Helicobacter pylori*	Bacterium	Peptic ulcer disease
1985	*Enterocytozoon bieneusi*	Parasite	Persistent diarrhea
1986	*Cyclospora cayetanensis*	Parasite	Persistent diarrhea
1988	Human herpesvirus 6 (HHV-6)	Virus	Exanthema subitum
1988	Hepatitis E	Virus	Enterically transmitted non-A, non-B hepatitis
1989	*Ehrlichia chafeensis*	Bacterium	Human ehrlichiosis
1989	Hepatitis C	Virus	Parenterally transmitted non-A, non-B hepatitis
1991	Guanarito virus	Virus	Venezuelan hemorrhagic fever
1991	*Encephalitozoon hellem*	Parasite	Conjunctivitis, disseminated disease
1991	New species of *Babesia*	Parasite	Atypical babesiosis
1992	*Bartonella henselae*	Bacterium	Cat-scratch disease; bacillary angiomatosis
1992	*Tropheryma whipplei*	Bacterium	Impaired absorption of nutrients, weight loss, joint pain, and anemia
1992	*Vibrio cholerae* O139	Bacterium	Cholera with wide-spectrum drug resistance
1993	Sin Nombre virus	Virus	Hantavirus pulmonary syndrome (HPS)
1993	*Encephalitozoon cuniculi*	Parasite	Disseminated disease
1994	Sabia virus	Virus	Brazilian hemorrhagic fever
1994	Henipaviruses (Hendra)	Virus	Encephalitic disease carried by fruit bats that can be transmitted from horses to humans (Hendra)
1995	Human herpesvirus 8 (HHV-8)	Virus	Associated with Kaposi's sarcoma in AIDS patients
1996	New variant Creutzfeldt–Jakob disease agent	Prion	Progressive degenerative neurologic disease
1997	H5N1 strain of avian influenza	Virus	Influenza transmitted from chickens to humans; often fatal
1999	Henipaviruses (Nipah)	Virus	Encephalitic disease carried by fruit bats that can be transmitted from pigs to humans
2001	Human metapneumovirus	Virus	Acute respiratory infections
2002	Vancomycin-resistant *Staphylococcus aureus*	Bacterium	First vancomycin-resistant *S. aureus* strain identified in the USA
2003	SARS coronavirus	Virus	Severe acute respiratory syndrome (SARS)
2003	*Clostridium difficile*, strain NAPI/027	Bacteria	Pseudomembranous colitis

Table 4.2 Newly identified microbial pathogens—cont'd

	Agent	Type	Disease
2005	Bocavirus	Virus	Associated with lower respiratory tract infections in children; discovered through molecular screening of respiratory tract samples
2007	New strain of Ebola (the fifth one identified)	Virus	Hemorrhagic fever
2008	Transplant-associated arenavirus related to lymphocytic choriomeningitis virus	Virus	Severe febrile illness
2008	*Plasmodium knowlesi* as a human pathogen	Parasite	Previously classified as a cause of simian malaria, this parasite is now known to be a cause of human malaria in Malaysia, sometimes misdiagnosed as *Plasmodium malariae*, a milder form of malaria
2009	Pandemic (H1N1) 2009 virus	Virus	Pandemic influenza (see Chapter 161)

Updated from World Health Organization.[7]

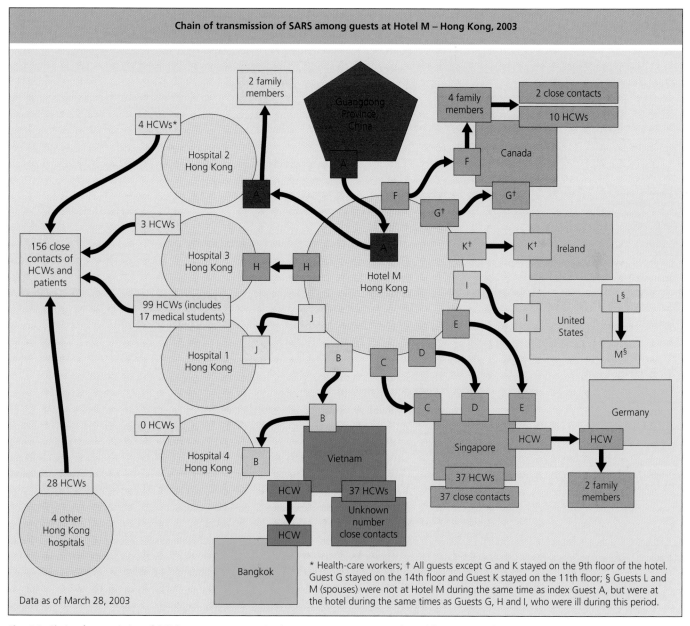

Fig. 4.2 Chain of transmission of SARS among guests at Hotel M – Hong Kong, 2003. Adapted from Centers for Disease Control and Prevention.[8]

Table 4.3 Resurging diseases

Disease or agent	Factors in re-emergence
Viral	
Rabies	Breakdown in public health measures; changes in land use; travel
Dengue and dengue hemorrhagic fever	Transportation; travel and migration; urbanization. Many countries reported high numbers of dengue infections in 2007; this trend continued in 2008, with a large outbreak of 120 570 cases reported in Brazil, including 75 399 cases in Rio de Janeiro
Yellow fever	Favorable conditions for growth of the mosquito vector. In June 2008, Paraguay reported the first identified yellow fever cases in more than 30 years, some of them near the capital city, Asuncion. The apparent re-emergence of urban yellow fever, which can spread rapidly through susceptible populations, has raised public health concerns in other countries in the region
Rift Valley fever	Infected humans, animals or mosquitoes that have traveled across East Africa to Saudi Arabia and Yemen
Polio	Cessation in vaccination campaigns or decline in average vaccine coverage
Chikungunya fever	A strain of chikungunya virus isolated during a 2005–2006 outbreak on Reunion Island (an island in the Pacific Ocean) has a mutation[1,2] that may facilitate transmission by *Aedes albopictus* (the Tiger mosquito), which is native to South East Asia, but is now present on all continents except Antarctica. Disease spread via travelers who visited chikungunya-affected areas in India, Mauritius or other islands in the Pacific Ocean apparently led to the first cases of local transmission in Italy (in 2007) and in Australia, Singapore and Malaysia (in 2008)
Parasitic	
Malaria	Drug and insecticide resistance; civil strife; lack of economic resources
Schistosomiasis	Dam construction, improved irrigation and ecologic changes favorable to the snail host
Neurocysticercosis	Immigration; agricultural practices
Acanthamebiasis	Introduction of soft contact lenses
Visceral leishmaniasis	War; population displacement; immigrations; habitat changes favorable to insect vector and increase in immunocompromised human hosts
Toxoplasmosis	Increase in immunocompromised human hosts
Giardiasis	Increased use of child-care facilities
Echinococcosis	Ecologic changes that affect the habitats of the immediate (animal) hosts
Trypanosomiasis (African sleeping sickness)	Breakdown in public health infrastructure
Bacterial	
Tuberculosis	Human demographics and behavior; international commerce and travel; breakdown of public health measures; microbial adaptation (i.e. multidrug-resistant tuberculosis [MDR-TB] and extensively drug-resistant tuberculosis [XDR-TB]); the HIV/AIDS pandemic
Trench fever	Breakdown of public health measures
Plague	Economic development; land use
Diphtheria	Interruption of immunization programs due to political changes
Pertussis	Refusal to vaccinate in some countries because of belief that pertussis vaccines are not safe
Salmonella	Industry and technology; human demographics and behavior; microbial adaptation; changes in food production
Pneumococcus	Human demographics; microbial adaptation; international travel and commerce; misuse and overuse of antibiotics
Cholera	International travel; long-term increases in sea surface temperatures and sea levels that may lead to higher concentrations of *Vibrio cholerae*, which grow on zooplankton that flourish in warm water

[1]Martin E. Epidemiology: tropical disease follows mosquitoes to Europe. Science 2007; 317(5844):1485.
[2]Tsetsarkin KA, Vanlandingham DL, McGee CE, Higgs S. A single mutation in Chikungunya virus affects vector specificity and epidemic potential. PLoS Pathog 2007;3(12):e201.
Adapted and updated from Lorber.[9]

Table 4.4 Selected infectious disease challenges, 1993–2008

1993	Hantavirus pulmonary syndrome (USA)
1994	Plague (India)
1995	Ebola fever (Zaire)
1996	New variant Creutzfeldt–Jakob disease (UK)
1997	H5N1 influenza (Hong Kong); vancomycin-intermediate resistant *Staphylococcus aureus* (Japan, USA)
1998	Nipah virus encephalitis (Malaysia, Singapore)
1999	West Nile encephalitis (Russia, USA)
2000	Rift Valley fever (Kenya, Saudi Arabia, Yemen); Ebola fever (Uganda)
2001	Anthrax (USA); foot and mouth disease (UK)
2002	Vancomycin-resistant *Staphylococcus aureus* (USA)
2003	Severe acute respiratory syndrome (SARS)
2003	Re-emergence of H5N1 influenza (beginning in South East Asia and spreading internationally)
2003	Monkeypox (USA)
2003	Highly virulent strain of *Clostridium difficile* (Canada, the Netherlands, UK, USA)
2005–2006	Multistate outbreak of mumps in the USA, involving 11 states (The widespread use of a second dose of mumps vaccine among US schoolchildren beginning in 1990 was followed by historically low reports of mumps cases, and it was hoped that the disease might be eliminated by 2010. However, a multistate outbreak of mumps – the largest US outbreak in two decades – occurred in 2006)
2004	Chikungunya fever outbreak associated with high fever and severe protracted joint pain in Lamu Island, Kenya
2007	New strain of Ebola (the fifth one identified), responsible for large outbreaks in Uganda and the Congo
2008	Measles outbreaks in Europe (Switzerland, Austria, Ireland and Britain), Israel and the USA (San Diego, California), associated with declining rates of measles vaccination
2008	Outbreak of Zika fever (a mosquito-borne illness similar to dengue) in the Yap Islands, Federated States of Micronesia
2009	Pandemic (H1N1) influenza. See Chapter 161.

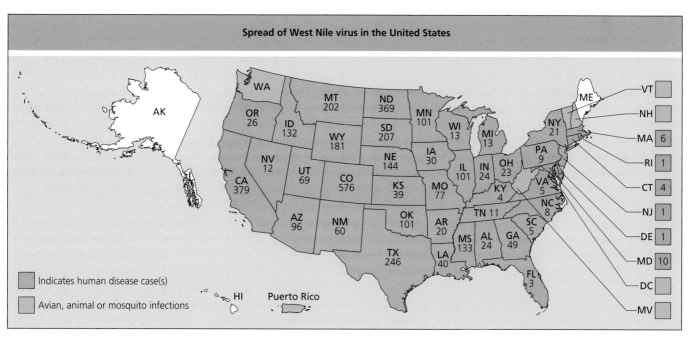

Fig. 4.3 Spread of West Nile virus in the United States. In the 8 years since West Nile virus was first reported in the USA (in New York City), human infections have been reported in 47 states. West Nile activity from January 1, 2007, to February 5, 2008, is indicated above. *Source:* Centers for Disease Control and Prevention. Adapted from: http://www.cdc.gov/ncidod/dvbid/westnile/Mapsactivity/surv&control107Maps.htm

of crows; the 1999 Nipah encephalitis outbreak, which was preceded by illness in pigs; and the 1996 outbreak of new variant Creutzfeldt–Jakob disease, which was preceded by the recognition of an epidemic of bovine spongiform encephalopathy (BSE) among cows.

Formal mechanisms have been developed to link public health disease monitoring with surveillance for diseases in agricultural animals, migrating birds and wild animals. They include the US-government-sponsored Global Avian Influenza Network for Surveillance (http://www.gains.org), which was established in 2006 in co-operation with the Wildlife Conservation Society (WCS) to monitor high pathogenicity avian influenza (HPAI) in wild birds. Within the USA, ArboNet tracks nationally notifiable arboviral diseases (including West Nile fever; see Fig. 4.3), and the National Antimicrobial Resistance Monitoring System (NARMS; http://www.cdc.gov/narms) continues to monitor the emergence of antimicrobial resistance in zoonotic bacteria (e.g. *Salmonella* and *Campylobacter*) that infect livestock. In addition, the federal, state and local public health laboratories are also linked with agricultural, wildlife and military reference laboratories through the Laboratory Response Network (LRN), which was founded in 1998 by the Centers for Disease Control and Prevention (CDC) in partnership with the Association of Public Health Laboratories and the Federal Bureau of Investigation (FBI).

In addition to protecting human health, rapid detection and control of animal diseases will benefit agriculture, help preserve wildlife species and avert economic losses due to expensive disease control measures (Box 4.1). The special challenges of understanding the ecologic factors that favor the emergence and spread of zoonotic diseases are discussed below.

Molecular diagnostics and outbreak detection

To ensure optimal medical care and disease control strategies, clinical diagnosis of unusual diseases must be confirmed by laboratory tests. Today's advances in microbial genomics, molecular immunology and bioinformatics are facilitating the development of accurate, rapid and sensitive diagnostics based on detection of microbe-specific or strain-specific nucleic acids or proteins. Molecular testing that involves amplification of genetic sequences using the polymerase chain reaction (PCR) technique is especially useful when unidentified pathogens are difficult to grow in the laboratory, making other types of testing difficult or impossible. In the future, advances in human genomics may also allow the identification of individuals with increased genetic susceptibility to certain diseases or to severe manifestations of those diseases (Table 4.5).[16,17]

Molecular testing has the potential not only to confirm clinical diagnoses but also to facilitate the detection of outbreaks. This function may be especially important when individual cases are not clustered geographically or by other easily identifiable risk factors. Examples include:

- food-borne pathogens transmitted simultaneously to many localities when a contaminated product is shipped to supermarkets or restaurants in several states or countries;
- disease agents dispersed by international travelers, such as the 2000 leptospirosis outbreak in Malaysian Borneo and the 2003 outbreak of SARS; and
- an unannounced and undetected (covert) release of a bioterrorist agent.

Public health tools are already in place in Europe and the USA to identify and trace the source of geographically dispersed food-borne

---

Box 4.1 Agricultural costs of controlling diseases carried by food animals

When a dangerous animal-borne disease threatens human health or food safety, a government may be forced to slaughter large numbers of food animals as a control measure, despite considerable economic costs. Recent examples include two zoonotic diseases (Nipah encephalitis and H5N1 influenza) and two veterinary diseases (foot and mouth disease and bovine spongiform encephalopathy (BSE; also called mad cow disease)). Ingestion of beef containing the causative agent of BSE (a prion) may result in the development of a fatal human neurodegenerative illness (new variant Creutzfeldt–Jakob disease) many years later.

Between 1997 and 2007, the culling of animals to control outbreaks of Nipah encephalitis, avian influenza, foot and mouth disease, and BSE cost the agricultural sector billions of dollars.

- *Nipah encephalitis.* In 1999 Malaysian health authorities were faced with an outbreak of encephalitis among farm workers, which had a nearly 50% mortality rate. The cause was a previously unknown paramyxovirus called the Nipah virus, which is carried by bats. To control the outbreak, approximately 1.1 million pigs were culled within a few weeks, severely harming the Malaysian meat industry.
- *Avian influenza (strain H5N1).* In 1997, a similar precautionary measure was taken by the government of Hong Kong, which arranged the culling of all 1.6 million chickens on Hong Kong Island and the New Territories to prevent chicken-to-human transmission of a virulent avian form of influenza.

The 2003 re-emergence of avian influenza A[H5N1] in South East Asia – and its consequent spread to Central Asia, Africa, Europe and the Middle East – has also had a significant economic impact. In South East Asia, for example, bird deaths due to disease and to bird cullings have caused severe losses to farmers in Vietnam and Thailand (whose poultry stocks declined by 15–20%), as well as to farmers in Indonesia, China, Cambodia and Laos. According to the World Bank, economic impacts in these countries have also affected poultry traders, feed mills and breeding farms (http://web. worldbank.org/WBSITE/EXTERNAL/COUNTRIES/EASTASIAPACIFICEXT/EXTEAPHALFYEARLYUPDATE/0,contentMDK:20708543~menuPK:550232~page PK:64168445~piPK:64168309~theSitePK:550226,00.html).

- *Bovine spongiform encephalopathy.* In 2006, the European Union lifted a 10-year ban on the export of live cattle and cattle products (other than milk) from the UK. Control measures, including the slaughter of affected cows, cost the UK government an estimated £3.5 billion sterling (about US$5 billion). The export ban cost the UK agricultural sector about £675 million a year.
- *Foot and mouth disease.* The costs of controlling an outbreak of foot and mouth disease in the UK and continental Europe in 2001 – estimated at £8.5 billion – dwarfed those of the BSE outbreak and devastated the centuries-old British livestock industry. Foot and mouth disease does not infect humans but can be spread by travelers who have contaminated soil on their shoes or clothing or who carry contaminated food products. The St Patrick's Day parade in Ireland was cancelled due to concerns about spreading the virus, and the British army was mobilized to help bury the carcasses of 7 million animals slaughtered because of potential exposure to the disease.

In August 2007, the European Union imposed a temporary ban on export of livestock, meat and milk from the UK, and the UK halted the internal movement of farm animals nationwide, to minimize the risk of spreading foot and mouth disease after cases were detected in Surrey. The outbreak, which affected about eight farms, was traced to an accidental release of an experimental vaccine strain from a high-security animal laboratory in rural England.

Table 4.5 Examples of genetic factors that influence susceptibility to disease or disease progression

- Alleles of the chemokine receptor gene CCR5 confer partial protection against HIV infection and the development of AIDS[1]
- Globin gene alleles (e.g. sickle globin and α- and β-thalassemias) confer partial protection against malaria[2]
- Lack of the Duffy blood group on red cells (due to a mutation in a chemokine receptor gene) confers complete protection against *Plasmodium vivax* malaria[3]
- Some vitamin D receptor (VDR) genotypes may reduce the risk of developing clinical tuberculosis[4]
- Blood group O is associated with severe cholera[5]
- Mutations in the cystic fibrosis gene may confer some protection against cholera[6]
- HLA alleles may influence susceptibility to – or course of infection of – HIV/AIDS, hepatitis B, measles, hantavirus pulmonary syndrome, malaria, tuberculosis, human papillomavirus infection and coccidioidomycosis[7]
- Mutations in the regulatory region of the PARK2 gene – the cause of early onset Parkinson's disease – and the co-regulated gene PARKCG are associated with increased susceptibility to leprosy[8]
- Heterozygosity at codon 129 of the prion protein gene might provide a measure of protection against sporadic and iatrogenic infection with Creutzfeldt–Jakob disease (CJD)[9]
- The apolipoprotein E, type ε4 allele (ApoEε4) – which is a marker for cognitive decline with Alzheimer's and cardiovascular diseases later in life – might play a protective role in the cognitive and physical development of children with heavy burdens of diarrhea in early childhood[10]

[1]Reiche EMV, Bonametti AM, Voltarelli JC, Morimoto HK, Watanabe MAE. Genetic polymorphisms in the chemokine and chemokine receptors: impact on clinical course and therapy of the human immunodeficiency virus type 1 infection (HIV-1). Curr Med Chem 2008;14(12):1325–34.
[2]Weatherall DJ. Thalassaemia and malaria, revisited. Ann Trop Med Parasitol 1997;91(7):885–90.
[3]Langhi DM Jr, Bordin JO. Duffy blood group and malaria. Hematology 2006;11(5):389–98.
[4]Roth DE, Soto G, Arenas F, et al. Association between vitamin D receptor gene polymorphisms and response to treatment of pulmonary tuberculosis. J Infect Dis 2004;190(5):920–7.
[5]Harris JB, Khan AI, LaRocque RC, et al. Blood group, immunity, and risk of infection with *Vibrio cholerae* in an area of endemicity. Infect Immun 2005;73(11):7422–7.
[6]Gabriel SE, Brigman KN, Koller BH, Boucher RC, Stutts MJ. Cystic fibrosis heterozygote resistance to cholera toxin in the cystic fibrosis mouse model. Science 1994;266(5182):107–9.
[7]Nikolich-Zugich J, Fremont DH, Miley MJ, Messaoudi I. The role of mhc polymorphism in anti-microbial resistance. Microbes Infect 2004;6(5):501–12.
[8]Mira MT, Alcaïs A, Nguyen VT, et al. Susceptibility to leprosy is associated with PARK2 and PACRG. Nature 2004;427(6975):636–40.
[9]Riemenschneider M, Klopp N, Xiang W, et al. Prion protein codon 129 polymorphism and risk of Alzheimer disease. Neurology 2004;63(2):364–6.
[10]Oriá RB, Patrick PD, Blackman JA, Lima AA, Guerrant RL. Role of apolipoprotein E4 in protecting children against early childhood diarrhea outcomes and implications for later development. Med Hypotheses 2007;68(5):1099–107.

outbreaks by comparing molecular fingerprinting data from clinical and public health laboratories. This is the operating principle behind PulseNet,[18] a molecular subtyping network that has used the pulse-field gel electrophoresis (PFGE) technique to detect several major multistate food-borne outbreaks. For example, PulseNet was used to detect an outbreak of *Escherichia coli* O157:H7 transmitted by fresh spinach sold in 26 states (in 2006) and an outbreak of *Salmonella* St Paul associated with jalapeno peppers sold in more than 40 states (in 2008). This technology is in use in many countries all over the world (http://www.pulsenetinternational.org). In the future, advances in genome sequencing and bioinformatics may lead to the development of increasingly sophisticated typing methods that will facilitate discovery of novel disease risk factors for hundreds of pathogens and help health authorities identify linkages among geographically dispersed cases of disease. For example, the CDC has proposed the development of an international database called Microbe. Net that could potentially match a pathogen isolated from an ill person in one country with an environmental microbe isolated in another.

Being prepared for the unexpected

Infectious pathogens are extraordinarily resilient and have a remarkable ability to evolve, adapt and develop resistance to drugs in an unpredictable and dynamic fashion. Because we do not know what new diseases will arise, we must always be prepared for the unexpected (see Table 4.4). In 2002, the first vancomycin-resistant *Staphylococcus aureus* strain was identified in the USA.[19] In 2003, SARS emerged from an animal reservoir in Guangdong province in China and quickly spread via travelers through South-East Asia and then to Toronto, Canada. Later in the same year, more than 30 people in the midwestern United States contracted monkeypox – a disease that resembles a mild case of smallpox – from rodents imported as pets that carried an orthopox virus known to infect people who live in remote villages near tropical rainforests in Central and Western Africa (http://www.cdc.gov/MMWR/preview/

mmwrhtml/mm5226a5.htm). In 2009, a new strain of pandemic influenza – the pandemic (H1N1) 2009 virus – emerged in North America and spread rapidly around the world (see later).

The unexpected may include intentional as well as naturally occurring outbreaks. In 2001, the USA experienced a multistate outbreak of anthrax that necessitated antibiotic prophylaxis for more than 30 000 people. Rapid medical, public health and law enforcement action limited the outbreak to 11 inhalational cases, 11 cutaneous cases and five deaths.

These examples of unforeseen outbreaks underscore the need to maintain a strong public health system that is supported by a well-informed and vigilant medical community.

Shifts in perspectives on infectious disease in the past 50 years

Over the past 50 years, there have been significant shifts in how infectious diseases are viewed by the medical and scientific world and by the public. In the years following the Second World War, it was widely believed that humans were winning the war against infectious microbes. Vaccines and antibiotics, coupled with earlier improvements in sanitation and water quality, had dramatically lowered the incidence of infectious diseases. Therefore, it became possible to imagine a world in which infectious pathogens would no longer prey upon humanity. In 1962, the Australian Nobel prize winner Frank Macfarlane Burnet stated:[20]

One can think of the middle of the twentieth century as the end of one of the most important social revolutions in history, the virtual elimination of the infectious disease as an important factor in social life.

Five years later, Surgeon General William H Stewart expressed the views of many US doctors and health experts when he stated that it was time to 'close the book on infectious illnesses', as long as we continue to prevent disease through vaccination'.[21] He encouraged the public health community to turn its attention to chronic diseases. Over the following years, biomedical research in the USA became increasingly focused on heart disease, stroke and the 'war on cancer', which was declared by President Richard Nixon in 1971. Local and federal programs aimed at monitoring and studying infectious diseases were greatly reduced or abolished.

New diseases continue to emerge and re-emerge

In spite of optimistic predictions, infectious diseases continued to cause serious problems. As early as the 1940s and 1950s, certain bacteria, such as *Staphylococcus aureus*, began to develop resistance to penicillin. In 1957 and 1968, new strains of influenza emerged in China and Hong Kong, respectively, and spread rapidly around the globe. In the 1970s there was a resurgence of sexually transmitted diseases in the USA (perhaps due in part to changes in human sexual behaviors and to the importation of antibiotic-resistant strains of gonorrhea by infected soldiers returning from Vietnam). The final blows to our complacent attitude toward infectious diseases came in the 1980s, with the appearance of AIDS and the re-emergence of tuberculosis, including multidrug-resistant strains.

By the early 1990s, many health experts no longer believed that the threat of infectious diseases was receding in the developed world. Growing concern about the threat of emerging infectious diseases was cogently expressed in a 1992 report issued by the Institute of Medicine (IOM) of the National Academies. The report, *Emerging Infections: Microbial Threats to Health in the United States*, emphasized the intimate links between US health and international health.[3] It described the major factors that contribute to disease emergence, including societal changes and microbial evolution (see Table 4.1). The report concluded that emerging infectious diseases are a major threat to US health, and it challenged the US government to take action.

In 1994, the CDC answered the challenge by launching a national effort to revitalize the US capacity to protect the public from infectious diseases. This ongoing effort is described in *Addressing Emerging Infectious Disease Threats: A Prevention Strategy for the United States* (http://www.cdc.gov/mmwr/PDF/rr/rr4305.pdf) and an updated version published in 1998 (http://www.cdc.gov/mmwr/preview/mmwrhtml/00054779.htm). In view of the public health importance of vector-borne and zoonotic diseases – which account for more than half of all emerging diseases[15] – CDC is working with medical partners (e.g. the American Medical Association [AMA]) and animal health partners (e.g. the World Organization for Animal Health [OIE], the American Veterinary Medical Association [AVMA] and the Wildlife Conservation Society [WCS]); see below to study ecologic aspects of disease emergence and develop prevention strategies that take into account human, veterinary, and environmental factors (see Fig. 4.1).

Looking back to the 1950s and 1960s it is useful to remember that very little was then known about how microbes evolve or develop drug resistance. In the 1970s and 1980s, with the development of molecular biology, biologists learned how resistance genes are carried on plasmids and transmitted from one bacterium to another. They also learned how quickly viruses can evolve by generating mutations with each round of replication, as well as by reassorting gene segments or jumping species barriers. As molecular tools became available, many new viruses (pathogenic and nonpathogenic) were discovered in humans, animals and plants.

CATEGORIES OF EMERGING AND RE-EMERGING INFECTIOUS DISEASES

For the purposes of this discussion, emerging and re-emerging threats may be grouped into five (sometimes overlapping) categories:

- drug-resistant diseases;
- food-borne and water-borne diseases;
- zoonotic and vector-borne diseases;
- diseases transmitted through blood transfusions or blood products; and
- chronic diseases caused by infectious agents.

Drug-resistant diseases

Drug-resistant pathogens are a growing menace to all people, regardless of age, sex or socioeconomic background. They endanger people in affluent, industrial societies such as the USA, as well as in less developed nations. Examples of clinically important microbes that are rapidly developing resistance to available antimicrobial agents include bacteria that cause pneumonia, ear infections and meningitis (e.g. *Streptococcus pneumoniae*), skin, bone and bloodstream infections (e.g. *Staphylococcus aureus*), urinary tract infections (e.g. *E. coli*), food-borne infections (e.g. *Salmonella*) and infections transmitted in health-care settings (e.g. enterococci) (Table 4.6).

Special concerns include health-care-associated and community-acquired methicillin-resistant *Staphylococcus aureus* (HA-MRSA and CA-MRSA) and extensively drug-resistant tuberculosis (XDR-TB; see below). A large study led by the CDC estimates that HA-MRSA was responsible for 94 360 serious infections and associated with 18 650 hospital stay-related deaths in the USA in 2005, making it the cause of more deaths in the USA each year than HIV/AIDS.[22]

Until recently, most MRSA cases were seen in hospitals. However, clusters of CA-MRSA skin infections are increasingly reported among athletes, military recruits, prisoners and groups of people who live in crowded conditions. Athletes at highest risk include those who participate in contact sports such as wrestling, football and rugby, probably because most MRSA infections begin with a cut, scratch or bruise.[23] However, MRSA infections have also been diagnosed among athletes in other sports such as soccer, basketball, field hockey, volleyball, rowing, martial arts, fencing and baseball. Risk factors for

Table 4.6 Examples of emerging resistance in bacterial pathogens

Gram-positive cocci	Methicillin-resistant and vancomycin-resistant *Staphylococcus aureus* Coagulase-negative staphylococci Penicillin-resistant pneumococci Macrolide-resistant streptococci Vancomycin-resistant enterococci
Gram-negative cocci	Penicillin-resistant meningococci Quinolone-resistant gonococci
Gram-negative bacilli	*Enterobacter* spp. and other Enterobacteriaceae with chromosomal β-lactamases Multidrug-resistant *Pseudomonas aeruginosa* *Stenotrophomonas maltophila* *Acinetobacter* spp. with novel β-lactamases, aminoglycoside-modifying enzymes and other resistance mechanisms Enterobacteriaceae with extended-spectrum β-lactamases Multidrug-resistant diarrheal pathogens (*Shigella* spp., *Salmonella* spp., *Escherichia coli*, *Campylobacter* spp.)
Acid-fast bacilli	Multidrug-resistant *Mycobacterium tuberculosis* (MDR-TB) Extensively drug-resistant *Mycobacterium tuberculosis* (XDR-TB) Multidrug-resistant *Mycobacterium avium* complex

these athletes may include contact with contaminated objects such as towels and sports equipment. It is also possible that other strains could emerge in farms where animals are fed antibiotics as growth promoters.[24]

Many other pathogens – including the bacteria that cause gonorrhea; the virus that causes AIDS; the fungi that cause *Candida* infections; and the parasites that cause malaria – are also becoming resistant to standard therapies. In the absence of effective action to address the problem of antimicrobial resistance, drug choices for the treatment of common infections will become increasingly limited, expensive and, in some cases, unavailable.

Reasons for the rapid development of antibiotic resistance include the ability of organisms to mutate and share genetic material. However, this process has been facilitated by:

- inappropriate prescription practices by physicians and veterinarians;
- administration of antibiotics to agricultural animals as growth promoters;
- unrealistic patient expectations that lead to requests for antibiotic treatment of nonbacterial infections;
- the economics of pharmaceutical sales; and
- increased use of sophisticated medical interventions that result in the administration of large quantities of antibiotics (e.g. transplant surgery and immunosuppressive and cytotoxic drug therapy).

Growing antibiotic resistance poses a substantial threat to modern gains in infectious disease control. About 70% of bacteria that cause infections in hospitals in many countries, including the US, are resistant to at least one of the drugs most commonly used to treat infections. The medical community must therefore join with patients and members of the agricultural and pharmaceutical industries in a common effort to promote appropriate use of antibiotics to safeguard their effectiveness for future generations. Steps to be taken by the European Union and the US government to facilitate this process are outlined in the *Copenhagen Recommendations* (http://www.im.dk/publikationer/micro98/recommen.htm) and *A Public Health Action Plan to Combat Antimicrobial Resistance*, respectively (http://www.cdc.gov/drugresistance/actionplan). In addition, the Infectious Diseases Society of America (IDSA) has issued *Bad Bugs, No Drugs* (http://www.idsociety.org/Content.aspx?id=5558) to call attention to the lack of new antibiotics in the pharmaceutical development pipeline.

Food-borne and water-borne diseases

Twentieth-century improvements in sanitation, food sterilization and processing, and water treatment have greatly reduced the burden of food-borne and water-borne illnesses in developed countries, nearly eliminating many diseases that remain major killers in the developing world (e.g. typhoid fever, cholera and dysentery). Now, in the 21st century, however, there is growing evidence that modern factors such as centralized food processing may pose challenges to food safety and water quality.

Food-borne diseases

Food-borne diseases cause an estimated 76 million illnesses, 325 000 hospitalizations and 5000 deaths in the USA each year.[25] As noted above, food-borne pathogens such as *Salmonella*, *Shigella*, *Cyclospora*, *Campylobacter* and *E. coli* O157:H7 can be transmitted via commercial products that are processed in large quantities and shipped to different states or nations. Although food processing techniques are very advanced, when contamination does occur it can affect many people in many different localities (see Table 4.5). A recent example is an outbreak of *E. coli* O157:H7 (transmitted via frozen hamburger patties) that affected people in eight US states and led to the recall of 21.7 million pounds of ground beef products. Six days after the recall, the company that marketed the beef went out of business (http://www.cdc.gov/ecoli/2007/october/100207.html).

Water-borne diseases

Microbial contamination of water can occur when animal or human sewage contaminates source water that is not adequately treated by filtration, chlorination or other methods. In addition, some parasites are resistant to routine water treatment methods. These include *Cryptosporidium*, the causative agent of a major disease outbreak in the Milwaukee drinking water system in 1993 that affected more than 400 000 people.[26] In 2006, series of articles reviewing current research on water-borne diseases was published in a special issue of the *Journal of Water and Health* (http://www.epa.gov/nheerl/articles/2006/waterborne_disease.html). This research was mandated by the Safe Drinking Water Act Amendments of 1996 and supported by the US Environmental Protection Agency (EPA) and the CDC. A workshop of experts from academia, the EPA and the CDC made recommendations for additional health studies related to microbial exposures in drinking water. Although associations between illness and water are often difficult to evaluate – since most people drink water every day, often from more than one source – the EPA estimates that there may be as many as 16.4 million cases of water-borne illness in the USA each year (http://www.epa.gov/nheerl/articles/2006/waterborne_disease/national_estimate.pdf).

Worldwide, approximately 1 billion people lack access to safe water and 2.6 billion lack access to basic sanitation. Water-borne diarrheal diseases cause 1.8 million deaths every year, most of them in children in developing countries with unsafe water supplies. In 2007, the World Health Organization (WHO) issued *Combating Waterborne Disease at the Household Level* (http://www.who.int/household_water/advocacy/combating_disease/en/index.html), which advocates the use of inexpensive point-of-use water quality interventions that can be used in the home in areas that lack access to safe drinking water.

Zoonotic diseases

Many of the novel human pathogens identified over the past decade are carried by animals. For example, Sin Nombre virus, which is carried by the deer mouse, was identified in 1993 in the USA as the cause of hantavirus pulmonary syndrome, and Hendra virus, carried by fruit bats, was identified in Australia in 1994 as a cause of encephalitis in humans and horses.[27] Nipah virus, which is also carried by fruit bats, was identified in 1999 in Malaysia as a cause of encephalitis in humans and swine and has since been reported in Bangladesh and India.[28–30] Like Sin Nombre virus, the Nipah and Hendra viruses (henipaviruses) are highly virulent, and there are as yet no drugs or vaccines for their treatment or prevention. Other examples include Marburg hemorrhagic fever virus, which is apparently maintained in cave-dwelling African fruit bats,[31,32] and the SARS coronavirus, which is associated with Chinese horseshoe bats.[33]

Zoonotic agents can become established in any geographic area that has a suitable animal reservoir. The arenavirus that causes lymphocytic choriomeningitis (first isolated in 1933) was probably introduced into the New World at the same time as its vector, *Mus musculus*, the common house mouse. Plague (which is both rodent-borne and vector-borne) was introduced into the USA in the early 1900s, via infected rats and fleas in ships that arrived at port cities. It quickly became established in the North American prairie ecosystem, infecting a wide range of animals, including native rodents and their fleas, which have been the most frequent sources of human infection. Like plague, newly emergent disease agents that are able to infect many animal species (e.g. Nipah and Hendra viruses and monkeypox virus) have the potential to spread worldwide.

Disease dispersion via insect vectors

Diseases that are carried by insect vectors (i.e. mosquitoes, fleas, ticks and other blood-sucking arthropods) can also spread into new geographic areas and infect new human populations. In 1999, for example, mosquito-borne transmission of three nonendemic diseases – malaria, dengue and West Nile fever – was reported in the USA. West Nile encephalitis may have entered New York City via an imported or migrating bird or a mosquito that 'hitch-hiked' on an airplane or (less likely) an infected traveler; dengue fever most likely arrived in Texas via both people and mosquitoes.

Asian tiger mosquitoes (*Aedes albopictus*) that can transmit dengue and Chikungunya fever arrived in the USA in Houston in 1987 in imported used-tire casings[34] and appeared more recently in California in commercial shipments of a Chinese ornamental indoor plant called 'lucky bamboo'.[35] During the 1990s, *A. albopictus* became established in Italy after mosquito eggs traveled to Italy in imported tires.[36] In 2007, when a traveler who had contracted Chikungunya in Kerala, India, fell ill after arriving in Ravenna, Italy, his disease was transmitted to others via the now-indigenous Italian *A. albopictus* mosquitoes, causing an outbreak that affected at least 204 people.[37]

While many cases of 'airport malaria' have been reported in Europe and North America (presumably involving small numbers of traveling mosquitoes), locally acquired malaria cases have also been identified that apparently involved at least one cycle of human-to-mosquito transmission. For example, a cluster of non-airport malaria cases was detected in Virginia in 2002 in a community that included immigrants from malarious countries who might have had asymptomatic malaria infections.[38] Another cluster was detected in 2003 in Palm Beach County, Florida.[39]

Another example of vector-borne disease spread is the recent identification of Rift Valley fever (previously seen only in Africa) in the Middle East.[40] Within a few years, Rift Valley fever (RVF) virus traveled from sub-Saharan Africa to northern Africa (Egypt and the Sudan) and then to Saudi Arabia and Yemen. Competent mosquito vectors for RVF, a febrile hepatitis associated with encephalitis, retinitis and hemorrhagic fever (among both humans and animals), are present throughout the world. Importation of RVF into the USA would constitute a major threat to the US livestock industry and to human public health.

Diseases transmitted through blood transfusions, blood products, or transplanted organs or tissues

Improvements in donor screening, serologic testing and transfusion practices have made the US blood supply one of the safest in the world, despite its size and complexity. However, because blood is a human tissue, it is a natural vehicle for transmission of infectious agents. During the 1980s, HIV was transmitted through clotting factor and blood transfusions, and during the 1990s, hepatitis C virus was transmitted by intravenous immunoglobulin. More recently, transmission of Chagas disease trypanosomes,[41] West Nile virus,[42] rabies virus,[43] Creutzfeldt–Jakob disease prions,[44] tuberculosis,[45] a new arenavirus related to lymphocytic choriomeningitis virus[46] and HIV virus (for the first time in the USA since 1986[47]) has been reported in patients who received organ transplants, grafts or blood from infected persons.

In recent years, there has been renewed interest in xenotransplantation – the transplantation of animal organs and tissues to humans – because of the shortage of human organs and tissues. The US Food and Drug Administration (FDA) is currently developing a comprehensive approach to the regulation of xenotransplantation to address public health concerns about potential infection of recipients with recognized or unknown zoonotic pathogens and possible subsequent transmission of these pathogens to close contacts and into the general population (http://www.fda.gov/cber/xap/xap.htm).

Infectious diseases also have implications for the availability of blood and blood products, because people who have traveled in countries where they may have been exposed to blood-borne diseases are often excluded as blood donors. Examples include individuals who have recently visited malaria-endemic countries and people who have stayed for 6 months or more in the UK, where they might have ingested beef from cows with BSE and acquired the prion that causes new variant Creutzfeldt–Jakob disease.

Chronic diseases caused or exacerbated by infectious agents

Several chronic diseases once attributed to lifestyle or environmental factors (such as some forms of cancer, diabetes, heart disease, arthritis and ulcers) are actually caused by or exacerbated by an infectious agent.[48-50] Three of the six major causes of cancer death in the world are caused by infectious agents: hepatocellular carcinoma by hepatitis B and C viruses, cervical cancer by human papillomavirus and gastric cancer by *Helicobacter pylori* bacteria (see below). Hepatitis B and C are also major causes of cirrhosis and end-stage liver disease, while *H. pylori* causes peptic ulcer disease in addition to stomach cancer. Moreover, Epstein–Barr virus is associated with nasopharyngeal carcinoma, Burkitt's lymphoma, B-cell lymphoma and post-transplant lymphoproliferative disease.

Current research suggests that some chronic cardiovascular, intestinal and pulmonary diseases may also have an infectious etiology. For example, Whipple's disease is caused by a bacterial infection (*Tropheryma whipplei*)[51,52] and tropical spastic paraparesis is caused by a viral infection (HTLV-1).[53] Potential associations are being investigated for many other illnesses and syndromes, including coronary artery disease (*Chlamydia* infection),[54] Paget's disease (paramyxoviridae infection),[55,56] Crohn's disease (mycobacterial infection)[57] and bronchiectasis (respiratory infections during early childhood).[58] There are also preliminary data suggesting that Wegener's granulomatosis responds to antibiotic therapy. These findings raise the possibility that some chronic conditions, including asthma, arthritis and heart disease, may someday be treated with antimicrobial drugs or prevented by vaccines.

INFECTIOUS DISEASES AND THE GLOBAL VILLAGE

As stressed in the Institute of Medicine reports in 1992 and 2003, US health and global health are inextricably linked.[3,4] Modern factors that connect us culturally, commercially and physically such as air travel and the globalization of the food supply (see Table 4.5) put us at risk of exposure to microbes that are endemic in other countries, whether we live in large cities or small rural hamlets. As the HIV/AIDS epidemic has illustrated, a disease that emerges or re-emerges anywhere in the world can spread far and wide. This concern is reflected in the most recent (2005) version of the WHO International Health Regulations (http://www.who.int/csr/ihr/en), which require reporting not only of some specific diseases, as in the 1969 version, but also of 'all events that may constitute public health emergencies of international concern' – including outbreaks caused by previously unidentified microbes, by microbes that appear in new, drug-resistant forms, or by bioterrorism. The list of specific notifiable diseases (which used to consist of cholera, plague and yellow fever) now includes a single case of smallpox, polio due to wild-type poliovirus, human influenza due to a new subtype and SARS.

Several diseases of global public health importance – including epidemic-prone diseases, newly emerging or re-emerging diseases, vaccine-preventable diseases and diseases slated for regional elimination or worldwide eradication (e.g. polio) – have resurged in recent years, spreading across countries and (sometimes) continents (see Table 4.3). HIV/AIDS, tuberculosis, malaria and measles continue to be major infectious causes of death worldwide, along with acute lower respiratory infections and diarrheal diseases (Fig. 4.4). Globally important diseases that continue to be of special domestic concern to the USA and other developed countries include HIV/AIDS, tuberculosis and pandemic influenza.

HIV/AIDS

HIV/AIDS incidence in the USA increased rapidly through the 1980s and early 1990s, with the peak of new diagnoses occurring after the expansion of the AIDS surveillance case definition in 1993.[59]

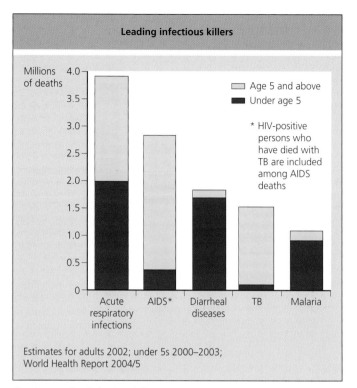

Fig. 4.4 Leading infectious killers.

Malaria

Forty-one percent of the world's population lives in areas where malaria is transmitted (e.g. parts of Africa, Asia, the Middle East, Central and South America, Hispaniola and Oceania) and 350–500 million cases occur annually. More than one million people die of malaria each year, most of them young children in sub-Saharan Africa.

Malaria prevention efforts include treatment with artemisinin-containing drugs, mosquito control (insecticide-treated bed nets and/or indoor residual spraying) and prophylactic treatment of vulnerable populations such as pregnant women and children.

Tuberculosis

Tuberculosis is the attributable cause of one-third of all adult deaths in developing nations.[62] Once thought to be controlled in Western countries, tuberculosis has re-emerged in Europe and the USA, where multi-drug-resistant *Mycobacterium tuberculosis* (MDR-TB) has been reported in 45 of the 50 states,[63] and extensively drug-resistant *Mycobacterium tuberculosis* (XDR-TB) is present in 4% of cases. MDR-TB bacteria are defined as resistant at least to the two first-line drugs against TB (isoniazid and rifampin (rifampicin)), while XDR-TB bacteria are defined as resistant not only to isoniazid and rifampin but also to any fluoroquinolone and at least one of three injectable second-line drugs (capreomycin, kanamycin and amikacin).[64] Since 1998, the percentage of US-born patients with MDR-TB has remained at less than 0.7%. However, the frequency of resistant infections in foreign-born persons increased from 25% (103 of 407) in 1993 to 80% (73 of 91) in 2006 (http://www.cdc.gov/tb/statistics/reports/2007/default.htm).

HIV infection confers the greatest known risk for the development of TB, stimulating both the activation of latent infection and rapid progression to primary disease. UNAIDS estimates that approximately 30% of all AIDS deaths result directly from tuberculosis.[65]

After 1996, with the introduction of effective combination antiretroviral therapies, sharp declines were reported in AIDS incidence and deaths, while AIDS prevalence continued to increase. Currently, US disease prevention efforts are targeted primarily to young men who have sex with men, the group that currently exhibits the highest incidence nationally.[60,61]

Worldwide, an estimated 33.2 million people are living with HIV/AIDS (Fig. 4.5). In 2007, there were 2.1 million HIV-related deaths and approximately 2.5 million new infections.

Special challenges

Climate change and infectious diseases

Understanding the effects of climate change on specific diseases – especially those of major concern to developing countries, such as malaria, dengue and cholera – is currently an active area of research,

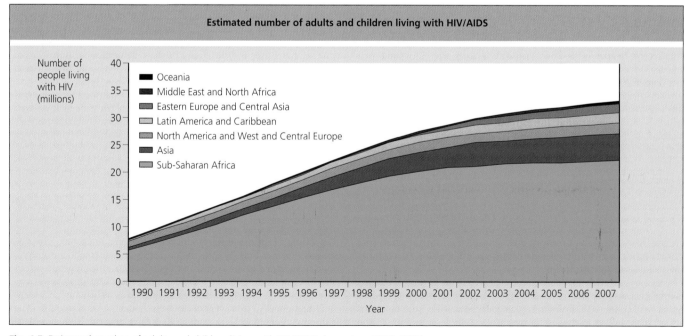

Fig. 4.5 Estimated number of adults and children living with HIV/AIDS, by region, 1990–2007.

which involves separating weather effects from other environmental factors that influence disease spread, such as land use, water management, urbanization and human behavior. From a public health point of view, the major challenge is to enhance surveillance for disease vectors and reservoirs, as well as for the diseases they carry, and to address all the factors that facilitate disease transmission. The potential introduction of disease vectors and reservoirs into new areas as weather patterns change is another reason why we need to be prepared for the unexpected. See Practice Point 1 for a further discussion on the relationship between health and climate change.

An ecologic approach to prevention and control of zoonotic and vector-borne diseases

The development of public health strategies to prevent and control zoonotic and vector-borne diseases – which include the great majority of new and re-emerging diseases[15] – requires an ecologic approach that takes into account the human, animal, microbial and environmental facts that influence disease emergence (see Fig. 4.1). In recognition of this fact, the Wildlife Conservation Society (WCS) has organized a series of *One World – One Health* symposia in New York, Thailand, China and Brazil to focus world attention on the 'essential link between human, domestic animal, and wildlife health' and the threat that animal diseases pose to people, food supplies and national economies.

A comprehensive approach to addressing these diseases would involve:

- new partnerships among experts in animal and human health, conservation biology, law and public policy;
- expansion of disease surveillance systems that integrate animal and public health data;
- routine availability of veterinary and entomologic expertise at public health departments; and
- development of an interdisciplinary research agenda to identify ecologic factors and interactions among animals, humans, and insects and their environments that influence disease emergence.

A better understanding of the ecologic factors that influence disease emergence will facilitate the development of innovative strategies for detection, control and prevention of zoonotic and vector-borne diseases such as the One Health Initiative (http://www.onehealthinitiative.com), as well as the creation of predictive models that indicate when outbreaks are likely to occur.

Infectious diseases as national security threat

From the end of the Cold War until 2001, US concerns about the impact of health issues on national security were focused primarily on events overseas[67] (Table 4.7). During the 1990s, security experts expressed particular concern about the destabilizing effects of HIV/AIDS in poor countries where high death rates among young adults have damaged economic, social, political, military and educational infrastructures and created vast numbers of orphans. In July 2000, the Group of Eight Industrialized Nations pledged to reduce deaths from HIV/AIDS, malaria, tuberculosis and vaccine-preventable diseases by supporting global health initiatives launched by the World Health Organization and other groups.[69] Combating HIV/AIDS and malaria was adopted by 189 nations as a Millennium Development Goal in 2000 (http://www.un.org/millenniumgoals), and the Global Fund to Fight AIDS, Tuberculosis and Malaria was established by the G8 in 2001 (http://www.theglobalfund.org/en). These ongoing international efforts reflect a growing consensus that global health security must be a shared responsibility.

Since the autumn of 2001, domestic security concerns have taken center stage, as they did in the 1950s, when the Epidemic Intelligence Service (EIS), the US training program for epidemiologists, was established in response to the Cold War threat of biologic warfare.[70] The anthrax attacks illustrated that the USA is vulnerable to bioterrorism,

---

Table 4.7 Biologic national security issues

- Diseases that spread across borders, crossing countries and continents (e.g. cholera, bacterial meningitis, measles, and pandemic influenza)
- The emergence of new and antibiotic-resistant diseases that arise in one region and spread throughout the world (e.g. AIDS and drug-resistant TB)
- Environmental issues that may have global effects (e.g. pollution, loss of biodiversity and global warming, which may affect the growth rate of insect vectors of disease)
- Population overgrowth that may lead to disease, war, famine, large-scale migration, and political instability
- Bioterrorism: the deliberate release of infectious agents by a terrorist or rogue nation

Adapted from Goldberg.[68]

---

stimulating renewed bioterrorism preparedness and response efforts. Of the 15 National Planning Scenarios developed by the White House Homeland Security Council to guide emergency preparedness exercises, five involve infectious disease threats (anthrax, pandemic influenza, plague, food contamination and disease of agricultural animals).

Physicians are one of the three cornerstones of the 'golden triangle' for bioterrorism preparedness, along with the health-care delivery system and public health officials.[71] All clinicians, regardless of their specialty, must have basic information about the clinical manifestations of such potential bioterrorist agents as variola virus (smallpox), *Yersinia pestis* (plague) and *Bacillus anthracis* (anthrax). They must have a high index of suspicion and know how to recognize unusual diseases and report them to local public health and law enforcement officials. The expertise and full engagement of the medical community are essential to the national effort to preserve health security. For further discussion of issues related to bioterrorism, see Chapter 71.

Pandemic influenza

New strains of influenza viruses can emerge unpredictably from animal reservoirs and spread rapidly and pervasively through susceptible populations, sometimes causing worldwide epidemics. This is due in large part to two features of the influenza virus: its ability to exchange genetic information between strains and its ability to occasionally 'jump' species barriers between avian and porcine (or other mammalian) hosts. Influenza pandemics typically cause major morbidity and mortality, with significant societal and economic impacts.[46]

The sudden and unpredictable emergence of a potential pandemic strain of influenza was illustrated in 1997 by an outbreak of avian influenza A (H5N1) in Hong Kong, which raised the specter of a worldwide epidemic similar to the one that killed 20–50 million people (including 500 000 Americans) in 1918. Epidemiologic studies suggested that the H5N1 virus was transmitted from chickens to people and only poorly (if at all) from person to person. Nevertheless, it was feared that the virus might reassort with a human influenza virus during the winter influenza season, creating a virulent strain capable of air-borne human-to-human transmission. To ensure that the H5N1 virus would have no opportunity to evolve, the Hong Kong government authorized the culling of all 1.6 million chickens in Hong Kong (see Box 4.1). Six years later (in 2003) influenza A (H5N1) re-merged in poultry in South East Asia and then spread to Central Asia, Africa, Europe and the Middle East, leading to a worldwide pandemic alert (http://www.who.int/csr/disease/avian_influenza/phase/en/index.html).

Unexpectedly, however, a different virus – unrelated to avian influenza A (H5N1) – has emerged as the cause of a new pandemic officially declared by WHO in June 2009. First detected in the United

States and Mexico, the pandemic (H1N1) 2009 virus was originally referred to as 'swine flu' virus because laboratory tests indicated that it contained genes similar to those of influenza viruses in North American pigs. However, further study has shown that this new virus is actually a 'quadruple reassortant' virus, which also contains gene segments from human, avian and Eurasian swine influenza viruses.

As of January 2010, the pandemic (H1N1) 2009 virus was the predominant influenza virus in circulation worldwide. Disease severity appeared to be generally similar to the severity of disease during recent influenza seasons, although different age groups have been predominantly affected, with most cases and most severe cases occurring in older children and adults less than 65 years of age (http://www.cdc.gov/h1n1flu/).

CONCLUSION

Now more than ever, global health and well-being depend on the vigilance of concerned and well-informed clinicians. Each and every clinician plays a critical role in the public health early warning system for unusual infectious diseases, whether they are new, rare, zoonotic, vector-borne, drug-resistant or intentionally caused. These efforts are essential to maintaining a strong and effective public health system.

REFERENCES

References for this chapter can be found online at http://www.expertconsult.com

Chapter | 5 |

Peter J White
Mark C Enright

Mathematical models in infectious disease epidemiology

The first mathematical model of infectious disease transmission was constructed by Bernoulli in 1760[1] to determine the effectiveness of variolation, a crude form of smallpox vaccination. Specifically he sought to calculate life tables for actuarial purposes assuming an eradication of smallpox in the population (for a review of Bernoulli's life and work, see Dietz & Heesterbeek[2]). Mathematical systems have been used extensively not only in the study of pandemic viral diseases such as AIDS, severe acute respiratory syndrome (SARS), influenza, smallpox and polio, but have also been successful in modeling transmission of bacterial pathogens including sexually transmitted infections (STIs) and methicillin-resistant *Staphylococcus aureus*, vector-borne diseases including malaria and diseases caused by macroparasites such as helminths.

Modern infectious disease epidemiology relies heavily on mathematical modeling to characterize the complex interactions between the biology and environment of human or animal hosts, the pathogens responsible for disease and, where present, vector species. Transmission models are vital for understanding the dynamics present in the spread of infectious agents in populations and for assessing the likely impact of public health interventions such as isolation, vaccination and chemotherapy. The defining characteristic of infectious diseases – that they are transmissible – means that an individual's risk of acquiring infection changes dynamically as levels of infection rise and fall in the population. Therefore vaccinating individuals or treating infectious individuals benefits not only the individual patient directly but also benefits others in the population indirectly by reducing their risk of acquiring infection through the reduction in levels of infection in the population. This was demonstrated by the effect of vaccination against pneumococcus: the incidence of infection with 'vaccine' serotypes fell in those who were older than the target group for vaccination who did not receive the vaccine, as well as those who were vaccinated.[3]

However, 'indirect' effects are not always beneficial and may even be harmful.[4] For example, whilst reducing levels of infection in the population through vaccination protects those who are not vaccinated as well as those who are vaccinated by reducing the overall rate of infection, those who do still get infected are older on average when they get infected and can suffer more severe disease outcomes, so vaccination can increase the overall rate of disease for a period, until infection is eliminated from the population.[4] Mathematical models can be constructed that can help predict these effects and aid the design of strategies to mitigate them.

Mathematical models of infectious disease transmission are increasingly being used to guide public health policy in the areas of naturally disseminated pathogens such as viruses, bacteria and fungi and in developing response measures to mitigate the human and environmental costs caused by the deliberate release of infectious agents, i.e. bioterrorism.[5] Examples include the control of an epidemic of foot-and-mouth disease in the UK in 2001,[6,7] the SARS outbreak of 2003,[8,9] planning control strategies for TB, HIV and STIs,[10–13] and planning for pandemic influenza,[14,15] as well as examining general principles of disease control.[16]

Importantly for infectious diseases, there is typically a complex nonlinear relationship between the size of an intervention and the benefits. This is due to the 'indirect' effects interventions have on those who are not treated by changing levels of infection in the population, which affects the risk of acquiring infection.

As the scale of an intervention (e.g. vaccination coverage or provision of treatment) increases from a low level, the benefits – reductions in levels of disease – increase faster than the costs, until disease has been reduced to a low level or even eliminated. This means that when health economic analyses are performed to determine the cost-effectiveness of interventions, it is essential that the models take account of the transmissible nature of infectious diseases and the 'indirect' effects of interventions.[17] One example is vaccination, where vaccinating only a small proportion of the population mostly benefits only those who receive the vaccine because it does little to interrupt transmission, i.e. the indirect effect is small. Vaccinating a large proportion of the population can prevent epidemics, providing a large indirect benefit to those who were not vaccinated in addition to the direct benefit. Another example is in the control of curable infections (e.g. STIs) through treatment: if treatment capacity is inadequate then there is a 'vicious circle' where failing to control transmission in the present results in more infections in the future, maintaining the inadequacy of treatment capacity.[13] Conversely, making a concerted effort to increase capacity can break this vicious circle and change it to a virtuous circle, where promptly treating a large enough proportion of infections reduces transmission rates, allowing a more intense focus on remaining disease and reducing future need for treatment, leading to significant cost savings.[13]

Infectious disease epidemiology is inherently multidisciplinary because the transmission of infection within a population is affected not just by the biologic characteristics of the infectious agent and its human host, but also by the patterns of contact between individuals, their use of health services, their response to public health interventions, etc. Mathematical models enable information from diverse sources, including social sciences, to be integrated. Infectious disease modeling is not a purely technical, 'mathematical' exercise – many modelers come from biologic or clinical backgrounds.

EPIDEMIOLOGIC DATA

The fundamental measures of the epidemiology of a pathogen in a population are the incidence and prevalence, which are sometimes confused in the nonspecialist literature. Incidence is the number of new infections arising per unit time, and is usually expressed at x% per year or x cases per 1000 per year or x cases per 100 000 per year.

Prevalence is the proportion of the population (usually expressed as a percentage) that is infected at a point in time and is measured by cross-sectional surveys. Incidence can be measured directly in longitudinal cohort studies, where a group of subjects is followed through time, or can be calculated from a series of cross-sectional prevalence surveys.[18] Case notifications are often used as a proxy measure for incidence; long-term datasets are available for a large number of infectious agents due to mandatory (notifiable) disease surveillance schemes in developed countries. Historical datasets containing valuable information on causes of death and age, in some cases going back for hundreds of years, are also available. These datasets are rather subjective but have been useful in examining epidemics such as the Black Death (plague) and smallpox.

Table 5.1 lists 30 disease agents that are currently notifiable by clinicians to the Health Protection Agency (HPA) in the UK and similar arrangements are in place with the Centers for Disease Control and Prevention (CDC) in the USA. In developed countries demographic and clinical information is collected by clinicians when examining patients and raw incidence data can therefore usually be stratified by sex, age, ethnicity, spatial location and other factors such as tobacco and alcohol consumption. This is important because incidence can vary markedly across different groups of people. Such stratified longitudinal studies, where populations are placed into discrete classes, are extremely useful in examining trends of infection rates. In many of these datasets the impact of vaccination on childhood infectious diseases is striking.

Models are tools used throughout science and medicine – they are used to derive diagnoses from observed signs and symptoms and test results. Formulating models mathematically facilitates rigorous analysis and allows quantitative predictions to be made of trends in disease burden and the impact of interventions. The benefit of quantitative analysis in research is that one can determine if a putative cause for an observed effect would have been strong enough to cause the effect – for example, a mathematical modeling analysis of the HIV epidemic in Uganda found that several modes of behavior change (delaying sexual debut, reducing numbers of sexual partners, increasing condom use) must have occurred to explain the observed decline in prevalence. This is because no single change was sufficient to account for the reduced disease burden observed.[19]

Crucially, models allow evaluation of the impact of interventions that have been implemented by allowing comparison with what would have happened in the absence of the intervention. Epidemics have 'natural dynamics', with incidence typically rising to a peak then declining in the absence of any intervention. Therefore, simply observing a decline in incidence following an intervention is not sufficient evidence to demonstrate its effectiveness.[19] Indeed, in some circumstances it is even possible to observe incidence continue to rise despite an effective intervention, due to an increase in the prevalence of infection.[20]

Another important use of models is in setting priorities for empiric research by determining the importance of different 'gaps' in knowledge. This is done by testing the 'sensitivity' of a model's behavior to changes in the value of parameters that are poorly estimated by current data – for example, there is uncertainty in the amount of protection that bacille Calmette–Guérin (BCG) vaccination offers against TB acquisition and against progression to disease in those who are infected. By testing how much varying these parameters affects a model's behavior we can determine how important it is to obtain more precise estimates of each parameter.

DYNAMICS OF INFECTIOUS DISEASE TRANSMISSION

The transmissibility of infectious diseases means that there is dynamic feedback between the prevalence of infection (or, more precisely, of infectious individuals) and the incidence of infection. This is why dynamic models are required for infectious diseases.

In a typical epidemic, the prevalence of infection rises initially as infection spreads. This causes an increase in the incidence of infection, which in turn causes prevalence to increase even faster – so the epidemic accelerates. Consequently, the supply of susceptible individuals becomes depleted (by their becoming infected) and the incidence falls, even though prevalence may continue to rise for a time. Eventually, the fall in incidence leads to a fall in prevalence because infections are 'lost' from the population (due to recovery, death or emigration) faster than they are replaced by the spreading of infection. In the longer term, the infectious agent may be able to persist in the population (i.e. become endemic) if there is a high enough rate of resupply of susceptible individuals due to birth, immigration, recovery from infection (if there is no lasting immunity) or waning of immunity (if applicable); otherwise the infectious agent will go extinct locally.

The key measure of an infectious agent's ability to spread in a population is the reproduction number (sometimes called the net reproduction number or effective reproduction number), $R(t)$, which is the mean number of new infections caused by a single infectious individual in the population of interest. (Note that '(t)' indicates that the value can change with time – see below.) A related quantity is the basic reproduction number R_0, which is defined as the mean number of new infections caused by a single infectious individual in a population of wholly susceptible individuals, i.e. the basic reproduction number is what the value of the reproduction number would be if the population were totally susceptible. It is important to understand that the reproduction number is specific to the particular infectious agent in the particular population at the particular time, and can be changed by interventions. The value of the reproduction number depends upon the average rate of transmission from an infectious individual and the average duration of infectiousness. An epidemic requires that $R(t)$ be greater than 1, so that the prevalence of infection increases because more than one new infection arises from the

---

Table 5.1 Infectious diseases notifiable to the United Kingdom Health Protection Agency

- Acute encephalitis
- Acute poliomyelitis
- Anthrax
- Cholera
- Diphtheria
- Dysentery
- Food poisoning
- Leprosy
- Leptospirosis
- Malaria
- Measles
- Meningitis
- Meningococcal septicemia (without meningitis)
- Mumps
- Ophthalmia neonatorum
- Paratyphoid fever
- Plague
- Rabies
- Relapsing fever
- Rubella
- Scarlet fever
- Smallpox
- Tetanus
- Tuberculosis
- Typhoid fever
- Typhus fever
- Viral hemorrhagic fever
- Viral hepatitis
- Whooping cough
- Yellow fever

average infected person before that person is 'lost' from the infected population. In the typical epidemic described above, depletion of the 'supply' of susceptible individuals causes $R(t)$ to fall, even though R_0 was not changing. In fact, $R(t)$ falls even as incidence rises; the increase in incidence is driven by the increase in prevalence, which initially 'overcomes' the effect of $R(t)$ falling.

Public health interventions aim to reduce and maintain $R(t)$ below 1, which may be achieved by reducing the average infectious period (e.g. through treatment or isolation) or the transmission rate (e.g. by closing schools and workplaces to combat SARS or influenza, or promoting condom use and reductions in numbers of sexual partners to combat STIs) or vaccinating people to remove them from the susceptible population. The higher the value of R_0, the harder an infection will be to control. In a homogeneous population (one where everyone has the same average risk of acquiring and transmitting infection) the relationship between R_0 and $R(t)$ is $R(t) = R_0 \times s$ where s is the proportion of the population that is susceptible. To prevent an epidemic by vaccination requires that s be reduced so that $R(t) <1$ (i.e. that s be reduced below $1/R_0$), thus the greater the value of R_0 the smaller s must be. The critical vaccination threshold is the proportion of the population that must be successfully immunized to prevent an epidemic; for childhood infections such as measles which have high typical R_0 values this is typically >90% or even >95%.

It is important to realize that R_0 alone does not provide complete information on the transmission dynamics of an infectious agent. A highly infectious agent that spreads rapidly but which has a short infectious period could have the same R_0 value as another infectious agent that is much less infectious but which has a longer infectious period – the latter agent would spread more slowly but for longer.

COMPARTMENTAL MODELS OF INFECTION

The most common approach used in mathematical modeling of disease transmission is to divide or compartmentalize the study population with regard to their infection status (Fig. 5.1). Note that the structure of the model depends upon the natural history of the infection and so differs amongst infections. Important characteristics of the natural history of an infection are the incubation period (the time from the point of infection until the appearance of symptoms) and the latent period (the time from infection to becoming infectious). These periods vary greatly (from days to years, depending upon the infection) and either can be longer than the other. For HIV and influenza the latent period is shorter than the incubation period, with people becoming infectious before they become unwell, but for pulmonary TB they can be the same, with people becoming infectious at the time they become unwell.

In modeling there is a trade-off between complexity/realism and the ability to understand the model's behavior. Since even simple models can have complex dynamics it is important to make the model as simple as possible, whilst still capturing the essential features of the infection. For example, for gonorrhea the incubation period is often omitted from models[13] because it is short relative to the infectious period – and so has little effect on the dynamics of infection – while HIV's incubation period is long compared with the symptomatic late-stage period and so it is usually incorporated into models.[21] In the case of TB, most people with infection never develop infectious disease (they remain latently infected) and so models distinguish between these states.[22]

For a directly transmitted pathogen such as influenza, where acquired immunity (to a particular strain) is lifelong, the host population can be represented by three compartments containing the number of susceptible, infected (and infectious) and recovered (immune, non-infectious) individuals. In this example, the latent period is ignored, so individuals become infectious as soon as they become infected. This so-called called 'Susceptible–Infected–Recovered' (or 'SIR') model approach was first developed by Kermack & McKendrick in 1927,[23] elaborated upon more recently by Anderson & May,[4] and now forms the basis for many modern-day models of epidemics.

We present a simple example of an SIR-type model (see Fig. 5.1), which we apply to data from an outbreak of influenza in a boarding school in England.[24] Since the time period of the outbreak is short, we effectively have a 'closed' population: no one enters or leaves the population and there was no mortality due to infection, which simplifies our analysis. (Usually, one has to consider people entering the population through immigration and birth and leaving through emigration and death – and if the infection being modeled causes mortality then infected individuals have an additional disease-induced mortality rate which must be considered.)

Each compartment has a state variable that 'keeps track' of the number of individuals in that compartment, and how that number changes through time. In this case, the state variables are $X(t)$ for the Susceptible individuals, $Y(t)$ for the Infected individuals and $Z(t)$ for the Recovered individuals, where '(t)' indicates that the values can change with time. The total population size is $N(t)$, where $N(t) = X(t) + Y(t) + Z(t)$. (In this particular example, $N(t)$ does not change because the population is closed and there is no mortality.) The model consists of a set of differential equations which describe the rates that individuals flow between different compartments as they become infected, recover, die (if applicable), etc. The net rate of change in $X(t)$ is described by the differential equation $dX(t)/dt$, the net rate of change in $Y(t)$ is described by the differential equation $dY(t)/dt$, etc. In this example, there are two processes: infection and recovery.

The rate of infection (the number of people becoming infected per day) in the population depends upon the force of infection, the risk per susceptible individual of acquiring infection per unit time; and the number of susceptible individuals available to become infected, $X(t)$. The force of infection depends upon the prevalence of infection, $Y(t)/N(t)$, and the transmission parameter, β, which is a combination of the rate of contact between people in the population and the probability of transmission upon contact between an infected person and a susceptible person. Therefore, the force of infection is $\beta Y(t)/N(t)$ and the transmission rate is $X(t) \times \beta Y(t)/N(t)$, which is conventionally written as $\beta X(t)Y(t)/N(t)$. Since infection transfers people from the susceptible compartment ($X(t)$) to the infected compartment ($Y(t)$), the term $\beta X(t)Y(t)/N(t)$ appears negatively in $dX(t)/dt$ and positively in $dY(t)/dt$. (Note that the transmission parameter, β, does not change with time; changes in the infection rate are due to changes in $Y(t)/N(t)$ and $X(t)$.)

The rate of recovery (the number of people recovering per day) depends upon the per capita rate of recovery, γ, and the number of people who are infected, $Y(t)$, and is $\gamma Y(t)$. Since recovery transfers people from the Infected compartment ($Y(t)$) to the Recovered compartment ($Z(t)$), the term $\gamma Y(t)$ appears negatively in $dY(t)/dt$ and positively in $dZ(t)/dt$. (Note that the per capita rate of recovery, γ, does not change with time; changes in the recovery rate are due to changes in $Y(t)$.)

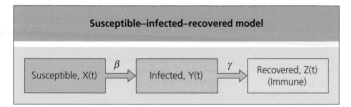

Susceptible–infected–recovered model

Susceptible, X(t) $\xrightarrow{\beta}$ Infected, Y(t) $\xrightarrow{\gamma}$ Recovered, Z(t) (Immune)

Fig. 5.1 The population is divided into three compartments according to whether they are Susceptible to infection, Infected (and infectious) or have Recovered from infection and are immune. Individuals who become infected move from the Susceptible compartment to the Infected compartment; the process of recovery subsequently moves them from the Infected compartment to the Recovered compartment. The parameters β and γ affect the rate of transmission of infection and the rate of recovery, respectively.

The equations of the model are:

$$\frac{dX(t)}{dt} = \frac{-\beta X(t)Y(t)}{N(t)}$$

$$\frac{dY(t)}{dt} = \frac{\beta X(t)Y(t)}{N(t)} - \gamma Y(t)$$

$$\frac{dZ(t)}{dt} = \gamma Y(t)$$

$$N(t) = X(t) + Y(t) + Z(t)$$

Note that this model is deterministic, i.e. random (stochastic) events are not considered. This is a common simplification that makes it much easier to gain insight into the fundamental dynamics of transmission because the effects of random chance, which cause fluctuations in the graph, are omitted. This model was fitted to data from an outbreak of influenza in a boarding school in England[24] (Fig. 5.2) by estimating values of β and γ.

The algebraic expression for R_0 depends upon the particular model. For this model, it can be derived simply. R_0 is the mathematical product of the transmission rate from a single infected individual in a wholly susceptible population and the average infectious period. The rate of transmission from a single infected individual when the population is wholly susceptible (i.e. when $Y(t) = 1$ and $X(t) = N(t)$; we ignore the fact that really $X(t) = N(t) - 1$ because one person is infected, because we assume that $N(t)$ is large) is:

$$\frac{\beta X(t)Y(t)}{N(t)} = \frac{\beta N(t).1}{N(t)} = \beta$$

The average infectious period is the reciprocal of the average recovery rate (the faster people recover, the shorter their infectious period), which is $1/\gamma$. Therefore $R_0 = \beta/\gamma$. The estimated values of β and γ obtained by fitting to the data were $\beta = 1.97$ per day, $\gamma = 0.47$ per day (corresponding to a mean infectious period of 2.12 days). Therefore the estimated R_0 value was 1.97 day^{-1}/0.47 day^{-1} = 4.18.

Note that there are other types of model used to represent infectious disease transmission, including stochastic compartmental models, individual-based network simulation models and spatial metapopulation models.[25]

EXAMPLES

Below we discuss SARS and influenza. Recent reviews of modeling of STIs and HIV[10,26,27] and TB[22] can be found elsewhere.

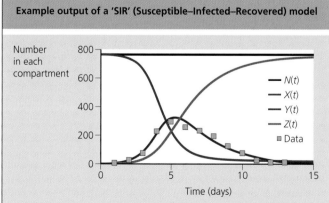

Example output of a 'SIR' (Susceptible–Infected–Recovered) model

Number in each compartment

— $N(t)$
— $X(t)$
— $Y(t)$
— $Z(t)$
▪ Data

Time (days)

Fig. 5.2 Example output of a Susceptible–Infected–Recovered (SIR) model applied to data from an outbreak of influenza. Model parameters were adjusted to fit the number of Infected individuals, $Y(t)$, to the observed data.

Severe acute respiratory syndrome

The huge rise in the volume of international travel and the huge growth in population densities in many cities, especially in Asia, offer new challenges in controlling the spread of new epidemics. The first such epidemic, 'the first severe and readily transmitted disease of the 21st century' was SARS.[28] On November 16, 2002 the first human case of SARS was identified in Guangdong province in China. From here the disease is known to have spread quickly to other parts of Asia, then to Europe, the Americas and elsewhere, infecting >8000 individuals in 29 countries and killing at least 774 people.[8,28] SARS is caused by a coronavirus (SARS-CoV) normally found in wild animals such as the palm civet cat and Chinese ferret badger.[29] Early cases are thought to have involved zoonotic infection from animal reservoirs, a jumping of the species barrier, but genetic changes in the coronavirus enabled human-to-human transmission which accounted for the vast majority of cases in the global pandemic of 2002/3.

The causative agent of SARS was identified at an early stage of the outbreak and its genome was sequenced in a timely effort involving a multinational collaborative effort.[30] The sequence, published on May 30, 2003, showed it to be a single-stranded RNA virus containing 11 presumptive genes (open reading frames). Other RNA viruses include influenza and HIV and these are thought to be particularly prone to mutation as they are not proofread by DNA polymerases before transcription. The WHO global alert of March 2003 alerted countries to the spread of SARS and accurate case definitions were communicated to identify symptomatic carriers worldwide which led to the rapid control of the disease. This effective collaboration between health-care professionals in different countries and the sharing of patient and demographic data informed public health policy which limited the scale of the epidemic so that more than half of the countries affected reported fewer than 10 cases.

Sophisticated mathematical models of the SARS epidemic of 2002/3 have been developed, providing estimates of the key epidemiologic quantities and showing how disease transmission was controlled by effective intervention. The mean incubation period of SARS was reported to be between 4 and 6 days in most patients with a generation time of 8–12 days. The number of reported cases in the epidemic with time were used to estimate the initial growth rate (r, the rate of exponential increase in new cases at the start of an epidemic) which is related to the basic reproduction number (R_0) and the generation time (Tg, the mean period of time from a host becoming infected to infecting another individual) by the equation $R_0 = rTg + 1$. Using data from the initial period (before control measures were introduced) of the SARS epidemic in Hong Kong the epidemic growth rate was shown to be approximately 0.15 cases per day[31] which, when used in the above equation with $Tg = 10$, gives an R_0 value of 2.5, an estimate close to that made by analyses of data from Singapore by Lipsitch et al.[32] of between 2.2 and 3.6 days. Wallinga & Teunis[33] analyzed incidence data from four countries before and after the WHO global alert and subsequent control measures of March 2003. Before and after the alert, average $Z(t)$ values for Hong Kong, Vietnam, Singapore and Canada were 3.6 before the alert (0.7 after), 2.4 (0.3), 3.1 (0.7) and 2.7 (1), respectively. The reduction in the reproductive number in each country reflects the effectiveness of control measures such as quarantine and travel restrictions in curbing the epidemic.

SARS transmission was linked to close contact with another case and most of these were hospital-acquired infections of health-care workers or patients.[8,34] The mortality due to SARS calculated from WHO figures of 8098 probable SARS cases and 774 deaths gives a crude case fatality rate (CFR) of approximately 10.5%; however, the actual CFR is strongly positively correlated with age, with mortality in those over 65 years old exceeding 50% in a number of studies reviewed in Donnelly et al.[8] Estimating the case fatality rate of newly emerged pathogens is difficult as defining true cases can be problematic. The CFR may be overestimated if many subclinical infections go uncounted. Alternatively, in epidemics where patients are hospitalized for lengthy periods, the CFR may be underestimated as patients can be recorded as cases before their outcome is known. In the 2003 SARS epidemic estimates of the CFR became more accurate as the fate of more patients became known but at the time this increasing CFR was wrongly taken as evidence that the virus was increasing in virulence.[8]

Influenza

In common with SARS, influenza is a disease that has been extensively modeled using data from past pandemics to predict the effectiveness of particular interventions in different disease scenarios. Influenza A is divided into subtypes based on differences in hemagglutinin (H) and neuraminidase (N) proteins. The 'Spanish flu' of the 1918 pandemic was an H1N1 lineage that was estimated to have caused up to 80 million deaths – many more than were killed in the First and Second World Wars combined. Small alterations to the influenza A genome occur by a process known as antigenic drift, where mutations increase in prevalence in the population driven by the selection of mutations in the viral genome in proteins exposed to the host immune system. These small changes lead to the differing severity of seasonal flu epidemics.

From a public health perspective the rarer phenomenon of antigenic shift is much more worrying. This results from the recombination of influenza genes to give novel combinations of virulence genes such as strains of avian flu of the H5N1 subtype that is widely feared to be the cause of the next pandemic wave of influenza. Past pandemic strains of influenza A are thought to have emerged from animal reservoirs following antigenic shifts that enabled them to become extremely pathogenic to humans, with surface proteins to which the host had little acquired immunity. Pandemic influenza differs from seasonal epidemic strains not only in the severity of infection but in other ways also. It is not restricted to the 'flu season' of the winter months and it tends to be most lethal in young children who presumably lack the immune memory of older patients.

In 2008 an epidemic of H5N1 influenza amongst Asian and African wild bird and poultry populations led to 385 cases of human disease resulting in 243 deaths – a case fatality rate of 63%.[35] These cases were overwhelmingly in individuals from Indonesia and Vietnam who had been in contact with poultry later shown to be infected with H5N1 strains. Control measures to destroy birds infected with H5N1 have been effective in limiting the number of human cases thus far but experts fear that a strain of highly pathogenic H5N1 will emerge that will acquire the ability to transmit between humans at high frequency which would lead to a global pandemic.

The 1918 influenza pandemic claimed between 50 and 100 million lives worldwide,[36] even although effective infection control procedures were in place in some areas (e.g. in some US cities). Bootsma & Ferguson[37] modeled the impact of infection control measures (such as the banning of mass gatherings, isolation, and improved hygiene and disinfection procedures) on transmission of the H1N1 epidemic in 16 US cities using historical datasets. The found that R_0 was reduced in cities with the most effective control measures (introduced at an early stage), which increased the length of the epidemic but reduced the overall and peak mortality. These data indicate that control measures may have a significant impact on a future H5N1 pandemic if introduced early in the course of the pandemic – in this case reducing mortality by 30–40%. The authors of this study caution against extrapolating data from the study too precisely on modern cities as family units and workplaces nowadays contain fewer people who are generally healthier. However, an H5N1 virus causing death in 14–33% of individuals infected would be expected to kill more individuals globally. This mortality could be mitigated by the rapid deployment of an effective H5N1 vaccine and the use of antiviral drugs such as neuraminidase and influenza A protein M2 inhibitors.[38]

Modeling pandemic influenza

A case fatality rate of 63% for avian influenza (from the number of cases and fatalities reported by WHO above) will be higher than the CFR during a pandemic as the number of cases reported so far will be an underestimate due to the non-inclusion of many nonfatal, mild and asymptomatic cases which will not be entered on the WHO reporting system. Additionally, some authors maintain that changes in the viral genome resulting in high rates of human-to-human transmission may cause a reduction in virulence in humans. From historical data the CFR for pandemic influenza A was calculated at between 0.1% (1957 and 1968 pandemics) and 2.5% (1918).[39] However, a recent article by Li et al.[39] suggests that a CFR of between 14% and 33% may be more realistic for a human transmissible H5N1 strain derived from an avian reservoir.

The examination of the SARS epidemic using mathematical models demonstrates some key qualities that enabled it to be contained effectively; however, when we compare these to features of past influenza epidemics and pandemics it appears that containing a future H5N1 pandemic will be much more difficult using similar containment/control measures. The generation time for influenza (4–6 days)[40] is much shorter than for SARS (8–12 days)[9,32] which means that influenza will spread much quicker than SARS given an overwhelmingly naive population (e.g. an H5N1 genotype epidemic). This will make a human transmissible H5N1 epidemic much harder to control than SARS. The R_0 of SARS of ~2.5 is similar if not higher than that estimated from reanalyses of pandemic influenza of 1.4–3.0,[40,41] but with a much higher expected CFR. In younger age groups in particular the impact of H5N1 would be expected to be much more costly not only in terms of disease but also from an economic viewpoint as a larger proportion and number of working-age individuals will be removed from the workforce by influenza.

One caveat about H5N1 that should be mentioned is that the factor that has primarily restricted transmission from birds to humans is that the sialic acid linkage favoured for binding to respiratory epithelium by highly pathogenic H5N1 is found primarily in the lower respiratory tracts of humans. This is one of the reasons that respiratory distress is such a common cause of death. The relative lack of these receptors in the upper respiratory epithelium causes much lower titers of virus to grow in nasal mucosa; hence, the virus is more pathogenic but much less transmissible by infected humans. In order to maintain its pathogenicity, the virus would need to maintain its tropism for the lower respiratory epithelial sialic acid receptor linkage and to acquire the ability to simultaneously bind to sialic acid linkages present in upper respiratory epithelium. It is quite possible (indeed likely) that the virus would have to compromise and be less pathogenic if it becomes more transmissible. Thus, a more highly transmissible H5N1 might be less transmissible than SARS and currently circulating strains of influenza A and less pathogenic than the strains that have to date been acquired directly from birds.

FUTURE RESEARCH

There is increasing integration between infectious disease modeling and empiric research in the field and laboratory. As noted above, models can be used to help set research priorities by determining which gaps in knowledge are most important epidemiologically. Increases in computing power make it possible to develop increasingly sophisticated simulation models and to use them in real-time to analyze outbreaks to determine whether interventions are working and to guide policymakers in their response. DNA finger-printing techniques are being used to identify clusters of transmission between individuals[42,43] and there is currently a lot of interest in synthesizing analysis of evolution and transmission dynamics, termed 'phylodynamics'.[44] Another area of research is in characterizing contact patterns between individuals in more detail[45] since this has important consequences for patterns of transmission. Finally, the use of modeling in planning and evaluating clinical trials has been advocated.[46]

REFERENCES

References for this chapter can be found online at http://www.expertconsult.com

Chapter | 6 |

Francesca Torriani
Randy Taplitz

History of infection prevention and control

In the United States, the hospital discipline of infection control was established in the 1950s in response to a nationwide epidemic of nosocomial *Staphylococcus aureus* and the recognition of the need for nosocomial infection surveillance.[1] As a concept, however, the epidemiology and prevention of infection has its roots in a time prior to the understanding of the germ theory of disease. In 1846 Semmelweis, a Hungarian physician, noted that the mortality from childbed fever among women who had babies delivered by midwives was lower than among mothers with babies delivered by physicians. After in-depth analysis of differences between the groups, Semmelweis concluded that the high rate of childbed fever was caused by cadaverous materials on the hands of medical students who came to the obstetric clinic directly from the autopsy chamber. A policy of hand washing in chlorinated lime solution before maternal contact was instituted, and the mortality rate among mothers cared for by physicians dropped.[2] John Snow, a British physician, applied statistics and epidemiologic approaches to determine and eradicate the source of a cholera outbreak in 1854 in London. The theories underlying the findings of both Semmelweis and Snow – that disease could be spread by hand contamination and fecal–oral transmission – were soundly rejected by the medical community in favor of the miasma or 'bad air' theory of disease causation. These two examples highlight not only some of the conceptual framework for medical epidemiology and infection control but also some of the challenges that face public health and infection control practitioners.

TRENDS AND COMPLEXITY OF CURRENT HEALTH CARE IN DEVELOPED COUNTRIES

Health-care-associated infections (HAIs) are a significant cause of morbidity and mortality in developed countries. It is estimated that between 5% and 10% of patients admitted to acute care hospitals acquire one or more infections. Using a multistep approach and three data sources, the Division of Healthcare Quality Promotion of the Centers for Disease Control and Prevention (CDC) estimated that the number of HAIs in US hospitals in 2002 was approximately 1.7 million. Thirty-two percent of all HAIs were urinary tract infections, 22% surgical site infections, 15% pneumonia and 14% bloodstream infections. The estimated number of deaths associated with HAIs in US hospitals in this study was approximately 99 000. The total number of deaths associated with HAIs by major site was highest for pneumonia (35 967) and bloodstream infection (30 655). The additional cost of patient care attributable to these infections was estimated to be $4.5–5.7 billion per year.[3,4] In the UK in 2000, it was estimated that 100 000 cases of hospital-acquired infection occurred in England with 5000 deaths, costing the National Health Services (NHS) as much as £1bn ($1.4bn) a year.[5]

In addition to the challenges posed by the numbers of HAIs, the complexity of these HAIs and the measures required to prevent them have become more complicated. Additional challenges that come under the umbrella of hospital infection prevention also continue to be identified. Such challenges include:

- controlling antimicrobial resistance and spread of multidrug-resistant pathogens;
- addressing emerging infections such as severe acute respiratory syndrome (SARS) and avian flu;
- providing constantly updated data for an increasingly sophisticated public;
- attempting to modernize surveillance and reporting systems, often with limited resources available;
- addressing the infectious consequences of ever more complicated medical procedures, with special populations such as highly immunosuppressed transplant patients, gene therapy, xenotransplantation; and
- maintaining a safe workplace in an ever more complex medical system.

ORGANIZATION OF INFECTION PREVENTION AND CONTROL

Infection prevention and control is a discipline in which epidemiologic and statistical principles are used in order to prevent or control the incidence and prevalence of infection. The primary role of an infection prevention and control program (IPCP) is to reduce the risk of acquisition of hospital-acquired infection, thereby protecting both patients and staff from adverse infection-related outcomes. In order to ensure that an infection control program is successful, the appropriate infrastructure and institutional support, both material and administrative, needs to be made available to hospital epidemiology staff.

The functions and structure of a hospital epidemiology program may vary between institutions. The critical functions that often fall under the umbrella of a hospital epidemiology program are listed in Table 6.1.[1,6,7]

Managing critical data and information
Developing, implementing and monitoring surveillance based upon an institution-specific risk assessment

The importance of surveillance as a part of hospital infection control programs was established by the 1976 Study on the Efficacy of Nosocomial Infection Control (SENIC). SENIC found that hospitals reduced their nosocomial infection rates by about 32% if their surveillance and control plan included the following components:

Table 6.1 Critical functions often managed by hospital epidemiology

- Managing critical data and information
  - Developing, implementing and monitoring surveillance based upon an institution-specific risk assessment
  - Reporting of surveillance results/infection rates to monitoring services, administration and regulatory bodies
- Developing and implementing policies and procedures to prevent or minimize infection risk (e.g. isolation precaution policies, etc.)
- Intervening to prevent disease transmission
  - Outbreak investigation and control
  - Education and training
- Collaborating with other programs to achieve common goals
  - Occupational and employee health
    - Postexposure prophylaxis in the health-care setting
    - Management of the infected health-care worker
  - Environmental health and safety
    - Construction infection control
    - Infectious waste management
    - Environmental cleaning service
    - Air and water handling
    - Respiratory protection
  - Disinfection and sterilization
  - Microbiology laboratory
    - Monitoring for isolation of sentinel organisms
    - Monitoring antibiotic resistance profiles
  - Pharmacy and therapeutics
    - Antibiotic utilization
  - Safety, quality and public reporting
  - Disaster preparedness committee
    - Bioterrorism preparedness

appropriate emphasis on surveillance activities and control efforts; appropriate staffing of the infection control program; and, for surgical site infections, feedback of wound infection rates to practicing surgeons.[8] Surveillance for nosocomial infection is critical for infection control programs, but must be paired with appropriate risk assessment at any given institution or setting, assessment of the need for intervention and strategies for implementation of control measures.[9]

Hospital infection surveillance should be a systematic, ongoing process to monitor identifiable events (such as surgical site infection) in a defined population. This will initially require a risk stratification to determine what the critical targets of surveillance should be. In the USA and other developed countries, many surveillance activities will be mandated by local or federal authorities, such as the Centers for Disease Control and Prevention (CDC), the American Hospital Association and the regulatory efforts of the Joint Commission (TJC). Other surveillance activities will vary, based on an understanding of the epidemiology and risk at a particular institution. For instance, surveillance for invasive aspergillosis in an institution undergoing new construction and with a large compromised host population might be rated a higher priority than the long-term monitoring of *Legionella* in an institution where *Legionella* has not been identified for years. Each hospital must tailor its surveillance activities based on risk assessment of the population as well as the available resources within the infection control team and hospital. Such 'targeted' surveillance should be defined for each hospital.[10]

A number of components are critical for an effective surveillance system.

1. Clear and uniform definitions of the infection or other outcome should be developed. Often, standardized definitions such as those defined by the CDC are the most useful so that comparisons can be made both within the system and with other institutions.[11]
2. Surveillance should be an active process that includes review of microbiologic data, clinical and nursing records, pharmacologic and pathologic data, readmission and reoperation data following surgery for selected procedures, etc. These data are made more easily accessible by computer-based patient records and

other electronic systems for data retrieval and coordination. Indeed, automated surveillance systems for infection control may provide a sensitive, specific, time-efficient and cost-effective mechanism for surveillance in many institutions.[12,13] The surveillance methodology should rely on metrics that are objective, standardized and risk adjusted. Case validation by the practitioners of the procedural area under evaluation should be avoided; in this setting the process may be prone to bias and lose objectivity, especially if financial incentives are involved. On the other hand, periodic review of the case definitions and feedback on the surveillance should include members of the practice team in order to provide insights not necessarily within the skill set of the infection control team and to devise corrective quality improvement actions adapted to that specific practice.

3. Whatever the system of surveillance is, both numerator and denominator data must be available for review. For instance, central line-associated bloodstream infections (CLABSI) are generally expressed as number of CLABSI/number of central line days × 1000. This allows the surveillance to be expressed as a rate such that trends can be tracked and compared within and between institutions.[14]
4. Appropriate benchmarking should be sought. Increasingly, health-care systems are being asked to compare their rates of events to other institutions. In the USA between 1992 and 2004 the National Nosocomial Infections Surveillance (NNIS) System collected data regarding targeted infections from participating tertiary care hospitals; this system was reorganized in 2005 under the National Health and Safety Network (NHSN). Data provided from this network can be used for benchmarking infections between hospitals. However, although standardized data may be useful for identifying areas deserving more intensive interventions within a given institution, differences in hospital size, patient mix and risk adjustment introduce complexity when comparing rates across the spectrum from smaller community hospitals to tertiary care and specialty hospitals.[15,16]
5. Reports describing the surveillance activities and findings should be prepared (using appropriate statistical analysis) and distributed to the appropriate groups, which should include the services associated with the monitoring process and the administrative liaison affiliated with the service.
6. After feedback to the particular service is provided, that service (generally in conjunction with the IPCP) should develop an action plan for process improvement, if needed. This plan, after approval by all relevant parties, should be implemented. If possible, the next surveillance cycle should be used to evaluate if improvements occurred associated with the action plan.

Develop and implement policies and procedures to prevent or minimize infection risk (e.g. isolation precaution policies, etc.)

Another critical role for the infection control unit within a health-care facility is to develop and implement evidence-based policies and procedures that are aimed at preventing HAIs. These policies need to be practicable and available as a written or online resource to users. In general, these policies will be adapted to institutional needs using resources available from the following:

- relevant published literature;
- Healthcare Infection Control Practices Advisory Committee (HICPAC), Society for Healthcare Epidemiology of America (SHEA) and Association for Professionals in Infection Control and Epidemiology (APIC) guidelines;
- professional practice guidelines;
- state and federal regulatory bodies;
- Occupational Safety and Health Administration (OSHA);
- Environmental Protection Agency (EPA), etc.

Institutional policies and procedures should be regularly reviewed and updated.

Intervene to prevent disease transmission

Outbreak investigation and control

An outbreak can be defined as an increase in the incidence of a disease/infection above the background rate in a given population. In a health-care setting, the 'background' rate may be provided by ongoing surveillance activities as described above. In the health-care setting, prompt identification of an outbreak and intervention on the part of the IPCP is critical in preventing adverse outcomes and accruing costs. Whether the outbreak under investigation is SARS or methicillin-resistant *Staphylococcus aureus* (MRSA), or an increase in the baseline rate of hip prosthesis infection, the same basic components of outbreak investigation are followed, as outlined in Table 6.2.[17,18] An example of a functional surveillance program laying the groundwork for an outbreak investigation would be as follows:

Hospital X performs a large number of hip joint replacements, and this is a procedure monitored by IPCP (Fig. 6.1). Standardized NHSN criteria are used to define surgical site infections (SSIs) for hip prosthesis. Hospital X's surveillance for hip prosthesis involves review of all microbiology data for all hip replacements done at the institution plus readmission data after hip replacement, as well as antibiotic utilization data for patients with hip replacement. Charts are then reviewed to evaluate if a hip infection occurred and at what level (superficial, deep or organ space, by NHSN criteria).

It is noted that in July, there was a large increase in the rate of hip infections that was two standard deviations above the institutional mean and over the 75th percentile for NHSN hip infection rate. Charts are reviewed to confirm, and an epidemic curve is generated suggesting that the increase in infection started in mid July. This information is reported back to Orthopedics as well as Hospital Administration. Patient data review indicates that the infections are with multiple different organisms, with procedures performed with multiple different surgeries in different ORs.

It is noted by one of the health-care workers interviewed that a new surgical scrub was put into place in late June in the orthopedic ORs, and the concern is raised that the increased infection rate may be associated with this. A review reveals that the new scrub is not being used per recommendations. A plan to develop and implement an educational module regarding surgical scrub is enacted, and by September infection rates in this procedure are back to baseline.

The role of the microbiology laboratory

The microbiology laboratory plays a critical role in both surveillance and outbreak investigation. Traditional roles have included detection, identification and susceptibility testing of microbes causing hospital infection. Rapid detection and reporting of key organisms with high potential to cause outbreaks such as *Clostridium difficile* or *Mycobacterium tuberculosis* are critical components of infection prevention, leading to appropriate implementation of control measures and reducing the risk of secondary spread.[19] For instance, at our institution, when a *C. difficile* toxin is identified in the microbiology laboratory, a report goes out simultaneously to the ward where the patient resides, so that the appropriate isolation can be ensured, including signage; to the infection control group to ensure that the isolation is logged in centrally; and to environmental services to ensure use of bleach cleaning for that room.

The development of an institutional antibiogram is a critical function that often results from collaboration between different groups, as will be discussed below.

Understanding pathogen distribution and relatedness in the hospital is an important component of both surveillance and outbreak investigation. Typing of microbial pathogens can help determine if isolates that appear to be epidemiologically linked are in fact genetically related and thus likely to have originated from the same strain. Typing can help distinguish extent and pattern of spread of 'epidemic' clones; it can also help assess the source of an outbreak (environmental, personnel, etc.). The incorporation of molecular typing methodologies along

---

Table 6.2 Steps in the investigation and control of a potential outbreak

1. Establish case definition(s).
2. Confirm that the cases are 'real' (case confirmation).
3. Establish the background rate of disease (in order to confirm the outbreak and determine the scope of the outbreak geographically and temporally).
4. Case finding.
5. Examine the descriptive epidemiology of the cases (e.g. define the age, sex, home/overseas travel, occupation, attendance at events) and plot an 'epidemic curve' of time of onset of disease.
6. Generate a hypothesis regarding the source and route of exposure.
7. Test the hypothesis by case control, cohort or intervention studies and by epidemiologic typing of representative samples if indicated and if possible.
8. Collect and test potential sources of infection such as environmental surfaces, patients, personnel, iv fluids, etc. as indicated; consider epidemiologic typing to establish an epidemiologic link to cases.
9. Devise and implement control measures.
10. Review results of investigation or report on ongoing investigations to administration and staff; consider consultation with local public health officials.
11. Follow-up surveillance to evaluate efficacy of control measures; generate reports for administration and staff.

---

with traditional epidemiologic surveillance has been shown in a number of studies to reduce the number of HAIs and to be cost-effective.[20] Typing can be done using phenotypic methods (such as biotyping and serotyping) or genotypic/molecular methods, such as pulsed field gel electrophoresis, plasmid analysis, southern blotting or various forms of polymerase chain reaction (PCR). Newer modalities, such as sequence-based molecular epidemiologic analysis (SLST or MLST), have been used for the evaluation and typing of some pathogens.

Education and training

One of the most critical functions of the IPCP is to provide education and training. Education for health-care providers includes instruction on isolation precautions, aseptic practice, prevention of blood and body fluid exposures, and appropriate usage of personal protective equipment and safety devices. Teaching of policies and procedures should be simple, reproducible and, if possible, innovative (e.g. combinations of computer technology and live) in order to make an impact and reach the greatest number of health-care workers.

An important component of teaching involves the measurement and subsequent feedback of infection control data to the staff. As an example, performance and infection rate feedback in a neonatal unit has been effective in sustaining hand hygiene compliance improvement and in reducing infection risk in neonates.[21]

Collaboration with other programs to achieve common goals

Occupational and employee health

An active employee health service and IPCP collaboration is critical in the protection of health-care workers and the control of hospital-acquired infections. Joint objectives generally include:

- education of personnel about the principles and importance of infection control;
- prompt diagnosis and appropriate management of transmissible diseases in health-care workers, such as respiratory syncytial virus or pertussis;
- assessing and investigating potential exposures and outbreaks among personnel;

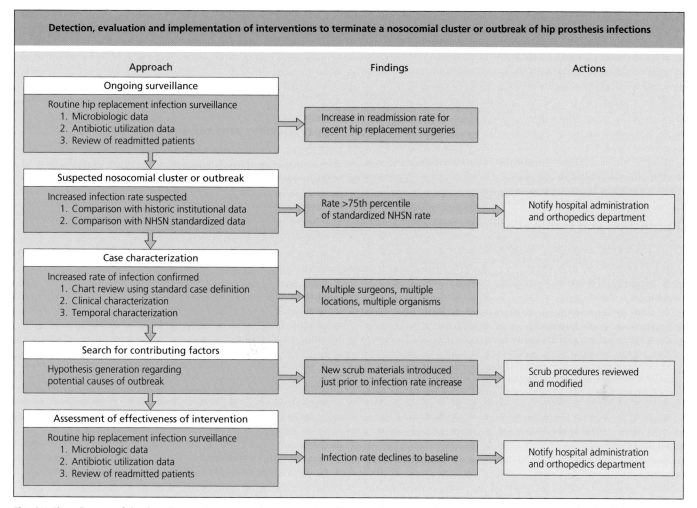

Detection, evaluation and implementation of interventions to terminate a nosocomial cluster or outbreak of hip prosthesis infections

Approach	Findings	Actions

Ongoing surveillance

Routine hip replacement infection surveillance
1. Microbiologic data
2. Antibiotic utilization data
3. Review of readmitted patients

Increase in readmission rate for recent hip replacement surgeries

Suspected nosocomial cluster or outbreak

Increased infection rate suspected
1. Comparison with historic institutional data
2. Comparison with NHSN standardized data

Rate >75th percentile of standardized NHSN rate

Notify hospital administration and orthopedics department

Case characterization

Increased rate of infection confirmed
1. Chart review using standard case definition
2. Clinical characterization
3. Temporal characterization

Multiple surgeons, multiple locations, multiple organisms

Search for contributing factors

Hypothesis generation regarding potential causes of outbreak

New scrub materials introduced just prior to infection rate increase

Scrub procedures reviewed and modified

Assessment of effectiveness of intervention

Routine hip replacement infection surveillance
1. Microbiologic data
2. Antibiotic utilization data
3. Review of readmitted patients

Infection rate declines to baseline

Notify hospital administration and orthopedics department

Fig. 6.1 Flow diagram of the detection, evaluation and implementation of interventions to terminate a nosocomial cluster or outbreak of hip prosthesis infections.

- identification and vaccination of workers susceptible to vaccine-preventable diseases;
- identifying work-related infection risks and instituting preventive measures; and
- surveillance of health-care workers for diseases such as tuberculosis.[22]

Detailed discussion of the role of employee health services is beyond the scope of this chapter. The CDC has published extensive guidelines and recommendations on immunization of health-care workers, occupational health guidelines and protection of health-care workers from blood-borne pathogens, including postexposure prophylaxis guidelines.[23-25] These are updated on a regular basis at http://www.cdc.gov.

Environmental health and safety and environmental services

The health-care facility environment is not commonly associated with disease transmission in competent hosts. Environmental Health and Safety and IPCP work together to ensure environmental safety and prevent exposure of patients and staff to environmental and airborne pathogens. The combination of infection control and environmental engineering strategies can help prevent such occurrences. These control measures include:

- adherence to ventilation standards for specialized care environments (e.g. airborne infection isolation rooms, protective environments or operating rooms) and to water-quality standards, including for hemodialysis;

- appropriate infectious waste management;
- appropriate use of cleaners and disinfectants; and
- appropriate use of precautions during construction.

Environmental Safety is often responsible, with Employee Health, for monitoring of pressure-negative airborne isolation rooms and N95 respirator fit testing.[26]

In this era of antibiotic resistant pathogens, the importance of environmental cleaning cannot be overstated. Environmental contamination of floors, beds, tables, faucets, doorknobs, blood pressure cuffs, thermometers, gowns, stethoscopes and computer terminals has all been well documented.[26,27] Among other factors associated with transmission, acquisition of drug-resistant organisms such as vancomycin-resistant *Enterococcus* (VRE) and MRSA may depend on room contamination, and the odds of acquiring antibiotic-resistant bacteria are increased by patient admission to a room previously occupied by a patient harboring the resistant organism.[27]

The cleaning and disinfection of all patient-care areas is important for frequently touched surfaces, especially those closest to the patient. Increased frequency of cleaning may be needed for compromised patients in a protective environment to minimize dust accumulation or in situations where environmental contamination is more likely (e.g. incontinent patients). During a suspected or proven outbreak where an environmental reservoir is suspected, cleaning procedures should be assessed and adherence should be monitored and reinforced.

In general, use of a US Environmental Protection Agency (EPA)-registered detergent/disinfectant (used according to the manufacturer's recommendations for amount, dilution and contact time) is sufficient to remove pathogens from surfaces of rooms of colonized or infected individuals. Certain pathogens (e.g. rotavirus, noroviruses, *C. difficile*) may be resistant to some routinely used hospital disinfectants. Since levels of spore production for *C. difficile* may be increased when exposed to nonchlorine-based cleaning agents, and the spores are quite resistant to commonly used surface disinfectants, many investigators have recommended the use of a 1:10 dilution of 5.25% sodium hypochlorite (household bleach) and water for routine environmental disinfection of rooms of patients with *C. difficile*. Many institutions also recommend bleach cleaning when faced with outbreaks of norovirus or rotavirus as well.

General and specific recommendations for disinfection and sterilization may be found in the CDC's *Guidelines for Environmental Infection Control in Health-Care Facilities*.[26]

Disinfection and sterilization

Numerous reports detailing infection outbreaks secondary to faulty or inadequately disinfected medical instruments highlights the critical importance of sterilization and disinfection of such items.[28] IPCP collaborates with sterile processing to help prevent such problems.

Medical equipment and instruments/devices must be cleaned and maintained according to the manufacturers' instructions to prevent patient-to-patient transmission of infectious agents. Cleaning to remove organic material must always precede high-level disinfection (a process that eliminates many or all pathogenic organisms except bacterial spores) and sterilization (complete elimination or destruction of all microbial life). Disinfection may be accomplished using physical, chemical or physiochemical strategies to denature proteins. Sterilization is most commonly performed by steam/heat sterilization; ethylene oxide or hydrogen peroxide gas or prolonged liquid sterilization is also sometimes used.

Noncritical equipment, such as commodes, intravenous pumps and ventilators, computers used in patient care, etc., must be thoroughly cleaned and low-level disinfected before use on another patient. Providing patients who are on transmission-based precautions with dedicated noncritical medical equipment (e.g. stethoscope, blood pressure cuff, electronic thermometer) may prevent pathogen transmission. If this is not possible, disinfection after use is recommended. Semicritical items come in contact with mucous membranes and intact skin. This includes respiratory therapy and anesthesia equipment. High-level disinfection after cleaning is an appropriate standard of treatment for heat-sensitive, semicritical medical instruments (e.g. flexible, fiberoptic endoscopes).[28] This process inactivates all vegetative bacteria, mycobacteria, viruses, fungi and some bacterial spores. Critical items are objects that enter sterile tissue or the vascular system and pose a high risk of infection if contaminated with micro-organisms. This includes surgical instruments, various catheters, implants, etc. These items should either be purchased sterile or undergo heat-based sterilization after cleaning prior to patient use.

Information detailing the specific agents and processing used in disinfection and sterilization of equipment has been extensively reviewed elsewhere[26,29] and is beyond the scope of this chapter.

Pharmacy and therapeutics

Infection with antibiotic-resistant bacteria has been associated with increased morbidity, mortality and costs of health care. The goals of an effective antimicrobial stewardship program (ASP) include optimizing clinical outcomes while minimizing both toxicity associated with antibiotic use and the emergence of resistance, and reduction of health-care costs while maintaining or improving quality of care. The Infectious Diseases Society of America recommends a multidisciplinary approach to an ASP, with an infectious disease physician and a clinical pharmacist with infectious diseases training as core members of the team. Collaboration with a clinical microbiologist, an information systems specialist, an infection control professional and

hospital epidemiologist is critical. Because such ASPs are important patient safety initiatives, they should function under the umbrella of quality assurance and patient safety and receive hospital administrative and fiscal support.[30-32] The ASP may also work with microbiology, pharmacy and the IPCP to create an institutional and unit-specific antibiogram, which can be accessible to all antibiotic prescribers in the health-care system.

Safety, quality and public reporting

Health-care-associated infections are one of the most common complications affecting hospitalized patients and are considered to be one of the more accurate indicators of the quality of patient care. Thus, the process and outcome data generated by infection control and other practitioners is relevant to patient safety and quality of care at the level of the institution, across institutions and extending to credentialing and governmental regulatory boards such as the Joint Commission (formerly JCAHO) and OSHA.[33] Ensuring the quality of care requires input from many groups, including infection control, quality improvement, risk safety and other committees.

Since 2002, seven states in the USA have enacted legislation that requires health-care organizations to publicly disclose HAI rates, and many others have submitted similar legislation for review. In the UK, mandatory health-care organization-based surveillance and public reporting of MRSA bloodstream infections have been in place since 2001.[34] Despite this movement toward public reporting of HAIs, little is known about its effectiveness in improving health-care performance. The CDC published consensus recommendations for public reporting in 2005,[35] which emphasize choosing standardized epidemiologic methodologies, promoting thoughtful choices of process and outcome measures depending on the nature of the institution, ensuring feedback to health-care providers and providing adequate infrastructure support. They recommended consideration of several process measures to evaluate, such as central line insertion practices, surgical antibiotic prophylaxis and influenza vaccination coverage of health-care workers and patients. The two outcome measures considered most appropriate for some hospitals to consider were rates of central line infections and surgical site infections for selected operations.

Disaster and bioterrorism preparedness

The anthrax letters in 2001, the SARS outbreak in 2002 and the continued concern about an avian influenza pandemic have all heightened awareness of the importance of disaster (natural or bioterrorism related) preparedness. Infection control plays an integral role in such a committee, in order to develop plans to minimize exposure of staff and the potential for nosocomial transmission (see isolation guidelines).

ISOLATION PRECAUTIONS

Standard and transmission-based precautions

Standard precautions

Standard precautions constitute a system of barrier precautions designed to be used by all health-care personnel on all patients, regardless of diagnosis, to reduce the risk of transmission of micro-organisms from both recognized and unrecognized sources. These sources include blood, all body fluids, secretions, excretions, intact and non-intact skin, mucous membranes, equipment and environmental surfaces. Standard precautions are part of the standard of care for all patients.

The use of barriers is determined by the care provider's 'interaction' with the patient and the level of potential contact with body substances. It is the responsibility of the individual to comply with all isolation precautions. Ongoing education concerning standard precaution principles will be given to newly hired employees involved directly or indirectly in patient care and as needed for dissemination of new information or for reinforcement of consistent practices.

Elements of standard precautions include hand hygiene and the banning of artificial nails. This is because most infections in the health-care environment are transmitted through contact with contaminated hands of the health-care workers. In 2002, the CDC published guidelines for hand hygiene.[36] These guidelines were adopted by the Joint Commission on Accreditation of Healthcare Organizations (JCAHO) in 2004 as part of the new National Patient Safety Goal 7A.[37]

Whenever possible and available, alcohol-based products will be the primary method used for decontaminating hands. Alcohol-based products are more effective for reducing microbes on the skin than soap or antimicrobial soaps and water, and should be the routine method for decontaminating hands if hands are not visibly soiled. Visibly soiled hands should be washed with soap or antimicrobial soap and water for 15 seconds.

Artificial nails are not permissible for personnel with any direct patient contact or with patient supplies, equipment or food. Studies have shown that long fingernails, both artificial and natural, are more likely than short natural nails to harbor bacteria that cause health-care acquired infections. The natural nails of health-care workers must be kept neatly manicured and should not extend 5 mm past the fingertips. Besides artificial nails, other nail enhancements must not be worn. This includes but is not limited to tips, wraps, appliqués, acrylics, gels and any additional items applied to the nail surface. Nail polish, provided it is not chipped, is the only enhancement that should be permitted on short natural nails.

Hand washing and hand antisepsis must occur before any direct patient contact and between patients, between tasks/procedures on the same patient to prevent cross-contamination of body sites, before donning gloves and performing an invasive procedure, after contact with patient's intact skin (e.g. taking a pulse, blood pressure or lifting a patient), after removing gloves or other personal protective equipment (PPE), after contact with body substances or articles/surfaces contaminated with body substances, and before preparing or eating food. Hands should be washed with soap and water after 7–10 applications of an alcohol-based product.

In the presence of *Clostridium* spores alcohol hand products should not be used because they are not killed by alcohol. In these situations, hands should be washed with soap and water. In addition, hands should be washed with soap and water after covering a sneeze, nose blowing or using the bathroom, all of which may contaminate and soil hands.

Gloves, masks, eye protection and face shields, aprons, gowns and other protective body equipment

Disposable gloves must be worn for anticipated contact with moist body substances, mucous membranes, tissue and non-intact skin of all patients, for contact with surfaces and articles visibly soiled or contaminated by body substances, during venous blood draws or other vascular access procedures (starting a venous line or blood draws) – in other words, in any situation where contamination of hands is anticipated. If the use of gloves is needed, gloves should be donned immediately prior to the task. Torn, punctured or otherwise damaged gloves must be replaced immediately. Gloves should be removed and disposed of after every task involving body substance contact and before leaving the bedside. Gloves should not be worn away from the bedside or laboratory bench, at the nursing station, to handle charts, when touching clean linen, clean equipment or patient care supplies, or in hallways or elevators. Hands have to be washed as soon as possible after glove removal or removal of other protective equipment. Gloves are not to be washed or decontaminated for reuse. An exception to this rule are utility gloves (not for direct patient care) used by house keepers, plumbers, etc. In this situation, gloves may be decontaminated and reused provided the integrity of the glove is not compromised.

Masks, in combination with eye protection devices (goggles or glasses with side shields) or chin-length face shields, should be worn during procedures or other close contact that are likely to generate droplets, spray or splash of body substances to prevent exposure to mucous membranes of the mouth, nose and eyes. This is particularly relevant in situations known to increase the risk of splash or splatter. Nonexhaustive examples are surgery, trauma care, newborn delivery, intubation and extubation, and suctioning, bronchoscopy and endoscopy, emptying bedpans and suction canisters into hopper or a toilet. Masks and eye protection devices should be used if caring for a coughing patient with suspected infection.

Plastic aprons or gowns and other protective body clothing are used during patient care procedures to prevent contamination of clothing and protect the skin of personnel from blood or body fluid exposure. In laboratory settings, laboratory coats should be used.

Additional protective equipment, including surgical caps, hoods and shoe covers or boots, may be used in surgical or autopsy areas. All protective body clothing should be removed immediately before leaving the work area.[26,36]

Transmission-based precautions

Transmission-based precautions are to be used in addition to standard precautions, in patients with documented or suspected infection or who are colonized with an organism that is transmissible and/or that is of epidemiologic significance. There are three types of transmission-based precautions: contact, droplet and airborne. A sign with the type of transmission-based precautions should be placed outside the room of the patient. In the USA, to comply with the Health Insurance Portability and Accountability Act (HIPAA), enacted by the US Congress in 1996, the name of the infecting organisms may *not* be written on the sign.

Waste disposal, spill management, linen and food trays should be handled in the same way for all patients, regardless of precaution category. Isolation trays are not required. After patient use, both linen and food trays are sent directly for cleaning and disinfection.[26,38,39]

Contact precautions

Contact precautions are initiated and maintained to interrupt the transmission of epidemiologically significant micro-organisms known to be spread by contact. These precautions are intended to reduce the colony count of bacteria on horizontal surfaces and in the immediate vicinity of the patient.

Contact precautions are to be instituted on a case-by-case basis at the discretion of the IPCP staff, infectious disease staff and/or medical or nursing staff. Examples of situations in which contact precautions are to be initiated are:

- when a patient is colonized and/or infected with multidrug-resistant organisms or organisms that are not treatable with the usual antibiotics, i.e. multidrug resistant Gram-negative rods, MRSA and VRE; and
- when a particular organism is identified as being potentially hazardous because of its pathogenicity, virulence or epidemiologic characteristics, e.g. rotavirus, *C. difficile*, *Salmonella* spp. and *Shigella* spp.

After hand hygiene, the key element of contact precautions is personal protective equipment (PPE). Upon entering the room of a patient placed in contact precautions, gown and gloves should be worn at a minimum. All PPE must be removed before leaving the room and hand hygiene must be done. Disposable gowns should be used at all times when entering the patient's room. Gowns may be worn one time only, and then should be disposed of in the regular (nonbiohazardous) waste before leaving the room.

The patient should be placed in a private room whenever possible. When a private room is not available, cohorting of patients with the same confirmed micro-organism (but with no other infection) is acceptable but IPCP should be notified. Because a negative air pressure room is not required, the door may remain open. When neither a private room is available nor cohorting is achievable, a space separation of at least 3 feet should be present between the infected patient and other patients or visitors.

To minimize contamination, equipment should not be shared (unless it is disinfected properly) between patients. Examples of dedicated equipment include, but are not limited to, electronic thermometer, blood pressure cuff, manometer, stethoscope, intravenous pole, wheelchair or gurney. For pediatric patients with fecal pathogens such as VRE or rotavirus and who require weighing, a dedicated scale should be placed in the room.

In the USA, hospital staff should use an EPA-approved detergent/disinfectant to wipe down high-touch (e.g. door knobs, bed rails) and horizontal surfaces (e.g. over bed table, night stand) as needed and at a minimum once a day. This cleaning should also include the surfaces of electronic equipment, respiratory therapy equipment and other items that come in physical contact with the patient.

In critical care units or units where there is a high endemic rate of the organism the wipe down should be repeated as needed and at minimum each shift. Cleaning cloths used in the room should not be used to clean other patients' rooms and equipment.

Traffic into the patient's room should be limited only to essential staff/visitors. All visitors shall be instructed in proper hand hygiene technique. Visitors that participate in direct patient care shall be instructed in gowning and gloving, if the patient is incontinent, diapered or has diarrhea or a draining wound. Visitors may be referred to infection control or given written educational material.

Droplet precautions

Droplet precautions are required when a patient is suspected or known to have a serious illness transmitted by large particle droplets or direct contact with respiratory secretions. Droplets are often 30–50 microns in size compared to aerosolized droplet nuclei which are less than 5 microns in size. They are often generated by a patient coughing, sneezing or talking, or during suctioning while in close contact with the patient. Droplet precautions include the use of barriers to prevent contact between infectious droplets and the mucous membrane of health-care providers and visitors. Organisms and diseases that require droplet precautions are listed in Table 6.3. After hand hygiene, the key element of droplet precautions is the use of a surgical mask with face shield or 'surgical masks with eye protection' for face to face contact within three feet of a symptomatic patient to prevent self-inoculation. A surgical mask should be donned upon entering the room. All PPE must be removed before leaving the room and hand hygiene must be done.

The patient should be placed in a private room whenever possible. Because a negative air pressure room is not required, the door may remain open. When neither a private room is available nor cohorting is achievable, a space separation of at least 3 feet should be present between the infected patient and other patients or visitors.

Patient movement should be limited to essential needs outside of room. Patients must wear a surgical mask while outside of room.

Visitors should be limited. If visitors are susceptible, they must wear a surgical mask with face shield. Visitors with upper respiratory symptoms should not visit, but special consideration may be given to close family members. Nursing staff must instruct family and visitors to wash hands after contact with patient secretions or contact with the immediate patient environment.

Airborne precautions

Airborne precautions are required when a patient is suspected or known to have a disease transmitted by airborne droplet nuclei. The evaporated droplets contain micro-organisms that remain suspended in the air and can be widely dispersed by air currents within a room or over a long distance. The diseases or infections requiring airborne precautions are listed in Table 6.4.

Strict hand hygiene after contact with patient or items contaminated with respiratory secretions is required. An OSHA-approved mask for tuberculosis, such as the N95 respirator that has been fit-tested or a powered air purifying respirator (PAPR), should be worn by health-care personnel.

In the USA, the patient should be placed in a designated private room with monitored negative air pressure in relation to surrounding areas, with a minimum of 12 air exchanges per hour for new construction and renovation and six air exchanges per hour for existing facilities. Air from the room must be discharged directly outdoors or recirculated through high-efficiency particulate air (HEPA) filters before being circulated to other areas in the hospital. The windows and the door to the patient's room must remain closed except for entry/exit. The patient is confined to the room unless a procedure outside the room is necessary. The patient must wear a tight-fitting surgical mask outside of the room when transported to another department and personnel accompanying the patient should wear an N95 respirator or a PAPR during transport. Patients who are discharged from the hospital but are still considered contagious must be instructed about the need to wear a surgical mask. Visitors should be limited to strictly necessary at all times. Visitors must wear a surgical mask that is secured and snugly fitted. Symptomatic household or other contacts of the patient should not visit until medically cleared. If a symptomatic contact must visit, a mask must be donned before entering the hospital and worn continuously while in the facility.

Table 6.4 Organisms and conditions requiring airborne transmission-based precautions

- Hemorrhagic fevers
- Lassa fever
- Marburg virus disease
- Mycobacteria, tuberculous
- Pneumonia
- SARS (coronavirus)
- Smallpox (variola)
- Smallpox vaccine (vaccinia) from UCSF
- Tuberculosis (TB) including multidrug-resistant tuberculosis (MDR-TB)
- Vaccinia

Table 6.3 Organisms requiring droplet transmission-based precautions

- Adenovirus infection
- Anthrax pneumonia
- Coronavirus infection, respiratory
- Croup (laryngotracheobronchitis)
- Diphtheria
- Ebola virus infection
- German measles (rubella)
- Herpes simplex
- Influenza
- Meningitis
- Meningococcal pneumonia
- Meningococcemia
- Mumps (infectious parotitis)
- *Mycoplasma* infections
- Parainfluenza
- Parvovirus B19
- Pertussis (whooping cough)
- Plague
- Rabies
- Respiratory infectious disease, acute (if not covered elsewhere)
- Respiratory syncytial virus (RSV) infection
- Rhinovirus infection, respiratory
- Rubella (German measles)
- Scarlet fever
- Streptococcus: Group A
- Whooping cough (pertussis)

Table 6.5 Organisms requiring airborne non-acid-fast bacillus transmission-based precautions
• Chickenpox (varicella) • Herpes zoster (disseminated) • Herpes zoster (shingles in immunocompromised) • Measles (rubeola) • Rubeola (measles) • Varicella (chickenpox)

Table 6.6 Hospital-acquired infection (HAI) groups

• Device-related infections
  • Central line-associated bloodstream infection (CLABSI)
  • Ventilator-associated pneumonia (VAP)
  • Foley catheter urinary tract infection (UTI)
  • Infection of a prosthetic device
• Nondevice-related infections
  • Health-care-associated pneumonia (HAP) other than VAP
  • Infections due to multidrug-resistant organisms (MDRO)
    – *Clostridium difficile* colitis
    – Methicillin-resistant *Staphylococcus aureus* (MRSA)
    – Vancomycin-resistant *Enterococcus* (VRE)
    – Gram-negative rods with MDRO pattern or extended spectrum β-lactamase (ESBL) producing
• Procedure-related infections
  • Transplant-associated infections
  • Surgical site infections (SSI)
  • Bloodstream infections
  • Septicemia

Vacating an airborne precautions patient room

If the patient is being ruled out for TB or diagnosed with TB and was in a room without negative pressure, the room must not be used for 1 hour after the patient has been discharged. If the patient is being ruled out for TB or is diagnosed with TB and was in a negative-pressure room, the room must not be used for 30 minutes after the patient has been discharged.

Airborne precautions are also required for patients with diseases that are highly communicable by the airborne route. Examples of diseases that fall into this category of precaution are listed in Table 6.5. Nonimmune staff or visitors are not allowed to enter the patient's room or provide care. Non immunity means either no history of the specific disease or no vaccination against that disease. Respiratory protection is not needed for immune healthcare workers.

HEALTH-CARE AND DEVICE-ASSOCIATED INFECTIONS

Health-care-associated infections (HAIs) are infections occurring as a result of treatment and after exposure to the health-care environment. Infections can be acquired in all health-care settings – ambulatory, inpatient or during emergency room visits. Duration and frequency of exposure appear to increase the risk of infection as does decreased immunity due to co-morbidities or treatments. Infections are considered health-care associated if they manifest 48 hours or more after admission to a hospital, within 30 days of discharge from a health-care facility or if a patient visited an outpatient medical facility within the past 6–12 months.[40,41]

Health-care-associated infections include those with hospital onset, which are diagnosed 48 hours or more after admission to the facility and those diagnosed with community onset in patients with previous health-care encounters. In contrast, community-associated infections are defined as infections manifesting and diagnosed within 48 hours of admission in patients without any previous encounter with health care. In this section, we will address HAIs.

A recent CDC report updated previous estimates of HAIs and related deaths in US hospitals.[42] This report was based on HAI surveillance outcome data submitted to the NNIS System. The NNIS was a voluntary collaborative network of 283 US hospitals with 100 or more beds performing HAI surveillance using standardized CDC definitions and methodologies.[43]

This report estimated that, in 2002, HAI accounted for 1.7 million infections and that 98 987 deaths were either associated or were caused by HAI. While the majority (1 195 142) of HAIs in adults and children occurred outside of an intensive care unit (ICU), 394 288 (23%) were among patients in an ICU, which were also associated with the highest rates of associated deaths, and 52 328 infections were in newborns residing in either a high risk or a well baby nursery. The calculated rates were 9.3 infections per 1000 patient days or 4.5 infections per 100 admissions in 2002.

In addition to the deaths, the morbidity associated with HAI is significant. Studies have demonstrated that HAI results in excess length of stay (LOS) and costs.[6] For example, the mean attributable cost of a catheter-associated bloodstream infection was $18 432 with a mean excess LOS of 12 days.[6] The cumulative excess cost of HAI based on the 2002 CDC data was recently estimated at $4.5–6.5 billion.[44]

Of all HAIs with an identifiable source, urinary tract infections (UTI) were the most frequent at 32%, followed by surgical site infections (SSI) at 22% (2% of all surgeries performed), pneumonias (PNA) at 15%, followed by bloodstream infections (BSI) at 14%. In the ICUs, 20–25% of all infections were caused by a UTI, PNA or a BSI. Outside the ICUs, 35% of HAIs were UTI, 11% were either BSI or PNA and 20% SSI. Thirty-six percent of deaths were attributed to PNA, 31% to BSI, 13% to UTI and 8% to SSI.[44]

Since the SENIC study,[45,46] HAI rates have decreased following implementation of infection prevention initiatives, but the proportion of truly preventable infections remains unclear. Based on a meta-analysis of infection control intervention studies, Harbarth and colleagues estimated this proportion to be between 10% and 70%, depending on preintervention HAI rate, hospital setting, study design, types of intervention and infection.[47] Interventions associated with the greatest reduction in a particular HAI have consistently been those aimed at prevention of central line-associated bloodstream infections (CLABSI).

HAIs can be divided into three broad, sometimes overlapping groups: device related, nondevice related and procedure related (Table 6.6).

Device-related HAI

Central line-associated bloodstream infections

Of all device-related HAIs, central line-associated bloodstream infections (CLABSI) are among the best studied. Vascular access is an essential part of care of patients and often extends beyond the inpatient stay into ambulatory care. Colonization of the device around the insertion site by bacteria or fungi on the skin are thought to constitute the most frequent first step of a central line infection. However, for invasion into the bloodstream to occur, bacteria have to adhere and incorporate into the biofilm,[48] multiply and then invade. Infection of the catheter hub and invasion of the lumen by coagulase-negative staphylococci is a known independent major risk factor for a central line infection that has been extensively researched.[49,50]

Bacteremia and septicemia secondary to contamination of the infusate occur much less frequently but are a recognized source of clusters or outbreaks of bloodstream infections with Gram-negative organisms.[51–53]

Risk factors for CLABSI include host factors (severity of illness, lack of skin integrity, type of immunosuppression), factors related to the device (catheter insertion and maintenance processes, type and size of catheter, number of lumens, insertion site) and finally factors related to the purpose of the catheter (function of catheter, duration of placement).[54,55]

CLABSI prevention initiatives and surveillance have been standardized internationally, have well-established definitions and methodologies and therefore can be easily linked to measurable process and outcome measures. Unlike other quality and safety measures, surveillance of CLABSI has proven very helpful in the objective evaluation of the efficacy of performance improvement initiatives.[4,36,56–59]

The significant reductions in CLABSI following adherence to simple infection control principles and surveillance observed in the SENIC study in the late 1970s have continued, with median CLABSI rates in adult critical care units now ranging from 0.6 to 4.0 CLABSI per 1000 line days.[4,60]

In 2002, a working group published guidelines for the prevention of intravascular device-related bloodstream infections. Among the key evidence-based recommendations were education and standardization of insertion and maintenance processes, the use of maximal sterile barrier precautions upon insertion, chlorhexidine skin preparation, antiseptic/antibiotic-impregnated central venous catheters for short-term use only when rates of infection are high, avoiding routine replacement of the line for the purpose of line-infection prevention and using standardized process metrics to measure compliance with these guidelines. However, it was not until the Institute for Healthcare Improvement (IHI) launched the '100 Thousand Lives' central line-associated bloodstream infection prevention initiative that these recommendations were widely adopted by health-care facilities in the USA in the ICU setting (http://www.ihi.org/IHI/Programs/Campaign). Following implementation of the IHI campaign, CLABSI rates have seen substantial and sustained drops not only in the ICU setting but also on acute care wards.[4]

Ventilator-associated pneumonia

Ventilator-associated pneumonia (VAP) develops in 9–27% of ICU patients who require mechanical ventilation.[61–63] To meet the criteria for VAP, the pneumonia has to manifest more than 48 hours after intubation.

Ventilator-associated pneumonia significantly increases the time on ventilator, the overall costs of care ($23 000–40 000) and length of stay in and after discharge from the ICU. The average length of stay is increased by 9.6 days in a patient who develops VAP.[6,64,65]

Moreover, VAP is the leading cause of death among HAIs and is associated with a doubling of mortality compared to ventilated patients with similar characteristics who do not develop VAP.[42,64,66–70]

Infection control/infectious diseases and critical care specialists have not come to full agreement on the definitions and methodology to be used for the diagnosis of VAP.[71,72] Diagnosis of VAP is challenging because patients requiring mechanical ventilation have underlying complex diseases and co-morbidities with similar and confounding symptoms and signs.[19,73]

Despite the lack of an uncontested gold standard for the diagnosis of VAP, the American Thoracic Society and the Infectious Diseases Society of America published guidelines in 2005 recommending that clinical signs and quantitative cultures of the bronchoalveolar lavage (BAL) fluid be used to diagnose and treat VAP.[74] In 2006, a large randomized trial of 740 patients on mechanical ventilation in 28 ICUs across the USA and Canada did not demonstrate any difference in outcomes and in antibiotic use between quantitative cultures of BAL and nonquantitative cultures of the endotracheal aspirate.[72] The development of institution-specific collaborative guidelines for the diagnosis and management of VAP have led to shorter antibiotic duration and improved antibiotic choice without affecting overall mortality.[75]

VAP prevention process measures are now better established and many are supported by randomized controlled trials. Preventive strategies are aimed at avoiding unnecessary intubation, decreasing the duration of ventilation, preventing aspiration, and minimizing inoculation and colonization of the lower respiratory tract with mouth, gastrointestinal and upper respiratory tract flora. When implemented fully, these measures have resulted in better patient outcomes and are cost-effective.[76,77]

Multidrug-resistant organisms

Many organisms can be potentially acquired in the health-care setting (Table 6.7).

As care has evolved and become more complex, new antimicrobials have increased antibiotic pressure and thus selection of drug-resistant mutants. As a result, organisms resistant to multiple classes of drugs have emerged worldwide.[65] Infections due to multidrug-resistant organisms (MDRO) represent a significant proportion of the both the HAI burden and the day-to-day work of the IPCP. A nonexhaustive list of MDRO associated with HAI is shown in Table 6.8.

Guidelines for metrics to be used to monitor, and processes to prevent, MDRO in health-care settings have just been published.[78–80]

While resistance definitions for Gram-positive organisms are well established, there is no standard definition for most Gram-negative

---

Table 6.7 Organisms that may be acquired in the health-care setting

- *Acinetobacter* species
- Blood-borne pathogens
- *Burkholderia cepacia*
- Chickenpox (varicella)
- *Clostridium difficile*
- *Clostridium sordellii*
- Creutzfeldt–Jakob disease (CJD)
- Ebola (viral hemorrhagic fever)
- Gastrointestinal infections
- HIV/AIDs
- Influenza
- Methicillin-resistant *Staphylococcus aureus* (MRSA)
- Mumps
- Norovirus
- Parvovirus
- Poliovirus
- Rubella
- Severe acute respiratory syndrome (SARS)
- *Streptococcus pneumoniae* (drug resistant)
- Tuberculosis
- Vancomycin-intermediate *Staphylococcus aureus* (VISA)
- Vancomycin-resistant *Enterococcus* (VRE)

Table 6.8 Multidrug-resistant organisms acquired in the health-care setting

- Drug-resistant *Staphylococcus aureus*
  - Methicillin-resistant *Staphylococcus aureus* (MRSA)
    - Healthcare-associated: acquired in hospital or outpatient health-care facilities
    - Community-associated: acquired in the community
  - Vancomycin-intermediate/resistant *Staphylococcus aureus* (VISA/VRSA)
- Other drug-resistant organisms
  - Vancomycin-resistant *Enterococcus* (VRE)
  - Gram-negative organisms with multidrug resistance (MDR) or extended spectrum β-lactamase (ESBL) producing
  - MDR *Acinetobacter* spp.
  - Penicillin-resistant *Streptococcus pneumoniae*
  - MDR *Pseudomonas* spp.
  - MDR *Mycobacterium tuberculosis*
- *Clostridium difficile*-associated disease (CDAD)

MDRO.[81,82] For the purpose of this chapter, Gram-negative MDRO are defined as organisms resistant to one or more classes of antimicrobial agent.[83]

Infections caused by MDRO are particularly prevalent in intensive care, transplant and human immunodeficiency virus units, where patients are most susceptible to invasion by colonizing organisms because of the acuity of the primary disease and the co-morbidities with multiple potential portals of entry and high exposure to broad-spectrum antibiotics. In this setting, the inability to perform personal hygiene to decrease the bioburden and the forced immobilization exponentially increase the potential for acquiring pathogens from the contaminated environment or the health-care worker's hands.

New guidelines for the prevention of MDRO in the health-care setting underscore the importance of well-described evidenced-based infection prevention measures and coordinated antimicrobial stewardship programs.[78]

REFERENCES

References for this chapter can be found online at http://www.expertconsult.com

Chapter | 7 |

Pierre-Edouard Fournier
Didier Raoult

Bacterial genomes

SUMMARY

Within just a decade, genomics has become an irreplaceable source of insight into the genetic diversity, pathogenesis, evolution, diagnosis and treatment of bacteria. To date, 883 genomes have been completed, including those of all major human pathogens, and the development of high-throughput sequencing methods in parallel with improved analysis tools should boost this field, as highlighted by more than 2600 announced projects. Herein, we summarize the current achievements in bacterial genomics, with emphasis on their applications to clinical microbiology and infectious diseases.

INTRODUCTION

Two decades ago, the availability of a complete genome sequence was a dream. In 1995, scientists at The Institute for Genomic Research (TIGR) opened the road of bacterial genomics by sequencing the *Haemophilus influenzae* genome.[1] This pioneering work generated major enthusiasm from scientists worldwide and bacterial genome sequencing subsequently experienced considerable development, with the annual number of sequenced genomes nearly doubling every 2 years since 2000 (Fig. 7.1).

Initially, genome sequences were mostly used to address fundamental questions in research, notably for studying bacterial evolution. However, the development of high-throughput sequencing technologies,[2] computational assembly of sequences and functional inferences gave access to a tremendous source of information and revolutionized basic aspects of microbiology. In particular, genome size boundaries between viruses, bacteria and eukaryotes are less clear than initially thought. As a matter of fact, *Mimivirus*, the largest known virus to date, has a genome of 1.18 Mb, larger than those of 54 bacterial and two eukaryotic genomes, the latter two genomes, from protists, being smaller than all but four bacterial genomes.

Genome analysis, also known as genome mining or in-silico analysis, now constitutes an irreplaceable research tool for various aspects of microbiology. In particular, the availability of genomes from virtually all bacterial human pathogens has opened perspectives in the fields of diagnosis, epidemiology, pathophysiology and treatment.[3]

A major advantage of genome sequences over phenotypic methods is that data can be deposited in online databases and thus are easily comparable among laboratories. The main three databases are the

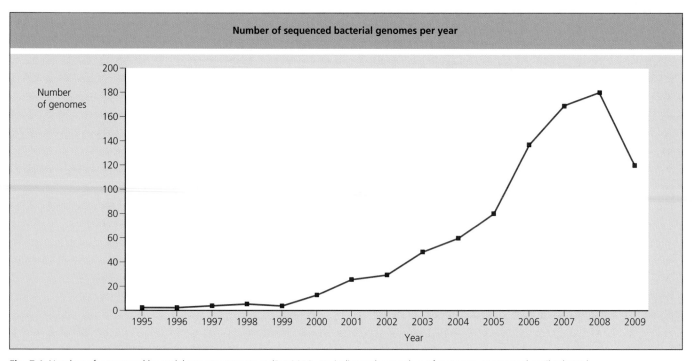

Fig. 7.1 Number of sequenced bacterial genomes per year. (For 2009, we indicate the number of genomes sequenced until July 28.)

National Center for Biotechnology Information (NCBI, http://www.ncbi.nlm.nih.gov/), the DNA Data Bank of Japan (DDBJ, http://www.ddbj.nig.ac.jp/) and the European Bioinformatics Institute (EBI, http://www.ebi.ac.uk/). In addition to offering complete microbial genome sequences with links to corresponding publications, these databases provide online tools for analyzing genome sequences. As of July 28, 2009, 883 genome sequences from 573 bacterial species are available online (http://www.genomesonline.org/, http://www.ncbi.nlm.nih.gov/genomes/static/eub_g.html). The discrepancy between the number of genome sequences and bacterial species is explained by the fact that genomes from several individual strains have been sequenced for 68 species. Sequenced genomes include almost every significant human bacterial pathogen, covering all the phylogenetic domains of bacteria. In addition, more than 2600 sequencing projects are ongoing (http://www.genomesonline.org/). Moreover, new sequencing technologies are making possible the sequencing of random community DNA and single cells of bacteria without the need for cloning or cultivation.

There are multiple applications for genome sequences:

- They may be used as target sources for molecular detection or genotyping.
- Following the critical step of genome annotation which consists of identifying gene functions by analogy with other bacteria and is facilitated by comparison to databases such as Clusters of Orthologous Groups (http://www.ncbi.nlm.nih.gov/COG/) or Kyoto Encyclopedia of Genes and Genomes (http://www.genome.ad.jp/kegg/), specific phenotypic traits may be deduced from the genotype. Resulting applications include development of specific culture media, identification of antibiotic resistance mechanisms and virulence factors, and exploration of host–pathogen interactions.
- Within the deduced proteome, antigens may be selected for serologic applications, development of monoclonal antibodies or development of vaccines (Fig. 7.2).

SEQUENCING STRATEGIES

With the development of ultrahigh-throughput applications of genomics, such as metagenomics, conventional capillary sequencing, also named Sanger sequencing, is no longer the technology of choice. Over recent years, new high-throughput sequencing methods, termed 'next generation sequencing', 'flow cell sequencing' or 'massively parallel sequencing', have opened new perspectives in genomic studies (Table 7.1).

Sanger sequencing

In 1977, Sanger et al.[4] developed a DNA sequencing method using di-deoxynucleotides as chain terminators; this became the reference sequencing method worldwide for the next 27 years. Most recent developments of this method use capillary sequencers, with a maximum output of 0.44 Mb every 7 hours. The Sanger technology, used for sequencing most of the 883 bacterial genomes available to date, produces 650–800 bp reads.

Pyrosequencing

In 2004, the Roche (454) company commercialized a high-throughput pyrosequencer, the GS-20, later upgraded as GS-FLX. Each of the strands obtained by shearing the template DNA is hybridized to the surface of a distinct agarose bead and then amplified by emulsion polymerase chain reaction (PCR). The sequence of the fragment from each individual bead is subsequently obtained by iterative pyrosequencing, whereby the pyrophosphate molecule released on nucleotide incorporation by DNA polymerase initiates a set of reactions that ultimately produces light from the cleavage of oxyluciferin by luciferase[5] (an explanation of the technology is available at http://www.roche-applied-science.com/publications/multimedia/genome_sequencer/flx_multimedia/wbt.htm). The GS-FLX instrument produces an average read length of ~250 bp per sample, with a combined throughput of ~100 Mb of sequence data per 7-hour run.

Sequencing by synthesis

Commercialized by Illumina (Solexa), the 1G analyzer uses a glass substrate with covalently attached oligonucleotides that are complementary to specific adapters previously ligated onto DNA library fragments. In-situ amplification is obtained using an isothermal polymerase and sequencing proceeds by synthesis using Sanger-like but reversible four-color fluorescence terminator nucleotides. An explanation of the technology is available at http://www.illumina.com/media.ilmn?Title=Sequencing-By-Synthesis%20Demo&Cap=&Img=spacer.gif&PageName=illumina%20sequencing%20technology&PageURL=203&Media=1. Sequencing by synthesis produces ~40–50 million sequence reads of 32–40 bp simultaneously.

Ligation-based sequencing

The Supported Oligonucleotide Ligation and Detection (SOLID) instrument by Applied Biosystems uses a sequencing process catalyzed by DNA ligase. In this technology, oligonucleotide adapter-linked DNA fragments are coupled with magnetic microbeads that are covered with complementary oligonucleotides. Each bead-bound DNA fragment is amplified by emulsion PCR and ligation-based sequencing is obtained using a thermostable ligase and four color dye-labeled oligonucleotides. The method includes a quality check in which each base sequenced is verified twice, which provides greater overall accuracy. An explanation of the technology is available at http://marketing.appliedbiosystems.com/images/Product/Solid_Knowledge/flash/102207/solid.html. Sequencing by ligation produces 3–4 Gb of sequence data with an average read length of 25–35 bp.

Advantages, drawbacks

Sanger sequencing suffers major drawbacks, including its financial cost and the need for a substantial quantity of DNA (several micrograms), and requires that DNA fragment libraries be clonable in Escherichia coli. The latter constraint is particularly limiting because some bacterial genes were demonstrated to be highly unclonable in E. coli.[6]

In contrast, next-generation sequencing methods, although readily outperforming capillary sequencing in terms of higher output and lesser DNA quantity required and cost, see their applications limited by short read lengths (25–250 bp), small numbers of samples that can be run simultaneously, limited paired-end and targeted sequencing, and difficult sequence assembly, especially to disambiguate repeat regions. In addition, the Roche technology, although producing 250-bp reads, is impaired by homopolymers in the template DNA, in particular those made of more than four nucleotides. Other issues include misincorporation of excess nucleotides that are incompletely eliminated after a previous cycle, beads with mixed templates and multiple copies of the same template on different beads. The Illumina and Applied Biosystems technologies only produce 25–40 bp reads. The Applied Biosystems technology requires that reference genome sequences be converted into 'color space' format prior to analysis.

As a consequence, next-generation sequencing may currently be preferred for genome resequencing than for de novo assembly, although a combination of Sanger sequencing and next-generation sequencing has been proposed as a valuable alternative for this latter purpose.

Single cell genome sequencing

A recently developed technique allows genomic DNA sequencing from single microbial cells. This strategy is especially valuable for microorganisms that cannot be cultivated. Prior to sequencing, genomic

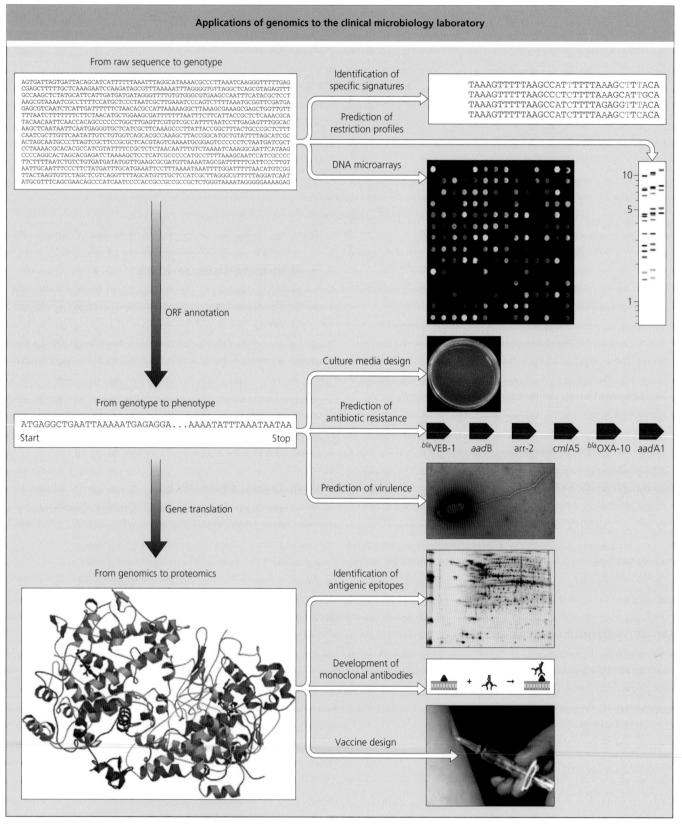

Fig. 7.2 Applications of genomics to the clinical microbiology laboratory.

DNA is amplified from a single bacterial cell, using three potential methods. These include primer extension preamplification, degenerate oligonucleotide primed PCR and multiple displacement amplification (MDA).[7] The best method, MDA, is based on isothermal strand displacement synthesis, i.e. a highly processive DNA polymerase repeat-edly extends random primers on template DNA and concurrently displaces previously synthesized copies. MDA was used successfully for *E. coli* and *Bacillus subtilis*[8] and may be of particular interest for complex floras. However, to date, MDA may not recover the entire genome from a single bacterial cell, and some DNA rearrangements may occur

Table 7.1 Currently available sequencing methods

	Sanger di-deoxy nucleotide sequencing	Pyrosequencing	Sequencing by synthesis	Ligation-based sequencing
Platform	Capillary sequencers	Roche (454) GS-FLX	Illumina genome analyzer	Applied Biosystems SOLID
Mb/run	0.44	100	1300	3000
Time/run	7 hours	7 hours	4 days	5 days
Read length (bp)	650–800	250	30–40	35
Limits	Cost	Limited paired-end and targeted sequencing, difficult sequence assembly, especially to disambiguate repeat regions		
	Need for high DNA quantity Cloning step	Low sensitivity in homopolymer sequencing Misincorporation of excess nucleotides Beads with mixed templates Redundancy		Specific sequence format

during the DNA amplification reaction; rather, a complete genome sequence may be obtained from the combination of data from several single cell MDA reactions.

Following genome amplification, sequencing may be obtained by any of the above-described methods, although an upcoming single molecule platform, the HeliScope by Helicos, should help solve single molecule sequencing challenges.

ANALYSIS OF GENOME SEQUENCES

Data analysis

The huge number of sequences produced at low cost by new sequencing methods created an increasing need for computational hardware and expertise. In particular, the assembly challenge posed by the short read length suggests that the software developed for Sanger sequencing cannot be applied to new sequencing methods.

Another major issue of genomics is sequence annotation.[9] In fact, the results from computational studies of hundreds of genomes depend directly on annotation quality. Genome annotation may be obtained using sequence similarity searches, calculated directly from the predicted gene and protein sequences or derived from comparisons of gene order between species, with some annotation systems being fully automated.[10] However, genomic annotations available in the above-cited databases may vary in several features (gene designation, level of detail, operons, repeats, etc.). To date, there is no consensus on annotation method and standardization of genomic data. Such an effort will be necessary to facilitate future studies.

Genetic diversity

A bacterial genome is a dynamic structure influenced by several events, including gene acquisition, duplication or loss, and/or genome reduction or rearrangement. Genome sequence comparison enabled the identification of many biologic patterns such as gene fusions, pseudogenes or non-coding RNAs, and ORFans. Such findings suggested that the mosaic of bacterial genomes would be more complex than expected. Indeed, the availability of several hundreds of bacterial genome sequences shed light on the great genetic diversity of the bacterial world, with genome sizes ranging from 0.159 Mb for

Candidatus 'Carsonella ruddii' to 13 Mb for *Sorangium cellulosum*. For example, among bacteria, members of the order Rickettsiales experienced a strict intracellular association with eukaryotic cells. This particular lifestyle paralleled a reductive genome evolution marked by the paradoxic expansion of genetic elements such as plasmids, repeats and gene duplications.[11] An extreme example of repeat expansion is the *Orientia tsutsugamushi* genome that contains the highest concentration of repeats (46.7%) for a bacterial genome.[12]

The study of the genetic diversity of bacteria using genomic sequences might also include phylogeny. Such an approach may limit the risk of biases linked to the selection of specific genes. The problem is to define adequate tools that would enable comparison of such large amounts of sequences. Recently, 8362 signature genes were identified that may served as targets for genome-based bacterial phylogeny.[13]

Pan-genome

Although a genome sequence gives access to a tremendous amount of information for a given strain, it may not reflect the genetic diversity at the species level. Recent studies have shown that intraspecies diversity in gene content may vary greatly. Therefore, the gene pool of some bacterial species may be far larger than that of a single genome, in part because of the frequency of homologous recombination and lateral gene transfer.[14] For *E. coli*, *Streptococcus agalactiae* and *Strep. pyogenes* it was estimated that an average 441, 33 and 27 new genes, respectively, would be unveiled by every new sequenced genome.[14] Such intraspecies variations might be linked to niche adaptation. Bacteria living in niches with limited access to the global microbial gene pool, such as *Bacillus anthracis*, *Chlamydia trachomatis* and *Mycobacterium tuberculosis*, have a much smaller intraspecies genomic diversity. The most extreme example of genome homogeneity is *Buchnera aphidicola* which experienced neither genome rearrangement nor gene duplication or transfer.[15]

The availability of several genomes for a given species led to the concepts of 'universal' minimal genome and species being challenged. Each bacterial species is composed of a 'core genome' containing genes present in all strains, a 'dispensable genome' made of genes present in two or more strains and genes unique to single strains. According to their structural and metabolic requirements, distinct species might have distinct minimal gene sets that would be different from the set of shared orthologs.

Metagenomics

Direct cloning and sequencing of DNA from complex floras, or metagenomics, has provided a unique access to the microbial species and genes present in these environments. Initially, metagenomic sequencing was performed using a random shotgun method following purification of any DNA. Metagenomic studies have been greatly facilitated by the development of new sequencing methods (described above) that enable the sequencing of random community DNA without the need for cloning or cultivation. In recent years, metagenomics nearly doubled the number of identified proteins and unveiled community-wide patterns in gene and taxa distributions among various habitats. In addition, when compared to the 883 bacterial genomes sequenced to date, metagenomic studies have demonstrated that the majority of the biologic diversity in the bacterial world remains unexplored.

To date, the metagenomic approach has been used to study the human microbiome, in particular the oral, lower intestinal and vaginal floras. In the gastrointestinal tract, 395 distinct bacteria were demonstrated; 62% of these were not previously known and 80% were uncultivated.[16] In addition, microbial genes outnumbered human genes 100 times, suggesting that the human microbiome may play a major role in human physiology.[16] Unexpectedly, this study demonstrated great intersubject variability and significant differences between stool and mucosal community compositions. Subsequently, other metagenomic studies allowed the identification of an imbalance in the distal gut flora of obese individuals compared to lean subjects, thus demonstrating that metagenomics may have medical applications.[17]

Aside from the human body, metagenomic studies are ongoing in several important ecosystems, including global soil, deep mines and the ocean. Ten grams of soil sample were estimated to contain 10^7 distinct bacterial species out of approximately 10^{10} cells.[18] In contrast, when applied to extremely simple microbial communities, metagenomic sequencing may enable genome reconstruction of their predominant members.

USING GENOME SEQUENCES

DNA sequences

The main limitation of molecular detection and sequence-based identification techniques is selection of target sequences, which can alter the reliability of results in terms of sensitivity and specificity of detection, as well as ability to discriminate between species and strains. Genome sequences offer the possibility of rational selection of targets depending on the desired objective. Their use has been demonstrated to be extremely valuable for fastidious pathogens that have poorly characterized genetic systems.

Detection of bacterial pathogens

Initially, the choice of PCR primers was empirical. 16S rRNA, the first 'universal' target gene, was widely used and enabled the first identification of the agents of bacillary angiomatosis[19] and Whipple's disease.[20] However, use of this gene was limited by a high risk of contamination, usage difficulties associated with polymicrobial specimens and insufficient discriminatory power.

The availability of genome sequences enables a rational choice of DNA signatures that may serve as PCR targets, according to the objective and degree of specificity required.[21] On the one hand, a PCR assay targeting a gene common to all bacteria may allow detection of any species. On the other hand, if the objective is to detect a unique or limited number of bacteria, it is possible by comparison of phylogenetically close genomes to identify DNA fragments that are specific for a genus, a species or a group of strains that exhibit, for example, specific virulence or antimicrobial resistance phenotypes. Such an approach was used to identify species-specific targets for Borrelia burgdorferi for example.[22] However, the specificity of in-silico identified genomic

targets should always be verified by comparison with databases, in particular GenBank (http://www.ncbi.nlm.nih.gov/Genbank).

In addition, the study of genomic sequences enabled the optimization of the sensitivity of detection, either by selecting a gene or fragment of noncoding DNA present as several copies in the genome[23] or by designing nested PCR assays with a reduced risk of contamination such as 'suicide PCR'.[24]

Molecular genotyping

Various genotyping methods may benefit from the study of genomic sequences.

- First, nonsequence-based methods that include in-silico design of macro restriction profiles for rare cutter enzymes may serve for restriction fragment length polymorphism (RFLP)-based analyses. Genomes may also be screened for single nucleotide polymorphisms (SNPs) or for tandem repeats, whose number and length are used in the variable number of tandem repeats (VNTR) method.[25]
- Second, several sequence-based genotyping methods have incorporated data from genome sequences or been designed on the basis of genome sequences. These include multilocus sequence typing (MLST) and multispacer typing (MST). MLST is based on sequencing several housekeeping genes, and genome sequences offer the possibility to select better candidate genes to be used in MLST approaches. MST relies on the assumption that intergenic spacers, undergoing less evolutionary pressure than coding sequences, are more variable between strains than genes. This is the first typing method to be entirely designed based on genomic data.
- Third, DNA microarrays have the advantage of allowing a simultaneous comparison of strains at the whole genome level with the sensitivity to detect subtle differences that are not detected by other methods. Another advantage of microarray technology is its ability to be facilitated by the development of automation. Chips may comprise up to 20 000 300–800 bp shotgun fragments or PCR products of one or several whole genome(s), specific sets of genes or as many as 600 000 50–70 bp oligonucleotides.[26] DNA microarrays have been used for genotyping bacterial strains in molecular epidemiologic studies.[25] DNA microarrays may also be used to detect and identify microorganisms in complex flora. Microarray-based typing methods can potentially identify new genes by including sequences derived from related bacteria or identifying polymorphisms that would still be detectable by oligonucleotide hybridization. In addition to genotyping applications, DNA microarrays may be used for detection of pathogens in clinical specimens, identification of vaccine candidates and detection of virulence factors or antibiotic resistance.[25]

Phenotype prediction

Development of specific culture media

Cultivation of the causative agent remains a priority during the diagnosis of bacterial infections. Genomic sequences thus constitute a unique source to identify incomplete metabolic pathways as well as the essential nutrients that a bacterium is unable to produce. It is thus theoretically possible to compose specific media by incorporating metabolites that bacteria cannot produce. Websites such as KEGG allow identification of anomalous pathways by comparison with previously analyzed genomes (http://www.genome.ad.jp/kegg/).

The first 'uncultivable' pathogenic bacterium whose genome analysis permitted axenic culture was Tropheryma whipplei, the causative agent of Whipple's disease.[27] However, the counter-example of M. leprae that cannot be grown axenically, despite the identification of many important lacking metabolic activities, highlighted the fact that the genomic identification of deficient metabolic pathways may not always provide all the clues to the growth of fastidious bacteria.

Detection of resistance to antimicrobials

The rapid acquisition of antibiotic resistance by pathogenic bacteria is a major public health problem. Genome sequencing has the potential to identify the various resistance determinants of a bacterium and allow for discovery of new arrangements of known resistance genes or new putative resistance markers. Genomic findings have identified resistance-causing genes or mutations that may be easily detected by PCR of clinical isolates and may serve as targets for routine detection tools.[28]

Another situation demonstrating the value of genome sequencing is during identification of resistance mechanisms in fastidious bacteria, for which phenotypic testing of antibiotic resistance is difficult or impossible, as in *Tropheryma whipplei* where the genome revealed the presence of mutated *gyrA* and *parC* genes, which explains resistance to fluoroquinolones.[29] Genome sequencing may also allow the identification of the mechanism of action and target genes of new antimicrobial compounds.

Identification of virulence factors

Virulence genes are potential targets for risk assessment and intervention strategies. The identification of virulence genes may lead to the development of rapid screening tests in order to proceed with effective isolation measures in hospitalized patients or delay hospitalization after carriage decontamination. Comparative sequence analyses provide insight into pathogenic mechanisms of bacteria, allowing identification of known virulence proteins with conserved sequences or motifs, as well as putative new virulence proteins.

There are three main methods for identifying virulence genes in a genome sequence:

- method 1 is based on homology searches of known virulence factor-encoding genes in the same or other species;
- method 2 identifies genes that are likely to result from lateral gene transfer (such genes are often localized in pathogenicity islands);
- method 3 identifies virulence genes by comparing the genomes of strains with different pathogenicity profiles.

Significant advances in understanding the pathogenic mechanisms of bacteria have been facilitated by genome sequence analysis, in particular by comparison of closely related species or strains with different virulence traits. For example, genome comparison allowed identification of pathogenicity islands in *H. influenzae*, *E. coli*, *Salmonella enterica* serovar Typhimurium and *Staphylococcus aureus*. In addition, various virulence mechanisms were found by genome comparison in *Bacillus cereus*, *Campylobacter upsaliensis*, *Chlamydia trachomatis*, *Francisella tularensis*, *Helicobacter pylori*, *Listeria monocytogenes*, *M. tuberculosis*, *Strep. pyogenes*, *Strep. agalactiae*, *Treponema pallidum* and *Yersinia pestis*.

In addition to allowing a better understanding of bacterial pathogenesis, identification of virulence factors in genomes may also allow the design of new potential antimicrobials in addition to allowing the identification of antimicrobial targets.

Exploration of host–pathogen interactions

The potential of genome sequence analysis for the exploration of host–pathogen interactions was recently demonstrated in *Strep. pyogenes*, for which an M3 protein variant was shown to alter the phagocytosis of human leukocytes, and *Neisseria meningitidis* for which a vaccine candidate protein was identified.

Proteome prediction

Development of serologic tools

Genome analysis offers the possibility of identifying all putative protein-encoding genes of a given bacterium. This exhaustive approach may be completed by expression of the corresponding proteome, testing immunoreactive characteristics of selected proteins, and use of the best antigens for the development of serologic tools. This strategy allowed the identification of a representative panel of antigens for *Treponema pallidum* and *M. leprae*. Conversely, the genome may serve to identify antigens that have been detected within the proteome of a bacterium by immunoblotting and mass spectrometry. This strategy was used for *Tropheryma whipplei* and resulted in identification of 17 proteins specifically reacting with patients' antibodies.

Development of specific monoclonal antibodies

Monoclonal antibodies are widely used for the diagnosis of infectious diseases, with many applications in serology and pathology. However, the usual strategy of monoclonal antibody production relies on the use of the entire bacterium or proteins selected empirically, which makes it difficult and expensive. In contrast, genomic analysis allows for identification of all potential antigenic proteins of a bacterium. One can, then, limit the number of candidate antigens by selecting those that are genus-, species- or strain-specific. In addition, it is possible to focus selection on protein fragments large enough to contain valuable epitopes but small enough for expression in *E. coli*. The genomic approach of monoclonal antibody production has been used successfully for *M. tuberculosis*, *N. meningitidis* and *Treponema pallidum*.

Vaccine design

The availability of complete bacterial genome sequences offers unprecedented access to its complete proteome, with the possibility of rational selection of vaccine candidates rather than empiric testing of antigens one at a time. This strategy, named reverse vaccinology, may be completed by functional immunomics for optimal epitope prediction and may result in DNA vaccines. It has been used successfully to identify potential vaccine targets for *Bacillus anthracis*, *Chlamydophila pneumoniae*, *Leptospira interrogans*, *M. tuberculosis*, *N. meningitidis*, *Porphyromonas gingivalis*, *Rickettsia prowazekii*, *Strep. agalactiae*, *Strep. pneumoniae* and *Strep. pyogenes*. However, the major drawback of reverse vaccinology for vaccine development is that the strain under investigation does not represent the genetic diversity of its species. This risk has been highlighted by the comparison of genome sequences from several strains of *Strep. agalactiae*. In this species, the core genome is constituted by only approximately 80% of genes, with each new genome exhibiting ~18% new genes. This finding motivated the design of a 'universal anti-*S. agalactiae*' vaccine made up of four antigens, none of which was present in all strains but the combination of which was protective against all strains.[30]

This example, together with accumulating evidence that a single genomic sequence may not be sufficient to represent the variability of bacterial populations within a species, suggests that genome sequences from multiple strains of a species might be necessary to identify an efficient vaccine formulation.

CONCLUSIONS AND PERSPECTIVES

In 1995, the outcome of bacterial genome sequencing promised breakthroughs in microbiology and infectious disease research. Since then, 883 bacterial genomes have been sequenced. The multiplication of genome sequencing projects, together with extensive metagenomic studies, will provide a much more complete picture of the bacterial world. As we move towards cataloging the sequences of all bacterial genomes, we are facing new potential but also new challenges. The potential of this inestimable source of information has already allowed scientists to reconsider the fields of bacterial virulence, host–bacteria interactions, microbiologic diagnosis and human microbial ecology. However, among the challenges is the need to develop new programs able to handle the specific characteristics of new sequencing technologies and the continuously growing number of genomic sequences, with a need in calculation capacity following an exponential growth, the difficulty of sequencing the genomes of uncultivated bacteria identified by metagenomics, and the large proportion of genes that still need a function assignment, which warrant wide open future research. The ability to sequence DNA from individual cells is also likely to have a significant impact on microbiology.

REFERENCES

References for this chapter can be found online at http://www.expertconsult.com

Health consequences of a changing climate

Climate change has direct and indirect consequences for human health. Heat waves affect health directly and are projected to take an increasing toll in developed and developing nations. Climate constrains the range of infectious disease vectors and agents, while weather affects the timing and intensity of outbreaks.

INTRODUCTION

In 1989 Alexander Leaf, in his prescient *New England Journal of Medicine* paper, explored the pantheon of ills that climate change portends[1]. Twelve years later, the Third Assessment Report of the United Nations' Intergovernmental Panel on Climate Change[2] – the world's most ambitious international scientific collaboration to date, involving over 2000 scientists from 100 nations – concluded:

- climate is changing;
- humans are contributing;
- weather patterns have become more extreme; and
- biologic systems on all continents are responding to warming.

The combustion of fossil fuels – coal, oil and natural gas – and deforestation are the principal producers of heat-trapping greenhouse gases, above all carbon dioxide (CO_2).

Since 2001 we've learned a great deal more:

- the pace of atmospheric accumulation of CO_2 and warming is quickening;[2]
- polar and alpine ice sheets are melting at rates not thought possible just several years ago;[3]
- global warming is retarding the repair of the 'ozone shield'; and, most ominously
- circumpolar westerly winds are accelerating in both hemispheres.[2]

The underlying physics of warming is driving changes in climate, i.e. changes in global temperatures and weather patterns. The ocean is the repository of the last century's global warming, and having warmed 22 times more (as measured in exajoules) as has the atmosphere.[4,5] Warming of the world ocean accelerates Earth's hydrologic cycle: water is warming, ice is melting and water vapor is rising. Enhanced evapotranspiration over land parches some regions, while tropical-like downpours fall elsewhere. When drought is followed by heavy rainfall, the dry, cracked, less-absorbent soil increases the potential for flooding.

Heavier rainfalls are becoming more frequent. In the USA, from the 1970s to the 1990s, rainfall increased 7%, while 2-inch a day rains increased 14%, and 4-inch a day rains increased 20%. Indeed, 6-inch a day precipitation has increased 27%[6] and more winter precipitation is falling as rain at high latitudes.

Signs of climate instability are most evident in the ice. West Antarctica's 'rivers of ice' are flowing faster towards the sea and, in Greenland, melt water is seeping through crevasses to lubricate the base of outlet glaciers, accelerating their slippage. One large outlet glacier on the western shelf – the Jakobshavn Isbrae – was slipping at a rate of 12 km a year in 2006, double the speed of the previous decade.

While loss of the entire West Antarctic or Greenland ice sheets are not projected to occur any time soon (each would raise sea levels 7 meters), slippage of portions of ice sheets at either pole is becoming more likely. The sudden collapse of West Antarctic Peninsula ice shelves (floating) in 2005 demonstrated that ice sheets can disintegrate precipitously.

As ice cover retreats (decreasing reflectivity or albedo), open seas absorb more heat (decreasing albedo), opening more water to absorb more heat, etc. The loss of albedo is therefore a 'positive feedback', amplifying warming. Moreover, the change in albedo could reach a threshold or tipping point, triggering an abrupt phase-state change in the climate.[7]

The observed changes in climate and biologic responses have occurred with only 1°F warming, while temperatures are projected to increase by 3–12°F (1.4–5.8°C) – or even up to 52°F (11°C) by some simulations – over this century (depending, primarily, on society's response).[2] Earth has experienced neither the current level of CO_2 nor the projected temperature changes since *Homo sapiens* evolved. We have truly entered uncharted seas.

EMERGING INFECTIOUS DISEASES

For interconnected sets of social and environmental reasons, we are in an era of the emergence, resurgence and redistribution of infectious diseases on a global scale. Since 1976, 40 diseases new to medicine have emerged.[8] Approximately half of these are antibiotic-resistant microbes associated with medical and farming practices. Changing social conditions, such as the growth of 'mega-cities' and widespread ecologic change, overwhelming Earth's carrying capacity (i.e. exhausting Earth's finite resources and generating wastes at rates beyond the ability of biogeochemical cycles to recycle them), are also contributing to the spread of infectious diseases. As climate changes, the warming and associated weather extremes are playing a growing role in the generation and spread of emerging infectious diseases.

For communicable diseases, land-use changes, species extinctions, global transport, wars and widening social inequities have conspired to unleash a barrage of emerging infectious diseases in the last three decades,[9] afflicting humans, wildlife, livestock, crops, forests and marine life. Multiple disturbances are contributing to this renegotiation between microbial and 'macrobial' communities: as climate changes, warming and wider weather fluctuations are playing expanding roles in the emergence, re-emergence and redistribution of infectious disease.

CLIMATE CHANGE AND EMERGING INFECTIOUS DISEASE PREVALENCE

Temperature constrains the range of vector-borne diseases (VBDs), while weather affects the timing, intensity and location of outbreaks.

Most insects are highly sensitive to temperature change: ants even run faster in warmer weather. Mosquitoes are especially sensitive to changes in temperature: warming (within their viable range) increases their activity, biting and reproductive rates, prolongs the breeding season and shortens the maturation of microbes (the extrinsic incubation rate or EIP) within them. Provided there is adequate moisture, warming can increase the populations of insects, although excessive heat decreases their survival. Between the limits of too hot and too cold there lies an optimum viability range in which warmth enhances metabolism, growth and the opportunities for disease transmission.

Findings from paleoclimatic (fossil) studies demonstrate that changes in temperature (and especially in winter temperatures; temperature minimums or TMINs) were closely correlated with geographic shifts of beetles near the end of the last glacial maximum about 10 000 years ago. Indeed, fossil records indicate that when changes in climate occur, insects shift their range far more rapidly than do grasses, shrubs and forests, and move to more favorable latitudes and elevations hundreds of years ahead of larger animals: 'Beetles', concluded one climatologist, 'are better paleo-thermometers than bears.'

THE VARIABLES

Three outcome variables are central to the question of changes in infectious disease range with warming: (1) shifts in altitude; (2) shifts in latitude; and (3) changes in seasonality. While models can project the changing envelope of *conditions conducive* to these shifts, their occurrence is a function of temperature and additional factors (e.g. previous exposure and immunity, drug-resistance, forest cover and preventive measures).

Another climate-related variable is the impact of extreme weather events on clusters of outbreaks and impacts on human nutrition.

Assessing range change

Mountain ranges are sentinel regions for monitoring global climate change and the biologic responses. Precisely because of their verticality, one can move quickly from desert to tropical to polar ecosystems. Adaptive shifts for plants and animals responding to warming (or cooling) occur much faster with regard to elevation than they do with respect to latitude. Due to the 'adiabatic lapse rate' (~1°F cooling for every 200 feet rise in elevation) the ratio is 1/600 for comparable cooling as one moves north or south.[10] For example, a plant moving 1 km up a mountain in response to warming would have to move 600 km north or south to adjust to the same shift in freezing isotherms – the line depicting the altitude or latitude at which the ground is permanently frozen all year round.

There are several concurrent changes occurring at high altitudes: (1) accelerating melt of alpine glaciers; (2) upward migration of plant communities; (3) appearance of disease vectors and/or diseases at high altitudes; and (4) the upward shift in the freezing isotherm as measured with weather balloons.[11]

Some examples of the shifts in disease vectors and diseases follow.
- Dengue fever – previously limited to about 1000 m in elevation in the tropics by the 10°C winter isotherm – has appeared at 1700 m in Mexico.
- *Aedes aegypti* mosquitoes – vectors for yellow, dengue, Rift Valley and chikungunya fevers – have been reported at 2200 m in the Andes, where temperature once restricted them to 1000 m.

- Dengue fever is now found in highland regions of Vietnam.
- Since the 1980s high-elevation malaria outbreaks have occurred in:
  - Rwanda at 1700 m
  - Ethiopia, Uganda and Kenya[12]
  - Nairobi, a mile-high city, where malaria is now circulating
  - Zimbabwe, where roughly 45% of the population is currently at risk for malaria (with warming, the area suitable for transmission will envelop the nation later this century)
  - the highlands of Papua New Guinea
  - high elevations in Bolivia.

Changes in the ranges of disease vectors in some areas may, in part, be attributable to local changes in habitat, vector ecology, pathogen and insect resistance. Climate affects not only the movement of animal populations, but can also provoke humans to migrate. Meanwhile Lafferty[13] argues that the belt of VBD transmission may shift but not expand due to excess heat and changes in hydrologic regimes. However, the disproportionate warming at night and winter, and the exaggeration of this rise in TMINs as one moves toward the poles, means that conditions at the southern end of vector ranges are not changing as fast as those at northern boundaries. Thus the conditions conducive to changes in the potential range of many vectors are expanding. Tick populations have not only shifted north in Sweden[14] with each warm winter, they have become more abundant in the areas they previously inhabited (the Stockholm Archipelago).

In addition, weather extremes can create conditions conducive to large outbreaks, and this may have as much or more to do with the location of outbreaks as the warming itself. Moreover, the changes are often nonlinear: in Honduras conditions in the south (around Choluteca) have become so hot and dry (due to climatic change, deforestation and wetland destruction that have altered the regional hydrologic cycle) that malaria has died out and agriculture has suffered greatly. Thus, people have also out-migrated, settling in the forested north where malaria is still rife.

The global pattern of physical, zoologic and botanical data is consistent with model projections, constituting an internally consistent 'fingerprint' of climate change. The set of changes occurring in the Americas (Andes, Sierra Nevada), the East African highlands, European Alps and in Asia (India and Nepal, Papua New Guinea and Irian Jaya) provides a consistent picture of changing conditions conducive to the transmission of VBDs at high altitudes.

Changes in latitude

On land, with spring arriving 1–2 weeks earlier in the Northern Hemisphere (depending on latitude) than in the 1961–1990 baseline period, birds are arriving and laying eggs earlier, butterflies are shifting in latitude and altitude, some pollinators are arriving (too) early, and plants are flowering and shedding pollen and seeds earlier.[2] In Antarctica – where the West Antarctic Peninsula has warmed 6°C since 1950 – a wholesale shift of the sub-Antarctic ecosystems poleward has occurred (as indicated by shifts in fish, penguin and seal populations), replacing polar ecosystems.

Today, ticks in Sweden are moving north with each warm winter and models project a similar shift in the USA and Canada. Meanwhile, declining predators of deer and competitors of mice, plus living patterns that fragment habitat, also contribute heavily to the propagation of Lyme disease.[15]

Computer models of global greenhouse warming project increased temperatures that will, in turn, favor the spread of VBDs into more temperate latitudes. While 42% of the globe presently offers conditions that can sustain the transmission of malaria, the fraction could rise to 60% with a global increase of a few degrees centigrade (Fig. PP1.1).

In the marine environment, the outbreak of *Vibrio parahaemolyticus* gastroenteritis from oysters harvested in warmed Alaskan waters (the mean daily water temperatures exceeding the threshold of 63°F/15°C) extended the northernmost documented source of oyster consumption causing *V. parahaemolyticus* illness by 1000 km (600 miles).

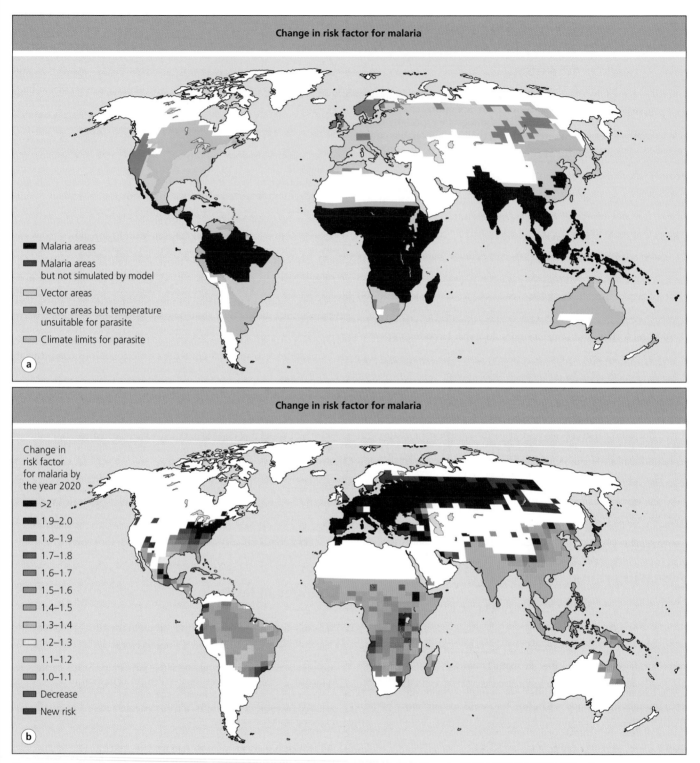

Fig. PP1.1 Projected change in risk factor for malaria by the year 2020 (1999 forecast). Reproduced with permission from Martens.[16]

Projected changes in seasonality

Models for conditions in sub-Saharan Africa project longer seasons (as measured in person-months) during which malaria may circulate. This variable needs monitoring in endemic areas.

A new variable: variability

Although weather always varies, increased variability, with rapid temperature fluctuations, altered precipitation patterns and wide swings in weather are characteristics of an unstable climate. Variability is most often considered the 'noise' about a trend; something to be cancelled out by using multi-year running averages. But for ecosystems (and humans) increased variability can be a disturbance. In the study of global climate change, variability is itself a signal – an outcome variable with multiple implications for health.

Increased variability can influence health via several pathways:

- increased seasonal and daily variability may have consequences for travel and ambulatory risks (see Health consequences of extreme weather events, below);

- increased seasonal and daily variability can affect winter cold and summer heat mortality, perhaps by weakening host defenses;
- climate instability can increase ecologic instability, altering the ratios of predators and prey (that can be pests) and populations of competitors (e.g. mice), constituting biodiversity that can 'dilute' pathogens:[15]
  - opportunistic *r*-strategists (e.g. micro-organisms, insects and rodents) rapidly proliferate with disturbances (pests and pathogens tend to be generalists and *r*-strategists)
  - specialist *K*-strategists reflect the carrying capacity of the environment (the resources used and wastes generated) and fare well under stable environmental conditions (large predators tend to be *K*-strategists)
  - increased climate variability (along with habitat fragmentation and excess chemicals) can alter *K*-to-*r* ratios, allowing the prey (insects, rodents) to escape their predators (bats, birds, damselflies, owls and kestrels) to become pests that can carry pathogens.

Increased interannual variability has been observed,[2] and the trend toward heavier precipitation events[2] (see below) and more winter precipitation falling as rain at high latitudes are indicative of increased seasonal and day-to-day variability.

Health consequences of extreme weather events

Floods frequently lead to disease 'clusters'. Heavy rains drive rodents from burrows, create mosquito-breeding sites, foster fungi and flush pathogens, nutrients and chemicals into waterways.[17] In the USA, water-borne disease outbreaks are highly correlated with heavy rains and flooding. Milwaukee's *Cryptosporidium* outbreak followed the 1993 Mississippi floods and outbreaks of *Escherichia coli* O157:H7 have most often occurred following intense rains, with sewage contaminating fresh water supplies. Floods in Europe have also been associated with outbreaks of noroviral, rotaviral and *Campylobacter* infections. Warming and extreme events can both contribute to diarrheal illness in underdeveloped nations.

Heavy rainfall along coasts can flush nutrients (chemicals and micro-organisms) into rivers, estuaries and bays, and trigger harmful algal blooms ('red tides') which can be toxic, harbor pathogens (e.g. *Vibrio* spp.) and contribute to the over 350 hypoxic 'dead zones' that affect marine coastal zones worldwide.

Flooding can also create breeding grounds for mosquitoes. The enormous outbreak of Rift Valley fever (RVF) in East Africa in 1998 occurred in the wake of heavy rains, in which the impact of the strongest El Niño event of the past century was compounded by exceptionally warm Indian Ocean sea surface temperatures; RVF also resurged in 2007 in the wake of intense East African flooding. Rift Valley fever causes a viral hemorrhagic fever in humans and its impact on animals affects nutrition, trade and livelihoods. Remote sensing and climate forecasting can generate health early warning systems for RVF,[18] facilitating timely veterinary vaccination programs.

Prolonged droughts can have severe health consequences. Droughts promote wildfires, leading to injuries, burns, respiratory illness and the loss of life. Drought can also set the conditions for infectious disease outbreaks. Water-borne diseases can stem from inadequate water supplies and hygiene, and stored water about houses can become breeding grounds for *Aedes aegypti* mosquitoes, carriers of dengue, yellow and chikungunya fevers. The recent Indian Ocean outbreak of over 500 000 cases of CHIK fever in Mauritius, the Comoros, Reunion and coastal Kenyan cities was associated with drought.

The outbreak of chikungunya fever in Italy was transmitted from an Indian traveler by *Aedes albopictus*, the cold-hardy Asian tiger mosquito introduced into Europe and the USA in old tires. This outbreak of a tropical disease in a temperate, developed region has been suggested to be a sign of global warming, and warmth may have played a role in the proliferation of mosquitoes and acceleration of the EIP of the chikungunya virus within them. On the other hand, the explosive appearance and spread of chikungunya in nations ringing the overheated Indian Ocean may have more to do with the extremes of temperatures and recurrent drought accompanying global warming.

Droughts also favor epidemics of meningococcal meningitis in the Sahel (Sahel rainfall has already fallen 25% in the past 30 years). The transmission of this person-to-person infection is presumably favored when dried mucous membranes allow colonized organisms to invade through weakened respiratory tracts. The 'meningitis belt' spans 14 nations: Ethiopia, Kenya, Sudan, Uganda, Burkina-Faso, Democratic Republic of Congo, Niger, Mali, Chad, Nigeria, Côte d'Ivoire, Ghana, Togo and Benin.

For Africa, the climate prognosis is dire. A United Nations report projects continued drying of the continent, with increasing consequences for health, crop yields, livelihoods, refugees and conflict.

The Institute of Medicine/National Academy of Sciences report *Global Climate Change and Extreme Weather Events: Understanding the Contributions to Infectious Disease Emergence* (2008) provides an excellent introduction to the impacts of weather extremes on pests and pathogens threatening humans, livestock, wildlife, forests, crops and coastal marine life.[19]

Case studies

West Nile virus

The means by which West Nile virus (WNV) was introduced into New York City in 1999 remains unknown; however, based on analysis of outbreaks of St Louis encephalitis (SLE) in the USA and WNV in Europe, some meteorologic conditions appear conducive to large epidemics. SLE first appeared in the US midwest during the Dust Bowl and outbreaks for the next four decades were associated with drought. (Once established in wildlife, rains and warmth can increase populations of 'bridge vectors'.) Outbreaks of WNV in Russia and Romania in the 1990s were also associated with drought.

The New York City epidemic occurred following a prolonged spring and summer drought along the Atlantic seaboard, and a 3-week heat wave in July. Urban, drain-dwelling, bird-biting *Culex pipiens* mosquitoes survive in warm winters and thrive in shallow pools of foul water that collect during spring droughts. Meanwhile, warm temperatures shorten the EIP and accelerate viral development, helping to boost the mosquito–avian and viral transmission cycle. Drought eventually yielded to heavy rains at the end of August (flooding New York subways and leading to an outbreak of *E. coli* O157:H7 at an upper New York State Fair) and Hurricane Floyd in mid-September.

During the hot, dry summer of 2002 (absent snow pack in the Rockies, thus no spring runoff) WNV raced across the North American continent, stopping in 44 states and reaching California and five Canadian provinces, resulting in the infection of 230 species of animals, including 37 species of birds.

Rodent-borne ills

The emergence of hantavirus pulmonary syndrome (HPS) and the explosive debut of WNV in the USA were both influenced by extreme weather. In the case of HPS, 6 years of drought in the American southwest is reported to have reduced rodent predators (owls, snakes and coyotes), while early downpours in 1993 produced a bounty of piñon nuts and grasshoppers, food for the rodents. The resulting mismatch hatched legions of white-footed mice, precipitating the explosive appearance of HPS in the Americas.

NATURE'S ILLS

A still greater threat to human health comes from the rash of illnesses stalking natural systems. The Millennium Ecosystem Assessment, involving 1300 scientists worldwide, found that 60% of the 'ecological services' they examined were being degraded or used unsustainably. The resulting biologic impoverishment has profound consequences for the control of pests and pathogens and for the quality of air, food and water.

Wildlife and livestock are developing new diseases and are increasingly suffering from old ones. Blue tongue disease, carried by *Culicoides* midges, has increased its range in Europe, threatening sheep and other ruminants.

The victims of WNV include raptors, such as owls, hawks, eagles, accipiters and kestrels. Improved monitoring of population-level impacts is needed, since these birds of prey help rein in rodent populations that can spread hantaviruses, arenaviruses, plague, *Leptospira* and Lyme-infected ticks. Most emerging infectious diseases are zoonoses.

Climate change, crop pests, nutrition and food security

Crops face a number of growing stresses, including vanishing pollinators, more volatile weather and the proliferation of agricultural pests, pathogens and weeds.[20] One fungal disease, Asian soybean rust (ASR) – believed to have entered the USA on the wings of Hurricane Ivan (one of the four to batter Florida in 2004) – is now present in over a dozen US states. Warm, moist conditions will favor the spread of ASR, a disease already widespread in Brazil and China, the other major producers of soybeans, a major staple used as food for humans and feed for animals.

- Climate change poses risks for food security and the reliability of crops used for feed, fiber and fuel.
- Warmer winters, more extreme weather events, and alterations in the timing, location and intensity of precipitation have already begun to reduce yields globally.
- Today 42% of growing and stored crops are lost annually due to pests, pathogens and weeds (equaling losses of ~$300 billion/year).
- Warming and extremes are conducive to crop pests and pathogens:
  - warming allows their overwintering and potential range;
  - floods foster fungi, the primary cause of crop blights; and
  - droughts favor aphids, geminivirus-injecting whiteflies and locusts.
- Agricultural weeds – like ragweed – are strengthened by rising CO_2 levels.
- Cassava plants grown in elevated CO_2 have increased cyanide and decreased yields (R Gleadow, Monash University, Australia, personal communication, 2009):
  - cyanide poisoning from cassava consumption during droughts has caused permanent neuropathy in children in Mozambique, Uganda and several West African nations.
- Higher atmospheric levels of CO_2 also change carbon-to-nitrogen ratios, forcing leaf-eating pests to consume more biomass (increasing herbivory) to obtain the nitrogen they need for growth.
- More pests, pathogens and weeds will, in turn, require higher use of pesticides, fungicides and herbicides that harm insectivores (spiders, ladybugs and birds), and can be carcinogenic, neurotoxic and harmful to reproductive health.
- Together, climate change and weather extremes, pests, pathogens and weeds may have 'nonlinear' impacts on agricultural yields, i.e. sudden, widespread losses.
- The potential for such extensive losses goes beyond the direct effects of changing growing seasons and shifting ecotones, with implications for nutritional health, biofuel reliability and political stability.

Climate change and resource scarcity can exacerbate strife, increasing refugees, malnutrition and disease.

Water

In many regions of the globe, ground water systems are being overdrawn and underfed. Shifting weather patterns further jeopardize water quality and quantity, and most montane ice fields will disappear this century – removing a primary source of water for humans, livestock, crops and hydropower for many nations.

In the last half of the 20th century the hydrologic cycle in the western USA changed significantly, affecting this arid region with a large and growing population. Barnett and colleagues find that warming winters, changes in precipitation and river flow, and diminished snow pack – 60% of which is attributable to anthropogenic greenhouse gas-induced warming – 'portend … a coming crisis in water supply for the western United States'.[21]

With current usage levels, an increase in environmentally displaced persons and a changing water cycle, the number of people suffering water stress and scarcity today is projected to triple in two decades.

PUBLIC HEALTH RECOMMENDATIONS

Climate forecasting and satellite images can provide early warnings of conditions conducive to disease outbreaks. During El Niño events, extreme weather conditions occur often and in relatively predictable geographic locations. Given scarce resources, the alerts can help communities target timely, environmentally friendly, health-protecting measures to the most vulnerable areas and populations. The measures include:

- distribution of antimalarials, impregnated bed nets and insecticides;
- breeding site (source) reduction;
- introducing the Western mosquito-fish (*Gambusia affinis*) into ponds;
- vaccination campaigns for bacterial meningitis; and
- preparation of oral rehydration therapy solutions and facilities for cholera.

Clean energy and development

Consistent energy supplies are necessary for development. Where grids are inadequate, stand-alone power generators – using solar, wind, geothermal and human power (hand- and bicycle-driven power) – can desalinate, decontaminate and pump water; irrigate land; power clinics; light homes; and drive small-scale enterprises. Clean distributed generation is necessary for meeting the Millennium Development Goals,[22] including adequate health care, agricultural productivity and provision of livelihoods.

Ultimately, however, governments must provide the infrastructure and financial incentives to enable large shifts in private investments, and the level of international cooperation needed to drive the clean energy transformation and preservation of the world's forests is unprecedented.

CONCLUSION

Just as we underestimated the rate at which climate would change, we have underestimated the breadth of biologic responses to those changes. Treating climate-related ills will require preparation, and early warning systems forecasting weather extremes can help to reduce casualties and disease spread. But primary prevention involves halting the extraction, mining, transport, refining and combustion of fossil fuels – a transformation that carries innumerable health and environmental benefits and is necessary to stabilize the climate.

Health professionals helped curb nuclear proliferation and focused world attention on the health implications of stratospheric ozone depletion. Now the public health community must focus its attention on the proposed energy solutions to ensure that safe technologies and practices are chosen.

The good news is that we may have also underestimated the economic benefits of the challenge ahead. With properly aligned rewards, rules and regulations, the clean energy transformation can become the driving engine for the international economy in the 21st century, laying the basis for a healthier, more equitable and sustainable future.

REFERENCES

References for this chapter can be found online at http://www.expertconsult.com

Section | 2 |

Jos WM van der Meer, Didier Raoult & Jack D Sobel

Syndromes by Body System

Chapter | 8 |

Adilia Warris
Frank P Kroon

Viral exanthems

INTRODUCTION

An exanthem or rash in a patient with fever can offer the clinician an additional clue to the etiology of the disease. The age, the immune state of the patient, geographic location and season will narrow the list of this broad differential diagnosis. A systematic history of immunizations, past childhood illnesses, exposure to other patients, animals including insects, sexual contacts, travel history and use of medications is essential. The appearance of the rash including the characteristics of a single lesion, the distribution on the skin and mucosa, the appearance and progression in relation to the development of the fever in combination with the medical history will guide the clinician. In this chapter we will focus on the viral diseases frequently accompanied by an exanthem. For an extensive review of the clinical presentation, pathogenesis, complications and treatment of the individual infections the reader is referred to the specific chapters elsewhere in this book. Viral causes of rash are outlined in Table 8.1.

Classic Viral Exanthems

VARICELLA

Varicella is an exanthematic disease with a characteristic vesicular appearance. It is caused by varicella-zoster virus (VZV), which is a member of the Alphaherpesvirinae with an enveloped linear, double-stranded DNA genome. Like other herpesviruses, it causes a primary infection (varicella or chickenpox) with seroconversion and subsequent lifelong latency. Reactivation causes localized neurologic disease with an associated skin eruption (herpes zoster or shingles). VZV is transmitted by droplets and by direct contact with the contents of the vesicles and is highly contagious. Virus shedding starts 2 days before the onset of the rash. The incubation period is 11–20 days. The peak age of infection is between 1 and 8 years.[1]

Table 8.1 Viral exanthems

Erythematous maculopapulous	Papulovesiculous	Vesiculobullous	Petechial and purpuric
Morbillivirus	Hepatitis B virus	Varicella-zoster virus	Cytomegalovirus (congenital)
Rubella	Gianotti–Crosti syndrome	Herpes simplex virus	
Human herpesvirus 6		Variola virus	Rubella (congenital)
Human herpesvirus 7	Asymmetric periflexural exanthem	Vaccinia virus	Enterovirus
Parvovirus B19		Monkeypox virus	PPGSS[†]
Epstein–Barr virus		Cowpox virus	Flaviviruses
Cytomegalovirus		Enteroviruses	Viral hemorrhagic fevers
Enteroviruses			
HIV			
Alphaviruses*			
Flaviviruses			
Menangle virus			

*Alphaviruses: Chikungunya virus, O'nyong-nyong virus, Sindbis virus, Ross River virus, Mayaro virus.
†Papular–purpuric gloves and socks syndrome

Clinical features

The lesions of varicella begin as papules, but progress within hours to clear vesicles surrounded by a variable halo of erythema. Vesicles are often oval, with the long axis parallel to skin creases, and are commonly pruritic (Fig. 8.1). New lesions appear progressively over 5–7 days. The head and upper trunk are affected first and most densely, whereas the limbs have fewer lesions and these appear later. The vesicular fluid opacifies, and in 2–3 days a central dimple appears. A crust then forms from this center outward, and falls off after about 5 days. Prodromal symptoms of malaise, headache and loss of appetite are mild and more common in adults. Unless secondary infection of the skin has occurred, scarring is limited to faint, pale outlines. Indicators of severe disease include confluence of the rash, multiple lesions in the mouth, pharynx, esophagus, trachea and mucosa of the genital tract.

Herpes zoster is heralded by pain in the dermatome served by the affected sensory root. Groups of papules then appear at the sites where the cutaneous nerves reach the skin. The skin eruption will be restricted to one dermatome unilaterally in the immunocompetent host; in the immunocompromised patient multidermatomal skin eruptions or generalization may occur. The papules progress to vesicles, pustules and crustae but, unlike varicella, lesions may become confluent and form large, flaccid bullae that rupture to leave weeping bare areas (Fig. 8.2). Uncomplicated lesions can heal in 4–6 days, but severe rashes may take 3–5 weeks. Nevertheless, skin depigmentation is often the only sequel. Scarring is rare.

Complications

Secondary bacterial skin infection is the commonest complication of varicella infection and occurs in 5–10% of the patients. The usual pathogens are *Streptococcus pyogenes* or *Staphylococcus aureus* (Fig. 8.3). Bacterial infections of individual spots cause pain, induration and often abscess formation. Local extension can cause cellulitis or erysipelas; necrotizing fasciitis is rare. Children are particularly prone to staphylococcal or streptococcal toxic shock syndrome. Secondary bacterial infection can also complicate herpes zoster, especially when severe and in the elderly. Varicella pneumonia which occurs in immunocompromised patients and pregnant women is a complication which is beyond the scope of this chapter (see Chapters 75 and 155.).

Postherpetic neuralgia is defined by persisting pain after an episode of herpes zoster and older patients are at risk of developing postherpetic neuralgia. Average duration in those aged over 60 years is 60 days, but may persist much longer.

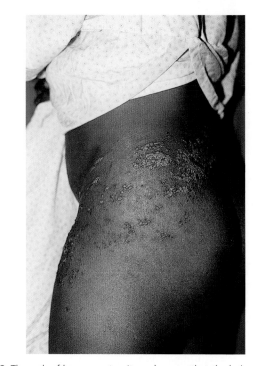

Fig. 8.2 The rash of herpes zoster. It can be seen that the lesions occur in groups, with coalescence of lesions in the larger groups. Courtesy of Barbara A Bannister, MD.

Management

Antiviral treatment has minimal impact on mild childhood infections and is not recommended. In adolescents and adults, aciclovir shortens the duration of VZV infections and may reduce the risk of complications. Valaciclovir, a prodrug of aciclovir, has an enhanced bioavailability and is the preferred oral antiviral drug. Intravenous aciclovir (10 mg/kg q8h) is the treatment of choice for VZV infections in immunocompromised patients or for severe and complicated VZV infections.

In herpes zoster, antiviral treatment started in the first 48 hours after the onset of the skin eruption reduces the duration of the rash and ameliorates zoster-associated pain, but does not prevent postherpetic neuralgia.[2,3] Prevention of herpes zoster and postherpetic neuralgia in elderly persons has been shown by immunization with the live attenuated Oka VZV vaccine. A reduction in the incidence of herpes zoster

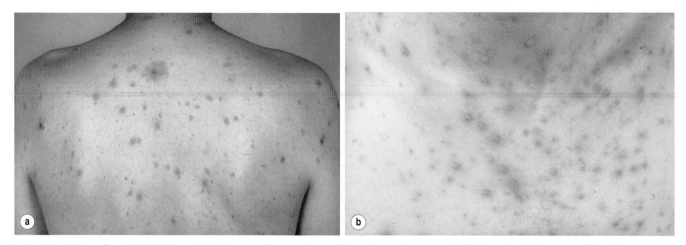

Fig. 8.1 The lesions of varicella (chickenpox). At the same time papules, vesicles and pustules, some of which are beginning to crust from the center, are seen.

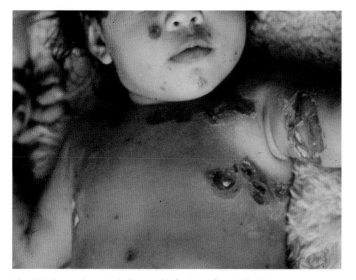

Fig. 8.3 Secondary staphylococcal infection of varicella lesions. Staphylococcal pyrogenic exotoxin has caused a 'scalded skin' type of lesion surrounding the infected spots. Courtesy of Dr MG Brook.

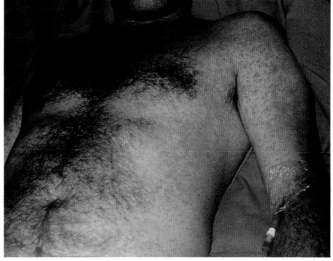

Fig. 8.4 The acute rash of measles. Marked conjunctivitis accompanied the maculopapular skin lesion in this unimmunized adult. Courtesy of Barbara A Bannister, MD.

and consequently the development of postherpetic neuralgia was seen by 61.1% and 66.5%, respectively, in adults more than 60 years of age.[4] Secondary bacterial skin infections should be treated promptly with antibiotics with activity against *Strep. pyogenes* and *Staph. aureus*. Postherpetic neuralgia responds poorly to analgesics. Amitriptyline or antiepileptic drugs may give some relief in patients with persistent postherpetic neuralgia.

MORBILLI

Morbilli is an exanthematic disease caused by the measles virus, genus Morbillivirus, member of the Paramyxoviridae, a family of enveloped, negative, single-stranded RNA viruses.

In most populations the majority of adults and children are immune due to exposure to the measles virus or vaccination. In resource-poor countries, where the vaccination coverage is low, measles is still a significant cause of morbidity and mortality. In countries where measles vaccination is included in the pediatric vaccination program, measles has become a rare disease and is often diagnosed as a disease imported by nonimmune individuals from endemic countries. Furthermore, sporadic epidemics of measles occur in religious communities where vaccination is not accepted. Humans are the only known reservoir of measles. The infection is highly contagious and is spread airborne, by droplets. The virus replicates in the respiratory mucosa and spreads (primary viremia) in leukocytes to endothelial and epithelial cells, monocytes and macrophages, which will release large amounts of virus several days after the first viremia, resulting in a secondary viremia. The asymptomatic incubation period of measles lasts 10–14 days. During the second viremia, symptoms of malaise, fever, anorexia, followed by conjunctivitis, coryza and cough, occur. This prodromal phase lasts for 2–3 days, sometimes up to 8 days. The period of contagion ranges from 5 days before to 4 days after the appearance of the rash. Maximum contagion is probably during the late prodromal phase, when the patient develops fever and respiratory symptoms.[5]

Clinical features

During the late prodromal phase, patients may develop an enanthem known as Koplik's spots. Koplik's spots are 1–3 mm grayish or bluish elevations with an erythematous base, seen on the buccal mucosa usually opposite the molars or sometimes on the labial mucosa. They have been described as 'salt grains on a red background'. Koplik's spots

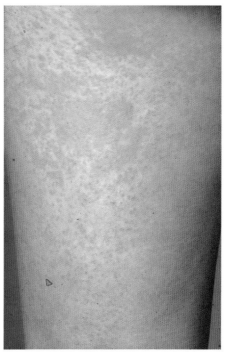

Fig. 8.5 The generalized confluent maculopapular rash as seen in measles.

occur approximately 48 hours before the measles exanthem occurs. Koplik's spots disappear by the second day of the exanthem. The characteristic rash is maculopapular and blanches, beginning on the face and spreading to the neck, upper trunk, lower trunk and extremities (Figs 8.4, 8.5). The lesions may become confluent, especially in areas such as the face. The palms and soles are rarely involved. The cranial-to-caudal progression of the measles rash is characteristic. Unlike Koplik's spots, the rash of measles is not pathognomonic. The rash begins to fade 3–4 days after it first appears, and changes to a purplish brownish color which is sometimes followed by fine desquamation. Clinical improvement ensues within 48 hours of the appearance of the rash.

The differential diagnosis of the measles exanthem includes human herpesvirus 6 (HHV-6) infection, rubella, infectious mononucleosis, scarlet fever, Kawasaki disease, toxic shock syndrome, dengue, Rocky Mountain spotted fever and drug allergy. Measles

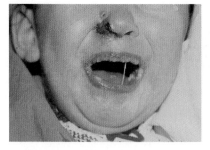

Fig. 8.6 Secondary infections complicating measles. Perioral infection and paranasal herpes simplex lesion in a 2-year-old girl. Courtesy of Barbara A Bannister, MD.

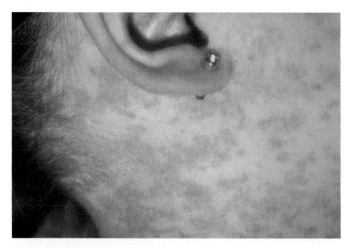

Fig. 8.7 Presenting rash with pink-red macules and papules on the face and neck as seen in rubella.

can usually be distinguished clinically from rubella, erythema infectiosum (parvovirus B19 infection), roseola and enteroviral infection by the intensity of the measles rash, its brownish coloration and the combination with other physical findings (e.g. coryza and conjunctivitis).

Complications

When poor hygiene, crowding or malnourishment exist, severe infection of macerated perioral or perinasal skin (cancrum oris) may be caused by pyogenic organisms, often accompanied by herpes simplex and/or anaerobic mouth flora (Fig. 8.6). Postinfectious encephalitis and subacute sclerosing panencephalitis are rare complications that are beyond the scope of this chapter.

Management

After introduction of the live attenuated measles vaccine in the 1960s this epidemic disease was rapidly controlled. Due to the inverse relationship between serum retinol concentrations and measles mortality, oral vitamin A is advised at diagnosis in areas where health care and nutrition are suboptimal. There is no specific treatment.

RUBELLA

Rubella, also known as German measles, is caused by the rubella virus, a member of the Togaviridae, which is a single-stranded RNA virus. The virus is transmitted from person to person by respiratory secretions. The infectious period starts 7 days before the onset of the rash and continues for another 2 days. Most shedding of infectious virus occurs before the onset of the rash. The incubation period is 15–20 days. In susceptible populations, the peak age of infection is between 5 and 9 years.[6]

Clinical features

Prodromal symptoms such as malaise are minimal in children, although the lymph nodes begin to enlarge 3–4 days before the onset of the rash. Large tender lymph nodes high in the occipital region are typical of rubella. Adults may suffer 3–4 days' prodrome with low-grade fever, muscle pains and headache. Conjunctivitis and coryza, if present, are usually minimal and accompany the rash. The rash presents with pink-red macules and papules on the face and spreads to the chest and peripheries over 1–2 days (Fig. 8.7). The exanthem begins to fade after 1–2 days in order of appearance and disappears completely in 2–3 days. There is often an enanthem with punctate erythematous spots scattered over the hard and soft palate and uvula, called the Forchheimer sign. It mimics the rashes of parvovirus infection, echovirus infections and mild scarlet fever or early Kawasaki disease, although it does not desquamate on healing.

Rubella in pregnant women may lead to the congenital rubella syndrome with a wide range of anomalies, and ongoing virus replication and inflammation after birth (see Chapter 52). Newborns with

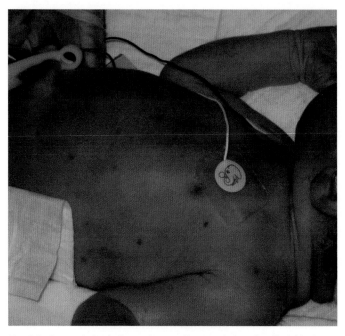

Fig. 8.8 Congenital rubella syndrome. Characteristic rash called 'blueberry muffin spots' in a newborn with congenital rubella.

congenital rubella syndrome show a completely different exanthem. The rash consists of petechial/purpuric-like lesions scattered over the skin (Fig. 8.8). Due to its appearance this characteristic exanthem is referred to as 'blueberry muffin spots'. These spots are thought to be the consequence of extramedullary dermal erythropoiesis.[7,8] Congenital cytomegalovirus (CMV) infection should be in the differential diagnosis when confronted with a neonate with 'blueberry muffin spots'.

Management

The illness is mild and self-limiting; specific treatment is not available. An excellent live attenuated rubella vaccine has been available since 1968 and is used in many parts of the world in childhood immunization programs. The efficacy of the rubella vaccine has been shown by a marked reduction in the prevalence of congenital rubella syndrome.

INFECTION BY PARVOVIRUS B19 (ERYTHEMA INFECTIOSUM)

Erythema infectiosum is caused by human parvovirus B19, which belongs to the Erythrovirus genus, and is the only member of the Parvoviridae family pathogenic to humans. The Parvoviridae are very small, nonenveloped, single-stranded DNA viruses. Parvovirus B19 infection occurs worldwide. Cases can be sporadic or can occur in clustered outbreaks. Most individuals become infected during their school years. More than 70% of adults have parvovirus B19-specific IgG antibodies. Approximately 25% of the infections are asymptomatic, 50% will have nonspecific flu-like symptoms and 25% will present with the classic symptoms of parvovirus B19 infection including rash and/or arthralgia. Parvovirus B19 infections are transmitted from person to person via respiratory secretions. It has an incubation period of 4–14 days. Furthermore, vertical transmission, resulting in congenital infection, and transmission by the administration of blood or blood products containing parvovirus B19 may occur.[9]

Clinical features

The childhood infection usually manifests itself as erythema infectiosum (fifth disease or slapped cheek syndrome), a mild febrile illness with rash.

In the first week after infection the viremia is accompanied by a nonspecific flu-like illness, with symptoms of fever, malaise, myalgia, headache and pruritus. Between 2 and 5 days later (i.e. 1–2 weeks after infection) the classic erythematous malar rash appears (the so-called slapped cheek rash) with circumoral pallor (Fig. 8.9). This facial rash is often followed by a maculopapular exanthem on the trunk and extremities, which confluences into a lacy, reticular pattern. The rash in adults is less characteristic than the rash in children. By the time the rash develops, viremia and symptoms have resolved. The rash disappears within a week.

Parvovirus B19 infection has been associated with other types of rash including morbilliform, confluent and vesicular. Moreover, parvovirus B19 has been linked in more than half of the reported cases of papular–purpuric gloves and socks syndrome (see below).

Complications

Severe outcomes may occur in immunocompromised patients and patients with hemoglobinopathies. Infection in these patient groups can cause a serious prolonged chronic anemia (pure red cell aplasia) owing to persistent lysis of red blood cell precursors.

Parvovirus B19 infection during pregnancy can result in fetal complications including miscarriage, intrauterine fetal death and/or nonimmune hydrops fetalis.

Management

Treatment of parvovirus B19 infection is symptomatic.

HUMAN HERPESVIRUS 6 INFECTION (ROSEOLA INFANTUM)

Roseola infantum is caused by human herpesvirus 6 (HHV-6), a double-stranded DNA virus, a member of the (beta) Herpesviridae family, genus Roseolovirus.[10] Worldwide the HHV-6 seroprevalence rates in adults vary from 20% to 100%; in industrialized countries rates of seroprevalence range from 72% to 95%. Ninety percent of cases occur in children younger than 2 years with a peak between 7 and 13 months of age. The most common route of HHV-6 transmission appears to be via saliva from mother to child. Perinatal transmission is also possible; approximately 2% of pregnant women shed low levels of virus in genital secretions. The incubation period is estimated at 5–15 days.

Clinical features

The classic manifestation of HHV-6 infection in children (roseola infantum, exanthema subitum, sixth disease) is an abrupt onset of fever that may exceed 104°F (40°C) and will lasts for 3–5 days, often accompanied by irritability, although most children appear well. Furthermore, malaise, palpebral conjunctivitis, edematous eyelids, uvulo-palatoglossal junctional macules or ulcers (sometimes called Nagayama spots), upper and lower respiratory symptoms, vomiting,

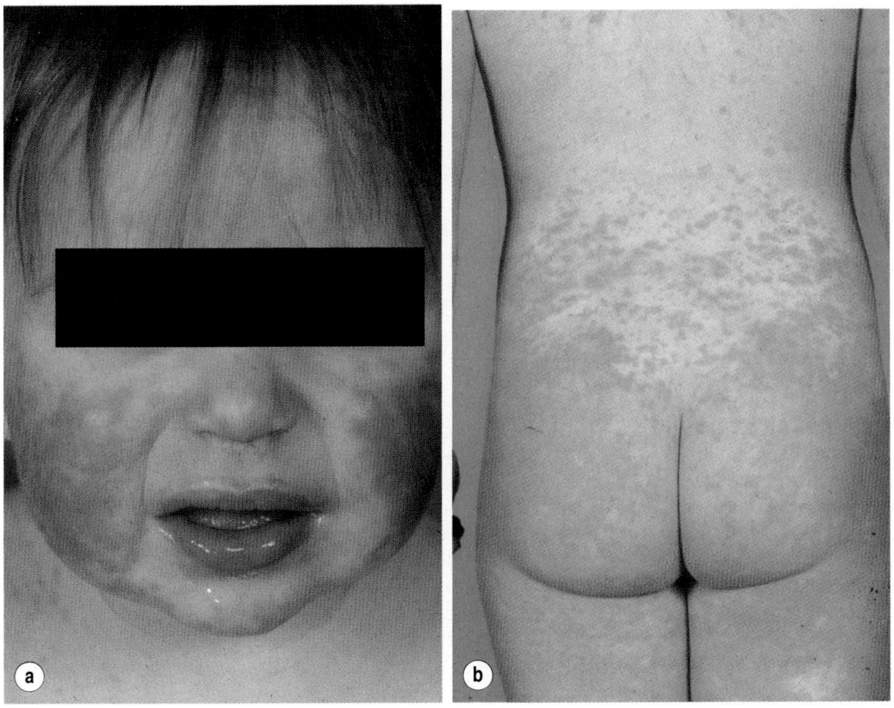

Fig. 8.9 Parvovirus B19 infections. Characteristic skin abnormalities of the 'slapped cheeks', circumoral pallor and a maculopapular exanthem on the trunk.

diarrhea and a bulging fontanel may be present. As the fever subsides, a blanching macular or maculopapular nonpruritic rash develops, starting on the neck and trunk and spreading to the face and proximal extremities. Sometimes this rash is vesicular. The rash usually persists for 1–2 days, but can disappear within several hours. Acute HHV-6 infection can also present as a febrile illness without a rash.

Cervical, postauricular and/or occipital lymphadenopathy are also common but later findings. Primary infection with HHV-6 in adults is rare. However, a mononucleosis-like syndrome of varying severity (with or without an exanthem) with prolonged lymphadenopathy has been described in adults.

The rash can be easily misdiagnosed as a drug allergy. Furthermore, the differential diagnosis of the exanthem as seen in roseola infantum includes rubella (rash and fever occur simultaneously), rubeola (rash and fever occur simultaneously), erythema infectiosum (slapped cheeks in school-aged children) and scarlet fever (rash may be confluent, which may be preceded by pharyngitis).

Complications

HHV-6 infections have been associated with the Gianotti–Crosti syndrome (see below) and the papular–purpuric gloves and socks syndrome (see below). HHV-6 infections have been associated with seizures, either secondary to the high fever or to the infection itself. Panencephalitis of variable severity can occur as the primary manifestation of HHV-6. HHV-6 remains latent in host cells after primary infection and can be reactivated in immunocompromised patients such as after solid-organ or hematopoietic stem cell transplantation. The majority of HHV-6 infections in these patients are asymptomatic. However, clinical syndromes associated with HHV-6 reactivation include unexplained fever, rash, hepatitis, pneumonitis, encephalitis and bone marrow suppression.

Management

Most cases are benign and self-limiting. Treatment is supportive.

Nonclassic Viral Exanthems

EPSTEIN–BARR VIRUS INFECTION (INFECTIOUS MONONUCLEOSIS) (SEE CHAPTER 155)

Infectious mononucleosis is caused by Epstein–Barr virus (EBV) or human herpesvirus 4, a member of the Herpesviridae family. Primary infection results from exposure to the oral secretions of seropositive individuals. EBV shares the properties of lifelong latency and persistence with other members of the herpesvirus family. The incubation period is 2–8 weeks in adolescents and young adults but probably shorter in younger children.

Clinical features

Classic infectious mononucleosis is characterized by fever (mean duration of 2 weeks), angina with tonsillitis, malaise and cervical lymphadenopathy. The age of the patient has a profound influence on the clinical presentation. In children, primary infection is often asymptomatic. A rash, which may be macular, petechial, scarlatiniform, urticarial or erythema multiforme-like, is present in about 10% of the cases between days 4 and 6 of the illness and is localized mainly on the trunk and upper extremities. The administration of penicillins (especially ampicillin and amoxicillin) produces a pruritic maculopapular to morbilliform eruption in 90–100% of the patients.[11,12] This rash has a prolonged duration (up to 10 days). Streptococcal pharyngitis/tonsillitis, CMV infection, thrombocytopenic purpura,

lupus erythematosus and malignancies might give a comparable clinical picture to that seen in infectious mononucleosis.

Complications

Epstein–Barr virus infections are also associated with the Gianotti–Crosti syndrome, Sweet's syndrome, Stevens–Johnson syndrome and persistent erythema multiforme.[13–15]

Management

Specific treatment is not available.

ACUTE CYTOMEGALOVIRUS INFECTION

Cytomegalovirus, belonging to the Herpesviridae family, is a beta-herpes virus and is the largest virus infecting human beings. Infection is common in all human populations. Disease in humans is varied, ranging from no disease in normal hosts to life-threatening infections in immunocompromised patients. Secondary infection represents activation of latent infection or re-infection in a sero-positive immune person. Congenital infection of the neonate is almost always the result of primary infection of the mother during pregnancy.

Clinical features

Most primary infections are subclinical during childhood although in young adults an infectious mononucleosis syndrome with fever and lymphadenopathy can be seen. A maculopapular and rubelliform rash may occur in the setting of CMV mononucleosis.[16] These rashes may develop after administration of penicillins and are thought to result from immunologic reactions to cellular antigens that are uncovered or expressed in association with acute CMV infection. CMV mononucleosis needs to be differentiated from EBV infection and malignancies.

Congenital infections in newborns can present with a petechial/purpuric rash, comparable to the so-called 'blueberry muffin spots' seen in congenital rubella syndrome.[7]

Complications

Skin manifestations of acute CMV infections are usually mild but can occasionally be severe, ranging from erythema multiforme to epidermolysis.[17,18]

Management

CMV infections in immunocompetent patients are self-limiting and specific treatment is not indicated. In contrast, CMV infections in immunocompromised patients can be life-threatening and need to be treated with (val)ganciclovir (see Chapter 52). Congenital CMV infections can be treated in the neonate with ganciclovir for 6 weeks and has been shown to be effective in preventing hearing loss[19] (see Chapter 52).

ACUTE HIV INFECTION

Acute HIV infection may present with a skin rash (see Chapter 89). HIV is a single-stranded RNA virus, a member of the Retroviridae family, genus Lentivirus.

HIV is transmitted via unprotected sexual intercourse, vertical transmission and incidents with blood–blood contact, such as needlestick incidents. Due to screening of blood and blood-derived products, transmission via transfusion is now extremely rare.

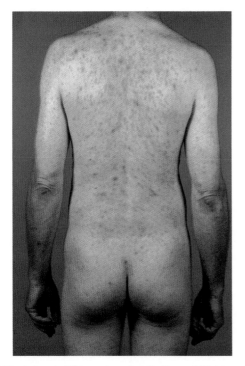

Fig. 8.10 The lesions in HIV are characteristically small (5–10 mm), well-circumscribed, oval or round, pink to deeply red colored macules or maculopapules.

Clinical features

The majority of patients with an acute HIV infection appear to be symptomatic (40–90%).[20] The usual time from HIV exposure to the development of symptoms is 2–4 weeks. Acute HIV infection is characterized by an abrupt onset of symptoms; the clinical syndrome develops within 24–48 hours and lasts 1.5–2 weeks. The most common findings are fever (range 100–104°F/38–40°C), lymphadenopathy, mild hepatosplenomegaly, sore throat, painful mucocutaneous ulceration (mouth, esophagus, penis, anus), myalgia/arthralgia, diarrhea, headache, nausea/vomiting, weight loss, dry cough and hepatitis. The presence of mucocutaneous ulcers is suggestive of the diagnosis.

The exanthem, occurring in 40–80% of symptomatic patients, typically occurs 48–72 hours after the onset of fever and persists for 5–8 days. The upper thorax, collar region and face are most often involved though the scalp and extremities, including the palms and soles, may be affected. The lesions are characteristically small (5–10 mm), well-circumscribed, oval or round, pink to deeply red colored macules or maculopapules (Fig. 8.10). Vesicular, pustular and urticarial eruptions have also been reported.

The differential diagnosis of acute HIV infection includes mononucleosis due to EBV or CMV, toxoplasmosis, rubella, syphilis, viral hepatitis and other viral infections.

Management

There is ongoing debate as to whether starting antiretroviral therapy during an acute HIV infection will improve prognosis by preserving the HIV-specific immune response. At the moment, no consensus has been reached on whether patients with primary HIV infection should be treated (see Chapter 89).

VIRAL HEMORRAGHIC FEVERS

Viral hemorrhagic fevers are discussed in detail in Chapter 126.

HAND, FOOT AND MOUTH DISEASE

Hand, foot and mouth disease (HFMD) is caused by enteroviruses, members of the picornavirus group (single-stranded RNA, nonenveloped) and is most commonly associated with Coxsackie virus A16 or enterovirus 71. This disease was described for the first time in 1957 in Toronto. The UK shows an epidemic course every 3 years. These epidemics seem to be associated with the warmer seasons (summer and early fall). Sporadic cases caused by Coxsackie viruses A4–7, A9, A10, B1–3 and B5 have been reported.

HFMD is highly contagious and is spread by oral–oral and fecal–oral routes. Fecal shedding may last for 4–6 weeks but its relevance in transmission is unknown. It typically affects children under 10 years of age. The incubation period is 3–6 days.[21]

Clinical features

A brief 12–36-hour prodrome of low-grade fever, malaise, cough, anorexia, abdominal pain and sore mouth occurs. Patients may present with either exanthem or enanthem but most manifest both. Painful ulcerative lesions in the oral cavity are most commonly found on the hard palate, tongue and buccal mucosa. The enanthem begins as 2–8 mm erythematous macules and papules, which progress through a short vesicular stage to form a yellow-gray ulcer with an erythematous halo. Lesions may coalesce, the tongue may become red and edematous (Fig. 8.11). Pain may interfere with oral intake. The oral lesions resolve spontaneously in 5–7 days.

The skin rash is characterized by 2–3 mm erythematous macules or papules with a central gray vesicle; these usually appear shortly after the oral lesions, with the hands more commonly involved than the feet (Figs 8.12, 8.13). The sides of the fingers and dorsal surfaces are more often involved than the palms and soles. Lesions appear elliptical, with the long axis running parallel to skin lines, and may be asymptomatic or painful. They crust and gradually disappear over 5–10 days without scarring. In addition, one-third of the cases show a maculopapular exanthem on the nates.

Stomatitis caused by herpes simplex virus is clinically indistinguishable from the oral lesions seen in HFMD, although the former is not followed by an exanthem. Other differential diagnostic considerations are herpangina, EBV infections, morbus Behçet and syphilis in adults.

Management

The illness is mild and self-limiting. Specific treatment is not available, but the lesions can be painful or tender and simple analgesics may help this.

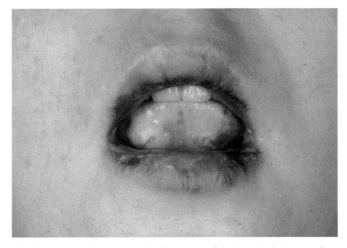

Fig. 8.11 Hand, foot and mouth disease. Painful ulcerative lesions on the tongue and buccal mucosa.

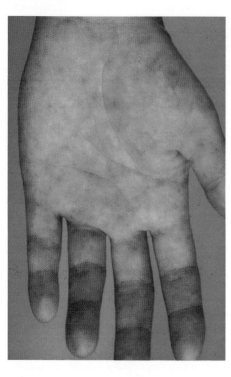

Fig. 8.12 Hand, foot and mouth disease. The skin rash is characterized by erythematous macules or papules, with the hands more commonly involved than the feet.

Table 8.2 Viral and bacterial infections and immunizations associated with the Gianotti–Crosti syndrome

Viral infections	Hepatitis A, B and C virus, Epstein–Barr virus, cytomegalovirus, human herpes virus 6, Coxsackie virus (A16, B4, B5), adenovirus, rotavirus, parvovirus B19, respiratory syncytial virus, parainfluenza virus, rubella virus
Bacterial infections	Group A streptococci, *Mycobacterium avium intracellulare* (HIV+), *Mycoplasma pneumoniae*
Immunizations	Measles–mumps–rubella, polio, influenza, diphtheria, pertussis, hepatitis B

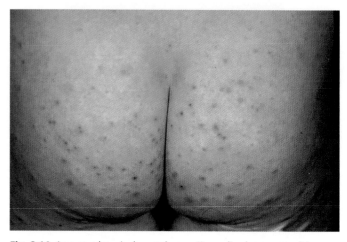

Fig. 8.14 Acropapulovesicular syndrome. Generalized monomorphic exanthem consisting of erythematous papules and papulovesicles distributed symmetrically.

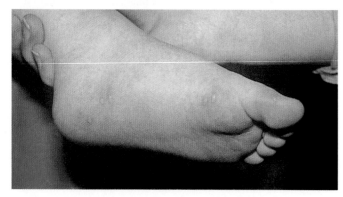

Fig. 8.13 Hand, foot and mouth disease. Typical vesicles are seen on the foot of a 3-year-old child. Courtesy of Barbara A Bannister, MD.

ACROPAPULOVESICULAR SYNDROME

Papular acrodermatitis of childhood or acropapulovesicular syndrome is a papular or papulovesicular skin eruption localized on the limbs. This syndrome was described for the first time by Gianotti in Milan, Italy and is also named Gianotti–Crosti syndrome. Initially, this syndrome was diagnosed in association with anicteric hepatitis B infection. It is well known that several viruses and some bacteria can cause this syndrome, and a number of reports suggest that it may also be associated with immunizations (Table 8.2).[22–24] The pathogenesis is still unclear. It mainly affects children between 2 and 6 years of age.

Clinical features

The rash is characterized by a monomorphic exanthem consisting of skin colored to erythematous papules and papulovesicles with a diameter of 2–4 mm distributed symmetrically on the cheeks, nates and the extensor side of the limbs (Fig. 8.14). Larger plaques of confluent papules can be seen on the elbows and knees. The nonitching exanthem develops within a week and disappears in 2–4 weeks; however, cases have been described in which the skin abnormalities lasted for 4 months. General

symptoms are usually mild. Malaise, lymphadenopathy, hepatosplenomegaly and low-grade fever may accompany the rash.[25]

Henoch–Schönlein purpura, erythema multiforme, hand, foot and mouth disease, pityriasis lichenoides and asymmetric periflexural exanthem of childhood may mimic the Gianotti–Crosti syndrome. Papular urticaria can also give a comparable exanthem.

Management

Specific treatment is not indicated. Symptomatic treatment of the pruritus with antihistamine drugs may give some relief. Due to the association (although sporadic) of hepatitis B virus infections, it is recommended to perform serology to exclude this disease.

UNILATERAL LATEROTHORACIC EXANTHEM OF CHILDHOOD

In 1962 a new localized exanthem was reported[26] and in 1992 was described as laterothoracic exanthem.[27] Because this exanthem is not only laterothoracically located, the term asymmetric periflexural exanthem is preferred. It is most likely caused by a virus, with a human herpesvirus considered to be the most likely cause. The peak age of infection is 2 years.

Clinical features

The rash consists of an erythematous papular, sometimes vesicular or squamous exanthem with a mild pruritus, localized around a skin fold such as the axilla or groin (Fig. 8.15). The skin fold itself is not affected. The exanthem consists of 1 mm erythematous pap-

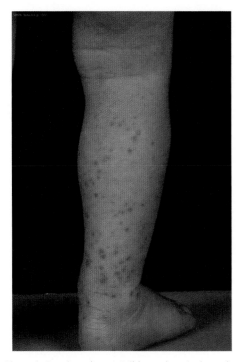

Fig. 8.15 Gianotti–Crosti syndrome. Mild papulovesicular rash on the lower extremities in a young boy. (Illustration kindly provided by the Department of Dermatology, Radboud University Nijmegen Medical Center, the Netherlands.)

ules that are often surrounded by a pale halo, followed by eczematous patches separated by normal skin. Centrifugal progression of the lesions can be seen for 8–15 days, with spontaneous recovery within 4 weeks. A mild upper respiratory illness or prodrome is often associated with the rash. Lymphadenopathy can be found but is not obligatory.[28]

The exanthem has to be differentiated from allergic contact eczema, miliaria, scarlet fever, pityriasis rosea (affecting mainly adolescents) and Gianotti–Crosti syndrome.

Management

Symptomatic treatment for the pruritus may be necessary. Complications are not known.

PAPULAR–PURPURIC GLOVES AND SOCKS SYNDROME

It has been suggested that papular–purpuric gloves and socks syndrome (PPGSS) is a manifestation of an underlying immunologic mechanism that may be induced by viral or drug-related antigens. Reported etiologies include parvovirus B19 (more than half of the cases),[29] measles virus, EBV, CMV, HHV-6, Coxsackie B6 and hepatitis B. PPGSS occurs most commonly in young adults during the spring and summer.[30]

Clinical features

Symmetric erythema and edema of the hands and feet progress to petechial and purpuric macules and papules that are followed by desquamation (Fig. 8.16). A sharp demarcation is seen at the wrists and ankles. Very seldom the rash extends to nonacral sites. Occasionally, complaints of pruritus or pain may accompany the skin eruption.[31] A polymorphous enanthem, including hyperemia, aphthae, petechiae and erosions on the palate, pharynx and tongue, are seen in the majority of patients.

The differential diagnosis includes erythema multiforme, HFMD, Gianotti–Crosti syndrome, Kawasaki disease and Rocky Mountain spotted fever, although the defined acral distribution generally allows differentiation from other exanthems.

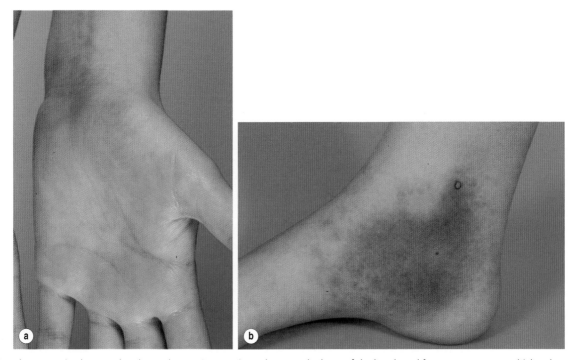

Fig. 8.16 Papular–purpuric gloves and socks syndrome. Symmetric erythema and edema of the hands and feet progress to petechial and purpuric macules and papules.

Complications

The rash resolves spontaneously in 1–2 weeks without any known sequelae.

Management

Symptomatic treatment with moisturizers and antihistamines may be indicated.

REFERENCES

References for this chapter can be found online at http://www.expertconsult.com

Cellulitis, pyoderma, abscesses and other skin and subcutaneous infections

INTRODUCTION

Infections of the skin and/or subcutaneous tissues are highly diverse in respect to etiologic organisms, incidence, clinical manifestations, severity and complications. They may occur as single or recurrent episodes. Many cases are mild or self-limited, but some progress to cause scarring, loss of digits or limbs, or even death.

The terminology can be confusing because several different names, which are often not precisely defined, may be used to describe the same condition. Nomenclature for the most common infections is summarized in Table 9.1.

When a patient presents with soft tissue infection, the clinician faces the challenge of establishing a specific diagnosis and prescribing definitive treatment. Important points in diagnosis are:

- the patient's symptoms;
- the general appearance of the infected site;
- historic clues such as contact with insects or animals, especially involving bites, travel to specific geographic areas, occupation or use of a hot tub (see Folliculitis, furuncles and carbuncles, below);
- the immune status of the host;
- chronicity; and
- anatomic distribution.

If the diagnosis cannot be established based upon the history, symptoms and signs, then needle aspiration, biopsy or surgical exploration may be necessary to obtain specimens for appropriate staining and culture.

As the antimicrobial susceptibility of these microbes varies greatly, treatment (particularly for severe infections) should be based upon the results of microscopy, Gram stain and culture whenever possible.

Table 9.1 Nomenclature, location and etiology of some common skin and subcutaneous infections

Terminology	Subgroups	Location	Etiology
Pyoderma	Impetigo (impetigo contagiosa)	Skin	*Streptococcus pyogenes*, *Staphylococcus aureus*
	Bullous impetigo	Skin	*Stap. aureus* with group II phage
	Folliculitis (pustulosis)	Skin, hair follicles	*Staph. aureus*
	Folliculitis (sycosis) barbae	Skin, hair follicles of the beard	*Strep. pyogenes*, *Staph. aureus*
	Hot tub folliculitis	Skin	*Pseudomonas aeruginosa*
Abscesses	Furuncle (boil, subcutaneous abscess)	Subcutaneous tissue	*Staph. aureus*
	Hydradenitis suppurativa	Multiple furuncles in sweat glands: axilla, groins	*Staph. aureus* and other bacteria, including Gram-negative bacilli and anaerobes
	Carbuncle	Dense group of furuncles in areas of thick skin: back of neck, shoulders, buttocks	*Staph. aureus*
Cellulitis		Skin and subcutaneous tissue	*Staph. aureus*, *Strep. pyogenes*, group C and G streptococci, *P. aeruginosa*, *Haemophilus influenzae* or Gram-negative bacilli; fungi can cause cellulitis in immunocompromised hosts
	Erysipelas	Skin	*Strep. pyogenes*
Ecthyma		Skin and subcutaneous tissue	*Strep. pyogenes*, *Staph aureus* or both; other bacteria *P. aeruginosa*
	Ecthyma gangrenosum	Skin and subcutaneous tissue in neutropenic patients	

EPIDEMIOLOGY

Although the exact incidence of these infections in the general population is unknown, they are among the most common infections occurring in all age groups. Some are age related; for example, impetigo is more common in children, erysipelas is more common in older adults.

Infections of the skin and soft tissues can be caused by bacteria (including rickettsiae), fungi, viruses, parasites and spirochetes. Although there are hundreds of possible etiologic agents (Tables 9.1–9.4), two common species of Gram-positive cocci are the predominant causes of skin and soft tissue infections – *Staphylococcus aureus* and *Streptococcus pyogenes*. Skin and soft tissue infections caused by newly recognized or previously rarely encountered microbes are continually being described in immunocompromised patients, especially those who have AIDS.

Several noninfectious diseases can mimic infection of the soft tissues. For example, patients who have contact dermatitis, pyoderma gangrenosum, gout, psoriatic arthritis with distal dactylitis, Reiter's syndrome, relapsing polychondritis or mixed cryoglobulinemia secondary to immune complex disease from chronic hepatitis C or B virus infection may present with erythematous rashes, with or without fever.

PATHOGENESIS

The integument is an organ that reacts to noxious, infectious, external and internal stimuli in a limited number of ways. It is therefore not surprising that infection can be mimicked by noninfectious inflammatory conditions. The rich plexus of capillaries beneath the dermal papillae provides nutrition to the stratum germinativum and the dermatocytes, which are bound together by tight junctions and form the barrier to microbial invasion. Once microbes have penetrated this barrier through a hair follicle, cut or bite, the dermal plexus of capillaries delivers the components of the host's defense – oxygen, complement, immunoglobulins, macrophages, lymphocytes and granulocytes – to the site of infection.

Table 9.3 Differential diagnosis of bullous skin lesions

Clinical condition	Etiology
Bullous impetigo	*Staphylococcus aureus* carrying group II phage
Erysipelas	*Streptococcus pyogenes*
Staphylococcal scalded skin syndrome	*Staph. aureus* producing exfoliative toxin
Necrotizing fasciitis	Type I: mixed aerobic and anaerobic bacteria
	Type II: *Strep. pyogenes*
Gas gangrene	*Clostridium perfringens, C. septicum*
Halophilic vibrio sepsis	*Vibrio vulnificus*
Pemphigoid	Immune-mediated
Toxic epidermal necrolysis	Drug-induced

Table 9.4 Differential diagnosis of crusted skin lesions

Clinical condition	Etiology
Impetigo	*Staphylococcus aureus, Streptococcus pyogenes* or both
Ringworm	Dermatophytic fungi (e.g. *Tinea rubrum*)
Systemic fungal infections	*Histoplasma capsulatum Coccidioides immitis Blastomyces dermatitidis*
Cutaneous mycobacterial infection	*Mycobacterium tuberculosis M. marinum*
Cutaneous leishmaniasis	*Leishmania tropica*
Nocardiosis	*Nocardia asteroides*

Table 9.2 Probable etiology of soft tissue infections associated with some specific risk factor or setting

Risk factor or setting	Likely etiologic agent
Cat bite	*Pasteurella multocida*
Dog bite	*P. multocida, Capnocytophaga canimorsus* (DF-2), *Staphylococcus intermedius*
Tick bite followed by erythema chronicum migrans rash	*Borrelia burgdorferi*
Hot tub exposure	*Pseudomonas aeruginosa*
Diabetes mellitus or peripheral vascular disease	Group B streptococci
Periorbital cellulitis (children)	*Haemophilus influenzae*
Saphenous vein donor site cellulitis	Groups C and G streptococci
Fresh water laceration	*Aeromonas hydrophila*
Sea water exposure, cirrhosis, raw oysters	*Vibrio vulnificus*
Cellulitis associated with stasis dermatitis	Groups A, C and G streptococci
Lymphedema	Groups A, C and G streptococci
Cat scratch	*Bartonella henselae, B. quintana*
HIV-positive patient with bacillary angiomatosis	*B. henselae, B. quintana*
Fishmongering, bone rendering	*Erysipelothrix rhusiopathiae*
Fish tank exposure	*Mycobacterium marinum*
Compromised host with ecthyma gangrenosum	*P. aeruginosa*
Agammaglobulinemic patient with 'erysipelas'	*Campylobacter jejuni*
Human bite	*Eikenella corrodens, Fusobacterium* spp., *Prevotella* spp., *Porphorymonas* spp., *Streptococcus pyogenes*

Perhaps the first clue available to the immune system to the presence of foreign material in the deep tissues is provided by the organisms themselves. Virtually all bacteria are comprised of proteins whose N-terminal amino acid sequence begins with an N-formyl-methionine group and these proteins are chemoattractive to phagocytes such as macrophages and granulocytes. Other microbial cell wall components such as zymosan of yeast, endotoxins of Gram-negative bacteria and peptidoglycans of Gram-positive bacteria activate the alternative complement pathway,[1] yielding serum-derived chemotactic factors. Chemotactic factors are therefore promptly produced at the site of infection by multiple mechanisms.

The efflux or diapedesis of phagocytes through endothelial cell junctions is dependent upon the orchestrated sequential expression of adherence molecules on the surface of the polymorphonuclear leukocyte (PMNL)[2,3] such as L-selectin and CD11b/CD18 in association with counter-receptors (adhesins) on the endothelial surface.[4] *In vivo*, surface expression of these molecules results first in 'rolling' of PMNLs along the endothelial surface, followed by tethering, and finally firm adhesion of the PMNLs onto the surface of endothelial cells. Phagocytes actually leave the capillary through endothelial cell interstices bound by peripheral endothelial cell adherence molecules, which are found only at these junctional sites.

Once diapedesis has occurred, the PMNL follows the gradient of chemotactic factors derived from the bacteria and serum to the site of active infection. Recent studies suggest that the activated endothelial cells also produce chemotactic cytokines, such as interleukin (IL)-8. Finally, activated granulocytes synthesize leukotriene B_4 from arachidonic acid, and this too is a potent chemoattractant for leukocytes.

Production of proinflammatory cytokines such as IL-1, IL-6 and tumor necrosis factor results in an augmentation of the immune functions described above. These cytokines induce fever, prime neutrophils, and increase antibody production and the synthesis of acute phase reactants, such as C-reactive protein.[5,6] Cytokine-driven stimulation of endothelial cells also results in the generation of nitric oxide and prostaglandins, both of which cause vasodilatation. The net physiologic effect is greater blood flow to the tissue. These processes result in the cardinal manifestations of inflammation:

* heat;
* swelling;
* erythema; and
* tenderness or pain.

At some locations, factors such as pressure, thrombosis or drugs may reduce or stop blood flow, resulting in inadequate oxygenation. Compounds such as corticosteroids, which inhibit phospholipase A_2 activity (necessary for releasing arachidonic acid from cell membranes), and nonsteroidal anti-inflammatory agents, which inhibit cyclo-oxygenase (the endogenous enzyme necessary for the synthesis of prostaglandins from arachidonic acid), reduce local blood flow to tissues. These drugs are therefore useful in the treatment of noninfectious inflammatory conditions because they reduce pain and swelling. However, if the inflammation is secondary to undiagnosed bacterial infection, these drugs may predispose the patient to more severe infection or mask the clinical signs, so delaying the correct diagnosis.

If tissue perfusion is moderately attenuated, tissues may remain viable, but the threshold for progression of infection may be lowered. Predisposing conditions in this category include:

* peripheral vascular disease affecting large arteries;
* diabetes mellitus causing microvascular disease; and
* chronic venous stasis causing postcapillary obstruction.

Necrosis of the skin and deeper tissue may occur if there is severe hypoxia. Two examples are:

* pressure necrosis resulting in decubitus ulcers; and
* compartment syndromes resulting in hypoxia and then necrosis in muscles confined within tight fascial bundles.

When the host is physiologically, structurally and immunologically normal, only certain pathogens such as *Staph. aureus* and group A streptococci are able to cause disease by virtue of their potent virulence factors, such as toxins, capsules or dermonecrotic enzymes, which confer ability to withstand the barrage of host defenses and to induce clinical disease. This statement is supported by the observation that normal skin, although constantly exposed to many indigenous and exogenous microbes, rarely becomes infected.

In contrast, patients who have compromised skin integrity (e.g. patients with burns), vascular defects (e.g. those who have diabetes mellitus or pressure ulceration) or immunologic deficits may become infected with either virulent organisms (e.g. staphylococci or streptococci) or microbes that are usually saprophytic, such as *Pseudomonas aeruginosa*, *Escherichia coli*, enterococci or *Fusarium* spp. Defects such as neutropenia attenuate the host response and once the invading pathogen has breached the skin could predispose to worse outcomes.

PREVENTION

Avoidance of cuts, scratches and other forms of trauma that disrupt the natural barrier function of the skin helps to prevent skin and soft tissue infections. For example, stopping shaving may prevent recurrent folliculitis in the beard area (sycosis barbae). Prompt cleansing, debridement and disinfection of such lesions are important for preventing infection, particularly in the case of bite wounds. Treatment of eczema reduces the risk of secondary bacterial infection.

Prevention of recurrent folliculitis or furunculosis is difficult to achieve, but there has been some success using intranasal applications of bacitracin or mupirocin ointment. Chlorhexidine scrub may be tried to eliminate or reduce staphylococcal carriage in adults.[7] Prophylaxis with systemic antibiotics is of doubtful efficacy and can result in the emergence of resistant strains; it should be tried only for severe cases (see Folliculitis, furuncles and carbuncles, below).

Recurrent bacterial cellulitis of the lower extremities can often be prevented by topical antifungal treatment for dermatophyte infections such as tinea pedis because even minor or inapparent superficial fungal infection can serve as a portal of entry for Gram-positive cocci.

CLINICAL FEATURES, DIAGNOSIS AND MANAGEMENT OF SPECIFIC SOFT TISSUE INFECTIONS

Folliculitis, furuncles and carbuncles

Pustules or abscesses can develop when organisms permanently or transiently resident on the skin surfaces are introduced into deeper tissues (Fig. 9.1). Pathogens can also seed the skin from hematogenous sources such as bacteremias, for example associated with staphylococcal endocarditis (Fig. 9.2) or by contiguous spread from infectious foci in the lung or gastrointestinal tract. Most commonly,

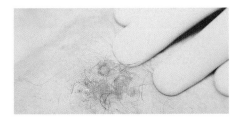

Fig. 9.1 Cutaneous infection at the previous insertion site of an intravenous catheter. Organisms from the skin were likely introduced into the dermis and subcutaneous tissue at the time of catheter insertion. Many of these infections remain superficial, but in this patient suppurative thrombophlebitis with bacteremia ensued.

111

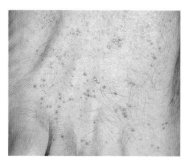

Fig. 9.2 Diffuse skin involvement. Petechial lesions in a patient with *Staphylococcus aureus* bacteremia, endocarditis and acute aortic insufficiency.

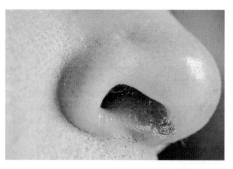

Fig. 9.4 Staphylococcal nasal carriage. This patient had a small staphylococcal abscess beneath the mucosa of the nose, illustrating how *Staphylococcus aureus*, which colonizes the nares, can infect skin and submucosa. Intact mucosa is highly resistant to infection; such infections usually occur as a result of defects in the mucosal membranes or via hair follicles inside the nose.

small focal abscesses develop in the superficial layers of the skin, where hair follicles serve as the portal of entry. Such lesions are called folliculitis. *Staphylococcus aureus* accounts for most of these infections, but many different bacterial species can occasionally cause localized folliculitis.

Folliculitis can progress to form subcutaneous abscesses, called furuncles or boils, which usually drain and resolve spontaneously, but may progress to form a large, exquisitely painful group of contiguous furuncles, called a carbuncle (Fig. 9.3). Carbuncles require surgical drainage as well as antibiotic treatment.[6]

Recurrent furunculosis

Certain individuals seem to be predisposed to recurrent *Staph. aureus* skin infections (recurrent furunculosis). Although it has been suggested that diabetic patients are especially prone to boils and carbuncles, few data support this concept. In contrast, it is well established that patients with Job's syndrome, who have high levels of serum IgE antibody and often a congenital defect of the STAT3 signaling pathway, are strongly predisposed to these focal *Staph. aureus* infections. However, most patients do not have immunologic or metabolic abnormalities, and the greatest predisposing factor has been the colonization of the anterior nares with *Staph. aureus* (Fig. 9.4). Thus, touching the nose or nasal secretions and then rubbing or scratching the skin results in autoinoculation and abscess formation. Breaking the cycle can be useful to prevent recurrences; however, it is important to document nasal colonization by appropriate techniques.

Administration of intranasal mupirocin or bacitracin ointment for the first 5 days of each month has been shown to decrease colonization and reduce the frequency of recurrent infection by about 50%.[8] Treatment of recurrent furunculosis may also require surgical incision and drainage as well as antistaphylococcal antibiotics such as oral dicloxacillin or parenteral nafcillin. In general, surgical drainage alone is successful, unless the patient has fever, leukocytosis or the lesions are greater than 5 cm in diameter. Community-acquired methicillin-resistant *Staph. aureus* (CA-MRSA) which harbors Panton–Valentine

leukocidin (PVL) has been associated with epidemics of these types of infection among prisoners, athletes and children in day-care centers.

Predisposing factors

Superficial dermal trauma such as insect bites or abrasions can result in cutaneous abscesses. Eczema may also serve as a portal of entry. Superinfected eczema may be difficult to distinguish from eczema itself because both result in crusted lesions, exudation and cutaneous erythema. The presence of lymphangitis, pustules or fever suggests infection. Because *Staph. aureus* is the most common cause of infected eczema, treatment with an oral antistaphylococcal antibiotic such as dicloxacillin or trimethoprim–sulfamethoxazole (for CA-MRSA) is warranted.

Sebaceous glands empty into hair follicles; if the ducts become blocked they form sebaceous cysts, which may resemble staphylococcal abscess or become secondarily infected. Chronic folliculitis is uncommon except in acne vulgaris in which normal flora (e.g. *Propionibacterium acnes*) may play a role.

Recurrent folliculitis is most common in black males and associated with trauma from shaving (folliculitis barbae). Hidradenitis suppurativa occurs in either acute or chronic forms and can lead to recurrent axillary, periareolar, perineal or pudendal abscesses. Although the exact pathogenesis of recurrent hidradenitis is not understood, it is considered to be due to abnormal apocrine sweat glands.

Diffuse folliculitis

Diffuse folliculitis occurs in two distinct settings. The first – 'hot tub folliculitis' – is associated with water maintained at a temperature between 98.6 and 104°F (37 and 40°C) that is insufficiently chlorinated and is caused by *P. aeruginosa*. The infection is usually self-limited, although serious complications of bacteremia and shock have occasionally been reported.

The second form of diffuse folliculitis – swimmer's itch (Fig. 9.5) – occurs when the skin is exposed to water infected with avian freshwater schistosomes. Warm water temperatures and alkaline pH are suitable for mollusks, which are the intermediate host between birds and humans. Free-swimming cercariae readily penetrate human hair follicles or pores, but quickly die. This triggers a brisk allergic reaction, causing intense itching and erythema. The infestation is self-limited, secondary infection is uncommon and antipruritics and topical corticosteroid cream promptly relieve the symptoms.

Staphylococcal scalded skin syndrome

Staphylococcal scalded skin syndrome has been described in all age groups, but it is usually seen in children under 5 years of age,

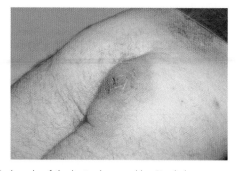

Fig. 9.3 Carbuncle of the buttock caused by *Staphylococcus aureus*. This large carbuncle developed over the course of 7–10 days and required surgical drainage plus treatment with antibiotics. The patient had previously experienced numerous episodes of *Staph. aureus* cutaneous abscesses. He carried the staphylococci in his anterior nares.

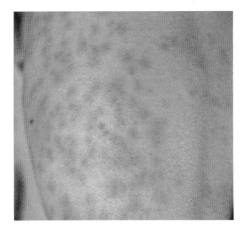

Fig. 9.5 Swimmer's itch. Diffuse folliculitis can be caused by *Pseudomonas aeruginosa* (hot tub folliculitis), schistosomes (swimmer's itch) or *Staphylococcus aureus* (folliculitis). This young man had been fishing in an alkaline lake in the western part of the USA. He had been fishing from a 'float tube' and had exposed only his hands and arms to the water. The rash was associated with severe itching. Although his white blood count was not elevated 35% of the white cells were eosinophils.

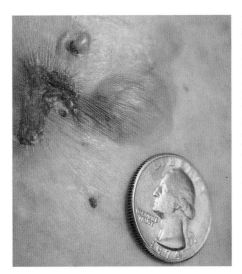

Fig. 9.6 Staphylococcal scalded skin syndrome. Flaccid bullae occur as single or multiple lesions. Examination of a frozen tissue section reveals that the cleavage plane is at the stratum corneum. This disease must be distinguished from toxic epidermal necrolysis (see Fig. 9.7).

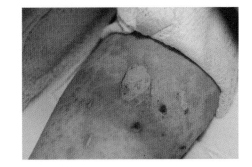

Fig. 9.7 Toxic epidermal necrolysis. This picture shows a skin slough (Nikolsky's sign), which resulted when lateral pressure was applied by the thumb in a plane parallel to the skin surface. This disorder is more common in adults, has a high mortality rate and is usually caused by medications.

including neonates.[9] The characteristic features are a faint erythematous rash with the formation of flaccid bullae (Fig. 9.6). *Staphylococcus aureus* of phage group II is the causative organism. These organisms produce the toxin exfoliatin, which appears to affect the cell junctions of young dermal cells. Specifically, there is intraepidermal cleavage at the level of the stratum corneum. A classic clinical feature is Nikolsky's sign, in which lateral pressure on the skin results in shearing off of the top layer of skin (Fig. 9.7). The mortality of staphylococcal scalded skin syndrome is low, and fluid loss from the skin is minimal. Appropriate antibiotic therapy is the main component of treatment.

Staphylococcal scalded skin syndrome must be distinguished from toxic epidermal necrolysis, a condition that is more common in adults, is usually secondary to a drug reaction and is associated with a high mortality rate (see Fig. 9.7). Frozen section examination of a punch biopsy readily distinguishes these two entities:

- staphylococcal scalded skin syndrome shows a cleavage at the level of the stratum corneum; and
- toxic epidermal necrolysis shows deeper cleavage at the stratum germinativum.

Impetigo

Impetigo contagiosa is a form of superficial pyoderma caused by streptococci and/or staphylococci. Currently, about half of impetigo cases are caused by *Staph. aureus*, including CA-MRSA.[9] Staphylococci and group A streptococci can be co-isolated from impetiginous lesions in many cases. Group A streptococci alone currently cause less than half the cases. Staphylococcal impetigo tends to occur sporadically, whereas epidemics of impetigo caused by group A streptococci have been well described. Epidemics occur throughout the year in tropical areas or during the summer months in more temperate climates. Impetigo caused by group A streptococci is sometimes complicated by the development of poststreptococcal glomerulonephritis. This important nonsuppurative complication is more likely to occur during epidemics of impetigo caused by certain M types such as M type 49 (see Chapter 166).

Impetigo is characterized by thick-crusted lesions with rounded or irregular margins (Fig. 9.8a), often located on the face.[10] Streptococcal pyoderma frequently has a golden brown or honey color, resembling a plaque of dried serum. Children between 2 and 10 years of age are most commonly infected. Impetigo is often associated with poor socioeconomic conditions and poor hygiene.

Initially, colonization of unbroken skin occurs either exogenously from other infected persons (hence the term impetigo contagiosa) or endogenously by contamination of the skin with organisms carried in the anterior nares or oropharynx. The development of impetiginous lesions takes 10–14 days and likely is initiated through lesions such as minor abrasions and insect bites, which serve as a means of intradermal inoculation. Initially, impetigo may appear as vesicular lesions, which then evolve into crusts (Fig. 9.8b).

Patients with group A streptococcal impetigo should receive penicillin treatment, particularly when numerous sites of the skin are involved, although treatment may not prevent poststreptococcal glomerulonephritis. Topical treatment with an agent effective against Gram-positive bacteria, such as bacitracin or mupirocin, is also effective.

Bullous impetigo

Bullous impetigo is caused by strains of *Staph. aureus* harboring a group II bacteriophage that contains genetic elements coding for a toxin, which causes cleavage in the epidermis. This results in separation of the cellular planes at the level of the stratum corneum and this is responsible for the superficial flaccid bullae that characterize this condition. Several of these lesions may coalesce and spread to form large reddish plaques, usually involving the neck, face or chin. The superficial flaccid bullae are easily ruptured and may not be apparent at the time when the patient is first seen. Because of the superficial

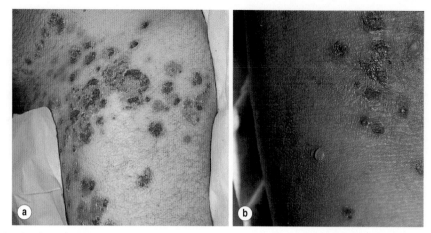

Fig. 9.8 Impetigo. (a) Impetigo in a homeless man. Both *Staphylococcus aureus* and group A streptococci were cultured from these lesions. (b) Impetigo, with initial vesicles changing to crusts.

nature of these infections, scarring does not occur. Appropriate treatment is an antistaphylococcal antibiotic, which may be given orally.

Ecthyma, paronychia and blistering distal dactylitis

Ecthyma, like impetigo, is characterized by dry crusted lesions of the skin and may be caused by *Staph. aureus*, group A streptococci or both. Unlike impetigo, this lesion extends into the dermis and may therefore lead to post-treatment scarring.[9]

Paronychia is an infection between the nail plate of a digit and the cuticle. It is associated with sucking of the fingers and occupations or hobbies involving prolonged immersion of the hands in water. Herpetic whitlow (see below) may resemble paronychia. Paronychia may occur in some immunocompromised patients. Staphylococci are the most common etiologic agents, although oral anaerobes and streptococci may also be isolated. *Candida albicans* and fungi such as *Fusarium* spp. may be isolated from paronychias in immunocompromised patients. Drainage is best accomplished between the nail plate and the cuticle. Antimicrobial agents are rarely needed in otherwise healthy individuals.

Blistering distal dactylitis is characterized by painful blisters on the fingerpads of digits. It is most common in children. *Streptococcus pyogenes* is the most common organism isolated, although *Staph. aureus* can cause a similar lesion. Incision and drainage may be useful, in conjunction with an antibiotic appropriate for *Staph. aureus* or *Strep. pyogenes*.

Erysipelas

Erysipelas is a specific variant of cellulitis caused by a toxin of *Strep. pyogenes*, and occasionally by streptococci of groups B, C and D.[11,12] It is characterized by an abrupt onset of fiery red swelling of the face or extremities. Distinctive features are well-defined margins, particularly along the nasolabial fold, rapid progression and intense pain (Fig. 9.9). Flaccid superficial bullae may develop during the second to third day of the illness, but extension to deeper soft tissues is rare. Since it is a toxic reaction in the skin, cultures of skin biopsies are generally negative.

Surgical debridement is rarely necessary, and treatment with penicillin is effective. Swelling may progress for a time despite appropriate treatment, even while fever, pain and the intense red color are diminishing. Desquamation of the involved skin occurs after 5–10 days.

Erysipelas is most common in elderly adults, and the severity of systemic toxicity can vary from region to region. Local lymphedema (e.g. after mastectomy) predisposes to recurrent erysipelas. It seems to be less common and less severe now than in the past. A rare form of erysipelas is caused by *Campylobacter jejuni* and *Campylobacter fetus*,

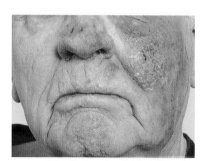

Fig. 9.9 Erysipelas. This form of cellulitis is caused by *Streptococcus pyogenes* and is most common in the elderly. Unique characteristics include a fiery red or salmon color, well-demarcated edges, desquamation after 5–7 days and location on the face or lower extremities. This picture was taken 48 hours after treatment with penicillin when the brilliant red salmon color had evolved to a reddish blue color. On the second day of treatment patients usually have less pain and fever subsides, but swelling may be more extensive.

especially in patients with agammaglobulinemia and occasionally in patients with AIDS.

Cellulitis

The term 'cellulitis' is commonly used by physicians, but is not well defined in the literature. It is a localized area of soft tissue inflammation characterized by:

- leukocytic infiltration of the dermis;
- capillary dilatation; and
- proliferation of bacteria.

Clinically cellulitis is recognized as an acute inflammatory condition of the skin characterized by localized pain, erythema, swelling and heat.[6] The area of erythema is a paler pink than the flaming red of erysipelas, and has indistinct margins (Fig. 9.10).

Cellulitis caused by *Staphylococcus aureus* and *Streptococcus pyogenes*

Cellulitis is most commonly caused by indigenous flora such as *Staph. aureus* and *Strep. pyogenes* which colonize the skin and appendages. Bacteria may gain access to the epidermis through cracks in the skin, abrasions, cuts, burns, insect bites, surgical incisions and intravenous catheters.

Cellulitis caused by *Staph. aureus* spreads centripetally from a central localized infection such as an abscess (Figs 9.11, 9.12), folliculitis or foreign body (e.g. a sliver, prosthetic device or intravascular catheter).

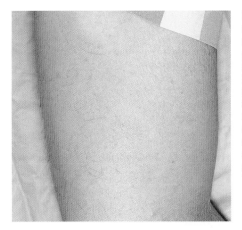

Fig. 9.10 Cellulitis. In contrast to erysipelas, cellulitis is a pink color rather than brilliant red and has indistinct margins. *Staphylococcus aureus* and group A, C and G streptococci are the most common etiologies. Many other bacteria may cause cellulitis (see Table 9.1).

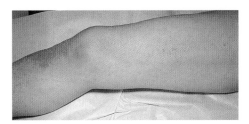

Fig. 9.13 Lymphangitis. Cellulitis caused by group A streptococci began below the knee and rapidly spread; about 4 hours later lymphangitis had spread up the inner aspect of the thigh.

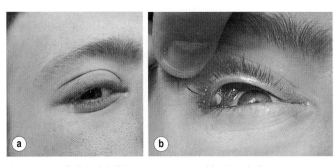

Fig. 9.11 Cellulitis. (a) This case was caused by *Staphylococcus aureus* and is spreading centripetally from a central localized focus of infection. The redness and swelling characteristic of cellulitis are apparent over the upper eyelid. (b) The cellulitis has developed from a localized staphylococcal abscess formed in a meibomian gland (chalazion).

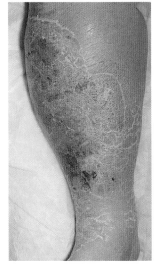

Fig. 9.14 Cellulitis of the lower leg associated with chronic venous insufficiency. Streptococci of groups A, B, C and G are the most common isolates. Group B streptococci seldom cause cellulitis in previously healthy hosts, but should be considered in people who have peripheral vascular disease or diabetes mellitus.

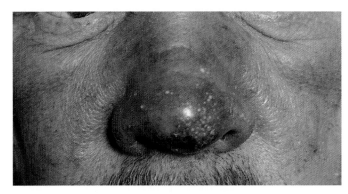

Fig. 9.12 *Staphylococcus aureus* cellulitis of the nose. The focal lesion began in a hair follicle inside the nose, with redness, swelling and pain. Rarely, such lesions on the nose are complicated by extension into the cavernous sinus via veins draining the central part of the face.

In contrast, cellulitis due to *Strep. pyogenes* is a more rapidly spreading diffuse process, frequently associated with lymphangitis (Fig. 9.13) and fever.[13]

Recurrent cellulitis

Recurrent streptococcal cellulitis of the lower extremities may be caused by group A, C or G streptococci in association with skin lesions such as chronic venous stasis (Fig. 9.14), saphenous venectomy for coronary artery bypass surgery[14] or healed burns, especially if the skin is colonized by dermatophyte fungi. Streptococci also cause recurrent cellulitis/erysipelas among patients with chronic lymphedema resulting from irradiation, lymph node dissection, Milroy's disease or elephantiasis.

Recurrent staphylococcal cutaneous infections occur in individuals who have Job's syndrome (see above) and among chronic nasal carriers of staphylococci.

Cellulitis associated with predisposing conditions

A number of other conditions predispose to infection by endogenous or exogenous pathogens (see Table 9.2). For example:
- *Streptococcus agalactiae* cellulitis occurs in patients who have diabetes mellitus or peripheral vascular disease; and[15]
- *Haemophilus influenzae* causes periorbital cellulitis in children in association with sinusitis, otitis media or epiglottitis and will presumably become less common, as has *Haemophilus* meningitis, due to the impressive efficacy of the *H. influenzae* type b vaccine.

Cellulitis associated with bites

Many other species of bacteria can cause cellulitis. These often occur in special settings, and the history can provide useful clues to the diagnosis (see Table 9.2). Bites of various types may introduce specific organisms into the deeper tissues, resulting in soft tissue infections. For example, cellulitis associated with cat bites and, to a lesser degree, dog bites is commonly caused by *Pasteurella multocida*, although in the latter case *Staphylococcus intermedius* and *Capnocytophaga canimorsus* (DF-2) must also be considered. Cellulitis and abscesses associated with dog and human bites also contain a variety of anaerobic organisms.[16] *Pasteurella multocida* is resistant to dicloxacillin and nafcillin, but sensitive to all other β-lactam antimicrobials as well as quinolones, tetracycline and erythromycin. Ampicillin–clavulanate, ampicillin–sulbactam or cefoxitin are good choices for treating animal or human bite infections.

Soft tissue infections may result from the bites of mosquitoes, horse flies and spiders; usually they cause only local allergic reactions with itching, swelling and erythema. Similarly, brown recluse spider bites may resemble acute infection at first, but later there is primary tissue destruction and central necrosis due to the action of dermonecrotic toxins. These infections may resemble pyoderma gangrenosum or may become secondarily infected with skin organisms. Mosquito bites may serve as portals of entry for skin organisms such as *Staph. aureus* or *Strep. pyogenes*. Such infections are not uncommon in clinical practice, but given the number of individuals bitten by insects, infection is a relatively rare complication.

Cellulitis associated with water exposure and exposure to fish

Aeromonas hydrophila causes a highly aggressive form of cellulitis in tissues surrounding lacerations that were sustained in fresh water lakes, rivers and streams. This organism is sensitive to aminoglycosides, fluoroquinolones, chloramphenicol, trimethoprim–sulfamethoxazole (co-trimoxazole) and third-generation cephalosporins, but is resistant to ampicillin.

Vibrio vulnificus can cause cellulitis or necrotizing fasciitis and is associated with swimming in the Gulf of Mexico or South Atlantic Ocean. In addition, patients who have cirrhosis of the liver may develop severe soft tissue infection after ingestion of oysters from these areas.

Streptococcus iniae is a newly recognized cause of cellulitis among workers handling tilapia fish.

Fish food containing the water fleas of the genus *Daphnia* can be contaminated with *Mycobacterium marinum*, which may cause cellulitis or granulomas on skin surfaces exposed to the water in aquariums or following injuries in swimming pools. Rifampin (rifampicin) plus ethambutol has been an effective treatment for some, although no comprehensive studies have been carried out. In addition, some strains of *M. marinum* are susceptible to tetracycline or trimethoprim–sulfamethoxazole.

There are four types of soft tissue cellulitis caused by *P. aeruginosa* and other Gram-negative bacteria:

- ecthyma gangrenosum in neutropenic patients;
- hot tub folliculitis;
- burn wound sepsis; and
- cellulitis following penetrating injury.

In the last of these *P. aeruginosa* is often introduced into the deep tissues by stepping on a nail, a scenario referred to as the 'sweaty tennis shoe syndrome'.

Treatment includes surgical inspection and drainage, particularly if the injury also involves bone or joint capsule. Choices for empiric treatment pending antimicrobial susceptibility data include aminoglycosides, third-generation cephalosporins such as ceftazidime, cefoperazone or cefotaxime, semisynthetic penicillins such as ticarcillin, mezlocillin or piperacillin, or fluoroquinolones. (The quinolones are not approved in children under 13 years of age.)

Cellulitis caused by Gram-negative bacilli, including *P. aeruginosa* as described above, is most common in hospitalized immunocompromised hosts. Recently, *Stenotrophomonas maltophilia* has emerged as an important cause of nosocomial cellulitis in patients who have cancer.[17] The bacterium has been isolated from incubators, nebulizers, humidifiers and tap water in hospitals. The cellulitis may be related to intravenous catheters and in some circumstances may be metastatic via the bloodstream.

Trimethoprim–sulfamethoxazole, or ticarcillin–clavulanic acid, with or without ciprofloxacin are reasonable treatment choices, although cultures and sensitivities are important because of the high prevalence of antibiotic-resistant organisms in the health-care environment.

Other causes of cellulitis

The Gram-positive aerobic rod, *Erysipelothrix rhusiopathiae*, which causes cellulitis in bone renderers and fishmongers, remains susceptible to erythromycin, clindamycin, tetracycline and cephalosporins, but is resistant to sulfonamides and chloramphenicol.

Differential diagnosis

The etiology of cellulitis can be suspected on the basis of the epidemiologic data supplied above. If there is drainage, an open wound or an obvious portal of entry, Gram stain and culture can often provide a definitive diagnosis (Table 9.5). In the absence of these findings, the bacterial etiology of cellulitis may be difficult to establish. Even with needle aspiration from the leading edge or punch biopsy of the cellulitis itself, cultures are positive in only 20% of cases.[18] This suggests that relatively low numbers of bacteria may cause cellulitis and that the expanding area of erythema within the skin may be the direct result of extracellular toxins or the soluble mediators of inflammation elicited by the host.

Antibiotic treatment

Because many different microbes can cause cellulitis, the choice of initial empiric antibiotic therapy depends upon the clinical features described above. Once cultures and sensitivities are available, the choice is easier and more specific. The physician must first decide whether the patient's illness is severe enough to require parenteral treatment, either in hospital or on an outpatient basis. Because of the virtual epidemic of MRSA infections worldwide, severe soft tissue infections should be treated with agents that have a high level activity against these strains. Local antibiograms are thus crucial for rational treatment.

Presumed streptococcal or staphylococcal cellulitis

For presumed streptococcal or staphylococcal cellulitis, nafcillin, cephalothin, cefuroxime, vancomycin and erythromycin are good choices. Cefazolin and ceftriaxone have less activity against *Staph. aureus* than cephalothin, although clinical trials have shown a high degree of efficacy. Ceftriaxone is a useful choice for outpatient treatment because it can be given once daily. Similarly, teicoplanin, like vancomycin, has excellent activity against *Strep. pyogenes* and both *Staph. aureus* and *Staph. epidermidis* and may be given once daily by intravenous or intramuscular injection. Because MRSA has recently increased in prevalence throughout much of the world, vancomycin, tigecycline, daptomycin or linezolid should be used empirically in patients with severe soft tissue infections who are toxic or in those who have recently been hospitalized or received antibiotics.[19]

For patients being treated with oral antibiotics, dicloxacillin, cefuroxime axetil, cefpodoxime, erythromycin, clarithromycin and azithromycin are all effective treatments.

For known group A, B, C or G streptococcal infections, penicillin or erythromycin should be used orally or parenterally. For serious group A streptococcal infections such as necrotizing fasciitis or streptococcal toxic shock syndrome, clindamycin is more efficacious than penicillin.[20]

Table 9.5 Differential diagnosis of ulcerative skin lesions

Clinical condition	Etiology
Anthrax	*Bacillus anthracis*
Cutaneous diphtheria	*Corynebacterium diphtheriae*
Ulceroglandular tularemia	*Francisella tularensis*
Bubonic plague	*Yersinia pestis*
Buruli ulcer	*Mycobacterium ulcerans*
Primary syphilis	*Treponema pallidum*
Chancroid	*Haemophilus ducreyi*
Lucio's phenomenon	*Mycobacterium leprae*
Decubitus (pressure) ulcer	Mixed aerobic and anaerobic bacteria
Leishmaniasis	*Leishmania tropica*
Ecthyma gangrenosum	*Pseudomonas aeruginosa*
Tropical ulcer	Idiopathic and nonspecific; mixed bacterial species

This is probably because in this type of infection where there are large numbers of bacteria, streptococci are in a stationary growth phase and do not express a full complement of penicillin-binding proteins.[21] In contrast, the activity of clindamycin is not affected by inoculum size or growth phase. In addition, clindamycin suppresses the synthesis of many streptococcal exotoxins and surface proteins.[22,23]

Other types of cellulitis

For cellulitis associated with *Eikenella corrodens* useful antibiotics are penicillin, ceftriaxone, trimethoprim–sulfamethoxazole, tetracyclines and fluoroquinolones. Interestingly, this organism is resistant to oxacillin, cefazolin, clindamycin and erythromycin.

Cellulitis associated with cat bites may fail to respond to treatment with oral cephalosporins, erythromycins and dicloxacillin. Reasons for failure include resistance of *P. multocida* to oxacillin and dicloxacillin and the inadequate serum and tissue levels attained with older oral cephalosporins and erythromycins.

Erysipelas-like skin lesions caused by *Campylobacter* spp. in patients with agammaglobulinemia may not respond to antibiotics alone; supplementation with IgM (by infusion of fresh plasma) may be necessary to obtain bactericidal serum.[24]

Cutaneous ulcers

Infectious ulceration of the skin results from either:
- direct destruction of dermal cells by bacterial products; or
- an intense inflammatory reaction.

Cutaneous anthrax

This is an example of direct destruction of dermal cells by toxins produced by *Bacillus anthracis* (see Table 9.5). This disease is traditionally contracted by direct inoculation of the skin of animal handlers, especially goat and sheep herders or hide processors,[25] but recent cases have occurred as the result of deliberate bioterrorism (see Chapter 71). The lesion begins as a papule, which evolves into a bulla and then ulcerates (Fig. 9.15). Sepsis may occur. The diagnosis is established by aspiration of the leading edge of the lesion, Gram stain and culture. Penicillin is appropriate therapy.

Cutaneous diphtheria

Since 1980 cutaneous diphtheria has been recognized in homeless individuals who present with chronic nonhealing ulcers with an overlying dirty gray membrane. These lesions may mimic those of psoriasis, eczema or impetigo, but have a deeper base. Appropriate cultures of the ulcer are mandatory because organisms growing from routine cultures may be misidentified as diphtheroids.[26]

Cutaneous tularemia (ulceroglandular tularemia)

Cutaneous tularemia occurs following a tick bite or handling of infected rodents or lagomorphs (rabbits). It most commonly presents with regional lymphadenopathy associated with suppuration and fever, although pneumonic, oculoglandular, oropharyngeal and typhoidal forms have also been described. The characteristic lesion is a small ulceration with an eschar, which develops 2–10 days after exposure. Treatment with streptomycin or gentamicin has been successful, and doxycycline, chloramphenicol or a fluoroquinolone are alternatives.

Buruli ulcer

Buruli ulcer is caused by *Mycobacterium ulcerans*. It presents as a shallow ulcer, which slowly expands centripetally. It is uncommon in the USA and Europe, but is endemic in tropical climates, particularly Africa. Diagnosis is easily established by biopsy, acid-fast staining or culture. The organism is susceptible to isoniazid, rifampin and *para*-aminosalicylic acid (PAS). Oral treatment with isoniazid and rifampin for 2–3 months is usually successful.

Leishmaniasis

Leishmaniasis also presents as shallow ulcers with an expanding margin (Fig. 9.16). Diagnosis should be suspected in patients residing in or returning from Central or South America. A biopsy from the raised edge stained with Giemsa or Wright's stain demonstrates the amastigote stage of *Leishmania tropica*. Treatment with antimony compounds is effective, but requires prolonged administration over 4–6 months.

Other causes of cutaneous ulcers

The differential diagnosis of cutaneous ulcers in genital areas should include:
- syphilis;
- chancroid;
- lymphogranuloma venereum; and
- herpes simplex virus infection.

Noninfectious causes of cutaneous ulceration include:
- Behçet's syndrome;
- cutaneous vasculitis, including lupus erythematosus;
- toxic epidermal necrolysis;
- pressure necrosis; and
- brown recluse spider bites.

Solitary shallow ulcers of skin and mucous membranes have also been described in disseminated histoplasmosis.

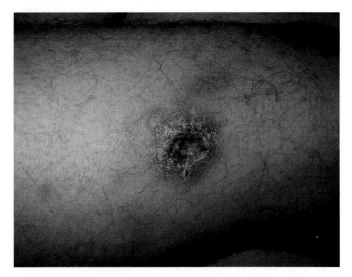

Fig. 9.16 Leishmaniasis. Typical crusted edge with central necrosis suggesting leishmaniasis. A history of travel to Central or South America or Iraq should be ascertained. Biopsy of the ulcer crater with Giemsa staining revealed amastigotes of *Leishmania tropica*. Courtesy of M Keuter.

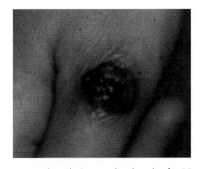

Fig. 9.15 Cutaneous anthrax lesion on the thumb of a 23-year-old Turkish woman. The lesion developed after wounding herself on the teeth of a slaughtered sheep. Microbiologic tests yielded *Bacillus anthracis*. She recovered after treatment with penicillin. Courtesy of IC Gyssens and D Weyns.

Herpes simplex can cause primary or recurrent cutaneous infections of the digits (herpetic whitlow) or head and neck. This viral infection is often misdiagnosed and mistreated as a bacterial condition, and occurs in those who are exposed to inoculation of the skin from oral secretions, such as from dentists, dental hygienists, nurses, anesthesiologists and wrestlers.

Orf is caused by a DNA virus similar to smallpox. It causes development of shallow ulcers (in general only one lesion) on the digits of animal handlers working with sheep or goats that harbor open mucous membrane lesions.[25]

Bacillary angiomatosis (see also Chapter 96)

Bacillary angiomatosis is a primary infection of endothelial cells that has important cutaneous manifestations.[27] The lesions may appear as purple nodules resembling Kaposi's sarcoma. They may also appear as scaly or ulcerated lesions and may have the appearance of superficial pink papules or plaques in black people. This disease usually occurs in people who have HIV infection and is caused by *Bartonella henselae* or *B. quintana*. The organisms can be acquired from cat bites and scratches or from cat fleas. The course and extent of infection is highly variable and depends upon the host's immune status.

Histopathology reveals capillary proliferation. The organisms can be visualized using Warthin–Starry silver stain or electron microscopy. Bacteriologic identification requires a special culture technique: lysed blood centrifugate or digested tissue is plated onto chocolate or Columbia agar and incubated for 10–14 days at 95 °F (35 °C) in 5–7% carbon dioxide. Small dry adherent oxidase-negative colonies of Gram-negative curved rods with twitching motility can be identified as *Bartonella* spp. by fluorescent antibody, gas–liquid chromatography or biochemical tests.[28]

Resistance to penicillin, cephalosporins, sulfonamides and vancomycin has been described. The recommended therapy is erythromycin 500 mg q6h.[23]

Cutaneous manifestations of infections of deep soft tissues

Staphylococcal infections of deeper tissues may also cause superficial redness, warmth and swelling of the skin, even though the skin itself is not infected (Fig. 9.17). Examples include olecranon bursitis

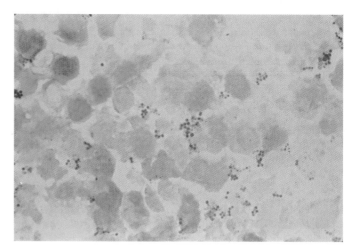

Fig. 9.17 Gram stain of purulent material demonstrating *Staphylococcus aureus*. The microbial etiology of cellulitis may be suspected based upon signs, symptoms and history; however, definitive diagnosis requires Gram stain and culture. If there is no portal of entry, aspiration or even punch biopsy of cellulitic skin yields a positive culture in only 20% of cases.

(Fig. 9.18), septic arthritis, osteomyelitis, staphylococcal parotitis and other deep infections of the head and neck, such as anaerobic infections, actinomycosis and tooth abscesses (Fig. 9.19).

Further information regarding the diagnosis and treatment of common and uncommon skin and soft tissue infections, including those in compromised hosts can be found in 'Practice guidelines for diagnosis and management of skin and soft-tissue infections'.[29]

REFERENCES

References for this chapter can be found online at http://www.expertconsult.com

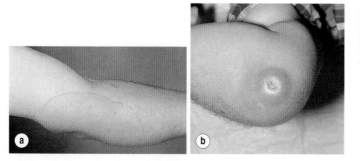

Fig. 9.18 Cellulitis at the elbow associated with olecranon bursitis. (a) Pale pink erythema on the inner aspect of the elbow. (b) Careful inspection demonstrates a focal infection over the point of the elbow. Fluid aspirated from the olecranon bursa yielded a pure culture of *Staphylococcus aureus*.

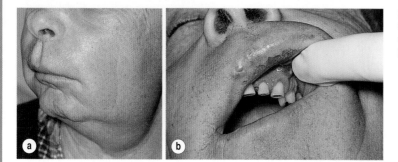

Fig. 9.19 Erythema and swelling of the face due to a tooth abscess. (a) Swelling of the face, on inspection resembling periorbital cellulitis. (b) Further inspection reveals a gingival abscess above the patient's left upper canine tooth.

Dennis L Stevens
Michael J Aldape
Amy E Bryant

Chapter | **10** |

Necrotizing fasciitis, gas gangrene, myositis and myonecrosis

INTRODUCTION

The spectrum of infections of the deep soft tissues ranges from localized bacterial, viral and parasitic lesions to rapidly spreading, tissue-destructive infections such as necrotizing fasciitis and myonecrosis. For example, pyomyositis, which is common in the tropics but rare in temperate zones, is a focal infection of skeletal muscle that is usually caused by *Staphylococcus aureus*; it generally remains localized and rarely causes systemic complications. In contrast, necrotizing fasciitis and myonecrosis may be caused by single or multiple pathogens and often give rise to extensive tissue loss, bacteremia, organ failure, shock and death. Even the experienced clinician may have difficulty distinguishing between the different forms of deep soft tissue infection during the early stages. Finally, despite early diagnosis and appropriate treatment, some patients will lose tissue, even limbs, whereas others will succumb to systemic complications. This chapter emphasizes the clinical clues that help to make early, specific diagnoses.

EPIDEMIOLOGY

Until the middle of the 20th century, wartime injuries were commonly complicated by gas gangrene caused by *Clostridium* spp. During the Civil War in the USA, nearly 50% of soldiers who sustained gunshot wounds developed infection and many of these developed gas gangrene. Clostridial gangrene is typically a sporadic infection but during the Civil War apparent epidemics of 'hospital gangrene' were described. Contributing factors included severe trauma, grossly contaminated wounds, crowded and dirty conditions, application of soiled dressings (often recycled from patients who had just died of infection) and primitive surgical techniques for debridement and fixation of open fractures. Group A streptococci undoubtedly caused some of these infections but other major bacterial pathogens, including *Clostridium perfringens*, Gram-negative bacteria and mixed aerobic–anaerobic bacteria, also contributed.

Gas gangrene was also common during the First World War, particularly in the European theater, where the soil was rich and well fertilized with animal feces containing large numbers of vegetative spores of clostridia. In contrast, in North Africa, cases of gangrene following gunshot wounds were far less common, presumably because the desert sand contained few clostridial spores.[1] Gas gangrene has become uncommon in modern warfare because wounded soldiers are evacuated rapidly to well-equipped hospitals for surgical intervention, arterial reconstruction and antibiotic treatment, all of which have greatly reduced the prevalence of this feared disease.

In modern times, these serious deep soft tissue infections have become less common. Sporadic cases in the general population most often occur as occasional complications of penetrating trauma, compound fractures or septic abortions. For the first time in history, spontaneous gas gangrene caused by *Clostridium septicum* may be more common than trauma-associated gas gangrene caused by *C. perfringens*, *C. histolyticum* or other *Clostridium* spp. (see Chapter 173). Recently, severe soft tissue infections caused by *C. perfringens*, *C. sordellii* and *C. novyi* have been described among intradermal ('skin popping') and intravenous drug users.[2,3]

Necrotizing fasciitis is a life-threatening form of soft tissue infection. It can occur in association with gas gangrene as a part of generalized tissue necrosis or as a separate clinical entity.[4] Two types of necrotizing fasciitis are recognized. Type I occurs in patients who have diabetes mellitus or severe peripheral vascular disease, or both;[5] it is usually caused by mixed aerobic and anaerobic bacteria. Although the risk for an individual diabetic patient is low, this type of necrotizing fasciitis is most common in the general population, because the total number of people who have diabetes is very large.

Type II necrotizing fasciitis, formerly called streptococcal gangrene, is caused by group A streptococci. Since the mid-1980s, this disease has been recognized with increasing frequency in many parts of the world, at a current annual incidence of 3–3.5 cases per 100 000.[6]

Morbidity and mortality

Before the availability of antibiotics, gas gangrene was usually fatal. Since then, mortality rates from gas gangrene caused by *C. perfringens* have improved, owing to aggressive antibiotic therapy, aggressive surgical therapy employing better surgical techniques and, possibly, hyperbaric oxygen therapy. The most important factors in improving outcome, reducing the need for amputations and preventing shock have been earlier recognition and aggressive treatment.

The mortality and morbidity of group A streptococcal necrotizing fasciitis have evolved differently. In the pre-antibiotic era this infection carried a mortality rate of about 25% when treated with surgery (such as 'bear claw' fasciotomies) alone.[7] In modern times, mortality due to group A streptococcal necrotizing fasciitis has not decreased and continues to range from 30% to 70% despite antibiotics, appropriate surgical debridement and intensive supportive care. This suggests that more virulent strains have emerged.

CLINICAL FEATURES

Pain, either generalized or localized, is the most common reason patients with deep-seated infection seek medical care (Fig. 10.1). Early in the course of necrotizing fasciitis caused by group A streptococci, patients may have a viral-like prodrome with nausea, vomiting, diarrhea and fever; however, later in the course of the disease, patients seek medical assistance because of increasingly severe localized pain with continuing fever.

Differential diagnosis of infections involving muscle and fascia

Clinical feature	Necrotizing fasciitis type I	Necrotizing fasciitis type II	Gas gangrene	Pyomyositis	Myositis due to viruses or parasites
Fever					
Diffuse pain					Note 1
Localized pain		Note 2			
Systemic toxicity					
Gas in tissue					
Obvious portal of entry		Note 3	Note 4		
Diabetes mellitus					

Note 1: Pain with influenza is diffuse myalgia. Pleurodynia may be associated with severe localized pain (i.e. devil's grip). Pain with trichinosis may be severe and localized.

Note 2: Severe pain is present in necrotizing fasciitis associated with group A streptococcal necrotizing fasciitis. Necrotizing fasciitis type I is commonly seen in people who have diabetes mellitus who have peripheral neuropathy; hence the pain may not be severe.

Note 3: Fifty percent of patients who have necrotizing fasciitis caused by group A streptococci may not have an obvious portal of entry.

Note 4: Gas gangrene associated with trauma may be caused by *Clostridium perfringens*, *Clostridium septicum* and *Clostridium histolyticum* and there is always an obvious portal of entry. Spontaneous gas gangrene caused by *Clostridium septicum* is usually not associated with an obvious portal of entry. Organisms lodge in tissue as a result of bacteremia originating from a bowel portal of entry.

Fig. 10.1 Differential diagnosis of infections involving muscle and fascia. Red, severe; orange, moderate; yellow, mild-to-moderate; blue, mild; white, none.

A portal of entry can be defined in the majority of cases of deep bacterial soft tissue infections such as type I necrotizing fasciitis and traumatic gas gangrene. In type I necrotizing fasciitis, infection begins at the site of a surgical incision, at a mucosal tear or at sites of skin breakdown in patients who have diabetes mellitus or peripheral vascular disease. Similarly, traumatic gas gangrene occurs at the site of major trauma such as crush or penetrating injuries severe enough to cause arterial damage. In these cases, the clinician has reason to suspect infection as a cause of fever or increasing pain. In contrast, patients who have either type II necrotizing fasciitis or spontaneous gas gangrene may have no apparent portal of entry.[8] Early in the course of infection in such patients, the only physical signs of infection may be fever and localized pain. Fever and localized pain are the cardinal clues to this diagnosis but in some cases clinical evidence of localized infection may not become apparent until after the development of systemic signs such as hypotension or organ failure.

Early in the course of type II necrotizing fasciitis associated with a defined portal of entry there is generally evidence of localized inflammation such as swelling, redness, warmth and tenderness. At that point the process may resemble simple cellulitis, which can be caused by any of a multitude of bacteria (see Chapter 9). In type I necrotizing fasciitis there is generally gas in the tissue, as there is in gas gangrene. Where there is no apparent portal of entry, the leading diagnoses to be considered are infection with group A streptococci (type II necrotizing fasciitis), *C. septicum* (spontaneous gangrene) or *Vibrio vulnificus*. The presence of gas in the tissue favors clostridial infection.

Gas may be detected by physical examination (crepitus) or by imaging (radiography, MRI or CT scan). Group A streptococci should be suspected if there is fever and severe pain and a history of blunt trauma or muscle strain. *Vibrio vulnificus* should be suspected in a patient who has cirrhosis of the liver, a history of ingestion of raw oysters or exposure to seawater.[9] Later, erythema is superseded by violaceous bullous lesions, massive local swelling becomes apparent and signs of systemic toxicity develop rapidly (see Chapter 171).

SPECIFIC TYPES OF DEEP SOFT TISSUE INFECTION

Necrotizing infections

Necrotizing infections of the skin and underlying soft tissues share the features of fulminant destruction of tissue and severe systemic signs of toxicity associated with high mortality (see Fig 10.1). Many different and confusing names have been used to describe infectious processes that share common pathologic features:

- extensive tissue destruction;
- thrombosis of blood vessels;
- abundant bacteria spreading along fascial planes; and
- relatively few acute inflammatory cells, although small collections of polymorphonuclear leukocytes or microabscesses have been described (Fig. 10.2).

For patients who have evidence of an aggressive localized soft tissue infection, prompt surgical exploration of that site is of extreme importance to determine whether a necrotizing process is present. The same is true for patients who have milder local features associated with severe systemic toxicity. In addition, although the clinical entity referred to as necrotizing fasciitis may occur alone, there is commonly also evidence of necrosis extending up to the dermis and down to underlying muscle (myonecrosis). Despite these common features, it is worth reviewing the many different types of necrotizing soft tissue infections that have been described in the literature because this may point to clinical clues leading to earlier surgical intervention and therefore an earlier diagnosis.

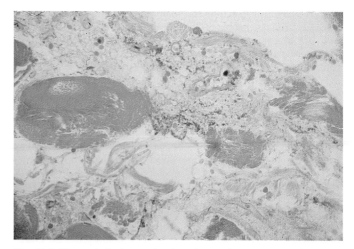

Fig. 10.2 Histopathologic examination of tissue from a patient who has necrotizing fasciitis with extension into the underlying musculature. Note the absence of acute inflammatory cells in the area of muscle necrosis. When present, infiltrating granulocytes can be seen at the interface between normal and necrotic tissue and are often massed within small postcapillary venules.

Necrotizing fasciitis

Necrotizing fasciitis is a deep-seated infection of the subcutaneous tissue that results in progressive destruction of fascia and fat, although it may spare the skin itself.[10] Two clinical types exist.

Type I necrotizing fasciitis

Type I necrotizing fasciitis is a mixed infection caused by aerobic and anaerobic bacteria. It occurs most commonly after surgical procedures, in diabetic patients or in those who have peripheral vascular disease (see Fig. 10.1). Nonclostridial anaerobic cellulitis and synergistic necrotizing cellulitis are both variants of the same syndrome. It may not be important to distinguish these entities from one another because all occur in diabetic patients and are caused by mixed anaerobic and aerobic bacteria.

Clinical features

These infections most commonly occur on or about the feet, with rapid extension along the fascia into the leg. Although cellulitis also occurs commonly in diabetic patients, necrotizing fasciitis should be considered in those who have cellulitis and systemic signs of infection such as tachycardia, leukocytosis, acidosis or marked hyperglycemia. In addition to its spontaneous occurrence in diabetic patients, type I necrotizing fasciitis may also develop as a result of a breach in the integrity of mucous membranes from surgery or instrumentation. In the head and neck region, bacterial penetration into the fascial compartments can result in a related syndrome known as Ludwig's angina (Fig. 10.3) or it may develop into necrotizing fasciitis. Group A streptococci (but also anaerobes such as *Fusobacterium necrophorum*) may cause necrotizing fasciitis or a peritonsillar abscess, which can extend into the deep structures of the neck (Fig. 10.4).

Diagnostic tests

The first goal of management is to determine the depth and extent of the infection. MRI or CT scans are invaluable in this regard to determine whether the infection is localized or spreading along fascial planes. The second goal is to determine whether surgical intervention is necessary. Because of the proximity to vital structures of the neck, surgical consultation is of major importance because exploration, drainage and debridement may be necessary to prevent airway obstruction, to determine the level of soft tissue involvement and to establish which bacteria are involved.

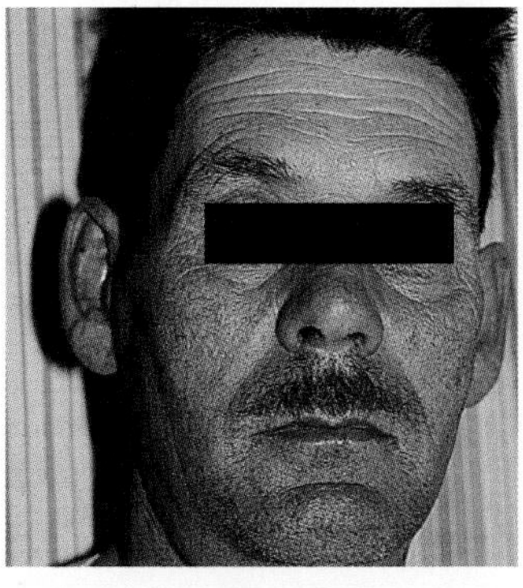

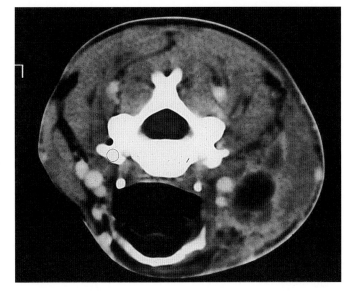

Fig. 10.4 CT scan of a soft tissue infection of the neck. This infection is caused by group A streptococci, which invaded as a rare complication of a previous 'strep throat'. Surgical drainage yielded a pure culture of group A streptococci and established a diagnosis. The patient was treated with intravenous penicillin for 10 days and made a good recovery.

Treatment

Both Ludwig's angina and necrotizing fasciitis of the head and neck are usually caused by mouth anaerobes such as *Fusobacterium* spp., anaerobic streptococci, *Bacteroides* spp. and spirochetes. Either penicillin or clindamycin is effective treatment, largely because the Gram-positive aerobic cocci and anaerobes of the oropharynx are generally susceptible to both. In contrast, type I necrotizing fasciitis below the diaphragm requires ampicillin plus clindamycin and a fluoroquinolone to cover the *Bacteroides* spp. and Enterobacteriaceae.

Type II necrotizing fasciitis

Type II necrotizing fasciitis is caused by group A streptococci and was previously called streptococcal gangrene.[5] In recent years, there has been a dramatic increase in the number of invasive infections, including necrotizing fasciitis, caused by group A streptococci. In contrast to type I necrotizing fasciitis, type II may occur in any age group and among patients who do not have complicated medical illnesses. Predisposing factors include:

- a history of blunt trauma;
- muscle strain;
- childbirth;
- chickenpox;
- nonsteroidal anti-inflammatory agents;[11]
- intravenous drug abuse; or
- penetrating injury such as caused by a laceration or a surgical procedure.

In penetrating injuries, it is the skin rather than the mucous membranes that serves as the portal of entry for the streptococci. In contrast, among patients who do not have a defined portal of entry, hematogenous translocation of group A streptococci from the throat (asymptomatic or symptomatic pharyngitis) to the site of blunt trauma or muscle strain probably occurs.[12] Another, highly conjectural possibility is that group A streptococci reside in a dormant state in the deep tissue and trauma of various types reactivates their growth.

Group A streptococci are contagious microbes that have caused epidemics of pharyngitis and scarlet fever in schools, rheumatic fever in military recruits and surgical wound infections in hospitalized patients. Thus, close contacts of a patient who has type II necrotizing fasciitis have a high likelihood of becoming colonized with a virulent strain.

Fig. 10.3 Ludwig's angina. Infection begins with a break in the mucosal lining in the oropharynx; oral bacterial flora invade the soft tissues at the base of the tongue and penetrate through the floor of the mouth and into soft tissue of the neck. The floor of the mouth is elevated and patients talk as though they have a 'hot potato' in their mouth. Potential airway obstruction is a major concern. Although patients usually respond to penicillin, surgical consultation should be obtained and CT or MRI scans are useful for determining whether a necrotizing process is present.

Clearly, the risk of developing a secondary case of fulminant necrotizing fasciitis is very low, but it is probably 50-fold higher than it is in the general population. In evaluating the risk to family members and hospital workers, the physician should consider the degree of exposure and the susceptibility of the host. Those contacts with conditions such as open wounds or chickenpox, as well as those family members and health-care workers with frequent or continuous contact with a case of necrotizing streptococcal infection, should be treated with an agent to which the strain is sensitive (e.g. penicillin).

Pathogenesis

Pyrogenic exotoxins can bind simultaneously to the major histocompatibility complex (MHC) class II portion of antigen-presenting cells, and specific Vβ segments of the T-cell receptor in the absence of classic antigen processing.[13] Thus, pyrogenic exotoxins are superantigens that can cause rapid proliferation of T cells bearing specific Vβ repertoires (see Chapter 2). This is associated with production of both monokines [tumor necrosis factor (TNF), interleukin (IL)-1 and IL-6] and lymphokines (IL-2, interferon and TNF).[14] Production of these cytokines in vivo probably contributes to shock, organ failure and tissue destruction.[15]

Clinical features

Necrotizing fasciitis exhibits a remarkably rapid progression from an inapparent process to one associated with extensive destruction of tissue, systemic toxicity, loss of limb or death.[8,12,16] Unexplained pain that increases rapidly over time may be the first manifestation of infection.[8,12] The early signs and symptoms of infection may not be apparent, particularly in patients who have postsurgical infection, gunshot or knife wounds, or diabetes. In patients who have diabetes, the absence of pain may be related to neuropathy and anesthesia at the site of infection. In surgical patients, patients who have traumatic injuries and postpartum patients, the increasing pain may be assumed to be part of the normal convalescence rather than to be due to acute infection. Such a delay in diagnosis may allow the disease to progress to later stages before appropriate antibiotics and surgical invention are initiated.

In addition to pain, there may also be fever, malaise, myalgias, diarrhea and anorexia during the first 24 hours; erythema, which may be diffuse or local, may also be present. However, in most patients excruciating pain in the absence of any cutaneous findings may be the only clue of infection. Within 24–48 hours, erythema may develop or darken to a reddish-purple color, frequently with associated blisters and bullae. Conversely, erythema may be absent and the characteristic bullae may develop in skin of normal appearance. The bullae are initially filled with clear fluid and rapidly take on a blue or maroon appearance (Fig. 10.5). When the bullous stage is observed, there is already extensive necrotizing fasciitis (Fig. 10.5) and patients usually exhibit fever and systemic toxicity.

Although many different M-types of group A streptococci have been associated with necrotizing fasciitis in the past, M types 1 and 3 have been the strains most commonly isolated from patients throughout the world.[12] These strains can produce one or more of the pyrogenic exotoxins A, B and C.[8,17] Necrotizing fasciitis caused by these strains is frequently associated with 'streptococcal toxic-shock syndrome'.[8] The hallmarks of this syndrome are the early onset of shock and multiple organ failure (see Chapter 166).

Diagnosis

Laboratory tests such as creatine phosphokinase, aspartate aminotransferase and serum creatinine are usually elevated, and, together with leukocytosis with marked left shift, these findings should be sufficient to prompt surgical exploration.[8] Some experts have advocated punch biopsy and frozen section to establish the diagnosis; however, there may be false-negative findings if the deep tissue is not adequately sampled. Routine soft tissue radiographs, MRI and CT scans show soft tissue swelling.[18] Gas is not present and abscess formation is not apparent. These radiographic abnormalities are not unusual in uninfected patients who have trauma or in postsurgical or postpartum patients (Fig. 10.6). Surgeons may not be interested in surgical exploration with such imaging findings, yet a toxic patient with the above laboratory abnormalities should provide the impetus to at least inspect the deep tissue. Direct surgical exploration will usually demonstrate that necrotizing fasciitis is present. At the same time, thorough debridement of necrotic tissue and suitable material for Gram stain and culture can be obtained.

Management

The three main themes in treatment are surgical debridement, appropriate antibiotics and intensive supportive care. Some patients require mechanical ventilation and others need hemodialysis. Because of intractable hypotension and diffuse capillary leak, massive amounts of intravenous fluids (10–20 liters per day) are often necessary, although anasarca is a common complication. In some patients blood pressure

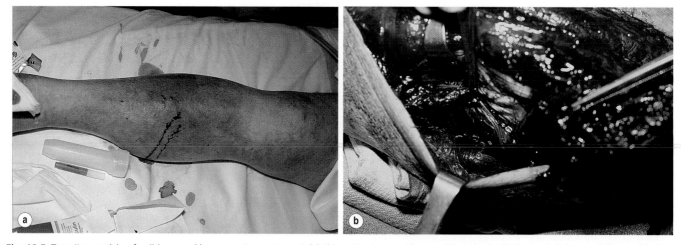

Fig. 10.5 Type II necrotizing fasciitis caused by group A streptococci. (a) This patient was a 60-year-old man who had type 2 diabetes mellitus and who had a 3-day history of malaise, diffuse myalgia and low-grade fever. Over the course of 2–3 hours the pain became excruciating and was localized to the calf. During this time the calf swelled. Note that the skin over the anterior shin looks relatively normal, but that two small purple bullae are present. (b) Extensive necrotizing fasciitis was present on surgical exploration. In addition, myonecrosis was present beneath the fascia. The patient developed profound hypotension, acute respiratory distress syndrome and renal failure. He died despite aggressive surgical and medical management. There was no definable portal of entry, yet group A streptococci were grown from deep cultures and from blood.

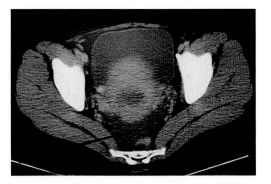

Fig. 10.6 Postpartum sepsis due to group A streptococci. The patient was a 24-year-old woman who delivered a normal child. Thirty-six hours after delivery she developed fever, leukocytosis with marked left shift and increasing low abdominal pain. This MRI demonstrates swelling of the uterus, although not out of proportion for a recent delivery. There was no gas in the tissue. An emergency laparotomy revealed necrosis of the mucosa of the uterus, necrotizing fasciitis and myonecrosis of the uterus.

improves with intravenous fluid alone. Pressors such as dopamine may be useful, but there is little controlled information from clinical or experimental studies in this specific infection. Although potent vasoconstrictors such as adrenaline (epinephrine) may improve blood pressure, symmetric gangrene may ensue, partly as a result of the drug and partly as a result of poor perfusion caused by the bacteria, toxins and endogenous mediators.

Antibiotic selection is difficult in patients who have rapidly progressing infection. Recent studies suggest that clindamycin is superior to penicillin for treatment of experimental necrotizing fasciitis or myonecrosis caused by group A streptococci.[19] It seems likely that penicillin failure is due to the reduced expression of critical penicillin-binding proteins during the stationary phase of bacterial growth.[20] Clindamycin may be more efficacious because:

- it is not affected by inoculum size or stage of growth;
- it suppresses toxin production;
- it facilitates phagocytosis of *Streptococcus pyogenes* by inhibiting M-protein synthesis;
- it suppresses the production of regulatory elements that control cell wall synthesis; and
- it has a long post-antibiotic effect.[21]

Neutralization of circulating streptococcal toxins is a desirable therapeutic goal and is advocated by some experts.[22–25] There seems little question that some batches of intravenous gammaglobulin contain neutralizing antibodies against some streptococcal toxins.[24] On the basis of two case reports[22,23] and a report of a nonrandomized clinical trial, there is a suggestion that this treatment may affect the mortality and morbidity of this fulminant infection.[25]

Fournier's gangrene

In the perineal area, penetration of the gastrointestinal or urethral mucosa by bacteria may cause 'Fournier's gangrene', an aggressive infection caused by aerobic Gram-negative bacteria, enterococci and anaerobic bacteria such as *Bacteroides* spp. and peptostreptococci. These infections begin abruptly with severe pain and may spread rapidly to the anterior abdominal wall and the gluteal muscles; in males, infection frequently extends to the scrotum and penis (Fig. 10.7).

Surgical inspection, placement of drains and appropriate surgical debridement are necessary for both diagnosis and treatment. Antibiotic treatment should be based upon Gram stain, culture and sensitivity information when available. An appropriate empiric regimen would be either ampicillin or ampicillin and sulbactam combined with either clindamycin or metronidazole. Broader Gram-negative coverage might be advisable if the patient has had prior hospitalization or if antibiotics have been used recently. This could be accomplished by substituting ticarcillin–clavulanic acid or piperacillin–tazobactam for ampicillin or by adding a fluorinated quinolone or an aminoglycoside.

Meleney's synergistic gangrene

This rare variant occurs in postsurgical patients. The lesion is a slowly expanding, indolent ulceration that is confined to the superficial fascia. It results from a synergistic interaction between *Staph. aureus* and microaerophilic streptococci. As in other forms of necrotizing infection, antibiotic therapy, together with surgical debridement, are the mainstays of treatment.

Nonclostridial anaerobic cellulitis

In nonclostridial anaerobic cellulitis, infection is associated with mixed anaerobic and aerobic organisms that produce gas in tissues. Unlike clostridial cellulitis, this type of infection is usually associated with diabetes mellitus and it often produces a foul odor. Surgical exploration is required to distinguish this condition from necrotizing cellulitis, myonecrosis and necrotizing fasciitis by *Clostridium* spp.

Clostridial cellulitis

In clostridial cellulitis, infection is usually preceded by local trauma or recent surgery. *Clostridium perfringens* is the most common species causing this entity. Gas is invariably found in the skin; the fascia and deep muscle are spared. Although clostridial cellulitis differs from

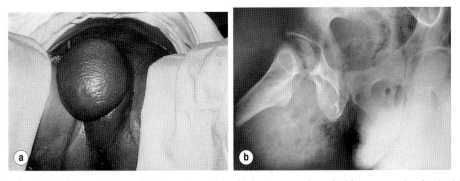

Fig. 10.7 Type I necrotizing fasciitis. A 24-year-old man had been in good health but was awakened with severe perineal pain. (a) This photograph was taken 3 hours later. Note the massive swelling of the scrotum. (b) Soft tissue radiograph shows gas in the tissues of the thigh, buttocks, scrotum and anterior abdominal wall. Surgical inspection revealed brownish fluid in the scrotum, with gray, dull-colored, friable fascia but normal underlying musculature. Cultures grew *Enterococcus faecalis*, *Bacteroides fragilis*, *Escherichia coli* and anaerobic streptococci. The patient was treated with ampicillin, clindamycin and gentamicin for 3 weeks and surgical drains were placed in the scrotum, buttocks, thigh and anterior abdominal wall. There was an excellent clinical response. In some cases, surgery of a more radical nature may be necessary.

clostridial myonecrosis in that there is less systemic toxicity, it is mandatory that thorough surgical exploration and debridement be performed to distinguish these entities. MRI or CT scans as well as a serum creatinine phosphokinase assay may also be useful for determining whether muscle tissue is involved. Treatment is discussed below under gas gangrene.

Clostridial gas gangrene

Three types of clostridial soft tissue infections have been defined:[1]
- simple wound contamination or colonization;
- anaerobic cellulitis; and
- clostridial gas gangrene.

The first type, simple wound contamination or colonization, does not progress to true infection for various reasons (e.g. there may be insufficient devitalized tissue to promote infection or there may be effective host responses or effective medical and surgical management). Contamination is a very common occurrence; 30–80% of open traumatic wounds contain clostridial species.[26]

The second type, anaerobic cellulitis, occurs when there is devitalized tissue in a wound, sufficient for growth of *C. perfringens* or other strains. Although gas is produced locally and extends along fascial planes, bacteremia and invasion of healthy tissue do not occur. Appropriate medical and surgical management, including prompt removal of the devitalized tissue, is all that is necessary for cure and mortality is generally nil.[1]

The third type is clostridial gas gangrene or myonecrosis. This is defined as an acute invasion of healthy living muscle that is undamaged by previous trauma or ischemia.[26] It is divided into three different subtypes:
- traumatic gas gangrene;
- spontaneous or nontraumatic gas gangrene; and
- recurrent gas gangrene caused by *C. perfringens*.

Traumatic gas gangrene is the most common subtype. It develops when a deep, penetrating injury that compromises the blood supply (e.g. knife or gunshot wounds, crush injury or car accident) creates an anaerobic environment that is ideal for clostridial proliferation. This type of trauma accounts for about 70% of cases of gas gangrene. *Clostridium perfringens* is found in about 80% of such infections;[1] the remaining cases are caused by *C. septicum, C. novyi, C. histolyticum, C. bifermentans, C. tertium* and *C. fallax*. Other conditions associated with traumatic gas gangrene are bowel and biliary tract surgery, intramuscular injection of adrenaline (epinephrine), illegal abortion, retained placenta, prolonged rupture of the membranes and intrauterine fetal demise or missed abortion in postpartum patients.

Spontaneous or nontraumatic gas gangrene is less common. This is often caused by the more aerotolerant species *C. septicum*. As described below, most of these cases occur in patients who have a gastrointestinal portal of entry such as adenocarcinoma.

Third, and least common, is recurrent gas gangrene caused by *C. perfringens*. This has been described in people who have nonpenetrating injuries at sites of previous gas gangrene; residual spores of *C. perfringens* may remain quiescent in tissue for periods of up to 20 years, and then germinate when minor trauma provides anaerobic conditions suitable for growth.[27]

Traumatic gas gangrene

Pathogenesis

The initiating trauma introduces organisms (either vegetative forms or spores) into the deep tissues and produces an anaerobic niche with a sufficiently low redox potential and acid pH for optimal clostridial growth.[1,26] Necrosis progresses within hours. At the junction of necrotic and normal tissues few polymorphonuclear leukocytes are present, yet pavementing of these cells along the endothelium is apparent within capillaries and in small arterioles and postcapillary venules.[28,29] Later in the course of the illness there is leukostasis within larger vessels. Thus, the histopathology of clostridial gas gangrene is opposite to that

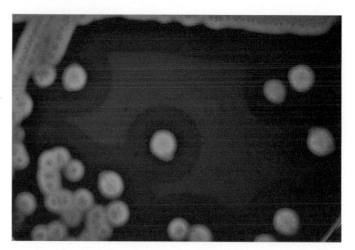

Fig. 10.8 Colonies of *Clostridium perfringens* growing on an anaerobic blood agar plate. Theta toxin causes the clear zone of hemolysis closest to the colony. A second area of partial hemolysis is caused by α-toxin, an enzyme with phospholipase C activity.

seen in soft tissue infections caused by pyogenic organisms such as *Staph. aureus*, in which an early luxuriant influx of polymorphonuclear leukocytes localizes the infection without adjacent tissue or vascular destruction. Recent studies suggest that theta toxin (Fig. 10.8), when elaborated in high concentrations at the site of infection, destroys host tissues and inflammatory cells.[30] As the toxin diffuses into surrounding tissues or enters the systemic circulation, theta toxin promotes dysregulated adhesive interactions between polymorphonuclear leukocytes and endothelial cells and primes leukocytes for increased respiratory burst activity.[30]

Alpha toxin (see Fig. 10.8), a phospholipase C, directly suppresses myocardial contractility *ex vivo*[31] and may contribute to profound hypotension via a sudden reduction in cardiac output.[32] Experimentally, alpha toxin induces a profound and irreversible defect in perfusion as measured by laser Doppler blood flow.[33,34] Simultaneously, there is rapid appearance of circulation aggregates of platelets and neutrophils bound together by the platelet surface receptor GPIIb/IIIa.[33] These actions lead to vascular leukostasis, endothelial cell injury and regional tissue hypoxia. Such perfusion deficits expand the anaerobic environment and contribute to the rapidly advancing margins of tissue destruction that are characteristic of clostridial gangrene.[1] In experimental models, theta toxin (a cholesterol-binding cytolysin) causes 'warm shock', defined as a markedly reduced systemic vascular resistance combined with a markedly increased cardiac output.[31,32] It is clear that theta toxin accomplishes this indirectly by inducing endogenous mediators that cause relaxation of blood vessel wall tension, such as the lipid autacoids prostacyclin or platelet-activating factor.[35] Reduced vascular tone develops rapidly and, in order to maintain adequate tissue perfusion, a compensatory host response is required; this either increases cardiac output or rapidly expands the intravascular blood volume. Patients who have Gram-negative sepsis compensate for hypotension by markedly increasing cardiac output; however, this adaptive mechanism may not be possible in shock induced by *C. perfringens* due to direct suppression of myocardial contractility by alpha toxin.[31] The role of other endogenous mediators such as cytokines (e.g. TNF, IL-1, IL-6) as well as the potent endogenous vasodilator bradykinin have not been elucidated.

Prevention

Aggressive debridement of devitalized tissue and rapid repair of compromised vascular supply greatly reduce the frequency of gas gangrene in contaminated deep wounds. Intramuscular adrenaline (epinephrine), prolonged application of tourniquets and surgical closure of traumatic wounds should be avoided. Patients who have compound fractures are at particular risk of gas gangrene if the wound is surgically closed. Patients who have contaminated wounds should receive prophylactic antibiotics.

Clinical findings

The first symptom is usually the sudden onset of severe pain at the site of recent surgery or trauma.[2,24] The mean incubation period is less than 24 hours, but it ranges from 6–8 hours to several days, probably depending on the degree of soil contamination or bowel contents spillage and the extent of vascular compromise.

The skin may initially appear pale, but it quickly changes to bronze then purplish red, becoming tense and exquisitely tender (Fig. 10.9). Bullae develop; they may be clear, red, blue or purple.

Gas in tissue may be obvious from physical examination, soft tissue radiographs, CT scan or MRI. None of these radiographic procedures has proved to be more specific or more sensitive than the physical finding of crepitus in the soft tissue.[10] However, radiographic procedures are particularly helpful for demonstrating gas in deeper tissue such as the uterus.

Signs of systemic toxicity develop rapidly; these include tachycardia, fever and diaphoresis, followed by shock and multiple organ failure. Shock is present in 50% of patients at the time they present to the hospital.[36] Bacteremia occurs in 15% of patients and may be associated with brisk hemolysis. In one patient, the hematocrit fell from 37% to 0% over a 24-hour period.[37] Subsequently, despite transfusion with 10 units of packed red blood cells over 4 hours, the hematocrit never exceeded 7.2%.[37] Alpha and theta toxins contribute to this marked intravascular hemolysis. Not all cases of C. perfringens bacteremia have been associated with gas gangrene[38] but 90% of C. perfringens and 100% of C. septicum isolates from blood were associated with clinically significant infection.[39]

Additional complications of clostridial myonecrosis include jaundice, renal failure, hypotension and liver necrosis. Renal failure is largely due to hemoglobinuria and myoglobinuria, but it may be a result of acute tubular necrosis caused by hypotension. Renal tubular cells are probably directly affected by toxins.

Diagnosis

Increasing pain at a site of previous injury or surgery, together with signs of systemic toxicity and gas in the tissues, support the diagnosis. Definitive diagnosis rests on demonstrating large, Gram-variable rods at the affected site (Fig. 10.10). Note that although clostridia stain Gram-positive when obtained from bacteriologic media, when visualized from infected tissues they often appear both Gram-positive and Gram-negative. In fresh specimens C. perfringens may appear to be encapsulated.[40,41]

The affected muscles appear edematous, may be an abnormal reddish-blue to black color and do not bleed or contract when stimulated. Usually, some degree of necrotizing fasciitis and cutaneous necrosis is also present. Microscopic evaluation of biopsy material (see Fig. 10.10) demonstrates organisms among degenerating muscle bundles and characteristically an absence of acute inflammatory cells.[26,42]

Management

Penicillin, clindamycin, tetracycline, chloramphenicol, metronidazole and a number of cephalosporins have excellent in vitro activity against C. perfringens and other clostridia. No controlled clinical trials have ever been conducted to compare the efficacy of these agents in humans. Based strictly on in-vitro susceptibility data, most textbooks state that penicillin is the drug of choice.[43,44] However, experimental studies in mice suggest that clindamycin has the greatest efficacy and penicillin the least.[45,46] Other agents with greater efficacy than penicillin include erythromycin, rifampin (rifampicin), tetracycline, chloramphenicol and metronidazole.[45,46] Slightly greater survival was observed in animals receiving both

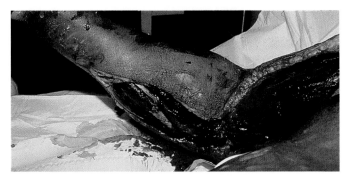

Fig. 10.9 Extensive gas gangrene of the arm due to *Clostridium perfringens*. A 35-year-old man sustained a knife wound to the forearm. He did not seek medical care, but 36 hours later experienced severe pain in the upper arm and came to the emergency room. There was extreme tenderness of the arm and crepitus was easily demonstrated. A radiograph also demonstrated gas in the deep soft tissues. Surgical debridement and antibiotics were instituted, but later amputation at the level of the shoulder was necessary. A pure culture of *C. perfringens* was grown from the deep tissues.

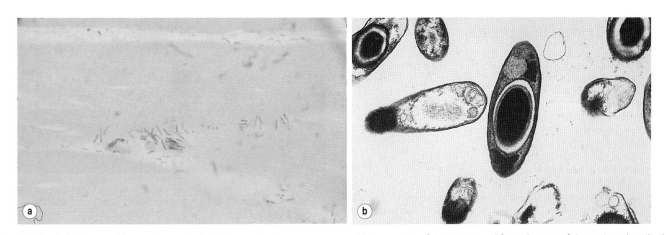

Fig. 10.10 *Clostridium perfringens* in a patient who has extensive gas gangrene. (a) Gram stain of tissue removed from the arm of the patient described in Figure 10.9. Note that the bacteria are rod shaped but Gram variable. Note also that there are few if any acute inflammatory cells at the site of infection. (b) Transmission electron micrograph of *C. perfringens*. Note the endospores.

clindamycin and penicillin; in contrast, antagonism was observed with penicillin plus metronidazole.[46] Because between 2% and 5% of strains are resistant to clindamycin, a combination of penicillin and clindamycin is warranted. Based on his experimental studies and his vast clinical experience with gas gangrene, the late Dr William Altemeier recommended tetracycline and penicillin.[47] Thus, given an absence of efficacy data from a clinical trial in humans, the best treatment would appear to be clindamycin or tetracycline combined with penicillin. The failure of penicillin in experimental clostridial myonecrosis may be related to continued toxin production and filament formation rather than lysis.[48] In contrast, the efficacy of clindamycin and tetracycline may be related to their ability to inhibit toxin synthesis rapidly.[48]

Aggressive and thorough surgical debridement is mandatory to improve survival, preserve limbs and prevent complications.[43,44] The use of hyperbaric oxygen (HBO) is controversial, although some non-randomized studies have reported good results with HBO therapy when combined with antibiotics and surgical debridement.[36,49,50] Experimental studies in animals have demonstrated that HBO alone can be effective treatment if the inoculum is small and treatment is begun immediately.[51] In contrast, other studies have demonstrated that HBO was only of slight benefit when combined with penicillin.[52] However, survival was better with clindamycin alone than with either HBO alone, penicillin alone or HBO plus penicillin together.[52] The benefit of HBO, at least theoretically, is to inhibit bacterial growth,[53] to preserve marginally perfused tissue and to inhibit toxin production.[54] Interestingly, Altemeier did not use HBO and was able to realize a mortality rate of less than 15% using surgical debridement and antibiotics (tetracycline plus penicillin) alone.[47]

Specific antitoxin antibodies for adjunctive treatment are no longer available. Future strategies may target endogenous proadhesive molecules such that toxin-induced vascular leukostasis and resultant tissue injury are attenuated.

Prognosis

Patients presenting with gas gangrene of an extremity have a better prognosis than those who have truncal or intra-abdominal gas gangrene, largely because it is difficult to debride such lesions adequately.[43,44,55] Hyperbaric oxygen could be useful in such patients. In addition to truncal gangrene, patients who have associated bacteremia and intravascular hemolysis have the greatest likelihood of progressing to shock and death. In one study, of those patients who developed shock at some point in their hospitalization, 40% died, compared with 20% mortality in the group as a whole.[36] In another study, those who were in shock at the time of diagnosis had the highest mortality.[55]

Spontaneous, non-traumatic gas gangrene due to *Clostridium septicum*

Pathogenesis

Predisposing factors include:[55–57]
- colonic carcinoma;
- diverticulitis;
- gastrointestinal surgery;
- leukemia;
- lymphoproliferative disorders;
- cancer chemotherapy;
- radiation therapy; and
- AIDS.

Cyclic or other forms of neutropenia are also associated with spontaneous gas gangrene due to *C. septicum* and in such cases necrotizing enterocolitis, cecitis or distal ileitis are commonly found. These gastrointestinal pathologies permit bacterial access to the bloodstream; consequently, the aerotolerant *C. septicum* can become established in normal tissues.[1]

Clostridium septicum produces four toxins:
- α-toxin (lethal, hemolytic, necrotizing activity);
- β-toxin (deoxyribonuclease);
- γ-toxin (hyaluronidase); and
- δ-toxin (septicolysin, an oxygen-labile hemolysin).

Clostridium septicum also produces a protease and a neuraminidase.[1]

The *C. septicum* α-toxin does not possess phospholipase activity and is thus distinct from the α-toxin of *C. perfringens*. Active immunization against α-toxin significantly protects against challenge with viable *C. septicum*.[58] The mechanism by which α-toxin contributes to *C. septicum* pathogenesis is unknown; however, the recent cloning and sequencing of this toxin should facilitate studies in this area (see Chapter 173).

Clinical features

The onset of disease is abrupt, often with excruciating pain, although the patient may sense only heaviness or numbness.[1,28,55–57] The first symptom may be confusion or malaise. Extremely rapid progression of gangrene follows. Swelling advances and bullae appear; these are filled with clear, cloudy, hemorrhagic or purplish fluid. The skin around such bullae also has a purple hue (Fig. 10.11), perhaps reflecting vascular compromise resulting from bacterial toxins diffusing into surrounding tissues.[55] Histopathology of muscle and connective tissues includes cell lysis and gas formation; inflammatory cells are notably absent.[55]

Diagnosis

Unlike the situation in traumatic gas gangrene, bacteremia precedes cutaneous manifestations by several hours. In the absence of the usual cutaneous manifestations of gas gangrene, other causes of fever and extremity pain such as deep vein thrombophlebitis or cellulitis are naturally considered first, delaying appropriate diagnosis and treatment, and, as a consequence, increasing mortality.

Management

No comparative human trials have evaluated the efficacy of antibiotics or HBO for treating clinical cases of spontaneous gas gangrene. *In-vitro* data indicate that *C. septicum* is uniformly susceptible to penicillin, tetracycline, erythromycin, clindamycin, chloramphenicol and metronidazole. The aerotolerance of *C. septicum* may reduce the likelihood that HBO therapy would be effective.[53]

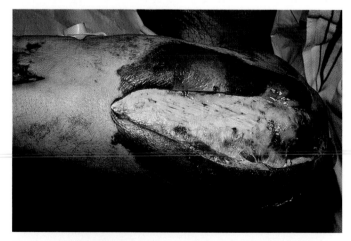

Fig. 10.11 Spontaneous necrotizing fasciitis due to *Clostridium septicum*. This patient developed sudden onset of severe pain in the forearm. Swelling rapidly ensued and he sought medical treatment. Crepitus was present on physical examination and gas in the soft tissue was verified with routine radiographs. Immediate surgical debridement revealed necrotizing fasciitis but sparing of the muscle. Note the purple-violaceous appearance of the skin. See also Figure 10.12.

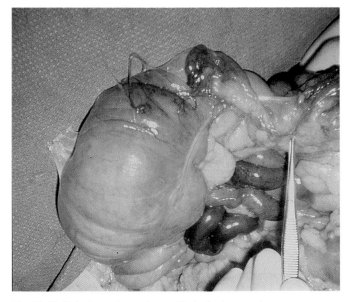

Fig. 10.12 Colonic carcinoma in a patient who has spontaneous gas gangrene caused by *Clostridium septicum*. The patient described in Figure 10.11 was found to have a mass in the colon. Surgical resection revealed an adenocarcinoma, which probably served as a portal of entry for the *C. septicum* bacillus. Hematogenous seeding of the forearm resulted in spontaneous gas gangrene.

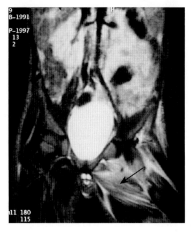

Fig. 10.13 MRI scan showing high-signal STIR sequence (consistent with marked edema) in the adductor muscles of the left leg in a patient with *Staphylococcus aureus* bacteremia (arrow). At operation, necrotic and infected muscle was decompressed and debrided. This represents the 'woody' stage, prior to muscle liquefaction and the formation of frank abscesses.

Prognosis

The mortality of spontaneous clinical gangrene ranges from 67% to 100%, with the majority of deaths occurring within 24 hours of onset. Unfavorable factors include underlying malignancy and compromised immune status. All patients who survive bacteremia or spontaneous gangrene caused by *C. septicum* should have appropriate diagnostic studies of the gastrointestinal tract (Fig. 10.12). Occasionally, this has led to detection and cure of an unsuspected malignancy that might otherwise have been fatal.[55]

Clostridium sordellii infections

Patients who have *C. sordellii* infection present with unique clinical features including edema, absence of fever, leukemoid reaction, hemoconcentration and later shock and multiple organ failure.[45] Often *C. sordellii* infections develop after childbirth or after gynecologic procedures,[59,60] and most represent endometrial infection. Rarely, other cases have occurred at sites of minor trauma such as lacerations of the soft tissues of an extremity. Recently, outbreaks of *C. sordellii* and *C. novyi* infections have been described among intravenous drug users in Scotland, Ireland and England. Patients have presented with severe soft tissue infections with shock with a case fatality rate of 20–30%.[3] Interestingly, the mortality rate of women who acquire postpartum *C. sordelli* has been 100%.[61]

Unlike *C. perfringens* and *C. septicum* infections, pain may not be a prominent feature of *C. sordellii* infections. The absence of fever and the paucity of signs and symptoms of local infection make early diagnosis difficult.[44] The mechanisms of diffuse capillary leak, massive edema and hemoconcentration are not well established but clearly are related to elaboration of a potent toxin or toxins. Aldape recently demonstrated that a crude toxin preparation caused leakiness of endothelial cells in tissue culture.[62] Hematocrits of 75–80% have been described and leukocytosis of 50 000–100 000 cells/mm³ with a left shift is common.[42,59]

Recent studies have demonstrated that a neuroaminadase of *C. sordellii* is responsible for proliferation of bone marrow progenitor cells that likely contributes to the leukemoid reaction.[61]

Clostridium tertium infections

Clostridium tertium has been associated with spontaneous myonecrosis; however, it more commonly causes bacteremia in compromised hosts who have received long courses of antibiotics. Bacteremia probably arises from bowel sources, and the presence of the organism in the bowel may be partly related to its relative resistance to penicillin, cephalosporins and clindamycin. *Clostridium tertium* is, however, usually quite sensitive to chloramphenicol, vancomycin and metronidazole. Because this organism can grow aerobically, it may be mistakenly disregarded as a contaminant such as a diphtheroid or a *Bacillus* sp.[43,44]

Pyomyositis

Most cases of pyomyositis occur in tropical areas; however, recent reports of pyomyositis have documented a large increase in cases in temperate climates caused by methicillin-resistant *Staph. aureus* (MRSA).[62] Local trauma, muscle strain and overuse are common predisposing factors. Initially, seeding of traumatized muscle occurs and physical findings are not usually helpful. Within 10–20 days, fever, chills, muscle pain and tenderness are manifest (see Fig. 10.1). Most patients seek medical care at this stage and a diagnosis can be established by appropriate imaging studies (Fig. 10.13), needle aspiration or exploration. Patients in whom a diagnosis has not been made may progress to shock and organ failure, though these complications are uncommon. *Staphylococcus aureus* is the most common cause of pyomyositis in tropical and nontropical areas, and among HIV-positive patients. Hospitalized immunocompromised patients who are HIV negative occasionally develop pyomyositis caused by Gram-negative bacteria.

Surgical drainage of the abscess and empiric administration of parenteral antibiotics such as nafcillin or cephalosporins are reasonable treatments since most cases are caused by *Staph. aureus*. Definitive treatment can then be established based on cultures and sensitivities. Due to an increase in the prevalence of MRSA, it may be necessary to use vancomycin or linezolid empirically pending sensitivity results.[63]

REFERENCES

📄 References for this chapter can be found online at http://www.expertconsult.com

Arthropods and ectoparasites

Arthropods

INTRODUCTION

The phylum Arthropoda, which includes the insects and the arachnids, is the largest and most varied of all the animal phyla, containing more than one million described species. Although only a small number of these directly or indirectly affect human health, arthropod species are responsible for considerable morbidity and mortality (Table 11.1). Arthropods can cause illness in a number of different ways. These include parasitization (usually as ectoparasites), envenomation, vesication, mechanical transmission of infection, acting as biologic vectors, and as agents of a variety of allergic respiratory and dermatologic conditions. In addition, arthropod parasites of domestic animals may contribute to food shortages and enforced population movement. This section concentrates on the clinical problems caused by arthropods which are *not* true parasites of man.

ENVENOMATION

A variety of ectoparasite orders and species are responsible for envenomation of humans, either through bites or stings. These attacks are usually part of the self-defense behavior of the animal, and are distinct from the feeding bites inflicted by true parasites of man (see below). The severity of the reaction to envenomation varies enormously depending on the nature of the toxin, the location of the wound and the individual host response, which may itself depend in part on previous exposure.[1,2] Even relatively harmless toxins, which produce transient local symptoms in most people, may cause severe systemic reactions (including anaphylaxis) in highly sensitized individuals.[3–5]

Bees, wasps and ants

These social insects, members of the order Hymenoptera, usually attack humans to defend either themselves or their nests. Bees and wasps inject venom using a modified ovipositor, while some species of ant, notably the fire ant and the bulldog ant, have evolved a venomous sting in addition to their bite.[3,6] The resulting envenomation usually causes relatively minor and transient local inflammation.

Scorpions

Scorpions use their sting to inject a neurotoxic venom, which is primarily intended for hunting prey but may also be used in self-defense. Many are relatively harmless, causing symptoms similar to a bee sting,

but some species have a far more dangerous toxin which may even be fatal. Scorpion stings kill more than 1000 people each year (mainly children) in Africa, Europe, and the Middle East.[7]

Spiders

Spiders also use their venom mainly for hunting, injecting it through fang-like chelicerae in their mouth parts. Fortunately, although most spiders are venomous, few have chelicerae capable of penetrating human skin. Even those that can bite humans (such as tarantulas and wolf spiders) usually cause no more than transient local pain and swelling. However, a few species can cause much more serious illness, due to production of powerful neurotoxins or venom which triggers serious tissue necrosis.

Widow spiders (genus *Latrodectus*) inject a potent neurotoxin which is capable of causing myalgia, paralysis, convulsions and occasionally death. Mortality rates are reported to be between <1% and 6%, depending to some extent upon what treatment is available, but deaths due to widow spider bites are rare in developed countries. There are no accurate figures for the annual number of deaths in less developed areas. *Latrodectus* species are found worldwide, with *L. mactans* (the black widow) and *L. geometricus* (the brown widow) the best known. The females of all species are distinguished by a characteristic red or orange hourglass-shaped marking on the back (Fig. 11.1). Other potentially dangerous producers of neurotoxins include the funnel web spider (genus *Atrax*) in Australia and the armed spider (genus *Phoneutria*) in South America.[2,8]

Necrotic arachnidism occurs worldwide, and is most commonly due to the bite of one of the recluse spiders (genus *Loxosceles*). These small brown spiders have a dark, fiddle-shaped marking on their back (hence the common names fiddleback or violin spiders), and tend to lurk in quiet undisturbed areas. The bite is initially painless, but after a few hours the area becomes red, swollen and painful. Necrotic enzymes in the venom cause progressive tissue death and sloughing over the subsequent days, and occasionally lead to systemic toxicity including hemolysis and renal failure. The skin lesions can be very slow to heal, and are prone to secondary infection.

Other spider genera implicated in producing necrotic arachnidism include the hobo spider *Tegenaria agrestis* in Europe and the Pacific Northwest of North America, crab spiders (genus *Sicarius*) in Africa and sac spiders (genus *Chiracanthium*), which are found worldwide.[1]

Other envenoming arthropods

A number of other types of arthropod produce defensive toxins which may cause minor symptoms in humans. Centipedes inoculate venom through their pincers, and the larger species may be capable of penetrating human skin to cause local tissue reactions. Some caterpillars

Table 11.1 Arthropods and their medical importance

Class	Subclass	Order	Pathogenic potential
Insecta (insects)		Anoplura (sucking lice)	Biting pests Local hypersensitivity Biologic vectors
		Siphonaptera (fleas)	Biting pests Local hypersensitivity Biologic vectors Superficial tissue invasion (*Tunga penetrans*)
		Dictyoptera (cockroaches)	Mechanical vectors Allergies
		Hemiptera (bedbugs, kissing bugs)	Biting pests Local and rarely systemic hypersensitivity Biologic vector (kissing bugs)
		Hymenoptera (bees, wasps, ants)	Envenomation Local and systemic hypersensitivity including anaphylaxis
		Coleoptera (beetles)	Mechanical and biologic vectors Urticating hairs (larvae), vesicating fluids (adults)
		Lepidoptera (moths, butterflies, caterpillars)	Urticating hairs and venomous spines (larvae) Urticating hairs and scales (adults)
		Diptera (flies, mosquitoes, biting midges)	Biting pests Local hypersensitivity Mechanical and biologic vectors Tissue invasion (myiasis)
Arachnida (arachnids)	Scorpiones (scorpions) Araneae (spiders) Acari (ticks, mites)		Envenomation with neurotoxins Envenomation with neurotoxins and necrotoxins Biting pests Local and systemic hypersensitivity Allergies (mites) Biologic vectors Superficial tissue invasion (*Sarcoptes scabiei*) Neurotoxins (ticks)
Diplopoda (millipedes)			Vesicating fluid
Chilopoda (centipedes)			Envenomation Local and rarely systemic hypersensitivity
Crustacea (crustaceans)		Copepoda (copepods, water fleas) Decapoda (crabs, crayfish)	Biologic vectors Biologic vectors
Pentastomida			Tissue and body cavity infection

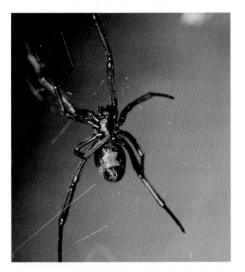

Fig. 11.1 Female *Latrodectus mactans*, the black widow spider. Note the characteristic red hourglass marking on the underside of the abdomen. With permission from New England Journal of Medicine 1994;331:777.

(larvae of moths and butterflies) possess hairs which inject a toxin when touched. In the vast majority of cases these cause minor local symptoms, but severe systemic reactions have been reported.[8]

Management

Most envenomation injuries require no specific treatment, although local symptoms may be alleviated with antihistamines. Anaphylaxis is life threatening, requiring immediate treatment with adrenaline (epinephrine) and/or bronchodilators. It may in some cases be possible to desensitize people with severe hypersensitivity reactions using very low doses of venom, but the success of this technique is variable. Specific antitoxins are available for certain spider and scorpion venoms.[9]

VESICATION

Some arthropods are capable of producing an irritant, blister-inducing (vesicating) chemical which is secreted or sprayed from specialized glands. As with envenomation, vesication is usually a self-defense reaction. The most common culprits are the so-called blister beetles and some species of millipede. Although beetles are best known as pests of agricultural crops, some species can give a painful bite, and others, especially the blister beetles, can exude vesicating fluids, including cantharidin, that cause dermatitis or blister formation. Cantharidin is the chief component of the aphrodisiac known as 'Spanish Fly'. The local irritation caused by these chemicals does not usually require specific treatment.[10]

MECHANICAL TRANSMISSION OF INFECTION

Arthropod species have been implicated as mechanical vectors of infection, carrying micro-organisms on their bodies and mouthparts. Flies play a major part in the transmission of trachoma (*Chlamydia trachomatis*) and can also spread a wide variety of gastrointestinal infections. Cat and dog fleas, which may be swallowed inadvertently, are intermediate hosts for the tapeworm *Dipylidium caninum* and less frequently for *Hymenolepis diminuta* and *H. nana*. The role of biting insects in the mechanical transmission of blood-borne viruses is considered below.

OTHER DERMATOLOGIC AND RESPIRATORY CONDITIONS

In addition to envenomation, vesication and parasitization, arthropods can cause skin problems through other mechanisms. So-called storage mites are small predatory arachnids which live in stored products such as grain, straw, flour, dried fruit, and cheese. They may migrate to humans who come into contact with their habitat, crawling onto exposed skin and getting underneath the horny layer of the skin. Here they can cause an acute dermatitis, with erythema and small vesicles: this condition, which is often related to occupation, is known by a variety of descriptive names such as 'grocer's itch', 'barley itch', and 'grain shoveler's itch'.[11]

Cheyletiellid mites are ubiquitous tissue-feeding parasites of domestic dogs and cats. Bites follow close contact with infected animals and lesions are usually seen on the thighs and abdomen after a pet has sat on someone's lap. Itchy papules similar to other arthropod bites result and the diagnosis is made by finding mites on the animal. Some hematophagous animal mites also attack humans, causing typical lesions in areas that depend on the form of contact with the animal. Poultry, cage birds, wild and domestic rodents and snakes have all been incriminated. In all these cases management is by removal or treatment of the principal animal host, with environmental acaricide if necessary.[11]

Demodex folliculorum, the follicle mite, is a tiny organism that lives in the pilosebaceous glands where it feeds on cell contents. The mites are found in areas of high sebum production: the forehead, cheeks, nose, and nasolabial folds. The role of follicle mites in skin disease is controversial: they are very common, and unless they are present in large numbers they do not appear to cause problems. However, they have been described as a cause of papulopustular eruptions in children and immunocompromised subjects, and have been implicated in the pathogenesis of skin conditions such as pityriasis folliculorum and rosacea.[12]

House dust mites (*Dermatophagoides* spp.) are cosmopolitan free-living mites that feed principally on human and animal skin detritus. Their main medical importance is as a cause of allergic rhinitis and bronchospasm.

MISCELLANEOUS

Pentastomes

Pentastomes or tongue worms are arthropods of uncertain affinities that possess few distinctive morphologic characteristics. Larval stages resemble mites and have occasionally been reported to cause liver and lung infections in humans in Asia and Africa. Adult stages are worm-like organisms that live in the nasal passages of certain predatory reptiles, birds and mammals; they have been recovered from the nasopharynx of individuals from the Middle East and Africa where they are responsible for an obstructive condition known as halzoun.[13]

Crustaceans

Crustaceans, most notably crabs, crayfish and microscopic copepods, are of medical importance by serving as hosts and vectors for larval stages of several different helminths (see Table 11.2).

Ectoparasites

INTRODUCTION

Parasites depend on their host for sustenance; an ectoparasite is a parasite that lives or feeds on the surface of that host. Most ectoparasites are hematophagous, but a few feed on living skin cells and tissue. Some spend their entire life on one host, while others move from host to host as they develop, and many simply alight on the host in order to feed. In this chapter the definition of 'ectoparasite' is extended to include those parasites that burrow into the epidermis as well as those that remain on the surface. The vast majority of ectoparasites are members of the phylum Arthropoda.

Humans are the preferred or only hosts of some ectoparasites, but the majority are less specific in their choice, or turn to humans only when their primary host is unavailable. Ectoparasites can cause human disease in a number of different ways. Local skin disease can be the direct result of the parasite bite, or may arise from secondary infection or hypersensitivity. Allergens or toxins introduced during feeding can cause systemic illness, and transient ectoparasites can act as vectors for a wide range of viral, bacterial, and parasitic infections. This section reviews the clinical syndromes caused by ectoparasites, outlining the key features associated with each.

SKIN PROBLEMS

Transient ectoparasites

Clinical and pathologic features

The most common feature of ectoparasite infection is local reaction to the bite of a blood-feeding arthropod. Numerous species of insects and arachnids rely on blood meals from vertebrate hosts. Although the behavior and feeding methods differ by species, most uncomplicated arthropod bites produce a similar local reaction.

Initial contact in an unsensitized person may produce little or no response. After repeated bites, typical raised pruritic lesions (papular urticaria) appear within 24–48 hours (Fig. 11.2), although delays of more than 1 week have been reported. Occasionally, these lesions are bullous. With further exposure and increased sensitization, an immediate wheal skin response may be seen, followed after some hours by papular urticaria. Some hypersensitive people may develop a pronounced immediate reaction with large areas of superficial edema. After prolonged and frequent biting, the delayed reaction often diminishes and eventually there is no response to further bites. The term papular urticaria is also used to describe a condition (usually seen in children) in which widespread papular lesions occur distant from but temporally related to insect bites; this may represent reactivation of previously sensitized bite sites.

The lesions of papular urticaria consist of pruritic papules, often with a central puncture marking the site of the bite. Superficial erosion and ulceration resulting from scratching is common. Unlike

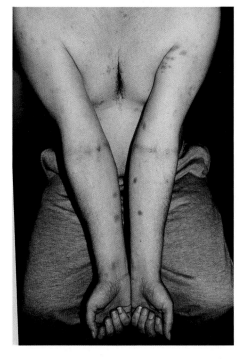

Fig. 11.2 Typical lesions of papular urticaria, caused in this case by bedbug bites.

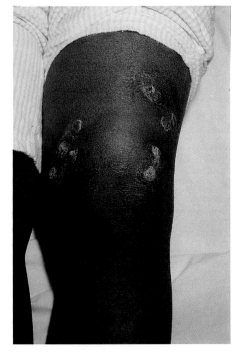

Fig. 11.3 Mosquito bites with secondary staphylococcal and streptococcal infection.

most other types of urticaria, papular lesions may persist for several days, although this period tends to decrease with regular exposure. Histologically there is intense inflammatory infiltrate with a predominance of T cells; the response is thought to be a type 1 IgE-mediated reaction.[14] A variety of vasodilators, anticoagulants and other substances have been isolated from arthropod saliva; in some species a specific allergen has been identified as the cause of local hypersensitivity, but in others the stimulus remains obscure.

Treatment of uncomplicated bites is usually unnecessary, although severe pruritus may be relieved by systemic antihistamines. Caution is needed with terfenadine and astemizole, which can cause prolongation of the cardiographic QT interval and have a synergistic cardiotoxic effect with certain antimalarial drugs. Secondary bacterial infection is common in hot moist climates (Fig. 11.3) and this may require antibiotic therapy; infection is usually due to gram-positive cocci. Local lesions caused by various blood-feeding arthropods are usually indistinguishable, and diagnosis of the precise cause relies either on epidemiologic knowledge or on detection and identification of the parasite. This may sometimes be necessary in order to eradicate the source of infection.

The major types of transient-feeding ectoparasites responsible for this type of bite are discussed below.

Flies

Insects of the order Diptera are characterized by the presence of a single pair of membranous wings. They vary enormously in size and appearance. Of all the arthropods, the flies are responsible for the greatest share of human disease as a result of blood feeding, transmission of infection, and myiasis (which is discussed below). Mosquitoes, blackflies, horseflies, sandflies, and midges are ubiquitous, whereas tsetse flies are essentially tropical. Only certain species of each family tend to attack humans, and in all except the tsetse fly only the females are blood feeders. Culicid mosquitoes usually feed by inserting their proboscis directly into the capillary, whereas other species feed by inflicting local tissue damage and sucking the resultant blood (pool feeding). This may explain the relatively more severe irritation that complicates bites by some species, although host factors also play a significant part. Some of the biting flies are important biologic vectors of infection (Table 11.2).

Fleas

Fleas (order Siphonaptera) are small (1–2 mm), laterally compressed, wingless insects with muscular back legs which enable them to jump great distances. They include both transient blood-sucking pests (some of which are also important vectors of infection; see Table 11.2), and the locally invasive jigger flea. Fleas occur worldwide and are a common cause of pruritic bites in humans. They are free living, only approaching their host in order to feed. The human flea, *Pulex irritans*, is found mainly in crowded and unhygienic living conditions and is relatively uncommon in the developed world. However, many species of animal and bird fleas will also feed on humans, and household infestations with cat and dog fleas (*Ctenocephalides felis* and *C. canis*) are increasing in frequency (Fig. 11.4).

Flea bites provoke typical papular urticaria, although there may be a more severe reaction with bulla formation. The distribution of the lesions reflects the source of the infestation; for example, bites on the lower leg are usually due to cat and dog fleas, at least in adults. Diagnosis can be difficult; fleas are rarely seen on the human victim and excoriation may mask the original nature of the lesions. If flea bites are suspected, careful inspection of the home environment is needed, although other sources of exposure (e.g. school, the workplace) should be considered. Household pets and their bedding should be checked thoroughly for fleas and droppings. Flea bites need no specific treatment unless there is secondary infection. Prevention depends on identifying the source of the infestation; in the case of pets, insecticides must be applied to both the animal and its environment. Because larvae of these species often develop in an animal's bedding or in carpets and furniture, eradication may require fumigation and cleaning of these articles.

Bugs

The bugs, or Hemiptera, are one of the largest and most diverse orders of insect. Although a number of bug species are blood feeders, only two families include significant ectoparasites of humans. The Reduviidae (kissing bugs) are large (1–3 cm) insects with a cone-shaped head and often conspicuous body markings. The bite of the kissing bug is relatively painless, although hypersensitivity can develop with repeated exposure. They are important principally as the vector of South American trypanosomiasis. Cimicidae (bedbugs) are flattish, wing-

Table 11.2 Important ectoparasite vectors of human infection

Ectoparasite	Vector genus/species	Infective organism	Disease	Distribution
Flies (Diptera)				
Mosquitoes	*Anopheles* spp. *Anopheles* spp. *Culex* spp. *Aedes* spp.	*Plasmodium* spp. *Wuchereria bancrofti*	Malaria Lymphatic filariasis	Tropics and sub-tropics Tropics
	Anopheles spp. *Mansonia* spp. *Aedes* spp.	*Brugia* spp.	Lymphatic filariasis	Southern Asia
	Aedes spp. *Culex* spp. *Anopheles* spp.	Arboviruses	Dengue, yellow fever, Japanese encephalitis, West Nile virus, St Louis encephalitis, etc.	Specific to each disease
Blackflies	Simuliidae	*Onchocerca volvulus* *Mansonella ozzardi*	Onchocerciasis Mansonelliasis	Sub-Saharan Africa, Central and South America Amazon basin
Sandflies	*Phlebotomus* spp. *Lutzomyia* spp.	*Leishmania* spp. Bunyaviridae *Leishmania* spp. *Bartonella bacilliformis*	Visceral and cutaneous leishmaniasis Sandfly fever Visceral and cutaneous leishmaniasis Bartonellosis (Oroya fever, Carrion's disease, verruga peruana)	Sub-Saharan Africa, Asia, Mediterranean Europe Central Asia, Mediterranean, North Africa Central and South America South America
Biting midges	*Culicoides* spp.	*Mansonella perstans* and *Mansonella ozzardi*	Mansonelliasis	Sub-Saharan Africa and Amazon basin
Tsetse flies	Glossinidae	*Trypanosoma* spp.	African trypanosomiasis	Sub-Saharan Africa
Deer flies	*Chrysops* spp.	*Loa loa* *Francisella tularensis*	Loiasis Tularaemia	West Africa Western USA
Fleas (Siphonaptera)				
E.g. tropical rat flea	Various species (notably *Xenopsylla*) Various species	*Yersinia pestis* *Rickettsia typhi* (*mooseri*)	Plague Murine typhus	Worldwide (patchy) Worldwide (patchy)
Bugs (Hemiptera)				
Kissing bug	Reduviidae	*Trypanosoma cruzi*	South American trypanosomiasis	Central and South America
Lice				
Body louse Body louse Head louse	*Pediculus humanus corporis* *P. h. corporis* *P. h. capitis*	*Rickettsia prowazeki* *Bartonella quintana* *Borrelia recurrentis*	Epidemic typhus Trench fever Louse-borne relapsing fever	Worldwide (patchy) Worldwide Worldwide (patchy)
Ticks				
Hard ticks (Ixodidae)	Numerous hard tick (ixodid) species	*Rickettsia* spp. *Borrelia burgdorferi* *Francisella tularensis* *Babesia* spp. Arboviruses *Ehrlichia* spp.	Tick typhus and various rickettsial spotted fevers Lyme disease Tularaemia Babesiosis Tick-borne encephalitis, Congo–Crimea hemorrhagic fever, etc. Ehrlichiosis	Worldwide USA, Europe, Far East, Australia USA, Europe, Japan USA, Europe Specific to each disease USA, Europe, North Africa, Far East

Table 11.2 Important ectoparasite vectors of human infection—cont'd

Ectoparasite	Vector genus/species	Infective organism	Disease	Distribution
Soft ticks (Argasidae)	*Ornithodoros* spp.	*Borrelia* spp.	Tick-borne relapsing fever	Africa, Central Asia, North and South America
Mites				
	Leptotrombidium spp.	*Orientia tsutsugamushi*	Scrub typhus	South East Asia, Pacific and (rarely) West Africa
	Liponyssoides sanguineus	*Rickettsia akari*	Rickettsial pox	USA, South Africa, Far East
Crustacea				
Crabs, crayfish Copepods	Decapods *Cyclops* spp.	*Paragonimus* spp. *Dracunculus medinensis* *Gnathostoma spinigerum*	Paragonimiasis Guinea worm Gnathostomiasis	Asia, Sub-Saharan Africa Sudan, Ghana Worldwide (patchy)

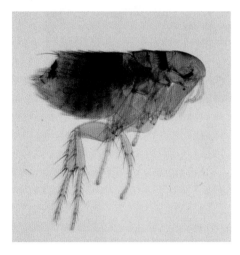

Fig. 11.4 Adult *Ctenocephalides canis*, the dog flea. Note the strong muscular hind legs. Courtesy of Thomas R Fritsche.

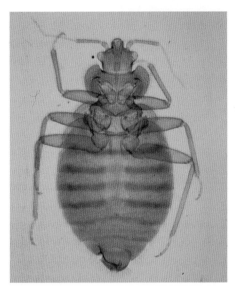

Fig. 11.5 Adult bedbug *Cimex lectularius*. With permission from ASM Press. Courtesy of Thomas R Fritsche.

less insects about 5 mm in length (Fig. 11.5). Bedbugs live and reproduce in crevices in walls and furniture, only approaching the host to feed (usually at night). They are found worldwide, the tropical bedbug (*Cimex hemipterus*) parasitizing humans in hot climates and the common bedbug (*C. lectularius*) in other areas. Bites cause papular lesions similar to those of other arthropods, but in unhygienic conditions infestations can be very heavy and secondary iron deficiency anemia has been reported. Personal insect repellants and permethrin-impregnated bed nets provide some protection, but decontamination of the environment with residual insecticides may be necessary.

The role of bedbugs as potential vectors of infection remains controversial. Viable infective hepatitis B virus and other pathogens have been found in the gut of bedbugs weeks after their last blood meal. However, community-based studies have failed to confirm that bedbugs have a significant role in hepatitis B transmission,[15] and attempts at transmitting infection among a group of chimpanzees using bedbugs were unsuccessful when the bugs fed normally.[16] Although HIV has been isolated from bedbugs up to 8 days after feeding on heavily infected blood under experimental conditions, there is no evidence to suggest transmission to humans by this route.[17]

Ticks

Ticks, which are arachnids rather than insects, are cosmopolitan ectoparasites of mammals, birds and reptiles. They are hugely important in the transmission of animal as well as human disease. Ticks

pass through four stages of development – egg, larva, nymph, and adult – with a blood meal required for progression. All stages of tick attach to vertebrate hosts in order to feed: some spend their entire life cycle on a single animal (one-host ticks), while others drop off before molting and then seek out a new host (multihost ticks). When not attached to feed, ticks are usually found in scrub or grassland in close proximity to their preferred hosts, or in the burrow or nest. Although ticks are relatively host-specific, most will attack humans in appropriate circumstances: this usually occurs when humans stray into the tick's home environment. Adult ticks are usually 2–5 mm in length: larvae and nymphs are smaller, and are easily missed on the skin. All stages swell enormously as they feed. Hard ticks (family Ixodidae) have a hard plate or scutum covering their back (Fig. 11.6), while soft ticks (family Argasidae) have a soft, leathery body (Fig. 11.7).

Most adult and immature ixodid ticks remain attached to the host for several days unless removed; argasid ticks feed more rapidly and may detach themselves after a few hours. The bite is often not irritating, and may pass unnoticed, especially in the early stages of attachment, which is an important factor in the role of the tick as a vector. In some cases, presumably when the host has been presensitized, tick bites can cause itchy papular lesions with evidence of a type 1 hypersensitivity reaction. Elevated levels of specific IgE against tick saliva can be demonstrated in such people.[18] Local skin reactions may occur

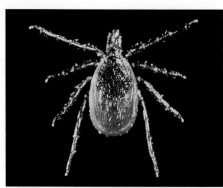

Fig. 11.6 Non-engorged adult female *Ixodes scapularis*, the black-legged tick or deer tick, of the family Ixodidae (hard ticks). With permission from Northwest Infectious Disease Consultants. Courtesy of Thomas R Fritshe.

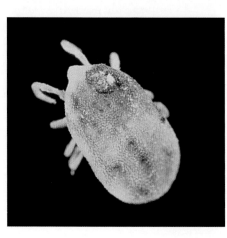

Fig. 11.7 Non-engorged adult *Ornithodoros hermsi*, of the family Argasidae (soft ticks). With permission from Northwest Infectious Disease Consultants. Courtesy of Thomas R Fritshe.

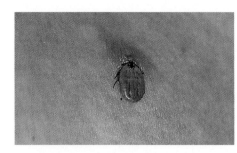

Fig. 11.8 Engorged tick after feeding on the host for several days.

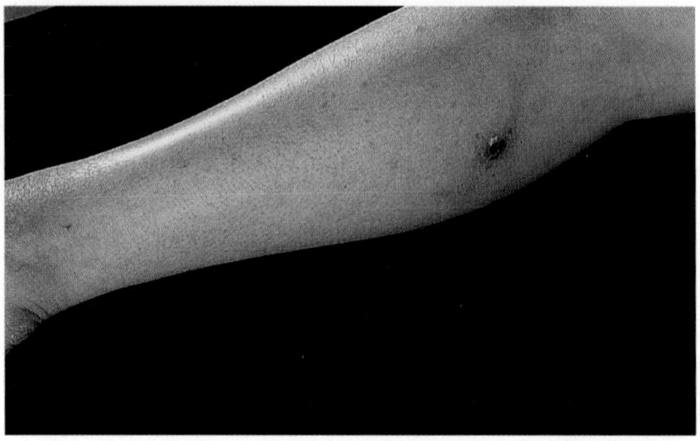

Fig. 11.9 Tick-bite eschar associated with African tick typhus.

when tick attachment is prolonged (Fig. 11.8). Hypersensitive people may experience more generalized urticarial skin reactions and even systemic features of anaphylaxis (see below).

A characteristic necrotic lesion may be seen when the tick bite is associated with the transmission of certain rickettsial infections – the so-called eschar or *tâche noire* (Fig. 11.9). Ticks are biologic vectors of a number of viral and bacterial infections (see Table 11.2).

Avoidance and management of tick bites

Ticks usually prefer certain specific types of vegetation and most species are more commonly found during the spring and summer. In adults, ticks are generally found on the lower body, while children are often bitten on the head, neck and axillae. Some species of tick also have preferential sites of attachment. A knowledge of the epidemiology of local tick species, as well as the wearing of long trousers and the use of permethrin-impregnated clothing, can decrease the incidence of tick bites and their complications (see below).

Most ectoparasite vectors of infection feed rapidly, and length of time on the host probably does not influence the likelihood of infection. Ixodid ticks, by contrast, can spend many days feeding and the risk of transmission of some infections appears to be directly related to the duration of the bite. Tick paralysis is also dependent on prolonged feeding and both infectious agents and toxins may be inoculated into the host by careless removal, which can also leave the barbed mouthparts embedded in the skin. As well as predisposing to bacterial infection this can also generate a chronic granulomatous response; in some cases local surgical excision is needed to relieve the symptoms. Early detection and appropriate detachment of ticks is therefore essential, especially in regions where tick-borne diseases are endemic. The ideal method of removal is to grasp the tick mouthparts as close to the skin as possible with fine forceps or tweezers and gently lever the creature off. The body should not be squeezed, in order to prevent further inoculation. Any retained fragments should not be dug out, but the site

cleaned and antiseptic applied. This method of removal is associated with a significantly lower incidence of rickettsial and borrelial infection following tick bites.[19,20]

In the particular case of Lyme disease, early antibiotic therapy after infection with *Borrelia burgdorferi* may provide some protection against the development of disease (see also Chapter 43.). Tick bites are very common, and even in areas where the majority of vector species are infected, the rate of human infection is very low.[20] However, risk of infection rises dramatically once the tick has been feeding for more than 72 hours (from about 1% at less than 72 hours to 20% at 72 hours or more).[21] The approximate duration of attachment of the tick can be estimated from an index of tick engorgement (the scutal index). There is some evidence that antibiotic prophylaxis following a tick bite in hyperendemic areas may decrease the incidence of clinical Lyme disease:[22] this is particularly likely to be justified in cases where the tick has been feeding for more than 72 hours. Other attempts at predicting high-risk groups following tick bites (e.g. by testing the tick for *B. burgdorferi* infection) have not proved successful.[21] There is no evidence that empiric antibiotic prophylaxis following tick bites has a role in the prevention of rickettsial infections such as Rocky Mountain spotted fever.[23]

Mites

Mites are tiny (≤1 mm) arachnids, most of which are free living in the environment. Many feed on other insects and larvae, but some parasitize larger animals including humans. The most important of these are trombiculid mites ('chiggers'), which are found worldwide. The adult and nymphal stages are free-living predators, but the larvae parasitize many animals, including humans. The mites inhabit areas of transitional vegetation, hence the alternative name of 'scrub mite', often forming localized 'mite islands' in areas inhabited by a host species. Larval mites climb onto a human host who is passing through the vegetation and crawl over the host's body to find a suitable area of skin to bite, such as the axillae or groins or areas of skin that are constricted by clothing. They feed for several days if undisturbed and then drop to the ground. The resulting lesions are similar to those caused by tick bites; the methods of prevention are also similar.

In certain parts of the world (principally Asia) trombiculid mites are the vector of scrub typhus.[24] Scabies and other resident parasitic mites are described below.

Infestations of resident hematophagous parasites

Most blood-feeding arthropods that attack humans are transient ectoparasites, alighting to feed and then moving on. A few stay on or close to the human host for their entire life cycle, living and breeding in the hair or clothing, and feeding frequently and repeatedly in the same area. The lifestyle of these resident parasites can cause a different and more chronic pattern of disease.

Lice

The sucking lice (order Anaplura) are dorsoventrally flattened wingless insects with characteristic claws at the end of each leg, allowing them to cling to hair or clothing. All species suck blood, and although single bites will cause typical papular lesions, repetitive feeding combined with chronic scratching and exposure to louse saliva and feces can cause a more generalized dermatitis. Head lice (*Pediculus humanus capitis*) and body lice (*P. humanus corporis*) are morphologically almost indistinguishable (Fig. 11.10), but they each tend to keep to their own territory on the host, and only the latter acts as a biologic vector of infection. Body lice cling to, and deposit eggs on, clothing fibers rather than hair shafts. They parasitize those who do not wash or change clothing, unlike the head louse which is not associated with poor hygiene alone. Pubic lice are distinctly different from the other species, and are usually confined to the pubic region.

Head lice

Children are more commonly infected with head lice than adults, and women are more commonly affected than men, at least in Western cultures. This is because the vast majority of infections are acquired by direct head-to-head contact, which is more likely in these groups. Overcrowding is also an important risk factor, but hair length is not. Head lice are more common in late summer, which probably reflects

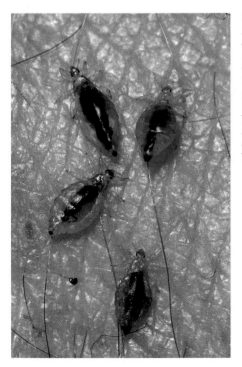

Fig. 11.10 Adult *Pediculus humanus corporis* (the body louse) feeding. Courtesy of Dr H Lieske. With permission from Peters W, Pasvol G. Tropical medicine and parasitology, 5th ed. London: Mosby-Wolfe; 2002.

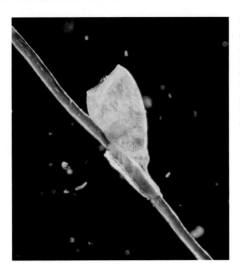

Fig. 11.11 Egg or nit of human head louse attached to a hair shaft. Note that the operculum is missing indicating previous emergence of the larval louse. Courtesy of Thomas R Fritsche.

the need for high ambient temperature to hatch eggs. The role of fomites in transmission is controversial; there is little evidence that hats and brushes are important. The main feature of head louse infestation is scalp itching, although secondary bacterial infection is not uncommon, and louse infection should be looked for in cases of scalp impetigo. Chronic infection can produce cervical lymphadenopathy. The definitive diagnosis can only be made by finding live adult lice in the hair. The presence of empty egg-cases ('nits') stuck to the base of hair follicles indicates recent infection, but nits may still be seen in successfully treated cases (Fig. 11.11). In heavy infestations, developing eggs, nymphs and adult lice may all be seen: the highest concentration of eggs is usually in the occipital and parietal regions.

Traditional combing methods (either wet or dry) can be effective, but they are very time consuming and require good technique and several repetitions to be of any benefit. Several insecticides are available for the treatment of head lice (Table 11.3).[25,26] The acetylcholinesterase inhibitors malathion and carbaryl both have reasonable ovicidal and pediculicidal activity, although some resistance has been seen. Malathion, unlike carbaryl, has a residual action of several weeks, but two applications 10 days apart are necessary whichever agent is used. The synthetic pyrethroids, such as permethrin, also have good activity, although there are concerns about the rapid development of resistance to these compounds. Topical ivermectin has also been used with good effect, although there is little evidence to suggest that it is preferable to other agents. Dimeticone kills lice by physically coating them rather than by a toxic effect, and is therefore not susceptible to the development of resistance.[27] It appears to have greater efficacy and fewer adverse events than malathion.[28]

Malathion and carbaryl need to remain on the scalp for 8–12 hours before they are washed off and they are degraded by high temperatures (e.g. as occurs during the use of a hair dryer). Pyrethroids need only a short application. Lotion or mousse preparations are generally preferable to shampoos, although some commercial preparations contain inadequate concentrations of active compound and are not recommended.[26] There are numerous trials comparing different drugs and preparations, but it is very difficult to draw general conclusions.[29,30] Several of the available treatments have reasonable efficacy and safety profiles,[31] but current British guidelines recommend using one of three agents: dimeticone, phenothrin or malathion.[26] The practice of rotating the locally recommended treatment to prevent resistance is not effective and should no longer be used. Systemic therapy has occasionally been used to treat head lice. Trimethoprim–sulfamethoxazole and ivermectin have been reported to be effective, although repeated doses are necessary because they affect only the feeding stages of the parasite. In most cases topical treatment should be adequate. Older drugs, such as organochlorines and mercury-based preparations, are less effective and more toxic.

Table 11.3 Commonly used topical preparations for the treatment of ectoparasite infestations

Class	Agent	Uses	Toxicity	Comments
Acetylcholinesterase inhibitors	Malathion	Scabies Head lice* Pubic lice		Good residual protection Recommended for pubic lice infestation of eyelashes Safe in pregnancy Prescription only in the UK
	Carbaryl	Head lice Pubic lice	Carcinogenic in animals; minimal risk to humans in therapeutic doses	
Organochlorines	Lindane	Head lice Pubic lice	Neurotoxic (potential for systemic absorption)	Increasing resistance No longer available in the UK
Natural pyrethroids	Pyrethrin	Head lice Pubic lice		Less evidence of efficacy than synthetic pyrethroids
	Phenothrin	Head lice* Pubic lice		
Synthetic pyrethroids	Permethrin	Scabies Head lice Pubic lice	Rarely rash and local edema	Probably safe in pregnancy and breast-feeding (limited data)
Others	Dimeticone	Head lice*		Physically coats lice rather than toxin More effective than malathion in randomized controlled trial No resistance
	Benzyl benzoate	Scabies	Skin irritation	Limited safety data in pregnancy; avoid in breast-feeding
	Ivermectin	Head lice Scabies		Available for topical and systemic use
	Crotamiton	Head lice Scabies		Relatively poor efficacy Avoid in pregnancy
	Mercury preparations	Head lice	Contact dermatitis Systemic toxicity	Available over the counter in some European countries
	Monosulfiram	Scabies	'Antabuse' effect (alcohol should be avoided)	No longer available in the UK
	Sulfur ointment	Scabies	Skin irritation	Cheap, safe, reasonably effective

*Recommended treatments for head lice in the United Kingdom.[26]

Body lice

Body lice are associated with poor hygiene and unwashed clothing and are principally parasites of vagrants and refugees. They can be found worldwide, but are more common in cooler climates where clothing is rarely removed. Transmission is by direct body-to-body spread or by sharing infected clothing. Initially the bites are similar to those of other hematophagous ectoparasites, but the prolonged and persistent nature of the infestation leads to widespread excoriation and secondary infection, and eventually to the hyperpigmented chronic skin condition known as 'vagabond's disease' or morbus errorum.

Body lice are important vectors of infection (see Table 11.2), and have been responsible for major outbreaks of disease such as typhus amongst refugees, soldiers and displaced populations. The diagnosis is made by finding lice and eggs in the clothing (particularly along seams), and treatment should be directed at the clothing rather than the patient. High-temperature washing, tumble-drying and malathion dusting powder are all effective at clearing garments of lice; permethrin-treated clothing may be protective for those at risk of infestation.

Pubic lice

Pthirus pubis (often written as *Phthirus pubis*) is morphologically different from *Pediculus humanus* and is unique to humans (Fig. 11.12).

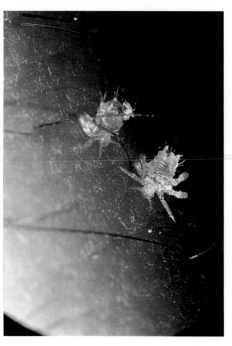

Fig. 11.12 The 'crab louse', *Phthirus pubis*, infests not only the pubic region but also other sites, including the eyelashes. Courtesy of Dr H Lieske. With permission from Peters W, Pasvol G. Tropical medicine and parasitology, 5th ed. London: Mosby-Wolfe; 2002.

Infection is usually confined to the pubic region, although lice and eggs are sometimes found in axillary and facial hair, eyelashes, eyebrows and (especially in children) the scalp. Infection is transmitted by close, usually sexual, contact and may be associated with other sexually transmitted diseases.

The main symptom is itching of the affected area, especially at night, although there may be few visible skin lesions. Close inspection may reveal eggs that are attached to the hair shafts, with adult lice clinging on close to the skin. Treatment is with the same insecticides as for head lice, with the proviso that alcohol-based preparations may irritate sensitive skin and mucous membranes. This is particularly true for the eyes, and eyelash infestations should always be treated with an aqueous formulation. It is usually advisable to treat the whole trunk and limbs in view of the possible spread to other hairy areas; where appropriate, sexual contacts should also be treated.[32]

Locally invasive ectoparasites

Strictly speaking the term 'ectoparasite' is reserved for those organisms which stay on the surface of the skin. However, there are a few arthropod parasites which spend some or all of their life cycle burrowing within or beneath the superficial layers of the skin, and the definition can usefully be stretched to include these locally invasive species. In some cases (e.g. the myiatic flies), only a specific and limited part of the life cycle is spent as a parasite, while in others such as the scabies mite the entire life cycle takes place within the host skin.

Myiatic flies

The house fly, *Musca domestica*, has no requirement for developing in mammalian tissue, but is occasionally found in dead tissue or under plaster casts. Facultative myiasis is most often caused by blowflies and flesh flies, which ordinarily feed on dead tissues, but may move into adjacent viable tissues or infest exposed ulcers or traumatic wounds. Risk factors in developed countries include homelessness, alcoholism and peripheral vascular disease,[33] and myiasis may occasionally complicate chronic otitis media in children[34] and neglected oral lesions.[35] The beneficial effects of larval therapy have been known to battlefield surgeons for centuries. Deliberate use of such 'biosurgery' is becoming increasingly acceptable to clean difficult wounds, including those that are complicated by multidrug-resistant bacterial infection. The flies most often used are the facultative calliphorids, with the greenbottle blowfly (*Lucilia sericata*) being the most widely used species.[36]

A few species of fly are specifically adapted to parasitize living flesh. These myiatic flies are confined to specific geographic locations, mainly in the tropics, and are quite often found in travelers returning from these areas.[37] Myiatic flies are of major veterinary importance and cause significant mortality in domestic livestock.

There are two main species of fly causing invasive human myiasis: the Tumbu or mango fly (*Cordylobia anthropophaga*) which is extensively distributed in sub-Saharan Africa, and the human botfly (*Dermatobia hominis*) which is found in Central and South America. Various other species which are primarily animal parasites may occasionally infect humans, such as the screwworm, *Cochliomyia hominivorax*. The modes of infection for the two common species are different. The eggs of *C. anthropophaga* are laid on the ground, or sometimes on bedding or clothing that has been left on the ground. Once hatched, the larvae seek out warm skin which they can rapidly penetrate. Infection can thus be avoided by not lying on, or laying out clothing on, potentially contaminated ground, or by ironing clothes that have been exposed. In contrast, the eggs of *D. hominis* are laid on the body of certain species of biting fly, and infection occurs when the host takes a blood meal: prevention of infection is thus more difficult.

The clinical features of furuncular myiasis are similar for all species. A small red papule develops within about 24 hours of infection, and gradually swells over the next few days as the larva develops. A dermal cavity containing the maggot is surrounded by an intense inflammatory response, which may be very itchy and painful. A hole appears at the centre of the swelling, through which the posterior tip of the larva (including its breathing spiracle) can be seen. After about 2 weeks in the case of *C. anthropophaga*, but up to 4 or more weeks in *D. hominis*, the mature larva forces its way out and drops to the ground. If there is no secondary infection the wound rapidly heals.

The diagnosis of myiasis is clinical, based on the appearance and history. Traditional methods of removal include blocking the surface hole with petroleum jelly, pork fat or nail varnish (which is useful in difficult to reach areas such as the scalp) and then grabbing the parasite as it pushes its spiracle out of the hole (Fig. 11.13). This is more effective for *C. anthropophaga*, but less successful for botfly infections, as the larva is flask-shaped and difficult to extrude. Minor surgery under local anesthetic is often needed to remove these (Fig. 11.14). Ivermectin has been used in refractory cases.[35] Secondary infection may necessitate antibiotic treatment. Tetanus has occasionally been reported as a complication of myiasis.

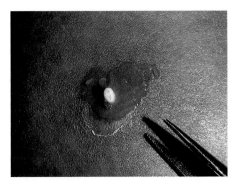

Fig. 11.13 Extracting a larva of *Cordylobia anthropophaga* after covering it with paraffin. The pair of black spiracles can just be seen in the center of the posterior tip of the larva. Courtesy of Professor A Bryceson. With permission from Peters W, Pasvol G. Tropical medicine and parasitology, 5th ed. London: Mosby-Wolfe; 2002.

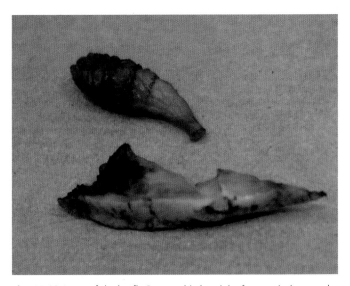

Fig. 11.14 Larva of the botfly *Dermatobia hominis* after surgical removal from the leg of a patient who had visited Belize (preserved specimens). Note flask shape of maggot, with bulbous portion at base of wound.

Jigger fleas

The jigger (or chigoe) flea, *Tunga penetrans*, has a wide distribution in Central and South America, Africa and parts of the Indian subcontinent. Unlike all other species of flea, the female jigger flea incubates her eggs while living within the dermis of a mammalian host. The gravid flea burrows into the skin until only the posterior end, bearing the respiratory spiracles, is protruding. While the flea feeds and grows the egg sac develops and gradually releases its contents back onto the ground.

Infection with *T. penetrans* results in small painful nodules, most commonly found on the sole of the foot or under a toenail. Multiple lesions are common. A small black spot can often be seen at the centre of the swelling: this is the site of the projecting spiracles. Secondary bacterial infection is common, and tetanus is a particular hazard. The diagnosis is made on the basis of appearance and epidemiology, although the lesions may sometimes be mistaken for plantar warts. The fleas can sometimes be shelled out carefully with a moderately sharp instrument such as a toothpick, but care should be taken not to disrupt the flea, and surgical excision under local anesthetic may be required (Fig. 11.15).

Scabies and pseudoscabies

Some infesting arthropod ectoparasites do not feed on blood at all, but cause disease in other ways. The most important of these is *Sarcoptes scabiei*, the human scabies mite, which is found worldwide in conditions of poor hygiene (Fig. 11.16). This skin-burrowing mite is not a blood feeder, but ingests predigested dermal cells as it tunnels through the epithelium. Female mites live in small burrows in the skin, which they extend by 2–3 mm daily, leaving a trail of eggs and feces behind them. The burrows are intensely itchy and are responsible for the features of scabies. They are usually found around the wrists, web spaces, toes and genitalia, although they may be more widespread; small papules are sometimes seen at the distal end adjacent to the female mite. Infestations are usually relatively light, with an average of 12 adult females found on an infected patient. Crusted scabies (also known as Norwegian scabies), in which there is heavy mite infestation and gross hyperkeratosis, may be seen in the elderly and in immunocompromised and institutionalized patients (Fig. 11.17). (See also Chapter 95.) Conversely, symptoms of scabies may be masked in some patients taking steroids.[38,39]

Diagnosis based on history and clinical features alone can be difficult and should be confirmed whenever possible by identification of mites. This is usually done by extracting parasites with a needle or in skin scrapings, but these techniques require operator experience and visible burrows. Newer methods of diagnosis include high-magnification videodermatoscopy, epiluminescence microscopy and polymerase chain reaction but none of these is widely available.[40] Treatment should be given if scabies is suspected, even if the diagnosis cannot be confirmed.

Scabies is usually treated with topical acaricides (see Table 11.3). Comparative trials suggest that 5% permethrin is the most effective treatment, with 0.5% malathion the second choice; permethrin is considerably more expensive.[32,41] Oral ivermectin has been increasingly used in recent years, especially in crusted or recurrent infections. It is well tolerated and appears to be highly effective, although a second dose may be needed 1 week after the first. Although unlicensed, oral ivermectin is probably the treatment of choice in recurrent cases, institutional outbreaks, and crusted scabies; combining systemic treatment with a topical preparation may give the best results in hyperkeratotic disease.[42,43] There is clinical and molecular evidence of emerging resistance to ivermectin and 5% permethrin, with renewed interest in the role of traditional remedies such as tea tree oil and other alternatives.[40] Crusted scabies is highly contagious, and can cause large nosocomial outbreaks of infection in staff and other patients. Inpatients should be nursed in isolation, and contact with other immunosuppressed people should be avoided. Bedding and clothing should be boil-washed or treated.

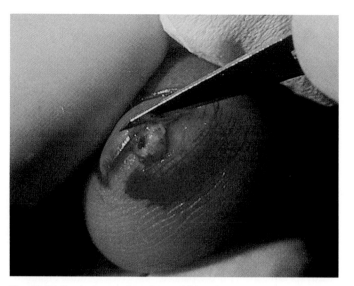

Fig. 11.15 Surgical extraction of a gravid female *Tunga penetrans*. Care must be taken not to disrupt the abdomen and release the eggs. Courtesy of Professor C Curtis. With permission from Peters W. A colour atlas of arthropods in clinical medicine. London: Wolfe Publishing Ltd; 1992.

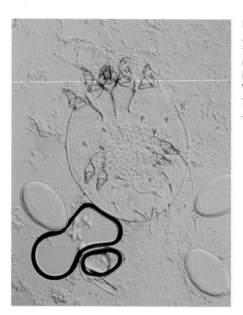

Fig. 11.16 Adult *Sarcoptes scabiei*, the human itch or mange mite, seen in skin scrapings. With permission from New England Journal of Medicine 1994;331:777.

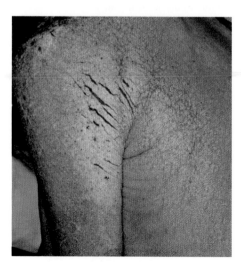

Fig. 11.17 Crusted Norwegian scabies in a patient who has AIDS. With permission from New England Journal of Medicine 1994;331:777.

Sarcoptid mites are relatively host-specific and mites acquired from animals do not usually cause prolonged infestations of humans. However, people in close contact with infected livestock (notably pigs, cows and dogs) may acquire temporary infestation, causing pruritic lesions but lacking the typical burrows of human scabies. In most cases no treatment is required except for avoidance of the source of infection.

NONINFECTIVE SYSTEMIC PROBLEMS

Tick paralysis/toxicosis

Paralysis and death of domestic animals and occasionally humans following tick bites has been documented in Australia and South Africa since the end of the 19th century and more recently it has been observed in North America and Europe. This syndrome is not, as once thought, an infective process, but is caused by a toxin in the saliva of the pregnant females of certain ixodid species. Children are more often affected than adults and the condition is most commonly seen in spring and early summer.

Tick paralysis almost always results from bites on the head, typically behind or within the ear, where the tick may not be noticed. Symptoms appear only after the tick has been feeding for at least 48 hours. The usual presentation is an ascending flaccid paralysis, frequently with cranial nerve involvement, although atypical features such as isolated nerve lesions and cerebellar signs are occasionally seen. There is no sensory loss or decrease in consciousness; however, if the condition is untreated, death from respiratory failure can supervene. In the North American form the paralysis starts to improve within a few hours of removing the tick, but in the Australian form of the disease deterioration may continue for a further 24–48 hours.[44]

The neurotoxin involved probably varies between different tick species. It has not been fully characterized, but there are many clinical and neurophysiologic similarities to the effects of botulinum toxin.[44] The essential treatment is to remove the tick carefully to prevent further transfer of toxin, followed by supportive care until the neurologic signs resolve. Although rare, the diagnosis should be considered in any progressive flaccid paralysis in an endemic area.[45]

Tick anaphylaxis

The local allergic urticarial reactions to tick bites have already been discussed. Rarely, in hypersensitive people, anaphylaxis can follow a bite, with bronchospasm, edema, and hypotension. This is an IgE-mediated response to tick salivary antigens, which can occur soon after the tick first bites or following careless removal.[46] Treatment is as for any form of anaphylactic reaction and sensitive people in tick-infested areas may benefit from carrying adrenaline (epinephrine) for inhalation or self-injection.

Delusional states

Patients with delusions of parasitosis present a difficult challenge. These people believe they are infested with a variety of bugs, and often give graphic descriptions of sensations of things crawling under their skin and/or emerging from their body. They appear in the clinic with a sample of the offending item, which invariably turns out to be fibers, hairs, pieces of tissue paper or bits of skin.[47,48] This is a monodelusional state that has a poor prognosis and may continue for years. Chronically affected patients often have multiple lesions of nodular prurigo, sparing areas of the skin that they cannot reach. A variant of this syndrome has acquired quasi-respectability under the name Morgellon's disease, in which the patient describes small fibers extruding from the skin.[49]

Management requires a sympathetic approach, with careful microscopic examination of the supposed ectoparasites and explanation that they are not genuine parasites. However, it is extremely difficult to persuade patients that they are not infested, and multiple consultations with successive specialists are common. Treatment with psychotropic agents such as risperidone or pimozide (under careful supervision) is often effective, but this approach is rarely acceptable to the patient.[50]

ECTOPARASITES AS VECTORS OF INFECTION

Although arthropod ectoparasites directly cause a wide variety of local and systemic illnesses, their principal medical importance is as biologic vectors of infection. Through blood feeding (and occasionally other routes) ectoparasites can transmit a range of viral, bacterial and protozoan parasites, including some of the most globally significant infectious diseases of humans: these are listed in Table 11.2. Details of the infections themselves, and of the biologic role of the parasite in their transmission, will be found in the relevant chapters.

PREVENTION OF BITES

Principles of prevention are directed at limiting skin and mucous membrane exposure to crawling and flying arthropods, by avoiding locations serving as their habitat, such as gardens, fields, orchards or unclean picnic areas that attract bees, wasps, and yellowjackets; crawl spaces, wood sheds or outdoor privies, which may harbor venomous spiders or scorpions; domiciles conducive to cockroach, bedbug, or kissing bug habitation; and outdoor environments known to be a source of ticks and biting diptera.

Remaining indoors during evening hours lessens the risks associated with exposure to night-biting mosquitoes. Light-colored clothing, especially long trousers, long-sleeved shirts and closed-toed shoes when working outdoors or pursuing outdoor recreation is less attractive than dark clothing, short pants, short-sleeved shirts and opened-toed shoes to flying insects, and allows the wearer to more readily recognize the presence of ticks and other crawling arthropods. In tick-infested areas, trousers should be tucked into socks to reduce tick access, and can be dusted with pesticides.

A variety of chemical repellents are available.[51] Those containing DEET (*N,N*-diethyl-M-toluamide) are among the most widely used and come in a variety of preparations for use on clothing and skin in concentrations varying from about 10% to 50%. DEET repellents should not be used on babies younger than 2 months. Fifty per cent strength DEET repellents can be used by pregnant or breast-feeding women, and on babies and children older than 2 months. Alternative repellents using synthetic compounds, such as picaridin and natural ingredients such as lemon eucalyptus oil are available for those who prefer not to use DEET products. In all cases, the user should read the manufacturer's instructions and follow them carefully. There is no evidence to support the use of garlic or vitamin B.

The introduction of permethrin-impregnated bed nets has revolutionized the control of malaria in both highly endemic and moderately endemic areas of the world and is a major feature of current control programs.[52,53] This has been shown to reduce maternal and infant mortality[54] and also reduces the prevalence of other nuisance arthropods such as bedbugs.[55] Permethrin also kills sandflies, which are small enough to get through the mesh of bed nets. Knock-down sprays and mosquito coils are also useful to kill mosquitoes in the room, but electronic buzzers are useless.[56]

Practical, detailed advice on bite avoidance measures for travelers is readily available from several travel health websites.[57,58]

REFERENCES

📖 References for this chapter can be found online at http://www.expertconsult.com

Anthony C Chu
Danielle T Greenblatt

Chapter | **12** |

Dermatologic manifestations of systemic infections

INTRODUCTION

The skin is the largest and most visible organ of the body. In addition to its role as a barrier separating the body from the external environment and its role in temperature regulation, the skin has a complex immune system that recognizes and attacks foreign antigens and microbes.

The skin may be affected by systemic infections in three ways:
- by direct involvement by the infectious agent;
- by specific reaction to an infection; and
- by nonspecific reaction to an infection.

In addition, there are a number of inflammatory dermatoses that can mimic skin infections.

DIRECT INVOLVEMENT OF THE SKIN BY AN INFECTIOUS AGENT DURING A SYSTEMIC INFECTION

Viral infections

Chickenpox

Viral infection of the skin as part of a systemic infection is well demonstrated by chickenpox. After an incubation period of 14–21 days the patient develops 1–2 days of fever and malaise. This is followed by crops of unilocular vesicles, which quickly become pustular, appearing over 2–4 days. After the acute infection the virus persists in dorsal root nerve ganglion cells and on reactivation of the residual latent virus, herpes zoster or shingles develops.

Hand, foot and mouth disease

Hand, foot and mouth disease is caused most commonly by coxsackievirus A16 and enterovirus 71.[1] It occurs predominantly in children in both sporadic and epidemic forms. After an incubation period of 5–7 days the patient develops painful stomatitis with oral vesicles that ulcerate. Small, thin-walled vesicles may later develop on the fingers and toes. Onychomadesis is a rare complication due to nail matrix arrest leading to nail shedding from the proximal portion.[2] Disease related to coxsackievirus infection is generally mild and self-limiting; however, cardiopulmonary failure and neurologic sequelae may follow enterovirus 71 infection.[3] Viral particles can be identified in the vesicles on electron microscopy.

Bacterial infections

Gonococcal infection

In disseminated gonococcal infection caused by *Neisseria gonorrhoeae*, characteristic skin lesions (called septic gonococcal dermatitis) may be observed. One or more crops of three or four macules or papules develop often over the extremities; these then become pustular or bullous. Occasionally, gonococci can be cultured from the skin lesions.

Tuberculosis

In tuberculosis, skin involvement may occur as the result of contiguous involvement of the skin from underlying lymph nodes, joints or bones, a condition called scrofuloderma.[4] A bluish-red nodule develops over the affected bone, joint (Fig. 12.1) or lymph node and multiple fistulae develop. Diagnosis must be confirmed by biopsy, which shows tuberculous granulation tissue. *Mycobacterium tuberculosis* can often be cultured from involved tissue.

Cutaneous involvement in tuberculosis may also occur secondary to hematogenous dissemination, so-called tuberculosis cutis miliaris disseminata.[5] In miliary tuberculosis, hematogenous dissemination of bacilli to the skin can produce profuse crops of bluish papules, which may become vesiculopustular and finally necrotic, leading to ulceration.

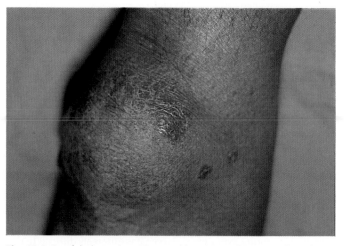

Fig. 12.1 Scrofuloderma in a 60-year-old patient. A biopsy confirmed tuberculoid granulation tissue and the patient responded to antituberculous therapy.

Chronic hematogenous dissemination of tubercle bacilli in patients with moderate or high degrees of immunity may present as one of the tuberculides, which are regarded as localized hypersensitivity reactions to *Mycobacterium tuberculosis*:

- papulonecrotic tuberculid, in which there are symmetric crops of necrotic papules predominantly affecting the extremities;
- lichen scrofulosum, in which minute lichenoid papules appear predominantly on the trunk rather than on the limbs;
- erythema induratum (or Bazin's disease), in which persistent or recurrent nodular lesions appear in the calves of the legs and may lead to ulceration (Fig. 12.2); and
- nodular tuberculid, a more recently described form in which nonulcerating red or bluish nodules present on the lower limbs. This form is considered a hybrid between papulonecrotic tuberculid and erythema induratum with distinctive histologic features.[6]

The tuberculides respond rapidly to antituberculous therapy.

Spirochetal infections

Disease caused by spirochetes tends to affect the skin as part of the primary manifestation, but it may also involve the skin during subsequent, disseminated disease.

Syphilis

In syphilis, the primary lesion or chancre is cutaneous or mucosal, occurring at the site of inoculation. Secondary syphilis starts approximately 3 months after the primary infection and gives rise to non-irritating, coppery red symmetric lesions, which start as macules and become papular. Secondary syphilis is the 'great pretender'[7] and lesions of secondary syphilis can mimic acne, psoriasis and a number of other nonspecific dermatoses. Characteristically, the palms and soles are affected. When mucosal surfaces are involved, 'snail track' ulcers may develop. Later, condylomata may occur perianally and on the vulva or penis. Patchy hair loss is a characteristic sign of secondary syphilis, giving rise to a moth-eaten appearance of the scalp.

Late or tertiary syphilis occurs after a latent period of up to 20 years. Both skin and mucous membranes may be affected. Nodular syphilides present as nodular subcutaneous lesions appearing in groups and tending to develop a circinate arrangement. These are more common on the extensor surfaces of the arms, the back and the face (Fig. 12.3), but they may occur in the oral cavity. Gummas are masses of syphilitic granulomatous tissue; they may originate in the subcutis, underlying bone or muscle. These masses ulcerate to produce punched-out cutaneous defects.

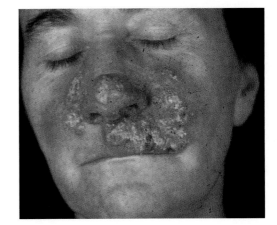

Fig. 12.3 Tertiary syphilis on the face of a 56-year-old woman.

Yaws

Yaws is caused by the spirochete *Treponema pertenue*. The primary lesion of yaws produces a cutaneous erythematous papule, which becomes papillomatous and resembles a raspberry, giving rise to its name, 'frambesia'. After 2–4 months the secondary eruption of yaws occurs, with multiple small papules developing into exudative papillomas (Fig. 12.4). Mucosal involvement does not occur in yaws. After 6 months to 3 years, tertiary yaws occurs; this is characterized by ulcerated nodular and tuberous cutaneous lesions and keratoderma of the palms and soles.

Pinta

Pinta is caused by the spirochete *Treponema carateum*. The initial eruption starts in the skin as multiple erythematous papules and plaques. This is followed after months or years by generalized cutaneous lesions, where the skin becomes pale, pigmented or erythematosquamous. The late phase occurs 2–5 years after primary infection with irregular pigmentation, which can be grayish, steely or bluish in color. Areas of leukoderma, particularly around the elbows, knees, ankles and wrists, may develop. Hyperkeratosis occurs, particularly on the legs and arms, and is associated with areas of atrophy, particularly around the large joints.

Lyme disease

In infections with *Borrelia burgdorferi*, the primary lesion occurs at the site of the Ixodes tick bite, with a characteristic eruption: erythema migrans.[8] The macular erythema starts up to 36 days after the bite and

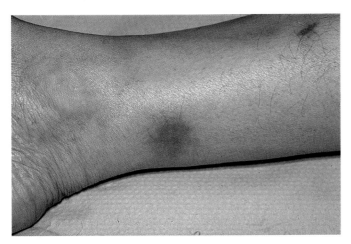

Fig. 12.2 Erythema induratum on the back of the leg of a 45-year-old woman.

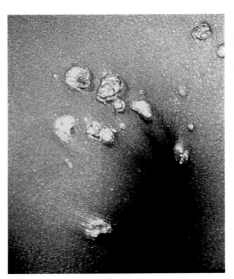

Fig. 12.4 Secondary yaws showing papular and vegetative lesions on the anterior chest wall.

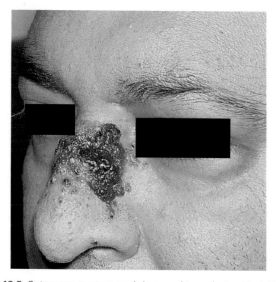

Fig. 12.5 Cutaneous cryptococcosis in a renal transplant patient. These lesions started as nodules that then rapidly ulcerated. CT scan of the patient's brain showed no abnormality but *Cryptococcus neoformans* was isolated from cerebrospinal fluid.

slowly increases in size by several centimeters each week. Subsequent dissemination in untreated patients leads to Lyme disease with involvement of the nervous system, heart and joints.[9]

One year or longer after the original infection, a late cutaneous manifestation may occur: acrodermatitis chronica atrophicans.[10] As the name suggests, this typically affects the hands and feet, but the elbows and knees may also be affected. Erythematous plaques develop, slowly enlarge and become atrophic. *B. burgdorferi* may be cultured from skin biopsies in this condition, though often with difficulty. Diagnosis therefore relies on clinical features supported by serologic testing and detection of *B. burgdorferi*-specific DNA in lesional skin biopsies by polymerase chain reaction.[8]

Fungal infections

A number of deep fungal infections may have cutaneous involvement in the course of systemic disease. These include blastomycosis, coccidioidomycosis, paracoccidioidomycosis, histoplasmosis, cryptococcosis and disseminated candidiasis.

Cutaneous manifestations tend to be nonspecific, with papules, nodules and ulcers developing on different parts of the skin. In disseminated blastomycosis cutaneous lesions start as papules or nodules, which then ulcerate and evolve into serpiginous lesions with raised warty borders. Disseminated coccidioidomycosis may result in cutaneous abscesses, granulomas and discharging sinuses, often on the face.

Disseminated cutaneous cryptococcosis is observed in immunocompromised patients, particularly those with AIDS. It presents as erythematous papules and nodules, which become exudative and eventually ulcerate (Fig. 12.5). Molluscum contagiosum-like lesions are a recognized feature of this disease in AIDS patients. These typically occur around the nose and mouth and punched-out ulcers with rolled edges may develop.

SPECIFIC SKIN REACTIONS RESULTING FROM SYSTEMIC INFECTIONS

Systemic infections with viruses and bacteria can occasionally cause specific cutaneous reactions. These skin reactions can establish the diagnosis of the specific systemic infections and it is thus very important to recognize them.

Viruses

Roseola infantum and pityriasis rosea

Infection with human herpesvirus 6 (HHV-6) and HHV-7, usually in the first 3 years of life, gives rise to a specific dermatitis: roseola infantum (exanthem subitum).[11,12] After an incubation period of 10–15 days, fever starts abruptly and lasts for 3–5 days. Ulcers at the uvulopalatoglossal junction may be an early sign of roseola infantum.[13] As the fever subsides, a maculopapular eruption, which is characteristically rose pink in color, develops on the neck and trunk. This later spreads to the proximal extremities and face. The skin eruption subsides after 1–2 days, leaving no pigmentation or scaling of the skin. In common with other herpesviridae, latency is established. Reactivation in the immunocompromised host is linked to various diseases, including encephalitis.

A similar eruption, known as pityriasis rosea, is observed in adults. There is generally no prodromal syndrome but patients develop a single erythematous macular lesion, which may reach several centimeters in diameter, most commonly on the trunk, thigh or upper arm. The macule has a characteristic collarette of fine scale. This herald patch is followed after 5–15 days by a widespread eruption of small erythematous, scaly macules, which typically form a Christmas-tree pattern on the trunk and eventually spread down the limbs, usually resolving after 6 weeks. A viral etiology is suspected in this condition, although the roles of HHV-7 and to a lesser extent HHV-6 remain controversial.[14]

Cutaneous changes associated with HIV infection are discussed in Chapter 95.

Bacterial infections

Specific bacterial infections may also cause a variety of cutaneous syndromes as a result of toxin production.

Scarlet fever

Scarlet fever complicates acute infections by group A β-hemolytic streptococci that produce pyrogenic exotoxins. Production of the exotoxin depends on the presence of a temperate bacteriophage and is exclusive to group A streptococci. Three antigenically distinct exotoxins can be produced: types A, B and C. After an incubation period of 2–5 days, fever develops with localized signs at the portal of entry (e.g. tonsillitis and lymphadenopathy or tenderness at a wound site).

The eruption of scarlet fever occurs on the second day of infection. It begins on the upper trunk with punctuate erythema that becomes generalized over a few hours to 3–4 days. A characteristic sign, known as Pastia's lines, results from capillary damage and is characterized by transverse red streaks at the sites of skin folds. The face is erythematous but with a characteristic perioral pallor. After 7–10 days the eruption subsides with desquamation of the palms and soles.

Staphylococcal scalded skin syndrome

Staphylococcal scalded skin syndrome is a blistering skin disorder caused by epidermolytic toxins produced by *Staphylococcus aureus*. Two major exfoliative toxin serotypes (ETA and ETB) have been identified.[15] Studies have shown that exfoliative toxins cleave desmoglein 1, resulting in loss of keratinocyte cell to cell adhesion within the epidermis.[16] Histologically, the epidermis is cleaved below the granular cell layer, resulting in the typical scalded skin appearance. The eruption usually starts suddenly with erythema and tenderness of the skin. Flaccid blistering occurs, which often rubs off, leaving raw exudative areas. This syndrome usually carries an excellent prognosis with resolution in 7–14 days following antibiotics.

The disease is one of infants and children. In the few reports of adults who have staphylococcal scaled skin syndrome there is generally an underlying medical problem, such as renal failure or immunosuppression, and it is thought that reduced clearance of the toxin by the kidneys in these patients may be important in the development of the disease.

Toxic shock syndrome

The toxic shock syndrome is recognized as a complication of toxic shock syndrome toxin-1 (TSST-1) production by selected strains of *S. aureus*. Cases have been reported following tampon use, and postcontamination of surgical or traumatic skin wounds and burns. Involvement of the skin, oral mucosa and conjunctiva is common. Dermatologic manifestations include diffuse erythema, punctate lesions and petechiae with subsequent palmoplantar desquamation and occasional nail loss.

Rheumatic fever

Rheumatic fever is caused by an abnormal immunologic reaction to previous infection with group A β-hemolytic streptococci. A specific (although now rare) cutaneous manifestation of rheumatic fever is erythema marginatum rheumaticum.[17] This consists of rings or arcs of pale, dull red erythema, which are either macular or slightly thickened. The rings make up a discrete or enlarged polycyclic pattern. These rings characteristically fade over a few hours or days and appear in recurrent crops, usually at different sites, over many weeks.

Sepsis

Sepsis caused by a variety of bacteria can cause disseminated intravascular coagulation. This results in hemorrhagic skin lesions, particularly of dependent areas, followed by purpura and cutaneous necrosis. In acute meningococcal sepsis, so-called purpura fulminans predicts poor outcome and signifies rapidly progressive infection.[18] Septicemia and purpura fulminans may also uncommonly be caused by infection with *Capnocytophaga canimorsus* following a dog bite. This Gram-negative bacterium is part of the normal oral flora of dogs and septicemia in adults most often occurs in the setting of immunocompromise – usually because of previous splenectomy, alcoholism or glucocorticoid use[19] (Fig. 12.6).

Henoch–Schönlein purpura

Henoch–Schönlein purpura (HSP) is an acute small vessel vasculitis, seen mainly in children and often following an upper respiratory tract infection. Although most cases are not directly linked to streptococcal infection, a substantial minority of patients with HSP have coexistent or previous streptococcal infection, as evidenced by positive throat culture (up to 30%) and raised anti-streptolysin O (up to 50%).[20] Henoch–Schönlein purpura has a characteristic appearance, with palpable purpuric papules developing on the lower legs and buttocks. This may be associated with arthritis, gastrointestinal syndromes and renal disease. Histologically, there is a leukocytoclastic vasculitis and characteristic deposition of IgA within the walls of affected blood vessels.

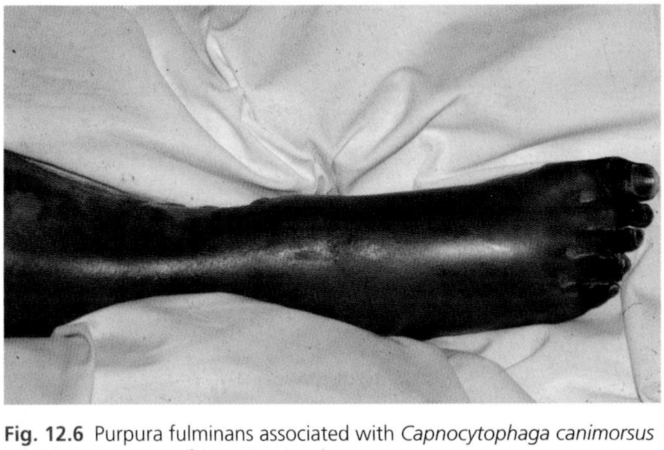

Leprosy

Mycobacterium leprae affects the skin in all forms of leprosy. In tuberculoid leprosy (paucibacillary) the skin lesions tend to be few or solitary. They are often hypopigmented but they may have an indurated coppery color or a purple border. These patches tend to be hypoesthetic and dry with loss of hairs. In lepromatous leprosy (multibacillary) multiple small macules, papules and nodules develop in a symmetric manner in all sites apart from the hairy scalp, the axillae and the groin, where the temperature tends to be higher. Patients often develop leonine facies because of diffuse involvement of the facial skin (Fig. 12.7). Borderline types of leprosy have clinical features between these extremes of immunologic reaction to the causative agent.

Two types of immunologically mediated inflammatory reactions can occur during the course of leprosy. Type 1 leprae (reversal) reactions occur in borderline disease and are associated with upgrading of cell-mediated immunity. Existing skin lesions may become more inflamed, ulcerated and new lesions may appear. This is associated with acute or insidious pain and tenderness of affected nerves. Type 2 leprae reactions occur in patients who have lepromatous leprosy and borderline leprosy. Immune complexes form and a systemic inflammatory reaction ensues. The most common cutaneous manifestation is that of erythema nodosum leprosum, in which painful red nodules occur in the skin, most commonly on the face and extensor surfaces of the limbs.[21] Individual lesions may ultimately ulcerate. Erythema nodosum leprosum may be accompanied by uveitis, myositis, lymphadenitis, neuritis, dactylitis, arthritis and orchitis.

The Lucio phenomenon is another type 2 leprae reaction. Here, a deep cutaneous necrotizing vasculitis leads to infarction of overlying skin. Irregular erythematous patches develop and these may necrose to leave deep painful ulcers.[22]

Ecthyma gangrenosum

Ecthyma gangrenosum is an uncommon cutaneous manifestation of *Pseudomonas aeruginosa* septicemia, usually occurring in immunocompromised or debilitated patients. Erythematous or purple macules initially develop on extremities or the anogenital region. Lesions subsequently become bullous and hemorrhagic, and rupture to leave a

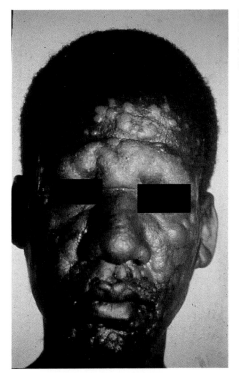

Fig. 12.7 Lepromatous leprosy, with multiple symmetric lesions on the face, causing a leonine facies.

Fig. 12.6 Purpura fulminans associated with *Capnocytophaga canimorsus* infection. Courtesy of Jos WM Van der Meer.

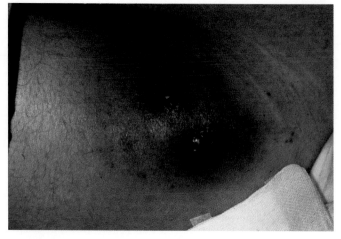

Fig. 12.8 Ecthyma gangrenosum in the setting of *Pseudomonas aeruginosa* septicemia. Courtesy of WM van der Meer.

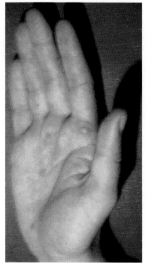

Fig. 12.9 Erythema multiforme showing target lesions and bullous lesions on the palms of the hands.

gangrenous ulcer with central black eschar (Fig. 12.8). The surrounding tissue is painful and inflamed. Histologically, a necrotizing hemorrhagic vasculitis is present and the Gram-negative organism may be seen within the walls of deeper vessels. When the diagnosis is suspected, culture and biopsy of skin lesions is essential, together with blood and urine cultures. Immediate treatment directed towards *P. aeruginosa* is indicated.

NONSPECIFIC CUTANEOUS SIGNS OF SYSTEMIC INFECTIONS

Erythema multiforme

Erythema multiforme (EM) may occur at any age although young adults are most commonly affected. The most common trigger for EM is herpes simplex infection but a variety of other infectious agents, including *Mycoplasma pneumoniae*, have also been implicated (Table 12.1).

The lesions are usually asymptomatic and start as dull red macules and papules that occur on acral sites (particularly the hands) and

then spread more centrally. Typical target lesions occur; these have a central area of damaged skin (dusky-hued, blistering or eroded) and a raised edematous border (Fig. 12.9). Less commonly, the feet, elbows, knees, face, neck and trunk are affected. Oral lesions may be present and severe involvement of the lips may occasionally mimic the crusting seen in Stevens–Johnson syndrome, although these conditions are now considered distinct in adult patients.[23]

Erythema nodosum

Erythema nodosum is a type IV delayed hypersensitivity reaction to a number of different stimuli. The skin and subcutaneous fat are affected with a septal panniculitis. Clinically, there may be a short prodrome of mild fever, myalgia and malaise. Erythematous nodules develop on the shins and more rarely on the arms, face and neck; these may extend up to several centimeters in diameter (Fig. 12.10). The hallmark of erythema nodosum is pain and exquisite tenderness of the lesions. Initially, lesions are bright red but as they subside over the next 3 weeks or so, they undergo a bruise-like change, becoming dusky in color with mild scaling of the skin.

A number of infectious agents have been implicated in the etiology of erythema nodosum (Table 12.2).[24] These vary with the age of the patient and the country of residence. Streptococcal infections (particularly upper respiratory tract) are the commonest infectious cause in both adults and children, and tuberculosis is still a common cause in endemic areas. Infections with *Chlamydia psittaci* have been responsible for small outbreaks of erythema nodosum in adults in the UK, where contact with birds and poultry may be an important clue in

Table 12.1 Infections and vaccines associated with erythema multiforme

Viral	Herpes simplex virus Human immunodeficiency virus Hepatitis B and C viruses Cytomegalovirus Epstein–Barr virus Coxsackie virus Poxviruses – including orf, milker's nodules Varicella-zoster virus Adenovirus Poliomyelitis virus
Bacterial	*Mycoplasma pneumoniae* *Treponema pallidum* *Legionella* spp. *Mycobacterium tuberculosis* *Rickettsia* spp.
Fungal	*Histoplasmosis capsulatum* *Coccidioides immitis* Dermatophytes
Vaccines	Diphtheria–tetanus–pertussis Hepatitis B Smallpox

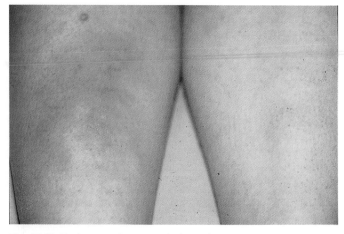

Fig. 12.10 Erythema nodosum on the lower legs.

Table 12.2 Infections associated with erythema nodosum

Bacterial	Streptococci *Mycobacterium tuberculosis* *Yersinia* spp. *Mycoplasma pneumoniae* *Chlamydia* spp. *Campylobacter* spp. Rickettsiae *Salmonella* spp. *Bartonella* spp. Treponema pallidum *Leptospira* spp. *Neisseria gonorrhoeae* *Franciscella tularensis*
Fungal	*Histoplasma capsulatum* *Coccidioides immitis* Blastomycoses
Viral	Herpes simplex virus Epstein–Barr virus Hepatitis B and C viruses Human immunodeficiency virus Parvovirus B19
Parasitic	*Entamoeba histolytica* *Giardia lamblia*

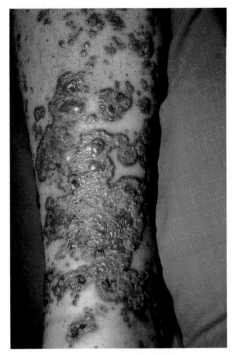

Fig. 12.11 Acute leukocytoclastic vasculitis showing bullous lesions on the lower leg. This patient was found to have a high antistreptolysin titer.

source identification. Infection with *Yersinia* spp. has been reported to cause erythema nodosum in France and Finland but is rare in other countries. Gonorrhea and varicella have been reported as rare causes of erythema nodosum in Singapore.[25]

Erythema nodosum may be related to inflammatory tinea capitis in children, particularly in association with kerion formation.[26] Deep fungal infection, particularly coccidioidomycosis, blastomycosis and histoplasmosis, has been associated with erythema nodosum. More rarely, erythema nodosum has been reported in association with tularemia, salmonellosis, *Campylobacter* spp. infection and leptospirosis.

Cutaneous vasculitis

The clinical features of cutaneous vasculitis depend on the size of the blood vessels affected and on whether the vasculitis is acute or chronic. Acute leukocytoclastic vasculitis is caused primarily by immune complex deposition in cutaneous blood vessels with complement fixation and damage caused by neutrophil infiltration and activation. This vessel wall injury is highly regulated by adhesion molecules and selectins, which are upregulated at sites of vasculitis.[27] The targeted blood vessels tend to be small and superficial, and the clinical signs are of a purpuric macular or papular eruption on the lower legs and dependent areas; these eruptions may become bullous and ulcerate (Fig. 12.11).

Cutaneous vasculitis is associated with underlying infection in approximately 15–20% of cases.[28] A variety of infectious agents including bacteria, viruses, fungi, protozoa and helminths have been associated with vasculitis (Table 12.3). Hepatitis B and C viruses may cause both cutaneous leukocytoclastic vasculitis and specific systemic vasculitis syndromes; hepatitis B virus is associated with polyarteritis nodosa and hepatitis C with cryglobulinemic vasculitis.[29]

Gianotti–Crosti syndrome

Gianotti–Crosti syndrome (GCS) is a self-limited cutaneous dermatosis, characteristically seen in children aged between 6 months and 12 years. It was first described in Europe associated with hepatitis B virus (HBV) infection; however, Epstein–Barr virus now appears to be the

Table 12.3 Infections associated with cutaneous vasculitis

Viral	Hepatitis virus A, B and C Human immunodeficiency virus Herpes simplex virus Varicella-zoster virus Hantavirus Cytomegalovirus Human T-cell lymphotrophic virus (HTLV-1)
Bacterial	Streptococci Staphylococci *Chlamydia* spp. *Mycobacterium* spp. *Treponema pallidum* *Neisseria* spp. *Rickettsia rickettsii* *Brucella* spp. Salmonellae
Fungal	*Candida* spp. *Cryptococcus neoformans*
Protozoal	*Acanthamoeba* *Plasmodia*

commonest cause.[30] This may relate to the increased use of anti-HBV immunizations worldwide. Many other viruses have been linked to GCS including cytomegalovirus, coxsackieviruses A16, B4 and B5, human herpesvirus 6, echovirus, rotavirus, respiratory syncytial virus, hepatitis A or C viruses and parainfluenza virus. There are rare reports of bacteria triggering GCS.

The eruption presents acutely with dull red papules of 5–10 mm diameter. These develop symmetrically over 3–4 days, starting on the buttocks and thighs and spreading to the arms and face. The papules may become vesicular or purpuric and are often mildly itchy. Axillary and inguinal lymphadenopathy is often present and may persist for several months after the eruption has settled, which generally occurs within 2–8 weeks to leave mild scaling but no scarring.

Kawasaki disease

Kawasaki disease (KD) is an acute vasculitis affecting medium-sized vessels, including the coronary arteries. Generally, children between 6 months and 4 years are affected. Although the etiology remains unknown, there is epidemiologic evidence that KD may be triggered by a response to an infectious agent.[31] Proposed but unproven causes of KD include adenovirus, herpesvirus, Epstein–Barr virus, streptococci, staphylococci and *Rickettsia* spp., a newly described human coronavirus [32] and human bocavirus.[33] In most cases no agent is identified. The incidence is highest in Japan although it has been reported worldwide.

The disease is acute in onset with fever lasting more than 5 days. The conjunctivae become injected and the lips and tongue are red. At the onset of fever, a generalized polymorphic eruption develops on the trunk and proximal limbs; this is associated with redness and induration of the palms and soles. Cervical lymphadenopathy develops in about three-quarters of children. As the fever subsides, the skin scales and the patient may develop arthralgia and arthropathy. Coronary artery aneurysms develop in up to 30% of untreated patients and myocardial infarction occurs in approximately 2% of those with coronary lesions.[31]

INFLAMMATORY DERMATOSES MIMICKING INFECTION

Acute febrile neutrophilic dermatosis (Sweet's syndrome)

Acute febrile neutrophilic dermatosis was first described by Sweet in 1964.[34] It is characterized by an explosive cutaneous eruption of raised violaceous plaques in association with constitutional symptoms and fever. Sweet's syndrome (SS) is now classified in three groups: classic (or idiopathic), malignancy associated and drug induced. Malignancy is present in approximately 20% of all patients with SS. Both hematologic malignancy and solid tumors occur but acute myelogenous leukemia is most commonly associated. Drug-induced SS is well described following administration of granulocyte-colony stimulating factor, as well as a number of other agents.[35] Uncommon or rare associations include streptococcal, *Salmonella* and nontuberculous mycobacterial infections, vaccination,[36] inflammatory bowel disease and pregnancy.

Clinical presentation is an acute eruption of dull red elevated inflammatory nodules and plaques, which may pustulate in later stages or clear centrally to give an annular appearance. The majority of patients have a persistent fever and neutrophilia with an elevated erythrocyte sedimentation rate. Diagnosis may be confirmed by cutaneous biopsy, which reveals a florid dermal polymorphonuclear cell infiltrate. Cases respond rapidly to systemic corticosteroid therapy, which is usually required for several weeks.

Toxic epidermal necrolysis

Toxic epidermal necrolysis (TEN) is a serious drug-induced skin disorder, which clinically may be difficult to distinguish from staphylococcal scalded skin syndrome (SSSS). Both conditions are characterized by an acute, widespread cutaneous erythema with sloughing of the epidermis in sheets. As described, SSSS occurs mainly in childhood and is caused by staphylococcal toxin-mediated superficial cleavage of the epidermis below the granular layer. It has an excellent prognosis if appropriately treated. In comparison, TEN is usually a drug-induced phenomenon causing full-thickness necrosis of the epidermis, with subsequent impairment of cutaneous barrier function and a high mortality (30%).[37]

Stevens–Johnson syndrome (SJS) and TEN are now recognized as variants of a single entity, with TEN being of greater severity.[23] The precise pathogenesis is poorly understood, although increased circulating levels of fasL, a ligand for the fas keratinocyte death receptor, have been identified in patients with TEN. Perforin and granzyme, proteins contained within lytic granules of cytotoxic T cells, have also been shown to induce keratinocyte apoptosis in TEN.[37]

The most commonly implicated drugs in TEN are antibiotics, particularly sulfonamides, and anticonvulsants, allopurinol and non-steroidal anti-inflammatory drugs. Nevirapine and lamotrigine have also recently been shown to be strongly associated with TEN.[38] TEN may be distinguished from SSSS by histologic examination of biopsied skin, allowing assessment of the level of epidermal splitting and identification of the presence or absence of micro-organisms. Treatment outcome is improved by intensive nursing in a specialist burns unit and by prompt withdrawal of all potential precipitants. No specific treatment has been unequivocally proven to be effective; however, intravenous immunoglobulins and plasmapheresis have been used.

Oral ulceration

Oral ulceration is a frequent clinical funding, with a wide differential diagnosis including infectious disease.

Primary herpes simplex gingivostomatitis usually occurs in early childhood. Fever is followed by development of painful vesicles on the lips, buccal mucosa, tongue and palate, with tender regional lymphadenopathy. Later in life, recurrences are usually less severe and lesions fewer in number.

Aphthous ulceration is common, painful and often occurs in crops. Minor aphthous ulcers are 2–4 mm in diameter with a gray–white surface and red margin. Commonest on the lips, buccal mucosa or floor of the mouth, they rarely occur on the gingiva, palate or dorsal tongue. Major aphthous ulcers may exceed 1 cm in diameter and occur anywhere in the mouth. They are more painful and protracted and often heal with scarring. Herpetiform aphthous ulceration produces painful vesicles and multiple tiny ulcers less than 2 mm in diameter. These coalesce to produce larger lesions and tend to recur frequently. This syndrome resembles herpetic gingivostomatitis, although there is no evidence of viral etiology.

Behçet's syndrome is characterized by the presence of recurrent oral and genital ulcers, and ocular disease. Other features which may be present include central nervous system disease, arthropathy, skin lesions (e.g. pustules, pathergy, erythema nodosum) and vascular disease.[39] Oral lesions in Behçet's syndrome start as small erythematous papules or pustules, which erode to form ulcers. Pain is variable. Recurrent ulceration may predate the syndrome by months or years.

Pemphigus vulgaris affects the oral mucosa in almost all patients and is the presenting feature in 50–70%. Bullae are fragile and therefore rarely seen. Ruptured bullae form painful large irregular erosions on any part of the oral mucosa. Most patients will also go on to develop flaccid cutaneous bullae which rupture easily.[40]

Eosinophilic cellulitis (Wells' syndrome)

Eosinophilic cellulitis is a rare syndrome which may closely mimic bacterial cellulitis or bullous erysipelas.[41] The etiology is unknown. It is characterized by development of indurated areas of erythema, usually on a distal limb, which may be single or multiple. Systemic illness is unusual, although associated fever has been reported and peripheral eosinophilia is common. Early lesions are often pruritic, infiltrated and may blister but then resolve without scarring within a few weeks. Diagnosis is suggested on skin pathology by the demonstration of marked dermal eosinophilia with areas of granulomatous change surrounding aggregates of eosinophilic material, known as 'flame figures'. The condition responds to oral corticosteroid therapy.

REFERENCES

References for this chapter can be found online at http://www.expertconsult.com

David W Warnock
Tom M Chiller
Katarina G Chiller

Chapter | **13** |

Superficial fungal infections

INTRODUCTION

This chapter reviews the different fungal diseases of the skin, nails and hair. The most common of these diseases are dermatophytosis, candidiasis and pityriasis versicolor. Other, less frequent infections of the skin and hair include tinea nigra and piedra. In addition, there are a number of nondermatophytic molds that can cause nail disease (onychomycosis). Superficial fungal infections, such as dermatophytosis and onychomycosis, have become an important problem in persons infected with HIV, transplant recipients and other immunocompromised host groups. Prompt diagnosis of these infections is important as they may lead to more severe complications; however, this can be difficult because of atypical clinical manifestations. Furthermore, in such patients, skin and nail infections can be difficult to treat because the disease is often more extensive and severe.

EPIDEMIOLOGY

The organisms that cause dermatophytosis are molds belonging to the genera *Trichophyton*, *Microsporum* and *Epidermophyton*.[1,2] Many of the 40 or so species that are recognized at present are worldwide in distribution, but others are confined to particular regions.[3] About 10 species are common human pathogens. The dermatophytes can be split into three ecologic groups depending on whether their usual natural habitat is the soil (geophilic species), animals (zoophilic species) or humans (anthropophilic species). Members of all three groups can cause human infections, but their different natural reservoirs have important implications in relation to the acquisition, site and spread of the disease. Infections originating from the soil are the least common. Infections having animal origins are more frequent and particular species are often associated with particular animal hosts. Anthropophilic dermatophytes account for most human infections; these species are contagious and are readily transmitted from person to person.

Tinea capitis (dermatophytosis of the scalp) is a common infection in children. The predominant etiologic agents differ from continent to continent, but the anthropophilic species *Trichophyton tonsurans* has replaced *Microsporum audouinii* as the dominant cause of this disease among urban populations in North, Central and South America.[4] Infections with this organism have also become much more common in the UK, particularly among black African or black Caribbean school children in London. The cause of this rise in anthropophilic infection rates is difficult to ascertain, but it is possible that it is associated with increased migration. In France, and in particular Paris, the main anthropophilic dermatophytes associated with tinea capitis are those that originate from Africa, particularly *Trichophyton soudanense*. Other less common causes of tinea capitis include the animal species

Microsporum canis and *Trichophyton verrucosum*. Tinea pedis (dermatophytosis of the feet) is a contagious condition and is easily spread from person to person. The predominant agent is the anthropophilic species *Trichophyton rubrum*, but this disease can also be caused by *Trichophyton mentagrophytes* var. *interdigitale*. Transfer within households has been reported, but the main spread occurs in communal baths and showers.[5]

Cutaneous candidiasis is a less common disease than dermatophytosis. *Candida albicans*, the predominant etiologic agent, is a commensal organism found in the mouth and gastrointestinal tract of a significant proportion of the normal population. It is seldom recovered from normal skin, being much less prevalent than *Candida parapsilosis*, but it is a frequent colonizer of moist or damaged skin and nails.

Malassezia spp. are common commensal organisms that colonize the normal skin of the head and trunk during late childhood.[6] In certain circumstances, such as hot humid climatic conditions, these lipophilic organisms produce the disease pityriasis versicolor. In the tropics, up to 50% of the population may be affected. *Malassezia* spp. can be transmitted from person to person, either through direct contact or through contaminated clothing or bedding. In practice, however, infection is endogenous in most cases and spread between individuals is uncommon.

Tinea nigra is a chronic infection of the palms and soles. The disease is rare but has a worldwide distribution, although it is more common in the tropics and subtropics. The etiologic agent, *Phaeoannellomyces werneckii*, is a saprobic mold that is found in the soil and in decomposing vegetation. Human infection is thought to follow traumatic inoculation.

Black piedra is an uncommon hair infection that occurs in humid tropical regions. The natural habitat of the etiologic agent, *Piedraia hortae*, has not been identified. There are some reports of familial infection. White piedra is less common than black piedra. It is found worldwide, but is more prevalent in the tropics and subtropics. The etiologic agents, *Trichosporon* spp., have a widespread natural distribution and are sometimes found on normal skin.

Onychomycosis is a nonspecific term used to describe fungal disease of the nails; tinea unguium is a more specific term used to describe dermatophyte nail infection. At least 80% of fungal nail infections and 90% of toenail infections are due to dermatophytes, in particular *Trichophyton rubrum*.[7] Between 5% and 10% of nail infections are due to *Candida* spp. and the remainder are attributable to nondermatophytic molds. Most prominent among these are *Scopulariopsis brevicaulis*, *Scytalidium dimidiatum* (*Hendersonula toruloidea*), *Aspergillus* spp. and *Fusarium* spp.[7] Unlike the dermatophytes, these molds are not contagious. Onychomycosis is more prevalent in older people and men are more commonly affected than women. Toenails are more frequently involved than fingernails.

PATHOGENESIS AND PATHOLOGY

The dermatophytes are keratinophilic fungi that are normally found growing only in the dead keratinized tissue of the stratum corneum, within and around hair shafts, and in the nail-plate and keratinized nail-bed. The clinical appearances of dermatophyte infections are the result of a combination of direct damage to the tissue by the fungus (mainly in the case of hair and nail infections) and of the immune response of the host. The damage to tissue is due to a combination of mechanical forces and enzymatic activities. Dermatophytes produce a number of keratinolytic proteinases that function best at an acidic pH and these have been recognized as important virulence factors.[1]

The immune response to dermatophytes has been studied in human infections as well as in animal models.[8] The humoral response does not appear to help in the elimination of infection; the highest levels of antibodies are often found in patients with chronic dermatophytosis. Rather, it is the cell-mediated response that is important in ridding the stratum corneum of the infection.[9] Dermatophytes vary in their host interactions. Zoophilic species, such as *Trichophyton verrucosum*, often elicit intense inflammation in humans. This leads to enhanced epidermal proliferation and can result in spontaneous cure.[10] In contrast, anthropophilic species such as *Trichophyton rubrum* often produce chronic or recurrent lesions. Chronic dermatophytosis in otherwise healthy people may be mediated by fungal cell wall components, such as mannan, that diminish the local immune response.[11]

Except for neonatal infections, most cases of superficial candidiasis result from infection of the host from his or her own commensal flora. This shift in the host–fungus relationship results from a number of influences, of which host factors appear to be the most important. Local tissue damage is a critical factor in the pathogenesis of cutaneous candidiasis; most infections occur in moist, occluded sites and follow maceration of the tissue. Chronic mucocutaneous candidiasis is a rare condition that results from inherited defects in the cell-mediated immune response.[12]

Malassezia spp. are present on the normal skin from late childhood. Hot, humid environmental conditions are among the factors that predispose to the development of the cutaneous lesions of pityriasis versicolor.

PREVENTION

Prevention of dermatophytosis must take into account the site of the infection, the etiologic agent and the source of the infection.

Anthropophilic tinea capitis is a common fungal infection in children. It is easily spread from child to child, both in the home and at school. To prevent this, contacts of children infected with *Microsporum audouinii* can be examined for infected fluorescent hairs with Wood's light (a source of ultraviolet light filtered through nickel oxide glass). In the more common nonfluorescent infection with *Trichophyton tonsurans*, detection is more difficult, but the scalp brush sampling method is often helpful in detecting subclinical disease.[13] All those found to be infected must be treated and the importance of good personal hygiene should be stressed. It is seldom practical to exclude infected children from school.

In the case of tinea capitis and tinea corporis caused by zoophilic species, such as *Microsporum canis* and *Trichophyton verrucosum*, it is important to locate the animal source. *Microsporum canis* infection of cats and dogs can often be detected with Wood's light examination. The subsequent course of action will depend upon the value placed on the infected animal. It is more difficult to detect and eliminate *Trichophyton verrucosum* infection in cattle, because infected hairs are not fluorescent and because the fungus can survive for long periods on hairs and scales that have been deposited on the walls of buildings and gates. Fungicidal washes have sometimes been effective in controlling this infection.

Tinea pedis is a contagious condition and is easily spread from person to person. Transfer within households has been reported, but the main spread occurs in communal baths and showers.[5] Educating infected people not to expose others to their infection by not walking barefoot on the floors of communal changing rooms and by avoiding public baths and showers can help to reduce the spread of this disease. Frequent hosing of the floors of public baths and antifungal foot dips near communal baths are helpful preventive measures. Prompt treatment of tinea pedis and the use of separate towels are sensible measures that can help to prevent tinea cruris, tinea manuum and tinea unguium.

Intertriginous candidiasis of the fingernails is often seen in people whose occupation necessitates frequent wetting of the hands. Wearing protective gloves can help to prevent this infection. This condition is also seen in diabetic patients and good glucose control is important in prevention and control.

Good personal hygiene is important in preventing the spread of piedra. Infected people should not share hair brushes or combs with others.

CLINICAL FEATURES

The dermatophytes are the predominant causal organisms of fungal disease of the scalp, toe clefts, soles, palms and nails. In the temperate, developed countries, tinea pedis is the most common form of dermatophytosis. By contrast, in the tropics, tinea capitis and tinea corporis are the most prevalent.

Tinea capitis

The clinical manifestations of tinea capitis are varied and depend on the species of dermatophyte involved and the degree of host response (Table 13.1). The appearance of the lesions can range from mild scaling and hair loss with minimal inflammation to severe inflammation with kerion formation.

In *Microsporum audouinii* infection the lesions consist of well-demarcated patches of partial alopecia. Inflammation is minimal, but fine scaling is characteristic. Most of the hairs in these lesions are broken off near the surface of the scalp. In *Microsporum canis* infection the picture is similar, but there is usually more inflammation. In both these infections the hair surface is coated with small arthrospores (ectothrix infection). The affected hairs show green fluorescence under Wood's light.

In *Trichophyton tonsurans* and *Trichophyton violaceum* infections the lesions are often inconspicuous and inflammation may be minimal. The typical lesions are irregular patches of scaling. The affected hairs often break off at the surface of the scalp, giving a 'black-dot' appearance. The hairs are filled with arthrospores (endothrix infection) and do not fluoresce under Wood's light.

The most florid form of tinea capitis is a kerion. A kerion is a painful inflammatory mass in which the hairs that remain are loose. Thick crusting with matting of adjacent hairs is common. Pus may be discharged from one or more points. A kerion may be limited in extent, but a large confluent lesion may develop (a severe form of kerion) that involves most of the scalp. In most cases this violent reaction results from infection with an animal dermatophyte such as *Trichophyton verrucosum* or *Trichophyton mentagrophytes* var. *mentagrophytes*. However, geophilic or anthropophilic organisms are sometimes involved. In *Trichophyton verrucosum* infections the hairs are covered with chains of large arthrospores but they do not fluoresce under Wood's light.

Favus is now rare, but it is still a distinctive form of fungal scalp infection. The causal organism is *Trichophyton schoenleinii*, an anthropophilic dermatophyte noted for its persistence. Favus presents with hair loss and the formation of cup-shaped crusts known as scutula. These give off a fetid odor and can amalgamate to form dense mats on part or all of the scalp. Longstanding favus can lead to permanent patches of cicatricial alopecia. Infected hairs give off a dull green fluorescence under Wood's light.

Table 13.1 Some characteristics of common dermatophytes causing scalp infection

Organism	Arthrospore size	Arthrospore arrangement	Fluorescence under Wood's light
Microsporum audouinii	Small (2–3 μm)	Ectothrix	Yes
Microsporum canis	Small (2–3 μm)	Ectothrix	Yes
Trichophyton mentagrophytes	Small (3–5 μm)	Ectothrix	No
Trichophyton soudanense	Large (4–8 μm)	Endothrix	No
Trichophyton tonsurans	Large (4–8 μm)	Endothrix	No
Trichophyton verrucosum	Large (5–10 μm)	Ectothrix	No
Trichophyton violaceum	Large (4–8 μm)	Endothrix	No

Tinea capitis must be distinguished from seborrheic dermatitis, psoriasis, bacterial folliculitis and cicatricial alopecia.

Tinea barbae

The animal species *Trichophyton verrucosum* and *Trichophyton mentagrophytes* var. *mentagrophytes* are the principal causes of dermatophyte infection of the beard and mustache areas of the face. *Microsporum canis* is a less common cause. The characteristic appearance is of a highly inflammatory pustular folliculitis (Fig. 13.1). Some infections are less severe and consist of circular, erythematous, scaling lesions.

Tinea faciei

The more common causes of dermatophyte infection of the face are *Trichophyton rubrum* and *Trichophyton mentagrophytes* var. *mentagrophytes*, but many other species may be involved, including *Trichophyton tonsurans* and *Microsporum canis*. The typical annular lesions are erythematous, but scaling is often absent. The lesions are often pruritic and exacerbation after exposure to the sun is common.

Tinea corporis

The clinical manifestations of tinea corporis are varied and often depend on the species of the infective organism. The disease often follows contact with infected animals, but occasional cases result from contact with contaminated soil. *Microsporum canis* is a frequent cause of human infection and *Trichophyton verrucosum* infection is common in rural districts. Infections with anthropophilic species, such as *Trichophyton rubrum*, often follow spread from another site, such as the feet. Infections with *Trichophyton tonsurans* are sometimes seen in children with tinea capitis.

The characteristic lesion is an annular scaling plaque with a raised erythematous border and central clearing. In their most florid form the lesions can become indurated and pustular (Fig. 13.2). This is more common in infections with zoophilic organisms. The differential diagnosis includes discoid eczema, impetigo, psoriasis and discoid

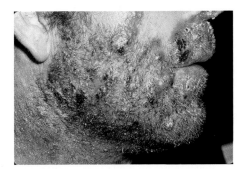

Fig. 13.1 Tinea barbae due to *Trichophyton verrucosum*.

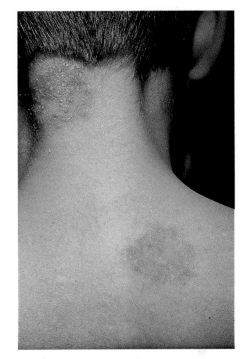

Fig. 13.2 Tinea corporis due to *Trichophyton mentagrophytes* var. *mentagrophytes*.

lupus erythematosus. Of note, formation of perifollicular pustules (Majocchi's granuloma) is indicative of deep-seated follicular involvement and requires systemic therapy.

Tinea cruris

Infection of the groin and the perianal and perineal regions is more common in men. The predominant causes are the anthropophilic species *Trichophyton rubrum* and *Epidermophyton floccosum*. The infection often follows spread from another site in the same person (e.g. feet or nails), but person-to-person spread (e.g. through contaminated clothing) is not uncommon.

In color, the lesions are erythematous to brown. They have raised scaling margins and radiate from the groin down the inner border of the thigh. Patients often complain of intense pruritus. The differential diagnosis includes intertriginous *Candida* infection, bacterial intertrigo, psoriasis and seborrheic dermatitis.

Tinea imbricata

This is a chronic infection that is characterized by the development of homogeneous sheets or concentric rings of scaling that can spread to cover large parts of the affected person. Most reports of tinea imbricata have come from the Pacific Islands and Melanesia but there have been occasional reports from South East Asia and Central and South America. The etiologic agent is the anthropophilic species *Trichophyton concentricum*.

Tinea pedis

Infection of the feet is the most common form of dermatophytosis in the UK and North America. The main organisms involved are the anthropophilic species *Trichophyton rubrum* and, less commonly, *Trichophyton mentagrophytes* var. *interdigitale*.

The most common clinical presentation is interdigital maceration, peeling and fissuring, mostly in the spaces between the fourth and fifth toes. Itching is a common symptom.

Another common presentation associated with *Trichophyton rubrum* is hyperkeratosis of the soles, heels and sides of the feet. The affected sites are pink and covered with fine, white scales. This form of the disease is often chronic and resistant to treatment. If there is extensive involvement of the foot, then the term 'moccasin tinea pedis' is often applied (Fig. 13.3). This presentation is frequently associated with nail infection.

A third form of tinea pedis, associated with *Trichophyton mentagrophytes* var. *interdigitale*, is an acute vesicular infection of the soles. This severe form of the disease may resolve without treatment, but exacerbations tend to occur under hot humid conditions. There is often associated hyperhidrosis.

Tinea pedis can be difficult to distinguish from other infectious causes of toe web infection, such as *Candida* intertrigo and erythrasma. Noninfectious conditions that mimic tinea pedis of the soles include psoriasis and contact dermatitis.

Tinea manuum

Tinea manuum is usually unilateral, the right hand being more commonly affected than the left. Lesions on the dorsum of the hand appear similar to those of tinea corporis, with a distinct border and central clearing. Infection of the palms is more common. This presents as a diffuse scaling hyperkeratosis, with accentuation of the fissuring in the palmar creases. *Trichophyton rubrum* is the most common cause of tinea manuum. The differential diagnosis includes contact dermatitis, eczema and psoriasis.

Tinea unguium

The most common causes of dermatophyte infection of the nails are *Trichophyton rubrum* and *Trichophyton mentagrophytes* var. *interdigitale*, but many other species may be involved. Three clinical forms of tinea unguium are recognized. Distal (or lateral) subungual disease is the most common presentation (Fig. 13.4). This usually begins as a discoloration and thickening of the nail and it can result in destruction of the entire nail-plate and separation of the nail from the nail-bed (Fig. 13.5). In superficial white onychomycosis, crumbling white lesions are evident on the nail surface, particularly the toenails. This condition

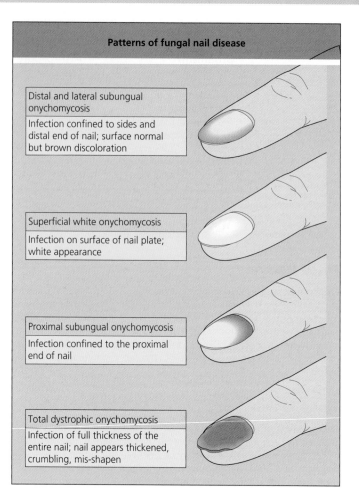

Patterns of fungal nail disease

Distal and lateral subungual onychomycosis
Infection confined to sides and distal end of nail; surface normal but brown discoloration

Superficial white onychomycosis
Infection on surface of nail plate; white appearance

Proximal subungual onychomycosis
Infection confined to the proximal end of nail

Total dystrophic onychomycosis
Infection of full thickness of the entire nail; nail appears thickened, crumbling, mis-shapen

Fig. 13.4 Patterns of fungal nail disease.

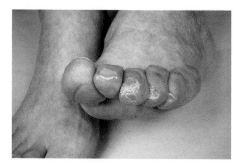

Fig. 13.5 Total dystrophic onychomycosis due to *Trichophyton rubrum*.

is most commonly caused by *Trichophyton mentagrophytes* var. *interdigitale*. Proximal subungual disease is the least common presentation of dermatophyte nail infection. In the USA *Trichophyton rubrum* is the principal cause of proximal subungual onychomycosis.

The differential diagnosis includes eczema, lichen planus and onychogryphosis. Unlike dermatophytosis, *Candida* infections of the nails often begin in the proximal nail-plate and are associated with nail-fold infection.

Candidiasis

The lesions of cutaneous candidiasis (intertrigo) tend to develop in warm, moist sites such as the folds of the skin under the breasts and the groin. The infection is more common in overweight or diabetic people. The initial lesions are papules or vesicopustules that later enlarge and

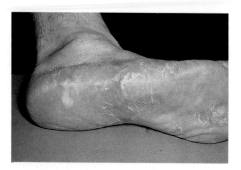

Fig. 13.3 Moccasin tinea pedis due to *Trichophyton rubrum*.

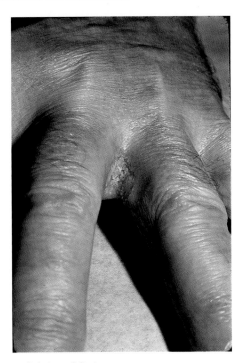

Fig. 13.6 Interdigital candidiasis.

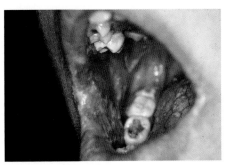

Fig. 13.7 Chronic mucocutaneous candidiasis of the mouth. Courtesy of Jos W M van der Meer, MD, PhD FRCP.

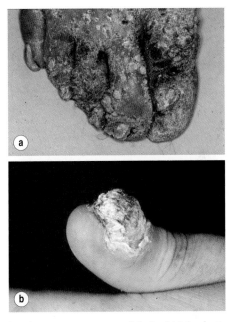

Fig. 13.8 Chronic mucocutaneous candidiasis of (a) the foot and (b) the thumb. Courtesy of Jos W M van der Meer, MD, PhD, FRCP.

become confluent. The larger lesions are erythematous and have an irregular margin. Smaller, satellite lesions are often present. Soreness and itching are usual. The differential diagnosis includes dermatophytosis, seborrheic dermatitis, bacterial intertrigo and psoriasis.

Infection of the skin between the fingers or toes can also occur. Infection of the webs of the fingers presents as a macerated, erythematous lesion (Fig. 13.6). It is often uncomfortable and may be painful. This condition is usually seen in people whose occupations necessitate frequent immersion of the hands in water. Infection of the webs of the toes mimics tinea pedis and many cases do occur in conjunction with this form of dermatophytosis.

Chronic mucocutaneous candidiasis is a rare condition that affects people with underlying endocrinologic or immunologic disorders. The disease often develops during the first 3 years of life. The mouth is usually the first site to be affected (Fig. 13.7), but lesions then appear on the scalp, hands, feet and nails (Fig. 13.8). In some patients, disfiguring hyperkeratotic lesions develop on the scalp and face.

Three forms of *Candida* nail infection are recognized: infection of the nail-folds (paronychia), distal nail infection and total dystrophic onychomycosis. The last is a manifestation of chronic mucocutaneous candidiasis. Infection of the nail-folds is more common in women than in men. The periungual skin is raised and painful and a prominent gap develops between the fold and the nail-plate. White pus may be discharged. The infection usually starts in the proximal nail-fold, but the lateral margins are sometimes the first site to be affected. The nail-plate may be invaded.

Distal *Candida* nail infection presents as onycholysis and subungual hyperkeratosis. It is often difficult to distinguish from dermatophytosis, but candidiasis tends to affect the fingernails rather than the toenails. In patients with chronic mucocutaneous candidiasis, the nail-plate is invaded from the outset, causing gross thickening and hyperkeratosis.

Pityriasis versicolor

Pityriasis versicolor is a disfiguring but otherwise harmless condition. The characteristic lesions consist of patches of fine brown scaling that are found particularly on the upper trunk, neck, upper arms and abdomen. In light-skinned people the affected skin may appear darker than

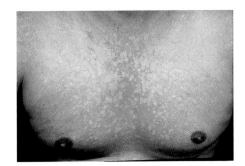

Fig. 13.9 Pityriasis versicolor showing depigmented lesions.

normal. The lesions are light pink in color but grow darker, turning a pale brown shade. In dark-skinned or tanned people, the affected skin becomes depigmented (Fig. 13.9).

Hyperpigmented lesions must be distinguished from erythrasma, seborrheic dermatitis, pityriasis rosea and tinea corporis. Hypopigmented lesions can be confused with pityriasis alba and vitiligo.

Malassezia folliculitis

In addition to pityriasis versicolor, *Malassezia* spp. are also associated with two other cutaneous disorders, folliculitis and seborrhoeic dermatitis. There are two main forms of *Malassezia* folliculitis. The first, which is most common in young adults, consists of small, scattered, itching and erythematous follicular papules that develop on the back, chest or upper arms, and slowly enlarge to become pustular. These often appear after sun exposure or antibiotic or immunosuppressive treatment. These patients do not usually have seborrhoeic dermatitis. This condition is often overlooked and may easily be confused with common acne.

In the second form, which is seen in some patients with seborrhoeic dermatitis, there are numerous small follicular papules scattered over the upper and lower chest and back. The rash is more florid and particularly marked on the back.

Tinea nigra

The lesions of tinea nigra, which are found on the palm or sole, consist of one or more flat, dark brown or black, nonscaling patches with a well-defined edge. Inflammation is absent. The lesions, which are small at first, expand and become confluent. The disease is asymptomatic and may remain undiagnosed for long periods. Tinea nigra must be distinguished from malignant melanoma and chemical stains.

Piedra

Black piedra is most often seen on the scalp hair. Small, brown or black, hard nodules, which are difficult to remove, are formed on the distal hair shafts. The appearance of white piedra is similar, but the nodules are softer and pale in color. This condition affects the hairs of the beard and moustache. Less commonly, it involves the scalp or pubic hair.

Onychomycosis

Up to 5% of cases of onychomycosis are due to nondermatophyte molds. With the exception of *Scytalidium dimidiatum*, these molds usually affect nails that have previously been diseased or damaged. This may account for the fact that these infections often affect only one nail. There is nothing specific about the clinical appearance of the lesions (Fig. 13.10). Distal subungual hyperkeratosis with onycholysis of the distal nail-plate is common (see Fig. 13.4). Superficial white lesions are another presentation.

Superficial fungal infections in immunocompromised patients

In general, fungal infections, such as dermatophytosis and onychomycosis, are no more common in immunocompromised persons than in immunocompetent individuals.[14,15] The clinical manifestations of dermatophytosis in the immunocompromised patient are often similar to those seen in normal individuals. However, the clinical presentation can be atypical, particularly in patients with T-cell defects, such as organ transplant recipients and persons who have AIDS. The major features of dermatophytosis in these groups are loss of obvious lesions, minimal scaling and the presence of follicular papules or pustules. In addition, the lesions can be more extensive than normal.

Tinea pedis has been described in both organ transplant recipients and persons who have AIDS. The lesions are often indistinguishable from those seen in normal individuals but can be extensive, with involvement of the dorsum of the foot. In tinea corporis and tinea cruris, the lesions can be extensive but the inflammation is mild and the margin is indistinct. Facial dermatophytosis has been noted in persons who have AIDS, where it can be confused with seborrheic dermatitis. This is because the rash is diffuse and can spread across both cheeks.

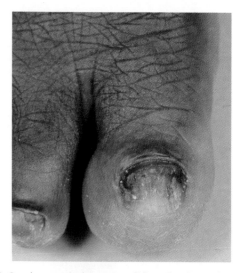

Fig. 13.10 Onychomycosis due to *Scytalidium dimidiatum (Hendersonula toruloidea)*.

Although proximal subungual onychomycosis is the most infrequent form of fungal nail disease in the general population, it is common in persons who have AIDS and has been considered a useful clinical marker of HIV infection.[16] Infection of the toenails is much more frequent than fingernail infection. *Trichophyton rubrum* is the usual etiologic agent. In AIDS patients, it can spread rapidly from the proximal margin and superior surface of the nail to produce gross white discoloration of the plate without obvious thickening.

Malassezia infections of the skin can take a number of different clinical forms in immunocompromised persons, including pityriasis versicolor, *Malassezia* folliculitis and seborrheic dermatitis.[14,15] The clinical manifestations of pityriasis versicolor in immunocompromised persons are similar to those seen in normal individuals. However, the lesions are usually more erythematous and may appear raised. *Malassezia* spp. can also cause folliculitis in immunosuppressed individuals. This is characterized by multiple itching follicular papules and pustules on the trunk and face, and is often associated with severe seborrhoeic dermatitis.

Seborrheic dermatitis is chronic relapsing scaling dermatosis of the face, scalp and trunk. It is the commonest cause of dandruff (scalp scaling). The role of *Malassezia* spp. in the pathogenesis of seborrheic dermatitis is controversial and is based on the fact that most cases respond to azole antifungal treatment. Improvement is associated with disappearance of the organisms and relapse with recolonization. Seborrheic dermatitis is a common and troublesome problem, estimated to occur in up to 80% of persons with HIV infection. The lesions take the form of an erythematous scaling rash on the scalp, face, ears, chest and upper back. Scaling of the eyelid margins and around the nasal folds is a common presentation. The rash is often more extensive than in other individuals.

DIAGNOSIS

Superficial fungal infections often present with characteristic lesions but where this is not the case, mycologic investigation can assist in diagnosis. Material should be collected from cutaneous lesions by scraping outward from the margin. Cleansing the site with 70% alcohol before sampling will increase the likelihood of detecting fungus on direct microscopic examination. Nail specimens should be taken from discolored or dystrophic parts of the nail and should include the full thickness of the nail. If distal subungual lesions are present, debris should be collected from underneath the nail. If there is superficial nail-plate involvement, the scrapings should be taken from the nail surface. Specimens from the scalp should include hair roots and skin scales. Wood's light can sometimes be useful for the selection of sites of active infection, especially if the lesions are inconspicuous or atypical.

Direct microscopic examination of skin and nail material is often sufficient for the diagnosis of a dermatophyte infection, but it gives no indication as to which species is involved. With hair specimens, the size and disposition of the arthrospores can give some indication as to the etiologic agent (see Table 13.1).

Culture is a more reliable method of diagnosis than microscopic examination. It permits the species of dermatophyte to be determined and this can aid the selection of the most appropriate form of treatment. If possible, both microscopic examination and culture should be performed on all specimens. If, however, there is insufficient material for both, microscopic examination should be performed.

Cutaneous candidiasis is often difficult to diagnose if the lesions are other than typical in appearance. Isolation of *Candida albicans* from scrapings is of doubtful significance because the organism is a common colonizer of cutaneous lesions in moist sites. Microscopic demonstration of the organism in scrapings is much more significant. Isolation of *Candida albicans* from nails is seldom significant unless the organism is seen on direct microscopic examination.

Microscopic examination of scrapings from lesions will permit the diagnosis of pityriasis versicolor if there are clusters of round or oval cells together with short broad filaments (which are seldom branched). Because this appearance is pathognomonic for pityriasis versicolor, and because *Malassezia* spp. are part of the normal skin flora, their isolation in culture is not helpful. Direct microscopic examination and culture of scrapings or epilated hairs will permit the diagnosis of tinea nigra and piedra.

It is not unusual to isolate molds other than dermatophytes from abnormal nails cultured on media from which cycloheximide has been omitted. In many cases, these molds are casual, transient contaminants and direct microscopic examination of the material is negative. However, if filaments are seen on microscopic examination but no dermatophyte is isolated, it is possible that the mold is the cause of the infection.

MANAGEMENT

There is now a good selection of topical and systemic agents for the treatment of superficial fungal infections. The choice of treatment and its duration depends on the causative organism, the site of infection and the extent of the disease, as well as on other factors for each individual patient, such as concurrent disease and medication. Topical agents can be used for localized skin infections, but they are seldom successful for sites with a thick keratin layer or when follicular structures are involved. The palms and soles and certainly the nails and hair often require systemic antifungal treatment. Although they respond well to many topical and systemic antifungal agents, persons who have AIDS often suffer from recurrent episodes of superficial fungal infections. If the disease is chronic and extensive, systemic treatment is required.

Tinea capitis

Topical treatment is ineffective on its own in tinea capitis. Terbinafine 250 mg/day and itraconazole 100 mg/day are both effective oral treatments for scalp infection. In adults, either agent should be given for 2–4 weeks. Terbinafine is licensed in some countries for use in children and it appears to be a safe and effective agent in this group.[17] In other countries, the older drug griseofulvin must still be used in children. The recommended dose is 20–25 mg/kg/day for at least 6–8 weeks. A confirmatory culture is often done at 5–6 weeks to determine if longer courses are needed.

Tinea corporis and tinea cruris

The choice of topical or systemic treatment in these conditions depends on the extent of the disease. Localized lesions can be treated with topical antifungal preparations. Numerous imidazoles and allylamines are available in different formulations. These agents should be applied morning and evening for 4–6 weeks. To prevent relapse, treatment should be continued for at least 1 week after the lesions have cleared.

If the disease is widespread or follicular structures are involved (i.e. pustules), or the patient fails to respond to topical preparations, oral treatment is usually indicated. Terbinafine 250 mg/day for 2–4 weeks and itraconazole 100 mg/day for 2 weeks are more effective than griseofulvin 10–20 mg/kg/day for 4–6 weeks. Unlike itraconazole, oral terbinafine has a low potential for drug interactions, making it a useful agent for the treatment of dermatophytosis in persons who have AIDS and other immunocompromised individuals. Terbinafine has been reported to be a safe and effective drug for tinea corporis and cruris in these patient groups.[18,19]

Tinea pedis

Tinea pedis is a chronic infection that seldom clears if left untreated. Infection of the webs of the toes will often respond to topical terbinafine, applied morning and evening for 1–2 weeks. Topical imidazoles can also be used, but they are less effective and must be applied for at least 4 weeks.[20] The recurrence rate following topical treatment is quite high and it is not uncommon for chronic infection to persist despite treatment.

If the disease involves the soles or if there is acute inflammation, oral treatment should be given. Terbinafine 250 mg/day for 2 weeks has been shown to be effective in tinea pedis. Itraconazole 100 mg/day is an alternative, but it must be given for 4 weeks.[21] Chronic tinea pedis is often associated with nail infection. Inadequate treatment of onychomycosis may result in reinfection of the feet. Terbinafine has been reported to be a safe and effective drug for tinea pedis in persons who have AIDS.[18,19]

Tinea manuum

Local treatment with an imidazole or an allylamine will often suffice to clear tinea manuum. In cases that fail to respond to topical preparations, oral treatment is usually indicated. Infections of the palms are difficult to clear with griseofulvin, but oral terbinafine 250 mg/day for 2–6 weeks has been shown to be highly effective.[22] Itraconazole 100 mg/day for 4 weeks is an alternative.

Candidiasis

Most patients with cutaneous candidiasis will respond to topical treatment with terbinafine or an imidazole such as clotrimazole or miconazole, applied for 2–4 weeks. However, relapse is common if any underlying problem is not controlled. If the infection is associated with an underlying skin disease, such as flexural eczema or diaper dermatitis, treatment with a combination preparation containing an azole agent together with hydrocortisone is often helpful.

Long-term treatment with itraconazole or fluconazole has helped many patients with chronic mucocutaneous candidiasis. However, protracted treatment has led to the development of azole-resistant strains of *Candida albicans* in some cases.[23]

Pityriasis versicolor

If left untreated, pityriasis versicolor will persist for long periods. Most patients with this disease respond to topical treatment with terbinafine, azole agents or selenium sulfide shampoo, but more than half relapse within 12 months. Oral treatment with itraconazole 200 mg/

day for 1 week or ketoconazole 400 mg once weekly for 2 weeks is indicated for extensive or recalcitrant lesions. Oral terbinafine and griseofulvin are ineffective.

Malassezia folliculitis

Treatment with a topical imidazole or selenium sulfide is often effective, but oral treatment with ketoconazole 200 mg/day for 1–2 weeks may be required in patients with extensive or recalcitrant lesions. To prevent relapse, maintenance treatment may be given once or twice per week.

Seborrheic dermatitis

This is a difficult condition to treat in persons who have AIDS. Milder forms can often be managed with topical ketoconazole 2% cream with or without a topical corticosteroid. Terbinafine cream may also be effective. Patients with inflamed lesions often benefit from topical application of combined hydrocortisone 1% and antifungal drugs. However, relapse is common once treatment is discontinued.

Tinea nigra

Benzoic acid compound ointment or 10% thiabendazole solution can be applied morning and evening for 3–4 weeks. Topical imidazoles are also effective.

Piedra

Black piedra can be treated with a topical salicylic acid preparation or an imidazole cream. However, relapse is common. Shaving or clipping the affected hairs is often sufficient to clear white piedra. To help prevent recurrence, an imidazole lotion can be applied to the scalp after shampooing.

Onychomycosis

Topical agents should only be used where the infection is confined to the distal ends of the nails. Topical applications of tioconazole, amorolfine or ciclopirox solution should be continued for at least 6 months for fingernails and 12 months or longer for toenails.

Oral terbinafine is the treatment of choice for proven dermatophyte infections of the nail (tinea unguium).[24] However, it is not appropriate for *Candida* infections, nondermatophytic mold infections or mixed infections.[25] Pulsed treatment with terbinafine is at least as effective as continuous treatment while offering potential improvements in patient compliance and cost-effectiveness.[26,27] Pulsed therapy with terbinafine consists of 250 mg twice daily for 1 week each month for 3–4 months. If continuous treatment is given, the dose is 250 mg/day for a period of 6–12 weeks for fingernails and 3–6 months for toenails. Treatment with oral terbinafine will also clear any associated skin infection without the need for additional topical treatment. Terbinafine 250 mg/day for 3 months has been proven to be effective in the treatment of dermatophyte infections of the nail in persons who have AIDS. No drug interactions or significant adverse effects related to the drug have been reported.[28]

Itraconazole is also licensed for the oral treatment of nail infections at a dose of 200 mg/day for 3–6 months. Pulsed treatment with itraconazole has also been advocated because it is as effective as continuous treatment. Itraconazole has a broader spectrum than terbinafine and is more appropriate for patients who present with nondermatophyte or mixed nail infections.[25] However, itraconazole interacts with a number of other drugs and this can limit its usefulness in certain situations. It is not recommended for simultaneous use with protease inhibitors in persons who have AIDS. Fluconazole is not licensed for use in fungal nail disease, but it is sometimes useful in severe *Candida* nail infections.

Oral griseofulvin is only effective in dermatophytosis. It is no longer regarded as a first-line choice for toenail infections, but it works quite well in fingernail infections if given over a 6–9-month period. It must be taken until the affected nail has fully grown out. It should be borne in mind that it has a number of side-effects and can interact with other medications.

Other interventions include chemical dissolution of the nail using 40% urea paste and, in rare instances, surgical removal of the nail. Surgical removal is a painful and disfiguring procedure that should be reserved for cases where there are either contraindications to the use of systemic antifungal agents or a drug-resistant fungus is present.

Oral antifungal treatment of onychomycosis can be followed with topical terbinafine or ciclopirox nail solution in an attempt to prevent recurrence.

REFERENCES

References for this chapter can be found online at http://www.expertconsult.com

Approach to the acutely febrile patient who has a generalized rash

INTRODUCTION

In assessing patients who have fever and rash, the following five points are essential.
- Is the patient well enough to give a further history?
- Is immediate cardiorespiratory support required?
- From the nature of the rash, does the patient require isolation precautions?
- Is immediate empiric antimicrobial therapy required?
- How rapidly did the clinical picture evolve?

The history obtained should give the following information:
- drugs taken within the past month;
- geographic itinerary of travel;
- immunizations;
- occupational exposure;
- sexually transmitted disease exposure and risk factors for HIV;
- the immunologic status of the patient;
- whether the female patient is pregnant;
- any history of valvular heart disease;
- recent exposure to other ill febrile patients;
- stay in a crowded situation (e.g. soldier dormitory);
- exposure to wild or rural habitats and wild animals;
- exposure to domestic animals (bites);
- prior medical history including allergies; and
- sun exposure.

PATHOGENESIS

Virtually any class of microbe can induce a local skin rash with fever if the microbes are allowed to penetrate the stratum corneum. The systemic effects of micro-organisms on the skin, however, can also produce cutaneous eruptions by:
- multiplying in the skin;
- toxin-mediated effects;
- inflammatory responses; and
- altering the vasculature of skin.

MICROBIOLOGY

The range of organisms causing systemic infections with prominent cutaneous manifestations is described in Table PP2.1(see Chapters 8, 9 and 12). There are other noninfectious causes of fever with a generalized rash and these need to be borne in mind.

CLINICAL FEATURES

Physical examination should include the following:
- vital signs including blood pressure;
- general appearance;
- signs of toxicity;
- evidence of adenopathy;
- presence of mucosal, genital or conjunctival lesions;
- presence of hepatosplenomegaly;
- evidence of arthropathy; and
- signs of meningismus or neurologic dysfunction.

The rash should be assessed with regard to:
- its distribution;
- its pattern of progression;
- the timing of its development relative to the onset of illness and fever (Table PP2.2); and
- its characteristics.

The morphology of skin lesions includes macules, papules, plaques, nodules, vesicles, bullae and pustules. Skin lesions are also characterized by their color and particularly by the presence or absence of hemorrhage. Lesions may also be hyperpigmented or hypopigmented. Blanching erythematous lesions are due to vasodilatation, whereas nonblanching erythemas may be due to extravasation of blood. Purpuric lesions are hemorrhages into the skin and they may be small, petechial or large and ecchymotic. Lesions of erythema multiforme usually begin as round or oval macules and papules that vary in size and have central erythema surrounded by a narrow ring of normal skin, which is also surrounded by another thin ring of erythema to form target lesions. Most cases are idiopathic, but the common infective causes are shown in Table PP2.3. The lesions of erythema nodosum are characterized by tender, erythematous nodules that vary in diameter from 1 cm to several centimeters. Infectious agents are a major cause of this lesion (Table PP2.4).

INVESTIGATIONS

Establishing the microbiologic diagnosis is of great importance in managing the patient. Blood cultures should form part of the essential investigations, along with full blood count and differential white cell count, platelet count, liver function tests, renal function tests and acute phase reactants (e.g. C-reactive protein). Rapid changes (e.g. fall of platelets) are ominous. Skin lesion aspirates or biopsy should be considered, particularly for the identification of meningococcal, staphylococcal and gonococcal infections. A punch biopsy of the

Table PP2.1 Microbiology of cutaneous manifestations associated with systemic infections

Macular or papular rash		Vesicobullous eruptions	
Viruses	Adenovirus Measles virus (atypical) Colorado tick fever Coxsackie viruses Cytomegalovirus Dengue virus Echoviruses Epstein–Barr virus Hepatitis B virus HIV-1 Human herpesvirus 6 Lymphocytic choriomeningitis virus Parvovirus B19 (erythema infectiosum) Rubella virus (German measles) Rubeola virus (measles)	Viruses	Coxsackie viruses Echoviruses Herpes simplex virus (disseminated) Vaccinia virus Varicella-zoster virus (varicella and disseminated zoster) Variola virus (smallpox)
Bacteria	*Bartonella bacilliformis* *Bartonella henselae* *Bartonella quintana* *Borrelia burgdorferi* (Lyme disease) *Borrelia* spp. (relapsing fever) *Chlamydia psittaci* *Francisella tularensis* *Leptospira* spp. *Mycobacterium haemophilium* *Mycoplasma pneumoniae* *Pseudomonas aeruginosa* *Rickettsia akari* (rickettsial pox) *Rickettsia prowazekii* (epidemic/louse-borne typhus) *Rickettsia rickettsii* (Rocky Mountain spotted fever) *Rickettsia tsutsugamushi* (scrub typhus) *Rickettsia typhi* (endemic/murine typhus) *Salmonella typhi* *Spirillum minus* (rat-bite fever) *Staphylococcus aureus* *Streptobacillus moniliformis* (rat-bite fever) Streptococci group A (scarlet fever) *Treponema pallidum* (secondary syphilis)	Bacteria	*Listeria monocytogenes* *Mycoplasma pneumoniae* *Rickettsia akari* (rickettsial pox) *Vibrio vulnificus*
		Petechial purpuric eruptions	
		Viruses	Adenovirus Atypical measles Cytomegalovirus (congenital infection) Coxsackie viruses Dengue virus Echoviruses Epstein–Barr virus Rubella virus (German measles) Viruses causing hemorrhagic fevers Yellow fever virus
		Bacteria	*Borrelia* spp. (relapsing fever) *Capnocylophaga canimorsus* *Neisseria gonorrhoeae* *Neisseria meningitidis* *Rickettsia prowazekii* *Rickettsia rickettsii* *Staphylococcus aureus* *Streptobacillus moniliformis*
Fungi (disseminated)	*Blastomyces dermatitidis* *Candida* spp. *Coccidioides immitis* *Cryptococcus neoformans* *Fusarium* spp. *Histoplasma capsulatum*	Protozoa	*Plasmodium falciparum* (malaria)

maculopapular skin lesion of disseminated candidemia is sometimes diagnostic. Occasionally, a Gram stain of a routine buffy coat may reveal the responsible organisms (e.g. staphylococci, meningococci or *Candida* spp.) in a septic patient. Isolation of the causative organisms may be difficult, particularly with viruses and some bacteria. Serologic methods (e.g. serologic test for syphilis, paired viral complement fixation tests), molecular techniques (e.g. polymerase chain reaction for dengue fever virus, cytomegalovirus, HIV and other hemorrhagic fevers) and immunofluorescence microscopy are useful methods for establishing the difficult culturable organisms.

Table PP2.2 Skin lesions and systemic infections

Lesion	Common pathogens	Time of appearance after onset of illness
Toxic erythema	*Staphylococcus aureus* *Streptococcus pyogenes*	At presentation
Rose spots	*Salmonella* spp.	5–10 days
Purpuric lesions (in critically ill patients)	*Neisseria meningitidis* *Rickettsia* spp. *Capnocytophaga canimorsus* Gram-negative bacteria	12–36 hours
Macronuclear lesions	*Candida spp.* *Cryptococcus neoformans* *Histoplasma capsulatum* *Fusarium* spp.	Days
Erythema multiforme, bullous lesions, ecthyma gangrenosum	*Pseudomonas* spp. *Vibrio vulnilicus* Gram-negative bacteria	Days

Table PP2.3 Infective causes of erythema multiforme

- Adenovirus
- *Chlamydia trachomatis*
- *Chlamydia psittaci*
- *Coccidioides imitis*
- Enterovirus
- Epstein–Barr virus
- *Franciscella tularensis*
- Hepatitis B virus
- Herpes simplex virus
- Histoplasma
- HIV
- *Legionella* spp.
- Mumps virus
- *Mycobacterium tuberculosis*
- *Mycoplasma pneumoniae*
- Orf
- Poliomyelitis virus
- *Pseudomonas aeruginosa*
- *Rickettsia* spp.
- *Salmonella typhi*
- *Streptococcus pyogenes*
- *Treponema pallidum*
- Vaccinia virus
- *Yersinia* spp.

Table PP2.4 Infections associated with erythema nodosum

- Blastomycosis
- Campylobacteriosis
- Cat-scratch disease
- Coccidioidomycosis
- Gonorrhea
- Hepatitis C
- Histoplasmosis
- Inflammatory dermatophyte infections
- Leptospirosis
- Lymphogranuloma venereum
- Psittacosis
- Salmonellosis
- Streptococcal infections
- Tuberculosis
- Tularemia
- Upper respiratory tract viruses
- Yersiniosis

FURTHER READING

Further reading for this chapter can be found online at http://www.expertconsult.com

Practice point | 3 |

Sajeev Handa

Management of foot ulcer

INTRODUCTION

Foot ulceration is a relatively common problem in clinical practice and one that sometimes poses difficult diagnostic and therapeutic dilemmas. Major complications are infection and, in more severe cases, the development of dry and wet gangrene. In certain cases making a determination of superinfection versus colonization can try even the most astute clinician.

PATHOGENESIS

The pathogenesis depends on the type and etiology of foot ulcer. The differential diagnosis includes:

- ischemic arterial ulceration;
- venous ulceration due to increased venous hydrostatic pressure causing local edema with its low exchange of oxygen and metabolites; edematous tissue (particularly skin) is more vulnerable to trauma than healthy tissue and is far less able to combat infection;
- neuropathic ulcers caused by diabetes, tabes dorsalis, leprosy, syringomyelia or hereditary sensory (radicular) neuropathy; the protective pain sensation is ablated, resulting in loss of awareness of trauma, which can cause further deterioration of the ulcer;
- vasculitis;
- infection, including acute pyogenic infections, tuberculous infections, tropical ulcer (chronic phagedenic ulcer secondary to Vincent's organisms), syphilis and yaws;
- patient disabilities, such as reduced vision, limited mobility and previous amputation(s); and
- health-care system failures, such as inadequate patient education, monitoring of glycemic control and foot care.

CLINICAL FEATURES

The ischemic arterial ulcer is typically located on the toes, heel, dorsum of the foot or lower third of the leg. The pain is severe and persistent and worsens at night. The ulcer is generally 'punched out' with a pale or necrotic base.

Venous ulcers are located in the 'gaiter' distribution around the ankle, especially around the medial malleoli. They are less painful, more diffuse and shallow and usually have some evidence of granulation tissue at the base.

Diabetic ulcers are usually located in the plantar or lateral aspect of the foot. They resemble arterial ulcers morphologically but are characteristically painless. Diabetic neuropathy (sensory, motor and autonomic),

microvascular and macrovascular lesions, and diminished neutrophil function all conspire to generate diabetic foot ulcers.

Diabetic foot ulcers may be classified under Wagner's grades as follows.

Grade 0	No ulcer in a high-risk foot
Grade 1	Superficial ulcer involving the full skin thickness but not the underlying tissues
Grade 2	Deep ulcer, penetrating down to the ligaments and muscle but not involving the bone and no formation of an abscess
Grade 3	Deep ulcer with cellulitis or abscess formation, often with osteomyelitis
Grade 4	Localized gangrene
Grade 5	Extensive gangrene involving the whole foot

All ulcers may become secondarily infected. Features of infection range from minimal cellulitis with lack of systemic toxicity to extensive cellulitis with associated lymphangitis, purulent drainage, sinus tract formation, osteomyelitis, septic arthritis, abscess formation and sometimes the development of gangrene. Systemic signs and symptoms often occur late and suggest severe infection.

INFECTED ULCER – DIAGNOSIS

A peripheral blood count may demonstrate a leukocytosis (this may be absent in severe cases, especially in diabetes); the erythrocyte sedimentation rate is usually raised. Blood cultures may be positive, especially if the patient is febrile and has not received prior antibiotic treatment.

Obtaining a swab culture of the ulcer itself is an unreliable means of establishing the causative organism(s) in superinfected ulcerations. Ulcers are typically colonized by a multitude of organisms that may or may not be pathogenic. Deep tissue cultures that avoid contact with the ulcer surface or other draining lesions are preferable. In osteomyelitis, bone cultures obtained by percutaneous biopsy or surgical excision are the best specimens for determining the etiology provided the incision site is away from the ulceration itself.

Plain radiographs of the affected area are useful in determining the presence of foreign bodies or air in the soft tissues, which may suggest the presence of gas-forming bacteria. CT scanning and MRI are useful for looking for abscesses as well as early osteomyelitis. The performance of technetium bone scanning for the diagnosis of osteomyelitis in the impaired foot is poor and a 24-hour indium-111 leukocyte scan is more sensitive than a bone scan in diagnosing osteomyelitis associated with a diabetic foot. However, this test is expensive and less specific than MRI and may be difficult to interpret in the presence of local soft tissue inflammation (Chapter 41). High resolution ultrasonography may also be helpful for detecting soft tissue abscesses or sinus tract formation.

MICROBIOLOGY

Mild ulcers may be infected by single organisms. Organisms frequently involved include:

- *Staphylococcus aureus*;
- *Streptococcus pyogenes*; and
- facultative Gram-negative bacilli and anaerobic organisms (which are isolated infrequently).

Severe ulcers, especially the diabetic foot, are usually polymicrobial with aerobic and anaerobic bacterial isolates, including:

- *Staphylococcus aureus*;
- coagulase-negative staphylococci;
- aerobic streptococci and enterococci;
- Enterobacteriaceae (e.g. *Escherichia coli, Klebsiella* spp. and *Proteus* spp.);
- *Pseudomonas* spp.;
- *Corynebacterium* spp.;
- *Bacteroides fragilis* and other Bacteroidaceae; and
- *Clostridium perfringens* and other clostridial spp.

THERAPY

Antibiotics are the mainstay of treatment (Chapter 9) and are recommended in the presence of a surrounding cellulitis, a foul-smelling lesion, fever or deep tissue infection. Empiric antibiotics are necessary until culture results are available (see Table PP3.1). The clinician should assume that *Staphylococcus aureus* is resistant because of the current high prevalence of community-associated methicillin-resistant strains (CA-MRSA). Compared with health-care-associated strains, CA-MRSA strains produce more toxins and appear more virulent. Agents effective against CA-MRSA such as vancomycin, linezolid or daptomycin should therefore be utilized. Step-down treatment with minocycline or trimethoprim–sulfamethoxazole may be feasible based on susceptibility test results and clinical response.

The optimal duration of therapy is unclear; however, for infections that are limited to soft tissue, intravenous therapy may be administered for 7–10 days followed by oral therapy for an additional 14 days. For those in whom osteomyelitis is identified, a minimum of 6–8 weeks' parenteral therapy is recommended if the offending tissue is not removed in its entirety (Chapter 41). Limb-threatening infections require immediate hospitalization, bed rest and a strict nonweight-bearing regimen, even if signs and symptoms of systemic infection are absent. Although medical stabilization, metabolic and glycemic control (in diabetic patients) and antimicrobial therapy are important, debridement should not be delayed. Failure to debride necrotic infected tissue and to drain purulent collections increases the risk of amputation. The initial debridement must be performed independently of the status of the arterial circulation and revascularization should be postponed until sepsis is controlled (Chapter 10).

Surgical consultation for intervention should be considered in infections accompanied by a deep abscess, extensive bone or joint involvement, crepitus, substantial necrosis or necrotizing fasciitis.

Table PP3.1 Selected empiric antimicrobial regimens for infected foot ulcers

Non-limb-threatening infection	
Oral regimens	Trimethoprim–sulfamethoxazole double strength (ds) Minocycline plus penicillin VK Cephalexin, cefprozil, cefuroxime, cefdinir, cefpodoxime or a fluoroquinolone Amoxicillin–clavulanate extended release plus trimethoprim–sulfamethoxazole ds or a fluoroquinolone Alternative: clindamycin plus a fluoroquinolone

Limb-threatening infection	
Parenteral regimens	Vancomycin plus ampicillin–sulbactam, piperacillin–tazobactam or ticarcillin–clavulanate Vancomycin plus ertapenem, imipenum or meropenem Daptomycin, linezolid or tigecycline may be substituted for vancomycin and ciprofloxacin, levofloxacin, moxifloxacin plus metronidazole for the β-lactam/β-lactamase inhibitor combination If methicillin-sensitive *Staphylococcus aureus* is identified then vancomycin may be switched to oxacillin, nafcillin or cefazolin The activity of clindamycin against CA-MRSA is geographically variable and is not recommended for use as a sole agent for severe infections Rifampin (rifampicin) is highly active against CA-MRSA and is commonly used in combination with trimethoprim–sulfamethoxazole or doxycycline but should never be used alone. It is particularly useful in patients with ulceration complicated by abscess formation

It should be noted that definitive management of the ulcer will require treatment of the underlying cause. For example, up to 60% of diabetic patients with nonhealing ulcers have associated arterial insufficiency. Therefore, the arterial circulation must be critically evaluated in all diabetics presenting with a foot ulcer. Once the ulcer has healed, a lifelong program of proper footwear, education and close follow-up for routine callus and nail care must be maintained. In addition, tetanus vaccination status must be ascertained in all patients presenting with ulceration or infection.

FURTHER READING

 Further reading for this chapter can be found online at http://www.expertconsult.com

Managing the patient with recurring skin infections

BACKGROUND

Skin infections come in many forms. Most commonly, troublesome skin infection is synonymous with cellulitis, an entity that perfectly illustrates the cardinal signs of inflammation. Cellulitis is therefore an acute, usually noncontagious inflammation of the connective tissue of the skin, resulting from bacterial infection and characterized by localized warmth, erythema, pain and tenderness, swelling and reluctance to mobilize the affected area (Fig. PP4.1). When such a problem is recurrent, this can become extremely tiresome and even disabling for the afflicted individual.

Cellulitis is usually consequent upon a break developing in the skin surface or its appendages, such as a laceration, cut, fissure, puncture wound, insect bite, animal or human bite, scratch, abrasion, blisters or friction burn, such as might occur with shoes that are too tight. Organisms normally confined to the skin surface are admitted to the dermis where they proliferate and lead to cellulitis.

Erysipelas is a specific form of cellulitis usually caused by group A streptococci. The skin is red and very tender with a raised, well-demarcated area of inflammation often on the lower extremities or face. It is thought to be toxin mediated with intense superficial inflammation and lymphatic involvement. This can result in lymphatic obstruction and make the patient susceptible to recurrent episodes. Direct microbiologic cultures of skin and aspirate are often negative.

RECURRENT CELLULITIS

Recurrent cellulitis implies that factors facilitate the recurrent entry of organisms into the dermis. Effective management of recurrent cellulitis involves identifying these factors and, if possible, remedying them. Recurrent cellulitis may cause local persistent lymphedema, resulting in permanent hypertrophic fibrosis.

With respect to location, most often it is the lower limbs that are involved in recurrent cellulitis. The site may be the arm if, for example, the patient has received radiotherapy to the axillary area as part of breast cancer treatment. Other sites, such as the vulva and perianal region (sometimes in association with *Enterobius vermicularis*) can also be problematic.

To make matters more complex, cellulitis of the lower extremities is more likely to be complicated by thrombophlebitis in elderly patients, which in turn can encourage recurrence of cellulitis.

A number of clinical scenarios and risk activities render patients particularly vulnerable to recurrent episodes of cellulitis. These include:

- tinea pedis or onychomycosis;
- fissures between toes;
- diabetes mellitus – there may be a family history;
- peripheral vascular (arterial) disease – there may be a history of smoking, angina pectoris or hypertension;
- ischemic or venous ulceration of the skin (including sickle cell disease);
- post-deep venous thrombosis;
- eczema and dermatitis;
- immunodeficiency states, for example patients with HIV infection (who may be more prone to recurrent staphylococcal skin sepsis), neutropenia (granulocytopenia), Job's syndrome (hyper IgE syndrome with recurrent staphylococcal cellulitis) or use of immunosuppressive or corticosteroid drugs – always establish the medication history;*

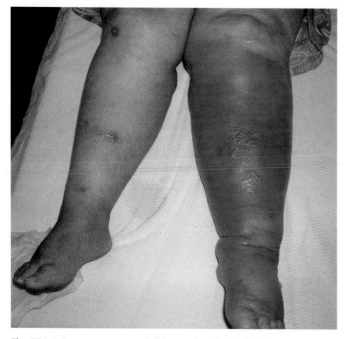

Fig. PP4.1 Severe recurrent cellulitis associated with obesity.

*Unusual organisms such as *Campylobacter jejunii* may cause an erysipelas-like cellulitis in patients with hypogammaglobulinaemia, probably as a result of a lack of serum bactericidal activity. Reference should be made to patients with agammaglobulinemia who develop *Campylobacter jejunii* cellulitis because of a lack of serum bactericidal effect (see Kerstens *et al.* in Further reading). *C. fetus* gives a similar picture in patients with deficient cell-mediated immunity.

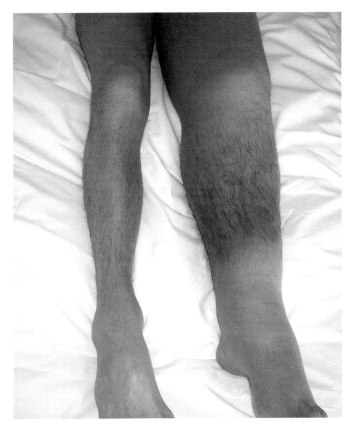

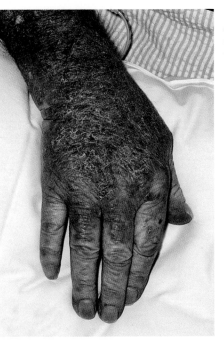

Fig. PP4.3 Mixed *Aspergillus* and *Prototheca* cellulitis in a neutropenic patient.

Fig. PP4.2 Severe recurrent cellulitis in a lymphedematous leg following radical surgery for rhabdomyosarcoma.

- lymphatic obstruction, for example post-radiotherapy (e.g. post-mastectomy), post-block dissection of lymph nodes for cancer (Fig. PP4.2), elephantiasis (e.g. due to infections by *Wuchereria bancroftii, Brugia malayi, Onchocerca volvulus*) or Milroy's disease;
- scar cellulitis (e.g. previous burn or skin graft sites and in areas from which veins were harvested for coronary artery bypass grafting);
- trauma related, for example cosmetic piercings (studs, rings), intravenous drug users, recurrent localized trauma, self-harm or Munchausen's syndrome;
- nasal carriage of staphylococci;
- lepromatous leprosy;
- underlying occult osteomyelitis;
- very poor personal hygiene (e.g. associated with alcoholism); and
- morbid obesity – largely associated with recurrent lower limb cellulitis (see Fig. PP4.1).

MICROBIOLOGY

In immunocompetent individuals, cellulitis is usually the result of Gram-positive aerobic cocci, particularly *Staphylococcus aureus* and *Streptococcus pyogenes*, or sometimes a combination of both. It can be clinically difficult to decide which of them is causing the problem.

A minority of *Staph. aureus* strains may produce the Panton–Valentine leukocidin toxin (PVL), a cytotoxin that causes leukocyte destruction and tissue necrosis. Outbreaks of recurrent cellulitis, boils and abscesses have been reported within families by this strain. Awareness of the high transmissibility and virulence of the PVL-producing strain is crucial in avoiding recurrence, eradicating reservoirs and preventing severe complications such as necrotizing pneumonia.

Non-group A streptococci, particularly groups B, C and G, are sometimes implicated in cellulitis, occurring in patients with lymphatic obstruction or post-vein harvesting for coronary artery bypass grafting.

Recurrent cellulitis due to streptococci may be seen in association with chronic lymphedema (e.g. from lymph node dissection, post-irradiation, Milroy's disease, elephantiasis).

Neutropenic patients may develop cellulitis due to other organisms, such as Gram-negative bacilli (e.g. *Proteus, Serratia, Enterobacter* spp.) and fungi. Rarely, the infection can be mixed with fungal and algal species (e.g. *Aspergillus* and *Prototheca* spp., Fig. PP4.3). *Campylobacter* species may cause both septicemia and cellulitis in hypogammaglobulinemic patients. The organism is often isolated from tissue biopsies and blood cultures.

Other organisms may be involved as part of a mixed picture, depending upon the source of the organisms. Incontinent patients may contaminate their lower limbs with urine and feces while intravenous drug users can inoculate their own tissues (Fig. PP4.4) with a variety of organisms from contaminated needles. Patients whose cellulitis is the result of deliberate self-harm may also yield multiple organisms on culture. This is an extremely difficult diagnosis to make and requires the highest levels of clinical acumen. For example, self-inoculation with milk has been reported as the cause of recurrent cellulitis.

IS IT REALLY CELLULITIS?

Sometimes the apparent recurrent cellulitis problem may not in fact be cellulitis, and the following should be considered:
- acute gout can resemble recurrent cellulitis and certain diuretics may predispose to gout;
- recurrent deep venous thrombosis;
- migratory necrolytic erythema associated with underlying neoplasia, particularly glucagonoma of the pancreas;
- inflammatory carcinoma of the breast, which produces a picture of localized cellulitis unresponsive to antibiotics;
- herpes zoster, which can cause recurrent rash that may be complicated by superinfection;
- erythema nodosum, especially if it recurs;

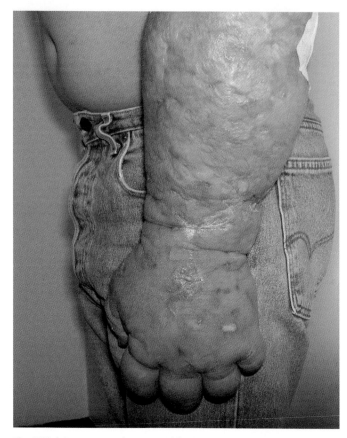

Fig. PP4.4 Intravenous drug user with severe recurrent cellulitis of the left arm.

- palmoplantar pustulosis and pyoderma gangrenosum, such as that associated with inflammatory bowel disease, can be mistaken for cellulitis;
- scurvy and pellagra; and
- fixed drug eruptions.

ASSESSMENT AND DIAGNOSIS

Unless pus has formed or an open wound is present, it is often difficult to isolate the responsible organism from a case of cellulitis. Aspiration of material from the advancing edge of the lesion, skin biopsy and blood cultures yield potential pathogens in only about 25% of cases. The etiology of most cases of cellulitis will usually be *Staph. aureus* and/or *Strep. pyogenes*.

In unusual circumstances, such as patients who are immunocompromised or those not responding to empiric therapy, or indeed whenever the clinical history points toward other infective or noninfective diagnostic options, further investigations may be warranted. This may become particularly important where the patient is suffering recurrent attacks. For example, among those with peripheral vascular disease or diabetes mellitus, minor injuries or cracked skin in the feet or toes can serve as an entry point for recurrent infection.

Attention should accordingly be directed toward establishing the presence or absence of factors that might be supporting the development of recurrent cellulitis and might be amenable to correction. The following range of tests can be applied selectively according to circumstances:

- microbiologic – samples for microscopy, Gram staining, culture and sensitivity, swabs from areas of abscess or bullae formation, needle aspiration of the advancing edge of cellulitis, full skin biopsy, interdigital skin and/or nail scrapings

(especially where tinea pedis is present), blood culture (positive in only a few patients), nasal swabs (especially for *Staph. aureus* carriage, including methicillin-resistant *Staph. aureus*, MRSA), perianal cellophane tape (for *Enterobius* ova), throat swab (for *Strep. pyogenes* in those with erythema nodosum) and bullous fluid (for immunofluorescence antibody test for varicella-zoster);

- imaging – tissue scanning (plain radiographs, ultrasound, CT, MRI and indium leukocyte scanning) may identify collections of pus meriting drainage, foreign bodies or underlying osteomyelitis (if gas is seen in the tissues, the differential diagnosis then includes gangrene and fasciitis, which are generally considered to be surgical emergencies), Doppler scans (which may assist in identifying deep venous thrombosis or peripheral arterial disease);
- hematologic and immunologic – blood films (macrocytosis associated with alcohol excess and microfilaria in suspected filariasis), differential white cell count (to identify neutropenia, eosinophilia, e.g. in filariasis), hemoglobin electrophoresis in sickle-cell disease, immunoglobulin levels and subsets, complement levels, T-cell subsets;
- serology – HIV-1 and HIV-2, antistreptolysin titer (may point toward erythema nodosum as the diagnosis), hepatitis C, hepatitis B (may point toward occult intravenous drug abuse), filariasis, onchocerciasis if the patient is at risk;
- biochemistry – blood glucose, urate levels, liver function tests; and
- skin biopsy – may help with rarer causes of cellulitis.

MANAGEMENT

Managing the acute phase of recurrences

Tissue penetration sufficient to achieve adequate local antibiotic concentrations can be problematic. For acute exacerbations, intravenous therapy may therefore be necessary. Useful combinations include (flucl)oxacillin–benzylpenicillin, (flucl)oxacillin–amoxicillin and clindamycin–ciprofloxacin.

Other antibiotics may be indicated, depending upon the clinical scenario:

- where allergy to β-lactam drugs is an issue – macrolides, levofloxacin or moxifloxacin;
- where MRSA is an issue – doxycycline and rifampin (rifampicin) can be given orally; vancomycin remains the first choice for parental therapy although linezolid, quinupristin–dalfopristin and more recently daptomycin and tigecycline are alternative options;
- where anaerobes are an issue – metronidazole, clindamycin or quinupristin–dalfopristin; and
- where *Campylobacter* spp. are an issue – macrolides, quinolones or carbapenems, with treatment according to sensitivities; regarding *Campylobacter*, macrolides, quinolones and imipenem are dependent on susceptibility with plasma treatment.

Surgical care includes debridement of devitalized tissue. Incision and drainage may be indicated if suppuration occurs. Treat local effects of cellulitis by elevating the affected limb.

Prevent recurrences

Adequate patient education and training are essential.

Skin and foot care for tinea pedis and onychomycosis includes:

- patient training regarding proper skin hygiene and suitable footwear;
- treating affected toe webs or feet with topical antifungals;
- consideration of oral antifungals such as itraconazole or terbinafine for severe chronic tinea pedis or onychomycoses; and
- expert podiatry – cuts and fissures should be washed and kept clean while healing.

For cases caused by edema, treat any underlying cause (e.g. cardiac failure) and relieve edema using support stockings, specialized bandaging and nocturnal elevation of the affected area. Diuretics may have a role.

Immunocompromised patients will remain vulnerable to recurrent infections and therefore may need prolonged antibiotics until their immune status improves.

There is no convincing evidence for the value of antibiotic prophylaxis and there is a risk of antibiotic resistance. Penicillin, erythromycin and clindamycin have all been advocated. Early institution of antibiotics may help in cellulitis of the lower extremities. The patient must be trained to spot the early signs of a recurrence, and given a supply of antibiotics (such as amoxicillin or flucloxacillin) to take. They should be advised to seek medical advice as soon as possible.

Nasal carriage of *Staph. aureus* can be treated with mupirocin if it is thought to be associated with recurrent disease.

CONCLUSION

Recurrent cellulitis is responsible for much morbidity. Diagnosis is not always straightforward and it presents a significant management challenge.

FURTHER READING

Further reading for this chapter can be found online at http://www.expertconsult.com

Chapter | **14** |

Ethan Rubinstein
Itzchak Levi
Bina Rubinovitch

Lymphadenopathy

INTRODUCTION

The body has approximately 600 lymph nodes, but only those in the cervical, submandibular, axillary or inguinal regions may normally be palpable in healthy people. Lymphadenopathy is a change in the size and/or consistency of a lymph node or lymph node group (regional lymphadenopathy), or may be generalized involving multiple sites and multiple lymph node groups. The lymph node system is the major component of the body's surveillance system against foreign invaders and functions as a filter to trap micro-organisms, tumor cells, immune complexes and foreign material.

The lymphoid system grows rapidly during childhood and achieves twice the adult size in early adolescence. Thereafter it starts regressing, reaching adult maturity at about the age of 20–25 years. Lymphadenopathy, particularly peripheral, is thus a common finding in childhood, adolescence and young adulthood.[1] Lymphadenopathy may be divided into acute and chronic lymphadenitis, i.e. inflammatory lymphadenopathy, lymphadenopathy that accompanies lymphoproliferative diseases, infiltrative lymphadenopathy secondary to malignant disease and reactive lymphadenopathy that may be infectious or noninfectious. Table 14.1 summarizes the differential diagnosis of lymphadenopathy.

PATHOGENESIS AND PATHOLOGY

The normal lymph node

Lymph nodes are widely distributed throughout the human body, particularly at potential portals (Fig. 14.1). The normal lymph node is an oval, encapsulated, soft structure, 1–2 cm in diameter with an average weight of approximately 1 g.

Histologically the lymph node can be divided into three regions (Fig. 14.2):[2]
- the cortex, the outmost layer, which is composed mainly of B lymphocytes and macrophages arranged in primary follicles;
- the paracortical region, underneath the cortex, which is composed mainly of T lymphocytes and dendritic cells; and
- the medulla, the innermost region, which has fewer lymphocytes than the other two regions but more plasma cells that secrete immunoglobulins.

Afferent lymphatic vessels empty the lymph drained from the tissues into the subcapsular sinus; from there the lymph flows through the cortex, paracortex and medulla, allowing phagocytic and dendritic cells to trap any foreign material. The efferent lymphatic vessels carry lymph rich in lymphocytes and antibodies into the circulatory system.

The lymph node has two functions:
- it acts as a defensive barrier; and
- it serves as a factory for lymphocyte maturation and differentiation and as an antibody production site during antigenic challenge.

Lymphadenitis

Lymphadenitis is an inflammation of the lymph node. The initial phase of an acute inflammation consists of swelling and hyperplasia of the sinusoidal lining cells and infiltration by leukocytes and edema. This leads to distention of the node's capsule which causes local pain. The process may progress to abscess formation causing the node to become fluctuant depending on the causative micro-organism and the host response. The node may break into the skin and produce a draining sinus. Following the infection the node resumes its normal architecture or, if severely damaged, may obliterate completely. Acutely inflamed lymph nodes are most commonly caused by entrapped microbes.

Chronic lymphadenitis is typically a proliferative process with either follicular hyperplasia or paracortical lymphoid hyperplasia depending on the cause of the inflammation; such nodes are nontender.

EPIDEMIOLOGY

In children the cause of lymphadenopathy is apparent in most cases. In approximately 80% of the cases it is benign, mainly reactive–infectious in origin. In contrast, lymphadenopathy in adults more often reflects serious disease. One study revealed a 0.6% annual incidence of unexplained lymphadenopathy in the general population. Of 2556 patients with unexplained lymphadenopathy, 3.2% required a biopsy but only 1.1% had a malignancy. The probability of a neoplasm affecting enlarged peripheral lymph nodes increases steadily with age; in those older than 50 years who are referred for biopsy because of longstanding enlarged lymph nodes, more than 60% of cases of lymphadenopathy are due to a malignancy.[2,3] In contrast, in primary care settings, patients 40 years of age and older with unexplained lymphadenopathy have about a 4% risk of cancer versus a 0.4% risk in patients younger than age 40.[4] In tropical and subtropical regions leading causes may include parasitic diseases as well as infections.

Lymphadenopathy is defined as generalized whenever three or more anatomically discrete groups of lymph nodes are involved. The different infectious etiologies of generalized lymphadenopathy are shown in Table 14.1. Occasionally lymph nodes that are not palpable may be involved as is the case with lymph node involvement in anthrax or typhoid (abdominal), sarcoidosis and tuberculosis (mediastinal).

Table 14.1 Differential diagnosis of lymphadenopathy			
Etiology	**Regional**	**Generalized**	**Suppurative/caseating**
Infectious lymphadenopathy			
Bacterial (acute)			
Streptococcal	+		+
Scarlet fever	+	+	
Staphylococcal	+		+
Diphtheria	+		
Ludwig's angina	+		
Tuberculosis	+	+	+
Syphilis	+	+	
Chancroid	+		
Plague	+		+
Tularemia	+		+
Rat-bite fever	+*		
Anthrax	+		
Melioidosis		+	
Glanders	+		+
Cat-scratch disease	+	+	
Typhoid fever		+	
Rickettsial			
Boutonneuse fever	+*		
Scrub typhus	+		
Rickettsialpox	+		
Chlamydial			
Lymphogranuloma venereum	+		+
Viral			
Measles		+	
Rubella		+	
Infectious mononucleosis		+	
HIV/AIDS		+	
Cytomegalovirus infection		+	
Dengue		+	
West Nile fever		+	
Lassa fever		+	
Genital herpes	+	+	
Epidemic keratoconjunctivitis (adenovirus)	+		+
Pharyngoconjunctival fever (adenovirus)	+		
Mycotic			
Histoplasmosis		+	+
Coccidioidomycosis	+		

(Continued)

Table 14.1 Differential diagnosis of lymphadenopathy—cont'd

Etiology	Regional	Generalized	Suppurative/caseating
Paracoccidioidomycosis	+		
Cryptococcosis	+	+	
Protozoan			
Kala-azar		+	
Leishmaniasis	+		+
African trypanosomiasis	+	+	
Chagas disease		+	
Toxoplasmosis	+	+	
Helmintic			
Loa loa	+		+ (Bubo)
Onchocerciasis	+		+ (Bubo)
Filariasis		+	
Noninfectious lymphadenopathy			
Sarcoidosis		+	
Connective tissue disorders		+	
Kawasaki disease	+	+	
Rosai–Dorfman disease	+	+	
Kikuchi's disease	+	+	
Castleman's disease	+	+	
Drug hypersensitivity		+	
Silicone breast implant	+		
Infiltrative malignant			
Metastatic carcinoma	+	+	
Metastatic melanoma	+		
Leukemia		+	
Infiltrative nonmalignant			
Lipid storage disease		+	
Amyloid		+	
Primary lymphoproliferative			
Lymphoma		+	
Angioimmunoblastic lymphadenopathy		+	
Lymphomatoid granulomatosis		+	
Malignant histiocytosis		+	
Drug induced			
Allopurinol, atenolol, captopril, carbamazepine, cephalosporins, gold, hydralazine, penicillin, phenytoin, primidone, pyrimethamine, quinidine, sulfonamides, sulindac		+	

*Ulceroglandular.

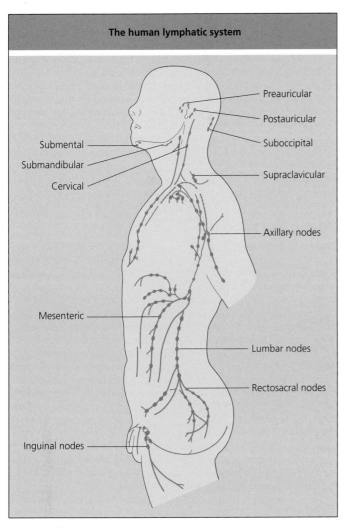

Fig. 14.1 The human lymphatic system.

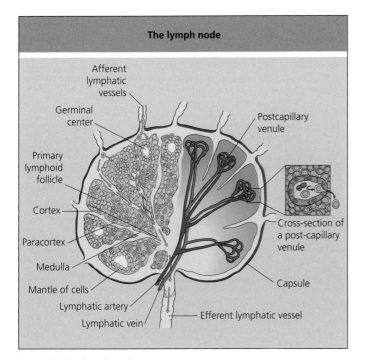

Fig. 14.2 The lymph node.

Viral diseases are the major cause of generalized lymphadenopathy. The bacterial diseases that may cause generalized lymphadenopathy include tuberculosis, typhoid fever, brucellosis and leptospirosis. In the differential diagnosis of generalized lymphadenopathy important parameters are the age of the patient, epidemiologic factors, relevant traveling, contact with sick individuals, accompanying signs and symptoms (rash, splenomegaly), and laboratory findings.

CLINICAL FEATURES

Regional lymphadenopathy and lymphadenitis

Acute suppurative lymphadenitis

Acute suppurative lymphadenitis is commonly caused by pyogenic infections, arising from draining of the organisms causing the initial focus of infection (especially *Staphylococcus aureus* or group A streptococci). The most commonly involved sites are the submandibular, cervical, inguinal and axillary lymph node groups.

The affected lymph node is extremely tender and firm, although it may be fluctuant, and the overlying skin may be red and warm. There are usually systemic manifestations. Acute cervical lymphadenitis due to a pyogenic infection is more common in children than adults. In both children and adults it is commonly due to staphylococcal infections of the face or neck and, uncommonly, it may be a complication of streptococcal pharyngitis.[5] In adults, anaerobic bacteria, of which the predominant species are *Prevotella* spp., *Peptostreptococcus* spp., *Propionibacterium acnes* and *Fusobacterium* spp., are recovered in 30% of cervical lymphadenitis, 13% are anaerobes alone and 17% are mixed anaerobic–aerobic bacteria.[6]

Acute pyogenic cervical lymphadenitis is unilateral. In contrast, acute bilateral cervical lymphadenitis is commonly due to viral upper respiratory infection, infectious mononucleosis, streptococcal pharyngitis or localized periodontal infections. Acute suppurative axillary lymphadenitis is a severe infection with prominent systemic manifestations and axillary pain that radiates to the shoulder and down to the arm. The axilla, arm, shoulder and supraclavicular and pectoral areas are markedly edematous, but there are no signs of skin infection or lymphangitis. The portal of entry of the infecting bacteria (group A streptococci or *S. aureus*) is often a traumatic lesion of the arm.[7] Rapidly enlarging lymph nodes may be accompanied by systemic manifestations, including toxic shock syndrome, without obvious genital or skin lesions.[8,9]

Patients who have chronic granulomatous disease experience recurrent pyogenic infections, of which the most common manifestations are lower respiratory tract infections, suppurative lymphadenitis, subcutaneous abscesses and hepatic abscesses.[10] The infecting pathogens are catalase-positive organisms such as *S. aureus*, *Serratia marcescens*, *Burkholderia* (*Pseudomonas*) *cepacia* and *Aspergillus* spp. The histologic appearance of the lymph node is one of inflammation with granuloma formation and necrosis.[10,11]

Cat-scratch disease

Cat-scratch disease typically manifests after a cat scratch or bite as regional lymphadenopathy distal to the involved lymph node. The mode of transmission is presumably direct contact with the causative agent, primarily *Bartonella henselae*. The disease occurs worldwide, with healthy children and adolescents being most frequently affected.[12] A history of a trivial cat scratch or a bite by a kitten can be elicited in most cases.[13] Rarely, a dog or monkey is implicated. Occasionally, typical cat-scratch disease cases can be caused by other pathogenic *Bartonella* sp. (i.e. *Bartonella clarridgeiae*).[14]

Tender lymphadenopathy develops within 1–3 weeks after inoculation. Commonly, an erythematous papule at the site of inoculation precedes the development of lymphadenopathy and may last for

Table 14.2 Oculoglandular syndromes		
Disease	**Infecting organism**	**Features**
Cat-scratch disease	*Bartonella henselae*	Parinaud's sign in 3%, conjunctivitis in 6%
Tularemia	*Francisella tularensis*	Parinaud's sign in 5%
Lymphogranuloma venereum	*Chlamydia trachomatis*	Parinaud's sign in <1%
Pharyngoconjunctival fever	Adenovirus 3, 7	Common in children
Epidemic keratoconjunctivitis	Adenovirus 8, 19, 37	Occasionally seen in adults
Chagas disease	*Trypanosoma cruzi*	Romaña's sign

several weeks. Regional lymph node enlargement is the sole manifestation in one-half of the patients. Most commonly the cervical, axillary or epitrochlear lymph nodes are involved, but any peripheral nodes at multiple sites may be enlarged. In one-third of the patients, low-grade fever is present, and about 15% have systemic manifestations such as malaise, headache, splenomegaly and sore throat. Unusual clinical manifestations occur in 10% of patients; the most frequent of these is the oculoglandular syndrome of Parinaud,[13,15] which is conjunctivitis with ipsilateral preauricular lymphadenitis (Table 14.2). The adenopathy subsides spontaneously within several months. Occasionally, aspiration of a suppurative lymph node is needed to relieve pain.

The diagnosis is based on epidemiologic exposure and can be confirmed by detection of serum antibody to *B. henselae*.[13] Occasional cat-scratch disease cases caused by other pathogenic *Bartonella* may, however, be serologically negative.[14]

In atypical presentations or whenever a neoplastic or mycobacterial process is suspected, a lymph node biopsy or aspirate may be needed.

Mycobacterial lymphadenitis

This is the most common form of extrapulmonary tuberculosis in the Western world.[16] Tuberculous cervical lymphadenitis is caused by spread of *Mycobacterium tuberculosis* from a lung infection. Scrofula often presents as a one-sided red, painless mass, located along the upper border of the sternocleidomastoid muscle or in the supraclavicular area or axilla. In areas in which both tuberculosis and HIV are prevalent, tuberculous lymphadenitis may be the presenting sign in 50% of young children and is often associated with intrathoracic disease[17] (Fig. 14.3). Currently most tuberculous lymphadenitis is caused by *M. tuberculosis* and atypical mycobacteria, particularly *M. scrofulosum* and *M. avium* complex (MAC).[18] The process is indolent and slowly progressive and is not accompanied by systemic symptoms.

If systemic signs appear, or the process is outside the cervical lesion, miliary tuberculosis should be suspected. With *M. bovis* infection the primary focus is usually the tonsil or the pharynx.

The diagnosis of mycobacterial lymphadenitis is confirmed microbiologically and with histology of the afflicted lymph node. Fine needle aspiration frequently reveals the presence of granuloma but only rarely yields smears that are positive or material that is culture positive.[18] Microbiologic and histologic examinations are complementary as *M. tuberculosis* has been isolated from lymph nodes not showing granuloma, and granulomata have occasionally grown atypical mycobacteria. Acid-fast bacilli are only rarely seen in smears except in HIV co-infected patients. New diagnostic techniques such as DNA hybridization, PCR and blotting techniques hold promise for more accurate and rapid diagnosis[19] (see Chapter 174).

Plague and tularemia

Both these infections are zoonoses that produce rather similar manifestations, mostly fever and regional lymphadenitis.[20] Plague and tularemia may be used as bioterrorism agents as they are highly infectious when dispersed by the airborne route.[21,22]

Plague is caused by *Yersinia pestis* (see Chapter 120). Most human cases are in the bubonic form transmitted by the bite of infected fleas. After an incubation period of 2–8 days patients develop sudden fever, chills, malaise and headache. Usually by the same time or within a few hours, a painfully swollen regional lymph node appears in the draining region of the inoculation site, commonly in the axilla, neck or groin. The primary lesion is occasionally found at the bite site and may develop into an area of cellulitis or an abscess. Over the next few days, the discrete lymph nodes become matted together to form the characteristic bubo with extensive surrounding edema (Fig. 14.4). The matted lymph nodes are exquisitely tender. Isolation of *Y. pestis* from an aspirated bubo, blood, bone marrow and multiple organs is possible but bacterial growth is slow; rapid identification can be accomplished by a characteristic Gram or Wayson stain. Such patients should be immediately isolated, reported and treated.[22]

Tularemia (see Chapter 121) occurs only in the northern hemisphere. Over 80% of infections are acquired by handling infected animals or by tick or deer fly bites. In the Western world most cases are sporadic, whereas in other parts of the world large water-borne, arthropod-borne and airborne outbreaks have been reported. Infection commonly manifests as an ulceroglandular or oculoglandular syndrome.[21] The most common portals of entry are the skin and the conjunctiva, with an ulcer or a pustule, or in the case of the conjunctiva or eyelid, conjunctivitis, a papule or an ulcer, developing 1–10 days after exposure. Regional lymphadenopathy follows and the enlarged lymph nodes may suppurate. Systemic manifestations are common

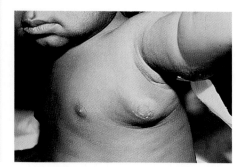

Fig. 14.3 Tuberculous lymphadenitis of the axilla.

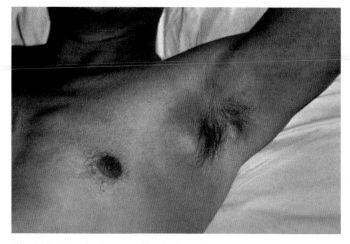

Fig. 14.4 Bubonic plague, axillary bubo and accompanying edema.

Table 14.3 Differential diagnosis of infectious inguinal lymphadenopathy

Sexually transmitted diseases	Other diseases
Syphilis	Pyogenic infections
Lymphogranuloma venereum	Cellulitis
Chancroid	Plague
Genital herpes	Filariasis
Granuloma inguinale	Onchocerciasis

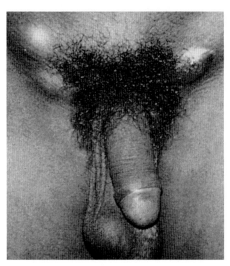

Fig. 14.5 Groove sign of lymphogranuloma venereum. There is cleavage of extensive lymphadenopathy by the inguinal ligament.

but systemic toxicity and prostration is absent. Presumptive diagnosis is made on epidemiologic grounds and confirmed by specific serologic tests.[23]

Inguinal lymphadenopathy

Sexually transmitted diseases (STDs) and metastatic genital neoplastic disease are the most common causes of inguinal lymphadenopathy. The differential diagnosis of infectious inguinal lymphadenopathy is shown in Table 14.3.

Chancroid

Chancroid is caused by *Haemophilus ducreyi* and in some parts of the world (e.g. Thailand) it is one of the most common causes of genital ulcer with inguinal lymphadenopathy (see Chapter 60). The chancroid ulcer is a painful, nonindurated lesion that appears 1 day to several weeks after inoculation. Inguinal lymphadenitis occurs in between one-third and one-half of untreated cases. The lymph nodes are enlarged, painful and tender. The process is most commonly unilateral and, without treatment, can progress to suppuration with periadenitis and involvement of the overlying skin (bubo).

Culture provides the definitive diagnosis; however, *H. ducreyi* is a fastidious organism and immediate direct inoculation into specific culture media is required for bacterial growth and isolation. Chemotherapy is sufficient in most uncomplicated cases but abscesses that are more than 5 cm in diameter may need surgical drainage[24] (see also Chapter 60).

Lymphogranuloma venereum

Lymphogranuloma venereum is a rare STD caused by *C. trachomatis* serovars L1, L2 and L3. The typical vesicular lesions appear 1–2 weeks after inoculation but the incubation period varies between 5 and 20 days. The lesions often go unnoticed by the patient. Inguinal lymphadenopathy appears 1–6 weeks after the vesicles disappear. The lymphadenopathy is most commonly unilateral but is bilateral in 30–40% of patients. The nodes are painful and the groove sign (cleavage of the enlarged nodes by the inguinal ligament) is seen in 25% of patients (Fig. 14.5). The involved lymph nodes frequently coalesce to form a bubo. If untreated, the nodes, which are filled with bacteria, rupture and a nonhealing fistula is formed.

The anorectal syndrome, which occurs mainly in women and homosexual men, results from involvement of the pelvic lymph nodes. In the male, abscess formation may occur in the dorsal lymphatic of the penis and cause tissue destruction and elephantiasis of the penis. *Chlamydia trachomatis* can be isolated from both blood and aspirates of lymph nodes in approximately 30% of cases. Incision of the bubo is not warranted for diagnosis and positive serologic tests (complement fixation antibody test or microimmunofluorescence test) in the appropriate clinical setting are highly sensitive and specific for the diagnosis[25] (see Chapter 60).

Syphilis

The lymphadenopathy of primary syphilis is easily differentiated from chancroid and lymphogranuloma venereum because nodes involved in syphilis are firm, only moderately enlarged, nonsuppurative and painless. The classic primary chancre appears 14–30 days after inoculation and is a nonexudative, painless ulcer. In the immunocompetent patient only one chancre appears but in the immunocompromised patient, especially in patients who have AIDS, multiple chancres may be seen. In women and homosexual men, the chancre may be located in the perianal region or in the anal canal. Regional painless lymphadenopathy is characteristic at this stage of disease. The chancre usually heals and disappears after 3–6 weeks, but the lymphadenopathy may persist for longer. The symptoms of secondary syphilis appear 2–8 weeks after the chancre has healed, with generalized lymphadenopathy and various skin lesions in the majority of patients. Epitrochlear lymphadenopathy suggests the diagnosis.[26]

Genital herpes

The typical vesicles associated with inguinal lymphadenopathy usually suggest the correct diagnosis. Rarely, lymph node enlargement may appear before the rash develops.[27]

The lymphadenopathy associated with primary herpes is either unilateral or bilateral; in severe cases generalized lymphadenopathy may also occur. Genital lesions and lymphadenopathy are common in genital herpes in the immunocompetent host; however, massive lymphadenitis is frequently seen in the immunocompromised patient. The diagnosis is based on isolation of herpes simplex virus from a skin lesion, preferably from a vesicle[28] (see also Chapter 58).

Granuloma inguinale

Granuloma inguinale (donovanosis) is caused by *Calymmatobacterium granulomatis*. The disease is rare in the Western world but is a major cause of genital ulcer in south-east India, Brazil and some parts of Africa. The penile papules of granuloma inguinale appear within days of inoculation and rapidly ulcerate to form a red, granulomatous, painless ulcer with a characteristic surface that bleeds easily on contact. Subcutaneous spread into the inguinal region results in swellings (pseudobuboes) that are not a true adenitis. Lymphedema and elephantiasis occasionally result from scarring and blockage of the lymphatics. Granuloma inguinale should be differentiated from other genital ulcerative lesions with inguinal lymphadenopathy. The diagnosis is established through the demonstration of the typical intracellular Donovan bodies in stained smears obtained from the lesions[29] (see Chapter 60).

Parasitic lymphadenopathy

Toxoplasmosis

Lymphadenopathy is an important clinical sign of acquired primary toxoplasmosis in the immunocompetent and occurs in up to 84% (mean 64%) of cases in different studies. Lymphadenopathy is typically found in the neck, most commonly in the posterior and anterior cervical regions, followed by the suboccipital region, the axillae and then the groins. It is usually found at single sites in adults (in 90%), but multiple sites are more common in children. Retroperitoneal or mesenteric lymphadenopathy may occur occasionally and cause abdominal pains. Toxoplasmic lymphadenopathy has been described in unusual sites such as the lung hilus, the mammary gland, parotid gland and chest wall.[30] Lymphadenopathy may be the only symptom of toxoplasmosis but generally there are additional symptoms – often fever and rarely splenomegaly and/or hepatomegaly. In approximately 15% *Toxoplasma* lymphadenopathy is associated with fever, headache, myalgia and sore throat that may mimic infectious mononucleosis.

On palpation, the lymph nodes are usually discrete, of varying firmness, and may or may not be tender; they rarely suppurate or ulcerate. A chronic lymphadenopathy fluctuating in size over several months has also been described.[30] The histologic appearance should be differentiated from lymphoma, cat-scratch disease and Kikuchi's lymphadenitis.

Enlarged glands will usually resolve within 1–2 months in 60% of patients. However, 25% of patients take 2–4 months to return to normal, 8% take 4–6 months and in 6% the enlarged lymph nodes do not return to normal until much later.

The diagnosis of toxoplasmosis cannot be made solely on clinical grounds. Histologic features in lymph node biopsies are suggestive of toxoplasmosis but are not diagnostic.[30]

Antibodies to *Toxoplasma gondii* are usually detectable within 2 weeks of infection and reach a peak within 2 months. *Toxoplasma* lymphadenopathy in immunocompetent patients normally resolves without treatment.

Acute infection by *Toxoplasma gondii* is common worldwide. The prevalence of seropositivity by the fourth decade of life in North America is 30–50% and higher than 90% in certain European countries.[31]

Toxoplasmosis has been estimated to cause between 3% and 7% of clinically significant lymphadenopathy. Of major importance is the diagnosis in pregnant women, because of the consequences to the fetus and in infected HIV patients, because of the accompanying central nervous system (CNS) disease. In other immunocompromised patients (e.g. transplant recipients) disseminated toxoplasmosis may occur. In addition, differential diagnosis of *Toxoplasma* from lymphoma may, on occasion, save unnecessary invasive diagnostic workup.

Leishmaniasis (see Chapter 117)

Enlarged lymph nodes occur in the majority (77%) of people with confirmed cutaneous leishmaniasis in South America and in patients who have *Leishmania major* acquired in equatorial Africa.[32,33] Lymphadenopathy may precede the cutaneous lesion by some 2 weeks in two-thirds of the cases. Cultures of the lymph nodes obtained by aspiration or biopsy are more frequently positive (86%) than cultures obtained from the skin lesions. In Brazil a lymphadenopathy (whether localized or generalized) may often be the first, and sometimes the only, symptom of cutaneous leishmaniasis.[34,35] Lymph node histology may show necrotizing or suppurative granulomas, sometimes with discharging sinuses. Patients who have leishmanial lymphadenopathy often have fever, hepatomegaly, splenomegaly, intense skin reaction and lymphocyte proliferation when exposed to suitable antigenic stimulation, but fewer previous infections. In an endemic area, therefore, an unexplained lymphadenopathy should prompt an investigation for leishmaniasis.

African trypanosomiasis (see Chapter 105)

Human African trypanosomiasis, or sleeping sickness, is an illness endemic to sub-Saharan Africa, caused by the flagellate protozoan, *Trypanosoma brucei*, which exists in two morphologically identical subspecies: *Trypanosoma brucei rhodesiense* (East African or Rhodesian African trypanosomiasis) and *Trypanosoma brucei gambiense* (West African or Gambian African trypanosomiasis). Both of these parasites are transmitted to human hosts by bites of infected tsetse flies (*Glossina* species), which are found only in Africa. Humans are infected following a fly bite, which occasionally causes a skin chancre at the site. These injected trypomastigotes further mature and divide in the blood and lymphatic system, causing symptoms of malaise, intermittent fever, rash and wasting. Eventually, the parasitic invasion reaches the CNS, causing behavioral and neurologic changes, such as encephalitis and coma.

In the first stage of the disease the major findings are painless skin chancre that appears about 5–15 days after the bite, intermittent fever (refractory to antimalarials), general malaise, myalgia, and headache usually 3 weeks after the tsetse fly bite, accompanied by generalized lymphadenopathy, pruritus, urticaria and facial edema (minority of patients). Axillary and inguinal lymphadenopathy is noted more often in patients with the East African form; cervical lymphadenopathy is more commonly observed in patients with the West African form. The classic Winterbottom sign is clearly visible (i.e. enlarged, nontender, mobile posterior cervical lymph node) (Fig. 14.6). Fevers, tachycardia, irregular rash, edema and weight loss ensue. Lymphadenopathy has to be differentiated from tuberculosis lymphadenitis, HIV and cancer, all of which are common in this part of the world. A definitive diagnosis of infection requires detection of trypanosomes in blood, lymph nodes, cerebrospinal fluid, skin chancre aspirates or bone marrow.

The standard serologic assay to diagnose West African trypanosomiasis is the card agglutination test for trypanosomiasis (CATT), results of which are available in only 10 minutes. It is highly sensitive (96%) but less specific because of cross-reactivity with animal trypanosomes. Commercial antibody tests for East African trypanosomiasis are not available. For early- and late-stage disease, treatment usually results in resolution of symptoms and rapid clearance of parasitemia on repeat blood smears. Most patients experience full recovery following treatment.[36,37]

American trypanosomiasis (Chagas disease)[38] (see Chapter 118)

Lymphadenopathy appears in around two out of three patients with the acute disease; additional signs and symptoms also occur. An enlarged

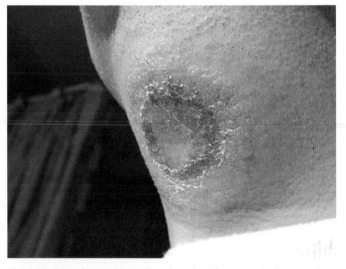

Fig. 14.6 Winterbottom's sign: lymph node enlargement in the posterior neck, a sign of African trypanosomiasis.

liver and spleen are mainly observed in children, whereas generalized lymphadenopathy is observed in 60% of all patients. Subcutaneous edema, either generalized or localized to the face and/or lower extremities, is observed in 30–50% of cases.

Filariasis[39] (see Chapter 115)

The most common symptoms of filarial lymphatic disease include fever, inguinal or axillary lymphadenopathy, distinctive lymphangitis spreading retrogradely from the lymph node where the filaria reside to the periphery, testicular and/or inguinal pain, skin exfoliation, and limb or genital swelling. Such attacks last for 3–7 days and recur between 6 and 12 times per year. Attacks subside spontaneously without specific therapy. Affected lymph nodes are enlarged and painful, and the surrounding lymph vessels also appear inflamed and indurated. With the continuation of lymphangitis and lymphadenitis, pitting edema of the skin appears; this is transformed into brawny edema of the involved area causing thickening of the subcutaneous tissue and hyperkeratosis. Coarsening of the skin ensues with deep fissuring and nodular and papillomatous hyperplastic skin changes. Occasionally local lymphedema appears causing penile, testicular, labial or limb enlargement. In some patients passage of cloudy milk-like urine may denote chyluria. Occasionally local thrombophlebitis may complicate the clinical picture. With an infection by *Brugia malayi* an abscess of the local lymphatic apparatus may develop leaving characteristic scars.

Onchocerciasis[40]

This infection is also known as hanging groins, leopard skin, river blindness or sowda. The major manifestations of the disease are dermatitis, onchocercoma, lymphadenitis and visual impairment or blindness. Mild to moderate lymphadenopathy is common, particularly in the inguinal and femoral areas. Involved nodes are characteristically firm and nontender; at times they may reach gigantic proportion and be associated with lymphedema causing elephantiasis (hanging groins). Itching skin and chronic papular onchodermatitis with depigmentation are bothersome, sometimes accompanied by lymphadenopathy in conjunction with secondarily infected skin lesions.

Wuchereria bancrofti infection[41]

Lymphadenopathy is the striking feature of infection with *Wuchereria bancrofti*. Filaria are frequently found in the enlarged lymph node. While the peripheral blood smear and involved organs are characterized by intense eosinophilia, the histology of the lymph node may not reveal in parallel eosinophilic infiltration. At times, the genitalia may be involved with funiculitis, epididymitis, scrotal pain and skin changes and disfiguration of the penis. Scrotal lymphedema, hydrocele and elephantiasis may be present. In addition, characteristic gigantic swelling of the leg below the knee and of the arm below the elbow described as elephantiasis may develop as a result of lymphatic involvement. Occasionally obstruction of the retroperitoneal lymphatics occurs, leading to rupture of lymphatic vessels into the kidney and appearance of chyluria.

Viral lymphadenopathy

HIV

Lymphadenopathy is very common in HIV-infected individuals and may occur at any stage of HIV infection. Generalized lymphadenopathy was one of the characteristic manifestations of the AIDS epidemic, even before its etiology was recognized.[42] In the San Francisco Men's Health Cohort Study marked lymphadenopathy was present in 29% of seropositive men[43] and 29.2% among 1616 HIV-positive persons in India.[44] Acute retroviral syndrome is often associated with generalized lymph node enlargement (see Chapter 89). In the

majority of cases it usually appears during the second week of the illness. The lymphadenopathy commonly involves the cervical, axillary and inguinal regions.[45] In the early stage of the infection the lymph nodes are characterized histopathologically by pronounced follicular hyperplasia that, with progression of the disease, evolves into a pattern of follicular involution.[46]

Lymph node enlargement in patients with HIV, especially with immunosuppression, may indicate a serious local or systemic condition, and should be evaluated carefully. Rapid enlargement of a previously stable lymph node or a group of nodes requires evaluation to identify the cause and to determine whether treatment is needed. Similarly, nodes that are abnormal in consistency, tender to palpation, fluctuant, asymmetrical, adherent to surrounding tissues or accompanied by other symptoms should be evaluated promptly.

A multitude of opportunistic infections and malignancies can cause lymphadenopathy in patients with HIV (see Chapter 91). The likely causes of lymphadenopathy, and thus the diagnostic workup, will depend in part on the patient's degree of immunosuppression (Table 14.4). Sudden enlargement, pain or tenderness of a lymph node warrants further diagnostic procedures.

In the evaluation of patients with HIV with lymph node enlargement, the history should include accompanying symptoms, particularly constitutional symptoms such as fever, sweats, fatigue and unintentional weight loss. In addition, the patient should be asked about travel history, country of origin, disease exposures (e.g. tuberculosis) and risk behaviors (e.g. sexual activity). A comprehensive physical examination should be done with emphasis on lymph node distribution, size, mobility and consistency. The size and consistency of the spleen and liver should also be examined. In patients with a CD4 cell count >200 cells/µl a tuberculin skin test should be done. Laboratory studies should include complete blood count, including a careful evaluation of the peripheral blood smear. CD4 cell count should be done as early as possible since the whole differential diagnosis will depend on this number. Evaluation of hepatic biochemistry, renal function and urine analysis are useful to identify underlying systemic disorders that may be associated with lymphadenopathy. Additional studies, such as lactate dehydrogenase (LDH), uric acid, calcium and phosphate, may be indicated if malignancy is suspected. Tests for specific organisms (e.g. *Bartonella henselae*) should be done according to clinical assessment.

Imaging studies should include chest X-ray and, when appropriate, tomography. Mediastinal or hilar lymphadenopathy is not a part of the persistent generalized lymphadenopathy (PGL) syndrome and whenever isolated intrathoracic lymphadenopathy is detected, a thorough investigation for mycobacterial disease is recommended. In such cases tuberculosis is found in more than half of the patients.[47]

Table 14.4 Causes of lymphadenopathy in HIV-positive patients

Generalized lymphadenopathy	Localized lymphadenopathy
HIV (acute or persistent generalized lymphadenopathy)	Local infection
Viral diseases (Epstein–Barr virus, cytomegalovirus, hepatitis B virus, hepatitis C virus)	Tuberculosis
	Fungal disease (histoplasmosis, coccidioidomycosis, etc.)
Tuberculosis	Lymphogranuloma venereum, chancroid
Syphilis (secondary)	
Bartonella henselae	Lymphoma or other malignancy
IRIS (immune reconstitution syndrome)	Castleman's disease
	Kaposi's sarcoma
Drugs (e.g. abacavir)	
Multicentric Castleman's disease	

Fine needle aspiration biopsy (FNA-B) is a worthwhile procedure and may allow a rapid diagnosis, obviating the need for surgery and enabling swift treatment to be undertaken in both adults and children.[48,49] If FNA-B is nondiagnostic (false-negative results are relatively common), an open biopsy for definitive evaluation should be done. Biopsy specimens should be sent for (myco)bacterial and fungal cultures, acid-fast staining for mycobacteria and cytologic examination.

Most patients with PGL will not require any treatment. In most patients highly active antiretroviral therapy (HAART) will reduce viral load and lymphadenopathy will subside. When a specific diagnosis is made, specific therapy should be instituted.

Human T-lymphocyte leukemia virus 1 (HTLV 1)[50]

Generalized lymph node enlargement is the most common manifestation of HTLV-1 infection. Additional characteristic findings include skin lesions, hepatosplenomegaly, hypocalcemia, lymphocytosis with abnormal circulating lymphocytes and hyperimmunoglobulinemia. Geographic-dependent findings are tropical spastic paraparesis and myelopathy in some tropical areas. Untreated, the disease undergoes rapid clinical deterioration.

Infectious mononucleosis (see Chapter 155)

Infectious mononucleosis is a disease of teenagers and young adults. It is classically characterized by fever, tonsillopharyngitis, lymphadenopathy, splenomegaly and atypical lymphocytes on peripheral blood smear. Epstein–Barr virus (EBV) is the cause in 80–90% of cases, followed by cytomegalovirus (CMV; 8–16%) and toxoplasmosis (1–2%).[51] It is usually a benign and self-limiting process. Patients exhibit generalized lymphadenopathy and localized lymph node enlargement with or without systemic manifestations. Lymphadenopathy is observed in the vast majority of children and young adults with infectious mononucleosis but only in approximately 45% of patients older than 40 years.[52] Lymph nodes are usually moderately enlarged and not very tender; they can be found at the posterior cervical, axillary, epitrochlear, submandibular, submental and groin regions. Lymph node histology demonstrates paracortical immunoblastic proliferation as seen in many viral infections.[53]

Serious complications of infectious mononucleosis include meningoencephalitis with seizures, myelitis, peripheral neuropathy, splenic rupture, upper airway obstruction, interstitial pneumonitis and severe hepatitis with liver failure. Death is rather rare.

Rarely, a progressive fatal disease develops in patients who have X-linked lymphoproliferative disorder and in other immunocompromised patients.[54] Another infrequent outcome is severe chronic active Epstein–Barr virus infection (SCAEBV).[55] Most often, complete recovery occurs within 1–26 weeks after onset of the disease although in some cases chronic fatigue syndrome may follow and remain for a prolonged period, even years (see Chapter 70).

MANAGEMENT

Lymphadenopathy may be the presenting sign in many diseases. The physical examination of a patient needs to include a description of the most important lymph node groups (cervical, clavicular, axillary, inguinal) and a search for lymph node enlargement of unconventional sites (suboccipital, scalenal, epitrochlear, popliteal, etc.) when indicated.

In adults, small lymph nodes, the size of a small olive, can be normally palpated in the inguinal region and in children in the suboccipital and submental regions. Enlarged and certainly persistent supraclavicular, scalenal, axillary and epitrochlear lymph nodes will usually require investigation, including aspiration or a biopsy of the node.

Mode of presentation

In acutely ill patients who have a tender enlarged lymph node, bacterial etiology is most likely, frequently but not always caused by Gram-positive cocci. A thorough ear, nose and throat examination is mandatory in lymphadenitis or lymphadenopathy of the cervical, submental and head regions. In endemic regions, plague, anthrax and tularemia should be suspected. An acutely ill patient found to have generalized lymphadenopathy (more than three sites) should be evaluated for systemic infections including infectious mononucleosis, typhoid fever, rickettsiosis, leptospirosis, miliary tuberculosis and tularemia, as well as disseminated streptococcal and staphylococcal infections. In mildly symptomatic younger individuals and in symptomatic transplant patients with generalized lymphadenopathy the most likely etiologies will be EBV, CMV and HIV; all of these require special laboratory investigations.[56]

Disease progression

Lymphadenopathy of long duration (>1 month) mandates a thorough investigation. While lymphadenopathy caused by the agent of cat-scratch disease, *Bartonella henselae*, and by *Toxoplasma gondii* can persist for several months, the presumed etiology may be in doubt if the enlarged lymph nodes persist for more than 6 months; in such cases a biopsy of the lymph node is indicated. Fine needle aspiration has replaced the previously often used open surgical biopsy, and is suitable for most diagnostic purposes (except for the diagnosis of lymphoma). The average rate of diagnosis of a biopsied lymph node is 50–60%. Among patients in whom a diagnosis cannot be established through a lymph node biopsy, 25% will develop a lymphoma within 1 year. Therefore patients who undergo a nondiagnostic lymph node biopsy need to be followed up.

The role of age

As mentioned above, lymphadenopathy is exceedingly common in the pediatric age group and represents a benign process in approximately 80% of cases. As such, a trial of antibiotics is justified prior to an extensive workup. In adults, particularly if over 50 years of age, lymphadenopathy (regional or generalized) that persists for several weeks requires a thorough evaluation and consideration for biopsy.

Physical characteristics of the enlarged lymph node

The size, consistency and relation to surrounding and underlying tissues are important clues to the diagnosis of enlarged lymph nodes. Lymph nodes involved by an infective process tend to be large, soft and tender. Signs of local inflammation may be present and draining sinuses may be seen in tuberculous cervical lymphadenitis; inguinal draining sinuses are occasionally seen in lymphogranuloma venereum and chancroid. Nodes involved by lymphoma are characterized as rubbery, matted together and usually nontender. Metastatic lymph nodes due to carcinoma are usually firm, nontender and fixed to the surrounding tissues.

Location

Specific locations of enlarged lymph nodes are frequently associated with specific etiologies (Table 14.5). As intrathoracic and intraabdominal lymph nodes are usually not palpable, appropriate imaging studies are necessary (ultrasound, CT).

Head and neck lymphadenopathy

The oropharyngeal cavity (including the teeth) is the most common cause for head and neck lymphadenopathy, followed by the nasal cavity and the skin covering the head and neck. In children and young adults enlarged lymph nodes must be differentiated from epidermoid

Table 14.5 Location of enlarged lymph node and associated disease

Site of enlarged lymph node	Associated disease or condition
Occipital	Scalp infections, insect bites, head lice, allergy to hair shampoo
Posterior auricular	Rubella, infected ear piercing, otitis externa, HIV infection
Anterior auricular	Eye and conjunctival infection, tularemia
Posterior cervical	Toxoplasmosis
Submental	Dental and oral cavity infections
Anterior cervical and submandibular	Oral cavity infections, infectious mononucleosis, cytomegalovirus, HIV, tuberculosis
Supraclavicular	Neoplasia
Mediastinal	Sarcoidosis, tuberculosis, histoplasmosis, blastomycosis, anthrax, neoplasia (lymphoma, metastasis)
Axillary	Cat-scratch disease, pyogenic infections of the arm, neoplasia
Epitrochlear	Viral diseases, cat-scratch disease, tularemia, hand infections, secondary syphilis
Abdominal/retroperitoneal	Tuberculosis, yersiniosis, neoplasia
Inguinal	Genital herpes, syphilis, lymphogranuloma venereum, granuloma inguinale, filariasis, pediculosis pubis, neoplasia

cysts, thyroglossal cysts, branchial cysts and parotid and submental enlarged glands. Symmetric lymph node enlargement is usually benign and of viral etiology in most instances; unilateral lymph node enlargement raises a wider differential diagnosis list including viral etiology. The most common causes of unilateral enlargement include inflammation of a draining lymph node of a local (bacterial) infection, cat-scratch disease, toxoplasmosis and neoplasia. If asymmetrical cervical lymph node enlargement persists beyond a few weeks and serologic tests for toxoplasmosis and cat-scratch disease are negative, a biopsy, usually with a fine needle, is indicated. An abnormal chest radiograph with associated unilateral cervical lymph node enlargement is highly suspicious (in 80% of patients) of neoplastic etiology or granulomatous disease, and in such instances a lymph node surgical biopsy may be more accurate than fine needle aspiration. Supraclavicular adenopathy, particularly in adults, is most likely to be neoplastic, frequently secondary to gastric cancer. Rare situations that may cause cervical lymphadenopathy include Kimura disease (eosinophilic hyperplastic lymphogranuloma) and Gianotti–Crosti syndrome (hepatitis B-associated lymphadenopathy in children).

Axillary lymphadenopathy

Infections causing unilateral axillary lymphadenopathy include local infectious processes of the arm and hand, hidradenitis suppurativa, cat-scratch disease, HIV, toxoplasmosis and tularemia, streptococcal and staphylococcal lymphadenitis, sleeping sickness and African trypanosomiasis. Postvaccinational lymphadenopathy was regularly seen following smallpox vaccination and occurs occasionally following anthrax vaccination. It is also seen post measles vaccination where characteristic Warthin–Finkeldey multinucleated giant cells are seen on biopsy. Bacille Calmette–Guérin (BCG) vaccination is also occa-

sionally accompanied by an enlarged local lymph node from which *M. bovis* may be isolated. Asymptomatic unilateral axillary lymph node enlargement is suspicious of being of neoplastic etiology. Bilateral axillary lymph node enlargement can be practically caused by all etiologies: viral, bacterial, protozoal, neoplastic, allergic and noninfectious inflammatory diseases.

Thoracic lymphadenopathy

Major etiologies causing thoracic lymphadenopathy include neoplasia, tuberculosis, sarcoidosis, endemic mycosis and anthrax. In children, mediastinal lymphadenopathy, uni- or bilateral with or without visible lung X-ray findings, is characteristic for primary tuberculosis; malignant lymphoma, however, may also present in this manner. The tuberculin test is usually positive in tuberculosis; however, if negative, it should be repeated in 14 days. If still negative a lymph node biopsy is indicated. Occasionally disseminated atypical mycobacterial infection (e.g. *M. cheloni*, *M. avium-intracellulare*) may also manifest as thoracic or generalized lymphadenopathy.

In adults, unilateral mediastinal and hilar lymphadenopathy without any other symptoms or signs suggests a neoplastic etiology and a biopsy to confirm the diagnosis is required. An exception may be the patient with HIV, or a person who arrives from an area endemic for tuberculosis or endemic fungal infection (such as cryptococcosis, histoplasmosis and coccidioidomycosis). Bilateral hilar lymphadenopathy in the asymptomatic young adult is commonly caused by sarcoidosis. In patients who have parenchymal involvement in addition to the hilar lymphadenopathy, a search for tuberculosis needs to be undertaken with sputum investigations (smear and culture) and, if necessary, bronchoscopy. Bronchoscopy increases the yield for *M. tuberculosis* in sputum-negative patients by 50–75%. The presence of an ulcerating granuloma on bronchoscopy will augment the positive rate even further.

Abdominal lymphadenopathy

Infectious etiologies of abdominal lymphadenopathy are few and include mesenteric and intestinal tuberculosis, *Yersinia enterocolitica* infection, Whipple's disease and intestinal anthrax; occasionally Crohn's disease will be accompanied by enlarged mesenteric lymph nodes. More commonly enlarged abdominal lymph nodes are of neoplastic etiology. Occasionally abdominal lymph node enlargement can be seen during attacks of familial Mediterranean fever (FMF) and similar disorders, such as Muckle–Wells syndrome, chronic infantile neurologic cutaneous articular syndrome (CINCA/NOMID), tumor necrosis factor (TNF) receptor-associated periodic syndrome (TRAPS) and hyperimmunoglobulinemia D with periodic fever syndrome (HIDS).[57]

Inguinal lymphadenopathy

Inguinal lymph node enlargement is very common in a variety of sexually transmitted diseases, namely syphilis, chancroid, lymphogranuloma venereum, granuloma inguinale, genital herpes, pediculosis pubis and HIV. In women there may be inflammation of the Bartholin or Skene glands of the labia, but also cat-scratch disease, purulent infections of the upper and lower leg (streptococcal and staphylococcal), Kikuchi's disease and toxoplasmosis. In endemic areas or in travelers or immigrants returning from endemic areas the differential diagnosis should include filariasis, Bancroftian filariasis, onchocerciasis and human plague.

REFERENCES

References for this chapter can be found online at http://www.expertconsult.com

Evaluation and management of the solitary enlarged lymph node

INTRODUCTION

The conditions resulting in enlargement of lymph nodes have been reviewed in Chapter 14. Lymph node enlargement should first be differentiated from other masses that originate from nonlymphoid tissue. The differential diagnosis of solitary lymph node enlargement is similar to that of generalized lymphadenopathy although the frequency of viral and protozoal infections is decreased in the former. The proportions of the different causes depend on the patient's age and the anatomic location of the lymph node; in histologic studies reported in the literature malignant causes are over-represented but this does not seem to be the 'real world'. Overall, staphylococcal and streptococcal infections are the most common causes of localized lymphadenopathy, especially when the enlarged nodes are cervical or axillary. In 17% to over 40% the etiology of solitary lymph node enlargement is not established; this is probably an underestimate since these figures are based on cases in which biopsy was deemed necessary.

In general, a lymph node will increase in size in response to several processes, the most frequent being:

- infiltration by malignant cells;
- infiltration by inflammatory cells in response to an infectious agent being filtered from afferent lymphatics or blood; and
- proliferation of lymphocytes in response to antigenic stimuli.

In most infections the histologic changes in an enlarged lymph node are nonspecific, while a few show a distinctive histologic appearance. Caseating necrosis suggests mycobacterial or fungal etiology, and granulomatous inflammation without necrosis is typical for several infectious and noninfectious processes, among which cat-scratch disease, Kikuchi's disease, sarcoidosis, tularemia and lymphogranuloma venereum are the leading causes. In most cases, however, the histologic features are insufficient to determine the exact infectious etiology.

Kikuchi's disease affects younger women and may be accompanied by constitutional symptoms suggesting lymphoma or a systemic infection. Lymph node biopsy reveals infiltration by plasmocytoid cells and histiocytes and coagulative necrosis (Fig. PP5.1). These findings, as well as the other symptoms, make it difficult to distinguish Kikuchi's disease from lymphoma and systemic lupus erythematosus. The course of Kikuchi's disease is usually self-limited with a favorable prognosis.

Noninfectious causes of an enlarged lymph node can be divided to two broad categories, inflammatory and infiltrative, with further subdivision into immunologic and lymphomyeloproliferative in the former and metastatic and storage in the latter (see Table PP5.1).

The infectious causes of solitary lymph node enlargement include viruses, bacteria, rickettsia, fungi and protozoa. Many of these agents are capable of causing generalized as well as localized lymphadenopathy. Table PP5.2 summarizes the infectious etiologies of solitary lymph node enlargement.

CLINICAL MANIFESTATIONS

Enlarged lymph node(s) may lead the patient to seek medical care or may be an incidental finding. Not every palpable lymph node has an underlying defined pathologic process – inguinal lymph nodes of up to 2 cm in diameter are considered normal for adults and axillary lymph nodes are commonly palpable in laborers. Enlarged cervical and submandibular lymph nodes are commonly found in infants and children and may indicate subclinical dental and oropharyngeal infections or are remnants of past infections.

Evaluation of the enlarged lymph node includes a detailed history that includes the duration of the lymphadenopathy; presence of pain, drainage, skin or mucosal lesions; and any associated local infections. Any accompanying systemic symptoms, history of travel, sexual behavior, occupation, exposure to animals, previous vaccinations and tattooing may provide useful clues and guide the diagnostic approach.

The physical examination should assess the size, texture, adherence to surrounding tissues, tenderness, discharge and fluctuance. Careful examination of the skin, mucous membranes and genitalia is of extreme importance in patients with regional adenopathy. All major lymph node groups should be palpated and examination of the abdomen should include assessment of the size of the liver and spleen.

INVESTIGATIONS

The history and the physical examination guide the diagnostic and therapeutic approach. A history of skin breakdown and a fluctuant lymph node make staphylococcal infection the most likely diagnosis; in other cases, however, the etiology may not be apparent. Basic tests include complete blood count and blood film, and swabs from skin lesions, ulcers and pharynx in the case of cervical adenopathy. A fluctuant node should be aspirated and stained with Gram, Ziehl–Neelsen, silver stain (when indicated) and potassium hydroxide (KOH). Specimens should be cultured for bacteria, mycobacteria and fungi, with additional specific tests according to clinical need. Blood cultures should be obtained from febrile patients. Serologic tests assist the diagnosis of some bacterial pathogens (antistreptolysin O, VDRL, treponemal tests, etc.); a tuberculin skin test may provide helpful information. Images of the chest, abdomen and pelvis are indicated when a systemic cause of infectious or noninfectious lymphadenopathy is suspected. Histology with specific staining for mycobacteria, fungi and cat-scratch disease is indicated when culture does not establish a diagnosis or when there is no response to empiric therapy.

Excisional biopsy is usually preferred to needle aspirate and is the mainstay of diagnosis for entities such as nontuberculous lymphadenopathy. The application of 16S DNA gene amplification as well as

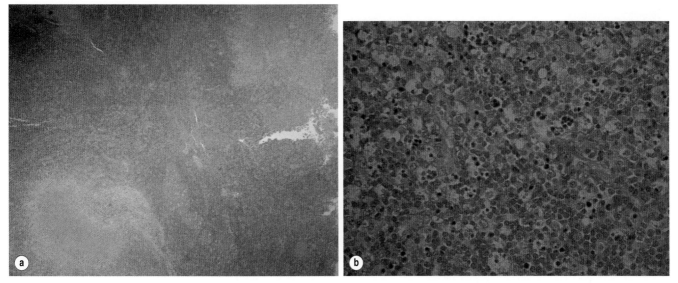

Fig. PP5.1 Kikuchi's disease. (a) Section of a lymph node with extensive paracortical area of coagulative necrosis (H & E). (b) Lesion with infiltrating of histiocytes intermingled with small lymphocytes, immunoblasts, apoptotic bodies (arrowhead) and foamy macrophage (arrow) (H & E). Courtesy of Doron Rimar and Yaaov Schendler.

specific target gene amplification are promising diagnostic methods for *Bartonella*, *Coxiella burnetii* and *Tropheryma whipplei*. However, further studies are needed in order to establish the role of these tests in the diagnosis of lymphadenopathy.

MANAGEMENT

Ideally, management should be guided by the findings of clinical and laboratory investigations. Identifying the causative organism leads to targeted therapy. Cervical adenopathy associated with pharyngitis or odontogenic infection can be treated with penicillin. When suppurative lymphadenopathy is accompanied by lymphangitis, or when a skin infection is thought to be the portal of entry, staphylococcal and streptococcal infections are the most likely diagnoses and penicillinase-resistant penicillin is an appropriate choice. The increasing incidence of community-acquired methicillin-resistant *Staphylococcus aureus* (MRSA) in some geographic areas should be kept in mind if patients fail to respond to β-lactam-based antistaphylococcal therapy. Cat-scratch disease is self-limited and no antimicrobial therapy is required. Aspiration may relieve pain and aid diagnosis, obviating the need for excisional biopsy.

If no specific diagnosis is evident after a detailed history, physical examination and laboratory tests, the course of action is determined by clinical suspicion. A node of less than 1 cm in a person under 40 years of age with no features suggesting malignancy (hard, fixed node) can be observed for a few weeks and in many cases spontaneous resolution will occur. If the disease process does not become apparent, the node is larger than 2 cm, or enlarges during the observation period or fails to respond to empiric therapy, a biopsy is indicated.

Table PP5.1 Noninfectious causes of lymphadenopathy

Inflammatory	Immunologic	Rheumatoid arthritis Systemic lupus erythematosus At the site of vaccination Sarcoidosis Drugs (anticonvulsants) Local allergic reactions
	Lymphomyeloproliferative	Leukemia Lymphoma Castleman's disease Sinus histiocytosis with massive lymphadenopathy (Rosai–Dorfman disease) Kikuchi's disease
Infiltrative	Metastatic malignancy	Skin, melanoma, head and neck, breast, sarcoma
	Storage	Gaucher's disease Niemann–Pick disease

Table PP5.2 Infectious etiologies of solitary lymph node enlargement

Infectious agent	Example	Site	Generalized adenopathy	Comments
Bacteria Pyogenic	Group A streptococci *Staphylococcus aureus* *Corynebacterium diphtheriae*	Cervical Regional Regional		

Table PP5.2 Infectious etiologies of solitary lymph node enlargement—cont'd

Infectious agent	Example	Site	Generalized adenopathy	Comments
Mycobacteria	Mycobacterium tuberculosis Mycobacterium scrofulaceum Nontuberculous mycobacteria	Regional Cervical Regional	+	
Treponema	Syphilis Endemic treponema, yaws	Regional Regional	+	
Other	Francisella tularensis Bacillus anthracis Yersinia pestis Burkholderia pseudomallei, mallei Bartonella Streptobacillus moniliformis, Spirillum minus Haemophilus ducreyi	Regional Regional Regional Regional Regional Regional Regional	+	
Rickettsia/Chlamydophila	Rickettsia tsutsugamushi Rickettsia akari Rickettsia africae, sibirica, australis, honei Rickettsia slovaca Rickettsia mongolotimonae Chlamydia trachomatis (lymphogranuloma venereum)	Regional Regional Regional Cervical Regional Regional	+ +	Lymphangitis-associated rickettsiosis
Fungi	Histoplasma capsulatum Coccidioides immitis Paracoccidioides brasiliensis	Regional Regional Regional		
Protozoa	Toxoplasma gondii Trypanosoma brucei Leishmania spp. (cutaneous)	Cervical Cervical	+	L. braziliensis regional lymphadenopathy may precede skin lesions
Helminths	Filariasis Loa loa Onchocerca volvulus		+	
Viruses	Herpes simplex virus type 2 Human herpesvirus 8 Adenoviruses HIV	Inguinal Cervical, preauricular	+ +	Mucocutaneous lesion may be absent Kaposi's sarcoma Especially types 3 and 7 pharyngoconjunctival fever Usually generalized; localized lymphadenopathy may be the presenting symptom of immune reconstitution

FURTHER READING

Further reading for this chapter can be found online at http://www.expertconsult.com

Conjunctivitis, keratitis and infections of periorbital structures

Conjunctivitis

Conjunctivitis is the inflammation of the conjunctiva, with bacterial conjunctivitis being the eye disease most commonly seen by general practitioners. The incidence of infectious conjunctivitis presented to general practitioners in the Netherlands was measured to be 13.9 per 1000 person-years.[1] Recent reports have confirmed that bacterial conjunctivitis has an excellent prognosis with a high frequency of spontaneous remission. Infectious conjunctivitis must be differentiated from noninfectious conjunctivitis, due to dry eye and acute and chronic inflammatory conditions of the conjunctiva such as Stevens–Johnson syndrome or mucous membrane pemphigoid. Exogenous causes include pollution and medication (conjunctivitis medicamentosa). Rarely conjunctival or eyelid tumors can cause conjunctivitis (masquerade syndrome). Molluscum contagiosum lesions near the eye can shed viral particles into the eye and cause a reactive follicular conjunctivitis, without evidence of conjunctival infection. Large crops of periocular molluscum lesions can be seen in patients with AIDS.

The distinction between noninfective and infectious causes is usually clear from the history. Except for chlamydial conjunctivitis, infectious conjunctivitis rarely lasts longer than 3 weeks, beginning to resolve after 10 days. Conjunctivitis medicamentosa can be a difficult condition to diagnose and may follow an infectious conjunctivitis. Clues include a history of initial improvement on starting a new type of eye drop, followed by worsening and complaints that the eye drops sting. Thorough history taking is essential because patients may not recall all the different eye drops that they have been using during an episode of conjunctivitis. Withdrawal of all topical medication and reassessment 2 or 3 days later is helpful.

COMMUNITY-ACQUIRED INFECTIOUS CONJUNCTIVITIS

Conjunctivitis in neonates

In neonates, infectious conjunctivitis is named ophthalmia neonatorum in the first 3 weeks of life. It occurs worldwide, but is uncommon where there is adequate infant eye prophylaxis. The most serious cause is *Neisseria gonorrhoeae* (gonococcal conjunctivitis), while more common causes are *Chlamydia trachomatis*,[2] chemical irritation and herpes simplex virus. Globally gonococcal ophthalmia neonatorum is an important cause of blindness. The risk of ophthalmia neonatorum for a child born to an infected mother is 30–50% for gonorrhea[3] and 15–35% for chlamydial infection.[4] Transmission usually occurs in the birth canal.

Gonococcal conjunctivitis presents as a hyperacute conjunctivitis 24–48 hours after birth and earlier after premature rupture of membranes. Lid edema, chemosis and profuse purulent secretion rapidly progress to corneal opacities and ulceration, and endophthalmitis may occur. Chlamydial conjunctivitis presents 5–12 days after birth with a watery discharge, which becomes purulent more slowly. Follicles are absent because the conjunctival lymphoid tissue in infants is immature. Untreated the condition usually resolves in 3–4 weeks, but can take up to a year. Rarely membranes and micropannus form, resulting in significant stromal scarring in later life. Pneumonitis, rhinitis, vaginitis and otitis can follow the conjunctivitis.

Conjunctivitis in infants

Brazilian purpuric fever is caused by a rare invasive clone of *Haemophilus influenzae* biogroup *aegyptius*. Systemic disease occurs in children 1–3 weeks after an episode of conjunctivitis. It is seen over a widespread area in Brazil and there is a case mortality of 70%. The clinical picture is similar to that of meningococcal sepsis.

The Brazilian purpuric fever clone of *H. influenzae* biogroup *aegyptius* is resistant to trimethoprim but is sensitive to chloramphenicol and ampicillin. During epidemics, systemic rifampin (rifampicin) (20 mg/kg/day for 2 days) may be used as prophylaxis against Brazilian purpuric fever for children who have conjunctivitis.

Conjunctivitis in adults

Bacterial conjunctivitis is ubiquitous and is more common in warmer months and regions. It is transmitted by contact with ocular or upper respiratory tract discharges of people who have the infection, fomites, medical equipment or shared cosmetics. In some areas insect vectors are involved. Tearing, irritation and sticky discharge without preauricular lymphadenopathy are early clinical features. The conjunctiva is pink (not red). The lids may be stuck together by a mucopurulent exudate on awakening.

Chlamydial infection results in three distinct clinical pictures:
Neonatal chlamydial conjunctivitis is described above.
Trachoma is a scarring condition of the conjunctiva and cornea in adults caused by recurrent childhood infection with *C. trachomatis*.[2] Trachoma occurs worldwide and is endemic in poorer rural areas of developing countries. Blindness due to trachoma is still common in parts of the Middle East, northern and sub-Saharan Africa, parts of the Indian subcontinent, South East Asia and China. There are pockets of infection in South America, among Australian Aborigines, in the Pacific islands and in native American reservations in southwest USA.

The acute chlamydial conjunctivitis is characterized by a diffuse follicular reaction in the conjunctiva of the superior tarsal plate and at the limbus with soft follicles. Papillary hypertrophy is a nonspecific sign.

With resolution of the follicles there is subconjunctival scarring and a loss of conjunctival mucin-producing goblet cells. Blinding complications result from chronic re-infection,[5] severe dry eyes and entropion leading to corneal scarring, bacterial superinfection and ulceration.

Adult inclusion conjunctivitis is an acute condition associated with sexually transmitted chlamydial infection; it presents with a mucopurulent discharge after a 4- to 12-day incubation period. It is often monocular and develops into a chronic follicular conjunctivitis, often with epithelial keratitis and limbal follicles. Tender preauricular lymphadenopathy is common. Untreated the disease has a chronic course and may progress to keratitis and possibly iritis.

VIRAL CONJUNCTIVITIS

Viral conjunctivitis is common and occurs worldwide. Epidemics frequently occur and may be propagated by eye clinics. Transmission is by direct or indirect contact with ocular or upper respiratory tract secretions. Airborne transmission occurs. Viral particles can remain infectious on surfaces for more than 1 month. The incubation period is from 2 days to 2 weeks, and infected people remain contagious for up to 2 weeks after the symptoms begin.

The main patterns of viral conjunctivitis are:

* epidemic keratoconjunctivitis (EKC);
* pharyngoconjunctival fever (PCF);
* acute hemorrhagic conjunctivitis (AHC).

The symptoms and signs of these patterns of infection are similar, but vary in degree. All of these patterns present as an acute follicular conjunctivitis, with watering, grittiness, redness, ecchymosis and lid edema, often with flu-like symptoms. Preauricular lymphadenopathy and bilateral involvement are common.

In EKC most patients have some focal epitheliopathy and photophobia by 2 weeks. Subepithelial opacities appear after 2 weeks in 50% of patients and occasionally impair vision. These lesions cause occasional recurrences of grittiness. The natural history is of slow resolution, which can take more than 1 year. In PCF there is a similar ophthalmic picture, but the systemic features are more pronounced.

In AHC ecchymosis is more prominent and the onset of symptoms more rapid. Rarely a polio-like radiculopathy follows AHC.

Diagnosis of infectious conjunctivitis

Microbiologic investigation is necessary only in neonatal, hyperacute, severe, unusual or chronic cases. Microscopy of conjunctival smears can be useful, and conjunctival swabs are cultured on blood agar and (especially in children) chocolate agar. *Haemophilus influenzae* biogroup *aegyptius* and *Streptococcus pneumoniae* are common causes. *Haemophilus influenzae* type b, *Moraxella* spp., *Branhamella* spp., *Neisseria meningitidis* and *Corynebacterium diphtheriae* are also involved.[6,7] The diagnosis of trachoma is made on clinical grounds in endemic areas.

Expressed follicles have a characteristic microscopic appearance involving macrophages (Leber's cells), plasma cells and lymphoblasts. *Chlamydia trachomatis* types A–C are involved. Secondary bacterial superinfection is common and causes severe disease. Antibodies to *C. trachomatis* can be demonstrated in the tears and serum. Enzyme-linked immunoassay or immunofluorescent monoclonal antibody stains of conjunctival scrapings are rapid and convenient ways to make the diagnosis of chlamydial conjunctivitis.[8] Most methods available for typing the viruses that cause acute conjunctivitis are polymerase chain reaction (PCR)-based.

Most epidemics of viral conjunctivitis are caused by adenoviruses, commonly serotypes 8, 19 and 37 for EKC, and types 3 and 8 for PCF. Picornaviruses such as enterovirus type 70 and Coxsackie virus type A24 cause AHC. Conjunctivitis can be a feature of many other viral diseases, including influenza, rubella, rubeola, chickenpox and glandular fever.

Prevention of infectious conjunctivitis

Topical prophylaxis was described in 1881 by Credé. His silver nitrate eye drops substantially reduced the incidence of gonococcal conjunctivitis; however, they are inactive against chlamydia, and toxicity is common. Recently, 2.5% aqueous povidone-iodine has been shown to be safer, cheaper and more effective.[9] Maternal treatment before birth is the best prevention.

Control of epidemics associated with eye clinics involves setting up a triage system for those suspected of viral conjunctivitis. These patients are seen in a separate room with dedicated personnel. The use of gloves and noncontact examination techniques are strongly recommended. Staff infected with viral conjunctivitis should be furloughed until 2 weeks after the start of symptoms, by which time they are considered to be no longer contagious.

Trachoma is transmitted by contact with ocular or nasopharyngeal secretions, either directly through fomites or insect vectors (the flies *Musca sorbens* in Africa and the Middle East and *Hippelates* spp. in the Americas). Untreated active lesions can be infectious for years. Prevention of transmission is the most important public health measure.[10] Education about personal hygiene and regular washing of the face is very important, and these hygiene measures require only a tiny amount of water. There has been mass treatment of the population with topical tetracycline or erythromycin in hyperendemic areas.

Management of acute conjunctivitis

Topical broad-spectrum antibiotic drops are used 2-hourly until the symptoms subside, which should occur rapidly. In Europe, chloramphenicol is used; in the USA, neomycin, polymyxin and bacitracin are used. Gentamicin and tobramycin are useful against Gram-negative organisms, but cause a higher rate of local toxic reactions. Erythromycin or the quinolones may also be used.

Treatment of chlamydial ophthalmia neonatorum comprises 2 weeks of erythromycin 10 mg/kg every 12 hours for the first week and every 8 hours for the second week of life. The Brazilian purpuric fever clone of *H. influenzae* biogroup *aegyptius* is resistant to trimethoprim but is sensitive to chloramphenicol and ampicillin. During epidemics systemic rifampin (rifampicin) (20 mg/kg/day for 2 days) may be used as prophylaxis against Brazilian purpuric fever for children who have conjunctivitis.

The drug of choice for treating *N. gonorrhoeae* and *N. meningitidis* is an extended-spectrum cephalosporin such as ceftriaxone 1 g (25–40 mg/kg) every 12 hours for 3 days. Repeated irrigation of the conjunctival sac is recommended to reduce inflammatory microbial mediators to the cornea. Treatment of chlamydial conjunctivitis is oxycycline 100 mg every 12 hours or erythromycin stearate 500 mg every 6 hours. Topical treatment is relatively ineffective.

The management of viral conjunctivitis is supportive, with warm or cold compresses reducing symptoms of itch, plus lubrication and cycloplegics if there is an element of keratitis (see below). Antibacterial prophylaxis is probably unnecessary and can cause an allergic or toxic conjunctivitis.

Neonates who have a purulent discharge are presumed to have gonococcal infection and are treated with ceftriaxone 25–50 mg/kg intramuscularly or intravenously to a maximum of 125 mg. Frequent irrigation removes bacteria and microbial products. A single intramuscular dose of 125 mg of ceftriaxone is effective therapy for gonococcal ophthalmia neonatorum.[11] Parents should be screened for sexually transmitted diseases.

Keratitis

Infectious keratitis can be caused by bacteria, viruses, fungi or parasites[12] and can be suspected in various clinical situations, herein classified as community-acquired keratitis, contact lens-related keratitis and health care-associated keratitis. Infectious keratitis is a medical emergency and improper management can lead to loss of vision. Noninfectious keratitis is important in that it can be confused with infectious keratitis.

COMMUNITY-ACQUIRED KERATITIS

Typical acute microbial keratitis is the major syndrome. Patients present with a corneal epithelial defect and a stromal infiltrate (Fig. 15.1). The other main clinical problems are herpesvirus infections, with recurrent inflammation leading to scarring, and infection in a 'compromised' cornea (i.e. after local or systemic immunosuppression, injury

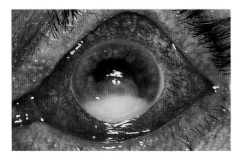

Fig. 15.1 Typical microbial keratitis. Note accumulation of inflammatory cells at the dependent part of the anterior chamber of the eye (hypopyon) and mid-corneal defect. Courtesy of Myron Yanoff.

or chronic disease). Algorithms for the initial division of keratitis into the main clinical situations are shown in Figure 15.2. Microbial keratitis is responsible for 30% of cases of blindness in some developing countries. In hot climates fungal infection is more frequent, although bacterial keratitis still accounts for 60% of cases.[13]

Surgery, particularly corneal grafts and corneal sutures, and concomitant use of topical corticosteroids increase the risk of infection. Other than vitamin A deficiency, systemic predisposing conditions are relatively unimportant clinically. Vitamin A deficiency is particularly important in children who are malnourished and who have a concomitant infection, especially measles, in which keratomalacia (corneal melting) can occur suddenly. *Staphylococcus* and *Micrococcus* spp., *Streptococcus* and *Pseudomonas* spp. and the Enterobacteriaceae (*Citrobacter, Klebsiella, Enterobacter, Serratia* and *Proteus* spp.) accounted for 87% of cases of bacterial keratitis in one series.[14]

Pseudomonas infection is recognized for its swift suppurative course to perforation, secondary to proteolytic enzyme release. It is particularly common in contact lens wearers (hard and soft). *Serratia marcescens* corneal ulcers have been associated with the wearing of contact lenses and with contaminated eye drops. *Neisseria gonorrhoeae, Corynebacterium diphtheriae, Haemophilus* spp. and *Listeria* spp. are capable of penetrating an intact corneal epithelium. Other bacteria and fungi produce disease only after a loss of corneal epithelial integrity. *Mycobacterium tuberculosis* is a rare cause of keratitis in the course of tuberculous scleritis.[15] Also, *Nocardia* spp. can cause keratitis with amikacin being the drug of choice for treatment.[16]

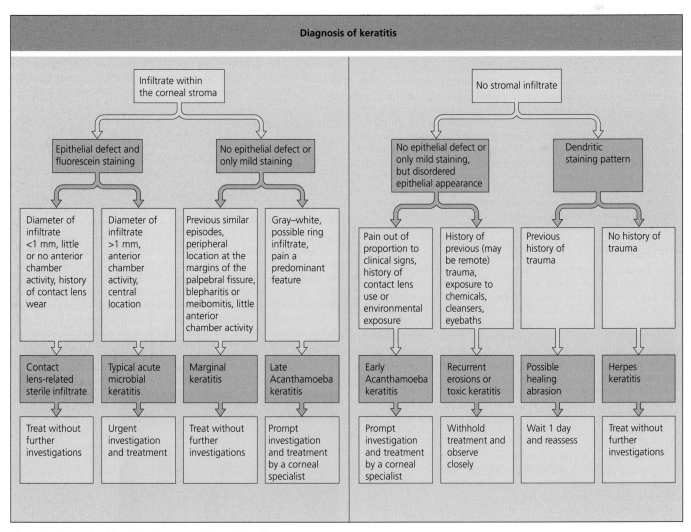

Fig. 15.2 Diagnosis of keratitis. Courtesy of Myron Yanoff.

If the clinical picture progresses after a 2-day treatment, the patient should be admitted to hospital for supervised treatment. If after the first week there is no response to therapy, consider stopping therapy and reculturing or switching to a different antibiotic guided by antibiotic sensitivity testing.

Viral keratitis: herpes simplex virus type 1 or 2

Epidemiology

Herpes simplex keratitis has an annual incidence of new cases of 8/10 000. The incidence peaks at ages 5–10 years and 35–40 years. Males are affected twice as often as females. Approximately 50% of patients have a history of herpes labialis. Primary ocular infection occurs in 5%.[17] Corneal infection is usually with herpes simplex virus type 1 (in 98% of cases), except in neonatal herpes infection, when 80% of cases are due to herpes simplex virus type 2.

Pathogenesis and pathology

The pattern of dendritic ulcers is caused by direct infection of corneal epithelium. It is thought that delayed-type hypersensitivity to viral antigens causes the inflammation that leads to disciform keratitis.[18] Recurrent herpes simplex virus keratitis has been described in the course of Alport's syndrome.[19]

Clinical features

Primary ocular infection is usually asymptomatic, although a vesicular reaction may be seen. Occasionally there is a follicular conjunctivitis. Corneal damage is caused by recurrent disease.

Recurrence occurs in around 10% of cases at 1 year and 50% by 20 years. Triggers include fever, trauma and ultraviolet light. Recurrence is a consequence of latency.[20] Latency develops as virus spreads to a sensory ganglion and remains dormant there. It is thought that infection can spread across a ganglion, for instance from the mandibular to the ophthalmic division of the trigeminal nerve, and hence from lip to eye. Spread from eye to eye is uncommon except in atopic patients in whom delayed-type hypersensitivity is impaired. These patients are at risk of bilateral disease, larger geographic ulcers and disseminated infection. With each recurrence corneal scarring increases, and it is thought that viral particles remaining within the cornea cause the continuing inflammation and edema seen in disciform keratitis.

Management

Either gentamicin 1.5% with cefuroxime 5% or the fluoroquinolones ofloxacin 0.3% or ciprofloxacin 0.3% are effective against 90% of expected isolates in most clinical settings.[21,22]

Aminoglycosides are toxic to the epithelium in moderate doses and quinolones are preferred as monotherapy. In cases in which streptococci are likely (e.g. chronic ocular surface disease, children) there may be quinolone resistance, and combination with cefuroxime 5% is recommended. There are increasing reports of quinolone resistance in some settings.[23]

Initial treatment is with drops every hour day and night for 2 days, followed by review.[24] If the clinical picture has improved or not worsened, treatment is then reduced to drops every hour by day for 3 days. After this time the ulcer should be sterile. Treatment is reduced to prophylactic levels every 6 hours until the epithelium has healed. One trap for the inexperienced is that intensive treatment with ciprofloxacin 0.3% can cause a white ciprofloxacin precipitate to form in the corneal stroma adjacent to an epithelial defect. This may be confused with progression of the infection.

Untreated herpes simplex keratitis usually resolves within 1–2 weeks, but it can progress, resulting in the development of geographic ulcers. Resolution is more rapid if the dendritic ulcer is debrided.

Antiviral treatment also speeds up resolution, and no benefit has been shown for a combination of debridement and antiviral agents when compared with the use of antiviral agents alone. The choice of antiviral agent depends on availability. In Europe aciclovir 3% ophthalmic ointment five times a day is almost universally preferred because it is effective and has a low incidence of toxicity.[25] In the USA, trifluridine 1% 2-hourly is used.

Oral aciclovir or famciclovir is effective but comparatively expensive. It may be useful when there is a desire to reduce corneal exposure to topical agents. Systemic antiviral treatment is recommended as prophylaxis against encephalitis for infants who have primary infection.

Prophylactic treatment with oral aciclovir 400 mg every 12 hours reduces the recurrence rate of stromal (severe) disease from 28% to 14%.[26]

The management of the chronic sequelae of herpes simplex keratitis may require topical corticosteroid therapy under close ophthalmic supervision. Topical antiviral treatment reduces recurrence rates in these patients.[27]

Viral keratitis: herpes zoster ophthalmicus

Epidemiology

The varicella-zoster virus is a herpesvirus that causes chickenpox as a primary infection and shingles on recurrence. Around 90% of adults are seropositive for varicella-zoster virus. The rate of recurrence increases with age, and second recurrences can occur in those who have impaired immunity.

Pathogenesis and pathology

Reactivated virus replicates in the ganglion, producing local inflammation and premonitory pain before it travels down peripheral nerves to the skin or eye. A perineuritis and vasculitis occurs, and in the eye a disciform keratitis, iritis and cyclitis are common manifestations.

Clinical features

The clinical appearance is typical. Symptoms of eye involvement include photophobia and decreased vision. Hutchinson's sign, a rash on the side of the nose, is associated with ocular inflammation (Fig. 15.3).

Management

Oral aciclovir 800 mg five times a day for 7 days accelerates skin healing and reduces the incidence of episcleritis, keratitis, iritis, postherpetic neuralgia and probably acute pain.[28] The newer antivirals famciclovir and valaciclovir have improved bioavailability and are increasingly used instead of aciclovir. There is little role for topical antivirals. Systemic corticosteroids used with antiviral therapy have some benefit in shortening the clinical syndrome, but they do not reduce the incidence of postherpetic neuralgia.[29] There is no clinical consensus on whether the benefits of treatment outweigh the risks.

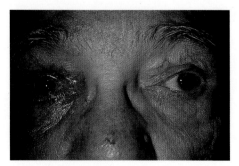

Fig. 15.3 Herpes zoster ophthalmicus. Inflamed right periorbital skin, with conjunctivitis and a lesion on the nose. Courtesy of Myron Yanoff.

Disciform keratitis, iritis and cyclitis respond to conventional topical corticosteroid treatment, but prolonged therapy, sometimes for years, is required.

AIDS: varicella-zoster epithelial keratitis

A chronic, painful epithelial keratitis has been described in patients with AIDS and severe immunodeficiency. Clinically characterized by a variable dendrite-like keratitis, the associated severe, burning pain is the most dramatic feature. Response to treatment is variable; some patients have responded to oral or topical aciclovir, but such patients tend to relapse when treatment stops.[30]

Fungal keratitis

Fungal infections are seen in two distinct clinical settings. In hotter climates the cornea is inoculated with infected vegetable matter as a result of agricultural or other trauma. Infection can then occur in otherwise healthy eyes. In temperate climates infection most often occurs in association with chronic ocular surface disease or prolonged corticosteroid use.

The main cause of fungal keratitis worldwide is trauma. In the developed world risk factors include protracted epithelial ulceration, therapeutic wearing of soft contact lenses, corneal transplant and topical corticosteroid therapy. Patients who have exposure keratitis and a history of previous herpes simplex or herpes zoster keratitis are at risk.

The septate filamentous fungal species, especially *Fusarium* and *Aspergillus* spp., are the most common cause of fungal keratitis. With increasing distance from the equator the relative incidence of candidal infection increases. Dematiaceous filamentous fungi such as *Curvularia* spp. are of low virulence and cause indolent infections.

Clinical features

Fungal keratitis usually presents as a typical microbial keratitis. It is not possible to diagnose the type of infection on clinical grounds. Clinical context is the most important guide to appropriate investigation and therapy. In filamentary fungal keratitis the corneal surface is gray or dull. Satellite lesions are common in the surrounding stroma and may be seen with an intact epithelium (Fig. 15.4). Candidal lesions appear in corneas that are already abnormal. They are often quite localized at first with a collar button configuration.

CONTACT LENS-RELATED KERATITIS

The wide use of contact lenses has led to increased prevalence of specific opportunistic pathogens including *Pseudomonas* spp., nontuberculous mycobacteria such as *Mycobacterium chelonae*,[31] fungi such as *Fusarium*[32] and free-living *Acanthamoeba* amebae.[33] The wearing of contact lenses increases the risk of developing bacterial keratitis.[34]

The annual incidence is 5/10 000 for daily wear of soft lenses and 20/10 000 for overnight wear of soft lenses, although estimates 10-fold

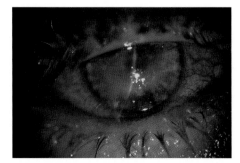

Fig. 15.4 Fungal keratitis. The corneal surface looks rough, and there are several satellite lesions best seen here at the periphery on the left side of the cornea. Courtesy of Myron Yanoff.

higher than this have been made. The largest risk factor is the overnight wearing of soft lenses. This increases the risk fivefold compared with the daytime wearing of lenses and 20-fold compared with the wearing of rigid lenses.[35] One particular situation is microbial keratitis associated with orthokeratology, with *Pseudomonas aeruginosa* and *Acanthamoeba* spp. being the leading causes; cases have been mostly reported in East Asian patients.[36] The incidence of fungal keratitis associated with contact lenses steadily increased up to >50% in Florida.[37] Higher incidence has been noted in the 2004–2006 multicountry *Fusarium* keratitis epidemic[38] which has been associated with the use of particular soft contact lenses and contact lens solutions. *Fusarium* keratitis evolves towards corneal ulceration.[39]

Acanthamoeba keratitis is a painful, vision-threatening infection, which can lead to ulceration of the cornea, loss of visual acuity and eventually blindness and enucleation. *Acanthamoeba* keratitis is associated with trauma to the cornea and contact lens wear; the use of contaminated saline solution is the major risk factor for *Acanthamoeba* keratitis. Approximately 10–15% of cases are associated with agricultural and other trauma, but most are associated with contact lens use. Poor lens hygiene by soft contact lens wearers and the use of homemade saline- or chlorine-based disinfection systems are risk factors.

A 360° or paracentral stromal ring infiltration is a characteristic of *Acanthamoeba* keratitis. A nonhealing corneal ulcer is often the first clue to *Acanthamoeba* keratitis. In early epithelial disease there may be punctate keratopathy, pseudodendrites, epithelial wrinkling, diffuse or focal subepithelial infiltrates and radial perineural infiltrates. Ring infiltrates and corneal ulceration may present later.[40,41] Pain out of proportion to the clinical signs is common, but not constant. The clinical picture may resemble herpetic or fungal keratitis, and a high index of suspicion is warranted in contact lens wearers who have apparent herpetic disease. Bacterial co-infection or superinfection in late disease occurs in around 10% of cases and causes an atypical presentation.

The clinical course of *A. histolytica* keratitis is prolonged. Early diagnosis is important, but treatment started before proper diagnostic tests are carried out only confuses the clinical picture. Unlike bacterial keratitis, there is no justification for starting therapy without investigation. A delay of 1–2 days while a patient is referred for expert opinion and investigation is less harmful than early inappropriate therapy. The grave prognosis of *A. histolytica* keratitis in the past was due to the slow inexorable progression of disease rather than fulminant corneal destruction.

Diagnosis

In some parts of the world broad-spectrum therapy is used without initial investigation and it has been suggested that this practice could be extended.[42] The laboratory diagnosis of infectious keratitis relies on culture-based and PCR-based detection of the pathogen in a suitable ocular specimen. A 'keratitis kit' has been developed in order to standardize both the clinical specimens and laboratory tests. Moreover, corneal scraping also debrides the ulcer, allows antibiotics to enter the base of the ulcer and provides microbiologic data (provided that antimicrobial therapy has not been given within the previous 24 hours). The cornea is anesthetized with nonpreserved amethocaine 1%, five or six drops at 2-minute intervals. Using a slit-lamp, necrotic material is removed from the center of the ulcer. A 23 gauge needle tip is scraped parallel to the cornea to remove infected tissue. A fresh needle is used for each specimen. If a slit-lamp is not available, scraping with a scalpel blade is safer than using a needle. The diagnostic yield is greater from the sides of the ulcer than from necrotic areas.

Slides should be made for Gram stain and Giemsa stain, and appropriate bacterial cultures (and fungal cultures if suspected) should be prepared directly from the needle. Bending the tip of the needle before use facilitates this. The sharp side is used to scrape the cornea and the smooth surface is used to plate out the specimen without penetrating the surface of the agar. For amebal analysis, specimens can be plated on non-nutrient agar, which is later overlain with *Escherichia coli* in the laboratory.[43] Tracks of bacterial clearing show where the amebae have been grazing. Bacterial and fungal cultures should also be obtained. In contact lens wearers the lenses and the lens case should be cultured.

Microscopy techniques vary. Fluorescent microscopy can be carried out using calcofluor white (which stains the walls of cysts), with acridine orange or with an immunofluorescent antibody. Confocal microscopy of a wet preparation can be used to identify motile trophozoites, which have a large karyosome and a contractile vacuole. Biopsy specimens should also be stained with hematoxylin and eosin, periodic acid-Schiff and methenamine silver to demonstrate *A. histolytica* cysts.

Definitive diagnosis of *Acanthamoeba* keratitis is made by microscopic observation of amebal trophozoites and cysts in corneal scrapings or biopsy, or on their cultivation from infected tissues. Confocal microscopy has been used as an aid in the diagnosis.[44] Also, PCR-based molecular tests applied to corneal specimens and tear fluid allow us to identify and genotype *Acanthamoeba* by 18S rDNA sequencing.[45] MALDI-TOF mass spectrometry is a promising rapid method, not only for the identification of isolates, but also the detection/identification of amebae in corneal specimens.[46] A real-time PCR assay[47] and a multiplex real-time PCR assay[48] have also been developed for the rapid detection of most, but not all, the *Acanthamoeba* spp. genotypes involved in keratitis. As for bacterial keratitis, microscopic examination of Gram-stained corneal smears or biopsy may reveal bacteria.[49] Acid-fast bacteria may be observed in cases of *Mycobacterium* spp. and *Nocardia* spp. keratitis.[49]

Viral culture or immunofluorescence[50] can be used to confirm infection, but in practice the diagnosis is clinical. In epithelial disease there is a characteristic dendritic ulcer (Fig. 15.5). Corneal sensation is often impaired, and there is usually a history of similar attacks in the past.

Management

The diamidines, propamidine isethionate 0.1% and hexamidine 0.1%, and the cationic antiseptics, polyhexamethyl biguanide (PHMB) 0.02% and chlorhexidine 0.02%, are probably the most effective medications,[41,51] although availability can be a problem. Local manufacture of chlorhexidine or PHMB may be possible from 20% disinfectant preparations. The azoles (clotrimazole, fluconazole, ketoconazole and miconazole) have also been suggested for use as a third agent, as for amebal keratitis.

Initial treatment starts immediately after the epithelium is debrided using a cationic antiseptic and a diamidine, each hour day and night for 48 hours, then hourly by day for 3 days. Dosage is then reduced to

3-hourly to reduce local toxicity. If toxicity is suspected, the frequency of the diamidine should be reduced. It may take 2 weeks to achieve a response to treatment. Pain relief with systemic nonsteroidal anti-inflammatory agents in cycloplegia is very important. The use of corticosteroids in controlling inflammation is controversial. Some authorities say that they are contraindicated at any stage. Others advocate the use of a weak topical corticosteroid to control inflammation after at least 2 weeks of antiamebic therapy, emphasizing the importance of continued antiamebic therapy until several weeks after the corticosteroid is stopped.

Historic data are the best guide to selecting antifungal therapy.[52] The greatest experience in the use of antifungals for keratitis comes from India. However, this experience may not apply to situations where there is a local or systemic disorder of immunity. No currently available antifungal agent has a favorable profile of activity and toxicity. Response to antifungal treatment is poor compared with that to antibacterial treatment. Surgical management (corneal transplant) may be necessary. Combined topical and systemic therapy is often used and is usually prolonged. Corneal drug penetration is helped by daily scraping of the epithelium and necrotic stroma. The choice of antifungal agent is often dictated by availability. Most topical antifungal agents must be made locally from tablets or intravenous preparations.

Among the polyenes, amphotericin B is fungicidal, but is toxic to the eye in high concentrations. It is used diluted in sterile water at 0.1–0.15% two to four times every hour for the first 1–2 days. Natamycin 5% has poor corneal penetration, but is useful for superficial filamentary fungal infections.

Among the pyrimidines, flucytosine 1% can be prepared from a commercially available intravenous or tablet form and is used in combination only (early resistance occurs) with amphotericin B for candidal keratitis. Concomitant systemic use may be helpful.

Among the imidazoles, miconazole 10 mg/ml in polyethoxylated castor oil (intravenous preparation) was effective in more than 60% of cases in a prospective trial in India[53] when used topically every 2 hours. Ketoconazole 2% prepared as an aqueous solution from tablets is probably effective against *Aspergillus flavus*, but not *Aspergillus fumigatus* or *Fusarium* spp. Systemic and topical administration is often combined. Econazole 1% is used topically in combination with systemic itraconazole, and clotrimazole 1% vaginal cream has also been used. Fluconazole is given systemically or as a 0.2–0.5% topical aqueous solution. Itraconazole used orally has some activity against filamentous fungi (see Chapter 149). It has poor tissue penetration, but a good clinical response when used against candidal infections. *Fusarium* spp. respond less well. Silver sulfadiazine 1% is used for antibiotic prophylaxis in patients who have burns. It has moderate antifungal activity *in vitro*, but has been widely used in developing countries as a topical antifungal with good rates of success, particularly against *Fusarium* spp.

Chlorhexidine gluconate 0.2% solution is at least as effective as natamycin in treating fungal infections and is suggested as an inexpensive agent for use in the developing world.[54]

Initial treatment for fungal keratitis depends upon local experience. In London, UK we use topical econazole 1% (or amphotericin B 0.15 or 0.3%) hourly for 48 hours, then 2 hourly for 72 hours and then reduce the dosage depending upon the initial response. Long-term treatment is required. Systemic treatment is used as an adjunct: itraconazole 200 mg daily initially, reduced to 100 mg for longer term use, or fluconazole 200 mg daily for *Candida* infections. If surgical debridement is performed, a 2 mm clear margin is advised. The inflammatory reaction results from live organisms and fungal debris. Because most antifungal agents are fungistatic, reduction of inflammation also depresses local immunity so that the organisms are not killed. Concomitant corticosteroid use is therefore not recommended for fungal keratitis.

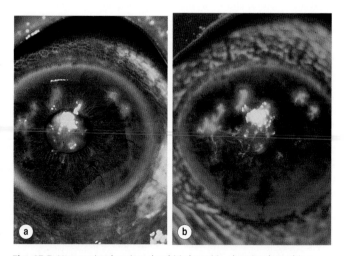

Fig. 15.5 Herpes simplex virus dendritic keratitis, showing branching epithelial lesions seen (a) without staining and (b) with rose bengal staining. Rose bengal stains the devitalized cells at the edges of the dendritic lesions. Courtesy of Myron Yanoff.

Prevention

Good lens hygiene, the use of hydrogen peroxide 3% for at least 3 hours[55] and avoidance of tap water in contact lens care are important preventive measures.[36] The role of mechanical rubbing is still debated.[56]

KERATITIS FOLLOWING OCULAR SURGERY

Penetrating keratoplasty has been complicated by *Gemella haemolysans* keratopathy[57] diagnosed by corneal biopsy. In children, penetrating keratoplasty may be complicated by bacterial keratitis in up to 1–3% of patients due to Gram-positive bacteria, chiefly *Streptococcus pneumoniae*.[58]

Laser *in situ* keratomileusis (LASIK) may be complicated by infectious keratitis. A three-patient cluster of *Nocardia asteroides* keratitis was traced to inappropriate use of the same blade and microkeratome in all patients.[49] *Propionibacterium acnes* has been recovered in one case.[59] Notably, several nontuberculous, rapidly growing mycobacteria caused post-LASIK keratitis including *Mycobacterium chelonae*.

Methicillin-resistant *Staphylococcus aureus* keratitis has been described following refractive surgery.[60] *Staphylococcus aureus* and *Streptococcus pneumoniae* in developing countries, and *Staphylococcus epidermidis* in developed countries, are responsible for infectious keratitis following keratoplasty.[61] Also, outbreaks of viral keratoconjunctivitis have been reported in ophthalmology departments.[62]

Infections of Periorbital Structures

PERIORBITAL CELLULITIS

The orbit is the bony structure surrounding the eye. Infection of the contents of the bony orbit is called orbital cellulitis. Orbital infection commonly occurs as a result of contiguous spread from adjacent structures. Periorbital cellulitis is divided into preseptal or postseptal (orbital) depending on the site of infection. Orbital cellulitis is sight-threatening and occasionally life-threatening.

Preseptal cellulitis is 5–10 times more common than orbital cellulitis in infants and toddlers and is not sight-threatening or life-threatening, but it can, rarely, spread to become orbital cellulitis. It is commonly caused by *H. influenzae* or *Streptococcus* spp. and follows an upper respiratory tract infection. In adults it is most often seen after minor trauma such as an infected bite or scratch. One case of *Tropheryma whipplei*, the Whipple's disease bacterium, orbital manifestation has been reported.[63]

The source and agents of infection causing orbital cellulitis vary with age. The paranasal sinuses (the ethmoid, maxillary and frontal sinuses) are the main sources. Orbital cellulitis is uncommon in neonates, but when it occurs it is usually secondary to conjunctivitis or a developmental abnormality such as a ruptured dacryocele. In infants respiratory tract infections may cause preseptal cellulitis; in older children and adults dental abscesses and trauma become important causes. Endogenous orbital cellulitis is rare.

Clinical features

In adults there is frequently a history of sinusitis, headache or recent tooth extraction or abscess. Children often have an antecedent upper respiratory tract infection. Preseptal cellulitis is characterized by eyelid swelling and edema, which is usually unilateral and mainly involves the upper lids. Lower lid swelling occurs when the cellulitis is secondary to dacryocystitis. Edematous conjunctiva can prolapse between the lids.

In orbital cellulitis features of preseptal cellulitis are variably present, but there is also proptosis, decreased ocular mobility and even decreased vision or a relative afferent pupil defect. These signs are caused by increased intraorbital pressure due to edema or abscess. If a subperiosteal abscess forms there may be nonaxial displacement of the globe and a palpable fluctuant mass in the orbit. Headache, fever and leukocytosis are common.

Diagnosis

Blood and local cultures are mandatory. A CT scan can distinguish between preseptal and orbital cellulitis and show the site of an orbital or subperiosteal abscess:[64]

- preseptal cellulitis produces edema of the lids and tissues anterior to the orbital septum;
- orbital cellulitis produces edema of the orbital tissues and proptosis.

Orbital cellulitis is often associated with signs of primary or secondary sinus disease.

Staphylococcus and *Streptococcus* spp. and, in those under 4 years of age, *H. influenzae* are the main pathogens that cause preseptal and orbital cellulitis in children. In subperiosteal abscesses in children over 9 years of age and adults there is often a mixed infection of aerobes and anaerobes[65] from extending sinus or dental infections.

Management

Preseptal cellulitis responds well to systemic antibiotics. One or more broad-spectrum agents that cover *Staphylococcus* and *Streptococcus* spp. and *H. influenzae* should be used. A response is usual within 24 hours.

Orbital cellulitis requires prompt diagnosis and inpatient treatment with intravenous antibiotics. Monitoring of vision, pupillary reaction, extraocular movements and central nervous system function should be carried out during the first 1–2 days until the infection begins to resolve. If a subperiosteal abscess or sinusitis is identified and the clinical picture is not improving after 24 hours, surgical management is required. Orbital or brain abscesses are less common and should be drained immediately.

LACRIMAL SYSTEM INFECTIONS

Dacryoadenitis

Dacryoadenitis is usually due to a viral infection of the lacrimal gland. Patients present with adenopathy, fever, malaise and leukocytosis. The causes include infectious mononucleosis, herpes zoster, mumps, trachoma, syphilis, tuberculosis and sarcoidosis. Dacryoadenitis occasionally occurs in dehydrated patients as an ascending staphylococcal infection associated with a purulent discharge. On CT scanning there is diffuse lacrimal gland swelling without bony defects.

Diagnosis

The condition is usually self-limiting. Investigation other than CT scanning is reserved for chronic dacryoadenitis, and such patients should be referred for specialist investigation to exclude neoplasia.

Management

Treatment is generally symptomatic. Corticosteroids can help speed up resolution. It can be difficult to distinguish dacryoadenitis from idiopathic lacrimal gland inflammation (pseudotumor), although the presence of enlarged preauricular lymph nodes makes a viral diagnosis more likely.

Canaliculitis

There are chronic and acute forms. Acute dacryoadenitis may be caused by herpes simplex or herpes zoster and is often unrecognized except as a conjunctivitis and by its sequelae: scarred closed canaliculi and a punctum.

Chronic canaliculitis is usually unilateral and is characterized by pain or tenderness at the inner canthus. A chronic conjunctivitis may mask the more specific signs. The lacrimal punctum may pout and 'sulfur granules' may be expressed. These sulfur granules are pathognomonic of infection with *Actinomyces israelii*, an anaerobic Gram-positive branching filamentous bacterium. Less common causes are *Aspergillus* and *Candida* spp.

Treatment is by incision of the infected canaliculus and wash-out of all 'sulfur' material, usually with a penicillin-containing irrigation fluid.

Dacryocystitis

Pathogenesis and pathology

This condition occurs in chronic and acute forms. In infants it is usually an indolent condition resulting from incomplete development of the lacrimal drainage system. There is a mucopurulent discharge and recurrent conjunctivitis. Colonization is usual with *H. influenzae, Streptococcus pneumoniae,* staphylococci and *Klebsiella* and *Pseudomonas* spp. In adults an acquired blockage of the lacrimal drainage system can cause an acute or chronic infection. An acute infection can be precipitated by instrumentation for investigation of a suspected blocked lacrimal duct. For this reason, mucoceles or chronic dacryocystitis should not be probed or syringed. Acute dacryocystitis presents with a painful swelling over the lacrimal sac.

Treatment is with warm compresses and systemic antibiotics. A large abscess should be drained by a stab through the skin or inferior fornix conjunctiva. A dacryocystorhinostomy will prevent recurrence.

REFERENCES

References for this chapter can be found online at http://www.expertconsult.com

Michel Drancourt
Michael Whitby

Chapter | **16** |

Endophthalmitis

Endophthalmitis is fortunately an uncommon condition; however, it may result in severe visual impairment or loss of an eye.

EPIDEMIOLOGY

Definition and nomenclature

Endophthalmitis is an infection within the vitreous and may involve the cornea and, in severe cases, the sclera (panophthalmitis). A number of classifications of this condition have been published but from a practical point of view, categorization by the clinical setting, taking into account such factors as the events preceding infection and the time to diagnosis, is most appropriate. Categories include postoperative endophthalmitis (acute within 2 weeks of operation), delayed onset (more than 2 weeks after operation), conjunctival filtering bleb associated, post-traumatic endophthalmitis and endogenous endophthalmitis. Each of these subtypes may have characteristic clinical features and a spectrum of common causative pathogens (Table 16.1). This classification fits with the clinical classification of uveitis.[1]

Incidence and prevalence of endophthalmitis

Although recent eye surgery is the most common cause of endophthalmitis, accounting for more than 70% of cases, the incidence of infection after cataract extraction, the most commonly performed eye surgery, is very low, at 0.07–0.13%.[2,3] Endophthalmitis may occur after any other form of ocular surgery, but appears to be more common after glaucoma filtering procedures. Nontuberculous mycobacteria are emerging agents in this situation.[4] It has been estimated at 1:5233 consecutive bevacizumab intravitreal injections.[5]

Endophthalmitis after penetrating ocular trauma is common, representing 7–30% of all endophthalmitis cases; 3–26% of penetrating eye injuries develop infection. It is more common when trauma is associated with a retained intraocular foreign body or when the injury is contaminated with vegetable matter.[6] The leading organisms in this setting are staphylococci, especially *Staphylococcus aureus*, and *Bacillus* spp. Endogenous bacterial and fungal endophthalmitis are the least common forms, accounting for less than 2–8% of cases; they usually follow bloodstream spread of organisms and are commonly associated with a number of chronic medical conditions, such as diabetes mellitus, chronic renal failure, chronic immunosuppression, invasive medical procedures (including urinary catheterization and intravascular central lines) and intravenous drug abuse.

Table 16.1 Microbial etiology of endophthalmitis

Category of endophthalmitis		Common causative organisms
Postoperative	Acute	Coagulase-negative staphylococcus *Staphylococcus aureus* *Streptococcus* spp. Gram-negative bacilli *Pseudomonas* spp.
	Delayed	*Staphylococcus epidermidis* *Propionibacterium acnes* *Candida* spp.
	Filtering bleb	*Streptococcus* spp. *Haemophilus influenzae* *Staphylococcus aureus*
Post-traumatic	Bacterial	*Staphylococcus aureus*; other staph. spp. *Bacillus* spp. *Pseudomonas* spp. Other Gram-negative bacilli; anaerobes; corynebacteria; streptococci
	Fungal	*Penicillium* spp.; *Fusarium* spp.; *Acremonium* spp; other filamentous fungi
Endogenous	Bacterial	Enteric Gram-negative bacilli Fungi (including *Candida albicans*, *Aspergillus* spp.) *Streptococcus* spp.
	Fungal	Yeasts (*Candida albicans*, *Cryptococcus* spp.) Filamentous fungi (*Aspergillus* spp., *Acremonium* spp., *Fusarium* spp., *Paecilomyces* spp.)

PATHOGENESIS AND PATHOLOGY

Although a broad range of organisms can cause endophthalmitis, the most common causative infectious agents are bacteria. Virtually any bacterium, including those usually accepted as saprophytes, can cause infection, although members of the normal ocular microflora are the most commonly implicated.

Acute and delayed-onset postoperative endophthalmitis

Infecting organisms are usually introduced into the eye via incisions at the time of surgery. Nosocomial outbreaks of endophthalmitis caused by contaminated irrigation fluids, intraocular lenses and donor corneas have been recognized. Contaminated phacoemulsification probe was demonstrated as a source of nosocomial endophthalmitis following phacoemulsification cataract extraction surgery.[7] Infiltration of pathogens in the immediate postoperative period may be associated with inadequately buried sutures, suture removal or the presence of vitreous wicks.

In over 70% of cases, the pathogenic organism is a Gram-positive bacterium. *Staphylococcus epidermidis* and other coagulase-negative staphylococci are now the most frequently isolated bacteria from postsurgical endophthalmitis, representing 50–55% of all culture-positive cases.[8] *Staphylococcus aureus* and *Streptococcus* spp. are cultured from 10–30% of postoperative infections, whereas Gram-negative organisms, including *Pseudomonas* spp., *Proteus* spp. and *Citrobacter* spp., are implicated in only 7–20%. The change in prevalence of *Staph. epidermidis* probably represents, at least in part, a past failure to recognize coagulase-negative staphylococci as potential ocular pathogens.

Delayed-onset endophthalmitis is often caused by *Staph. epidermidis*, *Corynebacterium* spp. and *Candida* spp. A specific syndrome of chronic localized infection may occur with *Propionibacterium acnes*. Filtering bleb endophthalmitis is frequently caused by streptococci (60%) and *Haemophilus influenzae* (20%), although *Staph. aureus* remains a prominent pathogen.[9] Fungal endophthalmitis is usually observed as a cluster of cases caused by the use of contaminated irrigating solution,[10] intraocular lens,[11] ventilation system[12] and hospital construction activity[13] but sporadic cases have also been observed.[14] Postoperative fungal infection is very rare; a 27-case series has been observed over a 5-year period of time.[14] In this series, endophthalmitis was caused mainly by *Aspergillus* spp. with a median 10.5-day latent period.[14]

Post-traumatic endophthalmitis

Post-traumatic infection may be polymicrobial (10–40%), caused by anaerobic organisms, especially *Clostridium* spp. *Staph. aureus* remains a common agent, although saprophytes such as *Bacillus* spp., especially associated with intraocular foreign bodies, may induce fulminating endophthalmitis.[15] Spread of organisms through corneal abrasions and penetrating corneal ulcers, particularly those involving *Staph. aureus* or *Pseudomonas aeruginosa*, may lead to endophthalmitis.

Endogenous endophthalmitis

Endogenous infection may be associated with a recognizable infective focus elsewhere in the body and this may provide an indication as to the likely causative organism. Ocular involvement, however, may also be the first and only manifestation of systemic infection, particularly in the course of endocarditis. The diagnosis of endogenous endophthalmitis should prompt investigation (three blood cultures, serology for fastidious bacteria and echocardiography) to eliminate endocarditis.[16,17] More recently, *Streptococcus* spp. other than *Strep. pneumoniae*, *Staph. aureus* and Enterobacteriaceae from gastrointestinal sources have become more prominent.[18] Intravenous drug use may be associated with infection with *Candida* spp., *Aspergillus* spp. and *Bacillus cereus*, although more common pathogens, including *Staph. aureus*, may be involved. Exceptionally, late-onset endophthalmitis may develop after bacille Calmette–Guérin (BCG) immunotherapy for bladder carcinoma.[19] Other mycobacterial organisms are also exceptional, including *Mycobacterium haemophilium*.[20]

Fungal endophthalmitis

Fungal endophthalmitis may occur as exogenous or endogenous infection. After trauma, fungal endophthalmitis may represent up to 10% of cases, particularly if penetration with vegetable matter has occurred.[21]

Extension of a fungal corneal ulcer may also lead to endophthalmitis. Fungi most commonly identified in this situation are usually saprophytic and may include *Aspergillus* spp., *Fusarium* spp., *Acremonium* spp. and *Paecilomyces* spp.

Endogenous fungal endophthalmitis has been seen with increasing frequency over the past two decades, concurrent with an increased recognition of systemic fungal infections. *Candida albicans* is the most frequently reported causative agent after hematogenous dissemination from other infected body sites, particularly infected central venous catheters, and often in immunocompromised patients.[22] Direct intravenous inoculation as a result of narcotic abuse or contaminated infusion solutions has also been reported. Other fungi less commonly implicated in endogenous fungal endophthalmitis include *Cryptococcus neoformans*, *Aspergillus* spp. and *Paecilomyces* spp.

PREVENTION

The prevention of endophthalmitis is based on identification and pre-treatment of high-risk patients, and reduction in the conjunctival commensal flora.

Preoperative precautions

High-risk patients

Host factors that lower resistance to infection, such as chronic immunosuppression or diabetes mellitus, have been reported as significant risk factors for postoperative endophthalmitis. Reduction in immunosuppressive medications, when possible, and optimal control of blood glucose are essential in such groups. Pre-existing infection of external ocular tissue, for example chronic blepharitis, conjunctivitis and lacrimal outflow obstruction, should be identified and treated with appropriate topical antibiotics.

Antimicrobial prophylaxis

The aim of preventive treatment is to reduce eyelid and ocular surface microflora; this may be achieved by using topical antibiotics, topical antiseptic agents or subconjunctival antibiotics at the time of surgery.

Topical antibiotics

Although there is no consensus as to the optimal use of preoperative topical antibiotics in intraocular surgery, several studies have demonstrated significant falls in bacterial colonization of the conjunctiva with the application of topical antibiotics and have thus suggested a reduction in the incidence of postoperative endophthalmitis with the use of such antibiotics preoperatively. Topical antibiotics have been reported to be most effective in decreasing conjunctival bacterial colony counts when administered 2 hours before surgery.[23]

Until the early 1980s, gentamicin (3 mg/ml) was consistently found to be the most effective antibiotic in this situation compared with other agents such as chloramphenicol (5 mg/ml), bacitracin (10 mg/ml), neomycin (5 mg/ml) and polymixin (2.5 mg/ml).[24] However, the increase in gentamicin resistance among *Staph. epidermidis*, now the most common cause of postoperative endophthalmitis, suggests that it may no longer be the optimal agent for prophylaxis.[25] Vancomycin, when used prophylactically, has been shown to be active against staphylococci, but the potential risk of emerging resistance in enterococci and to a lesser extent in methicillin-resistant *Staph. aureus* has led some authorities to discourage this practice. Although no specific recommendations have been developed for ophthalmology, it seems appropriate to restrict the use of vancomycin to the treatment of, for example, serious keratitis, endophthalmitis or orbital cellulitis caused by β-lactam resistant Gram-positive organisms or alternatively to the treatment of enterococci and *Staph. aureus* in patients unable to tolerate β-lactam antibiotics. More recently, fluoroquinolones (all compounded at a concentration of 3 mg/ml) have been shown to be very effective in reducing conjunctival and eyelid bacterial flora when used preoperatively.[26]

Subconjunctival antimicrobials

Subconjunctival antibiotics can be administered after intraocular surgery based on the rationale that, at the completion of the ocular procedure, it is appropriate to inhibit growth of any bacteria that may have gained entry into the eye during surgery. During routine cataract surgery, aqueous fluid samples have been demonstrated to be culture positive in up to 43% of cases.[27] Conflicting results as to the value of this modality have been reported and penetration into the vitreous is relatively poor.

Topical antiseptics

Application of 5% aqueous povidone–iodine solution alone has been shown to be nontoxic and to decrease perioperative conjunctival bacterial colony counts and reduce the incidence of postoperative endophthalmitis significantly. In combination with topical antibiotics, povidone–iodine has been found to sterilize the conjunctiva in more than 80% of treated patients.[28]

Intraoperative precautions

Although the judicious use of preoperative antibiotics can reduce infection rates considerably, they do not replace meticulous aseptic technique in intraocular procedures. An appropriate operating room environment, with efficient ventilation to reduce bacterial contamination, is essential; surgical techniques should be modified to minimize entry of ocular surface microbes into the eye during the surgical procedure, and adhesive-backed plastic drapes to isolate the eyelids and lashes from the operative field are recommended.

Implantation of intraocular lenses with prolene haptics appears to increase the risk of endophthalmitis, probably because coagulase-negative staphylococci bind well to this particular plastic. Binding to polymethylmethacrylate material is less, and therefore its use may reduce risk.[29] Care must be taken to minimize contact with the external eye during insertion of an intraocular lens to prevent contamination with conjunctival flora. A foldable lens insertion device has been developed to facilitate this. There is always the threat of infection from personnel and equipment in the operating room, and from contaminated irrigation solutions.

CLINICAL FEATURES

Clinical signs of endophthalmitis vary greatly depending on the preceding events, the nature of the infecting organism, the degree of tissue inflammation and the duration of disease. Early diagnosis requires the maintenance of a high index of suspicion as classic features of infection may be absent.

Acute postoperative endophthalmitis

Acute postoperative endophthalmitis usually occurs within 2 weeks of surgery, whereas the presentation of infection after penetrating trauma will often be more rapid. As a general principle, the more rapid the onset of symptoms, the more virulent the organism, with *Staph. aureus*, *Streptococcus pyogenes*, *Bacillus* spp. and Gram-negative bacilli being implicated in very rapid onset of infection within 24–72 hours of surgery. This presentation is characterized by marked anterior chamber inflammation, by the rapid development of a fibrinous anterior chamber exudate with hypopyon (which produces severe pain, more prominent than general postoperative discomfort) and by a progressive decrease in visual acuity. A marked vitreous inflammatory reaction, often obscuring visualization of the retina, frequently follows (Figs 16.1–16.3). Associated features may include marked conjunctival, lid and corneal edema, but systemic features are virtually never seen.

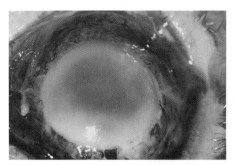

Fig. 16.1 Corneal edema and fibrinous anterior chamber exudate in a traumatic foreign body-induced endophthalmitis. Any posterior vitreal or retinal view is obscured by the anterior corneal and aqueous haze.

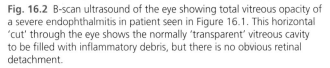

Fig. 16.2 B-scan ultrasound of the eye showing total vitreous opacity of a severe endophthalmitis in patient seen in Figure 16.1. This horizontal 'cut' through the eye shows the normally 'transparent' vitreous cavity to be filled with inflammatory debris, but there is no obvious retinal detachment.

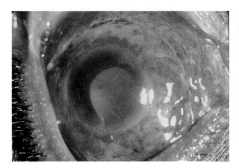

Fig. 16.3 A dense vitreous abscess in advanced endophthalmitis. This partially treated postoperative endophthalmitis has vitreous cellular and protein deposits obscuring the retinal view.

Delayed-onset postoperative endophthalmitis

Delayed-onset endophthalmitis has a more insidious course and frequently overlaps with acute postoperative endophthalmitis if less virulent organisms are implicated. Symptoms may not manifest until weeks or even months after surgery, although early mild clinical features with progressive worsening over time are not uncommon (Fig. 16.4). When delayed-onset endophthalmitis is caused by *P. acnes*, it usually develops months after cataract extraction; patients will often have a history of corticosteroid-responsive postoperative inflammation with a fluctuating course over many months. The most common clinical signs are posterior capsular deposits and chronic iridocyclitis.[30]

Fungal infection may also have a delayed clinical onset. Anterior chamber reaction is seen with progressive white infiltrates, often adherent to the iris and posterior corneal surface (Figs 16.5, 16.6). Fluffy white fungal ball infiltrates ('string of pearls') occurring in the vitreous are characteristic (Fig. 16.7). Patients who have chronic postoperative endophthalmitis caused by coagulase-negative staphylococci may present with a hypopyon and diffuse vitritis, which occasionally obscures the view of the fundus. Visual loss is usually more severe than that in endophthalmitis caused by *P. acnes* or fungi.

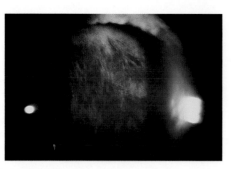

Fig. 16.4 The typical posterior capsular opacities seen in a late-onset *Staphylococcus epidermidis* endophthalmitis. These deposits are actual coccal colonies, which are frequently removed at subsequent vitrectomy surgery to open up the capsular bag to intraocular antibiotics.

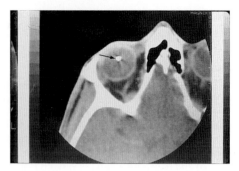

Fig. 16.8 Horizontal CT scan section of eye seen in Figures 16.1 and 16.2 revealing a metallic intraocular foreign body in the vitreous cavity (arrow). This CT scan demonstrates that the vitreous opacity seen by ultrasound is 'invisible' to this investigation.

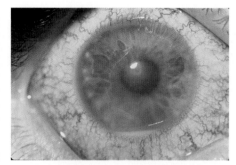

Fig. 16.5 A 'quiet' endogenous fungal endophthalmitis with small hypopyon. This eye is relatively quiet with little chemosis, injection or pain, but has a small hypopyon and some small fungal 'balls' on the temporal iris.

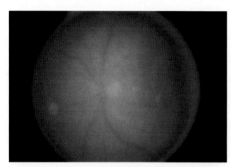

Fig. 16.6 The degraded ophthalmoscopic retinal view obtained in the patient seen in Figure 16.5. The corneal edema and anterior chamber activity make vitreous and retinal observation difficult.

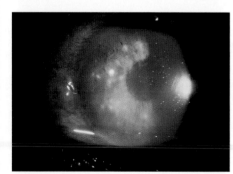

Fig. 16.7 Fungal 'fluff balls' on the iris seen in a fungal endophthalmitis. Although these are not pathognomonic, their appearance raises the real possibility that the infection is of fungal origin.

Filtering bleb endophthalmitis

A conjunctival filtering bleb is a collection of fluid under the conjunctiva resulting from the formation of a fistula at operation through the sclera from the anterior chamber in an endeavor to reduce pressure in the anterior chamber. Endophthalmitis associated with a conjunctival filtering bleb is actually an acute presentation of endophthalmitis, but may occur months to years after the operation with rapid development of symptoms. Intraocular spread occurs from an initial bacterial penetration through the mucosa of the bleb, often in association with bacterial conjunctivitis. Infection is often associated with late bleb leakage and is facilitated by antimetabolites (e.g. 5-FU or mitomycin) used to ensure bleb survival.[6] A purulent discharge and an injected bleb are commonly seen, ultimately in association with typical signs of endophthalmitis. Viridans streptococci, *H. influenzae*, *Staph. aureus* and *Moraxella* spp.[31] are commonly implicated.

Post-traumatic endophthalmitis

Presentation will vary depending on the nature and severity of the ocular trauma or the type of retained foreign body, for example steel or vegetable matter, and the virulence and concentration of the organism initially deposited into the intraocular tissues (Fig. 16.8). The more virulent this organism, including *Staph. aureus* and *B. cereus*, the more rapid the onset of pain and associated ophthalmic features of infection. *B. cereus*, fungi and to a lesser extent *Nocardia* spp. and atypical mycobacteria should be considered when injury to the eye is related to plant or vegetable matter.[32]

Endogenous endophthalmitis

Endogenous endophthalmitis usually has an insidious onset with a slow decrease in visual acuity caused by vitritis and localized areas of chorioretinitis. It may be suspected when other systemic symptoms of infection are present or in certain groups of patients, including those in whom bacteremia or fungemia is common, such as those with infective endocarditis and those with intravascular or urinary catheters, or patients who abuse intravenous drugs. Rarely, a fungal endophthalmitis, with a predilection for *Paecilomyces* infection, may occur in otherwise healthy individuals with no antecedent trauma.[33]

Differential diagnosis

The differential diagnosis of postoperative inflammation includes sterile uveitis related to retained lens cortex; operative complications such as vitreous loss, hemorrhage and iris trauma; pre-existing uveitis; and toxicity of foreign material such as irrigation solutions introduced during surgery. These presentations are often difficult to distinguish from similar symptoms caused by infective endophthalmitis and careful sequential monitoring of such eyes or intraocular sampling for culture is appropriate to facilitate early diagnosis and treatment.

DIAGNOSIS

Microbiologic investigations in endophthalmitis

Confirmation of the diagnosis of infective endophthalmitis is essential to rational management. Because most postoperative infections are caused by normal ocular flora, there is some correlation between the results of external swabs of the eyelid margins and conjunctivae with intraocular isolates.[34] These should not be used to determine causative pathogens; routine preoperative cultures have a low predictive value and are not recommended. The optimal specimen for laboratory processing in endophthalmitis is an intraocular aspirate; aqueous and vitreous specimens should be obtained, although the latter appears more reliable, as some 30–55% of concomitant aqueous specimens are negative in the presence of positive vitreous isolates.[35] In the case of late endophthalmitis, aqueous vitreous and some capsule material should also be cultured. Foreign bodies should be processed in traumatic endophthalmitis, whereas a swab of the bleb may assist in bleb-associated infections.

Because specimen volumes are often very limited, the traditional approach of direct inoculation onto culture media for aerobic and anaerobic bacteria and fungi remains important. Rapid results by microscopy of Gram stains are useful, with positive results occurring in some 50–70% of well-collected vitreous aspirates.[36] An appropriate clinical history should accompany specimens to the laboratory so that culture can be prolonged for fastidious organisms and so that skin commensals such as *P. acnes* are not routinely discarded as contaminants.

Polymerase chain reaction (PCR)-based detection of the 16S rRNA gene for detection of bacteria, and of the 18S rRNA gene for the detection of fungi, are of great help in the diagnosis of endophthalmitis.[37–40] These techniques are particularly helpful when the patient received intraocular antibiotic/antifungal treatment prior to intraocular sampling.[41] Previous methods based on the analysis of restriction profile[42] are now being replaced by direct sequencing of the PCR product.[40,41] Because of the high risk of contamination, nested PCR[37] should be replaced by real-time PCR, targeting specific pathogens such as *Neisseria meningitidis*.[43]

MANAGEMENT

Antibiotic chemotherapy

Early institution of antimicrobial therapy is essential to optimal outcome in the management of infective endophthalmitis. Controversy continues as to the best therapeutic approach.

Intravitreal antibiotics

Intravitreal injection of antibiotics is the most effective way of rapidly achieving high intraocular antibiotic levels. Direct intravitreal injections of nonpreserved (i.e. intravenous) formulations of antibiotics are now the recommended route of administration in endophthalmitis treatment. The rationale of such therapy is that, although antibiotics when administered topically, subconjunctivally or systemically may attain therapeutic concentrations in the anterior chamber, concentrations in the vitreous are much lower. Intravitreal injections may produce significant retinal toxicity, although single injections have been shown to be safe and effective.

The optimal combination of antibiotics in empiric therapy normally covers Gram-positive and Gram-negative organisms. Over recent years, vancomycin has replaced first-generation cephalosporins for Gram-positive activity because of the increasing incidence of *Staph. epidermidis* infection resistant to methicillin and other β-lactam drugs. Reports of retinal toxicity caused by gentamicin led to the use of amikacin to cover Gram-negative organisms, as this latter antibiotic was believed to be less toxic. Amikacin has now been used widely in controlled and uncontrolled clinical situations. However, more recently, gentamicin and amikacin have been associated with macular infarction[44] and this has led to increased use of other broad-spectrum Gram-negative antimicrobial agents, particularly ceftazidime. An initial single injection of 0.2 mg vancomycin maintains therapeutic concentration for at least 3 days and a repeat injection at that time for at least 4 days.[45] Repeat injections of aminoglycosides should be avoided,

except in severe cases. Intravitreal amphotericin B injections (1–5 µg) can be utilized in fungal endophthalmitis, with a single repeat inoculation after 72–96 hours in progressive infection; again, however, toxicity limits longer duration of therapy.

Subconjunctival antibiotics

The data regarding subconjunctival antibiotic penetration are conflicting, possibly because of varying degrees of inflammation in the eye or poor and variable sampling techniques. Penetration is affected by the transscleral and transcorneal permeability of the agent, but high aqueous levels can be achieved with vancomycin, gentamicin and β-lactam antibiotics for up to 4 hours; however, vitreous concentrations are generally poor. Subconjunctival injections are an irritant and are painful, thus limiting the duration of this form of therapy to a few days.

Topical antibiotic therapy

The efficacy of topical antibacterial applications in endophthalmitis is not well studied, although significant concentrations of antibiotics in the anterior segment can be obtained with frequent administration of highly concentrated (fortified) solutions. A combination of vancomycin and fortified gentamicin (e.g. 1.5%) provides broad-spectrum cover, but solutions must be prepared by a qualified pharmacist as they are not commercially available. Third-generation cephalosporins (such as cefotaxime and ceftazidime) and fluoroquinolones (such as ciprofloxacin) may be used to replace gentamicin to provide appropriate Gram-negative cover. The use of collagen shields to produce frequent topical application of antibiotic solutions has been explored, but is limited by potential corneal toxicity. Iontophoresis also increases anterior chamber concentrations, but its efficacy remains unproved.

Systemic antibiotics

In humans, intraocular penetration of systemically administered antibiotics is generally poor. However, intravenous antibiotics are a common adjunctive therapy in endophthalmitis, justified in that they may enhance concentrations of antibiotics achieved with intravitreal agents and extend the duration of therapeutic activity. Intraocular inflammation and/or performance of a vitrectomy may alter the blood–retina barrier to allow improved intraocular penetration.

Posterior chamber concentrations of newer and broad-spectrum agents, including ceftazidime, imipenem and ciprofloxacin, appear improved, particularly in terms of efficacy against Gram-negative bacilli such as *Pseudomonas* spp. However, none is reliably active against *Staph. epidermidis*, the most common cause of postoperative endophthalmitis, and resistance may develop rapidly.

A multicenter randomized trial, the Endophthalmitis Vitrectomy Study (EVS), sponsored by the National Eye Institute of the National Institutes of Health, followed a cohort of 420 patients who had clinical evidence of endophthalmitis within 6 weeks after cataract surgery or secondary intraocular lens implantation.[24] Patients were randomly assigned to therapy, with or without pars plana vitrectomy and with or without systemic antibiotics (ceftazidime and amikacin), but each patient underwent intravitreal injection of vancomycin and amikacin. When outcome was assessed 9–12 months after the operation, no difference in final visual acuity or media clouding between groups with and without systemic antibiotics could be determined. Well conducted as this study was, a number of questions remain unanswered, particularly in relation to generalization of the results. Do the results, for example, extrapolate to Gram-negative infection or to other categories of ocular surgery? Moreover, a significant percentage of coagulase-negative staphylococci and *Streptococcus* spp., the most common Gram-positive pathogens, are resistant to ceftazidime and amikacin, although vancomycin was active against all.

Duration of therapy is very variable. In spite of the presence of an ocular foreign body such as an intraocular lens, endophthalmitis caused by *Staph. epidermidis* will settle rapidly with appropriate management.

Length of therapy can be assessed by a reduction in cellular activity in both the anterior and posterior chambers and by improvement in visual acuity.

Guidelines have been published for the treatment of fungal endophthalmitis.[46] Itraconazole, a lipophilic antifungal imidazole, has been shown to be efficacious in *Aspergillus* endophthalmitis. Fluconazole, a hydrophilic imidazole, achieves useful concentrations in intraocular tissue and has also proved successful in *Candida* endophthalmitis. Voriconazole, a newer broad-spectrum antifungal with intraocular penetration, has been used successfully.[46,47] Amphotericin B, often the only available therapy in filamentous fungal infections other than those caused by *Aspergillus* spp., does not achieve significant concentrations in intraocular tissue. Nevertheless, it is widely used in both conventional and liposomal formulations in fungal endophthalmitis with some evidence of success.

Specific recommendations

Endophthalmitis may cause irreparable visual loss within 24–48 hours. Initial therapy must frequently be empiric, because of the low sensitivity of Gram stain film and the 24–48 hour delay until culture results become available. Antibiotic therapy should be chosen to cover the spectrum of pathogens likely to be implicated. In this situation classification of endophthalmitis by clinical setting provides useful information. Suggested initial antibiotic therapy for acute postoperative, filtering bleb and post-traumatic endophthalmitis is illustrated in Table 16.2.

Localized bleb infection without endophthalmitis can usually be managed initially with topical therapy. Because of the increased prevalence of *H. influenzae* in this infection, a combination of antibiotics that covers this pathogen and provides broad-spectrum activity against Gram-positive and Gram-negative organisms should be chosen. New combinations have been recently reviewed.[48]

Adjunctive therapy

Vitrectomy

The place of pars plana vitrectomy remains a controversial issue in the management of endophthalmitis. The theoretic rationale for such a procedure is that it offers a reduction in organism load, a reduction in traction effect on the retina with less potential for detachment, collection of adequate culture material and possibly improved distribution of intravitreal antibiotics. Evidence for its efficacy has been conflicting, often as a result of poorly controlled studies. The EVS was designed to determine definitively the value of vitrectomy in the presence of intravitreal antibiotics. The final conclusions of this study were that visual acuity was improved significantly in patients treated with vitrectomy only if the initial vision was light perception, but not if initial vision was hand movements or better; that is, the most severe cases on presentation benefited most from vitrectomy.[49]

Corticosteroids

The use of corticosteroids to reduce the inflammatory response to infection and thus preserve ocular tissue is widely practiced with administration by several routes, including intraocular, periocular, topical and systemic, but its place in therapy remains contentious. Experimental animal studies demonstrate superior outcomes utilizing corticosteroids with antibiotics even in endophthalmitis caused by pseudomonads and fungi. In general, clinical studies do not report deterioration in outcomes if corticosteroids are used in combination with antibiotics, at least at the ocular level.[50]

Management of intraocular lens

In most cases of acute postoperative pseudophakic endophthalmitis, removal of the intraocular lens is not necessary and does not influence outcome. In fact, it may be hazardous and predispose to anterior

Table 16.2 Initial empiric recommendations for antimicrobial therapy of endophthalmitis*

Category of endophthalmitis		ANTIMICROBIAL THERAPY		
		Topical	Intravitreal	Systemic
Postoperative	Acute	Cefazolin (5 mg/ml) + gentamicin (8–15 mg/ml) or amikacin (25–50 mg/ml) Vancomycin (50 mg/ml) + gentamicin or amikacin or ceftazidime (5 mg/ml) or ciprofloxacin (3 mg/ml)	Cefazolin (2.25 mg) + amikacin (400 μg) Vancomycin (1 mg) + amikacin or ceftazidime (2.25 mg)	Cefazolin (2 g q8h) + gentamicin (4–5 mg/kg q24h)† or amikacin (15 mg/kg q24h)† Vancomycin + gentamicin or amikacin or ceftazidime (2 g q8h) or ciprofloxacin (400 mg q12h)
	Delayed	Vancomycin + gentamicin or amikacin or ceftazidime or ciprofloxacin	Vancomycin + amikacin or ceftazidime	Vancomycin + gentamicin or amikacin or cefotaxime (2 g q6h) or ceftazidime or ciprofloxacin
	Filtering bleb	Vancomycin + ceftazidime or ciprofloxacin	Vancomycin + ceftazidime	Vancomycin +/or cefotaxime, ceftazidime, ciprofloxacin
Post-traumatic		Vancomycin + gentamicin or amikacin or ceftazidime or ciprofloxacin	Vancomycin + amikacin or ceftazidime	Vancomycin + gentamicin or amikacin or ceftazidime or ciprofloxacin

*Dosages given in brackets apply to all citations of each specific drug within the relevant column.
†Dosages must be adjusted to reflect the patient's age, body weight and renal function.

segment hemorrhage and retinal detachment. Exceptions may occur when the pathogen is a fungus and in cases of late-onset endophthalmitis caused by *P. acnes* when conservative treatment with intravitreal vancomycin and corticosteroids is unsuccessful. In such cases, complete capsulectomy and lensectomy may be necessary to provide cure.

Outcome

Up to 50% of patients who have endophthalmitis suffer major visual loss within 24–48 hours of onset, emphasizing the essential need for early diagnosis and prompt treatment.[50] Approximately 30% of patients in recent studies of endophthalmitis achieved a final visual acuity of 20/60 or better after treatment.[51,52]

Certain factors are highly correlated with poor visual outcome; these include severity of infection, delay in time to diagnosis and institution of treatment, virulence of infecting organisms and intraocular complications such as vitreous hemorrhage and retinal detachment. Poor vision at the time of diagnosis correlates with either a virulent organism, such as *Bacillus* spp., *Streptococcus* spp. or Gram-negative bacilli or fungi, or a delay in diagnosis even with a low-virulence organism. Normally, however, *Staph. epidermidis* endophthalmitis has an excellent outcome, although even in this situation some 10% of patients develop blindness.[53] Culture-negative cases of endophthalmitis generally have a better visual outcome than do culture-positive groups, which may relate to the lower virulence of more fastidious organisms or to the veracity of diagnosis.

The outcome of post-traumatic endophthalmitis and endophthalmitis related to a conjunctival filtering bleb is poor, probably because of the intrinsic virulence of organisms implicated; however, for converse reasons, prognosis in delayed ophthalmitis, including that caused by *P. acnes*, is usually more favorable.

The primary complication of endophthalmitis is retinal detachment that may occur at any time before, during or after treatment. Prognosis in this situation is poor, although surgical repair can salvage useful vision in a substantial number of patients.[54]

REFERENCES

References for this chapter can be found online at http://www.expertconsult.com

Infectious retinitis and uveitis

INTRODUCTION

Strictly speaking, uveitis is inflammation of any etiology in one or more parts of the uveal tract of the eye which includes the choroid, the iris and the ciliary body. In practice, however, uveitis has come to mean any inflammation of the intraocular structures. Inflammation localized to certain structures can be denoted by more specific terms. For example, inflammation of the iris (iritis) or ciliary body (cyclitis) is called anterior uveitis. Inflammation of the vitreous (vitritis), retina (retinitis) or choroid (choroiditis) is called posterior uveitis. Inflammation of the entire globe is called panuveitis. Inflammation localized to the outer coats of the eye or optic nerve without accompanying intraocular inflammation (e.g. scleritis, keratitis, optic neuritis) is not considered a uveitis.

The anterior segment of the eye consists of the cornea, anterior chamber, lens, iris, posterior chamber and ciliary body; the posterior segment refers to the vitreous cavity and posterior structures including the retina and optic nerve (Fig. 17.1).

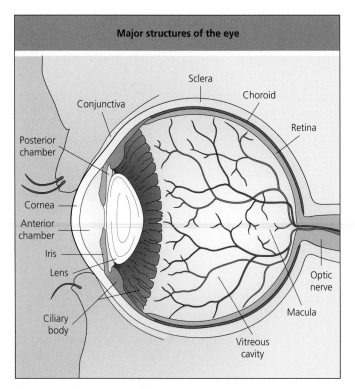

Major structures of the eye

Sclera

Choroid

Conjunctiva

Retina

Posterior chamber

Cornea

Anterior chamber

Iris

Lens

Optic nerve

Macula

Ciliary body

Vitreous cavity

Fig. 17.1 Major structures of the eye.

The location, distribution and ophthalmoscopic appearance of inflammatory lesions is useful to the ophthalmologist in suggesting likely causes of uveitis (Table 17.1).[1] Intermediate uveitis centers about the equator of the eye between the anterior and posterior parts of the uveal tract, whereas anterior uveitis involves the anterior chamber and posterior uveitis involves the posterior segment of the eye.

A diagnosis of retinal vasculitis is made by finding inflammatory sheathing of the retinal vessels on ophthalmoscopic examination and leakage of dye from the involved vessels on intravenous fluorescein angiography (Fig. 17.2).[1] Retinal vasculitis is sometimes isolated, but more commonly occurs in conjunction with posterior uveitis. It is a nonspecific finding and can occur in ischemic conditions as well as infection. Endophthalmitis, although overlapping to some degree with uveitis and retinitis, is considered separately (see Chapter 16).

There are many known causes of uveitis, including infections, autoimmune disorders, various other systemic diseases and trauma. Many cases of uveitis remain of uncertain origin despite extensive investigation. In trying to determine the cause of any particular case of uveitis, the ophthalmologist considers a number of features, including the distribution and morphologic characteristics of the lesions, the chronicity of the disorder and the presence of underlying systemic diseases. In select cases, invasive diagnostic testing in the form of anterior chamber paracentesis, vitreous biopsy or even retinal biopsy may be necessary to rule out an infectious etiology.

This chapter describes the major manifestations of uveitis and retinitis, with an emphasis on the infectious causes of these syndromes. Uveitis and retinitis in immunosuppressed patients and neonates are considered separately because the causative agents differ from those in immunocompetent and adult patients. Only the infectious aspects pertinent to the eye will be discussed.

EPIDEMIOLOGY

Uveitis and retinitis are uncommon in clinical practice. In Minnesota, USA, the annual incidence of new cases of uveitis has been found to be 17/100 000 population,[2] though it has been estimated that in the Western world uveitis accounts for approximately 10% of the visual handicap.[3] Typically, a general ophthalmologist is likely to see only a dozen patients with uveitis each year. The majority are anatomically 'anterior uveitis', accounting for 50–60% of all uveitis cases in a tertiary care center and 90% in primary care settings.[4] A specific etiology can be identified in only about half of the patients with uveitis. In some instances, uveitis provides the first evidence of an underlying systemic disease. HLA-B27 and its associated seronegative spondyloarthropathies are the most commonly identifiable causes of anterior uveitis in the Western world.[5] Uveitis and retinitis can occur at any age and the incidence is about equally divided between the sexes. In one study, the mean age of patients with uveitis was 45 years.[1]

Table 17.1 Anterior, intermediate and posterior uveitis. Definitions and common symptoms.

	Anterior uveitis	Intermediate uveitis	Posterior uveitis
Ophthalmoscopic signs that define the type of uveitis	Inflammatory cells in the anterior chamber with or without keratic precipitates or iris lesions	Inflammatory cells more highly concentrated in anterior vitreous than in anterior chamber	Inflammation of retina, choroid, retinal vessels, posterior vitreous humor, or a combination of these
Additional clinical signs	Ciliary flush (perilimbal injection of the sclera) Posterior synechiae	Macular edema Inflammatory exudate on pars plana	Retinal vasculitis Optic disk edema Macular edema
Symptoms	Pain Redness Photophobia	Floaters	'Floaters' Blurred vision

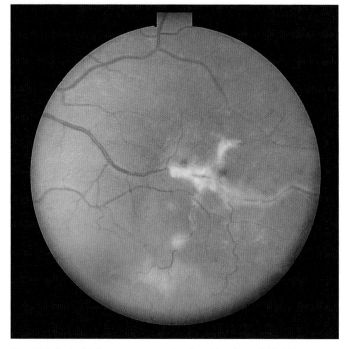

Fig. 17.2 Retinal inflammatory vascular sheathing (vasculitis). This case occurred secondary to sarcoidosis.

Infectious uveitis or retinitis in neonates is almost always the result of congenital infection – toxoplasmosis, rubella, cytomegalovirus (CMV), herpesvirus (i.e. the TORCH syndrome, see Chapter 52). Each of the TORCH agents can involve the uvea or retina. Among immunosuppressed patients, uveitis or retinitis is found most commonly in patients who have AIDS. However, hematogenous fungal endophthalmitis occurs primarily in patients with other forms of immunosuppression.

Although uveitis does not appear to be more prevalent in any particular part of the world, there is geographic variation in the underlying causes. For example:

- acquired ocular toxoplasmosis is quite common in Brazil, but rare in the rest of the world;
- Behçet's disease is prevalent in Turkey and the Middle East, but unusual elsewhere;
- leprosy has been eradicated in most developed countries, but can still be found in less developed regions;
- human T-cell lymphotropic virus type-1 (HTLV-1)-associated uveitis is commonly found in Japan;
- CMV retinitis associated with AIDS and a CMV-associated vitritis secondary to highly active antiretroviral therapy (HAART) occurs in patients from developed countries but is rarely seen in developing areas of the world; and

- onchocerciasis (river blindness), which primarily affects the cornea, but can produce retinitis and choroiditis, is seen only in equatorial Africa and Central America.

CLINICAL FEATURES

Common symptoms of intraocular inflammation, irrespective of the cause, are ocular pain, photophobia, 'floaters' (specks that appear to float in the visual field) and impaired vision (see Table 17.1). Both eyes may be affected simultaneously, but unilateral involvement does not rule out a systemic cause. Anyone with these symptoms should have an ophthalmologic evaluation with pharmacologic dilatation of the pupil with examination by slit lamp and indirect ophthalmoscopy. The findings allow the process to be characterized as anterior, intermediate or posterior uveitis, or panuveitis (see Table 17.1).

Additional clinical signs include conjunctival injection, anterior segment cells and 'flare' (protein floating in aqueous fluid, seen on slit lamp examination), keratic precipitates (white cells adherent to the posterior cornea), iris nodules (granulomas), posterior synechiae, posterior segment cells (Fig. 17.3), optic disk edema, retinal vasculitis, retinitis and choroiditis. A hypopyon refers to layered inflammatory

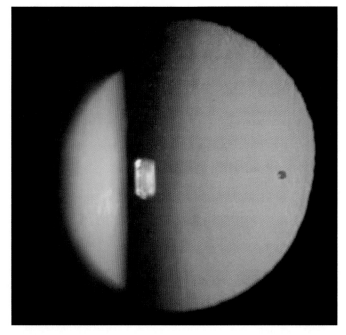

Fig. 17.3 A retroillumination view through the dilated pupil highlights the inflammatory cells suspended in the vitreous.

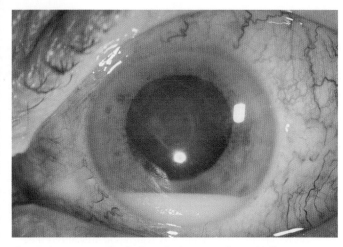

Fig. 17.4 Hypopyon. The finding of a hypopyon (layered inflammatory cells in the anterior chamber of the eye) usually denotes a severe anterior uveitis.

center only 50–60% of uveitis was anterior, with posterior uveitis and panuveitis significantly more prevalent.[4] In both settings, a specific diagnosis could be made in only about half of patients from data gathered at the initial visit. An infectious cause was documented in 21% of the referred patients and 14% of the community-based patients. The uveitis was attributed to a systemic disease, usually rheumatologic, in a smaller number of patients. The most common causes of uveitis in both settings were:

- HLA-B27-associated anterior uveitis;
- CMV retinitis;
- herpesvirus-associated uveitis, caused either by herpes simplex virus (HSV) or varicella-zoster virus (VZV); and
- *Toxoplasma* retinochoroiditis (see Table 17.2).

Thus, three of the four most common identified causes of uveitis were infectious, but infectious causes accounted for well under half of all cases of uveitis in either setting. Anterior uveitis is much more common than posterior uveitis, and the specific cause is more likely to be identifiable.

PATHOGENESIS AND PATHOLOGY

Most of the infectious agents discussed in this chapter gain access to the ocular structures via hematogenous spread of micro-organisms from other sites. The uveal tract is highly vascular, offering a ready target for seeding by blood-borne microbes. Some organisms (e.g. herpesviruses, *T. gondii*) have a propensity for the retina itself. Furthermore, circulating inflammatory cells and mediators of inflammation have a potent impact on the uveal tract and adjacent structures. In some types of infectious uveitis (e.g. tuberculous and possibly spirochetal uveitis), the inflammation may be produced by a combination of microbial

cells that settle gravitationally in the inferior aspect of the anterior chamber (Fig. 17.4). In cases of severe acute uveitis, there may be so much intraocular inflammation that a cloudy media results. Ocular ultrasonography should be performed in such cases.

The characteristic causes and clinical presentations of uveitis seen in a general community-based ophthalmologic practice and in a tertiary referral center have been found to differ (Table 17.2).[1] In the community ophthalmic practice, about 90% of uveitis was anterior and most cases of anterior uveitis were acute. By contrast, in the tertiary referral

Table 17.2 Uveitis in community-based and tertiary ophthalmology centers*		
	Patients in community-based ophthalmology practice	**Patients in tertiary referral center**
Mean age of patients (y)	46	45
Males (%)	49	52

Percentage with:
  Anterior uveitis
  Intermediate uveitis
  Posterior uveitis
  Panuveitis and other
	
	91
	1
	5
	3
		
		60
		12
		15
		13

Percentage of cases of anterior uveitis that are chronic	9	63
Percentage in which specific diagnosis was made	47	58
Percentage attributable to infection	14	21
Percentage associated with systemic disease (including infections)	13	9
Most common causes of uveitis	HLA-B27-associated anterior uveitis (15%) CMV retinitis (7%) Traumatic uveitis (5%) VZV uveitis (4%) *Toxoplasma* retinochoroiditis (4%)	CMV retinitis (33%) HLA-B27-associated anterior uveitis (8%) Pars planitis syndrome (6%) HSV-associated uveitis (5%) *Toxoplasma* retinochoroiditis (4%)
Most common causes of posterior uveitis	CMV retinitis *Toxoplasma* retinochoroiditis	CMV retinitis *Toxoplasma* retinochoroiditis

*The characteristics of uveitis seen in a community-based ophthalmology practice and in a tertiary referral center. The figures for the proportion of cases in which a specific diagnosis was made are based on data gathered at, or requested at, the first visit; cases of CMV retinitis and 'masquerade' syndrome are omitted. The figures for the proportion of cases associated with systemic disease include cases due to varicella, candidiasis, coccidioidomycosis and syphilis. Data from McCannel *et al*.[1]

invasion and immunologic mechanisms. Occasionally, uveitis occurs as a 'sympathetic' reaction to an adjacent infection (e.g. anterior uveitis in patients with HSV keratitis). It is hypothesized that other infections gain access to the eye by spreading along nerves, such as the acute retinal necrosis (ARN) syndrome associated with VZV.

The eye is unique among organs in showing a neovascular response to certain stimuli, especially prolonged inflammation. New vessels may form in the cornea, iris, retina, optic nerve and choroid, presumably as a result of the production of various protein growth factors such as vascular endothelial growth factor (VEGF). These newly formed, acquired vessels themselves can cause severe loss of vision. Together with specific treatment of the underlying cause, laser photocoagulation, corticosteroids or intravitreal injection with anti-VEGF agents may be needed to treat ocular neovascularization.[6]

PREVENTION

Patients who have systemic infections associated with an appreciable risk of intraocular infection should be screened by an ophthalmologist for early detection and treatment. An example is the periodic examination of patients who have HIV infection and a low CD4+ lymphocyte count to detect CMV retinitis. Likewise, patients who have HIV infection who develop ophthalmic zoster are at risk of developing necrotizing herpetic retinitis and are candidates for ophthalmologic screening examination. Patients who have *Candida* fungemia merit ocular examination to detect metastatic retinitis. Neonates who have congenital HSV infection must be screened carefully for ocular lesions, which may first appear up to several months after birth.

MOLECULAR DIAGNOSTICS

Molecular diagnostic techniques are playing an increasing role in the care of infectious uveitis and retinitis. The polymerase chain reaction (PCR) was first used to identify *T. gondii* DNA in ocular tissue in 1990.[7] Since then PCR of intraocular fluids has been utilized in the diagnosis of HSV, VZV, CMV, fungi (including *Fusarium*, *Candida* and *Aspergillus*) mycobacteria, protozoal eye disease and infectious bacterial endophthalmitis.[8] PCR is considered a helpful diagnostic adjunct, particularly when sample sizes are small and inadequate for culture, complementing other diagnostic processes including enzyme-linked

immunosorbent assay (ELISA), cytology and culture. Protocol refinement, including the use of a nested PCR protocol followed by restriction enzyme digestion, has led to the amplification and characterization of diverse mycobacterial species. It has also been used to identify immunoglobulin H rearrangements in lymphomatous uveitis. More recently 16s ribosomal DNA typing has been employed to identify bacteria in vitreous samples.[9] Internal transcribed spacer 1 (ITS1) and ITS2 5.8S ribosomal DNA typing has also been used to diagnose fungal endophthalmitis.[10] Most microbiologic techniques have difficulty identifying active disease. Reverse transcription PCR (RT-PCR) techniques hold promised for identifying active versus latent infections.

MANAGEMENT

There are two major principles of therapy for intraocular infections. The first is to treat the infection. Drugs for the treatment of ocular diseases may be given by topical administration, periocular injection, systemic administration (orally or intravenously, or both) and intravitreal injection.

The second principle is to suppress intraocular inflammation, lest there be persisting damage to the retina and other crucial structures. This is usually accomplished by using corticosteroids, which may be given by similar topical, oral, periocular or intravitreal routes. Rarely systemic immunosuppression is employed.

Uveitis in immunocompetent adults and children

Viral causes of uveitis

Uveitis, especially anterior uveitis, may occur in the course of many viral infections, most commonly those caused by rubeola virus and the herpesvirus family (Table 17.3). The uveitis is generally self-limited and does not require treatment.

Measles often causes conjunctivitis and keratitis; the keratitis rarely leads to bacterial ulceration and perforation of the cornea. Other rare complications are chorioretinitis or neuroretinitis; these may occur, together with measles encephalitis, 1–2 weeks after the onset of the rash.

The ocular lesions of rubeola are generally self-limited and no specific treatment is available. Involvement of the optic disk (optic neuritis)

Table 17.3 Viral causes of retinitis and uveitis*

Viral infection	Systemic infection	Features of retinitis or uveitis	Other ocular disease
Measles	Uveitis occurs 1–2 weeks after onset of rash	Common: anterior uveitis Rare: chorioretinitis or neuroretinitis	Common: conjunctivitis, keratitis Rare: optic neuritis
SSPE (see Fig. 17.6)	Uveitis occurs some years after infection	Chorioretinitis involves macula	Papillitis; motility disturbances
Herpes simplex virus	Primary infection; lids and conjunctiva	Common: anterior uveitis Rare: posterior uveitis, retinitis, ARN	Dendritic corneal ulcer common
Varicella-zoster virus	Convalescence from varicella or trigeminal zoster (often with nasociliary branch involved)	Common: mild, anterior uveitis, self-limited; rarely, chorioretinitis or ARN	Granulomatous keratic precipitates; synechiae; glaucoma, cataract
Epstein–Barr virus	Infectious mononucleosis	Rare: mild anterior uveitis or chorioretinitis	Common: follicular conjunctivitis
Influenza, adenovirus, mumps	Systemic infection usually evident	Rare: bilateral, mild, self-limited, anterior uveitis Rare: neuroretinitis or optic neuritis	None

*These ocular problems are seen in immunocompetent adults and children.

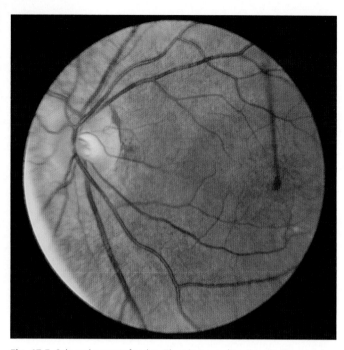

Fig. 17.5 Salt-and-pepper fundus. The pigment alterations in the macula give a 'dirty' appearance to the retina. The lesion occurred following congenital rubella infection. The vertical black line across the fovea is a focusing stick.

may cause severe visual loss, but this may improve spontaneously over subsequent months. There may be residual pigmentary retinopathy with the salt-and-pepper appearance (Fig. 17.5).

Subacute sclerosing panencephalitis (SSPE), which results from measles infection in very early life, commonly causes chorioretinitis, usually about the time that the neurologic signs of the disease become evident. The chorioretinitis is often focal, involving the macula, and there is mild vitritis (Fig. 17.6). Cortical blindness may occur. The prognosis of the ocular lesions is poor. There is no specific treatment.

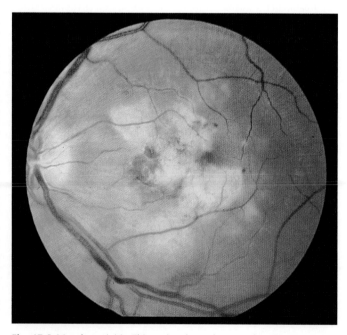

Fig. 17.6 Macular retinitis. This patient has subacute sclerosing panencephalitis.

Herpes simplex virus infection of the eye in children and adults usually presents as recurrent keratitis with characteristic dendrites (see Chapter 155). There may be an associated or isolated anterior uveitis and it has been estimated that 9% of anterior uveitis is attributable to HSV.[11] Rarely, HSV keratitis may spread along the axons to produce retinitis and posterior uveitis (see below).

Varicella, especially in the convalescent stage, may cause a mild, self-limited anterior uveitis. A more serious lesion, keratitis, may develop in patients who have trigeminal zoster, especially during convalescence from zoster that has involved the nasociliary branch of the trigeminal nerve. It may be accompanied by anterior uveitis which may be treated with 1% trifluridine ophthalmic drops or oral aciclovir or valaciclovir. Rarely, trigeminal zoster may lead to chorioretinitis and a form of necrotizing herpetic retinitis referred to as the ARN syndrome (see below). Cases have been reported with primary varicella infection of childhood (chickenpox).[12]

During infectious mononucleosis caused by Epstein–Barr virus (EBV) infection, a bilateral, mild, follicular conjunctivitis may be seen. Rarely, a mild anterior uveitis can occur as well. Recently, a choroiditis resembling that seen with histoplasmosis, but with vitritis, has been ascribed to acute or chronic EBV infection.[13]

Other viral infections may produce uveitis on occasion. Influenza virus infection may cause a mild, transient, bilateral anterior uveitis. Mumps virus infection may cause a mild, evanescent, bilateral anterior uveitis, which may appear up to 4 weeks after the onset of clinical infection. Optic neuritis, sometimes with neuroretinitis, may occur after mumps infection, but nearly always resolves spontaneously.

HLA-B27-associated uveitis

An autoimmune form of recurrent, bilateral anterior uveitis is common in patients who harbor the HLA-B27 antigen. It has been estimated that 55% of Caucasian patients with acute anterior uveitis are HLA-B27 positive versus 8–10% of the general population.[14] HLA-B27-associated uveitis is the most common type of nonidiopathic anterior uveitis.[5] Although usually considered immune-mediated rather than infectious, it may be triggered by systemic infection with Gram-negative bacteria, *Mycoplasma pneumoniae*, *Bartonella henselae* or *Chlamydia trachomatis*, as seen in Reiter's syndrome. Reiter's syndrome consists of the triad of conjunctivitis, urethritis and uveitis.[15] Several serologic studies from Scandinavian countries and Australia suggest that *Yersinia* infections may be important contributors.[16] Other data recently implicated *Helicobacter pylori* as a possible inciting agent.[17]

A recent retrospective cohort study found the average age of onset for HLA-B27 uveitis patients to be 36 years and was slightly more common in males. Bilaterality occurred in 21% and was more common in females. At the time of uveitis diagnosis, 33% of males had a systemically associated disease (most commonly ankylosing spondylitis) versus 17% of females. However, after the onset of uveitis the risk of developing systemic disease was statistically similar in males and females. At 10-year follow-up, the long-term visual prognosis of HLA-B27 uveitis was good.[18]

Bacterial causes of uveitis

Many bacterial species are associated with ocular infections (Table 17.4). Ocular lesions are common in the course of syphilis (*Treponema pallidum* infection). In the primary stage it may manifest as eyelid or conjunctival chancres. In the secondary stage, 1–3 months later, patients may develop a bilateral (though occasionally asymmetric) anterior uveitis, sometimes with iris nodules (granulomas). Less commonly is a choroiditis with large, white, 'geographic' lesions. There may also be retinal vasculitis, vitritis and papillitis.[19] Conjunctivitis, scleritis and episcleritis have also been reported.[20]

Uveitis remains the most common ocular finding in tertiary syphilis, affecting 2.5–5% of patients.[21] In addition to the Argyll Robertson pupil that may be present, other ophthalmic findings including papillitis, periphlebitis, vitritis and serous retinal detachment. One recent

Table 17.4 Bacterial causes of retinitis and uveitis*

Bacterial infection	Systemic infection	Features of retinitis or uveitis	Other ocular disease
Yersinia spp.	Infection occult, not proven	Suggested important cause of anterior uveitis in patients with HLA-B27 antigen	None
Borrelia burgdorferi	Features of extraocular Lyme disease	Nonspecific anterior or posterior uveitis	Conjunctivitis
Treponema pallidum	Uveitis usually during secondary syphilis; interstitial keratitis is delayed manifestation of congenital syphilis	Common: bilateral anterior uveitis Rare: choroiditis (large white lesions), retinal vasculitis, papillitis	Acute bilateral interstitial keratitis (age 5–10 years, after congenital infection)
Bartonella spp. (see Fig. 17.7)	Nonspecific systemic symptoms antedate ocular symptoms	Bilateral papillitis: optic disk edema, white retinal lesions, vitritis	None
Metastatic endophthalmitis	Often extraocular source is evident	Often bilateral: focal or diffuse uveitis or retinitis	None

*These ocular problems are seen in immunocompetent adults and children.

evaluation of the clinical findings in tertiary syphilis described a group of patients with an acute syphilitic posterior placoid chorioretinitis.[22] In the setting of HIV, early syphilis tends to be associated with a florid uveitis and VDRL-positive syphilitic meningitis. Late syphilis produces a chronic posterior uveitis with associated subclinical neurosyphilis;[23] this transition to the tertiary stage is often accelerated in those with HIV. Syphilis should be considered in the differential diagnosis of any posterior segment inflammation or any bilateral anterior segment inflammation. The diagnosis is made serologically and treatment is according to the stage of the syphilis (see Chapter 57).

Bartonella henselae in immunocompetent patients has been reported as a cause of stellate neuroretinitis, also known as macular star (Fig. 17.7). Cats are thought to be an important reservoir of *B. henselae*, and most infections have occurred in patients with a history of exposure to cats.[24] *Bartonella* infection should be suspected in any patient with optic disk edema and intraocular inflammation, especially if retinal lesions are seen.

Borrelia burgdorferi infection may cause a wide variety of ocular problems. Conjunctivitis and keratitis occur commonly in the early stages of infection. In the later stages of Lyme disease there may be iridocyclitis, retinal vasculitis, exudative retinal detachment, vitritis and optic disk edema. Orbital pseudotumor and orbital myositis have also been described.[25] The treatment is with systemic antibiotics appropriate for the stage of the disease (see Chapter 43).

The infectious agent of Whipple's disease, *Tropheryma whipplei*, is associated with a multisystem disorder, which can include panuveitis, retinitis and choroiditis. The diagnosis can be made by biopsy of affected tissue.[26]

Rarely, other bacterial infections have been associated with uveitis distinct from endogenous endophthalmitis. The list includes *Nocardia* infection (see Fig. 17.10), leptospirosis, brucellosis and tularemia.

Mycobacterium tuberculosis infection can cause anterior uveitis, posterior uveitis or isolated choroiditis. This infection should be a consideration in every case of nonspecific uveitis of unknown cause, though data from the USA suggest a tubercular etiology in less than 0.5% of patients managed in a tertiary care uveitis service.[27] If eye-related pathology is present, there is nearly always active extraocular disease. The anterior uveitis may be acute or chronic, unilateral or bilateral, and there may be granulomatous keratic precipitates. A periphlebitis resembling that seen in sarcoidosis may occur, along with choroidal infiltrates; these infiltrates represent miliary tubercles. More recently PCR analysis of the aqueous has become a popular aid to diagnosis. A recent analysis suggested that one-third of those with suspected TB-related anterior uveitis and two-thirds with posterior disease had a PCR-positive aqueous aspirate.[28] TB-associated uveitis usually improves within 2 weeks of the start of specific antituberculous treatment.

Bacterial endophthalmitis is considered in detail in Chapter 16.

Fungal causes of uveitis

The most common fungal species that cause metastatic endophthalmitis are *Candida* spp. (Table 17.5), especially *C. albicans*. The hallmark lesion is a yellow-white, fluffy patch of retinitis with indistinct borders (Fig. 17.8), almost always associated with vitritis. Some cases of *Candida* endophthalmitis have an indolent course and some even improve spontaneously. Treatment of *Candida* infections is discussed in detail in Chapter 149.

Whereas metastatic *Candida* infection usually occurs in a setting of active fungemia, *Histoplasma* ocular infection usually occurs without evident extraocular infection (see Table 17.5). The lesions arise from previous hematogenous spread to the choroid, producing a granuloma that usually becomes an inactive scar. Disk edema with optic neuritis can occur acutely. As a late complication, choroidal neovascular membranes can emanate from old choroidal scars, leading to retinal edema, hemorrhage and permanently decreased central vision.

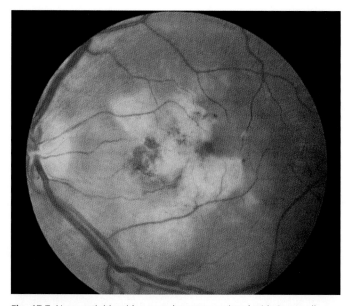

Fig. 17.7 Neuroretinitis with a macular star associated with *Bartonella* infection. Note the swelling of the optic disk with hard exudate in the macula in the so-called 'stellate' pattern.

Table 17.5 Fungal causes of retinitis and uveitis*

Fungal infection	Systemic infection	Features of retinitis or uveitis	Other ocular disease
Candida spp. (see Fig. 17.8)	Risk factors for candidemia	Whitish fluffy patch of retinitis and some vitritis	Anterior segment cells with hypopyon; corneal abscess
Histoplasma capsulatum (see Fig. 17.9)	History of residence in an endemic area; no extraocular infection evident	Choroidal granulomas, scars; optic neuritis; no vitritis	No anterior segment inflammation

*These ocular problems are seen in immunocompetent adults and children.

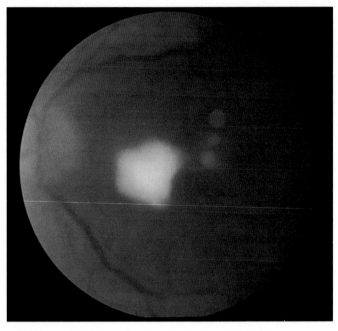

Fig. 17.8 A focal area of superficial retinitis and vitritis. This occurred secondary to *Candida albicans*.

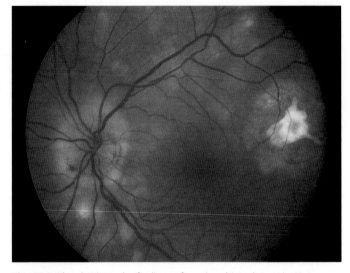

Fig. 17.9 The classic ocular findings of previous histoplasmosis. Note the peripapillary atrophy and punched-out yellowish chorioretinal scars. An old choroidal neovascular membrane is present in the center of the histoplasmosis scar temporal to the macula.

A diagnosis of ocular histoplasmosis is suspected by finding the characteristic choroidal lesions (Fig. 17.9) in a patient who has resided in an area endemic for the fungal infection. Serologic or skin tests for histoplasmosis are usually positive but do not prove the diagnosis. The primary visual risks are associated with late neovascular vessel growth from the chorioretinal scars. Laser photocoagulation and intravitreal administration of anti-VEGF agents are the primary treatment modalities. There is no indication for antifungal treatment.

Rarely, other fungi such as *Coccidioides*, *Blastomyces* and *Aspergillus* spp. and *Cryptococcus neoformans* may cause chorioretinitis by hematogenous spread. *Nocardia* spp. (Fig. 17.10) also occasionally cause chorioretinitis.

Parasitic causes of uveitis

Toxoplasma gondii infection is a common cause of posterior segment infection in children and adults (Table 17.6). It has been estimated to afflict 1.26 million individuals in the USA alone.[29] In the immunocompetent, it represents the most common cause of infectious posterior uveitis worldwide. In many countries, most cases of ocular toxoplasmosis are thought to represent reactivations following primary intrauterine infection (see Chapter 52). However, in some countries, such

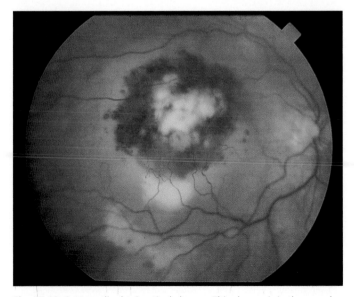

Fig. 17.10 A *Nocardia* chorioretinal abscess. This abscess is in the macula of a patient on systemic immunosuppression following heart transplant.

Table 17.6 Parasitic causes of retinitis and uveitis*

Parasitic infection	Systemic infection	Features of retinitis or uveitis	Other ocular disease
Toxocara canis (see Fig. 17.11)	Children 6 months to 4 years of age; no extraocular infection	Usually unilateral; pale granulomatous mass or focal retinitis; traction bands; vitritis	No anterior segment inflammation
Toxoplasma gondii (see Figs 17.12, 17.13)	Usually acquired in utero but not evident systemically	Recurrent self-limiting attacks of chorioretinitis and vitritis ('headlight in the fog')	May be keratic precipitates (granulomatous reaction) in anterior chamber
*These ocular problems are seen in immunocompetent adults and children.			

as Brazil, postnatally acquired infection is the more common antecedent of ocular toxoplasmosis. Postnatally acquired toxoplasmosis is followed by ocular toxoplasmosis in fewer than 5% of cases.

The lesions of ocular toxoplasmosis are found preferentially in the nerve fiber layer of the retina, but can affect any layer including the choroid.[30] Healed lesions of congenital toxoplasmosis are flat, atrophic, variably pigmented chorioretinal scars that have a propensity for the macular area of the fundus (Fig. 17.11). There may be recurrent bouts of uveitis, caused by the rupture of cysts, releasing trophozoites. Most patients have their first reactivation before 30 years of age and it has been estimated that recurrence occurs in 79% of patients.[31] Ophthalmoscopic examination shows vitritis and one or more white retinal lesions that are usually round or oval and up to 5 mm in diameter. There may be many such lesions surrounding an old scar (Fig. 17.12). Aggregates of vitreous cells over the active lesions are the rule. The appearance of the vitreous haze and the white granuloma has been likened to a 'headlight in the fog'. There may be retinal hemorrhages, sheathing of arterioles and venules, and papillitis. In the anterior segment, there may be a granulomatous reaction in the anterior chamber with keratic precipitates and conjunctival injection.

A diagnosis of ocular toxoplasmosis is based on the characteristic appearance of the lesions together with a positive serum antibody test for *T. gondii* (see Chapter 183). PCR of vitreous aspirates has also been utilized (see above). Other possible causes of localized necrotizing retinitis with vitritis, such as syphilis or tuberculosis, should be considered (Table 17.7).

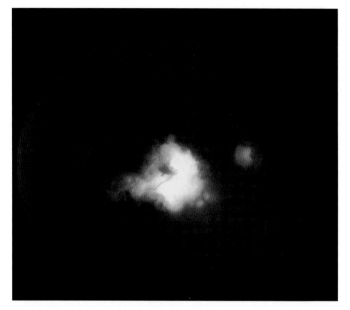

Fig. 17.12 A reactivated area of retinal toxoplasmosis. The lesion is the area of whitening in the macula of the right eye. Overlying vitritis creates the classic appearance of a 'headlight in the fog'.

In otherwise healthy persons, flare-ups of ocular toxoplasmosis tend to be self-limited over a period of weeks to months. Not all active lesions need to be treated. The highest priority for treatment is for lesions that threaten the fovea, the optic nerve or large areas of the nerve fiber layer, as well as those that produce enough vitritis to impair vision. Once the fovea is directly involved, visual acuity is usually permanently compromised. Severe vision loss (visual acuity ≤20/200) in at least one eye has been described in up to 24% of ocular toxoplasmosis patients.[31]

There is no consensus among uveitis specialists on treatment because evidence is sparse. Typically, treatment is the same as for other systemic forms of toxoplasmosis – pyrimethamine, sulfadiazine and clindamycin (see Chapter 150), though the use of antiparasitics does not affect visual outcome.[31] Many ophthalmologists avoid pyrimethamine initially because of its marrow-suppressive effects, preferring to rely on the other two agents. Others have advocated the use of trimethoprim–sulfamethoxazole alone and in combination with clindamycin and suggested similar efficacy.[32] Corticosteroids are often used concomitantly, but not without the anti-infective drugs. Laser photocoagulation may be used for active lesions unresponsive to medication and pars plana vitrectomy may be used to clear vitreous opacities.

Ocular infection by *Toxocara canis*, the dog roundworm, occurs in young children, especially boys, aged from 6 months to 4 years (see Table 17.6). *Toxocara cati*, the cat roundworm, has also been implicated, but the organisms have never been positively identified

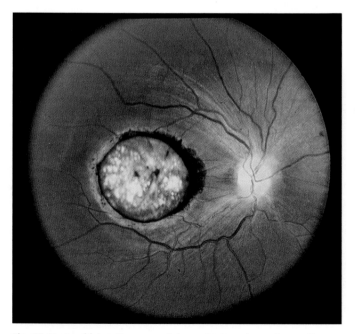

Fig. 17.11 An old, inactive congenital macular toxoplasmosis scar. The patient's vision was 20/400.

Table 17.7 Characteristics of some infections causing posterior uveitis/retinitis without extraocular manifestations

	Usual number of lesions	Appearance of lesions	Distribution of lesions	Accompanying vitritis
Toxoplasma gondii (see Figs 17.12, 17.13)	One to a few	'Headlight in fog'	Random, but heavier in macular area	Almost always
Toxocara canis (see Fig. 17.11)	One	Granuloma	Macula, optic disk or periphery	Always
Histoplasma capsulatum (see Fig. 17.9)	Multiple	Choroidal granulomas	Various	Almost never
Treponema pallidum	Diffuse retinochoroiditis	Bilateral anterior uveitis; large white geographic choroidal lesions	Random	Always
Borrelia burgdorferi	Focal or diffuse	Anterior uveitis, retinal vasculitis, exudative retinal detachment	Random	Usually
Mycobacterium tuberculosis	One or a few	Retinitis or chorioretinitis	Random	Usually

in the human eye. The typical presenting complaint is decreased vision, strabismus or leukocoria (a whitish lesion in the pupil). *Toxocara* infection is acquired by the ingestion of soil contaminated with embryonated eggs (see Chapter 184). The larvae are believed to reach the eye by hematogenous spread. The ocular findings are generally unilateral.

There are several ophthalmoscopic presentations of ocular toxocariasis (Fig. 17.13). The features they have in common are a whitish or yellowish retinal mass, representing a granuloma surrounding the larva, and the eventual formation of traction bands between the vitreous and the granuloma, which may result in retinal folds and exudative retinal detachment. There may be diffuse posterior uveitis, sometimes called nematode endophthalmitis. Unlike bacterial endophthalmitis, there is little pain and no anterior segment inflammation. Other presentations include localized retinitis affecting the macula or the peripheral retina, and acute optic neuritis, in which the granuloma overlies the optic disk. A macular star (neuroretinitis) may be seen as a result of leakage from vessels in the optic disk.

The major differential diagnoses of ocular toxocariasis are noninfectious diseases such as retinoblastoma and Coats' disease, a congenital vascular disorder. Retinoblastoma should always be considered and ruled out. Peripheral blood eosinophilia is rare in ocular toxocariasis.

A serum ELISA antibody titer to the parasite of 1 to 8 or more supports the diagnosis. A positive ELISA titer of the intraocular fluid, which may be found even if the serum titer is negative, is highly indicative of the infection. Treatment is directed toward stemming the intraocular inflammation, clearing any media opacity and preventing permanent distortion in the retinal architecture. Corticosteroids, usually applied locally in the eye, and cataract and/or vitrectomy surgery are the mainstays of treatment.

Diffuse unilateral subacute neuroretinitis has been attributed to two nematodes which invade the subretinal space and induce inflammation, *Ancylostoma caninum* (definitive host is dog, found in the southeast USA) and *Baylisascaris procyonis* (definitive host is raccoon, found in the northwest USA). Early in the clinical course, vitritis, grayish outer retinal lesions and optic disk edema are noted. Later in the course of the disease the retina takes on a 'retinitis pigmentosa'-like appearance with pigment epithelial changes, arteriolar attenuation and optic nerve atrophy. In 25% of cases, a worm is visualized on clinical examination. The condition is treated by applying laser photocoagulation directly to the visualized nematode, which if achieved early may arrest the severe vision loss that results.

Rarely, uveitis occurs in other parasitic infections such as cysticercosis, myiasis and onchocerciasis.

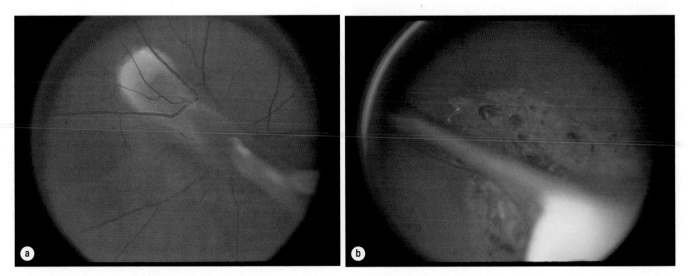

Fig. 17.13 Ocular toxocariasis. (a) The posterior pole of a left eye affected by toxocariasis. There is severe macular distortion and dragging of the retina toward a granuloma in the inferotemporal retinal periphery. (b) The periphery of the inferotemporal retina in the same eye showing the granuloma.

Table 17.8 Infectious retinitis and uveitis in neonates

	Systemic infection	Features of uveitis/retinitis	Other ocular disease
Viral infections			
Herpes simplex virus	Disseminated infection usually evident	Anterior uveitis early; optic neuritis, retinal hemorrhages and necrosis later; sparing of choroid	Conjunctivitis, keratitis common
Varicella-zoster virus	Features of congenital varicella-zoster (rare)	Chorioretinitis	Microphthalmia; cataracts
Cytomegalovirus (CMV)	Features of congenital CMV infection	Retinitis in 20–25% of infants with symptomatic CMV infection; resembles that seen in adults with AIDS	None
Rubella	Congenital rubella syndrome	Mild, self-limiting chorioretinitis & vitritis in 25–50% with congenital rubella syndrome; unilateral or bilateral; eventual salt-and-pepper fundus	None
Bacterial infections			
Treponema pallidum	Stigmata of congenital syphilis	Salt-and-pepper fundus; occasionally optic atrophy, retinal vascular sheathing	Delayed manifestation: acute interstitial keratitis (5–10 yrs)
Fungal infections			
Candida spp. (see Fig. 17.8)	Candida fungemia; risk factors	Whitish fluffy patch of retinitis, some vitritis	None
Parasitic infections			
Toxoplasma gondii (see Figs 17.12, 17.13)	Rarely, encephalitis, hydrocephalus at birth	Rarely, chorioretinitis at birth	None

Uveitis in neonates

There are several causes of uveitis in neonates (Table 17.8).

Herpes simplex virus

Congenital infection by HSV is usually acquired directly from the infected birth canal. Ocular findings may first appear from 1 week to several months after birth. About 80% of isolates are HSV-2 and this strain is associated with more severe ocular infections.

Congenital HSV infection may cause a wide variety of ocular lesions. Conjunctivitis and keratitis are most common, and are usually seen in the acute phase of the infection. Posterior segment changes tend to occur later in the infection. Retinal involvement ranges from scattered hemorrhages to widespread retinal necrosis similar to that seen in the ARN syndrome. Residual changes include pigment migration and clumping (salt-and-pepper appearance), macular chorioretinal scars, optic atrophy and preretinal neovascularization. Systemic treatment is required.

Cytomegalovirus

Congenital infections by CMV are usually asymptomatic (see Chapter 52). With symptomatic infections, retinitis occurs in 20–25% of cases. If retinitis is not evident at birth, it is unlikely to occur later. The retinitis resembles that seen in adult patients with HIV infection (see below).

Rubella

In the congenital rubella syndrome, ocular manifestations occur in 25–50% of affected children. The classic finding is a mild, self-limited chorioretinitis that may be unilateral or bilateral. Vision is usually not impaired. A common sequela is a salt-and-pepper fundus caused by changes in the retinal pigment epithelium (see Fig. 17.5).

Syphilis

The most common ocular manifestation of congenital syphilis (see Chapter 57) is a salt-and-pepper fundus. The lesions are almost always bilateral, but may be sectoral or exclusively peripheral. They are the result of chorioretinitis, which may be evident at birth or appear in the first few years of life. Visual acuity is rarely affected. In more severe cases, there may be diffuse sheathing of the retinal vessels, optic atrophy and migration of the retinal pigment epithelium in a manner resembling retinitis pigmentosa. Acute interstitial keratitis is a delayed manifestation of congenital syphilis. It may be accompanied by anterior uveitis and secondary glaucoma may develop. The lesions of keratitis are self-limited, but treatment of the syphilitic infection is indicated. Hutchinson's triad in congenital syphilis consists of peg-shaped teeth, deafness and interstitial keratitis.

Other causes

Candida spp. may cause retinitis and vitritis in neonates. Risk factors are prematurity, low birth weight, sepsis, malnutrition and treatment with broad-spectrum antibiotics. The clinical presentation and treatment are the same as for adults (see Chapter 149).

Toxoplasma chorioretinitis is usually acquired in utero. Although the ocular complications usually present long after the neonatal period, they are sometimes evident at birth in the TORCH syndrome (see above, and Chapter 52). Manifestations include encephalitis, hydrocephalus and bilateral chorioretinitis. Treatment is described in Chapter 150.

Endogenous spiroplasma infection has also been described in neonates, typically manifesting as anterior uveitis and unilateral cataract.

Acute retinal necrosis syndrome

The ARN (acute necrotizing herpetic retinitis) syndrome is a recently described, rare syndrome of vaso-obliterative retinal and choroidal vasculitis, diffuse retinal necrosis and vitritis. It typically affects healthy immunocompetent people and has no predilection for race or sex. ARN is bilateral in one-third of patients (BARN), although the two eyes need not be affected simultaneously and involvement in the fellow eye may occur years later. Although reported in children as young as 8 years of age, it occurs most often in adults with a bimodal age distribution with peaks at 20 and 50 years of age. Conclusive evidence now exists that VZV is the primary cause; HSV is less common.[33] Patients infected with HIV who develop herpes zoster of the first division of the trigeminal nerve appear to have a high risk of subsequent ARN, often bilateral, over the next few weeks to months.[34]

Recent immunologic research suggests that specific human leukocyte antigens (HLAs) may predispose to ARN. Some 55% of Caucasian ARN patients were found to have the HLA-DQw7 antigen versus 19% of controls. More aggressive and fulminant disease has been associated with HLA-DR9.[35]

Acute retinal necrosis causes diffuse arteritis and phlebitis with sheathing of the retinal vessels and striking white areas of full thickness retinal necrosis (Fig. 17.14). Broad areas of the peripheral retina are often involved early and the macula is usually spared initially. There is often mild inflammation of the anterior segment. As the disease progresses there is increasing vitritis. Optic neuropathy with disk edema may appear. Diagnosis is typically based on the characteristic clinical presentation though PCR of intraocular aspirates may be helpful.

Retinal detachment follows in up to 75% of patients. The detachments are notoriously difficult to repair. Previous prophylactic laser treatment of healthy retina posterior to the areas of necrosis reduces the incidence of retinal detachment.

The mainstay of treatment for ARN is aciclovir, given in high dosage intravenously (e.g. 12–15 mg/kg q8h for 7–14 days). Oral aciclovir or one of its prodrugs should be continued for at least 2–3 months to lessen the risk of fellow eye involvement. Systemic corticosteroids are employed to decrease inflammation, but never prior to the institution of antiviral therapy. Retinal detachments require complex vitreoretinal surgery for successful repair, often with silicone oil placement. It has been suggested that patients who have AIDS and who develop ophthalmic zoster should be given long-term oral prophylaxis with aciclovir, but there is no proof of benefit from this approach.[34]

Uveitis and retinitis in immunosuppressed patients

Because of the AIDS pandemic, ophthalmologists encounter a variety of intraocular infections that were previously either unknown or extraordinarily rare.

Cytomegalovirus retinitis

The most common ocular infection in HIV-positive adult patients is CMV retinitis. In developed countries prior to 1996, CMV retinitis occurred in about 35% of adult patients who had AIDS. Since HAART has become widely available in developed countries, the incidence of CMV retinitis has dropped dramatically. CMV retinitis rarely occurs in patients who have CD4+ lymphocyte counts over 50 cells/mm[3].[36] Pediatric patients who have AIDS have a much lower incidence of CMV retinitis than adults.

'Floaters' and blurred vision are the most common complaints, if any. Often, an active infection is noted incidentally on routine ophthalmologic screening examination. In 40% of patients with CMV retinitis, the lesions are bilateral at presentation. Nearly 75% of patients present to the ophthalmologist with disease that is considered immediately sight-threatening. Pain, redness or more than a mild anterior uveitis are unusual with CMV retinitis.

The hallmark lesion of CMV retinitis is a necrotizing, full-thickness retinitis resulting in retinal cell death (Fig. 17.15). Retinal tissue adjacent to major retinal blood vessels or the optic disk is often affected initially. The areas of active retinitis have a granular appearance and are dirty-white in color. Hemorrhage is common, owing to damage to vascular endothelial cells. The appearance has been likened to a 'brush fire' and to 'ketchup and cottage cheese'. The retinitis spreads contiguously as well as by producing satellite lesions. It is common to see areas of healed retinitis alongside areas of active necrosis. Areas of burned-out necrosis show an absence of retinal tissue while the underlying retinal pigment epithelium assumes a salt-and-pepper appearance.

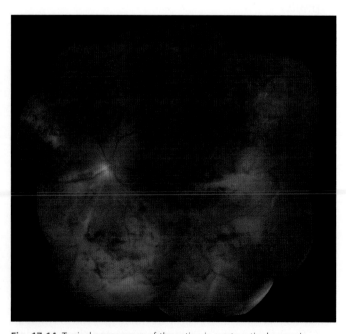

Fig. 17.14 Typical appearance of the retina in acute retinal necrosis syndrome. There is dense peripheral retinal whitening with a geographic border. Satellite lesions are common. The view is hazy owing to vitritis.

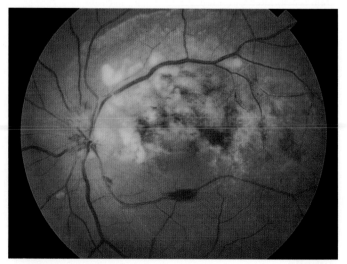

Fig. 17.15 Cytomegalovirus infection with granular retinal whitening along the major blood vessels with mild hemorrhage. The view is clear because there is only mild vitritis.

Loss of vision occurs because of both the death of retinal cells and retinal detachment. About 10–20% of eyes with CMV retinitis can be expected to suffer a detached retina. The risk is time dependent; after 1 year the risk approaches 50%. Although vitreous surgery to repair the detached retinas is anatomically successful in more than 90% of instances, visual results are often limited by the underlying disease process.

Treatment of HIV-associated CMV retinitis is discussed in detail in Chapter 91. Immunologic improvement with antiretroviral therapy may result in an immune recovery uveitis in patients with prior or undiagnosed CMV disease (see Chapter 92). It has been hypothesized to be secondary to a reaction to CMV antigens typically occurring 2–16 weeks (median 4 weeks) following an increased CD4 count. Treatment with corticosteroids has not been shown to reactivate CMV retinitis.[37,38]

Other causes of uveitis and retinitis

About 75% of patients with HIV-1 infection have a non-sight-threatening retinopathy that may be caused by the HIV-1 itself.[39] The lesions consist of multiple, bilateral, cottonwool spots and scattered retinal hemorrhages (Fig. 17.16). If there is concern that such lesions may be due to CMV, close observation over a period of days to weeks with documentation by photographs is recommended.

Opportunistic infections with *Pneumocystis jirovecii*, *Histoplasma capsulatum*, *Cryptococcus neoformans* and atypical mycobacteria may produce multifocal choroiditis in patients who have AIDS. These infections are rarely sight threatening, but they should alert the clinician to the presence of a systemic infection. Unfortunately, it is generally not possible for the ophthalmologist to distinguish between these possible opportunistic infections on the basis of the eye examination alone.[39]

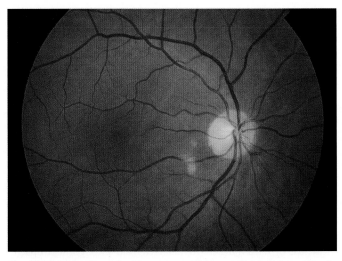

Fig. 17.16 HIV retinopathy. There are multiple superficial white patches in the retina (cottonwool spots). These do not affect vision and typically wax and wane over time.

Other important posterior segment infections that can occur in HIV-positive patients include toxoplasmosis, syphilis and infection with HSV and VZV. Whereas toxoplasmosis in immunocompetent patients produces a slowly progressive, focal, relapsing chorioretinitis, in immunocompromised patients it can produce a severe diffuse retinitis. Serologic testing may be helpful. Nearly one-third of patients who have AIDS and *Toxoplasma* retinitis have concurrent toxoplasmosis of the central nervous system. Ocular syphilis can also mimic CMV retinitis, but the lesions of secondary syphilis are usually a choroiditis, rather than a retinitis.

Acute retinal necrosis syndrome

The ARN syndrome (see above) occurs in both healthy and immunosuppressed people, including those with AIDS. Acute retinal necrosis differs from CMV retinitis in that the lesions of ARN are typically peripheral and the course is much more rapid. In addition, significant vitreous cells are a prominent feature of ARN, but not of CMV retinitis. Patients who have HIV infection and who develop zoster of the first division of the trigeminal nerve appear to have a high risk of subsequent ARN, which is often bilateral, over the next few weeks to months.[34] Therefore, when a rash of ophthalmic zoster appears, patients who have AIDS should be followed carefully for signs of ARN.

A specific type of rapidly progressive ARN is progressive outer retinal necrosis (PORN). PORN is secondary to VZV infection and has been described in patients who have AIDS and a low CD4[+] lymphocyte count.[40] Without aggressive therapy, PORN results in bilateral loss of vision within days to weeks. The recommended treatment is a combination of foscarnet and either ganciclovir or aciclovir, given intravenously or via intravitreal injection.

Perhaps the most common cause of noninfectious anterior uveitis in HIV-positive patients is a dose-related reaction to rifabutin. Patients receiving rifabutin for prophylaxis against *Mycobacterium avium-intracellulare* in conjunction with another agent that interferes with the metabolism of rifabutin (such as clarithromycin or ritonavir) and patients weighing less than 65 kg who are receiving 600 mg of rifabutin are at particular risk. The incidence of rifabutin-induced uveitis is 20% among AIDS patients taking the medication, but it has been reported in HIV-negative patients as well. Treatment with corticosteroids and discontinuation of the medication usually results in prompt reversal of the inflammation. Systemic cidofovir has also been reported to cause uveitis in patients who have AIDS.

REFERENCES

References for this chapter can be found online at http://www.expertconsult.com

Management of red eye

Red eye is a common sign of ocular infections (etiologies are presented in Chapters 15–17) and noninfectious conditions, some of which are vision-threatening etiologies requiring same-day referral to an ophthalmologist.

WHEN TO REFER THE PATIENT TO THE OPHTHALMOLOGIST?

Clinical interview and examination are required to identify the affected eye segment and select situations requiring same-day referral to an ophthalmologist (Table PP6.1). Such situations include a history of trauma and contact lens wear, severe ocular pain, impaired vision, foreign body sensation, corneal opacity or infiltrate at penlight examination and hypopyon (layer of white cells in the anterior chamber). In addition, unilateral red eye associated with nausea and vomiting, suggestive of acute angle-closure glaucoma, and masquerade syndromes due to malignant etiologies including B cell lymphoma and metastases of cancer such as breast cancer[1] (see Table PP6.1) should be referred.

WHICH OCULAR SEGMENT IS AFFECTED?

Conjunctivitis

Conjunctivitis is usually a benign, self-limited condition and probably the most common cause of red eye in the community setting. Conjunctivitis is responsible for diffuse or localized redness (episcleritis) in one or both eyes. Patients complain of morning crusting and daytime redness and discharge. Morning watery discharge of viral conjunctivitis contrasts with day-long purulent discharge in the course of bacterial conjunctivitis. Viral conjunctivitis, a self-limited infection, most often bilateral, typically caused by adenovirus, may be part of a viral prodrome followed by adenopathy, fever, pharyngitis and upper respiratory tract infection, or the eye infection may be the only manifestation of the disease.

Neisseria gonorrhoeae causes a hyperacute bacterial conjunctivitis that is severe and sight threatening, requiring immediate ophthalmologic referral. The eye infection is characterized by a profuse purulent discharge with redness, irritation and tenderness with chemosis, lid swelling, and tender preauricular adenopathy.

Conjunctivitis is the major clinical manifestation of active trachoma, a disorder that is largely limited to endemic areas in developing countries. Adult inclusion conjunctivitis is a chronic (weeks to months), indolent follicular conjunctivitis caused by certain serotypes of sexually transmitted *Chlamydia trachomatis*. Concurrent asymptomatic urogenital infection is typically present.

Keratitis

Keratitis is responsible for red eye along with photophobia and foreign body sensation. In addition, herpes simplex keratitis produces watery discharge. There may be a faint branching gray opacity on penlight examination, best visualized with application of fluorescein. Epidemic keratoconjunctivitis is a particularly fulminant cause of keratitis due to adenovirus types 8, 19 and 37. Multiple corneal infiltrates are barely visible with a penlight to the skilled observer but fluorescein staining reveals multiple punctate staining lesions.

Overnight wear of contact lenses is associated with a higher incidence of bacterial keratitis characterized by a corneal opacity or infiltrate (typically a round white spot) seen with a penlight in association with red eye, photophobia and foreign body sensation. Mucopurulent discharge is typically present. Fulminant cases may present with an associated hypopyon (layer of white cells in the anterior chamber). Amebal keratitis is also associated with contact lens wearing.[2]

Anterior uveitis

Anterior uveitis (or iritis) may be responsible for red eye (Fig. PP6.1; Table PP6.2). Patients with iritis may present in a similar fashion to those with an active corneal process but there is no foreign body sensation per se. The cardinal sign of iritis is ciliary flush: injection that gives the appearance of a red ring around the iris. Typically, there is no discharge and only minimal tearing. Patients with iritis should be referred to an ophthalmologist within a matter of days.

Toxoplasmosis is a surprisingly common cause of uveitis in the normal host, suspected on the basis of a very typical chorioretinal

Table PP6.1 Clinical signs and symptoms indicating same-day referral to an ophthalmologist in patient with red eye

Medical history	Contact lens wearing Ocular surgery Ocular trauma
Symptoms	Nausea, vomiting Severe ocular pain Impaired vision Foreign body sensation
Signs	Corneal opacity Corneal infiltrate Hypopyon (white cells in the anterior chamber)

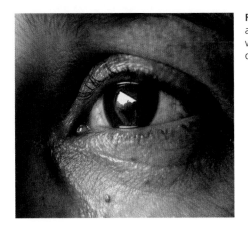

Fig. PP6.1 Red eye in a patient diagnosed with Whipple's disease uveitis.

Table PP6.2 Major groups of conditions responsible for the differential diagnosis of red eye

Aetiology	Associated clinical signs/symptoms
Acute angle-closure glaucoma	Nausea, vomiting
Conjunctivitis Viral Bacterial Allergic	 Morning – watery discharge Fever, pharyngitis Day-long purulent discharge Watery discharge
Keratitis Viral Bacterial Amebal	 Photophobia Impaired vision Foreign body sensation Corneal infiltrate Corneal opacity Hypopion
Anterior uveitis Viral Bacterial Parasite Masquerade syndromes Mycoses	

lesion. Most chorioretinal scarring from toxoplasmosis is due to infection during gestation, but scarring is increasingly being recognized as a result of primary infections as well. Other etiologies recognized after extensive investigations include viruses and fastidious bacteria of spirochetes, *Borrelia* and *Bartonella* spp.[3]

WHEN TO PERFORM MICROBIOLOGICAL SAMPLING?

The question then arises of when, how and which specimens to sample? Cultures are not necessary for the initial diagnosis and therapy of conjunctivitis except for patients with symptoms of hyperacute conjunctivitis in whom Giemsa and Gram stains may be helpful to identify Gram-negative diplococci suggestive of *Neisseria gonorrhoeae*. A point-of-care rapid test for adenoviral conjunctivitis has been favorably evaluated by modeled cost-effectiveness analysis.[4] The diagnosis of adult inclusion conjunctivitis can be confirmed with Giemsa or direct fluorescent antibody staining of conjunctival smears, by culture or by polymerase chain reaction (PCR) of swabbed specimens.

Keratitis lesions are sampled for microbiologic diagnosis based on culture and PCR-based detection of major pathogens including herpesvirus, bacteria and amebae.

In patients with uveitis of unknown etiology which is bilateral, recurrent, sight threatening or nonresponsive to therapy will require extensive evaluation for etiology. Vitreous humor should be sampled to exclude ocular lymphoma by cytology and interleukin 10 measurements and to search for selected pathogens (see below).

WHEN TO PROVIDE ANTI-INFECTIOUS TREATMENT?

Viral conjunctivitis is a highly contagious, self-limited process for which there is no specific antiviral agent.

Bacterial conjunctivitis is also likely to be self-limited in most patients, although treatment probably shortens the clinical course and reduces person-to-person spread of this highly contagious condition. Appropriate choices for bacterial conjunctivitis include erythromycin ophthalmic ointment, sulfa ophthalmic drops or polymyxin/trimethoprim drops. These agents cover the most common pathogens responsible for bacterial conjunctivitis, and patients should respond to this treatment within 1–2 days. Patients who do not respond should be referred to an ophthalmologist. The fluoroquinolones are effective and well tolerated; they are the treatment of choice for corneal ulcers and are extremely effective against *Pseudomonas*. However, fluoroquinolones are not first-line therapy for routine cases of bacterial conjunctivitis because of concerns regarding emerging resistance and cost. The exception is conjunctivitis in a contact lens wearer; once keratitis has been ruled out, it is reasonable to treat these individuals with a fluoroquinolone due to the high incidence of *Pseudomonas* infection.[5] A contact lens wearer with a red eye should discontinue contact lens wear. If the diagnosis is conjunctivitis, contact lens wear can resume when the eye is white and has no discharge for 24 hours after the completion of antibiotic therapy. The lens case should be discarded and the lenses subjected to overnight disinfection or replaced if disposable. Systemic therapy with doxycycline, tetracycline, erythromycin or azithromycin is required to eradicate adult inclusion conjunctivitis.

The duration of symptoms in patients with herpes simplex keratitis is reduced with treatment with topical or oral antiviral agents. Immunocompromised patients may require topical and systemic treatment, and longer duration of therapy. A small percentage of patients develop chronic or recurrent inflammation, or recurrent viral keratitis, both of which are treated with prophylactic oral antiviral agents. Some patients also benefit from treatment with topical corticosteroid agents, used in conjunction with antiviral prophylaxis. Fortified topical antibiotics and fluoroquinolones are still the mainstay of bacterial keratitis therapy, and new antimycotic agents such as voriconazole could be used for treating amebal keratitis.

Specific anti-infectious treatment will be prescribed in addition to steroids in cases of uveitis, in collaboration between the ophthalmologist and the infectious disease/clinical microbiology practitioner.

REFERENCES

🖱 References for this chapter can be found online at http://www.expertconsult.com

Acute and chronic meningitis

INTRODUCTION

Meningitis is an infection of the meninges and subarachnoid space, but can also involve the cortex and brain parenchyma (meningo-encephalitis) because of the close anatomic relation between the cerebrospinal fluid (CSF) and the brain. Inflammatory involvement of the subarachnoid space with meningeal irritation leads to the classic triad of headache, fever and meningism, and to a pleocytosis in the CSF. Involvement of the brain cortex and parenchyma may result in behavioral changes, focal neurologic abnormalities and impairment of consciousness. Although these latter signs are classically considered to be encephalitis, the meningitis and encephalitis should rather be seen as a continuum. Thus, although somewhat artificial, this chapter will be limited to those infections in which the meninges are inflamed. For a treatise of encephalitis the reader is referred to Chapter 19.

Acute Bacterial Meningitis

EPIDEMIOLOGY

The incidence of acute bacterial meningitis is 5–10/100 000 persons per year in high-income countries, resulting in 15 000–25 000 cases in the USA annually.[1,2] Vaccination strategies have substantially changed the epidemiology of community-acquired bacterial meningitis during the past two decades. The routine vaccination of children against *Haemophilus influenzae* type b has virtually eradicated *H. influenzae* meningitis in the developed world.[1] As a consequence, *Streptococcus pneumoniae* has become the most common pathogen beyond the neonatal period and bacterial meningitis has become a disease predominantly of adults. The introduction of conjugate vaccines against seven serotypes of *S. pneumoniae* that are among the most prevalent in children aged 6 months to 2 years has reduced the rate of invasive pneumococcal infections in young children and in older persons.[1] The integration of the meningococcal protein–polysaccharide conjugate vaccines into vaccination programs in several countries further reduced the disease burden of bacterial meningitis in high- and medium-income countries.[3]

Streptococcus pneumoniae affects all ages and causes the most severe disease in the very young and the very old.[4] Of the more than 90 pneumococcal serotypes, a few dominate as the causes of meningitis. The increase of drug-resistant strains of *S. pneumoniae* is an emerging problem worldwide. The prevalence of antibiotic-resistant strains in some parts of the USA is as high as 50–70% with important consequences for treatment.[5]

Neisseria meningitidis is mainly responsible for bacterial meningitis in young adults; it causes sporadic cases and epidemics.[6] Its incidence shows a peak in winter and early spring and varies greatly around the world. Small outbreaks typically occur in young adults living in close quarters, such as dormitories of military camps or schools. Major epidemics have occurred periodically in sub-Saharan Africa (the so-called 'meningitis belt'), Europe, Asia and South America. During these epidemics, attack rates can reach several hundred per 100 000, with devastating consequences.

The group B streptococcus (*S. agalactiae*) is a pathogen of neonates and often causes a devastating sepsis and meningitis.[7] It colonizes the maternal birth canal and is transmitted to the child. The colonized newborn can develop group B streptococcal disease of early onset (developing at less than 7 days of age; median 1 day) or late onset (developing later than 7 days of age).

Listeria monocytogenes causes meningitis preferentially in neonates, in adults with alcoholism, immunosuppression or iron overload, and in pregnant women.[8] There is often an encephalitic component to presentation, with early mental status alterations, neurologic deficits and seizures.

Haemophilus influenzae causes meningitis in young children. In countries with routine vaccination against *H. influenzae* type b it has become a rare disease.[9]

Bacterial meningitis also occurs in hospitalized patients ('physician associated meningitis' or 'nosocomial meningitis'). In a large city hospital, almost 40% of cases may be nosocomial.[10] Most cases occur in patients undergoing neurosurgical procedures, including implanting of neurosurgical devices, and in patients with focal infections of the head. The organisms causing nosocomial meningitis differ markedly from those causing community-acquired meningitis and include Gram-negative rods (*Escherichia coli*, *Klebsiella* spp., *Pseudomonas aeruginosa*, *Acinetobacter* spp., *Enterobacter* spp. and others), staphylococci and streptococci other than *S. pneumoniae*.[11,12]

PATHOPHYSIOLOGY AND PATHOLOGY

Specific bacterial virulence factors for meningeal pathogens include specialized surface components that are crucial for adherence to the nasopharyngeal epithelium, the evasion of local host defense mechanisms and subsequent invasion of the bloodstream (Fig. 18.1).[13] In pneumococcal disease, presence of the polymeric immunoglobulin A receptor on human mucosa, which binds to a major pneumococcal adhesin, CbpA, correlates with the ability of pneumococci to invade the mucosal barrier. Viral infection of the respiratory tract may also promote invasive disease.[4] From the nasopharyngeal surface, encapsulated organisms cross the epithelial cell layer and invade the small subepithelial blood vessels. Binding of bacteria to upregulated receptors (e.g. platelet activating-factor receptors) promotes migration through the respiratory epithelium and vascular endothelium, resulting in invasive disease.

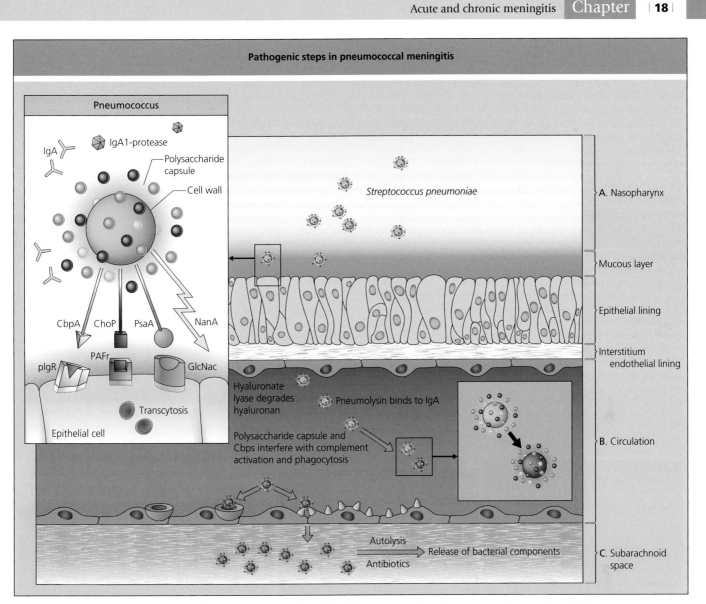

Pathogenic steps in pneumococcal meningitis

Pneumococcus

IgA1-protease
IgA
Polysaccharide capsule
Cell wall
CbpA ChoP PsaA NanA
pIgR PAFr GlcNac
Transcytosis
Epithelial cell

Streptococcus pneumoniae

A. Nasopharynx
Mucous layer
Epithelial lining
Interstitium endothelial lining

Hyaluronate lyase degrades hyaluronan
Pneumolysin binds to IgA
Polysaccharide capsule and Cbps interfere with complement activation and phagocytosis

B. Circulation

Autolysis
Antibiotics
Release of bacterial components

C. Subarachnoid space

Fig. 18.1 Pathogenic steps in pneumococcal meningitis. Neuraminidase (NanA) decreases viscosity of the mucus and exposes *N*-acetyl-glucosamine (GlcNAc)-receptors on epithelial cells, which interact with pneumococcal surface-associated proteins (such as PsaA). IgA1 proteases cleave opsonizing host IgA. Cytokines stimulate cell-surface expression of platelet-activating-factor receptors (PAFr). Binding to PAFr via cell-wall phosphocholine (ChoP) induces internalization and migration (transcytosis) of pneumococci through the epithelial barrier, which is facilitated by binding of choline-binding protein A (CbpA) to the polymeric Ig-receptor (pIgR). After penetrating the mucosal epithelium, hyaluronate lyase facilitates bacterial spreading by degrading hyaluronan, an important component of the interstitial matrix. Once in the bloodstream the polysaccharide capsule and Cbps enhance intravascular survival by interfering with activation of the complement cascades and phagocytosis. Pneumolysin reduces serum opsonic activity by binding to IgG. By changing the composition of surface components (phase variation) pneumococci adapt to the host environmental conditions and migration through the blood–brain barrier. Attachment to endothelial cells occurs to several glycoconjugates. Activated endothelial cells upregulate PAFr and thereby enable pneumococci (mainly transparent phase variants) to invade the subarachnoid space via transcytosis. The poor local host defenses in the subarachnoid space facilitate multiplication of bacteria, which undergo autolysis (mediated by autolysins or antibiotics) and release bacterial compounds. Reproduced with permission from Weisfelt *et al.*[4]

In the bloodstream, bacteria must survive host defenses, including circulating antibodies, complement-mediated bactericidal mechanisms and neutrophil phagocytosis. Encapsulation is a shared feature of the principal hematogenous meningeal pathogens. To survive the various host conditions they encounter during infection, pneumococci undergo spontaneous and reversible phase variation, which involves changes in the amount of important surface components.[4,14] The capsule is instrumental in inhibiting neutrophil phagocytosis and complement-mediated bactericidal activity. Several defense mechanisms counteract the antiphagocytic activity of the bacterial capsule. Activation of the alternative complement pathway results in cleavage of C3 with subsequent deposition of C3b on the bacterial surface, thereby facilitating opsonization, phagocytosis and intravascular clearance of the organism.[15] Impairment of the alternative comple-

ment pathway occurs in patients with sickle-cell disease and those who have undergone splenectomy, and these groups of patients are predisposed to the development of pneumococcal meningitis. Functional deficiencies of several components involved in the activation and function of complement-mediated defenses have been identified (i.e. mannose-binding lectin, properdin, lack of terminal complement components), which increase the susceptibility for invasive meningococcal infections.[16]

The blood–brain barrier is formed by cerebromicrovascular endothelial cells, which restrict blood-borne pathogen invasion. Cerebral capillaries, as opposed to other systemic capillaries, have adjacent endothelial cells fused together by tight junctions that prevent intercellular transport.[17] Bacteria are thought to invade the subarachnoid space via transcytosis. Nonhematogenous invasion of the CSF by bacteria occurs in situations of compromised integrity of the barriers surrounding the brain. Direct communication between the subarachnoid space and the skin or mucosal surfaces as a result of malformation or trauma gives rise to meningeal infection. Bacteria can also reach the CSF as a complication of neurosurgery, spinal anesthesia or ventriculostomy placement.

Physiologically, concentrations of leukocytes, antibodies and complement components in the subarachnoid space are low, which facilitates multiplication of bacteria. Pneumococcal cell-wall products, pneumolysin and bacterial DNA induce a severe inflammatory response via binding to Toll-like receptor (TLR)-2.[18] Once engaged, this signaling receptor transmits the activating signal into the cell, which initiates the induction of inflammatory cytokines.[19] Endotoxin is a major component of the outer membrane of the meningococcus and is crucial in the pathogenesis of sepsis and meningitis.[6] The host responds to bacterial endotoxin with proinflammatory gene expression and activation of coagulation pathways.

The subarachnoid inflammatory response is accompanied by production of multiple mediators in the central nervous system (CNS). Tumor necrosis factor (TNF), interleukin 1β and interleukin 6 are regarded as the major early response cytokines that trigger the inflammatory cascade, which induces various pathophysiologic alterations implicated in pneumococcal meningitis (Fig. 18.2).[13] TNF and interleukin 1β stimulate the expression of chemokines and adhesion molecules, which play an important part in the influx of leukocytes from the circulation to the CSF. Upon stimulation with bacterial components, macrophages and granulocytes release a broad range of potentially tissue-destructive agents, which contribute to vasospasm

and vasculitis, including oxidants (e.g. peroxynitrite) and proteolytic enzymes such as matrix metalloproteinases.[20] Matrix metalloproteinases, zinc-dependent enzymes produced as part of the immune response to bacteria that degrade extracellular matrix proteins, also contribute to the increased permeability of the blood–brain barrier.

The major element leading to increased intracranial pressure in bacterial meningitis is the development of cerebral edema, which may be vasogenic, cytotoxic or interstitial in origin. Vasogenic cerebral edema is a consequence of increased blood–brain barrier permeability.[21] Cytotoxic edema results from an increase in intracellular water following alterations of the cell membrane and loss of cellular homeostasis. Cytotoxic mechanisms include ischemia and the effect of excitatory amino acids. Secretion of antidiuretic hormone also contributes to cytotoxic edema by making the extracellular fluid hypotonic and increasing the permeability of the brain to water. Interstitial edema occurs by an increase in CSF volume, either through increased CSF production via increased blood flow in the choroid plexus, or decreased resorption secondary to increased CSF outflow resistance.

The exact mechanisms that lead to permanent brain injury are incompletely understood. Cerebral ischemic necrosis probably contributes to damage to the cerebral cortex (see Fig. 18.2). Cerebrovascular complications occur in 15–20% of patients with bacterial meningitis.[22] Other abnormalities include subdural effusion or empyema, septic sinus thrombosis, subarachnoid hematomas, compression of intracranial structures due to intracranial hypertension, and herniation of the temporal lobes or cerebellum. Gross changes, such as pressure coning, are rare.[23]

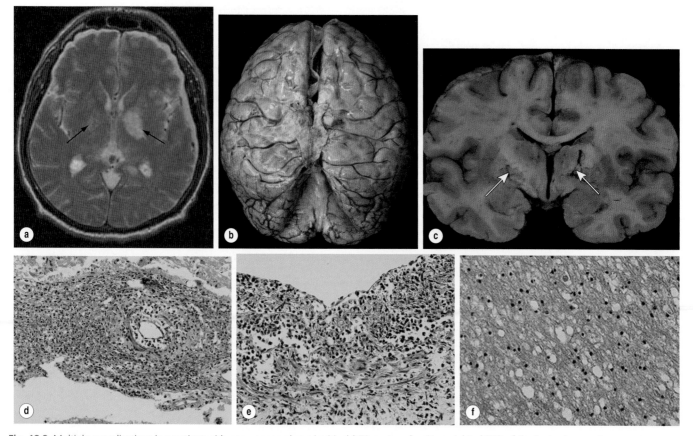

Fig. 18.2 Multiple complications in a patient with pneumococcal meningitis. (a) T2-proton-density-weighted MRI of the brain shows a transverse view of a hyperintense signal (arrows) in the basal ganglia that indicates bilateral oedema. (b) A post-mortem view of the brain of the same patient shows yellowish-coloured meninges as a result of extensive inflammation. (c) Confirmation of the bilateral infarction of the basal ganglia (arrows). The microscopic substrate in the same patient shows a meningeal artery with (d) lymphocytic infiltration in and around the vessel wall, (e) extensive subpial necrotizing cortical inflammation, and (f) edema in the white matter. Reproduced with permission from van de Beek et al.[21]

There is diffuse acute inflammation of the pia-arachnoid, with migration of neutrophil leukocytes and exudation of fibrin into the CSF. Pus accumulates over the surface of the brain, especially around its base and the emerging cranial nerves, and around the spinal cord. The meningeal vessels are dilated and congested and may be surrounded by pus (Fig. 18.3). Pus and fibrin are found in the ventricles and there is ventriculitis, with loss of ependymal lining and subependymal gliosis. Infection may block CSF circulation, causing obstructive hydrocephalus or spinal block. In many cases death may be attributable to related septicemia, although bilateral adrenal hemorrhage (Waterhouse–Friederichsen syndrome) may well be a terminal phenomenon rather than a cause of fatal adrenal insufficiency as was once imagined. Patients with meningococcal septicemia may develop acute pulmonary edema.

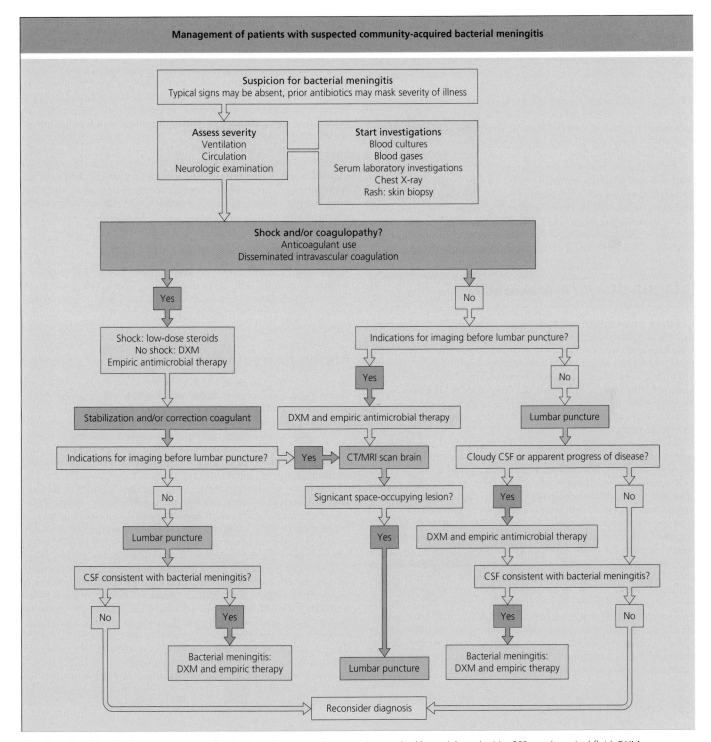

Fig. 18.3 Algorithm for the management of patients with suspected community-acquired bacterial meningitis. CSF, cerebrospinal fluid; DXM, dexamethasone. This material was previously published by van de Beek et al as part of an online supplementary appendix of reference 22. Copyright 2006 Massachusetts Medical Society. All rights reserved.

CLINICAL FEATURES

The clinical presentation of a patient with bacterial meningitis may vary depending on age, underlying conditions and severity of illness.[7,22] Clinical findings of meningitis in young children are often minimal, and in childhood bacterial meningitis and in elderly patients classic symptoms such as headache, fever, nuchal rigidity and altered mental status may be less common than in younger and middle-aged adults. Infants may become irritable or lethargic, stop feeding, and are found to have a bulging fontanel, separation of the cranial sutures, meningism and opisthotonos, and they may develop convulsions.

A meta-analysis of 845 patients aged over 30 years showed poor sensitivity and specificity for symptoms predicting community-acquired bacterial meningitis such as headache, nausea and vomiting.[24] A prospective study of 696 adults with community-acquired bacterial meningitis found an incidence of 44% for the classic triad of fever, neck stiffness and change in mental status (Glasgow Coma Scale ≤14).[2] However, 95% of patients with culture-proven bacterial meningitis presented with at least two signs or symptoms of headache, fever, neck stiffness and alterations in mental status. Purpuric rash is one of the hallmarks of meningococcal disease, but can be subtle.[6]

At physical examination, Kernig's sign, Brudzinski's sign and meningismus lack adequate sensitivity to be used in isolation to exclude bacterial meningitis. In a prospective study of 297 adults, Kernig's sign and Brudzinski's sign had poor sensitivity (5%) with high specificity (95%) in predicting meningitis.[25] Naturally, physicians do not rely on a single test for diagnosis and combine a number of historical and physical examination findings to form a clinical impression.

DIAGNOSIS AND MANAGEMENT

Given the high mortality of acute bacterial meningitis, starting treatment and completing the diagnostic process should be carried out simultaneously in most cases. The first step is to evaluate vital functions, obtain two sets of blood cultures, and start antimicrobial therapy and adjunctive dexamethasone when indicated (Fig. 18.3). At the same time, the severity of the patient's condition and the level of suspicion for the presence of bacterial meningitis should be determined. Performance and contraindications of lumbar puncture are covered in Practice Point 6.

Retrospective studies suggest a link between delay in the administration of antimicrobial therapy and adverse outcome.[23] In a prospective study involving 156 patients with pneumococcal meningitis who were admitted to the intensive care unit, a delay of more than 3 hours after presentation to the hospital before the initiation of antimicrobial therapy was associated with an increased 3-month mortality.[26]

In patients with suspected bacterial meningitis in whom lumbar puncture is postponed because of coagulation disorders (e.g. disseminated intravascular coagulation) or severe septic shock, or in whom cranial imaging is indicated before lumbar puncture, blood cultures should be drawn and antimicrobial therapy should be initiated without delay (see Fig. 18.3). In patients who have not undergone prior imaging and in whom disease progression is apparent, therapy should be started directly after lumbar puncture, as well as in all patients with cloudy CSF (suggestive of bacterial meningitis). In patients without apparent progress of disease and no cloudy CSF on lumbar puncture, antimicrobial therapy should be initiated after early CSF analysis (e.g. Gram stain, leukocyte count) confirms the diagnosis.

CSF analysis

When CSF analysis shows increased white blood cell counts, confirming a diagnosis of meningitis, many clinicians would like to determine who has life-threatening bacterial meningitis and who the less concerning viral meningitis. The CSF abnormalities of bacterial meningitis

include raised opening pressure in almost all patients, polymorphonuclear leukocytosis, decreased glucose concentration and increased protein concentration. In bacterial meningitis, the white blood cell count is typically >1000 cells/μl, while in viral meningitis it is <300 cells/μl, although there is considerable overlap.[23] The neutrophil count is higher in bacterial than in viral meningitis. More than 90% of cases present with CSF white cell counts of >100/μl. In immunocompromised patients, CSF white blood cell counts may be lower, although acellular CSF is probably rare, except in patients with tuberculous meningitis.[27] The normal CSF glucose concentration is between 2.5 and 4.4 mmol/l which is approximately 65% of the serum glucose. In bacterial meningitis the glucose concentration is usually <2.5 mmol/l or <40% of the serum glucose. The CSF protein in bacterial meningitis is usually >50 mg/dl.[2,28]

Gram stain is positive in identifying the organism in 50–90% of cases and CSF culture is positive in 80% of untreated patients.[2,28] Gram staining of CSF permits the rapid identification of the causative organism (sensitivity 60–90%; specificity >97%).[22] Latex particle agglutination tests that detect antigens of *N. meningitidis*, *S. pneumoniae*, *H. influenzae* and *S. agalactiae* can provide diagnostic confirmation but are not routinely available. Increasingly, laboratories are offering broad-range polymerase chain reaction (PCR) that can detect small numbers of viable and nonviable organisms in CSF. When the broad-range PCR is positive, a PCR that uses specific bacterial primers to detect the relevant pathogens can be done. However, although these tools are promising, further refinements are needed before PCR can be routinely recommended.

Skin biopsy

Microbiologic examination of skin lesions is routine diagnostic workup in patients with suspected meningococcal infection. It differentiates well between meningitis with and without hemodynamic complications and the result is not affected by previous antibiotic treatment.[22,29,30]

Antibiotic treatment

Empiric antibiotic treatment should be based on the most common bacterial species that cause the disease according to the patient's age or clinical setting and on antibiotic susceptibility patterns of the pathogens. Neonatal meningitis is largely caused by group B streptococci, *E. coli*, and *L. monocytogenes*.[7] Initial treatment, therefore, should consist of penicillin or ampicillin plus a third-generation cephalosporin (cefotaxime or ceftriaxone), or penicillin or ampicillin and an aminoglycoside (Table 18.1).[31,32]

Due to the emergence of multidrug-resistant strains of *S. pneumoniae*, vancomycin is often added to the initial empiric antimicrobial regimen in adult patients. Although intermediate penicillin resistance is common in some countries, the clinical importance of penicillin resistance in the meningococcus has yet to be established. In countries with low rates of pneumococcal penicillin resistance (such as The Netherlands),[33] penicillin is still recommended as a first-line agent. In the UK, the addition of vancomycin is also not considered necessary and is not recommended unless the patient presents from one of the geographic regions associated with high-level ceftriaxone resistance, such as Spain, southern Africa and the USA. In addition, in patients aged >50 years, treatment with ampicillin should be added to the above antibiotic regimen for additional coverage of *L. monocytogenes*, which is more prevalent among this age group.[22]

Recommendations directed at common specific organisms in adults are described below and general recommendations based on the isolated micro-organism are listed in Table 18.2.

Antibiotic prophylaxis

Prophylaxis is indicated for intimate contact of patients with meningococcal meningitis, which covers those eating and sleeping in the

Table 18.1 Recommendations for empiric antimicrobial therapy in suspected community-acquired bacterial meningitis

Predisposing factor	Common bacterial pathogens	Initial intravenous antibiotic therapy
Age		
<1 month	*Streptococcus agalactiae, Escherichia coli, Listeria monocytogenes*	Ampicillin plus cefotaxime or an aminoglycoside
1–3 months	*Streptococcus pneumoniae, Neisseria meningitidis, S. agalactiae, Haemophilus influenzae, E. coli, L. monocytogenes*	Ampicillin plus vancomycin plus ceftriaxone or cefotaxime*
3–23 months	*S. pneumoniae, N. meningitidis, S. agalactiae, H. influenzae, E. coli*	Vancomycin plus ceftriaxone or cefotaxime*
2–50 years	*N. meningitidis, S. pneumoniae*	Vancomycin plus ceftriaxone or cefotaxime*
>50 years	*N. meningitidis, S. pneumoniae, L. monocytogenes,* aerobic Gram-negative bacilli	Vancomycin plus ceftriaxone or cefotaxime plus ampicillin†
With risk factor present‡	*S. pneumoniae, L. monocytogenes, H. influenzae*	Vancomycin plus ceftriaxone or cefotaxime plus ampicillin†

*In areas with very low penicillin-resistance rates monotherapy penicillin may be considered.
†In areas with very low penicillin-resistance and cephalosporin-resistance rates, combination therapy of amoxicillin and third-generation cephalosporin may be considered.
‡Alcoholism, altered immune status.

European randomized controlled trial showed that dexamethasone, given before or with the first dose of antibiotics, met with a 0.59 relative risk of unfavorable outcome in adults with bacterial meningitis and 0.48 relative risk of mortality. This effect was most apparent in pneumococcal meningitis, in which mortality was decreased from 34% to 14%.[35] The benefits were not undermined by an increase of severe neurologic disability in survivors or by corticosteroid-induced complications. In a post-hoc analysis of pneumococcal meningitis patients who died less than 4 days after admission, the mortality benefit was due to reduced mortality from septic shock, pneumonia or acute respiratory distress syndrome; there was no significant reduction in mortality due to neurologic causes.[36]

A subsequent review in adults, which included five clinical trials, confirmed the corticosteroid-associated reduction in mortality and neurologic sequelae.[37] The reduction in case fatality in patients with pneumococcal meningitis was 21%. In meningococcal meningitis, mortality and neurologic sequelae were not significantly altered. Adverse events were equally divided between the treatment and placebo groups. Treatment with dexamethasone did not worsen long-term cognitive outcome.[38] Based on these results, dexamethasone has become routine therapy in adults with suspected bacterial meningitis.

An updated Cochrane analysis showed that corticosteroids were associated with lower case fatality (RR 0.83) and less severe hearing loss (RR 0.65) and long-term neurologic sequelae (RR 0.67). In children the beneficial effect was less convincing than in adults.[34] Subsequently, randomized studies in adults with pyogenic meningitis showed no significant benefit in Malawi,[39] and significant benefit in mortality (RR 0.43) in Vietnamese patients with pyogenic meningitis.[40]

Use of dexamethasone in bacterial meningitis remains controversial in certain patients. First, there seems to be no clear benefit in patients in the Malawi setting. Secondly, patients with septic shock and adrenal insufficiency benefit from corticosteroid therapy in physiologic doses and for more than 4 days; however, without adrenal insufficiency, corticosteroids may be detrimental. A review of nine studies in sepsis or septic shock showed a trend towards increased mortality with corticosteroid administration.[41] Animal studies of bacterial meningitis suggest that the initiation of steroid therapy before or with the first dose of antibiotics is more effective than after the first dose of antimicrobial therapy, but the time point at which dexamethasone loses effects is unknown. Thirdly, by reducing permeability of the blood–brain barrier, steroids can impede penetration of antibiotics into the CSF, as was shown for vancomycin in animal studies, and lead to treatment failures, especially in drug-resistant pneumococcal meningitis. However, an observational study in suspected pneumococcal meningitis showed appropriate concentrations of vancomycin in CSF when steroids were used.[42]

Intensive care management

Monitoring in an ICU is recommended to recognize changes in consciousness and the development of new neurologic signs, monitor for subtle seizures and treat severe agitation. Bacterial meningitis may be associated with septic shock, which is an important predictor of outcome. Patients with bacterial meningitis are at risk of hyponatremia, although often mild.[43] Hyponatremia may be a result of cerebral salt wasting, the syndrome of inappropriate antidiuretic hormone secretion, or aggressive fluid resuscitation. It is a dilemma whether intravenous fluids should be restricted in hyponatremia. Hypernatremia is predictive of unfavorable outcome and mortality.[44] Severe brain injury in meningitis rarely leads to decreased antidiuretic hormone secretion resulting in diabetes insipidus. Whether adequate fluid management improves prognosis is still uncertain.

Decline in consciousness

In patients with a decline in consciousness or failure to improve upon antimicrobial therapy, brain imaging is indicated. A decline in

same dwelling as well as those having close social and kissing contacts, or health-care workers who perform mouth-to-mouth resuscitation, endotracheal intubation or endotracheal tube management.[22] Patients with meningococcal meningitis treated with monotherapy of penicillin or ampicillin should also receive chemoprophylaxis, since carriage is not reliably eradicated by these drugs. Recommendations for prophylactic therapy are listed is Table 18.2.

Adjunctive dexamethasone treatment

Animal models of bacterial meningitis showed that bacterial lysis, induced by antibiotics, leads to subarachnoid inflammation (Fig. 18.4). The severity can be attenuated by treatment with steroids. Several trials were done to assess adjunctive steroids in bacterial meningitis. Dexamethasone is a glucocorticosteroid with excellent penetration in the CSF. In a meta-analysis of randomized trials dexamethasone reduced meningitis-associated hearing loss in children with influenzal meningitis.[34]

Most available studies on dexamethasone therapy in adults with bacterial meningitis suffered from methodologic flaws. In 2002, a

Table 18.2 Specific antimicrobial therapy in community-acquired bacterial meningitis based on CSF culture results and *in-vitro* susceptibility testing

Micro-organism, susceptibility	Standard therapy	Alternative therapies

Streptococcus pneumoniae
Penicillin MIC
   <0.1 mg/l
   0.1–1.0 mg/l
   >2.0 mg/l
	Penicillin G or ampicillin
	Cefotaxime or ceftriaxone
	Vancomycin plus cefotaxime or ceftriaxone*
		Cefotaxime or ceftriaxone, chloramphenicol
		Cefepime, meropenem
		Fluoroquinolone[†]

Cefotaxime or ceftriaxone MIC >1.0 mg/l	Vancomycin plus cefotaxime or ceftriaxone[‡]	Fluoroquinolone[†]
Neisseria meningitidis Penicillin MIC <0.1 mg/l 0.1–1.0 mg/l	Penicillin G or ampicillin Cefotaxime or ceftriaxone	Cefotaxime or ceftriaxone, chloramphenicol Chloramphenicol, fluoroquinolone, meropenem
Listeria monocytogenes	Penicillin G or ampicillin[¶]	Trimethoprim–sulfamethoxazole, meropenem
Group B streptococcus	Penicillin G or ampicillin[¶]	Cefotaxime or ceftriaxone
Escherichia coli and other Enterobacteriaceae	Cefotaxime or ceftriaxone[¶]	Aztreonam[¶], fluoroquinolone, meropenem[¶], trimethoprim–sulfamethoxazole, ampicillin[¶]
Pseudomonas aeruginosa	Ceftazidime[¶] or cefepime[¶]	Aztreonam[¶], ciprofloxacin[¶], meropenem[¶]

Haemophilus influenzae
   β-Lactamase negative
 	
   β-Lactamase positive
	Ampicillin
	
	Cefotaxime or ceftriaxone
		Cefotaxime or ceftriaxone, cefepime, chloramphenicol, fluoroquinolone
		Cefepime, chloramphenicol, fluoroquinolone

Chemoprophylaxis[§] *Neisseria meningitidis*	Rifampin (rifampicin), ceftriaxone, ciprofloxacin, azithromycin	

CSF, cerebrospinal fluid; MIC, minimum inhibitory concentration.
*Consider addition of rifampin (rifampicin) if dexamethasone is given.
[†]Gatifloxacin or moxifloxacin; no clinical data on use in patients with bacterial meningitis.
[‡]Consider addition of rifampin (rifampicin) if the MIC of ceftriaxone is >2 mg/l.
[¶]Consider addition of an aminoglycoside.
[§]Prophylaxis is indicated for close contacts who are defined as those with intimate contact, which covers those eating and sleeping in the same dwelling as well as those having close social and kissing contacts; or health-care workers who perform mouth-to-mouth resuscitation, endotracheal intubation or endotracheal tube management. General recommendations for intravenous empiric antibiotic treatment have included penicillin, 2 MU q4h; amoxicillin or ampicillin, 2 g q4h; vancomycin, 15 mg/kg q8h; third-generation cephalosporin: ceftriaxone, 2 g q12h, or cefotaxime, 2 g q4–6h; cefepime, 2 g q8h; ceftazidime, 2 g q8h; meropenem, 2 g q8h; chloramphenicol, 1–1.5 g q6h; fluoroquinolone: gatifloxacin, 400 mg q24h, or moxifloxacin, 400 mg q24h, although no data on optimal dose needed in patients with bacterial meningitis; trimethoprim–sulfamethoxazole, 5 mg/kg q6–12h; aztreonam, 2 g q6–8h; ciprofloxacin, 400 mg q8–12h; rifampicin (rifampin) 600 mg q12–24h; aminoglycoside: gentamicin, 1.7 mg/kg q8h. The preferred dose for chemoprophylaxis: rifampin (rifampicin), 600 mg po q12h for 2 days; ceftriaxone, 250 mg im; ciprofloxacin, 500 mg po; azithromycin, 500 mg po.

consciousness in bacterial meningitis is compatible with meningoencephalitis (see Fig. 18.4). Proinflammatory mediators in the subarachnoid space contribute to an increased permeability of the blood–brain barrier, cerebral edema and increased intracranial pressure. On neuroimaging, early signs of brain edema are the disappearance of Sylvian fissures and a narrowing of ventricular size. In an advanced stage of brain edema and raised intracranial pressure, basal cisterns and sulci may become obliterated.

Seizures occur in about 20% of patients with bacterial meningitis.[45] These patients tend to be older, are more likely to have focal abnormalities on brain CT and to have *S. pneumoniae* as the causative microorganism, and they have a higher mortality. If a patient with a falling conscious level has a normal brain CT and normal serum electrolytes, then an electroencephalogram (EEG) should be performed to look for seizure activity. The high mortality warrants a low threshold for starting antiepileptic therapy in those with clinical suspicion of seizures.

In bacterial meningitis a purulent exudate forms over the cerebral hemispheres where it interferes with CSF absorption by the arachnoid villi, resulting in communicating hydrocephalus.[21] When the inflammatory exudate involves the basal cisterns and surrounds the cranial nerves at the base of the brain (basilar meningitis), it may block CSF flow at the foramina of Luschka and Magendie, resulting in obstructive hydrocephalus. Obstructive hydrocephalus may also complicate infratentorial subdural empyema.[46] In patients with communicating hydrocephalus, lumbar punctures can be performed (with measurement of CSF pressure) or the temporary insertion of a lumbar drain. In patients with mild enlargement of the ventricular system without clinical deterioration, spontaneous resolution may occur and 'watchful waiting' may be justified. Acute obstructive hydrocephalus requires ventricular drainage.

Focal neurologic abnormalities

In meningitis, focal cerebral abnormalities (hemiparesis, monoparesis or aphasia) are most commonly caused by stroke or seizures, or a combination of the two. Activation of inflammation and coagulation are closely related and interdependent. In a patient with rapid deterioration, subdural empyema should be considered. Clues to the diagnosis are the presence of sinusitis and mastoiditis (and recent surgery for either of these disorders).[46] Abnormalities of the cranial nerves are caused by the meningeal inflammatory process or by an increase

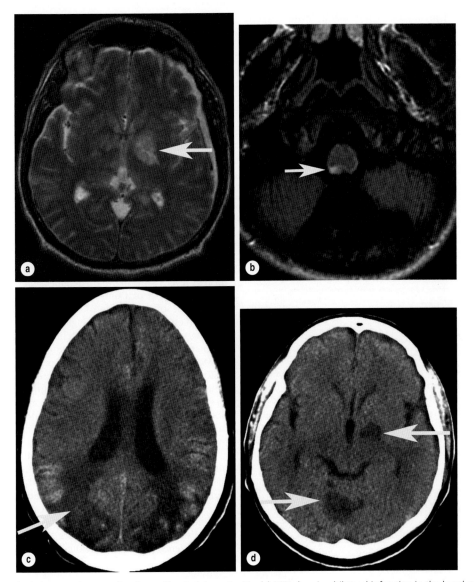

Fig. 18.4 Neuroimaging of cerebrovascular complications of bacterial meningitis. (a) MRI showing bilateral infarction in the basal ganglia causing decline in consciousness. (b) MRI showing a focal zone of signal abnormality in the right dorsal aspect of the medulla oblongata, which had restricted diffusion, suggestive of cerebral infarction. (c) CT showing bilateral occipital brain oedema indicating infarction. (d) CT showing hypodense areas in left basal ganglia and cerebellum consistent with infarction.

in CSF pressure. The most frequent cranial nerve abnormality is the involvement of the eighth cranial nerve, which is reflected in a hearing loss in 14% of patients.

Arthritis

The coexistence of bacterial meningitis and arthritis has been described in several studies; it occurs in 7% of patients overall, more in meningococcal meningitis (12%).[47] It is caused either by hematogenous bacterial seeding of joints (septic arthritis) or by immune-complex deposition in joints (see Chapter 40).

Recurrent bacterial meningitis

Recurrent bacterial meningitis occurs in 5% of community-acquired bacterial meningitis cases; predisposing conditions are head injury and CSF leak, and occasionally humoral immundeficiency.[48,49] The high prevalence of remote head injury and CSF leakage justifies an active search for anatomic defects and CSF leakage. Detection of β-2 trans-ferrin in nasal discharge is a sensitive and specific method to confirm

a CSF leak and thin-slice CT of the skull base is best to detect small bone defects. The detection of a small bone defect does not prove CSF leakage. Surgical repair has a high success rate.

When to repeat a lumbar puncture

A repeat CSF analysis should only be carried out in patients whose condition has not responded clinically after 48 hours of appropriate antimicrobial and adjunctive dexamethasone treatment. It is essential when pneumococcal meningitis caused by penicillin-resistant or cephalosporin-resistant strains is suspected. Gram staining and culture of the CSF should be negative after 24 hours of appropriate antimicrobial therapy.

OUTCOME

Community-acquired bacterial meningitis in adults is a severe disease with high fatality and morbidity rates. Meningitis caused by *S. pneumoniae* has the highest case fatality rates, reported from 19% to 37%.[7,22] Whereas neurologic complications are the leading cause of death in younger patients, elderly patients die predominantly from systemic complications.[50] Of those who survive, up to 50% develop neurologic sequelae, including cognitive impairment.[51] For meningococcal meningitis mortality is around 5%.[52] The strongest risk factors for an unfavorable outcome in bacterial meningitis are impaired consciousness, low CSF white cell count and infection with *S. pneumoniae*.[2,53]

POST-TRAUMATIC BACTERIAL MENINGITIS

This is often indistinguishable clinically from spontaneous meningitis. However, in obtunded or unconscious patients with a recent or previous head injury, few clinical signs may be present. Fever and deterioration in the level of consciousness or loss of vital functions may be the only signs of meningitis. The rare finding of a CSF leak supports the possibility of meningitis. The range of bacteria causing meningitis in these patients is broad and consideration should be given to broad-spectrum antibiotics including metronidazole for anaerobic pathogens.[31]

Viral Meningitis

EPIDEMIOLOGY

Acute viral meningitis and meningoencephalitis represent the majority of viral CNS infections and frequently occur in epidemics with a seasonal distribution.[54] Enteroviruses cause an estimated 90% of cases in countries that immunize against mumps, while arboviruses constitute the majority of the remaining reported cases in the USA.[55] Most cases occur from late spring to autumn, reflecting the increased incidence of enteroviral and arboviral infections during these seasons.

PATHOPHYSIOLOGY AND PATHOLOGY

The pathogenesis of meningitis and meningoencephalitis are similar and requires that viruses reach the CNS by hematogenous or neuronal spread. Viruses most frequently access the CNS after a high-titer secondary viremia and cell-free or cell-associated CNS entry. Other than direct entry via cerebral vessels, virus can initially infect the meninges and then enter the parenchyma across either ependymal cells or the pial linings. Viruses exhibit differences in neurotropism and neurovirulence.

CLINICAL FEATURES

Clinical manifestations of patients presenting with viral meningitis vary with age, immune status and viral etiology. The clinical examination of a patient with suspected meningitis has been described previously in this chapter.

Epidemiologic features such as the season of the year, prevalent diseases within the community, travel, recreational activities (e.g. caving or hiking), occupational exposures and animal contacts (e.g. insect or animal bite) may provide helpful clues to the diagnosis. Late summer and early fall are seasons when enteroviral infections are encountered in temperate climates. Similarly, during warm summer months, mosquito propagation may enhance the likelihood of transmission of arthropod-borne viruses.

Patients with enteroviral meningitis often present with nonspecific symptoms such as fever of 3–5 days' duration, malaise and headache.[56] Nuchal rigidity and photophobia are the hallmark sign and symptom for meningitis, but 33% of patients with viral meningitis have no evidence of meningismus.[57] Children may present with seizures secondary to fever, electrolyte disturbances or the infection itself. In the immunocompromised host, enteroviral infection is both a diagnostic quandary and a potentially life-threatening disease. While physical examination of the patient usually does not suggest an etiologic diagnosis, a few considerations are essential.

Patients with herpes simplex virus (HSV) meningitis are infected with HSV type 2 and present with a rather benign disease. This is in contrast with herpes simplex encephalitis (HSE) caused by HSV type 1 which is a serious illness with significant risks of morbidity and death (Chapter 155). Patients with herpes meningitis typically have recurrent episodes.[58]

LABORATORY FINDINGS

Initial CSF samples, while frequently suggestive of the diagnosis, are neither sensitive nor specific enough to differentiate viral from bacterial meningitis.[23] The CSF in patients with viral meningitis typically exhibits pleocytosis with 10–500 leukocytes and a slightly elevated protein level (>100 mg/dl). The glucose level in the CSF is typically greater than 40% of a simultaneously drawn serum sample.

Cultures of specimens of body fluids other than CSF may be useful in establishing the etiologic diagnosis in selected patients with meningoencephalitis.[31] Specific clinical findings should also direct other sites for culture (e.g. stool, skin, sputum).

Molecular techniques have advanced identification of viral agents. PCR provides a rapid and reliable test for verifying the etiology of certain types of meningitis. These techniques provide results within 24–36 hours and therefore may limit the duration of hospitalization, antibiotic use and excessive diagnostic procedures. For other infections, molecular techniques are the standard for diagnosing viral meningitis.

Diagnostic serologic assays have simplified the diagnosis of viral infections of the CNS. The ELISA assay that detects IgM antibodies in the CSF from patients with presumed Japanese encephalitis (JE) is both sensitive and specific, as most patients have antibodies at the time of hospitalization and virtually all acquire them by the third day of illness.[59] Unlike herpesviruses, which are ubiquitous agents with generally high basal seroprevalence levels in the general population, seroprevalence levels for individual arboviruses are generally low.

ANTIVIRAL TREATMENT

Antiviral therapy exists for HSV-1, HSV-2, varicella-zoster virus (VZV), cytomegalovirus (CMV) and human immunodeficiency virus (HIV).[60–62] The introduction of aciclovir has resulted in a sharp decline in mortality and morbidity from HSE.[62] Most authors recommend the use of intravenous aciclovir for HSV meningitis, although no definitive clinical trials have been conducted. There are no data on benefit of antiviral treatment or on suppressive therapy for recurrent HSV meningitis.

In the normal host, viral meningitis is a relatively benign self-limited disease. A prospective study in children less than 2 years of age, for example, found that even in the 9% of children who develop evidence of acute neurologic disease (complex seizures, increased intracerebral pressure or coma) long-term prognosis is excellent. During follow-up (42 months), children with acute CNS complications performed neurodevelopmental tasks and achieved developmental milestones as well as did children with an uncomplicated course.[63,64]

In case reports, immunoglobulin preparations, given systemically or intrathecally, retarded mortality and morbidity in agammaglobulinemic patients with enteroviral meningitis. Enteroviral infections in neonates frequently produce overwhelming viremia and CNS disease. A blind, randomized controlled trial did not demonstrate clinical benefit for enterovirus-infected neonates with severe life-threatening disease who received intravenous immunoglobulin.[65,66]

Pleconaril, an inhibitor of enterovirus replication, was tested in two placebo-controlled clinical trials. Of 607 randomized patients in a multicenter, double-blind, placebo-controlled study of pleconaril, 240 patients were confirmed to have enterovirus infection.[67,68] Resolution of headache in patients with concomitant moderate to severe nausea at baseline occurred at a median of 9.5 days in the absence of therapy and was reduced to 7.0 days for pleconaril recipients ($p = 0.009$). Over 50% of untreated patients had a persistent headache that was greater than 1 week in duration. Pleconaril shortened the course of illness compared to placebo recipients, especially in the early disease course. However, the benefit was achieved only modestly in a subgroup analysis of patients with more severe disease after adjusting for confounding variables.

SUPPORTIVE THERAPY

After establishing a presumptive diagnosis and instituting therapy, the clinician must also vigilantly anticipate and treat complications associated with the viral CNS disease or the therapeutic interventions,[55] as described in this chapter for patients with bacterial meningitis. Seizures secondary to direct viral CNS damage, inflammatory vasculitis and electrolyte changes require anticonvulsant therapy.

Chronic Meningitis

CLINICAL FEATURES

Chronic meningitis is defined by symptoms of meningeal inflammation with CSF pleocytosis that persist for more than 4 weeks. Symptoms and signs of chronic meningitis evolve over several days to weeks. Patients complain of headaches, often associated with signs of infection (fever, anorexia). Nuchal rigidity may be subtle or absent. Many forms of chronic meningitis involve the base of the brain and lead to cranial nerve palsies, often affecting eye movements and facial musculature. As the syndrome progresses, signs of brain involvement with seizures, mental status changes, confusion or hallucinations, and focal neurologic deficits develop. Hydrocephalus and increased intracranial pressure may accompany the syndrome.

TUBERCULOUS MENINGITIS

One of the most common causes of chronic meningitis is *Mycobacterium tuberculosis* (Table 18.3). Tuberculous meningitis (TBM) results from the rupture of a tubercle into the subarachnoid space. It is the most

Table 18.3 Microbial causes of chronic meningitis

Pathogen		Predominant type of CSF pleocytosis	Predisposition and risk factors	Associated clinical manifestations
Bacteria	*Actinomyces* spp.	Neutrophils	Mouth and ear lesions	CNS lesions, endophthalmitis
	Borrelia burgdorferi (Lyme disease)	Lymphocytes	Tick bite	Cranial nerve palsy (VII nerve)
	Brucella spp.	Lymphocytes, neutrophils	Unpasteurized dairy products	Undulant fever, hepatomegaly
	Leptospira spp.	Neutrophils	Exposure to urine of infected animals	Hepatomegaly, hepatitis, thrombocytopenia
	Mycobacterium tuberculosis	Neutrophils, monocytes, lymphocytes	Immunodeficiency, high endemic prevalence	Cranial nerve palsy (VI nerve)
	Nocardia spp.	Neutrophils	Immunodeficiency	Abscesses
	Treponema pallidum	Eosinophils, lymphocytes	Sexually transmitted diseases	Cranial nerve palsy (VII and VIII nerves)
	Tropheryma whipplei	Neutrophil	Gastrointestinal Whipple disease	Cognitive decline, gait ataxia, supranuclear gaze palsy
Viruses	Cytomegalovirus	Lymphocytes; neutrophils (in HIV)	Immunodeficiency	Fever, retinitis
	Echovirus	Lymphocytes	Agammaglobulinemia	Dermatomyositis
	Lymphocytic choriomeningitis virus	Lymphocytes	Exposure to rodents	Orchitis, leukocytopenia, thrombocytopenia
	Mumps virus	Neutrophils	No vaccination	Parotitis, orchitis, oophoritis
	HIV	Lymphocytes	HIV risk factors	Mononucleosis-like illness
Fungi	*Aspergillus* spp.	Lymphocytes or neutrophils	Immunodeficiency, surgery	Lung involvement
	Candida spp.	Neutrophils	Antibiotics, surgery, immunodeficiency	Disseminated disease
	Coccidioides spp.	Lymphocytes	Endemic areas	Lung involvement
	Cryptococcus spp.	Lymphocytes	Immunodeficiency	Encephalitis, headache
	Histoplasma spp.	Lymphocytes	Endemic areas, immunodeficiency	Fever, oral lesions, hepatosplenomegaly
	Pseudallescheria spp.	Neutrophils	Immunodeficiency	Skin lesions, endophthalmitis
	Sporothrix spp.	Neutrophils	Immunodeficiency	Skin lesions, endophthalmitis
Parasites	*Taenia solium*	Eosinophils	Endemic areas	Elevated intracranial pressure, calcified lesions on head imaging
	Angiostrongylus spp.	Eosinophils	Raw seafood	Fever

important cause of chronic meningitis. In the less developed world TBM remains a common cause of bacterial meningitis, particularly in populations with a high prevalence of HIV infection.[27]

Most patients with TBM have progressive headache and signs of meningeal irritation, followed by cranial nerve involvement, other neurologic deficits and progressive mental status changes over a period of weeks.[27,69] These prodromal symptoms can last from 2 to 8 weeks until the classic features of meningitis become more apparent. Patients commonly present to hospital, when the infection is well established. They will usually complain of headache and vomiting; many will present confused or comatose. Examination reveals neck stiffness in most, although rarely as marked as in pyogenic meningitis. Cranial nerve palsies (especially third, sixth and seventh nerves) are found in 25% of patients. Ten percent of patients will present with a mono- or hemiparesis. Rarely, TBM presents as an acute meningoencephalitis that can be difficult to distinguish from pyogenic bacterial or viral meningitis.[69] Seizures are rare in adults with TBM, but more common in children. HIV infection does not appear to alter the clinical presentation of TBM, although evidence of other extrapulmonary disease is more likely in HIV-infected patients.

Tuberculous meningitis may be a consequence of either primary infection or reactivation of disease. The diagnosis can be confirmed by a positive CSF culture; however, *M. tuberculosis* is recovered from the CSF in only 38–88% of cases.[27] A moderate lymphocytic pleocytosis is most common. The glucose can be very low; the protein is often very high. CSF smears for acid-fast bacilli are positive in only a minority of cases (10–20%). Tuberculin skin tests are frequently negative in TBM.

The treatment of TBM follows the model of short course chemotherapy of pulmonary tuberculosis (Table 18.4): an 'intensive phase' of treatment with four drugs, followed by a prolonged 'continuation phase' with two drugs. When there is no suspicion of multidrug resistance, the first 2 months of treatment should be with isoniazid, rifampicin, pyrazinamide and either streptomycin, ethambutol or ethionamide.[27] The British Thoracic Society (BTS) and the Infectious Diseases Society of America (IDSA) favor ethambutol as the fourth drug, although they acknowledge the lack of evidence from controlled trials. British and American guidelines suggest between 9 and 12 months total antituberculosis treatment for TBM, although a recent systematic review concluded that 6 months might be sufficient provided the likelihood of drug resistance is low.

The use of steroids in the treatment of TBM was first reported in the early 1950s.[70] Continued research supports the use of steroids while adequately treating with multiple antimycobacterial drugs in TBM.

A meta-analysis of 595 patients found that the use of adjunctive steroids led to fewer deaths and reduced incidences of death and disability.[70,71] A randomized, double-blind, placebo-controlled trial of 545 patients found that patients receiving dexamethasone had a reduced risk of death (RR 0.69) that was consistent across subgroups of differing clinical severity.[72] Although there were significantly fewer serious adverse events in the patients receiving dexamethasone, this study did not report an associated reduction in the proportion of patients who developed severe disabilities, and the lack of neurosurgical intervention might limit the generalizability of the results.

The largest randomized study recommend a stratified dexamethasone treatment regimen in patients with TBM.[72] Under this protocol, patients with a Glasgow Coma Scale score of less than 15 or who have a focal neurologic deficit are treated with intravenous dexamethasone for 4 weeks (0.4 mg/kg per day in week 1, 0.3 mg/kg per day in week 2, 0.2 mg/kg per day in week 3, and 0.1 mg/kg per day in week 4), followed by a taper of oral dexamethasone (4 mg/day, 3 mg/day, 2 mg/day and 1 mg/day, each for a period of 1 week). Patients with a normal mental status and no neurologic findings receive intravenous dexamethasone for 2 weeks (0.2 mg/kg per day in week 1, then 0.1 mg/kg per day in week 2), followed by the same oral taper as described above. It is recommended that the steroid treatment should start as soon as possible after initiation of first-line antituberculous drugs.

Tuberculous meningitis leads to severe CNS inflammatory processes with secondary damage; mortality of up to 50% has been reported.[27]

OTHER INFECTIOUS CAUSES OF CHRONIC MENINGITIS

Secondary syphilis may cause chronic meningitis.[73] The disease is slowly progressive, and generally symptoms have been present for more than 1 month before presentation. Cranial nerve palsies are common; the facial and acoustic nerves are the most frequently affected. Diagnosis is based on a positive VDRL test in CSF. Treatment consists of high-dose penicillin (see Table 18.4).

The diagnosis of meningitis associated with Lyme disease, caused by *Borrelia burgdorferi*, should be considered in patients who live or have traveled through endemic regions, particularly those with a history of a tick bite or erythema chronicum migrans.[74,75] Meningitis may persist for weeks and may be associated with cranial nerve palsies and peripheral neuropathies. Syphilis, other spirochetal diseases and collagen vascular diseases

Table 18.4 Treatment recommendations for common treatable causes of chronic infectious meningitis

Agent	Therapy	Dose	Route
Herpesviruses	Aciclovir	10 mg/kg q8h	iv
Mycobacterium tuberculosis	Isoniazid Rifampin (rifampicin) Ethambutol Pyrazinamide	10 mg/kg/q24h (up to 300 mg/q24h) 10 mg/kg/q24h (up to 600 mg/q24h) 25 mg/kg/q24h 25 mg/kg/q24h (up to 2.5 g/q24h)	po or iv po or iv po or iv po or iv
Brucella spp. (>8 years)	Doxycycline plus gentamicin	100 mg q12h 1.7–2 mg/kg q8h	po iv
Brucella spp. (<8 years)	Trimethoprim– sulfamethoxazole plus gentamicin	5 mg/kg trimethoprim q12h 25 mg/kg sulfamethoxazole q12h 2 mg/kg q8h	po po iv
Treponema pallidum	Penicillin G	2 g q4h	iv
Borrelia spp.	Ceftriaxone	2–3 g q24h	iv
Cryptococcus spp.	Amphotericin B plus flucytosine	0.5–0.8 mg/kg/q24h 37.5 mg/kg q6h	iv po
Coccidioides spp.	Fluconazole	400–600 mg/q24h	po

may result in a false-positive Lyme serology. Treatment consists of high-dose ceftriaxone, although a clinical trial showed oral doxycycline to be equally effective in European adults with mild neuroborreliosis.[74–76]

Whipple's disease is a rare, systemic infectious disease caused by the bacterium *Tropheryma whipplei*.[77] Neurologic manifestations occur in three situations: neurologic relapse of previously treated Whipple's disease, neurologic involvement in classic Whipple's disease, and isolated neurologic symptoms due to *T. whipplei* without evidence of intestinal involvement. Many patients have systemic symptoms, such as fever, weight loss, peripheral lymphadenopathy and arthralgia. The predominant symptoms include cognitive impairment, ophthalmoplegia, ataxia and upper motor neuron disorder. A review summarized outcomes for 30 patients described in the literature: 18 (60%) had improvement and 10 died (33%); in 1 patient, the disease stabilized. Treatment consisted of high-dose ceftriaxone, followed by maintenance therapy with co-trimoxazole or hydroxychloroquine in combination with doxycycline.[78]

Presentations of chronic meningitis caused by *Cryptococcus neoformans* range from a subacute meningoencephalitis to fever of unknown origin.[79] People at highest risk are those with defects in cellular immunity such as occurs in AIDS, hematologic malignancies and prolonged use of high-dose corticosteroids. CSF shows moderate lymphocytic pleocytosis; however, in patients who have AIDS, inflammation may be virtually absent. Cryptococcal antigen latex agglutination is positive in more than 90% of cases, whereas microscopy of India ink preparations to visualize the yeast in CSF is less sensitive (but may be more readily available). Treatment recommendations are provided in Table 18.4 (see also Chapter 91).

Coccidioides immitis grows in the dry sandy soils of the south-west USA, and Central and South America.[80] Acute infection is acquired by inhalation of the spores, and meningitis develops within a few months. There are few distinguishing features of the disease; some patients who have generalized disease have erythema nodosum; hydrocephalus is a common complication. CSF eosinophilia in patients who have lived or traveled through endemic regions should alert the clinician to the possibility of *Coccidioides* meningitis. Complement-fixing antibodies are present in the CSF in 75–95% of cases and CSF cultures are positive in more than 50%. Treatment is usually with an azole or amphotericin B, depending on the clinical manifestations and the immune status of the host.

Histoplasma meningitis is a rare complication of histoplasmosis.[81] The diagnosis should be considered in patients who live or have traveled through endemic regions – the Ohio River Valley of the USA, the Caribbean and South America. CSF cultures are positive in 27–65% of cases. Blood should be cultured and a buffy coat of the blood should be examined for the presence of the fungus. *Histoplasma* polysaccharide antigen is found in the urine, blood or CSF in 61% of patients and in an even higher proportion of patients who have AIDS. Adequate and prolonged antifungal therapy is indicated in all cases of CNS histoplasmosis.

Neurocysticercosis is endemic in Mexico, South America and Asia. Infection is acquired by eating food contaminated with eggs of *Taenia solium*.[82] Seizures are the most common manifestation. Intraventricular and basilar cysts (racemose cysticercosis) may present with signs of obstructive hydrocephalus. The CSF shows a lymphocytic pleocytosis with eosinophils. CT scans of the head show multiple calcified lesions. Serology of blood and CSF may provide support for the diagnosis. Treatment should be tailored according to the type of neurocysticercosis and may consist of albendazole, steroids, analgesics, antiepileptic drugs, surgical resection of lesions and placement of ventricular shunts.

Angiostrongylus cantonensis, the rat lung worm, is most prevalent in Asia and the Pacific Islands and is acquired by the ingestion of raw or inadequately cooked shellfish or snails.[83] Symptoms are typical of chronic meningitis, and rash with pruritus is also common. Infection results in peripheral eosinophilia and chronic eosinophilic meningitis, which resolves spontaneously within 2 months. There is no effective therapy.

Other even less common causes of infectious chronic meningitis are organisms that usually cause abscesses, which may leak into the subarachnoid space to cause chronic meningitis. These conditions include blastomycosis, paracoccidioidomycosis, phaeohyphomycosis, mucormycosis, actinomycosis, nocardiosis and toxoplasmosis. Less common fungi causing this syndrome include *Sporothrix schenckii*, chromoblastomycoses and *Aspergillus* spp.

REFERENCES

References for this chapter can be found online at http://www.expertconsult.com

Chapter | **19** |

Karen C Bloch
Carol A Glaser
Allan R Tunkel

Encephalitis and myelitis

INTRODUCTION

Encephalitis is defined by the presence of an inflammatory process in the brain, associated with clinical evidence of neurologic dysfunction. It is one of the most challenging syndromes for clinicians to diagnose and manage, particularly because a specific pathogen is identified in fewer than 50% of cases.[1] Diagnostic difficulties in establishing an etiology include the vast number of infectious causes of encephalitis, the many noninfectious etiologies that present with syndromes suggestive of encephalitis, and the confusion regarding the role of molecular versus serologic testing. Guidelines for the diagnosis and management of encephalitis have recently been published and address many of these issues.[2]

Myelitis refers to inflammation of the spinal cord, as a result of a direct infectious process or through postinfectious or other mechanisms;[3] in association with encephalitis, this syndrome is often referred to as encephalomyelitis. Encephalitis and myelitis are often considered together because there is overlap in terms of epidemiology, microbiology and approach to management. The current chapter will focus on the syndromes of encephalitis and myelitis in immunocompetent hosts, with a more detailed discussion of pathogen-specific infections in the chapters dedicated to these microbes.

EPIDEMIOLOGY

Encephalitis causes significant morbidity and mortality, and represents a significant burden on the health-care system. The average duration of hospitalization for patients with encephalitis is 12 days, with a cumulative cost for hospitalization exceeding $650 million per year in the USA alone.[4] The case-fatality rate among patients with encephalitis varies from 3.8% to 7.4% and is significantly higher in patients also infected with human immunodeficiency virus (HIV).[5,6] These aggregate data mask the fact that in some infections, such as those caused by rabies virus or *Naegleria fowleri*, the mortality rate is almost 100%. Additionally, these estimates of disease burden do not take into account the significant morbidity among survivors of encephalitis, with the resultant loss of productivity and need for prolonged rehabilitation or skilled nursing care.

Limited data exist on the incidence and epidemiology of encephalitis. A county-wide, population-based study of encephalitis diagnosed between 1950 and 1981 in Minnesota reported an incidence of 7.4 cases per 100 000 person-years;[5] similar rates have been reported in population-based studies in Finnish children.[7,8] A more recent study evaluating US hospital discharge survey data between 1988 and 1997 identified approximately 19 000 encephalitis hospitalizations annually, for a rate of 7.3 encephalitis hospitalizations per 100 000 US population.[4] While these studies of disparate populations have shown strikingly similar rates, these data predate the introduction of West Nile virus (WNV) in the USA, which in recent years accounted for 1000–2000 cases annually during summer and early fall.[9] Outside of the USA, there are many important viruses, such as measles, rabies and Japanese encephalitis virus (JEV), that contribute significantly to the disease burden in these areas (Fig. 19.1). For instance, JEV causes 20 000 illnesses each year worldwide; 20–30% of these infections result in death, and over 50% of survivors have neurologic sequelae.[10]

Several factors appear to increase the risk of encephalitis regardless of etiology. Rates of encephalitis are higher in males than females, and are highest at the lower and upper age ranges.[4,5] One study reported a rate of encephalitis in children <1 year of age of 18.4/100 000 child-years, almost double that seen in older children.[8] HIV co-infection is present in 15% of cases in population-based studies of encephalitis.[4] Furthermore, HIV-infected and other immunocompromised hosts are at risk for a broader array of pathogens than those found in the general population. While encephalitis does not appear to follow a seasonal pattern, specific pathogens, particularly those transmitted by arthropods, have well-defined temporal patterns. Other exposures or risk factors associated with specific infectious causes of encephalitis, and myelitis, are listed in Table 19.1.

MICROBIOLOGY

Infectious causes of encephalitis and myelitis are diverse and include viruses, bacteria, fungi and parasites. The spectrum of agents has shifted in recent years, primarily as a result of a decrease in vaccine-preventable conditions such as measles, mumps, rubella and varicella.[8,11] While the specific etiologies have changed, the overall incidence has remained stable due to increasing rates in other previously under-recognized or emerging pathogens.[8,12] Examples of emerging causes of encephalitis and myelitis worldwide in the last decade include WNV,[9] Nipah virus,[13,14] enterovirus 71,[15] *Balamuthia mandrillaris*[16,17] and Chandipura virus.[18]

A useful paradigm for organizing the vast number of causative agents is to categorize them based on the strength of association with encephalitis and myelitis. The most commonly identified etiologies in the USA are herpes simplex virus 1 (HSV-1), WNV and the enteroviruses, followed by other herpesviruses (Table 19.2). Other agents may be highly endemic regionally (e.g. La Crosse virus) or internationally (e.g. rabies virus, JEV). Bacterial agents, including *Ehrlichia* spp. and *Rickettsia rickettsii* are potentially treatable causes of encephalitis and myelitis, and prompt administration of antimicrobial therapy may be lifesaving.[19,20]

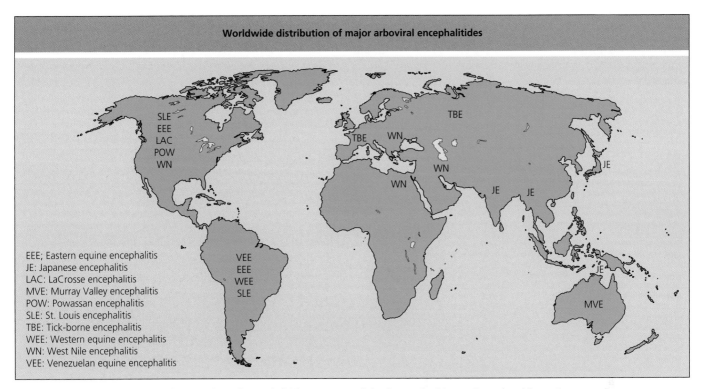

Fig. 19.1 Worldwide distribution of major arboviral encephalitides. Courtesy of the Centers for Disease Control and Prevention.

A second category includes agents less commonly identified, but which are neurotropic and are well-associated causes of sporadic encephalitis and myelitis (Table 19.3). These agents fall into two categories:

- uncommon pathogens with prominent central nervous system (CNS) symptoms (e.g. Eastern equine encephalitis and Venezuelan equine encephalitis viruses); and
- relatively common infections in which meningoencephalitis occurs in a minority of cases (e.g. *Borrelia burgdorferi*, *Coxiella burnetii*).

A number of these have well-defined geographic distributions (e.g. Chandipura virus in India, Nipah virus in Malaysia) and consideration of these agents is indicated if there is travel to or residence in an endemic area.

Most problematic is the third category of agents, those anecdotally associated with encephalitis and myelitis but with minimal neurotropism and limited laboratory data confirming direct CNS invasion (Table 19.4). For instance, *Mycoplasma pneumoniae* is the most common agent identified, usually by serology, in several large case series of encephalitis and myelitis.[21–23] However, the significance of serologic diagnosis of acute *M. pneumoniae* infections is unknown since *Mycoplasma* infections are relatively common and most serologic testing lacks specificity;[22] detection of bacteria in cerebrospinal fluid (CSF) by culture or by nucleic acid amplification tests, such as polymerase chain reaction (PCR), is diagnostic of CNS infection, but is rarely found. Other organisms associated with encephalitis, but with similar difficulties in establishing causality, include influenza virus,[24] rotavirus,[25] human herpes virus-6,[26] parvovirus[27] and others listed in Table 19.4.

Perhaps the most challenging aspect of encephalitis for patients, families and clinicians is that, despite the multitude of causal organisms, no pathogen is identified in the majority of cases. Studies conducted in geographically distant sites on disparate populations consistently report that between 50% and 70% of cases remain unexplained.[4,7,28,29] One of the most recent and ambitious studies of encephalitis performed prospective testing on 1570 well-defined cases over a 7-year period using a standardized diagnostic algorithm including extensive molecular testing. Despite this rigorous approach, no etiologic cause

was identified in 63% of patients.[30] Furthermore, approximately 10% of patients initially thought to have an infectious cause of encephalitis were ultimately diagnosed with a noninfectious condition.

CLINICAL FEATURES

Encephalitis is infrequently confirmed by pathologic means. Therefore, signs and symptoms of neurologic dysfunction are used as surrogate markers; these are often nonspecific. Encephalopathy, defined by a disruption of brain function in the absence of direct brain inflammation, may mimic encephalitis, although fever is less common and there is usually minimal CSF pleocytosis. Causes of encephalopathy include metabolic disturbances, hypoxia, ischemia, intoxications, organ dysfunction, paraneoplastic syndromes or systemic infections.

Encephalitis can present with purely parenchymal findings, but more commonly has associated meningeal inflammation, representing an overlap syndrome termed meningoencephalitis; for the purposes of this chapter, these terms are used interchangeably. The clinical signs and symptoms of encephalitis are determined by the specific area of the brain involved and by the severity of the infection. Some organisms show neurotropism for particular anatomic sites; for example, HSV-1 infection almost universally involves the temporal lobe and the presentation typically includes temporal lobe seizures.[31] Diffuse brain involvement, as is frequently seen with arboviral infections, is associated with global impairment in neurologic function and coma.

Fever and headache frequently precede the onset of altered mental status, which can range from mild confusion to obtundation. Rarely, patients with inflammation localized to extracerebral portions of the CNS may have intact cognition. For instance, primary varicella infection is associated with cerebellar inflammation, with findings of ataxia and nystagmus but no cognitive deficits.[32] Other neurologic manifestations may include behavioral changes (such as psychosis), focal paresis or paralysis, cranial nerve palsies, or movement disorders such as chorea.[30] The frequency of seizures varies based on the pathogen; generalized seizures are common with *Bartonella* (cat scratch) encephalopathy[33] but are noted in less than 10% of cases of WNV encephalitis.[34]

Table 19.1 Exposures associated with agents causing encephalitis and myelitis

Risk factor/exposure	Agent
Arthropods	
Mosquito bite*	Alphaviruses (Western equine encephalitis virus, Eastern equine encephalitis virus, Venezuelan equine encephalitis virus) Flaviviruses (West Nile virus, Japanese encephalitis virus, St Louis encephalitis virus) Bunyaviruses (California/La Crosse virus)
Tick bite	Powassan virus, *Anaplasma phagocytophilum*, *Ehrlichia* spp., *Rickettsia rickettsii*, tick-borne encephalitis virus, *Borrelia burgdorferi*
Sandflies	*Bartonella bacilliformis*, Chandipura virus (India)
Tsetse flies	*Trypanosoma brucei gambiense*, *Trypanosoma brucei rhodesiense* (Africa)
Wild/domestic animals	
Bats	Rabies virus, Nipah virus, *Histoplasma capsulatum*
Dogs	Rabies virus
Cats	*Bartonella hensalae*, *Toxoplasma gondii*, rabies virus
Rodents*	Lymphocytic choriomeningitis virus, *Leptospira* spp.
Raccoon	*Baylisascaris procyonis*, rabies virus
Sheep/goats	*Coxiella burnetii*
Birds*	*Cryptococcus neoformans*, *Chlamydia psittaci*
Old world monkeys	B virus
Horses*	Hendra virus (Australia)
Swine	Nipah virus (South East Asia)
Skunks	Rabies virus
Parturient animals (especially farm animals)	*Coxiella burnetii*
Fresh water	*Naegleria fowleri*, *Leptospira* spp.
Soil (aerosolized or ingestion)	*Balamuthia mandrillaris*, *Baylisascaris* procyonis, endemic fungi
Undercooked freshwater fish, chicken or pork	*Gnasthostoma* spp. (South East Asia, Mexico)
Raw or undercooked fresh water prawns, crabs or frogs, or unwashed produce (with snails/slugs)	*Angiostrongylus cantonensis* (South East Asia, Pacific Islands, Caribbean)
Unpasteurized milk	*Coxiella burnetii*, tick-borne encephalitis virus, *Listeria monocytogenes*
Season	
Fall	Enteroviruses, arthropod-borne pathogens (see above)
Winter	Influenza virus
Spring	Enteroviruses, arthropod-borne pathogens (see above)
Summer	Enteroviruses, arthropod-borne pathogens (see above)
Recreation	
Camping/hunting	Arthropod-borne pathogens (see above)
Spelunking	Rabies virus, *Histoplasma capsulatum*
Sexual activity	HIV, syphilis, herpes simplex virus 2

*Rodents, birds and horses may serve as reservoir hosts for arboviruses, but transmission to humans is generally from an arthropod vector.

Rabies infections deserve special mention because of their severity and worldwide importance. Rabies virus infections, with few exceptions, are fatal illnesses, and the time to progression from onset of symptoms to death is typically less than 2 weeks.[35] Symptoms initially are nonspecific, but may include fever, headache, pharyngitis and weakness. The diagnosis should be considered in any patient with a rapid progression of illness, particularly if hydrophobia, autonomic instability, extreme agitation and seizures are present. Paresthesia at the inoculation site is a unique feature of rabies.

Table 19.2 Relatively common causes of encephalitis and myelitis in immunocompetent patients

Etiology	Epidemiology	Clinical features	Diagnosis
Viruses			
Enteroviruses (includes coxsackieviruses, echoviruses and enterovirus 71)	Peak incidence in late summer and early fall; enterovirus 71 a cause of large outbreaks in Asia, with children primarily affected	Range from aseptic meningitis (most common) to encephalitis; enterovirus 71 causes rhombencephalitis	CSF PCR or culture. Stool or throat swab PCR or culture suggestive, but not diagnostic, of CNS involvement
Epstein–Barr virus	Either during acute infection or reactivation, primary CNS lymphoma	Infectious mononucleosis symptoms during acute infection, cerebellar ataxia, sensory distortion ('Alice-in-Wonderland' syndrome)	CSF PCR (may be falsely positive through detection of latently infected macrophages), serology (IgM positive in acute infection)
Herpes simplex virus (HSV) 1 and 2	HSV-1 accounts for 5–10% of encephalitis, typically reactivation disease; HSV-2 seen in neonates	Temporal lobe seizures (apraxia, lip smacking), behavioral abnormalities	CSF PCR, CSF serologies if >1 week of symptoms
Japanese encephalitis virus (JEV)	Mosquito-borne, most common worldwide cause of encephalitis, endemic throughout Asia; vaccine preventable	Seizures, Parkinsonian features, acute flaccid paralysis variably seen. MRI classically with thalamic and basal ganglia involvement	Serology, CSF IgM, CSF antigen (cross-reacts with other flaviviruses)
La Crosse virus	Mosquito-borne, endemic in midwestern and eastern USA; peak incidence in school-aged children	Varies from subclinical illness to seizures and coma	Serology
Rabies virus	Vaccine preventable; most common vector is bat, and bites often unrecognized; dogs important in developing countries; worldwide distribution	Often with numbness or neuropathic pain at site of bite, progressing to hydrophobia (with drooling), agitation, delirium, autonomic instability, coma; paralytic form with ascending paralysis in 30%	Antibodies (serum, CSF), PCR of saliva or CSF, IFA of nuchal biopsy or CNS tissue; coordinate testing with local health department
St Louis encephalitis virus (SLE)	Mosquito-borne, endemic to western USA, with periodic outbreaks in central/eastern USA; peak incidence in adults >50 years	Tremors, seizures, paresis, urinary symptoms, SIADH variably present	Serology (cross-reacts with other flaviviruses)
Tick-borne encephalitis virus	Transmitted via tick or ingestion of unpasteurized milk; endemic to Eastern and Central Europe, Far East	Weakness ranging from mild paresis to acute flaccid paralysis	Serology
Varicella-zoster virus	Acute infection (chickenpox) or reactivation (shingles)	Vesicular rash (disseminated or dermatomal), cerebellar ataxia, large vessel vasculitis	DFA or PCR of skin lesions, CSF PCR, serum IgM (acute infection)
West Nile virus (WNV)	Mosquito-borne, emerging cause of epidemic encephalitis throughout USA, Europe; endemic in Middle East; peak incidence adults >50 years	Weakness and acute flaccid paralysis, tremors, myoclonus, Parkinsonian features, MRI with basal ganglia and thalamic lesions	CSF IgM, paired serology (cross-reactivity with WNV and SLE)
Bacteria			
Bartonella henselae (and other *Bartonella* spp.)	Typically follows scratch or bite from cat or kitten; highest incidence in children	Encephalopathy with seizures (often status epilepticus), with rapid recovery; often peripheral lymphadenopathy noted; CSF usually paucicellular	Serology (acute usually diagnostic), PCR of lymph node, CSF PCR rarely positive
Mycobacterium tuberculosis	Most common in developing countries; disease in extremes of age or immunocompromised	Subacute basilar meningitis, lacunar infarcts, hydrocephalus; CSF formula often with low glucose, high protein; often have associated pulmonary findings	CSF AFB smear, culture, PCR; respiratory cultures highly suggestive
Ehrlichia/Anaplasma	Tick-borne bacteria causing human monocytotrophic and human granulocytotrophic ehrlichiosis, respectively; former endemic to southern and central USA, latter to northeast USA and Midwest	Acute onset of fever and headache; rash seen in <30% of cases of *Ehrlichia* in adults; leukopenia, thrombocytopenia and elevated LFTs frequent manifestations	Morulae in white blood cells, PCR of whole blood, serology (seroconversion may occur several weeks after symptoms)
Rickettsia rickettsii	Tick-borne infection found throughout North America, with peak incidence in southeast and south central USA	Acute onset of fever and headache; petechial rash in 85% of cases beginning 3 days after onset of symptoms	Serology (seroconversion may occur several weeks after symptoms), PCR or IHC staining of skin biopsy of rash

AFB, acid-fast bacilli; CSF, cerebrospinal fluid; DFA, direct fluorescent antibody; IFA, indirect fluorescent antibody; IHC, immunohistochemical; LFTs, liver function tests; PCR, polymerase chain reaction; SIADH, syndrome of inappropriate antidiuretic hormone secretion.

Table 19.3 Less common causes of encephalitis and myelitis in immunocompetent patients

Etiology	Epidemiology	Clinical features	Diagnosis
Viruses			
Eastern equine encephalitis virus	Coastal states (Atlantic and Gulf); children and elderly disproportionately affected	Ranges from subclinical to fulminant; mortality 50–70%	Serology
Hendra virus	Endemic in Australia; associated with horse exposure	Nonspecific	Contact local health department or Special Pathogens Branch at CDC
B virus	Transmitted by bite of old-world macaque	Vesicular eruption at site of bite followed by neurologic symptoms, including transverse myelitis	Culture and PCR of vesicles and CSF
Lymphocytic choriomeningitis virus	Peak incidence in fall and winter	Orchitis, parotitis	Serology
Measles virus	Vaccine-preventable illness; measles inclusion body encephalitis onset 1–6 months after infection; subacute sclerosing panencephalitis (SSPE) a late manifestation (>5 years after infection)	Measles encephalitis nonspecific; SSPE has a subacute onset with progressive dementia, myoclonus, seizures and ultimately death	CSF antibodies, brain tissue PCR; EEG changes often diagnostic
Mumps virus	Vaccine-preventable illness	Parotitis, orchitis; hearing loss frequent	Serology, throat swab PCR, CSF culture or PCR
Murray Valley encephalitis virus	Peak incidence in aboriginal children; indigenous to Australia and New Guinea	Nonspecific presentation; case fatality 15–30%	Serology (may cross-react with other flaviviruses)
Nipah virus	Epidemics in South East Asia	Myoclonus, dystonia, pneumonitis	Serology (Special Pathogens Branch, CDC)
Powassan virus	Tick-borne; endemic in New England states and Canada	Nonspecific	Serology
Rubella virus	Vaccine-preventable illness	Neurologic findings typically occur at same time as rash and fever	Serology, CSF antibodies
Vaccinia	Infection or vaccination as precipitating event; thought to be autoimmune phenomenon	Vaccinia rash (localized or disseminated)	CSF antibodies, serum IgM (natural infection)
Venezuelan equine encephalitis virus	Central/South America; rarely in border states of USA (Texas, Arizona)	Myalgias, pharyngitis, upper respiratory symptoms variably present	Serology, viral cultures (blood, oropharynx), CSF antibody
Western equine encephalitis virus	Summer and early fall onset; Western USA and Canada, Central and South America	Nonspecific	Serology
Bacteria			
Borrelia burgdorferi	Tick-borne infection, with encephalitis in early disseminated Lyme disease, encephalopathy in late disease	Facial nerve palsy (often bilateral), meningitis, radiculitis; may be associated with or follow erythema migrans rash	Serology (serial EIA and Western blot), CSF antibody index, CSF PCR
Coxiella burnetii	Animal exposures (particularly placenta and amniotic fluid)	Nonspecific	Serology
Treponema pallidum	Sexually transmitted disease, with meningoencephalitis seen in early disseminated disease and progressive dementia in late disease	Protean manifestations including temporal lobe focality (mimics herpes simplex virus), general paresis, psychosis, dementia	CSF VDRL (specific but not sensitive), serum RPR with confirmatory FTA-ABS
Tropheryma whipplei	–	Progressive subacute encephalopathy; oculomasticatory myorhythmia pathognomonic; variably enteropathy, uveitis	CSF PCR, PAS-positive cells in CSF, small bowel biopsy

Table 19.3 Less common causes of encephalitis and myelitis in immunocompetent patients—cont'd

Etiology	Epidemiology	Clinical features	Diagnosis
Protozoa			
Balamuthia mandrillaris	Central America (natives and immigrants)	Subacute progressive disease characterized by space-enhancing lesions, often with cranial nerve palsies and hydrocephalus (similar to tuberculosis)	Serology (research laboratories), brain histopathology
Naegleria fowleri	Summer months; children and adolescent boys at highest risk; swimming in fresh water, and particularly water sports, a risk factor	Anosmia, progressive obtundation; typically a neutrophilic pleocytosis	Motile trophozoites on wet mount of warm CSF, brain histopathology
Helminths			
Baylisascaris procyonis	Pica, particularly near raccoon latrine	Obtundation, coma; typically with significant CSF and peripheral eosinophilia	CSF and serum antibodies (Perdue Department of Veterinary Pathology)

CSF, cerebrospinal fluid; EIA, enzyme immunoassay; FTA-ABS, fluorescent treponemal antibody absorption; PAS, periodic acid-Schiff; PCR, polymerase chain reaction; RPR, rapid plasma reagin; SSPE, subacute sclerosing panencephalitis.

Table 19.4 Selected pathogens of unknown neurotropic potential that are anecdotally associated with encephalitis and myelitis

Etiology	Epidemiologic and clinical features	Diagnosis
Viruses		
Adenovirus	Sporadic cases; children and immunocompromised at greatest risk; variably associated respiratory symptoms	Viral culture or PCR from respiratory site, CSF, or brain tissue
Human herpes virus 6	Most commonly reported in immunocompromised, particularly bone marrow transplant recipients; latent infection of neural tissues making significance of detection in brain tissue difficult to determine	CSF PCR
Hepatitis C	Hepatitis C seropositive patient	CSF PCR
Human metapneumovirus	Newly described pathogen almost exclusively in children	Respiratory tract PCR
Influenza virus	Sporadic disease in children, with most reports from Japan and South East Asia; upper respiratory symptoms; acellular CSF, 10% with bilateral thalamic necrosis; high mortality	Respiratory tract culture, PCR or rapid antigen; CSF and brain PCR infrequently positive
Parvovirus B19	Sporadic cases, variably associated with skin rash	IgM antibody, CSF PCR
Rotavirus	Typically children, winter months, usually with diarrhea	Stool antigen, CSF PCR (CDC)
Bacteria		
Chlamydia spp.	Anecdotal reports with *C. psittaci* and *C. pneumoniae*	Nasopharyngeal swab; respiratory or CSF PCR
Mycoplasma pneumoniae	In some pediatric series, the most common cause of encephalitis; respiratory symptoms variably present, but pneumonia rare; often with white matter involvement consistent with ADEM	PCR of nasopharyngeal swab or respiratory culture; serum IgM, CSF PCR rarely positive

ADEM, acute disseminated encephalomyelitis; CSF, cerebrospinal fluid; PCR, polymerase chain reaction.

Myelitis may occur in patients with or without concomitant encephalitis. Myelitis is specifically characterized by motor weakness, rising sensory deficit, and early bowel and bladder involvement.[3,36] The motor weakness may be of the upper motor neuron type (manifested as spasticity, hyperreflexia, and extensor plantar reflexes) or the lower motor neuron type (manifested as flaccid weakness and decreased or absent deep tendon reflexes). Acute flaccid paralysis is seen in a number of viral causes of myelitis, including infection caused by enteroviruses (e.g. poliovirus and enterovirus 71) and flaviviruses (e.g. WNV, JEV and tick-borne encephalitis virus).[2,36,37] However, in most cases a specific viral cause is never determined. Chronic myelitis is often caused by retroviruses;[3,36] human T-cell leukemia virus 1 (HTLV-1) causes disease primarily in the thoracic spinal cord with resultant progressive spastic paraparesis, and HIV may cause spastic paraparesis and sensory ataxia.

When both halves of the spinal cord are affected, the entity is referred to as transverse myelitis.[3,36] Patients with transverse myelitis present with a syndrome mimicking transection of spinal cord with involvement of the motor, sensory and autonomic pathways; virtually all patients have paresthesias, numbness or radicular dysesthesias with an associated sensory level. Autonomic symptoms can include constipation, bowel or bladder incontinence, and urinary retention. Transverse myelitis may be produced by direct invasion of the spinal cord with organisms such as viruses or *Borrelia burgdorferi*; vasculitis of the anterior spinal artery caused by varicella-zoster virus (VZV), tuberculosis and syphilis may also lead to transverse myelitis. In most cases, there is no identifiable cause.

Evidence of inflammation or infection at sites distant from the CNS may be useful in making a microbiologic diagnosis in patients with encephalitis and myelitis. For instance, rickettsial diseases, VZV and WNV often have associated skin manifestations. Stomatitis and ulcerative lesions in the mouth or an exanthem in a peripheral distribution might suggest enterovirus infection. Patients with tuberculous and fungal meningoencephalitis may have suggestive pulmonary findings. Regional lymphadenopathy is typically present in patients with *Bartonella* encephalopathy. Diarrhea may be seen with enterovirus, adenovirus or rotavirus infections.

A syndrome frequently misclassified as encephalomyelitis, based on the similar clinical presentation, is postinflammatory encephalomyelitis, occurring days to weeks after an infectious illness or immunization. The most widely cited example is acute disseminated encephalomyelitis (ADEM), seen primarily in children and adolescents, and characterized by poorly defined white matter lesions on MRI that enhance following gadolinium administration (Fig. 19.2).[38,39] Postinflammatory encephalomyelitis is presumed to be mediated by an immunologic response to an antecedent antigenic stimulus, and is thought to account for 5–15% of cases.[4,40] As many as 90% of patients report an infectious illness, or receipt of an immunization, in the weeks before onset of ADEM.[39] Viral infections associated with ADEM include measles, mumps, rubella, varicella-zoster, Epstein–Barr, cytomegalovirus, herpes simplex, hepatitis A and Coxsackie virus. Immunizations temporally associated with ADEM include vaccines for JEV, yellow fever, measles, influenza, smallpox, anthrax and rabies virus; however, a direct causal association with these vaccines is difficult to establish. Onset of ADEM generally begins between 2 days and 4 weeks following the antigenic stimulus, with rapid onset of encephalopathy, with or without meningeal signs;[39] neurologic features depend upon the location of the lesions.

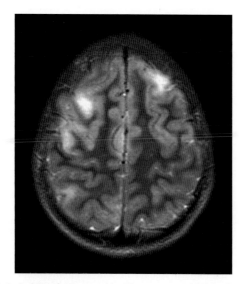

Fig. 19.2 Brain MRI of a 3 year old with new onset seizures showing increased T2 signal affecting the white matter in diffuse regions of the cerebral cortex consistent with acute disseminated encephalomyelitis.

PATHOLOGY AND PATHOGENESIS

Most viruses and other infectious agents that cause encephalitis and myelitis gain access to the CNS via the hematogenous route, causing diffuse neurologic dysfunction. The initial site of entry and replication varies depending on the organism and may include the respiratory tract (e.g. measles virus), gastrointestinal tract (e.g. enteroviruses) or skin (e.g. arboviruses). Following local infection, a viremia follows, leading to invasion and replication with the CNS.[41] Why certain viruses are more neurotropic than others is unknown, although it has been postulated that the small size of the arboviruses allows them to escape clearance by the reticuloendothelial system; arboviruses likely enter the CNS via cerebral capillaries, with vascular endothelial cell infection preceding infection of the neural parenchyma.[42] Recent studies have identified hypertension as a risk factor for the development of WNV neuroinvasive disease, suggesting that defects in the blood–brain barrier may be a risk factor for the development of WNV encephalitis.[43]

Another mechanism that organisms such as rabies virus and polioviruses use to gain access to the CNS is retrograde spread through neuronal networks. After introduction through the skin, usually via a bite, rabies virus replicates in the skeletal muscle and travels to the CNS via the peripheral nerves. In cases of prolonged incubation periods, the rabies virus likely remains close to the site of viral entry.[44] After spread of the virus to the brain via peripheral nerves, rabies virus disseminates rapidly throughout the CNS. Despite the high fatality rate, rabies CNS infection causes relatively benign neuropathologic changes without evidence of neuronal death.

A third pathogenic mechanism that organisms use to gain entry into the CNS is exemplified by free-living amebae such as *Naegleria fowleri*. These organisms enter transnasally and pass through the cribriform plate with invasion into the frontal lobes of the brain.[45]

The pathogenesis of herpes simplex encephalitis (HSE) is incompletely understood.[46–48] Serologic studies suggest that one-third of cases are the result of primary infection and two-thirds are a result of reactivation.[49] For primary HSE, theorized routes of entry into the CNS include hematogenous dissemination, migration from the nasopharyngeal mucosa through the cribriform plate, or retrograde spread from viral-infected ganglion to the brain tissue.[50] In cases of HSV reactivation, one theory is that the virus replicates in the trigeminal ganglion and spreads to the frontal and temporal lobes via the tentorial nerves.[46]

In acute viral encephalitis, the classic histopathologic findings include perivascular mononuclear cell inflammation, neuronal destruction, neuronophagia and microglial nodules.[40] Most of the pathology occurs in the gray matter. In contrast, the white matter is primarily affected in postinfectious encephalitis where there is perivenular mononuclear inflammation, edema and demyelination of brain tissue with a relative sparing of the axons.[9]

Infectious agents can also cause a clinical syndrome of encephalitis without CNS parenchymal involvement. For example, tuberculous and fungal meningitis can lead to hydrocephalus and cranial nerve palsies, causing symptoms similar to encephalitis. Alternatively, agents causing vasculitis lead to infarcts of the brain with resultant focal neurologic deficits mimicking encephalitis.

In patients with encephalomyelitis following infection or vaccination (i.e. as in ADEM), perivascular inflammation of mononuclear cells (T cells and macrophages) and perivascular demyelination are observed.[39] Other histopathologic features that have been described include varying degrees of cerebral edema, perivascular lymphocytic infiltrates with fibrin deposition and perivascular hemorrhagic necrosis.

DIAGNOSIS

Although many cases of encephalitis and myelitis remain undiagnosed, and many of the causes are not treatable, a thorough diagnostic evaluation is important. Identification of a specific agent may allow for the discontinuation of potentially toxic antimicrobial therapy and may be useful for prognosis, potential prophylaxis for contacts, counseling of patients and families, and initiating public health interventions.[2]

The initial laboratory testing of an individual should include a complete blood count, tests of renal and hepatic function, and coagulation studies. Results of these studies are often nonspecific but may suggest a particular etiology. For example, a low white blood cell count, low platelet count and elevated liver transaminases might suggest *Ehrlichia* or *Anaplasma* infection. A baseline chest radiograph should be obtained, as a focal infiltrate would be suggestive of particular pathogens (e.g. fungal or mycobacterial infections), and might prompt further diagnostic studies such as bronchoscopy.

Neuroimaging studies are important to perform in all patients with encephalitis; MRI is more sensitive at detecting abnormalities than CT, and is the preferred study.[2] Diffusion-weighted MRI is superior to conventional MRI for the detection of early signal abnormalities in viral encephalitis caused by HSV, enterovirus 71 and WNV. In addition, some neuroimaging patterns may suggest infection caused by certain organisms (Table 19.5). In patients with herpes simplex encephalitis, there may be significant edema and hemorrhage in the temporal lobes. Patients with flavivirus encephalitis may display characteristic patterns of mixed intensity or hypodense lesions on T1-weighted images in the thalamus, basal ganglia and midbrain. In patients with ADEM, MRI generally reveals multiple focal or confluent areas of signal abnormality in the subcortical white matter. MRI of the spine is abnormal in about 90% of patients with transverse myelitis,[3] commonly manifested as an area of increased T2-weighted hyperintensity in the central region of the spinal cord occupying two-thirds or more of the cross-sectional area; swelling of the spinal cord is seen in about 50% of patients.

Electroencephalography (EEG) should also be performed in patients with encephalitis. Although findings of the EEG are rarely specific for a given pathogen, results can be helpful in identifying the degree of cerebral dysfunction, detecting subclinical seizure activity, and may provide information about the specific area of the brain involved. For example, many patients with herpes simplex encephalitis demonstrate a temporal lobe focus with periodic lateralizing epileptiform discharges (PLEDs).

Lumbar puncture with CSF analysis (cell count and differential, glucose and protein) and a measurement of the opening pressure should universally be performed unless there is a specific contra-indication.[51] Mild to moderate CSF abnormalities are characteristic of most patients with viral encephalitis. Most patients have a mononuclear cell pleocytosis with cell counts ranging from 10 to 1000/mm^3.[40] Early in the disease process, CSF pleocytosis may be absent or there may be an elevation in neutrophils. The CSF protein concentration is typically elevated, but usually less than 100–200 mg/dl, while the CSF glucose concentration is typically normal. Neutrophilic pleocytosis (particularly when the total WBC count is >1000/mm^3, CSF protein >200 mg/dl or CSF glucose less than two-thirds of serum concentrations) suggests a bacterial, mycobacterial, fungal, parasitic or noninfectious etiology, and is distinctly unusual in patients with viral infections. CSF viral cultures are of limited value in patients with viral encephalitis because of low sensitivity and are generally not recommended.[52] Although of low yield, CSF cultures for bacteria, fungi and mycobacteria should be performed as identification of a pathogen has significant implications for treatment.

Brain biopsy, previously considered instrumental in the etiologic diagnosis of encephalitis, has largely been replaced by CSF molecular tests.[2] Histopathology of brain tissue, however, may help confirm whether a patient has encephalitis as opposed to another CNS process. For certain types of infection, brain biopsy may be diagnostic. In rabies infections, for example, Negri bodies are a distinctive histopathologic feature. Intranuclear eosinophilic amorphous bodies surrounded by a halo may be seen in such diseases as herpes simplex encephalitis. Pathologic examination of the brain may also be very helpful in the diagnosis of *Balamuthia mandrillaris* and other free-living amebic infections; amebic trophozoites and cysts can be detected by hematoxylin-eosin stained sections of necrotic regions of brain tissue.

In addition to the above studies, there are often epidemiologic clues that can help guide specific diagnostic testing, such as season of the year, geographic locale, prevalence of disease in a community, travel history, hobbies and recreational activities, occupation, insect and animal exposure, and vaccination history (see Table 19.1). Specific clinical findings should also direct other sites for culture or other diagnostic tests. For example, respiratory viral cultures should

Table 19.5 Possible etiologic agents of encephalitis based on neuroimaging findings

Neuroimaging finding	Possible infectious agents
Arteritis and infarctions	Varicella-zoster virus, Nipah virus, *Rickettsia rickettsii*, *Treponema pallidum*
Calcifications	Cytomegalovirus (cortical), *Toxoplasma gondii* (periventricular), *Taenia solium*
Cerebellar lesions	Varicella zoster virus, Epstein-Barr virus, *Mycoplasma pneumoniae*
Hydrocephalus	*Mycobacterium tuberculosis*, *Cryptococcus neoformans*, *Coccidioides immitis*, *Histoplasma capsulatum*, *Balamuthia mandrillaris*
Focal lesions in basal ganglia, thalamus and/or brain stem	Epstein–Barr virus, Eastern equine encephalitis virus, Murray Valley encephalitis virus, St Louis encephalitis virus, Japanese encephalitis virus, West Nile virus, enterovirus 71, influenzae virus (acute necrotizing encephalopathy), human transmissible spongiform encephalopathies
Space-occupying lesions	*Toxoplasma gondii*, *Balamuthia mandrillaris*, *Taenia solium*
Subependymal enhancement	Cytomegalovirus
Temporal and/or frontal lobe involvement	Herpes simplex virus, varicella-zoster virus, human herpesvirus 6, West Nile virus, enteroviruses, *Treponema pallidum* (medial lobes)
White matter abnormalities	Varicella zoster virus, cytomegalovirus, Epstein–Barr virus, human herpesvirus 6, HIV, Nipah virus, JC virus, measles virus (subacute sclerosing panencephalitis), *Baylisascaris procyonis*, acute disseminated encephalomyelitis

This is not meant to be a comprehensive list to detail all etiologic agents based on neuroimaging finding, but to suggest that certain etiologies have been associated with findings on neuroimaging studies.

be performed if patients have respiratory symptoms. If the patient has a rash, skin lesions should be cultured or biopsied.

Testing for specific agents includes various laboratory methods, such as antigen detection, culture, serology and molecular diagnostics.[2] The optimal method varies, depending both on the particular agent and the duration of symptoms. For instance, for many of the herpesviruses, molecular testing of CSF is the assay of choice, while serology is the preferred methodology for many of the arboviruses. However, very early in the course of disease, PCR may be positive for arboviruses, while after several weeks, there is evidence of HSV intrathecal antibody production.

More in-depth discussion of diagnostic testing is provided in the agent-specific chapters; however, there are some pathogens that should be routinely considered in all patients with encephalitis. Herpes simplex encephalitis is a treatable and relatively common cause of encephalitis, and an HSV PCR should be performed on the CSF of all patients with a clinical diagnosis of encephalitis. False-negative PCR tests can occur within the first 72 hours of onset, and if herpes simplex encephalitis is strongly suspected (e.g. in a patient with temporal lobe involvement), a repeat HSV PCR on a second sample of CSF from later in the disease course is recommended.[53,54] Enterovirus and varicella PCR should be done on CSF since these are also common causes of encephalitis.[30] Testing for M. pneumoniae deserves special mention since it is one of the leading agents identified serologically among pediatric patients with encephalitis;[21,22] diagnostic testing should include IgM on acute serum and IgG on paired samples, with attempts to amplify the bacteria from CSF and nasopharyngeal swabs in suggestive cases.

Testing for other agents should be individualized for each patient, with consideration of the patient's exposures, travel, season of the year and clinical and laboratory characteristics (see Tables 19.1–19.4). Many infections require acute and convalescent (i.e. paired) serum samples to determine a diagnosis.[2] Although results of paired serologies are not available during the acute presentation, analysis may be useful for the retrospective diagnosis of an infectious agent; therefore, a serum specimen collected during the acute phase of the illness should be stored and tested in parallel when the convalescent serum sample is drawn. Since arboviruses are a leading cause of encephalitis, testing for geographically relevant viruses should be considered during the appropriate season. Recently, IgM and IgG capture ELISAs have become useful and widely available for the diagnosis of arboviral encephalitis.[55,56] For WNV, detection of intrathecal IgM antibody is both a specific and a sensitive method for diagnosis.[57] It is important to realize that there is substantial cross-reactivity among the flaviviruses (e.g. WNV, SLE and JEV); plaque-reduction neutralization assays may be helpful in distinguishing which flavivirus is involved in the event of elevated titers.

Serologic testing for Rickettsia, Ehrlichia and Anaplasma spp. should be performed in all encephalitis patients during the appropriate season and with travel to, or residence in, endemic areas, especially since these are treatable etiologies. Empiric therapy should not be withheld in patients with a compatible clinical presentation, however,

since antibodies are not always present early in the course of illness.[20] Detection of antibodies against free-living amebae (e.g. Balamuthia) in patients with compatible clinical and laboratory findings is suggestive of amebic meningoencephalitis.[16,17]

MANAGEMENT

One of the most important first steps in management of patients with encephalitis is to consider treatable causes of encephalitis. Specific antiviral therapy is generally limited to infections causes by herpesviruses (especially HSV-1 and VZV) and HIV.[2] Aciclovir (10 mg/kg intravenously q8h in children and adults with normal renal function; 20 mg/kg intravenously q8h in neonates) should be initiated in all patients with suspected viral encephalitis and continued until HSV-1 has been excluded by PCR. Empiric therapy for acute bacterial meningitis should be initiated when clinical and laboratory testing is compatible with bacterial infection.[51] If rickettsial or ehrlichial infections are suspected, empiric doxycycline should also be used. Clinicians should consider conditions that mimic infectious encephalitis, particularly if no etiology is identified in the first week of illness.

In patients suspected to have postinfectious encephalomyelitis (i.e. ADEM), steroids or other immunotherapies are often recommended.[2] High-dose intravenous corticosteroids (methylprednisolone 1 g intravenously daily for at least 3–5 days, followed by an oral taper for 3–6 weeks) are generally recommended for ADEM; plasma exchange should be considered in patients who respond poorly to corticosteroids. Although there is no clear evidence of effective therapy for transverse myelitis, intravenous methylprednisolone (followed by oral prednisone) may shorten the duration of illness and improve outcome;[3] one study, however, did not confirm this benefit.[58] Some subsets of patients may also receive clinical benefit from plasma exchange or cyclophosphamide,[59] although more studies are needed.

In addition to directed therapy for patients with encephalitis, aggressive supportive care is critical, and minimizing secondary brain injury should be made a high priority. Complications of encephalitis include elevated intracranial pressure, hydrocephalus, stroke and seizures; these should be managed expectantly, often in an intensive care setting.[60]

REFERENCES

References for this chapter can be found online at http://www.expertconsult.com

Chapter 20

Itzhak Brook
Gregory C Townsend

Brain abscess and other focal pyogenic infections of the central nervous system

Focal pyogenic infections of the central nervous system (CNS) include brain abscess, spinal cord abscess, subdural empyema, epidural abscess and suppurative intracranial phlebitis. These conditions are characterized by the presence of one or more localized and well-defined collections of purulent material within the cranial vault or the paraspinal space. They exert their effects largely by direct involvement and destruction or encroachment of the brain or spinal cord parenchyma, by elevation of intracranial pressure or by interference with flow of blood or cerebrospinal fluid (CSF).

Infections in contiguous structures generally lead to infections relating to their anatomy (Fig. 20.1). The frontal and ethmoidal paranasal sinuses underlie the anterior cranial fossa and often lead to infections in or near the frontal lobe. The sphenoid sinuses adjoin the sella turcica, temporal lobes and cavernous sinuses; sphenoid sinusitis may lead to infections in the frontal or temporal lobes or pituitary gland or to cavernous sinus thrombosis. Middle ear infections and mastoids may spread to the temporal lobe, cerebellum or brain stem. The focal nature of these infections often manifests by focal neurologic deficits, rather than global CNS dysfunction.

Brain Abscess

Brain abscess is a focal suppurative process of the brain parenchyma. The diagnosis and management of brain abscess have undergone considerable changes during the past several years resulting from the availability of noninvasive radiographic diagnostic techniques, the use of antimicrobials that penetrate across the blood–brain barrier and into abscesses, and the refinement of minimally invasive surgical procedures.

EPIDEMIOLOGY

Brain abscess is uncommon The lifetime incidence is approximately 1.3 per 100 000 person-years, although the overall incidence decreased from 2.7 per 100 000 person-years in 1935–44 to 0.9 per 100 000 person-years in 1965–81. The highest rates were observed in children 5–9 years old and adults over 60 (approximately 2.5 per 100 000 person-years each).[1] Brain abscesses account for approximately 1 in 10 000 hospital admissions in the USA.[2]

The patients' predominant age varies with the predisposing factors; brain abscesses following otitis media are most common among young children and older adults, while those due to paranasal sinusitis are commonly among older children and young adults.[2–4] Brain abscesses are approximately two to three times as common among males as among females.[2]

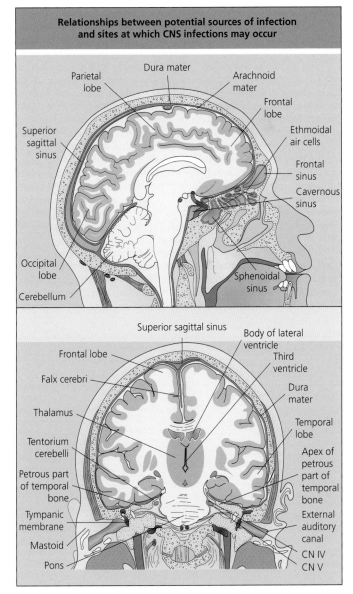

Relationships between potential sources of infection and sites at which CNS infections may occur

Parietal lobe — Dura mater — Arachnoid mater — Frontal lobe — Ethmoidal air cells — Frontal sinus — Cavernous sinus — Superior sagittal sinus — Occipital lobe — Cerebellum — Sphenoidal sinus

Superior sagittal sinus — Body of lateral ventricle — Third ventricle — Frontal lobe — Falx cerebri — Dura mater — Temporal lobe — Thalamus — Apex of petrous part of temporal bone — Tentorium cerebelli — Petrous part of temporal bone — External auditory canal — Tympanic membrane — Mastoid — CN IV — CN V — Pons

Fig. 20.1 Anatomic relationships between potential contiguous sources of infection and sites at which focal pyogenic central nervous system infections may occur.

The major predisposing factors are:

- an associated contiguous focus of infection (e.g. sinusitis, subacute or chronic otitis media and mastoiditis);
- trauma (e.g. penetrating head injury, post-neurosurgery);
- hematogenous spread from a distant focus (e.g. in association with pulmonary, skin, abdominal and pelvic infections, endocarditis, cyanotic heart disease and esophageal dilation or sclerosis of varices); and
- cryptogenic (no recognized focus).

Brain abscesses associated with a contiguous focus account for approximately 40–50% of the total; the percentage of cases without an identified predisposing factor has been reduced to approximately 15% with the use of newer, more sensitive imaging procedures. In addition, abscesses have been reported in immunocompromised individuals or after a cerebrovascular accident.

The commonest underlying conditions in developed countries are otitis media and mastoiditis.[4] However, the role of these conditions has declined in association with early antimicrobial therapy for ear infections. The current risk of brain abscess in cases of otitis media is less than 0.5%.[5] Brain abscess is also associated with cyanotic heart disease and trauma.[6] Other associated head and neck infections include paranasal and dental infections. A report from Turkey observed bacterial meningitis to be the most common predisposing factor in children.[7]

Brain abscesses associated with otitis media and mastoiditis are most common in the temporal lobe and cerebellum (Table 20.1). Brain abscesses associated with sinusitis occur primarily in the frontal or the temporal lobes. The frontal lobe is also most commonly affected following dental infections. Abscess can occur following complicated neurosurgical procedures. Post-traumatic abscesses usually occur with a penetrating wound, but also occur in closed head injuries such as facial trauma. Bullet and shrapnel wounds to the brain can result in necrotic tissue leaving metal fragments that can become a nidus for infection. Injuries include penetrating pencil tip and lawn dart injuries in children. Abscess presentation can occur months to years after the precipitating event. In one study, the median time to development of brain abscess was 113 days[8] and can occur up to 52 years after war-related penetrating head injuries.[9]

Abscesses occurring in a distant primary site following hematogenous spread are often multiple; approximately 10–15% of patients with brain abscesses have multiple abscesses. They tend to occur in the distribution of the middle cerebral artery at the junction of the gray and white matter, where microcirculatory flow is poorest. Cyanotic congenital

heart disease and chronic pyogenic lung diseases (e.g. lung abscess, bronchiectasis) are common predisposing factors. Hereditary hemorrhagic telangiectasia (Osler–Weber–Rendu disease) is also associated with brain abscess; it is thought that in these cases pulmonary arteriovenous malformations allow septic microemboli to bypass the normal pulmonary filter and gain access to the cerebral circulation. Abscesses can follow dental extractions and other manipulations, dilatation of esophageal strictures and endoscopic sclerosis of esophageal varices.

PATHOGENESIS AND PATHOPHYSIOLOGY

The main pathogenetic factors are a source of virulent organisms and the presence of ischemic or devitalized brain tissue. The vulnerability of compromised tissue to brain abscess is evidenced by their occurrence after trauma or cerebrovascular accident, in association with cyanotic heart or lung disease and in areas of poor local perfusion such as the junction of gray and white matter.

Experimental models demonstrated differences in the abilities of various organisms to induce brain abscesses. There are two main postulated mechanisms by which brain abscess may occur in association with a contiguous focus of infection:

- direct extension through infected bone; and
- hematogenous spread through emissary or diploic veins or spread through local lymphatics.

Infections associated with otogenic infections may also spread through the internal auditory canal, between suture lines or through cochlear aqueducts. Abscesses developing after trauma or neurosurgical procedures may follow deep wound injury with direct inoculation into the brain parenchyma or may be a result of extension of a superficial infection through compromised tissue.[10,11]

The sites most commonly involved by solitary brain abscess are the frontal and temporal lobes, followed by the frontoparietal region, the parietal, cerebellar and occipital lobes.[12] These areas are those most likely to be associated with a contiguous focus or hematogenous seeding. Although rare, abscesses may occur in other areas, such as the pituitary gland, thalamus, basal ganglia and brain stem, and may be associated with specific predisposing conditions. For example, abscesses of the pituitary are often associated with pre-existing pituitary adenomas and with sphenoidal sinusitis.

Experimental animal data, surgery and autopsy findings and radiographic examinations indicate that brain abscesses develop in a four-stage process:[13] an early and late cerebritis (days 1–3 and 4–9, respectively) and an early and late capsule formation (days 10–13 and day 14 and later, respectively). These represent a continuum rather than discrete steps. The evolution of this process is dependent upon the causative organism(s), local factors, host immunologic status and antimicrobial therapy.

The microbiology depends upon the site of the initiating infection, the patient's underlying condition and the geographic locale (Table 20.2).[14–18] The organisms most commonly isolated are anaerobes, streptococci, the Enterobacteriaceae, *Staphylococcus aureus* and fungi; approximately 30–60% are polymicrobial. The predominate bacteria are anaerobes that generally are members of the oropharyngeal flora and are associated with otorhinolaryngeal infections. However, anaerobes of gastrointestinal and female genital origin can also spread hematogenously and cause an abscess. The anaerobes most commonly isolated include anaerobic streptococci, *Bacteroides* (including *B. fragilis*), *Prevotella*, *Porphyromonas*, *Clostridium*, *Propionibacterium*, *Fusobacterium*, *Eubacterium*, *Veillonella* and *Actinomyces* spp. The aerobic pathogens include aerobic and microaerophilic streptococci which include alpha-hemolytic streptococci, *Streptococcus milleri* and *Streptococcus pneumoniae*. Aerobic Gram-negative rods are common following neurosurgery or head trauma and the common ones are *Klebsiella pneumoniae*, *Escherichia coli*, *Pseudomonas* spp. and *Proteus* spp. *Staph. aureus* is common after trauma.

High frequency of brain abscess due to *K. pneumoniae* is mainly seen in South East Asia.[19] It was found with or without meningitis and as

Table 20.1 Site of brain abscess based on predisposing condition

Predisposing condition	Site
Otitis media or mastoiditis	Temporal lobe Cerebellum
Paranasal sinusitis	Frontal lobe Temporal lobe
Dental infection/manipulation	Frontal lobe
Trauma/neurosurgery	Related to wound
Meningitis	Cerebellum Frontal lobe
Cyanotic heart disease	Middle cerebral artery distribution
Pyogenic lung disease	
Bacterial endocarditis	
Gastrointestinal source	
T-cell deficiency	
Neutropenia	

Table 20.2 Likely pathogens and suggested empiric therapy for brain abscess based on predisposing condition

Predisposing condition	Likely pathogens	Empiric therapy
Otitis media or mastoiditis	Aerobic, anaerobic and microaerophilic streptococci Anaerobic Gram-negative bacilli (i.e. *Prevotella* spp., *Bacteroides* spp.) *Staphylococcus aureus* Enterobacteriaceae *Pseudomonas aeruginosa*	Third-generation cephalosporin + metronidazole ± antistaphylococcal penicillin or a penicillin
Sinusitis	Aerobic, anaerobic and microaerophilic streptococci Anaerobic Gram-negative bacilli (i.e. *Prevotella* spp., *Bacteroides* spp.) Enterobacteriaceae *Haemophilus* spp. *Fusobacterium* spp.	Penicillin or third-generation cephalosporin + metronidazole
Trauma or post-neurosurgery	*Staphylococcus aureus* Coagulase-negative staphylococci Enterobacteriaceae *Streptococcus* spp. *Pseudomonas aeruginosa* *Clostridium* spp.	Vancomycin + third-generation cephalosporin ± metronidazole
Congenital heart disease	Aerobic and microaerophilic streptococci *Staph. aureus* *Haemophilus* spp.	Third-generation cephalosporin + vancomycin
Pyogenic lung disease	Streptococci *Nocardia asteroides* *Actinomyces* spp. *Fusobacterium* spp. Anaerobic Gram-negative bacilli (i.e. *Prevotella* spp., *Bacteroides* spp.) *Nocardia* spp. Alpha-hemolytic streptococci *Enterococcus* spp. *Haemophilus* spp.	Penicillin or third-generation cephalosporin plus metronidazole Trimethoprim-sulfamethoxazole Vancomycin + ampicillin and gentamicin + antistaphylococcal penicillin
Gastrointestinal source	Enterobacteriaceae *Bacteroides fragilis*	Third-generation cephalosporin + metronidazole
T-cell deficiency	*Toxoplasma gondii* *Nocardia* spp. *Mycobacterium* spp. *Listeria monocytogenes* *Cryptococcus neoformans*	Variable
Neutropenia	Enterobacteriaceae *Pseudomonas aeruginosa* Fungi, especially *Aspergillus*, *Mucor* and *Candida*	Third- or fourth-generation cephalosporin, meropenem Amphotericin B

a metastatic infection that is associated with community-acquired primary liver abscess. Fungi were the organisms most commonly isolated in a report from Saudi Arabia[20] and are particularly common causes of brain abscesses in immunocompromised patients; *Aspergillus* spp. are especially common in patients who have bone marrow and solid organ transplants.[21] Patients with T-cell immunity defects (including AIDS patients) are predisposed to infections with intracellular organisms such as *Toxoplasma gondii*, *Nocardia* spp., *Cryptococcus neoformans*, *Mycobacterium* spp. and fungi.[15]

Parasites that can cause brain abscess or infection include *Taenia solium* (cysticercosis), *Entamoeba histolytica*, *Schistosoma japonicum* and *Paragonimus* spp.[22]

PREVENTION

The appropriate use of antibiotics in patients with predisposing infections such as otitis media and mastoiditis is the primary means of prevention. Other measures include surgical correction of cyanotic congenital heart disease, maintenance of dental hygiene, management of pyogenic lung infections and attention to proper sterile techniques during neurosurgical procedures. In patients who have underlying T-cell defects, measures to prevent exposure to *T. gondii* are recommended.[17]

CLINICAL FEATURES

The clinical manifestations are due largely to the presence of a space-occupying lesion.[12,23] The most common symptoms are headache (75% of patients), which is usually hemicranial, altered mental status, focal neurologic findings (especially hemiparesis) (>60%), fever (50%), nausea and vomiting (25–50%) and seizures (usually generalized) (30%). Nuchal rigidity may occur if the abscess is near the meninges. Vomiting often develops in association with increased intracranial pressure.

Other signs and symptoms vary depending on the abscess stage, size and anatomic location:

- abscesses of the frontal lobe are characterized by headache, drowsiness, global mental status changes, inattention, hemiparesis with unilateral motor signs and expressive speech disturbances;
- temporal lobe abscesses may present with ipsilateral headache and aphasia (if the abscess involves the dominant hemisphere) and a visual field defect;
- cerebellar abscesses are associated with vomiting, ataxia, nystagmus and dysmetria; and
- brain stem abscesses generally present with headache, facial weakness, hemiparesis, vomiting and dysphagia.

Papilledema is present in the older child and adults, and bulging fontanels may be present in the younger infant. Rapid deterioration with nuchal rigidity suggests the possibility of abscess rupture into the intraventricular or subarachnoid space. A ruptured abscess may produce purulent meningitis associated with signs of neurologic damage.

Laboratory findings may include a peripheral leukocytosis and a left shift, but approximately 40% of patients have normal leukocyte concentrations. Serum sodium levels may be lowered resulting from inappropriate antidiuretic hormone production. Platelet counts may be high or low. The erythrocyte sedimentation rate is often elevated. An elevated C-reactive protein is both sensitive (77–90%) and specific (77–100%) when used to distinguish brain abscess from cerebral neoplasms.

The differential diagnosis of brain abscess includes subdural empyema, epidural abscess, bacterial meningitis, cerebral neoplasm, cranial osteomyelitis, mycotic aneurysm, suppurative thrombophlebitis, venous sinus thrombosis, cerebrovascular infarct or hemorrhage, headace and migraine, and encephalitis.

DIAGNOSIS

Radiographic imaging with contrast-enhanced CT or MRI has contributed greatly to diagnosis and management of brain abscess.[24,25] Plain skull radiographs are insensitive but the presence of air indicates the need for further evaluation. Technetium-99 (^{99m}Tc) brain scanning is very sensitive and is the procedure of choice where CT or MRI is unavailable; there is some evidence that ^{99m}Tc scanning may be more sensitive than CT in the early cerebritis stage. ^{99m}Tc-HMPAO labeled leukocyte single photon emission CT (SPECT) has been examined as a potential means of distinguishing brain abscess from other focal cerebral parenchymal lesions, such as neoplasms. Ultrasonography may also be used if other techniques are unavailable.

CT scanning, preferably with contrast, provides a rapid means of detecting the size, the number and the location of abscesses, and has become the mainstay of diagnosis and follow-up care. It is used to confirm the diagnosis, to localize the lesion, and to monitor the progression after treatment. However, CT scan results can lag behind clinical findings. The characteristic appearance of brain abscess on CT scan varies with the stage of the disease.[26] During the cerebritis stage, cerebral edema is prominent; no abnormalities may be seen in the early cerebritis stage. As capsule formation progresses, the abscess appears as a lesion with a hypodense center composed of necrotic debris surrounded by ring enhancement, which may in turn be surrounded by hypodense cerebral edema (Fig. 20.2). Although highly sensitive, CT scanning is not specific. These findings may also be seen in patients with cerebral neoplasms, cerebrovascular accidents or granulomas.

Many authorities consider MRI to be the first method for diagnosis. It permits accurate diagnosis and excellent follow-up because of its superior sensitivity and specificity. Compared with CT scanning, it offers better ability to detect cerebritis, greater contrast between cerebral edema and the brain, and early detection of satellite lesions and the spread of inflammation into the ventricles and subarachnoid space. MRI is more sensitive than CT in the early cerebritis stage of brain abscess, where it appears as slightly low intensity on T1-weighted

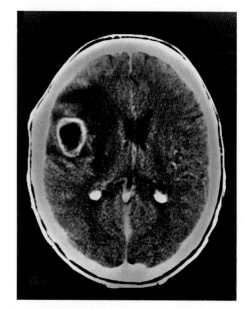

Fig. 20.2 Contrast-enhanced CT scan of the head in the coronal projection of a 43-year-old man with an atrial septal defect that persisted after attempts at surgical repair. The patient presented with seizures after undergoing dental work for which he did not receive antimicrobial prophylaxis. Note the ring-enhancing lesion in the right frontoparietal region with edema and mass effect.

images and very low intensity on T2-weighted images, and may be more sensitive in diagnosing lesions in the posterior fossa due to the absence of bone artifact[24,25] (Fig. 20.3). It may allow distinction of abscess fluid from cerebrospinal fluid, which may be important if intraventricular rupture is suspected. Enhancement with gadolinium-DTPA allows evaluation of disruption of the blood–brain barrier and permits greater distinction of the radiographic appearance of the central abscess, capsule and surrounding edema. Examination by ^{1}H magnetic resonance spectroscopic imaging has been proposed as a means of distinguishing brain abscess from other focal cerebral parenchymal lesions.

It must be noted that the appearance of edema and contrast enhancement on CT and MRI may be diminished or absent in immunocompromised patients, possibly due to poor host inflammatory response.

Lumbar puncture should be avoided in patients who have known or suspected brain abscess. The yield of CSF culture is low (less than 10% positive) and the risk of herniation is considerable (approximately 15–30%). The number of white blood cells is generally elevated. It reaches 100 000/µl or higher when a rupture of the abscess into the CSF occurs. Many red blood cells are generally observed at that time, and the CSF lactic acid level is then elevated above 500 mg/l. In patients in whom both diagnoses are considered, blood cultures should be obtained and appropriate empiric therapy should be initiated, after which an imaging procedure should be performed. Lumbar puncture may be performed if there is no evidence of a mass lesion or signs of raised intracranial pressure.

Serologic testing for anti-Toxoplasma IgG antibody in blood and anticysticercal antibodies on CSF specimens can aid in the diagnosis of toxoplasmosis or neurocysticercosis. These may be of value in the immunocompromised patient.

Specimens obtained during surgery or stereotactic CT-guided aspiration should be sent for aerobic, anaerobic, mycobacterial and fungal culture and, when indicated, for protozoa. In one study, the Gram stain revealed organisms in 82% of cases and the culture was positive in 88%.[24] Special stains should be performed which include fungal stains (e.g. methenamine silver, mucicarmine), an acid-fast stain for mycobacteria and a modified acid-fast stain for Nocardia spp. In patients with HIV infection, polymerase chain reaction (PCR) examination of CSF may be useful in diagnosing tuberculous abscesses.

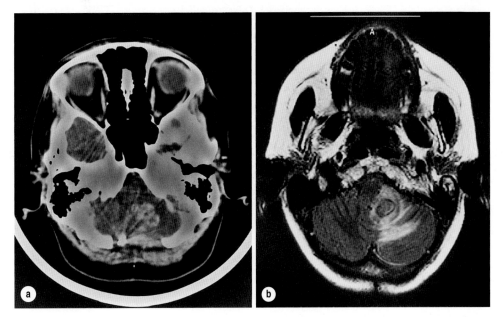

Fig. 20.3 Contrast-enhanced CT and MRI scans of the head in the coronal projection of a 43-year-old woman with headaches after a recent fall on her head. (a) CT scan image reveals a cystic ring-enhancing lesion in the left cerebellum. Note the prominent bone artifact. (b) T1-weighted MRI scan image reveals an enhancing cystic lesion in the left cerebellum with significant surrounding edema. Bone artifact is absent. Both CT and MRI scans were felt to be most consistent with a primary or metastatic neoplasm, but culture of material obtained at stereotactically guided aspiration grew *Staphylococcus aureus*.

MANAGEMENT

Before abscess encapsulation and localization, antimicrobial therapy, accompanied by measures to control increasing intracranial pressure, are essential.[27] Once an abscess has formed, surgical excision or drainage combined with prolonged antibiotics (usually 4–8 weeks) remains the treatment of choice. Some neurosurgeons advocate complete evacuation of the abscess, while others advocate repeated aspirations as indicated. The procedures used are aspiration through a burr hole and complete excision after craniotomy. In addition to its therapeutic effect, drainage permits microbiologic evaluation of abscess material, which guides antimicrobial therapy. Since aspiration is as effective as excision in most cases and is less invasive, it has become the procedure of choice. Stereotactic CT-guided aspiration permits accurate access even to areas that had been difficult to reach by aspiration, such as the brain stem, cerebellum and thalamus,[28] and multiple abscesses may be drained. Neuroendoscopic aspiration has also been used with success in a small number of patients.

Emergency surgery should be performed if a single abscess is present. Abscesses larger than 2.5 cm are excised or aspirated, while those smaller than 2.5 cm or are at the cerebritis stage are aspirated for diagnostic purposes only. In cases of multiple abscesses or in abscesses in essential brain areas, repeated aspirations are preferred to complete excision. High-dose antibiotics for an extended period may be an alternative approach in this group of patients.

A number of factors should be considered when trying to decide the appropriate approach to therapy.

Knowledge of the etiologic agent(s) by recovery from blood, CSF, abscess or other normally sterile sites is essential because it allows for the most appropriate selection of antimicrobials.

The duration of the symptoms before diagnosis is an important factor. Antibiotic therapy during the early stage, before expanding mass lesion exists, may prevent progress from cerebritis to abscess. Patients who have symptoms for less than 1 week have a more favorable response to medical therapy than patients with symptoms persisting longer than 1 week.

Growing evidence suggests that under certain circumstances brain abscess may be treated without surgical drainage. Small abscesses (less than 2.5 cm diameter) and abscesses in the cerebritis stage may respond to antimicrobial therapy alone. Medical therapy alone may also be indicated if the patient is a poor surgical candidate. In these cases, prolonged courses of antibiotics (at least 8 weeks of parenteral therapy) and close monitoring with sequential CT or MRI scans are necessary; MRI may be especially useful here because of its lack of ionizing radiation. Patients treated with medical therapy alone usually demonstrate clinical improvement before significant changes in the CT scan are observed. CT scanning and MRI should eventually show a decrease in the size of the lesion, a decrease in accompanying edema, and a lessening of the enhancement ring. Improvement on CT scans is generally observed within 1–4 weeks (average, 2.5 weeks) and complete resolution in 1–11 months (average, 3.5 months). Radiographic abnormalities may persist for months after successful therapy (Fig. 20.4).

The antimicrobial treatment of the brain abscess is generally long (6–8 weeks) because of the prolonged time needed for brain tissue to repair and close abscess space. The initial course is through an intravenous route, often followed by an additional 2–6 months of appropriate oral therapy. A shorter course (3–4 weeks) may be adequate in patients who had surgical drainage. Because of the difficulty involved in the penetration of various antimicrobial agents through the blood–brain barrier, the choice of antibiotics is restricted, and maximal doses are often necessary.

Initial empiric antimicrobial therapy should be based on the expected etiologic agents according to the likely predisposing conditions, the primary infection source and the presumed pathogenesis of abscess formation. Antibiotics should be parenteral, have activity against the likely pathogens, penetrate into abscess fluid (and the site of any underlying infection) in adequate concentrations and be bactericidal. The combination of penicillin or a third-generation cephalosporin (cefotaxime or ceftriaxone) plus metronidazole is effective as empiric therapy in most cases (see Table 20.2). An antistaphylococcal penicillin (such as flucloxacillin, nafcillin or oxacillin) should be used if staphylococci are suspected. Vancomycin should be used instead if methicillin-resistant *Staph. aureus* (MRSA) is suspected or identified, or if the patient is allergic to β-lactam antimicrobials. Cefepime or ceftazidime are administered to treat *Pseudomonas aeruginosa*. Patients with HIV infection may require therapy for toxoplasmosis.

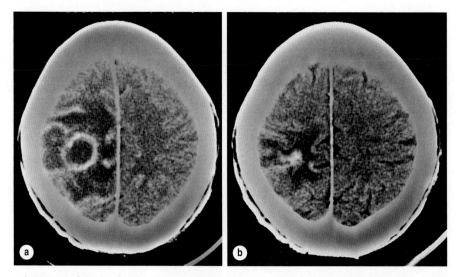

Fig. 20.4 Contrast-enhanced CT scans of the head in the coronal projection of a 66-year-old woman with a group B streptococcal brain abscess demonstrating evolution of the abscess during and after surgical and antimicrobial therapy. (a) The original scan demonstrates a hypodense necrotic center surrounded by an enhancing capsule and hypodense edema. (b) Seven weeks later, after stereotactically guided aspiration and a full course of antimicrobial therapy, the central cavity can no longer be seen, although the enhancement and surrounding edema persist to a small degree.

Open craniotomy with debridement, intraventricular lavage and intraventricular as well as intravenous antibiotics are recommended after intraventricular rupture of brain abscess. Changes in therapy should be guided by results of microbiologic examination and by clinical and radiographic progress.

Adjunctive therapy with corticosteroids, mannitol and hyperventilation may be indicated where there is evidence of increased intracranial pressure. Corticosteroid use is controversial. Steroids can retard encapsulation, increase necrosis, reduce antibiotic penetration into the abscess, alter CT scans and can produce a rebound effect when discontinued. If used to reduce cerebral edema, therapy should be of short duration. The appropriate dosage, timing and any effect of steroid therapy on the course of the disease are unknown. The routine use of corticosteroids in the absence of increased intracranial pressure cannot be recommended.

Prognosis has improved considerably, particularly since the introduction of CT scanning. Mortality is now less than 30%. Long-term sequelae may occur in about one-third of patients and include mental retardation, seizures and focal neurologic deficits. Poor prognostic factors include delayed or missed diagnosis, multiple lesions, deep-seated lesions, intraventricular rupture, severe impairment of mental or neurologic status (including coma), fungal etiology and extremes of age.

Subdural Empyema and Intracranial Epidural Abscess

Subdural empyema and epidural abscess are focal collections of purulent material between the dura mater and arachnoid mater, and outside the dura mater, respectively. Subdural empyema accounts for approximately 15–20% of all focal intracranial infections.

EPIDEMIOLOGY

Subdural empyema in adults is most often a complication of acute or chronic bacterial paranasal sinusitis, otitis media or mastoiditis.[29] It is the most common intracranial complication of sinusitis, accounting for approximately 60% of such cases.[30] The frontal and ethmoidal sinuses are the foci in over half of the cases. Hematogenous spread from a distant source may also occur. In children the most common predisposing condition is bacterial meningitis. Other predisposing conditions include trauma, neurosurgical procedures, infection of a pre-existing subdural hematoma, ethmoidectomy, polypectomy and nasal surgery. Hematogenous spread from a distant location (mainly from the lung) is uncommon. As with brain abscess, there is a male predominance.[31]

Most cases of intracranial epidural abscess in the past were due to paranasal sinusitis (particularly frontal), otitis media, mastoiditis or cranial trauma. Currently many cases occur after neurosurgical procedures. Males are again more commonly afflicted.[32]

PATHOGENESIS AND PATHOPHYSIOLOGY

As with brain abscesses, extension of infection into the epidural or subdural space from a contiguous focus may occur by extension through infected bone or by hematogenous seeding through emissary veins. Intracranial epidural abscess is generally associated with subdural empyema and overlying osteomyelitis, and usually consists of a localized lesion with a central collection of pus surrounded by a wall of inflammatory reaction that may calcify. These abscesses rarely spread downwards into the spinal canal because the dura is very tightly attached around the foramen magnum. In patients with subdural empyema, infection can spread rapidly through the subdural space until limited by its natural boundaries. These include the falx cerebri, tentorium cerebelli, base of the brain, foramen magnum posteriorly and the anterior spinal canal. Within the compartments defined by these boundaries, the progressing infection behaves as an expanding mass lesion.

As the lesion expands, intracranial pressure increases and the cerebral parenchyma is compromised. Interference with flow of blood or of CSF may cause cerebral edema and hydrocephalus. Septic thrombosis of veins within the affected subdural or epidural space may lead to thrombosis of cavernous sinuses or cortical veins, leading to infarction of brain tissue.

Organisms commonly isolated from adult patients with subdural empyema and intracranial epidural abscess include anaerobes, aerobic streptococci, staphylococci, *Strep. pneumoniae*, *Haemophilus influenzae* and other Gram-negative bacilli. Polymicrobial infections are common; in one study, more than 50% of infections were polymicrobial.[31,33] In children, the most common agents are those that are responsible for the underlying meningitis. In the past, this has been *H. influenzae* in children outside the neonatal age; however, as the relative frequency of *H. influenzae* meningitis declines, its role in subdural empyema may diminish as well. Anaerobes were identified in children in cases associated with sinusitis.[34]

Organisms commonly isolated from epidural abscesses associated with paranasal sinuses or ears are microaerophilic or anaerobic streptococci, *Propionibacterium*, *Peptostreptococcus* and *Prevotella* spp. When isolated associated with neurosurgery, the most likely organisms are staphylococci, especially *Staph. aureus*, and aerobic Gram-negative bacteria. The infection can also spread inward from osteomyelitis of the skull or be introduced by fetal monitoring probes during delivery.[35]

CLINICAL FEATURES

The signs and symptoms result from the infection and the slowly expanding intracranial mass. The most prominent early symptoms associated with subdural empyema and intracranial epidural abscess are fever and headache. The headache is often focal at onset but may become generalized. These symptoms are usually followed by papilledema and focal neurologic defects. Abscesses near the petrous portion of the temporal bone may be associated with palsies of cranial nerves V and VI, causing unilateral facial pain and lateral rectus muscle weakness. Periorbital edema and subgaleal abscess (Pott's puffy tumor) may be found in up to about one-third of patients. Signs of increased intracranial pressure (such as vomiting, gait disturbances and mental status changes) and meningeal irritation may follow and may be accompanied by seizures, hemiparesis and hemisensory defects.[31] Epidural abscess complicating sinus infections can cause purulent nose or ear drainage.[36]

DIAGNOSIS

CT and MRI scanning are the diagnostic procedures of choice. Imaging reveals a hypodense lesion with displacement of the arachnoid mater in both entities, with accompanying displacement of the dura mater noted in patients who have subdural empyema. Mass effect is more common with subdural empyema than with epidural abscess (Fig. 20.5). Capsule formation with contrast enhancement may be seen in either condition, but is more common with epidural abscess (Fig. 20.6). Cranial osteomyelitis may also be noted in patients who have underlying contiguous foci of infection. Gadolinium-enhanced MRI may detect lesions not noted on CT (because the lesions may be isodense with the cerebral tissue on CT). As with brain abscess, lumbar puncture is contraindicated in patients with known or suspected subdural empyema or epidural abscess (see Practice Point 6). Clinical deterioration was reported in 33 of 280 patients (11.3%) who underwent lumbar puncture with subdural empyema[31] and in 1 of 12 patients (8.3%) with epidural abscess.[32]

The differential diagnosis of epidural abscess includes metastatic tumors, disc and bony disease (including vertebral discitis and osteomyelitis), meningitis and early stage of herpes zoster.

MANAGEMENT

Treatment requires a combination of drainage and antibiotic therapy. Surgical evacuation is necessary for management of most patients. It can provide immediate decompression and specimens for microbiologic studies and should be accomplished by craniotomy or by the use of burr holes. Although the optimal surgical procedure has not been established, in one study of 699 patients with subdural empyema, the use of limited procedures such as burr holes was associated with a worse prognosis than more extensive procedures such as craniotomies.[37] It may also be necessary to debride the primary infection. Samples should be submitted for

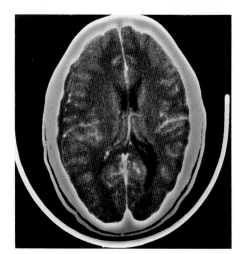

Fig. 20.5 Contrast-enhanced CT scan of the head in the coronal projection of a 23-year-old man with fever and headache. There is a small isodense extra-axial fluid collection in the subdural space on the right, with significant mass effect shown by right-to-left midline shift and effacement of the right lateral ventricle. There was also opacification of the frontal and ethmoid sinuses, suggesting sinusitis as the source of this subdural empyema.

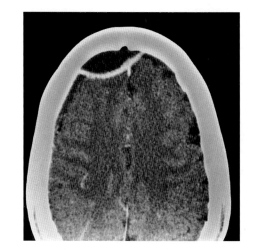

Fig. 20.6 Contrast-enhanced CT scan of the head in the coronal projection of a 19-year-old man with otitis media who presented with sinus congestion 1 week earlier. Plain films of the sinuses revealed opacification of the right maxillary and ethmoidal sinuses and an intracranial air–fluid level. Note the intracranial gas in the right frontal region abutting a hypodense region in the epidural space with ring enhancement and surrounding edema, representing an intracranial epidural abscess.

Gram stain and aerobic and anaerobic cultures. Antimicrobial therapy alone may be used for a limited number of patients with very small fluid collections.[31,32]

The choice of empiric antimicrobial therapy depends upon the patient's age, predisposing conditions and the primary infection site (Table 20.3). Antimicrobial choice should be guided and eventually be specific after the results of Gram stain of aspirated material and cultures are available. In adults, the wide variety of possible pathogens and the potential for polymicrobial infection dictate the use of broad-spectrum therapy. In children, therapy should be directed against the likely causes of meningitis. Parenteral antimicrobial therapy should be continued for 3–6 weeks, with close monitoring of clinical status and radiographic appearance.

Table 20.3 Pathogens and suggested empiric antibiotic regimens for subdural empyema and intracranial epidural abscess based on underlying condition

Predisposing condition	Likely pathogens	Empiric therapy
Sinusitis	Aerobic, anaerobic and microaerophilic streptococci Anaerobic Gram-negative bacilli (i.e. *Prevotella* spp., *Bacteroides* spp.) *Staphylococcus aureus* Enterobacteriaceae *Haemophilus influenzae* *Streptococcus pneumoniae*	Third-generation cephalosporin + metronidazole ± antistaphylococcal penicillin or a penicillin
Otitis media or mastoiditis	Aerobic, anaerobic and microaerophilic streptococci Anaerobic Gram-negative bacilli (i.e. *Prevotella* spp., *Bacteroides* spp.) *Staph. aureus* Enterobacteriaceae *Haemophilus influenzae*	Third-generation cephalosporin + metronidazole ± antistaphylococcal penicillin or a penicillin
Trauma	*Staph. aureus* Coagulase-negative staphylococci Enterobacteriaceae *Pseudomonas aeruginosa*	Vancomycin + third-generation cephalosporin
Dental infection	Aerobic, anaerobic and microaerophilic streptococci *Fusobacterium* spp. Anaerobic Gram-negative bacilli (i.e. *Prevotella* spp., *Bacteroides* spp.)	Penicillin or third-generation cephalosporin + metronidazole
Neonate	Enterobacteriaceae Group B streptococci *Listeria monocytogenes*	Third-generation cephalosporin + ampicillin
Infant or child	*Streptococcus pneumoniae* *Haemophilus influenzae* *Neisseria meningitidis*	Third-generation cephalosporin ± vancomycin

Suppurative Intracranial Phlebitis

Suppurative intracranial phlebitis is inflammation of the blood vessels within the cranium resulting from infection.[38]

EPIDEMIOLOGY, PATHOGENESIS AND PATHOPHYSIOLOGY

These usually follow infections of the paranasal sinuses, middle ear, mastoids, face, oropharynx and, in particular, the nasal furuncle. They may be associated with subdural empyema, epidural abscess or bacterial meningitis. Conditions associated with increased blood viscosity or hypercoagulability increase the risk of nonsuppurative thrombosis of the intracranial venous sinuses as well as of suppurative intracranial phlebitis

Spread generally occurs along emissary veins. The venous sinuses most commonly involved are the cavernous sinus, lateral sinus and superior sagittal sinus. If there is sufficient involvement of the vasculature, then cerebral edema and hemorrhagic infarction may result. The infarcts tend to occur in venous watershed regions. Involvement of the superior sagittal sinus or of the lateral sinuses may block CSF reabsorption and lead to hydrocephalus and increased intracranial pressure. Involvement of contiguous structures can lead to brain abscess, subdural empyema, epidural abscess or meningitis, or distant seeding and infection of the lungs and other organs.

The microbiology of suppurative intracranial phlebitis is similar to that of subdural empyema and intracranial epidural abscess, with *Staph. aureus*, streptococci and anaerobes being most commonly identified.

CLINICAL FEATURES

Clinical manifestations vary with the location of the involved venous sinuses or cortical veins.

Cavernous sinus thrombosis is associated with palsies of cranial nerves III, IV, V and VI, producing loss of corneal reflexes, ophthalmoplegia and hypesthesia over the upper part of the face. Papilledema and visual loss may result from obstruction of retinal venous return.

Lateral sinus thrombosis involves cranial nerves V and VI, resulting in altered facial sensation and lateral rectus muscle weakness. Obstruction of venous CSF resorption may cause communicating hydrocephalus and increased intracranial pressure. Cranial nerves IX, X and XI may also be affected.

Involvement of the superior sagittal sinus may also diminish CSF resorption. In addition, obstruction of venous drainage from the motor cortex region of the cerebral hemispheres may lead to weakness of the legs.

Cortical vein thrombosis may be neurologically silent or produce only transient defects if collateral venous drainage can compensate for thrombosis. If collateral flow is inadequate, the lesion will manifest as progressive neurologic defects. The precise nature of the defects depends on the location of the veins involved. Unilateral or bilateral extremity weakness, hemiparesis, aphasia, seizures and mental status changes may be seen.

DIAGNOSIS

MRI is more sensitive than CT and is the diagnostic procedure of choice. The appearance on MRI is that of increased signal within the

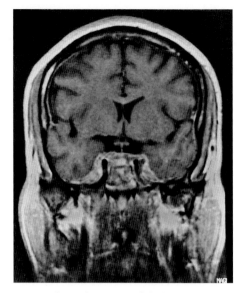

Fig. 20.7 Contrast-enhanced MRI scan of the head in the sagittal projection of a 29-year-old man with sinus congestion and headache. There is non-uniform signal intensity of the cavernous venous sinuses, indicating cavernous sinus thrombosis. The sphenoid, ethmoidal and maxillary paranasal sinuses also demonstrated abnormal signal intensity.

involved vessel (Fig. 20.7). Sensitivity of MRI can be enhanced by the use of magnetic resonance imaging angiography. CT may be used when MRI is unavailable. If CT or MRI is unremarkable and suppurative intracranial phlebitis is still suspected, angiography should be performed.

MANAGEMENT

Empiric antimicrobial therapy is similar to that employed for subdural empyema and intracranial epidural abscess (see Table 20.2). Control of increased intracranial pressure may be necessary with adjunctive measures such as corticosteroids, hyperosmolar agents and hyperventilation. Anticoagulant therapy has been used with some success, but carries the risk of hemorrhagic infarction. Surgery may be required for drainage of associated abscesses.

Spinal Epidural Abscess

Spinal epidural abscess is a focal infection of the paraspinal epidural space. It requires prompt recognition and appropriate management to avoid potentially serious complications.

EPIDEMIOLOGY

Spinal epidural abscess is rare and occurs in 2–25 patients per 100 000 admitted to hospital.[39] The increased sensitivity and accuracy of diagnosis, aided by the use of MRI, has increased the rate of diagnosis of this infection over the last 30 years.[40] The incidence is similar in males and females and the median age of onset is approximately 50 years.

PATHOGENESIS AND PATHOPHYSIOLOGY

Spinal epidural abscess may be secondary to epidural catheter placement (risk of 0.5–3%)[41] and contiguous source of infection, such as

vertebral osteomyelitis, pyogenic infectious discitis, penetrating trauma or decubitus ulcers, or may arise by hematogenous spread from a distant source.[29,40–43] The use of face masks when epidural catheters are placed has been recommended as a means to reduce spinal abscesses after epidural catheter placement.

A history of back trauma, spinal and paraspinal procedures, diabetes mellitus, alcoholism, intravenous drug use, HIV infection, tattooing, acupuncture, local spinal injections, and contiguous bony or soft tissue infection are common risk factors.[42] In addition to pulmonary infections, endocarditis and bacteremia as seen in patients who have brain abscess and subdural empyema, possible sources for hematogenous seeding of the spinal epidural space include cutaneous, intra-abdominal, pelvic and genitourinary infections. Spread from these sources occurs via the paravertebral venous plexus. In about a third of patients no identifiable source for the infection can be found.

The abscess can extend longitudinally in the epidural space, damaging the spinal cord by direct compression, interruption of the arterial blood supply and local vasculitis, thrombosis and thrombophlebitis of nearby veins, and by bacterial toxins and mediators of inflammation. Longitudinal extension is common in infection arising in the epidural space. The average extent is three to five spinal cord segments, but the whole length of the spinal column may be affected.

In the acute stage the abscess may have pus, but after about 2 weeks it may contain only granulation tissue.

In most cases in adults, the thoracic spine is involved, while cervical and lumbar involvement are more common in children. There is a male predominance.[43]

The organism responsible for the majority of cases is *Staph. aureus*, accounting for almost three-quarters of all cases in a meta-analysis of 915 cases reported.[43] The rate of proportion of infections due to MRSA is steadily rising, reaching 40% of all *Staph. aureus* in one report.[42] Other staphylococci, aerobic and anaerobic streptococci, *Escherichia coli* and *P. aeruginosa* are also common.[43] Polymicrobial infections may occur, but are uncommon. *Mycobacterium tuberculosis* can cause up to 25% of the cases.[44]

CLINICAL FEATURES

There are four clinical stages:
- fever and focal back pain;
- nerve root compression with nerve root pain;
- spinal cord compression with accompanying deficits in motor, sensory, and bowel and bladder sphincter function; and
- paralysis.

Respiratory compromise may also be present if the cervical cord is involved.[45]

Progression tends to be rapid with infection due to direct hematogenous spread, and may be accompanied by severe pain. Progression to the second stage tends to occur slowly in those with abscesses secondary to vertebral osteomyelitis, but may accelerate after that. Headache, meningismus and focal tenderness are common signs and symptoms.

DIAGNOSIS

Clinical suspicion is essential, as the presentation may not be typical. A recent study showed that the mean duration of symptoms between onset of symptoms and the first emergency room visit or admission was 5 and 9 days, respectively, and the median number of visits to the emergency room before admission was two (1–8).[46] Sedimentation rate is usually elevated and the leukocyte count may be elevated or normal.[46]

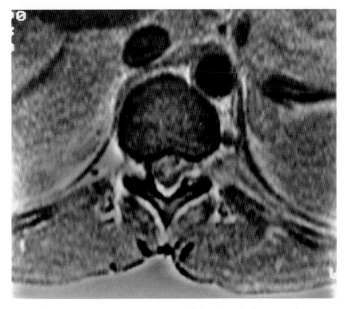

Fig. 20.8 Contrast-enhanced MRI scan of the spine in the coronal projection of a 28-year-old man with a 1-week history of headache, fever and sweats. Physical examination demonstrated meningismus but no focal neurologic deficits. Scans in the sagittal section demonstrated a substance nearly isointense with the spinal cord and running nearly the length of the cord. This scan clearly demonstrates impingement and anterior displacement of the cord by the spinal epidural abscess.

Plain radiographs may reveal changes of osteomyelitis or discitis. Gadolinium-enhanced MRI has supplanted CT and myelography as the diagnostic procedure of choice for spinal epidural abscess[47,48] (Fig. 20.8). MRI is highly sensitive (91%) and can identify osteomyelitis and intramedullary spinal cord lesions. It also enables early detection of an abscess while it is still small prior to spinal cord compression. If MRI is not available, myelography should be performed.

Recovery of etiologic organism(s) from blood, abscess contents or CSF is important. CSF may show high protein and pleocytosis. Gram stain is usually negative and cultures are positive in less than a 25% of the specimens.[42]

The differential diagnosis includes many conditions that cause back pain and neurologic deficits, including disc and bony disease, discitis, osteomyelitis, meningitis, malignancy and early stage herpes zoster.

MANAGEMENT

Urgent decompression and surgical drainage or aspiration plus parenteral antimicrobial therapy are indicated for the management of most patients.[49] Decompression and drainage are ordinarily achieved by laminectomy, but CT-guided aspiration may be performed in selected patients. Two studies reported the outcome in patients who received only medical therapy to be similar to those who had surgery.[50,51] The use of a nonsurgical conservative approach is rarely used but may be attempted in those individuals with significant surgical risk who have an identified pathogen (through blood culture or aspiration). Close neurologic monitoring and follow-up MRI that demonstrates reduction and resolution of the abscess are needed in these cases. If there is neurologic deterioration, surgery should be performed without delay.

An antistaphylococcal penicillin should be instituted as empiric therapy in all patients; vancomycin may be used in patients who are allergic to penicillin and those with MRSA. Antibiotics effective against Gram-negative organisms (i.e. third-generation cephalosporins) and anaerobes (i.e. metronidazole) should be added in patients whose underlying source might have been an intra-abdominal, pelvic or genitourinary infection. The usual duration of parenteral therapy should be at least 3–4 weeks; if osteomyelitis is present, it should be continued for 8 weeks. Therapy length can be adjusted according to resolution of the abscess on MRI. Follow-up MRI is generally performed at about 4 weeks if the patient is improving, or earlier if clinical deterioration occurs.

Spinal Cord Abscess

This is a rare condition defined as a focal suppurative processes of the spinal cord parenchyma. It usually involves the thoracic segment of the spinal cord and is generally hematogenous in origin. The lungs are usually the source of infection and it can occur in intravenous drug users and secondary to congenital dermal sinuses. The predominant pathogens are *Staph. aureus*, streptococci, *Listeria monocytogenes* and *Burkholderia cepacia*.[52] Symptoms mimic those of spinal epidural abscess. Diagnosis may be made by CT, MRI or myelography. Treatment consists of surgical debridement and prolonged antimicrobial therapy. Antibiotics should be directed against *Staph. aureus* and possibly Gram-negative bacilli.

REFERENCES

References for this chapter can be found online at http://www.expertconsult.com

Tetanus and botulism

Tetanus and botulism are completely preventable diseases that nevertheless continue to cause serious morbidity and mortality, especially in the developing world. Both are caused by members of the genus *Clostridium*; in both cases, disease is caused by exotoxins that conform to an A–B model, each being composed of an enzymatic (A) portion and a binding (B) portion. The biologic activity resides in the A portion, whereas the B subunits may bind to target cells but are biologically inactive. Common to both toxins described, A and B are domains of a single protein that is cleaved by proteolytic activity of the bacterium (Fig. 21.1). Tetanus is caused by tetanospasmin (TS), a neural toxin that predominantly interferes with the inhibition of spinal cord reflexes, and is produced by the obligate anaerobic bacterium *Clostridium tetani*. Botulism is caused by one of several neurotoxins (types A, B, E and F cause human disease) produced by *C. botulinum* (Table 21.1). There are three forms of the latter illness: food-borne botulism from ingestion of preformed toxin; wound botulism; and botulism from intestinal colonization, usually seen in infants.[1,2]

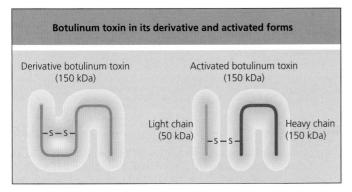

Botulinum toxin in its derivative and activated forms

Derivative botulinum toxin (150 kDa)

Activated botulinum toxin (150 kDa)

Light chain (50 kDa)

Heavy chain (150 kDa)

—S – S—

—S – S—

Fig. 21.1 Clostridial toxins as produced by the bacteria (left) and after nicking to produce light and heavy chains linked by a disulfide bond.

Table 21.1 Characteristics of groups of *C. botulinum* and the toxins that produce human disease

Group	Toxins produced	Proteolysis	Heat resistance of spores	Disease severity
Group I	A, B, F	Yes	High	Severe
Group II	B, E, F	No	Low	Less severe

EPIDEMIOLOGY

Tetanus is still common in developing tropical countries, where it is an important cause of death, particularly in neonates. The World Health Organization estimated in 2002 that about 180 000 newborns died worldwide from tetanus. In the developed world, however, active immunization and better hygiene, wound care and management of childbirth have meant that the disease is now rare. The annual incidence of tetanus has fallen from nearly 4 to 0.2 per million population in the USA since 1947 (Fig. 21.2); mortality has dropped even more, with the death:case ratio falling from about 50% to below 30%.[3] In England and Wales there were 175 cases of tetanus (and 19 deaths) in the period from 1984 to 2000.[4]

Neonatal tetanus usually occurs within 3–14 days of birth in infants delivered under nonsterile conditions to nonimmunized women. The umbilical cord stump is the usual portal of entry, particularly if cultural practices dictate the application of animal dung to the stump. At other ages acute wounds are the portal of entry for *C. tetani* in about 80% of cases, with the remainder associated with chronic decubitus ulcers, gangrene, abscesses or parenteral drug abuse. Tetanus is more likely to occur in the summer months when gardening and other pastimes bring people into contact with soil.

All three forms of botulism occur throughout the world, but for food-borne botulism, the causative strains, the responsible foods and the resulting illness vary in different geographic areas. Accurate data about the incidence of botulism are difficult to obtain but it is estimated that, in France, there were about 300 food-borne outbreaks between 1979 and 1988, and in the USA there were 474 outbreaks (a large proportion from Alaska) involving nearly 1050 persons between 1950 and 1990. Outbreaks were most frequent in the summer or autumn. In the UK the incidence is much lower than in Europe or the USA, with only nine outbreaks between 1922 and 1988. In 1989 the largest ever outbreak of food-borne botulism in the UK affected 27 people who had eaten hazelnut yoghurt. The illness was caused by type B toxin formed by bacteria growing in canned hazelnut conserve used to flavor the yogurt and that had been inadequately heat treated.[5]

Nearly 1000 cases of infant botulism (roughly equally divided between type A and type B *C. botulinum*) were reported in the USA between 1976 and 1990. Almost half the cases were reported from California, with an incidence of 7 per 100 000 live births. Cases occur most frequently in the second month of life and 95% of cases are in infants less than 6 months old.[1]

Most cases of food-borne botulism are associated with home-preserved meats, fish and vegetables but the common vehicles are often idiosyncratic to a country or culture.[6] In the USA (apart from Alaska), Spain, Italy and China most cases follow consumption of home-preserved vegetables (home-canned asparagus, beans and peppers in the USA, home-fermented bean curd in China) contaminated

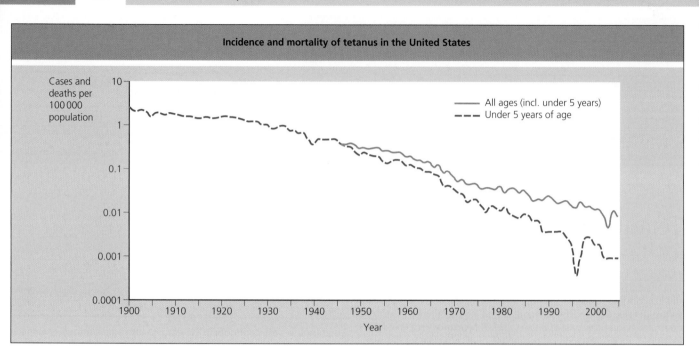

Fig. 21.2 Incidence and mortality of tetanus in the United States. From the US Centers for Disease Control and Prevention.

with type A *C. botulinum*. In Alaska, Japan, Canada and Scandinavia cases are usually due to type E toxin and follow eating fermented foods or preserved fish products; in central continental Europe cases typically arise from home-cured meats and are caused by nonproteolytic strains of type B *C. botulinum*. Commercially prepared foods are only rarely implicated. There is a significant association between infant botulism and ingestion of honey.

Occasionally, botulism follows wound infections with *C. botulinum*. The wounds are often compound fractures or penetrating wounds; cases have also been reported in intravenous drug users[7] and complicating sinusitis in chronic cocaine sniffers.

PATHOGENESIS AND PATHOLOGY

Tetanus

The clostridia are Gram-positive, anaerobic, spore-forming bacilli. In tetanus, spores of *C. tetani* contaminate a wound and germinate under anaerobic conditions. The proliferating organisms elaborate the tetanus toxin TS, one of the most potent of the known poisons, with an estimated lethal dose of 2.5 ng/kg. It is produced by a plasmid-encoded gene and is synthesized as a 151 kDa polypeptide. As with botulinum and diphtheria toxins, this polypeptide is then split by clostridial proteolytic cleavage into the light (L) chain (approximately 50 kDa and containing the enzymatic (A) domain) and the heavy (H) chain (approximately 100 kDa and containing the binding (B) domain).

From the standpoint of pathogenesis, the important difference between tetanus and botulinum toxin is that botulinum toxin remains outside of the central nervous system, while tetanus toxin enters the central nervous system and exerts most of its activity in the brain stem and spinal cord. The activity of each toxin at the cellular level is very similar, although the subunit of the transmitter release mechanism targeted by each toxin type varies.

Most of the tetanus toxin gets into the bloodstream, and then enters the central nervous system (CNS) via neurons to exert its toxicity (Fig. 21.3). The effect of each toxin is via a three-stage process: binding, internalization and induction of paralysis.[8] The H chain interacts with the ganglioside GT1 of neurons at neuromuscular junctions, both locally and distally (via the bloodstream), and enables the L chain to enter the cytoplasm of the neuron. The tetanospasmin is then transported intra-axonally at 75–250 mm/day in a retrograde manner to the cell body in the ventral horns of the spinal cord and the motor nuclei of cranial nerves and then, via trans-synaptic spread, to other neurons within the CNS. Within the neurons tetanospasmin acts as a zinc-dependent protease that cleaves synaptobrevin, a protein component of synaptic vesicles,[9] and prevents release of neurotransmitters at the presynaptic membrane. Inhibitory interneurons in the spinal cord (using glycine as a transmitter) and descending inhibitory projection neurons from the brain stem (using γ-amino butyric acid; GABA) are most severely affected, but cells of the autonomic nervous system are also involved.

There are no gross or histologic abnormalities in tetanus. Any changes described in fatal cases reflect terminal hypoxia and autonomic dysfunction.

Botulism

Food-borne botulism follows ingestion of preformed toxin, but in other forms of the disease toxin is produced *in vivo* and released when vegetative cells lyse. The toxin is not released from spores. Botulinum toxins are the most poisonous substances known, and are synthesized as a polypeptide of molecular weight 150–165 kDa, which is then broken into a heavy chain of about 100 kDa and a light chain joined by a disulfide bond. The mechanism of action is similar or identical to that of tetanospasmin, resulting in cleavage of synaptobrevin and inhibition of release of acetylcholine at peripheral cholinergic synapses. The heavy chain binds rapidly to the membrane of the presynaptic α motor neuron and then some (or all) of the toxin molecule translocates through the membrane. Finally, there is a slow paralytic step that may partially depend upon temperature and activity of the neuron. The process is slowly reversible and the synapse is inactivated for a long time. Initial recovery of function depends upon the budding and growth of new presynaptic end-plates, but the original synapse eventually can regain activity.

Infant botulism results from colonization of the infant's gastrointestinal tract with as many as 10[8] proteolytic *C. botulinum* organisms

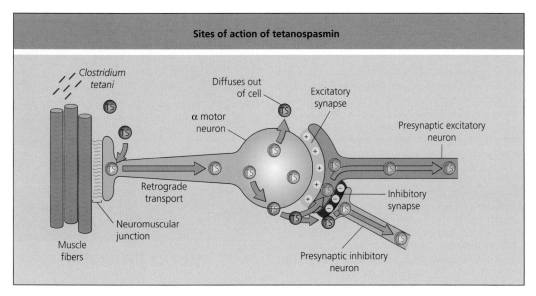

Fig. 21.3 Sites of action of tetanospasmin. Tetanospasmin (TS) is produced by *Clostridium tetani* at the site of the wound and binds and internalizes at the neuromuscular junction into the α motor neuron. It then travels by retrograde axonal flow to the cell body and diffuses out into the synapses and extracellular space of the CNS. It enters other neurons and travels further into the CNS. Its major effect is to inhibit transmitter release from the glycinergic presynaptic inhibitory neuron but it can also inhibit release of transmitters at the excitatory synapses and of acetylcholine at the neuromuscular junction.

per gram of feces.[10] The mechanisms that relate to colonization and toxin absorption from the infant gut are unclear, and both the organism and toxin may sometimes continue to be excreted in the feces for several months after the illness has resolved. Wound botulism typically results from soil contamination of severe head wounds, as occurs in warfare, or following the subcutaneous injection of contaminated material.

Death results from respiratory paralysis; there are no specific pathologic findings on gross or histologic examination in any of the forms of botulism.

PREVENTION

Tetanus

Tetanus is a completely preventable disease. Generally, concentrations of antibody to tetanospasmin as low as 0.01 IU/ml are regarded as protective against clinical tetanus, although cases have occurred in patients who have antibody concentrations at least 10-fold higher than this. Active immunization with tetanus toxoid is extremely effective. A primary series of three doses of tetanus toxoid given in infancy, either with diphtheria toxoid and acellular or whole cell pertussis (DTaP or DTP) or diphtheria toxoid alone (DT), with a booster at school entry, is virtually 100% effective for 5–10 years. Another dose should be given to school leavers. Older children and adults should receive the appropriate combined vaccine (TDaP) every 10 years.[11] Immunity wanes in the elderly, who should be specially targeted for booster immunization.[12] Neonatal tetanus can be prevented by ensuring that all pregnant women are immune.

The need for both active and passive immunization against tetanus, with toxoid and specific human tetanus immunoglobulin (HTIG), should be reviewed after any injury that brings an individual to medical attention (Table 21.2).[13]

Clean, minor wounds do not need any special treatment. Previously nonimmunized persons over 7 years of age should receive a three-dose series of TDaP, the first two doses 4–8 weeks apart and the third after 6–12 months. All other wounds, including frostbite, burns and others, should be considered to render the patient prone to tetanus. Foreign bodies and ischemic tissue should be removed. If the patient has not received a primary series then the age-appropriate tetanus vaccine and HTIG (250 IU intramuscularly), or equine tetanus antitoxin if HTIG is not available within 24 hours, should be given.

Botulism

The key to preventing botulism is adequate processing and storage of food to destroy spores and prevent their germination and toxin production. Spores are not killed by boiling at 212°F (100°C) but are

Table 21.2 Recommendations for use of tetanus prophylaxis in wound management				
History of tetanus toxoid administration	**CLEAN, MINOR WOUNDS**		**ALL OTHER WOUNDS**	
	Tetanus toxoid*	**Immunoglobulin**	**Tetanus toxoid***	**Immunoglobulin**
Unknown or less than three doses	Yes and proceed with basic immunization	No	Yes and proceed with basic immunization	Yes (250 IU HTIG or 3000 IU equine tetanus antitoxin)
Three or more doses	No, unless >10 years since last dose	No	No, unless >5 years since last dose	No
*Administered as Td (i.e. low dose of diphtheria toxoid) in adults.				

destroyed by heating at 250°F (121°C) for 2.5 minutes (the type of temperature achieved under pressure processing of low-acid foods). Once toxin is formed, it can be inactivated by boiling or heating at 176°F (80°C) for 30 minutes.

Toxin production by strains of *C. botulinum* is inhibited at a pH below 4.6, in saline, and at low temperatures (below 38°F (3.3°C)); the respective values differ somewhat for different strains. Commercial canneries pay particular attention to less acid (pH >4.6) fruit and vegetables; the canning and curing of meats relies on a reduced heat treatment to kill vegetative bacteria and sodium chloride and nitrite to inhibit spore growth. Vacuum packaging of food may encourage the growth of anaerobes and there are concerns that botulinum toxin may be produced before spoilage is obvious. Toxin has been detected in mushrooms and coleslaw kept in modified atmosphere packaging. This should be preventable by piercing the packaging of fresh vegetables with air holes to allow sufficient oxygen to be present.

Honey has been associated with infant botulism and honey is not recommended as a food for infants less than 1 year old. However, other dietary sources of spores are involved, as the incidence of infant botulism has only declined by about half after the association with honey was discovered and publicized.

CLINICAL FEATURES

Tetanus

Although tetanus can occur at any age, those over 60 are at greatest risk in the developed world since they have lowest immunization levels; elderly women are at greatest risk since they are less likely to have been immunized during earlier military service.

The incubation period to the first symptom ranges from 1 day to several months but most cases start between 3 and 21 days after an acute injury. There is a correlation between the distance of the injury from the CNS and the duration of the incubation period. The time between the first symptom and the first reflex spasm is termed the period of onset. There are four clinical forms of tetanus – neonatal, localized, cephalic and generalized – depending on the predominant site of toxin action.[14]

Localized tetanus consists of fixed muscle rigidity and painful spasms, sometimes lasting weeks or months, confined to an area close to the site of the injury. It is rare and generally mild but may herald generalized tetanus. Cephalic tetanus is a particular form of localized tetanus associated with wounds to the head or face or with chronic otitis media, and manifested by atonic palsies involving the motor cranial nerves. The incubation period is often only 1–2 days and generalized tetanus may follow.

Generalized tetanus (which is by far the most common form) typically starts with rigidity and spasm of the masseter muscles, causing trismus or lockjaw and the characteristic risus sardonicus – a grimace through clenched teeth and closed mouth with wrinkled forehead and raised eyebrows (Fig. 21.4). Other muscles, first in the neck, then the thorax, back and extremities, become rigid and go into spasms, producing opisthotonos, abdominal rigidity and apnea. Tetanic spasms are intermittent, irregular and unpredictable, although they are often triggered by external stimuli, sometimes very trivial such as a sudden noise or puff of cold air, or even the internal stimulus of a distended bladder or bowel. Each spasm is sudden, painful and generalized, resulting in opisthotonos, leg extension and arm flexion; pharyngeal spasm causes dysphagia and spasm of the glottis may cause immediate asphyxiation and death. Cognitive functions are not affected. Severe tetanus is accompanied by abnormalities of the autonomic nervous system, including hypo- or hypertension, arrhythmias and flushing.

Neonatal tetanus typically starts with poor sucking and irritability, followed by trismus and tetanospasms. It has a higher death:case ratio than tetanus at other ages.

With intensive care the death rate from tetanus (which is due to respiratory dysfunction or autonomic cardiovascular instability) may

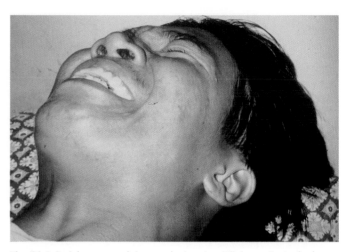

Fig. 21.4 Facial spasm and risus sardonicus in a Filipino patient who has tetanus.

be as low as 10–20%, with higher rates in infants and in the elderly. A rating scale for the severity and prognosis of tetanus may be used (Table 21.3). In general, the more rapid the evolution of symptoms and signs, the worse the prognosis but the belief that a short incubation period leads to a worse prognosis has been challenged.[14]

Complications related to spasms include vertebral and long bone fractures, glottic obstruction and asphyxia, and intramuscular hematomas. Rhabdomyolysis is common in generalized tetanus. Other complications are those related to general debility and prolonged intensive care.

Botulism

Food-borne botulism usually develops 12–36 hours after ingestion of the toxin, although the interval may be as short as 6 hours or as long as 10 days. Patients who have type E toxin-mediated disease tend to have shorter, and those with type B tend to have longer incubation periods. Wound botulism occurs at a mean of 7.5 days (range 4–18 days) after the injury.[15]

Table 21.3 Rating scale for severity and prognosis of tetanus

Score 1 point for each of the following

- Incubation period <7 days
- Period of onset <48 hours
- Acquired from burns, surgical wound, compound fracture, septic abortion
- Narcotic addiction
- Generalized tetanus
- Pyrexia >104°F (40°C)
- Tachycardia >120 beats/min (>150 beats/min in neonates)

Total score provides indication of severity and prognosis

Score	Severity	Mortality
0–1	Mild	<10%
2–3	Moderate	10–20%
4	Severe	20–40%
5–6	Very severe	>50%

Note: Cephalic tetanus is always scored as severe or very severe, and neonatal tetanus as very severe.

Table 21.4 Frequency of symptoms in types A, B and E food-borne botulism[16]

Symptoms	Type A disease (% of cases)	Type B disease (%)	Type E disease (%)
Dysphagia	25–96	77–100	63–90
Dry mouth	26–83	96–100	55–88
Diplopia	50–90	57–100	85
Dysarthria	25–100	69–100	50
Fatigue	8–92	69–100	Not known
Weakness of arm	16–86	64–86	Not known
Constipation	73	17–100	25–38
Weakness of leg	16–76	64–86	Not known
Dyspnea	35–91	34	88
Vomiting	70	50–100	88–100
Dizziness	8–86	30–100	63
Diarrhea	35	8–14	10
Paresthesiae	20	12–14	Not known

Typically, botulism first affects the muscles supplied by the cranial nerves with disturbances of vision and difficulties in swallowing and speech, followed by descending weakness of muscles of the trunk and extremities that is bilateral but not necessarily symmetric. Cardiovascular, gastrointestinal and urinary autonomic dysfunction may follow. The presentation may be related to the type of toxin: autonomic symptoms occur earlier and are more prominent in intoxication with type B and E toxins.

Common presenting symptoms are diplopia, dysphagia, dysarthria, dry mouth and fatigue (Table 21.4).[16] Ptosis and ophthalmoplegia are common physical signs, together with facial weakness and a decreased gag reflex. The pupils are dilated or fixed in less than 50% of cases. Frequently, there is weakness of the extremities, although deep tendon reflexes are usually normal. Patients are usually afebrile and have no sensory deficits. Patients who have wound botulism have a similar presentation but acute gastrointestinal symptoms are lacking.

Constipation is the first sign of infant botulism, with neurologic signs developing either concurrently or up to several weeks later. The neurologic signs progress in a similar fashion to those in other forms of botulism but they may be overlooked by the parents, who merely note the infant is irritable, lethargic or unable to suck. There is a wide range of clinical illness associated with infant botulism; 50% of cases develop ventilatory failure.

DIAGNOSIS

Tetanus

The diagnosis of tetanus depends upon clinical features, and epidemiologic history and laboratory tests are usually unhelpful. There is often a moderate leukocytosis, but the CSF is normal, except for increased intracranial pressure associated with increased muscle tone (raising intrathoracic pressure, which is then transmitted). Neither electroencephalography nor electromyography is helpful. Occasionally, characteristic Gram-positive bacilli with terminal or subterminal spores may be visualized in aspirates from a wound but anaerobic cultures are rarely positive and the organism may be grown from wounds in the absence of disease. However, neither stains nor cultures of wounds are diagnostically useful.

Botulism

Routine laboratory tests are not helpful in the diagnosis of botulism. The diagnosis is best confirmed by assay of botulism toxin in the patient's blood, gastric washings or feces by means of toxin neutralization tests in mice. Toxin may also be demonstrated in the incriminated food. This test takes anything from 6 to 96 hours to perform and the initial diagnosis must therefore be based on clinical findings. *Clostridium botulinum* may be cultured or the toxin detected by an enzyme-linked immunosorbent assay in the patient's feces, particularly in infant botulism and other cases resulting from intestinal colonization.

Electrophysiologic studies show normal nerve conduction velocities, but the electromyogram is often abnormal with facilitation (an incremental increase) of the amplitude evoked in the muscle when high-frequency (20–50 per second) repetitive stimuli are applied to the relevant nerve. Testing at this frequency is uncomfortable and is usually not performed unless the electromyographer is specifically asked to examine for botulism. These abnormalities may persist for several months after the onset of illness.

DIFFERENTIAL DIAGNOSIS

Tetanus

Strychnine poisoning is the only true mimic of tetanus, although there are several other diseases that may overlap to some extent. Strychnine poisoning develops more rapidly than tetanus and there is usually no muscle rigidity between spasms; serum analysis for strychnine should be performed in suspect cases. Other causes of trismus include dystonic reactions to phenothiazines (which may be ruled out by administration of benztropine 1–2 mg intravenously or diphenhydramine 50 mg intravenously) and dental abscesses. Tetany from hypocalcemia or alkalosis tends to affect the extremities rather than the axial muscles and there is no trismus.

Botulism

The diseases most often confused with botulism are Guillain–Barré syndrome (particularly the Miller–Fisher variant, predominantly affecting the cranial nerves), myasthenia gravis and the Eaton–Lambert myasthenic syndrome, other forms of food poisoning and tick paralysis. Guillain–Barré syndrome frequently has sensory complaints and the Miller–Fisher syndrome includes prominent ataxia. Myasthenias lack autonomic dysfunction and are less fulminant than botulism. In tick paralysis a careful search will reveal the Dermacentor tick still attached.

MANAGEMENT

Tetanus

A detailed guide to the general management of the patient with tetanus is available.[14] Human tetanus immune globulin (HTIG), 500 IU as a single intramuscular injection should be given at the time of diagnosis in order to prevent further circulating toxin from reaching the CNS.[13,17] The use of intrathecal HTIG to neutralize toxin that has entered but is not yet fixed to nervous tissue[18] has not been consistently beneficial and is not routinely recommended; injections are potent stimuli for tetanic spasms.

The source of toxin should be removed by wound debridement and removal of foreign bodies. Only vegetative forms of *C. tetani* will be susceptible to antibiotics. Therapy with metronidazole (15 mg/kg intravenously followed by 20–30 mg/kg/day intravenously for 7–14 days) should be used to eradicate *C. tetani*, even though antibiotics are not likely to penetrate into the anaerobic conditions that support growth of the organism.[19] Penicillin is less suitable (it is a central GABA antagonist).

A benzodiazepine (midazolam administered intravenously at 5–15 mg/h is suitable) should be used to produce sedation, decrease rigidity and control spasms. Airway protection during spasms is paramount. If ventilation is compromised, the patient should be sedated, intubated, provided with a soft nasal feeding tube and transferred to a quiet and darkened area. A tracheostomy may be needed, and is often advisable as the patient may require much higher doses of sedation to tolerate an endotracheal tube than a tracheostomy tube. If benzodiazepines do not adequately control the spasms then the patient will need long-term neuromuscular blockade.

The management over the next few weeks is that of any ventilated patient plus specific therapy for autonomic nervous system complications and control of spasms.[20] Sympathetic hyperactivity is treated with combined α- and β-blockade or morphine. Intrathecal baclofen has been shown to be effective in controlling muscle rigidity.[18] Epidural blockade with local anesthetics may be needed. Hypotension requires fluid replacement and noradrenaline (norepinephrine) administration. Parasympathetic overactivity is rare, but if bradycardia is sustained then a pacemaker may be needed.

Clinical tetanus does not induce immunity against further attacks of the disease and all patients should be fully immunized with tetanus toxoid (in the form appropriate for their age) during convalescence.

Botulism

Elimination of any unabsorbed toxin from the gastrointestinal tract should be encouraged in patients who have suspected botulism. Administration of an emetic or gastric lavage is recommended if ingestion of the suspect food has occurred within the preceding few hours and (unless there is a paralytic ileus) purgation or high enemas should be administered even several days after food ingestion.

The mainstay of therapy for botulism is meticulous supportive care. Patients should be admitted to an intensive care unit and their respiratory function monitored by repeat vital capacity measurements. Intubation should be performed if vital capacity falls below 12 ml/kg.

Equine antitoxin, containing antibodies to types A, B and E toxin, is available through public health services in many countries. There are few data concerning its use in humans but it is clearly effective in experimental animals. It has to be given as early as possible in the course of the illness but its use needs careful consideration in view of the risk of serious anaphylaxis or serum sickness. A test dose is administered into the skin or the conjunctiva. If there is no hypersensitivity, then one vial is given intravenously and one vial intramuscularly for an average adult; further doses may be given 2–4 hours later if the symptoms persist. Human botulinum immune globulin is available for infants through the California Department of Public Health (http://www.infantbotulism.org).

Antibiotics do not help except as part of meticulous debridement of the wound in wound botulism.

The relevant public health authorities should be notified promptly of a suspected case of botulism so that the necessary investigation may be conducted.

The severity and duration of food-borne botulism are related to the amount of toxin ingested. Respiratory failure occurs in 20–35% of patients; the mean duration of respiratory support is 7 weeks for those requiring mechanical ventilation. Recovery from botulism is usually complete but persistent dysphagia, diplopia and prolonged weakness are rare complications of severe cases.[21]

There has been a steady decline in mortality associated with botulism over the past century; the rate was about 70% in the period 1910–19 and about 9% during 1980–89. Mortality is higher in type A disease than in type B.[6] The prognosis for infants hospitalized with botulism and given meticulous supportive care is very good, with less than 1.3% case fatality and full recovery.

REFERENCES

References for this chapter can be found online at http://www.expertconsult.com

Chapter | **22** | Simon Mead
Sarah J Tabrizi
John Collinge

Prion diseases of humans and animals

The prion diseases or transmissible spongiform encephalopathies are a group of closely related transmissible neurodegenerative conditions of humans and animals. In recent years prion diseases have captured the public attention with the evolving epidemic of bovine spongiform encephalopathy (BSE) in Europe, and the subsequent appearance of a novel phenotype of Creutzfeldt–Jakob disease (CJD), variant CJD (vCJD) in humans, which is experimentally linked to dietary exposure to BSE. Recently, the transmission of vCJD by blood transfusion has generated concern about secondary transmission.

The nature of the transmissible agent in these diseases has been a subject of intense controversy. The understandable initial assumption that the agent must be some form of virus was challenged by the failure to directly demonstrate such a virus (or an immunologic response to it), and by the remarkable resistance of the transmissible agent to treatment expected to inactivate nucleic acids (such as ultraviolet radiation or treatment with nucleases). Such findings had led to suggestions by Alper and others that the transmissible agent may be devoid of nucleic acid,[1] and led Griffith to suggest in 1967 that the transmissible agent might be a protein.[2] Progressive enrichment of brain homogenates for infectivity resulted in the isolation of a protease-resistant sialoglycoprotein, designated the prion protein (PrP), by Prusiner and co-workers in 1982.[3] This protein was the major constituent of infective fractions and was found to accumulate in affected brains and sometimes to form amyloid deposits. The term prion (from *pro*teinaceous *in*fectious particle) was proposed by Prusiner in 1982 to distinguish the infectious pathogen from viruses or viroids.[3] Prions were defined as 'small proteinaceous infectious particles that resist inactivation by procedures which modify nucleic acids'.

The unifying hallmark of the prion diseases is the aberrant metabolism of the prion protein (PrP), which exists in at least two conformational states with different physicochemical properties. The normal form of the protein, referred to as PrP^C, is a highly conserved cell surface protein attached via a glycosylphosphatidylinositol (GPI) anchor (Fig. 22.1). It is expressed in a wide range of cell types, and particularly in neuronal cells. PrP^C is a sialoglycoprotein of molecular weight 33–35 kDa with a high content of α-helical secondary structure that is sensitive to protease treatment and soluble in detergents (Fig. 22.1). The disease-associated isoform, referred to as PrP^{Sc}, is found only in infected brains as aggregated material, is partially resistant to protease treatment and insoluble in detergents, and has a high content of β-sheet secondary structure.

Due to its physicochemical properties, the precise atomic structure of the infectious particle or prion is still undetermined but considerable evidence argues that prions are composed largely, if not entirely, of an abnormal isoform of PrP. According to the protein-only hypothesis of prion replication, PrP^{Sc} recruits PrP^C into the infectivity-associated isoform, an event that is central to prion propagation (Fig. 22.2).

EPIDEMIOLOGY

Animal prion diseases

Scrapie is the prototypic prion disease (Table 22.1). It has been recognized as an enzootic disease of sheep and goats for more than 250 years. Present in many countries, its prevalence in the UK has been

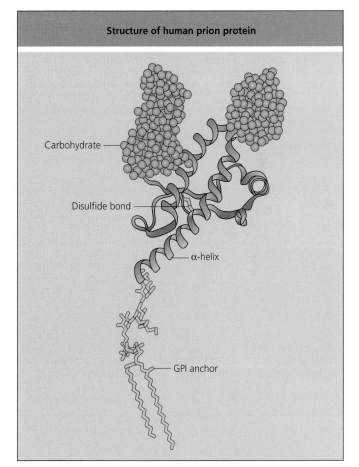

Fig. 22.1 Structure of the human prion protein. Model of glycosylated human prion protein indicating positions of *N*-linked glycans (blue), the single disulfide bond linking helixes 2 and 3, and the glycosylphosphatidylinositol (GPI) anchor to the outer surface of the cell membrane. Courtesy of Dr Richard Sessions and Mr Ray Young.

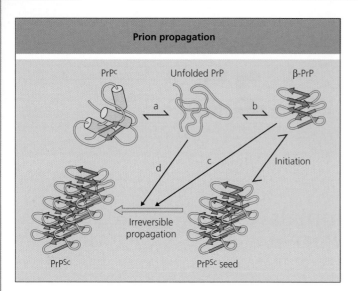

Prion propagation

PrP^C Unfolded PrP   β-PrP

a   b

d   c   Initiation

Irreversible propagation

PrP^{Sc} PrP^{Sc} seed

Fig. 22.2 Prion propagation. Schematic representation of a possible mechanism for prion propagation. The predominantly α-helical form of the normal prion protein (PrP^C) proceeds via an unfolded state (a) to refold into a predominantly β-sheet form (β-PrP) (b). Prion replication may require a critical 'seed' size. Further recruitment of β-PrP (c) or unfolded PrP (d) occurs as an essentially irreversible process. Courtesy of Prof Tony Clarke and Mr Ray Young.

Table 22.1 Animal prion diseases

Disease	Host	Etiology
Scrapie	Sheep and goats	Thought to involve both horizontal and vertical transmission
Transmissible mink encephalopathy	Captive mink	Probably food-borne, although the origin of infectious prions is uncertain
Chronic wasting disease	Captive and free-ranging mule deer and Rocky Mountain elk	Origin unknown. There is evidence for horizontal transmission
Bovine spongiform encephalopathy (BSE)	Cattle	Food-borne in the form of contaminated meat and bone meal
Feline spongiform encephalopathy	Domestic and zoo cats	Feed contaminated with bovine spongiform encephalopathy prions
Exotic ungulate encephalopathy	Captive bovidae	Feed contaminated with bovine spongiform encephalopathy prions

estimated that over 2 million cattle were infected with BSE in the UK.[5] Smaller epidemics have also been described in Switzerland, Ireland, Portugal and France, and cases have been reported in Japan, Canada and the USA. Epidemiologic studies point to contaminated offal used in the manufacture of meat and bone meal and fed to cattle as the source of prions responsible for BSE.[6] Because the UK has a relatively large sheep population in which scrapie is endemic, it was hypothesized that scrapie-contaminated sheep offal was the initial source of BSE. An alternative view is that BSE prions originated spontaneously in cattle and that infection was subsequently amplified by recycling of infected cattle that had subclinical disease. The host range of BSE appears to be unusually wide, affecting many other animal species (Table 22.1). Rare atypical forms of BSE were first identified in 2004 in Italy and France on the basis of an apparently higher (BSE-H) or lower (BSE-L) molecular mass of partially protease-digested PrP^{Sc} compared with typical BSE.[7,8] The pathogenicity of atypical BSE in humans is predicted by transgenic studies.[9]

Prion disease of wild and captive cervids, known as chronic wasting disease (CWD), has been increasingly documented in the USA and Canada, principally Colorado and Wyoming.[10] Deposition of PrP^{Sc} is widespread in peripheral cervid tissues, offering a mechanism for horizontal transmission through environmental contamination by carcasses.[11] Several polymorphisms of the cervid PrP gene are known to influence susceptibility to CWD.[10] Although CWD will have been consumed by humans, no atypical prion strains have been detected in hunters or local populations,[12] and transgenic studies with 'humanized' mice support the existence of a strong barrier to transmission between cervid and human.[13]

Human prion diseases

The human prion diseases are unique in biology in that they manifest as sporadic, genetic and infectious diseases (Table 22.2). The majority of cases of human prion disease occur sporadically as Creutzfeldt–Jakob disease (sporadic (s) CJD) at a rate of roughly 1 per 10^6 population across the world, with an equal incidence of disease in men and women. The etiology of sCJD is unknown, although hypotheses include somatic mutation of the PrP gene (referred to as *PRNP*), and the spontaneous conversion of PrP^C into PrP^{Sc} as a rare stochastic event. There is a common coding polymorphism at codon 129 of *PRNP* encoding either methionine or valine (Fig. 22.3). Homozygosity at this position (denoted 129MM or 129VV) predisposes people to the development of sporadic and iatrogenic CJD.[14,15] Additionally, susceptibility single nucleotide polymorphisms have been identified near to *PRNP*, indicating additional genetic effects at the locus which presumably act through altered expression of the gene.

Approximately 15% of human prion diseases are inherited with an autosomal dominant mode of inheritance. Inherited human prion diseases have been shown to segregate with more than 30 different missense and insertion mutations in the coding sequence of *PRNP* (see Fig. 22.3).[16] Although the human prion diseases are experimentally transmissible, the acquired forms have, until recently, been confined to rare and unusual situations. For example, kuru was caused by cannibalism among the Fore linguistic group of the Okapa district of the Eastern Highlands in Papua New Guinea.[17] The disease had its origins at the beginning of the 20th century and was the leading cause of death in this population by the middle of the century, killing over 3000 people in the total population of 30 000. Mainly adult women as well as children of both sexes were affected, to give an annual disease-specific mortality of approximately 3%. It is thought that the roughly sevenfold higher incidence of disease in adult women than adult men was the result of higher exposure of women to infectious brain material. Since the cessation of cannibalistic practices around 1956, the disease has all but died out, with only a handful of cases currently occurring in older people who were presumably exposed to kuru as young children, indicating an incubation time in these cases of greater than 50 years.[18] In kuru, all codon 129 genotypes were affected as the epidemic evolved, with codon heterozygotes (129MV) having

estimated as 0.5–1% of the sheep population. The etiology of natural scrapie has been the subject of intense debate for many years, but it is now clear that it is an infectious disease,[4] for which susceptibility is genetically modulated by the host.

Following its discovery in 1985, BSE reached epidemic proportions, with over 180 000 confirmed cases in UK cattle, and much smaller numbers in many other European countries. It has been

Table 22.2 Human prion diseases

Disease	Incidence	Etiology	Age of onset or incubation period and duration of illness
Sporadic Creutzfeldt–Jakob disease (CJD)	1 case per 1 million population	Unknown but hypotheses include somatic mutation or spontaneous conversions of PrP^C into PrP^{Sc}	Age of onset is usually 45–75 years; age of peak onset is 60–65 years; 70% of cases die in under 6 months
Inherited prion diseases (CJD, FFI, GSS)	10–20% of cases of human prion disease	Autosomal dominant *PRNP* mutation	Onset tends to be earlier in familial CJD compared to sporadic CJD. Can be wide phenotypic variability between and within families
Kuru	>2500 cases among the Fore people in Papua New Guinea	Infection through ritualistic cannibalism	Incubation period 5–>40 years; duration of illness 12 months
Iatrogenic Creutzfeldt–Jakob disease	About 90 cases to date	Infections from contaminated human growth hormone, human gonadotropin, depth electrodes, corneal transplants, dura mater grafts, neurosurgical procedures	Incubation periods of cases from human growth hormone 4–30 years; duration of illness 6–18 months
Variant Creutzfeldt–Jakob disease	Over 200 predominantly young adults in the UK and France*	Infection by bovine spongiform encephalopathy-like prions	Mean age of onset 26 years; mean duration of illness 14 months

*To October 2000.
FFI, fatal familial insomnia; GSS, Gerstmann–Straussler–Scheinker syndrome; *PRNP*, prion protein gene; PrP^C, normal form of prion protein; PrP^{Sc}, disease-associated isoform of prion protein.

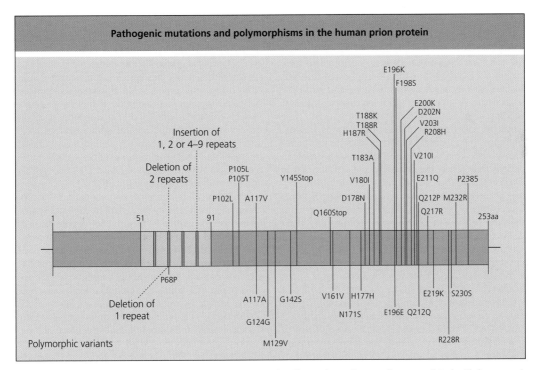

Fig. 22.3 Pathogenic mutations and polymorphisms in the human prion protein. The pathogenic mutations associated with human prion disease are shown above the PrP coding sequence. These consist of 4–9 octapeptide repeat insertions within the octarepeat region between codons 51 and 91, a deletion of two octapeptide repeats; and various point mutations causing missense amino acid substitutions. Point mutations are designated by the wild-type amino acid preceding the codon number, followed by the mutant residue, using single-letter amino acid conventions. Polymorphic variants are shown below the PrP coding sequence. Deletion of one octapeptide repeat is not associated with disease.

the longest mean incubation time.[19] Elderly women survivors of the epidemic of kuru are overwhelmingly codon 129MV, supporting the concept that kuru imposed strong balancing selection on the Fore.

Other examples of acquired human prion diseases have resulted from iatrogenic transmission of CJD during corneal transplantation, contaminated electroencephalographic (EEG) electrode implantation and surgical operations using contaminated instruments or apparatus. In addition, iatrogenic CJD has occurred as a result of implantation of dura mater grafts and treatment with growth hormone or gonadotropin derived from the pituitary glands of human cadavers.[20]

The appearance of CJD cases in teenagers and young adults in the UK during the mid-1990s prompted considerable concern that they might have acquired the illness as a result of exposure to BSE. By March 1996, it became clear that the unusual clinical presentation and neuropathology was remarkably consistent in these new cases.[21] Up until February 2008 there have been 163 deaths from probable or pathologically confirmed vCJD in the UK, predominantly teenagers and young adults, and over 200 deaths worldwide. Molecular strain typing, which focuses on the biochemical properties of PrP^{Sc} from the brains of BSE-infected cattle and patients who have CJD, has demonstrated that vCJD is different from sporadic CJD but similar to BSE.[22,23] Moreover, the incubation times and profile of neuropathologic lesions of vCJD and BSE prions are indistinguishable in inbred lines of mice.[24] These data argue that BSE and vCJD are the same strain. All reported cases of vCJD have been 129MM, a genotype shared by ~40% of the British Caucasian population.

Polymorphisms in the human *PRNP* gene are not the sole genetic influence on disease susceptibility and incubation time. Studies with inbred lines of mice show that large differences occur even with the same amino acid sequence of the prion protein, suggesting that other genes may contribute to the observed variation. Studies of quantitative trait loci (QTL) linked to prion disease incubation periods in mice have identified susceptibility loci on chromosomes 2, 4, 8, 11, 12 and 15.[25] These QTL studies provide strong evidence that genetic loci other than the coding region of *PRNP* have a major influence on scrapie incubation time in experimental prion disease.

Iatrogenic secondary transmission of vCJD has now occurred by blood transfusion from preclinical vCJD.[26–28] Three patients have been identified from a cohort of 23 who have survived more that 5 years after receiving vCJD-implicated blood. In 2004 a 62-year-old patient was diagnosed with vCJD post-mortem, 6.5 years after transfusion of a single unit of red cells.[27] Later in 2004 an elderly patient who died of an unrelated cause 5 years after transfusion of a single unit of red cells was found to have PrP^{Sc} deposition in lymphoreticular tissues consistent with vCJD infection.[26] In 2006 a patient was confirmed to have vCJD at autopsy, having received a unit of vCJD-implicated red cells 6 years earlier.[28] This patient was diagnosed whilst alive and had PrP^{Sc} deposition in tonsillar tissue. At an early stage of his disease, MRI was negative for the pulvinar sign. Both clinically affected patients were genotype 129MM, but the subclinically infected patient was 129MV, indicating for the first time the potential of individuals with this genotype to replicate vCJD prions. The fact than no PrP^{Sc} was detectable in the tonsil of this patient may reflect the selection of a novel strain in 129MV or alternatively relate to the amount and distribution of PrP^{Sc} seen at an early stage of infection. With an average of around 6 years, the shortest incubation times of secondary vCJD are, as expected, considerably shorter than the shortest incubation times of primary vCJD of around 12 years. Six thousand patients have been notified of their exposure to vCJD-implicated blood products.

As there is no blood test for pre- or subclinical carriers of vCJD, estimates of the prevalence of the carrier state rely on screening of surgical lymphoreticular tissue.[29,30] The larger study, conducted on 12 674 anonymized surgical appendectomy specimens, identified three positive samples, resulting in an estimated prevalence of vCJD infection of 237/million (95% CI 49–692). Subsequent genetic analysis of two of these positive samples identified 129VV genotypes, found in around 10% of the UK population.[31] A large prospective longitudinal study of surgical tonsil samples is currently being undertaken in the UK to clarify prevalence and obtain fresh tissue for strain type analysis.

CLINICAL FEATURES

The human prion diseases can be divided etiologically into inherited, sporadic and acquired forms with CJD, Gerstmann–Straussler–Scheinker syndrome (GSS) and kuru now seen as clinicopathologic *syndromes* rather than individual disease entities. The identification of one of the pathogenic *PRNP* mutations in a patient with neurodegen-

erative disease allows the diagnosis of an inherited prion disease and subclassification according to mutation. Over 30 pathogenic mutations have been described in two groups:

- point mutations resulting in amino acid substitutions in PrP or production of a stop codon resulting in expression of a truncated PrP;
- alteration of integral copies of an octapeptide repeat present in a tandem array of five copies in the normal protein (see Fig. 22.3).

They are all autosomal dominantly inherited conditions. Kindreds with inherited prion disease have been described with phenotypes of classic CJD and GSS, together with a range of other neurodegenerative disease phenotypes. Some families show remarkable phenotypic variability which can encompass both CJD- and GSS-like cases, as well as other cases which do not conform to either CJD or GSS phenotypes. Such atypical prion diseases may lack the classic histologic features of a spongiform encephalopathy entirely, although PrP immunohistochemistry is usually positive. Progressive dementia, cerebellar ataxia, pyramidal signs, chorea, myoclonus, extrapyramidal features, pseudobulbar signs, seizures and amyotrophic features are seen in variable combinations. *PRNP* analysis is also used for presymptomatic genetic testing in affected families.

Classic CJD is a rapidly progressive dementia accompanied by myoclonus. Decline to akinetic mutism and death is rapid and often occurs within 3–4 months. Cerebellar ataxia, extrapyramidal and pyramidal features and cortical blindness are also frequently seen. The electroencephalogram (EEG) may show characteristic pseudo-periodic sharp wave activity which is helpful in diagnosis but present only in around 70% of cases. To some extent, demonstration of a typical EEG is dependent on the number of EEGs performed and serial EEG is indicated to try and demonstrate this appearance. Cerebrospinal fluid (CSF) immunoassay for the neuron-specific 14-3-3 protein may be helpful. A combination of both 14-3-3 CSF analysis and EEG is recommended in the investigation of suspected classic CJD cases to increase the sensitivity of pre-mortem case definition. A raised 14-3-3 protein is not, however, specific for classic CJD and is raised in viral encephalitis or recent stroke; rather it is a marker of rapid neuronal injury and loss. More concerning with respect to the differential diagnosis is that it may also be raised in rapidly progressive forms of Alzheimer's disease, which may be confused with CJD. MRI scanning, particularly the use of diffusion weighted sequences, is highly sensitive in classic CJD. Caudate and putamen hyperintensity is well known, but cortical ribbon hyperintensity and thalamic high signal in 129MV patients is increasingly recognized. Atypical cases of classic CJD are well-recognized however, and can still present diagnostic difficulties.

The clinical features of kuru consist of a progressive cerebellar ataxia accompanied by dementia in the later stages and death, which usually occurs within 12 months. Iatrogenic prion disease arising from intracerebral or optic inoculation usually manifests clinically as classic CJD, whilst that arising from a peripheral route of inoculation, such as pituitary growth hormone, commonly presents like kuru with a progressive ataxia. GSS commonly presents as a chronic cerebellar ataxia with pyramidal features; dementia occurs much later in the clinical course which is longer than that seen in classic CJD. Fatal familial insomnia (FFI) is characterized by progressive untreatable insomnia, dysautonomia and dementia and selective thalamic degeneration, and is most commonly associated with a missense mutation at codon 178 of *PRNP*. The FFI phenotype has also been described occurring sporadically with no causative mutation in *PRNP* identified.

The early clinical presentation of vCJD resembles kuru more than classic CJD and consists of behavioral and psychiatric disturbances, peripheral sensory disturbance and cerebellar ataxia. Common early psychiatric features include dysphoria, withdrawal, anxiety, insomnia and apathy. Neurologic symptoms preceded psychiatric symptoms in 15% of cases studied, and were present in combination with psychiatric symptoms in 22% of cases from the onset of disease. No common early neurologic features were noted, but paresthesiae and/or pain in the limbs is seen in around half of the cases. However, a significant proportion of patients exhibited neurologic symptoms within 4 months of clinical onset, and these included poor memory, pain, sensory symptoms, unsteadiness of gait and dysarthria. Disorientation, hallucinations, paranoid ideation, confabulation, impaired self-care and the commonest neurologic features (cerebellar signs, chorea, dystonia, myoclonus, upper motor neuron signs and visual symptoms) developed late in the course of the illness. The duration of disease is longer in vCJD, with mean patient survival times of about 13 months, compared with about 4 months for classic CJD. Moreover, whereas classic CJD is predominantly a late-onset disease, with a peak onset between 60 and 65 years, the median age of onset of vCJD is 26 years.

The EEG is not helpful in the diagnosis of vCJD; whilst generalized slowing is usually present, the characteristic periodic changes associated with classic CJD are not. The CSF 14–3–3 protein is less helpful, and may often be negative. MRI, however, is useful in the diagnosis of vCJD; in the majority of cases high signal is noted in the posterior thalamus (pulvinar) bilaterally on dual echo (T_2- or proton density-weighted) MRI (Fig. 22.4). Other common MRI features of vCJD are medial thalamic and periaqueductal gray matter high signal, and the notable absence of cerebral atrophy. All cases to date are *PRNP* 129MM (unpublished data).

vCJD can be diagnosed by detection of characteristic PrP^{Sc} immunostaining on tonsil biopsy. Importantly, PrP^{Sc} is only detectable in tonsil and other lymphoreticular tissues in vCJD, and not other forms of human prion disease, indicating that it has a distinctive pathogenesis.[32,33] The PrP^{Sc} type detected on Western blot in vCJD tonsil has a characteristic pattern designated type 4, by the London classification. Tonsil is the tissue of choice for diagnostic biopsy in the investigation of possible vCJD. Tonsil biopsy is well tolerated with minor discomfort, and has, so far, shown 100% sensitivity and specificity.[32] If the tonsil biopsy is positive with the specific vCJD banding pattern (Fig. 22.5), then a more invasive brain biopsy becomes unnecessary.

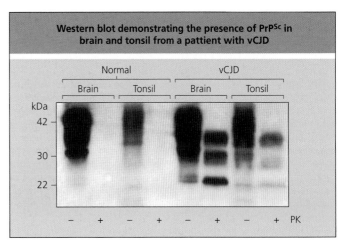

Fig. 22.5 Western blot demonstrating the presence of PrP^{Sc} in brain and tonsil from a patient with vCJD. The presence of PrP^{Sc} is revealed after proteinase K (PK) treatment, which digests the normal form of PrP (PrP^{C}) but not the pathologic form (PrP^{Sc}). Courtesy of Ms Susan Joiner and Dr Andy Hill.

PATHOGENESIS AND PATHOLOGY

Molecular strain typing

The marked clinical heterogeneity observed in sporadic CJD has yet to be explained. However, it has been clear for many years that distinct isolates, or strains, of prions can be propagated in the same host and these are biologically recognized by distinctive clinical and pathologic features in experimental animals (for review, see[34]). It is therefore likely that a proportion of the clinicopathologic heterogeneity in CJD, and other human prion diseases, relates to the propagation of distinct human prion strains. The identification of these prion strains would allow an etiology-based classification of CJD by typing of the infectious agent itself.

The existence of prion strains has been difficult to accommodate within the protein-only model of prion propagation. As they can be serially propagated in inbred mice with the same *PRNP* genotype, they cannot be encoded by differences in PrP primary structure. Furthermore, strains can be re-isolated in mice after passage in intermediate species with different PrP primary structures. Conventionally, distinct strains of conventional pathogens are explained by differences in their nucleic acid genome. However, in the absence of such a scrapie genome, alternative possibilities must be considered. A wealth of experimental evidence now suggests that PrP^{Sc} itself may encode strain-specific phenotypic properties. Different subtypes of PrP^{Sc} were associated initially with two strains of transmissible mink encephalopathy in hamsters.

Several human PrP^{Sc} types have been identified which are associated with different phenotypes of CJD.[22,35,36] The different fragment sizes seen on Western blots, following treatment with proteinase K, suggest that there are several different human PrP^{Sc} conformations, referred to as 'molecular strain types'. These types can be further classified by the ratio of the three PrP bands seen after protease digestion, representing di-, mono- and unglycosylated fragments of PrP^{Sc}. By the London classification system, sporadic CJD is associated with PrP^{Sc} types 1–3, while type 4 human PrP^{Sc} is uniquely associated with vCJD and characterized by glycoform ratios which are distinct from those observed in classic CJD.[22,35]

Importantly, these biochemical changes in PrP^{Sc} are transmissible to the PrP in a host. This has been demonstrated in studies with CJD isolates, with both PrP^{Sc} fragment sizes and the ratios of the three PrP glycoforms maintained on passage in transgenic mice expressing human PrP.[22] Furthermore, transmission of human prions and bovine

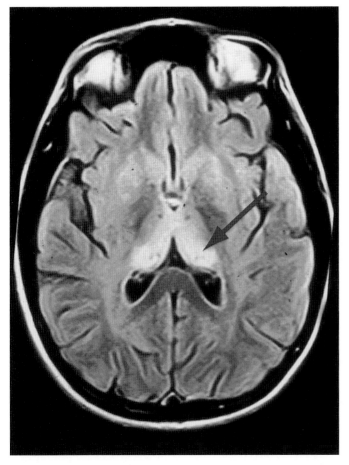

Fig. 22.4 Axial T_2-weighted MRI brain demonstrating high signal bilaterally in the posterior thalamus (arrowed) – the 'pulvinar sign' in a patient with vCJD.

prions to wild-type mice results in murine PrP^{Sc} with fragment sizes and glycoform ratios which correspond to the original inoculum.[22] Variant CJD is associated with PrP^{Sc} glycoform ratios which are distinct from those seen in classic CJD. Similar ratios are seen in BSE, and BSE when transmitted to several other species.[22]

BSE and vCJD have now been propagated in *PRNP*-null transgenic mice expressing the human prion protein modeling three different codon 129 genotypes. Transgenic mice for human 129MM propagate either type 2 or type 4 PrP^{Sc} with respective neuropathologies consistent with human sporadic CJD or vCJD, whereas transgenic mice homozygous for human 129VV either propagate novel type 5 PrP^{Sc} and a distinct pattern of neuropathology, or develop clinical prion disease in the absence of detectable PrP^{Sc}. Transmissions to human 129MV mice were complex, with four distinct phenotypes, including the propagation of type 4 PrP^{Sc} in the absence of florid plaques.

These findings argue that primary BSE prion infection, as well as secondary infection by iatrogenic routes, may not be restricted to a single disease phenotype, including extensive transmission as a subclinical carrier state. Further, these studies raise the possibility that some humans infected with BSE prions may develop a clinical disease indistinguishable from classic CJD associated with type 2 PrP^{Sc}. All these data strongly support the 'protein only' hypothesis of infectivity and suggest that strain variation is encoded by a combination of PrP conformation and glycosylation pattern.

Pathology

The animal and human prion diseases share a number of characteristic features, the most consistent being the neuropathologic changes that accompany disease in the central nervous system. Indeed, it was the neuropathologic similarities between scrapie and kuru which strongly suggested that the two diseases might be closely related, and that kuru, like scrapie, might also be transmissible by inoculation. Subsequently, brain extracts from patients who have kuru produced a progressive neurodegenerative condition in inoculated chimpanzees after a prolonged incubation period of 18–21 months. The neuropathologic similarities between kuru and CJD prompted similar transmission experiments from CJD patients.

Although the brains of patients or animals who have prion disease frequently show no recognizable abnormalities on gross examination, microscopic examination of the central nervous system typically reveals characteristic histopathologic changes, consisting of neuronal vacuolation and degeneration, which gives the cerebral gray matter a microvacuolated or 'spongiform' appearance (Fig. 22.6b) and a

reactive proliferation of astroglial cells (Fig. 22.6b), which is often out of all proportion to the degree of nerve cell loss. Although spongiform degeneration is frequently detected, it is not an obligatory neuropathologic feature of prion disease; astrocytic gliosis, although not specific to the prion diseases, is more constantly seen.

The lack of an inflammatory response is also an important characteristic. Although it is by no means a constant feature, some examples of prion disease are characterized by deposition of amyloid plaques composed of insoluble aggregates of PrP. Amyloid plaques are a notable feature of kuru and GSS but they are infrequently found in the brains of patients who have classic CJD.

Although there is wide variation in the neuropathologic profiles of different forms of human prion disease, the histopathologic features of vCJD are remarkably consistent and distinguish it from other human prion diseases. Large numbers of PrP-positive amyloid plaques are a consistent feature of vCJD but they differ in morphology from the plaques seen in kuru and GSS in that the surrounding tissue takes on a microvacuolated appearance, giving the plaques a florid appearance (Fig. 22.6a).[21]

vCJD is clearly very different in its pathogenesis from other human prion diseases, and this is reflected in the tissue distribution of PrP^{Sc} in vCJD. As mentioned, it is readily detectable in lymphoreticular tissue, and using highly sensitive immunoassays, PrP^{Sc} has been found in retina, optic nerve, rectum, adrenal gland and thymus in vCJD postmortem tissue (Fig. 22.7).[33]

Pathogenesis

Detection of PrP^{Sc} in brain material by immunohistochemical or immunoblotting techniques is considered to be diagnostic of prion disease (Fig. 22.6c). However, certain examples of natural and experimental prion disease occur without accumulation of detectable protease-resistant PrP^{Sc}, and the time course of neurodegeneration is not equivalent to the time course of PrP^{Sc} accumulation in mice expressing lower than normal levels of PrP^{C}.[37] Moreover, PrP^{Sc} is not toxic to cells that do not express PrP^{C}, and although mice expressing PrP without a glycosylphosphatidylinositol anchor to the cell membrane may be infected with prions, they do not develop neurodegeneration. Additional evidence that PrP^{Sc} may not be the neurotoxic species has been demonstrated in mice inoculated with ^{Sc}237 hamster prions. These mice replicate prions to high levels in their brains but do not develop any signs of clinical disease during their normal lifespan.

Recently, PrP^{Sc} fractionation experiments suggest that the most infectious entity of prion disease is an oligomer (about 14–28-mer) of misfolded PrP, analogous to the oligomers implicated as the prime cause

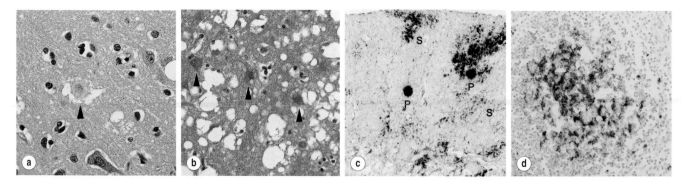

Fig. 22.6 Neuropathology of prion disease – histopathologic findings in vCJD. (a) Florid plaques, a characteristic feature of vCJD pathology. They consist of a round amyloid core (arrowed) surrounded by a ring of vacuoles (hematoxylin and eosin stain). (b) Spongiform degeneration in prion disease. This area shows severe vacuolization (spongiosis); there is severe neuronal loss and many strongly reactive astrocytes (arrowed) (hematoxylin and eosin stain). (c) Immunostaining of the pathologic prion protein. The specimen is pretreated to denature the normal PrP and staining with a prion protein antibody reveals the presence of plaques (P) and synapses (S) staining positively for PrP^{Sc}. (d) Detection of pathologic prion protein in the follicular dendritic cells in a tonsil. Accumulation of prion protein in lymphoreticular organs, such as spleen, tonsils or appendix, is a specific finding in vCJD and is not present in other forms of CJD. Therefore tonsillar biopsies can be used to specifically diagnose vCJD when clinical symptoms are only emerging. Courtesy of Dr Sebastian Brandner.

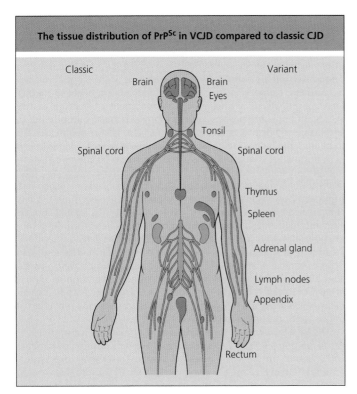

The tissue distribution of PrP^{Sc} in VCJD compared to classic CJD

Fig. 22.7 The tissue distribution of PrP^{Sc} in vCJD compared to classic CJD. In vCJD PrP^{Sc} is found in lymphoreticular tissue as well as brain and spinal cord. Using highly sensitive immunodetection methods, PrP^{Sc} has also been found in the optic nerve, retina, adrenal gland and rectum. Courtesy of Dr Jonathon Wadsworth and Mr Ray Young.

of disease in other neurodegenerative conditions such as Alzheimer's and Parkinson's disease. However, more precise characterization of the infectious and toxic entity of prion disease will require the synthesis of prion from recombinant substrates. Although there has been some success, synthetic prions have only been generated in such low concentrations that analysis of molecular structure is impossible.[34]

The essential role of host PrP^C for prion propagation and pathogenesis is demonstrated by the fact that mice in which the PrP gene has been disrupted (referred to as *Prnp*^{0/0}) are resistant to scrapie infection,[37] and that re-introduction of the murine PrP^C transgene restores susceptibility to infection.

Gene-targeted *Prnp*^{0/0} mice have also been studied to probe the normal function of PrP^C. Two independently generated lines of gene-targeted *Prnp*^{0/0} mice developed normally and appeared to suffer no gross phenotypic abnormalities. The relative normality of these PrP null mice was thought to result from effective adaptive changes during development. However data from *Prnp* conditional knockout mice suggest this is not the case; these mice undergo ablation of neuronal PrP expression at 9 weeks of age. The mice remain healthy without evidence of neurodegeneration or an overt clinical phenotype, demonstrating that acute loss of neuronal PrP in adulthood is tolerated, and that the pathophysiology of prion diseases is not due to loss of normal PrP function. The normal function of PrP is not known but evidence from PrP knockout mice reveals defects in neurophysiologic and biochemical function. Electrophysiologic studies have demonstrated that fast inhibition and long-term potentiation mediated by δ-aminobutyric acid receptors were impaired in hippocampal slices from *Prnp*^{0/0} mice,[38,39] and that calcium-activated potassium currents were disrupted.[40]

These abnormalities of synaptic inhibition are reminiscent of the neurophysiologic defects seen in patients who have CJD and in scrapie-infected mice,[38] and suggest a direct role for PrP in the modulation of neuronal excitability. Normal PrP has also been shown to

bind copper ions,[41,42] with femtomolar affinity,[43] and a role for PrP in copper metabolism or transport has also been suggested. Other suggested functions include as a nerve growth factor[44] or self-renewal of hemopoietic stem cells.[45]

Thus, it appears that neither accumulation of PrP^{Sc}, nor loss of normal PrP function, is the cause of the neurodegeneration in prion diseases. It is possible that a toxic intermediate species is produced in the conversion of PrP^C to PrP^{Sc}, and that the steady state level of such an intermediate could then determine the rate of neurodegeneration.[34]

Although the pathologic consequences of prion infection occur in the central nervous system, and experimental transmission of these diseases is most efficiently accomplished by intracerebral inoculation, most natural infections do not occur by these means. Indeed, administration to sites other than the central nervous system is known to be associated with much longer incubation periods, which may extend to 20 years or more. Experimental evidence suggests that this latent period is associated with clinically silent prion replication in the lymphoreticular tissue, whereas neuroinvasion takes place later.

The *M* cells in the intestinal epithelium mediate prion entry from the gastrointestinal lumen into the body, and follicular dendritic cells (FDCs) are thought to be essential for prion replication and for accumulation of disease-associated PrP^{Sc} within secondary lymphoid organs. Inhibition of the lymphotoxin (LTβ) signaling pathway with a soluble receptor that depletes FDCs abolishes prion replication in spleens and prolongs the latency of scrapie after intraperitoneal challenge. B-cell deficient mice are resistant to intraperitoneal inoculation with prions, possibly because of impaired FDC maturation. Opsonization by complement system components may also be important in peripheral neuroinvasion, as mice that are genetically engineered to lack complement factors, or mice deleted of the C3 complement component by the administration of cobra venom, are resistant to peripheral prion inoculation. Recent evidence suggests that infection of organs may play an important role in shedding of prions in milk (mastitis) or urine (nephritis).

PREVENTION

Because there are currently no treatments for these invariably fatal diseases, prevention is particularly important. Perhaps the most effective example of prevention was the cessation of cannibalistic practices among the Fore people of Papua New Guinea in the 1950s, which resulted in the disappearance of kuru. The replacement of growth hormone derived from the pituitary glands of human cadavers with recombinant growth hormone was implemented to avoid the continued iatrogenic transmission of CJD to young children who have growth hormone deficiency. Similarly, because CJD has resulted from the use of prion-contaminated surgical instruments or apparatus after neurosurgical or ophthalmic procedures, it is advised that surgical instruments be incinerated in cases where CJD is confirmed so as to avoid future iatrogenic transmission of prion disease. Current policy in the UK is to quarantine surgical instruments until a suspected diagnosis is confirmed (see http://www.advisorybodies.doh.gov.uk/acdp/tseguidance/index.htm). Experimental studies have confirmed that prions adhere readily to metal following a contact time with infected brain of as little as 5 minutes.[46]

When it was realized that BSE was caused by feeding prion-contaminated foodstuffs to cattle, a number of preventive measures were introduced in the UK. In July 1988 a ban on feeding ruminant-derived protein to other ruminants was introduced to break the cycle of infection via feed. A ban on specified bovine offals was introduced in the UK in 1989 to prevent inclusion in the human food chain of bovine tissues thought to contain the highest titer of prions; these included tissues from the lymphoreticular system and the central nervous system. The European Union imposed a worldwide ban on the export of British cattle, products derived from them (with the exception of products for technical uses) and mammalian meat and bone meal in March 1996 after the announcement that BSE and vCJD might be linked. Since then, more than 1.35 million cattle over 30 months old have been culled in the UK in a further attempt to limit human exposure to BSE. The 'over thirty month' (OTM) rule is one of the UK BSE controls to prevent further BSE-infected cattle from entering the human food chain because cattle over 30 months are more likely to develop BSE than younger animals. Therefore, since 1996 there has been a ban on selling meat in the UK from slaughtered cattle over 30 months old. The cost of tackling BSE to the British and European taxpayer has been estimated at over £7000 million. These measures appear to have been effective in reducing the incidence of BSE in the UK and the number of newly identified BSE cases has declined sharply. The EU-imposed worldwide ban on British beef exports was lifted in late 1999 after the EU were satisfied that appropriate measures had been taken to counteract the likelihood of BSE-infected animals getting into the human food chain.

Prior to the realization of blood transmission of vCJD, the UK government decided in 1998 that all blood donations should be leukodepleted. Since then the majority of European countries have followed this strategy. The UK National Blood Transfusion Service now imports all plasma and plasma derivatives from BSE-free countries, and blood donors are screened to exclude anyone with a blood relative with classic CJD or vCJD. Several countries have instituted policies of deferral of blood donors who have resided in the UK for a cumulative period of 6 months or more from 1980 until the end of 1996. In view of the potential exposure to the vCJD agent in other European countries in addition to the UK, the US Food and Drug Administration has a blood donation deferral policy of a cumulative 10-year residence in France, Portugal and Ireland. The American Red Cross Blood Banks have adopted a deferral policy of 3 months residence in the UK and 6 months residence in any other European country. The efficacy of these risk reduction procedures is not known, and a screening test for blood infectivity is urgently needed.

Transmission of classic CJD has occurred on surgical instruments as prion infectivity is resistant to conventional sterilization.[47] Surgery may be an epidemiologic risk factor for classic CJD.[48,49] The presence of vCJD in peripheral tissues commonly involved in routine surgery has raised concerns about this mechanism of secondary transmission. A three-stage detergent/enzymic procedure has now been demonstrated to be effective at decontamination of prions and is used by some NHS Trusts.[50]

An effective assay for low concentrations of prion may lead to a useful blood test. The new methodology implements a cyclical amplification and sonication of PrPSc derived from brain homogenates in a dilution of normal brain homogenate. This promising technique is known as protein misfolding cyclic amplification (PMCA).[51] It is likely that refinements will continue to take place over the ensuing years.[52]

DEVELOPMENT OF THERAPIES

Prion diseases are invariably fatal, and whilst curative therapies for prion infection are conceivable, such therapies, if developed, will not be available for some years.[53] Such approaches are likely to involve targeting PrP itself.[53] However, the development of neuroprotective agents, and pre- and post-exposure prophylaxis are also important. In addition, early firm diagnosis will be crucial to allow such treatments to be initiated before extensive brain damage occurs.

A number of compounds have been shown to be effective at clearing PrPSc in cell culture systems. These include the acridine and phenothiazine derivatives quinacrine and chlorpromazine, Congo-red, sulphated polyanions and anti-PrP antibodies (reviewed in[54]). A few compounds have been shown to prolong survival in animal models after intraperitoneal inoculation with prions. These include pentosan polysulphate, cyclic tetrapyrroles and CpG oligodeoxynucleotides. Treatment of mice with anti-prion monoclonal antibodies results in delay of clinical onset beyond 300 days (control animals were affected after about 190 days) after intraperitoneal administration of mouse prions.[55] However, clinical duration was not prolonged when treatment was started after neurologic onset, and there was no effect if prions were administered intracerebrally.

The PRION-1 trial of quinacrine in the UK has been completed.[56] Pentosan polysulphate has been used in a small number of patients with various human prion diseases, in many cases with direct intracerebral delivery. However, given the very small sample size, several adverse events and lack of placebo group, it is very difficult to conclude whether this treatment has any benefit (see http://www.cjd.ed.ac.uk/bone.pdf for details).

Currently, an international research effort is underway to develop therapies aimed at both pre- and post-exposure prophylaxis, in addition to neuroprotective agents that may slow down disease progression.

REFERENCES

References for this chapter can be found online at http://www.expertconsult.com

Infections in hydrocephalus shunts

Hydrocephalus shunts drain excess cerebrospinal fluid (CSF) from the cerebral ventricles, usually to the peritoneal cavity (ventriculo-peritoneal, VP) or to the right cardiac atrium (ventriculoatrial, VA) (Fig. 23.1).

EPIDEMIOLOGY

The incidence of infection varies according to the age at which the shunt is inserted. Up to 25% of operations in premature infants with hydrocephalus after periventricular hemorrhage result in infection, whereas in older children the incidence is 3–8%.[1,2] Although the incidence of shunt infections has generally fallen, it is still unacceptably high. Some centers have reported rates of infection near to zero[3,4] but this is rare.

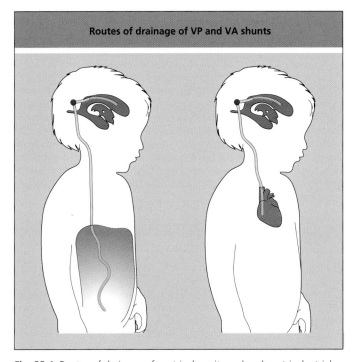

Fig. 23.1 Routes of drainage of ventriculoperitoneal and ventriculoatrial shunts. Ventriculoperitoneal shunts drain CSF from the cerebral ventricles to the peritoneal cavity via catheter tubing implanted superficially over the rib cage. The lower end of the peritoneal catheter lies free in the abdomen. Ventriculoatrial shunts drain CSF via a convenient neck vein such as the jugular and the superior vena cava to the right atrium.

PATHOGENESIS AND PATHOLOGY

The source of the organisms is almost invariably the patient's skin, from which they gain access to the device during its insertion.[5,6] Where there is a serious breakdown in surgical asepsis or where the operating room environment or air is grossly contaminated, these may be alternative sources. Although the bacterial population on the surface of the patient's skin can be reduced to almost zero by thorough skin preparation, resident bacteria in follicles remain and recolonization by resident bacteria occurs rapidly. It is therefore not unusual to find coagulase-negative staphylococci (CoNS) in the incision during the procedure. In nonimplant surgery these are irrelevant, but where a shunt is inserted they are highly likely to adhere to and colonize its inner surfaces. *Staphylococcus epidermidis* predominate in shunt infections. After adhering to the shunt material, they multiply and produce copious amounts of exopolysaccharide ('slime'), enabling the formation of a biofilm. Because of nutrient depletion, growth is very slow and this accounts for the often long periods between surgery and clinical presentation of infection. *Staphylococcus aureus* causes a different clinical picture and is more frequently involved in external shunt infections (Fig. 23.2). Unlike *Staph. epidermidis*, it produces toxins which evoke a very active inflammatory response, leading to erythema and suppuration.

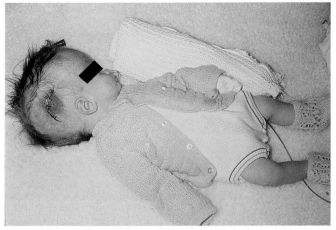

Fig. 23.2 External shunt infection in a premature infant with poor nutritional status. The infection can be caused by organisms introduced at surgery or they may gain access through minor skin abrasions and pressure necrosis. Differing from the more common internal shunt infections, they are usually caused by *Staphylococcus aureus* and constitute a wound infection enhanced by a foreign material.

Table 23.1 Clinical features of ventriculoatrial and ventriculoperitoneal shunt infections of surgical origin

	VA shunts	VP shunts
Time from surgery to presentation	Weeks, months, several years	<9 months
Intermittent fever	75%	<50%
Anorexia, lassitude, poor sleep pattern	>80%	>50%
Shunt obstruction	<1%	≥75%
Other features	Chills, rigors: 20% Arthralgia: 50% [late onset cases (1–15 years)] Rash: 70% [late onset cases (1–15 years)] Nephritis: 30% [late onset cases (1–15 years)]	Abdominal pain, bloating: ~75% Swelling, erythema over shunt tubing: ~60% Headache, vomiting, etc. (i.e. recurrence of hydrocephalus): ≥75%

Percentages indicate the approximate proportion of cases in which features are present. It is important to realize that each case is different and that many of these features may be absent or modified.

The clinical presentation of infection in VA shunts differs from that in VP shunts (Table 23.1). In the former, bacteria from the shunt enter the bloodstream directly to cause intermittent fever which, in infections caused by *Staph. epidermidis*, propionibacteria or coryneforms, may continue for months or years with little other evidence of infection. However, antibody to bacterial components is produced in large quantities and immune complex disease may ensue, with deposits of C3, C4, IgG and IgM on the synovial and glomerular basement membranes. Hypertension, renal failure (shunt nephritis) and arthropathy may result.[7] In contrast, in VP and lumboperitoneal (LP) shunt infections, the bacteria are discharged into the peritoneal cavity, provoking the greater omentum to seal off the distal catheter. This and associated adhesions give rise to shunt obstruction and raised CSF pressure (Fig. 23.3). Occasionally, peritoneal

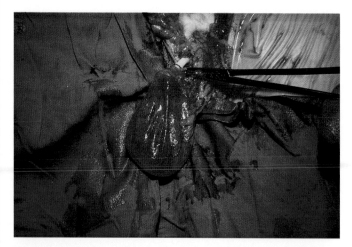

Fig. 23.3 Cystic obstruction of a ventriculoperitoneal shunt caused by shunt infection with *Staphylococcus epidermidis*. Bacteria and bacterial products entering the peritoneal cavity via the shunt catheter evoke an inflammatory response involving the greater omentum, which seals off the catheter outlet. The resulting cyst fills with CSF, giving rise to recurrence of the hydrocephalus. Cystic obstruction can occur from noninfective causes but unlike those cases caused by infection, which present within 6–9 months of surgery, they can arise at any time.

abscesses are seen, and the absorptive capacity of the peritoneum may be lost. In both VP and VA shunts ventriculitis is seen in most cases, although the inflammatory response is usually feeble.

Only a few shunt infections are due to causes other than surgery. In babies or adults whose nutritional status is poor, erosion of the skin over the shunt can take place, leading to secondary infection with *Staph. aureus* or Gram-negative bacteria. An unusual but well-documented cause of VP shunt infection is visceral perforation by the distal catheter, which results in polymicrobial infection of the cerebral ventricles.[8] However, peritonitis from this cause is rare. Following the increasing use of VP shunts in the elderly with normal pressure hydrocephalus, mixed enteric infections arising from diverticulitis may be seen.

Cerebrospinal fluid shunts, including VA, appear to be unusually free of risk from hematogenous spread, and no cases have been documented from such sources as dental surgery. However, VP shunts can become infected during abdominal surgery or continuous ambulatory peritoneal dialysis.

PREVENTION

Studies have shown that understanding of the causes of shunt infections and surgical experience are very important and shunt surgery should be carried out only by experienced personnel or by fully supervised trainees. In view of the source of infection, most attempts at prevention have been targeted at the surgical procedure. Povidone-iodine or chlorhexidine, both alcohol based, should be used for skin preparation, the latter having the greater activity. Assiduous surgical aseptic technique is extremely important, with attention to 'no touch' techniques and glove changing. The use of prophylactic antibiotics might appear to be reasonable, but they have not been found to have a statistically significant beneficial effect in properly designed trials unless the infection rate exceeds 15%.[9] Those who feel obliged to use them despite this are advised to administer 10 mg vancomycin hydrochloride and 3 mg gentamicin in 1–2 ml sterile water for injection intraventricularly[10] as soon as the ventricular catheter is inserted (this should be inserted first), and 1.5 g cefuroxime (25 mg/kg for children) intravenously at induction of anesthesia. Intravenous antibiotics alone are not recommended.

Because of the general lack of success in further reducing the infection rate beyond acceptable minima, an innovative process (Bactiseal, Codman & Shurtleff Inc.) has been developed for treatment of shunts in order to reduce bacterial colonization and infection. In preclinical tests high-level protection of all shunt surfaces has been demonstrated for approximately 2 months. Antibacterial activity is undiminished in the presence of high CSF protein levels such as those found after hemorrhage or meningitis.[11] While the six clinical trials carried out so far vary considerably in design and quality, all except one (where there was no randomization and no case definition for infection) show a reduction in infection rate.[12]

CLINICAL FEATURES

The clinical features of VA shunt infection differ considerably from those of VP and LP shunts (see Table 23.1). Although the shunt lumen becomes colonized at implantation, in VA shunts symptoms considered serious enough to warrant specialist medical attention may not appear for months or years.[7] Many patients have intermittent low-grade fever, but some do not. Some report chills and occasionally rigors. Transient rashes are common. Sore throat and muscular and joint pains are common complaints. Anemia is almost universally found and there is increasing lassitude, anorexia, irritability and poor sleep. Dyspepsia may also be a problem. In later stages, arthralgia becomes more common. Unfortunately, these features are nonspecific and are often mistaken for those of other conditions. As the disease progresses, nephritis and vasculitis may appear. The vasculitic rash is usually confined to the lower extremities and can be frankly hemorrhagic and can ulcerate. Nephritis is indicated by hypertension, hematuria and proteinuria, edema and often loin pain. Endocarditis has been reported only rarely.

In contrast, infections in VP and LP shunts almost always present within 6 months of surgery.[13,14] Fever is present in fewer than 50% of cases and is usually intermittent and mild. Chills and rigors are rare. There may be abdominal discomfort, bloating, pain or tenderness and occasionally persistent flatulence. In cases presenting within 1 or 2 weeks of surgery, there may be failure of the abdominal wound to heal, with CSF leak and sometimes catheter protrusion. In LP shunts there is often spinal pain. However, the most constant symptoms are those of hydrocephalus caused by obstruction at the distal end and the differential diagnosis is between infective and noninfective shunt obstruction. In the former there is often erythema and tenderness over the lower shunt track, whereas these features are absent in noninfective obstruction. In addition, distal VP shunt obstruction occurring more than 9 months after shunt surgery is very unlikely to have an infective cause.[14,15] A very small number of cases present as acute abdomen, with fever, abdominal pain and tenderness suggesting appendicitis or peritonitis.[16] These may present at any time and may lead to unnecessary laparotomy. The tenderness is not necessarily associated with the location of the shunt tip.

Ventriculoperitoneal shunt infections can also present at any time after perforation of the bowel, vagina or other organ.[17] The distal catheter often protrudes from the anus or vagina and CSF leaks from these sites. Presentation is usually as meningitis rather than shunt obstruction or peritonitis, with few abdominal features. Considering the often large numbers of bacteria seen in the CSF in these cases, the patients are not usually severely ill and recovery is often uneventful after shunt removal, without need for laparotomy.

DIAGNOSIS

Blood should be drawn for culture in all cases of suspected shunt infection. However, in infected VP and LP shunts the positive culture rate is less than 5%, except where *Staph. aureus* or Gram-negative bacilli are involved. In VA infections the positivity rate is much higher and blood should be drawn for culture on several occasions. However, in longstanding infections blood cultures may remain negative, possibly because of high antibody and opsonin titers. All isolates, however doubtful, should be saved until a definitive diagnosis is made. Attempts should be made to compare consecutive isolates, by antibiograms and by proprietary kits such as API Staph, or by molecular typing techniques if available. Differentiation between contaminants and pathogens, however, remains a problem. Critical evaluation of tests for 'slime' production shows that these tests, as currently formulated, are of no value in the diagnostic laboratory.[18]

Aspiration of CSF from the shunt reservoir carries little risk of introducing infection. The CSF sample should be examined promptly and a portion should be centrifuged for Gram film and culture, whatever the cell count, because bacteria are not infrequently found in the absence of a significant cellular response. As with blood cultures, isolates should be kept and identified, although the isolation of an organism from a shunt aspirate, particularly if it is also seen on Gram film, is diagnostic of shunt infection. It is important to realize that no isolate should be disregarded, whatever its identity. Gram film is essential to detect *Propionibacterium acnes*, which will require anaerobic incubation for up to 2 weeks.

It should be noted that the shunt might be infected only distal to the reservoir. In such cases reservoir aspiration may yield normal CSF that is culture negative.

In the presence of symptoms and a suggestive history, negative blood and CSF cultures cannot rule out shunt infection completely and a high index of suspicion should be retained. If symptoms persist, consideration should be given to removing the shunt empirically

and it is then imperative that it is sent immediately to the laboratory in a sterile container for Gram stain and culture. Cultures should be incubated for at least 5 days. The Gram stain is very important; where organisms are isolated on culture without being seen on microscopy they are almost invariably contaminants, except where antimicrobials have been given immediately before shunt removal.

In view of the difficulties both of laboratory and clinical diagnosis, serologic tests have been developed. For example, a whole-cell agglutination test using *Staph. epidermidis* has proved useful in diagnosing VA shunt infections.[7] The agglutinin titer in individuals without shunts rises with age. In patients who have VA shunt infection caused by coagulase-negative staphylococci, the titer rises before symptoms appear and, over several months, it can rise to 15–30 times the normal level for age. It can therefore be used as a screening test. When used in this way, shunt nephritis is not seen because a diagnosis is invariably made sufficiently early for it to be avoided.[7] Ventriculoperitoneal and LP shunts do not discharge directly into the bloodstream, which may explain why the agglutination test is not useful in these cases. The plasma C-reactive protein (CRP) can be helpful in distinguishing between infective and noninfective distal VP shunt obstruction. For VP shunts, if symptoms of obstruction appear within 6–9 months of surgery, and the plasma CRP is raised with no other cause, shunt infection is likely and should be confirmed by CSF aspiration.

MANAGEMENT

Three factors are important in the antimicrobial chemotherapy of shunt infections. The first is the mode of growth of the organisms in the shunt lumen. The concentration of antimicrobials required to kill biofilm organisms is often several logs higher than the conventional minimum inhibitory concentration.[19]

The second is the inherent multiresistance of many strains of coagulase-negative staphylococci. Almost all are resistant to penicillin and at least 50% are resistant to methicillin and therefore to cephalosporins. Resistance to aminoglycosides is also common. However, only rare clinical isolates of *Staph. epidermidis* are resistant to vancomycin, although some strains of *Staph. haemolyticus* and a few of *Staph. epidermidis* are resistant to teicoplanin. Similarly, the incidence of resistance to rifampin (rifampicin) and lincosamines is low in most centers.

The third factor is the lack of a vigorous inflammatory response in the CNS to most shunt infections, so that most systemically administered antimicrobials fail to penetrate the CSF, this being particularly true of aminoglycosides, β-lactams, glycopeptides and streptogramins. Of the few drugs that give acceptable CSF concentrations in such circumstances, chloramphenicol is bacteriostatic and ineffective in treating shunt infections; rifampin is highly active against most organisms causing shunt infections but cannot be given alone because of rapid development of resistance; and trimethoprim is active against fewer Gram-positive bacteria than rifampin. However, linezolid is active against bacteria commonly found in shunt infection, including those that are methicillin resistant, and it has good CSF penetration even in the absence of meningeal inflammation.[20]

These factors explain the generally disappointing results achieved whenever attempts are made to treat shunt infections without shunt removal. The shunt should therefore be removed early and an external ventricular drain (EVD) inserted to control CSF pressure (Table 23.2). This course of action is supported by many reports, clearly indicating that shunt retention is associated with a greater chance of relapse, a longer hospital stay and a greater risk of death. However, a recent report has claimed success in *Staph. epidermidis* shunt infections using intraventricular vancomycin and intravenous or oral rifampin without shunt removal.[21] The success of the regimen appears to depend on early diagnosis, the elective placement of a contralateral reservoir for antibiotic therapy, and *Staph. epidermidis* as the cause.

Table 23.2 Treatment of shunt infections caused by *Staphylococcus epidermidis*, other coagulase negative staphylococci and other susceptible Gram-positive bacteria

- Shunt removal, insertion of external drain with ≥5 cm tunnel
- Intraventricular vancomycin 20 mg q24h plus intravenous/oral rifampin (rifampicin) 15 mg/kg q24h (pediatric) or 600 mg q24h (adults), both in two divided doses
- After 7–10 days of treatment, if clinical response and if CSF cultures negative, re-shunt if necessary. Stop both antibiotics on day of re-shunting

Antimicrobials should be begun as soon as the diagnosis is confirmed. Vancomycin is recommended for CoNS, *Staph. aureus*, coryneforms and for those enterococci that are susceptible. As the drug does not give adequate CSF concentrations when given intravenously,[22] it should be given intraventricularly via a reservoir or through the clamped EVD tube. A Rickham reservoir should be incorporated in the system if the chosen EVD does not have a reservoir or injection port. Alternatively, an Ommaya reservoir can be inserted contralaterally.[21] The standard dose of intraventricular vancomycin is 20 mg daily, although this should be reduced to 10 mg daily for those with small ventricles. It should be noted that the dose depends on ventricular volume rather than on age or body weight. The vancomycin should be diluted in 1–2 ml sterile water for injection. In addition to vancomycin, rifampin should be given intravenously in a total dose of 15 mg/kg per day (two divided doses) for children or 300 mg every 12 hours for adults along with intravenous or intramuscular flucloxacillin (250–500 mg every 6 hours or 60–125 mg every 6 hours for children) or oxacillin (500 mg every 6 hours; for children >40 kg body weight, use adult dose, <40 kg 25–50 mg/kg every 4 hours). The intravenous drugs can be given orally in most cases after a few days. Alternatively, trimethoprim can be given intravenously, 3 mg/kg every 8 hours for children and 250 mg every 12 hours for adults. Teicoplanin offers no obvious advantage over vancomycin.

Intraventricular vancomycin given in the doses recommended above leads to CSF concentrations that commonly reach 5–10 times the expected plasma concentrations, but no toxicity has been encountered. Attempts should not be made to titrate the dose to keep the CSF concentrations below the toxic plasma levels. There is no indication for the use of intravenous vancomycin in addition to that given by the intraventricular route except in the case of methicillin-resistant *Staph. aureus* shunt infections, for which vancomycin might be the only available agent. The drug may be given by the intravenous route alone if the CSF cell count and protein concentration are sufficiently raised to indicate a vigorous inflammatory response, but this is the case only with *Staph. aureus* infections.

Using this regimen, CoNS should no longer be detectable in the CSF on microscopy or culture by day 4 and any fever should have resolved. A new shunt, if needed, can be inserted by day 7–10 of the regimen, the last dose of antibiotics being given on that day. It is unwise to wait for a few days after stopping treatment, as this is the period of greatest risk for secondary infection from the EVD. Using this regimen for CoNS, *Staph. aureus*, coryneforms and propionibacteria, successful eradication and re-shunting within 10 days without relapse can be expected in almost all cases.[23]

For shunt infections caused by Gram-negative bacilli, the shunt should again be removed and the treatment for Gram-negative meningitis (Chapter 18) instituted.

A notable exception to the rule of shunt removal is community-acquired bacterial meningitis in shunted persons. Such patients should be treated in the same way as those without shunts and can be expected to respond at least as well. On no account should these patients be subjected to shunt removal.[24]

REFERENCES

References for this chapter can be found online at http://www.expertconsult.com

When to do a lumbar puncture for the evaluation of meningoencephalitis

Lumbar puncture, with removal of cerebrospinal fluid (CSF), is an essential procedure in the evaluation and proper management of patients with meningitis and encephalitis. In patients with suspected bacterial meningitis, for example, CSF analysis allows assessment of whether the cell count and biochemical profile are consistent with the diagnosis (i.e. neutrophilic pleocytosis, elevated protein and decreased glucose) and permits performance of tests, such as Gram stain and culture, to establish the bacterial etiology.[1] Furthermore, the CSF profile may suggest other etiologies, and allow discontinuation of antibacterial therapy or management of other treatable infections or conditions. In patients with suspected encephalitis, performance of specialized tests on CSF (e.g. virus-specific IgM and nucleic acid amplification tests, such as polymerase chain reaction) can help determine the etiology of encephalitis and verify continuation of appropriate empirical therapy or allow discontinuation of therapy based on negative results; identification of a specific etiology may also be important for prognosis, potential prophylaxis, counseling of patients and family members, and public health interventions.[2]

Despite the benefits of CSF analysis in the management of patients with meningitis and encephalitis, lumbar puncture is sometimes not performed in an expeditious manner, or not performed at all, because of concerns of potential adverse events. Complications associated with lumbar puncture have ranged from mild alterations in comfort to life-threatening brain herniation.[1] The most common complication of lumbar puncture is headache, generally occurring in 10–25% of patients. Headache results from continued leakage of CSF at the site of the procedure, and is usually absent when the patient is supine, appearing rapidly when the patient stands. The risk of headache can be reduced with use of small-gauge, atraumatic needles and reinsertion of the stylet before needle removal.[3] Other complications of lumbar puncture include painful paresthesias, infection, local bleeding, and spinal subdural or epidural hematoma.

However, the most important potential complication following lumbar puncture is brain herniation (Fig. PP7.1).[4] In patients who undergo lumbar puncture, there is normally a transient lowering of lumbar CSF pressure as a result of removal of CSF and continued leakage of CSF from the opening made in the arachnoid membrane; this lowering of CSF pressure is rapidly communicated throughout the subarachnoid space.[5] In patients who happen to have an intracranial mass lesion, there is already a relative pressure gradient with downward displacement of the cerebrum and brain stem that can be further increased by lumbar puncture. This can then precipitate brain herniation. Furthermore, brain herniation can occur in patients with acute bacterial meningitis as a result of the development of cerebral edema and increased intracranial pressure. The exact incidence of brain herniation following lumbar puncture is unknown, but the possibility is such that patients should

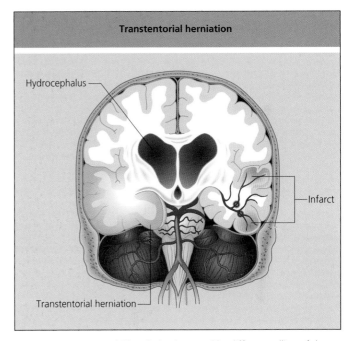

Fig. PP7.1 Transtentorial herniation is caused by diffuse swelling of the brain, or hydrocephalus; the herniation may be asymmetrical when lateral focal lesions are present. From van de Beek *et al*.[4]

be carefully evaluated, always with an appropriate clinical examination and sometimes with a neuroimaging study such as CT scan of the head, to reduce the likelihood of precipitating this devastating complication.

In one study of 301 adults with bacterial meningitis,[6] an attempt was made to determine the clinical characteristics at baseline prior to CT that could be used to identify patients who would have abnormalities on neuroimaging. These were:

- age ≥60 years;
- a history of central nervous system (CNS) disease (e.g. mass lesion, stroke, focal infection);
- an immunocompromised state (e.g. HIV infection, immunosuppressive therapy, transplantation);
- a history of seizure ≤1 week before presentation; and
- specific neurologic findings (i.e. an abnormal level of consciousness, an inability to answer two consecutive questions correctly or to follow two consecutive commands, gaze palsy, abnormal visual fields, facial palsy, arm drift, leg drift or abnormal language).

None of these features was present at baseline in 96 of the 235 patients who underwent CT scan of the head. Of these 96 patients, the CT findings were normal in 93, yielding a negative predictive value of 97%. Of the three patients who did not have normal findings, only one had mass effect on CT and all underwent lumbar puncture with no evidence of brain herniation. On the basis of these findings, and review of other literature and expert opinion, a panel of the Infectious Diseases Society of America developed guidelines for adult patients who should undergo CT of the head prior to lumbar puncture, which were as follows:[1]

- immunocompromised state;
- history of CNS disease;
- new onset seizure;
- papilledema;
- abnormal level of consciousness; or
- focal neurologic findings.

The decision of when to perform a lumbar puncture in patients with suspected meningitis or encephalitis is further complicated by the fact that a normal CT scan of the head does not necessarily mean that lumbar puncture is safe, and it has been suggested that in patients with clinical signs of impending herniation, it is best to delay lumbar puncture as the procedure may precipitate brain herniation.[7] These clinical signs include a deteriorating level of consciousness (particularly a Glasgow Coma Scale of ≤11), brain-stem signs (e.g. papillary changes, posturing, or irregular respirations) and a very recent seizure. These findings would argue against the use of lumbar puncture or, if performed, use of a 22- or 25-gauge needle in order to remove the smallest amount of CSF for essential studies to minimize leakage after the procedure.[5] This is followed by careful monitoring for any clinical signs of impending herniation.

Despite concerns regarding the potential risk of brain herniation, CSF analysis should continue to be performed in patients who are appropriately evaluated prior to lumbar puncture.

REFERENCES

References for this chapter can be found online at http://www.expertconsult.com

Approach to the patient who has fever and headache

INTRODUCTION

Fever and headache are common presenting symptoms with a wide differential diagnosis. The physician needs to be able to recognize the early features of meningitis and initiate appropriate treatment without delay as the consequences of a missed diagnosis or inadequate treatment can be fatal.

PATHOGENESIS AND MICROBIOLOGY

Inflammation of the meninges may result from a number of pathologic processes including infection, acute vasculitis, malignant infiltration and subarachnoid hemorrhage. Organisms can enter the meninges via local or blood-borne spread.

The organisms causing bacterial meningitis vary with age and geographic region (Table PP8.1). Meningococcal meningitis is most common in infants, children and young adults. Outbreaks of infection occur more frequently during the winter months and may affect nurseries, schools, universities and residential accommodation. The incidence of *Haemophilus influenzae* b and meningococcal types a and c meningitis has decreased dramatically since the introduction of conjugate vaccines; however, the current meningococcal vaccine does not protect against group b disease and there continue to be outbreaks of meningococcal infection in sub-Saharan Africa (type a) and the Hajj pilgrimage in Saudi Arabia (type W135). Pneumococcal meningitis may follow an initial otitis media, sinus infection or pneumonia. Most cases occur in infants with a second rise in incidence in the middle-aged and elderly.

Listeria monocytogenes is associated with pregnancy, advanced age and underlying immunosuppression or malignancy. If meningitis follows surgery or trauma the causative organisms may include Gram-negative and anaerobic bacteria. Tuberculous and fungal meningitis occur most frequently in patients who have resided in endemic areas or have had contact with infected cases and may be associated with immunosuppression, including underlying HIV infection.

Viral meningitis is predominantly caused by the enteroviruses (70%), but can also be caused by mumps, herpes simplex virus, varicella-zoster virus, measles virus, adenoviruses and Epstein–Barr virus.

CLINICAL FEATURES

The cardinal features of meningeal inflammation are headache, neck stiffness and photophobia. The speed of progression of the illness and any prodromal symptoms are often helpful in making the diagnosis.

The presence of intracranial shunts, previous head trauma or surgery, travel history, age of the patient and underlying immunosuppression will influence the range of potential pathogens. Symptoms and signs of meningitis may be nonspecific in very young or elderly patients. Fulminant meningococcal sepsis, when purpuric lesions and hypotension may be prominent, is often present without meningitis or meningeal signs.

The vital signs should be documented and careful examination may reveal the presence of a purpuric rash (meningococcus; Fig. PP8.1), viral exanthem or lymphadenopathy. Evidence of meningism should be sought, including presence of neck stiffness, photophobia and any focal neurology or papilledema. Kernig's and Brudzinski's signs are of limited diagnostic value.[1] Examination of the tympanic membrane may reveal an underlying otitis media. Urinary dipstick examination should be performed as a urinary tract infection may occasionally present with meningism.

Table PP8.1 Likely organisms causing bacterial meningitis	
Group of patients	**Likely organisms**
Neonates	Group B streptococci *Escherichia coli* *Listeria monocytogenes*
Children	*Neisseria meningitidis* *Streptococcus pneumoniae* *Haemophilus influenzae*
Adults	*Neisseria meningitidis* *Streptococcus pneumoniae* *Haemophilus influenzae* *Listeria monocytogenes*
Elderly persons/underlying malignancy	*Neisseria meningitidis* *Streptococcus pneumoniae* *Haemophilus influenzae* *Listeria monocytogenes* Gram-negative organisms
Post-traumatic surgery	*Streptococcus pneumoniae* *Haemophilus influenzae* *Escherichia coli* *Klebsiella pneumoniae* *Enterobacter* spp. *Pseudomonas* spp. *Staphylococcus aureus* Anaerobic organisms

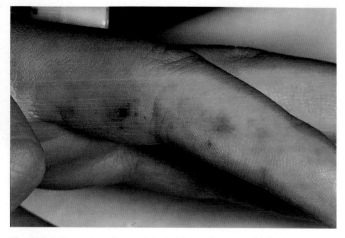

Fig. PP8.1 Purpuric rash associated with meningococcal infection.

INVESTIGATIONS

Routine investigations include blood count, biochemistry and clotting profile. Antigen detection and culture of body fluids – blood, sputum, urine, cerebrospinal fluid (CSF), throat swab and skin scrapings (particularly meningococcal-related purpura) – may reveal the causative pathogen. Meningococcal, tuberculosis, herpes simplex and enterovirus genome detection by the polymerase chain reaction (PCR) is available in many centers. Comparison of meningococcal antibody titers in acute and convalescent serum samples can yield a retrospective diagnosis. Chest radiograph may reveal underlying infection.

Examination of the CSF remains important in many cases. Acute bacterial meningitis is usually associated with polymorphonuclear leukocytosis in the CSF with raised protein and low glucose levels. Viral meningitis characteristically gives a lymphocytosis with normal protein and glucose levels. However, there is a wide differential diagnosis of a lymphocytic CSF (Table PP8.2). A low CSF glucose (<2/3 serum glucose) usually indicates a bacterial, fungal, tuberculous or carcinomatous cause.

Table PP8.2 Some causes of lymphocytic cerebrospinal fluid

Viruses	Enteroviruses Mumps virus Herpes simplex virus
Bacteria	Partially treated bacterial meningitis Early bacterial meningitis Cerebral abscess Tuberculosis Brucellosis Spirochaetes (treponemes, leptospirosis, *Borrelia* spp.)
Fungi	Cryptococcosis Histoplasmosis
Protozoa	Toxoplasmosis Amebiasis
Inflammatory conditions	Seropositive conditions (e.g. lupus) Seronegative conditions (e.g. Behçet's syndrome, Kawasaki's disease)
Chemicals	Irritants and drugs
Carcinomatous conditions	Usually secondary deposits Cerebral lymphoma

MANAGEMENT

Immediate management

If bacterial meningitis is suspected, immediate hospital admission should be arranged and blood cultures and intravenous antibiotic therapy instituted without delay. Resuscitation may be required and all patients who have suspected or confirmed bacterial meningitis should be closely monitored, preferably in a high-dependency or intensive care unit. There is compelling evidence that immediate empiric antibiotic therapy can improve the outcome of meningococcal sepsis and meningitis. Following admission and any immediate resuscitation the two major questions for the clinician managing the patient are whether to do a head scan (CT or MRI) or a lumbar puncture.

Role of head scanning

The indications for performing an urgent scan before lumbar puncture include focal neurologic signs, altered level of consciousness, papilledema or symptoms suggestive of raised intracranial pressure, convulsions and suspected subarachnoid hemorrhage. A CT or MRI head scan can identify the presence of cerebral edema, hydrocephalus or a mass effect, and exclude alternative diagnoses of intracranial hemorrhage, subdural collection or abscess formation (Fig. PP8.2).

Role and safety of lumbar puncture

Immediate lumbar puncture should be avoided in patients with fulminant meningococcal disease and a widespread purpuric rash as there is a significant risk of cerebral edema and coning. In other cases lumbar puncture remains a very important diagnostic investigation which is recommended in all patients with suspected meningitis, except where there is a clear contraindication.[2] It is safe to perform a lumbar puncture in uncomplicated suspected viral meningitis without prior scanning.[3] If the CSF is clear, further investigations should be performed to establish the cause of fever and headache.

Choice of empiric therapy

Empiric antimicrobial therapy should cover all likely pathogens; treatment can then be modified if any organisms are identified. The role of corticosteroids remains controversial. Early dexamethasone treatment has been shown to be associated with an improved outcome in

Fig. PP8.2 Post-contrast MRI scan showing cerebral abscesses.

meningitis caused by *Haemophilus influenzae* and *Streptococcus* pneumoniae,[4] but the effect of corticosteroids is less clear in other forms of bacterial meningitis. This is discussed in Chapter 18.

Management of the complications of meningitis

Bacterial meningitis may be accompanied by all the features of sepsis syndrome, with multiorgan failure requiring intensive care support. Early hemofiltration may be beneficial in seriously ill patients, but there are no controlled trials; there are anecdotal reports of the use of extracorporeal membrane oxygenation (ECMO).

Complications of meningitis can include cerebral abscesses and subdural empyema, secondary hydrocephalus and venous sinus thrombosis. Sensorineural deafness occurs in about 10% of patients who have pneumococcal meningitis and a smaller proportion of patients who have meningococcal meningitis. Audiologic assessment is recommended for all patients who have recovered from bacterial meningitis.

PUBLIC HEALTH ISSUES

Public health physicians should be notified immediately of any patients with known or suspected meningitis so that appropriate action can be taken, including provision of antibiotic prophylaxis to close contacts of patients with meningococcal or *Haemophilus* meningitis and more extensive prophylaxis and vaccination campaigns if these are indicated.[5]

REFERENCES

References for this chapter can be found online at http://www.expertconsult.com

Empiric antimicrobial therapy for suspected infection of the central nervous system

INTRODUCTION

The selection of an appropriate initial antimicrobial regimen for the management of infections of the central nervous system (CNS) is frequently empiric. The key clinical determinants that will guide this therapy include the patient's age, clinical presentation, immune status and medical history. The common utilization of vaccines against the most frequent bacterial pathogens in meningitis has made knowledge of a patient's vaccination record a key component of the history. Previous trauma or instrumentation of the CNS will also significantly impact the choice of antimicrobial therapy while cultures are pending. The clinical presentation of bacterial infections of the CNS can vary from rapidly life-threatening illnesses such as pneumococcal meningitis to more insidious infections such as neuroborreliosis. A detailed history including the use of immunosuppressive agents such as corticosteroids or disease-modifying agents utilized in the treatment of autoimmune illnesses is necessary to adequately assess a patient's risk of immune dysfunction. Use of these agents will result in an expanded list of potential pathogens and thus alter the selection of empiric therapy. A previously healthy adult who has acute bacterial meningitis poses different etiologic considerations from those of a patient with arthritis treated with a tumor necrosis factor-blocking drug. Similarly, surgical manipulation compromising the integrity of the blood–brain barrier, such as placement of a ventriculostomy or epidural pump, dictates empiric antimicrobial therapy targeted toward pathogens that gain entry by these routes.

PATHOGENESIS

The mechanisms of infection that account for most CNS infectious processes are well established. Bacteremia is the frequent cause of hematogenous seeding and acute meningitis. Direct extension of local infections, such as sinusitis and otitis, have been implicated as frequent causes of brain abscesses and surgical manipulation (such as the placement of a ventriculoperitoneal shunt) or trauma may allow direct seeding of the CNS.

MICROBIOLOGY

The most frequent pathogens associated with bacterial meningitis in a previously healthy host are *Streptococcus pneumoniae* and *Neisseria meningitidis*. Routine vaccination against *Strep. pneumoniae* in children as well as the use of licensed meningococcal vaccine in high-risk groups such as military recruits and college students is likely to result in a change in the frequency of these pathogens in the near future. *Haemophilus influenzae*, formerly a frequently encountered organism,

is now rarely implicated owing to routine pediatric immunization. The emergence of strains of *Strep. pneumoniae* highly resistant to penicillin and ceftriaxone has major implications in the selection of empiric treatment of meningitis. In neonates, *Strep. agalactiae* is frequently isolated. In elderly individuals, immunocompromised patients and patients with iron overload, *Listeria monocytogenes* must be included in the differential diagnosis of acute bacterial meningitis (Table PP9.1).

Patients with foreign bodies or who have undergone recent neurosurgical procedures are at increased risk for infections caused by Gram-positive pathogens such as *Staphylococcus aureus* and coagulase-negative staphylococci, although a host of other organisms including fungi have been reported. Common skin flora such as diphtheroids and coagulase-negative staphylococci may cause infection in patients undergoing procedures penetrating the CNS, including epidural injections. Aerobic Gram-negative bacilli have also been implicated in trauma and postoperative patients. A detailed review of bacterial meningitis is found in Chapter 18.

CLINICAL FEATURES

The most common presenting clinical features of acute bacterial meningitis are fever, headache and meningismus. This triad of symptoms is seen in over 85% of cases and should be easily recognizable to the experienced clinician. Confusion and altered sensorium are also frequently noted. Fever and a change in baseline mental status should always raise the potential diagnosis of meningitis and requires rapid evaluation.

Physical examination frequently reveals nuchal rigidity, a positive Kernig's or Brudzinki's sign (although see comment in Practice Point 8) and the presence of photophobia.

Table PP9.1 Common bacterial pathogens associated with predisposing factors for meningitis

Age of patient	Most common bacterial pathogens
0–4 weeks	*Streptococcus agalactiae*, *Escherichia coli*, *Listeria monocytogenes*, *Klebsiella pneumoniae*
4 weeks to 2 years	*Streptococcus agalactiae*, *Streptococcus pneumoniae*, *Haemophilus influenzae*
2–18 years	*Haemophilus influenzae* (decreasing), *Neisseria meningitidis*, *Streptococcus pneumoniae*
18–60 years	*Streptococcus pneumoniae*, *Neisseria meningitidis*
Over 60 years	*Streptococcus pneumoniae*, *Listeria monocytogenes*, others

Presumptive evidence of meningococcal meningitis may be apparent on physical examination. Of patients who have meningococcemia, with or without meningitis, 50% manifest a macular erythematous papular rash early in the course of the disease. This rash rapidly appears petechial and then becomes purpuric.

The presentation of acute bacterial meningitis in neonates may be subtle as meningismus is uncommon and irritability and temperature instability may be the only indications of meningitis. Refusal to feed, lethargy, a high-pitched cry, vomiting, diarrhea and respiratory distress should alert the clinician to this diagnosis.

An insidious onset is frequently noted in elderly patients and in patients with co-morbid disease, as well as immunosuppressed hosts. Fever is frequently absent and headache, confusion or altered level of consciousness may be the only clinical finding.

Other less common causes of meningitis may frequently present with varying clinical syndromes. The presentation of cryptococcal meningitis in an AIDS patient manifests as an insidious illness; persistent fever and headache over several days or even weeks is often the only clinical complaint. A CD4 count below 50 is typically noted with this syndrome. Lyme meningitis, more common in highly endemic areas, often presents as a subacute basilar meningitis with one or more cranial nerve palsies and radiculopathy. Tuberculous meningitis may also present in an insidious manner, necessitating a high index of suspicion for early recognition and successful treatment.

The clinical manifestations of a brain abscess are usually more attributable to the anatomic location and space-occupying effect of the lesion than to the actual infection or pathogen. The classic triad (fever, headache and a focal neurologic deficit) is seen in only 50% of patients. Headache, which frequently is moderate to severe, is the most common manifestation; the next most common is fever. Eventually, altered mental state, ranging from confusion to coma, ensues. Neurologic findings may be focal, but this depends on the size and location of the abscess. Seizures as well as papilledema are more common in brain abscess than in meningitis.

The clinical presentation of infections of the CNS in patients with recent neurosurgical manipulation, with foreign implanted devices or recent epidural injection will vary depending upon the etiologic agent. Patients with a foreign body infection caused by *Staph. aureus* will likely appear toxic with fever and other common signs of meningeal inflammation, while patients with infection from coagulase-negative staphylococci will likely present with a complaint of a mild headache over several days. Clinical obstruction of a previously functioning ventricular drainage shunt should raise suspicion for infection and warrants evaluation of the cerebrospinal fluid (CSF).

INVESTIGATIONS

Rapid diagnosis and initiation of appropriate antimicrobial therapy are essential in patients who present with clinical manifestations of acute CNS infection. A lumbar puncture should be performed in all patients unless there are specific contraindications to this procedure. Patients who present with papilledema or focal neurologic findings should undergo a CT scan before lumbar puncture to determine whether there is a space-occupying lesion under increased intracranial pressure; it will determine the presence of a brain abscess in most cases as well. Initiation of antibiotic therapy should not be withheld awaiting imaging studies when bacterial meningitis is suspected. In patients with a CSF shunt or reservoir, samples should be obtained from these sites.

CSF should be examined using a cytospin technique for the presence of bacterial and fungal pathogens utilizing appropriate stains. Glucose and protein levels in the CSF should be obtained, together with a simultaneous serum glucose level for comparison. Cultures of CSF for bacterial, fungal and mycobacterial organisms should be

obtained. If cryptococcal meningitis is suspected, a cryptococcal antigen assay should be performed on CSF as well an India ink stain. Bacterial latex agglutination tests are frequently used but are of limited benefit. Blood cultures should be sent in all cases because of the high rate of concomitant bacteremia. Other specimens, such as sputum, urine and sinus aspirates, should be obtained and evaluated when clinically appropriate.

MANAGEMENT

The rapid initiation of appropriate antimicrobial therapy in acute bacterial meningitis is imperative. As noted above, initiation of antibiotics should not be delayed while awaiting an imaging study before lumbar puncture. In general, the patient should receive the first dose of antibiotics within 30 minutes of arrival at the hospital if bacterial meningitis is suspected. Appropriate therapy should be based on the age, clinical presentation and predisposing factors, and therapy should be modified when identification of the pathogen and sensitivity testing become available.

In the past several years the incidence of resistance of community isolates of *Strep. pneumoniae* to penicillin has risen to the point where the author believes that vancomycin should be included with a third-generation cephalosporin (ceftriaxone or cefotaxime) as the initial empiric treatment of choice for acute bacterial meningitis in adults. In patients aged under 3 months or over 60 years, ampicillin should be included in the empiric regimen for the treatment of potential listeriosis. Therapy should be adjusted when antimicrobial sensitivities of the cultured isolate become available.

Patients who develop a CNS infection after trauma or postoperatively are at higher risk of Gram-negative bacillary infections. An antipseudomonal cephalosporin (ceftazidime or cefepime) or meropenem in combination with vancomycin is an appropriate empiric regimen. The frequent β-lactam resistance seen with coagulase-negative staphylococci, a common pathogen in this setting, dictates the use of vancomycin. This is also the empiric regimen the author suggests for patients who have foreign bodies in place. In patients with an indwelling reservoir, direct administration of vancomycin may be utilized (5–10 mg initially, diluted in preservative-free saline). In patients with organisms difficult to eradicate, intrathecal antimicrobial treatment should be considered.

Brain abscesses are typically caused by streptococci, Gram-negative bacilli and anaerobes and empiric antimicrobial therapy must target these pathogens and penetrate purulent collections. A third-generation cephalosporin (ceftriaxone or cefotaxime) in combination with metronidazole is appropriate in this clinical setting. Meropenem is another appropriate treatment option. The diagnosis and treatment of brain abscess is presented in detail in Chapter 20.

Although there are no controlled clinical trials, most clinicians treat acute bacterial meningitis for 7–14 days. The duration of therapy for brain abscesses is prolonged and determined by clinical and radiographic response. AIDS patients who are infected with cryptococcal meningitis require prolonged therapy followed by chronic suppression (see Chapter 178 for further discussion).

FURTHER READING

Further reading for this chapter can be found online at http://www.expertconsult.com

Rafik Bourayou
Valérie Maghraoui-Slim
Isabelle Koné-Paut

Chapter | **24** |

Laryngitis, epiglottitis and pharyngitis

Laryngitis

Croup is a common respiratory tract infection of infants and children younger than 6 years of age, with a peak incidence between 7 and 36 months.[1,2] It is characterized by varying degrees of inspiratory stridor (noisy breathing on inspiration), barking cough, and hoarseness as a result of laryngeal and/or tracheal obstruction. Before the advent of treatment with corticosteroids and racemic adrenaline (epinephrine) for severe croup, intubation, tracheotomy and death were typical outcomes. Nowadays, mortality from croup has become a rarity in developed countries. Most children can be managed in the primary care setting.

EPIDEMIOLOGY

Croup is the most common cause of stridor in children and accounts for up to 15% of emergency department and primary care visits for respiratory infections in the USA.[3] The disease mainly affects those aged between 6 months and 3 years, with a peak annual incidence in the second year of life of nearly 5%. However, croup does occur in babies as young as 3 months old and in adolescents.[1] There is a slight male preponderance (male:female ratio, 3:2). Although croup is observed throughout the year, the majority of cases occur with parainfluenza viral infections, typically in the autumn. Those with the respiratory syncytial virus present mainly in the winter. There is often a smaller spring peak. The generalization of treatment with oral corticosteroids and nebulized adrenaline during the 1990s reduced the rate of hospitalization. Nowadays, most cases of croup are managed in the primary care or emergency room setting, with 1.5–31% of patients requiring admission[4] and less than 5% requiring endotracheal intubation.[5]

PATHOGENESIS AND PATHOLOGY

Parainfluenza is the etiologic agent in 50–70% of patients who are hospitalized for croup.[6] Other pathogens causing croup include influenza virus, respiratory syncytial virus, metapneumovirus, adenovirus, rhinovirus, enterovirus and, rarely, measles virus and herpes simplex virus. When croup is caused by influenza virus, the clinical picture is usually more severe than that caused by a parainfluenza virus.[7]

A strong association has been described between both human metapneumovirus and coronavirus HCoV-NL63 infection and croup in children.[8,9] However, a likely possibility is that the increasing number of viruses seen in association with croup is merely a reflection of improvements in methods of detection.

Laryngeal diphtheria is now very rare in immunized populations. However, outbreaks have been reported in case series from Russia and India. Measles remains an important cause of croup in nonimmunized children. Treatment with vitamin A has been reported to be effective for prevention of secondary infections, especially croup, in children with severe measles.

In acute laryngotracheitis, there is erythema and swelling of the lateral walls of the trachea, just below the vocal cords. Histologically, the involved area is edematous, with cellular infiltration in the lamina propria, submucosa and adventitia. The infiltrate contains histiocytes, lymphocytes, plasma cells and neutrophils. In bacterial croup – laryngotracheobronchitis and laryngotracheobronchopneumonitis – the tracheal wall is infiltrated with inflammatory cells; in addition, ulceration, pseudomembranes and microabscesses are present. There is thick pus within the lumen of the trachea and the lower air passages. In spasmodic croup, there is non-inflammatory edema in the subglottic region.[3]

PREVENTION

Prevention of disease depends mainly on good hand washing and preventing the spread of oral secretions. Masks and handkerchiefs inoculated with antiviral drugs have been used in experimental trials; however, after several minutes of breathing, when the mask becomes wet, the protection seems to diminish.

Vaccines are available to prevent some of these diseases. Effective measles vaccines have been used for approximately 30 years, so the disease has decreased dramatically in most countries. Certain adenoviral vaccines have been used with some degree of success, mostly in military personnel. Vaccines against parainfluenza viruses would have the most impact in preventing laryngitis and croup; however, these are still experimental. The ability of influenza vaccine to prevent laryngitis has not been studied.

CLINICAL FEATURES

Croup usually begins with nonspecific respiratory symptoms, including rhinorrhea, sore throat and cough. Fever is generally low grade (38–39°C) but can exceed 40°C. Within 1–2 days, the characteristic signs of hoarseness, barking cough and inspiratory stridor develop, often suddenly, along with a variable degree of respiratory distress. Symptoms may fluctuate depending on whether the child is calm or agitated. They are perceived as worsening at night and most emergency department visits occur at night between 10 pm and 4 am. Croup symptoms are generally short lived, with about 60% of children showing resolution of their barky cough within 48 hours. However, a few children continue to have symptoms for up to 1 week. Spasmodic croup typically presents at night with the sudden onset of 'croupy' cough and stridor. The child may have mild upper respiratory complaints but more often appears completely well prior to the onset of symptoms.

The diagnosis of croup should be made clinically. The child's symptoms may range from minimal inspiratory stridor to severe respiratory failure secondary to airway obstruction. In mild cases, respiratory sounds at rest are normal; however, mild expiratory wheezing may be heard. Children with more severe infection have inspiratory and expiratory stridor at rest with suprasternal, intercostal and subcostal retractions. Air entry may be poor. Lethargy and agitation may be a result of hypoxemia. Warning signs of severe respiratory disease include tachypnea, tachycardia out of proportion to fever and hypotonia. Children may be unable to maintain adequate oral intake, which results in dehydration. Cyanosis is often a late ominous sign.

Determination of disease severity relies on clinical assessment. The most commonly used scoring system has been that of Westley et al.[10] (Table 24.1), which evaluates the severity of croup by assessing five factors: level of consciousness, cyanosis, stridor, air entry and retractions. This system has been extremely valuable in treatment trials but has little use in the routine clinical setting. However, the Alberta Clinical Practice Guideline Working Group has developed another clinically useful severity assessment table. Using this classification scheme, 85% of children in 21 general emergency departments in Alberta, Canada,[11] were determined to have mild croup and less than 1% had severe croup. The assessment is as follows:

- mild croup: occasional barking cough, no audible rest stridor, and either mild or no suprasternal or intercostal retractions;
- moderate croup: frequent barking cough, easily audible rest stridor, and suprasternal and sternal retractions at rest, with little or no agitation;
- severe croup: frequent barking cough, prominent inspiratory and, occasionally, expiratory stridor, marked sternal retractions, agitation and distress; and
- impending respiratory failure: barking cough (often not prominent), audible rest stridor, sternal retractions may not be marked, lethargy or decreased vigilance, and often dusky appearance with no supplemental oxygen.

DIAGNOSIS

Radiologic studies are not recommended in a child who has a typical history of croup and who responds appropriately to treatment. Plain films of the airway and a chest radiograph may be obtained to rule out findings suggestive of another etiology. Anteroposterior films may demonstrate symmetric subglottic narrowing ('steeple sign') (Fig. 24.1),[12] although this may be absent in up to 50% of cases and may be present in the absence of croup. If radiographs are justified by an atypical clinical picture, the child must be closely monitored during imaging by skilled personnel with appropriate airway management equipment, as airway obstruction can worsen rapidly.

Cardiorespiratory monitoring, including continuous pulse oximetry, is indicated in children with severe croup but it is not necessary in mild cases. Oxygen saturation may be near normal in severe croup and yet significantly lowered in some children with mild to moderate disease.[10] This apparent discrepancy may relate to the degree of lower airway disease present.

MANAGEMENT

Over the past 50 years, there has been considerable controversy regarding many therapies for croup, including the role of humidified air and the optimal type (warm versus cold) and the roles of corticosteroids and racemic adrenaline (epinephrine).[3] However, the marked success of corticosteroids in the outpatient management of croup and the effectiveness of nebulized adrenaline (epinephrine) in more severe cases have led to the resolution of many of the controversies. The general consensus is that children with croup should be made as comfortable as possible, and clinicians should take special care during assessment and treatment not to frighten or upset them because agitation causes substantial worsening of symptoms. Sitting the child comfortably in the lap of a parent or caregiver is usually the best way to lessen agitation.

Oxygen is the immediate treatment of choice for children with severe viral croup who have considerable upper airway obstruction with significant oxygen desaturation (SaO_2 <90%). This therapy has not been subjected to a randomized controlled trial and is unlikely ever to be. It is the initial treatment before the administration of pharmacologic treatment in the hospital setting.

During much of the 20th century, treatment with humidified air (mist therapy) was the cornerstone of the management of croup.[3]

Table 24.1 Westley croup score[10]

Symptom	Descriptor	Score
Stridor	None	0
	When agitated	1
	At rest	2
Retractions	None	0
	Mild	1
	Moderate	2
	Severe	3
Air entry	Normal	0
	Decreased	1
	Markedly decreased	2
Cyanosis in room air	None	0
	With agitation	4
	At rest	5
Level of consciousness	Normal	0
	Disoriented	5
Total score		0–17

Mild croup: scores 1–2; moderate croup: scores 3–8; severe croup: scores >8.

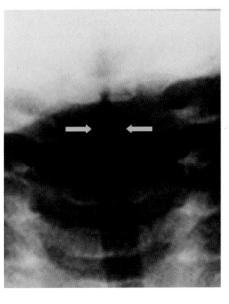

Fig. 24.1 Anteroposterior neck film demonstrating steeple sign (arrows) in a case of croup.

More recently, however, the effectiveness of mist therapy has been questioned. In a recent trial[13] comparing the effects of high humidity (100%), low humidity (40%), and blow-by humidity (in which a plastic hose is held near the child's nose and mouth) in children with mild croup, there were no significant differences in the croup score responses among the three groups; each group had significant improvement (about 33%) over baseline in the croup score 60 minutes after administration. In two other small trials, control subjects who received nebulized saline also had improvement in their croup scores over baseline values.[10] Since none of these studies included an untreated control group, it is not possible to determine whether or not the improvements were due to the moist air. A recent Cochrane Review of data from three other studies concluded that there was no evidence that inhalation of humidified air in children with mild-to-moderate croup resulted in a substantial improvement in the croup score.[14]

Corticosteroid therapy is now routinely recommended by all experts. In a cotton-rat laryngotracheitis model,[15] corticosteroids reduced the degree of inflammation and cell damage; although the viral load was increased, the duration of shedding was not prolonged. Meta-analyses of randomized trials[16] have consistently demonstrated significant improvement in patients treated with corticosteroids as compared with controls. For example, in a meta-analysis of 37 trials, patients who were given corticosteroids had significantly lower croup scores at 6 hours, a decrease in return visits and a decrease in time spent in emergency rooms or hospitals.[16]

Trials of corticosteroids in croup have involved a variety of drugs, dosages and routes of administration. The regimens studied most frequently have been single-dose dexamethasone (0.6 mg/kg of body weight given orally or intramuscularly) and nebulized budesonide (2 mg in 4 ml of water); some studies have involved additional doses (up to four doses of dexamethasone or nebulized budesonide given over a period of 2 days). No studies have directly compared the outcomes of single-dose therapy with the outcomes of 2-day treatment schedules. The 1992 recommendation by the Canadian Paediatric Society to use dexamethasone for treatment was followed by a marked decrease in hospitalizations for croup in Ontario, providing further support for the use of corticosteroids.[2] Similar findings were noted in Perth, Australia.

A potential concern with corticosteroids, however, is their immunosuppressive effects, which might predispose the patient to infectious complications. Trials have not been powered to assess these risks, but such complications would be expected to be rare with standard (single-dose) therapy.

Nebulized adrenaline (epinephrine) has been extensively studied for the treatment of croup. Early controlled trials demonstrated that the administration of 2.25% racemic adrenaline (epinephrine) (0.5 ml in 2.5 ml of saline) by intermittent positive-pressure breathing resulted in a significant reduction in the croup severity score,[10,17] but this benefit lasted for less than 2 hours. Later trials also showed that nebulized L-epinephrine diluted in 5 ml of saline at a ratio of 1:1000 was as effective as racemic adrenaline (epinephrine) in the treatment of croup.[18] In severe croup, repeated treatments with adrenaline (epinephrine) have been used and have often decreased the need for intubation.

GUIDELINES

The American Academy of Pediatrics has no guidelines for the management of croup. The Infectious Diseases and Immunization Committee of the Canadian Paediatric Society published a brief statement in 1992, recommending corticosteroid therapy for children admitted to the hospital with croup. The Alberta Medical Association published a guideline for the diagnosis and management of croup in 2004, which was updated in 2007.[11] An algorithm for the management of croup in the outpatient setting is shown in Figure 24.2.

Epiglottitis

Epiglottitis is an acute inflammation of the epiglottis or supraglottis that may lead to the rapid onset of life-threatening airway obstruction and is considered an otolaryngologic emergency. Since the widespread implementation of a conjugate vaccine for *Haemophilus influenzae* type b (Hib) nearly 2 decades ago, the incidence of epiglottitis has significantly declined in children. Securing the airway should be accomplished immediately in a controlled setting. Coordinated communication between the otolaryngologist, anesthesiologist, and intensive care physician is vital to the care provided to these critically ill patients.

PATHOGENESIS AND PATHOLOGY

Haemophilus influenzae type b (Hib) can colonize the pharynges of otherwise healthy children through respiratory transmission from intimate contact. These bacteria may penetrate the mucosal barrier, invading the bloodstream and causing bacteremia and seeding of the epiglottis and surrounding tissues. Bacteremia may also lead to infection of the meninges, skin, lungs, ears and joints.

Hib infection of the epiglottis leads to acute onset of inflammatory edema, beginning on the lingual surface of the epiglottis where the submucosa is loosely attached. Swelling significantly reduces the airway aperture. Edema rapidly progresses to involve the aryepiglottic folds, the arytenoids and the entire supraglottic larynx. The tightly bound epithelium on the vocal cords halts edema spread at this level. Aspiration of oropharyngeal secretions or mucous plugging can cause respiratory arrest.

Despite the dramatic decrease of Hib-related infections after the introduction of the vaccine, recent reports have shown that Hib may still cause epiglottitis despite adequate vaccination.[19,20] It should be noted, however, that vaccination failure may have prevailed with use of the older, purified polysaccharide vaccine.[19] Infectious agents in the postvaccination era associated with epiglottitis include group A *Streptococcus pneumoniae*, *Staphylococcus aureus*, *Klebsiella pneumoniae*, *Haemophilus parainfluenzae* and β-hemolytic streptococci.

EPIDEMIOLOGY

Traditionally, epiglottitis was most commonly caused by Hib and primarily reported in children aged 2–7 years. The introduction of the Hib conjugate vaccine in 1988 dramatically changed the epidemiology of acute epiglottis. At the Children's Hospital of Buffalo, a rate of 3.5 cases of epiglottis per 10 000 admissions in 1969–1977 decreased to 0.3 cases per 10 000 admissions in 1995–2003. Hib was the causative organism identified in 84% of the cases in the earlier years, but was completely absent in the later segment of the study.[21] A 5-year retrospective review of the incidence of epiglottitis at the Children's Hospital of Philadelphia indicated a frequency of 10.9 per 10 000 admissions before 1990. Only 1.8 episodes per 10 000 admissions were noted 5 years after introduction of the vaccine.[22] A Finnish study also demonstrated a decreased prevaccination era incidence of 50 and 60 cases annually in 1985 and 1986, respectively, to only two cases in 1992 after widespread administration of the Hib vaccine.[23] In a Swedish study, the incidence of epiglottitis also decreased substantially from 20.9 in 1987 to 0.9 in 1996 for children younger than 5 years.[24]

There is a male preponderance of acute epiglottitis, with male-to-female ratios ranging from 1.2:1 to 4:1. Most studies have not demonstrated a seasonal variation in the incidence of acute epiglottitis.

Mortality rates have decreased considerably since the introduction of the Hib vaccine and the consequent shift in disease from young children to adults. Death rates are now less than 1% for children but approach 7% for adults. When deaths have occurred, a large percentage transpired due to delay in diagnosis or shortly after arrival at a medical facility for appropriate care.[25]

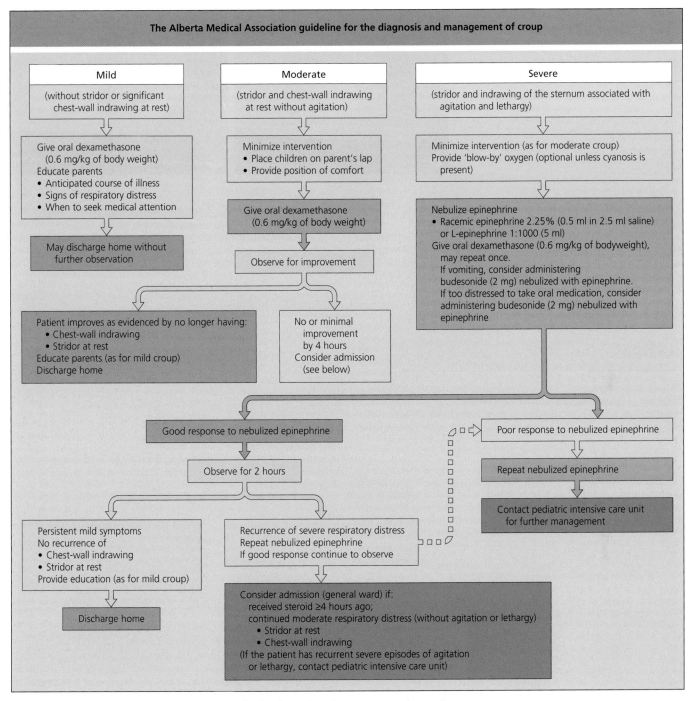

Fig. 24.2 The Alberta Medical Association guideline for the diagnosis and management of croup.[11]

PREVENTION

In the only study to date seeking specific risk factors for epiglottitis, day-care attendance was the strongest predictor for disease but the association was modified by whether the subject had had an upper respiratory illness in the previous 4 weeks. There was also the suggestion that northern European ancestry was a risk factor as well. Fortunately, the incidence of epiglottitis (and meningitis) has decreased markedly since the advent of the Hib vaccination. Whether the incidence of Hib disease in adults may change in the future is unknown, because long-term immunity from vaccination may prove to be either more or less effective than that due to natural infection.

CLINICAL FEATURES

Patients with epiglottitis often have an underlying illness, presumed to be viral. They then have sudden onset of fever, with the neck extended forward, drooling and air hunger. Affected children are anxious and lean forward to open their airway. The diagnosis is easily made by viewing the epiglottitis, which is swollen and red (Fig. 24.3). Intubation is often required. Culturing swabs from the epiglottis in children almost always obtains *Haemophilus influenzae* type b. Some children have been discharged without intubation after receiving only one dose of ceftriaxone when the epiglottis did not appear reddened, but subsequent epiglottic and blood cultures have been positive for Hib. They were

Fig. 24.3 Acute epiglottitis with views of the cherry red epiglottis on direct laryngoscopy.

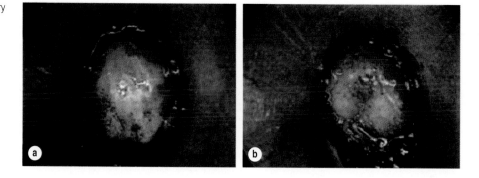

Fig. 24.3 Acute epiglottitis with views of the cherry red epiglottis on direct laryngoscopy.

cured completely. The duration of hospital treatment averages 3 days. Intubation is needed for less than 24 hours in most cases.[26]

In adults other pathogens may be obtained.[27] In most adults the disease is less severe and of slower onset. The airway obstruction occurs because of a progressive cellulitis of the supraglottic area. Thus at presentation, antibiotic treatment and intubation at the first sign of increasing respiratory compromise may avert the need for tracheotomy. The use of steroids to reduce inflammation and decrease the need for tracheotomy is appealing but unproven.

DIAGNOSIS

Visualization of the posterior pharynx is the best way to confirm the diagnosis of epiglottitis. Because airway obstruction is the most feared complication of this disease, this examination should be done in a manner and place where immediate intubation can be performed if necessary.

Lateral neck radiographs may demonstrate the classic thumb sign (Fig. 24.4). It is actually a rounded mass shadow of the normal leaf-like epiglottis resulting from the thickening and edema of the inflamed epiglottic tissue. Another radiologic feature of acute epiglottitis is the 'vallecula sign', which is the result of partial or complete obliteration of a well-defined air pocket bounding the base of the tongue and the epiglottis. The poor sensitivity (38%) and specificity (78%) of plain films limits the utility of this radiographic modality in the current age of technologic advances, whereby the larynx can be safely and accurately visualized with flexible laryngoscopy.[28]

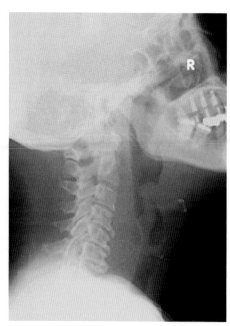

Fig. 24.4 Lateral neck film demonstrating thumb sign with edema of the epiglottis.

A complete blood cell count with differential, blood cultures and epiglottic cultures (when an artificial airway has been placed) are obtained after the airway is secure and the patient is stable. Elevated white blood cell counts are frequently present, but positive blood culture results are extremely variable (6–15%).

MANAGEMENT

Securing the airway is the initial step in the management of epiglottitis. Various studies have been performed to identify predictive factors for the need for airway intervention. A combination of features such as stridor, drooling, acute onset or rapid progression, hoarseness, respiratory distress, dyspnea, chest wall retractions and upright position have been associated with the need for airway intervention.[29]

Appropriate antibiotics include ceftriaxone, cefotaxime and cefuroxime (for non-meningitic infections). Ampicillin should not be used due to the high frequency of ampicillin-resistant strains of Hib. Steroids are commonly employed to decrease mucosal edema of the epiglottis, but no data exist in the literature to prove any benefit from their use.

Most children can be successfully extubated after 24 hours of antibiotic therapy and some extubate themselves before that time has expired. Family members and day-care contacts should receive rifampin prophylaxis (300 mg q12h for 2 days) to avoid secondary infection.

Pharyngitis

Pharyngitis is a very common inflammatory condition of the pharynx accompanied by a sore throat and occasionally difficulty in swallowing. It is usually viral but may be caused by bacterial or fungal infection. Gastroesophageal reflux disease (GERD) or particularly extraesophageal reflux (EER) can also cause an acid pharyngitis in adults and children. Serious complications of pharyngitis may include peritonsillar abscess or retropharyngeal abscess.

EPIDEMIOLOGY

Pharyngitis can be separated into one group of illnesses with associated nasal symptoms (which are most commonly viral in origin) and another that causes only pharyngitis. It is important to distinguish between these infections because rheumatic fever and acute glomerulonephritis may complicate untreated group A β-hemolytic streptococcal infections, but they can usually be prevented by appropriate antibiotic treatment.

Adenoviruses, rhinoviruses, coronaviruses, enteroviruses and parainfluenza viruses most frequently cause self-limiting viral infections. Other viral infections, such as respiratory syncytial virus (RSV) and Epstein–Barr virus (EBV), are less common but still frequently occur. Bacterial causes of upper respiratory infections are led by group A β-hemolytic streptococci (GAS) but can also be caused by *Haemophilus influenzae*, *Bordetella pertussis*, *Chlamydia pneumoniae*, *Corynebacterium haemolyticum*, *Mycoplasma pneumoniae* and *Yersinia enterocolitica* among others.

These upper respiratory infections are often difficult to differentiate and hence difficult to diagnose, frequently leading to futile overtreatment in many cases. Further complicating the issue is the fact that primary viral infections are often succeeded by secondary 'opportunistic' bacterial infections, making undertreatment a problem in a significant minority of infections. Additionally, individuals with allergies are sometimes more prone to secondary bacterial infections. The clinician is therefore challenged to weigh multiple factors involved in deciding whether an infection is viral or bacterial in origin, and whether antibiotic treatment is warranted.

Viral upper respiratory infections frequently occur in mini-epidemics (RSV, parainfluenza, influenza, varicella, measles). They are more common in the winter except for those caused by enteroviruses, which are more common in the summer.[30] Some viral infections occur year round, with no seasonal pattern (adenoviruses). Group A β-hemolytic streptococcal infections are more common in the winter, but many other nonviral respiratory infections do not appear to be seasonally linked (*Chlamydia* and *Mycoplasma* spp.). Some bacterial infections appear to be linked to preceding viral infections and hence occur more commonly in the winter. Pharyngeal colonization may occur throughout the year.

Influenza infections vary significantly from year to year. In the USA one subtype was predominant each year until about 1990, since which time both H3N2 and H1N1 strains have been circulating simultaneously. When there is a major shift in antigen type, significant excess morbidity occurs as the new strain infects the community. Increasing air travel has accelerated the rate at which the influenza viruses travel around the world and has perhaps been responsible for the increasing frequency with which the viruses are detected. The shifted strain outbreaks have most affected the elderly and children with congenital heart and lung disease. Minor influenza drifts have occurred also, but cause less disease. There has also been a recent decrease in the average age at which children acquire upper respiratory diseases because of the increasing use of day care for children. Although the long-term effect of this is unknown, in the short term it appears that it has been responsible for a significant increase in the number of ear infections in children less than 2 years old.[31]

Rheumatic fever, a complication of group A β-hemolytic streptococcal pharyngitis, has waxed and waned in importance.[32] After a century of prominence, the disease was in considerable decline in developed countries for 40 years. Recently, clusters of rheumatic fever cases have occurred, for example in Salt Lake City, Utah, USA, where it is hypothesized that the re-emergence of certain M types has been responsible.

PATHOGENESIS AND PATHOLOGY

The pathogenesis of the sore throat due to pharyngitis is poorly understood. Volunteers given rhinoviral infections produce bradykinin and lysylbradykinin, which are known inflammatory mediators that can excite nerve endings in the pharynx to cause pain.[33] There is also suggestive evidence from laboratory animals that adenovirus, RSV and other viral infections directly invade the pharyngeal cells and produce an inflammatory response. This leads to the well-described 'red, sore throat'. Additionally, adenovirus and EBV often produce lymphoid hyperplasia and tonsillar exudation. Herpes simplex virus (HSV) and coxsackievirus infections frequently lead to ulcerations of the oral mucosa. Herpes simplex virus ulcers are more common in the anterior part of the mouth and coxsackievirus ulcers occur more frequently in the posterior part of the pharynx, but this is only a guide and both viruses can cause ulcers in any part of the oropharynx. Herpes simplex often produces a significant gingivitis as well.

Streptococcal pharyngitis often involves the posterior pharynx, with petechiae on the uvula and soft palate.[34] When one sees this clinical sign, GAS is often isolated by throat culture. A confusing factor is that up to 10% of patients who have EBV infections will have a secondary group A β-hemolytic streptococcal pharyngitis during their illness. *Corynebacterium diphtheriae* can also cause pharyngitis, producing a characteristic gray membrane across the structures of the posterior pharynx. This is seldom seen today except in a few geographic areas where diphtheria outbreaks have occurred recently, such as Russia. There are also noninfectious causes of pharyngitis, such as Behçet's syndrome, Kawasaki disease, Marshall's syndrome and Stevens–Johnson syndrome.

PREVENTION

Preventing pharyngitis is desirable but difficult to achieve. Mostly aerosolized oral secretions, hand-to-mouth contact with multiple individuals and the use of common utensils, glassware, etc. spread viral pharyngitis. Certain viruses are known to be particularly resilient; RSV has been cultured from tabletops hours after being inoculated.[35] Measles has been known to be contracted from the air in a physician's waiting room, as long as 1 hour after the child with measles had left the room. Other viruses may be less durable and less contagious, but close contact is obviously not necessary to transmit many of these agents. Prevention of disease depends mainly on good hand washing and preventing the spread of oral secretions. Masks and handkerchiefs inoculated with antiviral drugs have been used in experimental trials, but after several minutes of breathing, when the mask becomes wet, the benefit seems to diminish.

There are vaccines available to prevent some of these diseases. Effective measles vaccines have been used for approximately 30 years, so the disease has decreased dramatically in most countries. Certain adenoviral vaccines have been used with some degree of success, mostly in military personnel. Vaccines for RSV and parainfluenza viruses are currently under development. These vaccines could have a significant effect on the population's health, particularly on that of the youngest children.

Transmission of streptococcal pharyngitis seems to require closer contact than for most viruses. Studies performed in the military during the Second World War showed that soldiers in barracks sleeping on either side of the index case were more likely to have disease than those further away.

To date, there are no immunizations available to prevent streptococcal disease, although trials evaluating group B and group A vaccines are under way. For patients who have had prior group A disease and subsequent rheumatic fever, penicillin prophylaxis is recommended. Most patients receive intramuscular benzathine penicillin, 1.2 million units, once per month; although oral regimens are acceptable, they have poorer compliance rates.

CLINICAL FEATURES

Pharyngitis is a ubiquitous infection. A 'sore throat' affects most people at least once every year. Most cases of viral pharyngitis are associated with an upper respiratory infection (nasopharyngitis). Generally nasopharyngitis has a prodrome that may include malaise, diaphoresis, fever, headache and general aches and/or pains. Coryza and sore throat then begin. Many infections will progress to produce a cough and/or laryngitis. Some viral infections produce predominantly coryza, others more pharyngitis, and others more cough or laryngitis. Coxsackieviruses often cause ulcers in the posterior pharynx along with a sore throat. Measles can cause a severe pharyngitis, but the associated symptoms of conjunctivitis, rash and Koplik's spots make the disease easily diagnosable. Parainfluenza and influenza viruses can give a particularly painful pharyngitis, with frequently associated symptoms of cough and laryngitis.

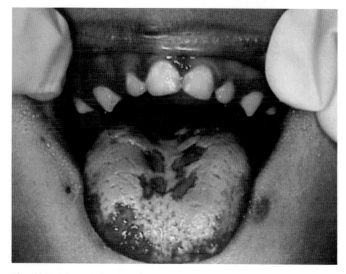

Fig. 24.5 Primary infection of HSV-1

The DNA viruses EBV, adenovirus, cytomegalovirus and HSV can produce significant pharyngitis. They also tend to last longer than the other viral causes of pharyngitis. These viruses produce other upper respiratory symptoms such as nontender cervical adenopathy of, in the case of HSV, tongue and mouth ulcers. Herpes simplex virus pharyngitis has been described as a disease in which 'the gums swell up and swallow the teeth' (Fig. 24.5). Rhinoviruses and RSV infections give upper respiratory symptoms as well as pharyngitis in infants.

The syndrome of acute HIV infection ('seroconversion illness') is well described and may cause symptoms in up to 50% of patients. It is a mononucleosis-like illness in which pharyngitis is a prominent feature. Patients will also have fever, lymphadenopathy, rash and myalgias. The symptoms are nonspecific.

It is important to diagnose bacterial causes of pharyngitis because, unlike viral causes, many can be treated specifically with antibiotics. Proper treatment can avoid significant morbidity and/or mortality. Pharyngitis caused by GAS is the most common infection causing significant pharyngeal edema, frequently with petechiae on the soft palate and uvula (Fig. 24.6). Tender cervical nodes are common. Small children may complain of abdominal pain, which may be due to mesenteric adenitis. Headache and raised temperature are also common. Some patients who have a streptococcal sore throat have a characteristic red 'scarlet fever' rash that begins in the groin and axillary areas and spreads over the body (Fig. 24.7). The rash is sandpaper-like and may itch. A strawberry tongue is also often present. Other patients have a characteristic rash on the face. Without treatment the illness usually resolves over 3 or 4 days, but rheumatic fever may ensue.

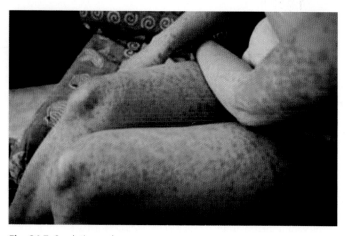

Fig. 24.7 Scarlatine rash.

The recommended treatment is penicillin, or clindamycin, erythromycin or azithromycin for those allergic to penicillin. There is concern about the recurrence rate of streptococcal pharyngitis in adequately treated patients but there is no evidence for microbiologic resistance to therapy. It is more likely that the organism is reacquired or sequestered in a sanctuary site and simply re-emerges after therapy is discontinued. Some have used rifampin at the end of therapy in an attempt to alleviate this possibility. While all therapies have similar response profiles, azithromycin has a higher culture-positive recurrence rate.

The risk of rheumatic fever without antibiotic treatment is difficult to assess. Wannamaker and colleagues documented rates as high as 3% in 1952;[36] however, more typical rates of 0.4% were found in a pediatric population in 1961.[37] Certainly M protein type, genetic susceptibility and previous infection play a part in this diversity of recurrence rates. Other β-hemolytic streptococcal infections (groups C, G and B) can cause pharyngitis but not rheumatic fever. For these, antibiotic treatment may provide symptomatic relief.

Occasionally, pharyngitis can be secondary to an abscess in the peritonsillar area. This is usually easily diagnosed by an asymmetry of the tonsillar pillars. The affected side is asymmetrically enlarged and protrudes anteriorly into the mouth. *Haemophilus influenzae* (nontypeable and types a–f) can cause pharyngitis and type b can also cause epiglottitis or meningitis. Many individuals are carriers but are not ill.

Corynebacterium diphtheriae causes diphtheria, which is easily diagnosed because of the gray pseudomembrane in the posterior pharynx along with pharyngitis (Fig. 24.8). The disease has recently become endemic in parts of the former Soviet Union. *Arcanobacterium* (previously *Corynebacterium*) *haemolyticum* is a common cause of pharyngitis and can also cause a scarlatiniform rash. It is the cause of many non-GAS throat infections.[38] *Neisseria gonorrhoeae* can also cause pharyngitis. The appearance of the pharyngitis is nondiagnostic, so heightened awareness is required to make this diagnosis.[39] *Chlamydia*

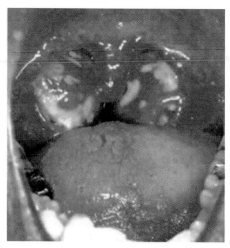

Fig. 24.6 GAS tonsillitis.

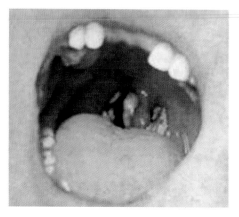

Fig. 24.8 Diphtheria pharyngitis with gray pseudomembranes in the posterior pharynx.

pneumoniae and *Mycoplasma pneumoniae* can cause pharyngitis, but generally will go on to cause cough also, often with wheezing and pneumonia.[40,41] *Candida albicans* can cause pharyngitis but normally only in the immunocompromised host. The pharyngitis is hyperemic, with white plaques on the buccal mucosa.

Aphthous stomatitis is a common feature of mouth ulcers. The etiology is unclear. Small painful ulcers appear on the buccal mucosa, but can also appear in the posterior pharynx. The ulcers are usually stress related and last approximately 1 week. Very extensive aphthous ulceration can also be seen as a complication of HIV infection. Behçet's syndrome may cause aphthous stomatitis. Kawasaki disease, most common in young children, can cause significant redness of the oral mucosa. Most children with Kawasaki disease also have fever, a strawberry tongue and, importantly, conjunctivitis. This condition is frequently confused with streptococcal disease. Stevens–Johnson syndrome can result in pharyngitis, stomatitis and perioral swelling and ulcerations. Marshall's syndrome or PFAPA (periodic fever, aphthous stomatitis, pharyngitis, cervical adenitis) syndrome is a pediatric periodic disease characterized by recurrent febrile episodes associated with head and neck symptoms.[42]

DIAGNOSIS

Prevalence of group A β-hemolytic streptococcus (GABHS) during school outbreaks of pharyngitis is between 15% and 50% in healthy school-age children. Since toddlers with GABHS respiratory tract infection may not present with classic symptoms, the diagnosis of GABHS pharyngitis among children should be based on laboratory tests in conjunction with the clinical findings. Culture isolation of GABHS from the pharynx is the gold standard, but 2 days are needed for it to be informative. On the other hand, the rapid antigen detection test (RADT) detects the presence of GABHS within a few minutes and has high sensitivity and specificity.

Rapid testing has many additional benefits: early treatment within 48 hours provides symptomatic relief for the child and limits spreading of the organism. In addition, it allows the practitioner to treat only those cases with GABHS, thus avoiding prescribing antibiotics for viral infections. Group B, C and G streptococci can also cause significant morbidity, but only group A leads to rheumatic fever, so the reason for treatment is not only to eliminate the pharyngitis but also to prevent the subsequent rheumatic disease. Viral causes of pharyngitis do not normally require specific diagnosis, but serologic tests are available for mononucleosis (EBV) and cytomegalovirus. Adenoviruses, RSV and parainfluenza viruses can be diagnosed using rapid antigen tests, which are available but rarely used in uncomplicated community-acquired infections.

MANAGEMENT

For group A streptococcal pharyngitis the recommended therapy is 6–10 days of oral penicillin or amoxicillin. Erythromycin and clindamycin are acceptable alternatives. There have been studies showing that one dose of ceftriaxone intramuscularly or oral azithromycin or cefaclor for 5 days is equally effective at eliminating carriage of GAS, but recurrent pharyngeal colonization occurs with all treatment regimens. Viral causes of pharyngitis can be most suitably treated with supportive measures: gargles, lozenges, etc. *Mycoplasma* and *Chlamydia* spp. infections can be treated with erythromycin or tetracycline (depending on age). Diphtheria and *Arcanobacterium* spp. infections should be treated with erythromycin or penicillin. *Legionella* spp. infections should be treated with tetracycline. *Haemophilus influenzae* type b and *Yersinia enterocolitica* infections should be treated with a third-generation cephalosporin.

REFERENCES

References for this chapter can be found online at http://www.expertconsult.com

Otitis, sinusitis and related conditions

Otitis

Otitis media (OM) is a frequent disease in early childhood and is the first reason for prescription of antibiotics in pediatric practice. Viruses are the leading cause and in 60–80% of cases OM resolves spontaneously within 48 hours. Overuse of antibiotics is due to current misunderstanding of the microbial ecology and is also explained by the fear of secondary complications. However, it is well known that unnecessary antibiotic treatment may favor the development of multiresistant pathogens. Appropriate prescription of antibiotics for OM is based on clinical findings, the patient's age and the bacterial ecology.

EPIDEMIOLOGY

Acute otitis media (AOM) is common in young children and is associated with upper respiratory tract infection.[1] The immaturity of the immune system plays a major role in its development but other risk factors – such as male sex, lower age (peak age of incidence is between 6 and 18 months),[2] family history and above all the early entry into day care[3] – are well known. The frequency of AOM increases with allergy and passive smoking that modify the ciliated respiratory membrane. Esophageal reflux can also favor AOM by way of throat inflammation.[4]

PHYSIOPATHOLOGY

The middle ear and rhinopharynx are covered by a ciliated respiratory mucous membrane. The middle ear communicates with the pharynx by the Eustachian tube that allows physiologic drainage of the mucus secreted by the middle ear. Viral aggression against the respiratory epithelium, so frequent in early childhood, decreases ciliary movement, favoring bacterial adhesion. At the same time, the inflammation provokes Eustachian tube obstruction. Together, these mechanisms facilitate bacterial proliferation in the middle ear, with the formation of pus.[1]

Acute otitis media develops into two phases:
* first, the congestive phase (red eardrums, not inflated with normal reliefs); and
* second, the purulent phase (tympanic inflammation and effusion behind the eardrum).

The principal causative pathogens are *Haemophilus influenzae* (HI), *Moraxella catarrhalis* (MC) and *Streptococcus pneumoniae* (SP), the last being associated with a more frequent risk of complications.

PREVENTION

Vaccination

Vaccination by the octavalent vaccine or 14-valent anti-SP vaccine in the 1980s reduced the frequency of AOM but only in children aged more than 6 months. Moreover, efficacy was limited to the first 6 months following vaccination.[5] The new anti-SP conjugated heptavalent vaccine (7-valent SP conjugate vaccine or PCV7) is effective against the invasive forms of diseases caused by SP in children who were immunized at 2, 4 and 6 months of age.[6] Immunized children had fewer episodes of AOM caused by the seven serotypes (4, 6B, 9V, 14, 18C, 19F, 23F) contained in the vaccine but had more episodes of AOM caused by the other serotypes. The use of PCV7 has a strong impact on penicillin nonsusceptible SP carriage in children with AOM.[7] Unfortunately, since the introduction of PCV7, a multiresistant serotype, 19A SP, not included in PCV7, has emerged in the USA.[8]

Prevention of respiratory viral infections

Viruses can be co-factors of AOM. AOM and sinusitis are the most common bacterial complications of upper respiratory tract infections in children.[9] The use of the vaccine against influenza reduced the frequency of AOM caused by influenza by 36%. However, the benefit of vaccination is low because influenza is responsible for only 5% of cases of AOM.[10] Respiratory syncytial virus (RSV) is closely associated with AOM. The use of anti-RSV immunoglobulins decreases the frequency of bronchiolitis but does not modify the frequency of AOM.

Antibiotic prophylaxis

Prophylaxis against AOM with antibiotics is not currently recommended as this favors the selection of multiresistant pathogens. However, in patients who had multiple episodes of AOM within 6 months and/or have proven immunodeficiency, amoxicillin or trimethoprim treatment may be considered.[11]

Tympanostomy tubes and adenoidectomy

The efficacy of these procedures in the prevention of AOM has not been demonstrated but they do avoid hearing disorders due to repeated episodes of AOM. They are beneficial in chronic otitis media with effusion.[11]

DIAGNOSIS AND CLASSIFICATION

The diagnosis of AOM is difficult and should be based on rigorous criteria. Indeed, according to the severity of symptoms and associated systemic signs, the child may (or may not) receive antibiotic treatment initially.[12] Otoscopic examination allows the diagnosis of AOM. However, the technique can be problematic due to issues that may arise during examination (e.g. small auditory canals, cerumen obstruction, child restlessness).[13] Rhinopharyngitis and/or child screams during examination induce congestion and hypervascularization of the eardrum.

Congestive otitis and purulent otitis are separate conditions:

- Congestive otitis (CO) is an acute inflammation of the middle ear. Eardrums are congested but reliefs are normal and there is no tympanic convexity. More often CO is caused by viral infection. Secondary bacterial infection is possible and justifies medical follow-up.
- Purulent otitis (PO) (Fig. 25.1) is an inflammation of the tympanic membrane associated with a retrotympanic effusion, which can sometimes be exteriorized by otorrhea. Common symptoms are severe ear pain (expressed in a young child by irritability, tears and sleeplessness), fever, asthenia and anorexia. Ear pain arising at night and fever are frequent but not mandatory. Associated nonspecific signs include gastrointestinal disorders, cough and rhinorrhea in the context of associated viral infection.

Some clinical associations indicate a diagnosis of bacterial otitis media – for example, otitis with conjunctivitis indicates HI; high fever with ear pain indicates SP. Acute otitis media without systemic signs is called seromucous otitis. External otitis must be distinguished from AOM with otorrhea, in which there is no perforation of the tympanic membrane and pain persists in spite of drainage of secretions.

BACTERIOLOGY

Bacteria are retrieved in 50–90% of cases of AOM.[14] The principal pathogens identified by aspiration and culture of middle ear fluid are SP (the most frequent, 20–35%), HI (nontypeable), MC and *Strep. pyogenes* (group A streptococcus). *Staphylococcus aureus* (less than 5%) and *Pseudomonas aeruginosa*, retrieved in few cases, may also cause chronic OM.[14] Since the use of PCV7, the cost of non-invasive pneumococcal diseases such as AOM has increased in the US population, as well as the frequency of HI AOM.[15] Moreover, PCV7 has reduced

the rate of vaccine-type-associated AOM by 57%.[16] *Strep. pyogenes* is more frequent in Europe than in the USA, especially in children more than 2 years old. Respiratory viruses (RSV and influenza mostly, but also enterovirus and rhinovirus) are also found alone or in association with bacteria in the auricular liquid.

In light of this information, the treatment of AOM remains empiric because the responsible pathogen is not identifiable in the majority of cases. Modification of the bacterial ecology over the past few years, as well as increasing resistance, may influence antibiotic treatment.

SP strains isolated in AOM can be resistant to β-lactams by modification of protein-linking penicillins (PLPs). Sensitivity decrease concerns G penicillin, amoxicillin and oral cephalosporins. The rate of penicillin-resistant SP is 12% in the USA and more than 30% in Asia.[14] More than 80% of AOM SP strains are resistant to macrolides. The major serotypes involved in AOM are 19A, 19F, 23F, 6B and 14; all are contained in the heptavalent-conjugated vaccine except 19A. Since the generalization of SP vaccination in USA, there has been an emergence of nonvaccinal serotypes with decreased sensitivity to β-lactams.[8] Nontypeable HI causes most cases of AOM. HI secretes β-lactamases, which inactivate amoxicillin and sometimes C1G. Occasionally there is modification in the target of β-lactams, the PLPs. These strains are called 'BLNAR' (β-lactamase-negative, ampicillin-resistant). They are fortunately sensitive to high-dose amoxicillin and to C3G. Macrolides are naturally only slightly active or inactive against HI. *M. catarrhalis* is resistant to amoxicillin due to secretion of β-lactamases. Amoxicillin–clavulanic acid, C2G and C3G are active against these strains.

Acute otitis media in children less than 3 months of age is caused by pathogens such as Enterobacteriae and *Staph. aureus* that may disseminate rapidly into systemic life-threatening infection. Treatment requires parenteral antibiotic therapy after thorough research of the pathogen by tympanocentesis.

TREATMENT

In March 2004 the American Academy of Pediatrics (AAP) proposed guidelines for treatment of AOM.[17] The goal of treatment is sterilization of the middle ear and reduction of pain. Prescription of antibiotics depends essentially on two factors: the age of the child (younger or older than 2 years) and the severity of systemic signs. For children younger than 2 years, initial antibiotic treatment is recommended. For children older than 2 years with few or no symptoms, symptomatic treatment only is recommended, with patient re-evaluation after 48–72 hours. This attitude is called 'watchful waiting' and is justified because immediate antibiotic treatment has only a modest effect on the course of AOM. For example, a study compared the safety, efficacy, acceptability and cost of non-antibiotic intervention for children with mild AOM versus amoxicillin treatment. Results showed the same parent satisfaction in both groups and no serious adverse events in patients who did not receive antibiotics.[18]

Antibiotics are not recommended for treatment of congestive otitis and seromucous otitis, unless symptoms last more than 3 days in cases of congestive otitis and more than 3 months in cases of seromucous otitis. Clinical studies comparing antibiotics versus placebo have shown that the majority of cases of AOM recover spontaneously. The spontaneous cure is more frequent when the child is more than 6 months old and is infected by HI. Conversely, most serious complications are more frequent before 2 years of age.

The goal of antibiotics is to treat the source of infection and to sterilize the middle ear to avoid systemic dissemination. Antimicrobial agents must be active against both HI and SP and must reach adequate levels in serum and the middle ear. Successful sterilization occurs when drug concentrations exceed minimum inhibitory concentration (MIC) by 50%. For this reason, the first choice is amoxicillin because of its efficacy against SP and nontypeable HI, as well as its safety and low cost. The dose of amoxicillin to administer raises controversies. Some recommend 40–45 mg/kg/day in two or three

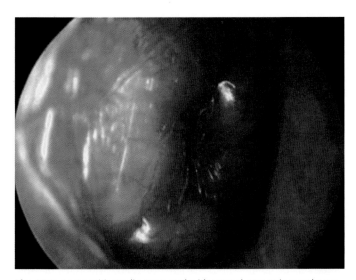

Fig. 25.1 Acute otitis media compared with normal tympanic membrane.

divided doses in children who have received more than three doses of PCV7, and 80–90 mg/kg/day in two doses in other children, including those recently treated with antibiotics. This higher dose is safe and appropriate for SP with reduced sensitivity to penicillin.[19] Other recommended antibiotics are the β-lactams: amoxicillin–clavulanic acid, cefpodoxime proxetil or cefuroxime axetil. If β-lactams are contraindicated because of the risk of failure due to current resistance to HI and SP, erythromycin–sulfafurazole or pristinamycin are suitable alternatives.

If antibiotic treatment is instituted, dosage and timing of administration must be strictly followed. Re-evaluation of patients within 48–72 hours must be undertaken if symptoms persist and to check the eardrum at the end of treatment in case of recurrent AOM or a past history of treatment failure. The duration of treatment should be as short as possible to reduce the cost and the risk for both development of resistant pathogens and drug-related adverse events.[20] In in-vitro and animal studies the middle ear is sterilized after 5 days on antibiotic treatment. However, there appears to exist a higher risk of recurrence following short-term treatment, with the effusion persisting for a longer period.[21] Thus, a short course of treatment (5 days) is recommended for children without the risk of SP multidrug resistance and for children more than 2 years of age. In children younger than 2 years a 5-day course of antibiotics is less efficient, especially for those in day-care centers, and an 8-day course is more effective.

Treatment is considered to have failed if symptoms persist after 48 hours on medication or if AOM recurs within 4 days following the end of treatment. Obtaining a bacterial sample is then necessary to adapt the treatment. Pathogen-resistant β-lactamases producing nontypeable HI or SP with reduced susceptibility to penicillin are likely to be identified.

Amoxicillin (100 mg/kg/day for 10 days) or ceftriaxone (50 mg/kg/day for 3 days) are treatments recommended in cases of SP with decreased sensitivity to amoxicillin. In cases of resistant HI, both oral and intravenous C3G have the same effect as amoxicillin–clavulanic acid.

Penicillin-resistant SP is emergent in South Africa, France and the USA, with an MIC to penicillin of more 2 mg/ml in children with AOM or sinusitis. Associated risk factors include recent antimicrobial treatment, children younger than 1 year and children in day care. High-dose amoxicillin (80/150 mg/kg/day), amoxicillin (40 mg/kg/day) and amoxicillin–clavulanic acid (45 mg/kg/day), ceftriaxone (50 mg/kg/day), amoxicillin–clavulanic acid (90 mg/kg/day) or clindamycin (50 mg/kg/day) can be used. In penicillin allergy there is significant cross-reactivity with other antimicrobial agents such as cephalosporins. Macrolides can be used against SP but are less effective against nontypeable HI and resistant SP. Trimethoprim–sulfamethoxazole (TMP–SMX) can be effective but resistance rates reach 20–50% against SP. The best choice is to combine TMP–SMX and macrolides. When cultures are negative (30–45% of cases), careful patient monitoring is recommended.

Therapeutic abstention is possible for children who will be examined by a doctor in case of persistent signs, for children more than 2 years old and if there are no systemic signs. Benefits of short-term antibiotic treatment versus longer treatment are equivalent in efficacy but there is better compliance, fewer adverse effects, improved parental satisfaction, less impact on emergence of resistant flora and lower costs. The adjuvant treatments include analgesics and antipyretics. Ibuprofen did not show better efficacy than paracetamol for treatment of pain in AOM and has more side-effects. Codeine can be used for severe pain. Auricular drops have no indication in AOM.

COMPLICATIONS

Some 60–80% of cases of uncomplicated AOM resolve within 24–48 hours without antibiotic treatment. Following treatment of AOM with antibiotics, the occurrence of mastoiditis, labyrinthitis, brain abscesses, facial nerve palsy and septic thrombophlebitis has become exceptional. However, some retrospective reviews have shown that the

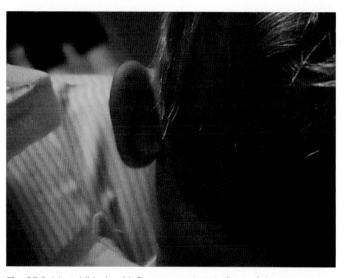

Fig. 25.2 Mastoiditis: local inflammatory signs in front of the mastoid.

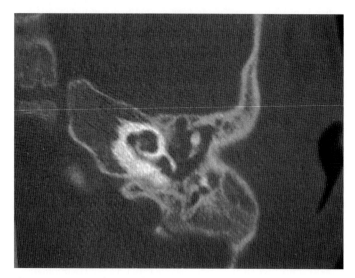

Fig. 25.3 CT scan of mastoiditis.

use of antibiotics to treat purulent AOM in children did not influence the development of acute mastoiditis.[22,23]

Mastoiditis particularly affects children younger than 2 years. Systemic signs are associated with local inflammatory signs in front of the mastoid (Figs 25.2 and 25.3). Virulent pathogens such as group A streptococcus, SP and type b HI in non-immunized subjects are commonly found. Mastoiditis may progress to cerebral abscess, central venous thrombosis, osteomyelitis and hydrocephaly. Staph. aureus and Enterobacteriae cause subacute mastoiditis. Parenteral antibiotic treatment is mandatory.

Another AOM complication is labyrinthitis caused by dissemination of infection in the inner ear. Vestibular syndrome is the key feature. Benign facial nerve palsy may also occur; this has a favorable outcome with antibiotic and corticosteroid treatment.

Sinusitis

Sinusitis refers to inflammation of the lining of the paranasal sinuses (infectious or noninfectious; bacterial or viral). Symptoms of acute sinusitis last less than 4 weeks, symptoms of subacute sinusitis last less than 4–8 weeks and symptoms of chronic sinusitis last more than 12 weeks. Sinusitis can be further classified according to the anatomic site (maxillary, ethmoidal, frontal and sphenoidal).

CLINICAL FEATURES

Sinusitis can cause different symptoms in children at varying ages. Younger children often present with persistent rhinorrhea (often purulent), cough and foul-smelling breath; fever is generally low grade. Facial pain and headaches are rare. The differential diagnosis with a viral upper respiratory tract infection (URTI) is difficult to establish and no single sign or symptom has strong diagnostic value. However, sinusitis should be considered in patients who present with symptoms of a viral URTI of more than 10 days' duration.[24]

During a viral throat infection, there is inflammation of the mucous membrane and a continuum between the ordinary cold, acute viral congestive rhinosinusitis and acute bacterial sinusitis characterized by the presence of pus in the paranasal sinuses.

In older children and adults, signs are more localized and the most frequent symptoms are facial pain, headaches, fever, nasal congestion or obstruction and daytime cough. Clinical examination may reveal facial tenderness or swelling over the maxillary or frontal sinuses.

In chronic sinusitis (signs present for at least 12 weeks), cough is prominent. This cough is usually present throughout the day and occasionally precipitates emesis, especially after wakening. Chronic headache may also be present: the pain is often dull in nature and radiates to the top of the head or in temporal regions. Purulent or mucopurulent nasal discharge often completes this cluster of signs.

The localization of sinusitis varies according to age because of the chronology of development of the sinuses: patients between 6 months and 5 years develop ethmoidal sinusitis; those older than 3 years develop maxillary sinusitis and those older than 10 years develop frontal sinusitis. Sphenoid sinusitis is exceptional among children. Maxillary sinusitis is common in children older than 3 years and resolves spontaneously in most cases.

Two clinical pictures can be distinguished:
- acute purulent maxillary sinusitis with fever >39°C lasting more than 3 days, headaches, purulent rhinorrhea and sometimes periorbital edema; and
- subacute maxillary sinusitis with cough, purulent rhinorrhea and nose obstruction, which may last more than 10 days without amelioration.

Headaches, prolonged fever associated with morning cough and purulent sputum are clear signs of bacterial sinusitis. Frontal sinusitis is rare. It particularly affects children older than 10 years and teenagers. The pain is located above the eye socket, is unilateral and throbbing in nature, and is increased by anteflexion of the head. Complications can be serious (eyes, osteomyelitis of the cranial bones). Most cases of sinusitis are caused by bacterial or viral infections but may also be related to allergy.[25] Between 97.8% and 99.5% of sinusitis is viral initially.[26] Bacterial sinusitis starts with a viral disease or an allergic rhinitis with secondary bacterial infection. Persistent obstruction of the sinus ostium by inflammatory edema causes secondary bacterial colonization. In addition, there is a diminution of mucociliary transport which may impair the normal secretion flow, creating an optimal environment for bacterial multiplication.[27] The American Academy of Pediatrics (AAP) defines acute bacterial sinusitis as a bacterial infection of the paranasal sinuses lasting less than 30 days in which symptoms resolve completely.[28]

Microbiologic diagnosis of sinusitis is difficult and requires a sample of sinus secretions not contaminated by the resident bacterial flora of the nose. This sample may be obtained by a needle puncture of the sinus. This is an invasive procedure, which may explain the lack of data concerning bacterial pathogenic agents of sinusitis in children. The most common infectious agents are SP (30–66%), HI (20–30%) and MC (12–28%). Conjugate vaccines have been developed to target SP and HI. Since the introduction of these vaccines, a significant decrease in the frequency of SP has been observed and the bacterial

data have changed, with predominance of non-b HI (41%), SP (25%), MC (14%), *Strep. pyogenes* (12%) and *Staph. aureus* (8%). There is also a decrease of SP resistant to penicillin from 44% in 1997 to 27% in 2005 and an increase of HI with β-lactamase (37% versus 44%), although these differences are not statistically significant.[29]

Rare cases of sinusitis of dental original must be considered in patients with pain following recent dental procedures. In most cases, anaerobic bacteria of the oropharynx colonize necrotic dental tissue and then colonize the sinuses. Treatment with antibiotic therapy is essential.[30] Finally, some studies explore the link between gastro-esophageal reflux and chronic sinusitis.[4]

DIAGNOSIS

The diagnosis of sinusitis is clinical. Plain film radiographs may help when diagnosis is difficult (the radiograph shows an opaqueness of the sinus, which may be unilateral or the sinus shape is asymmetrical, and thickening of the mucous membrane is greater than 4 mm; liquid levels are exceptional). Radiography must be interpreted according to age. In fact, in young children only maxillary and ethmoidal sinuses are aerated. However, opacification of the sinus or a mucous thickening may be present even if the child is asymptomatic. CT scan (computed tomography) is used in cases of sphenoidal sinusitis (not seen on standard radiography), ethmoiditis and complicated maxillary sinusitis (Fig. 25.4).[31]

COMPLICATIONS

Sinusitis may be severe in children. The AAP published recommendations about sinusitis in the child and advocated the use of antibiotics.[32] Complications of sinusitis are caused by bacterial spread to nearby structures such as the orbit, bone or central nervous system via the venous system. Although extremely rare, bacterial spread by hematogenous dissemination can cause distant site infections.[33] Orbital cellulitis is the most common complication, especially in ethmoidal sinusitis.

Purulent acute ethmoiditis (exteriorization of ethmoiditis in the orbit wall which is very tenuous) represents a real pediatric emergency, which can occur in children aged more than 1 year. This diagnosis must be considered in a child presenting with edema of the superior eyelid associated with swelling of the internal corner of the eye and nose root (Fig. 25.5). It is a severe complication of an apparently common viral rhinopharyngitis, with a high fever in the presence of general signs. The etiologic agents are *Staph. aureus* and Hib (before generalization of vaccination). *Staph. aureus* is suspected if there is a

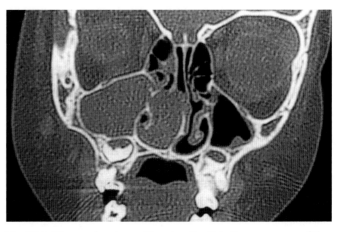

Fig. 25.4 CT scan of acute maxillary sinusitis. Note the opaqueness of the right maxillary sinus.

Fig. 25.5 Acute ethmoiditis. (a) Swelling of the internal corner of the eye and nose root. (b) Edema of superior eyelid.

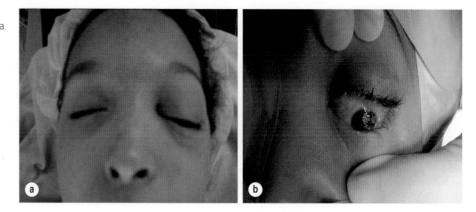

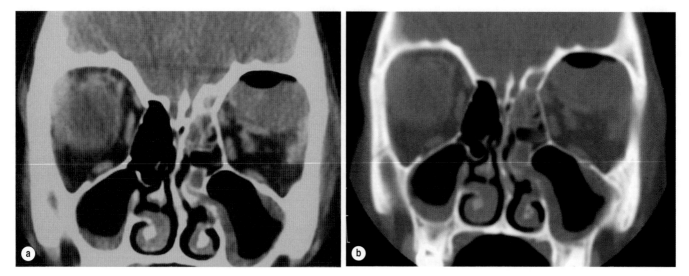

Fig. 25.6 (a, b) CT scans of left acute ethmoiditis.

suggestion of facial trauma or cellulitis of the face. Complications are serious because of the nearness of the brain and its venous channels, i.e. vascular complications (thrombosis of the cavernous sinus) and neuromeningeal complications (purulent meningitis, brain abscess and cerebral empyema). Cerebral computed tomography must be ordered if any neurologic sign is present (Fig. 25.6). Visual involvement may include loss of vision or loss of eye-globe mobility.

Ethmoiditis requires parenteral empiric antibiotic therapy in a hospital setting. Nose pus swab and hemocultures may guide the antibiotic choice. The antibiotic must target HI and *Staph. aureus*. An intravenous third-generation cephalosporin, such as cefotaxime or ceftriaxone associated with an aminoglycoside, is active against *Haemophilus* and methicillin-sensitive staphylococci. Penetration and meningeal distribution are adequate. To cover methicillin-resistant *Staph. aureus*, a third-generation cephalosporin (e.g. fosfomycin) is advised because of the extensive meningeal and osseous distribution. Duration of treatment is 10 days in a hospital setting. In anaerobic infection, an antibiotic of the imidazole family will be added in first intention (e.g. metronidazole, ornidazole). Surgical intervention can be considered according to the efficacy of antibiotics, ophthalmologic involvement and CT data.

Intracranial complications are more common in older children and adults (e.g. cerebral abscess of the frontal lobe or subdural abscess).

These patients present with fever, neck rigidity and neurologic abnormalities. Osteomyelitis of the frontal bone may be observed in maxillary sinusitis.

MANAGEMENT

Antibiotic treatment is indicated in cases of purulent sinusitis and hospitalization may be required in severe forms of ethmoiditis. Most cases of mild maxillary sinusitis will resolve spontaneously without antibiotics. A meta-analysis of randomized controlled trials in 2008 assessed the efficacy of antibiotics in acute sinusitis compared with placebo. This study showed a higher success rate with antibiotics and faster symptom resolution; side-effects were higher with antibiotics, but complications and recurrence were comparable in both groups.[33]

A randomized, placebo-controlled trial of antimicrobial treatment for children with clinically diagnosed acute sinusitis showed that neither amoxicillin nor amoxicillin–clavulanate offered any clinical benefit compared with placebo.[34] However, for severe maxillary or frontal sinusitis, and for subacute forms in children with risk factors (asthma, heart disorder, etc.), antibiotics are indicated. For children without risk factors, antibiotics may be discussed – for example, symptomatic treatment with a follow-up visit after 3–4 days or antibiotics immediately. Treatment is the same as for AOM since the pathogenic agents are the same.

Amoxicillin is used as first-line therapy for uncomplicated acute bacterial sinusitis. Second-line antibiotics should be used in case of failure with amoxicillin: amoxicillin–clavulanic acid (80 mg/kg q8h), cefpodoxime proxetil (10 mg/kg/12h) or cefdinir (14 mg/kg/day). For penicillin-allergic patients, macrolides must be used (azithromycin, erythromycin–sulfisoxazole) or trimethoprim–sulfamethoxazole. Antibiotics may be continued for 7 days after symptom improvement.[35] Besides antimicrobial therapy, symptomatic treatment is necessary – analgesics, antipyretics and nasal obstruction management (nasal solution, iso- or hypertonic, and vasomotor treatment in children aged more than 30 months for less than 5 days).[36]

The benefits of anti-inflammatory drugs (steroids and NSAIDs) were not demonstrated. This treatment may reduce swelling of mucous membranes and sinus openings, allowing better air circulation and reducing bacterial multiplication that have been facilitated by oxygen decline.

Fungal Sinusitis

Fungi contribute to sinusitis in two ways. Invasive fungal infections affecting immunocompromised hosts, such as patients with neutropenia, diabetes mellitus and AIDS are discussed in Chapter 178. In contrast, allergic fungal sinusitis is believed to be an allergic reaction to aerosolized environmental fungi, including Aspergillus and dematiaceous species, in an immunocompetent host. Although not associated with invasive disease, systemic antifungals such as itraconazole may have a limited therapeutic benefit in some patients.

REFERENCES

References for this chapter can be found online at http://www.expertconsult.com

Bronchitis, bronchiectasis and cystic fibrosis

INTRODUCTION

Genetic, environmental and infectious factors can contribute to acute and chronic inflammation of the airways of the lung. The nature, severity and duration of these insults may produce acute or chronic inflammation with associated cough, dyspnea, sputum and obstructive lung disease. Clinically, these are classified as *bronchitis* (acute or chronic) when the main symptoms are cough and sputum production or *bronchiectasis* when the airways are structurally damaged and dilated, and abundant (>60 ml/day) sputum is expectorated. The diagnosis and clinical management of these various airways diseases are related to the underlying pathogenic processes and to differences among patients.

This chapter describes the pathophysiology, clinical features and management of bronchitis and bronchiectasis. Guidelines for diagnosis and therapy are provided. Cystic fibrosis (CF) is a common genetic disease that leads to progressive bronchitis and bronchiectasis. The molecular, cellular and organ-level pathogenesis of CF has been elucidated and new treatments are being developed. Some of these advances are applicable to bronchiectasis caused by other diseases. It must be emphasized that clinical outcomes are highly variable and treatment decisions must be based on the presentation and responses of the individual patient.

Bronchitis

EPIDEMIOLOGY

Bronchitis is defined as inflammation of the bronchial mucous membranes. Acute bronchitis is manifest by the development of a cough, with or without sputum, that typically occurs during the course of an acute viral illness. Such cough commonly develops in the first week of upper respiratory tract infections (URIs) induced by rhinoviruses in 30% of patients.[1] Acute bronchitis develops in 60% of patients during influenza A infections.[2] In the USA, over 34 million annual office visits are for acute sinusitis, bronchitis or URIs. A majority of these patients are treated with antibiotics and such prescriptions comprise 31% of the total antibiotic prescriptions written.[3]

Chronic bronchitis is defined by the clinical criteria of productive cough for more than 3 months per year for at least 2 years.[4] More than 12 000 000 Americans (about 5% of the population) have chronic bronchitis. The male-to-female distribution is about 2 to 1, but the prevalence is increasing in females. Chronic bronchitis is a major category of chronic obstructive pulmonary disease (COPD) and accounts for significant morbidity and mortality, especially in individuals over age 55. COPD accounted for nearly 83 000 deaths in 1989 and was the fifth leading cause of death in the USA.[5] COPD was also a contributing factor in death due to heart disease and other illnesses.

PATHOGENESIS AND PATHOLOGY

Acute bronchitis is most commonly due to infection of the respiratory epithelium with viruses, such as rhinoviruses, adenoviruses and influenza. Acute bronchitis may also be caused by infections with *Mycoplasma pneumoniae*, *Chlamydia pneumoniae* or *Bordetella pertussis*. The pathogenic effects of these organisms are incompletely understood, but they infect and directly damage airway epithelia, cause release of proinflammatory cytokines, increase production of secretions and decrease mucociliary clearance. Airways damaged by such infections may be more susceptible to irritation by inhaled toxins or bacteria. The role of secondary bacterial infections in the development of symptoms is not clear.

Chronic bronchitis develops as the result of a recurring or persistent injury and the resultant inflammatory responses. Cigarette smoking is the principal etiologic factor. Air pollutants such as sulfur dioxide or occupational exposures may also contribute. The pathologic effects are an increase in the proportion of goblet cells in the surface epithelium and an increase in the size of submucosal glands (Fig. 26.1). The distribution of these pathologic changes along the airway tree depends in part on the composition of the inhaled toxins and may involve peripheral bronchioles as well as central bronchi. There is an influx of polymorphonuclear leukocytes (PMNs), surface epithelial cell hyperplasia and metaplasia, and inflammatory mucosal edema. Genetic diseases that impair airway defenses may amplify these effects. Primary ciliary dyskinesia[6] decreases mucociliary transport secondary to altered ciliary structure and function. α_1-Antitrypsin deficiency produces an imbalance in the defenses against neutrophil elastase and leads to panacinar emphysema and bronchitis, particularly in smokers.[7]

PREVENTION

Chronic bronchitis primarily occurs in cigarette smokers. Avoidance of inhaled toxins, particularly cigarette smoke, is of paramount importance in reducing the incidence and progression of chronic bronchitis. The loss of lung function, as measured by spirometry, is more rapid in active cigarette smokers. Such individuals can gain significant benefits from stopping or significantly decreasing their cigarette consumption. Sputum production usually decreases within weeks. The accelerated decline of lung function seen in smokers slows to that of nonsmokers of the same age.[8] Thus, the importance of avoiding primary and secondhand cigarette smoke cannot be overemphasized.

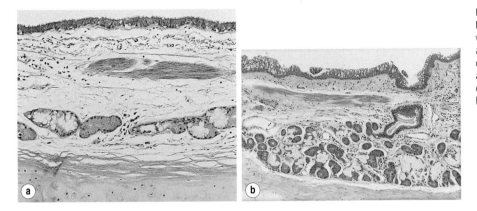

Fig. 26.1 (a) Bronchial wall from normal patient. Normal pseudostratified columnar epithelium with few goblet cells overlies smooth muscle and a submucosal gland. Cartilage is at the bottom of the figure. H&E stain. (b) Bronchial wall from a patient with chronic bronchitis. Hyperplastic epithelium with mucous cell metaplasia overlies a hypertrophied submucosal gland. H&E stain.

CLINICAL FEATURES

Acute bronchitis typically develops during the course of an acute URI. Pharyngitis, coryza, low-grade fever and malaise precede the development of a cough with scanty sputum. Dyspnea is rare. In the absence of other lung disease, most symptoms subside over several days, although the cough may persist for weeks to several months. The quantity of sputum and frequency of cough decrease with time and no long-term sequelae occur.

The key symptoms of individuals with chronic bronchitis are chronic cough, production of sputum, wheezing and exertional dyspnea. These symptoms develop insidiously, often over many years. Presentation for medical care typically occurs during an acute exacerbation. Upon direct inquiry, patients often recall persistent dyspnea and sputum production following URIs for several years prior to presentation. The sputum is purulent, yellow or green, and may be blood-streaked. The daily volume ranges from scanty up to about 60 ml. The cough and sputum are usually most severe soon after awakening. Exertional dyspnea and fatigue are first noticed during exacerbations and later become persistent.

Acute or subacute exacerbations are characterized by increases in cough, sputum production, dyspnea and wheezing.[9] These symptoms often follow acute URIs and tend to be more frequent during winter months. The sputum often changes in color to darker yellow or green. Sputum cultures may identify one of the bacterial pathogens listed in Table 26.1 but the pathogenic role of these microbes is not certain.[10,11] Pulmonary function decreases during such exacerbations and may lead to further complications. The progressive disease often leads to increasingly frequent exacerbations over time, further loss of lung function and worse symptoms.

Patients with severe obstructive airways disease may develop the serious complications of hypoxemic and/or hypercapnic respiratory failure.

Hypoxemia develops initially during exercise or sleep and may cause morning headaches. Prolonged hypoxemia may cause cyanosis, polycythemia, pulmonary hypertension and cor pulmonale. Secondary signs of right heart failure, such as jugular venous distention, hepatomegaly and peripheral edema develop in late disease and may become chronic. The respiratory acidosis that signals hypercapnic respiratory failure may be of gradual onset and be compensated by a metabolic alkalosis through renal retention of bicarbonate. Individuals with scanty sputum production and greater degrees of emphysema often achieve adequate oxygenation and ventilation until late in the course of the disease. Exacerbations in the setting of severe disease often produce superimposed acute respiratory failure that is life threatening and requires intensive care.

DIAGNOSIS

The history of persistent cough and daily sputum is essential to the diagnosis of chronic bronchitis. The extent and duration of cigarette smoking quantify the major risk factor. The presence of antecedent reactive airways disease (e.g. childhood asthma) may increase the risk for developing chronic bronchitis and COPD. Physical examination reveals tachypnea and late expiratory wheezes on auscultation. Patients with advanced disease develop hyperinflation of the lungs with increased anterior–posterior diameter of the thorax and a depressed diaphragm. In such patients, breath sounds and heart sounds are muted. Patients with severe disease may use accessory muscles of respiration and/or pursed-lip breathing. Medium or coarse inspiratory crackles appear in patients with bronchitis and excess airway secretions. Patients with severe disease may develop central and peripheral cyanosis or neck vein distention, hepatomegaly and peripheral edema as signs of hypoxemia and right heart failure.

Pulmonary function tests are essential to establish the diagnosis of obstructive lung disease, to measure the severity of airway obstruction and to follow the course of illness. Spirometry performed before and after inhaled β-adrenergic agonists often reveals decreased FEV_1 and decreased $FEV_1{:}FVC$ ratio. Improved flows following inhaled β-adrenergic agonists indicate the presence of reversible bronchoconstriction. Forced vital capacity (FVC) is also decreased in patients with very severe obstruction. In such individuals, lung volumes should be measured to distinguish restrictive and obstructive respiratory impairments and to quantify lung hyperinflation and gas trapping. The diffusing capacity for carbon monoxide (DLCO) may be reduced in patients with severe obstruction or emphysema. The chest X-ray shows increased lung volumes. In patients with emphysema the heart may appear small and the bronchovascular markings decreased. Patients with chronic bronchitis often have enlarged hearts, engorged apical vessels, bronchial cuffing and other signs of fluid overload. Arterial blood gases may reveal mild to severe hypoxemia. Patients with severe disease may develop respiratory acidosis and a compensatory metabolic alkalosis.

Table 26.1 Viral and bacterial pathogens in bronchitis

Common	Uncommon

Viruses: – rhinoviruses
         – adenoviruses
         – influenza A and B
         – parainfluenza
Haemophilus influenzae
Haemophilus parainfluenzae
Moraxella catarrhalis
Neisseria spp.
Streptococcus pneumoniae
	Chlamydia pneumoniae
	Klebsiella pneumoniae
	Mycoplasma pneumoniae
	Pseudomonas aeruginosa

The complete blood count may reveal polycythemia and the serum electrolytes a metabolic alkalosis. Sputum Gram stain and culture are important to assess the abundance of PMNs and to help identify bacterial pathogens that may be associated with acute exacerbations.

MANAGEMENT

The symptoms of acute bronchitis are best managed with symptomatic treatment. Nonsteroidal anti-inflammatory drugs and decongestants are useful for pharyngitis, sinusitis and coryza. Antibiotics are indicated for clinically significant bacterial bronchitis, but such a complication is difficult to distinguish from viral bronchitis. Antibiotics are prescribed for 53–66% of patients with acute sinusitis, bronchitis or URIs,[3] indicating excess usage. This practice promotes the development of antibiotic-resistant bacteria, which may lead to greater morbidity in the community. Therefore, antibiotics should be reserved for patients with acute bronchitis who have increased numbers of PMNs and numerous bacteria in Gram-stained sputum samples or who do not respond to symptomatic therapy.

The most important feature of managing chronic bronchitis is the avoidance of exposure to irritants, particularly cigarette smoke. Thus, smoking cessation is of primary importance for each individual. Support for smoking cessation can be provided by individual counseling, provision of smoking cessation literature or through smoking cessation groups. Nicotine gum or transdermal nicotine may be useful to reduce withdrawal symptoms.

No specific therapy is available to treat chronic bronchitis. Symptomatic therapy is directed at reducing mucosal edema, mucus hypersecretion, bronchial smooth muscle constriction and airway inflammation (Table 26.2). Inhaled β-adrenergic agonists and anticholinergic drugs may be of benefit to patients with reactive airways disease, as demonstrated on pulmonary function tests.[12] Theophylline may be useful in patients with nocturnal symptoms or severe hyperinflation and respiratory muscle fatigue. In addition to relaxing bronchial smooth muscle, β-adrenergic agonists enhance mucociliary clearance. Inhaled drugs with intermediate (4–6 hours) and long (8–12 hours) duration of action are available. These are generally preferred to systemic treatments. Metered dose inhalers (MDIs) appear to have comparable efficacy to nebulizers, but effective treatment requires coordination of actuation and the breathing cycle. The beneficial effects can be enhanced by the use of a spacer to improve deposition of drugs in the lungs. Dry powder inhalers (DPIs) can be easier to use and more effective. Anticholinergic drugs relax bronchial smooth muscle and have intermediate and long durations of action. Ipratropium bromide is available as an MDI and tiotropium as a DPI. The effects of anticholinergics and β-agonists appear to be roughly equivalent.[13] The responses of individual patients to such drugs must be assessed to determine the optimum treatment.

Systemic and inhaled corticosteroids provide a beneficial effect by reducing severity of airway inflammation. This typically results in decreased airway obstruction and decreased mucus secretion. Long-term use of systemic corticosteroids may be complicated by osteoporosis, central obesity and/or glucose intolerance. Once a beneficial steroid effect has been demonstrated with systemic therapy, these side-effects can be minimized by use of moderate to high doses of inhaled steroids. Typical drugs include beclometasone 800–1600 μg per day and fluticasone 88–1760 μg per day. Other forms of therapy such as cromolyn sodium, expectorants and chest physiotherapy have not been demonstrated to have significant effects in chronic bronchitis or COPD.

The role of bacterial infection in causing acute exacerbations of chronic bronchitis is controversial. It is likely that less than half the cases of acute exacerbation are due to bacterial infection. A number of controlled studies have failed to show significant benefit of antibiotic therapy.[14,15] Nevertheless, antibiotics have a role in patients who demonstrate a significant increase in the number of PMNs in expectorated sputum and dominant bacteria on Gram stain or in culture. Previous positive responses to antibiotic therapy may also support repeated use in individual patients. Antibiotics effective against the common bacterial species are listed in Table 26.3. Patients with exacerbations of sufficient severity to require hospitalization should be treated with

Table 26.2 Therapeutic options for acute exacerbations of chronic bronchitis

Class/agent	Examples	Notes
Bronchodilators		
β-Adrenergic agonists	Albuterol, salmeterol	Inhaled administration preferred
Anticholinergics	Ipratropium bromide	Inhaled administration mandatory
Theophylline		Second-line agent
Anti-inflammatory agents		
Corticosteroids	Prednisone, fluticasone	Administration by inhalation may reduce side-effects
Expectorants		
rhDNase	Dornase alpha	Efficacy in COPD not established
Iodinated compounds	Iodinated glycerol	Limited efficacy
Reducing agents	N-acetyl cysteine	Limited efficacy
Airway clearance measures		
Controlled coughing		Efficacy not established
Physical therapy		Efficacy not established
Supplemental oxygen		Corrects significant hypoxemia
Antibiotics		Indications and efficacy controversial

Table 26.3 Oral antibiotics for acute exacerbations of chronic bronchitis

Agent	Dose
Amoxicillin	250–500 mg q8h
Amoxicillin–clavulanic acid	875/125 mg q8h
Ampicillin	500 mg q6h
Azithromycin	500 mg day 1, then 250 mg q24h
Cefaclor	500 mg q8h
Cephalexin	500 mg q6h
Ciprofloxacin	500–750 mg q12h
Clarithromycin	500 mg q12h
Doxycycline	100 mg q12h
Erythromycin	500 mg q6h
Ofloxacin	400 mg q12h
Tetracycline	500 mg q6h
Trimethoprim–sulfamethoxazole	160/800 mg q12h

parenteral antibiotics with comparable antibacterial spectra, and the treatment modified based on sputum culture results.

Hypoxemia may be diagnosed by ambulatory, exercise or nocturnal pulse oximetry, as well as by arterial blood gases. Patients with significant hemoglobin desaturation (SaO_2 <90%) should receive supplemental oxygen. Nocturnal oxygen has been shown to improve survival[16] and continuous treatment has greater effects than nocturnal treatment alone.[17] Some patients with COPD also have obstructive sleep apnea and detailed sleep studies may be required to establish the effectiveness of oxygen and/or continuous positive airway pressure (CPAP) by nasal mask to prevent nocturnal hypoxemia.[18] Noninvasive assisted ventilation by nasal mask has been used for some patients with severe hypercapnic respiratory failure.[19] Patients with acute respiratory failure and significant respiratory acidosis or hypoxemia often require hospitalization, parenteral antibiotics, ICU care and mechanical ventilation.[20]

Bronchiectasis

EPIDEMIOLOGY

Bronchiectasis is defined as abnormal dilatation of the bronchi.[21,22] It typically involves medium-sized bronchi and results from destruction of the muscular and elastic components of the walls. Bronchiectasis is classified as cystic, cylindrical or varicose, based on the morphologic structure of the airways. Chronic airway inflammation is the essential pathologic feature, resulting from genetic abnormalities that impair airway defense mechanisms or from chronic respiratory infections.[23] Such infections have become relatively rare in the USA; the current prevalence of bronchiectasis is less than 1 in 10 000.

PATHOGENESIS

The principal diseases that cause bronchiectasis are listed in Table 26.4. The genetic diseases cause deficits in airway defense or immunologic mechanisms that permit the development of chronic bacterial infections in the airways. Bacterial and inflammatory cell-derived proteolytic and oxidative molecules cause progressive airway wall damage that eventually produces bronchiectasis. Immune

Table 26.4 Principal causes of bronchiectasis
Genetic
Cystic fibrosis
Immunoglobulin deficiency
Primary ciliary dyskinesia
Infectious
Bordetella pertussis
Tuberculosis
Nontuberculous mycobacteria (especially *M. avium* complex)
Inflammatory
Allergic bronchopulmonary aspergillosis (ABPA)
α_1-Antitrypsin deficiency
Bronchial obstruction
Other
Bronchopulmonary sequestration
Congenital cartilage abnormalities
Yellow nail syndrome

reactions to fungi can produce the central bronchiectasis that is associated with allergic bronchopulmonary aspergillosis (ABPA). Chronic infections with *Mycobacterium tuberculosis*[23] or nontuberculous mycobacteria (particularly *Mycobacterium avium* complex)[24] and *Bordetella pertussis* infections are recognized infectious causes. Bacteria that secondarily infect damaged airways following other injuries probably propagate airway damage, but the time course and relative contributions of the different organisms have not been established.

CLINICAL FEATURES

Daily cough and production of purulent sputum are the most typical symptoms of bronchiectasis. Sputum production can range from less than 10 ml to greater than 150 ml daily and tends to correlate with disease extent and severity. Bronchiectasis associated with cystic fibrosis, which becomes generalized and progresses relentlessly, is described in greater detail below. Occasional individuals have no discernible sputum production ('dry bronchiectasis'). The clinical course is usually of progressive symptoms and respiratory impairment. Airway obstruction progresses and leads to increasing exertional and resting dyspnea. Acute exacerbations may be precipitated by viral or newly acquired bacterial pathogens, as with chronic bronchitis. The main clinical differentiating feature is the quantity of sputum production. In addition to progressive respiratory failure, patients with bronchiectasis are prone to hemoptysis due to hypertrophied bronchial arteries that are closely apposed to the inflamed airways.[25] Hemoptysis from this source can be massive, even fatal.

DIAGNOSIS

Diagnosis is suggested by clinical symptoms and a physical examination with hyperinflated chest and medium- to low-pitched inspiratory crackles and sometimes expiratory wheezes. Chest X-ray may demonstrate hyperinflation and bronchiectatic cysts or dilated bronchi with thickened walls forming tram track patterns radiating from the lung hila. High-resolution chest CT scans readily demonstrate mild and severe forms of bronchiectasis. CT scans have largely replaced bronchography as a diagnostic examination.

Sputum culture may identify characteristic pathogens, including *H. influenzae*, *Strep. pneumoniae* and/or *Pseudomonas aeruginosa*. Sputum acid-fast bacilli (AFB) smears and cultures should be performed to evaluate mycobacterial disease. Spirometry is essential to determine the severity of airway obstruction and to evaluate the course of disease.

MANAGEMENT

Specific etiologies such as tuberculosis should be identified and treated whenever possible. Standard therapy includes measures to clear excess secretions from the airways. Chest physiotherapy based on chest percussion and postural drainage is accepted as the most effective technique. Alternatives such as pneumatic vests and aerobic exercise or flow interrupter valves may be effective, but their use must be individualized. Bronchodilators have a role in patients with objective spirometric or subjective clinical responses. Acute exacerbations are managed with intensification of airway clearance measures and the use of antibiotics directed at pathogens identified in recent sputum cultures. The use of prophylactic oral or inhaled antibiotics has been advocated to control the major symptoms of bronchiectasis and such treatment must be tailored to the individual responses. Surgical resection of localized bronchiectatic lung is occasionally indicated.[26]

Cystic Fibrosis

EPIDEMIOLOGY

Cystic fibrosis is the most common lethal genetic disease in Caucasians.[27] This autosomal recessive disease is caused by mutations in the cystic fibrosis transmembrane conductance regulator (CFTR) gene located on chromosome 7. The incidence is 1 in every 3300 live Caucasian births, with a gene carrier rate of 1 in 29. Other ethnic groups have lower carrier rates, with the Hispanic birth incidence being 1 in 9500, the Native American 1 in 11 200, the African-American one in 15 300 and the Asian 1 in 32 100 live births.

When cystic fibrosis was first described in 1938, survival past infancy was rare. Improved treatments for pancreatic insufficiency, lung infections and other complications have increased the median survival from less than 1 year to more than 36 years (Fig. 26.2). Over 24 500 CF patients have been identified in the United States.[28] The median survival in 2006 was 36.9 years. Adults (≥18 years old) now account for 44.5% of CF patients and survival can extend to 78 years.[28]

PATHOGENESIS

The CFTR gene encodes a 1480 amino acid protein, with 12 membrane-spanning regions, two nucleotide-binding folds and a regulatory ('R') domain (Fig. 26.3). This protein is localized to the apical membranes of epithelia lining the organs affected by the disease, particularly the airways, pancreatic duct, sweat gland duct, intestines and reproductive tract. CFTR protein acts as a Cl⁻ channel[29] and as a regulator of epithelial Na⁺ channels[30] and other Cl⁻ channels.[31] Over 1500 different mutations in the CF gene have been identified, encompassing several functional abnormalities (Fig. 26.4):

- Class I mutations prevent protein production.
- Class II mutations produce proteins that fail to traffic to the apical cell membrane. The most common CF mutation, ΔF508, is in this class; it accounts for 68% of US mutations.
- Class III mutations traffic properly but have defective regulation.
- Class IV mutations traffic properly but have defective Cl⁻ conductance.

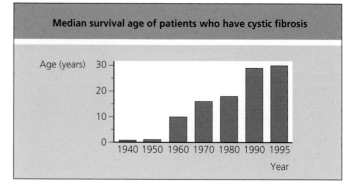

Fig. 26.2 Median survival age of patients who have cystic fibrosis. The median survival age has increased dramatically. Data from Cystic Fibrosis Foundation, Bethesda, MD.

- Some exon splice-site mutations have been labeled class V mutations and may permit transcription of some normal CFTR mRNA, conferring a less severe clinical phenotype.[32]

All classes of mutation alter Cl⁻ permeability and regulation of ion transport in the affected epithelial cells.

The pathogenesis of airways disease in cystic fibrosis is partially understood. CFTR mutations produce decreased Cl⁻ permeability and increased net Na⁺ absorption by bronchial epithelial cells. The effects on bronchiolar epithelial cells and on submucosal gland secretion are not fully defined. It has been suggested that CF mutations lead to relative dehydration of the airway surface liquid.[33] This impairs mucociliary clearance and leads to secondary bacterial infection and airways inflammation. This chronic infection and inflammation forms a vicious cycle that produces progressive airway obstruction, bronchiectasis and eventually respiratory failure. This scheme of pathogenesis is illustrated in Table 26.5. Some existing and potential treatments, directed at the specific pathogenic processes, are indicated.

CLINICAL FEATURES

Cystic fibrosis is classically recognized from the triad of bronchiectatic airways disease, exocrine pancreatic insufficiency and elevated sweat chloride. Most patients have onset of cough and chronic respiratory tract

Fig. 26.3 Representation of the CFTR model, based on structural, hydropathy and expression studies. The membrane-spanning domains are arranged in groups of six, each associated with a nucleotide-binding fold. These features are similar to those of the multidrug resistance 'P' glycoprotein. The 'R' domain is unique to CFTR.

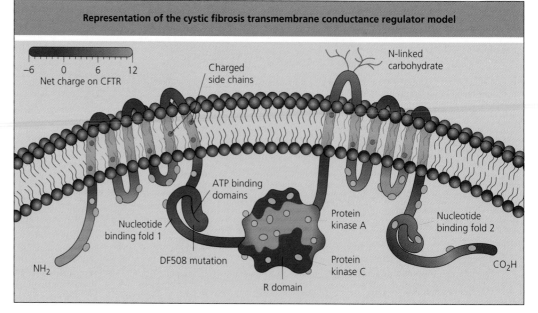

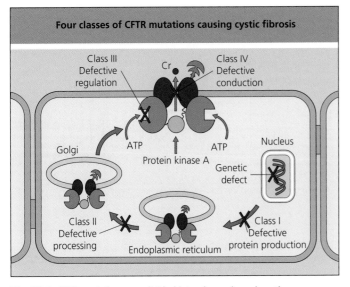

Four classes of CFTR mutations causing cystic fibrosis

Fig. 26.4 CFTR mutations are divided into classes based on the mechanisms of dysfunction. See text for detailed descriptions. Figure provided by Cystic Fibrosis Foundation, Bethesda, MD.

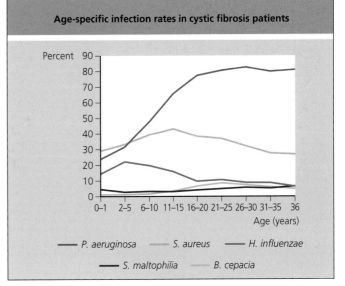

Age-specific infection rates in cystic fibrosis patients

Fig. 26.5 Age-specific infection rates in cystic fibrosis patients. Bacteria isolated from CF sputum samples vary with age and demonstrate the trend toward *Pseudomonas aeruginosa* as the dominant pathogen. Figure provided by Cystic Fibrosis Foundation, Bethesda, MD.

infections during infancy or childhood. Early respiratory tract pathogens include *Staphylococcus aureus* and *Haemophilus influenzae*. *Pseudomonas aeruginosa*, particularly mucoid variants, appears in greater prevalence with increasing age and becomes the dominant pathogen by the teenage years (Fig. 26.5). It is common to isolate several different bacteria from the sputum of adolescent and adult CF patients. *Burkholderia cepacia* has become a significant problem in some centers, and recently non-tuberculous mycobacteria has emerged as a new issue (see Practice Point 15). Pathologically, there is inflammation and obstruction of both bronchioles (Fig. 26.6) and bronchi, with submucosal gland hypertrophy (Fig. 26.7). Bronchiectasis tends to start in the upper lobes and becomes generalized. Chest X-rays show hyperinflated lungs, cystic bronchiectasis and occasionally upper lobe atelectasis (Fig. 26.8).

The clinical course of chronic cough, mucus hypersecretion and airway obstruction is progressive and is punctuated by acute exacerbations, characterized by the features listed in Table 26.6. When such exacerba-

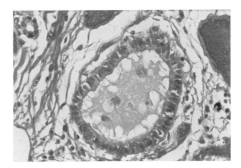

Fig. 26.6 A CF bronchiole is completely occluded by mucoid secretions and surrounded by fibrotic tissue. H&E stain.

Table 26.5 Treatment approaches to cystic fibrosis airways disease

		APPROACH	
Abnormality	**Solution**	**Available**	**Investigational**
Abnormal CF gene	Provide normal gene		Gene therapy
Abnormal CFTR protein	Provide normal protein. Activate mutant form		Protein therapy ?Phosphodiesterase inhibitors ?Phosphatase inhibitors ?Others
Abnormal salt transport	Block Na⁺ uptake. Increase Cl⁻ efflux		Amiloride UTP
?Abnormal mucus	Decrease viscosity	Dornase alpha (rhDNase) (*in vitro*)	Gelsolin
Impaired clearance	Augment ciliary action	Airway clearance techniques	
?*Pseudomonas* infection	Reduce bacterial count	Antibiotics	
Inflammatory response	Decrease host reaction	Anti-inflammatory drugs (corticosteroids, ibuprofen)	Antiproteases. Pentoxifylline. Intravenous immunoglobulin
Bronchiectasis	Replace irreversibly damaged areas	Lung transplantation	

The pathogenesis of cystic fibrosis lung disease is based on a vicious cycle of airway infection, inflammation and obstruction (first column). Treatment can be directed at different pathogenic mechanisms (second column). Currently available and proposed treatment options are shown in final columns. Table provided by Cystic Fibrosis Foundation, Bethesda, MD.

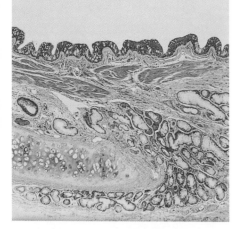

Fig. 26.7 A CF submucosal gland demonstrates marked hypertrophy and dilated gland ducts with mucoid secretions. The surface epithelium has marked goblet cell metaplasia. H&E stain.

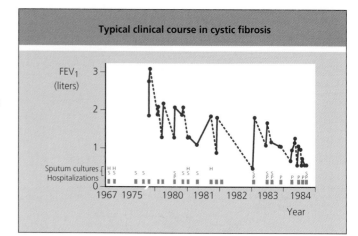

Fig. 26.9 Typical clinical course in CF. Serial pulmonary function measurements (FEV₁) demonstrate a typical clinical course. Measurements are connected by solid lines during therapy for acute exacerbations. The lower bars indicate periods of hospital treatment. Pulmonary function decreases and the exacerbations are more frequent and less responsive to treatment in advanced disease. H, Haemophilus; P, Pseudomonas; S, Staphylococci.

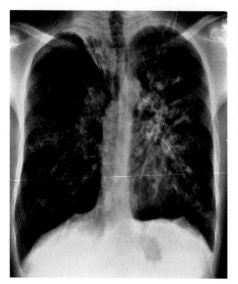

Fig. 26.8 A typical postero-anterior chest X-ray of a 24-year-old man with CF. The lungs are hyperinflated due to airway obstruction and bronchiectasis. The right upper lobe atelectasis is chronic.

and infection with typical bacterial pathogens; exocrine pancreatic insufficiency which occurs in more than 85% of CF patients; and elevated sweat chloride which occurs in more than 98% of patients. The diagnosis initially may be suggested by a family history of CF or by the presence of meconium ileus at birth, noted in 17% of cases. Of patients reported to the Cystic Fibrosis Foundation (CFF) Patient Registry, 51% presented with acute or persistent respiratory symptoms, 43% with failure to thrive or malnutrition, 35% with steatorrhea and 21% with meconium ileus or intestinal obstruction.

Developments in the understanding of the molecular and physiologic pathogenesis of cystic fibrosis have led to additional diagnostic criteria. CFTR mutational analysis is offered by several companies that test for up to 70 common mutations and can detect mutations in about 95% of CF cases. Abnormal CFTR function in airway epithelia can be assessed by *in-vivo* measurements of nasal electrical potential difference and its response to selected modulators of ion transport.[34] The clinical application of these tests has been summarized by a CFF-sponsored Consensus Committee.[35]

Table 26.6 Signs and symptoms of a cystic fibrosis pulmonary exacerbation

- Increased cough
- Increased sputum
- Increased dyspnea
- School or work absenteeism
- Reduced exercise tolerance
- Weight loss >1 kg or >5% of body weight
- Decreased FEV₁ (10% from baseline)
- New chest findings
  - Rales
  - Wheezes
- New radiographic findings

Table provided by Cystic Fibrosis Foundation, Bethesda, MD.

MANAGEMENT (see also Practice Point 15)

Exocrine pancreatic insufficiency and malnutrition are managed with oral pancreatic enzymes and dietary supplements. Pulmonary disease causes the major morbidity in CF and eventually death in 95% of patients. Daily clearance of airway secretions is essential (Table 26.7).[36] This can be accomplished by chest physiotherapy, which enhances sputum production and increases pulmonary function.[37] Physical exercise augments airway clearance and improves cardiovascular function. Special breathing techniques, including forced expiratory technique, autogenic drainage and active cycle of breathing,[38] have been useful in some individuals. Mechanical devices, including the flutter valve[39] and external thoracic compression devices, may improve patient independence, but their efficacy is less well established.

Antibiotics are used extensively. Acute exacerbations are treated with intravenous antibiotics directed at the major pulmonary pathogens, especially *Pseudomonas* species and *Staph. aureus*. Because of the high bacterial burden, two antibiotics with different mechanisms of action and with *in vitro* efficacy against each major bacterium are selected. Pharmacokinetic studies of β-lactams, aminoglycosides and

tions are effectively treated, pulmonary function may return to baseline levels. With more severe disease, exacerbations become more frequent and less reversible, culminating in fatal respiratory failure (Fig. 26.9).

DIAGNOSIS

The standard diagnostic criteria for cystic fibrosis are the combination of characteristic lung disease with airway obstruction, bronchiectasis

Table 26.7 Standard therapy for cystic fibrosis lung disease

Airway clearance
   Chest physical therapy
   Physical exercise
   Special breathing techniques
   Mechanical devices

Antibiotics
   Intravenous
   Oral
   Inhaled

Others
   Bronchodilators
   Supplemental oxygen
   Anti-inflammatory agents (ibuprofen, corticosteroids)
   Recombinant human deoxyribonuclease (rhDNase)

Table 26.8 Inhaled and parenteral antibiotics commonly used for cystic fibrosis

Parenteral (normally two effective agents against each bacterial isolate)	
Class/drug	**Pertinent efficacy**
Aminoglycosides*	
Gentamicin	*Staph. aureus, H. influenzae, Pseudomonas*
Tobramycin	*Staph. aureus, H. influenzae, Pseudomonas*
β-Lactams*	
Ceftazidime	*Pseudomonas*
Piperacillin	*H. influenzae, Pseudomonas*
Ticarcillin–clavulanate	*Staph. aureus, H. influenzae, Pseudomonas*
Monobactam	
Aztreonam	*Pseudomonas*
Carbapenem	
Imipenem–cilastatin	*Staph. aureus, H. influenzae, Pseudomonas*
Fluoroquinolones	
Ciprofloxacin	*Staph. aureus, H. influenzae, Pseudomonas*
Sulfa drugs*	
Trimethoprim–sulfamethoxazole	*Staph. aureus, B. cepacia*
Glycopeptides	
Vancomycin	Oxacillin-resistant *Staph. aureus*

Aerosolized	
Drug	**Common doses**
Tobramycin	80–300 mg q8–12h
Colistimethate sodium	75–150 mg q8–12h
Aztreonam	75 mg q8–12h

*Higher doses required because of increased clearance in cystic fibrosis.

sulfa drugs demonstrate increased clearance in CF patients, necessitating the use of higher doses. Typical antibiotic choices are listed in Table 26.8. Home intravenous antibiotic therapy has cost and convenience advantages,[40] but its clinical efficacy in this setting has not been rigorously established. The benefits of chronic oral antibiotics are controversial, but some aerosolized antibiotics have demonstrated efficacy.[41]

CF patients are particularly susceptible to the complications of massive hemoptysis and pneumothorax. Episodes of massive hemoptysis, defined as more than 240 ml blood per 24 hours, are managed with antibiotics, transient cough suppression and reduction in chest physiotherapy, and bronchial artery embolization.[42] Such therapy is usually effective and does not compromise candidacy for eventual lung transplantation. Large pneumothoraces are managed by chest tube drainage. Recurrent pneumothoraces may require repeated chest tubes or abrasion pleurectomy.[43] Hypoxemia is best treated with supplemental oxygen plus standard pulmonary therapy. Ventilatory assistance can be effectively provided by mask ventilation.[44,45]

Lung transplantation has become an effective form of therapy.[46] From the first heart–lung transplant for CF in 1983 to 2007, more than 3200 heart–lung or sequential double lung transplants (the preferred operation in the USA) for CF have been performed worldwide. Transplant evaluation is indicated when FEV_1 is less than 30% predicted or increasing functional impairment leads to frequent hospitalizations and less response to standard treatments. In May 2005 the United States changed from a waiting time list to the lung allocation score (LAS) that considers urgency and benefit.[47] The 1- and 5-year survivals after lung transplantation for CF are 81% and 55%, respectively. These are comparable to the survival of patients who received lung transplants for other diseases.[48] Deaths in the first year are primarily due to operative complications and infections. After 1 year most deaths are caused by obliterative bronchiolitis, the pathologic marker of chronic rejection.

CONCLUSION

Inflammatory airways diseases are highly prevalent, causing significant morbidity and mortality. Different pathogenic factors cause distinct patterns of disease, including bronchitis and bronchiectasis.

The ability to stop the progression of these diseases is often limited by chronic inflammation and by structural alterations in the airways. Nevertheless, antibiotics, anti-inflammatory drugs and other forms of therapy can modulate acute exacerbations and, potentially, the progression of these diseases. Elucidation of the pathogenic mechanisms, as is being done in cystic fibrosis, may uncover new and more effective means of treatment. The diagnostic tests, continued monitoring and choice of therapeutic options must be tailored to the individual clinical presentation and responses of each patient.

REFERENCES

References for this chapter can be found online at http://www.expertconsult.com

Chapter | **27** | *Michael S Niederman*

Community-acquired pneumonia

INTRODUCTION

Pneumonia is a respiratory infection of the alveolar space, which can vary from a mild outpatient illness to a severe illness necessitating hospitalization and intensive care. In 2004, pneumonia, along with influenza, was the eighth leading cause of death in the USA, the sixth leading cause of death in those over age 65, and the principal cause of death from infectious diseases.[1] When the infection occurs in patients who are living in the community it is termed community acquired pneumonia (CAP), while it is called nosocomial pneumonia if it arises in patients who are already in hospital.[2,3] However, the distinction between these two forms of infection is becoming increasingly blurred because of the complexity of patients who are now living outwith hospital, including those in nursing homes, those receiving chronic hemodialysis and those recently admitted to hospital, all of whom have contact with the health-care environment and may import multidrug-resistant (MDR) organisms when they come to the hospital with 'healthcare-associated pneumonia' (HCAP). Thus, the relationship between bacteriology and the site of origin of infection is a reflection of several factors, including the co-morbid illnesses present in the patient who develops pneumonia, their host-defense status and their environmental exposure to specific pathogens.[4] This discussion focuses on patients who develop pneumonia out of the hospital (including CAP and HCAP), who are not HIV infected and who do not have traditional immune suppression (cancer chemotherapy, immune suppressive medications).

The complexity of CAP management has increased in recent years, not only because of the presence of more co-morbid illness in at-risk individuals, but also because the etiologic pathogens are changing. Historically, CAP was regarded as a bacterial illness caused by one pathogen, *Streptococcus pneumoniae*, but now the number of identified pathogens has expanded to include not only bacteria, but also viruses (influenza), fungi and a number of other recently identified organisms (e.g. *Legionella* spp. and *Chlamydophila pneumoniae*). In addition to an expanding number of etiologies, the ability to treat CAP is being challenged by the rising frequency of antimicrobial resistance among many bacteria, including pneumococcus.

EPIDEMIOLOGY

In 1994, over 5.6 million people were diagnosed with CAP in the USA, but the majority, 4.6 million, were treated out of the hospital.[5] Data from 2005 showed that there were 1.3 million hospitalizations for pneumonia in the USA, more in females than males, and approximately 60% in those over the age of 65.[1] Community-acquired pneumonia has a seasonal variability, with a rise in frequency during the winter months, paralleling the times of influenza and viral infection,

illnesses which can interfere with host defense and predispose to secondary bacterial pneumonia. Certain pathogens, such as *Legionella* spp., are more common in the late summer and early fall, reflecting the water-borne sources of this organism.

The cost of care for patients with CAP in the USA was estimated to be over $40 billion in 2005, including both direct and indirect costs.[1] The elderly account for a disproportionate amount of this cost, largely because they often require inpatient treatment, reflecting a high frequency of co-morbid illness. Although those over age 65 account for only about one-third of all cases of CAP, they are responsible for 60% of those hospitalized with CAP.

The elderly have both an increased incidence of pneumonia and an increased mortality, compared to younger populations. The high frequency and enhanced mortality of pneumonia in older patients are well known, but controversy still continues about whether this is a consequence of aging itself or the result of the co-morbid illnesses that become increasingly common in the aging population.

PATHOLOGY AND PATHOGENESIS

Pneumonia is an infection of the gas exchanging units of the lung, most commonly caused by bacteria, but occasionally by viruses, fungi, parasites and other infectious agents. In the immunocompetent individual, it is characterized by a brisk filling of the alveolar space with inflammatory cells and fluid. If the alveolar infection involves an entire anatomic lobe of the lung, it is termed 'lobar pneumonia'. Multilobar illness can be present in some instances and may lead to more severe clinical manifestations. When the alveolar process occurs in a distribution that is patchy, and adjacent to bronchi, without filling an entire lobe, it is termed a 'bronchopneumonia'.

Pneumonia occurs when a patient's host defenses are overwhelmed by an infectious pathogen. This can happen because the patient has an inadequate immune response, often as the result of underlying chronic medical diseases (congestive heart failure, diabetes, renal failure, chronic obstructive lung disease, malnutrition), because of anatomic abnormalities (endobronchial obstruction, bronchiectasis), as a result of acute illness-associated immune dysfunction (as can occur with sepsis or acute lung injury) or because of therapy-induced dysfunction of the immune system (corticosteroids, endotracheal intubation). Some commonly used therapies may actually reduce the mortality risk of pneumonia, including angiotensin-converting enzyme (ACE) inhibitors and statins.[6] Admission hyperglycemia may increase mortality risk in CAP, but it is unclear if therapy can mitigate this risk.[7]

Pneumonia can even occur in patients who have an adequate immune system if the host defense system is overwhelmed by a large inoculum of micro-organisms, which can occur in a patient with massive aspiration of gastric contents. Patients with impaired gastro-intestinal or neurologic function may also aspirate, and this process involves failure to protect the lower respiratory tract from the entry of oropharyngeal secretions, which are often overgrown with potentially pathogenic Gram-negative bacteria.[8] In patients outside the hospital, a normal immune system can also be overcome by a particularly virulent organism to which the patient has no pre-existing immunity (such as certain bacteria or viruses) or to which the patient has an inability to form an adequate acute immune response. The epidemic spread of severe acute respiratory syndrome (SARS), due to a virulent virus, is one example of this phenomenon.

Bacteria can enter the lung via several routes, but aspiration from a previously colonized oropharynx is the most common mechanism for pneumonia.[9] Although most pneumonias result from microaspiration, some patients can also aspirate large volumes of bacteria if they have impaired neurologic protection of the upper airway (stroke, seizure) or if they have intestinal illnesses that predispose to vomiting. Other routes of entry include inhalation, which applies primarily to viruses, *Legionella pneumophila* and *Mycobacterium tuberculosis*; hematogenous dissemination from extrapulmonary sites of infection (right-sided endocarditis); and direct extension from contiguous sites of infection (such as liver abscess).

Based on these mechanisms, previously healthy individuals often develop infection with virulent pathogens such as viruses, *Legionella pneumophila*, *Mycoplasma pneumoniae*, *Chlamydophila pneumoniae* and *Strep. pneumoniae* (pneumococcus). On the other hand, chronically ill patients can be infected by these organisms, as well as by organisms that commonly colonize the oropharynx (primarily enteric Gram-negatives) but only cause infection when immune responses are inadequate. These organisms include enteric Gram-negative bacteria (*Escherichia coli*, *Klebsiella pneumoniae*, *Pseudomonas aeruginosa*, *Acinetobacter* spp.), as well as fungi.

Severe forms of pneumonia develop when the infection is not contained (inadequate immune response) or, alternatively, if the inflammatory response to infection is unable to be localized to the site of infection (excessive immune response) and it 'spills over' into the systemic circulation (sepsis) or to the rest of the lung (acute respiratory distress syndrome). The normal lung immune response to infection is generally 'compartmentalized' and thus most patients with unilateral pneumonia have an inflammatory response that is limited to the site of infection. In patients with localized pneumonia, tumor necrosis factor (TNF), interleukin (IL)-6 and IL-8 levels are increased in the pneumonic lung and generally not increased in the uninvolved lung or in the serum.[10] Patients with severe pneumonia have increased serum levels of TNF and IL-6. It remains uncertain why localization does not occur in all individuals, but it is likely that genetic polymorphisms in the immune response may explain some of these differences, with patients who have certain inherited patterns of response being more prone than others to severe forms of pneumonia, and even mortality from this illness.[11,12] For example, CAP severity is increased with genetic changes in the IL-10 1082 locus, which are often present along with changes in the TNF 308 locus.[11,12] Currently, there are a large number of genes that have been identified as being able to affect the severity and outcome of CAP, but the ability to use this information to impact patient management does not currently exist.

ETIOLOGY

Etiologic pathogens (overview)

An etiologic pathogen is identified in only about half of all CAP patients, reflecting the limited value of even extensive diagnostic testing and the likelihood that we do not know all the organisms that can cause this illness. For example, in the past three decades, a variety of new CAP pathogens have been identified, including *Legionella pneumophila*, *Chlamydophila pneumoniae*, hantavirus, metapneumoviruses and coronaviruses (including the SARS virus). In addition, antibiotic-resistant variants of common pathogens such as drug-resistant *Streptococcus*

pneumoniae (DRSP) and methicillin-resistant *Staphylococcus aureus* (MRSA) have become more prominent.

The number one pathogen for all patient populations with CAP is *Strep. pneumoniae*, or pneumococcus (including DRSP), and some studies have suggested that it may be responsible for many of the patients with no established etiologic diagnosis using standard diagnostic methodology.[13] In addition, atypical pathogens such as *M. pneumoniae*, *C. pneumoniae* and *Legionella pneumophila* are also common in patients with CAP, but may exist as co-pathogens, along with bacterial organisms.[14] Viruses may be present in up to 20% of all patients, particularly influenza, parainfluenza, adenovirus and respiratory syncytial virus.[15] Because a diagnosis of viral pneumonia requires specialized testing, usually acute and convalescent titers, this diagnosis is often not established. *Haemophilus influenzae* is a common organism in patients who smoke cigarettes and in those with chronic obstructive lung disease. Enteric Gram-negatives are not common causes of CAP, being found in only a few patients, and most of those with these organisms actually have HCAP which is treated similarly to nosocomial pneumonia.[3,16] Seasonal variations of pathogens may also be seen – pneumococcus and respiratory viruses are more common in winter in temperate countries.

In approaching management, it is important to stratify patients into different populations that are at risk for infection with specific pathogens (Table 27.1). The classification is based on the severity

Table 27.1 Common pathogens causing CAP and HCAP in specific patient populations (in order of decreasing frequency)

Outpatient, no cardiopulmonary disease or modifying factors	*Streptococcus pneumoniae*, *Mycoplasma pneumoniae*, *Chlamydophila pneumoniae* (alone or as mixed infection), *Haemophilus influenzae*, respiratory viruses, others (*Legionella* spp., *Mycobacterium tuberculosis*, endemic fungi)
Outpatient, with cardiopulmonary disease and/or modifying factors, or HCAP with no resistance risk factors	All of the above plus DRSP, enteric Gram-negatives and possibly anaerobes (with aspiration)
Inpatient, with cardiopulmonary disease and/or modifying factors, or HCAP with no resistance risk factors	*Strep. pneumoniae* (including DRSP), *H. influenzae*, *Mycoplasma pneumoniae*, *C. pneumoniae*, mixed infection (bacteria plus atypical pathogen), enteric Gram-negatives, anaerobes (aspiration), viruses, *Legionella* spp., others (*Mycobacterium tuberculosis*, endemic fungi, *Pneumocystis jirovecii*)
Inpatient, with no cardiopulmonary disease or modifying factors	All of the above, but DRSP and enteric Gram-negatives are unlikely
Severe CAP, with no risks for *Pseudomonas aeruginosa*	*Strep. pneumoniae* (including DRSP), *Legionella* spp., *H. influenzae*, enteric Gram-negative bacilli, *Staphylococcus aureus*, *Mycoplasma pneumoniae*, respiratory viruses, others (*C. pneumoniae*, *Mycobacterium tuberculosis*, endemic fungi)
Severe CAP, with risks for *P. aeruginosa*, or HCAP with resistance risk factors	All of the above pathogens, plus *P. aeruginosa*

DRSP, drug-resistant *Streptococcus pneumoniae*; HCAP, health-care-associated pneumonia.

of illness and the presence of clinical risk factors for specific pathogens, referred to as 'modifying factors'. Patients with severe CAP may have a slightly different spectrum of organisms, being commonly infected with pneumococcus, atypical pathogens (especially *Legionella* spp.), enteric Gram-negatives (including *P. aeruginosa*), *Staph. aureus* and *H. influenzae*. As mentioned, HCAP patients are often at risk for infection with MDR Gram-negatives and Gram-positives, but not all HCAP patients are at the same risk (Table 27.1). In fact, these organisms are only a consideration for the HCAP patient with at least two of three risk factors, which include severe illness, poor functional status and prior antibiotic therapy.[16] Table 27.2 shows that certain clinical conditions are associated with specific pathogens and these associations should be considered in all patients when obtaining a history. One common, and important, association is infection with MRSA in patients with recent influenza infection.[17]

Table 27.2 Clinical associations with specific pathogens

Condition	Commonly encountered pathogens
Alcoholism	*Streptococcus pneumoniae* (including DRSP), anaerobes, Gram-negative bacilli (possibly *Klebsiella pneumoniae*)
Chronic obstructive pulmonary disease/ current or former smoker	*Strep. pneumoniae, Haemophilus influenzae, Moraxella catarrhalis, Legionella* spp., enteric Gram-negatives
Residence in nursing home	*Strep. pneumoniae*, Gram-negative bacilli, *H. influenzae, Staphylococcus aureus*, anaerobes, *Chlamydophila pneumoniae*; consider *Mycobacterium tuberculosis*
Poor dental hygiene	Anaerobes
Bat exposure	*Histoplasma capsulatum*
Bird exposure	*Chlamydia psittaci, Cryptococcus neoformans, Histoplasma capsulatum*
Rabbit exposure	*Francisella tularensis*
Travel to south-west USA	Coccidioidomycosis, hantavirus in selected areas
Exposure to farm animals or parturient cats	*Coxiella burnetii* (Q fever)
Travel to South East Asia	*Mycobacterium tuberculosis, Burkholderia pseudomallei*, SARS virus
Suspected bioterrorism	Anthrax, smallpox, pneumonic plague
Endobronchial obstruction	Anaerobes
Post influenza pneumonia	*Strep. pneumoniae, Staph. aureus, H. influenzae*
Structural disease of lung (bronchiectasis, cystic fibrosis, etc.)	*Pseudomonas aeruginosa, P. cepacia* or *Staph. aureus*
Recent antibiotic therapy	Pneumococcus resistant to the class of agents to which the patient was recently exposed, enteric Gram-negatives

DRSP, drug-resistant *Streptococcus pneumoniae*; SARS, severe acute respiratory syndrome.

SPECIFIC ORGANISMS

Streptococcus pneumoniae

Streptococcus pneumoniae is the most common pathogen for CAP in all patient populations, possibly even among those without an etiology recognized by routine diagnostic testing. In one study, when no etiologic pathogen was defined by conventional testing, transthoracic needle aspirates, analyzed with polymerase chain reaction (PCR) probes, identified pneumococcus in half of the patients in whom the needle provided a diagnosis.[13] The organism is a Gram-positive, lancet-shaped diplococcus, of which there are 84 different serotypes, each with a distinct antigenic polysaccharide capsule, but 85% of all infections are caused by one of 23 serotypes, which are now included in a vaccine.

Infection is most common in the winter and early spring, which may relate to the finding that up to 70% of patients have a preceding viral illness. The organism spreads from person to person and commonly colonizes the oropharynx before it causes pneumonia. Pneumonia develops when colonizing organisms are aspirated into a lung that is unable to contain the aspirated inoculum. Patients at risk include the elderly; those with asplenia, multiple myeloma, congestive heart failure, alcoholism; after influenza; and in patients with chronic lung disease. Individuals with HIV infection develop pneumococcal pneumonia with bacteremia more commonly than in healthy populations of the same age.

The classic radiographic pattern is a lobar consolidation; however, bronchopneumonia can also occur and is a common pattern in some series. Bacteremia is present in up to 20% of hospitalized patients with this infection, and although the impact of this finding on mortality is uncertain, its presence probably does not lead to a worse outcome. Extrapulmonary complications include meningitis, empyema, arthritis, endocarditis and brain abscess.

Drug-resistant pneumococci (DRSP)

Since the mid-1990s, antibiotic resistance among pneumococci has become increasingly common in the USA and penicillin resistance, along with resistance to other common antibiotics (macrolides, trimethoprim-sulfamethoxazole, selected cephalosporins), is present in over 40% of these organisms, using older definitions of resistance. Fortunately, in the USA, a large number of penicillin-resistant organisms are of the sensitive and 'intermediate' type. In other parts of the world (e.g. the UK) rates of DRSP have remained low over the last decade. Recently, the definitions of resistance have changed for nonmeningeal infection, with sensitive being defined by a penicillin minimum inhibitory concentration (MIC) ≤ 2 mg/L, intermediate as an MIC of 4 mg/l and resistant as an MIC ≥ 8 mg/l.[18] While the clinical impact of resistance on outcomes such as mortality was hard to show using older definitions, with the new definitions of resistance very few pathogens will be defined as resistant; however, those that are may affect outcome. In fact, most experts believe that CAP caused by organisms with a penicillin MIC of ≥ 4 mg/l, still an uncommon finding, can lead to an increased risk of death.[19]

Later studies have shown that higher levels of resistance can affect outcomes such as mortality and the development of suppurative complications such as empyema. The relationship of resistance to illness severity is complex and in some studies severity of illness may be reduced in patients with resistant organisms, implying a loss of virulence among organisms that become resistant.

Resistance of pneumococcus has even been reported to the quinolones, which are ordinarily a reliable class of antibiotic for these organisms. In general, one important risk factor for resistance is repeated use of a given agent in the same patient. In fact, pneumococcal resistance to β-lactams (penicillins and cephalosporins), macrolides and quinolones is more likely if a patient has received the same agent in the past 3 months.[20] With these data in mind, new guidelines have suggested that CAP patients not receive the same antibiotic as in the recent past, with the cutoff of defining this time interval being within the past 3 months.

Atypical pathogens

Originally the term 'atypical' was used to describe the nonclassic clinical features of infection with certain organisms, but recent studies have suggested that the term does not accurately describe a unique pneumonia syndrome related to specific pathogens. However, the term has been retained to refer to a group of organisms which includes *M. pneumoniae*, *C. pneumoniae* and *Legionella*, a group of organisms that cannot be reliably eradicated by β-lactam therapy (penicillins and cephalosporins) but must be treated with a macrolide, a tetracycline or a quinolone. The frequency of these organisms as CAP pathogens has varied in studies, with recent data from North America and elsewhere suggesting that they may be present in up to 60% of CAP episodes, and that they can serve as co-pathogens, along with bacteria, in up to 40% of patients.[14] When mixed infection is present, particularly with *C. pneumoniae* and pneumococcus, it may lead to a more complex course and a longer length of stay than if a single pathogen is present. In patients with severe CAP, atypical pathogens can be present in almost 25% of all patients, but the responsible organism may vary over time. While atypical pathogens have been thought to be most common in young and healthy individuals, some population data have shown that they are present in patients of all ages, including the elderly in nursing homes.[21]

Studies reporting a high frequency of atypical pathogens have made the diagnosis with serologic testing, which may not be as accurate and specific as culture and antigen identification. The importance of atypical pathogens has been suggested by a number of studies of inpatients, including those with bacteremic pneumococcal pneumonia, showing a mortality benefit from therapies that include a macrolide or quinolone, agents that would be active against these organisms.[22,23] Atypical organism pneumonia may not be a constant phenomenon, and the frequency of infection may vary over the course of time and with geography. In one study, the benefit of providing empiric therapy directed at atypical pathogens was variable, being more important in some calendar years than in others.[23] Differing views about the importance of atypical pathogens have led to disparate recommendations about whether they should be covered by empiric therapy, with some CAP guidelines recommending routine coverage, while others, particularly from the UK and Europe, suggest otherwise.

Legionella pneumophila

This small, weakly staining, Gram-negative bacillus was first characterized after an epidemic in 1976, and can occur either sporadically or in epidemic form. At present, although multiple serogroups of the species *L. pneumophila* have been described, serogroup 1 is the most commonly diagnosed and can be identified with a urinary antigen test. The other species that commonly causes human illness is *Legionella micdadei*. *Legionella* is a water-borne pathogen that can emanate from air conditioning equipment, drinking water, lakes and river banks, water faucets, saunas and shower heads. Infection is more common in the summer and early fall, and is generally caused by inhalation of an infected aerosol generated by a contaminated water source. When a water system becomes infected in an institution, endemic outbreaks may occur, as has been the case in some nursing homes and hospitals. In its sporadic form, *Legionella* may account for 7–15% of all cases of CAP, being a particular concern in patients with severe forms of illness.

The varying incidence of *Legionella* infection among admitted patients is a reflection of geographic and seasonal variability in infection rates, as well as the extent of diagnostic testing. For a serologic diagnosis, it is necessary to collect both acute and convalescent titers. The urinary antigen test is the single most accurate acute diagnostic test for *Legionella*, but is specific to serogroup 1 infection. In recent years, most cases have been diagnosed with urinary antigen and there has been less reliance on serology and culture.[24] With this increased reliance on urinary antigen testing, the case fatality rate of *Legionella* has fallen, possibly reflecting diagnosis of less severe illness than in the past.[24]

It is difficult to identify the microbial etiology of CAP on the basis of clinical and radiographic features and a unique presentation of *Legionella* is uncommon. The classic clinical syndrome is characterized by high fever, chills, headache, myalgias and leukocytosis, along with a history of preceding diarrhea, early onset of mental confusion, hyponatremia, relative bradycardia and liver function abnormalities. Symptoms are rapidly progressive, and the patient may appear to be quite toxic, so this diagnosis should always be considered in patients admitted to the intensive care unit (ICU) with CAP.

Mycoplasma pneumoniae

Mycoplasma pneumoniae can cause CAP year-round, with a slight increase in the fall and winter. All age groups are affected, and although it is common in those less than 20 years of age, it is also seen in older adults. Respiratory infection occurs after the organism is inhaled and then binds via neuraminic acid receptors to the airway epithelium. An inflammatory response with neutrophils, lymphocytes and macrophages then follows, accompanied by the formation of IgM and then IgG antibody. Some of the observed pneumonitis may be mediated by the host response to the organism rather than by direct tissue injury by the organism. Up to 40% of infected individuals will have circulating immune complexes.

Although *Mycoplasma* causes pneumonia, the infection is often characterized by its extrapulmonary manifestations such as upper respiratory tract symptoms, including sore throat and earache (with hemorrhagic or bullous myringitis). Pleural effusion is seen in at least 20% of patients although it may be small. Other manifestations include neurologic illness such as meningoencephalitis, meningitis, transverse myelitis and cranial nerve palsies. The most common extrapulmonary finding is an IgM autoantibody that is directed against the I antigen on the red blood cell and causes cold agglutination of the erythrocyte. Although up to 75% of patients may have this antibody and a positive Coombs' test, clinically significant autoimmune hemolytic anemia is uncommon. The extrapulmonary manifestations may follow the respiratory symptoms by as long as 3 weeks.

Gram-negative bacteria

The most common Gram-negative organism causing CAP is *H. influenzae*, an organism seen in the elderly and in those who smoke cigarettes, or who have a history of alcoholism or chronic bronchitis. *H. influenzae* is a coccobacillary rod that can be either a typeable (encapsulated) or nontypeable organism, and can lead to bronchopneumonia and rarely empyema. Encapsulated organisms require a more elaborate host response and thus are more virulent than unencapsulated organisms. However, several studies have shown that in adults, particularly those with chronic obstructive pulmonary disease (COPD), infection with unencapsulated bacteria is common. The encapsulated type of organism may cause bacteremic pneumonia in some patients, particularly in those with segmental pneumonias as opposed to those with bronchopneumonia.

Enteric Gram-negatives are generally not common in CAP unless the patients are elderly and have chronic cardiac or pulmonary disease, have HCAP or are alcoholic. In one study, the identified risk factors for Gram-negative CAP were probably aspiration, prior hospitalization, prior antibiotic therapy and pulmonary co-morbidity.[25] In these patients, organisms such as *E. coli* and *K. pneumoniae* can be found. Although *P. aeruginosa* is an uncommon cause of CAP, it can be isolated from patients with bronchiectasis, in those with severe forms of CAP and in patients with pulmonary co-morbidity and prior hospitalization.[2,25] Gram-negative CAP was often a severe illness, with septic shock and hyponatremia, and occurred especially in patients with malignancy, cardiac disease and a history of cigarette smoking.[26]

While the frequency of enteric Gram-negatives in CAP has been controversial, many of the patients at risk for these organisms would now be re-classified as HCAP. It is still important to identify patients at risk, since infection with a Gram-negative increased the chance of dying by more than threefold, with a mortality rate of 32% in one study.[25] These patients also need ICU admission and mechanical ventilation more often than patients infected with other organisms. Patients with HCAP severe enough to require mechanical ventilation, admitted from a nursing home and with risk factors for aspiration (intestinal or neurologic risk factors), are particularly at risk for infection with enteric Gram-negatives, more than any other pathogens, including anaerobes.

Anaerobes

These organisms have always been a concern in patients with poor dentition who aspirate oral contents, and those at risk have been patients with neurologic or swallowing disorders, as well as individuals who abuse alcohol and opiate drugs. As mentioned, these patients may also be at risk for infection with enteric Gram-negatives and in the study cited above, many of the aspiration-prone patients who had anaerobes recovered, had them along with aerobic Gram-negatives and their presence did not correlate with poor oral hygiene. Many of these patients received inadequate therapy for anaerobes, yet most recovered, raising a question about whether these organisms really need to be treated. These findings suggest that anaerobes may not always be pathogens but may be colonizers in the institutionalized elderly, including those with aspiration risk factors.

Staphylococcus aureus

Community-acquired pneumonia can also be caused by this organism, which can lead to severe illness and to cavitary pneumonia. This organism can also seed the lung hematogenously from a vegetation in patients with right-sided endocarditis or from septic venous thrombophlebitis (from central venous catheter or jugular vein infection). When a patient develops postinfluenza pneumonia, *Staph. aureus* can lead to secondary bacterial infection, along with pneumococcus and *H. influenzae*. In the past several years, community-acquired strains of methicillin-resistant *Staph. aureus* (CA-MRSA) have emerged, primarily in skin and soft tissue infections, but also as a cause of severe CAP. CA-MRSA is a clonal disease, emanating from the USA 300 clone of *Staph. aureus*, and is clinically and bacteriologically different from the strains of MRSA that cause nosocomial pneumonia.[17] In addition, it can infect previously healthy individuals, and the classic clinical presentation of this pathogen causing CAP is as a complication of a preceding viral or influenza infection. The illness is characterized by a severe, bilateral, necrotizing pneumonia. Since the pathogenesis of pneumonia due to this organism may be related to toxin production by the bacteria, therapy may need to involve both an antibacterial agent and an antitoxin-producing agent.[27]

Viruses

Although the incidence of viral pneumonia is difficult to define, during epidemic times influenza should be considered as it can lead to primary viral pneumonia or to secondary bacterial pneumonia. One careful study of over 300 nonimmunocompromised CAP patients looked for viral pneumonia by paired serologies and found that 18% had viral pneumonia, with about half being pure viral infection and the others being mixed with bacterial pneumonia.[15] Influenza (A more than B), parainfluenza and adenovirus were the most commonly identified viral agents.

Although influenza A and B are the most common causes of viral pneumonia, they can be prevented to a large extent by vaccination. There are also other viruses that can cause severe forms of pneumonia, as evidenced by the recent experience with SARS, which demonstrated the potential of epidemic, person-to-person spread of a virulent respiratory viral infection.

CLINICAL FEATURES

Symptoms and physical findings

Patients with an intact immune system who develop CAP generally have 'typical' respiratory symptoms such as cough, sputum production and dyspnea, along with fever and other complaints. Cough is the most common finding and is present in up to 80% of all patients, but is less common in those with impaired immune responsiveness, such as the elderly, those with serious co-morbidity or individuals coming from nursing homes (HCAP).[4] Pleuritic chest pain is also a common symptom in CAP and its absence has been identified as a poor prognostic finding.[28]

When pneumonia occurs in elderly patients, it can have a non-respiratory presentation with symptoms of confusion, falling, failure to thrive, altered functional capacity or deterioration in a pre-existing medical illness, such as congestive heart failure. Patients with advanced age often have a longer duration of symptoms such as cough, sputum production, dyspnea, fatigue, anorexia, myalgia and abdominal pain than younger patients. In addition, they have delirium or acute confusion more often than younger patients. Very few elderly patients with pneumonia are considered well nourished, with kwashiorkor-like malnutrition being the predominant type of nutritional defect and the one associated with delirium on initial presentation.[29]

Physical findings of pneumonia include tachypnea, focal crackles, rhonchi and signs of consolidation (egophony, bronchial breath sounds, dullness to percussion). Other physical findings can be signs of pleural effusion, metastatic infection (arthritis, endocarditis, meningitis) or extrapulmonary manifestations that can occur with *M. pneumoniae* or *C. pneumoniae*. One of the most important physical assessments in CAP is a careful measurement of respiratory rate, which can have both diagnostic and prognostic relevance. In the elderly, an elevation of respiratory rate may be the initial presenting sign of pneumonia, preceding other clinical findings by as much as 1–2 days.[30] In general, tachypnea is the most common finding in elderly patients; it is present in over 60% of all patients, but occurs more often in the elderly than in younger patients with pneumonia. Measurement of respiratory rate also has prognostic significance and the presence of a respiratory rate greater than 30 per minute is one of several factors associated with increased risk of mortality.

Typical vs atypical pneumonia syndromes

In the past, the clinical and radiographic features of CAP were characterized as fitting into a pattern of either 'typical' or 'atypical' symptoms which could be used to predict a specific etiologic agent. The typical pneumonia syndrome, attributed to pneumococcus and other bacterial pathogens, is characterized by sudden onset of high fever, shaking chills, pleuritic chest pain, lobar consolidation and a toxic-appearing patient with the production of purulent sputum. The atypical pneumonia syndrome, which is characterized by a subacute illness, nonproductive cough, headache, diarrhea or other systemic complaints, can be the result of infection with *M. pneumoniae*, *C. pneumoniae*, *Legionella* spp. or viruses, but bacterial pneumonia can present in this fashion if the patient has an impaired immune response.

Recent studies have shown that this approach is not highly accurate and there is only a weak relationship between clinical features and the etiologic pathogen, primarily because host, as well as pathogenic, factors play a role in defining patient symptoms. Clinical features have been shown to be only about 40% accurate in differentiating pneumococcus, *M. pneumoniae* and other pathogens from one another.[2,31] The limitations of clinical features in defining the microbial etiology also apply to evaluations of radiographic patterns.

Clinical assessment of pneumonia severity

Careful evaluation of illness severity is necessary to guide decisions about whether to hospitalize a patient, and if so, whether to admit the patient to the ICU. Although a number of models have been developed to predict mortality, and they have been proposed to guide the admission decision, the decision to admit a patient to the hospital should be based on social as well as medical considerations and remains an 'art of medicine' determination. In general the hospital should be used to observe patients who have multiple risk factors for a poor outcome, those who have decompensation of a chronic illness or those who need therapies not easily administered at home (oxygen, intravenous fluids, cardiac monitoring).

Risk factors for a poor outcome include a respiratory rate ≥30/min, age ≥65 years, systolic blood pressure <90 mmHg, diastolic BP ≤60 mmHg, multilobar pneumonia, confusion, blood urea nitrogen (BUN) >19.6 mg/dl, Pao_2 <60 mmHg (on room air), $Paco_2$ >50 mmHg, respiratory or metabolic acidosis, or signs of systemic sepsis.[2] The two best-studied and most widely used prediction rules for pneumonia severity are the Pneumonia Severity Index (PSI) and the CURB-65 rule, a modification of a prognostic model developed by the British Thoracic Society.[28,32] The PSI uses multiple demographic and historic findings, physical findings and laboratory data, each assigned a point score, and the total score is used to categorize patients into one of five classes, each with a different risk of death. Although this tool has worked well to define mortality risk, it has had variable success in predicting site of care and is limited by its complexity and its failure to always recognize the most severely ill patients, especially if they do not have underlying co-morbid illness.[33] The CURB-65 rule is simpler, using only five assessments: Confusion (due to the pneumonia), blood Urea nitrogen >7 mmol/l, Respiratory rate ≥30/min, Blood pressure of <90 mmHg systolic or ≤60 mmHg diastolic, and age ≥65 years. Each of the five criteria receives 1 point, and the score falls between 0 and 5, with mortality risk rising with the score.

In recent studies, both tools have worked equally well to identify patients at low risk of dying, but the CURB-65 has been more discriminating in recognizing patients who need ICU care (score of at least 3) and who have the highest risk of death.[34] On the other hand, the CURB-65 does not account well for patients with decompensated chronic illness that results from the presence of CAP. This is because the PSI weights advanced age and chronic illness very heavily, whereas the CURB-65 model includes age as only one of several risk factors and co-morbid illness is not measured, but instead most of the score is based on acute physiologic abnormalities. Neither prediction model includes 'social factors' and clearly these issues need to be included in patient assessment, paying attention to whether the patient has a stable home environment for outpatient care, an ability to take oral medications, the absence of acute alcohol or drug intoxication, and stability of other acute and chronic medical problems.

There is no specific rule for who requires intensive care, but in general ICU admission (in the USA) is associated with a mortality rate of at least 30%, compared to a mortality rate of 12% for all admitted patients and a 1–5% mortality rate for outpatients.[35] When the ICU is used early in the hospital stay, the mortality rate is lower than if patients are first admitted to the ward, then deteriorate and move to the ICU.[36] Earlier studies that suggested a limited benefit from ICU admission generally found that patients were admitted too late in the course of illness to benefit, thus emphasizing the need for accurately assessing mortality risk when the patient is first evaluated.

Radiographic abnormalities

Most patients are diagnosed and treated for CAP after the physician obtains a chest radiograph which shows the presence of a new infiltrate, although not all outpatients have access to this evaluation. However, even when the radiograph is negative, if the patient has appropriate symptoms and focal physical findings, pneumonia may still be present. When CT scanning has been used in patients with clinical signs and symptoms of CAP, it can demonstrate abnormalities in some patients with a negative chest radiograph and the abnormalities

are generally more extensive on CT scan than on chest radiograph.[37] Thus, if a symptomatic patient has an initially negative chest radiograph, it should be repeated after 24–48 hours. It is uncertain why a chest film would initially be negative, but the idea that hydration, especially in the elderly, is the explanation is not proven and falls into the realm of anecdotal reports.

Numerous studies have documented that the pattern of radiographic abnormality cannot reliably be used to predict the etiology of infection. Pleural effusion may appear on the initial chest radiograph and if present, it is necessary to distinguish empyema from a simple parapneumonic effusion by sampling the pleural fluid.

DIAGNOSTIC TESTING

Recommended testing (Table 27.3)

History

Historic data should be collected to suggest the presence of specific unusual pathogens, in addition to the likely organisms[2] (see Tables 27.1 and 27.2). For example, if the presentation is subacute following contact with birds, rats or rabbits, then the possibility of psittacosis, leptospirosis, tularemia or plague should be considered. *Coxiella burnetii* (Q fever) is a concern with exposure to parturient cats, cattle, sheep or goats; *Francisella tularensis* is a concern with rabbit exposure; hantavirus with exposure to mice droppings in endemic areas; *Chlamydia psittacii* with exposure to turkeys or infected birds; and *Legionella* with exposure to contaminated water sources (saunas). Following influenza, superinfection with pneumococcus, *Staph. aureus* (including MRSA) and *H. influenzae* should be considered. The onset of respiratory failure after a preceding viral illness should lead to suspicion of a viral pneumonia. Endemic fungi, (coccidioidomycosis, histoplasmosis and blastomycosis) occur in well-defined geographic areas and may present acutely with symptoms which overlap with acute bacterial pneumonia.

Radiography

Once the clinical evaluation suggests the presence of pneumonia, the diagnosis should be confirmed by chest radiograph. Although a radiograph is recommended in all outpatients and inpatients, it may be impractical in some settings outside of the hospital. A chest radiograph not only confirms the presence of pneumonia, but can also be used to identify complicated illness and to grade severity of disease by noting such findings as pleural effusion and multilobar illness. As mentioned above, there is no specific radiographic pattern that can be used to define the etiologic pathogen of CAP but certain findings can be used to suggest specific organisms (see above).

Table 27.3 Recommended diagnostic testing for CAP

- Diagnose the presence of pneumonia with a chest radiograph and clinical data
- Look for specific pathogens that alter therapy, based on historic and epidemiologic clues
- Outpatient testing optional
- Blood cultures only with severe illness
- Sputum Gram stain and culture prior to therapy if good quality and rapid transport and processing in the laboratory (especially valuable if a drug-resistant or unusual pathogen is suspected, but not to narrow empiric therapy)
- *Legionella* and pneumococcal urinary antigen for severe CAP
- Endotracheal aspirate or sputum culture for severe CAP
- No routine serologic testing for atypical pathogens or viruses

Other testing

Even with extensive testing, at least half of all patients do not have an etiologic diagnosis established and thus therapy is usually empiric. In addition, recent studies have emphasized the mortality benefit of prompt administration of effective antibiotic therapy for those with moderate to severe illness, and therapy should never be delayed for the purpose of diagnostic testing. While several studies have shown that establishing an etiologic diagnosis does not improve the outcome of patients with severe CAP, diagnostic testing may have value for the purpose of narrowing and focusing therapy and for guiding management in the patient who is not responding to empiric therapy.[38]

Recommended testing for outpatients is limited to a chest radiograph and pulse oximetry, if available, with sputum culture being considered in patients suspected of having an unusual or drug-resistant pathogen. For admitted patients, current guidelines recommend that diagnostic testing should include a chest radiograph, assessment of oxygenation (pulse oximetry or blood gas, the latter if retention of carbon dioxide is suspected) and routine admission blood work. If the patient has a pleural effusion, this should be tapped and the fluid sent for culture and biochemical analysis. In addition, the patient should have blood cultures only in the presence of severe illness, while sputum Gram stain and culture have their greatest value when the sample is of good quality and can be transported to the laboratory rapidly. Culture is particularly valuable if the patient has risk factors for a drug-resistant or unusual pathogen. In the patient with severe CAP, an endotracheal aspirate should be obtained, along with urinary antigen testing for pneumococcus and *Legionella*.[2]

Although blood cultures are positive in only 10–20% of CAP patients, most often showing pneumococcus, they can be used to identify a specific pathogen and to define the presence of drug-resistant pneumococci. However, they should be limited to patients with a reasonable likelihood of having a true-positive result. If low-risk patients routinely have blood cultures, it is possible that the frequency of false-positives could exceed the true-positives and lead to inaccurate and unnecessary therapy. Thus, blood cultures are only recommended for patients who are severely ill, especially if they have not received antibiotic therapy prior to admission.[39]

The role of Gram stain of sputum to guide initial antibiotic therapy is controversial, but this test has its greatest value in guiding the interpretation of sputum culture and can be used to define the predominant organism present in the sample. The role of Gram stain in focusing initial antibiotic therapy is uncertain since the accuracy of the test to predict the culture recovery of an organism such as pneumococcus depends on the criteria used.[2] Even if Gram stain findings are used to focus antibiotic therapy, this would not allow for empiric coverage of atypical pathogens which might be present even in patients with pneumococcus as part of a mixed infection. However, Gram stain can be used to broaden initial empiric therapy by enhancing the suspicion for organisms that are not covered in routine empiric therapy (such as *Staph. aureus* being suggested by the presence of clusters of Gram-positive cocci, especially during a time of epidemic influenza).

Routine serologic testing for viruses and atypical pathogens is not recommended. However, in patients with severe illness, the diagnosis of *Legionella* can be made by urinary antigen testing, which is the single test that is most likely to be positive at the time of admission, but is specific only for serogroup 1 infection. Commercially available tests for pneumococcal urinary antigen have been developed and may have value to identify pneumococcus; however, as mentioned, the impact of a positive test on therapy choices is uncertain. Bronchoscopy is not indicated as a routine diagnostic test and should be restricted to immunocompromised patients and to selected individuals with severe forms of CAP.

THERAPY

Initial therapy should be focused on the administration of antibiotics and the use of supportive care. Since it is not possible to know the etiology of CAP on the basis of clinical and laboratory findings,

and because of the need to administer therapy as quickly as possible, once the diagnosis is made antibiotic choice is empiric, focusing on the pathogens most likely to be present for a given type of patient. Supportive care includes oxygen if needed, hydration, control of hyperglycemia and possibly chest physiotherapy, as well as administration of bronchodilators and expectorants. For more severely ill patients, the management is similar to severe sepsis, as CAP is a common cause of this syndrome. This means evaluating the need for vasopressors in the presence of hypotension, the use of corticosteroids if relative adrenal insufficiency is suspected and consideration of the use of drotrecogin alpha in selected patients. In addition, the routine use of corticosteroids in patients with severe pneumonia is advocated by some, because of limited data showing a survival benefit with this anti-inflammatory intervention.[40]

In the past 15 years, a variety of professional societies have developed guidelines for the management of CAP and included in the recommendations are antibiotic choice, along with other strategies. Several studies have shown that when therapy is concordant with guideline recommendations, outcomes such as mortality and rate of treatment failure are improved, while for severely ill patients duration of mechanical ventilation is reduced.[41-43] However, the presence of a guideline by itself is not usually enough to lead to these benefits because the guideline requires an implementation strategy in order to be successful. In one study, the benefit of a guideline to reduce length of stay in the hospital was greatest when an implementation strategy was employed that relied on real-time intervention with case managers who identified variances from recommended management.[44]

Antibiotic therapy

Initial empiric therapy for CAP is selected by categorizing patients on the basis of place of therapy (outpatient, inpatient, ICU), severity of illness and the presence or absence of cardiopulmonary disease or specific 'modifying' factors that make certain pathogens more likely.[2] By using these factors, a set of likely pathogens can be predicted for each type of patient (see Table 27.1) and this information can be used to guide therapy. If a specific pathogen is subsequently identified by diagnostic testing, then therapy can be focused. In this scheme, it is also important to identify patients with HCAP and to exclude them from CAP management, as these patients require their own management approach.[2,3,16]

In choosing empiric therapy of CAP, certain principles should be followed. However, the principles that guide therapy in North America are not the same as those used in parts of Europe and the UK.[2,45-47] Although in general guidelines emphasize an empiric approach (without extensive microbiologic testing) and treatment in the community rather than in hospital, the North American guidelines suggest broad-spectrum agents reflecting a recommendation for routine atypical pathogen coverage. In contrast, the UK and European guidelines generally recommend an initial use of penicillins, avoid routine quinolone use and do not advocate therapy for both 'typical' and 'atypical' pathogens except in more severely ill patients. These regional differences reflect variability in the frequency and importance of atypical pathogens and of DRSP, and differing concerns about the importance of empiric broad-spectrum CAP therapy to the rise in resistant health-care-associated infection such as MRSA and *Clostridium difficile* infection. Table 27.4 highlights the principles for CAP management for the North American and UK approaches.

In North American guidelines, for outpatients with no co-morbid cardiopulmonary disease and no history of recent antibiotic use, therapy can be with an advanced macrolide (azithromycin or clarithromycin) or doxycycline. If the patient has co-morbid illness or a history of recent antibiotic therapy (in the past 3 months), then DRSP is a concern and therapy should be with a selected oral β-lactam (amoxicillin, amoxicillin-clavulanate, cefuroxime or cefpodoxime) combined with a macrolide or doxycycline.[2] Alternatively, these patients at risk for DRSP can be treated with an oral fluoroquinolone as monotherapy (gemifloxacin, levofloxacin or moxifloxacin). If the patient has received an

Table 27.4 Principles of antibiotic therapy for CAP: differences between North American and UK guidelines for treatment

Clinical situation	North American approach	UK approach
Timing of antimicrobials	Administer initial antibiotic therapy as soon as possible, after firmly establishing the presence of pneumonia	Antibiotics should be given as soon as possible and within 4 h of clinical diagnosis
Initial choice of antimicrobials	Treat all patients for pneumococcus (including DRSP) and for the possibility of atypical pathogen co-infection (if endemic rates in the community support a role for these organisms)	Treat all patients for pneumococcus. Other pathogens should be considered only in more severe cases or specific clinical situations
Initial antibiotic choice for adults hospitalized with low-moderate severity CAP treated in the community	Use either a macrolide alone (selected patients with no cardiopulmonary disease or modifying factors) or for those outpatients with cardiopulmonary disease or 'modifying factors': • use monotherapy with a quinolone • *or* the combination of a selected β-lactam (cefpodoxime, cefuroxime, high dose ampicillin (3 g/24 h) or amoxicillin-clavulanate) • with a macrolide or tetracycline. A macrolide alone should only be used in outpatients or inpatients with no risk factors for DRSP, enteric Gram-negatives or aspiration	Most patients can be adequately treated with oral antibiotics Oral therapy with amoxicillin is preferred When oral therapy is contraindicated, recommended parenteral choices include iv amoxicillin or benzylpenicillin, or clarithromycin
Initial antibiotic choice for adults hospitalized with moderate severity CAP	Provide initial therapy for hospitalized patients with an iv agent, or if oral only, use a quinolone because of its high bioavailability For inpatients at risk for DRSP: • use quinolone monotherapy • *or* the combination of a selected iv β-lactam (ceftriaxone, cefotaxime, ertapenem, ampicillin-sulbactam) • with a macrolide or tetracycline. Limit antipseudomonal therapy to patients with risk factors	Oral therapy with a combined β-lactam/macrolide regimen is recommended When oral therapy is inappropriate, parenteral amoxicillin or penicillin G are alternatives to oral amoxicillin, with clarithromycin, q12h, as the preferred macrolide for parenteral therapy Levofloxacin iv once daily or a combination of iv second- (e.g. cefuroxime) or third- (e.g. cefotaxime or ceftriaxone) generation cephalosporin with iv clarithromycin are also appropriate alternative choices
Initial antibiotic choice for adults hospitalized with severe CAP	If no pseudomonal risk factors use a selected β-lactam plus a macrolide or antipneumococcal quinolone New antipneumococcal quinolones, in order of decreasing antipneumococcal activity are: gemifloxacin (oral only), moxifloxacin (oral and intravenous), levofloxacin (oral and intravenous) In the combination regimens for severe CAP, consider a quinolone rather than a macrolide for suspected or proven *Legionella* infection For those with pseudomonal risk factors, use an antipseudomonal β-lactam *plus* either ciprofloxacin/high-dose levofloxacin *or* the combination of an aminoglycoside with *either* a macrolide or antipneumococcal quinolone (antipseudomonal β-lactams include cefepime, imipenem, meropenem, piperacillin-tazobactam) Never use monotherapy (including with a quinolone) for patients with severe CAP Empiric therapy for CA-MRSA should be confined to patients with severe pneumonia and evidence of necrotizing infection, particularly after a viral infection Consider using an antitoxin-producing agent with an antibiotic, either vancomycin combined with clindamycin or linezolid monotherapy	Patients with high severity pneumonia should be treated immediately after diagnosis with parenteral antibiotics An iv combination of a broad-spectrum β-lactamase stable antibiotic such as amoxicillin-clavulanic acid together with a macrolide such as clarithromycin is preferred Alternatively, in penicillin-allergic patients, a second- (e.g. cefuroxime) or third- (e.g. cefotaxime or ceftriaxone) generation cephalosporin can be used instead of co-amoxiclav, together with clarithromycin If *Legionella* is strongly suspected, consider adding levofloxacin

CA-MRSA, community-acquired methicillin-resistant *Staphylococcus aureus*; DRSP, drug-resistant *Streptococcus pneumoniae*.

antibiotic in the past 3 months, then ideally an agent from a different class should be chosen to avoid the risk of repeated use of the same agent, which can promote the emergence of pneumococcal resistance. In contrast to these recommendations, European and UK guidelines rely more on oral penicillins for these patients and place less emphasis on the need for macrolides, except for the more severely ill hospitalized patients, and discourage the routine use of quinolones (see Table 27.4).[45,46] As noted, this reflects different views on the frequency and importance of DRSP and atypical pathogens in the management and outcome of CAP.

The majority of inpatients will have cardiopulmonary disease or other risks for DRSP, and sometimes Gram-negatives, and North American guidelines suggest they should be treated with either a selected intravenous β-lactam (cefotaxime, ceftriaxone, ampicillin-sulbactam or ertapenem) combined with a macrolide or doxycycline; alternatively, they can receive monotherapy with an intravenous antipneumococcal quinolone (levofloxacin or moxifloxacin).[2] From the available data, either regimen is therapeutically equivalent, but an effort should be made to avoid repeating an agent in the same antibiotic class in the same patient, within a 3-month period. The antipneumococcal quinolones are being widely used in North America because as a single drug, given once daily, it is possible to cover pneumococcus (including DRSP), Gram-negatives and atypical pathogens. In addition, quinolones penetrate well into respiratory secretions and are highly bioavailable, achieving the same serum levels with oral or intravenous therapy. There are differences among the available agents in their intrinsic activity against pneumococcus and, based on MIC data, these agents can be ranked from most to least active as: gemifloxacin (available only in oral form), moxifloxacin and levofloxacin. Some data suggest a lower likelihood of both clinical failures and the induction of pneumococcal resistance to quinolones if the more-active agents are used in place of the less-active agents.[2,20] UK and European guidelines do not recommend fluoroquinolones as initial therapy in severe pneumococcal CAP because of residual concerns regarding the clinical effectiveness of these agents, as well as concerns about their contribution to healthcare-associated infection (e.g. *Clostridium difficile*). Although oral quinolones may be as effective as intravenous quinolones for admitted patients with moderately severe illness, most admitted patients should receive initial therapy intravenously to be sure that the medication has been absorbed. Once the patient shows a good clinical response, oral therapy can be started.

In the ICU population, all individuals should be treated for DRSP and atypical pathogens, but only those with appropriate risk factors (see above) should have coverage for *P. aeruginosa* (see Table 27.4). In addition, no ICU-admitted patient should receive monotherapy with any agent, including a quinolone. While patients with severe CAP can receive either a macrolide or a quinolone as a second agent, several studies have shown a remarkably high efficacy of levofloxacin and moxifloxacin for documented *Legionella* infection, and thus a quinolone may be the preferred agent if this organism is suspected or proven.[48]

In addition to the therapy regimens discussed, some patients with severe CAP need added coverage for *Staph. aureus*, including MRSA. However, not all patients with severe CAP require this therapy, but most experts recommend that this organism be targeted empirically only in patients with severe necrotizing CAP following a viral illness, particularly influenza. Optimal therapy has not been defined and vancomycin alone may not be sufficient, having led to clinical failure, presumably since it is not active against the PVL toxin that accompanies community-acquired MRSA. For that reason, it may be necessary to add clindamycin to vancomycin or to use linezolid, with rifampin (rifampicin) in severe illness, since both of these latter agents can inhibit toxin production.[27]

Patients with HCAP are a heterogeneous group, with some at risk for MDR Gram-negatives and MRSA, and others not. As discussed earlier, the risks for drug-resistant pathogens in this population include recent antibiotic therapy and poor functional status, as well as severe illness.[16] An HCAP patient (from a nursing home, dialysis center or a patient who was recently hospitalized) who is not severely ill, and who has no or only one risk factor for resistance, can still be treated as non-severe CAP. Similarly, an HCAP patient with severe illness, but 0–1 risk factors for MDR pathogens can be treated with a severe CAP regimen.[16] On the other hand, a patient with severe HCAP and two risk factors for MDR pathogens should be treated for drug-resistant Gram-negatives, MRSA and other pathogens seen in those with nosocomial pneumonia. For these patients, the therapy should be with an aminoglycoside (amikacin, gentamicin or tobramycin) plus an antipseudomonal β-lactam (cefepime, imipenem, meropenem or piperacillin-tazobactam) plus linezolid or vancomycin[2,16] (see Chapter 28 for management of nosocomial pneumonia). If the severely ill HCAP patient has come from a nursing home that is known to have patients with atypical pathogen infection, then additional coverage of these agents is needed.

Other therapy issues

In addition to the general approach to antibiotic therapy outlined above, there are several other therapeutic issues in the management of CAP as highlighted in Table 27.4. These include the need for timely administration of initial antibiotic therapy, the findings of improved outcomes when pneumococcal bacteremia patients receive dual therapy rather than monotherapy, especially in severely ill patients.

When a patient has CAP, administration of antibiotics as soon as possible has benefit for patient outcome and some retrospective data have suggested that mortality is reduced if the first dose of antibiotics is given within 4 hours of the patient's arrival to the hospital when compared to later administration.[49] These data led to widespread efforts in the USA to provide antibiotics as soon as possible to all CAP patients, with sometimes unintended consequences. While focus on this issue led to more patients receiving antibiotics sooner than before there was a focus on timely antibiotic administration, there was also more use of antibiotics before pneumonia was clearly known to be present, and in some instances patients without pneumonia were treated unnecessarily, occasionally leading to antibiotic-related complications such as *Clostridium difficile* colitis.[50,51]

As discussed, the antibiotic regimens used in North America provide routine therapy for atypical pathogens using either a macrolide or a quinolone, based on data that such an approach reduces mortality, especially in those with severe illness.[22,23] However, even in patients with documented pneumococcal bacteremia, the use of combination therapy (generally with the addition of atypical pathogen coverage to pneumococcal coverage) has been associated with reduced mortality compared to monotherapy.[52] In one study, the benefit of adding a second agent applied to those pneumococcal bacteremia patients who were critically ill, but not to other populations.[53] Rodriguez and colleagues found a benefit to adding a second agent for all patients with severe CAP and shock, and the benefit applied if the agent added was either a macrolide or a quinolone.[54]

For some patients, certain adjunctive therapies should be considered, including oxygen, chest physiotherapy (if at least 30 ml of sputum daily and a poor cough response are present), aerosolized bronchodilators and corticosteroids (if hypotension and possible relative adrenal insufficiency is suspected).

Response to therapy and duration of treatment

The majority of outpatients and inpatients will respond rapidly to empiric therapy, with clinical improvement usually occurring within 24–72 hours. Clinical improvement is measured by following the symptoms of cough, sputum production and dyspnea, along with documenting the ability to take medications by mouth and the presence of an afebrile status on at least two occasions 8 hours apart.[2] When a patient has met these criteria for clinical response, it is appropriate to switch to an oral therapy regimen and to discharge the patient, if he is otherwise medically and socially stable. Radiographic improvement lags behind clinical improvement and in a responding patient a chest radiograph is not necessary until 2–4 weeks after starting therapy.

There are few data about the proper duration of therapy in patients with CAP, especially those with severe illness. Even in the presence of pneumococcal bacteremia, short durations of therapy may be possible, with a rapid switch from intravenous to oral therapy in responding patients. Generally, CAP of unknown etiology and CAP due to *Strep. pneumoniae* can be treated for 5–7 days if the patient is responding rapidly, has been afebrile for 48–72 hours and has received accurate empiric therapy at the correct dose. The presence of extrapulmonary infection (such as meningitis and empyema) and the identification of certain pathogens (such as bacteremic *Staph. aureus* and *P. aeruginosa*) may require longer durations of therapy.[2] Traditionally, identification of *Legionella pneumophila* pneumonia prompted therapy for 14 days, although recent data have shown that quinolone therapy as short as 5 days with levofloxacin 750 mg may be effective.[48]

If the patient fails to respond to therapy in the expected time interval, then it is necessary to consider infection with a drug-resistant or unusual pathogen (tuberculosis, anthrax, *Coxiella burnetii*, *Burkholderia pseudomallei, Pasteurella multocida*, endemic fungi or hantavirus), a pneumonic complication (lung abscess, endocarditis, empyema) or a noninfectious process that mimics pneumonia (bronchiolitis obliterans with organizing pneumonia, hypersensitivity pneumonitis, pulmonary vasculitis, bronchoalveolar cell carcinoma, lymphoma, pulmonary embolus). The evaluation of the nonresponding patient should be individualized but may include CT scanning of the chest, pulmonary angiography, bronchoscopy and occasionally open lung biopsy.

PREVENTION

Prevention of CAP is important for all groups of patients but especially the elderly, who are at risk for both a higher frequency of infection and a more severe course of illness. Appropriate patients should be vaccinated with both pneumococcal and influenza vaccines and cessation of cigarette smoking should be a goal for all at-risk patients. Immunization can be effective even for the patient who is recovering from CAP and hospital-based immunization is an effective and efficient way to promote vaccine utilization.

Pneumococcal vaccine

Pneumococcal capsular polysaccharide vaccine can prevent pneumonia in otherwise healthy populations, as was initially demonstrated in South African gold miners and American military recruits. The benefits in those of advanced age or with underlying conditions in nonepidemic environments are less clearly proven and have been demonstrated in case–control studies rather than in randomized trials. In immunocompetent patients over the age of 65, effectiveness has been estimated to be 75%, while it ranges from 65% to 84% in patients with chronic diseases including diabetes mellitus, coronary artery disease, congestive heart failure, chronic pulmonary disease and anatomic asplenia.[2,55] Its effectiveness has not been proven in immunodeficient populations such as those with sickle cell disease, chronic renal failure, immunoglobulin deficiency, Hodgkin's disease, lymphoma, leukemia and multiple myeloma. A single revaccination is recommended in patients over age 65 who initially received the vaccine more than 5 years earlier and were under age 65 on first vaccination. If the initial vaccination was given at age 65 or older, repeat is only indicated (after 5 years) if the patient has anatomic or functional asplenia or has one of the immunocompromising conditions listed above.

The available pneumococcal vaccine is generally underutilized and the 23-valent pneumococcal vaccine carries the serotypes causing the majority of clinical infection seen in the USA. A protein-conjugated pneumococcal vaccine has been licensed and appears more immunogenic than the older vaccine; however, it contains only seven serotypes and although recommended for healthy children, it has not yet been shown to be effective in adults. Nonetheless, the vaccine has had benefit for adults, even when given only to children, demonstrating a 'herd immunity' effect. More recently, however, children who have received the 7-valent pneumococcal polysaccharide vaccine have developed infection with strains not included in the vaccine, leading to a higher frequency of severe necrotizing pneumonia, especially with serotype 3.[56]

Influenza vaccine

The current vaccine includes three strains: two influenza A strains (H3N2 and H1N1) and one influenza B strain. Vaccination is recommended for all patients over age 65 and for those with chronic medical illness (including nursing home residents) and for those who provide health care to patients at risk for complicated influenza. When the vaccine matches the circulating strain of influenza, it can prevent illness in 70–90% of healthy persons over age 65. For older persons with chronic illness, the efficacy is less, but the vaccine can still attenuate the influenza infection and lead to fewer lower respiratory tract infections and the associated morbidity and mortality that follow influenza.

REFERENCES

References for this chapter can be found online at http://www.expertconsult.com

Hospital-acquired pneumonia

EPIDEMIOLOGY

Definition

Hospital-acquired pneumonia (HAP) is defined as pneumonia occurring at least 48 hours after hospital admission, excluding any infection incubating at the time of admission.[1] Ventilator-associated pneumonia (VAP) is a particular subgroup of HAP for which the incidence, etiology, investigation and outcome are somewhat different. VAP is excluded from this chapter and is discussed in Practice Point 16. Recently[1] there has been an increasing awareness of health-care-associated pneumonia (HCAP) as a variant of HAP. Patients at risk for HCAP include:

- those receiving home intravenous antibiotics, home nursing or home wound care;
- residents in a nursing home or long-term care facility;
- those who have been hospitalized for more than 2 days in the past 90 days; and
- those who have received dialysis or intravenous therapy at a hospital-based clinic in the past 30 days.

The importance of recognizing this group is that these patients have an increased risk for multidrug-resistant (MDR) organisms and therefore require management more closely akin to VAP than community-acquired pneumonia.

Incidence and size of the problem

Pneumonia is the second most common infection acquired in hospital after urinary tract infection. In a European multicenter study on 10 000 patients, the prevalence of nosocomial pneumonias was reported at 10%, representing 47% of the infections acquired in the intensive care unit (ICU).[2] There is a decreasing risk of acquiring pneumonia during a hospital stay. For example, the risk of developing VAP is 3% per day until day 5, decreasing to 2% per day until day 10 and 1% at day 15.[3] HAP adds 5–9 days to the hospital stay of survivors and billions of dollars to health-care costs.[4] The incidence varies with the type of hospital and ward and the age of the patient. The incidence is lowest in district hospitals and in general medical and pediatric wards, and higher in teaching hospitals (presumably because of the increased complexity of medical cases) and in patients over 65 years of age.[4]

Mortality rate

The mortality rate of nosocomial pneumonias ranges from 13% to 55% depending on the author.[4] This disparity is in large part linked to the types of patient studied (medical, surgical, traumatic) and to the heterogeneity of the diagnostic criteria employed. The severity of the underlying disease is an essential factor and is often poorly evaluated in studies reporting mortality rates. The cause and effect ratio is difficult to determine. Thus, the studies centered on the prevention of VAP, either by selective digestive contamination or by the choice of gastric protector, reach the conclusion that the number of cases of VAP has diminished but that the mortality is unchanged. Likewise, the occurrence of VAP during acute respiratory distress syndrome does not modify the mortality.[5]

Few studies have been solely dedicated to the prognosis of nosocomial pneumonia. Leu et al.[6] reported a retrospective paired study of 74 pairs of patients. The mortality in each group was comparable with a nonsignificant difference: 20% with the presence of nosocomial pneumonia and 14% without nosocomial pneumonia. A study[7] of the mortality of patients with VAP documented by protected specimen brush (PSB) reported mortality in patients presenting VAP that was double that of the control patients (54% vs 27%). An absence of surmortality was noted in another work[8] with a similar methodology with 85 pairs of patients with a diagnosis of VAP also documented by PSB and where the mortality was 41% in both groups. On close examination of the differences between these two studies, one can note that the principal difference is in the pairing of the diagnosis. The study which reported an attributable mortality for VAP[7] was not based on pairing according to the type of surgery or the underlying disease. Very recently, an international study of 2897 patients reported no surmortality linked to the occurrence of VAP.[9] Even in trauma patients with head injuries or in patients presenting a cerebrovascular accident, the occurrence of VAP did not seem to modify the prognosis. On the other hand, it did appear to worsen the prognosis of ventilated patients who presented chronic respiratory failure of an obstructive nature.[10] The role of VAP in lengthening the duration of ventilation and ICU stay is not debated but nevertheless remains difficult to quantify. Finally, the costs generated by the appearance of VAP are very high, ranging from $12 000 to over $40 000 (€8000 to €27 000) per patient.[11]

Overall, the appearance of VAP does not appear to be an independent factor for mortality (except for patients presenting chronic obstructive respiratory failure) but appears to be especially linked to the underlying condition on which the pneumonia occurs and to associated co-morbidities.

PATHOGENESIS AND ETIOLOGIC AGENTS

Pathogenesis

Hospital-acquired pneumonia is usually caused by the aspiration into the lungs of bacteria that colonize the upper respiratory tract. The oropharynx of a debilitated patient becomes colonized rapidly by enteric Gram-negative bacteria (EGNB). These bacteria are not normally present in the upper respiratory tract and the frequency of colonization increases with the increasing severity of the underlying illness, the use of antibiotics and the duration of hospital stay. Microaspiration of pharyngeal secretions is usually clinically silent and even occurs in healthy subjects during sleep, but becomes very frequent in patients who have reduced consciousness.

In the healthy individual, aspirated secretions can be dealt with effectively by lung defenses, including mucociliary clearance and alveolar macrophages. When host defenses are impaired, bacteria are able to proliferate and cause pneumonia. Colonization of the lower respiratory tract is facilitated by changes in bronchial and alveolar epithelial cells that favor bacterial adherence. HAP is histologically characterized by the existence of infection sources made up of polymorphonuclear neutrophils present in the bronchioles and adjacent alveoli. A grading system of four successive stages based on histologic analysis of the lungs of 83 patients who were invasively ventilated and who died in the ICU has been proposed.[12] Owing to repeated seeding of the lower airways, these HAP lesions are very heterogeneous and can be associated with different lesional stages at the same time. It should be noted that the lesions are predominant in the right lung and in dependent lung segments. Less commonly, other mechanisms may be involved, including the hematogenous spread of infection to the lungs from a distant focus and inhalation of pathogens aerosolized either from contaminated respiratory equipment (e.g. ventilator or nebulizer equipment) or from the hospital environment (e.g. showers and water systems colonized with *Legionella* bacteria).

Causative organisms

The spectrum of potential pathogens associated with HAP differs from that of community-acquired pneumonia. The distribution of micro-organisms responsible for HAP (Table 28.1) is influenced by the existence of prior systemic antibiotherapy, by the type of patient (medical, surgical, or traumatic) and by the existence of co-morbidities.[4,13] The bacterial pathogens most frequently associated with HAP are EGNB and *Staphylococcus aureus*. Mixed infections are not unusual, particularly in VAP. The role of viruses has not been widely studied but is probably significant, not only at times of community outbreaks of viral infection, but also when staff and visitors may transmit viral infection to hospitalized patients. It has been admitted for 20 years that HAP is separated into early-onset pneumonia in patients who develop pneumonia early in their hospital stay (<5 days) and those who develop pneumonia later (≥5 days).[14] In general, the spectrum of causative organisms in patients who develop early pneumonia reflects community isolates – *Streptococcus pneumoniae*, *Haemophilus influenzae*, *Escherichia coli*, nonresistant EGNB, methicillin-sensitive *Staphylococcus aureus* (MSSA) – rather than highly resistant nosocomial organisms. On the other hand, patients who develop late-onset nosocomial pneumonia are more likely to have resistant organisms – *Pseudomonas aeruginosa*, *Acinetobacter* spp., other resistant Enterobacteriaceae, methicillin-resistant *Staphylococcus aureus* (MRSA) and viruses. As for *Candida* spp., it has been clearly demonstrated that there are no sure criteria outside of those found on a lung biopsy[15] and that the positivity of directed or nondirected samples has no value.[15] *Aspergillus* spp. are in question, especially in immunodepressed patients and particularly in oncohematology, and are generally considered as unusual in immunocompetent patients.

PREVENTION

General measures

Preferential use of noninvasive ventilation compared with first-intention invasive mechanical ventilation when possible reduces the incidence of nosocomial pneumonia.[16] The use of sedation and weaning protocols with noninvasive ventilation makes it possible to reduce the duration of invasive mechanical ventilation and therefore to reduce

Table 28.1 Micro-organisms responsible for hospital-acquired pneumonia[13]

Agent	Organism
Gram-positive cocci	*Staphylococcus aureus* *Streptococcus pneumoniae* Coagulase-negative staphylococcus
Gram-positive bacilli	*Corynebacterium* spp. *Listeria monocytogenes* *Nocardia* spp.
Gram-negative bacilli (lactose positive)	*Haemophilus influenzae* *Escherichia coli* *Klebsiella* spp. *Enterobacter* spp. *Proteus* spp.
Gram-negative bacilli (lactose negative)	*Pseudomonas aeruginosa* *Burkholderia cepacia* *Acinetobacter* spp. *Stenotrophomonas maltophilia*
Gram-negative cocci	*Neisseria* spp. *Moraxella* spp.
Anaerobes (cocci)	*Peptostreptococcus* *Veillonelia*
Anaerobes (bacilli)	*Bacteroides* spp. *Fusobacterium* spp. *Prevotella* spp. *Actinomyces* spp.
Intracellular micro-organisms	*Legionella* spp. *Chlamydia pneumoniae* *Mycoplasma pneumoniae*
Fungi	*Candida* spp. *Aspergillus* spp.
Viruses	Influenza, parainfluenza, adenovirus Respiratory syncitial virus Herpes simplex virus Cytomegalovirus
Other agents	*Pneumocystis jiroveci* *Mycobacterium tuberculosis* *Strongyloides stercoralis*

the incidence of HAP. Effective infection control measures include staff education, compliance with alcohol-based hand disinfection, and isolation to reduce cross-infection with MDR pathogens.[1]

Oral decontamination, selective digestive decontamination, antibioprophylaxis

Local oropharyngeal decontamination by antibiotherapy in the form of a paste or gel, or by chlorhexhidine[17] appears to be effective in the prevention of HAP. However, a recent multicenter American-European study examined the preventive effect of iseganan (an antimicrobial peptide active against bacteria and fungi) and concluded it was ineffective in the prevention of VAP.[18]

Selective digestive decontamination (SDD), given the coexistence of an oropharyngeal and a gastric colonization source, has long been proposed as a means to prevent VAP. It is generally made up of a combination of three anti-infectious agents with no or low systemic diffusion (amphotericin B, polymyxin, aminoglycoside), applied on the buccal mucosa and administered in the digestive tract by nasogastric tube associated with short parenteral systemic antibioprophylaxis. It was initially proposed[19] to institute systemic antibioprophylaxis using intravenous cefotaxime until negativity of microbiologic samples is confirmed. The first studies were principally on polytraumatized patients in whom the major risk of inhalation before and after intubation was known, as well as their particular susceptibility to early *Staphylococcus aureus* pneumonia. Numerous studies have reported a reduction in the incidence of VAP but in practice it would appear that this method is little used and not formally recommended in the latest international consensus conferences.[1,20]

Certain problems that are inherent in the use of SDD have been advanced. The aspiration of antibiotics in the lower respiratory tract accounts for a great number of sterile cultures or cultures that are inferior to the recommended thresholds, given the partial but insufficient activity on these pathogens by antibiotics administered orally and the theoretic impact that the extensive use of SDD could have on the ecology of ICUs and the emergence of MDR bacteria. However, recent studies could renew interest in this preventive method. A randomized prospective study on a large population reported a reduction in the incidence of VAP and a reduction in mortality in the group benefiting from SDD with, in addition, a reduction in Gram-negative bacteria,[21] while a randomized study of ICUs showed a decrease in mortality with SDD.[22]

Systemic antibioprophylaxis used alone without local decontamination increases the risk of the development of MDR bacteria and the data vis-à-vis its efficacy in the prevention of VAP are contradictory.[23]

Stress-ulcer prophylaxis

The use of gastric protectors that increase the gastric pH (anti-H_2, antiacids) expose the patient to the risk of gastric microbial development. Although the results in the literature are contradictory, sucralfate appears to present several advantages:

- it does not modify the gastric pH;
- it presents proper antibacterial efficacy;
- it does not require manipulation of perfusion lines for its administration; and
- it is much less expensive than other gastric protectors.

Nevertheless, the largest randomized study comparing sucralfate with ranitidine reported that the latter is more effective in the prevention of gastric bleeding and, in addition, did not increase the incidence of VAP.[24] Finally, a recent observational study has shown the futility of systematically prescribing a gastric protector,[25] so it would be better to reserve it for patients at risk. The latest consensus conference went in the same direction by reserving gastric protection only for patients at risk and preferably with anti-H_2.[20]

Enteral nutrition

Enteral nutrition is preferred over parenteral nutrition to reduce the risk of complications related to central intravenous catheters and to prevent reflux villous atrophy of the intestinal mucosa which could increase the risk of bacterial translocation. However, its use increases the risk of VAP.

Antibiotic policy

It would appear to be logical, although unproven, that the controlled use of antibiotics in the ICU, following protocols based on established and recognized recommendations, could in part prevent the appearance of MDR infections.[26] Monitoring of ICU infections in order to identify and quantify endemic and new MDR pathogens as well as the preparation of timely data for infection control to guide appropriate antimicrobial therapy in patients with suspected HAP or other nosocomial infections are recommended.

Respiratory physiotherapy

One study[27] has reported that respiratory physiotherapy appears to be independently associated with a reduction in the risk of VAP but a randomized study is required to confirm it.

Patient posture

The semirecumbent position makes it possible to limit inhalation in patients receiving enteral nutrition. The only randomized study evaluating the role of the position of the patient on the development of VAP has shown the protective effect of the semirecumbent position at 45°.[28] It should be noted that no benefit in terms of mortality was demonstrated between the two groups.

In all, the principal measurement and the only one currently recommended is a positioning of patients in the semirecumbent position between 30° and 45°,[1,20,28] especially when enteral nutrition is administered.

CLINICAL FEATURES AND DIFFERENTIAL DIAGNOSIS

The diagnosis of pneumonia may be obvious in a hospitalized patient not presenting a respiratory illness on admission and who develops the classic symptoms of fever, malaise, cough, purulent sputum, localized chest signs and consolidation on the chest radiograph. All too often, however, the situation is less straightforward, with numerous differential diagnoses. Hospital-acquired pneumonia should finally be considered in the context of an illness developing after hospital admission and characterized by fever, leukocytosis, purulent sputum or tracheobronchial secretions and new or persisting infiltrates on the chest radiograph. However, the accuracy of a clinical diagnosis is poor compared with a microbiologic or pathologic diagnosis.

DIAGNOSIS

General investigations (hematology, immunology and radiology)

Patients with suspected HAP should have a full blood count. Neutrophilia may point to infection. Biochemical tests are often indicated to assess the impact of pneumonia on the underlying condition and to assess renal and hepatic function. Oxygenation should be assessed by pulse oximetry or arterial blood gas estimation. The chest radiograph will show new or worsening lung shadowing, although it is not usually diagnostic of infection. Cavitation is suggestive of infection, particularly by EGNB, anaerobes or fungi. Multiple studies of biologic markers of infection have attempted to find a noninvasive, rapid and accurate means of determining who requires antibiotics for presumed HAP. Unfortunately, the results have largely been disappointing (procalcitonin, for example). More recently, measurement of a soluble triggering receptor expressed on myeloid cells (sTREM-1) that is upregulated in the setting of infection has been shown to have potential to improve our ability to accurately diagnose pneumonia. When compared with post hoc physician consensus, measurement of sTREM-1 by mini bronchial alveolar lavage (BAL) was shown to be 98% sensitive and 90% specific for the diagnosis of pneumonia in mechanically ventilated patients.[29] Although promising, additional studies are required before this test can be widely recommended.

General microbiologic investigations

Blood cultures should always be obtained. A positive culture identifies the pathogen and is associated with a worse prognosis. However, only about 8–20% of blood cultures from patients who have HAP are positive, indicating a low sensitivity.[1] Sources of the bacteremia, other than the lung, should always be considered. Pleural fluid should be sampled to identify impending empyema. Serologic tests for viral and atypical pathogens can be of some help. *Legionella* urinary antigen detection is a rapid, sensitive and specific test for nosocomial infection by *Legionella pneumophila* serogroup 1.

Special investigations and techniques to obtain lower respiratory tract samples

Ideally, there should be a widely available and accepted technique to obtain and culture uncontaminated secretions from the site of a lung infection that is simple, safe and inexpensive to perform, the results of which would differentiate infection from colonization and improve outcome. Although the past 25 years have seen a rapid expansion in the use of different techniques for sampling in HAP, none has fulfilled the above criteria and controversy continues among experts regarding the role of invasive and noninvasive investigations of HAP and VAP. The techniques can be broadly divided into noninvasive and invasive groups.

Noninvasive techniques

Expectorated sputum

The problems of sputum collection are well known and include contamination of the specimen by upper respiratory tract flora, making it unrepresentative of lower respiratory tract secretions. This is a particular problem in the nosocomial setting, when EGNB commonly colonize the upper respiratory tract and pathogens can be isolated with equal frequency in patients who have and do not have pneumonia. Only one-third to one-half of sputum cultures provide reliable information compared with blood cultures, transtracheal aspirates and PSB samples. Interest in tracheal aspiration in intubated patients with nonquantitative culture could be revived given the results of a recent North American multicenter study.[30] This study compared 741 patients with suspected VAP in a randomized and prospective manner, using quantitative BAL culture with nonquantitative tracheal aspirate culture, and demonstrated that mortality and targeted use of antibiotics were not different whatever the diagnostic strategy used. However, patients known to be colonized or infected with *Pseudomonas* spp. or MRSA were not included in this trial.

Bronchoscopic invasive techniques

Much has been published about the value of invasive techniques for managing HAP. However, the questions vis-à-vis in whom, when and how to perform these tests and the reliability of the results remain unresolved, as does the applicability of published results to everyday clinical situations. Fiberoptic bronchoscopy provides direct visual access to the lower airways. Bronchoscopic techniques are relatively simple to carry out in patients on mechanical ventilation. Invasive techniques could be considered in nonventilated patients who have moderate or severe HAP before antibiotic therapy is administered. In practice, immediate access to bronchoscopic techniques may be limited and the procedure itself could occasionally precipitate cardiorespiratory failure in a spontaneously breathing but hypoxic patient, necessitating ventilatory support earlier than anticipated.

Protected specimen brush

Protected specimen brush (PSB) consists of brushing the distal bronchial mucosa with a precision that requires the use of an endoscope. The low volume of secretions harvested (approximately 1 µl) explains a certain number of false-negatives as well as the difficulty of performing a direct examination and culture on the same brush. This technique, developed *in vitro* by Wimberley, was validated in ventilated patients by Chastre *et al.*[31] who studied the efficacy of this device

in 26 ventilated patients who died in the ICU. Human histologic studies[32-34] have reported sensitivity of PSB ranging between 33% and 57%. The accepted threshold of 10^3 cfu/ml can explain a certain number of false-negatives. Repeating PSB in cases of a negative result associated with an evocative radiologic-clinical picture has been proposed.[35] In fact, when the first PSB was borderline ($\geq 10^2$ and $<10^3$ cfu/ml), a subsequent PSB turned out to be positive at a threshold of 10^3 cfu/ml in 35% of the cases. This could be attributed to the heterogeneity of the pneumonia lesions and the low volume of secretions harvested. Finally, beginning at the 12th hour after administration of an effective antibiotic, the PSB was negative in almost one-third of the cases,[36] justifying a new sample collection before administration of any new antibiotherapy.

Bronchoalveolar lavage

For BAL, the bronchoscope is wedged into a subsegmental airway and the bronchoalveolar area is lavaged. Volumes of over 100 ml sterile normal saline are required to reach the distal alveoli. The advantage of this technique is that a large part of the lung is sampled and the specimen allows microscopic analysis to assess the presence of intracellular bacteria, neutrophils and cytologic evaluation. This can be particularly useful if the diagnosis of pneumonia is in doubt. Contamination of the BAL fluid in the bronchoscopic channel is one drawback and careful technique is required to avoid this. After wedging the tip of the bronchoscope in the relevant subsegment, 50 ml normal saline is instilled. This aspirate samples airways rather than the alveoli, is best referred to as a 'bronchial wash' and is more likely to be contaminated with bacteria present in the suction channel. This sample should therefore be processed separately from the second, third and, if necessary, fourth aliquots of 50 ml, which should be pooled. The sensitivity and specificity of quantitative BAL cultures have ranged from 42% to 100% and 69% to 100%, respectively, using threshold concentrations of at least 10^4 cfu/ml. When compared with PSB performed at the same time, BAL has greater sensitivity but a marginally reduced specificity.

Percutaneous invasive techniques

Percutaneous lung needle aspirate

Percutaneous lung needle aspirate (PLNA) has been used successfully to investigate nonventilated patients who have lung shadowing. The technique can be performed at the bedside with minimal equipment. The use of a 25-gauge ultrathin needle reduces the chance of pneumothorax. The sensitivity of PLNA in HAP is lower than its specificity and the pneumothorax complication rate is lower than 5% in spontaneously breathing patients. When compared with histologic diagnosis of pneumonia on lung biopsy immediately postmortem as a 'gold standard', PLNA had the lowest sensitivity but the highest specificity of the invasive techniques discussed.

Transtracheal aspiration

Transtracheal aspiration is now rarely used due to the ready availability of fiberoptic bronchoscopy. However, its value has been demonstrated for the investigation of patients who have suspected HAP in general medical and surgical wards.

Influence of quantitative cultures on the management of HAP

The literature supports the view that PSB, BAL and tracheal aspirate specimens cultured quantitatively can provide useful and reliable information about the likely presence and cause of HAP in patients who have the clinical features of pneumonia, particularly in the ICU. Their value is considerably diminished if the patient is already receiving antibiotics, which is the usual situation. There is controversy as to whether these tests improve patient management and outcome in routine clinical practice. Randomized studies have shown that invasive techniques lead to more antibiotic changes and increase costs, but do not affect mortality or morbidity.[37–39] Only one randomized study, from France, has shown a bronchoscopic strategy, including quantitative cultures of PSB and BAL specimens, to be superior to a clinical strategy using qualitative tracheobronchial aspirates in terms of 2-week mortality rate and overall morbidity.[40]

TREATMENT

Guidelines for empiric antibiotic therapy

The treatment of HAP is influenced by the availability of new anti-infectious agents, the development of micro-organism resistance and the willingness of clinicians to use therapies that have a reasonable cost-efficacy ratio. Since most cases of HAP are due to bacteria, empiric therapy or (even better) empiric antibiotherapy, oriented by the underlying condition, local microbiologic ecology and direct examination or the culture of routine tracheal aspirates, should be administered as soon as there are sufficient arguments to suspect a pneumonia. The selection of appropriate antibiotics for the initial management of HAP on the basis of time of onset of disease and risk for MDR pathogens as suggested by the American Thoracic Society/Infectious Diseases Society of America (ATS/IDSA) Consensus Conference is outlined in Tables 28.2 and 28.3. The key decision in initial empiric therapy is whether the patient has risk factors for MDR organisms. The adequate dosing of antibiotics for empiric therapy for MDR pathogens is summarized in Table 28.4. Ideally, this antibiotherapy must be administered after the performance of a series of hemocultures and respiratory samples (tracheal aspiration, PSB, BAL, etc.).[20] The recommended administration route is intravenous and, once the response to treatment is satisfactory, relayed by the oral route as soon as possible. Tracheal instillations or antibiotic aerosols are not recommended as a cure since the data in the literature are insufficient.[20] The latest ATS/IDSA Consensus Conference[1] proposed aerosols as a complementary treatment in cases of MDR Gram-negative bacilli if the systemic antibiotherapy appears to be insufficient.

Several observational studies have shown that administration of inappropriate initial antibiotherapy in patients with suspected pneumonia was associated with increased mortality.[41,42] This is not decreased by secondary adjustment of treatment after obtaining the results of microbiologic cultures.[41] The time period before antibiotherapy is administered is also important to consider. A period of 24 hours or more after the criteria for HAP have been collected is associated with increases in hospital mortality, duration of stay and cost.[43] The choice between mono- or bi-therapy has been discussed in only a few studies. The latest ATS/IDSA Consensus Conference[1] proposed a combination of antibiotics in cases of a multidrug-resistant patho-

Table 28.2 Initial empiric antibiotic therapy for HAP in patients with early onset HAP and no known risk factors for multidrug-resistant pathogens

Potential pathogen	Recommended antibiotic
Streptococcus pneumoniae *Haemophilus influenzae* Methicillin-sensitive *Staphylococcus aureus* Antibiotic-sensitive enteric Gram-negative bacilli • *Escherichia coli* • *Klebsiella pneumoniae* • *Proteus* spp. • *Serratia marcescens*	Ceftriaxone or Levofloxacin, moxifloxacin or ciprofloxacin or Ampicillin-sulbactam or Ertapenem

Table 28.3 Initial empiric therapy for HAP in patients with late-onset disease or risk factors for multidrug-resistant pathogens

Potential pathogen	Recommended antibiotic
Pathogens listed in Table 28.1 and multidrug-resistant organisms	Antipseudomonal cephalosporin (ceftazidime, cefepime) or
Pseudomonas aeruginosa	Antipseudomonal carbapenem (imipenem, meropenem, doripenem) or
Klebsiella pneumoniae (EBSL+)*	β-Lactam/β-lactamase inhibitor (piperacillin-tazobactam) plus
Acinetobacter spp.	
Methicillin-resistant *Staphylococcus aureus*†	Antipseudomonal fluoroquinolone (ciprofloxacin, levofloxacin)* or Aminoglycoside (gentamicin, tobramycin, amikacin) plus Vancomycin or linezolid

*If an ESBL+ strain, such as *K. pneumoniae*, or an *Acinetobacter* spp. is suspected, a carbapenem is a reliable choice. If *L. pneumophila* is suspected, the combination antibiotic regimen should include a macrolide (e.g. azithromycin) or a fluoroquinolone (e.g. ciprofloxacin or levofloxacin) should be used rather than an aminoglycoside.
†If MRSA risk factors are present or there is a high incidence locally.

Table 28.4 Initial intravenous adult doses of antibiotics for empiric therapy of HAP in patients with late-onset disease or risk factors for multidrug-resistant pathogens

Antibiotic	Dosage
Ceftazidime	2 g q8h
Cefepime	1–2 g q8–12h
Imipenem	500 mg q6h or 1 g q8h
Meropenem	1 g q8h
Piperacillin–tazobactam	4.5 g q6h
Gentamicin	7 mg/kg q24h
Tobramycin	7 mg/kg q24h
Amikacin	20 mg/kg q24h
Levofloxacin	750 mg q24h
Ciprofloxacin	400 mg q8h
Vancomycin	15 mg/kg q12h
Linezolid	600 mg q12h

gen and monotherapy, an approach mirrored by the British Society of Antimicrobial Chemotherapy.[44]

Finally, the choice of molecules is based on the suspected pathogen(s) depending on the underlying disease, the local microbiology, direct examination or cultures obtained in a systematic manner. After starting treatment, it is necessary to perform a careful clinical evaluation of the response to the treatment. Rapid deterioration or the absence of improvement after 72 hours of empiric treatment requires systematic re-evaluation. It should be noted that the absence

Table 28.5 Risk factors for multidrug-resistant pathogens causing HAP

- Antimicrobial therapy in previous 90 days
- Current hospitalization of 5 days or more
- High frequency of antibiotic resistance in the community or in the specific hospital unit
- Hospitalization for 2 days or more in the previous 90 days
- Residence in a nursing home or extended care facility
- Home infusion therapy (including antibiotics)
- Chronic dialysis within 30 days
- Home wound care
- Family member with multidrug-resistant pathogen
- Immunosuppressive disease and/or therapy

of a response to empiric treatment can be linked to a nonbacterial cause of infection (in particular viral) or to an extrapulmonary infection, or to the absence of an infectious problem requiring aggressive diagnostic measures which can go as far as a lung biopsy. In cases of favorable evolution, de-escalation of antibiotherapy is indispensable once the antibiogram is known. It is also necessary to know when to stop antibiotherapy that is useless owing to negative microbiologic samples (performed before the beginning of all antibiotherapy) if the patient is in a satisfactory clinical condition. Singh *et al.*[45] demonstrated that discontinuing antibiotics after 3 days of intubation in patients with a clinical pulmonary infection score <6 caused antibiotic usage to be reduced without compromising patient mortality rates. A French multicenter study has reported an equivalence in terms of efficacy between short antibiotherapy (8 days) and long antibiotherapy (15 days).[4] Antibiotherapy should be prolonged only in cases of *Pseudomonas aeruginosa* and bi-therapy maintained for at least the first 5 days. Antibiotic selection for each patient should be based on the risk factors for MDR pathogens summarized in Table 28.5.

REFERENCES

References for this chapter can be found online at http://www.expertconsult.com

Chapter | 29 |

Madhuri M Sopirala
Julie E Mangino

Lung abscesses and pleural abscesses

INTRODUCTION

Lower respiratory tract infections (LRTIs) are a major indication for antimicrobial therapy in developed countries. Although many LRTIs are self-limiting, those caused by necrotizing organisms are invariably serious; they may lead to abscess formation in the lung and can spread to the pleural space.

EPIDEMIOLOGY

The etiologies of lung abscess and pleural abscess, or empyema, vary in different parts of the world. The common denominator is usually aspiration pneumonia, acquired either in the community or in the hospital. Nosocomial or health-care-associated pneumonia is a major cause of morbidity and lengthened hospital stay, with enormous economic impact. Aspiration pneumonia leading to a necrotizing pneumonia or lung abscess, with or without empyema, is a continuum; any stage or all stages may be encountered. Underlying diseases, associated trauma or surgery and the timeliness of appropriate therapy are the major factors in determining the clinical presentation and prognosis.

Lung abscess

A lung abscess is arbitrarily defined as a localized area of pulmonary necrosis caused by infection, with a solitary or dominant cavity measuring at least 2 cm in diameter. When cavities are multiple and smaller than 2 cm, the infection is usually referred to as a necrotizing pneumonia.[1,2] Most abscesses are suppurative bacterial infections caused by aspiration.

Primary lung abscesses typically present in patients who have no predisposing disease other than a predilection to aspirate oral secretions; they are more common in males than in females. Secondary lung abscesses occur in patients who have an underlying condition such as a partial bronchial obstruction or lung infarct, or in those who are otherwise immunocompromised because of chemotherapy, malignancy, organ transplantation or HIV infection. Lung abscesses may be termed nonspecific or putrid, referring, respectively, to the often unclear etiology and the offensive odor of the sputum.[3]

Over the past five decades, the incidence of bacterial lung abscess in the USA has diminished considerably and the mortality rate has decreased from 30–40% to 5–10%. Factors associated with a worse prognosis include advanced age, prolonged symptoms, concomitant disease, nosocomial infection and (according to some studies) larger cavity size. In the past, tuberculosis was responsible for a higher proportion of lung abscesses. In recent years, more lung abscesses have been associated with pulmonary malignancies or other underlying conditions.[4–6]

Empyema

A pleural effusion associated with pneumonia, lung abscess or bronchiectasis is referred to as a parapneumonic effusion. These occur in up to 40% of people who have bacterial pneumonia; they are the most common cause of exudative pleural effusions in the USA.[7] Empyema, or pleural pus, is an infected parapneumonic effusion with characteristic changes in the composition of the pleural fluid. It has been declining in frequency and changing in etiology.[8] Mortality ranges from approximately 2% to 50%, with the lowest rates in young, healthy people and the highest rates in the elderly and immunocompromised. The prognosis is poorer when pathogens are resistant to antimicrobial drugs or when appropriate treatment is delayed.[7,9,10]

PATHOGENESIS AND PATHOLOGY

Micro-organisms gain access to the lower respiratory tract by a variety of routes, including inhalation of aerosolized particles, aspiration of oropharyngeal secretions and hematogenous spread from distant sites (Fig. 29.1). Less frequently, infection occurs by direct extension from a contiguous site. Lung abscess is caused only by organisms that cause necrosis, but empyema can result from infection by any pathogen that reaches the pleural space.

Lung abscess

Of the inhaled respiratory pathogens, only the mycobacteria (see Chapter 30) and the dimorphic fungi (see Chapter 31) commonly cause lung abscesses. Bacterial abscesses are usually caused by aspiration of oropharyngeal secretions or, occasionally, by hematogenous seeding.[1]

Aspiration of small quantities of oropharyngeal secretions occurs intermittently in everyone, particularly during sleep. Despite the frequency of aspiration, the airways below the level of the larynx are normally sterile. Highly efficient clearing mechanisms are in place; these include cough, a mucociliary system that carries particles cephalad to be swallowed, phagocytosis by alveolar macrophages and neutrophils aided by opsonizing antibodies and complement, and lymphatic trapping with sequestration in regional lymph nodes. Risk factors for pneumonia after aspiration include conditions that increase the inoculum of pathogenic organisms in aspirated secretions, conditions that increase the likelihood of aspiration and conditions that increase the volume of the aspirate (Table 29.1). Under these circumstances, aspirated oropharyngeal secretions are more likely to cause chemical irritation and infection. When an anaerobic pleuropulmonary infection occurs in an edentulous patient, the diagnosis of bronchogenic carcinoma should be considered.[1–3,11]

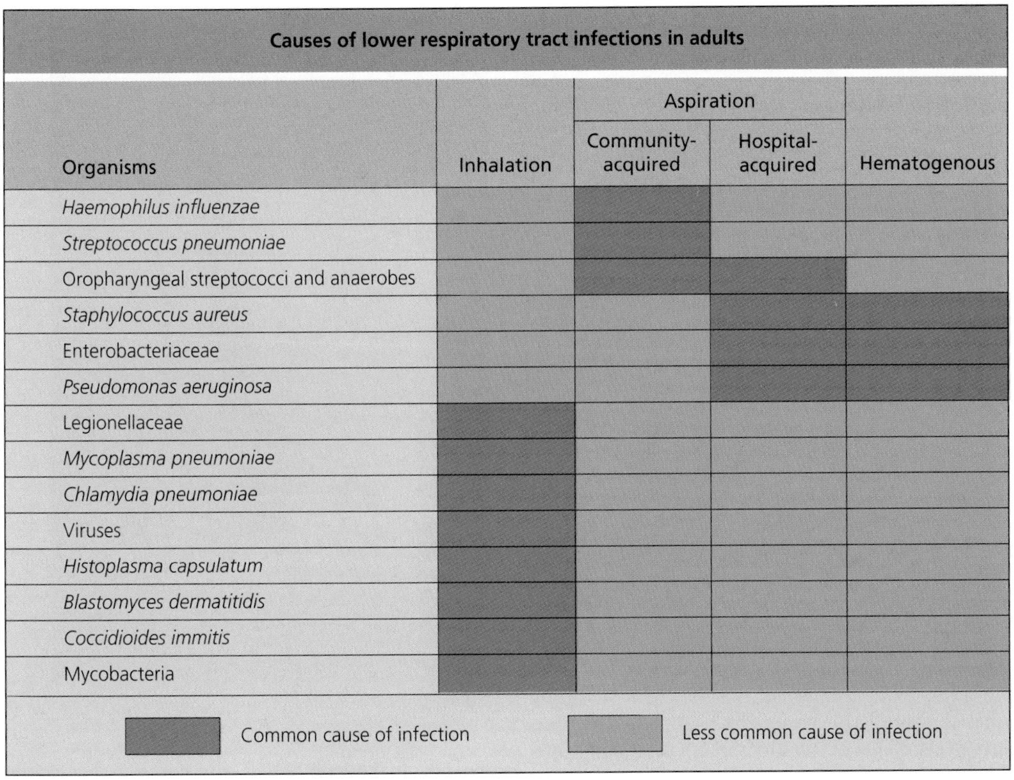

Organisms	Inhalation	Aspiration		Hematogenous
		Community-acquired	Hospital-acquired	
Haemophilus influenzae				
Streptococcus pneumoniae				
Oropharyngeal streptococci and anaerobes				
Staphylococcus aureus				
Enterobacteriaceae				
Pseudomonas aeruginosa				
Legionellaceae				
Mycoplasma pneumoniae				
Chlamydia pneumoniae				
Viruses				
Histoplasma capsulatum				
Blastomyces dermatitidis				
Coccidioides immitis				
Mycobacteria				

Causes of lower respiratory tract infections in adults

☐ Common cause of infection   ☐ Less common cause of infection

Fig. 29.1 Causes of LRTIs in adults. Oropharyngeal streptococci and anaerobes, *Staphylococcus aureus*, Enterobacteriaceae, *Pseudomonas aeruginosa*, the dimorphic fungi (*Histoplasma capsulatum*, *Blastomyces dermatitidis*, *Coccidioides immitis*) and mycobacteria frequently cause necrosis and subsequent abscess formation.

Table 29.1 Risk factors for aspiration pneumonia and lung abscess

Increased bacterial inoculum	Periodontal disease, gingivitis, tonsillar or dental abscess, drugs that decrease gastric acidity
Impairment of consciousness	Drugs, alcohol, general anesthesia, metabolic encephalopathy, coma, shock, cerebrovascular accident, cardiopulmonary arrest, seizures, surgery, trauma
Impaired cough and gag reflexes	Vocal cord paralysis, intratracheal anesthesia, endotracheal tube, tracheostomy, myopathy, myelopathy, other neurologic disorders
Impairment of esophageal function	Diverticula, achalasia, strictures, disorders of gastrointestinal motility, neoplasm, tracheoesophageal fistula, pseudobulbar palsy
Emesis	Nasogastric tube, gastric dilatation, ileus, intestinal obstruction

The composition of the oropharyngeal flora at the time of aspiration determines the potential etiologic agents for LRTIs. Those organisms that are most numerous or virulent proliferate and emerge as single or predominant pathogens. Although the classic non-necrotizing respiratory pathogens *Streptococcus pneumoniae* and *Haemophilus influenzae* can cause disease by this mechanism, normal oropharyngeal secretions contain many more streptococci of various species and more anaerobes (approximately 10^8 organisms/ml) than aerobes (approximately 10^7 organisms/ml). Some of the streptococcal species are microaerophilic (i.e. they require supplemental carbon dioxide to grow on artificial media).[12,13] The pneumonia that follows aspiration, with or without abscess formation, is typically polymicrobial with between two and four bacterial species present in large numbers. In general, 50% or more of these infections are caused by purely anaerobic bacteria, 25% are caused by mixed aerobes and anaerobes, and 25% or fewer are caused by aerobes only. Among hospitalized patients, progressive colonization with *Staphylococcus aureus*, Enterobacteriaceae and *Pseudomonas aeruginosa* occurs, and these aerobic organisms are frequent causes of health-care-associated aspiration pneumonia and lung abscess.[8,12,14,15] A retrospective evaluation of 90 adults with lung abscesses in Taiwan revealed that Gram-negative bacilli caused 36% of cases, whereas anaerobes accounted for 34% of cases. Twenty-five percent of the patients in this study had received antibiotics prior to culture, which could have made recovery of anaerobes even less likely.[16]

The anaerobic organisms that are associated with pleuropulmonary infection, using current nomenclature,[17,18] are shown in Table 29.2. The primary pathogens are *Streptococcus* spp., *Peptostreptococcus* spp. (now divided into four genera – *Anaerococcus*, *Finegoldia*, *Gallicola* and *Peptoniphilus*), *Fusobacterium nucleatum* and *Prevotella* spp. Additionally, *Porphyromonas* spp. are commonly associated with periodontal disease and may also be isolated. Although not consistently part of the normal oropharyngeal flora, members of the *Bacteroides fragilis* group of organisms are isolated from approximately 15% of patients.[2,11–14,17]

A variety of virulence factors associated with oropharyngeal streptococci and anaerobes have been identified. Properties that facilitate attachment include capsular polysaccharides, fimbriae, hemagglutinin and lectin. Tissue breakdown and the metabolic activity of organisms provide reducing substances and a low redox potential; these factors facilitate bacterial proliferation. Volatile fatty acids, sulfur compounds, indoles, amines and hydrolytic enzymes (hyaluronidase, chondroitin sulfatase and heparinase) produced by damaged tissue lead to subsequent abscess formation.[19]

Table 29.2 Anaerobic bacteria associated with pleuropulmonary infections

	Gram-negative bacteria	Gram-positive bacteria
Bacilli	*Bacteroides fragilis* group *Fusobacterium nucleatum* *Fusobacterium necrophorum* *Porphyromonas* spp.* *Prevotella* spp.	*Actinomyces* spp. *Bifidobacterium* spp. *Clostridium* spp. *Eubacterium* spp. *Lactobacillus* spp. *Propionibacterium* spp.
Cocci	*Veillonella* spp.	*Gemella morbillorum* *Peptostreptococcus* spp. *Streptococcus* spp.

*Note: *Porphyromonas* spp. include organisms previously named *Bacteroides melaninogenicus* subsp. *asaccharolyticus*, *B. endodontalis* and *B. gingivalis*. *Prevotella* spp. include organisms previously named *B. melaninogenicus* subspp. *melaninogenicus* and *intermedius*, *B. oralis* and *B. denticola*. *Gemella morbillorum* was previously named *Streptococcus morbillorum*. *Peptostreptococcus* spp. are now divided into four genera – *Anaerococcus*, *Finegoldia*, *Gallicola* and *Peptoniphilus*.

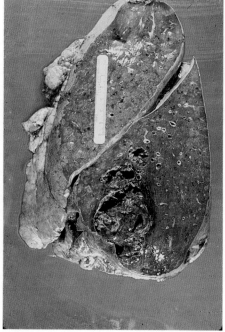

Fig. 29.2 Cross-section of a lung abscess.

The pathology of aspiration pneumonia is characterized by alveolar edema and infiltration with inflammatory cells. Foci of aspiration pneumonia most commonly develop in the subpleural regions of the gravity-dependent segments of the lungs, particularly the superior segments of the lower lobes and the posterior segments of the upper lobes. The right lung is the more frequent location, presumably because of the less acute angle in the take-off of the right main stem bronchus. In general, the right upper and lower lobes are most commonly involved, followed by the left lower lobe and right middle lobe.[1,3,20,21]

The degree and rate of progression of aspiration pneumonia vary considerably. These infections may be acute, subacute or chronic, depending on differences in the etiology, size of inoculum and host factors. If the process is indolent, fibrosis limits the spread of infection. Abscesses typically communicate with a bronchus, producing the familiar air-filled cavity, often with an air–fluid level that can be seen on radiographs. These are usually not apparent until the infection has been present for 1–2 weeks, when multiple adjacent microscopic abscesses filled with necrotic material (pulmonary gangrene) slough to form a gross cavity (Fig. 29.2).[4]

Although less common than aspiration, hematogenous seeding of the lung, or septic emboli, may also result in lung abscesses or necrotizing pneumonia. There may be a solitary infiltrate or cavity or, more often, multiple bilateral lesions. The most common etiologic agents are the health-care-associated pathogens *Staph. aureus* and aerobic Gram-negative bacilli (see Fig. 29.1). When the primary focus is in the abdomen, anaerobes, particularly *B. fragilis*, may be present.

Infective endocarditis (predominantly right-sided), intravenous drug injection and indwelling right atrial catheters placed for vascular access are commonly associated with septic pulmonary emboli. Any organism that is part of the skin flora or contaminants in injected material may be responsible. *Staph. aureus* and streptococci are the most common pathogens, but *P. aeruginosa* and *Candida* spp. may also be responsible, causing serious infections.[22]

Some uncommon causes of lung abscess should be considered in appropriate circumstances. Inhaled micro-organisms such as *Legionella* spp., *Chlamydia* spp., *Mycoplasma pneumoniae* and viruses are rare causes of lung abscesses. *Cryptococcus*, *Aspergillus* and *Rhizopus* spp. occasionally cause disease in normal hosts but are more commonly opportunistic pathogens. Patients who have advanced HIV disease may have cavitary lesions caused by atypical mycobacteria, particularly *Mycobacterium kansasii*, and other organisms such as *Rhodococcus equi* and *Nocardia asteroides*.[23] *Burkholderia pseudomallei* is endemic to South East Asia, particularly Thailand, and typically causes upper lobe

cavities. In endemic areas, the parasites *Paragonimus westermani* and *Entamoeba histolytica* may cause abscess by contiguous extension.

Empyema

The pleural space is normally sterile. It is most commonly contaminated by direct extension from a contiguous focus of infection, usually pulmonary, or by direct inoculation at the time of trauma or surgery (Table 29.3).[7,24,25] The pleural space may also become involved through hematogenous seeding from a distant focus of infection, particularly in the presence of hemothorax or pleural malignancy.

The initial stage in the pathogenesis of empyema associated with pneumonia is the development of a sterile parapneumonic effusion, which has varying characteristics depending on its stage of evolution (Table 29.4).[7,25] The effusion is initially transudative but rapidly becomes exudative with an influx of leukocytes and increasing permeability of the visceral pleura. Neutrophils, lactate dehydrogenase

Table 29.3 Causes of empyema

Pulmonary infection	Pneumonia Lung abscess Bronchiectasis
Mediastinal disease	Tracheal fistula Esophageal perforation
Subdiaphragmatic infection	Subphrenic abscess Hepatic abscess
Skeletal infection	Paravertebral abscess Vertebral osteomyelitis
Direct inoculation	Trauma Thoracentesis
Postoperative	Hemothorax (infected) Pneumothorax (infected) Bronchopleural fistula

Table 29.4 Characteristics* of pleural fluid associated with bacterial LRTI

| Pleural fluid characteristic | Transudate | EXUDATE | | Empyema |
		Uncomplicated parapneumonic effusion	Complicated parapneumonic effusion	
Appearance	Clear	Variable	Variable	Pus
White blood cell count (cells/ml)	<1000	Variable	Variable	>15000
Differential cell count	Variable	Neutrophils	Neutrophils	Neutrophils
Protein (g/dl)	<3.0	>3.0	>3.0	>3.0
Glucose (mg/dl)	Same as serum	>60	40–60	<40
pH	Greater than serum	>7.2	7.0–7.2	<7.0
Lactate dehydrogenase (units/ml)	<200	<1000	>1000	>1000
Bacteria	Absent	Absent	Absent	Absent

*The values may overlap. Complicated pleural effusions are those with fluid characteristics that indicate the potential need for tube drainage. When the glucose is 40–60 mg/dl or the pH is 7.0–7.2, repeat thoracentesis may be helpful. When the glucose is <40 mg/dl or the pH is less than 7.0, a chest tube is indicated even if bacteria are not present by smear or culture.
Data from Light[7] and Sokolowski et al.[26]

(LDH) and protein increase, and glucose and pH decrease. Fibrin is deposited on the pleural surfaces and loculations may occur. With time, a final organizing stage occurs in which pleural fibroblasts produce an inelastic membrane or pleural peel that encases the lung and restricts inflation. Invasion with bacteria accelerates the fibropurulent reaction. Empyema fluid is relatively deficient in opsonins and complement and it becomes progressively more acidic as the infection ensues. Occasionally, an empyema may spontaneously drain through necrotic lung tissue into a bronchus (bronchopleural fistula) or communicate through the chest wall (empyema necessitans).[7,10,25]

The various respiratory pathogens have different propensities to cause empyema. *Streptococcus pneumoniae*, the most common cause of pneumonia, is frequently associated with a parapneumonic pleural effusion, yet pneumococcal empyema is relatively uncommon.

Aspiration pneumonia more frequently progresses to empyema.[7] Empyema is also more common with organisms such as *Staph. aureus* and *P. aeruginosa* that produce potent extracellular enzymes that breach the integrity of the pleura, allowing penetration to the pleural space.

Overall, the relative frequencies of various organisms causing empyema have changed over time. Prior to the antibiotic era, most empyemas were caused by *Strep. pneumoniae* and, to a lesser extent, by *Staph. aureus* and *Strep. pyogenes*. Between 1955 and 1965, penicillin-resistant *Staph. aureus* was the predominant pathogen.[7,27] In the early 1970s, coinciding with a surge of interest in anaerobic infections, anaerobic empyemas were recognized more frequently (Table 29.5).[28,29] At that time, about 50% of empyemas were caused by aerobes, with Gram-positive cocci being more

Table 29.5 Frequency of organisms isolated from bacterial empyemas

| Organism | % OF ISOLATES | | |
	1971–1973[28] (n=214)	1969–1978[9] (n=93)	1973–1985[29] (n=343)
Haemophilus influenzae	<1	0	3
Streptococcus pneumoniae	2	7	20
Other streptococci (including microaerophiles)	13	22	8
Staphylococcus aureus	8	8	17
Enterobacteriaceae	9	10	11
Pseudomonas spp.	5	9	3
Other aerobes	5	2	2
Bacteroides spp.	11	14	8
Anaerobic cocci	15	9	10
Fusobacterium spp.	7	8	6
Prevotella spp.	6	4	6
Other anaerobes	19	7	6

common than Gram-negative bacilli. About 25% were caused by anaerobes and about 25% were mixed aerobic-anaerobic infections. *Streptococcus pneumoniae* was most frequent in young ambulatory patients, anaerobes were most frequent after aspiration, and *Staph. aureus* and aerobic Gram-negative bacilli were most frequent after thoracotomy.[9,12,30,31] Because one-quarter of all empyemas are now associated with trauma or surgery, there has been a relative increase in the proportion of staphylococcal infections and a decrease in anaerobic infections.[7] With the widespread use of *H. influenzae* type b vaccination, empyema due to this organism, previously common in children, has become rare.

PREVENTION

Minimizing the risks of aspiration in people who are unconscious, undergoing anesthesia or subject to seizures will reduce the incidence of pneumonia with subsequent abscess formation or empyema. If pneumonia does occur, the timely administration of appropriate antibiotics reduces the likelihood of progression. Pleural effusions should be aspirated for diagnosis and drained, if indicated, to abort progressive suppurative complications.

CLINICAL FEATURES

Lung abscess

Aspiration is usually subtle and unrecognized but may lead to pneumonia and lung abscess. If overt, it may be followed by symptoms and signs such as choking, cough, wheezing, cyanosis or asphyxia, which are related to the particulate, liquid and chemical nature of the material aspirated. Within hours, there may be fever, tachypnea, diffuse rales and hypoxemia.[11,31] If pneumonia develops, patients usually present within 1 week with a productive cough, a temperature over 102°F (38.9°C) and a leukocyte count of more than 15 000 cells/mm³.[31] Aspiration pneumonia is not readily distinguishable from pneumococcal pneumonia, although true rigors are uncommon in aspiration pneumonia and symptoms have usually been present for longer before presentation to medical care. A condition predisposing to aspiration is also more likely to be present. Among community-acquired cases, common conditions that predispose to aspiration are alcoholism, seizures and drug overdose. Among health-care-acquired cases, patients tend to have neurologic disorders, such as cerebrovascular accidents and brain tumors, or metabolic disorders that result in stupor or coma. Only a minority of patients who have aspiration pneumonia have putrid sputum, which, if present, tends to develop 1–2 weeks into the course when an abscess has formed.[8,12,14,31]

Lung abscesses may also present in a more indolent fashion with weeks to months of productive cough, malaise, weight loss, low-grade fever, night sweats, leukocytosis and anemia. The patient may become debilitated as if with tuberculosis. Findings that are suggestive of a suppurative lung abscess rather than tuberculosis include a shorter duration of symptoms, putrid sputum and leukocytosis. Lung abscess must also be distinguished from a necrotic neoplasm. Patients who have neoplasms often lack risk factors for aspiration, symptoms of respiratory infection, fever and leukocytosis. The possibility of tuberculosis or a noninfectious cause of a lung cavity (neoplasm, infarct or vasculitis) should be suspected in a patient treated for presumed lung abscess who does not respond to appropriate antimicrobial therapy.

In the pre-antibiotic era, lung abscess characteristically ran a chronic course with the potential for sudden, severe complications. These included brain abscess, massive hemoptysis, endobronchial spread to other portions of the lung, and rupture into the pleural space with the development of a bronchopleural fistula and pyopneumothorax. With modern antimicrobial therapy, these complications have become rare.

Empyema

Symptoms of empyema include fever, chills, cough, dyspnea and chest pain associated with a recent pulmonary or contiguous infection in the oropharynx, mediastinum or subdiaphragmatic area. The occurrence of persistent fever and leukocytosis with pleural effusion despite appropriate antibiotics should suggest the presence of empyema. There may also be severe constitutional manifestations such as shock, tachypnea, altered consciousness and respiratory failure. Typical findings on physical examination include diminished breath sounds, dullness to percussion and a pleural friction rub. Patients who have an empyema secondary to an aerobic pneumonia tend to present with an acute illness, whereas those who have an anaerobic pneumonia have subacute or indolent illness with findings such as putrid sputum to suggest the etiology.[1,4,31]

DIAGNOSIS

Radiography

Both lung abscess and empyema may be suspected from clinical symptoms but the chest radiograph is the primary tool for diagnosing these infections. Radiographs obtained soon after aspiration usually demonstrate localized or diffuse alveolar infiltrates within 1–2 days. There is nothing distinctive about the appearance of aspiration pneumonia except that infiltrates are usually in dependent segments of the lung. Multilobar involvement may suggest impairment of the host immune system.[32]

The characteristic appearance of a lung abscess is that of a density or mass with a cavity, frequently with an air–fluid level indicating communication with the tracheobronchial tree (Fig. 29.3). The time required for cavitation after a known episode of aspiration is about 1–2 weeks. With necrotizing pneumonia, multiple small lucencies in circumscribed areas of opacification may develop more rapidly.[1,4,33] Abscesses due to tuberculosis are less likely to have an air–fluid level and are more likely to have a dense fibronodular infiltrate that surrounds the cavities.[21] Those associated with a malignancy may be more sharply defined or have an eccentric-shaped cavity with a thick, irregular wall (Fig. 29.4).

A pleural effusion, visible on posterior-anterior and lateral upright chest radiographs, suggests the possibility of empyema. On a decubitus film, with the suspect side down, free pleural fluid can be visualized between the chest wall and the dependent lung. If the layer of pleural fluid is greater than 1 cm thick, it should be aspirated for diagnostic studies. A decubitus film with the suspect side up is also useful because it permits assessment of any underlying parenchymal infiltrate, less obscured by the effusion.[7,25]

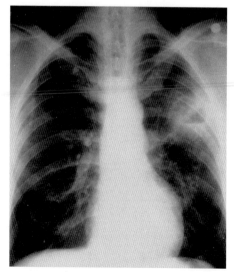

Fig. 29.3 A lung abscess showing an air–fluid level.

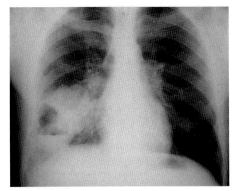

Fig. 29.4 A lung abscess associated with a multinodular bronchogenic carcinoma.

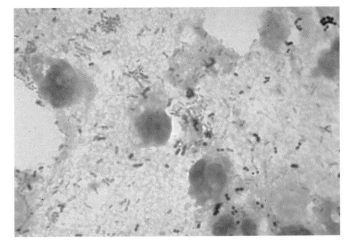

Fig. 29.6 Gram stain of lower respiratory tract secretions. The patient had a lung abscess caused by oropharyngeal streptococci and anaerobes.

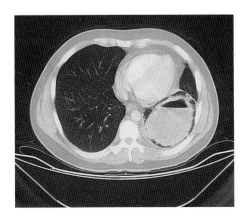

Fig. 29.5 CT scan of a lung abscess showing an air–fluid level.

Ultrasound and CT may be helpful in defining pleuropulmonary lesions. Ultrasound can define loculated collections of pleural fluid, and portable equipment is available for unstable or critically ill patients. CT can define abscesses that are not apparent on plain radiographs and can distinguish between parenchymal and pleural disease (Fig. 29.5). Loculated empyema with a bronchopleural fistula may resemble a lung abscess. Features on CT that tend to favor lung abscess are the presence of thick walls and lesions that are round or oblong, whereas empyemas have thinner walls with a smooth luminal margin and exterior.[34] Both ultrasound and CT may be used to guide aspiration of fluid from abscesses or the pleural space.

Investigations

The first step in determining the specific etiology of any LRTI is the evaluation of lower respiratory tract secretions by Gram stain. These are most likely to be useful if they are obtained before the administration of effective antimicrobial treatment. If stains of expectorated specimens show neutrophils and alveolar macrophages, without squamous epithelial cells (indicative of contamination with saliva), they are useful for defining the offending pathogen(s). In aerobic pneumonia there is usually a single predominant organism; in aspiration pneumonia there is usually a mixed flora, representing the diverse morphotypes of the oropharyngeal flora. Typically, there are various sizes of Gram-positive cocci and pleomorphic Gram-negative coccobacilli and bacilli, which may be tapered and are generally smaller and poorer staining than the Enterobacteriaceae (Fig. 29.6).[1,2,11,13,35] Although some of the individual organisms may resemble pathogenic aerobes such as *Strep. pneumoniae*, there is no predominant pathogen.

Invasive procedures, such as endotracheal aspiration and bronchoscopy, may be useful to obtain lower respiratory secretions for evaluation. Tracheal aspiration through the nose or the mouth is of limited use because these specimens are often contaminated with oropharyngeal flora. Bronchoscopy with bronchoalveolar lavage is useful

because large samples can be obtained with relatively little contamination. They can be concentrated by cytocentrifugation, permitting multiple microbiologic and cytologic evaluations. The bronchoscopic techniques of protected catheter aspiration and protected specimen brushing reduce contamination considerably but they provide relatively scanty specimens and rely on quantitative cultures to help distinguish the significance of cultures. In general, counts that indicate more than 10^5 cfu/ml of respiratory secretions for an appropriate organism (see Fig. 29.1, Table 29.2) are indicative of infection.[1,4,15,24]

Specimens of lower respiratory tract secretions that have passed through the mouth should be cultured for aerobes but not for anaerobes. Growth of recognized aerobic pathogens is helpful for interpreting Gram stains and for providing isolates for susceptibility testing. The absence of aerobic pathogens in specimens from untreated patients should indicate the possibility of anaerobic infection. When specimens are contaminated by saliva, the streptococci and anaerobes that comprise the normal oropharyngeal flora will always grow in culture, whether or not infection is present, and they provide no insight into the pathogenicity of the organisms isolated.

The problem of contamination of respiratory tract secretions by saliva can be avoided if specimens of lower respiratory secretions are obtained by transtracheal aspiration. A catheter is passed through the cricothyroid membrane and specimens are collected by suction.[1,12,14] Although rarely used today, this technique established the role of anaerobes in suppurative pleuropulmonary infections in the early 1970s. Another method for obtaining uncontaminated material for culture is percutaneous transthoracic needle aspiration (percutaneous abscess drainage). Today, this procedure is more frequently performed under fluoroscopic or CT guidance for the diagnosis of malignancy than to obtain material for culture. It can be used, however, to aspirate peripheral abscesses, particularly if bronchoscopy does not provide an adequate specimen for microbiologic diagnosis.

If appropriate specimens from the lower respiratory tract are obtained for culturing anaerobes, they should be expeditiously transported to the laboratory, with minimal exposure to air, for proper processing. If tuberculosis or fungal infection is in the differential diagnosis, appropriate smears and cultures should be requested. If a malignancy is suspected, cytologic stains should be performed. An amplified *Mycobacterium tuberculosis* direct test (MTD) can be useful for detection of smear-negative pulmonary tuberculosis cases.

In addition to lower respiratory tract secretions, blood and pleural fluid, if present, should also be sent to the laboratory for microbiologic evaluation. In anaerobic lung infections, blood cultures are rarely positive. Pleural fluid, if present, requires analysis of protein, LDH and glucose, and determination of pH, as well as microbiologic evaluation. With empyema, the Gram stain usually indicates the pathogens.[7]

With the advances in molecular diagnostics, rapid and accurate identification of anaerobic bacteria by the polymerase chain reaction-based method is possible. Even though there is an increasing trend toward molecular diagnostics of anaerobes, identification of infections caused by these bacteria currently relies on clinical findings, appropriate transport of specimens, laboratory identification of the organisms by morphology and biochemical tests.[37]

MANAGEMENT

Lung abscess

In the past, penicillin G was the preferred drug for treating aspiration pneumonia and lung abscesses, as well as for all anaerobic infections above the diaphragm caused by oropharyngeal flora. In a study of over 70 patients hospitalized with lung abscesses in the 1960s, nearly all responded to intravenous penicillin G. Oral penicillin V in a dose of 3 g/day was also effective and those rare patients who failed to respond to penicillin could be satisfactorily treated with tetracycline.[8]

In the 1970s, when transtracheal aspiration was used to define the microbiology of pneumonia and lung abscesses, concern over the use of penicillin was raised because of occasional therapeutic failures and the isolation of penicillin-resistant *B. fragilis* from some patients.[1,14] However, in one study that compared clindamycin, a drug that is active against *B. fragilis*, with penicillin G in the treatment of aspiration pneumonia and primary lung abscess, there was no difference in rates of defervescence, radiographic clearing or ultimate outcome. Notably, seven patients from whom *B. fragilis* was isolated responded to penicillin.[33]

Subsequently, in a prospective study published in 1983 of 39 patients who had lung abscess, there were 0/19 failures with clindamycin and 4/20 failures with penicillin G. Resolution of fever and putrid sputum was more rapid with clindamycin (4.4 days) than penicillin G (7.6 days). Patients who did not respond to penicillin G ultimately responded to clindamycin.[38] In a 1990 study of 37 patients who had lung abscess or necrotizing pneumonia,[39] only 1/19 patients failed to respond to clindamycin, whereas 8/18 failed with penicillin G. In this study, patients underwent transtracheal aspiration or protected specimen brushing to culture for anaerobes; 9/10 of the penicillin-G-resistant strains were β-lactamase producers. It is now recognized that there has been a change in the susceptibilities of the oropharyngeal Gram-negative anaerobes since the 1970s. Many, in addition to *B. fragilis*, are now β-lactamase producers and resistant to penicillin. In a study of 449 isolates, which included *Bacteroides* spp. other than *B. fragilis*, *Fusobacterium* spp., *Prevotella* spp. and *Porphyromonas* spp. from 28 US medical centers, 57.9% of isolates were β-lactamase producers.[40]

Today, transtracheal aspiration and other invasive procedures are rarely performed to determine the microbiologic etiology of aspiration pneumonia and lung abscesses in nonimmunocompromised patients. Treatment is usually empiric and largely effective.[8] Clinical outcome for most anaerobic infections seems to correlate with *in-vitro* data as broadly applied, and detailed study of individual cases does not seem to be necessary. Monitoring trends in susceptibility patterns and detailed study in problematic individual cases suffices.[31]

The *in-vitro* spectrum and clinical utility of antimicrobials for the treatment of lower respiratory tract bacterial infections is summarized in Figure 29.7. For community-acquired infections that result from aspiration, and where oropharyngeal streptococci and anaerobes are the likely pathogens, penicillin G (or ampicillin or amoxicillin) remains an excellent foundation for treatment, but the addition of a β-lactamase inhibitor or metronidazole is advisable owing to the frequency of β-lactamase production among Gram-negative anaerobes.[31,40,41] Clindamycin is also a primary therapeutic agent, despite *in-vitro* resistance among some *Bacteroides* and *Fusobacterium* spp. Resistance rates vary significantly in different geographic regions, so surveillance of resistance is important in assessing the utility in a given area.[5,8,35,41,42] Metronidazole alone is not effective because of its inactivity against the aerobic and microaerophilic streptococci.[8,41,43]

For health-care-acquired infections, where *Staph. aureus* and aerobic Gram-negative bacilli are common components of the oropharyngeal flora, piperacillin or ticarcillin (rather than penicillin or ampicillin) with a β-lactamase inhibitor provide better coverage of likely pathogens. Appropriate alternatives are imipenem alone, clindamycin plus an aminoglycoside or ciprofloxacin, or an expanded spectrum cephalosporin such as cefotaxime, ceftizoxime or ceftriaxone plus metronidazole. In health-care settings with a high incidence of methicillin-resistant *Staph. aureus* (MRSA) pulmonary infection, the addition of intravenous vancomycin or linezolid should be considered. Many cephalosporins, for example ceftazidime, have little or no activity against anaerobes and should not be used unless the etiology has been defined and found to involve aerobic Gram-negative bacilli.[8,10,43]

Tetracyclines, which were used for lung abscess and empyema in the 1960s, are no longer recommended for the treatment of aerobic/anaerobic pleuropulmonary infections because of high rates of resistance. Chloramphenicol has an excellent spectrum of activity but is rarely recommended because of potential hematotoxicity and the availability of alternative agents.[8,43] The macrolides and azalides have inconsistent *in-vitro* activity against oropharyngeal anaerobes and there is little clinical precedent for their use.[44] Aminoglycosides and quinolones should be used only for their activity against aerobic Gram-negative bacilli and need to be combined with a drug that is active against streptococci and anaerobes. A newer quinolone, such as moxifloxacin or gatifloxacin, has greater activity than ciprofloxacin or ofloxacin against oropharyngeal streptococci and anaerobes, and is more useful.[45,46] In the treatment of aspiration-associated pulmonary infections, moxifloxacin appears to be clinically as effective and as safe as ampicillin-sulbactam.[47] Ertapenem, a once-daily carbapenem, can be used if the oral route is precluded and if the infection does not include *P. aeruginosa*.[48] Other agents that have suboptimal or no activity against oropharyngeal streptococci and anaerobes include aztreonam and trimethoprim-sulfamethoxazole. The antistaphylococcal penicillins and vancomycin should be reserved for documented staphylococcal infections.

The duration of antimicrobial therapy necessary to treat pleuropulmonary infections is variable: 1–2 weeks may suffice for simple aspiration pneumonia but necrotizing pneumonia and lung abscesses may require 3–24 weeks. Parenteral therapy is generally employed until the patient is afebrile (most are afebrile in 7 days) and able to have a consistent enteral intake.[31] For most community-acquired infections, amoxicillin-clavulanate and clindamycin are excellent oral drugs that can be used for continued treatment after initial parenteral therapy. A less costly oral alternative is penicillin V plus metronidazole. If aerobic Gram-negative bacilli are present, oral treatment is more problematic and must be based on the results of susceptibility tests; ciprofloxacin or ofloxacin plus a penicillin or clindamycin may be appropriate. Prolonged therapy is advisable, with treatment continued until the cavity is gone or until serial radiographs show considerable improvement or a small stable residual scar (Fig. 29.8). The time to cavity closure depends largely on the size of the cavity when treatment is initiated and the condition of the patient.

Surgical drainage of lung abscesses is rarely indicated because drainage occurs naturally via the tracheobronchial tree. If spontaneous drainage is not adequate, even with the aid of postural drainage and percussion, clinical improvement is impeded; CT-guided percutaneous abscess drainage may then be beneficial.[49] The drainage catheter can be left in place until there is clinical improvement and drainage has diminished, usually within several days to 1 week. This technique may also be used to reduce the risk of endobronchial spread of infection to other areas of the lungs as well as in patients who are too ill to undergo lung resection to remove necrotic tissue, persistent cavities or nonfunctional lung. Other indications for drainage include large abscess cavity (>8 cm), abscess caused by resistant organisms, obstructing neoplasm impeding drainage and failure of medical treatment. Endoscopic drainage, when performed by an experienced operator, can also be useful for patients who are considered to be poor surgical candidates.[50]

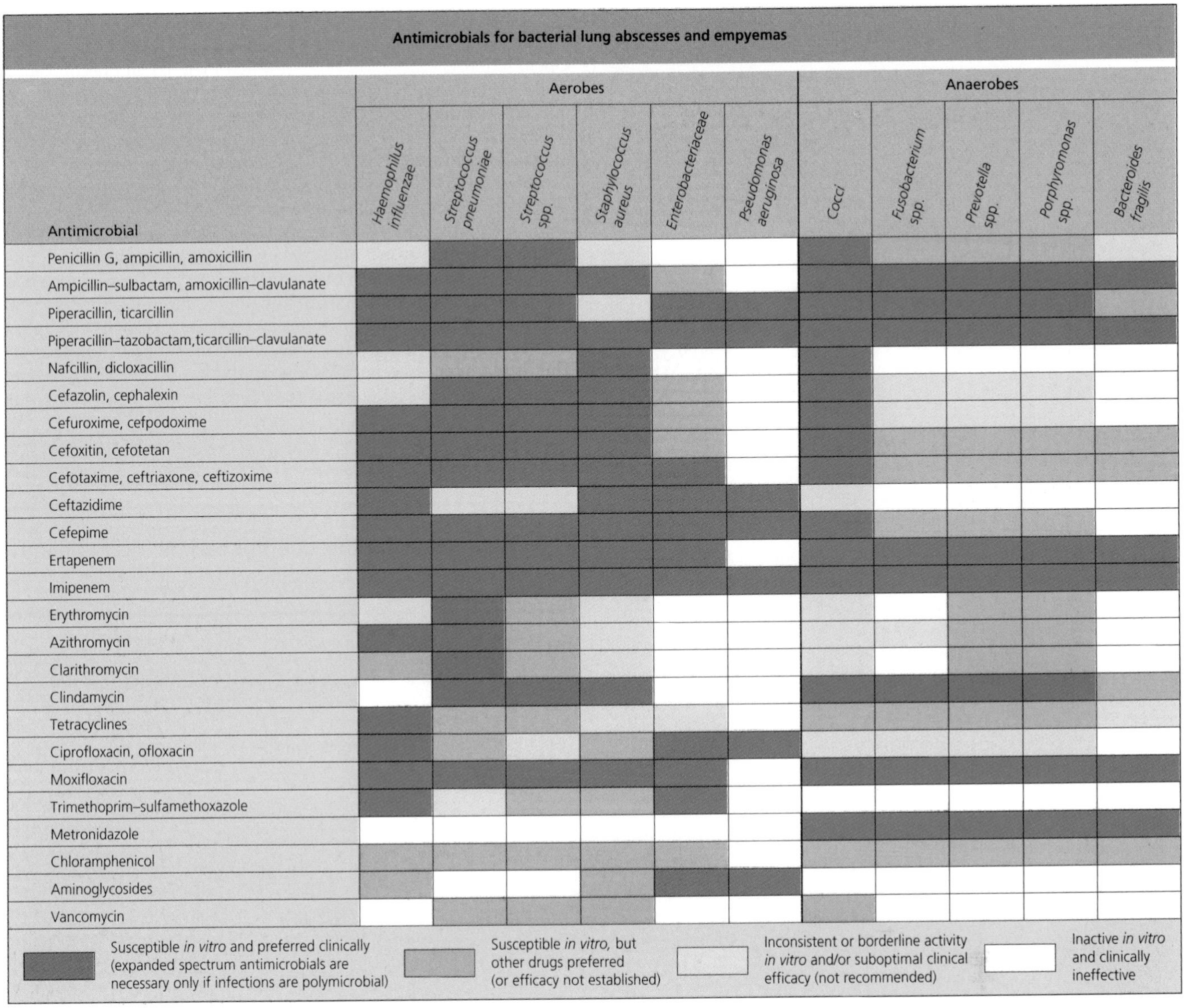

Antimicrobials for bacterial lung abscesses and empyemas

Antimicrobial	Aerobes						Anaerobes				
	Haemophilus influenzae	*Streptococcus pneumoniae*	*Streptococcus* spp.	*Staphylococcus aureus*	*Enterobacteriaceae*	*Pseudomonas aeruginosa*	*Cocci*	*Fusobacterium* spp.	*Prevotella* spp.	*Porphyromonas* spp.	*Bacteroides fragilis*
Penicillin G, ampicillin, amoxicillin											
Ampicillin–sulbactam, amoxicillin–clavulanate											
Piperacillin, ticarcillin											
Piperacillin–tazobactam, ticarcillin–clavulanate											
Nafcillin, dicloxacillin											
Cefazolin, cephalexin											
Cefuroxime, cefpodoxime											
Cefoxitin, cefotetan											
Cefotaxime, ceftriaxone, ceftizoxime											
Ceftazidime											
Cefepime											
Ertapenem											
Imipenem											
Erythromycin											
Azithromycin											
Clarithromycin											
Clindamycin											
Tetracyclines											
Ciprofloxacin, ofloxacin											
Moxifloxacin											
Trimethoprim–sulfamethoxazole											
Metronidazole											
Chloramphenicol											
Aminoglycosides											
Vancomycin											

Legend:
- Susceptible *in vitro* and preferred clinically (expanded spectrum antimicrobials are necessary only if infections are polymicrobial)
- Susceptible *in vitro*, but other drugs preferred (or efficacy not established)
- Inconsistent or borderline activity *in vitro* and/or suboptimal clinical efficacy (not recommended)
- Inactive *in vitro* and clinically ineffective

Fig. 29.7 Antimicrobials for bacterial lung abscesses and empyemas. Information for *Streptococcus pneumoniae* is for penicillin-susceptible strains – selected cephalosporins or vancomycin should be used for resistant strains. Information for *Staphylococcus aureus* is for methicillin-susceptible strains – vancomycin should be used for resistant strains. Vancomycin is the drug of choice for β-lactam-resistant Gram-positive organisms.

Empyema

The antimicrobial treatment of empyema is similar to that of aspiration pneumonia and lung abscess but single-organism infections with a defined etiology are more common, thus facilitating antibiotic choice. Antibiotics should be administered in full doses for 2–4 weeks. Therapy may need to be prolonged further, particularly if drainage is not optimal. Antibiotic levels in pleural fluid are comparable to those in serum, so standard systemic doses provide adequate pleural fluid levels.[25]

The proper assessment and management of parapneumonic effusions associated with LRTIs is critical for a successful outcome. Most small effusions clear with antimicrobial treatment and need not be drained. However, if fluid persists more than a few days or layers to more than 1 cm on a decubitus radiograph with the involved side dependent, it should be aspirated and analyzed. The characteristics of the fluid are used to determine the need for tube drainage (see Table 29.4).

Effusions are termed 'complicated' when characteristics indicate a potential need for tube drainage. Complicated effusions are termed 'empyemas' if they are frankly purulent and bacteria are present; tube drainage is mandatory. Chest tubes are placed using negative pressure until the lung is expanded, and then to an underwater drainage system until the fluid is scanty and clear, and then gradually withdrawn over a period of several days. Lack of prompt clinical improvement may indicate the need to reposition the tube to facilitate and continue drainage.

Chest tube drainage of complicated parapneumonic effusions is successful in most patients. It should not be delayed, because these effusions can progress from free-flowing to loculated fluid rapidly. When the fluid becomes loculated, drainage by repeated thoracentesis or tube insertion may not be adequate. The presence of loculated fluid should be suspected if the patient remains ill or febrile or has a persistent leukocytosis. After appropriate evaluation by ultrasound or CT, options for management include image-guided percutaneous drainage by an interventional radiologist[51] or instillation of thrombolytic agents (urokinase or streptokinase) through a catheter or chest tube.[52] If administered before fibrosis occurs, these agents attack the fibrin membranes causing the loculations. Successful therapy leads to an increase in the amount of drainage from the pleural space and can be administered for up to 2 weeks. Thoracoscopy to mechanically lyze adhesions and inspect the pleural cavity has also been used to assist in management.[7]

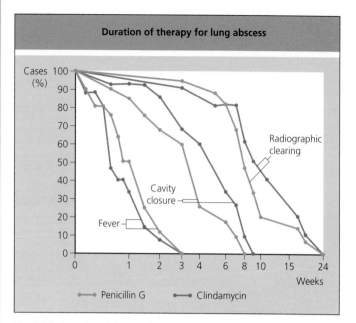

Duration of therapy for lung abscess

Radiographic clearing

Cavity closure

Fever

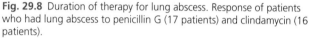

Penicillin G   Clindamycin

Fig. 29.8 Duration of therapy for lung abscess. Response of patients who had lung abscess to penicillin G (17 patients) and clindamycin (16 patients).

If patients do not respond to the above measures, contrast material can be injected into the chest tube to evaluate the empyema cavity. Open drainage, evacuation of all infected material and decortication of the pleura should be considered. This is a major surgical procedure that requires rib resection and may not be tolerated by debilitated patients. Open drainage, without decortication, may be better tolerated in these patients, but it is followed by a prolonged period of convalescence with an open chest wound.[7]

A serious complication of an empyema is a bronchopleural fistula. The presence of a peripheral air–fluid level radiographically suggests the presence of a bronchopulmonary fistula, although such an air–fluid level may occasionally be due to the presence of gas-forming bacteria. Adequate tube drainage is mandatory to minimize the spread of infection to other portions of the lungs. Empyema with a bronchopleural fistula after pneumonectomy is a disastrous surgical complication. The fistula often does not close with antibiotics, tube drainage and irrigation, and complex surgical procedures are usually necessary.[7]

REFERENCES

References for this chapter can be found online at http://www.expertconsult.com

Chapter | **30** | *Jon S Friedland*

Tuberculosis and other mycobacterial infections

Tuberculosis is the clinically most important of the mycobacterial infections and is the subject of the first section of this chapter; the second section covers other mycobacterial infections except for leprosy, which is dealt with in Chapter 103. Details of antimycobacterial drugs are to be found in Chapter 143. Tuberculosis and HIV co-infection is also covered separately in Chapter 93. The clinical microbiology of mycobacterial infections is discussed in Chapter 174.

Tuberculosis

Tuberculosis, a disease identified in skeletons over 6000 years old, remains the most prevalent infectious disease in the world. This chapter focuses on current understanding of pathophysiology, epidemiology and clinical aspects of tuberculosis.

EPIDEMIOLOGY

Worldwide incidence and prevalence

Mycobacterium tuberculosis is estimated to infect 1.6 billion people worldwide or approximately one-third of the world's population.[1] Usually infection is contained by the immune system so that about 14.4 million people have clinical disease at any one time. The World Health Organization (WHO) reported that there were approximately 9.2 million new cases and 1.7 million deaths from tuberculosis in 2006 (http://www.who.int/tb/publications/global_report/2008/en/index.html). Recent data on tuberculosis notification rates are shown in Figure 30.1. However, notification data may be incomplete with underreporting of cases. Confounding factors in global collection of incidence and prevalence data include effects of treatment, difficulties in identifying extrapulmonary disease and those associated with tuberculin testing.

Over 96% of tuberculosis-related deaths occur in the poorer nations of the world and the disease has huge social and economic costs. In wealthier nations, rates of tuberculosis have been falling over the last 50 years in part due to social improvements, development of effective treatments, active case finding and use of the bacille Calmette–Guérin (BCG) vaccine. Recently, this trend has been halted in some countries due to increased incidence of tuberculosis in high-risk population groups including poorer communities, migrants and patients with HIV infection. Levels of disease in homeless populations, intravenous drug users and prisoners in developed countries may also be high.[2] The worldwide prevalence of diabetes mellitus is increasing and increases the risk of tuberculosis.[3]

The impact of HIV

The WHO estimate that there were 709 000 new cases of tuberculosis associated with HIV in 2006. HIV-seropositive patients are more susceptible to infection by *M. tuberculosis*. Reactivation of tuberculosis occurs at least 10 times more frequently than in age-matched controls. The majority of people co-infected with tuberculosis and HIV live in sub-Saharan Africa (over 85%), the Indian subcontinent and South East Asia (Fig. 30.2). Patients tend to be sicker and in greater need of hospitalization. The relationship between HIV and tuberculosis is such that tuberculosis patients should be offered HIV screening. Diagnosis of dual infection may be difficult since HIV predisposes to atypical, nodal and extrapulmonary disease. The subject of HIV–tuberculosis co-infection is explored in depth in Chapter 93 and is not considered further here.

Spread of infection

Spread of infection is dependent on inhalation of aerosols from individuals with pulmonary infection. Proximity to and duration of association with an index case are critical factors. Up to 25% of household contacts of an index case may acquire infection although the extent to which individual genetic predisposition or immunologic impairment contributes to this is uncertain. Although contributory, the exact role of factors such as vitamin D deficiency and iron overload in the spread of tuberculosis is unknown. Spread of infection is separate to development of disease which occurs in less than 10% of infected persons and is significantly affected by impaired cell-mediated immunity. Congenital transmission of tuberculosis is not a significant factor in the natural spread of disease.

Transmission in closed institutions

Overcrowding contributes to the spread of tuberculosis amongst the poor. Close proximity to infected individuals is a significant issue in any closed institution and for health-care workers. Many countries have specific guidelines for tuberculosis control in institutions. In prisons, the situation is complicated by the fact that inmates have an increased incidence of HIV, are frequently moved to other prisons or back into the community with little warning and may be poorly managed in terms of health services. Since release of prisoners is often into poor circumstances and crowded hostels, the consequence of undetected or inadequately treated tuberculosis may be rapid spread of disease. Mass incarceration can lead to an increase in cases of tuberculosis and a rise in drug-resistant disease.[4] An effective public health program with an active community care component can overcome such problems.

Genetic techniques using restriction fragment length polymorphism (RFLP) analysis (often of the insertion sequence IS6110) to provide

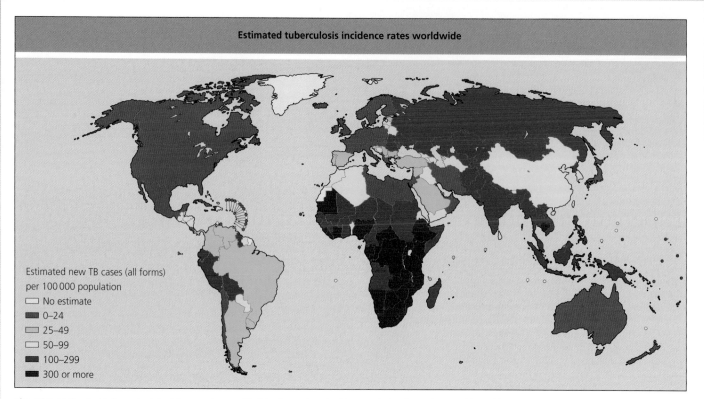

Estimated tuberculosis incidence rates worldwide

Estimated new TB cases (all forms)
per 100 000 population
- No estimate
- 0–24
- 25–49
- 50–99
- 100–299
- 300 or more

Fig. 30.1 Estimated tuberculosis incidence rates worldwide. Reproduced with permission from the World Health Organization, 2008.

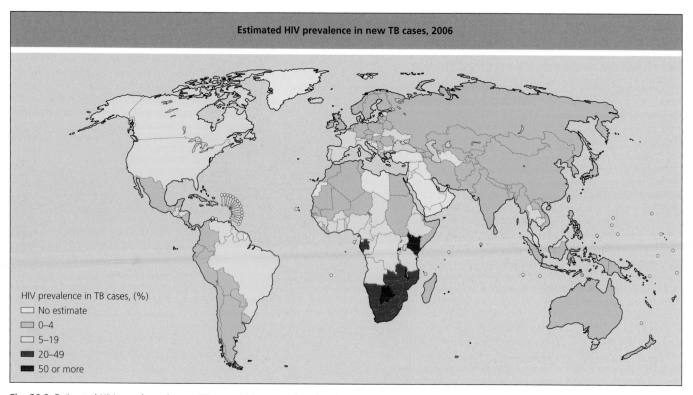

Estimated HIV prevalence in new TB cases, 2006

HIV prevalence in TB cases, (%)
- No estimate
- 0–4
- 5–19
- 20–49
- 50 or more

Fig. 30.2 Estimated HIV prevalence in new TB cases 2006. Reproduced with permission from the World Health Organization, 2008.

DNA fingerprints and spoligotyping have proved useful in documenting local outbreaks of tuberculosis including those involving drug-resistant organisms.[5] Recent analyses, using DNA sequencing, showed greater genetic diversity than had been previously recognized.[6]

PATHOGENESIS AND PATHOLOGY

The pathogen

Mycobacterium tuberculosis, discovered by Robert Koch in 1882, is characterized by a complex cell wall rich in mycolic acids, together with peptidoglycan and arabinogalactan, a complex polysaccharide molecule that surrounds the cell membrane. Many cell wall components, such as lipoarabinomannin, are of pathogenic significance. Mycobacteria contain diverse proteins associated with growth, virulence and intracellular survival. Amongst the most critical are the 10 kD, 65 kD, 70 kD and 90 kD families of heat shock proteins (HSPs) which are molecular chaperones involved in protein folding and assembly, and whose production is upregulated by environmental stress.

Host immune factors

The principal tissue immune response in tuberculosis is the formation of granulomas comprised of cells of the monocyte lineage including multinucleate giant cells, together with T lymphocytes and interdigitating stromal cells such as fibroblasts (Fig. 30.3). In the initial stages of the immune response, neutrophils are present whilst more advanced disease is characterized by caseous necrosis and eventually deposition of calcium. Granuloma formation is a consequence of a complex interaction between the organism, the immune system and local release of tissue factors and proteases. This process may be modulated by systemic or local production of hormones such as 1,25 dihydroxyvitamin D$_3$. Caseous necrosis, typical of mycobacterial granulomas, is probably due to the delayed type hypersensitivity response although it is not known why it is so very rare in nontuberculous granulomas.

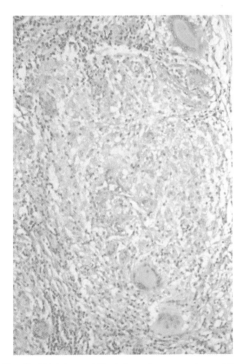

Fig. 30.3 Detailed histology of the tuberculous granuloma. Monocytic cells and smaller T cells are shown together with multinucleate giant cells.

Monocytes, macrophages and phagocytosis

Following inhalation, *M. tuberculosis* is phagocytosed by the alveolar macrophage; similar fixed tissue cells are present elsewhere in the body. Pulmonary surfactant protein may enhance the process of phagocytosis. The phagocytosing macrophage initiates the host immune response (Fig. 30.4). Phagocytosis of the pathogen may involve complement receptors CR1, CR3 and CR4 as well as mannose-binding and scavenger receptors and adhesion molecules. Intracellular *M. tuberculosis* partly inhibits phagolysosome fusion, arresting phagosome maturation and preventing acidification of the vacuole, thus maintaining a pH around 6.4.[7] Some mycobacterial components escape the phagosome, are detectable in the cytoplasm and are subsequently presented via major histocompatibility complex (MHC) class I molecules to T lymphocytes.

Phagocytosis and engagement with Toll-like receptors (TLRs) is a potent stimulus to gene expression and secretion of proinflammatory cytokines such as tumor necrosis factor (TNF), interleukin (IL)-1 and IL-6. TLR-2 and -4 are the principal pattern recognition receptors that have been associated with the proinflammatory responses in tuberculosis,[8] although additional data suggest involvement of TLR-6, -8 and -9.[9,10] The known consequences of TNF secretion include fever and cachexia, two prominent symptoms in tuberculosis. TNF has a pivotal role in granuloma formation and is found at sites of human infection. The clinical use of anti-TNF antibodies is associated with reactivation of disease in individuals with latent infection.[11] Macrophage-derived chemokines control cellular recruitment to the granuloma, regulate the extent of the proinflammatory response and may drive mycobacterial killing.[12] The granuloma in tuberculosis is well circumscribed and downregulatory cytokines such as IL-10 are involved in limiting inflammatory responses.

Infected macrophages drive the tissue damage characteristic of tuberculosis. Macrophages and stromal cells associated with granulomas secrete a number of proteases including collagenase, elastase and gelatinase which are matrix metalloproteinases (MMPs) whose action is normally opposed by tissue inhibitors of MMPs. Relatively unopposed MMP activity is found in tuberculosis and is associated with local tissue damage.[13] Other monocyte-derived proteins involved in tissue destruction include lysosomal proteases such as cathepsins which function best at acid pH and the plasminogen activator urokinase. Activation of plasminogen is followed by activation of the clotting system and laying down of fibrous tissue, a process in which macrophage-derived transforming growth factor beta (TGF-β) has a central role. The exact mechanisms by which monocytes and macrophages kill *M. tuberculosis* in man are not fully understood. Cathelicidins and similar molecules appear to have a central role and may be regulated in a vitamin D-dependent manner. Reactive oxygen may be involved in mycobacterial killing in man.

Lymphocyte responses in tuberculosis

Both αβ and γδ CD4$^+$ T cells are critical in immunity to tuberculosis. Patients with reduced T-cell function or numbers are at higher risk of clinical tuberculosis. *Mycobacterium tuberculosis* may impair macrophage antigen presentation to T lymphocytes by downregulating the co-stimulatory molecule B7-1. Cells of the T-helper 1 (Th1) subclass which secrete interferon gamma (IFN-γ) and IL–2 are central to control of infection in murine models. In human disease the situation is more complex, with Th1, Th2 (IL-4, -5, -6, -10 and -13 producing), Th17 and intermediate cell types detectable.[14] The dual presence of Th1 and Th2 cells may account for the fact that although tuberculosis is limited within the granuloma, the organism is not usually completely killed off by the immune response. IL-23, together with IL-12 with which it partly shares a receptor, are both involved in the protective IFN-γ response seen in tuberculosis.[15]

Other T-cell phenotypes involved in immunity to tuberculosis include CD8$^+$ cells and double-negative T lymphocytes lacking CD4 and CD8 which recognize mycobacterial lipoglycan antigens presented via CD1.[16] Many proteins, carbohydrates and lipids of *M. tuberculosis* contain epitopes that stimulate B lymphocyte antibody production. In terms of pathogenesis, it has proved difficult to identify specific antibody responses in sera of tuberculosis patients of importance in host defense.

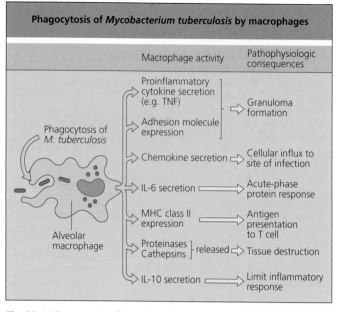

Phagocytosis of *Mycobacterium tuberculosis* by macrophages

Fig. 30.4 Phagocytosis of *Mycobacterium tuberculosis* by macrophages. Phagocytosis initiates many critical pathways involved in host defense to infection.

Host genetic factors

There is a genetic component to host resistance to *M. tuberculosis*. Human leukocyte antigen (HLA) haplotypes associated with susceptibility to tuberculosis include A8, A10, B8, Bw15 and DR2. Non-HLA linked genes, such as the natural resistance-associated membrane protein, are a determinant of disease susceptibility in certain populations.[17] Certain families that are susceptible to mycobacterial infections have deletions in the IFN-γ receptor gene.[18] A milder phenotype of mycobacterial susceptibility is found in patients with mutations affecting IL-12 signaling.[19] It is likely that although many genetic polymorphisms which have been described in tuberculosis and that are encoded in diverse cytokine and endocrine (including vitamin D) genes influence susceptibility to infection to varying degrees, environmental factors have a greater effect on disease presentation.

PREVENTION

Public health measures

Strategies to prevent spread of tuberculosis aim first to identify and promptly treat infectious patients and secondly to prevent infection by vaccination. Many countries have a system, often legally enforced, of infectious patient notification to a central body which traces infected contacts of index cases. In addition, high-risk patients or communities such as intravenous drug users may be screened in order to institute definitive or prophylactic therapy. In its simplest form, case finding involves examining sputum smears although radiologic examination may be a useful adjunct. However, sputum smear microscopy will miss about 50% of culture-positive patients who are highly infectious. Routine screening for latent infection may be appropriate in countries with low rates of infection or in subgroups of patients particularly likely to reactivate disease such as those who are immunosuppressed, including renal dialysis patients[20] and those about to receive immunosuppressive therapy. Prevention programs may require incentives for successful implementation; they should be linked to educational initiatives and involve social services.

Infectious patients and those who are suspected of infection should be isolated until either tuberculosis infection has been ruled out or effective treatment established. In the USA and other affluent nations, laminar airflow and negative pressure ventilation rooms are used for known or suspected tuberculosis, particularly in patients with multidrug-resistant disease. Extensive guidelines have been produced in the USA relating to control of tuberculosis but these are not universally applicable.[21] The use of an efficient personal protective mask is key although even this is not available in many parts of the world where tuberculosis is prevalent. In many instances, basic patient isolation and possibly specified, ventilated rooms for procedures which generate aerosols is all that is feasible. Shortwave ultraviolet illuminators to kill organisms in clinics and shelters are potentially useful. Appropriate control measures should be defined in advance in high-risk procedure rooms (e.g. bronchoscopy suites), during patient transport and in all at-risk institutions which range from health-care facilities through to shelters for the homeless.

Testing for exposure

The tuberculin skin test

The Mantoux test is still the commonest test used to screen for tuberculosis exposure and depends on the intradermal injection of a specified quantity of an internationally standardized purified protein derivative (PPD) of tuberculin. PPD solution should not be left in syringes since it may be variably adsorbed to their surface. Tuberculin positivity manifests as induration at the site of testing after 48 hours. Induration less than 5 mm diameter following a standard injection of 5 units PPD is regarded as negative and greater than 15 mm diameter as positive. PPD may have a booster effect on immunologic memory particularly in older persons which can cause confusion if re-testing occurs after a few months when an apparently positive result is not the result of new infection.

Induration in the 5–15 mm diameter range may be indicative of current infection, previous treated infection, exposure to nontuberculous mycobacteria, vaccination or disease in the immunosuppressed patient, all of which have unpredictable confounding effects on Mantoux testing. In the USA, induration greater than 5 mm is taken as positive in patients with HIV, a close contact with tuberculosis or a fibrotic chest radiograph; induration above 10 mm is positive in any other at-risk groups. Patients who are immunosuppressed such as those with HIV (particularly if the CD4+ T-cell count is below 400/mm³) or who have viral infections such as measles or sarcoidosis, have a strong tendency to anergy. Systemic illnesses, including miliary tuberculosis, are also associated with anergy. There is a poor relationship between general anergic responses to other antigens and tuberculin negativity. False-negative tests occur at the extremes of age, following use of inadequately stored tuberculin or due to poor injection technique.

The Heaf test involves placing PPD on the skin of a subject and then using a multiple puncture gun to piece the skin in six places. The response is then graded as described in Table 30.1. Heaf guns must

Table 30.1 The Heaf test grades

Heaf test grade	Response
0	No induration at puncture sites
1	Discrete induration at a minimum of four needle sites
2	Induration at needle sites merge to form ring but leave clear center
3	One large induration site seen (5–10 mm diameter)
4	Induration over 10 mm diameter

be resterilized between patients or a disposable head used. The Tine test is similar to the Heaf test except that the puncture needles (usually four not six) are precoated with tuberculin. There has been controversy as to the reliability of this technique and it has faded from general use.

Interferon gamma release assays (see also Chapter 174)

There are two main types of IFN-γ release assay (IGRA) in use and their main advantages are that they are not affected by previous BCG vaccination, are not confounded by boosting and do not require reading at 48 hours so can be arranged at a single clinic visit. Like skin tests, they cannot distinguish latent from active infection. They are relatively expensive compared to skin tests. IGRAs are stimulation assays and the current incarnations are based on immune responses to antigens encoded in the RD-1 region of the *M. tuberculosis* complex which make them specific for this organism. The first is a whole-blood enzyme-linked immunosorbent assay (ELISA)-based system and the second is an enzyme-linked immunospot (ELISpot)-based detection of IFN-γ.[22] Both use as antigens early secreted antigen target (ESAT)-6 and culture filtrate protein (CFP)-10.

The advantages of IGRAs mean that they are incorporated into national testing guidelines for screening and prevention of tuberculosis in a number of different countries including the UK (Clinical Guideline 33 from the National Institute for Health and Clinical Excellence; http://www.nice.org.uk/CG033) and the USA.[23] However, these tests do not necessarily replace the skin tests and have different sensitivities and specificities which may be population specific. There are many areas where their value is limited, unproven or confused, including diagnosis of active or early reactivating disease (when interferon responses can be suppressed) and use in immunosuppressed patients. There is a theoretic advantage in systems which use both skin tests and IGRAs although this still requires two clinic visits. IGRAs have use in excluding diagnosis of tuberculosis in children and in the context of occupational health screening. The negative predictive value of IGRAs is clinically useful. A negative test in a healthy patient excludes tuberculosis infection. However, as with other diagnostic tests, the positive predictive value depends on the prevalence of *M. tuberculosis* in the population that is being tested.

Chemoprophylaxis

Chemoprophylaxis is an important and arguably underused component of tuberculosis control programs which is misleadingly named since it is actually treatment of latent, nondividing organisms which can be undertaken with a single drug. Chemoprophylaxis may be primary in unexposed individuals or secondary in those exposed to *M. tuberculosis* who do not have clinical disease. Secondary prophylaxis is practiced most commonly and successfully in tuberculosis control programs in the USA. This approach, which is based on regular skin prick testing, is not possible where vaccination is common

or resources inadequate. Isoniazid 300 mg daily for 6–12 months is the usual preventive regimen and is given with vitamin B_6 to prevent neurologic side-effects. Since patients are well, chemoprophylactic regimens with a high incidence of side-effects such as isoniazid and pyrazinamide[24] are not acceptable. Chemoprophylaxis is advocated in HIV-seropositive patients because of the increased incidence of clinical disease in patients exposed to *M. tuberculosis*. Chemoprophylaxis should also be considered in patients with latent infection prior to the initiation of TNF inhibitors and all such patients should be screened. However, if diagnostic facilities are poor, there is a significant chance of inadvertently treating established tuberculosis and increasing isoniazid resistance. In contrast, use of chemoprophylaxis in potential transplant recipients is established. Chemoprophylaxis should be deferred in pregnant women, a group more prone to isoniazid hepatitis (see also Chapter 143).

Vaccines

The live-attenuated BCG vaccine, developed by Albert Calmette and Camille Guérin, was first used in 1921. Subsequently, many strains have been used clinically although the current reference type is the Pasteur strain. Vaccination leads to a local immune response and ultimately scar formation (Fig. 30.5). Adverse reactions other than local irritation are uncommon and anaphylaxis extremely rare. Local abscesses or ulcers usually reflect poor technique although keloid formation may arise in susceptible individuals. Adenitis, sometimes suppurative, is the most important complication, the incidence of which depends on many factors including vaccine strain and immune status of the host. Lupoid reactions, infected osteitis and disseminated BCG disease are very rare, the latter two necessitating therapy with rifampin (rifampicin) and isoniazid (BCG is resistant to pyrazinamide).

Extent of immunity following BCG vaccination depends on the strain used, environmental factors and the genetics of the population being vaccinated as well as individual host factors such as age. There is a poor correlation between tuberculin reactivity after vaccination which develops to maximal levels within 3 months, and protection against disease. BCG vaccine efficacy is about 60–80%[25] and is most efficacious in preventing serious disease in children. Giving BCG to infants gives significant protection from tuberculosis in household contacts.

There is great interest in a number of approaches to developing new tuberculosis vaccines. The first is to improve the efficacy of the BCG vaccine by genetic modification or to develop a new live attenuated vaccine by deletion of specific virulence factors. The second approach involves using subunit vaccines often given as a booster to a BCG or modified BCG vaccine. A vaccine based upon *M. tuberculosis* antigen 85 is in field trials.[26] Different antigens may be linked in subunit vaccines. The third approach is to use naked DNA vaccines encoding for immunogenic mycobacterial antigens which has been successful in animal models.[27] New vaccines have potential both to prevent infection and to treat established disease.

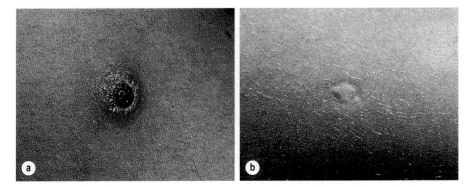

Fig. 30.5 BCG response at 6 weeks. (a) Clinical evidence of cell-mediated immune response is clearly apparent at 6 weeks. (b) The healed BCG scar. With permission from James DG, Studdy PR. A colour atlas of respiratory diseases, 2nd ed. London: Mosby; 1992.

CLINICAL FEATURES

In this section, the diverse clinical presentations of primary, pulmonary and miliary tuberculosis are reviewed, together with the characteristic changes found on radiologic examination. In addition, the principal extrapulmonary manifestations of tuberculosis are considered.

Primary and childhood infection

Primary tuberculosis is usually acquired by inhalation of infected particles in childhood, although in affluent countries the first encounter with tuberculosis may be as an adult. Although a single bacillus can cause disease, usually 50–200 organisms are required for development of active infection. Inhaled bacilli pass into the lung where damage is usually but not always confined to one segment with concurrent involvement of draining, frequently hilar, lymph nodes. This gives rise to the primary (ghon) complex. Clinical disease develops in less than 5% of people exposed to *M. tuberculosis*. After initial infection, the only sequela may be scar tissue which is often calcified and later identified on routine chest X-ray. After the first year of infection, there is a 3–5% lifetime chance of reactivation of disease in non-HIV infected individuals. Children aged 5–15 years develop active tuberculosis relatively infrequently.

Symptomatic patients present with cough with variable amounts of sputum and hemoptysis together with localized pleuritic chest pain and dyspnea. In addition, systemic features such as fever, night sweats, anorexia and weight loss occur. A minority of patients have retrosternal pain sometimes exacerbated by swallowing and increased by sternal pressure which is thought to relate to lymphadenopathy. Primary tuberculosis is seen as asymmetric hilar adenopathy and associated consolidation on chest X-ray. In children, isolated lymphadenopathy is more common. Less typical chest X-rays of primary infection include those which appear normal or have widespread disease, lobar consolidation and pleural effusions. An unusual complication of primary tuberculosis is bronchial obstruction due to pressure of a node on a main bronchus. This phenomenon, sometimes called epituberculosis, may lead to secondary bronchiectasis. Untreated primary disease may progress to involve the entire lung and disseminate. Symptoms are present at this stage and may be severe with continuous cough and sputum production, severe dyspnea, high fevers, drenching sweats and cachexia. Chest X-ray reveals widespread patchy consolidation with areas of collapse and cavitation.

Endobronchial tuberculosis is usually a complication of primary infection although it may occur during reactivation. It may follow adhesion of inflamed lung parenchyma or lymph nodes to bronchi or may arise via lymphatic or hematogenous spread of infection and even from direct seeding of inhaled bacilli. Endobronchial tuberculosis probably frequently goes undiagnosed since it was found in over 400 of 1000 consecutive autopsies. The classic clinical presentation is with a barking cough and wheeze but onset may be gradual, mimicking other respiratory diseases ranging from asthma to cancer. Sputum production may be exacerbated when the mucosa is breached and caseous material extruded. Parasternal pain, dyspnea, symptoms due to collapse and consolidation of distal lung tissue and systemic manifestations of tuberculosis may be found. The most important late complication of endobronchial infection is bronchiectasis.

Pulmonary infection

Risk factors for reactivation

The majority of cases of tuberculosis are due to reactivation of infection acquired years earlier. The stimulus to reactivation may be frank immunosuppression or may be more subtle when factors such as malnutrition and vitamin D deficiency may be involved. TNF inhibitors increase the susceptibility of patients to reactivation. The role of steroids in reactivation of tuberculosis has not been fully defined.

High doses may cause reactivation which often presents atypically or is detected belatedly since the symptoms of infection may mimic symptoms of the disease for which steroids were being prescribed. Tuberculosis does not appear more common in asthmatics maintained on daily low-dose prednisolone. Other conditions associated with reactivation of tuberculosis are end-stage renal disease, diabetes mellitus, silicosis, gastrectomy and transplantation when disease is usually due to immunosuppression although it has been transmitted with the implanted organ. Although tuberculosis and lung malignancy may coexist and the symptoms of tuberculosis may mimic those of cancer, tuberculosis is not a risk factor for lung cancer. However, lung malignancy is a systemic risk factor for reactivation of tuberculosis and may invade and disrupt old tuberculous lesions leading to active infection. Some workers have detected mycobacterial DNA in patients with sarcoid but others have not and whether there is any link between these diseases is unresolved.

Clinical presentation

In one prospective study, symptoms of reactivation of pulmonary tuberculosis were cough in 78% of patients, weight loss in 74%, fatigue in 68%, fever in 60% and night sweats in 55%.[28] Some patients have only mild feelings of nonspecific malaise. Hemoptysis occurs in up to a third of patients. It may be massive from either enlarged bronchial arteries around tuberculous cavities (Rasmussen's aneurysms) or more frequently from erosions involving other bronchial or pulmonary arteries. Dyspnea suggests extensive disease and is a late symptom. Pleuritic chest pain indicates inflammation in and possibly infection of adjacent pleura.

Clinical examination may be misleading in the early stages of reactivation and radiologically apparent changes of consolidation and cavitation hard to detect. Noninfectious complications of tuberculosis may be present (see below). Some patients with advanced disease present in acute respiratory failure progressing rapidly to the adult respiratory distress syndrome (ARDS).

Chest X-ray shows disease localized to apical and posterior segments of the upper lobes of the lung in over 85% of cases with other sites often secondarily affected. The apical segment of the lower lobe is also frequently involved. Infiltration and cavitation secondary to caseous necrosis may be associated with air–fluid levels. On treatment, most cavities heal completely leaving residual scarring, often calcific. Tuberculous chest X-rays frequently show upper zone shadowing with fibrotic changes, lobar atelectasis, elevation of hilar nodes and deviation of the trachea (Fig. 30.6). A wide range of less common findings are described such as pneumonic consolidation (Fig. 30.7). It is notoriously

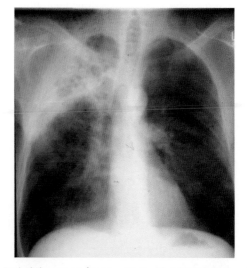

Fig. 30.6 Typical chest X-ray from a patient with tuberculosis showing upper lobe shadowing, elevation of hilar lymph nodes and deviation of trachea.

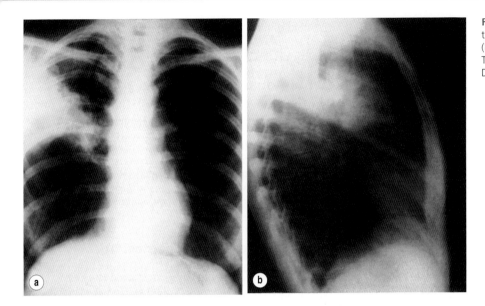

Fig. 30.7 Chest radiograph of pulmonary tuberculous pneumonia. (a) Posteroanterior and (b) lateral chest radiographs of a patient with TB presenting as a consolidation. Courtesy of Dr W Lynn, Ealing Hospital, UK.

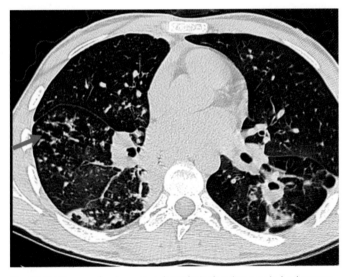

Fig. 30.8 CT scan of pulmonary tuberculosis showing tree-in-bud pattern (arrowed). Courtesy of Dr S Copley, Imperial College Healthcare NHS Trust, London, UK.

difficult to distinguish early reactivation from chronic healed lesions without follow-up. CT and MRI scan findings include cavitation with scarring as well as characteristic nodules and branching linear structures, sometimes referred to as a tree-in-bud pattern (Fig. 30.8).

Other investigations in pulmonary tuberculosis may reveal leukocytosis or more specifically but uncommonly a monocytosis. More commonly the leukocyte count is normal and more rarely, it is leukopenic. Anemia, generally normochromic and normocytic, is typical. An acute phase response is almost invariably present with elevated C-reactive protein (CRP) concentrations in plasma, raised erythrocyte sedimentation rate (ESR) and in more chronic cases, decreased serum albumin. Hyponatremia occurs in about 10% of patients due to antidiuretic hormone-like activity although may be a manifestation of concurrent extrapulmonary infection. A small number of patients have hypercalcemia, probably due to abnormal vitamin D processing by granuloma macrophages.[29]

Complications

The principal acute complications of pulmonary tuberculosis are hemoptysis (discussed above) and pneumothorax. Bronchopleural

fistulae may heal spontaneously or require tube drainage and sometimes surgery. Prognosis is good because of formation of scar tissue in tuberculosis. Chronic complications of lung tuberculosis relate to parenchymal damage and scarring. Aspergillomas may develop within healed cavitating lesions in up to 20% of cases; patients typically present with hemoptysis. Localized bronchiectasis (see Chapter 26) may only become clinically significant years later and is best defined by high-resolution CT scanning. Tissue destruction may be so great as to cause respiratory failure.

Pleural tuberculosis

Pleural tuberculosis classically occurs 3–6 months after primary disease but onset may be delayed and pleural disease may be the first sign of reactivation. Pleural disease may accompany lung infection or be the predominant feature. Tuberculosis and malignancy are the principal differential diagnoses of massive effusions which are exudates (protein concentration greater than 3 g/dl (30 g/l)). Effusions are usually straw colored but may be blood stained and occasionally frankly bloody. Glucose concentrations in tuberculous effusions are frequently, but not always, below 40 mg/dl (2.22 mmol/l). Pleural fluid lysozyme, lactate and pH may be elevated in tuberculous effusions, as in bacterial infections. Elevated adenosine deaminase (ADA), derived from CD4 lymphocytes, is characteristic. Low ADA levels are against a diagnosis of tuberculosis but high concentrations are nonspecific. The leukocyte count of tuberculous effusions is usually raised and may be as high as 5000 cells/mm³. Lymphocytes are generally the most prevalent cell type. Monocytes are also characteristic but mesothelial cells are scanty. Neutrophils may be present and even predominate in acute disease.[30]

Chest X-ray usually demonstrates a unilateral effusion, more often on the right. An effusion may be massive and bilateral effusions occur in approximately 10% of patients. Ultrasound may reveal loculated effusions containing fibrinous tissue reflecting activation of the fibrinolytic system. Ultrasound and CT or MRI scanning are useful to document underlying disease and to aid diagnostic and therapeutic aspirations.

Miliary tuberculosis

Miliary tuberculosis follows dissemination of *M. tuberculosis* and clinical presentation is varied. Factors involved in the development of miliary infection include delay in diagnosis, impaired immune responses, mycobacterial virulence factors, mycobacterial load and the number of organisms able to gain entry to the bloodstream. At least 50% of patients with miliary disease in developed countries are immunosuppressed, most commonly by alcohol. Diabetes, chronic renal failure, underlying malignancies and immunosuppressive drugs are other risk factors. Disseminated infection due to *M. bovis*, BCG strain, may follow installation of the organism into the bladder when it is used as an adjuvant to chemotherapy for malignancy.

Miliary tuberculosis may present as pyrexia of unknown origin or with symptoms attributable to involvement of one or more organ systems. Commonly there are widespread pulmonary granulomas and CNS disease and rarely cardiac involvement (although pericardial, myocardial and endocardial manifestations have all been reported). Differential diagnosis is often wide and clinicians must be alert to the possibility of miliary tuberculosis. Acute miliary tuberculosis presenting with shock and ARDS has a mortality which may approach 90%. In more chronic cases, cachexia is prominent and localizing features may be few. Widespread macular and papular skin lesions (tuberculosis miliaris disseminata) are suggestive of miliary infection. Choroidal tubercles 0.5–3.0 mm in diameter are essentially diagnostic of miliary disease (Fig. 30.9).

The chest X-ray of miliary tuberculosis has well-defined nodules less than 5 mm in diameter throughout both lung fields (Fig. 30.10). X-ray changes may only develop after a patient has been admitted to hospital, so patients must be reassessed frequently. Larger nodules and a pulmonary focus occur in approximately one-third of patients. CT or MRI scanning may show smaller nodules not apparent on X-ray. Ultrasound scanning may show increased echogenicity and focal lesions in the liver but is not diagnostic. Hematologic investigations are similar to those found in tuberculous pneumonia but a neutrophilia may be seen and should not put the diagnosis in doubt or cause empiric therapy to be restricted to antibacterials. Rarer abnormalities include disseminated intravascular coagulation and the hemophagocytic syndrome. Sterile

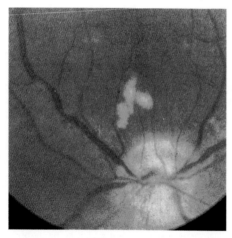

Fig. 30.9 Choroidal TB. Choroidal disease is a manifestation of TB which is highly suggestive of miliary disease. With permission from James DG, Studdy PR. A colour atlas of respiratory diseases, 2nd ed. London: Mosby; 1992.

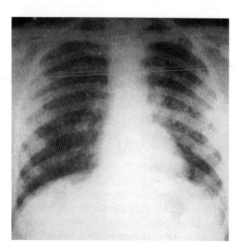

Fig. 30.10 Miliary TB. Chest radiograph of miliary TB showing characteristic mottled shadowing throughout both lung fields. Courtesy of Dr W Lynn, Ealing Hospital, UK.

pyuria and organisms in the absence of urinary leukocytes have been reported but the exact frequency of such renal manifestations is uncertain. Delay in diagnosis contributes to mortality.

Extrapulmonary tuberculosis

This section reviews extrapulmonary tuberculosis not considered in detail elsewhere and refers readers to other relevant chapters. The 2008 Annual Report of the Health Protection Agency (http://www.hpa.org.uk/web/HPAweb&HPAwebStandard/HPAweb_C/1225268885969) revealed that 44% of all cases of tuberculosis diagnosed in the UK was extrapulmonary. It is very likely that in resource-poor areas of the world, where the focus is on diagnosis of people who are potentially infectious, a large amount of extrapulmonary disease goes undetected.

Lymph node disease (see Chapter 14)

Lymphadenitis, also known as scrofula or the 'King's evil' (so called because in Europe the royal touch was thought to be curative in the Middle Ages), is a very common extrapulmonary presentation of tuberculosis. Peripheral nodes are usually infected following hematogenous spread of *M. tuberculosis* from the lung. The most commonly involved nodes are those in the cervical region, sometimes in association with axillary, inguinal or hilar lymphadenopathy. Patients may present with painless lymphadenopathy or with marked systemic symptoms. There may be associated sinuses and abscess formation. Hilar nodes may be associated with thoracic pain and untreated may infrequently result in esophageal erosion or a bronchoesophageal fistula. Unusual symptoms such as obstructive jaundice have been reported in specific association with anatomically defined local lymph nodes.

Tuberculosis of the head and neck

Aside from cervical node disease, tuberculosis of the head and neck is relatively uncommon and usually arises secondarily to pulmonary infection. Laryngeal tuberculosis may present with hoarseness, pain on speaking or swallowing, hemoptysis and respiratory obstruction. Cough may reflect lung disease or involvement of the superior laryngeal nerve. Untreated, widespread local tissue destruction may occur with secondary laryngeal stenosis. Chest X-ray may be suggestive but in one series radiographic changes were minimal in two-thirds of cases. In this study from a specialist center, coexistent squamous cell carcinoma of the larynx was present in 10% of cases. Therefore, all laryngeal lesions should be biopsied to exclude malignancy.

Tuberculosis rarely involves the middle ear when it may present with a local, painless discharge from which the organism may be cultured. There may be destruction of the ossicles, hearing loss and invasion of the facial nerve canal, sinuses and extension into the posterior cranial fossa. Secondary pyogenic infection may obscure the diagnosis. Tuberculosis of the nose, nasopharynx and adenoids is rare even in areas where infection is endemic and symptoms such as epistaxis reflect local tissue damage. Tuberculosis in the oral cavity generally presents as a solitary, often inflamed ulcer with irregular borders. There may be secondary infection of salivary glands.

Musculoskeletal infection

Vertebral infection (Pott's disease) is the commonest presentation of tuberculous osteomyelitis, accounting for about 50% of all cases of bony tuberculosis (Fig. 30.11). The male to female ratio is approximately 2:1. The thoracic spine is most frequently involved, followed by lumbar and then cervical regions. Presentation is usually with back or neck pain. Systemic symptoms tend to be less marked than in pulmonary disease. Neurologic symptoms such as weakness, numbness and disturbances of gait occur in about a third of cases. Some patients have an associated flank mass or other evidence of extraspinal

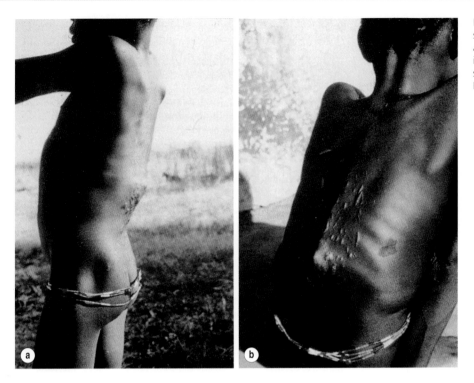

Fig. 30.11 Vertebral TB. Tuberculosis of the spine or Pott's disease. Kyphosis is secondary to anterior destruction of vertebral bodies resulting in wedging of adjacent vertebrae and loss of disk space clearly seen by radiography. Courtesy of Professor J Cohen, Brighton, UK.

tuberculosis. In more advanced cases, vertebral body collapse and gibbus formation lead to kyphosis of the spine. Destructive lesions with invasion of the joint space and deformity may be seen on plain X-rays, although CT or ideally MRI scanning is a better imaging modality for spinal pathology (Fig. 30.12).

Osteomyelitis is otherwise most frequently found in the metaphyses of long bones, although rib, pelvis and skull may be infected. In children in countries where tuberculosis is prevalent, osteomyelitis is a significant cause of crippling deformity. Direct extension from the ribs to the lung is rare, as is meningitis or tuberculomas in cases where there is skull involvement. Bony tuberculosis may be accompanied by sinus tracts or soft tissue masses. Diagnosis may be difficult since

lesions can appear osteolytic or sclerotic on X-ray and malignancy may be suspected at first. Like X-rays, ^{99m}technitium bone scans have no pathognomonic features. Trauma does not predispose to tuberculous osteomyelitis.

Tuberculous arthritis most frequently presents in the hips and other weight-bearing joints although any joint may be involved. Polyarticular disease occurs in less than 20% of patients but evidence of tuberculosis elsewhere, generally the lung, is present in about 50% of cases. Synovial fluid is usually turbid with a high leukocyte count and up to 60% may be neutrophils rather mononuclear cells. Organisms are found in less than a quarter of cases although positive cultures are more frequent. Ideally a synovial biopsy should be examined histologically and microbiologically. Prosthetic joints may be infected with *M. tuberculosis* following either hematogenous spread or contiguous reactivation of infection. Tenosynovitis is rare and is generally associated with adjacent osteomyelitis.

Tuberculous abscesses may form in most soft tissues including muscle and may be multiple (Fig. 30.13). This is usually secondary to contiguous spread of infection but may follow hematogenous dissemination. The classic abscess site is in the psoas muscle, which can present with or without localizing signs, and a high index of clinical suspicion is necessary for the appropriate imaging to be arranged prior to diagnostic aspiration.

Abdominal infection

The abdomen is a frequent site of tuberculosis, especially in patients from the Indian subcontinent, where rates are up to 50 times higher than those in Europe, and those immunosuppressed with HIV. Disease is usually secondary to hematogenous spread of mycobacteria but can be secondary to local invasion or ingestion of organisms. Tuberculosis frequently mimics other pathologies such as gastrointestinal malignancy and diagnosis is often delayed. In the gut, tuberculosis most frequently affects the ileocecal region, then the small bowel and then the colon, with involvement of the duodenum occurring in less than 2.5% of cases and the stomach and esophagus in less than 1% of patients. Approximately one-third of patients have evidence of tuberculosis elsewhere, usually in the lung.

Symptoms reflect the site of involvement but may be nonspecific with fever, weight loss, chronic abdominal pain, nausea and anorexia.

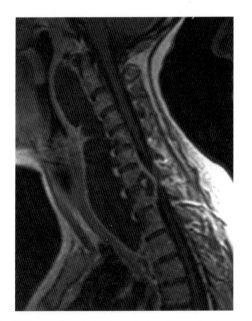

Fig. 30.12 MRI scan of cervical tuberculosis with massive paravertebral abscess which extends through the left C7 to T1 neural exit foramen causing an extradural collection compressing the spinal cord. Courtesy of Dr J Jackson, Imperial College Healthcare NHS Trust, London, UK.

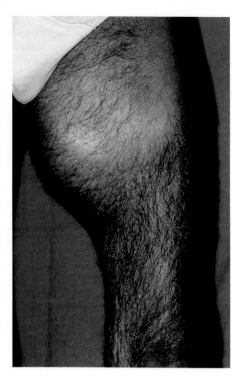

Fig. 30.13 Abscess formation in TB. This patient has multiple TB abscesses particularly affecting the psoas and quadriceps muscle groups.

Diarrhea occurs in less than 20% of cases and reflects either secondary overflow due to obstruction or stimulation of the gastrointestinal tract by cytokines. Ileocecal tuberculosis may present as an acute abdomen secondary to either obstruction of the bowel lumen or appendix or following bowel perforation. Any tuberculous lesion, particularly those in the colon, may present with massive gastrointestinal bleeding but this is rare. Lesions may be ulcerative or hypertrophic and can be associated with fistulas which are probably due in part to secondary bacterial involvement. Unusual sites of intra-abdominal tuberculosis include the pancreas and the adrenal glands where disease presents very rarely as an adrenal crisis but more commonly with an insidious onset of symptoms that may be difficult to distinguish from those associated with infection. Tuberculous peritonitis is an important manifestation of disease and is discussed in Chapter 37. Hepatobiliary infection is considered in Chapter 39. Tuberculosis of the urogenital tract is specifically explored in Practice Point 28.

Pericardial infection

Tuberculous pericarditis is potentially fatal and may present in diverse ways. Onset is often insidious although acute pericarditis may occur. Common symptoms include breathlessness, chest pain and nonspecific changes such as fever and weight loss. Signs of cardiac tamponade such as raised jugular venous pressure, hepatomegaly, ascites and edema may be present, and in a minority of cases develops acutely requiring urgent pericardiocentesis. ECG may show low voltage or ST elevation consistent with acute pericarditis. An effusion may be seen on chest X-ray but is better characterized by echocardiogram or CT scanning. Pericardial calcification occurs late and in less than 25% of cases although data are limited. Diagnosis may be extremely difficult; failure to identify the organism and to detect granuloma on biopsy specimens does not rule out infection. Constrictive pericarditis may develop after active infection has resolved or been treated.

Central nervous system and eye disease

Tuberculous meningoencephalitis and central nervous system tuberculomas are extremely important, carrying a high morbidity and mortality. These topics are considered further in Chapters 18 and 20.

Ocular tuberculosis is relatively uncommon but important since, if overlooked, blindness may result. The commonest manifestation is choroidal disease (see Fig. 30.9) secondary to hematogenous spread in the context of miliary tuberculosis which may rarely spread to the retina. Conjunctival tuberculosis may be due to accidental self-inoculation by an infected person, spread from skin or very rarely by direct spread from another infected individual. Infection may be ulcerative or nodular although occasionally focal tuberculomas, sometimes appearing polypoid, are seen. Tuberculosis of the sclera and cornea are rare as is uveitis.

Dermatologic disease

Lupus vulgaris is the best documented manifestation of dermatologic tuberculosis and details of the dermatologic manifestations of primary and miliary infection are to be found in Chapter 12.

Clinical manifestations in HIV-positive patients

The clinical manifestations of tuberculosis in HIV-seropositive and -seronegative patients are often similar and are reviewed in Chapter 93. However, as the CD4 T-lymphocyte count falls, tuberculosis may be more widespread, have more atypical features and is more often extrapulmonary. Many relatively unusual presentations of tuberculosis have been reported, bronchoesophageal fistula being one example.[31] *Mycobacterium tuberculosis* bacteremia is more frequent in HIV-seropositive patients. Nonspecific systemic features of tuberculosis such as fever, malaise and a prolonged acute phase protein response are also characteristic of HIV infection.

Noninfectious complications

Erythema nodosum is the most common noninfectious complication of primary tuberculosis although it may occur in other granulomatous diseases (e.g. leprosy, sarcoid). It is particularly associated with primary disease. Arthritis occurs in up to 1% of patients with acute infection and may also complicate reactivation. Poncet's disease is a reactive polyarthritis associated with tuberculosis which resolves with antimycobacterial chemotherapy. Bazin's disease is a vasculitic skin reaction to tuberculosis which usually manifests as a purpuric rash on the lower extremities. Another important immunologic complication of tuberculosis is renal interstitial nephritis. Eales disease is the association of tuberculosis with retinal vasculitis with or without neurologic symptoms. More common in patients from the Indian subcontinent, the retinal manifestations may occur before or after the development of clinically apparent tuberculosis.

Bronchogenic carcinoma was thought for many years to be more frequent in patients with tuberculosis but this has not been borne out in careful studies. Hypertrophic pulmonary osteoarthropathy, principally associated with bronchogenic carcinoma, has been reported in tuberculosis[32] although some attribute the finding to undiagnosed lung malignancy. The syndrome of inappropriate antidiuretic hormone secretion is more common in pulmonary and miliary disease.

DIAGNOSIS

Clinical approach

The definitive diagnosis of tuberculosis requires identification of the pathogen in a patient's secretions or tissues. Therapy is often initiated before a definitive diagnosis has been made but this should always be pursued to determine the drug susceptibility of the organism which guides individual treatment regimens. Sputum microscopy and culture has a high diagnostic yield, identifies the majority of infectious patients and is cheap to perform. Sputum should be collected on three separate occasions but additional specimens are not helpful.[33] Although induced sputum obtained in properly ventilated and isolated areas can be useful, bronchoscopy with alveolar lavage has the best diagnostic yield. *Mycobacterium tuberculosis* is infrequently seen on aspiration of pleural fluid and cultured in less than 50% of cases. Pleural biopsy reveals granuloma or results in culture of the pathogen in over 90% of cases. Thoracoscopy, in exceptional circumstances, may be indicated since it allows for visually guided biopsy of lesions. Elevated adenosine deaminase concentrations (in pleural fluid for example) support a diagnosis of tuberculosis but have limited specificity. 2-Fluorodeoxyglucose–positron emission tomography (FDG-PET) scans may be helpful in patients with tuberculosis but are also positive in other diseases such as malignancy (Fig. 30.14).

In extrapulmonary or miliary infection, appropriate body fluids and/ or tissues must be obtained for microbiologic and histologic examination, with the aid of ultrasound, CT or MRI scanning if available. Liver biopsy and bone marrow aspiration are useful investigations in disseminated or occult disease.[34] An acid-fast stain of buffy-coat leukocytes may be diagnostic in the immunosuppressed. For tuberculous lymphadenitis, fine needle aspiration (FNA) is the initial investigation of choice since it is easy to perform and has a high specificity and sensitivity when both microbiologic and cytologic specimens are collected. FNA does not preclude subsequent lymph node biopsy. In pericardial tuberculosis, aspiration of pericardial fluid may recover the pathogen but is frequently nondiagnostic and pericardial biopsy is often indicated.

Specimens from potentially infected patients are normally analyzed in local laboratories but drug sensitivity testing and more specialized facilities are ideally concentrated in centralized laboratories. All laboratories must be arranged to deal with hazardous, possibly drug-resistant pathogens. Safety measures include containment areas, approved safety cabinets and centrifuges, as well as gowns, gloves, sinks and facilities for disposal of contaminated waste and treatment of spillages. Staff training is essential and may be legally required.

Usual principles of microbiologic safety apply to collection of specimens into sterile containers. Tissue biopsies should be divided and a fresh specimen sent to microbiology and one in formalin to histology. Tissue is better for culture than necrotic material and old pus which may contain acids toxic to mycobacteria, a fact to be considered when selecting biopsy sites. Blood and bone marrow specimens can be injected directly into BACTEC bottles. Examination of cerebrospinal fluid for *M. tuberculosis* is usually an emergency investigation with the clinician forewarning the laboratory. Specimens from gastric lavage should be rapidly transported to the laboratory since stomach acidity may kill mycobacteria. Feces are not useful in the diagnosis of *M. tuberculosis* in HIV-negative patients.

If no diagnostic results are forthcoming in patients in whom tuberculosis is a possibility, the clinician may reasonably resort to a trial of therapy. Improvement of symptoms and a decrease in the acute phase response (monitored by ESR, CRP, etc.) are sufficient indication to move from the diagnostic trial to full therapy. A diagnostic trial of therapy should last a minimum of 2 weeks and ideally 4.

Microbiologic diagnosis

The standard method for staining clinical specimens for *M. tuberculosis* is that of Ziehl–Neelsen (Fig. 30.15) which requires application of heat whereas a modification, the Kinyoun method, does not. Both methods utilize the fact that the stained cell wall is resistant to decolorization by acid alcohol although the biochemical reason for this is unknown. Auramine staining has facilitated rapid screening of diagnostic specimens and has greater sensitivity (Fig. 30.16). Mycobacteria are often scanty and specimens should be reviewed by an experienced operator. Diagnostic microscopy is most successful in patients with extensive disease and cavitation on chest X-ray but only diagnoses about 50% of cases positive by culture. Culture of the organism with subsequent testing for drug sensitivity from clinical specimens is the cornerstone of diagnosis and ultimate treatment; this is particularly important with the emergence of drug-resistant TB, as 'blind' therapy in the absence of sensitivity testing may increase the risk of multi-drug resistance. The clinical microbiology of tuberculosis is reviewed in Chapter 174.

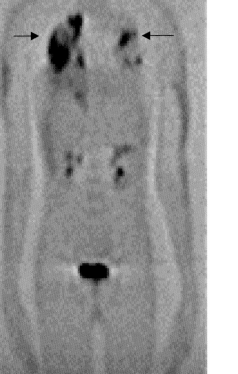

Fig. 30.14 2-Fluorodeoxyglucose–positron emission tomography (FDG-PET) scan in bilateral apical pulmonary TB (arrowed). Tracer is excreted via the renal tract and is seen in the bladder.

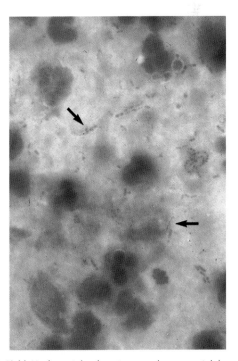

Fig. 30.15 Ziehl–Neelsen-stained sputum specimens containing *Mycobacterium tuberculosis*. Courtesy of Dr F Ahmed, Ealing Hospital, UK.

Fig. 30.16 *Mycobacterium tuberculosis* in sputum detected by auramine staining. Courtesy of Mr M Croughan, with permission from Edmond RTD, Rowland HAK, Welsby PD. A colour atlas of infectious disease. London: Mosby; 1992.

Genetic techniques

The polymerase chain reaction (PCR) has the potential to allow rapid detection of low levels of infection with the possibility of immediate probing for known drug-resistance genes. The usual target for DNA amplification is the insertion sequence IS6110 which is found in all the *M. tuberculosis* complex of organisms (*M. tuberculosis*, *M. bovis*, *M. africanum* and *M. microti*) or ribosomal RNA. Considerable methodologic problems with PCR have been encountered and sensitivity is still laboratory dependent outside recognized expert centers. PCR is potentially of most use in smear-negative culture-positive disease but sensitivity in pulmonary disease is no greater than culture. A problem is that PCR positivity in sputum may persist during treatment and after clinical cure.[35] PCR is potentially useful in diagnosing extrapulmonary tuberculosis but to date has been disappointing.

The major role of PCR is to determine drug sensitivities in culture and smear-positive specimens. In particular, detecting mutations in the *rpoB* gene which encode about 96% of resistance to rifampin is useful in identifying patients likely to have multidrug-resistant (MDR) TB. Line probe assay kits for detection of drug resistance (particularly to rifampin[36]) were approved by the WHO in 2008 for use in resource-poor countries although there is a severe shortage of well-resourced laboratories in many such countries.

Serodiagnosis

Serodiagnostic techniques do not perform well enough for routine use (http://www.stoptb.org/wg/new_diagnostics/assets/documents/jane_cunningham.pdf). Enzyme-linked immunoassays have been developed to detect a number of mycobacterial proteins and lipoarabinomannan but the sensitivity of antibody testing is not sufficiently high in ELISAs with adequate specificity. Local testing for antibodies at sites of infection such as in pleural effusions has also not proved to be useful. Antibody levels are often low in culture-negative individuals where alternative diagnostic approaches are needed. Alterations in antibody levels over time are not a useful guide to clinical response to treatment.

MANAGEMENT

First-line antimycobacterial drugs and their toxicities

This and the next section briefly outline the principal characteristics of the most important antituberculous drugs. These drugs are frequently used in fixed-dose regimens in various combination tablets in order to simplify regimens and improve patient compliance. More detail as to mechanisms, dosage regimens and complications are to be found in Chapter 143.

Isoniazid

Isoniazid (INH or isonicotinic acid hydrazide: $C_6H_7N_3O$) is a bactericidal drug (minimum inhibitory concentration generally <0.1 µg/ml) whose biologic activity resides in a pyridine ring and a hydrazine group. Isoniazid is well absorbed, minimally bound to plasma proteins, has a half-life of 1–3 hours depending on patient acetylator status and is excreted in urine. Concentrations achieved in most tissues are similar to those in serum with the important exception of the CNS where concentrations are approximately 20% of those in serum. Thus, the drug may be used at double the normal dose in CNS disease. Isoniazid enters *M. tuberculosis* by diffusion and by oxygen-dependent active transport where it inhibits mycolic acid synthesis, the nicotinamide adenine dinucleotide (NAD) pathway and interacts with the catalase–peroxidase enzyme system. Mutations in the *katG* gene encoding catalase–peroxidase confer resistance to isoniazid and account for approximately 25% of cases of drug resistance.[37]

The most important, potentially fatal side-effect of isoniazid is hepatotoxicity which is more common in patients older than 60 years, in the presence of coexisting liver disease and possibly in pregnancy. Asymptomatic, usually transient rises in transaminases occur in about 20% of patients. A greater than threefold increase in enzyme levels above the normal range is an indication to discontinue therapy. In practice, it is often impossible to separate isoniazid hepatotoxicity from that due to rifampin or pyrazinamide but interestingly, re-introduction of these drugs singly rather than in combination usually avoids a second episode of hepatotoxicity. The other major side-effect is a peripheral and rarely optic neuritis due to interference with niacin metabolism. This is prevented by concomitant administration of vitamin B_6 (pyridoxine 10 mg daily). Less serious side-effects include nausea, vomiting and arthralgia, while rare ones are hypersensitivity reactions, lupus-like reactions, cerebellar ataxia, convulsions, psychoses, hyperglycemia, agranulocytosis and in malnourished patients, pellagra.

Rifampin

Rifampin is a bactericidal drug which undergoes first-pass metabolism in the liver where it is deacylated, excreted into bile and then into the gut where there is a minor degree of enterohepatic circulation. Rifampin is a potent inducer of hepatic enzymes and therefore has many clinically significant interactions with other drugs (Table 30.2). Rifampin targets the RNA polymerase beta subunit blocking initiation but not elongation of mRNA transcripts.

Patients should be warned that rifampin turns all body secretions, including urine and tears, orange (Fig. 30.17). This is a useful side-effect in terms of monitoring compliance. Rifampin may cause hepatic injury, particularly in the presence of pre-existing liver disease. Gastrointestinal side-effects seldom necessitate stopping therapy and include anorexia, nausea, vomiting, abdominal pain and diarrhea. Pseudomembranous colitis due to *Clostridium difficile* toxin production is described. Immune-mediated problems associated with rifampin include rashes, urticaria, conjunctivitis and rarely hemolysis or thrombocytopenic purpura. A flu-like syndrome may

Table 30.2 Drug interactions with rifampin (rifampicin)*

Drug category	Example
Antibacterials	Chloramphenicol
Antifungals	Fluconazole
Antimalarials	Mefloquine
Corticosteroids	Prednisolone
Anticoagulants	Warfarin
Analgesics	Methadone
Immunosuppressive therapy	Ciclosporin
Ulcer-healing drugs	Cimetidine
Respiratory drugs	Theophylline
Cardiac drugs	
Beta-blockers	Propranolol
Calcium channel blockers	Diltiazem
Cardiac glycosides	Digitoxin (only member of class affected)
Antiarrhythmics	Disopyramide
Lipid-lowering drugs	Fluvastatin
CNS drugs	
Anti-epileptics	Phenytoin
Anxiolytics	Diazepam
Antidepressants	Tricyclic compounds
Antipsychotics	Haloperidol
Endocrine drugs	
Antidiabetics	Tolbutamide
Estrogens and progesterones	Combined and progesterone only contraceptive pill
Thyroid replacement	Thyroxine

*These are the principal classes of drugs for which metabolism is increased (plasma concentration decreased) when taken with rifampin (rifampicin). The examples are not exhaustive and clinicians should check interactions with related drugs in appropriate formularies. (Interactions with drugs used to treat HIV are considered elsewhere.)

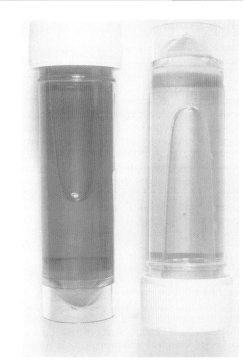

Fig. 30.17 Rifampin (rifampicin) urine testing. Patients should be warned that rifampin turns urine and other body secretions orange. This fact can be helpful in monitoring compliance with drug treatment. Courtesy of Dr W Lynn, Ealing Hospital, UK.

be troublesome, particularly in intermittent therapy regimens, and very rarely may be severe with circulatory collapse and respiratory failure.

Pyrazinamide

Pyrazinamide, a structural analogue of nicotinamide, is a bactericidal drug which is well absorbed via the gut and distributed widely including in the CNS where concentrations are the same as those in serum in patients with tuberculous meningitis. Serum half-life is about 10 hours and excretion is urinary. Pyrazinamide principally acts intracellularly at relatively acidic pH although it may also have some cidal action on extracellular bacteria. The drug penetrates macrophages where an enzyme from *M. tuberculosis* converts it into active pyrazinoic acid. Some strains of *M. tuberculosis* are resistant to pyrazinamide due to production of the enzyme pyrazinamidase.

Hepatotoxicity ranging from elevation of liver transaminases to frank jaundice and liver failure is the principal side-effect of pyrazinamide. More common are mild gastrointestinal problems and an arthralgia associated with raised serum urate concentrations secondary to inhibition of tubular secretion of uric acid by pyrazinamide. Classic gout is rare. Sideroblastic anemia has been reported.

Ethambutol

Ethambutol is a bactericidal drug which is rapidly and well (over 80% of the dose) absorbed in the gut, with peak serum levels occurring 2 hours after a dose. It is then rapidly excreted in urine. Ethambutol appears to alter both *M. tuberculosis* RNA synthesis and transfer of mycolic acids into the cell wall. Changes in cell wall lipids have been noted in organisms resistant to the drug.

The most important complication of ethambutol therapy is retrobulbar neuritis manifest by impaired visual acuity, color blindness and restricted visual fields. Except in patients with pre-existing ophthalmic disease, optic neuritis is extremely rare when ethambutol is used at standard doses (15 mg/kg). In affluent countries, it is appropriate to have patients assessed by an ophthalmologist prior to starting treatment but lack of this facility should not prevent use of ethambutol. Patients should be warned to report symptoms of visual change immediately and ethambutol should generally be avoided in children. Very rarely ethambutol may cause a peripheral neuritis.

Streptomycin

Streptomycin, the first clinically useful drug discovered in the fight against tuberculosis, is an aminoglycoside that has to be given intramuscularly. Streptomycin penetrates cerebrospinal fluid and other remote tissues (e.g. prostate and eye) poorly. There is an immediate and a delayed pathway of excretion via the renal tract. The persistence of the drug at low doses is one factor in the development of side-effects. Streptomycin binds to the 30S ribosomal RNA subunit which results in decreased protein synthesis and misreading of mRNA. Mutations including those in the 30S subunit arise readily in response to isolated streptomycin therapy and lead to drug resistance. The principal side-effects of aminoglycosides are ototoxicity and nephrotoxicity. Rarer ones are neuromuscular blockade and hypersensitivity reactions with maculopapular rashes, fever and eosinophilia.

Second-line drugs

Second-line agents are becoming increasingly important with the rise in drug-resistant organisms. Basic information about such drugs is provided in Table 30.3. Quinolones such as levofloxacin and moxifloxacin are emerging as potentially valuable tools in the fight against tuberculosis and they are being investigated as agents that may reduce the duration of therapy required for treatment of drug-sensitive disease. The value of proven efficacious drugs such as ethionamide is limited by toxicity. Side-effects such as Stevens–Johnson syndrome have effectively eliminated the use of thiacetazone. The potential second-line role of clofazimine, used in the treatment of *M. leprae*, is uncertain. There is evidence to suggest that there may be a role for some drugs not normally considered as useful treatment for tuberculosis such as imipenem[38] and linezolid.[39] More details concerning second-line agents can be found in Chapter 143.

Treatment regimens

Many trials, notably ones involving the British Medical Research Council, have established short-course chemotherapy as the preferred treatment of pulmonary, pleural, nodal and most other forms of tuberculosis. Such regimens are dependent on using the potent antituberculous drugs isoniazid and rifampin throughout a 6-month course as well as 2 months of initial treatment with pyrazinamide. A fourth drug (e.g. ethambutol or streptomycin) is now routinely used in the induction period to ensure that single-resistant organisms are effectively treated. The aim of multidrug therapeutic regimens is to kill *M. tuberculosis* whilst preventing the spontaneous emergence of drug-resistant mutants.

One standard treatment protocol is given in Table 30.4. Alternative regimens are essential in the presence of drug resistance and are possible when drugs are in short supply. For example, 6 months of isoniazid and ethambutol can substitute for isoniazid and rifampin in the period following 2 months of quadruple therapy. For sensitive organisms, drug therapy in compliant patients is very efficacious with cure rates approaching 100%. However, it may be 2 weeks before clinical improvement becomes apparent which is important in both empiric trials of therapy and for appropriate patient expectations. Radiologic improvement lags further behind and it may take 3–5 months before all that remains is residual scarring on chest X-ray. Drug therapy must be linked with the public health measures discussed above.

The necessary duration of treatment for extrapulmonary tuberculosis is debated. Limited trials in osteomyelitis, regarded as a difficult site to treat, indicate that 9 months of therapy is effective providing both isoniazid and rifampin are used. In miliary disease, the 6-month regimens have been very successful. Complications may develop during treatment of disease, partly as a result of the influx of inflammatory leukocytes. The consequences of this depend on the site of infection and include pneumothoraces, expansion of intracerebral granulomas or discharge from subcutaneous nodes.

Directly observed therapy

Compliance with therapy is critical for successful treatment and to limit development of drug-resistant strains. Many social, personal, public health and economic factors influence patient noncompliance with treatments. The WHO and others strongly advocate directly observed therapy, short-course (DOTS) regimens although their efficacy in diverse clinical settings is not completely established.[40] When patients are in hospital, normal treatment regimens may be used but for patients in the community intermittent therapy (Table 30.5) is preferred. DOTS as defined by the WHO is a five-point strategy involving political commitment, increased case detection, standardized and closely supervised treatment, an effective drug supply and an established monitoring and evaluation system (http://www.who.int/tb/dots/en).

Treating multidrug- and extensively drug-resistant organisms

Multidrug resistance is defined as resistance to at least isoniazid and rifampin and has become a major international problem. In the fourth

Table 30.3 Second-line therapy in TB (see also text and Chapter 143)

Drug (chemically closely related drug)	Mechanism of action	Toxicity	Usual initial adult dose
Para-aminosalicylic acid (PAS)	Competes with mycobacterial dihydropteroate synthetase May decrease proinflammatory immune responses	Gastrointestinal intolerance, hypersensitivity, hypothyroidism, crystalluria	12 g q24h (divided doses)
Ethionamide (prothionamide)	Inhibits cell wall mycolic acid synthesis	Gastrointestinal intolerance, hepatitis, hypersensitivity, convulsions, depression, alopecia	0.5–1.0 g q24h (divided doses)
Moxifloxacin (levofloxacin, ciprofloxacin)	Inhibits topoisomerase II	Gastrointestinal intolerance, crystalluria, tremor, convulsions, rash, hepatitis, renal failure	400 mg q24h
Capreomycin (viomycin)	Binds 30S and 50S ribosomes	Nephrotoxic, ototoxic, hypersensitivity	1 g q24h
Kanamycin	Binds 30S ribosome	Nephrotoxic, ototoxic, hypersensitivity	15 mg q12h*
Amikacin	Binds 30S ribosome	Nephrotoxic, ototoxic, rash, neuromuscular blockade, eosinophilia	7.5 mg/kg q12h*
Cycloserine	Competitive D-alanine analogue	Seizures, psychoses, various CNS effects	250 mg q12h

*Peak drug levels should be less than 3 mg/dl (30 mg/l) and trough less than 1 mg/dl (10 mg/l).

Table 30.4 Short-course chemotherapy regimen for treatment of TB and necessity for drug dose modifications in renal impairment

Drug	Adult dose (orally)	Duration of treatment	Modification of drug dose in renal failure
1. Isoniazid*	5 mg/kg (maximum 300 mg)	6 months	No
2. Rifampin (rifampicin)*	10 mg/kg (maximum 600 mg)	6 months	No
3. Pyrazinamide*	30 mg/kg (maximum 2.0 g)	2 months	↓ dose or ↑ dosage interval
4. Ethambutol	15 mg/kg †	2 month	↓ dose or ↑ dosage interval
or			
Streptomycin	15 mg/kg im (maximum 1.0 g)	2 months	↓↓ dose or ↑↑ dosage interval

*Isoniazid and rifampin (rifampicin) are marketed as a single combination tablet ± pyrazinamide which may facilitate compliance.
†Some authorities use ethambutol at 25 mg/kg for 2 months only (longer courses should be at 15 mg/kg).

Table 30.5 Intermittent chemotherapy for TB

Drug	3 times/week dose
1. Isoniazid	10 mg/kg for 6 months (maximum dose 900 mg)
2. Rifampin (rifampicin)	10 mg/kg for 6 months (maximum dose 900 mg)
3. Pyrazinamide	40 mg/kg for 2 months (maximum dose 3.0 g)
4. Ethambutol	30 mg/kg for 2 months
or	
Streptomycin	15 mg/kg for 2 months

global report on drug resistance released in 2008 and available on the web, the WHO estimate that there are about 500 000 new cases of MDR tuberculosis worldwide, with the greatest burden of such disease in the Russian Federation, China and India. This is a consequence of multiple factors including poor prescribing practice by doctors, patient noncompliance with treatment and the endogenous mutation rate of *M. tuberculosis*. Patients should never be prescribed fewer than three drugs initially and seldom fewer than four if there is any chance of resistance or a history of previous therapy irrespective of the sensitivity of the organism initially isolated.

In 2006, a large cohort of HIV-infected patients in South Africa with extensively drug-resistant (XDR) tuberculosis (MDR tuberculosis plus resistance to at least a quinolone and one injectable agent) and a high mortality was described.[41] It has rapidly become apparent that this is a worldwide problem not restricted to HIV-positive individuals and approximately 50 countries have reported patients with XDR tuberculosis. This is an alarming trend.

Treatment protocols for MDR and XDR disease must be designed for the individual but the aim is use as many of the first-line drugs as possible before adding in second-line drugs. The WHO Green Light Committee provides second-line drugs in many parts of the world. A second-line therapeutic regimen should be continued for 18–24 months after cultures are negative. It is critical that affected patients are adequately isolated. Treatment of MDR tuberculosis can be difficult and reported success rates vary in different parts of the world[42,43] (Fig. 30.18). A concern is the rise of secondary drug resistance in other pathogens such as the *Pneumococcus* normally treated with second-line antituberculous agents such as quinolones.[44]

The use of steroids (see also Practice Point 13)

Steroid therapy is often advocated but seldom proven to be of benefit in tuberculosis. In pericardial tuberculosis, steroids have been shown to decrease acute mortality from pericarditis and reduce the need for pericardiocentesis.[45] They do not appear to influence the long-term

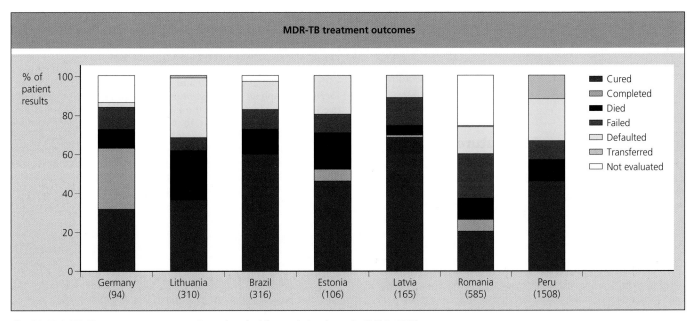

Fig. 30.18 MDR-TB treatment outcomes. Reproduced with permission from the WHO, 2008.

development of constrictive pericarditis. Steroids may have a role in pleural disease but further data are needed before they can be recommended.[46] Steroids are indicated during treatment of CNS tuberculomas to limit their expansion due to cellular influx and prevent raised intracerebral pressure and in tuberculous meningitis.[47] Retrospective studies investigating the role of steroids in miliary tuberculosis have shown no benefit. In all cases, steroid metabolism is increased by rifampin.

Pregnancy

Pregnancy probably does not alter the severity or reactivation rate of tuberculosis or responses to therapy.[48] However, there may be a significant increase in spontaneous abortions and labor difficulties. Congenital tuberculosis is very rare, presents with hepatosplenomegaly, respiratory distress and fever, and carries a high mortality.[49] Tuberculosis frequently requires treatment during pregnancy and this should not be deferred. Isoniazid, rifampin and ethambutol are not teratogenic but few data exist on pyrazinamide. Streptomycin is associated with fetal hearing loss and should be avoided. Little is known about second-line drugs in pregnancy except *para*-aminosalicylic acid (PAS) which appears to be safe. The presence of antituberculous drugs in breast milk is seldom a problem unless both mother and child are on treatment, in which case up to 20% more isoniazid than indicated may be taken by the child and bottle feeding is preferable. Breast-feeding children of mothers taking isoniazid require pyridoxine supplementation.

Surgery for tuberculosis

Surgical techniques such as artificial pneumothoraces, phrenic nerve paralysis, plombage and thoracoplasty are part of the history of tuberculosis before the era of chemotherapy. Now surgeons are most often involved in diagnostic rather than therapeutic procedures. However, resection of tissue may be very useful in patients with MDR or XDR tuberculosis and circumscribed disease.[50] Other indications include massive hemoptysis (after embolization has failed) and in the management of tuberculous empyema, draining sinuses and bronchopleural fistulae. Surgery has been widely used in the treatment of spinal tuberculosis but is only indicated in the presence of progressive neurologic abnormality and spinal instability and to drain large paravertebral abscesses where CT-guided drainage is not possible. Surgery may be required following destructive tuberculosis involving weight-bearing joints. Surgery may have an adjuvant role in nodal tuberculosis if a fluctuant mass persists. In pericardial disease, a pericardial window removes the need for repeated drainage. Pericardectomy may be required in constrictive disease which may develop in patients with previous or treated infection. The most appropriate timing of such surgery remains controversial. Success rates are greater if surgery is performed before extensive calcification develops. In laryngeal infection, temporary tracheotomy may be necessary and a few patients may require complex surgery such as partial laryngectomy.

Immunotherapy and the future

Drugs remain at the forefront in the treatment of tuberculosis but only a small number of new drugs are in development such as the diarylquinolines.[51] These may be insufficient to deal with the increasing amount and complexity of drug-resistant disease. The long-term aim must be to produce true short-course therapy of a few weeks' duration, rather than months, but study is hampered by inadequate biomarkers of disease. Increasing understanding of immune and inflammatory responses including the processes that drive tissue damage and development of cavitation may allow the development of novel therapies or treatment vaccines. Despite the increasing research funds being directed at tuberculosis, successes to date have been limited, in part due to inadequate *in vivo* models of this multifaceted disease of humans.

Nontuberculous Mycobacterial Infections

Nontuberculous mycobacteria (NTM) include all mycobacteria except for those in the *M. tuberculosis* group and *M. leprae*. This section briefly reviews the main pathogenic organisms focusing on clinical presentation and management.

EPIDEMIOLOGY

Nontuberculous mycobacteria are mainly environmental organisms although some are pathogens of other animal species. Many are found in soil and water including tap water. Transmission may be via the aerosol route as reported in *M. avium* complex infections or NTM may be ingested or infection may arise following direct exposure of broken skin. NTM are found worldwide. There are no good data on their incidence or prevalence as they are not notifiable diseases. Better diagnostic techniques are making their identification more frequent, rapid and accurate. Some NTM are more frequently though generally not exclusively reported from specific areas of the world such as *M. malmoense* from northern Europe and *M. fortuitum* complex from the USA. *Mycobacterium xenopi* which is relatively common in Europe is also frequently reported in Canada but is rare in the USA. *Mycobacterium ulcerans* is restricted to more tropical regions of Africa, South East Asia and Australia. In affluent countries, NTM infection, particularly by the *M. avium* complex, is associated with HIV (see Chapter 91) but this is not reported in sub-Saharan Africa, possibly in part because such patients die from other intercurrent illness including tuberculosis.

PATHOGENESIS

The noncaseating granuloma is the main host response to NTM. While there are many similarities, there are also subtle differences from the immune response to *M. tuberculosis* (see above). Granuloma formation may be poor to some NTM, particularly in the presence of immunodeficiency. There are diverse sites of infection, and in immunocompetent hosts with no structural abnormalities, the pathogen is often eliminated by the host response. NTM express virulence factors common to other mycobacteria whilst others seem relatively specific. Hemolysin has been identified as a virulence factor in disseminated *M. avium* infection.[52]

T lymphocytes have a key role in protection against NTM. NTM infection, particularly by the *M. avium* complex, is most common in HIV-seropositive patients when the CD4+ T-cell count falls below $50/\mu l$. *Mycobacterium ulcerans* infection is less strongly associated with HIV infection.[53] NTM infections are more common in patients with mutations in the IFN-γ and IL-12 pathways. TNF and granulocyte–macrophage colony-stimulating factor (GM-CSF) have both been implicated in driving the killing of NTM by monocytes and macrophages. There appear to be cross-immunologic responses between different types of mycobacteria but there is controversy as to whether infection by environmental NTM offers some protection against development of tuberculosis. In this context, it is interesting that repeated BCG vaccination in the Malawi population offered no protection against tuberculosis but decreased *M. leprae* infection rates.[54]

CLINICAL PRESENTATION

Mycobacterium avium complex

This complex includes the *M. avium* and *M. intracellulare* species. *Mycobacterium avium* infection may be disseminated in HIV-seropositive patients (see Chapter 91) whereas both species are associated with more focal lung disease which tends to present in non-HIV-infected patients, although it is found in association with HIV.[55] Clinical signs may be nonspecific (e.g. malaise, fever and weight loss). Such symptoms in patients with HIV should alert the physician to the possibility of *Mycobacterium avium* complex (MAC) infection although the differential is wide and includes tuberculosis.

Pulmonary symptoms include cough and sputum production in the majority of patients while hemoptysis and dyspnea are rarer. MAC infection is well described in older men with chronic obstructive airways disease secondary to smoking or other underlying pulmonary abnormalities. MAC infection is more common in patients with a high alcohol consumption. Scoliosis, pectus excavatum and mitral valve prolapse are associated with pulmonary NTM including MAC infection but specific immune deficits are not well characterized.[56] Cystic fibrosis is associated with NTM including MAC infection and this may increase disease progression as well as susceptibility to other pathogens. MAC is also reported in children who are otherwise well. Bronchiectasis may both predispose to and be a consequence of infection and this may be more common in elderly nonsmoking women (Lady Windermere syndrome). Cavitatory disease is common in MAC infection which may mimic tuberculosis (Fig. 30.19) and multiple infiltrates are often found on CT scanning (Fig. 30.20). MAC aerosols can cause a hypersensitivity pneumonia (hot tub lung) presenting with dyspnea and dry cough, and ground glass shadowing and nodular change on CT scan.

MAC may cause lymph node disease in children.[57] Patients are usually under the age of 5 years and cervical nodes are most commonly affected. Other sites of MAC infection are rare but diverse. Tenosynovitis, septic arthritis and osteomyelitis are well described and occur mainly in the immunocompromised. Diverse skin manifestations have been reported.

Mycobacterium kansasii

Patients with *M. kansasii* usually present with respiratory symptoms that may be associated with night sweats, fever, weight loss and malaise. Presentation may be as insidious and prolonged exacerbation of underlying chronic obstructive airways disease. Hemoptysis may be present in up to a third of patients. Cavitation is frequent and disease is often located in the upper zones of the lung on radiologic examination of HIV-negative patients[58] (Fig. 30.21). Mediastinal lymphadenopathy and pleural effusions are very unusual. Respiratory or disseminated infection may be found in HIV patients. Lymph node disease occurs uncommonly, mainly in children.

Mycobacterium ulcerans

Mycobacterium ulcerans is the cause of Buruli ulcer which is a chronic necrotizing skin infection that is associated with stagnant water and the bugs residing within it. Inoculation is believed to follow minor trauma including bites. Initially a painless swelling develops which becomes a shallow ulcer with a necrotic base and characteristic undermined margins. Ulcers can become very large and involve joints or develop satellite lesions. This organism appears unique amongst NTM in that pathology is largely due to a secreted immunomodulatory cytotoxin called mycolactone.[59]

Other slowly growing atypical mycobacteria

Other slowly growing mycobacteria are a diverse group including *M. xenopi*, the *M. simiae* complex, *M. szulgai*, *M. malmoense*, *M. haemophilum*, *M. scrofulaceum*, *M. celatum*, *M. paratuberculosis* and

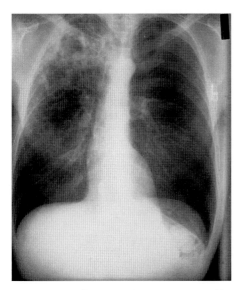

Fig. 30.19 Apical cavitary infiltrates similar to those caused by pulmonary tuberculosis in a 60-year-old male cigarette smoker with *Mycobacterium avium* complex lung disease.

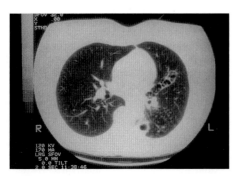

Fig. 30.20 *Mycobacterium avium* complex lung disease. Chest CT scan from a 52-year-old woman with MAC lung disease demonstrating three abnormalities that are common in MAC lung disease: bronchiectasis, a cavity and small (<5 mm) nodules.

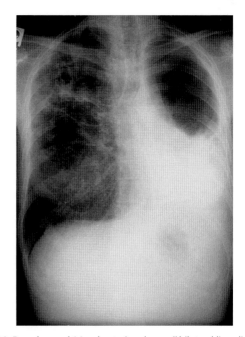

Fig. 30.21 Far advanced *Mycobacterium kansasii* bilateral ling disease in a 42-year-old male cigarette smoker with extensive cavity destruction of the left upper lobe.

M. genavense. M. marinum and *M. gordonae* which may grow somewhat faster are usually included within this group. Many members of this group grow optimally at lower temperatures, which for *M. marinum* is 30°C. This means that infection is usually localized to the skin, classically a single nodule on the skin which may spread along lymphatics to regional lymph nodes. Deep infections do occur but systemic spread and symptoms are rare. Minor trauma and exposure to water sports or hobbies may be found in *M. marinum* infections; this organism is also a fish pathogen.

In contrast, *M. xenopi* grows best at 43°C and has been recovered from hot water systems. It is a pulmonary pathogen in patients with underlying chronic lung disease. It may cause disease in patients immunosuppressed due to HIV or solid-organ transplantation. *Mycobacterium scrofulaceum* may cause lymph node disease but there is immunologic evidence that exposure to the organism is usually not associated with disease. Many of these organisms cause disseminated disease in HIV. They are also being increasingly recovered from patients with underlying lung disease although whether they are all of clinical significance is controversial. However, many would treat if there is evidence of increasing clinical symptoms with worsening changes on high-resolution CT scanning. Infection of skin, soft tissues, lymph nodes, indwelling plastic devices (including central lines) and bone, joint and tendon have all been reported. The number of mycobacteria associated with case reports of human disease, particularly in immunocompromised patients, is increasing and the list here is necessarily restricted.

Mycobacterium fortuitum complex and other rapid growers

The *M. fortuitum* group includes the named strain as well as *M. chelonae* and *M. abscessus*. There are many other rapidly growing mycobacteria, of which the *M. smegmatis* group (encompassing *M. smegmatis, wolinskyi* and *goodii*) is the best known. The *M. fortuitum* group of NTM is associated with both postsurgical infections and infections of indwelling catheters and shunts. They are also associated with skin infections or deep tissue infections which may be aggressive and disseminated. Infection can follow trauma including nail cutting.[60] These organisms are also more common in cystic fibrosis patients. *Mycobacterium fortuitum* has been found in deep CNS infections, sometimes following traumatic injury. *Mycobacterium smegmatis* organisms usually cause skin infections although lung infection and disseminated disease in a child with an IFN-γ receptor deficiency has been reported.[61]

DIAGNOSIS

The approach to diagnosis is similar to that in tuberculosis with the need to obtain a positive culture if at all possible. It is necessary for clinicians to be aware of the diagnostic possibility of NTM infection so that the correct samples are sent for the correct mycobacterial culture procedure. Alterations in high-resolution CT scans in patients with pulmonary disease may suggest the possibility of NTM and this is an important investigation in patients with potential NTM pulmonary disease. The diagnostic sample taken depends on the presentation of the infection and will range from sputum or bronchoscopic samples to lymph node biopsy. In childhood nodal disease fine needle aspiration is avoided to prevent the formation of discharging sinuses and scars. In systemic disease, particularly in the immunosuppressed, mycobacterial blood cultures are essential. NTM skin tests have no role. Genetic techniques are mainly used to determine whether smear- or culture-positive cases are due to NTM or the *M. tuberculosis* complex. PCR may be used to diagnose *M. ulcerans*. Drug sensitivity testing should be undertaken for NTM but not all laboratory breakpoints are well defined. In addition, there may be poor concordance between laboratory and clinical sensitivities.

In contrast to tuberculosis, the finding of a single positive sputum culture is not diagnostic of infection in the non-immunosuppressed patient but may represent contamination or colonization, although data concerning how and when colonization progresses to active infection are limited. In general, a single positive NTM sputum culture should be accompanied by progression of symptoms, ideally with worsening of findings on chest X-ray or high-resolution CT scan and exclusion of other diagnoses. Repeat sputum positives or growth of NTM from deeper bronchoscopic samples support a diagnosis of active disease. Expert advice should be sought on individual cases and even a positive diagnosis may allow an expectant strategy without initiation of therapy with toxic antimycobacterial drugs in some instances. A single positive diagnostic specimen in sites other than the lung is highly suggestive of active disease.

MANAGEMENT

Management of NTM is not well defined and in many areas, particularly for the less commonly detected organisms, there is a very weak evidence base. The situation is particularly obscure if two or more different mycobacteria are isolated. The threshold for active management may be influenced by co-morbidities such as cystic fibrosis. The American Thoracic and Infectious Diseases Societies have produced a useful consensus statement.[62]

Mycobacterium avium complex

Prophylaxis (see Chapters 90 and 91)

HIV-seropositive patients with a CD4 T-cell count less than 50/μl should be given clarithromycin 500 mg twice daily or azithromycin 1200 mg weekly. Rifabutin 300 mg weekly is an alternative, although the emergence of rifampin-resistant tuberculosis due an *rpoB* mutation in a patient taking rifabutin prophylaxis for *M. avium* complex infection raised concern.[63] Once the CD4 count rises above 100/μl prophylaxis may be stopped.

Treatment

MAC pulmonary disease is treated with 1 g clarithromycin or 500 mg azithromycin with 600 mg rifampin and 15 mg/kg ethambutol. In mild disease, alternate day or three times weekly regimens are sometimes used; in severe disease an aminoglycoside may be added. Treatment normally continues until 12 months after the last positive culture. Concurrent use of bronchodilators should be given as required but there are no data to support the use of steroids. In disseminated disease, therapy can be stopped when symptoms resolve and immune function is improved. Fluoroquinolones have good *in-vitro* activity against MAC but clinical data about their use are sparse. Additional positive cultures after a treatment course may represent infection by new strains rather than relapse. Macrolide-resistant organisms should only be treated in consultation with expert advice. Surgery has a very limited role in MAC infection. Successful management of the hypersensitivity syndrome requires removal of exposure to MAC antigens. Treatment of disseminated MAC infection in HIV disease is discussed in Chapter 91.

Mycobacterium kansasii

The best regimen and duration of therapy are not established. Ethambutol and rifampin are essential and isoniazid is normally added. A macrolide may be an effective alternative. The safest approach is to continue treatment until sputum cultures are negative for at least 12 months. Many isolates are sensitive to quinolones and amikacin but pyrazinamide resistance is the rule. Children with lymph node disease can be treated by excision alone.

Mycobacterium ulcerans

Surgical debridement is the main treatment for *M. ulcerans* infection which responds poorly to antimycobacterial drugs. Excision of pre-ulcerative lesions is advocated by some. Rifampin and streptomycin or amikacin for 2 months have been advocated for treatment or as an adjunct to surgery. Quinolones may also be active against *M. ulcerans*.[64]

Slowly growing atypical mycobacteria

The treatment for most members of this group is empiric, supported by available drug sensitivity data. Dual therapy often involving a macrolide is common and should continue for at least 3 months after resolution of symptoms. Lymph node disease in children may be treated by excision alone although a short course of clarithromycin has been advocated by some authorities. *Mycobacterium marinum* is usually treated by clarithromycin and ethambutol, with rifampin added for deeper infections. *Mycobacterium smegmatis* is typically resistant to isoniazid and rifampin. *Mycobacterium scrofulaceum* is frequently resistant to multiple antibiotics. *Mycobacterium xenopi* sensitivities may not transfer well to clinical responses but therapy with ethambutol, rifampin and a macrolide is one approach, with streptomycin and quinolones being potentially useful drugs. Surgical debridement or removal of focal infection should always be considered in such NTM. Treatment should involve physicians with an interest and expertise.

Mycobacterium fortuitum complex and other rapid growers

Mycobacterium fortuitum is relatively drug sensitive and may be treated with quinolones, amikacin, imipenem, doxycycline and macrolides according to sensitivities of a particular organism. However, as *M. fortuitum* (and *M. smegmatis*) may express an inducible macrolide resistance gene, therapy with clarithromycin is avoided. Removal of foreign bodies or infected lines and catheters is necessary and surgical debridement is often required (Fig. 30.22). *Mycobacterium chelonae* is sensitive to macrolides and 6 months of monotherapy with clarithromycin was effective in a study of 14 patients. In severe disease, a second agent such as tobramycin should be considered. *Mycobacterium abscessus* is relatively resistant to drugs other than macrolides which may be combined with intravenous amikacin. Surgical resection should always be considered for localized infection. Treatment should be for 12 months.

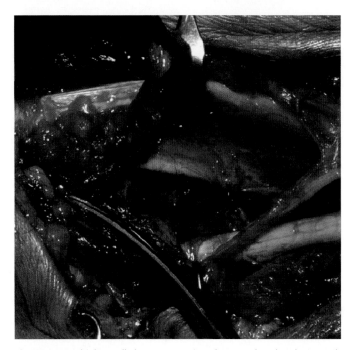

Fig. 30.22 Multiple small abscesses running along tendon sheaths caused by infection with *Mycobacterium fortuitum* following a fishing accident. Reproduced from Patel *et al.*[65] with kind permission of Springer Science and Business Media.

In general, susceptibility testing should be used to guide treatment in these rapidly dividing organisms. Linezolid may have useful activity against all members of the *M. fortuitum* complex although prolonged treatment is associated with side-effects.

REFERENCES

🖰 References for this chapter can be found online at http://www.expertconsult.com

Fungal pneumonias

INTRODUCTION

This chapter will focus on the pulmonary aspects of the endemic mycoses, those fungi that are geographically restricted and that have the capability to cause infection in healthy hosts. Most infections with these fungi are initiated with inhalation of the conidia from the mold phase, which exists in the environment, and thus the lungs play a major role in the pathogenesis and clinical presentation of these infections. Infections with the endemic mycoses in immunosuppressed individuals are usually more severe and are more likely to be disseminated.

Histoplasmosis

MYCOLOGY AND EPIDEMIOLOGY

The causative agent of histoplasmosis is *Histoplasma capsulatum*, a dimorphic fungus that exists as a mold in the environment but converts to a yeast form in tissues at 37°C. There are two human pathogens, *H. capsulatum* var. *capsulatum* and *H. capsulatum* var. *duboisii*. The latter organism is endemic in Africa and will not be discussed further. In the mold phase, *H. capsulatum* var. *capsulatum* (hereafter referred to as *H. capsulatum*) develops characteristic macroconidia and microconidia. *H. capsulatum* is found primarily in North America in the Ohio and Mississippi River valleys and in many countries in Central America; localized foci exist in countries surrounding the Mediterranean Sea and in South East Asia.

The environmental niche for *H. capsulatum* is soil that is enriched by the nitrogen contained in bird and bat guano. Abandoned buildings and areas under trees that serve as bird and bat roosts and caves with high bat populations are especially likely to have high concentrations of *H. capsulatum*. In the endemic areas, exposure to *H. capsulatum* is common and it is estimated that hundreds of thousands of persons are infected yearly. Most infections are sporadic, acquired during the course of daily living, but dramatic outbreaks have been documented, including the large outbreak in Indianapolis that infected over a hundred thousand persons;[1] many smaller outbreaks have been traced back to spelunking, demolition of buildings or other activities that disrupt contaminated soil.[2]

PATHOGENESIS AND PATHOLOGY

Infection begins when the microconidia of *H. capsulatum* are inhaled into the alveoli. Neutrophils and macrophages phagocytize the organism, which triggers conversion to the yeast phase. The organism survives within macrophages, is spread to the hilar and mediastinal lymph nodes, and subsequently disseminates hematogenously. Asymptomatic hematogenous dissemination likely occurs in most patients who are infected. Specific cell-mediated immunity against *H. capsulatum* develops in a few weeks, leading to macrophage activation and, ultimately, killing of the organism. Cell-mediated immunity is crucial for control of the infection. It is thought that organisms can remain in a dormant state, similar to that which occurs with *Mycobacterium tuberculosis*, and then reactivate years later should cellular immunity wane.

The extent of disease is determined both by the inoculum of conidia inhaled and the immune response of the host. A small inoculum can cause severe infection in markedly immunosuppressed hosts, especially those who have AIDS or have been treated with anti-tumor necrosis factor (TNF) agents.[3,4] Conversely, healthy individuals can develop life-threatening infection when exposed to a large inoculum of fungi. Re-infection is possible in persons previously infected with *H. capsulatum* if they are exposed to a heavy inoculum of the organism.

CLINICAL FEATURES

It is important to emphasize that most patients who become infected with *H. capsulatum* remain asymptomatic or at most have a self-limited 'flu-like' illness. In those patients who do have acute pneumonia, symptoms are usually fever, fatigue, dyspnea, cough, mild chest discomfort, arthralgias and myalgias. The chest radiograph reveals a patchy lobar or multilobar infiltrate; hilar lymphadenopathy, when present, is a clue to the possibility of a fungal pneumonia.[5] The initial diagnosis in almost all patients is an atypical bacterial pneumonia, and almost all have received antibiotics to no avail before the possibility of histoplasmosis is entertained. If several patients who were involved with a particular outdoor activity have the same symptoms and see the same physician, then fungal pneumonia assumes a more prominent position in the differential diagnosis.

A small minority of patients with acute pulmonary histoplasmosis develop severe pneumonia that can progress to acute respiratory distress syndrome (ARDS). This occurs most often in patients who are immunosuppressed or in those who had an overwhelming exposure to the organism. Diffuse infiltrates that often have a nodular component are noted on chest radiograph (Fig. 31.1). In immunosuppressed patients, severe diffuse pulmonary involvement is often one component of widespread disseminated infection.

Chronic cavitary pulmonary histoplasmosis almost always occurs in older adults who have underlying emphysema and clinically mimics reactivation tuberculosis. Symptoms include fever, fatigue, anorexia, weight loss, cough productive of purulent sputum, and hemoptysis. Chest radiographs show unilateral or bilateral upper lobe infiltrates and thick-walled cavities, and fibrosis is seen in the lower lung fields[5] (Fig. 31.2).

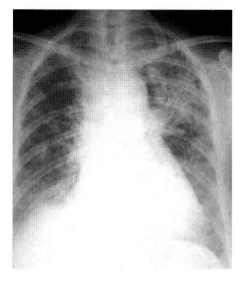

Fig. 31.1 Diffuse pulmonary infiltrates in a 40-year-old woman who had received a renal transplant 2 years before and who developed acute pulmonary histoplasmosis.

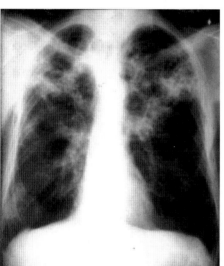

Fig. 31.2 Chronic cavitary pulmonary histoplasmosis in an elderly man who had severe underlying emphysema.

Many patients with disseminated histoplasmosis will have pulmonary manifestations. These may be subtle, as often occurs in older patients with chronic progressive histoplasmosis, but the pulmonary component may also be life threatening, which is noted most often in immunosuppressed patients. On presentation, some patients have chest radiographs that show diffuse pneumonia; in others, the primary manifestations are those related to other organ systems and pulmonary involvement is verified only later.

DIAGNOSIS

Histoplasmosis is definitively diagnosed by growth of the organism from samples taken from the infected site.[8] For pulmonary histoplasmosis, sputum, bronchoalveolar lavage (BAL) fluid, lung tissue or mediastinal lymph nodes are acceptable samples. *H. capsulatum* may take as long as 4–6 weeks to grow on Sabouraud's agar at room temperature in the mold form. Tentative identification can be made on seeing the characteristic tuberculate macroconidia; definitive identification is made with the use of a commercially available DNA probe that is highly specific for *H. capsulatum*.

Identification of the organism in tissue or fluid samples allows an early diagnosis while awaiting culture results. The organisms appear as uniform, 2–4 µm oval budding yeasts, most easily seen on tissue stained with methenamine silver or periodic acid–Schiff (PAS) stains or in smears or touch preparations stained with Giemsa stain (Fig. 31.3). For patients who have disseminated disease in addition to pulmonary manifestations, biopsy samples taken from bone marrow, lymph nodes or lesions on the mucous membranes or skin may reveal the organisms and avoid the need for bronchoscopy.

Serology plays an important role in the diagnosis of pulmonary histoplasmosis, especially chronic cavitary histoplasmosis and acute pulmonary histoplasmosis.[8] Both complement fixation (CF) and immunodiffusion (ID) tests are available. The ID test, which detects H and M antibodies, is slightly more specific than the CF test; however, the CF test has better sensitivity than the ID test. For patients with acute pneumonia, the initial studies may be negative but will show a fourfold rise over the subsequent few weeks. Antibody titers are almost always positive in patients with chronic cavitary histoplasmosis. In general, serology is not as useful in immunosuppressed patients who cannot mount an antibody response.

Antigen detection, using an enzyme immunoassay that measures a cell wall polysaccharide antigen of *H. capsulatum* in urine and serum, is useful in patients with acute pulmonary histoplasmosis, especially those with diffuse pneumonia, but is not useful for chronic cavitary histoplasmosis or mediastinal syndromes.[8] In those patients who

There are several complications of pulmonary histoplasmosis that can occur months to years after the initial infection. Mediastinal granuloma is characterized by persistent mediastinal and/or hilar lymphadenopathy.[6] Many patients are asymptomatic and the problem is discovered when a chest radiograph is performed for another reason. Others have symptoms of dysphagia, chest pain, dyspnea or nonproductive cough when the enlarged lymph nodes impinge on adjacent structures. CT scan usually reveals a confluence of lymph nodes that are surrounded by a fibrous capsule and that have central necrosis. Most patients have resolution of the lymphadenopathy, but fistula formation and compression of adjacent structures may require intervention. This syndrome does not progress to mediastinal fibrosis.

Mediastinal fibrosis is a rare complication of pulmonary histoplasmosis in which the host responds to histoplasmosis with excessive fibrosis that ultimately encases the great vessels and/or bronchi.[7] Obstruction of the superior vena cava and/or the vessels to one lung is most common. The disease is progressive and the symptoms include dyspnea, cough, wheezing and hemoptysis. CT scan reveals the extent of the fibrosis and angiographic studies pinpoint those vessels that are stenotic. When vessels to both lungs are involved, the disease is almost always fatal.

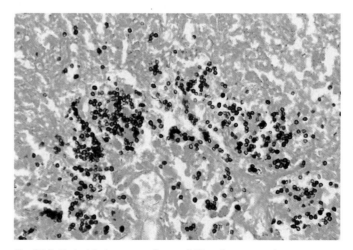

Fig. 31.3 Typical 2–4 µm yeast forms of *Histoplasma capsulatum* seen on a biopsy taken from an enlarged necrotic adrenal gland. The tissue is stained with Gomori methenamine silver stain.

have dissemination in addition to pulmonary involvement, the antigen assay has proved to be extremely useful. Cross-reactivity occurs with blastomycosis, coccidioidomycosis, paracoccidioidomycosis and penicilliosis.

MANAGEMENT

The Infectious Diseases Society of America has recently updated guidelines for the management of histoplasmosis.[9] Recommendations are based primarily on multicenter, nonrandomized, open-label treatment trials and case series from individual institutions. In general, patients with severe pulmonary histoplasmosis should be treated initially with an amphotericin B formulation. Lipid formulations are associated with fewer adverse effects, and in the only randomized treatment trial that was performed in AIDS patients who had severe disseminated histoplasmosis, liposomal amphotericin B was superior to amphotericin B deoxycholate.[10] For most patients, after a few weeks of amphotericin B therapy, step-down therapy to itraconazole is recommended.

Patients who have mild to moderate pulmonary histoplasmosis should be treated with itraconazole.[9] Fluconazole has proved to be less effective, and in a small number of AIDS patients resistance developed during fluconazole use.[11] Voriconazole and posaconazole both have *in-vitro* activity against *H. capsulatum*; however, there are only a limited number of case reports using these two azoles to treat histoplasmosis and they are currently reserved for therapy of patients who have failed therapy with other agents.[12,13] The echinocandins do not appear to have activity against *H. capsulatum* and should not be used.

Most patients with acute pulmonary histoplasmosis have self-limited infection and do not need to be treated with an antifungal agent. However, some patients remain symptomatic for weeks, and in these patients a short course of treatment with itraconazole 200 mg daily for 6–12 weeks is recommended.[9] Severe acute pulmonary histoplasmosis should be treated with lipid formulation amphotericin B, 3–5 mg/kg daily, or amphotericin B deoxycholate, 0.7–1.0 mg/kg daily. After the patient improves, step-down therapy to itraconazole can be initiated. Therapy should continue for at least 12 weeks and until all infiltrates have resolved. Many clinicians use intravenous methylprednisolone in addition to amphotericin B during the first 1–2 weeks in patients who are severely hypoxemic.[9]

Most patients who have chronic cavitary pulmonary histoplasmosis are chronically ill and can be treated with itraconazole, 200 mg twice daily for at least a year, and sometimes longer. The outcome is still dismal in many patients because of the degree of fibrosis and lung destruction that has occurred.

Patients with mediastinal granuloma do not require therapy with an antifungal agent. However, in symptomatic patients, many clinicians give a 6- to 12-week course of 200 mg itraconazole once or twice daily although there are no data showing this is effective.[9] Surgical resection of the granulomatous mass can be helpful in relieving compressive symptoms caused by encroachment on vital structures.

Mediastinal fibrosis should not be treated with an antifungal agent or with corticosteroids. Placement of stents in obstructed great vessels by an interventionalist who is experienced in the treatment of this rare disease has proved extremely useful in providing symptomatic relief.[14]

Patients who have pulmonary involvement as one manifestation of disseminated disease should always receive antifungal therapy. Patients who have mild to moderate symptoms can be treated with itraconazole, 200 mg twice daily for a year. Patients who have severe symptoms should be treated initially with lipid formulation amphotericin B, 3–5 mg/kg daily, that can be changed to itraconazole after a clinical response is noted.

Patients who have AIDS should receive chronic suppressive therapy with itraconazole, 200 mg daily as long as their CD4 counts remain below 200 cells/μl. It is safe to discontinue suppressive therapy if they have consistently taken antiretroviral agents and their CD4 count remains >200 cells/μl for at least 1 year (see also Chapter 91).[9]

Blastomycosis

MYCOLOGY AND EPIDEMIOLOGY

The causative agent of blastomycosis is *Blastomyces dermatitidis*, a dimorphic fungus that exists as a mold in the environment but converts to a yeast form in tissues at 37°C. The organism is found in North America, Africa and the Middle East. Most cases are reported from states that border the Mississippi River basin, the Canadian provinces of Ontario and Manitoba, and areas bordering the St Lawrence Seaway. There are occasional reports of cases that are associated with small microfoci that exist outside the typical endemic areas.

The environmental niche for this organism appears to be soil and decaying wood, especially along waterways. It is difficult to isolate the organism from the environment, but several outbreaks have been traced back to activities involving canoeing, camping and dismantling a beaver lodge.[15]

PATHOGENESIS AND PATHOLOGY

Blastomycosis begins with inhalation of the conidia of *B. dermatitidis* into the alveoli. The filamentous form converts to the yeast form in the lungs, and both neutrophils and cell-mediated immunity are important in the response to infection. It is likely that hematogenous dissemination occurs early in most patients, but clinical manifestations are uncommon. Weeks to months later, frequently after the pulmonary lesion has healed, patients can present with cutaneous or other organ involvement. It should be presumed that all extrapulmonary lesions represent hematogenous dissemination. The histopathologic picture is one of a mixed pyo-granulomatous process. Blastomycosis tends to be more severe in those with cell-mediated immune dysfunction;[16,17] these patients have minimal granuloma formation and mount mostly a neutrophilic response. Reactivation of prior infection with *B. dermatitidis* has been noted, but appears to be less common than noted with *H. capsulatum*.

CLINICAL FEATURES

Most patients with acute pulmonary infection with *B. dermatitidis* remain asymptomatic or have a mild 'flu-like' illness that is never diagnosed as blastomycosis. Those who have acute pneumonia manifest fever, cough, mild dyspnea, myalgias and arthralgias, and are noted to have a localized pulmonary infiltrate on chest radiograph. Most patients are given a diagnosis of an atypical bacterial pneumonia and are treated with antibiotics. Only when the infection does not respond to this therapy is a fungal infection considered and further diagnostic studies undertaken.

A small proportion of patients with acute blastomycosis develop overwhelming pulmonary infection with ARDS[18] (Fig. 31.4). This occurs

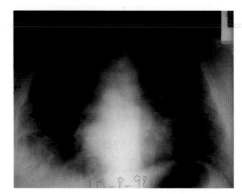

Fig. 31.4 Severe diffuse pneumonia with ARDS due to *Blastomyces dermatitidis* in a 50-year-old patient with no underlying illnesses.

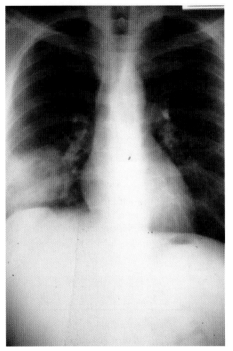

Fig. 31.5 Mass-like lesion in a 47-year-old man who was thought to have lung cancer until the biopsy revealed many granulomas and culture yielded *Blastomyces dermatitidis*.

more often in immunocompromised patients, but is also reported in previously healthy adults. The presumption in the latter group is that they inhaled an excessively large number of conidia that overwhelmed their immune response. The mortality rate is extremely high in this rapidly progressive form of pulmonary blastomycosis.

Pulmonary blastomycosis can also present as a mass-like lesion that is indistinguishable from lung cancer or with upper lobe cavitary lesions that resemble tuberculosis or histoplasmosis[19] (Fig. 31.5). Fever, night sweats, weight loss, fatigue, dyspnea and cough with purulent sputum and hemoptysis are often present for weeks before the patient seeks medical attention. Pleural effusions and hilar or mediastinal lymphadenopathy each occur in only about 20% of patients.

Cutaneous lesions are the most common manifestation of extrapulmonary blastomycosis; their appearance in a patient who has a nonresolving pneumonia can lead toward the diagnosis of blastomycosis. The lesions are frequently multiple and classically are well-circumscribed, plaque-like lesions that become verrucous and often show punctate draining areas in the center (Fig. 31.6). Less commonly, painful ulcerated lesions or multiple rapidly developing nodular lesions are noted.

Common noncutaneous manifestations of disseminated blastomycosis that can occur at the time the patient has pneumonia or after the pulmonary manifestations have resolved include osteomyelitis, septic arthritis and genitourinary tract infection, especially with prostatic involvement. Focal blastomycosis of other organs and central nervous system (CNS) infection manifested as chronic meningitis or brain abscess are well described.[20]

DIAGNOSIS

Blastomycosis is definitively diagnosed when the organism is grown on Sabouraud's agar from a sample taken from an infected site.[21] For pulmonary blastomycosis, sputum, BAL fluid and lung tissue are acceptable samples. *Blastomyces dermatitidis* takes several weeks to grow at room temperature in the mold form. Once growth occurs, identification can be made quickly with the use of a commercially available DNA probe that is highly specific for *B. dermatitidis*.

Prior to the growth of the organism, a preliminary diagnosis of pulmonary blastomycosis can often be made by examining sputum or BAL fluid treated with potassium hydroxide or calcofluor white or by examining a cytologic preparation stained with Papanicolaou stain.[22] The organisms are large (8–10 μm), thick-walled yeasts that have a single broad-based bud; this specific morphology distinguishes *B. dermatitidis* from other yeasts (Fig. 31.7).

If skin lesions are present in a patient with pulmonary infiltrates, biopsy should be performed and may yield a diagnosis of blastomycosis without having to perform bronchoscopy. The yeasts can be visualized in tissues with methenamine silver or PAS stains.

CF and ID antibody assays are neither sensitive nor specific for blastomycosis and are of little use for diagnosis. An enzyme immunoassay that detects a polysaccharide cell wall antigen of *B. dermatitidis* in urine and serum is commercially available and may prove useful for the diagnosis of blastomycosis.[23] There is a high degree of cross-reactivity between the antigen tests for *H. capsulatum* and *B. dermatitidis*.

MANAGEMENT

The Infectious Diseases Society of America has recently updated guidelines for the management of blastomycosis.[24] Recommendations are based on multicenter, nonrandomized, open-label treatment trials and case series from individual institutions. In general, all patients with symptomatic blastomycosis should be treated with an antifungal agent. Even patients who have acute pulmonary blastomycosis that

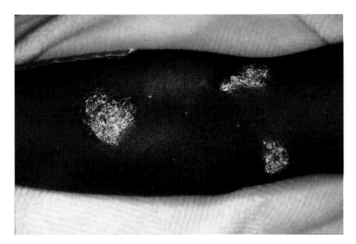

Fig. 31.6 Typical skin lesions of blastomycosis in a 24-year-old man. Courtesy of Dr Hector Bonilla.

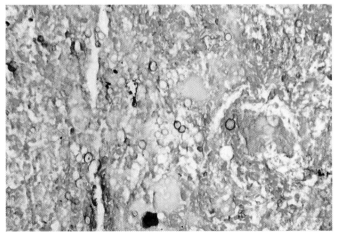

Fig. 31.7 Lung biopsy from a 54-year-old man who had a left upper lobe pulmonary infiltrate. Thick walled, broad-based, budding yeasts are seen with the periodic acid–Schiff stain.

appears to be resolving should be treated in order to decrease the risk for subsequent extrapulmonary infection.[24] Patients who have only a single cutaneous lesion or other focal manifestation should be treated because, by definition, they have disseminated blastomycosis. Mild-to-moderate blastomycosis should be treated with an azole agent; severe infection should be treated with an amphotericin B formulation as initial therapy.

Most cases of pulmonary blastomycosis can be treated with itraconazole.[24] The dosage is 200 mg once or twice daily. Second-line agents that can be used for patients who cannot tolerate itraconazole include high-dose fluconazole (800 mg daily), voriconazole (200–300 mg twice daily) and posaconazole (400 mg twice daily).[24-26] Fluconazole is not as effective as itraconazole for blastomycosis. *In-vitro* susceptibility studies show voriconazole and posaconazole to be active against *B. dermatitidis*, but there is little clinical experience with these agents to date. The echinocandins appear to have no activity against *B. dermatitidis* and should not be used.

Amphotericin B is reserved for those patients who have severe infection with *B. dermatitidis*; this includes those who have severe pneumonia, CNS involvement and widespread visceral infection, and most immunosuppressed patients. A lipid amphotericin B formulation, 3–5 mg/kg daily, or amphotericin B deoxycholate, 0.7–1 mg/kg daily, can be used.[24] After 1–2 weeks, if the patient's condition has improved, step-down therapy with oral itraconazole is recommended.

The length of time required for the treatment of blastomycosis depends on the extent of the infection and the clinical response of the patient. Most patients who have pulmonary blastomycosis should be treated for 6–12 months. If other sites of infection are noted, such as osteoarticular involvement, a minimum of 1 year of azole therapy should be planned. Immunosuppressed patients may require lifelong suppressive therapy with an azole.[24]

Coccidioidomycosis

MYCOLOGY AND EPIDEMIOLOGY

Coccidioides is a dimorphic fungus that exists as a mold in the environment and as a spherule *in vivo*. It differs from the other dimorphic fungi in that the dimorphism is not regulated by temperature. It has recently been verified that there are two species: *C. immitis* refers to isolates from California and *C. posadasii* to isolates from all other areas. *Coccidioides* species are generally found in the Lower Sonoran life zone, which is a desert environment that occurs in certain areas of South America, Central America and the south-western United States.

Most inhabitants of the endemic area are infected before they reach adulthood. An increasing number of infections are reported in older adults who moved to these warm climates at retirement and had never been exposed to this organism previously.[27] Catastrophic events, such as earthquakes, have led to the occurrence of coccidioidomycosis in areas beyond those normally seen, and environmental cycles of rain and drought in the desert are important in the natural history of *Coccidioides* spp.[28]

PATHOGENESIS AND PATHOLOGY

The mold form of *Coccidioides* develops arthroconidia that are easily dispersed and inhaled into the alveoli where the organism transforms into the spherule form. Spherules are large (20–80 μm), thick-walled structures that contain hundreds of endospores. The spherule ruptures when filled and releases many endospores, each of which is able to spread to form a new spherule.

The primary host defense against *Coccidioides* appears to be cell-mediated immunity. Neutrophils are present in most lesions, but they cannot eliminate spherules. It is likely that many patients experience silent hematogenous dissemination. *Coccidioides* species have the potential to

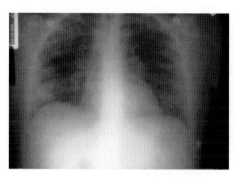

Fig. 31.8 Diffuse infiltrates in a patient with AIDS who developed pulmonary coccidioidomycosis.

reactivate years after the primary infection with the organism. For still unexplained reasons, dark-skinned races, especially African Americans and Filipinos, are at higher risk for dissemination and severe infection than white-skinned persons.[29] Pregnant women, especially those in the third trimester, are also at risk for severe disease.[30]

CLINICAL FEATURES

Most persons infected with *Coccidioides* species have no symptoms or have mild symptoms suggesting a 'flu-like' illness. Patients with acute coccidioidal pneumonia have fever, fatigue, myalgias, arthralgias, dry cough, anterior chest pain and dyspnea. Erythema nodosum frequently occurs, especially in women, and should raise the possibility of coccidioidomycosis. Chest radiographs show patchy pneumonitis, with or without hilar lymphadenopathy patients[31] (Fig. 31.8).

In patients who are immunocompromised, especially those with AIDS, transplant recipients and those treated with anti-TNF agents, and in those who had exposure to a large number of arthroconidia, severe pneumonia with progression to ARDS can occur.[31,32] Chest radiographs reveal diffuse reticulonodular infiltrates.

Approximately 5–10% of patients have pulmonary complications following acute coccidioidal pneumonia. These include benign coccidioidomas, which are persistent asymptomatic pulmonary nodules, and solitary, thin-walled cavities that can persist for months to years. Although many cavities will resolve, hemoptysis or cavity rupture into the pleural space can occur in some patients.[31] Chronic progressive pneumonia is characterized by thick-walled cavity formation, fibrosis, purulent sputum, hemoptysis and dyspnea. This form of coccidioidomycosis occurs mostly in those who are older and have chronic obstructive pulmonary disease and/or diabetes mellitus.[33]

Less than 1% of patients with symptomatic coccidioidomycosis will develop symptoms of disseminated infection. Almost always, these patients are either dark-skinned or are immunosuppressed. The sites involved, in addition to the lungs, are most often skin, subcutaneous tissues, osteoarticular structures and meninges, but any organ can be affected. Meningitis, which is a dreaded complication, can be the sole manifestation of dissemination or it can be present along with dissemination to multiple different organs.

DIAGNOSIS

Coccidioidomycosis is definitively diagnosed when the organism is grown in culture from involved tissues or body fluids. *Coccidioides* species grow as a white mold within a few days on most standard media. It is important to warn laboratory personnel if coccidioidomycosis is a possibility as the mold form is highly infectious. *Coccidioides* is classified as a bioterrorism agent and must be handled using biosafety level 3 precautions, which are not present in most laboratories.

The large spherules are readily identified using KOH or calcofluor white preparations on sputum or BAL fluid. Smears from skin lesions show the spherules, which are readily seen on standard hematoxylin

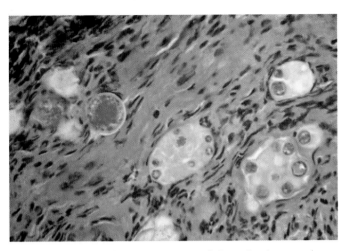

Fig. 31.9 Lung biopsy from the patient noted above showing several *Coccidioides* spherules containing endospores.

and eosin-stained tissue sections (Fig. 31.9). This is extremely helpful in establishing an early diagnosis before culture evidence is available.

Serology is helpful in the diagnosis of coccidioidomycosis, especially if a reference laboratory experienced in testing for coccidioidomycosis performs the tests.[34] Acute coccidioidomycosis can be diagnosed by finding IgM antibodies that are measured by an ID assay; IgG antibodies measured by CF appear later and persist longer. A positive CF antibody test for *Coccidioides* in CSF is diagnostic of coccidioidal meningitis.

MANAGEMENT

The Infectious Diseases Society of America has recently updated guidelines for the management of coccidioidomycosis.[35] Most of the recommendations are based on multicenter, nonrandomized, open-label trials and case series. There is one randomized, blinded comparative trial that showed an overall similar efficacy for fluconazole and itraconazole for the treatment of mild-to-moderate nonmeningeal coccidioidomycosis and a superior response with itraconazole for osteoarticular coccidioidomycosis.[36] There is little experience with the new azoles, but there are anecdotal reports of success with voriconazole[37] and several small series reporting on the use of posaconazole for patients with pulmonary and disseminated coccidioidomycosis.[38,39] The echinocandins appear to have no activity against *Coccidioides* species and should not be used to treat coccidioidomycosis.

Most patients with acute pulmonary coccidioidomycosis have a benign course and do not require therapy with an antifungal agent. However, patients who continue to have symptoms for 3–4 weeks with no improvement should be treated either with fluconazole, 400 mg daily, or itraconazole, 200 mg twice daily, for 3–6 months.[35] Patients who have underlying immunosuppression, those who are pregnant and patients who are African American or Filipino should be treated because of the high risk for dissemination in these groups.

Severe coccidioidal pneumonia should be treated initially with amphotericin B deoxycholate, 0.7–1.0 mg/kg daily, or a lipid formulation of amphotericin B, 3–5 mg/kg daily. After the patient has had a clinical response, therapy can be stepped down to itraconazole or fluconazole, given for 1–2 years.

Persisting thin-walled cavities can be observed, but surgical removal is reasonable for those that are adjacent to the pleura or that are noted to enlarge.[35] Chronic pulmonary coccidioidomycosis should be treated with itraconazole, 200 mg twice daily, or fluconazole, 400 mg daily, for 1–2 years. Persistent cavitary lesions that remain after adequate therapy should be evaluated for the feasibility of surgical removal.

Disseminated coccidioidomycosis is always treated. Severe infection is treated initially with amphotericin B deoxycholate, 0.7–1.0 mg/kg daily, or lipid formulation amphotericin B, 3–5 mg/kg daily.[32,35] After a clinical response is seen, therapy can be changed to an azole. Patients who have mild-to-moderate infection and are not immunosuppressed can be treated either with itraconazole, 200 mg twice daily, or fluconazole, 400 mg daily. The total treatment course is usually 1–2 years.

Coccidioidomycosis is the most difficult of the endemic mycoses to treat, and relapses are more common than with the other endemic mycoses. African Americans with disseminated coccidioidomycosis are at high risk for relapse, as are AIDS patients, and lifelong azole therapy is often required to prevent relapse.[32,35]

Paracoccidioidomycosis

MYCOLOGY AND EPIDEMIOLOGY

Paracoccidioidomycosis, or South American blastomycosis, is caused by *Paracoccidioides brasiliensis*, a thermally dimorphic fungus that in the environment is a mold and at 37°C, a yeast that has multiple buds. *Paracoccidioides brasiliensis* is endemic in humid areas in several countries in Central and South America; most cases are reported from Brazil.[40] The environmental niche is presumably soil and the disease is most often seen in middle-aged to elderly men who live in rural areas. Paracoccidioidomycosis is unique among the endemic fungi in that there is a strong sexual preference (male to female ratio 13:1). This imbalance can be partly explained by environmental exposure, but may also possibly be related to inhibitory effects of estrogens on the growth of the organism.[41,42]

PATHOGENESIS AND PATHOLOGY

Paracoccidioidomycosis is acquired by inhalation of conidia of *P. brasiliensis* into the alveoli where they are phagocytized by macrophages and convert to the yeast phase. It is likely that silent hematogenous dissemination occurs during most infections. Both neutrophils and cell-mediated immunity play a role in host defense although the latter is likely the more important. Patients who have deficient cellular immunity, especially those who have AIDS, have widespread disseminated infection and histopathologic examination reveals poorly formed granulomas.[43] Well-documented cases have occurred years after patients have left the endemic area, establishing reactivation of latent infection as a pathogenetic mechanism for this disease.[44] Many authors consider early childhood exposure the initial event and subsequent reactivation to be the cause of most cases of the chronic adult form of paracoccidioidomycosis.

CLINICAL FEATURES

Most cases of paracoccidioidomycosis occur in older men, are slowly progressive and are characterized as the chronic or adult form of the disease.[42] Pulmonary involvement is prominent; symptoms include fever, cough productive of purulent sputum, hemoptysis and dyspnea. Chest radiographs reveal nodular, interstitial or cavitary lesions that are more often seen in the middle and lower lung fields rather than the apices (Fig. 31.10). Progressive fibrosis is frequently seen, and is a major cause of death.[46] Most patients with this form of paracoccidioidomycosis have ulcerative or nodular mucous membrane lesions, primarily in the anterior nares and oral cavity, and papular, nodular or ulcerative skin lesions.

A less common form of paracoccidioidomycosis, the acute or juvenile form, also involves the lungs.[42] The hallmark of this form of paracoccidioidomycosis is widespread involvement of liver, spleen, lymph

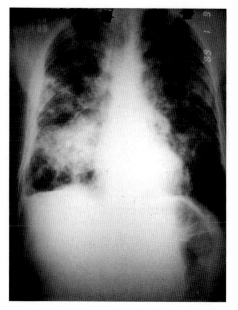

Fig. 31.10 Chest radiograph of an older man who had chronic paracoccidioidomycosis. Reproduced with permission from Kauffman.[45]

nodes, bone marrow, skin and lungs. Patients younger than 30 years of age, as well as immunosuppressed patients, especially those with AIDS, typically show this manifestation of paracoccidioidomycosis. The disease can progress rapidly and culminate with ARDS.

DIAGNOSIS

Growing *P. brasiliensis* from samples taken from infected sites, such as sputum, BAL fluid or lung tissue from those with pulmonary infection, establishes the diagnosis. The organism grows slowly in the mold phase at room temperature on Sabouraud's agar, and conversion to the yeast phase is necessary for firm identification.[40]

A presumptive diagnosis of paracoccidioidomycosis can be made if the organism can be visualized in smears with calcofluor white or KOH or in tissue sections stained with methenamine silver or PAS stains. The yeast cells are large (10–30 μm) and thick walled, and the budding daughter cells have a narrow base and remain attached around the circumference of the mother cell, creating a distinctive picture likened to a ship's steering wheel (Fig. 31.11).

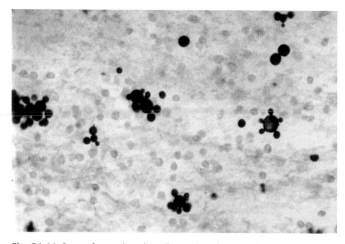

Fig. 31.11 Smear from a lymph node aspirate showing the typical captain's wheel configuration of budding daughter cells on the mother cell of *Paracoccidioides brasiliensis*. Reproduced with permission from Kauffman.[45]

Serology is less useful than culture techniques. Several different assays, including ID, counterimmunoelectrophoresis and CF, have been used, but none is commercially available and the sensitivity and specificity of each test has not been firmly established.

MANAGEMENT

Azole agents have assumed the primary role for the treatment of paracoccidioidomycosis. Itraconazole, 100 mg daily, for 6–12 months, is recommended most often.[47] Ketoconazole, 200–400 mg daily for 1 year, is still used because it is much less expensive than itraconazole; however, it is not as efficacious and has more adverse effects than itraconazole. Voriconazole appears to be efficacious and achieves superior levels in the CNS in those patients with disseminated infection.[48] Sulfonamides had been the treatment of choice used for years, but are less effective than the azoles and are used less frequently now.

For immunosuppressed patients who have widely disseminated *P. brasiliensis* infection, amphotericin B deoxycholate, 0.7–1.0 mg/kg daily is recommended;[42] there is little experience with lipid formulations of amphotericin B. After a clinical response is achieved, step-down therapy with itraconazole is appropriate. For patients who have HIV infection, lifelong suppressive therapy with itraconazole or trimethoprim–sulfamethoxazole is indicated.

Sporotrichosis

MYCOLOGY AND EPIDEMIOLOGY

Sporothrix schenckii is another dimorphic fungus that is a mold in the environment but assumes a yeast-like form at 37°C. Although found worldwide, most cases are reported from South America, North America and Japan. The organism can be found in soil, decaying wood and sphagnum moss, and outbreaks are described in association with exposure to contaminated moss or timbers.[49] Most cases are sporadic and related to exposure during activities, such as landscaping, farming, rose gardening or dirt biking. The organism can also be acquired from animals, with most cases being linked to cats that have the disease.[50,51]

PATHOGENESIS AND PATHOLOGY

In contrast to the other dimorphic fungi, *S. schenckii* causes disease in almost all cases by inoculation of the conidia through scratches or punctures from thorns, wood splinters or other sharp objects, rather than inhalation. It is likely that pulmonary sporotrichosis occurs when conidia are inhaled, but dissemination to lungs from skin lesions is also possible. The immune response to *S. schenckii* is a mixture of neutrophils and cell-mediated immunity. Patients with cellular immune deficiencies, such as AIDS, or those treated with immunosuppressive drugs are at risk of developing widespread dissemination, including pulmonary disease, when infected with *S. schenckii*.[52,53]

CLINICAL FEATURES

Sporotrichosis is primarily a localized lymphocutaneous infection and is discussed in depth elsewhere. Pulmonary sporotrichosis is rare and almost always occurs in patients with underlying chronic obstructive pulmonary disease and alcoholism.[49,54] The clinical picture is similar to tuberculosis or chronic cavitary histoplasmosis. Fever, night sweats, fatigue, cough with purulent sputum, hemoptysis and increasing dyspnea are noted in most patients. Chest radiographs show apical infiltrates with thick-walled cavities (Fig. 31.12). Even more uncommon,

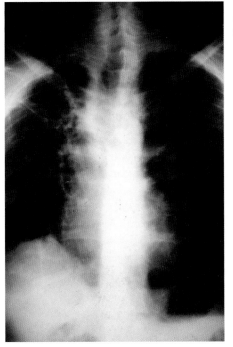

Fig. 31.12 Chronic cavitary pulmonary sporotrichosis in a 54-year-old man who had emphysema.

disseminated sporotrichosis in markedly immunosuppressed patients can have diffuse pulmonary infiltrates associated with dyspnea and hypoxemia.[53]

DIAGNOSIS

The diagnosis of sporotrichosis is based on growth of the organism from samples taken from involved tissues. In the case of pulmonary sporotrichosis, sputum, BAL fluid and lung tissue are appropriate samples for culture. The organism grows in days to weeks on Sabouraud's agar at room temperature as a mold with conidia arranged in a distinctive bouquet pattern on thin hyphae. Seeing this allows for presumptive identification, but definitive identification requires conversion to the yeast phase at 35–37°C. The yeasts are rarely seen in sputum or BAL fluid. They can be found in tissue using methenamine silver or PAS stains, but are often difficult to visualize.

If a patient has cutaneous lesions in addition to pulmonary disease, sampling a skin lesion is a simple way in which to make the diagnosis. However, as pulmonary sporotrichosis is sufficiently rare that one must be sure that the pulmonary infiltrate is not due to another etiology, most patients have sputum or BAL fluid cultures performed as well.

Serology has not proved useful and is currently not available.

MANAGEMENT

The Infectious Diseases Society of America has recently updated guidelines for the management of sporotrichosis.[55] Recommendations are based mostly on case series from individual institutions and a few multicenter, nonrandomized, open-label treatment trials. None of these reports specifically addresses the issue of pulmonary sporotrichosis.

Most patients with pulmonary sporotrichosis should be treated initially with amphotericin B, either a lipid formulation, 3–5 mg/kg daily, or amphotericin B deoxycholate, 0.7–1.0 mg/kg daily.[56] After improvement is noted, step-down therapy to itraconazole, 200 mg twice daily, for at least 1 year is recommended. If the patient is not seriously ill, itraconazole at the dosage and length of treatment noted above is recommended.[55] If surgical removal of the area infected is feasible, this should be carried out. Unfortunately, most patients have severe underlying pulmonary disease and surgery is not an option.

Fluconazole failure rates for pulmonary sporotrichosis are high, voriconazole has no activity and should not be used, and posaconazole, although active *in vitro*, has not been used to treat sporotrichosis. Drugs that are used for lymphocutaneous sporotrichosis, such as potassium iodide and terbinafine, are ineffective and should not be used for pulmonary sporotrichosis.

Penicilliosis

MYCOLOGY AND EPIDEMIOLOGY

Penicillium marneffei is a mold in the environment and a yeast in the tissues at 37°C. The yeast divides by septation and not budding in contrast to most other dimorphic fungi. *Penicillium marneffei* is endemic in rural areas in most south-eastern Asian countries, including Thailand, Vietnam, Laos and southern China. The environmental niche is presumably soil. Bamboo rats in these same areas are also frequently infected, but there is no evidence of transmission from rats to humans.[56]

PATHOGENESIS AND PATHOLOGY

Penicillium marneffei is presumed to cause infection after the conidia are inhaled into the alveoli. Pulmonary manifestations are usually silent and hematogenous dissemination is the rule. The most important host defense against this organism is cellular immunity. Healthy individuals rarely have symptoms, but those who have deficient cellular immunity, especially persons with AIDS, develop disseminated infection.[57] The pathologic features include both neutrophilic infiltration and granuloma formation.

CLINICAL FEATURES

Pulmonary manifestations of infection with *P. marneffei* are almost entirely seen in patients who have widespread disseminated infection. Fever, weight loss, lymphadenopathy, hepatosplenomegaly and skin lesions are common presenting symptoms. Pulmonary symptoms other than dyspnea are uncommon.[57,58] The chest radiograph usually shows diffuse infiltrates.

DIAGNOSIS

The diagnosis of penicilliosis is established by growing the organism from a tissue sample or body fluids. Most patients will have a biopsy taken from a skin lesion, a lymph node or bone marrow, and not samples from the respiratory tract. The organism grows as a mold at room temperature after a few weeks; production of red pigment on Sabouraud's agar allows a presumptive diagnosis before conversion to the yeast phase is accomplished to confirm identification.

Smears of body fluids or from a bone marrow aspirate can establish an early diagnosis if the characteristic yeast form of *P. marneffei* is identified. The yeasts are oval to sausage-shaped and have a central septum, unlike other small yeasts, such as *H. capsulatum*.

MANAGEMENT

Penicillium marneffei is susceptible to amphotericin B, 5-flucytosine, ketoconazole and itraconazole. Most studies have been performed in patients with AIDS. Both amphotericin B and itraconazole have been shown to be effective.[59] Amphotericin B is recommended for those patients who have severe illness; following a clinical response, step-down therapy with itraconazole, 200 mg twice daily, is recommended. For patients who have mild-to-moderate illness, itraconazole, 200 mg twice daily, is recommended. Long-term suppressive therapy with itraconazole is required to prevent relapse, and prophylaxis with itraconazole may also be useful in highly endemic areas.[60,61]

REFERENCES

References for this chapter can be found online at http://www.expertconsult.com

Investigation of pleural discharge/fluid

INTRODUCTION

The presence of pleural fluid, or parapneumonic effusion (PPE), is a common finding during bacterial pneumonia, occurring in 20–57% of cases. PPE usually consists of a small amount of fluid which disappears spontaneously with antimicrobial therapy. In 5–10% of patients, presenting late in the course of pneumonia or receiving inadequate antimicrobial therapy, the persistent eruption of bacteria into the pleural space leads to complicated PPE including thoracic empyema. The timing and indications for investigation of pleural fluid are crucial in the management of PPE in order to decrease the morbidity and mortality associated with the development of these complications.

PATHOGENESIS

Pleural effusion can be separated into three stages on the basis of the natural course of the disease.

1. Stage 1 (uncomplicated PPE) corresponds to an increase in production of interstitial lung fluid and capillary leakage which exceeds the pleural resorption capacity. At this stage, pleural fluid contains protein and neutrophils and is free from bacteria. This exudate usually resolves with pneumonia treatment and does not lead to pleural sequelae.
2. Stage 2 (complicated PPE) is related to the persistence of bacterial invasion within the pleural space and involves fibrinous adhesions. Neutrophil recruitment and lysis in the pleural space increases the lactate dehydrogenase (LDH) concentration and promotes the anaerobic metabolism of glucose with local acidosis.
3. Stage 3 corresponds to empyema and is defined by the presence of pus in the pleural fluid. Bacteria may be observed on a Gram stain but a positive culture is not required for diagnosis. Indeed, cultures are often negative due to inappropriate bacterial culture conditions, prior exposure to antibiotics or the presence of loculation.

Persistent inflammation of visceral pleura leads to fibrosis and lung entrapment requiring appropriate pleural drainage in all cases.

MICROBIOLOGY

All pneumonia-related pathogens can induce PPE, including typical bacteria, atypical bacteria and viruses. However, *Streptococcus* spp., *Staphylococcus* spp., Gram-negative bacilli and anaerobes are more likely to be associated with pleural effusion. The causative pathogens of empyema are aerobes in about 40% of cases, anaerobes in up to 30% and multiple organisms in around 30%.

PRESENTATION

Patients presenting with pleural effusion due to pneumonia do not differ clinically from those presenting without PPE. Seemingly, patients do not differ clinically according to the stage of pleural disease (complicated or not). Physical signs include unspecific fever, cough, shortness of breath, chest pain, chills and purulent sputum. Recrudescence or persistence of the symptoms of pneumonia should evoke the presence of empyema.

Chest radiography can suggest the presence of PPE. Ultrasonography is used to confirm and estimate the amount of liquid in the pleural space. It can also detect standing effusion or loculation, and be used for guided thoracocentesis. In the case of complicated pleural effusion, a thoracic CT scan with contrast is recommended to check for the presence of indirect signs of empyema, such as thickening of the parietal pleura, loculated pleural fluid and small air bubbles within the collection. It can be used to detect any underlying lung abnormalities (Fig. PP10.1).

PLEURAL FLUID ANALYSIS

Pleural fluid analysis should be performed early in the course of pneumonia, ideally before starting antimicrobial therapy, when pleural effusion is non-minimal (>10 mm on lateral decubitus), loculated or non-free-flowing. A specimen of at least 30 ml of pleural fluid should be collected. Appearance, biochemical (pH, LDH, glucose and protein), bacteriologic (Gram stain and culture) and cellular count analyses should be performed systematically (Table PP10.1). Pleural effusion for pH measurement should be collected using a heparinized syringe and pH measured with a blood gas analyzer.

To improve the yield of bacterial cultures, pleural fluid should be inoculated directly into bottle culture medium for aerobic and anaerobic bacteria, and on demand for mycobacteria, fungi and viruses. A cytologist should also examine the morphology and type of pleural cells in order to detect malignant effusion.

Depending on the appearance, pH, glucose, LDH and bacteriologic findings, the pleural effusion can be classified into three stages as summarized in Table PP10.1.

PROCEDURES FOR PLEURAL INVESTIGATION

Thoracocentesis is the simplest procedure to collect pleural fluid. It should be performed with patients sitting comfortably with their arms held straight upwards. The procedure should be explained to the patient and informed consent obtained. Sterile conditions should be maintained throughout the procedure.

Nosocomial pneumonia complicated by left lung abscess and empyema in an immunocompromised patient

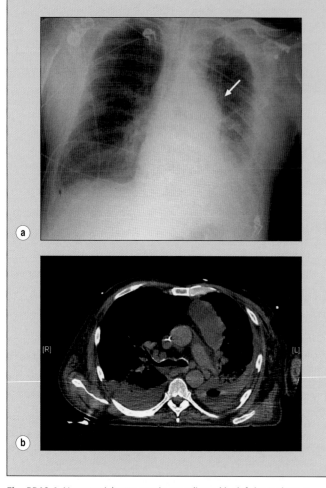

Fig. PP10.1 Nosocomial pneumonia complicated by left lung abscess and empyema in an immunocompromised patient. (a) Chest radiograph. (b) CT scan. White arrow indicates empyema.

The site of puncture is localized by percussion or ultrasonography and usually corresponds to the intersection between the hemithorax line and the sixth or seventh intercostal space. Local anesthesia should be administered to the upper side of the lower rib of the intercostal space until aspiration of pleural fluid into the syringe.

Insertion of a chest tube (from 16F to 28F) is recommended when a complicated PPE is diagnosed. Patients may be supine or semirecumbent. The ipsilateral arm should be placed behind the head. The safe zone for puncture corresponds to the intersection between the mammary and midaxillary line at the fourth to fifth intercostal space. The chest tube is introduced within the pleural space and directed towards the lower lobes. Aspiration of pleural fluid with a closed suction system is recommended at a depression range from -30 to $-100\,cmH_2O$. Complications of chest tube insertion include pain, pneumothorax, hemorrhage and subcutaneous emphysema.

Small-bore catheters (from 8F to 16F) are more comfortable for patients and offer fewer complications. They should be placed using ultrasound or CT for the drainage of small or multiloculated effusion but they have also been used successfully for the management of empyema. These procedures should not be performed in patients presenting with coagulation abnormalities (for further details, see Dev *et al.* and Thomsen *et al.* in Further reading).

MANAGEMENT OF PLEURAL EFFUSION

Management of PPE is mainly guided by the results of pleural fluid analyses, which should be performed without delay (Fig. PP10.2). Delivering early and appropriate antimicrobial therapy will largely prevent the development of PPE or avoid the progression of uncomplicated to complicated PPE. In patients who already have complicated PPE, antibiotics alone are not sufficient to eradicate the pleural sepsis and pleural drainage is required for recovery. The risks for poor outcome situations requiring pleural drainage have been addressed by the American College of Chest Physicians. These include radiographic findings of a large effusion (>50% of hemithorax), a loculated effusion, an air–fluid level and pleural thickening. The characteristics of the pleural fluid also guide the need for drainage in the presence of pus or when one of the criteria for complicated PPE is present.

Pleural space drainage can be performed by repeat thoracocentesis, standard chest tube or small-bore catheter. Drainage failure may be related to misplacement or malfunction of the chest tube and loculation. In the setting of inappropriate pleural drainage, persistent pleural sep-

Table PP10.1 Pleural fluid analyses at different stages of parapneumonic effusion

Characteristics	Uncomplicated parapneumonic effusion	Complicated parapneumonic effusion	Empyema
Appearance	Slightly turbid	Cloudy	Pus
pH	≥7.2	<7.2	NA
Glucose, g/l	>0.6	<0.4	NA
LDH, IU/l	<700	>1000	NA
Ratio pleural:serum LDH	>0.6	>0.6	NA
Ratio pleural:serum protein	>0.5	>0.5	NA
PMN leukocyte count, cells/µl	<15 000	>25 000	NA
Gram stain and culture	Negative	May be positive	May be positive

LDH, lactate dehydrogenase; NA, not applicable; PMN, polymorphonuclear.

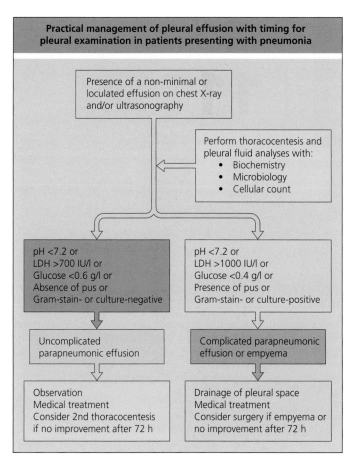

Practical management of pleural effusion with timing for pleural examination in patients presenting with pneumonia

Presence of a non-minimal or loculated effusion on chest X-ray and/or ultrasonography

Perform thoracocentesis and pleural fluid analyses with:
- Biochemistry
- Microbiology
- Cellular count

pH <7.2 or
LDH >700 IU/l or
Glucose <0.6 g/l or
Absence of pus or
Gram-stain- or culture-negative

pH <7.2 or
LDH >1000 IU/l or
Glucose <0.4 g/l or
Presence of pus or
Gram-stain- or culture-positive

Uncomplicated parapneumonic effusion

Complicated parapneumonic effusion or empyema

Observation
Medical treatment
Consider 2nd thoracocentesis if no improvement after 72 h

Drainage of pleural space
Medical treatment
Consider surgery if empyema or no improvement after 72 h

Fig. PP10.2 Practical management of pleural effusion with timing for pleural examination in patients presenting with pneumonia.

sis, multiple loculations or empyema, surgical options should be considered promptly. These include thoracoscopy, video-assisted thoracic surgery (VATS) and thoracotomy. VATS has been reported to improve the recovery rate in complicated PPE up to 86%. If VATS is unable to provide adequate pleural investigation, thoracotomy will be required.

Decortication is the optimal treatment, but this requires major surgery and cannot be performed in the most debilitated patients. It consists of stripping the visceral pleura, allowing the lung to fully expand into the parietal pleura. It is indicated in uncontrolled pleural sepsis or sometimes in restrictive ventilatory failure.

CONCLUSION

All patients with pneumonia should be screened to detect the presence of pleural effusion. If pleural effusion is more than minimal or loculated, thoracocentesis should be performed without delay. Examination of pleural fluid guides the management of PPE between observation, pleural drainage and surgery. It can discriminate uncomplicated from complicated PPE, providing information on the stage of the disease and the expected outcome. In nonpurulent effusion with pH <7.2, pleural drainage is recommended using either a small-bore catheter or a chest tube. Surgical options, starting with VATS, should be proposed in the presence of empyema or in ineffective pleural drainage. Decortication is a more invasive procedure which should only be performed in patients with uncontrolled pleural sepsis or unexpandable lung disease.

FURTHER READING

Further reading for this chapter can be found online at http://www.expertconsult.com

Managing postoperative fever

INTRODUCTION

Thermoregulation physiologists divide the body into core (deep chest and abdomen, central nervous system) and peripheral (arms, legs) thermal compartments. The core temperature is usually 2–4°C warmer than the peripheral compartments. Body temperature is tightly regulated by a complex system involving parallel positive- and negative-feedback loops. The system is located in nearly every part of the autonomic nervous system. Normal core temperatures typically range from 97.7°F to 98.6°F (36.5–37°C). Values less than 96.8°F (36°C) or greater than 100.4°F (38°C) are related to loss of control or a thermal environment so extreme that it overcomes thermoregulation defenses. In healthy individuals, the temperature varies by 0.5–1.0°C, according to circadian rhythm and menstrual cycle. In nursing home residents, the oldest are the coldest and fail to demonstrate a diurnal rise in body temperature.

DEFINITION

Fever is a rise of the normal core temperature exceeding the normal daily variation. The guidelines of the Society of Critical Care Medicine and the Infectious Diseases Society of America define arbitrary fever as a temperature of or above 100.9°F (38.3°C).[1] In neutropenic patients, fever is defined as a single oral temperature above 100.9°F (38.3°C) in the absence of an obvious environmental cause, or a temperature elevation above 100.4°F (38°C) for longer than 1 hour.

BRIEF PATHOPHYSIOLOGY

Fever is a normal adaptation in response to a pyrogenic stimulus resulting in the generation of cytokines and prostaglandins. Pyrogenic cytokines are released into the circulation by systemic mononuclear phagocytes that are activated by exogenous inflammatory agents. They are transported to the preoptic anterior hypothalamic area of the brain, where they act through prostaglandin E_2 activation.

In murine models of peritonitis, increasing core temperature from basal to febrile levels improves survival by accelerating pathogen clearance.[2] More conflicting results are found in models of pneumonia. The febrile response fails to improve survival despite affecting a profound reduction in pulmonary bacterial burden. Elsewhere, hyperthermia protects against pulmonary injury. Hence, antipyretic treatment should be administered in only a few situations where fever is irrefutably detrimental.

MEASURING BODY TEMPERATURE

Body temperature should be measured using the most accurate and reliable methods based on the clinical circumstances of the patient. The American College of Critical Care Medicine and the Infectious Diseases Society of America have provided guidelines for selecting the best sites and technologies for temperature measurement (Table PP11.1).[1]

Table PP11.1 Site and technology of temperature measurement

Order of sites accuracy	Limitations
Pulmonary artery thermistors	Pulmonary artery catheters not available
Urinary bladder thermistors	Costly Require urinary bladder catheter Should not prolong urinary bladder catheterization
Esophageal probe	Difficult placement Uncomfortable Risk of esophageal perforation
Rectal probe	Limitation due to patient position Spreading enteric pathogens Risk of trauma, perforation Perceived as unpleasant and intrusive
Oral probe	Requires alert and co-operative patients Local damage Should be avoided in neutropenic patients
Infrared ear thermometry	Conflicting results on accuracy Not accurate if auditory canal inflamed, tympanic membrane inflamed, external canal obstructed
Temporal artery thermometer	Impact of environmental temperature and sweating
Axillary thermometer	Lack of agreement with standard measurements
Chemical dot	Lack of agreement with standard measurements

ANESTHESIA- AND SURGERY-RELATED TEMPERATURE VARIATIONS

During anesthesia, patients are unable to activate behavioral responses.[3] Warm-response thresholds are elevated slightly, whereas cold-response thresholds are reduced. Manifestation of intraoperative fever is impaired by volatile anesthetics and muscle relaxants. Alfentanil reduces the febrile response to pyrogenic cytokines.[2]

The surgical procedure also interferes with postoperative fever incidence. Laparoscopic techniques have been associated with reduced incidences of postoperative fever, as compared with open techniques. Antibiotic prophylaxis and painkiller use are associated with reduced incidences of postoperative fever.

POSTOPERATIVE FEVER: INCIDENCE AND IMPACT

The incidence of postoperative fever ranges from 14% to 91%. Febrile patients are older, sicker, more likely to have undergone emergency surgery, more likely to develop organ dysfunction and more likely to die. On the first postoperative day after total hip arthroplasty, 44% of the patients are febrile. The number of febrile patients progressively decreases until the fifth postoperative day. The magnitude of postoperative fever is a determinant of mortality.

Fever is a nonspecific acute-phase response. An infectious cause is present in 40–60% of postoperative fevers. Fevers higher than 104.8°F (41°C) are more likely a result of noninfectious causes. Procalcitonin has been proposed to differentiate sepsis from other noninfectious causes of inflammation. Systematic reviews do not support the widespread use of the procalcitonin test in critical care settings.[4] One should note that a substantial proportion of infected patients may be euthermic or hypothermic, such as elderly patients, those with open abdominal wounds, patients with large burns, patients receiving extracorporeal membrane oxygenation or continuous renal replacement, and patients with congestive heart failure, end-stage liver disease or chronic renal failure.

STRATEGY FOR PATIENTS WITH POSTOPERATIVE FEVER

Fever occurring within two postoperative days does not need investigation beyond clinical assessment.[5] Surgical trauma is responsible for more than 70% of early postoperative fever episodes. Elsewhere, atelectasis (Fig. PP11.1) and medications are identified as causes of postoperative fever. β-lactam antibiotics, diphenylhydantoin and antiarrhythmics are commonly thought to induce fever in almost 10% of hospitalized patients. Other causes – including anesthetic drug effect on thermoregulation, transfusion of blood products, acalculous cholecystitis, local hematomas, deep venous thrombosis, pulmonary embolism, subarachnoid hemorrhage, fat embolism, hyperthyroidism and acute adrenal insufficiency (Fig. PP11.2) – can be responsible for postoperative fever. Thus, febrile patients should not be treated with antibiotics within two postoperative days. However, clinicians have to rule out pulmonary aspiration, myonecrosis and cellulitis. As suggested above, antipyretics should only be used if benefits exceed risks.

New or persistent fever occurring more than 72 hours after surgery suggests an infectious process. A systematic diagnostic approach helps to identify the potential source of infection (Fig. PP11.3).[5] Pneumonia is often suspected but remains diagnosed in less than 1% of postoperative patients. Clinical features, chest radiography showing

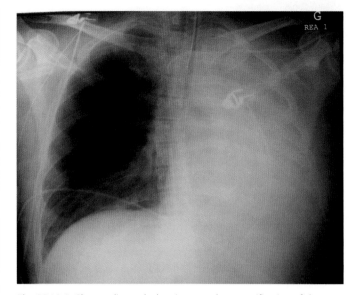

Fig. PP11.1 Chest radiograph showing complete opacification of the left hemithorax in a patient with postoperative fever. This suggests airway obstruction with whole-lung atelectasis. However, at first glance, ventilator-associated pneumonia cannot be ruled out. Fiberoptic examination will confirm this diagnosis. Another possible source is central line infection.

new or progressive infiltrate, and blood and sputum cultures are the commonest components in diagnostic assessment (see Fig. PP11.1). Antibiotic therapy should be initiated early with a broad-spectrum β-lactam antibiotic. A glycopeptide can be added if methicillin-resistant *Staphylococcus aureus* is suspected.

Urine cultures are positive in up to 30% of postoperative patients with a urinary bladder catheter *in situ*. However, as positive urine cultures are associated with sepsis in only 10% of patients, antibiotics should be used only after other causes of fever are ruled out. Wound infection is the second most common hospital-acquired infection. Subcutaneous abscesses are diagnosed by the presence of erythema, pus and tenderness of the surgical incision. Fascia and muscle can be involved. CT scan is useful in cases of deep infection (Fig. PP11.4). Deeper infections need early resuscitation, surgical debridement and antimicrobial therapy.

Catheter-related sepsis is another common cause of postoperative fever. The risk depends above all on the length of time since insertion. Central venous catheters inserted through the femoral vein are associated with a higher risk of infection than those inserted through the subclavian vein. Examination of catheter sites, blood cultures through the catheter and from peripheral venepuncture sites, and culture of suspected catheters lead to diagnosis. Removal of implanted sites should be discussed depending on the virulence of bacteria. Sinusitis, *Clostridium difficile* colitis, septic thrombophlebitis and fungal infection related to prolonged antibiotic use are less common causes of postoperative fever.

CONCLUSION

Fever is common after surgery and noninfectious causes are responsible for most episodes. Routine workup for early postoperative fever of low clinical yield adds cost. A rational approach is required for new or persistent fever arising more than 3 days after surgery. Among surgical patients with sepsis, fever-related infection seems protective, whereas excessive inflammatory response unrelated to infection predicts poor outcome.

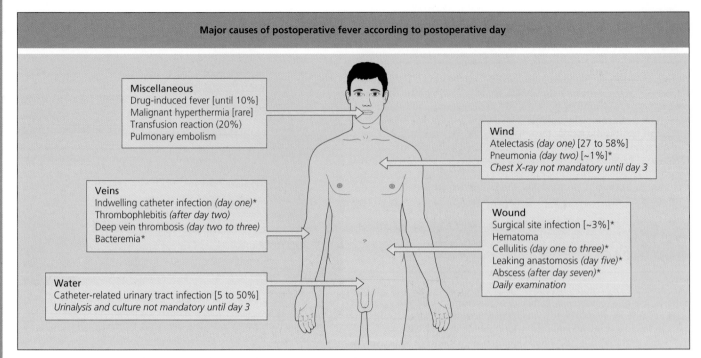

Fig. PP11.2 Major causes of postoperative fever according to postoperative day.

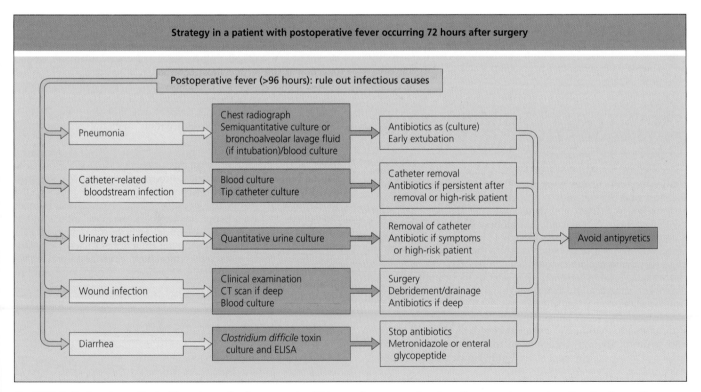

Fig. PP11.3 Strategy in a patient with postoperative fever occurring 72 hours after surgery. A systematic approach serves to rationalize the routine workups.

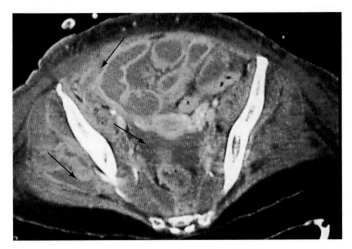

Fig. PP11.4 Persistent postoperative fever after gallbladder surgery. CT scan of the pelvic area shows several collections (arrows) requiring surgical drainage and prolonged antimicrobial therapy.

REFERENCES

References for this chapter can be found online at http://www.expertconsult.com

Use of antibiotics in common respiratory infections

INTRODUCTION

Respiratory infections are the most common infections encountered. Although acute bronchitis usually does not require antibiotics, antibiotics are essential in the management of community-acquired pneumonia (CAP). Some patients with acute exacerbation of chronic obstructive pulmonary disease (COPD) might benefit from antibiotics. It is essential to make a correct diagnosis before prescribing antibiotics. Clinical distinction between these three syndromes is sometimes difficult and might require radiologic examination.

TREATMENT OF ACUTE BRONCHITIS

Acute bronchitis is one of the most common causes of antibiotic abuse, although it is generally caused by a virus. Most reports show that more than 70% of patients with acute bronchitis who seek care are given antibiotics. This has resulted in campaigns in most countries to dissuade physicians from this practice through the use of guidelines. In fact, multiple studies show that patients with acute bronchitis do not benefit from antibiotics.

TREATMENT OF ACUTE EXACERBATIONS OF CHRONIC OBSTRUCTIVE PULMONARY DISEASE

It is estimated that 50–60% of exacerbations of chronic obstructive pulmonary disease (COPD) are due to respiratory infections. Most exacerbations caused by respiratory infections are thought to be viral, rather than bacterial. *Haemophilus influenzae, Moraxella catarrhalis* and *Streptococcus pneumoniae* are the bacteria most frequently isolated during exacerbations of COPD. Even if bacteria are identified, it is uncertain whether they actually caused the exacerbation or whether they were present as part of the flora before the exacerbation. Patients who can clearly benefit from antibiotics are those with severe exacerbations; there is no evidence of benefit in patients with mild or moderate disease.

The optimal antibiotic regimen for the treatment of exacerbations of COPD has not been determined. The antibiotic chosen should target *H. influenzae, M. catarrhalis* and *S. pneumoniae*, while taking into account local patterns of antibiotic resistance. The recommended first-line agents (amoxicillin, trimethoprim–sulfamethoxazole, doxycycline) now have limited *in-vitro* activity against these pathogens. These days, broad-spectrum agents such as amoxicillin–clavulanate, azithromycin, telithromycin, cephalosporins, macrolides and fluoroquinolones are preferred (Table PP12.1).

TREATMENT OF COMMUNITY-ACQUIRED PNEUMONIA

Community-acquired pneumonia (CAP) is a common and serious illness with considerable mortality and morbidity. CAP is of particular concern for elderly patients with significant co-morbidities, and risk factors for drug resistance (see below) need to be sought. In fact, a new syndrome – health-care associated pneumonia (HCAP) – has recently emerged and has been shown to affect a significant number of patients. Treatment of HCAP is as for nosocomial pneumonia.

Indications for hospitalization

Determination as to whether a patient with CAP can safely be treated as an outpatient or requires hospitalization is essential before selecting an antibiotic regimen. Severity of illness scores have been developed to assist physicians in the decision of site of care. The Pneumonia Severity Index (PSI, Table PP12.2) and the CURB-65 are the two best evaluated scores. The PSI is better studied and evaluated, but requires a more complicated assessment. The CURB-65 uses five prognostic values:
- Confusion;
- Urea greater than 7 mmol/l (blood urea nitrogen >20 mg/dl);
- Respiratory rate of 30 breaths per minute or greater;
- Blood pressure less than 90 mmHg systolic or diastolic blood pressure 60 mmHg or less;
- age **65** or older.

Patients with PSI <3 and CURB-65 <2 should be treated as outpatients.

Principles of antimicrobial therapy

The selection of antibiotics for empiric therapy is based upon a number of factors, including the most likely pathogens, clinical trials proving efficacy, risk factors for antimicrobial resistance, and medical co-morbidities that can influence the likelihood of a specific pathogen and may be a risk for clinical failure.

Drug resistance

Risk factors for infection with multidrug-resistant (MDR) pathogens include:
- treatment with intravenous antibiotics within the preceding 90 days;
- current hospitalization of >5 days;
- admission from a health-care-related facility (e.g. long-term care facility, dialysis unit);
- hospitalization for 2 days or more in the preceding 90 days;

Table PP12.1 Frequently used antibiotics for common respiratory infections

Antibiotic	Adults ≥60 kg	Adults <60 kg	Duration in CAP
Erythromycin (iv)	1 g q6–8h	30–40 mg/kg q24h in four equally divided doses (max 4 g)	Until afebrile for 2–3 days, minimum 5 days
Erythromycin (po)	500 mg q6h	30–40 mg/kg q24h in four equally divided doses (max 4 g)	Until afebrile for 2–3 days, minimum 5 days
Azithromycin (po)	500 mg day 1, then 250 mg q24h	5 mg/kg q24h (max 500 mg q24h)	5 days
Azithromycin (iv)	500 mg q24h	5 mg/kg q24h (max 500 mg q24h)	Until afebrile for 2–3 days, minimum 5 days
Clarithromycin (po)	500 mg q12h	7.5 mg/kg q12h (max 1 g q24h)	Until afebrile for 2–3 days, minimum 5 days
Telithromycin (po)	800 mg q24h	800 mg q24h	Until afebrile for 2–3 days, minimum 5 days
Doxycycline (po)	100 mg q12h	4 mg/kg q24h (max 200 mg) in two equally divided doses	7–10 days
Amoxicillin (iv/po)	1 g q8h	100 mg/kg q24h in three equally divided doses	Until afebrile for 2–3 days, minimum 5 days
Ampicillin–sulbactam (im/iv)	2 g ampicillin + 1 g sulbactam q6h	200 mg ampicillin/100 mg sulbactam/kg q24h in four divided doses (max 4 g sulbactam)	Until afebrile for 2–3 days, minimum 5 days
Amoxicillin–clavulanate (iv/po)	3–4 g q24h in two to four equally divided doses	80 mg/kg q24h in three equally divided doses (max 4 g/j)	Until afebrile for 2–3 days, minimum 5 days
Ceftriaxone (iv/im)	2 g q24h	50–75 mg/kg q24h (max 4 g q24h)	Until afebrile for 2–3 days, minimum 5 days
Cefotaxime (iv)	2 g iv q8h	150–200 mg/kg q24h in three or four equally divided doses (max 8–10 g q24h)	Until afebrile for 2–3 days, minimum 5 days
Gemifloxacin (po)	320 mg q24h	320 mg q24h	Until afebrile for 2–3 days, minimum 5 days
Levofloxacin (iv/po)	750 mg q24h	750 mg q24h	Until afebrile for 2–3 days, minimum 5 days
Moxifloxacin (iv/po)	400 mg q24h	400 mg q24h	Until afebrile for 2–3 days, minimum 5 days
Gatifloxacine (iv/po)	400 mg q24h	400 mg q24h	Until afebrile for 2–3 days, minimum 5 days

CAP: community-acquired pneumonia; iv, intravenous; po, per os.

- home infusion therapy;
- chronic dialysis;
- home wound care;
- family member with an MDR pathogen;
- immunosuppressive disease and/or therapy.

If one of these risk factors exists, pneumonia is no longer considered as community acquired, but as HCAP. Empiric treatment should be directed against MDR pathogens.

Treatment regimens for outpatients

No co-morbidities or recent antibiotic use

Two different approaches are used (Table PP12.3). The North American approach is to use first-line antibiotics that provide coverage for *S. pneumoniae* plus atypical pathogens. The macrolides, which are effective against atypical pathogens, are therefore recommended in the absence of significant risk factors for macrolide-resistant *S. pneumoniae* (e.g. recent use of macrolides). Erythromycin is not

recommended due to its frequent side-effects. In Europe, due to the high level of resistance of *S. pneumoniae* to macrolides, amoxicillin and telithromycin are the recommended first-line empiric antibiotics. In fact, treatment failures have been demonstrated with the use of macrolides for macrolide-resistant *S. pneumoniae*. Despite *in-vitro* resistance, penicillin-resistant *S. pneumoniae* may respond to higher-dose β-lactams.

Benefit of initial coverage of atypical pathogens in outpatients is currently unclear. The use of fluoroquinolones in ambulatory CAP is discouraged since there is concern that widespread use of fluoroquinolones may promote fluoroquinolone resistance among bacteria. Concern has been expressed regarding liver toxicity of telithromycin, thus limiting its use.

Co-morbidities or recent antibiotic use

Where there are significant co-morbidities (e.g. chronic obstructive pulmonary disease, liver or renal disease, cancer, diabetes, chronic heart disease, alcoholism, immunosuppression) and/or use of antibiotics

Table PP12.2 Calculation of the Pneumonia Severity Index (PSI)

Factor	PSI score
Patient age	Age in years (male) or age −10 (female)
Nursing home resident	+10
Coexisting illnesses	
Neoplastic disease	+30
Liver disease	+20
Congestive cardiac failure	+10
Cerebrovascular disease	+10
Renal disease	+10
Signs on examination	
Altered mental state	+20
Respiratory rate ≥30 per minute	+20
Systolic blood pressure <90 mmHg	+20
Temperature ≤35°C or ≥40°C	+15
Pulse rate ≥125 bpm	+10
Results of investigations	
Arterial pH <7.35	+30
Serum urea level ≥11 mmol/l	+20
Serum sodium level <130 mmol/	+10
Serum glucose level ≥14 mmol/IL	+10
Hematocrit <30%	+10
Po_2 <60 mmHg or O_2 saturation <90%	+10
Pleural effusion	+10

Mortality within 30 days according to PSI risk class

Risk class	Score	Mortality (%)
I	Score not calculated	0.1
II	≤70	0.6
III	71–90	0.9
IV	91–130	9.3
V	>130	27.0

Table PP12.3 First- and second-line antibiotics for common respiratory infections

Syndrome	First-line antibiotics	Second-line antibiotics
Acute bronchitis	No antibiotics	
Community-acquired pneumonia		
Non-severe pneumonia, no co-morbidities (outpatient, PSI 1–2)	USA: macrolide Europe: amoxicillin or telithromycin	Respiratory fluoroquinolones
Moderately severe pneumonia (PSI 3) or significant co-morbidities	Amoxicillin–clavulanate or third-generation cephalosporin, plus macrolide	Respiratory fluoroquinolones
Severe pneumonia (PSI 4–5)	Third-generation cephalosporin, plus macrolide or respiratory fluoroquinolone	Antipseudomonal antibiotics if risk factors for *Pseudomonas aeruginosa* (bronchiectasis or chronic obstructive pulmonary disease and frequent antimicrobial or corticosteroid use), plus vancomycin or linezolid if risk factors for methicillin-resistant *Staphylococcus aureus* (prior influenza or Gram stain of respiratory secretions suggesting *S. aureus*)

PSI, Pneumonia Severity Index.

against infection with more resistant pathogens, the preferred regimens are combination therapy with a β-lactam effective against *S. pneumoniae* or a third-generation cephalosporin plus a macrolide or doxycycline; an alternative is a respiratory fluoroquinolone.

Treatment regimens for hospitalized patients

Not in the ICU

Combination therapy with a third-generation cephalosporin plus a macrolide is recommended; an alternative is a respiratory fluoroquinolone.

In the ICU

Intravenous combination therapy with a third-generation cephalosporin plus either a macrolide or a respiratory fluoroquinolone is recommended. In patients who may be infected with *Pseudomonas aeruginosa* (particularly those with bronchiectasis or COPD and frequent antimicrobial or corticosteroid use), therapy should include agents effective against *P. aeruginosa*, *S. pneumoniae* and *Legionella* spp. For severely ill patients, empiric treatment should include vancomycin or linezolid if there are risk factors for methicillin-resistant *Staphylococcus aureus* infection (e.g. recent influenza-like illness or a Gram stain of respiratory secretions suggesting *S. aureus*).

Health-care associated pneumonia

HCAP should be treated as for nosocomial pneumonia with broad-spectrum antibiotics directed against potential MDR pathogens, including *P. aeruginosa*.

Delay in administering the first dose of antibiotics has been associated with higher mortality and longer length of hospital stay. The first dose of antibiotics for the hospitalized patient should be administered within 6 hours of admission. Antibiotics should be modified when results of diagnostic studies indicate a specific pathogen. Intravenous therapy should be switched to oral therapy when patients are hemodynamically stable, demonstrate some clinical improvement and are able to take oral medication. Antibiotic therapy should be modified based on microbiologic results.

The recommended duration of therapy in CAP is 48–72 hours after clinical improvement (defined as no more fever) with a minimum of 5 days. This should be extended if infection is due to *Chlamydia pneumoniae* (21 days) or *Legionella pneumophilia* (10–14 days), or if the patient had necrotizing pneumonia or empyema (minimum 21 days).

FURTHER READING

Further reading for this chapter can be found online at http://www.expertconsult.com

When to use corticosteroids in noncentral nervous system tuberculosis

INTRODUCTION

The use of corticosteroids in the management of noncentral nervous system tuberculosis is supported by much anecdote but little data from controlled trials. It has long been observed that the symptoms of tuberculosis often worsen after the start of treatment, a phenomenon that is believed to be caused by an exaggerated inflammatory response to dead or dying mycobacteria. It is hypothesized that corticosteroids suppress this response and thereby improve outcome. This hypothesis has never been clearly refuted or confirmed in any form of the disease, but remains sufficiently attractive to induce many physicians to start adjunctive corticosteroids, particularly when faced with a patient with severe or disseminated disease whose clinical condition deteriorates after the start of antituberculosis therapy.

EVIDENCE OF EFFICACY

The most convincing evidence for a beneficial effect of corticosteroids in noncentral nervous system disease exists for pericardial tuberculosis and stems primarily from two randomized controlled trials performed 25 years ago in South Africa.

- The first trial compared prednisolone with placebo in the treatment of 143 patients with active constrictive tuberculous pericarditis and showed that prednisolone increased the rate of clinical improvement, reduced the risk of death from pericarditis and reduced the need for pericardiectomy.
- The second trial studied 243 patients with tuberculous pericardial effusion and used a factorial design to compare the value of open complete surgical drainage with percutaneous pericardiocentesis as required; in addition, all patients were randomized to receive either prednisolone or placebo. Prednisolone reduced the risk of death from pericarditis and the need for repeat pericardiocentesis, but did not reduce the incidence of constrictive pericarditis. After 10 years of follow-up, the use of prednisolone was associated with a significant reduction in the risk of death from pericarditis of either form.

In the light of these data, treatment guidelines published in the UK and the USA recommended adjunctive prednisolone for the treatment of HIV-uninfected patients with pericardial tuberculosis. There is less certainty as to whether the same should apply for those with HIV infection, although a small randomized controlled trial from Zimbabwe suggested that 6 weeks of adjunctive prednisolone reduced the risk of death in adults with effusive tuberculous pericarditis and advanced HIV infection.

There is no convincing evidence that adjunctive corticosteroids benefits patients with other forms of noncentral nervous system tuberculosis, although few large randomized controlled trials have been conducted. Advocates of corticosteroids will point out that there is little evidence they do harm and appear to speed symptom resolution. Data from 12 controlled trials of corticosteroids for pulmonary tuberculosis support this view. Treatment with corticosteroids was associated with more rapid resolution of symptoms and chest radiographic appearances in many of the studies, although a reduction in the incidence of chronic restrictive lung disease or death was not observed. The beneficial effect on clinical condition was most pronounced in those with severe lung disease and it is probably only in these circumstances that adjunctive corticosteroids should be given for pulmonary tuberculosis. However, data from a large, well-conducted study published in 1983 strike an important note of caution: patients with bacteria resistant to two or more drugs who received prednisolone responded to treatment less well than those in the control group and bacteria could be cultured from the sputum for longer. Therefore, the risk of drug resistance should be carefully assessed before adjunctive corticosteroids are considered for any form of tuberculosis.

There is evidence that corticosteroids speed early symptom resolution in primary tuberculosis and tuberculous pleuritis and peritonitis, although their use does not appear to reduce the fibrotic complications of these diseases. Corticosteroids may also reduce mediastinal lymph node enlargement in primary tuberculosis and decrease the local obstructive complications, although the latter was not a recorded end point in the two published controlled trials. Unfortunately, there have been no controlled trials of the use of adjunctive corticosteroids in the treatment of cervical or inguinal tuberculous lymphadenitis, despite painful node enlargement occurring in one-third of patients after the start of treatment. Extrapolation of the effect of corticosteroids on mediastinal adenopathy suggests they might be of benefit and many physicians use them in patients with painful, swollen nodes that are threatening to rupture. A summary of the evidence and treatment recommendations for all forms of noncentral nervous system tuberculosis are presented in Table PP13.1.

USE OF ADJUNCTIVE CORTICOSTEROIDS IN TUBERCULOSIS AND HIV INFECTION

The safety and efficacy of adjunctive corticosteroids in patients with tuberculosis and HIV infection are unproven. HIV-infected adults with pericardial tuberculosis probably should receive prednisolone, but for all other forms of HIV-associated tuberculosis (with the exception of cerebral tuberculosis) there are no grounds to recommend their routine use. In addition, while there is little evidence that adjunctive corticosteroids are harmful to HIV-uninfected patients with drug-susceptible tuberculosis, this may not be true for those infected with HIV.

Table PP13.1 Summary of treatment recommendations and evidence for adjunctive corticosteroids in noncentral nervous system tuberculosis

Type of tuberculosis	Corticosteroids recommended by the National Institute for Health and Clinical Excellence (2006)	Corticosteroids recommended by the Infectious Diseases Society of America (2003)	Suggested corticosteroid regimens	Summary of the evidence from randomized controlled trials (RCTs)
Pulmonary	No	No		Twelve RCTs of variable size and quality suggest corticosteroids may speed resolution of symptoms and chest X-ray changes, but have no beneficial effect on long-term fibrotic complications or death. May be indicated in those with severe lung disease
Pericardial	Yes	Yes	Prednisolone 60 mg weeks 1–4 30 mg weeks 5–8 15 mg weeks 9–10 5 mg week 11. Then stop	Three RCTs (one involving HIV-infected adults) observed prednisolone was associated with faster resolution of effusions and lower mortality. Progression to constrictive disease not affected
Pleural	No	No		Four RCTs suggest prednisolone resulted in faster resolution of symptoms and effusion, but no impact on development of fibrosis, restrictive lung disease or death
Primary	No (except if evidence of bronchial obstruction)	No		Two RCTs suggest prednisolone may reduce mass effects of mediastinal lymphadenopathy, although one trial used very high doses (5 mg/kg) to achieve the effect
Lymph node	No	No		No evidence from controlled trials
Bone and joint	No	No		No evidence from controlled trials
Peritoneal	No	No		One RCT of 47 patients, using prednisolone 30 mg q24h for 3 months, reported no difference in symptom resolution between groups and a nonsignificant reduction in chronic fibrotic complications in the prednisolone group
Genitourinary	No	No		No evidence from controlled trials
Miliary	No	No		One RCT from China involving 55 patients (14 of whom also had meningeal disease) reported fewer deaths in the prednisolone group (not statistically significant)

A randomized controlled trial of prednisolone for HIV-infected adults with pleural tuberculosis in Uganda suggested the predniso-lone-treated group recovered faster but suffered from a significantly increased incidence of Kaposi's sarcoma. Peripheral blood CD4+ T-cell counts and viral loads increased in both treatment arms, but without any significant difference between them. Another study from the same centre of the immunoadjuvant properties of prednisolone in HIV-infected adults with pulmonary tuberculosis again observed a transient and worrying rise in peripheral blood HIV viral load in the predniso-lone group that fell when the drug was discontinued. Unlike the previous study, there was no observed increase in Kaposi's sarcoma or other opportunistic infections in those treated with prednisolone, although they suffered more fluid retention, hypertension and hyperglycemia than the controls. The study was not powered to detect a difference in clinical outcome and few data regarding clinical and radiographic progress are given. However, the authors report a faster time to sputum sterility in the prednisolone group, an intriguing observation that replicates the findings of studies performed 40 years previously in HIV-uninfected patients with pulmonary tuberculosis.

There are no controlled trial data from patients receiving highly active antiretroviral therapy and studies involving such patients are urgently required (see Chapters 92 and 93).

FURTHER READING

Further reading for this chapter can be found online at http://www.expertconsult.com

How to manage a patient on anti-TB therapy with abnormal liver enzymes

INTRODUCTION

Although isoniazid, rifampin (rifampicin) and pyrazinamide are all potentially hepatotoxic, when pyrazinamide is added to the other drugs there does not seem to be an increase in the incidence of hepatitis. However, in unselected cases outside clinical trials, pyrazinamide is the drug with the highest monthly rate of hepatitis.

The incidence of hepatic reactions to antituberculosis drugs depends on the drug itself, and the age and possibly sex and ethnic group of the patient. Hepatic reactions to antituberculosis drugs were reported in 4% of cases treated with isoniazid/rifampin with or without pyrazinamide in a UK trial, and in 3% in a large clinical series. The overall rate of adverse reactions increases with age. Liver function tests (LFTs), particularly serum bilirubin and transaminases – aspartate aminotransferase (AST) and alanine aminotransferase (ALT) – should therefore be checked before treatment. Pre-treatment liver function testing is not advised for children receiving treatment for latent infection (chemoprophylaxis) because of the very low incidence of reactions. This may, however, be required if rifampin/pyrazinamide for 2 months is used to treat latent infection in adults, a regimen not advised in the UK where rifampin/isoniazid for 3 months is the alternative to isoniazid.

TESTING OF LIVER FUNCTION

Regular monitoring of liver function is not required for those with no evidence of pre-existing liver disease and normal liver function pre-treatment. Patients and their family doctors should, however, be informed of possible side-effects and the indications for stopping medication and seeking medical advice, preferably in writing in their native language. Tests of liver function only need to be repeated (and treatment stopped) if fever, vomiting, jaundice, malaise or unexplained deterioration occur. In such circumstances virologic tests to exclude coexistent viral hepatitis (A or B) should also be considered.

MANAGEMENT OF ELEVATED TESTS OF LIVER FUNCTION

Modest elevations of hepatic transaminases (AST/ALT) are not uncommon in tuberculosis patients even without known liver disease. They are also to be expected in patients with chronic liver diseases, including alcoholism, chronic active hepatitis and cirrhosis, and in chronic carriers of hepatitis B or C. Monitoring of such patients should be as in Figure PP14.1. If the pre-treatment AST/ALT is more than twice normal, liver function should be monitored weekly for 2 weeks then

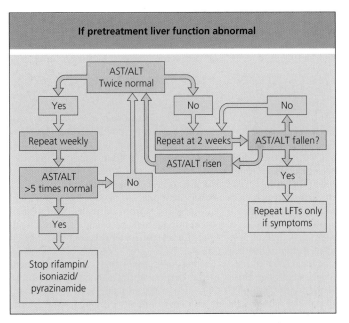

Fig. PP.14.1 Management of elevated tests of liver function if pretreatment liver function is abnormal. Derived from Ormerod LP, Skinner C, Wales J. Hepatotoxicity of antituberculosis drugs. Thorax 1996;51:111–13, with permission from BMJ Publishing Group.

2-weekly until normal. If the pre-treatment AST/ALT is less than twice normal, liver function should be repeated at 2 weeks. If the transaminase levels have fallen further, repeat tests are only needed for symptoms. However, if the AST/ALT rises to above twice normal, management should be as above (see Fig. PP14.1).

If the AST/ALT rises to above five times normal, or the bilirubin becomes elevated, then isoniazid, rifampin and pyrazinamide should be stopped. Immediate management then depends on the severity of the patient's illness and whether they are infectious as judged by positivity on sputum smear-microscopy within 2 weeks of treatment commencement (Fig. PP14.2). If the patient is not unwell and had a form of tuberculosis that is noninfectious, no treatment is needed until liver function returns to pre-treatment levels. If the patient is unwell or the sputum is smear-positive within 2 weeks of commencing a rifampin/isoniazid-based regimen, some form of drug treatment needs to be given until liver function returns to pre-treatment levels, preferably as an inpatient because of the monitoring required. In such cases a regimen of streptomycin and ethambutol with appropriate renal and visual checks is advised unless there are clinical

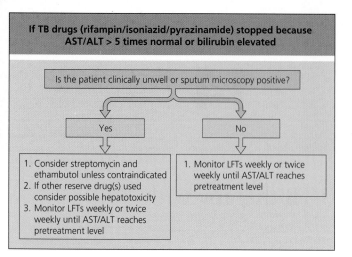

If TB drugs (rifampin/isoniazid/pyrazinamide) stopped because AST/ALT > 5 times normal or bilirubin elevated

Is the patient clinically unwell or sputum microscopy positive?

Yes →
1. Consider streptomycin and ethambutol unless contraindicated
2. If other reserve drug(s) used consider possible hepatotoxicity
3. Monitor LFTs weekly or twice weekly until AST/ALT reaches pretreatment level

No →
1. Monitor LFTs weekly or twice weekly until AST/ALT reaches pretreatment level

Fig. PP14.2 Management of elevated tests of liver function if antituberculosis drugs (rifampin/isoniazid/pyrazinamide) stopped because AST/ALT over five times normal or bilirubin elevated. Derived from Ormerod LP, Skinner C, Wales J. Hepatotoxicity of antituberculosis drugs. Thorax 1996;51:111–13, with permission from BMJ Publishing Group.

Table PP14.1 Order of re-Introduction* of antituberculosis agents following drug-associated hepatotoxicity

Start: Ethambutol (15 mg/kg) plus isoniazid 50 mg q24h for 2–3 days then plus isoniazid 150 mg q24h for 2–3 days then plus isoniazid 300 mg q24h for 2–3 days and continue
If no reaction then: Ethambutol (15 mg/kg) plus isoniazid 300 mg q24h plus rifampin (rifampicin) 75 mg q24h for 2–3 days then plus rifampin 300 mg q24h for 2–3 days then plus rifampin 450 mg q24h (under 50 kg) or rifampin 600 mg q24h (≥50 kg) for 2–3 days and continue
If no reaction then: Ethambutol (15 mg/kg) plus isoniazid 300 mg q24h plus rifampin 450/600 mg q24h and add sequentially: pyrazinamide 250 mg q24h for 2–3 days then pyrazinamide 1 g q24h for 2–3 days then pyrazinamide 1.5 g (<50 kg) or pyrazinamide 2 g (≥50 kg) for 2–3 days and then continue if no reaction
Ethambutol can then be withdrawn if not required on drug resistance probability grounds

*Re-introduction is carried out with daily monitoring of clinical condition and regular LFTs.
Derived from Ormerod LP, Skinner C, Wales J. Hepatotoxicity of antituberculosis drugs. Thorax 1996;51:111–13, with permission from BMJ Publishing Group.

contraindications or drug resistance to these agents is known or suspected. If second-line drugs are used, any potential hepatotoxicity (e.g. with macrolides, quinolones, prothionamide or ethionamide) should be considered. Occasionally patients with serious liver disease and active tuberculosis have very abnormal LFTs, with raised bilirubin and AST/ALT over five times normal pre-treatment levels. In these circumstances a risk/benefit analysis needs to be made, and often the risk of death (and infectivity) from untreated tuberculosis significantly exceeds that of additional hepatotoxicity. Standard treatment may then be appropriate under corticosteroid cover with regular monitoring of liver function.

Once liver function has returned to normal or pre-treatment levels, challenge doses of the original drugs can be re-introduced sequentially (Table PP14.1). Such re-introduction is best carried out in parallel with treatment with ethambutol 15 mg/kg to prevent the possible emergence of drug resistance during the re-introduction. The patient's condition should be monitored daily together with liver function. Sequential re-introduction of isoniazid, rifampin and pyrazinamide is advised. Isoniazid should be started initially at 50 mg/day, increasing to 150 mg/day after 2–3 days and then 300 mg/day after a further 2–3 days if no reaction occurs, which is then continued. After a further 2–3 days without reaction, rifampin at a dose of 75 mg/day can be added, increasing to 300 mg/day after 2–3 days, and then to 450 mg (<50 kg) or 600 mg (>50 kg) according to patient's weight after a further 2–3 days without reaction, and then continued. Finally, pyrazinamide can be added at 250 mg/day, increasing to 1.0 g after 2–3 days and then to either 1.5 g (<50 kg) or 2.0 g (>50 kg). If there is no further reaction, standard chemotherapy can be continued and any alternative drugs introduced temporarily may then be withdrawn. Ethambutol may need to be continued in the initial phase if indicated by local drug-resistance profile and national treatment guidelines.

MANAGEMENT OF FURTHER REACTIONS FOLLOWING RE-INTRODUCTION OF THERAPY

If there is a further reaction during the re-introduction, the offending drug should be excluded and an alternative regimen constructed. If pyrazinamide is the offending drug, then a regimen of rifampin and isoniazid for 9 months, supplemented by ethambutol for 2 months, will be required. For other drugs an alternative regimen may need to be on the advice of an experienced TB physician. Sometimes, for example because of drug resistance, the choice of drugs is so limited that if reactions occur, desensitization and re-introduction of the offending drug may be necessary using conventional protocols.

Such densensitization may need to be carried out under the cover of two other antituberculosis drugs to avoid the emergence of drug resistance.

FURTHER READING

Further reading for this chapter can be found online at http://www.expertconsult.com

Management of the infected cystic fibrosis patient

DEFINITION OF THE PROBLEM

The airways of persons with cystic fibrosis (CF) are chronically infected with bacteria, usually *Staphylococcus aureus* and *Pseudomonas aeruginosa* (typically mucoid strains). This persistent infection and the accompanying inflammatory response result in mucus hypersecretion with obstruction of smaller airways, bronchiectasis and the symptoms of chronic cough, sputum production and dyspnea. While chronic symptoms are slowly progressive, intermittently patients may have a more accelerated decline associated with increases in the bacterial burden in the airways with additional symptoms, usually referred to as an acute respiratory exacerbation. Optimal management of the infected CF patient necessitates strategies to combat both the chronic airway infection and acute exacerbations.

TYPICAL CASE

Persons with cystic fibrosis typically exhibit symptoms of chronic cough, sputum production and dyspnea on exertion when they develop more advanced obstructive lung disease. Exacerbations of their lung disease are usually characterized by an increase in cough and sputum production, a change in the color (to darker or more green) or character (thicker and more viscous) of the sputum, dyspnea and worsening exercise tolerance. These exacerbations may also be accompanied by generalized fatigue, fevers, decreased appetite, weight loss and, in diabetic patients, worsening glycemic control. Acute exacerbations may be highlighted by massive hemoptysis, a true medical emergency (Table PP15.1).

Physical examination may demonstrate new clinical findings such as wheezes or crackles, use of accessory muscles of respiration, tachycardia, cyanosis and decreased oxyhemoglobin saturation. Chest X-rays may reveal a new infiltrate or evidence of increased mucus plugging on a background of chronic bronchiectatic changes. Many patients with acute exacerbations will not demonstrate any change in their radiograph. On occasion the onset of an exacerbation may be insidious and occur over weeks. Under these circumstances patients may not fully appreciate the magnitude of their decline unless questioned carefully. In these cases pulmonary function testing (discussed below) will usually detect a significant change from the patient's baseline.

DIAGNOSIS

Diagnosis of an acute respiratory exacerbation of cystic fibrosis-related bronchiectasis is best made by a clinician experienced in the care of patients with CF. It is usually made when a patient presents with a combination of some or all of the above-mentioned signs and symptoms, in association with a decrease in their forced vital capacity (FVC)

Table PP15.1 Signs and symptoms of acute exacerbations of CF-related lung disease

- Increase in cough and sputum production
- Change in the color or character of sputum
- Dyspnea and worsening exercise tolerance
- Fatigue
- Fevers
- Decreased appetite
- Weight loss
- Worsening glycemic control
- Massive hemoptysis
- New wheezes or crackles
- Use of accessory muscles of respiration
- Tachycardia
- Cyanosis
- New radiographic infiltrate
- Decrease in FEV1

and forced expiratory volume in 1 second (FEV1). These pulmonary function tests or spirometry are the best objective measure of a patient's status and during exacerbations will usually demonstrate worsening airway obstruction and a decline of at least 10%. A significant decline in FEV1 even in the absence of worsening symptoms should result in an intensification of the patient's therapy.

MANAGEMENT OPTIONS

Optimal management of the infected patient with CF requires the identification of specific pathogens which infect the individual patient. Early in life infection with *S. aureus* and *Haemophilus influenzae* is common. While infection with oxacillin-sensitive and resistant *S. aureus* may persist as patients age, infection with *P. aeruginosa* and, less commonly, other Gram-negative organisms, such as *Achromobacter xylosoxidans*, *Stenotrophomonas maltophilia* and *Burkholderia cepacia*, predominates. Infections with *B. cepacia* can be especially difficult to treat, and have been associated with an accelerated decline in lung function in some patients and with epidemic outbreaks at some CF care centers. As this organism may not grow readily in culture, all respiratory samples from patients with CF should be cultured on media specific for this organism, in addition to the other organisms mentioned above. Increasing frequency of infection in CF patients with community-associated methicillin-resistant *S. aureus*, sometimes expressing the Panton–Valentine leukocidin (PVL) virulence factor, has recently been documented. This may be associated with acute invasive pulmonary infections and abscesses. When applied to lower respiratory tract secretions, techniques for molecular identification of pathogens may identify pathogens (including anaerobes) which are not typically associated with airway infection in CF. The significance of these pathogens remains to be determined.

Many patients will be infected with multiple organisms or multiple colony types of the same organism that may have different susceptibility patterns. It is therefore recommended that all organisms and their differing microcolonies be identified in culture and have their susceptibility patterns determined to facilitate selection of the optimal antibiotic regimen.

When treating acute exacerbations (Table PP15.2), selection of specific antimicrobials should be guided by results of sputum culture and sensitivity. Mild exacerbations may sometimes be treated with oral and/or inhaled antibiotics if effective agents are available. Response to therapy should be closely monitored and if ineffective, a switch should be made to parenteral therapy. More severe exacerbations should be treated parenterally and in general two antipseudomonal agents are chosen, usually a third- or fourth-generation cephalosporin or antipseudomonal penicillin, along with an aminoglycoside. Therapy should be modified based on culture results. The antipseudomonal penicillins or carbapenems may be more active against *Achromobacter xylosoxidans*, and carbapenems such as meropenem may have increased activity against *B. cepacia*. Infections with *Stenotrophomonas maltophilia* are sometimes best treated with trimethoprim–sulfamethoxazole, minocycline or ticarcillin–clavulanate. Since patients with CF often exhibit high volumes of distribution and increased antimicrobial drug clearance, higher doses of antibiotics should be utilized. Aminoglycosides should be administered on an 8-hour dosing schedule with target peak levels of 8–12 μg/ml and trough levels less than 2 μg/ml. Some have reported successful therapy with single daily dosing regimens. Typically 2–3 weeks of parenteral therapy is required.

Therapy of the chronically infected CF patient who is not in the midst of an acute exacerbation may include inhaled suppressive antibiotic therapy. In clinical trials, a preservative-free formulation of tobramycin (TOBI®) has been shown to improve lung function and decrease the risk of hospitalization in patients colonized with *P. aeruginosa* who inhaled this medication for three cycles of twice-daily administration for 28 days followed by 28 days off medication. Patients are often treated with other inhaled antibiotics such as colistin; however, the use of these agents is less well studied or standardized. Additional inhaled antibiotics with novel and more convenient delivery systems are currently in all stages of drug development and some should be available for use in the near future. A study of oral cephalexin prophylaxis in infants and young children with cystic fibrosis failed to demonstrate a clinical benefit.

In addition to antimicrobial therapy, airway clearance is an essential component in the management of the infected airways of patients with CF. This may be accomplished via traditional chest percussion and postural drainage or with the assistance of various devices such as percussors, pneumatic compression vests or handheld devices which provide oscillatory positive expiratory pressure to the airways such as the Flutter and Acapella devices. Bronchodilators facilitate airway clearance and decrease airway obstruction, and are commonly used by patients with CF. Dornase alpha (Pulmozyme®) degrades extracellular DNA which is present in airway secretions of patients with CF as a result of the neutrophilic infiltration of the lung. Daily inhalation of dornase alpha decreases the resulting increased viscoelasticity of the CF sputum to allow improved airway clearance and has been shown to improve lung function and decrease the need for parenteral antibiotics in patients with CF. Recent studies have shown that inhalation of hypertonic saline (4 ml of 7% saline twice daily) improves lung function and decreases exacerbation rates in patients with CF. The mechanism of action is either via restoration of the airway surface liquid volume which is diminished in CF, or by enhancing cough-mediated airway clearance.

When administered three times per week to patients with CF who are chronically infected with *P. aeruginosa*, the macrolide antibiotic azithromycin has been shown to improve lung function and decrease exacerbations when compared to placebo. The mechanism of action is unclear but could be related to anti-inflammatory effects of macrolides or disruption of biofilm formation. Care must be taken to screen patients for nontuberculous mycobacterial infection to prevent emergence of macrolide-resistant infection in these patients. A study evaluating the utility of this therapy in CF patients without *Pseudomonas* infection is underway.

As many as 13% of CF patients in the USA may become infected with nontuberculous mycobacteria, most commonly *Mycobacterium avium* complex and *Mycobacterium abscessus*. Since some patients may acquire these organisms without a clear effect on clinical status, deciding which patients to treat can be problematic, as treatment can be difficult and eradication may not be possible. Patients who grow these organisms on repeated culture, do not respond as expected to courses of routine antibacterial therapy, have evidence of new cavitary disease on chest X-ray or CT scan, or evidence of progressive changes on CT scan compatible with mycobacterial infection, should be considered for specific therapy.

Other adjunctive therapies for the infected CF patient include regular exercise and aggressive nutritional support to address the increased metabolic needs and malabsorptive problems which these patients may exhibit. Since the inflammatory response in the CF lung may contribute to the morbidity of the chronic airway infection, anti-inflammatory therapy may benefit some patients. Short courses of corticosteroids may benefit some patients; however, while long-term corticosteroid use may slow the decline in lung function, their benefit is outweighed by side-effects of the therapy. High-dose ibuprofen may slow the decline in lung function in young patients with mild disease but this therapy should be closely monitored. Identification and evaluation of more specific and less toxic anti-inflammatory agents is currently being actively researched.

Optimal management of infected CF patients requires an effective infection control strategy to prevent patient-to-patient transmission of virulent organisms. This strategy should include both the inpatient and outpatient settings and conform to local infection control guidelines. Frequent handwashing is extremely important. Patients infected with *B. cepacia* should be segregated from other CF patients who are not infected with this organism. Since children infected with *P. aeruginosa* have decreased lung function and survival when compared with children only infected with *S. aureus*, some advocate segregating these groups of patients.

CONCLUSION

Management of the infected patient with cystic fibrosis requires strategies to address both the chronic infection and acute exacerbations of infection. This necessitates routine symptomatic and physiologic evaluation of patients, along with frequent microbiologic surveillance of airway secretions. These should guide aggressive but appropriate use of oral, inhaled and parenteral antibiotics, along with adjunctive therapies such as bronchodilators, mucolytics, airway clearance, pulmonary rehabilitation and nutritional support. Finally, an effective infection control policy should be in place to prevent patient-to-patient transmission of potentially harmful organisms.

FURTHER READING

Further reading for this chapter can be found online at http://www.expertconsult.com

---

Table PP15.2 Management of acute exacerbations of CF-related lung disease

- Parenteral antimicrobial therapy based on respiratory culture results (typically two antipseudomonal agents)
- Enhanced airway clearance
- Bronchodilators
- Mucolytics
- Pulmonary rehabilitation
- Nutritional support

Diagnosis and management of ventilator-associated pneumonia

A ventilator-associated pneumonia (VAP) appears, by definition, after at least 48 hours of invasive mechanical ventilation and is recognized as the first cause of nosocomial infection in the ICU.

CLINICAL, RADIOGRAPHIC, AND BIOLOGIC DIAGNOSIS

Diagnosis is based on an association of an infectious syndrome (fever or hypothermia/leukopenia or hyperleukocytosis), a lung infiltrate on chest X-ray (appearance or modification), purulent bronchorrhea and worsening gas exchange. The clinical pulmonary infection score (CPIS) proposed by Pugin *et al.*[1] uses six of these different criteria. Its sensitivity and specificity for a threshold at 6 are acceptable (Table PP16.1).

Table PP16.1 Clinical pulmonary infection score	
Temperature	≥36.5° C and ≤38.4° C: 0 points ≥38.5° C and ≤38.9° C: 1 point ≤36° C or ≥39° C: 2 points
White blood cells	≥4 g/l and ≤11 g/l: 0 points <4 g/l or >11 g/l: 1 point If ≥0.5 g/l immature forms: + 1 point
Tracheal aspirations*	<14+: 0 points ≥14+: 1 point If purulence: + 1 point
Pao_2/Fio_2 ratio	>240 or ARDS: 0 points ≤240 without ARDS: 2 points
Chest X-ray	Absence of infiltrate: 0 points Diffuse infiltrate: 1 point Localized infiltrate: 2 points
Semiquantitative culture of tracheal secretions (0, 1, 2 or 3+)	Pathogenic bacteria ≤1+: 0 points Pathogenic bacteria >1+: 1 point Same bacteria as the Gram: + 1 point

ARDS, acute respiratory distress syndrome.
*For each aspiration, the nurses estimate the quantity of tracheal secretions harvested and assign a semiquantitative score (increasing from 0 to 4+). The total estimation is obtained by adding up all of the pluses noted for 24 hours. The total score ranges from 0 to 12. A score >6 is in favor of a ventilator-associated pneumonia with a sensitivity of 93% and a specificity of 100% compared with bronchoalveolar lavage, and a sensitivity of 72% and a specificity of 85% compared with lung histologic assessment.

Nonrespiratory microbiologic samples

A large number of micro-organisms have been implicated in VAP (Fig. PP16.1).

Blood cultures are insufficient but are nevertheless always recommended before administering antibiotherapy.[2] Antigenuria by chromatographic techniques enables the detection of *Streptococcus pneumoniae* and *Legionella pneumophila* serogroup 1 antigens, usually performed on urinary strip (or even in the alveolar liquid) within the framework of community-acquired pneumonia and can be useful with VAP. Serology for intracellular bacteria and viruses is only of retrospective interest given the waiting period for seroconversion. Cytomegalovirus (CMV) viremia or antigenemia confirms extensive cytomegalic infection and makes it possible for CMV to attack the lungs. Hepatic cytolysis must lead the clinician to suspect an active CMV infection within the framework of late VAP (at least 5 days of mechanical ventilation).

Nondirected respiratory samples (Table PP16.2)

Thanks to the contribution of quantitative cultures, tracheal aspirate (TA) has found its place among diagnostic methods. The predominance of the right side and the fact that one is dealing with bronchopneumonia with a bronchial component undoubtedly explains the interest of this technique in the diagnosis of VAP. When TA at a threshold of 10^5 cfu/ml was compared with protected specimen brush (PSB) or bronchoalveolar lavage (BAL), the sensitivity and specificity were 92.8% and 80%, respectively.

A protected double catheter (double-plugged catheter), protected by a glycol polyethylene plug, makes it possible to perform 'blind aspiration brushing' through an internal catheter or mini-BAL in which 20 ml of liquid are instilled and whose semiquantitative culture has revealed a sensitivity of 80% and a specificity of 66%.

Directed respiratory samples (Table PP16.2)

Bronchoalveolar lavage (BAL) is performed by instilling and recovering sterile saline solution through the internal channel of the fiberscope which is positioned in a third- or fourth-generation bronchus where only distal bronchioles and alveoli are sampled. No consensus has been established on the quantity to administer by aliquot, on the number of aliquots or on preserving or eliminating the first aliquot representing the bronchial fraction of BAL. A meta-analysis of 23 studies revealed the sensitivity of BAL at 73 ± 18% and its specificity at 82 ± 19% when VAP was diagnosed.[3]

The interest in BAL is based on the possibility of examining for other pathogens such as intracellular pathogens and their nucleic acid thanks to polymerase chain reaction (PCR) amplification which appears to be

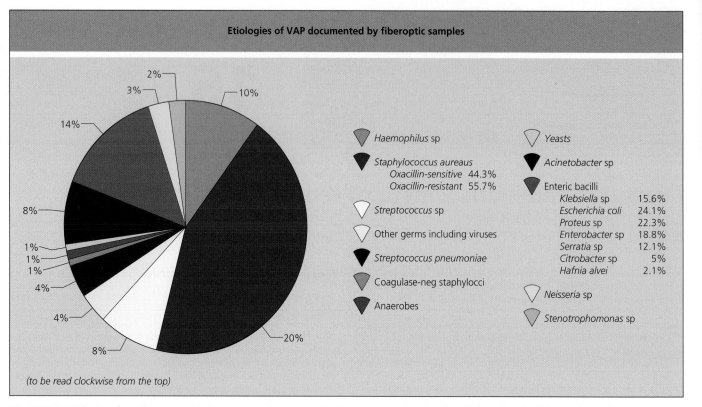

Etiologies of VAP documented by fiberoptic samples

Haemophilus sp		*Yeasts*
Staphylococcus aureaus		*Acinetobacter* sp
Oxacillin-sensitive 44.3%		
Oxacillin-resistant 55.7%		Enteric bacilli

Enteric bacilli
- *Klebsiella* sp 15.6%
- *Escherichia coli* 24.1%
- *Proteus* sp 22.3%
- *Enterobacter* sp 18.8%
- *Serratia* sp 12.1%
- *Citrobacter* sp 5%
- *Hafnia alvei* 2.1%

Streptococcus sp

Other germs including viruses

Streptococcus pneumoniae

Coagulase-neg staphylocci

Anaerobes

Neisseria sp

Stenotrophomonas sp

(to be read clockwise from the top)

Fig. PP16.1 Etiologies of ventilator-associated pneumonia documented by fiberoptic samples. Results of 24 studies of 1689 episodes and 2490 pathogens.

Table PP16.2 Microbiologic diagnostic tools and thresholds of significance that are usually retained

- Blind tracheal aspirate ≥10^5 or 10^6 cfu/ml
- Blind mini-bronchoalveolar lavage or blind protected double catheter brushing ≥10^3 cfu/ml
- Protected specimen brush under fibroscopy ≥10^3 cfu/ml
- Bronchoalveolar lavage under fibroscopy ≥10^4 cfu/ml

---

more effective than cultures which are difficult to perform. A viral diagnosis (herpes simplex virus, cytomegalovirus) can also benefit from PCR amplification parallel to classic or rapid cultures and cytologic analysis.

Protected specimen brush (PSB) is a double catheter sealed by a glycol polyethylene plug that enables brushing of the distal bronchial mucosa following insertion of an endoscope. The low volume of secretions harvested (approximately 1 µl) explains a certain number of false-negatives as well as the difficulty in performing a direct examination and culturing on the same brush. This technique, developed *in vitro* by Wimberley, provides a sensitivity ranging from 33% to 100%.

No consensus conference has decided among the different types of sampling although the choice should favor quantitative techniques.

TREATMENT

Since the great majority of ventilator-associated pneumonias are due to bacteria, empiric therapy or (even better) empiric antibiotherapy – oriented by the patient's health status, local microbiologic ecology and direct examination (with TA, BAL, mini-BAL) – must be administered as soon as there are enough clinical arguments. The consensus from the American Thoracic Society and the Infectious Diseases Society of America[2] proposes broad-spectrum empiric double antibiotherapy in case infection with multidrug-resistant bacteria is suspected (Tables PP16.3, PP16.4) and double or even mono narrow-spectrum antibiotherapy in other cases (Table PP16.4). This antibiotherapy must begin after performing a series of hemocultures and respiratory samples (tracheal aspirate, PSB, BAL, etc.). Antibiotics are given intravenously, and when the response to treatment is satisfactory, relayed by oral or enteral administration if possible. Tracheal or aerosol instillations of antibiotics are not recommended as a cure can be but complementary in the treatment of multidrug-resistant Gram-negative bacilli if systemic antibiotherapy appears to be insufficient.[2]

Several observational studies have shown that appropriate antibiotherapy administered as soon as possible was associated with a reduction in the mortality of patients with suspected VAP.[4] The choice of therapy must also take into account recent antibiotherapy received by the patient so that a different class of antibiotic is used to initiate treatment. For this choice, the latest consensus conference has proposed that the recommended guidelines, regularly updated, adapted to local microbiology and the availability of molecules within the structure be systematically used. Another method to orient initial antibiotherapy can be proposed. It is to administer antibiotherapy as soon as BAL has

---

Table PP16.3 Risk factors associated with an increased incidence of multidrug-resistant bacteria

- Antimicrobial therapy in preceding 90 days
- Current hospitalization of 5 days or more
- High frequency of antibiotic resistance in the community or in the specific hospital unit
- Hospitalization for 2 days or more in the preceding 90 days
- Residence in a nursing home or extended care facility
- Home infusion therapy (including antibiotics)
- Chronic dialysis within 30 days
- Home wound care
- Family member with multidrug-resistant pathogen
- Immunosuppressive disease and/or therapy

Table PP16.4 Empiric antibiotherapy proposed by the ATS/IDSA Consensus Conference

Empiric antibiotherapy in case of early-onset VAP (<5th day) and in the absence of multidrug-resistant bacterium risk factors	Empiric antibiotherapy in case of late-onset VAP (≥5th day) and/or the presence of multidrug-resistant bacterium risk factors
β-Lactamine/inhibitor of β-lactamase Or ceftriaxone Or levofloxacin or moxifloxacin Or ertapenem	Cefepime or ceftazidime Or imipenem or meropenem Or piperacillin–tazobactam *plus* Ciprofloxacin or levofloxacin Or gentamicin or tobramycin Or amikacin *plus* Linezolid or vancomycin*

*If suspicion or risk factors of methicillin-resistant *Staphylococcus aureus* (corticotherapy, recent antibiotherapy, mechanical ventilation >6 days).

been performed by making use of the tracheal aspirate results systematically performed twice a week in all patients under invasive mechanical ventilation (Fig. PP16.2). A study has shown that this method improves the appropriateness of treatment compared with the use of the recommended guidelines.[5]

In any case, rapid deterioration or the absence of improvement after 72 hours of empiric treatment imposes systematic re-evaluation. It should be noted that the absence of response to empiric treatment can be linked to a nonbacterial infection, particularly viral, or to an extrapulmonary infection, or to the absence of an infectious problem (for example, during the fibroproliferative phase of the acute respiratory distress syndrome) requiring aggressive diagnostic measures which can go as far as a lung biopsy. In case of improvement, reduction or even discontinuation of antibiotherapy is mandatory once sampling results are known and appear to be coherent.

Short antibiotherapy (8 days) is currently recommended except in cases of *Pseudomonas aeruginosa* where at least 15 days of antibio-therapy appear to be necessary with bitherapy maintained for the first 5 days.[6] The administration of antiviral treatment (ganciclovir for CMV, aciclovir for herpes simplex virus, and amantadine, rimantadine, oseltamivir or zanamivir for respiratory viruses) and antifungal agents (with recently available molecules such as voriconazole and caspofungin) is conditioned by diagnostic difficulties. Finally, immunity-modulating treatments are not recognized and only a sufficient nutritional contribution and respiratory physiotherapy can be recommended as adjuvant treatments.

REFERENCES

References for this chapter can be found online at http://www.expertconsult.com

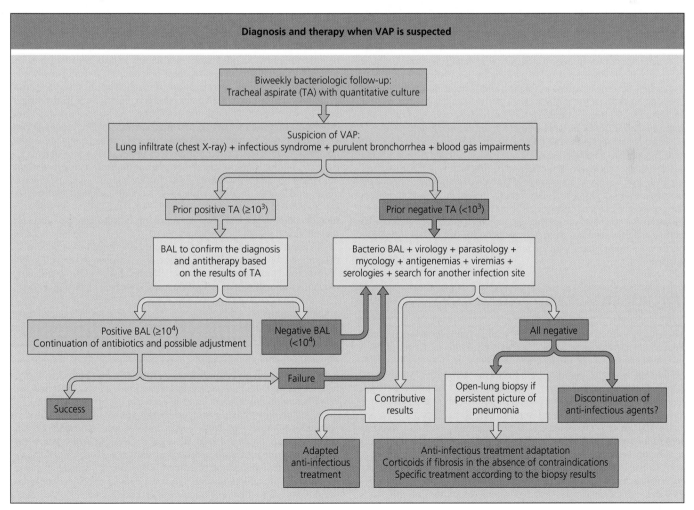

Fig. PP16.2 Decision tree proposed for diagnosis and therapy when ventilator-associated pneumonia (VAP) is suspected. BAL, bronchoalveolar lavage.

Orocervical infection

Infections of the oral cavity and neck include dental and periodontal infections, deep fascial space infections of the neck that are often odontogenic or caused by contiguous spread from pharyngeal foci, nondental oral infections, including ulcerative and gangrenous stomatitis, and infections of the salivary glands. Infections of the esophagus mostly occur in the context of severe underlying disease.

Dental and Periodontal Infections

EPIDEMIOLOGY

Dental caries is the commonest infectious disease in humans. Incidence is closely related to the use of derivatives of cane sugar and began to take on epidemic proportions in Europe in the 19th century. Dental caries first becomes evident in infancy and is most noticeable on the chewing surfaces of the molar teeth. The likelihood of dental caries is increased by high sugar intake, poor oral hygiene and any factors that reduce salivary flow – notably drugs (e.g. antidepressants).[1]

Periodontal disease, including gingivitis, is mainly related to poor oral hygiene and increasing age. Increased incidence of periodontal disease is also evident in diabetics and during hormonal disturbances, including puberty and pregnancy.[2] It is suspected that most periodontal disease arises from an inflammatory response to the accumulation of dental plaque in the gingival margin. Plaque contains mainly *Streptococcus* spp. and *Actinomyces* spp., which probably generate an early gingivitis, leading ultimately to periodontitis.[3] These processes occur over many years with incremental destruction of periodontal tissue.[4]

PATHOGENESIS AND PATHOLOGY

The indigenous oral flora includes a large number of aerobic and anaerobic bacteria and varies by site within the oral cavity. There are of the order of 10^{11} micro-organisms per gram wet weight of oral secretions, with the majority being obligate anaerobes. *Streptococcus* spp., *Peptostreptococcus* spp., *Veillonella* spp., *Lactobacillus* spp., *Corynebacterium* spp., *Bacteroides* spp., *Prevotella* spp. and *Actinomyces* spp. form the majority of oral flora.[5]

Dental caries is characteristically polymicrobial with no fixed pattern of microbial etiology, except that *Streptococcus mutans* has emerged as the only organism consistently isolated from carious teeth compared with normal teeth. In contrast, gingivitis has characteristic microbial specificity; the normal flora of the periodontium (i.e. *Streptococcus sanguis* and *Actinomyces* spp.) is replaced by anaerobic Gram-negative rods, notably *Prevotella intermedia*. With chronic gingivitis there is ulceration of the mucosa, loss of attachment of periodontal tissue, loss of enamel and necrosis of the dental pulp, and an increase in complexity of microbial flora with a preponderance of anaerobic Gram-negative rods, including *Porphyromonas gingivalis*.[2] When abscesses form, for example periapical abscesses, the flora is always polymicrobial with species such as *Fusobacterium*, pigmented *Bacteroides*, *Peptostreptococcus*, *Actinomyces* and *Streptococcus*.

In healthy individuals teeth are protected from decay by the cleansing action of the tongue and buccal secretions, the buffering effect of saliva and the acquired pellicle – the fluid microenvironment of the tooth surface. With poor dental hygiene the acquired pellicle is colonized and replaced by plaque that contains bacteria, notably *Strep. mutans*. This process is accelerated by intermittent exposure to carbohydrates and simple sugars. The presence of subgingival plaque leads to inflammation of the gingival epithelium and to destruction of the periodontium.[5] The normal resident polymicrobial flora provides an important defense against invasion of gingival epithelium by pathogenic bacteria. Normal saliva also protects the epithelium by irrigating it with enzymes, including lysozyme and lactoperoxidase, and other antimicrobial substances such as lactoferrin. Secretory IgA provides additional protection by aggregating organisms and preventing bacterial adherence. The importance of intact phagocytic defenses is reflected by the high prevalence of periodontal infections in patients who have cyclic neutropenia and chronic granulomatous disease.[3] Some oral micro-organisms involved in periodontal disease secrete IgA proteases.[6] Host factors credited with leading to periodontitis include psychosocial stress, diet, smoking, alcoholism and intercurrent disease.[7]

The usual cause of deep-seated odontogenic infection is necrosis of the pulp of the tooth, followed by bacterial invasion through the pulp chamber and into the deeper tissues.[8] If a pulp abscess is allowed to progress, infection will spread toward the nearest cortical plate (Fig. 32.1).

PREVENTION

Prevention of dental and periodontal infections includes interference with transmission and suppression of *Strep. mutans* colonization once it has occurred. There is a strong correlation between maternal salivary *Strep. mutans* infection and the presence of this organism in children. Acquisition of *Strep. mutans* by infants has been prevented by aggressive treatment of *Strep. mutans* infection in mothers.[9] Existing infections can be suppressed by regular cleaning with agents that include fluoride and antimicrobial substances such as chlorhexidine. Periodontal disease can be prevented by good oral hygiene and regular rinsing with chlorhexidine. Clinical trials of vaccines to prevent periodontitis have been conducted but vaccination has not yet entered current recommended practice.[10]

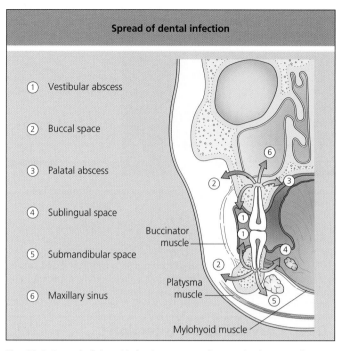

Fig. 32.1 Spread of dental infection. A spreading tooth abscess will encroach upon the nearest cortical plate and its subsequent spread depends on the relationship of that site to muscle attachment. Adapted from Peterson.[8]

Spread of dental infection

1. Vestibular abscess
2. Buccal space
3. Palatal abscess
4. Sublingual space
5. Submandibular space
6. Maxillary sinus

Buccinator muscle
Platysma muscle
Mylohyoid muscle

CLINICAL FEATURES

Subgingival dental caries is asymptomatic, but destruction of enamel results in invasion of the pulp with subsequent necrosis, eventually leading to a periapical abscess. The tooth becomes sensitive to temperature and pressure once the enamel is penetrated, and toothache results.

In simple gingivitis there is usually discoloration of the gum margin with occasional bleeding after brushing of the teeth. There may be halitosis. If gingivitis is allowed to become chronic there may be destruction of periodontal tissue with loosening of the teeth. This may be relatively asymptomatic or the patient may have itchy gums, temperature sensitivity and halitosis.

COMPLICATIONS

Dental pulp infections can lead to involvement of the maxillary and mandibular spaces (see Fig. 32.1). Spread of infection from maxillary (upper) teeth most commonly leads to vestibular abscesses (Fig. 32.2).

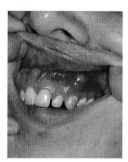

Fig. 32.2 Painful vestibular abscess. Courtesy of Professor I Brook.

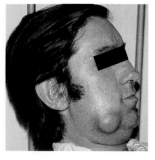

Fig. 32.3 Buccal space abscess originating from right lower molar infection. The buccal space lies between the buccinator muscle and the overlying skin and fascia. Courtesy of Professor I Brook.

Erosion of canine pulp abscesses can lead to canine space abscesses if the abscess points above the insertion of the levator labii superioris. This results in swelling lateral to the nose, which usually obliterates the nasolabial fold. Buccal space abscesses can result when pulp abscesses of the molar teeth erode above or below the attachment of the buccinator muscle; these point below the zygomatic arch and above the inferior border of the mandible (Fig. 32.3).

When infection spreads from mandibular (lower) teeth the commonest result is again vestibular abscess. Deeper abscesses may point into the sublingual and submandibular spaces. The sublingual space lies underneath the oral mucosa and above the mylohyoid muscle (see Fig. 32.1). Posteriorly, it communicates with the submandibular space. Infection within the sublingual space results in swelling of the floor of the mouth, which may spread to involve both sides and be sufficiently pronounced to lift the tongue. This space is involved if the infected tooth apex giving rise to the disease is superior to the insertion of the mylohyoid (e.g. premolars and first molars).

The submandibular space lies between the mylohyoid muscle and the skin. It becomes involved if the apex of the infected tooth is inferior to the insertion of the mylohyoid muscle (e.g. third molar). Clinically, infection in this space causes extraoral swelling (unlike sublingual space infections) that begins at the inferior lateral border of the mandible and extends medially to the digastric area. Occasionally the abscess may point spontaneously and rupture (Fig. 32.4).

Ludwig's angina refers to a severe cellulitis of the tissue of the floor of the mouth with involvement of the submandibular and sublingual spaces (Fig. 32.5). The source of infection is almost always the second and third mandibular molars. If the infection is allowed to continue there may be local lymphadenitis, systemic sepsis and extension of the disease to involve deep cervical fascia, with a cellulitis that extends from the clavicle to the superficial tissues of the face. Other potential complications include asphyxia, aspiration and mediastinitis. The disease is almost always polymicrobial, including α-hemolytic streptococci and anaerobes such as *Peptostreptococcus* spp., *Prevotella melaninogenica* and *Fusobacterium nucleatum*.[11]

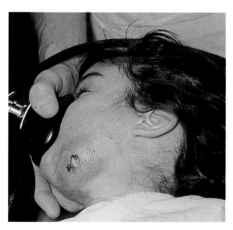

Fig. 32.4 Submandibular abscess originating from a 2nd molar tooth infection. Courtesy of University of Sheffield School of Dentistry, UK.

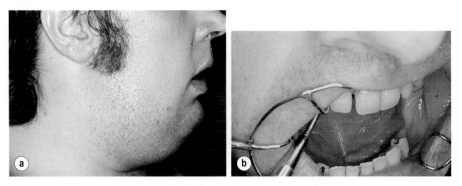

Fig. 32.5 Ludwig's angina. (a) This patient had painful cellulitis within the submandibular and sublingual spaces. (b) Brawny edema was present within the floor of the mouth, pushing the tongue upwards. Courtesy of University of Sheffield School of Dentistry, UK.

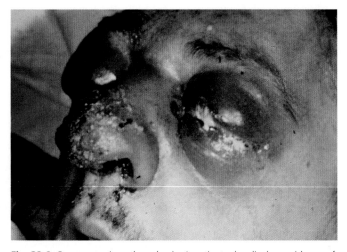

Fig. 32.6 Cavernous sinus thrombosis. A patient who displays evidence of severe orbital swelling caused by obstruction of orbital veins is shown. In this patient, the originating focus was infection of soft tissues of the nose. Courtesy of University of Sheffield School of Dentistry, UK.

Very rarely, spread of infection from maxillary teeth may cause orbital cellulitis or cavernous sinus thrombosis (see Chapter 20). The latter is distinguished by toxemia, venous obstruction within the eye and orbital tissues (Fig. 32.6), involvement of the III, IV and VI cranial nerves and meningismus.

MANAGEMENT

Treatment of dentoalveolar infections includes elimination of the diseased pulp and deep periodontal scaling or tooth extraction. Any dentoalveolar abscess present should be surgically drained. If drainage is not complete, antibiotic therapy is appropriate. Treatment of periodontal disease includes appropriate debridement and short-term antimicrobial therapy with oral metronidazole 400 mg q8h or oral phenoxymethylpenicillin 500 mg q6h. Periodontal and vestibular abscesses should be treated by drainage.

Treatment of maxillary and submandibular space infections should always be by surgical drainage of pus. Ludwig's angina is a life-threatening condition and the first aim of treatment is protection of the airway, if necessary by emergency intubation or occasionally tracheostomy. Intravenous antibiotics should be administered. Benzylpenicillin 1.2 g q4h plus metronidazole 400 mg q8h or clindamycin 450 mg q8h are appropriate.

Management of cavernous sinus thrombosis is by surgical decompression and high-dose intravenous antibiotics, the choice of which is influenced by whether the originating focus is dental or within soft tissues.

Deep Cervical Space Infection

Infections of the lateral pharyngeal space, the retropharyngeal space and the prevertebral space are uncommon but life-threatening problems. The lateral pharyngeal space is funnel shaped, with its base at the sphenoid bone at the base of the skull and its apex at the hyoid bone. It is bounded by the medial pterygoid muscle laterally and the superior pharyngeal constrictor medially. Posteromedially it extends to the prevertebral fascia and communicates with the retropharyngeal space. The carotid sheath and cranial nerves are within the posterior compartment of the space. The retropharyngeal space lies posteromedial to the lateral pharyngeal space, between the superior constrictor muscle and the alar portion of the prevertebral fascia. Superiorly, it extends from the skull base of the pharyngeal tubercle down to the level of C7 where the superior pharyngeal muscle and the prevertebral fascia fuse.[8]

Unlike the lateral pharyngeal space it has few contents apart from lymph nodes, but its importance as a site of infection relates to its proximity to the airway and to the contents of the superior mediastinum. The prevertebral space extends from the skull base inferiorly to the diaphragm. It is bounded by the two layers of prevertebral fascia: the alar and prevertebral layers.

EPIDEMIOLOGY AND PATHOGENESIS

Parapharyngeal infections can complicate peritonsillar abscess (see Chapter 24), but a larger proportion of infections are odontogenic or secondary to intravenous drug abuse. Rarer sources include parotitis, otitis and mastoiditis. The incidence of parapharyngeal infection has declined sharply in the antibiotic era and such infections now form less than 30% of all deep cervical infections.[11,12]

Infections of the retropharyngeal and prevertebral spaces most commonly result from lymphatic spread of infection in the pharynx or sinuses, with subsequent suppuration of the retropharyngeal lymph nodes. Retropharyngeal infections are therefore commonest in children, mainly because retropharyngeal lymph nodes are more numerous.[13] Occasionally retropharyngeal infections may be caused by accidental perforation of the pharynx, for example during emergency intubation. The bacteriology of deep cervical space infections reflects the microbial flora of the originating source. Thus, infections arising from the pharynx are often caused by *Streptococcus pyogenes*, whereas odontogenic infections are polymicrobial and include *Strep. mutans* and anaerobic pathogens such as *F. nucleatum*, *P. melaninogenica*, *Peptostreptococcus* spp., *Eikenella corrodens* and *Actinomyces* spp.

CLINICAL FEATURES

The characteristic feature of lateral pharyngeal space infection is severe trismus, which results from involvement of the pterygoid muscle and other muscles of mastication. There is also swelling of the lateral pharyngeal wall, which pushes the tonsil toward the midline. Occasionally there is lateral neck swelling below the angle of the mandible. The disease can be confused with peritonsillar abscess, although the latter should not produce trismus. The patient experiences fever, painful swallowing and pain that occasionally radiates to the ear. The infection tends to be severe and progresses rapidly. Posterior extension of the process into the carotid sheath can result in suppurative jugular thrombophlebitis, carotid artery erosion or interference with cranial nerves IX–XII. There is hyperacute sepsis, with rigors and high fever. There may be pain and swelling below the mandible, marked swelling of the lateral pharyngeal wall, torticollis and neck rigidity. There may be metastatic abscesses within the brain, lungs and bone. Suppurative thrombophlebitis of the internal jugular vein secondary to oropharyngeal infection was described by Lemierre and the syndrome bears his name.[14] The major organism associated with this complication is *Fusobacterium necrophorum*, which is usually obtained from blood cultures, but may require several days of anaerobic culture to grow.

Patients who have retropharyngeal abscess may present with fever and rigors that usually follow on from a streptococcal pharyngitis, but often there is no history of sore throat.[15] A child with a retropharyngeal abscess may be withdrawn and irritable. Adults may complain of sore throat, dysphagia, neck pain and dyspnea. The neck may be hyperextended, and there may be drooling and stridor. Examination of the throat by indirect laryngoscopy may reveal bulging of the posterior pharyngeal wall. Potential complications include upper airway obstruction as a result of anterior displacement of the posterior pharyngeal wall into the oropharynx, and spontaneous rupture of the abscess with aspiration pneumonia (which may complicate attempted insertion of an endotracheal tube). Other potential complications include purulent pleural effusion, pericardial effusion and posterosuperior mediastinitis.[16]

Patients who have AIDS, particularly intravenous drug users, have a higher incidence of deep neck infections, most commonly caused by *Staphylococcus aureus*, which is often methicillin resistant. In contrast to immunocompetent patients, there is often no leukocytosis.[17] Diabetics are also at increased risk of deep neck infections, and in addition to *Staph. aureus*, Gram-negative organisms, notably *Klebsiella* spp., may be isolated from these patients.[12]

DIAGNOSIS

If lateral pharyngeal space infection is suspected, the diagnosis is best confirmed by MRI or CT scanning. Plain radiographs are usually unhelpful. In contrast, a retropharyngeal space abscess can be diagnosed by a lateral radiograph of the neck (Fig. 32.7). The average width of the prevertebral soft tissue should be no more than 7 mm (average 3.5 mm) at C2 and no more than 20 mm (average 14 mm) at C6.[18] The neck should be fully extended during evaluation. The major clinical differential diagnosis of retropharyngeal abscess includes cervical osteomyelitis and meningitis. The latter can usually be discounted when there is obvious pharyngeal swelling, but cervical osteomyelitis may require MRI scanning of the cervical vertebral bodies for exclusion.

MANAGEMENT

In any patient with a suspected deep neck infection, maintenance of the airway is always the first consideration; up to one-third of patients who have retropharyngeal abscess will require tracheostomy. If pus is

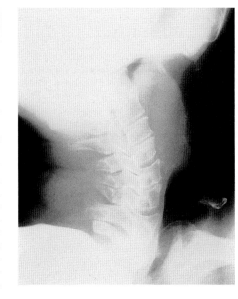

Fig. 32.7 Retropharyngeal abscess. Lateral radiograph of the neck in a patient who has a retropharyngeal abscess, showing gross expansion of prevertebral soft tissue. Courtesy of Mr R Bull.

shown to be present, incision and drainage of involved spaces should be performed and intravenous antibiotic therapy should be administered promptly in order to produce rapid and complete resolution of the infection with minimal likelihood of complications.[12] Radiologic evidence of gas within soft tissues increases the urgency, because expansion of lesions containing anaerobes is usually rapid.

Lateral pharyngeal and retropharyngeal abscesses can be drained by an incision along the anterior border of the sternocleidomastoid muscle followed by blunt dissection and drainage. Extensive surgery should be unnecessary if infections are treated promptly and high-dose intravenous antibiotics are used. Appropriate intravenous antibiotics include penicillin 1.2–1.8 g q3h plus clindamycin 300–600 mg q8h or metronidazole 400 mg q8h, plus ceftriaxone 2 g q12h. Alternatives include a carbapenem (e.g. imipenem or meropenem), or the combination of a penicillin (e.g. ticarcillin) and a β-lactamase inhibitor (e.g. clavulanate). Antimicrobial therapy can abort abscess formation if administered at an early stage of the infection.

Cervical Necrotizing Fasciitis

Cervical necrotizing fasciitis is a rare and extremely dangerous complication of odontogenic and deep cervical space infection. The disease is characterized by involvement of more than one neck space (usually bilaterally) and contiguously spreading necrosis of connective tissue, with cellulitis that extends below the hyoid bone to the chest wall, onto the face and into the mediastinum. Most cases are odontogenic, particularly after dental abscesses, but some cases follow on from tonsillar abscess or from surgical trauma to the oropharynx. Almost all cases are polymicrobial, often with a single aerobic isolate (e.g. *Streptococcus* spp.) plus two or more anaerobes (mostly *P. melaninogenica* and *F. nucleatum*), although any of the oral anaerobes can be involved.

The typical clinical presentation is usually with dental pain and submandibular swelling over a few days, followed by rapid evolution of fasciitis, which is extremely tender on palpation and usually associated with crepitus. Mediastinal extension can be clinically silent and detectable only by CT of the chest, but can lead to pericarditis, pneumonia or empyema. Predisposing conditions include diabetes mellitus, alcoholism and malignancy. Management includes surgical drainage via incision along the sternocleidomastoid muscle followed by blunt dissection of the neck.[19] Appropriate intravenous antibiotic therapy is benzylpenicillin 1.2–1.8 g q3h plus clindamycin 600 mg q8h, though rates of penicillin and clindamycin resistance of up to 40% of isolates from clinical cases have recently been shown.[20]

Actinomycosis

Actinomycosis is a chronic suppurative bacterial infection that principally affects the head and neck but can involve almost any system. It spreads directly through tissue, skin and bone, and therefore is able to form sinuses and fistulas.

EPIDEMIOLOGY AND PATHOGENESIS

The agents that cause actinomycosis are facultative anaerobic Gram-positive commensals of the mouth. *Actinomyces israelii* is the most common pathogen, but *Actinomyces naeslundii*, *Actinomyces viscosis*, *Actinomyces odontolyticus* and *Arachnia propionica* may also cause the disease. These agents commonly inhabit carious teeth, dental plaque and cavities and also the normal intestinal tract. Head and neck infection usually occurs in the context of dental disease or dentistry, during which the normal mucosal barriers are broken down. Thoracic involvement usually follows aspiration of infected oropharyngeal secretions in patients who have poor dentition. Lesions of actinomycosis consist of areas of acute inflammation surrounded by fibrosing granulation tissue. Such material contains 'sulfur granules' (colonies of organisms forming an amorphous center surrounded by a rosette of clubbed filaments); these usually contain associated organisms, including *Actinobacillus actinomycetemcomitans*, *Haemophilus* and *Fusobacterium* spp., which probably contribute to the pathogenesis of the disease.

Any age group can be infected, including infants and children. Males outnumber females by three to one.

CLINICAL FEATURES

The most common manifestation of actinomycosis is soft tissue swelling of the head, face or neck, usually over or underneath the mandible.[21] Occasionally the swelling is very extensive and waxes and wanes over many months, spreading to involve other parts of the head and neck, including the scalp, palate, eyes, larynx, salivary glands, middle ear and paranasal sinuses. Sinuses and tracts develop that open into the mouth and the skin (Fig. 32.8). Involvement of local bone (e.g. the mandible) can result in periosteal reaction or frank osteomyelitis.

DIAGNOSIS

The diagnosis is usually obvious in patients who have head and neck swelling, particularly in the context of poor dentition and discharging sinuses yielding sulfur granules. The granules can be trapped in gauze placed over the sinus opening or by injecting and aspirating saline from the sinus; by shaking the aspirate, the granules can be seen with the naked eye. Sulfur granules can also be seen in sputum on microscopic examination. Any material obtained can be cultured under anaerobic conditions. In formalin-fixed tissues, immunofluorescence can be used to identify species. There is no reliable serologic test; laboratory diagnosis depends on microscopy and culture of material from the patient.

MANAGEMENT

Most patients who have actinomycosis will respond to intravenous benzylpenicillin, 1.2–1.8 g q3h for 3–6 weeks, followed by oral penicillin V, 2–4 g/day for 6–12 months. Alternative treatments include intravenous amoxicillin or ampicillin, followed by oral amoxicillin. Chloramphenicol, erythromycin, tetracycline and clindamycin have also been used successfully. Prolonged treatment with penicillin results in complete resolution of the disease, although there may be some residual fibrosis or scarring (see Fig. 32.8). While intravenous benzylpenicillin has been the traditional treatment for this condition there have been reports of the use of intravenous agents that can be given in once-daily dosing for home therapy, including ceftriaxone, imipenem and fluoroquinolones.

Infections of the Oral Mucosa: Gangrenous Stomatitis

Acute necrotizing ulcerative gingivitis, or trench mouth, is an ulcerative necrosis of the marginal gingivae. The disease may spread to other oral structures, including the tonsils or pharynx, to cause Vincent's disease or may result in rapid necrosis and sloughing of facial structures, producing the classic features of cancrum oris (noma).

EPIDEMIOLOGY

The disease is mostly seen in developing countries in the context of severe debilitation and malnutrition. In addition, poor oral hygiene, HIV infection, measles, local irritation from food impaction and smoking are associated factors.[22]

PATHOGENESIS

Necrotizing gingivitis may begin as an aseptic necrosis secondary to mucosal capillary stasis. In infections in which the disease spreads superficially to involve the pharynx, it is most likely secondary to a combination of *F. nucleatum* and Gram-negative anaerobic organisms (*Bacteroides* subsp. *intermedius*). If the disease spreads deeper into facial tissues to cause cancrum oris, fusospirochetal organisms such

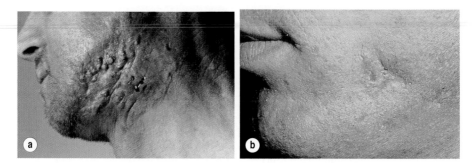

Fig. 32.8 Actinomycosis. (a) This patient had chronic disease over the mandible which (b) healed with several months of antibiotics, leaving a residual chronic sinus. Courtesy of Professor I Brook.

as *Borrelia vincenti* and *F. nucleatum* are consistently cultured. *Prevotella melaninogenica* may also be present. Biopsies of any advancing lesion often reveal a mat of predominantly Gram-negative, thread-like bacteria that cannot be positively identified.

CLINICAL FEATURES

The earliest feature is a small painful red lesion that may be vesicular on the attached gingiva and often in the premolar or molar region of the mandible, with sudden onset of painful gums (Vincent's disease; Fig. 32.9). The disease may then progress rapidly to produce halitosis and gingival bleeding. If there is involvement of the tonsils and pharynx (Vincent's angina) there is searing pain in the pharynx with high fever, regional lymphadenopathy and anorexia. If the disease spreads into deeper tissues (noma) a necrotic ulcer rapidly develops with painful cellulitis of the lips and cheeks, which often sloughs, exposing underlying bone, teeth and deeper tissues (Fig. 32.10).

DIAGNOSIS

Although the infection is usually polymicrobial, material should be obtained for Gram stain and aerobic and anaerobic culture. Debrided material is optimal for anaerobic culture. Gram stain may reveal fusospirochetal Gram-negative organisms as well as Gram-positive cocci and Gram-negative rods.

MANAGEMENT

In early acute necrotizing ulcerative gingivitis (Vincent's infection), treatment with oral penicillin V 500 mg q6h and metronidazole 400 mg q8h is usually sufficient. In patients who have noma, high doses of intravenous penicillin and metronidazole are required, with the dose being dependent on the age and size of the patient. An antibiotic to treat aerobic Gram-negative rods, such as ceftriaxone, may be necessary. Gangrenous tissues should be removed and loose teeth extracted. The patient should be carefully rehydrated. Once the infection has been controlled, reconstructive surgery is often necessary.

Infections of the Oral Mucosa: Primary Herpetic Gingivostomatitis

EPIDEMIOLOGY

Herpes simplex virus (HSV)-1 and HSV-2 can cause a primary infection of the oral cavity, although type 1 is much more frequently responsible. The disease can occur in infants, although this is becoming increasingly uncommon. Oral lesions caused by HSV-2 are seen in sexual contacts of patients who have genital herpes and are clinically indistinguishable from those caused by HSV-1.

CLINICAL FEATURES

The disease may be very mild, with a few painful ulcers and no systemic features, or it may be more severe with fever, sore throat, malaise, headache and regional lymphadenopathy. Oral lesions tend to appear 1–2 days after the onset of pain and lead to a painful, red gingiva or palate. These symptoms generally persist for approximately 2 days. The vesicles occur as 2–4 mm ulcers on a red background. When lesions coalesce they can resemble aphthous ulcers (Fig. 32.11). At this point the disease is highly infectious. The clinical course of unmodified primary herpetic gingivostomatitis usually lasts 2 weeks.

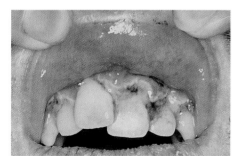

Fig. 32.9 Acute necrotizing gingivitis. Courtesy of Professor I Brook.

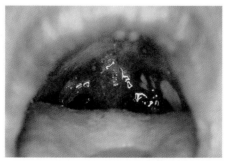

Fig. 32.11 Primary HSV-1 stomatitis.

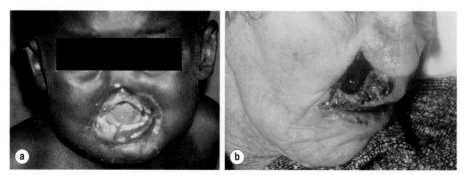

Fig. 32.10 Noma. This is a destructive process extending from oral structures, which is a sequel of necrotizing gingivitis and (a) is seen most commonly in patients in developing countries, although (b) occasionally it is seen in the elderly debilitated in developed countries. Courtesy of Professor I Brook.

361

DIAGNOSIS

The clinical differential diagnosis of oral herpetic gingivostomatitis includes herpangina, varicella, herpes zoster, and hand, foot and mouth disease. These diseases can usually be distinguished on the basis of concomitant cutaneous features. Primary herpes infection of the mouth can occasionally be recurrent and several other recurrent diseases have similar oral lesions – these include minor aphthous ulcers, Behçet's syndrome, cyclical neutropenia and erythema multiforme. A laboratory diagnosis of herpes can be verified by direct immunofluorescence or viral culture of material obtained by swabbing the ulcers.

MANAGEMENT

In primary herpetic gingivostomatitis oral aciclovir 200–400 mg q8h is appropriate therapy.

Other Infections of the Oral Mucosa

HERPANGINA

Herpangina produces characteristic oropharyngeal vesicles, generally at the junction of the hard and soft palates (Fig. 32.12). It primarily affects children and teenagers and generally occurs in epidemics during the summer. Several different coxsackieviruses, notably coxsackievirus A (types 1–10, 16 and 22) and less commonly coxsackievirus B (types 1–5), have been associated with this disease. Other enteroviruses, including echovirus, have been implicated.

Patients usually have mild disease, but they can complain of sudden fever, anorexia, neck pain, extremely sore throat and headache. The lesions are often more vesicular than herpetic, and consist of multiple small white papules with an erythematous base that appears less inflamed than that with herpetic lesions. These lesions usually spontaneously rupture within 2 or 3 days and seldom persist for more than 1 week. There may be cervical lymphadenopathy but this is unusual. A laboratory diagnosis can be obtained by culturing swabbed material from the lesions. Herpes simplex virus infection can usually be distinguished on clinical grounds, but can be rapidly excluded by direct immunofluorescence. Management consists of topical analgesia only.

HAND, FOOT AND MOUTH DISEASE

Hand, foot and mouth disease is caused by systemic infection with Coxsackie group A viruses (usually serotype 16) and primarily affects children, but occasionally adults. The disease consists of vesicular eruptions on the hands, wrists, feet and within the mouth. Lesions on the hands are almost always present, but oral lesions are present

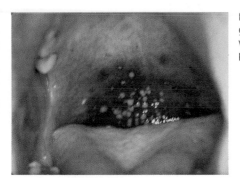

Fig. 32.12 Herpangina in a teenager with severe throat pain.

in 90% of patients and can occasionally be the only manifestation of the disease.[23] The oral vesicles are often on the palate, tongue and buccal mucosa and may range from a few isolated lesions to a marked stomatitis. In addition, patients may suffer fever, malaise, conjunctival injection, headache and abdominal pain and occasionally diarrhea. The lesions on the feet and hands are flaccid, grayish vesicles, most often on the sides of the fingers, instep and toes. If the disease is confined to the oral cavity it is almost indistinguishable from primary herpetic gingivostomatitis. Laboratory diagnosis of the disease can be confirmed by culture of feces or swabs obtained from the lesions.

Management is symptomatic. The disease is usually self-limiting and rarely persists for more than 2 weeks. However, hand, foot and mouth disease caused by enterovirus-71, associated with occasionally lethal encephalitis, has been occurring in outbreaks in South East Asia and China over recent years.[24]

APHTHOUS STOMATITIS

The cause of aphthous ulceration is unknown but a number of infectious agents, including viruses, have been implicated. It usually manifests as small ulcers of the buccal and labial mucosa, often affecting the floor of the mouth or the inferolateral aspect of the tongue, almost always within the anterior part of the oral cavity; the palate and pharynx are rarely involved. The ulcers are characteristically exquisitely painful, particularly during eating, and in the most severe form can lead to anorexia. Humoral and cytotoxic T cell-mediated immune responses to oral mucosa have been demonstrated in some patients, suggesting an autoimmune process. The lesions are usually raised and appear grayish yellow, but in severe cases they may be herpetiform with secondary bacterial infection and cervical lymphadenopathy. Major aphthous ulcers may persist for months, but minor lesions usually heal over 2 weeks. They often recur, with periods of remission lasting as long as a few years. Cultures of swabs from aphthous ulcers are negative on viral culture.

Treatment is usually symptomatic with mouth washes and anesthetic lozenges. Oral prednisolone has been used in some patients but is generally unhelpful. Severe aphthous ulcers have been successfully treated with oral thalidomide. The risk of teratogenicity precludes the use of this drug in women of child-bearing potential. Ulcers are particularly severe in HIV-infected patients.

PRIMARY SYPHILIS

Primary chancres can occur in the mouth approximately 3 weeks after oral sex. An ulcerating papule develops at the site of initial contact of *Treponema pallidum* with the oral mucosa. The papule is painless but is accompanied by significant regional cervical lymphadenopathy. At presentation patients are often seronegative, but darkfield microscopy of material obtained from the ulcer may reveal spirochetes, although care should be taken to avoid contamination of the material obtained with saliva because other *Treponema* species inhabit the mouth and may be easily mistaken for *T. pallidum*. Treatment is discussed in Chapter 57.

Candida Infections of the Mouth

Oral candidiasis is a common problem that usually signals local or generalized disturbance of host defenses.

EPIDEMIOLOGY

Most patients who have oral candidiasis are at the extremes of age, but any individual who has recently taken oral or inhaled steroids or broad-spectrum antibiotics is at risk. The disease is also seen in patients wearing dentures and patients who have diabetes mellitus.[25]

Between 1980 and 1989, rates of oropharyngeal candidiasis in hospitalized patients increased from 0.34 to 1.6 cases per 1000, caused mainly by the HIV epidemic.[26]

PATHOGENESIS

Yeasts are common colonizers of the oral cavity of healthy individuals. *Candida albicans* is the most common of oral yeast isolates (up to 50%).[27] *Candida albicans* can adhere to complement receptors, various extracellular matrix proteins and carbohydrate residues on oral epithelial cells and oral micro-organisms.[28] The organism exists in yeast and hyphal forms. Invasion of tissue is probably related to secreted hydrolytic enzymes and hyphal formation, each of which is possibly initiated by contact with epithelial cells. The immunopathology of mucosal candida infections is unclear, although suppression of normal oral microflora by antibiotics probably permits proliferation of yeasts. Salivary antibodies inhibit bacterial adherence to buccal epithelial cells and are protective in animal models.[29] Saliva also contains a number of antifungal proteins, including histatins and calprotectin, that protect the mouth in concert with local antibody and cell-mediated defense. A disturbance of cell-mediated immunity is partly responsible for overproliferation in patients who have HIV-1 infection and malignancy.

CLINICAL FEATURES

In patients using broad-spectrum antibiotics, or who suffer from candidiasis as a result of denture use, lesions are often erythematous with a burning sensation of the tongue, which displays diffuse redness of the entire dorsum. Most patients who have denture-related oral candidiasis are asymptomatic. Patients who have cell-mediated defects (i.e. diabetics, those on oral steroids or immunosuppressed patients) mostly have the characteristic syndrome of thrush, a pseudomembranous form of the disease in which there is a layer of white curd-like flecks of material that can be wiped off to leave an erythematous surface, beneath which there may be bleeding points.

DIAGNOSIS

The diagnosis is usually clinically obvious in patients who have thrush, but in patients who have erythematous lesions diagnosis can be made by scraping the mucosa and identifying characteristic ovoid yeasts with hyphal forms on microscopy. The organism can be cultured on Sabouraud's agar, but culture alone is insufficient to make the diagnosis since the organism can be recovered from the mouth of approximately 10% of completely normal individuals with no symptoms.

MANAGEMENT

In normal individuals the disease can usually be terminated by removing the cause – either inhaled steroids or broad-spectrum antibiotics – or by removing dentures at night. If necessary, patients can use 7–14 days of topical antifungal therapy, such as nystatin or clotrimazole, which is usually quite sufficient to ablate the infection. Immunocompromised individuals, particularly those with advanced immunosuppression, may require systemic therapy. For a full discussion of candidiasis in patients who have AIDS, see Chapter 91.

Other Oral Fungal Infections

Histoplasma capsulatum is endemic in the midwestern USA and Central and South America. The organism is generally associated with lower respiratory tract infection, but oral lesions can occur, particularly in elderly, debilitated patients who have disseminated disease. The lesions tend to appear as erythematous areas that may ulcerate.[30] Biopsy is usually required to establish a diagnosis. Because the infection is usually disseminated, systemic therapy with amphotericin B is generally required (see Chapters 31 and 178).

The dimorphic fungus *Paracoccidioides brasiliensis* is a major cause of systemic mycosis in Central and South America and should be considered in patients originating from these regions. Most patients have an oral mucosal ulcer with some surrounding edema. There may be perioral lesions that may be ulcerated or warty. Diagnosis can be made by smear and culture, and treatment with oral imidazole compounds is generally sufficient (see Chapters 149 and 178).

Oral Lesions in Patients Who Have Malignancy

A common problem among cancer patients undergoing chemotherapy or radiotherapy is severe mucositis and stomatitis that occurs approximately 1 week after the onset of chemotherapy.[31] At this point, destruction of oral epithelium is at its height with an accompanying disturbance of immune surveillance of oral mucosal micro-organisms. This leads to opportunist bacterial[32] or fungal infection. Patients nearly always complain of pain and tenderness in the mouth with or without formation of a pseudomembrane. Symptoms can persist long after chemotherapy has been terminated.

Management should include a vigorous search for a microbial etiology; a short course of metronidazole is sometimes helpful. Some prevention can be achieved by careful oral hygiene and effective management of xerostomia associated with chemotherapy. Once there is established mucositis, topical therapy with antiseptic and anesthetic preparations is indicated. Aluminum hydroxide gel can be used to provide symptomatic relief of painful inflammation.

HALITOSIS

Halitosis may affect up to 30% of the population. Oral malodor is the result of the production of volatile sulfur compounds by bacteria in the process of breaking down components of epithelial cells, salivary proteins and food debris. The main volatile compounds include methyl mercaptan, hydrogen sulfide and dimethyl sulfide. A wide range of oral anaerobes are associated with this, including *Porphyromonas* spp., *Prevotella intermedia*, *Treponema denticola*, *Fusobacterium nucleatum*, *Tannerella forsythensis* and *Eubacterium* spp. Most recently, halitosis has been linked to *Solobacterium moorei*.[33] Clinically, halitosis is mostly associated with periodontitis or with abnormal tongue coating.

Management is directed at reducing the bacterial load both in periodontitis and in tongue coating by oral hygiene measures, control of tongue flora by brushing or scraping, and occasionally the adjunctive use of antiseptic agents. Treatments have also been proposed to neutralize malodorous compounds by chemical agents such as zinc- and copper-containing compounds to mask the presence of the condition.[34]

Infections of the Salivary Glands

The most common cause of parotitis is mumps virus, but parotitis can occasionally be caused by bacteria or other viruses, including parainfluenza virus, coxsackievirus, echovirus, Epstein–Barr virus and HIV.

EPIDEMIOLOGY

The incidence of mumps has markedly decreased in the era of childhood measles, mumps and rubella (MMR) vaccination, which confers lifelong immunity. Despite this, mumps virus remains the most common cause of parotitis. It is highly contagious by air-borne droplet transmission. Mumps infections occur in late winter and early spring; enterovirus infections, including parotitis, are mostly seen in mid to late summer. Before the introduction of the MMR vaccine in the UK in 1988, the annual incidence of mumps was approximately 5 per 100 000 population; however, in the postvaccine era this has declined to less than 0.5 per 100 000.[35]

Most patients who have primary bacterial parotitis are over the age of 60 years and are frequently debilitated because of chronic illness or have underlying diseases such as diabetes. Patients who are dehydrated, whatever the cause, are at greatest risk. Medications that lead to xerostomia include anticholinergic and occasionally diuretic agents. Poor oral hygiene increases the chances of reflux of bacteria into the salivary gland.[36]

PATHOGENESIS

Mumps virus is a paramyxovirus and gains entry via the respiratory tract. The subsequent viremia allows access of the virus to tissues for which it has tropism, including salivary gland tissue, gastrointestinal tissue such as pancreas, testicular tissue and the central nervous system. The incubation period is 18–21 days.

Bacterial infection of the salivary glands is normally prevented by constant salivary flow, which removes contaminants from the ductal systems. Dehydration, xerostomia or obstruction of the ducts can lead to bacterial proliferation within the salivary glands and subsequent parotitis.

CLINICAL FEATURES

The most common clinical manifestation is gradual onset of painful swelling of either one or both of the parotid glands, which occurs 14–21 days after contact with an infected individual. Pain within the parotid gland can be initiated by salivation during meals, and the glands are tender. Occasionally, submandibular salivary glands are involved, but inflammation of sublingual glands is extremely rare. Orchitis is present in approximately 10–20% of individuals and is bilateral in 5%, but there is no firm evidence that it causes male sterility. Mumps meningoencephalitis may occur in concert with parotitis, but patients who have mumps meningitis often do not have parotitis. In the pre-MMR era mumps was a relatively common cause of viral meningitis in children less than 15 years old in whom

permanent unilateral deafness was a recognized complication. Pancreatitis is rare. On examination there is smooth tender swelling that obliterates the angle of the jaw and may raise the pinna. Rarely, the outlet of Stensen's duct may be inflamed. There may be generalized symptoms, including fever, arthralgia, malaise and headache, which generally persist for up to 1 week. Culturable virus is present in the saliva for up to 1 week after gland enlargement. Management is essentially symptomatic.

Recurrent episodes of glandular swelling, particularly of the parotid gland, can occur in children with a history of mumps. Clinical features include recurrent parotid swelling with general malaise and pain frequently after a meal. Viridans streptococci are usually cultured from exudate from the Stensen's duct.

In primary bacterial parotitis there is usually rapid onset of pain, swelling and induration of the involved gland (Fig. 32.13). Manual palpation of the gland is exquisitely painful and can result in discharge of pus from the duct. In addition, there are usually systemic features, including fever, rigors and a neutrophilia. The most frequently isolated organisms are *Staph. aureus*, *Strep. pyogenes*, viridans streptococci and *Haemophilus influenzae*.

HIV-associated salivary gland swelling most commonly occurs as a bilateral cystic enlargement of the parotid glands, occasionally in association with xerostomia, dry eyes and arthralgia. Salivary gland involvement can occur very early on in HIV infection but is most commonly seen in late disease. Histologically, there are numerous epithelium-lined cysts, some up to several centimeters in size, containing macrophages and lymphocytes. The commonest identified opportunist infection of salivary glands is cytomegalovirus (CMV); about 15% of post-mortem submandibular glands of all patients who have AIDS have evidence of CMV inclusion bodies.[37] In children, there is a strong association between HIV-parotid swelling and lymphocytic interstitial pneumonitis. Examination usually reveals smooth bilateral swelling. Uneven swelling should be biopsied because 10% of salivary gland disease in HIV-infected patients is caused by lymphoma.[38]

DIAGNOSIS

In mumps, this can be achieved by detection of salivary IgM or by culture of salivary washings or of viral throat swab. A convalescent rise in complement-fixing antibody occurs. In established viral parotitis there is elevation of serum salivary-type amylase. Rarely, there may be biochemical evidence of pancreatitis.

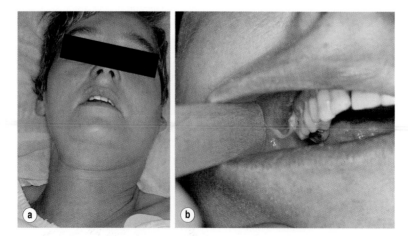

Fig. 32.13 Suppurative parotitis (a) in a diabetic patient who had a recent history of dehydration secondary to diabetic ketoacidosis. (b) Pus was manually expressed from Stensen's duct from which *Staphylococcus aureus* was cultured. Courtesy of Dr E Ridgway.

PREVENTION

The MMR vaccine consists of live attenuated measles, mumps and rubella viruses. Immunization provides protection for 90% of recipients for measles and mumps and over 95% for rubella. The antibody response to the mumps component is too slow for effective postexposure prophylaxis. After the first dose of MMR, malaise, fever or rash may occur about 1 week after immunization, although this syndrome usually self-terminates within 3 days. Febrile convulsions occur in approximately 0.1% of children between 1 and 2 weeks after administration of the vaccine (similar to the attenuated live measles vaccine), and by the fourth week parotid swelling is seen in approximately 1% of infants.[39]

MANAGEMENT

Management of viral parotitis is symptomatic. Bacterial parotitis can usually be managed by prompt fluid replacement and parenteral antibiotic therapy using amoxicillin–clavulanate 1.2 g q8h or intravenous cefuroxime 750 mg q8h. Drainage of the duct should be assisted by manual massage. Occasionally steroids are necessary to suppress inflammation and potentiate drainage. Surgical drainage of a salivary gland abscess is rarely necessary.

PAROTITIS CAUSED BY *MYCOBACTERIA* SPECIES

Nontuberculous mycobacterial infections of the parotid gland are now increasingly seen in children, in whom they present as unilateral painless indurated swellings that can be mistaken for neoplasm. Diagnosis can be made by fine needle aspiration with cytology and culture, which may reveal organisms such as *Mycobacterium scrofulaceum, Mycobacterium avium-intracellulare* or *Mycobacterium malmoense*. Management is conservative. *Mycobacterium tuberculosis* infection of the parotid gland is rare, but is one of the differential diagnoses of parotid tumor and should be rigorously excluded by histology of needle biopsy or fine needle aspiration cytology before unnecessary deforming surgery is undertaken.[40] The disease responds well to conventional antituberculous chemotherapy.

REFERENCES

References for this chapter can be found online at http://www.expertconsult.com

Gastritis, peptic ulceration and related conditions

INTRODUCTION

In 1983, Marshall and Warren described the bacterium now known as *Helicobacter pylori* (see Chapter 171) and suggested that it may be important in the pathophysiology of chronic active gastritis and peptic ulceration. In 2005, they received the Nobel Prize for Medicine for this discovery.[1] *H. pylori* infection is extremely common, affecting nearly half of the world's population. It invariably induces a chronic active gastritis, a histologically defined inflammation of the stomach which in itself is usually asymptomatic.[2] However, approximately 10–15% of infected people develop a duodenal or gastric ulcer in their lifetime and a much smaller proportion develop distal gastric adenocarcinoma or primary gastric lymphoma. *H. pylori* infection is now also thought to play a causal role in some cases of chronic anemia and possibly idiopathic thrombocytopenic purpura (ITP). At a population level, infection is protective against conditions caused by gastroesophageal reflux: reflux esophagitis, Barrett's esophagus and esophageal adenocarcinoma. Interesting but controversial recent reports suggest that it may also contribute to the 'hygiene hypothesis', i.e. that chronic infection may offer a degree of protection against conditions such as asthma, allergy and autoimmune diseases.

The term 'gastritis' is often erroneously applied to the macroscopic appearance of 'inflamed' (erythematous) gastric mucosa seen at endoscopy (Fig. 33.1a). However, these appearances correlate poorly with histologic inflammation, for which the term 'gastritis' should be reserved. Gastritis may be subtyped from the histologic appearance and distribution within the stomach, and these features often indicate etiology and risk of associated disease (Table 33.1). The main cause of gastritis is *H. pylori* infection. Two other helicobacters, namely *Helicobacter bizzozeronii* (formerly called *Helicobacter heilmannii* or *Gastrospirillum hominis*) and *Helicobacter felis*, are tight spiral bacteria present transiently in 2–6% of the population of a developed country and thought to be zoonotically acquired, as both commonly colonize domestic pets.[3,4] They usually cause mild gastritis and although there are case reports of associated disease and response to anti-helicobacter treatment, this is rare and a causal link is not well established.[3,4]

Peptic ulcers may be associated with some types of gastritis. A peptic ulcer is a macroscopic break in the gastric or duodenal mucosa with obvious depth and definite size (usually defined as greater than 0.5 cm; Fig. 33.1). Erosions are smaller breaks in the mucosal surface, which usually reflect the ulcer diathesis and should be managed similarly. Although gastric and duodenal ulcers share some characteristics, there are notable differences in their etiologies and pathogeneses (Table 33.2).

Gastric adenocarcinoma is the fourth most prevalent cancer in the world and the second most common cause of cancer deaths. The more prevalent distal form is now known to be caused by *H. pylori* infection, making *H. pylori* the leading infectious cause of human malignancy. Even the most conservative estimates place the attributable fraction of gastric adenocarcinoma to *H. pylori* at 60%.[5,6] Thus, primary prevention of *H. pylori* infection would more than halve gastric adenocarcinoma incidence.

EPIDEMIOLOGY

Prevalence and incidence

The age prevalence of *H. pylori* differs markedly between countries, but two broad patterns are found (Fig. 33.2).

- In group 1 countries (predominantly developing countries), there is a rapid rise in prevalence before 20 years of age, after which point prevalence stabilizes at above 80%, implying that *H. pylori* is acquired in childhood and persists throughout life.
- In group 2 (usually developed) countries, the prevalence of infection increases steadily with age at a rate of roughly 1%/year of life. Epidemiologic evidence suggests that this is largely the result of a birth cohort effect.[7] Thus, about 30% of 30-year-olds have acquired the infection in childhood, as compared with 60% of 60-year-olds, because of a changing incidence of infection in childhood over the past 60 years.

Associations

Aside from associations with age and geographic area, *H. pylori* is closely associated with socioeconomic conditions, particularly in childhood. This may explain the different prevalences of infection found in different ethnic groups within the same geographic area.[8] Markers of childhood socioeconomic status that have been correlated with prevalence of infection include general level of hygiene, water supply and sanitation, and level of crowding in the household. These associations further support the view that most *H. pylori* acquisition is in childhood, from when it persists throughout life in the absence of effective treatment.

Transmission

Helicobacter pylori is thought to be acquired by direct human-to-human contact in childhood. In developed countries it is usually acquired from the primary care giver but it may also be spread between children. Family members thus often, but not invariably, share the same strain, although this may evolve *in vivo* to change its pathogenicity. Although most infected adults became infected as children, there are well-documented examples of *H. pylori* being acquired de novo in adult life and several studies have suggested that crowding and poor sanitation are risk factors for this. However, marital status is only weakly associated with infection (and in some studies not associated), supporting the view that acquiring the infection *de novo* as an adult is rare.

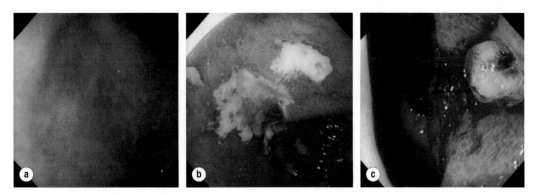

Fig. 33.1 Endoscopic pictures of the stomach and duodenum. (a) Erythema of the gastric antrum. This appearance correlates poorly with histologic gastritis and may be a normal finding. (b) Duodenal ulceration. (c) Gastric ulceration. Note the clot in the base indicating recent bleeding and high risk of rebleed and the endoscope in the stomach.

Table 33.1 Classification of chronic gastritis according to the updated Sydney system

Type of gastritis	Etiology
Nonatrophic	*Helicobacter pylori*

Atrophic
  Autoimmune
  Multifocal atrophic
	
	Autoimmunity
	H. pylori ± dietary and other environmental insults

Special forms
  Chemical
  Radiation
  Lymphocytic
 	
  Noninfectious granulomatous
  Eosinophilic
  Other infectious gastritides
	
	Aspirin/NSAIDs, bile and possibly other agents
	Radiation
	Idiopathic, overt or latent celiac disease, drugs (ticlopidine), possibly *H. pylori*
	Crohn's disease, sarcoidosis, vasculitides, foreign substances, idiopathic
	Food sensitivity, possibly other allergies
	Bacteria other than *H. pylori* (particularly *H. bizzozeronii* or '*H. heilmanii*' and *H. felis*, mycobacteria and syphilis), viruses (particularly cytomegalovirus), fungi (particularly *Candida* spp., *Histoplasma capsulatum* and Mucoraceae)

Non-helicobacter infectious gastritides are very rare, usually occur in immunocompromised patients and are not discussed in this chapter. Data from Dixon *et al.*, with permission.[2]

Table 33.2 Causes of duodenal and gastric ulceration (with estimated proportions)

Cause		Duodenal ulcer (% of cases)	Gastric ulcer (% of cases)
Infection	*Helicobacter pylori*	80	60–70
Drugs	Aspirin and NSAIDs	10–20	25–30
Neoplasms	Zollinger–Ellison syndrome Lymphoma Gastric adenocarcinoma Other adenocarcinoma Leiomyoma	Rare Rare – Rare –	Rare Rare 2–5 Rare Rare
Others	Crohn's disease Systemic mastocytosis Severe systemic illness	Rare Rare Rare	Rare Rare Rare

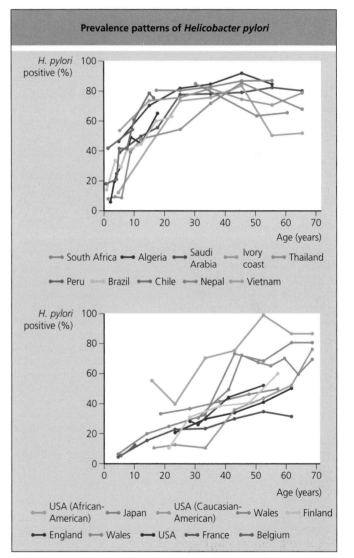

Prevalence patterns of *Helicobacter pylori*

H. pylori positive (%)

South Africa • Algeria • Saudi Arabia • Ivory coast • Thailand
Peru • Brazil • Chile • Nepal • Vietnam

USA (African-American) • Japan • USA (Caucasian-American) • Wales • Finland
England • Wales • USA • France • Belgium

Fig. 33.2 Prevalence patterns of *Helicobacter pylori*. Prevalence of *H. pylori* infection in 10 developing countries (Group 1) and 10 developed countries (Group 2). Adapted with permission from Pounder & Ng.[7]

Although monkeys and domestic cats may become infected, these are not an important reservoir for human infection. Although *H. pylori* DNA has been isolated from drinking water supplies in developing countries, *H. pylori* has not been cultured consistently from these sources and most data do not support an environmental source of infection. In transfer between humans, it is unclear whether *H. pylori* is transmitted by the fecal–oral or oral–oral route, or both. The bacterium has been cultured with difficulty from the feces of people who have *H. pylori* infection in both developing and developed countries, but it is more easily cultured from gastric refluxate into the mouth and from vomitus. However, it appears not to persist in the mouth as, although *H. pylori* DNA has been found in dental plaque, *H. pylori* culture from dental plaque is rarely successful. In past years, transmission of *H. pylori* has been documented following insufficient sterilization of endoscopy or gastric pH measuring equipment, although with adequate sterilization this is no longer a problem. Acute *H. pylori* infection by this route is thought to be the cause of the occasional outbreaks of epidemic acute hypochlorhydria[9] observed before the discovery of *H. pylori*.

PATHOGENESIS AND PATHOLOGY

Pathology and disease associations

Helicobacter pylori is primarily a gastric infection, although it may colonize areas of gastric metaplasia in the duodenum and esophagus, and rarely heterotopic gastric tissue elsewhere in the gastrointestinal tract. In the stomach, infection causes chronic active gastritis characterized by continuing neutrophil and lymphocyte infiltration, epithelial damage and thinning of the mucous layer (Fig. 33.3a). This is in contrast to gastritis caused by chemical agents, including nonsteroidal anti-inflammatory drugs (NSAIDs), which is characterized by regenerative epithelial changes and a paucity of inflammatory cells (Fig. 33.3b).

Most people infected with *H. pylori* remain asymptomatic and disease free throughout their lifetime, but some will develop an associated disease. These include:

- duodenal ulceration;
- gastric ulceration;
- gastric adenocarcinoma arising from the distal stomach; and
- primary gastric lymphoma.

There is controversy over whether *H. pylori* is the cause of symptoms in a subset of people with a microscopically normal upper gastrointestinal tract (so called 'functional dyspepsia'); treatment cures a small proportion of such patients. Longstanding *H. pylori* infection leads, in some people, to atrophic gastritis. This may be a precursor of gastric cancer, but also is increasingly recognized as an important cause, not just of vitamin B12 deficiency and its associated anemia, but also of iron deficiency anemia.[10] *H. pylori* is thought possibly to contribute to the reduced platelet count in a proportion of people with idiopathic thrombocytopenic purpura; treatment of *H. pylori* increases platelet count in some of these patients.[11] Finally, there is a weak association between *H. pylori* and atherosclerosis but it remains unclear whether this is a causal association or due to confounding, for example by social class.[12]

Less controversially, it is now clear that *H. pylori* infection, especially when associated with gastric atrophy, offers a degree of protection against complications of gastroesophageal reflux, including esophageal adenocarcinoma. Recent work also shows a negative association between *H. pylori* and autoimmune and allergic diseases, including asthma.[13] Again, it is unclear whether this is a causal relationship.

Pathogenesis

Whether an infected person develops disease is dependent on a combination of bacterial strain virulence, host genetic susceptibility and environmental co-factors.[14] Several bacterial virulence factors are found more prominently in ulcer- or cancer-associated strains than in nondisease-associated strains.[14] These include:

- the presence of the *cag* (cytotoxin-associated gene) pathogenicity island;
- production of an active vacuolating cytotoxin, VacA;
- the presence of other genes including the duodenal ulcer promoting gene A (*dupA*) and the outer inflammatory protein encoding gene A (*oipA*); and
- certain adhesins, most notably the blood group antigen binding adhesin A (BabA).

The *cag* pathogenicity island is a genetic region containing over 30 genes. The island encodes a type IV secretory apparatus, best thought of as a syringe, through which one *cag*-encoded protein, CagA, is 'injected' into epithelial cells where it stimulates a number of signaling pathways resulting in cytoskeletal changes and proliferation.[14] Soluble components of the peptidoglycan bacterial cell wall also leak across the syringe and are recognized by the intracellular receptor Nod1. Both pathways result in proinflammatory signaling.[15] CagA is also highly immunogenic and anti-CagA antibody detection can be used as a serum test for the presence of the *cag* island. About 70% of strains in the USA are *cag*+ and these strains colonize the gastric mucosa more densely, cause more inflammation and are more likely to be associated with ulcers and gastric cancer than are *cag*- strains.[14]

The vacuolating cytotoxin, VacA, is a pore-forming toxin that increases epithelial permeability and causes massive epithelial cell vacuolation *in vitro*. It is particularly suited to the stomach because it is activated by acid, then becoming acid and pepsin resistant.[16] Although only about 40% of strains isolated in the USA exhibit cytotoxin activity, all have *vacA*, the gene encoding the cytotoxin. However, only some *vacA* genotypes are associated with the toxigenic phenotype[17] and infection with strains of certain *vacA* genotypes is associated with increased prevalence of gastric cancer[18] and, in some reports, of peptic ulcer disease.

Host genetic susceptibility to disease amongst *H. pylori*-infected people is also becoming better understood. Polymorphisms in the interleukin-1β (IL-1β) gene which lead to more IL-1β expression in response to bacterial infections increase the risk of gastric cancer.[19] Many other polymorphisms in both cytokine genes and mediators of the innate immune response also affect disease risk. However, the risks confirmed by these polymorphisms differ in different worldwide human populations.

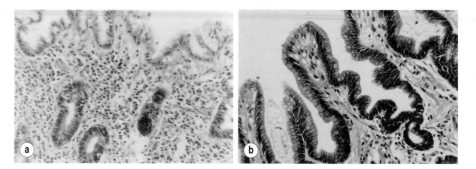

Fig. 33.3 Appearances of *Helicobacter pylori* and NSAID antral gastritis. (a) Antral gastritis in *H. pylori* infection with active (neutrophil) and chronic (lymphocyte) inflammation of the lamina propria and glands. The epithelial surface is typically ballooned. *Helicobacter pylori* organisms are not readily apparent on a hematoxylin and eosin stain. (b) Antral gastritis associated with NSAID use. Foveolar hyperplasia with a mild chronic inflammatory infiltrate and smooth muscle cells are seen in the lamina propria. Courtesy of Dr MM Walker.

Environmental co-factors are an important and underappreciated risk factor for disease. Amongst *H. pylori*-infected people, smoking is the most important determinant of whether duodenal ulceration will develop. Smoking and male sex are also important risk factors for gastric adenocarcinoma. High salt diets predispose to gastric cancer and diets high in fresh fruits and antioxidants are weakly protective.

Duodenal ulcer disease

The pathogenic link between infection in the stomach and ulceration in the duodenum is now reasonably well accepted. Duodenal ulcers arise in patients with antral-predominant gastritis. Infection of the gastric antrum leads to a reduction in somatostatin-producing D cells, resulting in hypergastrinemia, as somatostatin inhibits gastrin production.[20] Both inflammation and hypergastrinemia are more marked in infection with *cag*+ strains. High gastrin levels lead to increased stimulated acid output from parietal cells in the gastric corpus, which is most marked when the corpus is relatively spared of inflammation. The resulting increased acid load entering the duodenum leads to the formation of adaptive gastric metaplasia. This can be colonized by *H. pylori* and local inflammation and release of toxic bacterial products can lead to ulceration. What remains unclear is why only some people have antral-predominant inflammation in response to *H. pylori* and so are at risk of duodenal ulceration. Aspirin and NSAIDs can cause ulcers independently of *H. pylori* infection and further increase the risk of ulcers in people with *H. pylori*.

Gastric ulcer disease

Helicobacter pylori-associated gastric ulcers usually arise in junctional mucosa between antral- and corpus-type tissue, typically on the lesser curvature. They usually occur in patients with pan-gastritis rather than antral-predominant gastritis and are not associated with increased stimulated acid output. Although *H. pylori* infection is the most common cause of gastric ulceration, the proportion caused by aspirin and NSAIDs is higher than for duodenal ulcers.

Gastric adenocarcinoma

The World Health Organization has classified *H. pylori* as a type 1 or causal carcinogen.[21] It is a risk factor for *distal* adenocarcinoma with a relative risk of 4–9. The relationship of *H. pylori* with *proximal* gastric adenocarcinoma is interesting. Cancers in this region appear to have two etiologies: some are related to *H. pylori* infection and others are related to gastroesophageal reflux and therefore negatively associated with *H. pylori* infection.[22] Thus overall in most populations there is no association between *H. pylori* and gastric cardia cancer because the opposing risks in different individuals cancel each other out. Gastric adenocarcinoma usually arises in patients with pan-gastritis or corpus-predominant gastritis; patients who have previous duodenal ulceration (usually with antral-predominant gastritis) are less likely than others to develop gastric cancer. Both *cag*+ and cytotoxic strains are more likely to be associated with carcinoma than other strains.

The pathogenesis of gastric carcinoma is unclear and may differ between the two main types, intestinal and diffuse cancer. Intestinal-type gastric cancer is thought to occur by a step-wise process from superficial gastritis through atrophy to intestinal metaplasia, dysplasia and ultimately carcinoma.[23] One possibility is that the hypochlorhydria associated with pan-gastritis and with atrophy may allow survival of DNA-damaging oxygen and nitrogen free radicals produced by inflammatory cells or by other bacteria able to colonize the hypochlorhydric stomach. Hypergastrinemia may also be important in gastric carcinogenesis and is increasingly recognized as a risk factor for other gastrointestinal tract malignancies. Diffuse-type gastric cancer

occurs in younger individuals and may arise more directly from simple *H. pylori*-induced gastritis.

Gastric lymphoma

Primary gastric lymphomas arise in lymphoid tissue; this is only present in the stomach following *Helicobacter* infection. Low-grade B-cell mucosa-associated lymphoid tissue (MALT) lymphomas are particularly interesting as they are driven by chronic stimulation by *H. pylori* antigens. A majority of low-grade lymphomas regress following *H. pylori* eradication, but some, particularly those with a t(11;18) chromosomal translocation, do not.[24] All patients need careful monitoring after treatment and although these low-grade gastric lymphomas are rather indolent, many physicians treat those that do not respond to *H. pylori* treatment with gentle chemotherapy or low-dose radiotherapy.

Protection against gastroesophageal reflux disease (GERD)

There is increasing epidemiologic evidence that people with *H. pylori* infection, especially those with pathogenic strains, are less likely to develop GERD and its sequelae – Barrett's esophagus and esophageal adenocarcinoma.[25] This is of considerable interest because the incidence of these conditions is increasing rapidly in developed countries. Evidence suggests that reduced risk is associated with pangastritis and reduced gastric acid production, presumably because this makes gastroesophageal refluxate less damaging. In people with *H. pylori* infection, its treatment may improve, worsen or not affect GERD symptoms and esophagitis. Thus the possibility of affecting or inducing GERD symptoms should not deter physicians from treating *H. pylori*, where an indication exists.

Other diseases

H. pylori has been associated with iron deficiency anemia in the absence of other causes of blood loss.[10] This may be due to recurrent peptic ulceration in some cases but is more frequently thought to be secondary to reduced iron absorption due to low acid production in the stomach. This is not entirely due to gastric atrophy, as several studies have shown that *H. pylori* eradication normalizes the blood count in some patients and gastric atrophy responds extremely slowly (if at all) to *H. pylori* treatment. More controversially, *H. pylori* has also been associated with idiopathic thrombocytopenic purpura (ITP).[11] *H. pylori* is more prevalent in patients with ITP than in controls and eradication leads to increased platelet counts in some ITP patients.

PREVENTION

Prevention of *H. pylori* infection is an attractive public health aim as it should lead to a vast reduction in the incidence of gastric adenocarcinoma and peptic ulceration. It is unclear to what extent it might lead to an increase in GERD and its complications, or more controversially to other diseases of modern life such as autoimmune and allergic diseases. However, most authorities consider that the balance lies firmly in favor of a large benefit from *H. pylori* prevention.

In developed countries, *H. pylori* incidence is falling steadily already, due to improvements in living conditions and public health, and possibly widespread antibiotic use. Thus specific preventive measures may not be necessary. As the wealth of developing countries improves, similar falls in *H. pylori* incidence are likely to follow. However, this will take time. A good solution in the meantime would be immunization against *H. pylori*. However, although vaccine research in animal models is encouraging, whether an effective human vaccine can be developed remains uncertain.

CLINICAL FEATURES

Acute *Helicobacter pylori* infection

The clinical features of acute infection in the community are unknown. However, where high doses of *H. pylori* have been self-administered, upper abdominal discomfort and pain occurred 3 days after dosing, followed by vomiting and finally a resolution of symptoms by the end of the week.[26] A similar pattern of symptoms was observed in patients with acute epidemic hypochlorhydria,[9] an illness that occurred in volunteers undergoing nasogastric intubation for acid secretion studies in the 1970s and now shown to be due to iatrogenic acute *H. pylori* infection. *Helicobacter pylori* is most commonly acquired in childhood, but whether initial colonization is usually symptomatic or asymptomatic is not known.

Chronic *Helicobacter pylori* infection

Chronic *H. pylori* infection is characterized by chronic active gastritis, but this condition is asymptomatic. Chronic infection is therefore only manifest symptomatically if complications develop, such as duodenal ulceration, gastric ulceration or gastric cancer.

DIAGNOSIS

For all tests, other than serology, proton pump inhibitors should be stopped for at least 2 weeks and antibiotics for at least 4 weeks before testing or false-negative results may occur. Diagnosis of *H. pylori* infection can be made by noninvasive tests or endoscopic biopsy-based tests. Noninvasive tests include serology, the urea breath test (UBT) and the stool antigen test. These tests are useful in primary diagnosis in young patients with dyspepsia. The urea breath test and stool antigen test (but not serology) are useful in assessing the success of *H. pylori* treatment. In patients undergoing endoscopy, these tests are unnecessary, because tests for *H. pylori* can be performed on gastric biopsy specimens.

Following *H. pylori* treatment, whether and how to retest for *H. pylori* depends on the treatment indication. If the treatment is for uninvestigated dyspepsia, most physicians do not retest unless symptoms recur, as modern treatment regimens have a very high efficacy. Following gastric ulcer treatment, it is usual to repeat endoscopy to check mucosal healing as occasionally a gastric neoplasm can masquerade as an ulcer. In this situation, biopsy-based tests can be repeated, but importantly these tests must be delayed for at least 4 weeks after finishing treatment. In cases of duodenal ulceration, treatment success can be assessed noninvasively by the urea breath test or stool antigen test. Some physicians do not do this routinely unless symptoms recur, but it is recommended for patients with complicated or large ulcers and our practice is to check treatment success in all patients with definite peptic ulceration. Serologic tests are not suitable for checking the success of treatment as specific antibody levels fall only slowly.

Many patients require endoscopy to assess indications for treatment, and so tests for *H. pylori* can be performed at this time. The choice of endoscopic-based test depends upon the information required, cost and convenience; usually only a biopsy urease test is used. As infection is very likely in non-NSAID-associated duodenal ulceration, some regard testing for *H. pylori* in this context as unnecessary. Our practice, however, is to make a positive diagnosis before prescribing potentially harmful multiple antibiotic treatment regimens.

Endoscopic tests for *H. pylori*

Endoscopic tests are based on mucosal biopsy specimens. Infection may be patchy, and so if possible two biopsies should be taken from the usually more uniformly infected antrum to minimize sampling error. In some situations, notably after treatment, during acid-sup-pressive therapy or when intestinal metaplasia and atrophy are likely (e.g. in the elderly), the infection may be more marked in the corpus and at least two additional biopsies should be taken from there.

Culture

Helicobacter pylori can be cultured from gastric biopsies, although sensitivity is often low compared with that of other tests. Biopsies should be put into a sterile solution and transferred as soon as possible to the laboratory. Methods for culture and identification are discussed in Chapter 171. Cultured bacteria can be tested for antibiotic sensitivities and the main indication for culture is previous failed treatment.

Histology

Chronic superficial gastritis seen on standard hematoxylin and eosin staining is strongly indicative of *H. pylori* infection, but unless specialized stains are used (e.g. modified Giemsa, Gimenez (Fig. 33.4), Warthin–Starry or Genta) the infection may be missed. Histology is expensive, but sensitive in experienced hands, and may provide other useful information, such as the presence of epithelial dysplasia.

Biopsy urease test

In this test, two gastric biopsies or one large biopsy are placed in a gel or solution containing urea and a pH indicator. If *H. pylori* is present, its urease enzyme catalyzes urea hydrolysis and a color change occurs. These tests can be performed in the endoscopy room and are sensitive, specific, cheap, convenient and quick. A positive result can be obtained in a few minutes, although for most commercial tests a 24-hour wait is necessary to ensure that the test is negative.

Nonendoscopic tests

Urea breath tests

Several protocols exist, but in essence the patient drinks urea solution isotopically labeled with either stable ^{13}C or, more unusually nowadays, ultra-low-dose radioactive ^{14}C. If *H. pylori* is present, the urea is hydrolyzed and labeled carbon dioxide can be detected in breath samples. Both isotopes are safe, although it is sensible to avoid ^{14}C in pregnant women and children. The best UBT protocols are as specific as biopsy-based tests and are perhaps more sensitive as sampling error is avoided. The UBT is the most widely used and appropriate test to check for treatment success in situations where repeat endoscopy is unnecessary, but must be performed at least 1 month after any antibiotic, bismuth or proton pump inhibitor treatment.

Stool antigen tests

These newly described simple stool tests are an alternative to UBTs and indications for use are the same.[27] The stool antigen test may be simpler and more cost-effective than the UBT for community use, and

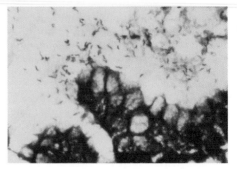

Fig. 33.4 *Helicobacter pylori* (Gimenez stain). Other special stains that can be used are the modified Giemsa stain or a silver stain such as Warthin–Starry stain. Courtesy of Dr MM Walker.

stool antigen tests are now accepted as appropriate in this setting.[6] However, the storage and handling of stool tests is crucial for their accuracy.

Serology

Although serology is cheap and convenient, a wide range of commercial tests are available and most of these are less accurate than the stool antigen test and UBT. Thus serology has rather fallen out of favor. However, serology should still be considered in patients where other tests may show a false-negative, such as patients with bleeding ulcers on proton pump inhibitors or patients with MALT lymphoma in whom other tests are negative. It may also be the best test for infection screening in primary care, provided appropriate cut-off values are employed and the best locally validated test is used.

MANAGEMENT

The clearest indications for *H. pylori* treatment are peptic ulcer disease (whether active or previous) and low-grade MALT lymphoma (unless it is known to be of the t(11;18) type). However, *H. pylori* treatment is now commonly given for other indications, including iron deficiency anemia (when no other cause is found) and more controversially for idiopathic thrombocytopenic purpura.

As discussed below, young patients with uninvestigated dyspepsia are often tested for *H. pylori* noninvasively and treated if they are positive.[28] Some physicians treat *H. pylori* in patients with dyspepsia even if an endoscopy shows no ulceration. This is because meta-analysis has shown that for 1 in 10–15 people symptoms will resolve following *H. pylori* treatment.[29]

Helicobacter pylori treatment is not normally recommended for the primary prevention of gastric adenocarcinoma, as treatment of established infection has not been shown to reduce cancer risk. However, in children and younger patients, successful treatment is likely to reduce cancer risk, so many physicians treat people in this age group if infection is found. Also, patients taking long-term proton pump inhibitors have an increased risk of developing accelerated atrophic gastritis, and although there is no evidence to date that this results in an increased risk of gastric adenocarcinoma, many physicians treat *H. pylori* in these patients.[6] Some also treat *H. pylori* where there is a family history of gastric malignancy.

Finally, in patients starting chronic or intermittent NSAID therapy (e.g. patients with chronic arthritis) there is good evidence that ulcer risk is reduced if *H. pylori* is treated. However, in high-risk patients, co-prescription of NSAIDs with a proton pump inhibitor is even more effective in preventing ulcers.

Peptic ulcer disease

Eradication of *H. pylori* not only heals ulcers but also prevents their recurrence. Therefore, once an ulcer is diagnosed by endoscopy or barium meal, *H. pylori* infection should be sought and, if found, treated (Fig. 33.5). This is usually done immediately, but if there is a delay in performing diagnostic tests for *H. pylori*, ulcer healing can be started with acid-suppressing drugs and *H. pylori* treatment can be added when the infection has been confirmed.

Uninvestigated dyspepsia

In young patients with dyspepsia, most national and other guidelines advocate a 'test and treat' approach: noninvasive testing for *H. pylori* (thus avoiding endoscopy) and treatment if positive.[6,28,30] This reduces the number of endoscopies performed (and therefore cost), is more comfortable and convenient for patients, and is equivalent for successful management of symptoms. The reason for performing endoscopy in older people is to avoid delay in diagnosing gastric cancer. Thus the age cut-off for deciding who should undergo endoscopy depends on the local incidence and demographics of this disease; it is usually set at

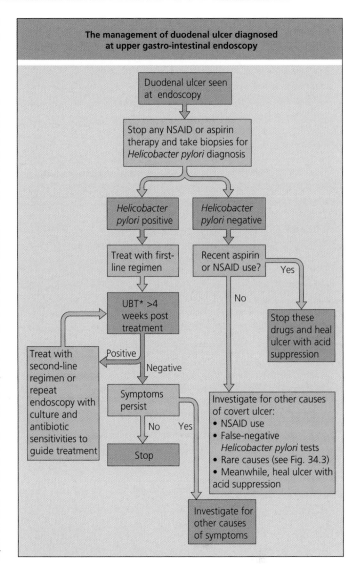

Fig. 33.5 Decision algorithm for the management of duodenal ulcer disease diagnosed at upper gastrointestinal endoscopy. UBT, urea breath test.

between 40 and 55 years. All patients with 'alarm' symptoms or signs such as weight loss, dysphagia, persistent vomiting, gastrointestinal bleeding, unexplained anemia, epigastric mass, previous gastric ulcer or gastric surgery should be referred for upper gastrointestinal endoscopy and/or other investigations regardless of age, both to exclude malignancy and to make a positive diagnosis.

Helicobacter pylori treatment regimens

First-line treatment is with 'low-dose triple therapy' consisting of either a proton pump inhibitor, clarithromycin and metronidazole, or a proton pump inhibitor, clarithromycin and amoxicillin (Table 33.3). Although 1 week is usually recommended, meta-analyses show that 2 weeks of treatment is slightly more effective; whether it is cost-effective and worth the increased side-effects remains controversial.[6] Knowledge of local antibiotic resistance patterns is helpful in choosing optimal *H. pylori* treatment as regimens are less effective if *H. pylori* has *in-vitro* resistance to a component antibiotic. Metronidazole resistance is a partial phenomenon; metronidazole-containing regimens retain some efficacy. Metronidazole resistance in *H. pylori* is common in:

- developing countries;
- in many ethnic populations within developed countries; and
- in individuals who have previously taken metronidazole for concurrent illnesses, even in the distant past.

Table 33.3 *Helicobacter pylori* treatment regimens

First-line treatments

Regimen 1	
Omeprazole 20 mg q12h*	
Clarithromycin 500 mg q12h†	} 7–14 days
Metronidazole q12h	
Regimen 2	
Omeprazole 20 mg q12h*	
Clarithromycin 500 mg q12h*	} 7–14 days
Amoxicillin 1 g q12h	

Second-line treatments‡

Regimen 1	
Omeprazole 20 mg q12h*	
Bismuth subcitrate§ 120 mg q6h	
Tetracycline HCl 500 mg q6h	} 14 days
Metronidazole 400 mg q8h	
Regimen 2	
Omeprazole 20 mg q12h*	
Levofloxacin 250 mg q12h	} 10 days
Amoxicillin 1 g q12h	

*Other proton pump inhibitors are equally effective or, in regimens 1 and 2, ranitidine bismuth citrate 400 mg.
†Several studies show 250 mg to be as effective as 500 mg in this regimen.
‡Most physicians in North America and Northern Europe prefer the more complicated first of these second-line treatments. It is thought less likely to increase risk of serious *Clostridium difficile* infection. Also resistance to quinolones occurs easily in *H. pylori*
§Bismuth subsalicylate may be used instead of bismuth subcitrate.

Clarithromycin resistance is potentially more serious as it renders clarithromycin completely ineffective. It is relatively uncommon but increasing in many countries as the antibiotic becomes more commonly used for respiratory tract infections. Amoxicillin resistance is very rare.

Recently there has been interest in 'sequential' eradication therapy where a proton pump inhibitor is given with amoxicillin for 5 days before standard low-dose triple therapy for a further 5 days. Most studies show increased eradication success with these sequential regimens, but further large scale studies are needed before this becomes standard practice.[31]

For any *H. pylori* treatment regimen, patients should be warned of the importance of compliance and of potential side-effects. Providing written instructions may be the most effective strategy. Close compliance is important as failure of complete compliance is, after antibiotic resistance, the most common cause of treatment failure. Treatment failure is serious because unsuccessful treatment often induces antibiotic resistance in the colonizing strain, making further treatment more difficult.

If first-line treatment fails, several second-line treatments are available (Table 33.3). If second-line treatment fails, the usual approach is to use a third-line treatment, most usually the other second-line treatment given in the table. However, an alternative third-line strategy (which we prefer) is to perform endoscopy for *H. pylori* culture and sensitivity testing and to give appropriate therapy guided by known antibiotic sensitivities.

REFERENCES

References for this chapter can be found online at http://www.expertconsult.com

Food-borne diarrheal illness

INTRODUCTION

Food-borne illness is defined by the World Health Organization (WHO) as a disease, either infectious or toxic in nature, caused by agents that enter the body through the ingestion of food; however, a more symptom-based case definition may be more useful.[1] Every person on the planet is at risk from food-borne illness but the risk varies geographically and also by age. Most food-borne illness results in vomiting and/or diarrhea and is commonly called food poisoning. In developed countries each adult consumes annually at least 500 liters of water and about 450 kg of meat and vegetables, along with other foodstuffs and liquids. Food production and distribution have become extremely complex in developed countries. It is now commonplace for food to be consumed long distances from its source and, often, a long time after its production. There is also an increasing tendency to eat food away from the home prepared by others. In the developing world consumption is less and food is usually produced and consumed locally. However, the lack of refrigeration and the problems of access to potable water create their own risks. This chapter will consider the causes of food-related diarrhea, its investigation and management.

EPIDEMIOLOGY

Food poisoning may be sporadic or may involve outbreaks; the latter are more common in developed countries because of the centralization of food production and the distribution of food over large distances. In the United States it is estimated that there over 76 million cases of food-borne illness per year, with as many as 300 000 hospitalizations and 3000 deaths. Laboratory-confirmed cases of food-related diarrhea in the United States occur with an incidence of 26 000 per 100 000 population and a mortality of 1.7/100 000.[2] In Europe, figures are 3400/100 000 in the UK and 1210/100 000 in France.[3] The French mortality rate is 0.9/100 000. The UK Food Standard Agency figures for the year 2000 showed 81 280 cases of culture-proven food-borne diarrhea, of which 62 209 were acquired in the UK and the rest abroad. Although responsible for much morbidity, the mortality from food-borne diarrhea is low in developed countries. The groups at the highest risk of death are the extremes of age, particularly the elderly. Studies in the United States suggest that *Salmonella* infections are most likely to lead to death compared with other causes of food poisoning.[4]

In developed countries, although most cases of food-related diarrhea occur sporadically, outbreaks from a point source are common and can affect many thousands of people. Ice cream contaminated with *Salmonella* affected 224 000 people in the United States in 1994.[5]

Salmonella was also responsible for 19 deaths in the Stanley Royd Hospital outbreak in the UK in 1984 and the subsequent finding of the risk of infected eggs led to changes in legislation relating to food.[6] Although *Campylobacter* is now the most common cause of food-borne diarrhea, *Salmonella* is more likely to be the cause of outbreaks. This may be because *Campylobacter* does not multiply well in food. Increasingly, outbreaks are related to illness in food handlers and, particularly in the case of norovirus, there may be person-to-person spread from an initial food-poisoning episode.[7]

Figures from developing countries are much more difficult to ascertain as there are rarely any reporting regulations and no routine surveillance of food-borne disease.[8] The lack of data, compounded by increasing antibiotic resistance in bacteria, can make disease control very difficult in these settings. Estimates put the annual number of deaths from diarrhea (most of which is due to food-borne illness) at 2.5 million in the tropics. Most of the burden falls on children with about 3.2 episodes of diarrhea per child per year.[9] Diarrheal illness accounts for 21% of all deaths in children under 5 years old in developing countries.

PATHOGENESIS

Pathogens causing food-borne diarrhea include bacteria, viruses and protozoa (Table 34.1). In order to cause disease, they must overcome the natural defenses of gastric acidity, intestinal mucus, normal intestinal bacterial flora, intestinal motility and the immune system. Some organisms are more pathogenic than others and this is reflected in the inoculum needed to cause disease (Table 34.2). Diarrhea due to these organisms results from two common mechanisms:

- there may be excessive secretion of fluid and electrolytes by the small bowel, usually caused by enterotoxins, that overwhelms the absorptive capacity of the large bowel and leads to watery diarrhea; or
- there may be inflammatory damage to the intestinal mucosa, typically occurring in the distal small bowel or the colon, and the inflammatory process causes diarrhea, often with blood in the stools.

Bacterial causes of diarrhea

One factor that is important in the survival of pathogenic bacteria in the gut is achlorhydria.[10] The widespread use of proton pump inhibitors (PPI) and, to a lesser extent, H_2-antagonists has rendered many people more prone to food-borne illness. In general, once bacteria have successfully reached the small bowel they usually have to adhere to intestinal mucosa and elaborate toxins or they need to invade the mucosa.

Table 34.1 Characteristics of selected food-borne illnesses associated with diarrhea (arranged by incubation period)

Organism	Incubation period in hours median (range)	Vomiting	Diarrhea	Fever	Other symptoms	Common vehicles
Histamine fish poisoning (scombroid)	5 min to 1 hour	+	+++	–	Headache, flushing, urticaria	Tuna, mackerel, bonito, mahi-mahi, bluefish
Staphylococcus aureus	3 (1–6)	+++	++	–		Ham, poultry, cream-filled pastries, potato and egg salad
Bacillus cereus (emetic syndrome)	2 (1–6)	+++	+	–		Fried rice
Ciguatera	2 (1–6)	+	++	–	Paresthesias, myalgias, headache, arthralgia	Barracuda, snapper, grouper, amberjack
Bacillus cereus (diarrheal syndrome)	9 (6–16)	+	+++	–	Abdominal cramps	Beef, pork, chicken
Clostridium perfringens	12 (6–24)	+	+++	–	Abdominal cramps	Beef, poultry, gravy
Vibrio cholerae non-O1	11 (5–96)	+	+++	+++	Abdominal cramps, bloody diarrhea (25%)	Fish, shellfish
Vibrio parahaemolyticus	15 (4–96)	++	+++	++	Abdominal cramps, headache, bloody diarrhea (rare)	Fish, shellfish
Norwalk virus	24 (12–48)	+++	+++	++	Headache, myalgias	Water, ice, shellfish, salads
Shigella spp.	24 (7–168)	+	+++	+++	Abdominal cramps, bloody diarrhea	Lettuce, street food
Enterotoxigenic Escherichia coli	36 (16–72)	+	+++	+	Abdominal cramps, headache, myalgias	Ice, water, produce
Vibrio cholerae O1	48 (6–120)	++	+++	+	Dehydration	Shellfish
Salmonella spp.	36 (12–72)	+	+++	++	Abdominal cramps, headache, myalgias	Beef, poultry, pork, eggs, dairy products, vegetables, fruit
Campylobacter jejuni	48 (24–168)	+	+++	+++	Abdominal cramps, bloody diarrhea, myalgias	Poultry, milk
Clostridium botulinum	18 (6–240)	++	++	–	Dysarthria, diplopia, dry mouth, paralysis	Canned food, fermented seafood, garlic under oil, dried salted fish

–, rare symptom (<10%); +, infrequent symptom (11–33%); ++, frequent symptom (33–66%); +++, classic symptom.

Table 34.2 Doses of viable organisms responsible for producing diarrheal disease (ID_{25})

Enteropathogen	ID_{25}
Shigella spp.	10–100
Giardia and *Cryptosporidium parvum*	30–100
Shiga toxin *Escherichia coli* O157:H7	10–100
Norwalk-like virus	100
Salmonella	10^3–10^5
Campylobacter	10^3–10^6
Vibrio cholerae	10^6
Enterotoxigenic *Escherichia coli*	10^8

Adherence

In order to produce disease, bacteria need to attach themselves to mucosal epithelial cells and colonize the mucosa. Bacteria have developed a variety of mechanisms for adherence and such adhesins are often referred to as colonization factor antigens (CFA) which are usually encoded by genes on plasmids and, thus, transferable to other pathogens.[11] Details of the mechanisms by which bacteria adhere to enterocytes have been worked out in most detail for various types of *Escherichia coli* but *Salmonella* and *Shigella* strains use similar mechanisms.[12]

Enterotoxins

The elaboration of enterotoxins by bacteria accounts for most cases of secretory, or watery, diarrhea. The classic example of this mechanism is the cholera toxin, the details of which were clarified some years ago.[13] This toxin has five B subunits that bind to the enterocyte, allowing the active A1 subunit to enter the cell and activate adenylate cyclase and increase cyclic AMP (Fig. 34.1). The

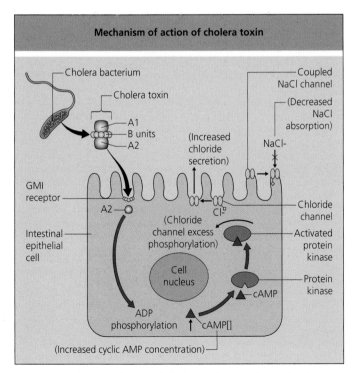

Fig. 34.1 Mechanism of action of cholera toxin. A similar mechanism occurs with enterotoxigenic *Escherichia coli* (ETEC) heat-labile (LT) toxin.

increase in cAMP results in increased secretion of chloride ions by crypt cells and also inhibition of absorption of coupled chloride and sodium ions. The net result is excessive secretion of fluid and electrolytes into the lumen of the bowel and an inability of the bowel to reabsorb this excess. Goblet cells are probably also affected by the cholera toxin as there is excessive mucus secretion as well. The mucus is responsible for the 'rice water' appearance of the stool.

Enterotoxigenic *E. coli* (ETEC) produces a toxin that is heat-labile, often referred to as LT.[14] It is very similar to cholera toxin in both structure and mode of action. Other bacteria, such as *Salmonella* and *Campylobacter jejunii*, can also produce LTs but these are rarely the sole factor in the pathogenesis of these two organisms. ETEC also produces a heat-stable toxin (ST) which leads to an increase in cAMP in the enterocyte and also results in net secretion into the gut lumen. Similar toxins may be produced by *Yersinia*, *Citrobacter* and some non-O1 strains of *Vibrio cholerae*.

Cytotoxins

Whereas true enterotoxins act by stimulating secretions, enteric cytotoxins produce inflammation in the bowel mucosa, usually through effects on protein synthesis. Cytotoxins primarily act on the distal small bowel and colon, producing an inflammatory colitis that can mimic inflammatory bowel disease. The classic cytotoxin is the Shiga toxin that is produced by *Shigella dysenteriae*.[15] This toxin has a B subunit that binds to cells and an active A subunit that disrupts protein synthesis in the 60S ribosome. Vascular endothelium may be the target, explaining the capillary lesions seen in the mucosa.

Enterohemorrhagic *E. coli* (EHEC), such as O157:H7, causes disease by cytotoxin production. This toxin is closely related to Shiga toxin and is known as Shiga-like toxin or verotoxin. Its mechanism of action is similar to Shiga toxin and often the disease is indistinguishable from dysentery.[16] It is now recognized that other serotypes of EHEC, in addition to O157, cause a similar illness and can also result in hemolytic–uremic syndrome (HUS).[17] Other bacteria, such as *Clostridium perfringens* and *Salmonella* strains, also produce cytotoxins that are similar to verotoxin.

Invasiveness

The classic bacteria that invade the mucosa of the intestine are *Shigella dysenteriae* and enteroinvasive *E. coli* (EIEC). There is local invasion and destruction of mucosal cells and the resulting inflammation leads to dysentery. The invasiveness relates to adhesion and invasion proteins that are probably carried on plasmids.[18]

Salmonella typhi and *S. paratyphi* also invade, but usually through Peyer's patches. Although there is local inflammation, most of the disease caused by these organisms relates to bacteremia following invasion. Occasionally, nontyphoidal *Salmonella*, *C. jejunii* and *Yersinia* spp. do the same and bacteremia is then a complication of the initial diarrheal illness.

Neurotoxins

Some bacteria involved in food poisoning elaborate toxins that work primarily on the emetic center in the central nervous system and on the autonomic nerves. As these toxins are ingested preformed, symptoms develop quickly. Here, the primary symptom is vomiting although diarrhea is also common. Food poisoning by *Staphylococcus aureus* is mediated by this mechanism so that vomiting occurs soon after ingestion of the preformed toxin in the food.[19]

Botulinum toxin is also ingested preformed and although the primary symptoms are neurologic, diarrhea and vomiting also occur. This toxin affects neuromuscular transmission, inhibiting the release of acetylcholine at peripheral synapses.

Other organisms and pathogenic mechanisms

Viruses that cause diarrhea, such as rotavirus, probably cause disruption of the tips of the villi.[20] Animal studies show that the virus replicates in mature enterocytes near the villus tip. Disruption of the villus may lead to some malabsorption of sugars and proteins that can be osmotically active and lead to diarrhea. In addition, a viral nonstructural protein, NSP4, may have toxin-like activity. NSP4 has been shown to stimulate crypt cells to increase secretion and lead to diarrhea in mice.

Protozoa infections may cause diarrhea by similar mechanisms. *Giardia lamblia* attaches to enterocytes on the villi by a ventral disk and may disrupt the brush border enzymes, leading to malabsorption. In addition, crypt cells may increase in number in response to infection, leading to excess secretion.[21] Chronic giardiasis leads to villus blunting, reducing the surface area available for absorption. *Entamoeba histolytica* may cause disease by the cytopathic effect of secreted cysteine proteinases that damage enterocytes and cause inflammation.[22]

PREVENTION

Sanitation

The most important factor in reducing food-borne infections is the provision of safe water for washing and drinking, and adequate sanitation arrangements for the safe disposal of human waste. Modern water supplies and sewage systems have dramatically cut the incidence of diarrheal diseases in developed countries, a point recognized two centuries ago by John Snow in London. Unfortunately, the lack of such amenities in developing countries leads to the consumption of contaminated food and water and explains the high prevalence of diarrheal disease, particularly in children in the tropics.

Food hygiene

Education about and knowledge of the safe handling of food is another critical factor in reducing food-borne diseases. Ensuring that potentially infected raw foods, such as poultry, do not contaminate other foods or work surfaces is fundamental, as is the appropriate cooking temperatures and times to ensure potential pathogens are killed.[23] Adequate refrigeration is also important so that foodstuffs are kept safely. These basic domestic safety issues need to be reinforced in restaurants and other commercial food preparation outlets by national food regulations.[24] In the UK, the Food Safety Act compels organizations to give due regard to food safety. Regulation has to be coupled with proper surveillance and public health involvement to ensure compliance, and to be alert to problems related to food safety.

Vaccines

The majority of food-borne illnesses are not preventable by current vaccines. Early cholera vaccines were not very effective but new, recombinant vaccines can be protective.[25] However, they are rarely available in the parts of the world where cholera is endemic. Typhoid vaccines, both recombinant oral and parenteral polysaccharide varieties, offer protection for travelers but, again, are rarely used in endemic countries.

The relatively new rotavirus vaccine may well have significant impact on the incidence of diarrhea in children in developed countries but will be more difficult to roll out to developing countries where the need is greatest.[26] More recently a promising vaccine that uses LT from *E. coli* in the form of a transdermal patch was shown to provide protection from travelers' diarrhea.[27]

There is some evidence that antibiotics can be used to prevent travelers' diarrhea but generally the risks outweigh the benefits. It may be reasonable to use such prophylaxis in high-risk travelers such as the immunocompromised or those with inflammatory bowel disease. A recent study of the use of a nonabsorbable agent, rifaximin, showed promise but, again, the risks and benefits are not clear cut.[28,29]

CLINICAL FEATURES

Food-borne diarrhea can present in a number of ways and often the timing of onset and the accompanying symptoms might help to focus on a particular likely pathogen. Pathogens that primarily affect the small bowel usually cause watery diarrhea, whereas those that lead to inflammation of the colon cause diarrhea that often contains white and red cells or can lead to frank dysentery. One of the common features in food-related diarrhea is dehydration which may be severe enough to warrant hospitalization for fluid replacement.

Early onset vomiting and diarrhea

When vomiting and diarrhea occur within a few hours of a meal, the likely cause is the ingestion of preformed toxins from either *Staph. aureus* or *Bacillus cereus*. Vomiting is usually the predominant symptom and can lead to rapid dehydration in severe cases. The duration of symptoms is usually less than 24 hours.

Very similar symptoms, with predominant vomiting, occur with viral infections such as norovirus. Because the vomitus and stool contain large numbers of virus particles, secondary cases are common from aerosol spread or from fomites. Thus, outbreaks of vomiting and diarrhea with these small round-structured viruses are common.[30] Particular problems arise in hospital wards, nursing homes and, sometimes, on cruise ships.[31] The symptoms usually abate after 2–3 days.

Diarrhea within 24 hours of eating

Ingestion of food containing *Clostridium perfringens* or *B. cereus* leads to diarrhea after about 8–16 hours. This is the time it takes for the multiplying bacteria to generate toxins *in vivo*. The diarrhea is usually watery and is often accompanied by abdominal cramps. Vomiting is not a major feature, unlike some *B. cereus* infections when toxin has already formed in the food before ingestion.

Diarrhea 1–2 days after eating

A large number of cases of food poisoning result in symptoms 24–48 hours after eating the infected food. *Campylobacter jejunii* is the most common cause identified in sporadic cases, whereas *Salmonella* species, such as *S. enteritidis*, are more common in outbreaks.[32] More recently recognized as causes of diarrhea are *Listeria monocytogenes*, *Aeromonas* spp. and *Plesiomonas shigelloides*.[33–35] Most cases have diarrhea which can be watery and is often associated with abdominal cramps. However, more severe cases of *C. jejunii and S. enteritidis* may lead to more inflammatory disease. *Yersinia enterocolitica* and invasive *E. coli* infections may cause similar symptoms. Vomiting occurs in less than 30% of cases but fever is common. Abdominal pain can be severe and bloody diarrhea may occur so that the differential diagnosis of inflammatory bowel syndrome needs to be entertained.

Bloody diarrhea several days after eating

Unlike the syndrome described above, infections with EHEC, such as *E. coli* O157:H7, may take a few days to evolve. These cases are characterized by bloody diarrhea where there is little or no fever. These infections carry the risk of the development of hemolytic–uremic syndrome. Most cases are sporadic but large outbreaks have been recorded with significant morbidity and mortality, including one linked to hamburger meat, a continuing risk with ground beef.[36,37]

Diarrhea with neurologic symptoms

Although rare, cases of botulism continue to occur, often associated with home-canning of fruit and vegetables.[38] Botulinum toxin in the contaminated food is predominantly a neurotoxin leading to paralysis but in the early stages vomiting and diarrhea occur, probably as a result of effects of the toxin on the autonomic nervous system. Symptoms usually start 18–36 hours after ingestion of the toxin. The delayed onset of the neurologic symptoms differentiates botulism from some of the syndromes associated with the ingestion of seafood (see below).

Noninfective food poisoning

There are a variety of circumstances where ingestion of certain foods leads to vomiting and/or diarrhea due to toxins in the food that do not originate from microbial pathogens. Most commonly these syndromes relate to the ingestion of seafood or mushrooms but it should be remembered that poisoning with heavy metals, such as cadmium, can cause severe gastric irritation and produce vomiting and abdominal pain within an hour or so of ingestion.

Scombroid poisoning

The ingestion of certain oily fish, such as tuna and mackerel (Fig. 34.2) is associated with a syndrome of flushing, vomiting and diarrhea within an hour of ingestion.[39] The symptoms relate to excess histamine ingestion. Poorly cleaned or stored fish contain bacteria that cause the breakdown of fish muscle and the build-up of histamine. The histamine is not affected by cooking the fish and if enough is ingested the symptoms come on soon after consuming the contaminated fish.

Paralytic shellfish poisoning

A variety of neurologic symptoms can result from eating contaminated shellfish. Dinoflagellates (algae) that are fed on by various shellfish produce saxitoxins that are harmless to the shellfish but are neurotoxic if ingested by humans. The symptoms come on within an hour of ingestion and range from partial paralysis to amnesia. Although usually short lived, some of the neurologic impairment can, occasionally, be permanent. Diarrhea and vomiting can occur early on but are often absent.

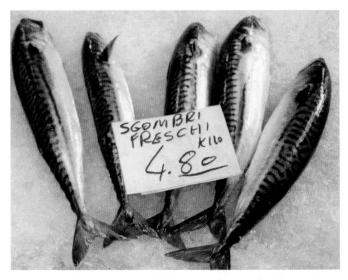

Fig. 34.2 Mackerel and other oily fish may lead to scombroid poisoning, a noninfective cause of food-related diarrhea.

Ciguatoxin poisoning

Some tropical fish, such as barracuda, may contain a toxin, ciguatoxin, which can lead to paraesthesia a few hours after ingestion. This toxin probably derives from dinoflagellates in the food chain and is heat stable; hence can be present in adequately cooked fish, even if previously frozen.[40] Early symptoms include abdominal cramps and diarrhea, with circumoral paraesthesia. Neurologic symptoms often take a few hours to develop and may remain for some days.

Mushroom poisoning

A variety of mushroom species may lead to illness if ingested by humans. Many of the more serious symptoms are neurologic, but nausea, abdominal pain and diarrhea often occur early on.[41] The most serious type of mushroom poisoning is that caused by *Amanita* spp. (e.g. *Amanita phalloides*). With these species diarrhea and abdominal cramps occur within a few hours; hepatorenal failure may occur a day or two later with significant risk of mortality.

SPECIAL CLINICAL SYNDROMES

Travelers' diarrhea

The most common infectious problem to befall travelers is gastroenteritis, particularly when travel is to less developed countries. Estimates are that attack rates of up to 50% occur in travelers and that as many as 11 million cases occur annually worldwide.[42] Although any of the pathogens described above may be the cause, the most common cause worldwide is ETEC.[43] This organism produces an enterotoxin which is structurally and immunologically related to cholera toxin. The result of infection is secretory, or watery, diarrhea. *Campylobacter jejunii* and *Salmonella* are responsible for a significant proportion of cases, as is norovirus in some settings.[44]

Risk factors include travel from a high income country to a less developed one, travel in the summer, staying in self-arranged accommodation, eating shellfish and gastric achlorhydria (usually resulting from the use of PPI drugs).[45] The highest risk regions of the world are South Asia, South East Asia, Central and South America and the poorer countries of sub-Saharan Africa.

Symptoms of travelers' diarrhea commonly start within 2–3 days of arrival and almost all cases occur within the first 2 weeks. In the majority of patients symptoms are short lived, lasting 3–5 days, but up to 40% may have to alter their itinerary due to diarrhea and around 1% require hospital treatment. Depending on the pathogen, most cases have watery diarrhea but some will develop dysentery with systemic features, such as fever. A small number of people may go on to have chronic diarrhea, some of which may be due to giardiasis. There is also a small risk (<10%) of irritable bowel syndrome developing after travelers' diarrhea.[46]

Diarrhea in those infected with HIV

The advent of highly active antiretroviral therapy (HAART) has dramatically altered the risk of gastrointestinal infections associated with HIV infection. In the pre-HAART era infectious diarrhea was a common problem, often with unusual pathogens.[47] Most of the disease occurs in those with CD4 lymphocyte counts <50 cells/mm³. *Cryptosporidium parvum* was a particular problem, frequently causing cholera-like diarrhea which became chronic and debilitating. In some cases, this was associated with cryptosporidial cholecystitis and a sclerosing cholangitis clinical picture. Although less of a problem now in developed countries, in parts of the world where HIV is a major problem and where HAART is not readily available, *Cryptosporidium* remains a major problem.[48] Other protozoal parasites causing diarrhea, but usually less severe than *C. parvum*, are *Isospora belli*, *Cyclospora cayetanensis* and microsporidia species.[49]

Again, more of an issue in the pre-HAART era is infection with *Mycobacterium avium-intracellulare* (MAI). This usually harmless mycobacterium is often ingested with water and sometimes food, and multiplies in Peyer's patches before becoming disseminated. Although the dissemination and mycobacteremia cause the most symptoms, diarrhea is a frequent clinical feature as the intestinal mucosa becomes densely infiltrated with the organism. Patients may also develop cytomegalovirus (CMV) colitis, characterized by fever, bloody diarrhea and abdominal pain, but this is not food borne. Sigmoidoscopy reveals mucosal ulceration and typical CMV inclusions are found in histologic sections.

DIAGNOSIS

Clinical features

Although the symptoms of diarrheal illness are usually obvious, the history needs to be clarified to ensure that there is increased stool frequency. Diarrhea is probably best defined as three or more bowel movements in 24 hours in which the stool is loose and takes the shape of its container. Diarrhea that is watery is likely to be a result of infections affecting the small bowel and is more likely with ETEC, *Cl. perfringens* or viral infections. Bloody diarrhea, often with abdominal pain, usually reflects large bowel infection and inflammation and can be due to *C. jejunii, S. enteritidis,* EIEC, etc. However, none of these clinical variations is specific.

Radiology

Radiographs are not useful in clarifying the etiology of gastrointestinal infections but may identify those that are severe and should be done in patients with bloody diarrhea or marked systemic symptoms. Infectious diarrhea that inflames the colon can lead to toxic megacolon that can mimic severe inflammatory bowel disease and this will be identified with a plain abdominal radiograph. CT scanning may also show severe inflammatory changes.

Endoscopy

Upper gastrointestinal endoscopy is not useful in food-borne infections but flexible sigmoidoscopy can be helpful in cases admitted to hospital, particularly if bloody diarrhea is a symptom. Some infectious cases may be indistinguishable from inflammatory bowel disease on endoscopy, although histology may be helpful. Cases of dysentery due to amebiasis often show discrete ulcers separated by areas of normal mucosa (Fig. 34.3). Biopsies from the ulcers will often reveal trophozoites in the tissue.

Nonspecific laboratory tests

In cases of diarrhea due to food poisoning there might be nonspecific indicators of inflammation, such as a raised white cell count in the peripheral blood or an elevated serum C-reactive protein (CRP). With severe dysentery, the hemoglobin may drop and with more chronic diarrhea the serum albumin will fall, partly as a result of protein loss in the stool.

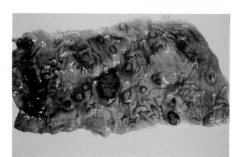

Fig. 34.3 Post-mortem specimen of colon showing discrete, 'flask-like' ulcers caused by amebic dysentery.

Stool microscopy and culture

Microscopy of stool samples in the investigation of infectious diarrhea is rarely diagnostic. The finding of white and red cells points to colonic involvement but their absence does not preclude a colonic source. Because the detection of fecal leukocytes can be helpful but often time-consuming, some studies have addressed the utility of testing stool for the presence of lactoferrin, a marker of leukocytes.[50,51] The assays are rapid and less labor intensive than microscopy but relatively expensive. However, there have been mixed reports concerning the usefulness of measuring lactoferrin and it is not commonly used. The main utility of stool microscopy is the identification of ova, cysts and parasites. *Giardia* trophozoites are rarely seen but cysts may be present. Although the ova of *Entamoeba* may be seen, some species, such as *Entamoeba dispar*, are nonpathogenic but indistinguishable from the pathogenic *E. histolytica*. The finding of *Entamoeba* trophozoites that have ingested red cells is, however, diagnostic of *E. histolytica*.

Stool culture is the mainstay of diagnosis of infectious diarrhea. Although bacteria remain the most common causes of food-borne diarrhea, cultures are positive in less than 40% of cases. Part of the reason for the low positivity rate is that various types of *E. coli* (EIEC, EHEC, ETEC, etc.) are not routinely identified in diagnostic laboratories. In the UK, since 2005, diagnostic laboratories have been required to screen stool specimens from cases of bloody diarrhea for *E. coli* O157:H7. This laborious process involves picking colonies from plates with selective media (MacConkey–sorbitol); this serotype, unlike most *E. coli* in the gut, does not ferment sorbitol. Identification by serologic or molecular tests confirms the diagnosis.

Blood cultures

Most cases of food poisoning lead to diarrhea without much in the way of systemic upset. However, about 1% of cases of nontyphoidal *Salmonella* infections are associated with invasion and bacteremia, particularly in the elderly.[52] It is sensible, therefore, to obtain blood cultures in those patients with diarrhea and fever and those with bloody diarrhea. Blood cultures are also mandatory in returning travelers with diarrhea and fever as enteric fever due to *Salmonella typhi*, although classically associated with constipation, can present with diarrhea.

Nonculture methods for detecting pathogens

These days, very few laboratories culture viruses routinely and although electron microscopy (EM) was used until recently to identify viruses causing food-borne illnesses (Fig. 34.4), molecular methods and antigen detection systems are more commonly used now.

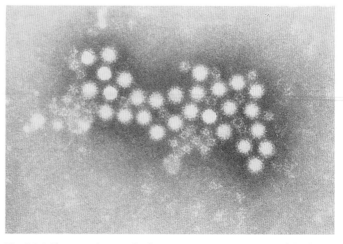

Fig. 34.4 Electron micrograph of norovirus, a common cause of diarrhea.

Because noroviruses are the most common viral causes of food-borne infections, many laboratories use a reverse transcriptase polymerase chain reaction (RT-PCR) assay to identify the virus rapidly.[53] Rotavirus detection is usually by latex agglutination tests or by enzyme immuno-assay (EIA).[54]

There are still no readily available molecular methods for identifying bacteria from stool samples in cases of food-borne diarrhea although PCR-based methods are used to type *E. coli* in reference laboratories. Although light microscopy is still the mainstay of diagnosis for parasitic intestinal infections, there are EIA and other rapid antigen detection assays for *G. lamblia* and for *C. parvum*.[55]

MANAGEMENT

Hydration

As the most common problem in diarrheal illness is dehydration, attention must focus on the state of hydration of the patient and the maintenance of the circulation. In many cases rehydration can be safely and adequately achieved with oral fluids. Oral rehydration has been promoted by the WHO for the primary and secondary care of diarrheal illness in the tropics (Table 34.3). The recommended oral rehydration solution (ORS) contains sodium and potassium (as chlorides) to replace losses, glucose to facilitate active transport of sodium and, hence, water across the mucosa, and citrate to correct the acidosis resulting from diarrhea and dehydration.[56] The WHO also recommends zinc supplementation of ORS for children because of the large zinc losses in childhood diarrhea.[57] Studies have shown that, for adults, rice water-based ORS reduces diarrhea volumes and, more recently, the addition of L-histidine to rice ORS brings further improvement.[58]

In some severe cases, and often in hospitals in developed countries, intravenous fluid replacement is used (Fig. 34.5). The emphasis is on volume replacement with crystalloid solutions that provide sufficient sodium, potassium and glucose. However, the dangers of overhydration in the elderly and the risk of nosocomial line-related infections should be borne in mind before embarking on intravenous therapy. The success of fluid replacement should be monitored clinically by assessing blood pressure, urine output, skin turgor and, in some cases, central venous pressure measurement. Laboratory monitoring of renal function and plasma electrolytes should also be carried out.

Nutrition

Malnutrition secondary to diarrhea is a serious problem in the tropics and is responsible for considerable morbidity and mortality. Feeding in these settings is important to ensure both protein and calorie intake is adequate. In developed countries there are few trials of feeding in relation to food-borne diarrhea. Most clinicians recommend clear fluids orally initially, followed by a bland diet with starchy foods, such as rice or potatoes, until the diarrhea settles. Secondary lactose

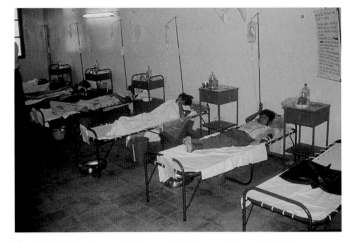

Fig. 34.5 Patients on a cholera ward in Peru receiving rehydration intravenously. (Courtesy of Dr J Sanchez.)

intolerance can be a problem after infections, such as giardiasis, that target the small bowel.

Antidiarrheal agents

There is considerable controversy about the use of antimotility agents in patients with food-borne diarrhea. An early study suggested that loperamide may increase the severity of illness in *Shigella* infections.[59] Although this has not been confirmed by other studies, this drug should probably be avoided if shigellosis is suspected or confirmed. Loperamide is the agent of choice, however, for adults with food-borne disease as it not only reduces intestinal motility but can also reduce secretion.[60] It has the advantage over codeine and other opiates in that it is not absorbed and thus relatively free of adverse effects. Bismuth subsalicylate has also been shown to be effective, even in viral gastroenteritis.[61] Trials have also shown that zaldaride, a calmodulin antagonist, can be effective but this has not found widespread use, probably because of cost and limited availability.[62]

Antibiotics

The vast majority of food-borne infections causing diarrhea can be treated symptomatically and antimicrobial agents are not required. However, there are some clinical scenarios where antimicrobials should be used or, at least, should be considered. Sometimes this is because a specific diagnosis has been made and the pathogen isolated is best eliminated with antibiotics; in other situations, there may be justification for empiric antibiotic therapy in an attempt to reduce symptoms and complications.

Specific antibiotic therapy

Randomized, controlled trials have shown that antibiotic therapy will reduce the duration of illness due to *Shigella* species. Quinolones remain effective in many instances but azithromycin is an alternative.[63] Infections with *C. jejunii* can also be affected favorably; however, in this infection, the duration of illness will only be shortened if treatment is given within 4 days of the symptoms starting.[64] Because of the dramatic increase in quinolone resistance in *Campylobacter*, erythromycin is the drug of choice and has been shown to shorten the duration of excretion.[65]

Most nontyphoidal *Salmonella* infections do not require therapy as treatment may only reduce symptoms by a day or so. However, because of the risk of bacteremia in certain patient groups, treatment is warranted for those at risk. The risk groups include children under 1 year of age, adults over the age of 60 and those who are immunocompromised.

Solute	Grams/liter	Mmol/liter
NaCl	2.6	Na 75; Cl 65
Glucose	13.5	7.5
KCl	1.5	K 20
Trisodium citrate	2.9	Citrate 10
TOTALS	20.5	245 osmolality

Table 34.3 Composition of oral rehydration solution recommended by WHO

As with *Campylobacter*, quinolone resistance is increasing in *Salmonella* spp., so azithromycin may be a better choice than a quinolone.

Although fluid replacement is the mainstay of treatment, cholera responds to antibiotic therapy and tetracycline and doxycycline are the drugs of choice in adults.[66] In addition to killing the bacteria, these drugs also help to diminish toxin production via their effects on protein synthesis.

The protozoan parasites that cause diarrhea usually require specific treatment although some immunocompetent individuals may clear the infections spontaneously. Giardiasis is best managed by metronidazole or tinidazole. If the diarrhea has been chronic, it may also be helpful to give a cysticide and to recommend a lactose-free diet, as secondary lactose intolerance is not uncommon. Infections with *Cyclospora cayetanensis* and *Isospora belli* can be treated with co-trimoxazole (trimethoprim–sulfamethoxazole). Amebic dysentery responds to metronidazole but, as with giardiasis, it is often wise to give a drug active against the cysts, such as diloxanide furoate. Although *Cryptosporidium* is rarely a serious problem in the immunocompetent,[67] it can cause severe diarrhea in the immunocompromised. Recent studies have shown that nitazoxanide is effective.[68] There have been some studies to suggest that microsporidial diarrhea can be managed with albendazole.[69]

Although Shiga toxin-producing *E. coli* such as O157:H7 may be sensitive to some antibiotics *in vitro*, there are concerns that antibiotic therapy may worsen outcomes and increase the risk of hemolytic–uremic syndrome.[70] As a consequence, guidelines recommend withholding antibiotics if this infection is known or suspected.[71]

Empiric antibiotic therapy

Some clinicians advocate the use of empiric antibiotic therapy in adults with diarrhea and evidence of inflammation. A number of studies have shown benefit but, generally, the duration of diarrhea is only reduced by 1 or 2 days. The potential benefits of empiric therapy must be weighed against the risks which include drug side-effects, prolonging excretion of the organism and infection with *Cl. difficile*. Quinolones are often used as empiric therapy but over the past decade there has been increasing quinolone resistance in enteric pathogens and, more recently, quinolone therapy has been associated with colitis due to *Cl. difficile*.[72]

Travelers' diarrhea

This is one condition for which empiric therapy can still be considered. Studies have shown that a number of antibiotics given empirically can reduce the duration of symptoms. Bismuth subsalicylate is effective but its use is limited by the volumes that need to be given and by the risk of developing a blackened tongue due to the bismuth. Doxycycline has been shown to be effective, as has a single dose of ciprofloxacin.[73] However, the studies showing efficacy of these drugs were done before the more widespread antibiotic resistance of enteric pathogens worldwide was recognized. It may be that single dose azithromycin may be more effective.[74] Some studies have shown that rifaximin, a nonabsorbable rifamycin, may be useful in travelers' diarrhea.[75]

PUBLIC HEALTH MANAGEMENT

All cases of food-borne diarrhea should be reported to the appropriate public health authorities. This can allow suspect food sources to be investigated and might also point to outbreaks, sometimes even when cases are geographically separated. Ideally, stool specimens and food samples should be collected and detailed food histories obtained from affected patients. However, in practice, many instances of food-related diarrhea go unreported and even outbreaks are poorly investigated.[76] Public health issues are particularly important in the era of bioterrorism as the threat to the food supply is an important one and measures need to be in place to prevent attacks but also to recognize outbreaks secondary to malicious intent.[77]

CONCLUSION

Food-borne diarrhea is extremely common and costly, both in human and monetary terms. Better food safety regulations, improved hygiene and sanitation, and proper surveillance all contribute to containing the problem. Increased public understanding of the issues concerned should also help to reduce the incidence of disease in developed countries, whereas continued improvement in access to safe water remains a priority in the tropics.

REFERENCES

References for this chapter can be found online at http://www.expertconsult.com

Acute diarrhea

INTRODUCTION

There is an increasingly recognized array of bacterial, parasitic and viral organisms associated with infection of the intestinal tract which can profoundly disrupt intestinal function with or without causing acute diarrhea. Acute diarrhea is a syndrome that is frequently not differentiated clinically by specific etiologic agent. The wide spectrum of evolution varies from self-limited disease to death. Death is mainly due to dehydration and children in developing countries pay the highest tribute to acute diarrhea. This chapter examines the viral and bacterial causes of acute diarrhea, clinically defined by the emission of three or more loose or watery stools per day or a definite decrease in consistency and increase in frequency based upon an individual baseline lasting for less than 2 weeks. Parasitic infections of the gastrointestinal tract will be presented in Chapter 109 and diarrhea associated with food poisoning will be presented in Chapter 34. When diarrhea lasts for 14 days it can be considered persistent; the term chronic generally refers to diarrhea that lasts for at least 1 month (see Chapter 36).

EPIDEMIOLOGY

Prevalence

Acute diarrheal diseases ranked seventh in the causes of mortality in the low- and middle-income countries in the global disease burden series, 2001, with an estimated 1.78 million deaths (3.7%).[1] Most of these deaths occur in children under the age of 5 years in developing countries and diarrhea accounted for 15% of all deaths among children younger than age 5 years, as tabulated in 2001.[1] However, diarrheal diseases ranked fourth in the causes of life-years lost to disability and premature death, just after lower respiratory tract infections, HIV-related deaths and unipolar depression.[2] The incidence of acute diarrhea in the general population could be estimated by prospective studies such as those organized in the Foodborne Disease Active Surveillance Network (FoodNet) in the USA. The network observed that 6% of interviewed people reported an acute diarrheal illness during the 4 weeks preceding the interview, i.e. an annualized rate of 0.72 episodes per person-year. Rates of illness were highest among children younger than 5 years (1.1 episodes per person-year) and were lowest in persons aged ≥65 years (0.32 episodes per person-year).[3] A study in 2000 that estimated the economic burden of both infectious and noninfectious gastrointestinal and liver disease in the USA found that the most prevalent diseases were non-food-borne gastroenteritis (135 million cases per year) and food-borne illness (76 million cases per year).[4] A report from the Centers for Disease Control and Prevention (CDC) found that food-borne diseases account for approximately 76 million illnesses, 325 000 hospitalizations and 5000 deaths each year in the USA based upon surveillance data from multiple sources.[5] In the Netherlands, the incidence of gastroenteritis was 45 per 100 person-years in a prospective study.[6]

Surveillance

Not all enteric pathogens are notifiable, depending on the country. Moreover, report may not be timeless and a recent study in six US states indicated that multiple steps between onset of food-borne illness and its investigation by a public health agency could take up to 3 weeks.[7]

Sources of pathogens

Enteric pathogens are mainly food-borne and water-borne pathogens. Gastroenteritis is commonly contagious and may be transmitted by hand or saliva. While acute diarrhea occurs in most cases of food-borne illness, there are other causes of acute diarrhea that would not be captured in this type of survey. Water-borne outbreaks associated with recreational water (e.g. swimming or wading pools) are another source of acute diarrhea. The outbreaks were associated most frequently with *Cryptosporidium* (50%) in treated water sources and with toxigenic *Escherichia coli* (25%) and norovirus (25%) in freshwater sources. Swimming pools have been demonstrated as a source of norovirus gastroenteritis outbreak.[8] Travel is increasingly reported as a circumstance for acute diarrhea including enterotoxigenic *E. coli* infection. Cruising appears to be an emerging circumstance for food-borne pathogen outbreak such as reported for norovirus.[9] *Aeromonas* infections have been traced to aquarium water.[10] As for nosocomial enteritis, patients with actual infectious diarrhea are the main source of infection and health-care workers suffering the same condition are a second source. Contaminated food is a potential source of food-borne *Salmonella enteritidis* outbreak and a contaminated inanimate hospital environment is a source for *Clostridium difficile* nosocomial acute enteritis.

PATHOGENESIS AND PATHOLOGY

Diarrhea reflects an increased water content of the stool, whether due to impaired water absorption or active water secretion by the bowel. In severe infectious diarrhea, the daily volume of stool may exceed 2 liters. Dehydration and loss of potassium (hypokalemia) are two life-threatening consequences of severe diarrhea. Water is mainly absorbed in small bowel (for about 8 liters a day in an adult) and further in the colon. By the time the initial 8 liters of fluid reaches the ileocecal valve, only about 600 ml remain, representing an efficiency of water absorption of 93%. By the time the remaining 600 ml of fluid reaches the anus, only about 100 ml of fluid remains, generally as formed feces. In the small intestine, water is absorbed by three basic mechanisms:

- 'neutral' sodium chloride (NaCl) absorption mediated by two coupled systems – one exchanges Na/H (cation exchanger) and the other exchanges Cl/HCO_3 (anion exchanger);
- 'electrogenic' sodium absorption where sodium enters the cell via an electrochemical gradient (this electrogenic sodium absorption mechanism is commonly damaged during acute enteric infection); and
- sodium co-transport.

Sodium absorption is coupled to the absorption of organic solutes such as glucose, many amino acids, and peptides. This co-transport mechanism remains intact during most acute diarrheal disorders. It is for this reason that oral rehydration is possible during acute diarrheal illness.

Osmotic diarrhea occurs when an absorbable solute, such as lactose, is not absorbed properly and retains water in the gut lumen. Infections that damage the intestinal epithelial cells either directly (rotavirus) or by a toxin (*Shigella* spp., *C. difficile*) can cause malabsorption and osmotic diarrhea. Secretory diarrhea results from an active, toxin-mediated secretion of water into the gut lumen. This is observed during cholera and infection by Shiga-toxin-producing *E. coli* and *Shigella* spp. Rotavirus also produces a viral enterotoxin, the nonstructural glycoprotein (NSP4).

Lastly, diarrhea can result from infection-mediated intestinal inflammation. After ingestion, an enteric organism colonizes the intestinal epithelium by adhering to an enterocyte. One of two pathways are generally followed depending upon the offending organism, either mucosal invasion or production of an enterotoxin.

ETIOLOGIES

As some enteric pathogens, such as *Vibrio cholerae*, are not ubiquitous, some pathogens are seasonal and some pathogens are responsible for epidemics, the prevalence of various pathogens responsible for diarrhea is variable. As for bacteria, the pathogens most frequently found are enteropathogenic clones of *E. coli*, *Shigella* spp., *Salmonella enterica* subsp., *Campylobacter* spp. and *Aeromonas* spp. As for viruses, the most frequent causes (outside local epidemics) include rotavirus, calicivirus (norovirus and saporovirus), astrovirus and enteric adenovirus. Less prevalent viruses include paramyxovirus, morbillivirus, rubivirus and reovirus. The prevalence of norovirus has recently been estimated to be 12% in children younger than 5 years hospitalized for severe diarrhea and 12% of mild and moderate diarrhea cases among patients of all ages.[11] These authors estimated that norovirus organisms were responsible for up to 200 000 deaths of children less than 5 years of age in developing countries.[11]

Nosocomial enteritis is due to *C. difficile*,[12] rotavirus and norovirus.[13] *Salmonella enteritidis*,[14] other Enterobacteriaceae pathogens and methicillin-resistant *Staphylococcus aureus*[15] are rare causes of nosocomial enteritis. In Canada, *C. difficile* enteritis has an incidence of 65 per 100 000 patient-days and a total attributable mortality of 5.7%.[12] The same incidence figure has been found in children with a median age of 4 years.[16]

CLINICAL FEATURES

Bacterial enteritis

Aeromonas infection

Aeromonas spp. are inhabitants of aquatic environments worldwide, including rivers and lakes as well as drinking water in plants and distribution systems. Also, most pathogenic *Aeromonas* spp. can be found in meat and dairy products. Some *Aeromonas* isolates encode enterotoxins, including an *alt* gene-encoded heat-labile and an *ast* gene-encoded heat-stable enterotoxin. *Aeromonas* enteric infection may range from, most commonly, an acute watery diarrhea to dysenteric illness. Symptoms may include abdominal cramps (70%), nausea (40%), vomiting (40%) and fever (40%). Infection is usually self-limiting and children may be rarely hospitalized because of dehydration. *Aeromonas caviae* is the most prevalent species. *Aeromonas veronii* can be associated with rare cholera-like illness and dysenteric diarrhea resembling shigellosis with bloody and purulent stools. One-tenth of patients are co-infected with a second enteric pathogen. Intermittent and persistent diarrhea may occur for years after initial infection. *Aeromonas* enteritis could be complicated by the hemolytic–uremic syndrome and kidney disease.[17]

Campylobacter infection

Campylobacter spp. comprise motile, Gram-negative, S-shaped, microaerophilic organisms responsible for zoonoses. Not only food animals such as poultry, cattle, sheep and pigs, but also domestic pets are reservoirs for worldwide human infections. Despite the incidence decreasing in the USA, *Campylobacter* spp. are still responsible for sporadic infections following improper manipulation of poorly cooked meat. Poultry is a major source of infection.[18] Unpasteurized dairy products and water have been found to be sources of limited outbreaks. The incidence of *Campylobacter* spp. infection is higher in developing countries than in developed ones and travelers to developing countries are at risk of *Campylobacter* infection.

The pathogenesis of *Campylobacter* infections is poorly understood. *Campylobacter jejunii* and *Campylobacter coli* are the most frequently encountered species responsible for diarrhea. Signs and symptoms vary from asymptomatic infections and may include fever, abdominal cramps and diarrhea with or without blood and fecal white blood cells. Although generally self-limited, relapses and chronic diarrhea are possible, as well as extraintestinal infection including bacteremia. *Campylobacter jejunii* infection is the most frequently recognized infection preceding the development of Guillain–Barré syndrome.[19] The mechanisms rely on the cross-reactivity between ganglioside-like motifs present in *Campylobacter jejunii* lipopolysaccharide and those of peripheral nerves. Also, this species has been associated with immunoproliferative small intestinal disease.[20] Species other than *Campylobacter jejunii* and *Campylobacter coli* are increasingly isolated from the stools of patients with diarrhea, including *Campylobacter fetus*, mainly isolated from extraintestinal sites, and *Campylobacter upsaliensis*. As both species are susceptible to cephalotin, an antibiotic usually incorporated in *Campylobacter jejunii*-selective media, their prevalence in stools and diarrhea may be underestimated by culture methods.

Clostridium difficile infection

Clostridium difficile is a sporulated Gram-positive anaerobe of the Firmicutes phylum. Spores are highly resistant in an inanimate environment which can be a source of infection. *Clostridium difficile* genome analysis indicated that this extremely variable genome encodes toxin A and toxin B[21] which are cytotoxic toxins implicated in the inflammatory intestinal lesions. Some *C. difficile* strains encode only toxin B and may be missed in laboratory tests detecting only toxin A. Also, emerging *C. difficile* clones have recently been identified as being responsible for both community-acquired and nosocomial severe enteritis due to the additional production of the iota toxin[22] or to the hyperproduction of toxin A and toxin B due to mutation in the regulator gene.[23]

Clostridium difficile is indeed responsible for episodes of community-acquired and nosocomial acute enteritis, some of them associated with the previous administration of a wide variety of antibiotics, with *C. difficile* being responsible for about 20% of antibiotic-associated diarrhea.[24] If the use of the offending antibiotic continues, *C. difficile* may cause severe enteritis and life-threatening pseudomembranous colitis.

Escherichia coli infection

Of the six *Escherichia* spp., *E. coli* organisms are common inhabitants of the intestinal tract of healthy people, yet a limited number of clones are responsible for acute diarrhea and extraintestinal infections. *Escherichia fergusonii* is frequently isolated from stools, yet its pathogenic role is unproven; *Escherichia albertii* is a possible agent of acute diarrhea.[25] There are five groups of *E. coli* organisms associated with acute diarrhea:

- Shiga-toxin producing *E. coli* (STEC), also termed enterohemorrhagic *E. coli* (EHEC);
- enterotoxigenic *E. coli* (ETEC);
- enteropathogenic *E. coli* (EPEC);
- enteroaggregative *E. coli* (EAEC); and
- enteroinvasive *E. coli* (EIEC).

STEC produce one or several Shiga toxins (also known as verocytotoxins) and are the most frequent *E. coli* organisms associated with acute diarrhea in developed countries. These organisms, comprising various *E. coli* O157 serotypes, are responsible for mild non-bloody and bloody acute diarrhea.[26] Non-O157:H7 STEC are associated with illnesses that differ from those caused by *E. coli* O157:H7. Most notably, they are found later and have a lower proportion of bloody diarrhea than in patients infected with *E. coli* O157:H7.[27] STEC are also responsible for an estimated 80% of hemolytic–uremic syndrome cases in about 4% of patients with enteric infection. Ground beef has been the major vehicle of transmission of O157 STEC, although other vehicles contaminated by bovine manure have been reported, including raw milk, sausage, apple cider, raw vegetables and nonchlorinated water supplies. Additionally, person-to-person transmission is responsible for outbreaks in communities.

ETEC produce heat-labile (LT) and heat-stable (ST) enterotoxins and are a frequent cause of acute diarrhea in developing countries, thus being a frequent cause of travelers' diarrhea. ETEC infection manifests as relatively mild watery diarrhea and abdominal cramps, but no vomiting or fever.

EPEC comprise organisms characterized by an adherence factor plasmid and the chromosomal locus of enterocyte effacement. These organisms are responsible for severe infantile diarrhea in developing countries associated with fever, vomiting and prolonged evolution. Chronic diarrhea may follow EPEC infection and be responsible for malabsorption, weight loss and growth retardation.

EIEC are responsible for an infection mimicking shigellosis. EAEC are responsible for worldwide, mild enteric infections with non-bloody diarrhea, abdominal pain and mild fever.

Salmonella infection

The genus *Salmonella* comprises motile enteric bacteria of problematic nomenclature. *Salmonella* comprises two species and the species *Salmonella enterica* comprises five subspecies. The vast majority of human infections are due to strains of *Salmonella enterica* subspecies I, also isolated from warm-blooded animals, while the other *Salmonella* organisms are isolated from the environment and cold-blooded animals. These organisms are further serotyped and serotype generally correlates with the food source of infection. Notably, *Salmonella enterica* serotype Typhi is the agent of typhoid fever. *Salmonella enterica* serotypes Enteritidis and Typhimurium are the most commonly isolated in developed countries. Salmonellosis outcome differs significantly with serotype.[28]

Nontyphoidal *Salmonella enterica* organisms are responsible for acute diarrhea with fever and abdominal cramps lasting for an average of 1 week. Rarely, these organisms are responsible for bacteremia and extraintestinal infections in immunocompromised patients. Contacts with animals and animal foods are the sources of infection, with the Enteritidis serotype being associated with chicken and egg products. Serotype Cholerasuis is adapted to pigs and serotype Dublin is adapted to cattle. Later serotypes harbor virulence traits in common with serotype Typhi, the typhoid fever agent. Typhoid fever is a life-threatening septicemia rarely observed in developed countries but still of public health concern in developing countries. The mortality rate in patients who did not receive appropriate therapy is more than 10% whereas it is less than 1% in patients who did receive appropriate antibiotic therapy.

Clinical presentation includes fever and headache without diarrhea and healthy carriers have been observed. Humans are the only known reservoir for serotype Typhi, which can be transmitted by direct person-to-person contact and contaminated water and food. A syndrome similar to typhoid fever is due to serotypes Paratyphi A, Paratyphi B and Paratyphi C.

Shigella infection

Although from a genetic standpoint, *E. coli* and *Shigella* spp. form a single bacterial species, four subgroups of *Shigella* have been taken as different species, i.e. *Shigella dysenteriae*, *Shigella flexneri*, *Shigella boydii* and *Shigella sonnei*.[29] Humans are the only known reservoir for *Shigella* spp. and transmission is by direct contact from person to person and by contaminated water and food. Sexual transmission has been observed in homosexual males. Most cases in developed countries are imported from developing countries. *Shigella* spp. are responsible for bacillary dysentery characterized by acute, bloody diarrhea accompanied by fever and abdominal cramps. Classic dysentery is characterized by the emission of scant stools containing mucus, pus and blood. Shigellosis is responsible for rectal and colonic ulcerations which do not develop beyond the lamina propria. Rare cases of septicemia have been observed but *Shigella* spp. are responsible for the hemolytic–uremic syndrome.

Vibrio infection

Vibrios are ubiquitously found in aquatic environments and are classified into more than 70 species responsible for trauma-related, extraintestinal infections and intestinal infections with diarrhea.[30] *Vibrio cholerae* is the etiologic agent of cholera. This is a motile, Gram-negative, facultative anaerobe bacterium which requires a small concentration of sodium for growth. *Vibrio cholerae* is primarily an aquatic inhabitant found in freshwater rivers and lakes as well as in estuarine and maritime environments. In these environments, *V. cholerae* is isolated from both inanimate environments and from plankton and various bivalves, crabs, shrimp and prawns. A viable-but-not-cultivable state has been described, the regulation of which may be phage-dependent.[31]

Vibrio cholerae comprises three major subgroups: *V. cholerae* O1, *V. cholerae* O139 and *V. cholerae* non-O1, widely distributed in tropical and subtropical areas, including the Gulf of Mexico for *V. cholerae* O1. The *V. cholerae* O1 chromosome contains a virulence cassette and pathogenicity islands, encoding virulence factors such as the pilus responsible for the attachment of *V. cholerae* O1 organisms to the intestinal epithelium and the cholera enterotoxin responsible for the large excretion of electrolytes and water in the intestinal lumen. Two biotypes, designated classic and El Tor, can be differentiated on the basis of simple laboratory tests including the hemolysis of sheep erythrocytes, the Voges–Proskauer test and the resistance to polymyxin, which are all positive in the El Tor biotype. The first six historical pandemics are though to be due to the classic biotype whereas the ongoing seventh pandemic (which started in 1961) is due to the El Tor biotype.

Vibrio cholerae O1 is the organism responsible for historic pandemics of cholera since 1816, including the current pandemics. Contamination may be hand transmitted through water drinking (and flies). Most patients contaminated with *V. cholerae* O1 have an asymptomatic or self-limited diarrhea (>75%), but massive contamination results in severe diarrhea with large volumes of 'rice water stools' and dehydration or infection in patients with neutral gastric pH. Clinical manifestations include loss of skin elasticity, watery eyes, painful muscle cramps and anuria. Dehydration leads to hypovolemic shock and death. Exceptional extraintestinal *V. cholerae* O1 bacteremia infections have been reported.

In 1992, cholera cases due to a new serogroup *V. cholerae* O139 (Bengal) were reported in India and Bangladesh and spread rapidly throughout Asia. The new serogroup probably resulted from the lateral gene transfer of novel capsule and somatic antigen genes to the El Tor strain. It causes disease similar to that caused by *V. cholerae* O1 except that adults are more frequently infected.

Some *V. cholerae* isolates do not agglutinate with anti-O1 and anti-O139 antisera and are therefore referred as *V. cholerae* non-O1 isolates. *Vibrio cholerae* non-O1 isolates do not produce the cholera enterotoxin and are responsible for mild watery diarrhea. Unlike *V. cholerae* O1 isolates, *V. cholerae* non-O1 isolates are responsible for extraintestinal infections, such as life-threatening septicemia, especially in patients with previous liver disease or hematologic malignancies. *Vibrio cholerae* non-O1 isolates have also been recovered from other anatomic sites.

Other *Vibrio* spp. responsible for diarrhea include *V. mimicus*, a species phenotypically related to *V. cholerae*, which is responsible for diarrhea after the consumption of raw seafoods; some strains harboring the cholera toxin can produce cholera-like symptoms. In Asia, *V. parahaemolyticus* is the leading cause of food-borne intestinal infections after the consumption of raw fish or shellfish. The species is responsible for watery diarrhea, rarely bloody diarrhea, and is particularly responsible for severe dehydration and death. The first pandemic clone, *V. parahaemolyticus* serotype O3:K6, emerged in 1996 in Taiwan and then spread throughout Asia to America, Africa and Russia. New serotypes emerged for a few years.

Vibrio vulnificus is primarily responsible for life-threatening septicemia and secondary skin infection with necrosis. It has an intestinal route of entry and is responsible for vomiting, diarrhea and abdominal cramps after the consumption of raw oysters in 95% of patients. Three biogroups have been defined in *V. vulnificus*, the vast majority of infections being due to biogroup 1. *Vibrio fluvialis*, *Vibrio furnisii* and *Grimontia* (*Vibrio*) *hollisae* cause sporadic cases of diarrhea worldwide.[32,33] *Vibrio alginolyticus* is seldom isolated from stools and there is little evidence for *V. alginolyticus* actually being responsible for intestinal infection and diarrhea.

Yersinia infection

Among the numerous members of the *Yersinia* genus, only *Yersinia enterocolitica* and *Yersinia pseudotuberculosis* have been associated with digestive tract infection. *Yersinia enterocolitica*, further divided into two subspecies *enterocolitica* and *palearctica* on the basis of 16S rDNA sequencing,[34] comprises more than 70 serotypes, five of them being associated with human infection. These strains encode for an enterotoxin and some strains harbor a chromosome-borne pathogenicity island which contains the yersiniabactin gene, providing the organisms with iron. *Yersinia enterocolitica* is primarily an environmental organism isolated from the gastrointestinal tract of numerous animals, most commonly swine, dogs and rodents. Its distribution is mostly in Northern Europe and northern states of the USA, reflecting its increased growth at cold temperatures. This species is responsible for gastroenteritis associated with the consumption of contaminated water and food, mainly poorly cooked pork.

The disease spectrum comprises self-limited, acute diarrhea to terminal ileitis and mesenteric lymphadenitis mimicking appendicitis. Prolonged shedding has been observed. Septicemia is an uncommon complication observed in patients with an increased iron pool such as thalassaemic patients in Western countries,[35] patients with liver disease or cancer and those undergoing steroid therapy. *Yersinia enterocolitica* is the bacterial organism most frequently associated with blood transfusion. Reactive arthritis is an uncommon sequel observed in HLA-B27 positive patients and immunocompromised patients; it is characterized by asymmetric involvement of multiple joints including the sacroiliac joint and the spine.

Yersinia pseudotuberculosis is rarely isolated as a cause of a self-limited acute diarrhea; it has been associated with outbreaks of gastroenteritis after consumption of contaminated fresh vegetables.[36,37]

Yersinia pseudotuberculosis is also responsible for pseudoappendicitis, and reactive arthritis may develop after infection with *Yersinia pseudotuberculosis* O3.[38]

Miscellaneous bacteria

Arcobacter are *Campylobacter*-like organisms seldom isolated from the stools of patients with diarrhea, including *Arcobacter butzleri*[39] and *Arcobacter cryaerophilus* DNA group 1B.[40] Particular culture conditions are required for proper isolation of these fastidious organisms, thus limiting their detection to a few studies.

Listeria monocytogenes has only recently been recognized as an agent of acute enteritis, mainly transmitted by milk, but it has now been associated with several enteritis outbreaks.[41] Enteritis typically occurs after ingestion of a large inoculum and is self-limited after a few days' evolution.[42]

Klebsiella oxytoca is found in the environment but its principal reservoir is the human gastrointestinal tract; it has been associated with *C. difficile*-negative antibiotic-associated colitis.[43] *Klebsiella oxytoca* organisms cause experimental colitis and exhibit cytotoxicity against HEp-2 cultured cells.[43] Its culture is not routinely performed and requires a specific isolation agar medium.

Laribacter hongkongensis is a facultative anaerobic Gram-negative bacillus initially reported as being responsible for acute diarrhea in Asian patients.[44] A case-controlled study indicated that eating fish and travel were associated with *L. hongkongensis* acute diarrhea.[45]

Dysgonomonas capnocytophagoides (formerly CDC group DF-3)[46] are *Captocytophaga*-like organisms isolated from the stools of immunocompromised patients.[47–49]

Viral enteritis

Rotavirus infections

Rotaviruses are RNA viruses presenting as 70 nm particles with a wheel-like appearance (Fig. 35.1). Based on group-specific antigens of the major viral structural protein VP6, rotavirus can be classified into six groups, A–G. Groups A–C infect humans; the other groups are found in animals. Human rotaviruses are responsible for severe acute diarrhea with dehydration associated with childhood death in developing countries. In Europe, children with rotavirus-positive acute gastroenteritis were more likely to have lethargy, fever, vomiting and dehydration, and, therefore, more severe disease than were children with rotavirus-negative acute gastroenteritis. Dehydration was up to 5.5 times more likely in children with rotavirus-positive acute gastroenteritis than in those with rotavirus-negative acute gastroenteritis.[50] Acquisition of rotaviruses is likely from subclinical infection in parents or siblings but rotavirus infection can be a zoonosis. Rotaviruses are resistant in inanimate environments which may be implicated as a source of infection, including nosocomial outbreaks. Rotavirus infection is seasonal, with a peak incidence in winter/spring in temperate countries. Clinical symptoms include acute diarrhea for 2–3 days, fever, vomiting and anorexia.

Calicivirus infections

The family Caliciviridae comprises norovirus and saprovirus, both responsible for enteritis. These RNA viruses appear as <40 nm non-enveloped particles. Norovirus comprises five genotypes: genotypes I, II and IV are responsible for human infections, genotypes III and V are animal associated. Likewise, saprovirus comprises five genotypes; genotypes I, II, IV and V are responsible for human infections. These highly contagious human viruses reside in inanimate environments comprising contaminated surfaces, water and food. Direct evidence for animals as a reservoir for human infection is still lacking.

Noroviruses are the most prevalent cause of nonbacterial acute enteritis worldwide.[51] These viruses cause large outbreaks and provoke incapacity for a few days; they have therefore been included in List B

The direct diagnosis of acute diarrhea in the microbiology laboratory

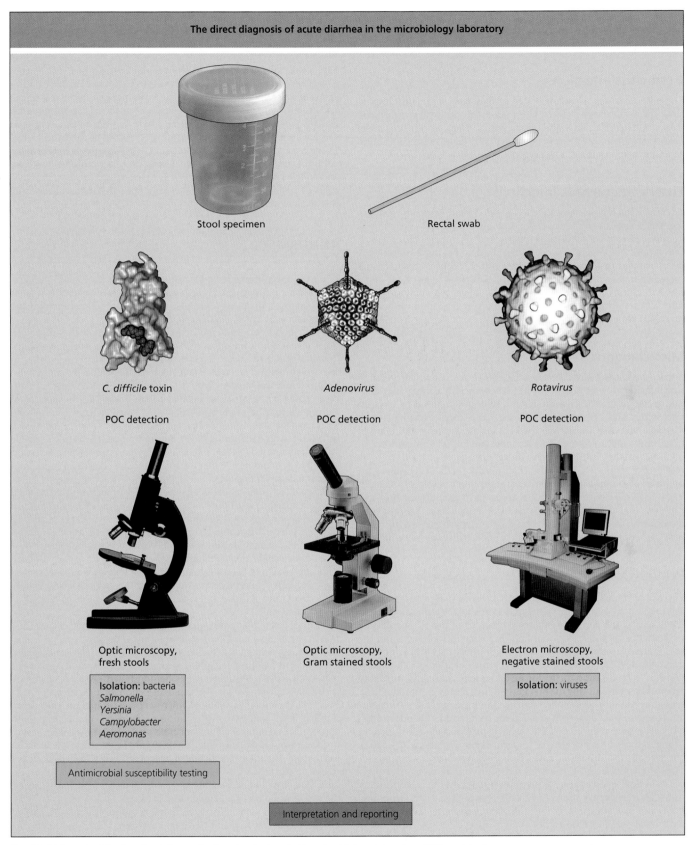

Stool specimen

Rectal swab

C. difficile toxin

Adenovirus

Rotavirus

POC detection

POC detection

POC detection

Optic microscopy, fresh stools

Optic microscopy, Gram stained stools

Electron microscopy, negative stained stools

Isolation: bacteria
Salmonella
Yersinia
Campylobacter
Aeromonas

Isolation: viruses

Antimicrobial susceptibility testing

Interpretation and reporting

Fig. 35.1 Flow-chart for the direct diagnosis of acute diarrhea in the microbiology laboratory. POC, point of care.

of potential bioterrorism agents by the US National Institute of Allergy and Infectious Diseases (NIAID). Outbreaks mainly occur in institutions, health-care centers and cruise ships.

Astrovirus infections

These RNA viruses, averaging 30 nm in diameter, are mainly responsible for acute diarrhea in children, although outbreaks in military troops and hospitals have also been reported. These worldwide viruses are responsible for 2–10% of pediatric cases of acute diarrhea. Clinical signs and symptoms are nonspecific.[52]

Enteric adenovirus infections

Adenoviruses are nonenveloped, 100 nm round particles containing DNA and are responsible for human infections. Adenoviruses are divided into 51 different serotypes and six subgroups, of which only two serotypes – Ad40 and Ad41 (subgroup F) – have been clearly demonstrated to be agents of acute diarrhea. Clinical characteristics include a higher prevalence in children less than 4 years of age and a mean duration of disease of 5–10 days, i.e. longer than that caused by other viruses. Prolonged diarrhea has been observed in immunocompromised patients.[53]

Miscellaneous viruses

A few other viruses have been associated with acute diarrhea, yet their role remains to be firmly established. These include coronavirus, definite agents of diarrhea in animals and seldom visualized by electron microscopy and isolated in culture from the stools of patients with diarrhea. Likewise, toroviruses are responsible for acute human gastroenteritis and are responsible for nosocomial cases. Aichi virus, a member of the family Picornaviridae, has been characterized by reverse transcriptase-polymerase chain reaction (RT-PCR) during an outbreak of enteritis following the consumption of oysters in Japan.[54] Picobirnaviruses have been detected in stools of animals and humans; however, their significance remains to be established. Recently, cardioviruses closely related to Theiler's murine encephalomyelitis virus have been detected in stools in 1.2% patients with acute enteritis.[55]

Prevention

The global mortality from diarrhea declined from approximately 4.6 million annual deaths during the mid-1980s to 2.4 million deaths in 1990, and to the current estimate of 1.6–2.1 million.[1,56] The decline is generally attributed to global improvements in sanitation and the use of glucose–electrolyte oral rehydration therapy (ORT) which has dramatically reduced acute mortality from dehydration caused by diarrhea. In contrast to the fortunate decrease in mortality, morbidity remains as high as during the previous century. However, simple, cheap measures could be undertaken to make the incidence fall. A prospective study in India demonstrated that the promotion of hand washing with plain soap reduced by 53% the incidence of acute diarrhea (and of pneumonia and impetigo).[57] Indeed, hand washing with soap is effective against almost all enteritis-causing pathogens, whereas efficacy of alcohol against rotavirus and calicivirus remains controversial.[58] In developed countries, prevention relies on increased sanitary measures in collective sources of enteric pathogens such as swimming pools and recreational lakes for fishing and swimming, as well as better control over fresh foodstuffs. Patients should be isolated at home and children excluded from nurseries and school for the duration of the illness.

Another vaccine against ETEC, administered as a patch, is being evaluated.[59] A live oral vaccine against rotavirus has recently been licensed after a few previous attempts and its safety and preventive effects have been carefully evaluated.[60] Cost-effectiveness of vaccine against rotavirus has been evaluated favorably in the Netherlands.[61]

As for travelers, pre-travel prophylaxis relies on vaccines. There is currently only one vaccine available that provides protection against diarrhea caused by *Vibrio cholerae* and by ETEC. This vaccine is licensed in only a few Western countries. Protective efficacy against cholera is 85%, while protection against the heat-labile toxin of ETEC reaches 67%. Current studies show a protective effect of up to 43%. Vaccination against cholera and ETEC should be recommended for at-risk travelers, in particular those with high exposure at their travel destination or high personal risks through fluid loss.[62] Typhim Vi is a conjugate vaccine aimed at prevention of typhoid fever, and its safety and effectiveness have been favorably evaluated.[63,64] During travel, systematic administration of antibiotics including fluoroquinolones, cyclines and co-trimoxazole is controversial. Prophylaxis may rely on the basic rules of boiling fresh water or drinking bottled water, and ensuring that meat is well cooked.

DIAGNOSIS

There is no recommended serologic test for the microbiologic diagnosis of enteric pathogens and the laboratory diagnosis of diarrhea relies solely on direct diagnosis. Serologic testing is useful for epidemiologic investigation of *Campylobacter* spp. infections.[65]

Fresh stools should be collected in a clean container with a tight lid. Alternatively, a transport medium incorporating buffered glycerol in saline could be used. A rectal swab is an alternative specimen in selected situations. It is well established that hospitalized patients who did not enter the hospital with diarrhea are unlikely to develop diarrhea caused by bacterial agents other than *C. difficile*. As such, stool culture will not be performed in patients hospitalized for more than 72 hours (the 3-day rule) and rapid detection of *C. difficile* toxins will be alternatively performed.[66] For routine purposes, testing a single stool specimen has acceptable sensitivity; however, testing a second specimen is mandatory when the first one was subject to a more than 2-hour delay in transport.[67]

Several techniques have been developed for the point-of-care diagnosis of diarrhea including the rapid (<30 minutes) agglutination-based detection of rotavirus and adenovirus as well as the detection of *C. difficile* toxins. The rapid detection of *C. difficile* toxins A and B should be routinely performed for both inpatients and outpatients. Point-of-care detection of Shiga toxin-producing *E. coli* in children using EIA has not been evaluated favorably.[68] However, a commercially available *Campylobacter* antigen detection kit has been favorably evaluated,[69] and a dipstick test for the rapid detection of *Shigella* is under appraisal.[70]

Further detection of the causative organism relies on stool examination in the clinical microbiology laboratory. Direct microscopic examination may yield motile bacteria such as *Vibrio* and *Salmonella* spp. and parasites. Although Gram-staining analysis of stool specimens may not be done routinely, it has demonstrated 66–94% sensitivity and >95% specificity for the rapid detection of *Campylobacter* species.[71] We therefore recommend microscopic examination after Gram staining in all specimens in addition to Ziehl–Neelsen staining and appropriate staining for microsporidia and other parasites in immunocompromised patients. Specimens should be examined by electron microscopy for the observation of enteric viruses within 4 hours of receipt in the laboratory. Negative staining is a rapid and easy procedure. Rotavirus and adenovirus are readily detected, which may not be the case for calicivirus and astrovirus[72] (Fig. 35.2).

Culture of stools will focus on frequent pathogens and the systematic search for less frequent bacterial pathogens will be guided by the local epidemiologic situation. Pathogens routinely detected by culture of diarrheal stools include *E. coli* O157, *Shigella* spp., *Salmonella enterica* serotypes, *Campylobacter jejunii*, *Campylobacter coli* and *Aeromonas* spp. Stools in O157, O111 and O26 serotypes of *E. coli* can be enriched by using specific, commercially available magnetic beads. Sorbitol MacConkey agar can be used for the isolation of O157 STEC as these organisms do not ferment D-sorbitol, contrary to the vast majority of

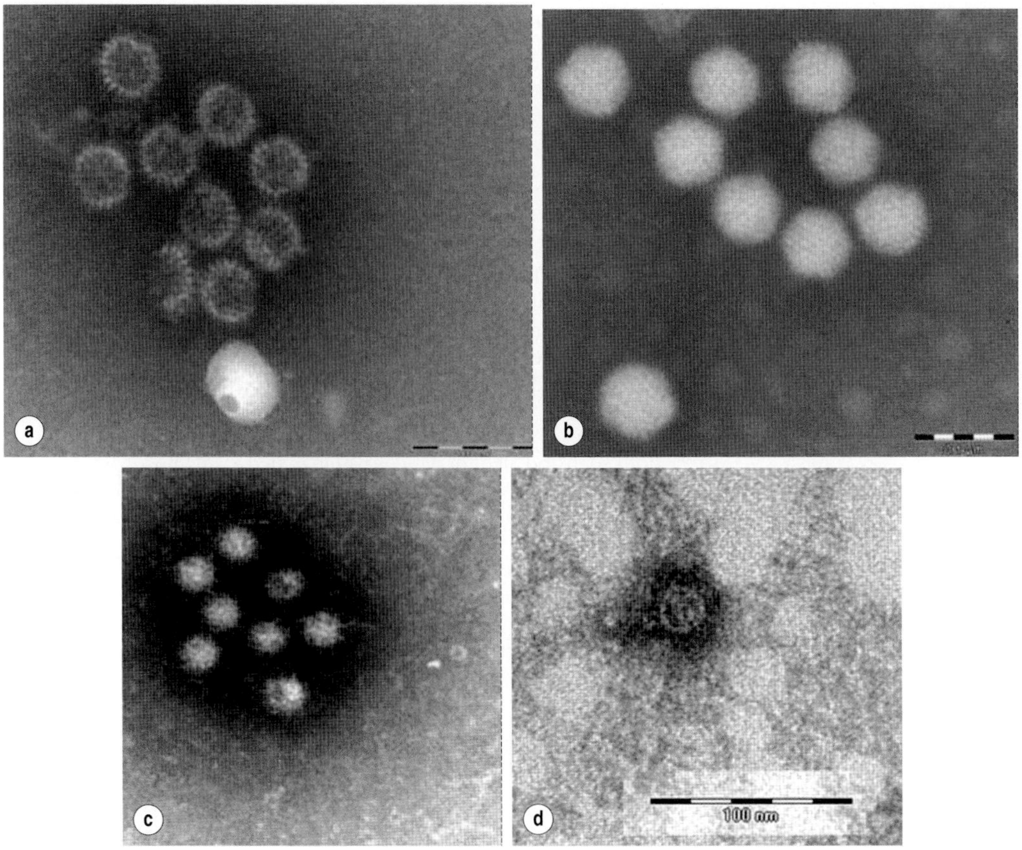

Fig. 35.2 Electron microscopy examination of diarrheal stools after negative staining shows the presence of enteric viruses responsible for acute diarrhea, such as (a) rotavirus, (b), adenovirus, (c) calicivirus and (d) enterovirus.

E. coli strains, and several chromogenic media have been developed for the selective isolation of O157 STEC. Although many rapid methods have been proposed for confirming the identification of O157 STEC, methods for the identification of ETEC, EPEC, EAEC and EIEC are most often available in reference laboratories only.

Salmonella enterica serotypes are better isolated by using an enrichment broth before plating onto selective media. Biochemical identification of *Salmonella* spp. and O (somatic), H (flagellar) and Vi (capsular) antigen serotyping should be performed in order to identify *Salmonella* enteritis Typhi (the typhoid fever agent, being capsular antigen Vi positive) and the most prevalent non-Typhi serotypes. The Vi capsular antigen is occasionally detected in non-Typhi, Dublin and Paratyphi C serotypes. O serotype determination is carried out by agglutination using pooled antisera while further H serotype determination is performed by tube agglutination tests using broth culture and testing the two phases of the flagellar antigens. MALDI-TOF mass spectrometry rapid analysis of *Salmonella enterica* isolates may resolve the serotype.[73]

Campylobacter spp. are recovered by using the filtration method in parallel to selective, blood-containing or non-blood-containing media and a microaerophilic atmosphere. Some *Campylobacter* spp. require 6% hydrogen in atmosphere. Incubation at 108°F (42°C) allows the growth of *Campylobacter jejuni* and *Campylobacter coli* but not all *Campylobacter* and *Aeromonas* spp. are recovered using blood agar incorporating 20 μg/ml ampicillin and produce β-hemolytic colonies. Further identification will be needed for oxidase-positive and indole-positive colonies. Modified cefsulodin-irgasan-novobiocin agar is also suitable for the isolation of *Aeromonas* spp. On this medium, *Aeromonas* colonies are undistinguishable from *Yersinia enterocolitica* colonies. Molecular identification should rely not only on 16S rDNA sequencing because of intragenomic heterogeneity and further identification based on *gyrB* and *rpoD* genes is mandatory. The interpretation of recovery of *Aeromonas* in stools must be cautious since there is

no strong evidence that all *Aeromonas* isolates from stools are responsible for diarrheal infection.[74]

Blood cultures are mandatory for the diagnosis of typhoid fever as well as bacteremia due to non-Typhi serotypes of *Salmonella*.

The systematic search for other enteritis pathogens will depend on local epidemiology including *Yersinia enterocolitica*, *Vibrio* spp., *Klebsiella oxytoca*, *Listeria monocytogenes* and *Plesiomonas shigelloides*. Growth of *Yersinia enterocolitica* from stools is enhanced by incubation on selective media (e.g. pectin agar) at 95°F (35°C) and the search for *Listeria monocytogenes* could be routinely done in certain laboratories. *Vibrio cholerae* will be visible as very motile, Gram-negative, slightly curved bacilli cultivated using a thiosulfate citrate bile salts sucrose (TCBS) agar after enrichment. Yellow colonies of oxidase-negative bacilli could be identified after electron microscopy observation, by 16S rDNA sequencing. In parallel with the search for pathogenic bacteria, the search for viruses should be done using electron microscope observation after negative staining as well as detection of rotavirus.

Although identification based on the observations of phenotypic traits after bacterial growth is the routine approach to the identification of bacteria responsible for diarrhea, novel techniques are warranted in order to speed the identification process in a timely fashion. Rapid and cheap identification by using mass spectrometry analysis of entire organisms has already been reported for *Vibrio* spp.[75]

MANAGEMENT

Community-acquired enteritis

Management of acute diarrhea should include the clinical evaluation of the patient, including risk factors for specific etiology and dehydration; rapid diagnosis of viral diarrhea; and treatment including rehydration, antibiotic therapy and symptomatic treatment. Rehydration is a major therapeutic measure; however, it should be borne in mind that patients on oral rehydration have a higher risk of paralytic ileus, and those on intravenous rehydration are exposed to risks of intravenous therapy. For every 25 children treated with oral rehydration one would fail and require intravenous rehydration.[76]

Rapid diagnosis of viral diarrhea is important in order to avoid unnecessary antibiotic treatment. Because of the absence of any antiviral drug effective against the viruses responsible for acute diarrhea, the management of viral diarrhea comprises the relief of symptoms and rehydration in cases of dehydration. Meta-analysis has confirmed that antibiotic treatment is useful to shorten the duration of signs and symptoms in travelers' acute diarrhea,[77] although most acute diarrheal episodes are self-limited and do not require antibiotic treatment. If an antibiotic is to be prescribed, fluoroquinolones are the drugs of first choice, including norfloxacin (400 mg q12h) or ciprofloxacin (500 mg q12h) and 1-day treatment is advocated except for *Campylobacter* and *Shigella* infection which should be treated for 3 days.[78] In the case of patients back from countries where fluoroquinolone resistance is prevalent,[79] such as *Campylobacter* spp. in Thailand, azithromycin (500 mg/day) could be used for 3 days.[80] Antimicrobial therapy for O157 *E. coli* enteritis or hemolytic–uremic syndrome remains a controversial issue because some studies reported a deleterious effect on the evolution of the latter syndrome. Antibiotic treatment of other serotypes by fluoroquinolones is advocated.

The increasing resistance of *Salmonella enterica* serotype Typhi to antibiotics, notably ciprofloxacin, makes the choice of first-line antibiotic treatment of typhoid fever more problematic. The majority of cases of *Yersinia enterocolitis* gastroenteritis do not require antibiotic treatment, contrary to systemic infection which could be treated using co-trimoxazole (no resistant strain reported) or fluoroquinolones, despite the fact that a few resistant strains have been reported.

Nosocomial enteritis

The main goal is to prevent nosocomial transmission of the etiologic agent in order to prevent and limit an extensive outbreak. The first step is to avoid the admission of patients diagnosed with diarrhea but without serious signs, and patients diagnosed at point-of-care as viral diarrhea. As for hospitalized patients, cohorting was not effective in the prevention of outbreaks. Patients suspected of infectious diarrhea should be treated in a single room, using standard precautions including hand washing and barrier protection using gloves and gowns. The duration of these precautions is for the duration of the illness.

Hand washing is the single most important measure in the control of nosocomial transmission of enteric pathogens. Because of concerns regarding the low virucidal activity of ethyl and isopropyl alcohols against naked viruses (rotavirus, norovirus, saporovirus)[81] and the lack of sporicidal activity (*C. difficile*), hand washing with soap in addition to alcohol is mandatory. The impact of improved hand hygiene using both soap and alcohol hand washing in decreasing nosocomial rotavirus infection has been proved.[82] Room environments should be carefully cleansed using sporicidal biocides in cases of *C. difficile* diarrhea.

There is no specific treatment for nosocomial viral enteritis. Cessation of the inciting antibiotic as soon as possible is the main management measure in case of *C. difficile* diarrhea. Patients should benefit from oral metronidazole (500 mg q8h) or vancomycin (125 mg q6h) for 10 days. The role of immunoglobulin for the treatment of severe *C. difficile* infection remains controversial.[83]

REFERENCES

References for this chapter can be found online at http://www.expertconsult.com

Chronic diarrhea

INTRODUCTION

Chronic diarrhea is a common symptom of many conditions with an estimated prevalence of 3–5%.[1–3] A current definition is the abnormal passage of three or more loose or liquid stools per day for more than 4 weeks and/or a daily stool weight greater than 200 g.[3] Indeed, a clinical definition of chronic diarrhea based on symptom reporting alone will lead to an overlap with functional bowel disorders such as irritable bowel syndrome, in which stool weight does not usually increase, and 'true' diarrhea. As irritable bowel syndrome affects 9–12% of the population, there is clearly the potential for inappropriate investigation of patients reporting diarrheal symptoms.[3] Conversely, new onset of diarrhea may reflect serious organic disease such as colonic neoplasia. Thus, chronic diarrhea continues to be a diagnostic challenge, largely because of the vast number of conditions included in its differential diagnosis as demonstrated in Table 36.1.

Most acute diarrheas are generally due to infectious etiologies, whereas symptoms persisting for longer than 4 weeks suggest a noninfectious etiology and occasionally might be due to microorganisms.[3] The main circumstances in which chronic infectious diarrhea is observed are in travelers, mainly in developing and tropical countries, or people living in such areas, in immunocompromised hosts, in hospitalized patients with *Clostridium difficile* and in patients with Whipple's disease.[4,5] In HIV-infected patients, chronic diarrhea is more common in patients with low CD4 lymphocyte counts (<200/mm³, especially those <50 cells/mm³).[6] The most essential component of any therapeutic strategy for an immunocompromised patient is restoration of the underlying immunologic defect such as highly active antiretroviral therapy (HAART) for HIV-infected patients.[6] Microorganisms observed are those which are capable of causing diarrhea in the immunocompetent population but also opportunistic such as *Cryptosporidium, Microsporidium, Cyclospora, Mycobacterium avium-intracellulare* and cytomegalovirus.[4,7]

In this chapter, bacterial, parasitic, fungal and viral causes of chronic diarrhea are reviewed and a general stepped strategy to explore chronic diarrhea (Fig. 36.1) is proposed. Obtaining a detailed medical history and stool characteristics should be the first step in defining a potential etiology and guiding appropriate choice of investigations. The second step should be based on the analysis of stool specimens, which is sufficient to establish the diagnosis of most infectious etiologies. Specific stepwise approaches for chronic diarrhea in travelers[8] (Fig. 36.2), HIV-infected patients[6] (Fig. 36.3) and patients suspected of Whipple's disease (Fig. 36.4)[9] are also proposed. Chronic (possibly infectious) diarrhea, such as tropical sprue and Brainerd diarrhea, is discussed, as well as perspectives to improve knowledge of chronic infectious diarrhea.

Table 36.1 Main causes of chronic diarrhea showing the place of infectious etiologies (shown in bold) among a broad spectrum of noninfectious etiologies

Colonic
Colon cancer, lymphoma
Ulcerative colitis, Crohn's disease
Microscopic colitis
Ischemic colitis
Radiation colitis
Gastrointestinal protozoans and helminths
Clostridium difficile
Ulcerating viral infections: cytomegalovirus and herpes simplex virus

Small bowel
Celiac disease
Crohn's disease
Whipple's disease
Other small-bowel enteropathies (tropical sprue, amyloid, intestinal lymphangiectasia)
Bile acid malabsorption
Disaccharidase deficiency
Mesenteric ischemia
Radiation enteritis
Lymphoma
Gastrointestinal protozoans and helminths
Small intestinal bacterial overgrowth

Pancreatic
Chronic pancreatitis
Pancreatic carcinoma
Cystic fibrosis

Endocrine
Hyperthyroidism
Diabetes
Hypoparathyroidism
Addison's disease
Hormone secreting tumors (gastrinoma, VIPoma, somatostatinoma, mastocytosis, carcinoid syndrome, medullary carcinoma of thyroid)

Others
Factitious diarrhea
Surgical causes (postresection diarrhea, internal fistula, postvagotomy diarrhea, postsympathectomy diarrhea)
Drugs
Alcohol
Autonomic neuropathy

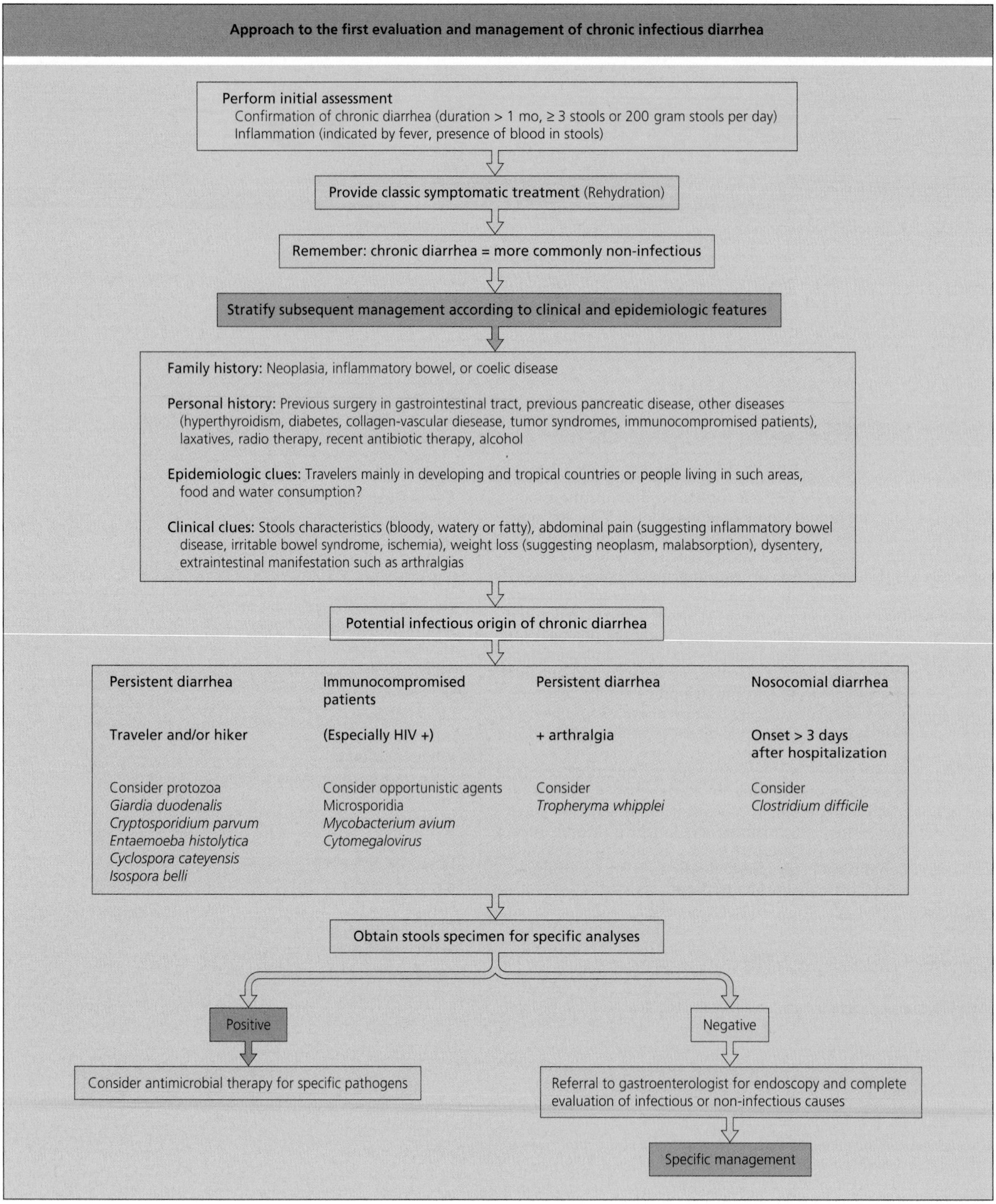
Approach to the first evaluation and management of chronic infectious diarrhea
Perform initial assessment
Confirmation of chronic diarrhea (duration > 1 mo, ≥ 3 stools or 200 gram stools per day)
Inflammation (indicated by fever, presence of blood in stools)
Provide classic symptomatic treatment (Rehydration)
Remember: chronic diarrhea = more commonly non-infectious
Stratify subsequent management according to clinical and epidemiologic features
Family history: Neoplasia, inflammatory bowel, or coelic disease
Personal history: Previous surgery in gastrointestinal tract, previous pancreatic disease, other diseases (hyperthyroidism, diabetes, collagen-vascular diesease, tumor syndromes, immunocompromised patients), laxatives, radio therapy, recent antibiotic therapy, alcohol
Epidemiologic clues: Travelers mainly in developing and tropical countries or people living in such areas, food and water consumption?
Clinical clues: Stools characteristics (bloody, watery or fatty), abdominal pain (suggesting inflammatory bowel disease, irritable bowel syndrome, ischemia), weight loss (suggesting neoplasm, malabsorption), dysentery, extraintestinal manifestation such as arthralgias
Potential infectious origin of chronic diarrhea
Persistent diarrhea
Traveler and/or hiker
Consider protozoa
Giardia duodenalis
Cryptosporidium parvum
Entaemoeba histolytica
Cyclospora cateyensis
Isospora belli
Immunocompromised patients
(Especially HIV +)
Consider opportunistic agents
Microsporidia
Mycobacterium avium
Cytomegalovirus
Persistent diarrhea
+ arthralgia
Consider
Tropheryma whipplei
Nosocomial diarrhea
Onset > 3 days after hospitalization
Consider
Clostridium difficile
Obtain stools specimen for specific analyses
Positive
Consider antimicrobial therapy for specific pathogens
Negative
Referral to gastroenterologist for endoscopy and complete evaluation of infectious or non-infectious causes
Specific management

Fig. 36.1 Approach to the first evaluation and management of chronic infectious diarrhea.

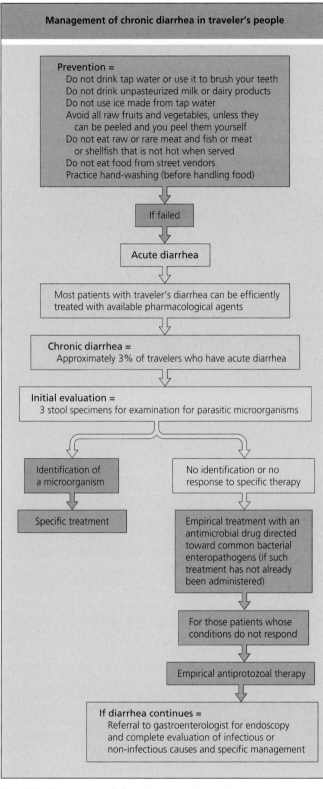

Management of chronic diarrhea in traveler's people

Prevention =
Do not drink tap water or use it to brush your teeth
Do not drink unpasteurized milk or dairy products
Do not use ice made from tap water
Avoid all raw fruits and vegetables, unless they
can be peeled and you peel them yourself
Do not eat raw or rare meat and fish or meat
or shellfish that is not hot when served
Do not eat food from street vendors
Practice hand-washing (before handling food)

If failed

Acute diarrhea

Most patients with traveler's diarrhea can be efficiently treated with available pharmacological agents

Chronic diarrhea =
Approximately 3% of travelers who have acute diarrhea

Initial evaluation =
3 stool specimens for examination for parasitic microorganisms

Identification of a microorganism

No identification or no response to specific therapy

Specific treatment

Empirical treatment with an antimicrobial drug directed toward common bacterial enteropathogens (if such treatment has not already been administered)

For those patients whose conditions do not respond

Empirical antiprotozoal therapy

If diarrhea continues =
Referral to gastroenterologist for endoscopy and complete evaluation of infectious or non-infectious causes and specific management

Fig. 36.2 Management of chronic diarrhea in travelers.

BACTERIAL CAUSES

Usual bacterial pathogens (*Salmonella* spp., *Yersinia enterocolitica*, *Campylobacter* spp., *Plesiomonas shigelloides* and *Vibrio parahaemolyticus*), which cause acute diarrhea in the immunocompetent population, produce more severe or prolonged infections in immunocompromised

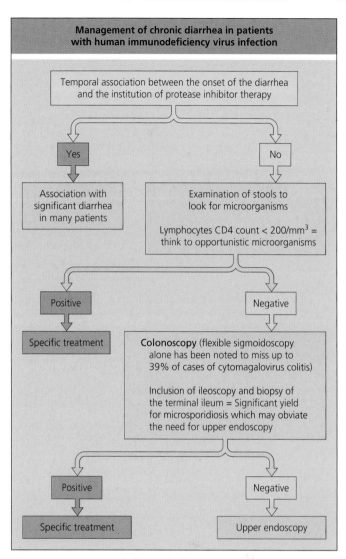

Management of chronic diarrhea in patients with human immunodeficiency virus infection

Temporal association between the onset of the diarrhea and the institution of protease inhibitor therapy

Yes

No

Association with significant diarrhea in many patients

Examination of stools to look for microorganisms

Lymphocytes CD4 count < 200/mm³ = think to opportunistic microorganisms

Positive

Negative

Specific treatment

Colonoscopy (flexible sigmoidoscopy alone has been noted to miss up to 39% of cases of cytomagalovirus colitis)

Inclusion of ileoscopy and biopsy of the terminal ileum = Significant yield for microsporidiosis which may obviate the need for upper endoscopy

Positive

Negative

Specific treatment

Upper endoscopy

Fig. 36.3 Management of chronic diarrhea in patients with HIV infection.[6] Knowledge of CD4 lymphocyte count and type of antiretroviral therapy is useful in management of patients.

people.[7,10] Gastrointestinal tuberculosis remains a problem in impoverished areas, immigrants from developing countries and HIV-infected patients.[11] *Mycobacterium avium-intracellulare* is also involved in chronic diarrhea in HIV-infected patients, mainly those with CD4 lymphocyte counts >50/mm³.[12] Clinical presentation, diagnosis and treatment for both mycobacteria are summarized in Table 36.2.

Other bacteria that are responsible for chronic diarrhea are *Clostridium difficile* and *Tropheryma whipplei*. Finally, small intestinal bacterial overgrowth is a condition that has been described for a long time but is still not clearly understood.[13,14]

Clostridium difficile infection

The anaerobic bacterium *Clostridium difficile* is an important nosocomial pathogen. Hospitalized patients may be rapidly colonized by *C. difficile* following admission.[15] It has been argued that any patient who develops diarrhea during hospital stay should be routinely tested for *C. difficile* infection.[15] Antibiotic therapy (mainly clindamycin, cephalosporins, quinolones) is the most significant risk factor for acquiring *C. difficile* infection.[15] *C. difficile* infection has a wide clinical range, from asymptomatic carriage to mild self-limiting diarrhea, chronic diarrhea and more severe pseudomembranous colitis.[16] Stools may be unformed or watery and

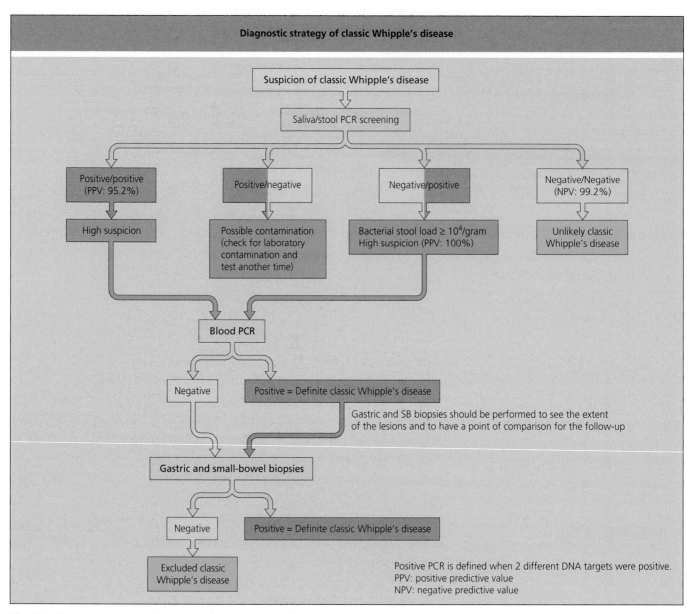

Fig. 36.4 Diagnostic strategy of classic Whipple's disease depending on quantitative real-time PCR results on saliva and stool specimens. (Adapted from Fenollar *et al.*[18])

rarely bloody.[15] Other common manifestations include abdominal pain and cramping, increased temperature and leukocytosis.

Many different tests are now available for the detection of *C. difficile* but most clinical laboratories use a commercial enzyme immunoassay for *C. difficile* toxin A or B, or both.[15] Colonic endoscopic examination may show classic pseudomembranes.[15] The most important therapeutic step is to immediately discontinue the agent responsible for provoking the disease.[15] In severe cases, or when the infection persists, metronidazole and vancomycin are the antibiotics of choice.[15]

Whipple's disease

Epidemiology

Whipple's disease (WD) is caused by the bacterium *T. whipplei*. The disease is considered as rare but there is no valid estimate of its actual prevalence.[17] The disease occurs worldwide; however, the typical patient is a middle-aged Caucasian male.[18] *T. whipplei* appears to be present in the general environment, though neither its source nor transmission is

well established. Studies using polymerase chain reaction (PCR) have demonstrated *T. whipplei* DNA in sewage plant effluent.[18]

It has been speculated that *T. whipplei* might be acquired via fecal–oral transmission.[19] One hypothesis concerning pathogenesis of WD is that although many people in a given population are exposed to *T. whipplei*, only some of those with predisposing immune factors, as yet undelineated, subsequently develop the disease.[18]

Clinical features

WD is characterized by a prodromal stage, marked mainly by arthralgia/arthritis, and a much later steady-state stage typified by weight loss and/or chronic diarrhea, and occasionally by other manifestations, since nearly all organs can be involved. The time between the prodromal and the steady-state stage averages 6 years; however, in patients on immunosuppressive therapy a more rapid clinical progression may occur.[18] Roughly 15% of cases lack classic signs and symptoms.[18] Currently, the spectrum of infections caused by *T. whipplei* is more complex than previously suspected.

Table 36.2 Bacterial, viral and fungal opportunistic pathogens associated with chronic diarrhea: presentation, diagnosis and treatment

Microorganisms	Clinical presentation	Diagnosis	Treatment
Bacterial causes			
Mycobacterium avium-intracellulare	Chronic diarrhea, abdominal pain, weight loss, night sweats, fever	Blood: – specific culture Stools and colonic biopsies: – acid-fast stain – culture – PCR	Clarithromycin 1 g, ethambutol 15 mg/kg and rifabutin 300 mg, all po q24h for 3–6 months *Secondary prophylaxis in lack of immune reconstitution*: rifabutin 300 mg po q24h
Mycobacterium tuberculosis	Chronic diarrhea, abdominal pain, weight loss, fever, night sweats Only 15–20% of patients have concomitant active pulmonary infection	Stools and colonic biopsies: – acid-fast stain – culture – PCR	Rifampicin 10 mg/kg and isoniazid 5 mg/kg, both po q24h for 9 months, plus Pyrazinamide 20 mg/kg and ethambutol 15 mg/kg, both po q24h for 2 months
Viral causes			
Cytomegalovirus	Chronic diarrhea, cramps, tenesmus, fever, abdominal pain, weight loss	Blood: – antigenemia – viremia Stools: PCR Colonic biopsies: – H&E – PCR – viral culture – electron microscopy	Ganciclovir 5 mg/kg and foscarnet 90 mg/kg, both iv q12h for 2–3 weeks *Secondary prophylaxis in lack of immune reconstitution*: valganciclovir 900 mg po q24h and foscarnet 120 mg/kg iv q24h
Herpes simplex virus	Chronic diarrhea, proctitis, distal colitis, tenesmus, rectal pain	Colonic biopsies: – H&E – PCR – viral culture – electron microscopy	Aciclovir 10 mg/kg po q8h for 2–3 weeks and valaciclovir 1 g po q12h for 2–3 weeks *Secondary prophylaxis in lack of immune reconstitution*: valaciclovir 1 g po q24h
Fungal cause			
Histoplasmosis	Diarrhea, hematochezia, weight loss, fever, abdominal pain	Stools: NA Colonic biopsies: – H&E – PAS stain – silver stain – fungal culture	*Severe cases*: amphotericin B 0.7 mg/kg iv for 2–3 weeks *Mild or moderate cases*: itraconazole 200 mg po q8h for 2–3 weeks *Secondary prophylaxis in lack of immune reconstitution*: itraconazole 200 mg po q24h

H&E, hematoxylin and eosin; iv, intravenous; PCR, polymerase chain reaction; po, per os (oral).

We can describe classic WD as marked by histologic lesions in the gastrointestinal tract in association with diverse clinical manifestations, with typical histologic lesions on periodic acid–Schiff (PAS) stains of small-bowel biopsies, localized infections due to *T. whipplei* without histologic digestive involvement (blood culture-negative endocarditis, neurologic infection, uveitis, etc.) and asymptomatic carriers. The main clinical manifestations of classic WD are summarized in Table 36.3.

In asymptomatic carriers, *T. whipplei* exists in stool, saliva and duodenal biopsies.[9] In stools, the estimated prevalence is from 1 to 11% in the general population. In sewage workers, this rate is higher, from 12 to 26%. Carriage in saliva (0.2% in the general population and 2.2% in sewage workers) is present only in people who are also carriers in stools. In duodenal biopsies, a carriage of 0.2% has been reported. Finally, asymptomatic neurologic involvement of patients with classic WD has been demonstrated by detecting DNA of the microorganism in cerebrospinal fluid (CSF) using PCR.[18]

Diagnosis

Several nonspecific findings are observed in blood samples. Increasing acute phase reactants, anemia, leukocytosis, thrombocytosis and evidence of malabsorption may be present at the time of diagnosis.[18] Thrombocytopenia and eosinophilia have also been reported.[18] In cases of classic WD, the endoscopic examination might show that the duodenum and jejunal mucosa are pale yellow, shaggy, eroded, erythematous or mildly friable.[20]

The usual tool for diagnosing classic WD is the light microscopic finding of magenta-stained inclusions within macrophages of the lamina propria on PAS stain of small-bowel biopsies (Fig. 36.5A). Depending on clinical manifestations, other tissues might be sampled and stained with PAS stain.[20] However, it is important to note that PAS stain is not pathognomonic of WD.[20] For example, PAS-positive cells are also seen in patients with *Mycobacterium avium-intracellulare*.[19] The presence of noncaseous granulomas composed of epithelioid cells, PAS-negative in 40% of cases, may be observed mainly in the gastrointestinal tract and the lymphatic tissues.[18]

Immunohistochemistry using antibodies directed against *T. whipplei* allows the detection of the microorganism in various fixed tissue fragments (even retrospectively), in body fluids and on blood monocytes, providing direct visualization of the bacilli (Fig. 36.5B).[18,21] This technique, which offers increased sensitivity and specificity as compared to PAS staining, is not yet widely available.

Table 36.3 Main clinical manifestations of patients with classic Whipple's disease

Frequent manifestations (>50%)
Chronic diarrhea
Arthralgia
Weight loss

Less frequent manifestations (<50%)
Adenopathy (mainly mediastinal and mesenteric)
Melanoderma
Fever

Neurologic manifestations
Cognitive change
Supranuclear ophthalmoplegia
Hypothalamic manifestations
Myoclonus
Oculomasticatory or oculo-facial-skeletal myorhythmia

Cardiovascular involvement
Endocarditis
Pericarditis
Myocarditis

Pulmonary involvement
Pleural effusion
Pulmonary infiltration

Ocular involvement
Uveitis

Noncaseating epithelioid and giant cell granulomas, most often lymph node granulomas

PCR may be performed to detect *T. whipplei* in samples from a variety of tissue types and body fluids, including gastric and small-bowel biopsies and stools.[18] Currently, quantitative real-time PCR assay targeting repeated sequences of *T. whipplei* using fluorescent labeled oligonucleotide hybridization probes for specific identification is the best tool to establish the diagnosis of WD.[18] A diagnostic strategy for classic WD using this tool and depending on results of saliva and stool specimens has recently been proposed (see Fig. 36.4).[9] It is also critical to include positive and negative controls systematically to validate each PCR run. Cultivation of *T. whipplei*, using mammalian cell cultures and axenic medium supplemented by amino acids from various specimens, including small-bowel biopsies and stools, has been achieved. However, this technique is not generally available. Serologic diagnosis of classic WD is not available.

Treatment

WD was fatal before the advent of antibiotics. Moreover, the treatment is still empirical. Current recommendations, which include oral administration of trimethoprim (160 mg) and sulfamethoxazole (800 mg) twice daily for 1–2 years, usually preceded by parenteral treatment with ceftriaxone (2 g daily) or streptomycin together with penicillin G (2 g and 1.2 million units daily, respectively) for 2 weeks, are not based on therapeutics trials or the susceptibility of *T. whipplei* to antibiotics.[18] The reported relapse rate is as high as 23% after antibiotic cessation.[18]

With the recent culture of *T. whipplei*, susceptibility tests and full genome sequencing have been achieved. Many antibiotics, including doxycycline and trimethoprim–sulfamethoxazole, are active *in vitro*.[18] In axenic culture, ceftriaxone and levofloxacin are active; in cell culture, however, cephalosporins (including ceftriaxone) and fluoroquinolones are not active. Genomic analysis has pointed out that *T. whipplei* lacks the coding sequence for dihydrofolate reductase, a trimethoprim target. *In-vitro* tests confirm that trimethoprim is not active, whereas sulfonamide compounds, such as sulfamethoxazole and sulfadiazine, are active.[18] Interferon gamma (IFN-γ) has been proposed for treatment of recurrent WD, and success lasted for at least 1 year after IFN-γ therapy was stopped.[18] A combined regimen of oral doxycycline (200 mg daily) and oral hydroxychloroquine (200 mg thrice daily), the only successful bactericidal regimen against *T. whipplei in vitro*, has been proposed in patients with WD without neurologic symptoms and negative PCR on CSF. In cases with neurologic involvement, high-dose oral sulfamethoxazole or sulfadiazine must be added to the regimen described above.

There is no established marker to determine treatment duration at the present time. By analogy with other chronic infections,[18] it would seem reasonable to use this regimen for at least 18 months. Only a long-term follow-up of patients, ideally during all-life, will allow determination of the best management of WD.

Small intestinal bacterial overgrowth

Small intestinal bacterial overgrowth (SIBO) is a condition caused by an abnormal number of bacteria in the small intestine.[13,14] Related symptoms are malabsorption and diarrhea.[13,14] This entity was first described in patients in the context of abnormal or

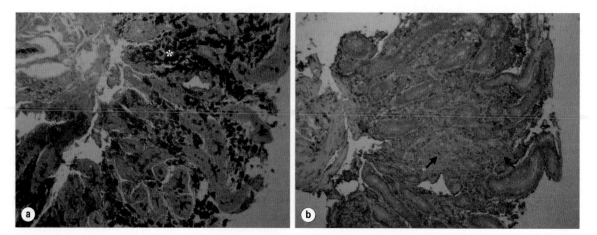

Fig. 36.5 Duodenal biopsies from a patient with classic Whipple's disease. (a) Duodenal biopsy specimen with reduced villous architecture and PAS-positive (asterisk) macrophages in the lamina propria. Periodic acid–Schiff stain. (b) Demonstration of *T. whipplei* by immunohistochemistry (arrows) in duodenal biopsy. Polyclonal rabbit anti-*T. whipplei* antibody used at a dilution of 1:2000 with hemalun counterstain. Courtesy of Hubert Lepidi.

postsurgical anatomy. The characteristic situation where SIBO was found to be most prevalent was the stagnant loop syndrome. Since then, there has been increasing suspicion of a bacterial overgrowth-like entity in many other diseases, adding to the confusion.[13,14] Indeed, currently, there is no adequately validated test for SIBO.[13,14] Although not widely accepted, the diagnosis may be suggested on small-bowel culture with a colony count >10^5/ml or on hydrogen breath test.[13,14] Thus, a better method for identifying SIBO accurately is needed.

The treatment of SIBO should address different aims: removal of the predisposing condition, nutritional support and suppression of the contaminating bacterial flora. Up to now, there has been no conclusive information on the most effective therapeutic approach.[22]

PARASITIC CAUSES

Parasitism and diarrhea are both endemic in areas with suboptimal sanitation.[23] Parasitic infections are mainly observed in travelers returning from developing countries and in immunocompromised people. The more frequent parasitic causes are *Giardia, Cryptosporidium* and *Entamoeba histolytica*.[5] In contrast to infection with intestinal protozoans, those with intestinal helminths are less common in returning travelers.[24]

To detect parasites, three or more stool samples should be examined. Special stains or concentration protocol may be required to look for some parasites that are also identified by appearance and

size. Testing by means of enzyme immunoassay is considerably better than older methods based on microscopic examination.[4] Recently, real-time PCR assays targeting various protozoan or helminthic DNA sequences have become available.[25–28] Stool samples mixed with ethanol allow the samples to be stored and transported at room temperature to laboratories with the appropriate facilities for DNA extraction and detection. Obviously, PCR will not be appropriate as a routine diagnostic tool in clinical settings in endemic areas where laboratory resources are often limited. Serologic tests for intestinal protozoans and helminths are not really useful or helpful. If stool analysis does not reveal the cause of the diarrhea, additional tests may include endoscopy. Main parasitic causes of chronic diarrhea with their more relevant epidemiologic, clinical, diagnostic and therapeutic characteristics are summarized in Table 36.4.

Protozoan parasites

Giardiasis

Giardiasis is caused by the flagellated protozoan *Giardia duodenalis* (former *G. lamblia* or *G. intestinalis*). *G. duodenalis* is one of the major causes of parasitic diarrhea worldwide. In the developing world, giardiasis is pandemic, with peak prevalence rates of up to 20% in children less than 10 years of age.[23] It is an important cause of chronic diarrhea in travelers returning from developing countries, with an infection rate of 1–3% in short-term visitors to endemic areas.[23] Major routes of transmission are consumption of contaminated water and food or by

Table 36.4 Main parasitic causes of chronic diarrhea with their more relevant epidemiologic, clinical, diagnostic and therapeutic characteristics

Microorganisms	Modes of transmission and common epidemiologic settings	Clinical features	Diagnosis	Treatment
Protozoans				
Giardia duodenalis	Fecal–oral route, IgA deficiency	Most infections are asymptomatic Watery diarrhea/malabsorption Abdominal pain	Stools; if negative, small-bowel aspiration or biopsies: – ME – immunofluorescence, ELISA methods – PCR	Treatment recommended in symptomatic and asymptomatic disease to reduce transmission: metronidazole 250–750 mg po q8h for 7 days
Cryptosporidium parvum	Fecal–oral route, immunocompromised host	Watery diarrhea/malabsorption Immunocompetent host: usually asymptomatic or mild self-limited gastroenteritis, occasionally lasting more than 1 month Immunocompromised host: chronic, more often severe diarrhea, dehydration, weight loss	Stools; if negative, small-bowel aspiration or biopsies: – ME with modified acid-fast stain – immunofluorescence, ELISA methods – PCR	Generally not necessary in immunocompetent individuals Severe disease/immunocompromised host: supportive therapy, no single effective therapy; nitazoxanide may be considered In patients with AIDS, HAART sufficient to achieve immunologic reconstitution is most effective
Cyclospora cayetanensis	Fecal–oral route, travel	Watery diarrhea/malabsorption	Stools; if negative, small-bowel aspiration or biopsies: ME with modified acid-fast stain	Trimethoprim–sulfamethoxazole (co-trimoxazole) 160–800 mg po q8h for 10 days

(Continued)

Table 36.4 Main parasitic causes of chronic diarrhea with their more relevant epidemiologic, clinical, diagnostic and therapeutic characteristics

Microorganisms	Modes of transmission and common epidemiologic settings	Clinical features	Diagnosis	Treatment
Entamoeba histolytica	Fecal–oral route Travel to tropical regions, recent emigration from such region	Asymptomatic colonization: ~90% Bloody diarrhea/dysentery	Stools; if negative, colonic biopsies: – ME – immunofluorescence, ELISA methods – PCR	Generally recommended for symptomatic and asymptomatic individuals to prevent transmission: metronidazole 750 mg po q8h for 5–10 days plus treatment for 7 days with paromomycin 500 mg po q8h
Isospora belli	Fecal–oral route, immunocompromised host	Watery diarrhea/malabsorption Immunocompetent host: acute-self-limited Immunocompromised host: chronic, occasionally severe diarrhea, dehydration, weight loss	Stools; if negative, small-bowel aspiration or biopsies: – ME with modified acid-fast stain – PCR	Trimethoprim–sulfamethoxazole (co-trimoxazole) 160–800 mg po q12h for 7–10 days
Microsporidia	Fecal–oral route, immunocompromised host	Watery diarrhea/malabsorption Immunocompetent host: rare cause of acute self-limited diarrhea Immunocompromised host: chronic diarrhea, dehydration, anorexia, weight loss	Stools; if negative, small-bowel aspiration or colonic biopsies: – ME with special stain – PCR	May be indicated in immunocompromised patients: albendazole 400 mg po q12h for 3 weeks In HIV-infected patients, HAART sufficient to achieve immunologic reconstitution is most effective
Balantidium coli	Fecal–oral route	Bloody diarrhea/dysentery	Stools: ME	Tetracyclines po for 10 days
Helminths				
Strongyloides stercoralis	Developing countries, immunocompromised host	Watery diarrhea/malabsorption Immunocompromised host (HTLV-1): chronic diarrhea	Stools; if negative, small-bowel aspiration or biopsies: ME	Ivermectin 200 µg/kg po q24h for 2 days
Trichuris trichiura	Fecal–oral route	Bloody diarrhea/dysentery	Stools; if negative, rectal biopsies: ME	Mebendazole 100 mg po q12h for 3 days Albendazole 400–600 mg po, single dose

ELISA, enzyme-linked immunosorbent assay; HAART, highly active antiretroviral therapy; ME, microscopic examination; PCR, polymerase chain reaction; po, per os (oral).

direct fecal–oral contact. Chronic infection has been associated with hypogammaglobulinemia, protein-calorie malnutrition, previous gastrectomy and use of immunosuppressive medication.[23] There is no particular increase in incidence among the HIV-infected population.[23]

The clinical spectrum of giardiasis ranges from asymptomatic carriage, through acute diarrhea to severe chronic diarrhea with intestinal malabsorption and growth failure in children.[29] Chronic infection is associated with profound malaise, lassitude, epigastric discomfort, headaches and steatorrhea.[23] Patients who develop recurrent diarrhea after treatment for giardiasis may have associated lactose intolerance rather than relapse of their infection.[23]

The most common method for diagnosis is microscopic examination of the stools for trophozoites using either wet mount or trichrome stain. Immunofluorescent- and enzyme-linked immunosorbent assay (ELISA)-based methods have been developed.[30] Highly sensitive and specific real-time PCR procedures have been validated for the detection of *G. duodenalis*.[25,26] In patients with negative stools, small-bowel aspiration or biopsies may be considered.

For treatment, the drug of choice is oral metronidazole.[23] The adult dose is 250 mg and for children 5 mg/kg three times daily for 7 days. Pregnant women may be treated with paromomycin.[23]

Cryptosporidiosis (see also Chapter 108)

Cryptosporidiosis in humans is most commonly due to *Cryptosporidium parvum*, a coccidian parasite. The number of cases has risen dramatically since the description of HIV infection. Cryptosporidiosis is described worldwide in both immunocompetent and immunocompromised hosts. When clinical stool specimens are examined for *Cryptosporidium* oocysts, approximately 1–3% are positive in North

America and Europe and 5–10% in developing countries. Risk factors for the acquisition of cryptosporidiosis include transmission via the fecal–oral route, contact with farm animals or pets, drinking contaminated water and eating contaminating food.[30]

The clinical manifestations depend on the host response. In immunocompetent hosts, the most commonly identified symptom is acute diarrhea, with watery stools that typically resolve in 10–14 days; prolonged disease is uncommon.[31,32] In immunocompromised hosts, disease onset is usually insidious. Watery diarrhea may gradually increase over weeks to months.[33] Weight loss, profound dehydration, abdominal pain and cramping are common. Symptoms typically persist unless there is improvement in the immunologic status.

Infection can be diagnosed by identification of oocysts in stools using modified Ziehl–Neelsen stain, immunofluorescence with monoclonal antibodies and commercially available ELISA.[30,34] Highly sensitive and specific real-time PCR procedures have been also validated for the detection of *Cryptosporidium* spp.[25,27] In patients with negative stools, small-bowel aspiration or biopsies may be considered.

Treatment of the immunocompetent host is supportive because cryptosporidiosis is self-limited.[30] Few options exists for HIV-infected patients in whom highly active antiretroviral therapy fails.[30] Monotherapy with spiramycin or paromycin has been reported to be active but efficacy has not been confirmed by controlled trials and a majority of patients relapse.[23,30] Nitazoxanide has been considered as a promising agent but clinical trials performed in the USA demonstrated little efficacy.[30]

Cyclosporiasis

Cyclosporiasis is caused by a coccidian parasite, *Cyclospora cayetanensis*.[23] Cyclosporiasis is described worldwide but more frequently in tropical countries. Its prevalence is unknown. Transmission occurs via the oral route, and local outbreaks have been traced to contaminated water or food supply.

C. cayetanensis is the cause of persistent diarrhea in immunocompetent and immunocompromised patients. Other common symptoms are abdominal pain, nausea, vomiting and anorexia. The duration of illness ranges from 4 to 107 days.[35] In HIV-infected patients, *C. cayetanensis* results in chronic diarrhea.[30]

Diagnosis is dependent on microscopic demonstration of morphologic characteristics, staining properties and autofluorescence under ultraviolet light.[35] In contrast to *Cryptosporidium*, staining is variable with the modified Ziehl-Neelsen stain. Measurement of oocysts is recommended to distinguish *C. cayetanensis* (8–10 μm) from *C. parvum* (3–5 μm).[30] In patients with negative stools, small-bowel aspiration or biopsies may be considered.

Trimethoprim–sulfamethoxazole (160–800 mg, twice daily) for 10 days is the treatment.[30]

Amebiasis (see also Chapter 110)

Amebiasis caused by *Entamoeba histolytica* and *Entamoeba dispar* is especially prevalent in Mexico, India, Africa and Central and South America. These species are morphologically indistinguishable but can be differentiated by monoclonal antibodies and DNA probes.[30]

Infections with *E. dispar* are characteristically asymptomatic, do not elicit a serologic response and are responsible for the majority of infections with *Entamoeba* species. In contrast, infections with *E. histolytica* result in symptomatic illness (80–98%) or invasive disease (2–20%) and the production of serum antibodies. In indigenous populations, asymptomatic carriage of *E. histolytica* is common. Major routes of transmission are consumption of contaminated water and food or by direct fecal–oral contact.[23] Individuals at highest risk for infection include persons who travel to developing nations, immigrants or migrant workers from areas of high endemicity, immunocompromised persons and persons housed in mental institutions.[23] *E. histolytica* is not a common cause of traveler's diarrhea but can be a cause of chronic diarrhea in travelers returning from developing countries.

Patients may be asymptomatic or present with colicky abdominal pain, frequent bowel movements and tenesmus.[23] Amebic dysentery is characterized by blood-stained stools with mucus occurring up to 10 times a day.[23] The duration of the dysentery can be very variable and may last for only a few days or for several months with concomitant weight loss.[23] Chronic amebic colitis is clinically indistinguishable from idiopathic inflammatory bowel disease.[30] Because corticosteroid therapy may result in perforation, stool examination for trophozoites should be performed prior to making a diagnosis of inflammatory bowel disease.[30]

Identification of *E. histolytica* cysts and trophozoites requires examination of a fresh stool sample and a trichrome stain.[30] New fecal antigen detection methods (monoclonal antibodies, ELISA) may also prove useful.[30,36] Real-time PCR procedures have been recently developed for the detection of *E. histolytica*.[25] In the presence of negative stool microscopy, colonic biopsies may sometimes be useful.

Invasive disease, such as severe colitis, should be treated with oral metronidazole (750 mg thrice daily) for 10 days, followed by an oral luminal agent such as diloxanide (500 mg thrice daily) or paramomycin (500 mg thrice daily) to prevent future invasion with any remaining cysts.[23]

Isosporiasis

Isosporiasis is caused by the coccidian parasite, *Isospora belli*. Infections have been described worldwide but with an increased prevalence in tropical and subtropical climates and in areas with poor sanitation.[30] Transmission is associated with contaminated water, although that route has not been proven.[30] Little is known about the prevalence of human infection. In a limited number of studies employing adequate techniques, 0.1–1.8% of stools were positive.[23] Isosporiasis is observed in HIV-infected patients with an incidence ranging from approximately 0.2 to 20% in tropical areas. *I. belli* has also been described in transplant patients (liver, renal) as well as in patients with lymphoblastic leukemia, adult T-cell leukemia, Hodgkin's and non-Hodgkin's lymphoma, either prior to or after chemotherapy, and in patients with human T-cell leukemia virus 1 (HTLV-1) infection.[37,38]

The predominant clinical symptoms are diarrhea-associated weight loss, abdominal pain and sometimes fever.[39,40] Stools are watery and foamy, suggesting malabsorption. While symptoms are usually self-limited in immunocompetent hosts, patients are often ill for 6 weeks to 6 months. In HIV-infected patients, isosporiasis presents with an insidious onset of diarrhea, weight loss and abdominal pain.[23]

Stool specimens frequently contain Charcot–Leyden crystals and fat. Peripheral eosinophilia is frequent.[30] Infection can be diagnosed by identification of oocysts in stools using acid-fast stains, such as the modified Ziehl–Neelsen method.[30] Real-time PCR has been recently developed.[28] If stool examination remains negative, even in cases of severe diarrhea, small-bowel aspiration or biopsies may be necessary to establish the diagnosis.

Isosporiasis responds promptly to oral trimethoprim–sulfamethoxazole (160–800 mg, four times daily) for 10 days in immunocompetent patients.[23] For HIV-infected patients, approximately half will relapse if not placed on secondary prophylaxis; therefore secondary prophylaxis should be maintained, using oral trimethoprim–sulfamethoxazole (160–800 mg) thrice weekly.[23]

Microsporidiosis

Microsporidiosis is caused by microsporidia, intracellular protozoan parasites belonging to the phylum *Microspora*.[23] Two species are associated with enteric infection, *Enterocytozoon bieneusi* and *Encephalitozoon intestinalis* (former *Septata intestinalis*). The former is more common. Little is known about the epidemiology of microsporidiosis. Serologic surveys suggest that infection with these organisms is widespread.[23] Spread of the organisms through environmental, person-to-person (fecal–oral, aerosolized respiratory secretions) and animal-to-person transmission have been postulated.[23] The prevalence of infection in selected groups of HIV-infected patients in different countries has a range of 1.7–30%.[30]

Microsporidia cause acute self-limiting diarrhea in immunocompetent persons and in patients who have immunodeficiency other than HIV infection.[41] In immunocompromised HIV-infected patients with CD4 lymphocyte counts <100 cells/mm³, E. bieneusi is responsible for chronic watery diarrhea.[23,42] E. intestinalis is a less commonly recognized cause of chronic diarrhea.[23]

Spores of microsporidia can be detected in stools and in small-bowel and colonic biopsy specimens using Giemsa, Weber's trichrome or fluorochrome stains (Calcofluor, Uvitex 2B), but identification of the specific species requires electron microscopy or PCR.[30,43]

No real therapeutic options exist for HIV-infected patients in whom highly active antiretroviral therapy fails.[30] Preliminary data suggest that albendazole may be of use in the treatment of infections with E. intestinalis but not for E. bieneusi.[23]

Balantidiosis

Balantidiosis is caused by Balantidium coli, the only ciliate associated with human infection.[23] It has a widespread distribution, but is only rarely found in human stools (<1% in all surveys).[23] Many cases are asymptomatic.[23] A chronic form has been described with loose movements, abdominal pain, tenesmus, mucus in the stools and weight loss.[23] Diagnosis is based on demonstration of the trophozoites in stools.[23] Tetracyclines for 10 days are recommended as treatment.[23]

Helminths and chronic diarrhea

Strongyloidiasis (see Chapter 108)

Strongyloidiasis is caused by Strongyloides stercoralis, a helminthic parasite of worldwide distribution.[24] The prevalence is 5–10% in tropical countries. Humans are usually infected from moist soil by transcutaneous penetration. The clinical behavior of this disease is believed to be largely dependent on the host's immune response.

S. stercoralis can be associated with persistent watery diarrhea, cramping abdominal pain and weight loss with evidence of malabsorption, particularly when there is hyperinfection or disseminated strongyloidiasis.[24] This massive invasion by S. stercoralis can be observed in people debilitated by concurrent disease or malnutrition, patients treated with immunosuppressive drugs harboring S. stercoralis, patients infected with HTLV-1 but not in HIV-infected patients.[44] Eosinophilia is a prominent feature of this infection.

Diagnosis depends on demonstration of S. stercoralis larvae in stools, or in small-bowel aspiration or biopsies. Culture can be also undertaken. Ivermectin (200 μg/kg/day) for 2 days is the treatment of choice.[24] Albendazole can also be used, but may be less effective.[24]

Trichuriasis

Trichuriasis caused by the whipworm Trichuris trichiura is prevalent worldwide, with approximately 400 millions persons infected.[24] When few worms are present there is little damage, but heavy infections (more than 200 adult worms recovered after antihelminthic expulsion) cause a clinical syndrome characterized by chronic dysentery, predisposition to rectal prolapse, anemia and digital clubbing.[45] Reduced childhood growth rates, reduced food intake, iron deficiency and gastrointestinal protein loss are seen in heavy infections.[24] T. trichiura has been also described as an unusual cause of chronic diarrhea in a renal transplant patient.[46]

Most symptomatic cases can be readily diagnosed by routine microscopic stool examination.[24] The diagnosis is made when numerous worms are seen on the rectal mucosa. Treatment with mebendazole (100 mg twice daily) for 3 days is highly effective, as well as albendazole in a single dose of 400–600 mg.[24]

Trichinosis

Trichinosis caused by Trichinella spiralis is widely distributed throughout the world, except in Australia and parts of the South Pacific.[24] The occurrence of diarrhea of short duration following the ingestion of infected meat has been well described.[24] Intestinal symptoms typically resolve spontaneously. There is no reliable therapy.

A new clinical syndrome has been reported in the Inuit population in northern Canada.[24] These patients presented with chronic diarrhea, lasting up to 14 weeks. They also had only mild and transitory myalgias without fever. These clinical manifestations differ considerably from those of classic trichinosis, suggesting that this may be due to a distinct strain of parasite.

Capillariasis

Capillariasis is caused by a small nematode, Capillaria philippinensis, initially described in patients from the Philippines.[24] Since then, Thailand has been found to be endemic for the disease, and a few cases have been identified in Japan, Taiwan, Iran, Egypt and India.[24] Human infection results from consumption of raw fish. C. philippinensis can cause chronic diarrhea and malabsorption.[47]

The detection of C. philippinensis is based on the recovery of eggs, larvae and/or adult worms in the stool of the patients. However, small-bowel aspiration or biopsies may be necessary to confirm capillariasis. Oral treatment with mebendazole 200 mg twice daily for 20 days or thiabendazole 25 mg/kg/day has been used successfully.[24] However, relapse can occur. Albendazole (400 mg/day for 10 days) is currently the drug of choice since it appears to act on adult as well as larval stages of the parasite, thus reducing relapse.[24]

Schistosomiasis (see Chapter 112)

Colorectal schistosomiasis (usually Schistosoma mansoni infection) can present with chronic bloody diarrhea, due to the resulting granulomatous inflammation of the colon seen during the chronic phase in patients with heavy infections.[47]

Fungus

Histoplasmosis is caused by Histoplasma capsulatum, a fungus that is endemic in America and Africa.[12] It is a soil fungus that proliferates especially in soil enriched by bat and bird droppings.[12] Infection occurs by inhalation of conidia, and it is confined initially to the respiratory system. Severely immunocompromised patients are susceptible to disseminated histoplasmosis, which may involve the digestive tract and cause diarrhea.[12] An isolated colonic histoplasmosis infection was recently reported in a man who presented in end-stage renal disease, for which he was on chronic hemodialysis.[48]

Histologic examination of PAS-stained or silver-stained gastrointestinal biopsies allow detection of the fungus.[48] Treatment is based on amphotericin or itraconazole. Clinical presentation, diagnosis and treatment for histoplasmosis are summarized in Table 36.2.

VIRAL CAUSES

Usual viral microorganisms (rotavirus, astrovirus, adenovirus, norovirus) responsible for acute diarrhea are not involved in chronic diarrhea except perhaps in specific immunocompromised hosts. Indeed, rotavirus and astrovirus diarrhea may continue for months in children who have defects in T-cell function (e.g. DiGeorge syndrome, cartilage–hair hypoplasia syndrome).[49] Adenovirus is also a cause of chronic diarrhea in patients with immunodeficiency, mainly HIV-infected patients, in whom the infection is commonly systemic.[12,50] Light microscopic examination of colonic biopsies can identify adenovirus colitis which is significantly associated with chronic diarrhea, and in addition may facilitate gastrointestinal co-infection with cytomegalovirus.[12] Finally, norovirus and adenovirus have also been identified as responsible for chronic diarrhea in a transplant child.[51]

Cytomegalovirus and herpes simplex virus are both specifically responsible for chronic diarrhea due to ulcerating chronic infection in immunocompromised patients, including HIV-infected patients and transplant recipients.

Cytomegalovirus

Cytomegalovirus is a herpesvirus and is the commonest viral cause of diarrhea in HIV-infected patients.[12] Cytomegalovirus is ubiquitous and endemic in humans. In individuals with normal immune systems, this organism is usually latent and asymptomatic. The occurrence of cytomegalovirus in the gastrointestinal tract, any part of which can be affected, is evidence of systemic infection and is related to failure of the dysfunctional immune system to maintain latency. It may cause enteritis, colitis, ulcers, appendicitis, ileocaecal obstruction, toxic megacolon, perforations and gastrointestinal hemorrhage.[12] Diagnosis and treatment are summarized in Table 36.2. (See also Chapter 91.)

Herpes simplex virus (HSV)

Although most humans are infected at some time in their lives by HSV-1 or HSV-2, diarrhea caused by these double-stranded DNA viruses are rare, virtually confined to individuals with impaired immunity.[12] Diagnosis and treatment are summarized in Table 36.2.

CHRONIC (POSSIBLY INFECTIOUS) DIARRHEA

Tropical sprue

Tropical sprue is associated with chronic diarrhea, malabsorption and nutritional deficiency in patients who live in or have visited tropical areas.[52] Pathogenesis is still unknown but an infectious cause is suspected.[52,53]

Tropical sprue starts with an acute intestinal infection (bacterial, viral or parasitic) which can affect predominantly the small or the large intestine.[52,53] Macrocytic anemia and hypoalbuminemia are present, together with progressive villus atrophy of the small intestine. Treatment with tetracycline, folic acid and nutritional support is generally effective but relapses after treatment are common.[52]

Brainerd diarrhea

A form of chronic diarrhea showing worldwide distribution and manifesting as outbreaks is Brainerd diarrhea from Brainerd, Minnesota.[54] The source is characteristically unpasteurized milk or untreated water. Despite intensive laboratory examinations, the cause of Brainerd diarrhea remains unknown. Extensive laboratory and environmental testing for bacterial, parasitic, mycotic and viral agents did not identify an etiologic agent.

Treatment with a wide variety of antimicrobial agents gives no significant clinical response. The prognosis is good, with diarrhea generally subsiding after 6 months to 1 year.

PERSPECTIVES

Research using modern techniques may be able to settle some of the unanswered issues and open new fields. For example, the advent of metagenomic sequencing has enabled systematic and unbiased characterization of microbial populations, including in children with acute diarrhea.[55] Thus, metagenomic approaches have the potential to define the spectrum of microorganisms, including novel microorganisms, present in stools during episodes of chronic diarrhea. The detection of novel or unexpected microorganisms would then enable investigations to assess whether these agents play a causal role in human chronic diarrhea.

REFERENCES

References for this chapter can be found online at http://www.expertconsult.com

Chapter | **37** |

P Ronan O'Connell
Gerard Sheehan

Intra-abdominal sepsis, peritonitis and pancreatitis

INTRODUCTION

Intra-abdominal infection is a common clinical problem that contributes significantly to surgical, intensive care and laboratory workloads. The severity of infection may vary from mild appendicitis with minimal systemic upset to feculent peritonitis with multiorgan failure. Pancreatitis, by initiating an inflammatory cascade, can mimic peritonitis and although the inflammatory process is initially sterile, it may progress to fulminant, life-threatening sepsis. Management of peritonitis, intra-abdominal sepsis and pancreatitis remains one of the most challenging and resource-consuming activities of modern critical care. Therapy of intra-abdominal sepsis requires surgery or percutaneous drainage, antimicrobial therapy and resuscitation. Each pillar complements the other, and failure to meet an adequate standard in one may undo the benefit of the others.

ANATOMY

The peritoneum is the largest cavity within the body with a surface area that approximates that of the skin. The parietal peritoneum is lined by a surface layer of mesothelial cells supported by a lamina propria and loose connective tissue which covers the inner surfaces of the abdominal wall, the diaphragm and the pelvis, and is reflected onto the external surfaces of the abdominal organs as the visceral peritoneum. The visceral peritoneum has no somatic innervation whereas the parietal peritoneum overlies a well-vascularized subserosa with extensive lymphatic drainage and somatic innervation.[1] The peritoneal cavity is separated by the lesser or gastrocolic omentum into the greater and lesser sacs, while the greater sac is divided by the great omentum into supra- and infracolic compartments. The greater sac is functionally further divided by the viscera it contains into subphrenic, subhepatic, paracolic and pelvic spaces. The latter comprises the rectovesical pouch in males and the rectouterine pouch (of Douglas) in females. Knowledge of peritoneal anatomy is of importance to the surgeon and interventional radiologist in planning treatment of intraperitoneal pathology.

The peritoneal cavity normally contains a small volume (approximately 50 ml) of fluid which provides lubrication and facilitates peristalsis and other movements of abdominal viscera. The peritoneal fluid is secreted throughout the peritoneal cavity but is primarily absorbed through the pelvic and subphrenic peritoneum. This reflects the effects of gravity, capillary attraction and changes in intra-abdominal pressure occasioned by respiration. It explains the propensity for infected peritoneal fluid to cause subphrenic and pelvic collections and the incidence of transcelomic spread of malignant cells to these areas. The luminal surface of the mesothelial cells has numerous microvilli which act to protect the delicate surface by entrapping water and serous exudates.[2]

MICROBIOLOGY

In health, the low pH of the stomach maintains the number of organisms at less than 10^3 bacteria per mm^3, with a microflora similar to that of the oral cavity and upper respiratory tract. Organisms present are usually viridans streptococci, lactobacilli or *Candida* species, all of low pathogenic potential. Proton pump inhibitors or other causes of achlorhydria may allow the microflora of the stomach to approximate that of the small bowel, with increasing numbers of facultative Gram-negative bacilli, such as *Escherichia coli*, and strict anaerobes. Many intubated and ventilated patients in intensive care units have an increase in bacterial density in stomach fluid, with a shift towards aerobic Gram-negative bacilli, including *E. coli*, *Pseudomonas aeruginosa* and also *Candida*. Nasogastric and percutaneous endoscopic gastrostomy (PEG) feeding tubes, malignancy and bariatric surgery cause similar alterations.

The density of the normal microflora progressively increases from the stomach to the colon. In the proximal small bowel there are $\sim 10^{4-5}$ bacteria per mm^3, whereas the terminal ileum contains $10^7 – 10^9$ organisms per mm^3. In the presence of intestinal pathology such as scleroderma, celiac disease or other conditions causing stasis or diverticula, the microflora of the small intestine often more closely resembles that of the colon. A similar phenomenon occurs in patients with decompensated cirrhosis. The terminal ileum in health is a transition zone with equal numbers of strict anaerobes and facultative or aerobic organisms.

The highest absolute numbers of bacteria are found in the colon, with in excess of 10^{11} bacteria/gram of feces and more than 400 species. Strict anaerobes outnumber facultative and aerobic bacteria by a ratio of 1000 to 1 or greater. These include large numbers of various species of *Bifidobacterium*, *Propionibacterium*, *Fusobacterium*, *Lactobacillus*, *Veillonella*, *Eubacterium* and *Clostridium*. However, with the exception of *Bacteroides fragilis*, other members of the *B. fragilis group*, *Fusobacterium* species and *Bilophila wadsworthia*, they generally contribute little to clinical intra-abdominal infection.

The genus Bacteroides is now limited to the *B. fragilis* group, which numbers greater than 20 species. The most common pathogen within the *B. fragilis* group is the *B. fragilis* species itself, which although comprising a minority (1–10%) of the group within the normal colonic microflora, is the most common anaerobic pathogen (31%) and the most virulent of the group. Other species of the group commonly isolated in intra-abdominal sepsis are *B. thetaiotaomicron* (15.4%), *B. ovatus* (10.9%), *B. vulgatus* (9.4%), *B. uniformis* (4.9%) and *B. distasonis* (10%) (renamed *Parabacteroides distasonis* in 2006).

Most intestinal aerobic Gram-negative bacilli are Enterobacteriaceae, which as facultative anaerobes can survive and multiply in the relatively anaerobic environment of the colon. *E. coli* is the most common of the Enterobacteriaceae; others include species of *Klebsiella, Enterobacter, Serratia, Proteus, Providencia, Morganella, Citrobacter* and *Hafnia*. Other Gram-negative but strictly aerobic bacilli such as *Pseudomonas aeruginosa* and *Acinetobacter* species are usually transient in the normal gastrointestinal flora of healthy humans and in most populations are uncommon pathogens in community-acquired intra-abdominal sepsis. However, their frequency increases after prolonged hospitalization, especially with exposure to antimicrobial agents and requirement for intensive care. *Enterococcus faecalis* is present in feces in large numbers, as high as 10^{10}/g.

Studies from the 1970s and 1980s using aerobic techniques in patients with proven intra-abdominal infection show a mean of 3.8 organisms per patient, about half anaerobes and the others aerobic or facultative. *Pseudomonas* made up only about 6% of the aerobes. The most common aerobic pathogen was *E. coli*, accounting for 30% of the aerobes. Other aerobic Gram-negative bacilli also comprised 30%. Enterococci and Group D streptococci made up 12% of aerobic organisms. The *B. fragilis* group comprised 36% of the anaerobes, with other anaerobic Gram-negative bacilli comprising 20%. Clostridial species made up 18% and anaerobic Gram-positive cocci, 10%.[1] Animal models of intra-abdominal infection have also shown that the initially diverse complex inoculum from the colonic microflora is simplified to a limited set of pathogens. *E. coli*, other Enterobacteriaceae and the *B. fragilis* group are predominant; enterococci are found in a minority. Other anaerobic organisms, although dominant numerically in the fecal flora, are rarely pathogens.

The role of enterococci remains controversial. The balance of clinical and experimental evidence suggests that enterococci are unimportant in community-acquired intra-abdominal sepsis. In animal models, antimicrobial agents directed against Enterobacteriaceae prevent mortality, agents active against anaerobes reduced the incidence of abscesses, but failure to cover enterococci had no effect. Randomized controlled clinical trials of antimicrobial regimens in which one arm was active against enterococci and the other was not, have consistently shown no benefit from anti-enterococcal coverage, including most recently a large trial comparing ertapenem (32% susceptible) to piperacillin–tazobactam (97% susceptible).[3] However, isolation of enterococcus from the initial drainage has been associated with a higher treatment failure rate than in patients without enterococcus (28% versus 14%).[4]

HOST DEFENCE

The lymphatic drainage is of primary importance in defense against the initial inoculum. In the first few minutes of peritoneal contamination, organisms are absorbed directly by the lymphatics or phagocytosed by resident macrophages and dendritic cells and quickly removed by the lymphatics to the lymph nodes of the mediastinum, the thoracic duct and the bloodstream. This is the dominant host defense mechanism in the first few hours, but at a cost of bacteremia and systemic sepsis. The peritoneal polymorphonuclear leukocyte (PMN) response begins at 1–2 hours and is maximal at 24–72 hours. Lipopolysaccharide (LPS) released by Enterobacteriaceae is the major mediator and is recognized by cells of the innate immune system via the LPS receptor complex consisting of CD14, Toll-like receptor 4 (TLR-4) and the myeloid differentiation protein 2 (MD-2). Spontaneous diffusion of LPS is very slow due to its amphiphile structure and tendency to form aggregates in aqueous solution. LPS binding protein (LBP) is an acute phase protein, the systemic levels of which are greatly increased in the first few days of sepsis. Local LBP in the peritoneal cavity greatly enhances the transfer of LPS to the CD14/TLR-4/MD-2 complex and augments the immediate response to LPS up to 1000-fold. This causes a release of cytokines and chemokines, and initiates the inflammatory response.

Encapsulated strains of *B. fragilis* are necessary for abscess formation, as *B. fragilis* strains without a capsule generally fail to induce abscess. Extracted capsular polysaccharide from *B. fragilis* induces a sterile abscess, histologically identical to that induced by live organisms. Athymic or T-cell depleted models show that T lymphocytes are required for the formation of intra-abdominal abscesses and large numbers of CD4+ T cells are present in the abscess wall. The proliferative response of T cells depends on amino acid (positively charged) and carboxyl or phosphate groups (negatively charged) on each repeating unit of the *B. fragilis* polysaccharide. These zwitterionic polysaccharides (ZPSs) are processed to low molecular weight carbohydrates by a nitric oxide-dependent mechanism in endosomes of antigen-presenting cells (APCs) and initially co-localize with HLA-DR MHC class II molecules on the endosomes and surface of the APCs. Co-stimulation via B7-2 and CD40 on the surface of the APC is required. This T-cell dependent abscess formation, unique to *B. fragilis*, *Staphylococcus aureus* and *Streptococcus pneumoniae* type 1, is an important exception to the general rule that the immune response to bacterial polysaccharide antigens is B-cell dependent and T-cell independent.[5,6] These models also demonstrated that adjuvant substances are critical through the induction of proinflammatory cytokines including tumor necrosis factor (TNF), interleukin (IL)-2, IL-18 and especially IL-17, produced by CD4+ T cells in the abscess wall.

PATHOPHYSIOLOGY

Injury to the peritoneum causes desquamation of the mesothelial cells and exposes the underlying extracellular matrix causing an innate inflammatory reaction characterized by release of matrix-bound proinflammatory cytokines (transforming growth factor beta (TGF-β), TNF and IL-1), chemoattractants (IL-8 and monocyte chemoattractant protein 1 (MCP-1)) and growth factors (TGF-β, IGF-1 and platelet-derived growth factor (PDGF)). Expression of tissue factor, the major initiator of the extrinsic pathway of coagulation, is upregulated by macrophages and mesothelial cells.[7] Activation of the extrinsic pathway leads to a fibrinous exudate which is organized by activated fibroblasts. Contact with adjacent tissue results in formation of fibrin bands, ultimately leading to adhesion formation. The process resolves with ingrowth of mesothelium to cover the injured surface and fibrinolysis driven by the enzyme plasmin, derived from its precursor plasminogen, a process regulated by tissue plasminogen activator (tPA). In the first 24 hours of peritonitis, tPA increases in the peritoneal fluid as high as 65-fold, and is critical to host defense by enhancing the migratory response of polymorphonuclear leukocytes.

The greater the injury to the peritoneal surface, the greater is the inflammatory response. Activation of the adaptive immune system takes longer to develop. Cytokines, released as part of the innate immune response, activate dendritic cells which in turn function as APCs to lymphocytes.[8] Exposure to bacteria leads to activation of Toll-like receptors, the most characterized of which is TLR-4, which recognizes LPS.[8] At least 10 different TLRs have been identified in humans that respond to different pathogen-associated molecular patterns.[9] TLRs are widely present in extracellular matrix and cell surfaces, particularly peritoneal mesothelial cells. In addition, endogenous agonists, such as heparin sulfate, a biologically active saccharide released from cell surfaces and extracellular matrices, also activate dendritic cells via a TLR-4 response. Prior release from constitutive inhibition by exposure to extracellular proteases such as elastase is required for TLR-4 activation.[10] Once activated, TRL-4 stimulates proinflammatory transcription factors such as nuclear factor kappa B (NF-κB) with resultant upregulation of proinflammatory genes. The resulting cascade produces the local and systemic manifestations of the systemic inflammatory response syndrome (SIRS) or sepsis in the presence of bacterial infection.

Whether the inflammation is contained and eradicated depends on the nature of the contamination, the concentration and virulence of infecting organisms and the immune competence of the individual.

The local inflammatory response, fibrin deposition and secondary intestinal ileus act to confine the area of inflammation. The greater omentum frequently becomes adherent, a process facilitated by local ileus. Thus a visceral perforation may 'seal' or contamination be confined and an abscess develop, as for example in diverticulitis. In the absence of continuing bacterial contamination, the host response may be sufficient to resolve the process; more often surgical or radiologic drainage is needed.

CLINICAL PRESENTATION

The history and physical examination define the urgency of intervention and guide decisions regarding diagnostic techniques. The history should determine how long the patient has been ill, where the pain is located, whether it has changed location or character, whether it is associated with anorexia, vomiting or obstipation, and whether the patient has been aware of fever or chills. A pertinent past medical history should include recent hospitalization, medications, especially antimicrobial exposure, chronic disease diagnoses and prior operations.

INVESTIGATION

Imaging and laparoscopy

An erect chest X-ray (Fig. 37.1) or lateral decubitus X-ray of the abdomen may show free intra-abdominal air, indicating perforation of a hollow viscus. Ultrasound examination of the biliary tree and pelvis and CT scans have superseded other diagnostic methods in assessing intra-abdominal sepsis (Figs 37.2, 37.3). The urgency is dictated by the degree of hemodynamic instability present; however, CT is the single best modality for fully evaluating the extent of disease.

Increasingly MRI is of use, particularly in patients who have been exposed to considerable radiation dosage in the course of their disease. Ultrasound is quite versatile and portable, allowing procedures to be performed in the ICU. Ultrasonography is limited by bowel gas, body habitus and lower sensitivity for retroperitoneal processes and parenchymal infection. In suspected biliary sepsis, ultrasound rapidly provides information concerning gallstone disease and biliary obstruction. Laparoscopy is a valuable diagnostic and potentially therapeutic tool in the management of localized peritonitis, particularly in suspected appendicitis, pelvic inflammatory disease, diverticulitis and tuberculous peritonitis.

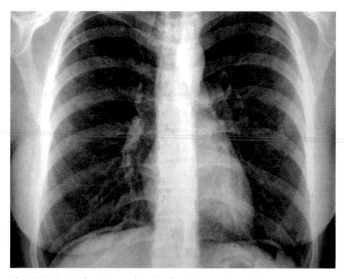

Fig. 37.1 Erect chest X-ray showing free intraperitoneal air.

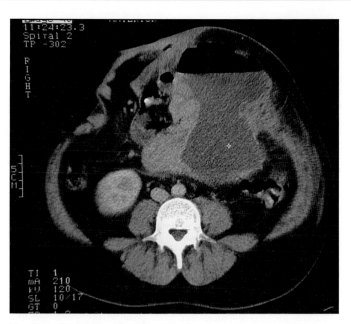

Fig. 37.2 CT abdomen showing a large intraloop abscess secondary to perforation from Crohn's disease.

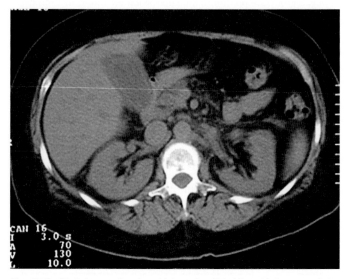

Fig. 37.3 CT abdomen showing thickened gallbladder with intramural air and pericholecystic fluid in a patient with biliary sepsis.

Microbiologic investigations

Blood cultures do not provide additional clinically relevant information for patients with community-acquired intra-abdominal infections. They are recommended in hospital-acquired complicated intra-abdominal sepsis, and when the patient presenting from the community is immunosuppressed or in shock, has a vascular access device, is an intravenous drug abuser or is otherwise at risk of bacteremia due to resistant organisms. With the exception of appendicitis, intra-operative cultures are recommended to detect resistant organisms, as failure rates are higher if therapy is not active against all Gram-negative facultative and anaerobic pathogens, and modifying the antibiotic regimen in response to the aerobic culture result improves outcome. A single sample of a least 0.5 cc of aspirated fluid or tissue is preferred to a swab. If anaerobic cultures are done, the specimen should be transported to the laboratory in an anaerobic transport system. If Gram staining is available in a timely manner then it may be valuable in health-care associated intra-abdominal infection in defining the need for specific therapy for methicillin resistant *Staphylococcus aureus* (MRSA) or vancomycin resistant enterococci (VRE).

ANTIMICROBIAL THERAPY

General considerations

In choosing the optimal antimicrobial regimen there is always difficulty between the need to cover all possible pathogens so as to minimize morbidity and mortality and the need to avoid the adverse effects of excessively broad-spectrum regimens. The latter include not only greater risk of *Clostridium difficile* superinfection, direct toxicities and cost, but also selection of resistant pathogens in the individual unit, hospital and broader community. The imperative of wise antimicrobial stewardship therefore applies, tempered by knowledge that failure to provide therapy active against the subsequently identified pathogens is associated with increased mortality.[11]

Patients who present from the community with a low risk of mortality should receive narrower spectrum regimens, primarily active against facultative Gram-negative bacilli such as *E. coli*. Agents with activity against the *B. fragilis* group are required for distal small-bowel and colon-derived infections and for more proximal gastrointestinal perforations, when obstruction is present. Enterococcal coverage is not required. Prolonged hospitalization, previous antimicrobial therapy and postoperative peritonitis are associated with more resistant microflora. In this context, and in patients with septic shock, multiorgan failure or high APACHE score, antimicrobial regimens should be both broad spectrum and informed by local nosocomial isolation and susceptibility patterns. This often requires the use of multidrug regimens such as combinations of an extended spectrum penicillin–β-lactamase inhibitor or a carbapenem, with an aminoglycoside, quinolone, tigecycline, vancomycin or antifungal agent.[12]

Timing and duration

Antimicrobial therapy should be initiated without delay, as deterioration to severe generalized peritonitis, septic shock and multiorgan failure can occur over a few hours. Administration of effective antimicrobial agents to patients with septic shock within the first hour of hypotension is associated with a survival of 80%, with each hour of delay causing an increment in mortality of 8% per hour over the first 6 hours.[13] Delay should be overcome, if necessary, by the physician administering the first dose.

Bowel injuries repaired within 12 hours, due to penetrating, blunt or iatrogenic trauma with intraoperative contamination, should be treated with antimicrobial agents for less than 24 hours. Acute perforations of the stomach, duodenum and proximal jejunum in the absence of antacid therapy or malignancy should also be treated for no more than 1 day. Similarly, acute appendicitis, without evidence of gangrene, abscess, perforation or peritonitis requires only 24 hours of an inexpensive regimen.[12]

Antimicrobial therapy for established intra-abdominal infection should be continued until resolution of clinical signs of infection occurs, including normalization of temperature and white blood cell (WBC) count and return of gastrointestinal function. When clinical features of infection persist or recur 5–7 days after definitive surgical and antimicrobial therapy, a thorough diagnostic effort should be undertaken, directed at potential abdominal and extra-abdominal sources. Investigations should include CT or ultrasonographic imaging, and antimicrobial therapy effective against the organisms initially identified should be continued. If a patient has persistent clinical symptoms and signs, but no evidence of a new or persistent infection is uncovered after careful investigation, termination of antimicrobial therapy is warranted.

Antimicrobial susceptibility in the *B. fragilis* group (see also Chapter 173)

Most clinical laboratories neither fully identify organisms to the species level within the *B. fragilis* group nor determine antimicrobial susceptibilities, as results are typically only available after the infection has resolved. Susceptibility testing of anaerobes is recommended when there is persistent isolation of the organism, when bacteremia is present, and when prolonged therapy is needed. Antimicrobial agents for anaerobic infections are selected empirically, based on multicenter surveys of the *B. fragilis* group. The largest of these was reported from 10 centers in the USA, with over 5000 isolates, over 8 years.[14] This reported only one isolate resistant to metronidazole (0.02%) and none resistant to chloramphenicol. The carbapenems and piperacillin–tazobactam had rates of resistance of 1% or less. Ampicillin–sulbactam (2.6%) and tigecycline (4.3%) had acceptable rates for empiric use but cefoxitin (10.3%), clindamycin (25.6%) and moxifloxacin (34.5%) did not. Tigecycline has potential as monotherapy, as *in vitro* it is active against anaerobes, most aerobic and facultative Gram-negative bacilli (except *Pseudomonas* and *Proteus* species), along with MRSA and VRE. However, other reports of higher rates of resistance to tigecycline in the *B. fragilis* group (19%)[15] give cause for concern.

Choice of antimicrobial regimen

A variety of narrower spectrum choices are appropriate for lower risk patients with community-acquired intra-abdominal sepsis. First- or second-generation cephalosporins cover *E. coli* and most other community Enterobacteriaceae. Metronidazole must be added when the *B. fragilis* group is a concern. Ampicillin–sulbactam or amoxicillin–clavulanic acid are active against almost all community-acquired Gram-negative bacilli and against almost all the *B. fragilis* group. Quinolones such as ciprofloxacin, ofloxacin, levofloxacin and moxifloxacin will also cover community-acquired Gram-negative bacilli. Metronidazole should be added when a quinolone is used if the *B. fragilis* group is a concern.

For patients at higher risk, piperacillin–tazobactam, ticarcillin–clavulanic acid or the carbapenems (namely imipenem–cilastatin, meropenem, ertapenem and doripenem) are all appropriate as monotherapy. However, generally carbapenems should be held in reserve to avoid selection of resistance against this important class. A third- (cefotaxime, ceftriaxone, ceftizoxime, ceftazidime) or fourth- (cefepime) generation cephalosporin, or a monobactam such as aztreonam, are also appropriate, but all must be combined with metronidazole. For health-care associated intra-abdominal sepsis, additional coverage against MRSA, VRE or a second agent for resistant Gram-negative bacilli may be warranted. Ceftobripole and ceftaroline are new cephalosporins with excellent *in-vitro* anti-MRSA and anti-enterococcal activity (including VRE), while maintaining activity against Enterobacteriaceae, other than extended-spectrum β-lactamase (ESBL) producers and *P. aeruginosa*. Their role in combination with metronidazole for intra-abdominal sepsis awaits the outcome of clinical trials.

Because aminoglycosides have narrow therapeutic ranges and cause nephrotoxicity and ototoxicity, they are no longer recommended as primary agents to cover facultative Gram-negative bacilli. Ototoxicity is irreversible, and is generally unappreciated as a risk. When antimicrobial therapy directed at enterococci is required, a penicillin (including piperacillin–tazobactam, ampicillin–sulbactam, ticarcillin–clavulanic acid or amoxicillin–clavulanic acid) or vancomycin is bacteriostatic, but sufficient. The addition of a low-dose aminoglycoside is required to render the regimen bactericidal only when enterococcal bacteremia has been demonstrated, when endocarditis is thought possible or when prosthetic cardiac valves are present. Cephalosporins and monobactams are not active against enterococci, with the exception of ceftobripole and ceftaroline. All carbapenems, except ertapenem, are active against *E. faecalis*. However, carbapenems are not active against other enterococcal species, such as *E. faecium*.

The extended-spectrum penicillins, when combined with a β-lactamase inhibitor (piperacillin–tazobactam or ticarcillin–clavulanic acid), are almost uniformly active against the anaerobic and facultative Gram-negative bacilli and enterococci, and are preferred choices as monotherapy for the sickest patients. Carbapenems should be chosen where ESBL-producing Gram-negative bacilli are recognized as a significant local problem. The chosen regimen should always cover enterococci for patients with septic shock, immunosuppression, prosthetic heart valves and postoperative peritonitis.

Intra-abdominal candidiasis

Candida is isolated from peritoneal samples in 20% of patients presenting in the community with acute perforation. However, this rarely progresses to invasive candidiasis so that specific antifungal therapy is unnecessary, unless the patient is immunosuppressed. Invasive intra-abdominal candidiasis is a significant complication of necrotizing pancreatitis and of postoperative peritonitis, especially in those with recurrent perforation or anastomotic leak. It carries a high mortality and manifests as peritonitis or abscess, with or without candidemia and disseminated candidiasis. It is difficult to confirm a diagnosis early, yet timely specific antifungal therapy is required in addition to drainage of abscess and surgical repair of perforation. Delay in antifungal therapy is associated with increased mortality.

The azole, fluconazole (800 mg load, 400 mg per day) is uniformly effective against *Candida albicans*. It is nontoxic, relatively inexpensive and effective by intravenous and oral routes. However, resistant non-albicans species such as *C. kruzei* and *C. glabrata* have become increasingly prevalent, especially in ICUs with considerable azole use. Fluconazole is the agent of choice for patients with mild to moderate disease, no previous azole exposure and not in a high risk group for *C. glabrata* (elderly, diabetics, cancer patients). In contrast to azoles, which are fungistatic, the echinocandins (caspofungin, anidulafungin, micafungin) are fungicidal, which is critical when cardiac or central nervous system involvement is suspected. Echinocandins may be superior to fluconazole and are clearly preferred as initial therapy for patients with moderate to severe disease and in those with recent exposure to azoles. In stable patients who are improving on an echinocandin, a switch to oral fluconazole should be considered when the isolate has been identified as a species susceptible to fluconazole (*C. albicans, C. paropsilosis, C. tropicalis*) or to oral voriconazole (*C. kruzei*). Fluconazole should be favored over echinocandins for *C. paropsilosis*, as resistance to echinocandins is a concern in this species. The duration of antifungal therapy is 14 days after resolution of clinical findings, drainage of abscess and correction of leaks.

Prophylaxis with fluconazole at 400 mg per day is justified in patients with necrotizing pancreatitis who are receiving broad-spectrum antibacterial therapy and in those with recurrent perforations or anastomotic leak. Empiric therapy with an echinocandin can be considered for critically ill patients with pancreatitis or intra-abdominal sepsis and no correctable cause of fever.

SURGICAL MANAGEMENT

The principles of surgical management of peritonitis are closure or removal of the perforated viscus and peritoneal decontamination, following appropriate preoperative resuscitation including antimicrobial therapy. In patients manifesting sepsis syndrome, resuscitation, prior to operative intervention, takes precedence over immediate laparotomy. The decision whether to re-anastomose following intestinal resection requires experienced assessment of risk factors. In general, anastomosis should not be undertaken in the presence of fecal peritonitis, hemodynamic instability or immunosuppression. Within these guidelines, primary anastomosis can be safely undertaken in patients

with perforated diverticular disease, avoiding the substantial postoperative morbidity of a Hartmann's procedure and the likelihood of a permanent colostomy.

In extreme circumstances, a damage control laparotomy may be performed with the object of arresting hemorrhage and preventing further contamination. Devitalized tissues and perforated bowel are either removed or exteriorized. No attempt is made to perform anastomosis and the abdominal wound is left open pending more definitive exploration 24–48 hours later. It is essential to avoid blood loss and hypothermia, both of which can lead to irretrievable coagulopathy. Handling of inflamed viscera is minimized to reduce the cascade of inflammatory mediators that are inevitably released into the systemic circulation, causing further hemodynamic instability.

Relaparotomy

Scheduled or 'second-look' relaparotomy became popular in the 1980s as a means of treating diffuse peritonitis. This was based on the concept that repetitive laparotomy would allow abdominal irrigation and prevent recurrent abscess formation. However, as experience accumulated, it became clear that mortality was not decreased and that there was a substantial increase in the incidence of intestinal fistulas. Relaparotomy has, in the main, been superseded by CT scanning, when clinically indicated, with percutaneous drainage of collections. Second-look laparotomy is now rarely used, except in the management of patients with mesenteric ischemia in whom doubt remains at first laparotomy concerning the viability of significant portions of small intestine.[16]

Wound closure

Wound closure is particularly problematic in the presence of peritonitis. By definition the wound is 'dirty' with a risk of postoperative wound infection that approximates 30% and subsequent wound dehiscence of 5–10%. The risks are increased in the elderly, malnourished, obese and diabetic, and in the presence of sepsis syndrome. Surgical options are to close the fascial layer and leave skin and subcutaneous tissue as an open wound that can be closed 5–7 days later (delayed primary closure) or left to close by secondary intention. In the latter situation, closure may be accelerated by use of a vacuum-type dressing as long as the fascial closure remains intact. Occasionally, intestinal distention and edema, particularly of the small bowel, preclude safe closure. In such circumstances, fascial closure is unwise and may lead to abdominal compartment syndrome with intra-abdominal pressures exceeding 25 mmHg. A number of surgical techniques are available to 'silo' abdominal contents until it is safe to close the peritoneal cavity. Postoperatively, abdominal distention and falling urinary output should raise suspicion of abdominal compartment syndrome, which can be confirmed by measuring intravesical pressure.

Postoperative peritonitis

Peritonitis following recent abdominal surgery poses a particular diagnostic and therapeutic challenge. It is usually due to a leak from a suture line and is typically discovered only after some delay, as a rule between the fifth and seventh postoperative days. The symptoms are often insidious and may mimic a cardiorespiratory complication, most commonly pulmonary embolism. A high index of suspicion must exist after intestinal anastomosis, particularly in patients who have undergone anterior resection or resection for Crohn's disease. In this situation, CT scanning is valuable but may not be diagnostic. The presence of free air within the peritoneal cavity is sometimes wrongly attributed to residual air following recent laparotomy. A high index of suspicion should lead to laparotomy, even in the absence of definitive radiologic evidence of anastomotic leakage. Where anastomotic leakage is confirmed, conventional wisdom dictates takedown of the anastomosis with a proximal stoma and closure of the distal stoma. Occasionally an experienced surgeon may choose to repair the defect and defunction the bowel proximally. Such a course can be considered only in a stable patient with minimal contamination.

Percutaneous drainage procedures

Percutaneous drainage and operative intervention are best viewed as complementary rather than competitive techniques. There are many situations for which percutaneous drainage is the definitive procedure of choice, others for which surgery alone is indicated and some for which both techniques are applicable, alone or in conjunction. Inflammation may manifest as a phlegmon (viable inflamed tissue), a liquefied abscess or infected necrotic (nonviable) tissue, or as a combination. Liquefied abscesses are drainable, whereas phlegmonous and necrotic tissue are not. Decisions regarding which modality to employ are largely based on CT findings.

Indications for percutaneous drainage have expanded significantly over the past decade and now include multiple and/or multiloculated abscesses, abscesses with enteric communication and infected hematomas. It is important that the drainage route does not cross a sterile fluid collection or other infected space due to the risk of cross-contamination. Crossing the pleural space for thoracic and upper abdominal drainage carries the risk of empyema formation. In most cases drainage is performed following fine needle (18–22 gauge) aspiration, with the aspirate being used to document infection, by Gram stain and culture and to determine the viscosity of the fluid. For most collections, a drain should be placed to ensure complete evacuation and minimize the chance of recurrence. The aspiration needle can be used for placement of a guide wire or as a guide for tandem insertion of the drain. If the patient is not already on antimicrobial therapy, this should be instituted prior to the drainage procedure to prevent bacteremia and minimize infection of sterile tissue.

The choice of catheter size is determined primarily by the viscosity of the fluid to be drained. In the majority of cases, 8–12F drains are sufficient. Larger drains may be needed for collections containing debris or more viscous fluid. Drains of larger caliber can be placed, if needed, by exchange over a guide wire. There is no limit to the number of drains that can be placed. While most abscesses can be drained with a single catheter, there should be no hesitation in placing as many drains as are needed to effectively evacuate the abscess(es).

Following catheter placement, the cavity should be evacuated as completely as possible and irrigated with saline until the fluid is clear. Initial manipulation of the catheter(s) and irrigation should be done as gently as possible to minimize the induction of bacteremia. Immediate imaging determines the need for repositioning of the catheter or for placing additional drains. For cavities that are completely evacuated at the initial drainage and for which there are no abnormal communications to viscera, simple gravity drainage is generally sufficient. For larger or more viscous collections and those with ongoing output due to fistulous connections, suction drainage with sump catheters is more effective. Presacral collections may be drained transrectally. Recent developments include endoscopically placed vacuum dressings mounted on a catheter delivery system.

Primary (spontaneous) peritonitis

Primary peritonitis is defined as infection of peritoneal fluid in the absence of causative intraperitoneal visceral pathology. It is almost always monomicrobial and bacterial, but herpes simplex virus and fungi, such as histoplasmosis and coccidioidomycosis, have also been described. Almost all cases occur in patients with ascites and cirrhosis and are then termed spontaneous bacterial peritonitis (SBP). Other underlying pathologies include nephrotic syndrome and congestive cardiac failure. The most common organisms cultured from SBP are *E. coli* and *K. pneumoniae*, which translocate from the bowel to the mesenteric lymph nodes and then to the ascitic fluid via to the

bloodstream. An increasing proportion is now due to viridans streptococci, MRSA along with quinolone-resistant and ESBL-producing Gram-negative bacilli due to the use of prophylactic quinolones and cephalosporins in patients with severe ascites.

Historically, *Streptococcus pneumoniae* was the most commonly recognized cause of primary peritonitis and remains a significant cause in patients with cirrhosis, in whom it usually arises as a bacteremic complication of respiratory tract infection. Pneumococcal peritonitis can also arise by the ascending route through the fallopian tubes in both healthy women of reproductive age and in premenarchial girls. *Aeromonas hydrophila* has recently emerged as an important cause of SBP in East Asia. It is usually a summer infection, preceded by diarrhea, and may originate from shellfish consumption.

New onset abdominal pain and distention with evidence of systemic sepsis in a patient with chronic ascites suggests SBP, but this presentation is not typical. More usually the presentation is subtle, with acute deterioration in renal function, unexplained encephalopathy and borderline fever. A low threshold for paracentesis is thus appropriate in patients with chronic ascites, who have unexplained nonspecific alteration in their clinical state. Ascitic fluid will yield >250 neutrophils/mm^3; this, combined with a monobacterial-positive culture, defines SBP. An ascitic fluid pH of less than 7.35 or a blood–ascitic fluid pH gradient >0.10 supports the diagnosis. Inoculation of blood culture bottles at the bedside with ascitic fluid improves the culture yield.

Culture-negative ascites with >250 neutrophils/mm^3 is termed culture-negative neutrocytic ascites (CNNA); it responds to antimicrobial therapy. Patients with positive ascites cultures, but with <250 neutrophils/mm^3 (bacterascites), should be treated if symptomatic, as some will progress to SBP. An ascitic fluid protein >1 g/dl, a low ascitic fluid glucose (<50 mg/dl) or an ascitic fluid lactate dehydrogenase (LDH) greater than serum level and especially polymicrobial infection, all point to the possibility of secondary peritonitis and the need for emergency imaging to detect gastrointestinal perforation.[17] Early diagnosis and treatment significantly improve prognosis. A third-generation cephalosporin, a quinolone or amoxicillin–clavulanic acid are all appropriate choices for 7 days. Repeat diagnostic paracentesis is indicated at 48–72 hours if there is no clinical improvement.

Treatment failure (10%) is associated with a mortality of 50–80% and is either due to delay in treatment initiation or to resistant organisms. Albumin infusions (1.5 g/kg day 1, 1 g/kg day 3) have been shown to reduce acute renal failure and mortality in those with pre-existing renal impairment and are recommended for all patients with SBP. Long-term secondary prophylaxis with a quinolone is recommended for all patients after an episode of SBP, despite the selection of quinolone-resistant Gram-negative bacilli, and higher rates of MRSA colonization and *C. difficile* diarrhea.

Short prophylaxis with a quinolone or a third-generation cephalosporin for up to 7 days in patients with variceal hemorrhage, irrespective of the presence of ascites, also improves patient survival. Survival benefit with long-term primary prophylaxis (before a first episode of SBP) has been demonstrated in two small studies,[18,19] which selected higher risk patients with low ascitic fluid protein. A low ascitic fluid protein of <10 g/dl and poor hepatic function, such as in those awaiting transplantation, identify a subset of patients who are at higher risk for developing SBP and in whom primary prophylaxis can be justified.

PERITONITIS ASSOCIATED WITH CHRONIC AMBULATORY PERITONEAL DIALYSIS (CAPD)

CAPD peritonitis carries a 1–6% mortality risk per episode, with an incidence that varies from 0.2 to 1.3 per patient per year.[20] Repeated bouts may result in sclerosing peritonitis, with resultant failure of dialysis and sometimes intestinal obstruction. Organisms gain entry most commonly by touch contamination, but a significant minority are caused by a prior exit-site infection and possibly by translocation from the bowel. The causative organisms are coagulase-negative staphylococci (22%), *S. aureus* (15%), Gram-negative bacilli (28%), fungi (2.5%) or anaerobes (2.5%), with up to 20% culture-negative. There has been a decline in numbers due to *S. aureus* and coagulase-negative staphylococci, related to improved exit-site care and to newer techniques.

Diagnosis is suggested by a cloudy peritoneal effluent, usually with abdominal pain and fever, and confirmed by >100 WBC/mm^3 in the effluent, with greater than 50% polymorphonuclear cells. Initial empiric antimicrobial therapy should cover both Gram-positive and Gram-negative organisms. A combination of cefazolin and gentamicin is generally preferred, but a vancomycin–gentamicin combination is preferred in centers with significant rates of MRSA. Intraperitoneal administration is superior to the parental route and achieves equivalent blood levels. Duration is for 2–3 weeks.

Eradication of the infection and continuation of CAPD is usual in 80–85% of the episodes. Approximately 10–15% of patients require catheter removal and transfer to hemodialysis. Early removal of the peritoneal catheter should occur for episodes due to *P. aeruginosa*, fungi, mycobacteria and vancomycin-resistant enterococci. The catheter should also be removed in patients who fail to respond to appropriate therapy within 4 days and in those who develop recurrent peritonitis with the same organism.

TUBERCULOUS PERITONITIS

Tuberculous peritonitis is now rare in developed countries with just 136 cases reported in the USA in 1999 (compared with 26 800 cases of ovarian cancer in 1997). However, it is common in the developing world and in emigrant communities. In sub-Saharan Africa it is the most common cause of exudative ascites. In the anti-tuberculous therapy era, mortality has varied from 15% to 52%, depending on the proportion of patients with underlying conditions.[21]

It is the great pretender or mimic, because it presents with non-specific, highly variable clinical findings. Investigations lack sensitivity and specificity with the exception of laparotomy or laparoscopy and possibly adenosine deaminase levels in ascitic fluid. Other conditions such as peritoneal metastatic malignancy and culture-negative neutrocytic peritonitis (CNNP) closely resemble it. Definitive diagnosis is often delayed due to the prolonged time required for mycobacterial culture. Furthermore, even culture of ascitic fluid may lack sensitivity, and although positive in the majority of modern reports, sensitivity in the past has been as low as 20%.

The proportion of all TB cases presenting as peritonitis has increased in some countries, in part related to a higher incidence amongst patients receiving CAPD and those with chronic ascites due to cirrhosis. Diagnosis in these groups is particularly challenging due to the difficulty in distinguishing TB peritonitis from the more common complications of CAPD peritonitis and spontaneous bacterial peritonitis. The triad of abdominal swelling, pain and fever is present in only 60% of patients, mainly due to a lack of fever in patients with advanced liver and renal failure.[21,22] The classic finding of doughy, tender abdominal masses occurs in only a small minority. Weight loss is common, but often obscured by weight gain from ascites. Peritoneal fluid is classically a lymphocytic exudate. However, especially in patients with cirrhosis or on CAPD, protein levels are commonly <25 g/dl. A significant minority of cases have >250 polymorphonuclear leukocytes/dl, suggestive of SBP in cirrhotic patients or of CNNP when bacterial cultures are negative.

Particularly in settings of high TB prevalence, care should be taken to exclude TB peritonitis using adenosine deaminase ascitic fluid levels (when available) or laparoscopy, before diagnosing CNNP. If measured, CA-125 levels can be markedly elevated in tuberculous peritonitis, leading to a false impression of ovarian carcinoma. Glove hypersensitivity, food-starch granulomatous peritonitis and pseudomyxoma peritonei are very rare conditions that may mimic TB peritonitis.

Although a tuberculin skin test (or QuantiFERON test) is often negative, a positive result in the presence of abdominal findings should heighten suspicion of tuberculous peritonitis. Abdominal CT scanning may show peritoneal or omental nodules or thickening, suggestive of carcinoma. Microscopy of ascitic fluid using Ziehl–Neelsen (ZN) staining is positive in zero to 6% of cases, while polymerase chain reaction (PCR) is positive in only a minority.[21] Adenosine deaminase is both highly sensitive and specific, when applied in countries of high prevalence. However, it had lower sensitivity (60%) when applied in a small study in the USA.

Direct inspection of the peritoneal cavity by laparoscopy, mini-laparotomy or full laparotomy, with detection of tubercles macroscopically and granulomata microscopically, is diagnostic in patients presenting with ascites of unknown cause.[21,23] Uniform nodules of less than 0.5 cm with adhesions are virtually diagnostic, while hemorrhagic inflammation, with either adhesions or nodules, is highly suggestive of tuberculous peritonitis. Tissue samples free of formalin, along with ascitic fluid, should be sent for mycobacterial culture, which is especially important to detect multidrug-resistant TB (MDRTB). Empiric treatment for TB peritonitis should be considered while awaiting definitive diagnosis, using four drugs initially, consisting of rifampicin, isoniazid, pyrazinamide and ethambutol. In areas with significant rates of MDRTB, a quinolone and amikacin should be added while awaiting the results of full sensitivities. Delay in treatment is associated with greater mortality. (See also Chapter 30.)

A minority of survivors may have recurrent intestinal obstruction from multiple chronic adhesions. There is suggestive evidence that corticosteroids will diminish this morbidity, but by abrogating the host response, the patient's demise may be hastened in the event of MDRTB. Adjunctive corticosteroids should be considered in patients in whom the diagnosis of tuberculous peritonitis is certain and in whom there is little concern about MDRTB. If used, corticosteroid doses should be sufficient to abrogate the granulomatous response. The authors favor prednisone or prednisolone at 1 mg/kg/day for 2 months with a slow wean over the following 2 months. (See also Practice Point 13.)

BILIARY SEPSIS

Biliary sepsis is usually associated with gallstone disease, pancreatic or bile duct malignancy or previous biliary tract surgery that has resulted in bile duct obstruction with secondary infection. The organisms involved are usually Enterobacteriaceae. Enterococci are uncommon and anaerobes are involved only if there is a bile duct to bowel anastomosis or previous biliary tract surgery. Acute cholecystitis is often an inflammatory but noninfective condition. If infection is suspected because of clinical and radiologic findings, antimicrobial therapy should be directed solely at facultative Gram-negative bacilli. Enterococcal coverage is not required and anaerobic coverage is necessary only in patients with bile duct–bowel anastomoses and in patients who have had previous biliary tract surgery. Infection in the biliary tree (cholangitis) typically presents with a triad of fever, rigors and jaundice (Charcot's triad).

Ultrasound is the best modality to confirm dilatation of bile ducts and the level of obstruction, usually at the lower end of the common bile duct or intrahepatic ducts. Magnetic resonance cholangiogram is particularly useful for delineation of biliary anatomy. Treatment is with antimicrobial agents and urgent decompression of the obstructed system. The technique used to decompress depends on the site of obstruction. Endoscopic retrograde cholangiopancreatography (ERCP) with stent insertion is used for common bile duct lesions, whereas percutaneous transhepatic cholangiography (PTC) with stenting, with or without external drainage, is used for intrahepatic or hilar lesions. Occasionally, both techniques are used simultaneously in a so-called 'rendezvous procedure'.

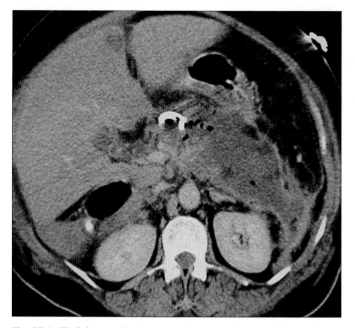

Fig. 37.4 CT abdomen showing extensive pancreatic necrosis.

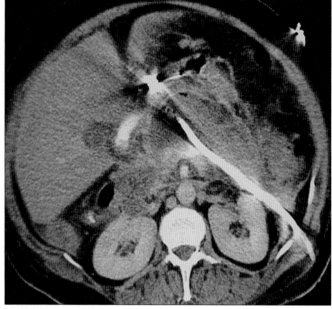

Fig. 37.5 CT drainage of pancreatic necrosis shown in Fig. 37.4.

PANCREATITIS

Severe acute pancreatitis occurs in about 25% of patients with acute pancreatitis. The severity of pancreatitis is related to development of SIRS, multiorgan failure and necrotizing pancreatitis.[24] The mortality in severe pancreatitis is bimodal, with a peak in the first week related to multiorgan failure, while a second peak occurs at 3–4 weeks related to pancreatic necrosis and retroperitoneal sepsis. Development of early multiorgan dysfunction and pancreatic necrosis (as determined by the presence of nonviable pancreatic tissue on CT scan) are highly predictive of subsequent later pancreatic and retroperitoneal sepsis. Infection complicating necrotizing pancreatitis is usually polymicrobial and resembles that occurring after colonic perforation.[25] There has been considerable surgical interest in whether early surgical intervention to debride the pancreas might favorably alter the course of necrotizing pancreatitis and reduce the incidence of late multiorgan failure, sepsis and death. Patients with extensive (>50%) sterile necrosis are at high risk of infection and progressive multiorgan failure.

Surgical debridement of necrotic pancreatic tissue is technically difficult and is associated with high perioperative complication rates. Frequently more than one exploration of the abdomen is required, leading to considerable difficulties in wound management and risks enteric and/or pancreatic fistula development. An aggressive early surgical approach advocated in many institutions has been replaced by a more conservative approach guided by the clinical course, sequential CT imaging (Fig. 37.4) and percutaneous wide bore catheter drainage (Fig. 37.5).[26] When a minimally invasive approach does not adequately evacuate the necrotic pancreatic and peripancreatic tissue, then either open or laparoscopic debridement may become necessary in the face of ongoing or worsening multiorgan dysfunction. Where possible, a retroperitoneal approach should be used to minimize risks of enteric injury leading to fistula.

There have been conflicting results concerning the role of prophylactic antimicrobial agents in preventing later pancreatic and retroperitoneal sepsis in patients with severe pancreatitis. Initially, a number of studies suggested a survival advantage and a decrease in pancreatic sepsis for the antibiotic treatment groups; however, a more recent meta-analysis[27] has shown no decrease in pancreatic sepsis but still a decrease in overall mortality was observed with treatment. However, a large multicenter, double-blinded trial of the use of intravenous meropenem in preventing or delaying pancreatic or peripancreatic infection in patients with a confirmed diagnosis of necrotizing pancreatitis has demonstrated no difference between treatment groups with respect to infection, mortality or requirement for surgical intervention.[25] This study leads to the conclusion that early prophylactic antibiotic use for patients with necrotizing pancreatitis is not supported.[26]

REFERENCES

References for this chapter can be found online at http://www.expertconsult.com

Stephen D Ryder

Chapter | **38** |

Viral hepatitis

INTRODUCTION

The clinical syndrome of acute hepatitis has been recognized since antiquity and is characterized by jaundice, usually after a prodromal illness. Acute hepatitis may cause severe sequelae, including fulminant hepatitis, but the major impact on human health is chronic liver disease and hepatocellular carcinoma resulting from chronic infection.

The nomenclature of the hepatitis viruses is somewhat eclectic, being based on the time of discovery of new or putative agents rather than on any consideration of modes of transmission or clinical problems associated with that agent. There are at present five primary human hepatotropic viruses, A, B, C, D and E, which are well characterized and known to account for approximately 90% of acute and 95% of chronic viral hepatitis. Other viruses may cause human disease (see Chapter 154).

EPIDEMIOLOGY

Hepatitis A virus

Hepatitis A virus (HAV) is distributed throughout the world and causes outbreaks of infection, usually in association with direct fecal–oral contact[1] or contaminated water supplies.[2] Most food-related outbreaks of HAV infection are sporadic and due to poor food hygiene measures; however, contamination of shellfish caused by sewage pollution is well described[3] and represents a continuing problem because mollusks are able to retain and concentrate viruses from water. Homosexual men and those working with newly imported nonhuman primates are high-risk groups for HAV infection. In the 1980s the proportion of cases of hepatitis A spread by blood contact increased to 19% of reported cases in the USA; this appears to have been due to intravenous drug use.[4]

In the developed world, the proportion of people who have immunity to HAV has declined over the past two decades owing to improved sanitary conditions in childhood. Travelers from low-risk geographic areas to high-risk areas are at substantial risk of acquiring HAV infection.[5] In the developing world, infection rates are as high as 95% by the age of 16 years. Early infection usually produces a less severe clinical illness and immunity to future infection. The incubation period is short, ranging from 15 to 50 days (mean 30 days).

Hepatitis B virus

Hepatitis B virus (HBV) is one of the most common chronic viral infections in the world, with estimates of approximately 170–350 million chronically infected people.[6] Hepatitis B virus infection is relatively rare in developed countries, with an incidence of 1 per 200 population in the UK and North America. Even in areas like the UK, where acute infection is relatively uncommon, up to 2% of the population show evidence of past infection. In high-risk areas such as South East Asia and sub-Saharan Africa up to 20% of the population have evidence of previous infection.[7] A major mode of spread in high-endemicity areas is vertical transmission from carrier mother to child, and this may account for 40–50% of all HBV infections in such areas.[8] This mode of transmission is highly efficient; more than 95% of children of carrier mothers are infected and develop chronic viral infection themselves. In low-endemicity countries the mode of spread in acute HVB is predominantly by sexual transmission or blood-borne transmission through intravenous drug use, whereas in most of northern Europe immigration accounts for a substantial proportion of new chronic cases of hepatitis B infection presenting to the health-care services. Many migrants are from areas of the world where hepatitis B infection is very common. It is estimated that in the UK 90% of new hepatitis B diagnoses are in migrant populations with chronic infection acquired in childhood. Between 5% and 10% of acutely infected adults develop chronic viral infection. Certain groups in the Western world are known to be at higher risk of HBV exposure; these include intravenous drug users, hemodialysis patients, homosexual men and institutionalized people, particularly those with mental handicap. Males are more likely to become chronic HBV carriers than females, for reasons that are unclear. The incubation period ranges from 28 to 160 days (mean 80 days).

Hepatitis C virus

Hepatitis C virus (HCV) infection is common, with an estimated 350 million cases worldwide. Unlike infection with HBV, this infection is very common in the developed world, with 0.3–0.7% of the UK population infected. The virus is spread almost exclusively by blood contact. Since the introduction of screening of blood products in 1990/1991, intravenous drug use has become the almost exclusive mode of hepatitis C transmission in Northern Europe and North America. In the early 1990s, 35% of cases in northern Europe had a past history of blood transfusion and a further 40% had used intravenous drugs. Of new cases seen in the late 1990s, intravenous drug use accounted for over 75% of cases. Sexual transmission does occur, but is unusual; less than 5% of long-term sexual partners become infected.[9] Vertical transmission also occurs, but again is unusual. It is certainly not the predominant mode of spread of HCV, with the frequency of infection in children of viremic mothers less than 5%. The mode of delivery does not affect infection rates and breast feeding is safe.[10] The rate of infection in children of infected parents may rise in the first 10 years of life but it seems relatively difficult to acquire this viral infection from close household contact.

This leaves a substantial minority of those identified in whom no specific risk factor is present. This proportion may be up to 20% of cases. It has been postulated that this group may have acquired the infection from medical interventions. This is based on the high prevalence of infection in areas such as southern Italy, where military vaccination programs were undertaken in the period immediately after the Second World War, and in Egypt, where up to 20% of the population has HCV markers in certain geographic areas and treatment for diseases such as schistosomiasis is commonly given by injection. Hospitalization for whatever reason appears to be a risk factor for HCV infection. The incubation period varies between 14 and 60 days (mean 50 days).

Hepatitis D virus

Hepatitis D virus (HDV) or delta virus is an incomplete RNA virus that uses hepatitis B surface antigen (HBsAg) to enable replication and transfer from cell to cell. Hence, its epidemiology is closely linked to that of HBV. There are, however, considerable differences in the frequency of delta infection or superinfection in different patient groups. Intravenous drug users have a relatively high incidence of HDV infection whereas homosexual men, a high-risk group for the sexual spread of HBV, have a low incidence of delta infection. The reason for this epidemiologic paradox is unknown. Transmission of HDV is parenteral,[11] either via transfusion or close personal contact. Screening of blood products for HBsAg effectively excludes HDV-positive donors. The commonest risk factor for the acquisition of HDV infection in the Western world is intravenous drug use, with between 17% and 90% of HBsAg-positive addicts also testing positive for HDV.[12] In developing countries, HDV infection generally parallels HBV infection, although there are exceptions, particularly in areas of Asia, where HDV is rare despite a high level of HBV carriage. In general, approximately 5% of people with chronic HBsAg carriage will be co-infected with HDV, giving an estimated worldwide figure in excess of 10 million. The incubation period is quite variable.

Hepatitis E virus

Hepatitis E virus is transmitted by the fecal–oral route. Its epidemiology correlates with the presence of contaminated water. It is responsible for outbreaks of epidemic-type hepatitis in the Indian subcontinent, but sporadic cases are seen throughout the world. The incubation period is short, ranging between 15 and 45 days (mean 40 days).

PATHOGENESIS AND PATHOLOGY

The molecular structure of the hepatitis viruses is considered in Chapter 154. The mechanisms of pathogenicity of the hepatitis viruses are complex and involve viral and host immune factors. The basis of any hepatitis is hepatocyte death, usually immunologically mediated in order to eliminate infected cells and to prevent further viral replication. It is highly likely that the mechanisms involved vary depending on the virus. Further differences in either the virus or the host response are involved in the development of chronic infection with HBV or HCV. Because these are the major cause of liver disease, these two viruses are considered in detail in this chapter.

Hepatitis B virus

Hepatitis B virus enters the hepatocyte by binding of determinants that are present on HBsAg. The virus replicates mainly in the hepatocyte (Fig. 38.1), although HBV DNA has been found in extrahepatic tissues, including skin, pancreas, kidneys, bone marrow and peripheral blood mononuclear cells. Hepatitis B virus has a highly unusual genetic structure, with a circular, partially ssDNA genome. When internalized in the hepatocyte, the genome is released and the negative strand is converted by ligation to a closed circular supercoiled form.[13] This form is present in the hepatocyte nucleus and forms the template for HBV RNA synthesis. Hepatitis B virus is almost unique in that its DNA is synthesized

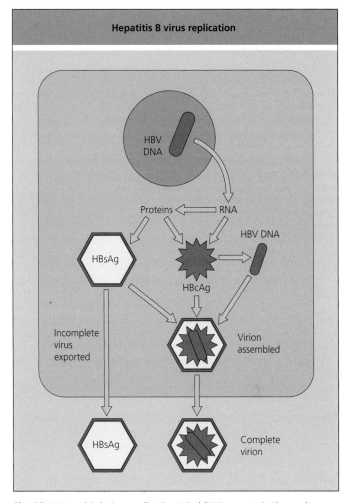

Fig. 38.1 Hepatitis B virus replication. Viral DNA present in the nucleus is transcribed to RNA, which then acts both as a template for protein synthesis (viral coat-HBsAg and viral proteins essential for infectivity and replication-HBcAg). Viral particles are then assembled and secreted from the cell cytoplasm. For every complete virion a large number of incomplete particles derived from HBsAg alone are exported. HBV, hepatitis B virus; HBsAg, hepatitis B surface antigen; HBcAg, hepatitis B core antigen.

via an RNA intermediate; the same molecules are therefore used for protein synthesis and for reverse transcription to DNA.

The HBV RNA template is encapsulated in hepatitis B core antigen (HBcAg) particles and reverse transcribed to produce negative-strand DNA. This is then used to synthesize an incomplete positive DNA strand and the virion is encapsulated with HBsAg before excretion from the cell.

There are a number of host mechanisms deployed to prevent initial infection and then to remove infected hepatocytes. Hepatitis B virus is not thought to be directly cytopathic except in highly specific circumstances, such as fibrosing cholestatic hepatitis seen in re-infection of liver grafts, when the host is immunosuppressed. Liver cell damage in both acute and chronic HBV infection is thought to be immunologically mediated.

Cell-mediated and humoral immune responses occur in HBV infection, and both are probably important in limiting and eliminating infection. There is invariably a humoral immune response directed against HBcAg and usually against HBsAg,[14] but this response alone is not the cause of hepatitis as evidenced by liver disease in agammaglobulinemic patients. The responses of human leukocyte antigen (HLA) class I restricted cytotoxic T lymphocytes are thought to be the major mechanism of liver cell injury.[15] The fact that patients with production of HBsAg alone in hepatocytes usually have little inflammatory liver disease suggests that the target of this attack is likely to be core antigen.

Acute HBV infection can be self-limiting with complete clearance of the virus or it can develop into chronic infection with the potential for the development of cirrhosis and primary liver cell cancer.

Chronic HBV infection can be thought of as occurring in phases, depending on the degree of immune response to the virus. This is particularly true of patients infected in the first few weeks of life. If infected when the immune response is 'immature', there is initially little or no immune response to HBV. The levels of HBV DNA in serum are very high and the hepatocytes contain abundant HBsAg and HBcAg, but little or no ongoing hepatocyte death is seen on a liver biopsy because of the defective immune response. This state persists for a variable period of time; usually the degree of immune recognition increases over some years. When immune recognition starts to occur, the level of HBV DNA tends to fall and the liver biopsy shows increasing inflammatory liver disease. This inflammation and hepatocyte death produces hepatic fibrosis. Once this phase of infection is initiated there are two major possible outcomes: either the immune response is adequate and the virus is inactivated and then removed from the system or the attempt at removal results in extensive fibrosis, distortion of the normal liver architecture and death from the complications of cirrhosis.

A third phase of hepatitis B virus infection is now recognized. This occurs late in the natural history of the immune response against HBV. In situations where the wild-type virus is inactivated but not eradicated, characterized by hepatitis B surface antigen positivity, e antigen negativity and undetectable levels of HBV DNA, there is still virus present in hepatocytes. This virus will be present in a number of forms, with viral mutants commonly produced. It is now well recognized that some of these mutant species can replicate in the presence of an adequate immune response against wild-type virus. This leads to re-emergence of HBV DNA in serum and

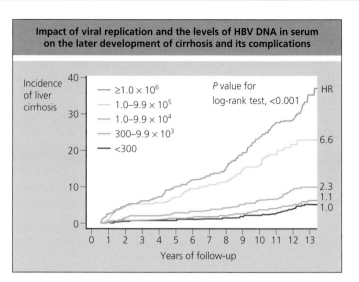

Impact of viral replication and the levels of HBV DNA in serum on the later development of cirrhosis and its complications

Fig. 38.3 Impact of viral replication and the levels of hepatitis B virus (HBV) DNA in serum on the later development of cirrhosis and its complications.

can lead to progressive liver injury (Figs 38.2, 38.3). These mutant stains may account for up to 60% of all replicating HBV infection in Europe. Recognition of this situation clinically is important because reactivation of HBV replication carries a significant risk of the development of hepatic fibrosis and cirrhosis and therapy is different from the usual 'wild type', e antigen-producing HBV. It is simple to recognize as abnormal transaminases and significant levels of HBV DNA are present in the serum in patients who are HBsAg positive but e antigen negative.

Hepatitis C virus

Chronic HCV infection has a long natural history, with most patients discovered in the presymptomatic stage. In the UK, most patients are now screened because of an identifiable risk factor (previous intravenous drug use or blood transfusion) or because of abnormal liver biochemistry.

The mechanism by which HCV causes human disease is unclear. A very high proportion (70–80%) of acute infections go on to become chronic and the prognosis from chronic infection is very variable. Some infected people have normal liver histology,[16] which indicates that HCV is not directly cytopathic for hepatocytes. Immune mechanisms are again thought to be important in determining outcome.

Hepatitis C virus is an RNA virus. It is highly variable, with six major genotypes.[17] Genotypes are frequently geographically restricted, such as type 4 in the Middle East, or may vary with time and mode of spread. This has been seen in Europe with genotype 1 occurring in older transfused individuals, with type 3 in younger drug users. There is some evidence that viral factors are important in the outcome of HCV infection. More severe fibrotic disease has been found in patients infected with genotype 1a or 1b than in those infected with other genotypes.[18] This is somewhat controversial as there are confounding factors, such as duration and mode of transmission, that make interpretation difficult.[19] The variability of the infecting HCV has also been postulated to affect outcome. The number of quasispecies present, a measure of genetic variability within a viral population, has been suggested as an important factor in evading the host immune response. Furthermore, quasispecies variability has been shown to be associated with increasing severity of liver disease,[20] whereas the number of quasispecies present in serum is higher in acute infection than in chronic infection.[21] More severe outcome appears to be correlated with selection of single species in the infecting HCV, which are presumably better adapted to survive in that particular immune environment.[22] The level of viremia in a patient with HCV infection can be determined using quantitative polymerase chain reaction (PCR) methods and is important in determining response to therapy.

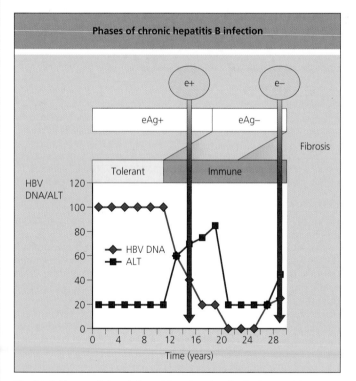

Phases of chronic hepatitis B infection

Fig. 38.2 Phases of chronic hepatitis B virus (HBV) infection. Initial infection is usually in childhood and has a long immune tolerant phase. Immune recognition then develops which can allow inactivation of HBV by either clearance of infected cells (with associated liver cell damage) or suppression of viral antigen expression on infected hepatocytes. This produces viral inactivation. In a significant proportion of patients where this has occurred, a third phase develops, where replication of HBV resumes due to viral escape mutants, leading to HBV DNA again appearing in serum and the risk of chronic liver disease. The two phases of liver injury where treatment may be required are indicated by the red arrows. ALT, alanine transaminase.

Evidence suggests that the host immune response is important in determining the outcome of HCV infection. There are HLA associations with viral clearance as evidenced by positive antibodies and negative tests for circulating viral genome. In addition, patients with combined HCV and HIV infections and patients who were infected with HCV as a result of contaminated immunoglobulin given for hypogammaglobulinemia have more severe and more rapidly progressive liver disease.

PREVENTION

Strategies are available to prevent some, but not all, hepatitis virus infections; a detailed discussion is provided in Chapter 154.

CLINICAL FEATURES

Acute hepatitis

Anicteric disease

A large proportion of infections with any of the hepatitis viruses are asymptomatic or anicteric illnesses. Hepatitis A virus typically causes a minor illness in childhood, with more than 80% of infections being asymptomatic. In adult life infection is more likely to produce clinical symptoms, although only 30% of a cohort exposed to contaminated water experienced icteric illness.[2] Infections with HBV, HCV and HDV can also be asymptomatic. With HBV infection this again depends on the mode and time of transmission. Vertical transmission of infection from mother to child is almost always asymptomatic, although it produces chronic infection in the child. Transmission of HBV by other routes is much more likely to produce a symptomatic illness; about 30% of cases transmitted by intravenous drug use are icteric.

Clinically apparent acute hepatitis

Acute hepatitis presents with jaundice or elevated liver enzymes, usually preceded by a prodromal illness. The clinical features give little indication as to the likely etiologic agent. A history from patients who are suspected to have an acute hepatitis should be aimed at identification of specific risk factors for viral or other liver disease (Table 38.1).

Common symptoms in the preicteric phase include myalgia, nausea, vomiting, fatigue and malaise. There is often a change in the sense of smell or taste, and right upper abdominal pain is common. Coryza, photophobia and headache are often seen, and cough may be prominent in hepatitis A. Diarrhea with transient pale stools and dark urine may occur.

A serum sickness-like illness occurs in about 10% of patients who have acute HBV infection and in 5–10% of patients who have acute HCV infection.[23] This is characterized by an urticarial or maculopapular rash and arthralgia, typically affecting the wrist, knees, elbows and

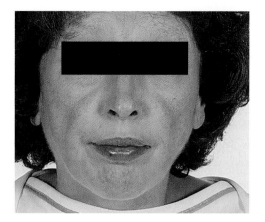

Fig. 38.4 Facial stigmata of chronic liver disease. This woman presented with serologically proven acute hepatitis A virus infection. She has multiple stigmata of chronic liver disease including facial spider nevi and was shown to have pre-existing cirrhosis.

ankles. This illness is due to immune complex formation and rheumatoid factor is frequently positive. It is almost always self-limiting and usually settles rapidly after the onset of jaundice.

Viral hepatitis may produce other clinical or subclinical problems. Acute hepatitis B is rarely associated with clinical pancreatitis in the acute phase of the illness, although elevation of amylase is present in up to 30% of patients and autopsy studies in patients who have fulminant hepatitis B show histologic changes of pancreatitis in up to 50%. Myocarditis, pericarditis, pleural effusion, aplastic anemia, encephalitis and polyneuritis have all been reported.

Physical examination in the preicteric phase is usually normal although mild hepatomegaly (10%), splenomegaly (5%) and lymphadenopathy (5%) may be seen. Stigmata of chronic liver disease should not be present in patients who have an acute illness, and their detection suggests either that the episode causing presentation is the direct result of chronic liver disease or that there has been an acute event superimposed on a background of chronic liver disease, as for example in HDV superinfection in an HBV carrier (Fig. 38.4).

The transaminase levels in acute hepatitis may reach 100 times normal.[24] Leukopenia is common, and in 10% of patients the white cell count may fall below 5000/mm³.[25] Both anemia and thrombocytopenia are described. Immunoglobulin levels may be nonspecifically elevated in viral hepatitis, with levels usually returning to normal within 2 weeks. In a small proportion of patients who have acute viral hepatitis, a profound cholestatic illness may occur. This is most frequently seen in patients who have hepatitis A and it may be prolonged, with occasional patients remaining jaundiced for up to 8 months.

Death from acute viral hepatitis is usually due to the development of fulminant hepatitis. This is usually defined as hepatic encephalopathy with an onset within 8 weeks of symptoms or within 2 weeks of onset of jaundice.[26] The risk of developing fulminant liver failure is generally low but there are groups with higher risks. Pregnant women with acute HEV infection have a risk of fulminant liver failure of around 15%, with a mortality of 10–40%.[27] The risk of developing fulminant liver failure in HAV infection increases with age[28] and with pre-existing liver disease.[29] Fulminant hepatitis B is seen in adult infection but it is relatively rare.

The primary clinical features of acute liver failure are encephalopathy and jaundice. Jaundice almost always precedes encephalopathy in acute liver failure, and the onset of confusion or drowsiness in a patient who has acute viral hepatitis is always a sinister development. The degree of the rise in transaminase values does not correlate with the risk of developing liver failure. Prolongation of coagulation is the

Table 38.1 Important points in the history of a patient who has suspected viral hepatitis

- Contacts with jaundiced patients
- Intravenous drug use
- History of blood transfusion
- Surgery or hospitalizations
- Family history of chronic liver disease
- Occupation

biochemical hallmark of liver failure; it is caused by lack of synthesis of liver-derived clotting factors. Prolongation of the prothrombin time in acute hepatitis, even if the patient is clinically well without signs of encephalopathy, should be regarded as sinister and monitored closely. Hypoglycemia is seen only in fulminant liver disease, when it can be profound.

Chronic hepatitis

The agents that cause chronic hepatitis are HBV, HCV and HDV. Chronic hepatitis has been defined as abnormality of transaminase values persisting for more than 6 months. This has generally been a useful concept in patients who present with an acute illness. In clinical practice, the vast majority of patients will present with either an asymptomatic biochemical or serologic abnormality or the complications of cirrhosis, and it is reasonable to assume chronicity in these clinical settings at the time of initial presentation. Chronic viral hepatitis is characterized by the presence of inflammatory infiltrates in the liver associated with hepatocyte death.

The risk of developing chronic infection varies greatly with the virus implicated. Hepatitis A virus never causes chronic viremia or chronic liver disease. Hepatitis B virus causes chronic liver disease in a proportion of infected patients; this rate varies depending on the mode of transmission. Patients who are infected at or around the time of birth via a chronic carrier mother have infection rates of almost 100%, with the vast majority becoming chronic carriers of the virus and therefore at risk of long-term liver damage.[30] If HBV is acquired in later life, the risk of chronic infection falls considerably, with only 5% of such patients remaining HBsAg positive at 5 years.[31] The difference in the rate of chronic infection is probably related to the maturity of the host immune response.

Infection with HCV has, overall, the highest risk of chronicity. Post-transfusion studies indicate that at least 50% of patients with icteric disease develop chronically abnormal transaminase values, and most studies suggest that up to 80% of acutely infected people remain viremic.[32]

Hepatitis D virus can cause chronic liver damage and there is evidence to suggest that the combination of HBV and HDV carries a particularly poor outlook.

Most patients who have chronic viral hepatitis either present with a complication of their viral liver disease or are detected by screening, either for viral serology or for abnormal biochemistry.

Symptoms

The majority of patients who have chronic viral hepatitis are asymptomatic and patients are often unaware of the infection. In HCV infection a number of symptoms are frequently reported by patients in the absence of severe liver disease. These include lethargy, inability to concentrate and pain over the liver. It is unclear if these symptoms are the direct result of the viremia or are related to depression as a result of the diagnosis. These symptoms, whatever their origin, contribute to a reduced quality of life for patients with hepatitis C compared to patients with chronic hepatitis B.[33] Other symptoms are due either to associated diseases affecting organs other than the liver or to end-stage liver disease.

Extrahepatic manifestations

Chronic hepatitis B can be associated with polyarteritis nodosa, with vasculitic rash, fever and polyarthralgia. Circulating HBsAg and anti-HBs complexes can be demonstrated, as can cryoglobins and HBsAg in blood vessel walls.[34] Glomerulonephritis is now known to occur with both HBV[35] and HCV infections.[36] This is a relatively rare association thought to be mediated by the deposition of immune complexes. The renal lesion improves on treatment of the responsible virus. Up to 60% of patients who have mixed essential cryoglobulinemia are anti-HCV positive;[37] the condition is again thought to be the result of

immune complex formation and antigen–antibody deposition in the vasculature. Successful therapy of the underlying hepatitis C produces remission.

Porphyria cutanea tarda is strongly associated with HCV infection, with up to 76% of Italian patients with porphyria cutanea tarda having antibodies to HCV.[38] Lichen planus is also associated with HCV infection.

Clinical signs

Patients who have decompensated cirrhosis caused by viral agents present with jaundice, encephalopathy, ascites or gastrointestinal bleeding as a result of portal hypertension (Fig. 38.5).

Cutaneous stigmata of chronic liver disease, spider nevi, leukonychia, gynecomastia, testicular atrophy and loss of body hair may be present. A late complication of chronic liver disease caused by HBV, HCV or HDV is hepatocellular carcinoma (Figs 38.6, 38.7).

Hepatocellular carcinoma may present as a sudden decompensation of previously stable chronic liver disease or as pain in the right upper quadrant of the abdomen, or there may be distant metastatic disease, with pulmonary or bone metastases being most common. Alpha-fetoprotein is often raised, although this is normal in up to 60% of small hepatomas.

All of these clinical signs occur late in the course of these viral infections and for most of the duration of infection no abnormal clinical signs will be present and the patient will be asymptomatic.

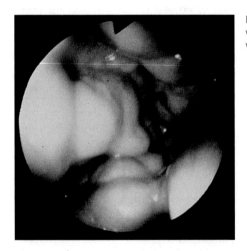

Fig. 38.5 Endoscopic view of esophageal varices.

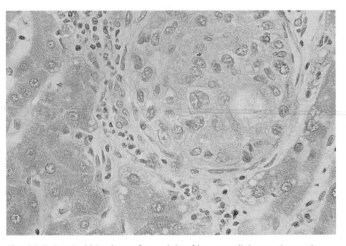

Fig. 38.6 Surgical histology of a nodule of hepatocellular carcinoma in a patient undergoing liver transplantation for hepatitis C cirrhosis.

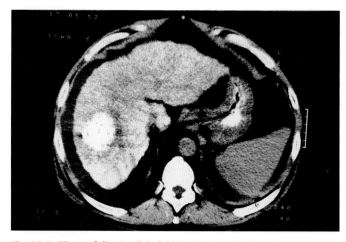

Fig. 38.7 CT scan following lipiodol injection into the hepatic artery showing hepatocellular carcinoma in the cirrhotic liver of a hepatitis B virus-positive male. Lipiodol is selectively retained in the tumor.

DIAGNOSIS

Acute hepatitis

Infection with HAV can be diagnosed by the presence of anti-HAV IgM with very high sensitivity and specificity.[39]

Infection with HBV is usually characterized by the presence of HBsAg. In acute HBV infection the serology can be difficult to interpret. The reason that an acute hepatitis develops is the immune recognition of infected liver cells, which results in T-lymphocyte-mediated hepatocyte killing. Active hepatocyte regeneration then occurs to replace those hepatocytes that have been lost. Because of the brisk immune response at the time of presentation with acute hepatitis B, viral replication may already have ceased and the patient may be HBsAg positive, hepatitis B e antigen (HBeAg) negative.

The diagnostic test is IgM antibody to HBcAg (IgM anticore; Fig. 38.8), which represents a sensitive and specific marker of acute HBV infection.[40]

Diagnosing past HBV infection or establishing immunity to vaccine is easy serologically. The levels of HBV-associated antibodies

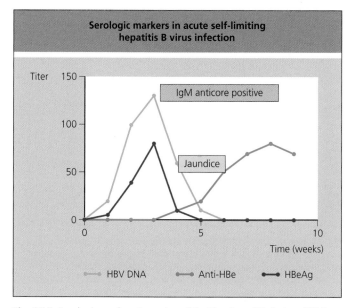

Fig. 38.8 Serologic markers in acute self-limiting hepatitis B virus (HBV) infection. HBeAg, hepatitis B e antigen. Measurements in arbitrary units.

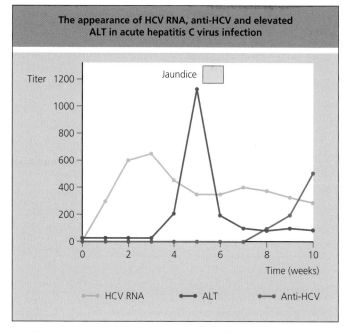

Fig. 38.9 The appearance of hepatitis C virus (HCV) RNA, anti-HCV and elevated alanine transaminase (ALT) in acute HCV infection. Measurements in arbitrary units.

decline with time. This is particularly true of anti-HBsAg. Despite this low level, immunity is still sufficient to prevent re-infection. Natural immunity is proven by the presence of IgG antibodies to HBcAg. These are a highly reliable marker of past infection and remain at detectable levels for a long period. Vaccine-induced immunity is directed purely against HBsAg epitopes, and hence a vaccinated person will have detectable levels of anti-HBsAg but no anti-HBcAg.

Acute hepatitis C cannot be reliably diagnosed by antibody tests because these frequently do not become positive for up to 3 months (Fig. 38.9).

Hepatitis C virus used to be the cause of more than 90% of all post-transfusion hepatitis in Europe and North America.[41] Acute HCV infection is now most commonly seen in intravenous drug users or in HIV-positive men who have sex with men where the risk of sexual transmission seems relatively high. If clinical suspicion is high and risk factors are present, testing of serum for HCV RNA is the only means of establishing the diagnosis (see Fig. 38.9). Identification of cases of acute HCV infection is important because there is strong evidence that early treatment with interferon alpha (IFN-α) may reduce the risk of chronic infection with HCV from around 80% to less than 10% with interferon monotherapy given for 6 months.[42]

Patients with HBV infection are at risk of delta virus infection either after HBV infection (superinfection) or simultaneously (co-infection). Co-infection is usually relatively benign; the determining factor for severity of illness is the HBV infection. As this is usually self-limiting, with loss of HBsAg after a relatively short interval, chronic infection with HDV is rare (about 2%).

Superinfection with HDV is a much more severe disease. The presence of large amounts of HBsAg allows rapid replication of the HDV and establishment of both acute and chronic infection. Chronic infection is common in this setting because the continued production of HBsAg allows the delta agent to continue replication. Diagnosis of delta hepatitis is by antibody testing and viremia is confirmed by the detection of HDV RNA in serum.[43]

A number of other viruses can cause hepatitis (Table 38.2). In the main, liver involvement is incidental and other features of the illness will suggest a diagnosis other than primary hepatitis. The exceptions are yellow fever, and disseminated herpes simplex and varicella-zoster infections in immunosuppressed patients, which in both cases may be associated with a severe hepatitis.

Table 38.2 Viral infections that may be associated with hepatitis

CMV, EBV	Both these viruses cause an acute mononucleosis-type syndrome in the normal host. Mild elevations of the liver transaminases may be seen but are usually of little consequence
CMV, HSV, VZV	All may cause hepatitis in the immunosuppressed host as part of a disseminated infection. CMV is the least severe
Flaviviruses	Yellow fever causes severe hepatitis
Measles, rubella, rubeola, Coxsackie B adenovirus	Mild hepatitis occurs occasionally

CMV, cytomegalovirus; EBV, Epstein–Barr virus; HSV, herpes simplex virus; VZV, varicella-zoster virus.

Chronic viral liver disease

Chronic viral liver disease may present with abnormal liver biochemistry (elevated transaminases), by serologic testing in at-risk groups without symptoms or as a result of the complications of cirrhosis. In contrast to the situation in acute infection, the rise in the transaminases is characteristically only two or three times the upper limit of normal. In HCV infection, the gamma-glutamyl transpeptidase values are also often elevated. The degree of abnormality of transaminases has little relevance to the degree of underlying hepatic inflammation. This is particularly true of HCV infection, in which the transaminase values are often normal despite active liver inflammation.

Further investigation in patients who have a positive serologic test for a hepatotrophic virus is to exclude other concomitant liver disease and assess the severity of liver damage. Table 38.3 shows the required baseline serologic tests required. In HCV infection, autoantibodies are frequently positive, antismooth muscle antibodies being detected in about 10% of patients and low-titer antinuclear antibodies in 15–20%. These autoantibodies do not appear to play a part in pathogenesis and would only alter management if a high titer were present with a raised IgG, suggesting a primary autoimmune hepatitis, in which interferon therapy may be contraindicated.

Chronic hepatitis B

The vast majority of patients who have hepatitis B will be HBsAg positive. There are viral mutants that do not produce HBsAg detectable by the usual serologic tests (Table 38.4), but these are very rare except in patients treated with interferon or after liver transplant.

The traditional classification of those individuals who have chronic hepatitis B has been based on the presence of HBeAg. All patients who have HBsAg can be regarded as infected but HBeAg has been regarded as a marker of infectivity. Hepatitis B e antigen is produced as a truncated version of core protein (Fig. 38.10).

Table 38.3 Tests required in asymptomatic patients who have elevated transaminase levels

- Hepatitis B surface antigen
- Hepatitis C virus antibodies
- Antismooth muscle, antinuclear antibodies
- Immunoglobulins
- Copper studies (if patient >50 years)
- Ferritin
- α_1-Antitrypsin phenotype (if indicated)

Table 38.4 Tests required for diagnosis in hepatitis B virus infection

- Hepatitis B surface antigen
- Hepatitis B e antigen
- Hepatitis B anticore antibody (HB total anticore)
- Hepatitis B DNA
- Hepatitis B IgM anticore

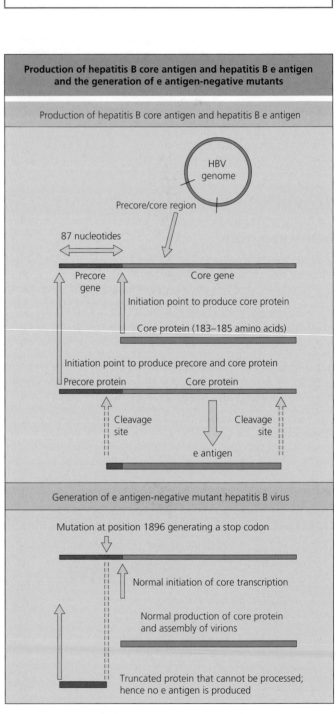

Fig. 38.10 Production of hepatitis B core antigen and hepatitis B e antigen and the generation of e antigen-negative mutants. Hepatitis B virus (HBV) has a closed circular genome that contains insufficient bases to produce all its required proteins. It therefore uses different start points for transcription, enabling it to use the same base sequence to produce different proteins. Two important proteins, e antigen and core antigen, are produced by transcription of the same region with overlap; e antigen is produced from the core protein by cleavage at a specific site.

Table 38.5 Investigations required in anti-hepatitis C virus-positive patients

Tests to assess hepatitis C virus	Tests to exclude other liver diseases
PCR for hepatitis C virus RNA Viral load Genotype	Ferritin Autoantibodies and immunoglobulins Hepatitis B serology Liver ultrasound

In the wild-type virus, HBcAg and HBeAg are transcribed together using overlapping bases. Hence HBeAg is an indirect marker of viral replication. The exact function of HBeAg is unclear but it appears to be involved in the downregulation of the T-lymphocyte response to HBV infection and may play a pivotal role in the development of the long phase of relative immunologic tolerance seen in chronic HBV infection acquired in childhood.

The discovery of HBeAg-negative mutant viruses has produced the need for a more specific marker of viral replication. The measurement of HBV DNA directly detects the circulating HBV genome.[44] This is the most sensitive measure of viral activity and is measured using PCR-based techniques, which can detect levels down to 40 IU/ml.

Patients who have persistence of HBsAg after 20 weeks of an acute episode can be assumed to have chronic infection. Spontaneous loss of HBsAg after this time is unusual, being seen in only 1–2% of patients a year. An apparently healthy person who is HBsAg positive can be regarded as chronically infected with HBV. The prognosis for that person is largely determined by the presence or absence of ongoing viral replication.

Chronic hepatitis C

Screening for HCV relies on antibody testing. Direct detection of viral RNA in peripheral blood using PCR provides evidence of ongoing viremia. Patients presenting with detectable antibodies to HCV should be investigated (Table 38.5) to exclude other causes of chronic liver disease and to assess the factors that will affect the outcome of therapy.

Chronic hepatitis D

Chronic infection with HDV has a high risk of producing severe liver disease. In the vast majority of cases of chronic infection, the HBV infection is nonreplicative as evidenced by HBeAg negativity and absence of HBV DNA.[45] This viral interference is seen in many combined viral infections (e.g. HBV and HCV infections) and it is rare to find patients with two replicating hepatotropic viruses. However, if the accompanying HBV is replicating, the prognosis is very poor, with rapid progression to cirrhosis over as little as 2 years.[45]

Diagnosis of chronic HDV infection is by antibody testing and viremia confirmed by delta RNA testing.

MANAGEMENT

Hepatitis B

Natural history of hepatitis B infection

Worldwide the majority of chronic HBV infections are in childhood. Infection in infancy with an immature immune system allows chronicity of infection. There are then two key factors in the outcome of that infection: viral replication and the inflammatory liver disease induced by the host in an attempt to clear infected hepatocytes from the liver. The virus is not itself cytopathic, other than in profound immunosuppression. The degree of immune recognition determines control of viral replication as well as causing liver injury.

There are a number of phases of infection with HBV determined by this immune response. Initially, there is high level viral replication in a host who has no immune recognition of the virus. At this stage there is no liver injury, hence alanine transaminase (ALT) is normal and if a liver biopsy were performed there would be no inflammatory liver disease. This phase of HBV infection lasts a variable time, from days to decades.

At some point, however, immune recognition of HBV-infected hepatocytes starts with the onset of liver injury. This phase of immune activation again is variable in its duration which is important in the risk of development of hepatic fibrosis, cirrhosis and its complications. If immune control is established rapidly it is likely that viral inactivation will occur (marked by the transition from e antigen to e antibody positivity) without the development of severe liver fibrosis; however, the opposite is also true, that a prolonged immune active phase may well result in the death of the infected patients from the complications of cirrhosis. Thus one of the key goals of therapy in e antigen-positive HBV is to reduce this phase of viral replication in the face of an immune response to reduce the risk of hepatic fibrosis. In most patients, with or without therapy, inactivation of HBV is marked by e antigen seroconversion and cessation of viral replication. With this control of viral replication liver injury also stops and transaminases return to normal. The patient remains infected with HBV and continues to be HBsAg positive. This was previously referred to as 'chronic carrier state' but this term is rather misleading and implies a benign process which is not always the case. The phase of immune control may last lifelong but is a dynamic situation, with the virus attempting to replicate and the host immune response providing control.

A final phase of HBV infection then ensues in approximately 40% of patients with the development of precore mutants of HBV which evade a previously adequate immune response and resume replication with concomitant liver injury.

Assessment of a patient who has chronic HBV infection should include ALT, e antigen and antibody status and HBV DNA levels. In patients who have no evidence of viral replication and normal liver enzyme levels and a normal liver ultrasound, liver biopsy is not usually required. Such patients have a very low risk of developing symptomatic liver disease or hepatocellular carcinoma. Reactivation of HBV replication has been described due to development of viral mutants which escape immune surveillance and patients who are HBsAg positive should be followed with yearly serology and liver enzyme estimations. The low risk of hepatocellular carcinoma does not justify screening in this group unless the patient is known to have cirrhosis. In patients who have abnormal liver biochemistry (even without detectable HBV DNA) or an abnormal liver texture on ultrasound, a liver biopsy is probably required, because such patients may either have superinfection with HDV or have had ongoing replication of HBV in the past, sustaining substantial liver damage in the process. It is estimated that around 5% of patients in developed countries who have only HBsAg carriage at presentation will have a posthepatic cirrhosis on liver biopsy. This finding is important because they are at risk of developing the complications of cirrhosis including variceal bleeding and hepatocellular carcinoma.

Patients with detectable HBV DNA in their blood are at risk of developing liver disease. There are a number of possible aims in HBV therapy, with the ideal being clearance of HBsAg. This is not commonly possible with current therapy and it is now generally accepted that the key aim is viral inactivation, with the hope that sustained suppression of viral replication will in time lead to viral eradication. There are two phases of HBV when therapy may be helpful: eAg positive immune-active phase and eAg negative reactivation (see Fig. 38.2).

Assessment of patients who have HBV replication is carried out by assessing the degree of liver inflammation and the stage of the underlying liver disease. Patients who are still in the tolerant phase of their infection usually have normal transaminase levels and high serum levels of HBV DNA (in excess of 10^8 IU/ml). As immune recognition increases, the HBV DNA levels fall, the degree of hepatic damage increases and the transaminases become abnormal. This is important in the selection of patients for therapy. Patients who have viral replication and abnormal transaminases should have a liver biopsy. The need for liver biopsy in a patient who has high levels of HBV DNA and repeatedly normal transaminases is less clear because it is very unlikely that the biopsy will show advanced liver disease or considerable inflammatory activity. Age and gender are important in the risk of immune tolerance persisting and a male of 40 has a high risk of liver injury compared to a female of 20. The normal ranges for transaminases are also probably incorrect, not reflecting the variability with age. A normal ALT for a 20-year-old female is probably less than 20. For all of these reasons, liver biopsy has played an increasing role in assessment of patients with HBV infection.

Therapy for hepatitis B

When assessing the need for therapy in HBV infection the phase of the infection and the natural history should be taken into account. There is now compelling evidence that HBV DNA levels predict both the progression to cirrhosis and complications of liver disease (see Fig. 38.3) and the risk of developing hepatocellular carcinoma, particularly so in patients outside the immunotolerant phase.[46] There are differences in both treatment type and aims in HBV infection in the e antigen positive and negative phases.

There are two types of licensed drug treatment for hepatitis B: IFN-α and nucleoside/nucleotide analogues. Although the agents used to treat hepatitis B vary considerably in their mode of action, the basic aim of treatment is the same – to stop viral replication. The concept of 'viral eradication' is not possible in hepatitis B, as it is clear that viral DNA remains present in infected individuals over their lifetime. This is exemplified by reactivation of HBV in patients undergoing chemotherapy or other profound immunosuppression in whom the only marker of infection is antibodies to core antigen. It is, however, clear that almost all the major sequelae of infection with HBV are a consequence of active viral replication. Individuals who remain HBsAg positive but have no ongoing viral replication are not at risk of developing significant hepatic fibrosis and consequently have a dramatically reduced risk of developing decompensated liver disease compared to those with ongoing viral replication. The only serious complication of HBV infection which is not entirely dependent on viral replication is cancer development where a risk remains, particularly in those with established cirrhosis. Even there, the risk of developing hepatocellular carcinoma is substantially greater in patients where replication continues. Consideration of therapy is therefore only appropriate in patients where HBV is active as evidenced by detectable levels of HBV DNA. The choice of therapy is then determined by a number of factors: the stage of infection, the level of HBV DNA, the presence of mutant virus as the predominant strain (as evidenced by the presence or absence of e antigen), the degree of inflammatory liver disease and the degree of hepatic fibrosis.

Interferon therapy

Interferon alpha in eAg-positive HBV

Interferon alpha (IFN-α) was first shown to be effective for some patients who have HBV infection in the 1980s and it remains an effective therapy.[47] There are a number of commercially available variants of IFN-α including natural interferon, recombinant interferons and consensus interferons. In HBV infection there is little evidence that the type of IFN-α used has any substantial difference in effect or side-effect profile. Pegylated interferons are more convenient for patients because of once rather than three times weekly administration and have become the standard form of IFN-α used in HBV infection despite no evidence of improved effectiveness. There are a number of factors that can help predict the likelihood of response to treatment with IFN-α in e antigen-positive disease, and these help in selection of patients who have the best chance of response to therapy (Table 38.6).

Overall, in e antigen-positive disease the probability of response to interferon therapy in chronic hepatitis B is between 25% and 40%. A response to therapy is loss of e antigen in blood, accompanied by

Table 38.6 Factors indicating the likelihood of response to interferon in chronic hepatitis B virus infection

Factor	High probability of response	Low probability of response
Age	<50 years	>50 years
Sex	Female	Male
Hepatitis B DNA level	Low	High
Activity of liver inflammation	High	Low
Country of origin	Europe, North America, Australasia	Asia
Co-infection with HIV	Absent	Present

the development of antibodies to e antigen and the cessation of viral replication; only a small number of patients lose all markers of infection with HBV (2%) and HBsAg usually remains in the serum. There is now good evidence that successful therapy with interferon, which renders the HBV nonreplicative, produces a sustained improvement in liver histology and a decrease in the risk of developing end-stage liver disease. The risk of developing hepatocellular carcinoma also appears to be reduced but is not abolished in those who remain HBsAg positive. The likely reason why a number of patients with apparently successful responses to interferon therapy go on to develop significant liver disease is the emergence of mutant HBV strains which resume viral replication and hence liver cell injury.

Interferon therapy has a number of drawbacks: it is not effective in many patients, it is expensive and it has a large number of side-effects (Table 38.7). In general, about 15% of patients on interferon therapy have no side-effects, 15% cannot tolerate therapy and the remaining 70% experience side-effects but are able to continue therapy. Most patients are able to continue at work during therapy but many require substantial support. Depression can be a major problem and both suicide and admissions with acute psychosis are well described. Early use of antidepressants and close monitoring are essential, especially if there is a preceding history of depression.

Treatment of hepatitis B in patients who have significant fibrotic liver disease is rewarding because they have a relatively high probability of response and have most to gain from cessation of viral replication. Many patients have a substantial improvement in liver function if viral replication is stopped, but treatment in such patients does carry an increased risk. Interferon therapy produces viral clearance, at least in part, by inducing immune-mediated killing of infected hepatocytes, and hence a transient hepatitis can cause severe decompensation requiring liver transplantation.

Table 38.7 Common side-effects of interferon-α therapy for viral hepatitis

Side-effect	Frequency (%)
Flu-like syndrome	80
Depression	20
Local inflammation at injection sites	25
Hypothyroidism	10
Arthralgia or arthritis	10
Hair loss	10

The optimal dose and duration of interferon for hepatitis B remains somewhat contentious, but most clinicians use pegylated interferons, with doses based on body weight for the 12 kDa molecule and a standard dose of 180 µg for the 40 kDa molecule for 6 months, even though trials with pegylated interferons were with 1 year's therapy. This practice is based on the extensive data using non- pegylated interferon where 6 months was as effective. No comparative data exist as to their relative effectiveness.

Patterns of response and special situations

The most frequent pattern of response to IFN-α is shown in Figure 38.11. The HBV DNA level falls rapidly after initiation of interferon therapy. This is followed by a marked rise in transaminase values. This represents immune-mediated clearance of virus, and HBV DNA levels quickly fall to undetectable levels. This is then followed within a few weeks by sero-conversion to HBeAg-negative, HBeAb-positive status with complete normalization of transaminases. This type of response is seen in 25% of treated patients. Hepatitis B surface antigen usually remains positive, with a small proportion of patients clearing all markers of viral infection either during interferon therapy (2%) or many months after it (6%).

Delayed responses to therapy occur in 10–15%, usually within 9 months of completion of therapy

Interferon alpha in eAg-negative HBV

Interferon therapy for e antigen-negative patients is less effective. In this phase of the disease there is no e antigen seroconversion and therefore end points of studies are based on virologic suppression. Although a good rate of initial response to interferon with disappearance of HBV DNA from serum can be achieved, patients very frequently relapse after cessation of treatment (Fig. 38.12). Giving interferon therapy for longer in such patients may improve the rate of loss of viral replication. A regimen of 6 000 000 units of standard interferon three times a week for 24 months has been shown to produce a loss of viral replication in 30% of patients.[48] Pegylated interferons given in a 12-month treatment schedule were shown to be more effective than lamivudine[49] 6 months after stopping therapy; however, this is probably not a realistic trial as the use of nucleoside analogues would not be short term. The study did, however, show that a durable response to pegylated interferon could be achieved with suppression of viral replication below 400 IU/ml in 18% of patients after 6 months off therapy. This study also confirmed that the combination of interferon and lamivudine did not add to overall response rates to interferon (Fig. 38.13).

Clearly while confirming that pegylated interferon can be effective in a minority, the side-effects of interferon will make it second-line therapy for most patients and clinicians in e antigen-negative chronic hepatitis B.

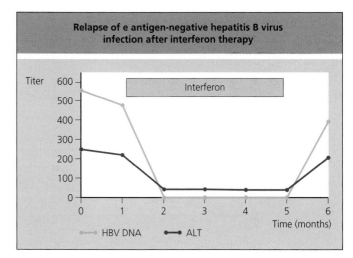

Fig. 38.12 Relapse of eAg-negative hepatitis B virus (HBV) after interferon therapy. ALT, alanine transaminase. Measurements in arbitrary units.

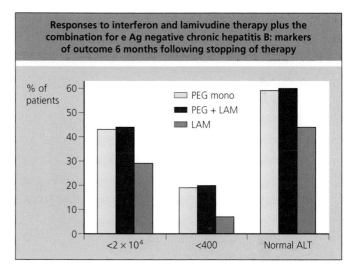

Fig. 38.13 Responses to interferon and lamivudine (LAM) therapy plus the combination for e Ag negative chronic hepatitis B: markers of outcome 6 months following cessation of therapy. The left columns are HBV DNA, either below a commonly accepted threshold for clinical significance or the limit of detection of the assay. ALT, alanine transaminase; mono, monotherapy; PEG, pegylated interferon. Redrawn from Marcellin et al.[49]

Nucleoside/nucleotide therapy

There are now a number of oral antiviral agents available for the treatment of HBV infection. The first of these, lamivudine, established the principle that these agents could improve the outcome in patients with serious liver disease by directly inhibiting HBV replication. A randomized study versus placebo in South East Asia showed a reduction in both progression of liver disease and cancer development in treated patients and hence no further placebo-controlled studies in HBV are ethical[50] (Fig. 38.14). Lamivudine also established the key feature of all oral antiviral agents active against hepatitis B, i.e. resistance. Initial descriptions of mutations in the tyrosine–methionine–aspartate–aspartate (YMDD) motif of the HBV DNA polymerase gene were rapidly confirmed and shown to result in reactivation of replication, albeit at a lower level, and resumption of liver injury as a result (Fig. 38.15).

Emergence of lamivudine-resistant HBV is increasingly common with prolonged treatment. Genotypic resistance is detectable in 14–32% of patients after 1 year and increases to 38%, 49% and 66%

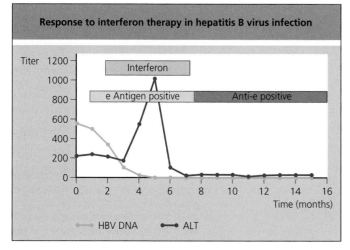

Fig. 38.11 Response to interferon therapy in hepatitis B virus (HBV) infection. ALT, alanine transaminase. Measurements in arbitrary units.

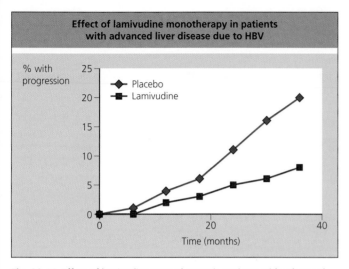

Fig. 38.14 Effect of lamivudine monotherapy in patients with advanced liver disease due to HBV. Progression was either points in Child–Pugh score or the development of hepatocellular carcinoma. Redrawn from Liaw et al.[50]

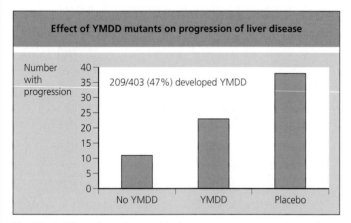

Fig. 38.15 Effect of tyrosine–methionine–aspartate–aspartate (YMDD) mutants on progression of liver disease, showing that resumption of viral replication leads to the development of progressive liver disease and confirms that YMDD mutant viruses are just as pathogenic. Redrawn from Liaw et al.[50]

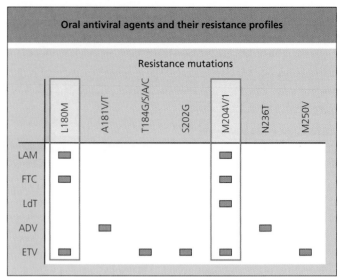

Fig. 38.16 Oral antiviral agents and their resistance profiles. The key feature is that most drugs share a resistance mutational profile with lamivudine (LAM) and cross-resistance is highly likely. Entecavir (ETV) shares this resistance but requires additional mutations for full resistance to develop. Adefovir dipivoxil (ADV) has a distinct resistance profile which it shares with tenofovir (not shown). FTC, emtricitabine; LdT, telbivudine.

therapy (see Fig. 38.17). A strategy of stopping drug when e seroconversion has occurred appears safe providing that sufficient time after seroconversion is given to consolidate the switch, probably 1 year. This is also with the caveat that HBV DNA should be completely suppressed. This may give the patient a significant time away from therapy but monitoring for reactivation remains mandatory. If the patient remains eAg positive after a year of therapy, then the drug therapy will have to be continued.

In Europe, up to 60% of all replicating hepatitis B infections now are in the late, e antigen negative, phase of infection. It is well described that these mutants are generally much less responsive to therapy with IFN-α and given the lack of a marker for immunologic control in this setting there will be a need for long-term therapy once initiated. Modeling of hepatocyte turnover suggests that with complete viral inhibition, and therefore a lack of new hepatocytes being infected, it may take more than a decade of continued viral suppression to clear all infected hepatocytes from the liver. The potential aims of therapy in patients on oral antiviral agents, both those with e antigen-positive disease who have not achieved short-term seroconversion and those with e antigen-negative disease, will be surface antigen loss. This will, however, require high levels of compliance with tablet taking over a decade or more to achieve – a significant challenge.

Lamivudine is not suitable for this task. Resistance rates are high and resumption of replication occurs in almost all patients given time. The newer agents are more effective, both in terms of potency and the genetic barrier to resistance. In terms of resistance profiles there are two classes of oral agent: lamivudine-like and adefovir-like (Table 38.8). There is no rationale for the use of sequential therapy with drugs of the same class; even entecavir, which requires a third mutation in the HBV DNA polymerase in addition to the two common ones which confer resistance to lamivudine, has been shown to have high rates of resistance if used in the presence of pre-existing lamivudine resistance mutants[52] (Fig. 38.17). This means that initial therapy must be with either a potent drug as monotherapy (entecavir or tenofovir), with the availability of a drug from the other class to act as rescue therapy if this fails, or with a combination of a drug from each class at the outset. National guidelines generally allow both strategies, and it will fall to individual clinicians and patients to decide, although the experience with HIV tends to suggest that combining drugs with differing resistance profiles may be the better strategy when 10 or more years of

after 2, 3 and 4 years, respectively.[51] There is no doubt that despite the lesser replication competence of YMDD mutant viruses as evidenced by the lower HBV DNA levels, they are still responsible for liver injury and once replication resumes liver disease resumes. This was demonstrated clearly in the study by Liaw and colleagues,[50] with patients with lamivudine resistance showing an increased risk of progression of their liver disease.

When assessing the oral agents now available there are key features that will predict their potency, i.e. the ability to rapidly and profoundly suppress viral replication. This is important as replication of the virus in the presence of drug is highly likely to select for mutant viral species which can survive in the presence of drug. The mutational resistance profile determines where changes in HBV DNA can select for drug resistance; thus if two drugs have a similar resistance profile then resistance to one is highly likely to predispose to resistance to the other. Currently available drugs and key resistance data are shown in Figure 38.16.

A small subgroup of patients with e antigen-positive chronic hepatitis B who would be eligible for short-duration therapy with oral agents are those who seroconvert from e antigen positivity to e antibody on

Table 38.8 Markers of response to therapy including eAg seroconversion rates after 1 year of therapy with existing anti-HBV agents

Outcome	DRUG			
	Lamivudine (%)	Adefovir (%)	Entecavir (%)	Pegylated interferon (%)
HBV DNA negative	44	21	67	25
eAg/AB seroconversion	18	12	21	34
Alanine transaminase normal	55	48	68	39
Durability	50–80	91	82	82

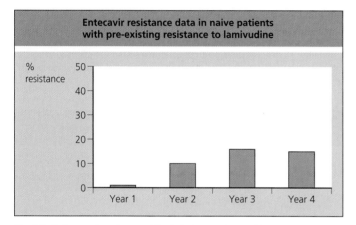

Fig. 38.17 Entecavir resistance (ETVr) data in patients with pre-existing resistance to lamivudine (LVDr). ETVr = LVDr (M204V & L180M) + T184, S2 and/or M250 substitutions plus virologic breakthrough (≥1 log increase from nadir) over 4 years of entecavir therapy in patients with prior lamivudine resistance. No resistance is seen at 4 years in non-lamivudine-resistant patients by comparison. Redrawn from Colonno et al.[53]

viral suppression is required to have any chance of cure. There are few significant side-effects of these agents, although renal impairment is a potential issue with tenofovir and monitoring is recommended.

Treatment of HIV and HBV co-infection (See Practice Point 44)

With the advent of improved antiretroviral therapy, patients with HIV infection have good immune reconstitution and excellent long-term survival. Co-infection with hepatitis viruses is common and liver disease is now a leading cause of death in HIV-infected people. Hepatitis B infection in this group is challenging to manage. Many patients have been exposed to lamivudine as part of their antiretroviral therapy and have high levels of replication with lamivudine-resistant HBV. In this setting interferon has only a limited role, as the altered immune environment rarely allows clinical response to this agent. In general the strategy in treatment-naive patients is to treat both HIV and hepatitis B. If the HIV requires therapy then it may be reasonable to give as part of that therapy two agents which will also suppress HBV, such as tenofovir and either lamivudine or emtricitabine (as Truvada in a single pill). If the HIV does not require therapy and the HBV does, a relatively unusual situation, the choices are difficult as most agents (including entecavir) do have activity against HIV which will incur resistance in that virus. In patients already on highly active antiretroviral therapy (HAART) for HIV who have HBV infection, significant HBV replication should lead to assessment of the liver and a change of therapy to cover HBV if significant liver injury is present.

Hepatitis C

Natural history of hepatitis C virus infection

In order to assess the need for treatment in a patient who has hepatitis C it is important to have a clear understanding of the natural history of this infection and of the factors that may predispose to more severe outcome. It is clear that HCV-related liver disease is usually slowly progressive, taking many years to produce significant hepatic fibrosis. The most definitive studies to date suggest that the average time from infection to the development of cirrhosis is 33 years.[54] The rate of progression is, however, very variable, with some 'rapid fibrosers' progressing to cirrhosis 11 years after infection and other 'slow fibrosers' who would take more than 40 years to progress to cirrhosis. The major factors associated with increased risk of progressive liver disease are age over 40 years at infection, high alcohol consumption and male sex (Fig. 38.18).

Therapy for hepatitis C

The current standard of care treatment for hepatitis C is a combination of pegylated IFN-α and ribavirin.

Interferon alpha was first used to treat non-A, non-B hepatitis in the 1980s. Since the identification of HCV in 1989, a large amount of information has become available about the effectiveness of interferon therapy in HCV infection and its drawbacks. These 'standard interferons' have been superseded by the advent of pegylated molecules, and these should now be regarded as the standard treatment for HCV infection when given in combination with ribavirin.

Defining response to therapy

There are three potential responses to interferon-based therapy in patients who have HCV infection:

- no response in virologic markers (nonresponders);
- a suppression of HCV RNA on therapy but relapse after cessation of therapy (relapsers); or

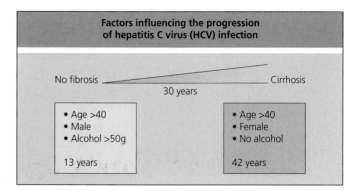

Fig. 38.18 Factors influencing the progression of HCV infection. Redrawn from Poynard et al.[54]

- a disappearance of HCV RNA that is maintained after stopping therapy (sustained responders).

In addition, the kinetics of viral disappearance in the responder groups also has prognostic significance, a rapid virologic response (RVR) being PCR negativity in serum using a sensitive assay (40 IU/ml) at week 4 of treatment, and early virologic response (EVR) being either PCR negativity or a 2 log drop in HCV RNA at week 12. The RVR is used as a predictor of high sensitivity to interferon-based therapy and may safely allow shortening of therapy and the EVR is used in a negative fashion, since failure to achieve this implies a poor response and early cessation of therapy.

Overall, the chance of sustained virologic response (SVR) to IFN-α as monotherapy in HCV infection was approximately 20%. Ribavirin (1-b-D-ribofuranosyl-1H-1,2,4-triazole-3-carboxamide) is an oral nucleoside analogue. Initial studies of ribavirin in chronic HCV infection showed a lowering of transaminase levels but no effect on viral load when given as monotherapy. A landmark study in 1998[55] showed that combining standard IFN-α (3 million units thrice weekly) with ribavirin (1–1.2 g/kg/day) increased overall cure rates from around 20% to 35–40%. This study in the USA and a parallel study in Europe[56] established the vital importance of hepatitis C genotype in the prediction of response to therapy, and these rules still hold true with the use of current standard therapy with pegylated interferon. Genotype (G) 1 or 4 infection is more difficult to treat and requires a longer duration of therapy to obtain the best results (Fig. 38.19).

While genotype of virus remains the major determinant of response to therapy, other factors continue to have an influence (Fig. 38.20). Ribavirin produces a hemolytic anemia in a substantial minority of patients treated. This effect is dose dependent, and it is possible to keep patients on therapy by the use of dose reduction (Fig. 38.21). The mechanism of ribavirin's effect on hepatitis C remains unknown. It appears that it acts predominantly by immunomodulation, rather than as a direct antiviral effect. Its major action seems to be to prevent patients with relatively interferon-sensitive hepatitis C infection relapsing once initial viral clearance has occurred.

Pegylated interferons have now superseded standard interferons. Peglyation involves the attachment of an inert polyethylene glycol molecule to the active molecule, in this case IFN-α. There are two pegylated IFN-α molecules available and they do have substantial differences in their chemistry, if not in clinical effect. Interferon alpha 2a (IFN-α$_{2a}$) has been pegylated to form a 40 kDa molecule whereas IFN-α$_{2b}$ is pegylated into a 12 kDa molecule. The 40 kDa molecule is excreted in bile and to a lesser extent renally, whereas the smaller molecule is cleared exclusively by the kidney. Overall half-life in plasma is around 5–7 days with both molecules (Fig. 38.22).

Initial studies with these agents as monotherapy showed that effectiveness was enhanced compared to standard interferon monotherapy (Fig. 38.23).[57] These and other studies also established that the fibrosis seen in patients with hepatitis C infection could reverse with

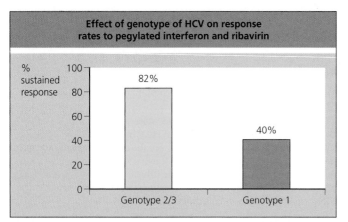

Fig. 38.19 Effect of genotype of HCV on response rates to pegylated interferon and ribavirin.

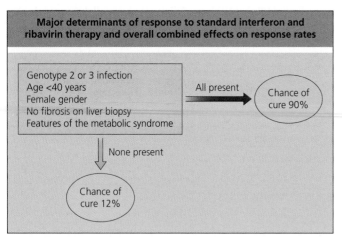

Fig. 38.20 Major determinants of response to standard interferon and ribavirin therapy and overall combined effects on response rates.

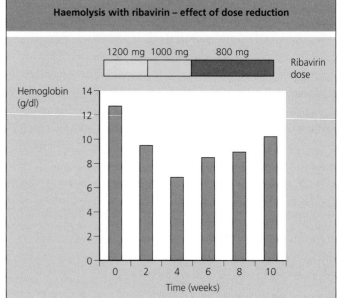

Fig. 38.21 Hemolysis with ribavirin – effect of dose reduction.

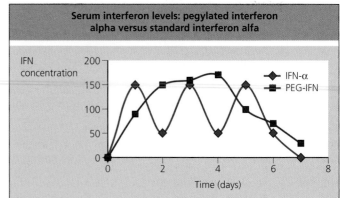

Fig. 38.22 Serum interferon levels: pegylated interferon alpha (PEG-IFN) versus standard interferon alpha (IFN-α).

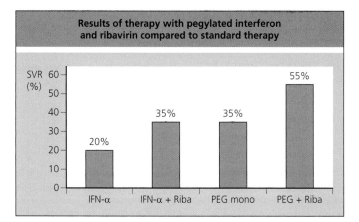

Fig. 38.23 Results of therapy with pegylated interferon (PEG) and ribavirin (Riba) compared to standard therapy. All based on 12 months duration of therapy. IFN-α, interferon alpha; mono, monotherapy.

successful therapy, underlining the fact that all patients with severe fibrotic liver disease should be considered for therapy.[58]

Both forms of pegylated interferon have been subjected to large trials and both seem equally effective, with sustained virologic responses seen in 55–60% of patients.[59,60] Response rates vary, with both host- and virus-related factors (Fig. 38.24) allowing reasonably accurate prediction of response rates in individual patients. Genotype remains the dominant response factor and cure rates in favorable genotypes (2 or 3) approach 80%. These high cure rates have markedly lessened the requirement for liver histology, although severe fibrosis remains a substantial factor predicting a negative outcome for therapy. The development of noninvasive markers of fibrosis, both in serum and using measures of liver stiffness (fibroscan), also allow reasonably reliable identification of patients with advanced fibrosis or those with no fibrosis.[61] These tests are less informative in the mid range of fibrosis and liver biopsy is still undertaken in many patients although most guidelines for therapy no longer include it as routine.

This great improvement in effectiveness of therapy has encouraged many patients to try treatment. The side-effect profile differs very little from standard interferon and ribavirin therapy, the only changes being

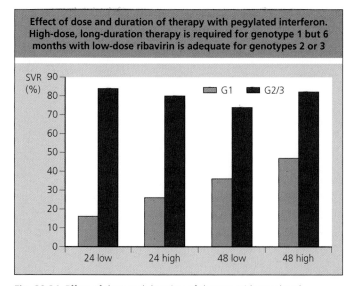

Fig. 38.24 Effect of dose and duration of therapy with pegylated interferon. High-dose, long-duration therapy is required for genotype 1 but 6 months with low-dose ribavirin is adequate for genotypes 2 and 3. SVR, sustained virologic response. Redrawn from Hadziyannis et al.[60]

a greater degree of injection site reactions. This remains a challenging therapy for patients to take. Compliance has been shown to be important. In an analysis of the 12 kDa molecule with ribavirin, patients who were able to comply with therapy (by taking 80% of their medication for 80% of the time[62]) had better response rates than those who did not. Hence encouraging patients to complete the intended duration of therapy is important. This is somewhat easier in patients with genotype 2 or 3 (G2/3) infection as they have a high chance of cure with only a 6-month course of treatment required. It is more difficult for genotype 1 or 4 infected patients who have to have 12 months of therapy to obtain best results. About 15% of patients will be nonresponders to pegylated interferon and ribavirin, and there is now good evidence to show that the results at week 12 of treatment are able to detect these individuals.

The viral kinetics of responders show an initial very rapid decline in viral load, often complete in the first week or two of therapy. In a proportion, this initial decline slows and a second phase of more gradual decline starts. With both pegylated interferons, if the virus has not disappeared from serum at week 12 or at least declined by 2 logs from pre-treatment samples, then the chance of a sustained response is almost nil (0% for the 12 kDa molecule, 2% for the 40 kDa molecule[63]). This allows patients who will not benefit from further therapy to be identified at the 3-month stage of treatment and therapy can be stopped. It also has the advantage of giving significant encouragement to patients who do make this cut-off, since if they have responded at this stage their overall chance of cure rises.

The high rates of response seen in G2/3 infected patients raised the possibility that shorter duration therapy may be effective based on viral kinetics. Patients with G2/3 who have a rapid virologic response have similar SVR rates with shorter therapy, 12 weeks for genotype 2 and 16 weeks for genotype 3.[64,65] It is important to stress, however, that all the short-duration therapy studies have been in patients without other patient-related adverse response factors, particularly advanced fibrosis. It seems prudent to restrict short-duration therapy to those without proven adverse response factors. The same RVR would theoretically apply to harder-to-treat patients, i.e. those with G1 infection. The registration studies of pegylated interferon and ribavirin showed that G1 low viral load patients do well with therapy, SVR rates of 70% being expected.[60] A study of 6 months' therapy in G1 low viral load patients showed that this was not sufficient, with SVR rates being below the expected; however, in the subgroup of G1 low viral load patients who had an RVR, response rates of 89% were achieved, showing this strategy can be successful.[66]

The dose–response relationship seen in G1 patients who are difficult to treat suggested that those patients who have unfavorable viral kinetics may benefit from extended-duration therapy. In genotype 1 patients with a 2 log drop at week 12 on therapy but who are not PCR negative, a trial has shown improved SVR with continuation of therapy for 72 weeks.[67] This remains a major undertaking for patients and motivation to continue such arduous therapy is clearly required.

In harder-to-treat populations there remains a need for improved therapy. Understanding of the HCV genome has allowed the identification of key components of the HCV replicative mechanism with the potential to act as targets for small molecule inhibitors. Most research has focused on the polymerase and protease genes of HCV in the NH3 and NS5 regions of the genome. Initial studies have established that these compounds have activity against HCV, with oral dosing leading to a drop in HCV RNA. When given as monotherapy, resistance rapidly developed with return to baseline HCV RNA levels in a period of 2 weeks, perhaps not surprising given the huge replication load in HCV infection where every base change compatible with viral viability will occur every day. The second issue limiting early drug development was toxicity, with a number of drugs falling at the preclinical or phase I stage. Phase II studies are now available for one agent which shows that in a group of genotype 1 high viral load patients treated with triple therapy (interferon, ribavirin and VX950) for 3 months, with a follow-on therapy of standard interferon and ribavirin, the SVR rate rose from 40% to 60% (Fig. 38.25), holding out promise that these agents

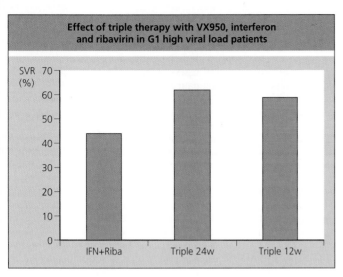

Fig. 38.25 Effect of triple therapy with VX950, interferon (IFN) and ribavirin (Riba) in G1 high viral load patients.

will improve the effectiveness of current therapies.[68] Other small molecule inhibitors of HCV are also in development as well as further modifications of interferon which have a longer half-life still and may allow dosing every 2 or even 4 weeks (albumin–interferon).

Special patient populations

Pegylated interferon–ribavirin in individuals co-infected with HIV shows a reduced SVR, on average some 10% lower than monoinfected patients. Immune reconstitution seems important in response; if CD4 counts are normal, response rates seem only slightly lower than non-HIV-infected patients but patients with CD4 counts below 200 do not respond well to therapy. The reduction in response rates is primarily due to the increased rate of side-effects on therapy, perhaps not surprising in a group already on HAART.[69] See Practice Point 46.

In renal replacement therapy units or after renal transplantation, treatment is difficult. Ribavirin is renally excreted and effectively contraindicated in this setting. Pegylated interferon monotherapy can be given and has a reasonable chance of success prior to renal transplant but carries significant risks of rejection if used post transplant.

Hepatitis D

Treatment of hepatitis D virus infection

Delta virus infection is uncommon and the mainstay of therapy is to inactivate HBV replication in those with active co-infection. For patients with negative HBV DNA, IFN-α therapy has been studied with only limited success. With standard interferon given at a dose of 3 million units three times per week, 29% will normalize ALT but most do not lose HDV RNA and relapse at the end of therapy. Higher dose treatment (9 million units three times per week) had a better biochemical and virologic response but again most patients relapsed.[70] It is clear that if interferon therapy is given for delta infection a long duration of therapy is required, which few patients can tolerate. There is a case report of resolution of HDV replication after 12 years on interferon,[71] but few patients will be so motivated. Studies of lamivudine[72] have shown no benefit. There are as yet no trials of pegylated interferon in delta hepatitis.

REFERENCES

References for this chapter can be found online at http://www.expertconsult.com

Hepatobiliary and splenic infection

Liver Abscesses

PYOGENIC ABSCESS

Pathogenesis and pathology

Bacteria can reach the liver via the portal vein, the systemic circulation, the biliary tree, through the skin (following trauma or transhepatic procedures such as liver biopsy) or directly following perforation of a viscus with an ingested fish bone or other sharp object (Fig. 39.1).[1] Small animal bones may not be visible on a plain X-ray and can erode through the stomach wall. Leakage from the associated gastric perforation can impinge locally on the liver and lead to abscess formation. A similar phenomenon has been reported with the accidental ingestion of toothpicks or parts of toothpicks. However pyogenic liver abscesses are usually associated with biliary tree obstruction or gastro-intestinal (GI) tract infection such as missed appendicitis, diverticulitis, perforated peptic ulcers, colonic carcinoma or following colonic surgery. The usual organisms are therefore from the GI tract or biliary tree. Liver abscesses are often polymicrobial with Enterobacteriaceae and enterococci predominating. *Streptococcus milleri* is increasingly seen in liver abscesses and staphylococci are not uncommon. There are reports in Taiwan and South Africa of an increasing incidence of infec-tion with an invasive strain of *Klebsiella pneumoniae* with liver abscesses and endophthalmitis.[2] *Actinomyces* spp.,[3] *Bartonella henselae*[4] and *Capnocytophaga* spp.[5] are more unusual isolates from liver abscesses; in immunosuppressed persons infections by *Nocardia* spp.,[6] mycobac-teria[7] and fungi such as *Aspergillus* spp. can cause abscess formation. Abscesses can be solitary or multiple and range in size from several centimeters in diameter to microabscesses identified histologically.

Clinical features

Pyogenic liver abscesses are classically seen in elderly patients with underlying GI disease. The patient may complain of right hypochon-drial discomfort that is insidious in onset or may present more acutely with feverishness or an acute confusional state. Interventions such as transarterial embolization and percutaneous laser ablation and other percutaneous approaches to hepatocellular carcinoma therapy can be complicated by liver abscess[8] and the diagnosis may be missed because fever and discomfort are not uncommon following the pro-cedure. The differential diagnoses include cholecystitis and pyelone-phritis. The clinical features of pyogenic and amebic liver abscesses are compared in Table 39.1.

Diagnosis

Abdominal ultrasound is the simplest way of making the diagno-sis. Single or multiple abscesses may be present and the ultrasound may also help identify the original source of the sepsis, such as an

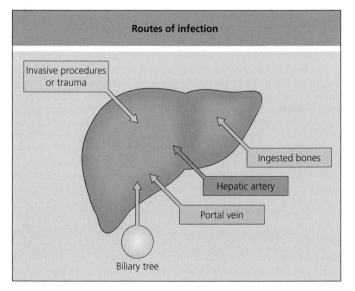

Fig. 39.1 Routes of infection.

Table 39.1 Features of pyogenic and amebic liver abscess

	Pyogenic	**Amebic**
Patients	Elderly, underlying gastrointestinal or biliary tract disease	Much more common in males than females
Imaging	Single or multiple abscesses	Solitary abscess right lobe
Pathogens	Polymicrobial, Enterobacteriaceae, enterococci	*Entamoeba histolytica*
Other tests	Blood cultures	Amebic immunofluorescent antibody test
Treatment	Broad-spectrum antimicrobials, aspiration	Metronidazole, diloxanide ± aspiration

obstructed biliary tree. Smaller abscesses not detected on ultrasound may be visible on CT scanning,[9] which can also help determine the source of sepsis if this is not apparent on the ultrasound. Aspiration of the abscess yields useful microbiologic material and is an important part of therapy. Cytologic examination of smears from the abscess are important to exclude underlying malignancy.

Blood cultures may also help with the microbiologic diagnosis. The white count is usually elevated and liver function tests may be deranged with elevation of alkaline phosphatase. The presence of a microcytic hypochromic anemia in an elderly patient, for example, may point to an underlying colonic carcinoma. The patient should also be screened for diabetes and iron overload syndromes should be considered when *Yersinia* spp. are identified.[10]

Management

Drainage of the abscess is important and the favored approach is needle aspiration under ultrasound guidance. This may need to be repeated on several occasions, particularly if there are multiple lesions. Percutaneous catheter drainage is another approach, but is generally only practicable if there is one large and accessible abscess.

Abscesses are often polymicrobial and broad-spectrum intravenous antibiotics are generally recommended. If the abscesses are thought to have occurred as a result of biliary sepsis it is advisable to give antibiotics that achieve good concentrations in bile. Positive blood cultures and cultures from the abscess should help direct antimicrobial chemotherapy. Piperacillin–tazobactam and the carbapenems are useful and metronidazole can be added if there is concern about possible amebic infection.

Although liver abscesses are more commonly seen in hospital practice the mortality rate has fallen considerably over the past 40 years,[11] attributed to advances in imaging and antimicrobial chemotherapy.

AMEBIC LIVER ABSCESS

See Chapter 110.

Diffuse Parenchymal Involvement

The liver may be involved in many systemic infections. Viral infection has been described elsewhere (Chapter 38), but acute hepatitis has been described with several bacterial pathogens including meningococci, *Salmonella typhi*, *Listeria*, *Campylobacter*, *Borrelia* and *Brucella* spp.[12,13] Septicemia and other causes of circulatory collapse can also cause hepatic ischemia, which can be associated with high transaminase values.[14] Infections account for many of the main causes of granulomatous liver disease (Table 39.2). Liver involvement and symptoms of liver disease can be a major part of the following infections.

MYCOBACTERIAL INFECTIONS

Tuberculosis of the liver

The liver is generally involved in miliary tuberculosis and the liver biopsy may help establish a diagnosis of tuberculosis in a patient with unexplained fever.

Pathology

Tuberculosis of the liver may present as an abscess[7] or more diffuse disease and liver biopsy may reveal nonspecific hepatitis or granulomatous liver disease. Rarely tuberculomas may be present or enlarged intra-abdominal lymph nodes can cause compression of the biliary tree and the patient presents with features of biliary tract obstruction.

Table 39.2 Major causes of granulomatous liver disease

Bacteria Mycobacteria (*Mycobacterium tuberculosis*, *Mycobacterium avium-intracellulare*, *Mycobacterium leprae*) *Brucella* spp. *Listeria* spp. *Tropheryma whipplei* *Yersinia* spp. *Treponema pallidum*
Viruses Cytomegalovirus Epstein–Barr virus Hepatitis A and C viruses
Rickettsiae *Coxiella burnetii* *Rickettsia conori*, *Rickettsia typhi*
Protozoa *Leishmania* spp.
Worms *Schistosoma* spp. *Toxocara* spp.
Fungi *Histoplasma* spp. *Coccidioides* spp.
Drugs
Primary liver disease (e.g. primary biliary cirrhosis)
Neoplasms (e.g. lymphoma)
Diseases of unknown cause (e.g. sarcoidosis, inflammatory bowel disease)

Clinical features

Fever and weight loss are the usual symptoms. The patient may appear wasted. Hepatomegaly may be evident, but massive hepatomegaly is unusual. In severe tuberculosis infection the patient may present with liver failure.

Diagnosis

Elevated alkaline phosphatase levels are usually present and the albumin levels may be low if the disease has been longstanding. Anemia and elevation of the erythrocyte sedimentation rate and C-reactive protein are common. A chest radiograph is important to exclude active pulmonary disease, which is evident in a minority of cases.[15] The abdominal ultrasound may demonstrate intra-abdominal lymphadenopathy or evidence of peritoneal involvement. Liver biopsy may be diagnostic, but caseating granulomas with acid-fast bacilli are demonstrable in less than 10% of cases. The appearances may be nonspecific and it is important to culture some of the liver biopsy material. Recently available blood tests such as enzyme-linked immunospot assay (ELISpot) may be helpful in this setting[16] and there is an increasing use of polymerase chain reaction testing of biopsy material.[17]

Management

Standard antimycobacterial therapy should be given (see Chapters 30 and 143). Liver function tests should be monitored as with standard therapy. As the patient improves the elevated alkaline phosphatase gradually returns to normal. Elevation in the transaminase level may be a sign of drug toxicity. Fever may persist for several weeks, but if the patient fails to improve then the possibilities of resistant *Mycobacterium tuberculosis* or atypical mycobacteria have to be considered.

Atypical mycobacteria

Atypical mycobacterial infection of the liver is usually seen in the setting of immunosuppression, particularly underlying HIV infection[18] or congenital immunodeficiency. Again culture of the biopsy material is important to establish the diagnosis, but the appearance of many organisms with poorly formed granulomas may be an important clue to atypical mycobacterial infection in an immunocompromised host.

SYPHILIS

The liver is involved with congenital, secondary and later stages of syphilis.

The standard screening tests usually confirm the diagnosis of congenital infection, but the diagnosis should also be considered in the setting of undiagnosed acute hepatitis in adults.[19] This is discussed in detail in Chapter 57.

LEPTOSPIROSIS (SEE ALSO CHAPTER 124)

Epidemiology

Several *Leptospira* species are associated with human disease, but *L. icterohaemorrhagiae* is specifically associated with Weil's disease. The main source of this pathogen is rat urine and it is therefore an occupational hazard for farm and sewage workers and those who use contaminated waters for recreational purposes such as rowing.

Pathology

The liver demonstrates cholestasis with swelling of hepatocytes, but very little necrosis. In classic Weil's disease renal disease is evident with acute tubular necrosis. There may be evidence of multifocal hemorrhage, particularly within skeletal and cardiac muscle.

Prevention

The use of protective clothing can help prevent occupational exposure and it has been recommended that sewage workers carry cards to remind clinicians of the possibility of leptospirosis should they become ill. Prophylactic antimicrobials such as doxycycline[20] have been suggested for those at risk of exposure through work or leisure activities such as canoeing, although this is not generally recommended.

Clinical features

The patient's occupation or leisure activities may point to the diagnosis.

In common with other spirochaetal infections there are several characteristic stages of the disease process. The severity varies from a minor influenza type illness to life-threatening multisystem failure. The incubation period ranges from 2 to 17 days.

The first (septicemic) stage is of a multisystem disease. It is abrupt in onset. Features may include:

- high fever
- myalgia (often severe)
- abdominal pain
- nausea
- vomiting
- severe headache and meningitis (cerebrospinal fluid leukocytosis and an elevated protein level)
- pneumonitis

- conjunctivitis
- hepatomegaly
- jaundice (said to be an ominous sign)
- bleeding (thought to be mainly related to capillary damage and leading to ecchymoses, gastrointestinal bleeding and on occasion intracerebral bleeding).

Urinalysis reveals proteinuria and bilirubinuria. The white count is usually elevated with mainly polymorphonuclear cells (it may be as high as 30 000/ml or 3 × 10^9/l). Thrombocytopenia may be present. The liver function tests demonstrate elevated levels of bilirubin and alkaline phosphatase. In contrast to fulminant viral hepatitis the transaminase values may be normal or moderately elevated.

During the second ('immune') stage the pyrexia generally resolves, but life-threatening disease may be evident. There may be signs of myocardial involvement with arrhythmias and nonspecific ECG changes. Blood tests confirm deteriorating liver function with evidence of muscle damage (elevated muscle enzymes). Worsening renal function is also a feature with elevations in the serum creatinine and proteinuria.

In the third (convalescent) stage a steady clinical and biochemical improvement occurs with resolution of the liver and renal failure and improved myocardial function. Minor relapses of symptoms can occur at this stage with further episodes of myalgia and spikes of fever.

Diagnosis

During the first stage of the disease *Leptospira* may be found on examination of the blood film or grown from blood cultures. By the second stage the blood cultures are likely to be negative. Leptospira may be evident on urine microscopy, but the diagnosis is more likely to be made from the serologic tests for anti-*Leptospira* antibodies, which are found in increasing titers in the convalescent stage of the disease.

At the time of the initial presentation, although the symptoms and jaundice may suggest a viral hepatitis, the high fever and leukocytosis would be unusual for viral etiology, but similar hepatic illnesses with or without renal failure have been described with hantaviruses.[21,22]

Management

Most patients with leptospirosis are not seriously ill, but for those with Weil's disease full supportive care may be required with support and hemodialysis in an intensive care unit. High-dose intravenous penicillin is the treatment of choice, but the dose may need modification according to the renal function. A febrile reaction, similar to the Jarisch–Herxheimer reaction, can occur.

Helminthic Parasites of the Liver

SCHISTOSOMIASIS (SEE ALSO CHAPTER 112)

Schistosomal ova can reach the liver via the mesenteric veins and portal system. Liver involvement is particularly seen with *Schistosoma japonicum* and *Schistosoma mansoni*, but can also occur with *Schistosoma haematobium*. In the early stages a granulomatous reaction is seen, but over years, if untreated, extensive collagen deposition can lead to portal fibrosis with the development of portal hypertension and splenomegaly (Fig. 39.2).

The diagnosis of schistosomal liver disease may only come to light when the patient presents with features of portal hypertension and, for example, has a variceal bleed.

Diagnosis

The diagnosis may be made from the serologic test – schistosomal enzyme-linked immunosorbent assay – or the histologic appearances of the granulomatous liver disease in the early stages and the fibrosis in the later stages. In the early stages a peripheral eosinophilia may be evident.

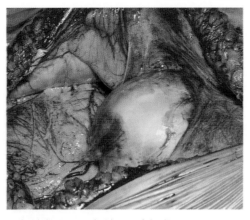

Fig. 39.2 Hydatid disease. Hydatid cyst of the liver.

Management

Praziquantel is the treatment of choice. Patients should be warned that an influenza-like illness can follow therapy. Supportive therapy is required for the patient with severe fibrosis and liver transplantation may be required in advanced cases.

HYDATID INFECTION (SEE ALSO CHAPTER 114)

Hydatid cysts can follow infection with the *Echinococcus* tapeworm.

Epidemiology

The disease is widespread and humans are typically infected by close contact with dogs which have become infected by the consumption of eggs from infected meat. Echinococcal infection is endemic in the main sheep farming areas of the world and is a particular concern throughout much of Europe, the Mediterranean littoral, Asia, South America and Kenya.

Pathology

The liver is the most frequent site for hydatid cysts (Fig. 39.3).

The ova enter the liver via the portal vein and lead to cyst formation within the liver parenchyma – classically involving the right lobe of the liver on the inferior surface. Rupture of a cyst, spontaneously or following trauma or surgical procedures, can lead to cardiovascular collapse. This is thought to be an inappropriate immune response to released hydatid antigens. Rupture of the cysts can also lead to infection in the biliary tree, the peritoneum, lungs and pleura.

Clinical features

Hydatid disease may be asymptomatic and liver cysts are found incidentally on ultrasound examination, as calcified lesions on plain abdominal radiographs or at autopsy. Hepatomegaly may be present. The cyst may be diagnosed after rupture or if secondary infection of the cyst occurs. Cysts can also be found within the brain, lungs, kidney and the heart (Fig. 39.4).

Diagnosis

The hydatid serology test is particularly useful although false-positive and -negative results can occur. A peripheral eosinophilia may be present. Several radiologic features can be helpful in making the diagnosis. Plain abdominal radiographs may reveal calcified spherical structures within the liver. Ultrasound examination can often reveal several forms of the cysts, which can be single, multiple, thin- or thick-walled. CT scanning can detect smaller lesions and the presence of calcification. It may difficult to differentiate a single cystic lesion from a tumor. Biopsy or aspiration of the cysts may be dangerous in view of the risk of antigen leakage and immune response and should be performed only when there is appropriate backup to treat circulatory collapse and laryngeal edema.

Management

The management of hepatic hydatidosis remains controversial and many approaches have been tried. It is recognized that by itself antimicrobial therapy with albendazole, mebendazole or praziquantel is generally ineffective and should be combined with a drainage procedure. Percutaneous drainage has the advantage of avoiding major surgery, but in open surgical procedures peritoneal contamination is thought to be minimized by packing the surgical field with povidone–iodine swabs, decompressing the cysts by aspiration and then removing the cyst contents. Some surgeons advocate the use of injecting formalin or hypertonic saline into the cysts following decompression. In one study,[23] 50 patients with hepatic hydatidosis were randomized to receive either percutaneous aspiration and albendazole or cystectomy. Similar efficacies were demonstrated in both treatment groups, but the open surgical procedure was associated with greater morbidity. Puncture, aspiration and the use of alcohol and polidocanol as sclerosing agents are being increasingly used.[24]

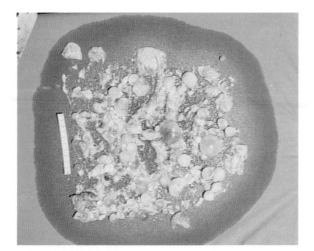

Fig. 39.3 Hydatid disease. Hydatid 'daughter cysts'.

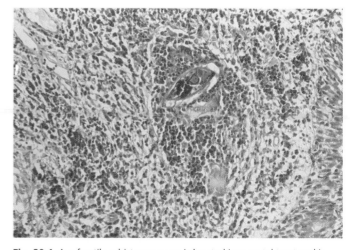

Fig. 39.4 A refractile schistosome ova is located in a portal tract and is associated with an eosinophil-rich granulomatous inflammatory reaction.

ASCARIASIS

Rarely the large *Ascaris* roundworm can migrate up through the bile duct and cause biliary obstruction. More commonly the liver is involved as a result of ova invading the liver via the portal vein and setting up a localized granulomatous reaction.

Liver involvement is usually asymptomatic unless rare complications such as biliary obstruction, hemobilia or liver abscesses develop.

Worms within the biliary tree may show up as motile linear lesions on ultrasound or endoscopic retrograde cholangiopancreatography (ERCP).

TOXOCARA

Toxocariasis is a further cause of hepatic granulomas. The recommended therapy is thiabendazole.

Liver Flukes

Liver flukes are thought to invade the liver from the peritoneal cavity and migrate through the liver parenchyma to the biliary tree where an inflammatory reaction develops.

CLONORCHIS SINENSIS

Infection with *Clonorchis sinensis* is usually associated with the consumption of raw or undercooked fish in Asia. The flukes live within capillaries of the biliary tree and the inflammatory reaction can cause obstruction and encourage cholelithiasis. Cholangitis is a common complication and the ongoing inflammation and fibrotic reaction is thought to predispose the patient to the development of cholangiosarcoma.[25]

Diagnosis

Flukes may be evident on radiologic imaging such as percutaneous transhepatic cholangiography or ERCP. This diagnosis must be considered when atypical cholangiopathy is diagnosed in patients of eastern origin. The diagnosis is confirmed by finding the ova on stool microscopy.

Management

Praziquantel is the treatment of choice. Surgical or endoscopic approaches may be required to deal with associated cholelithiasis and biliary obstruction.

FASCIOLA HEPATICA

Infection with this common sheep fluke can follow consumption of contaminated watercress and is recorded throughout Europe, South America, the Caribbean, Africa and China.

Pathology

The picture is usually of biliary tract infection and obstruction, but hepatic granulomatous reactions can also occur.

Clinical features

In the early stages of infection the patient may complain of fever and right hypochondrial pain. Hepatomegaly may be present. The migration of the flukes within the biliary tree can lead to inflammatory and fibrotic reactions. Cholelithiasis can occur and the clinical picture may be of a bacterial cholangitis. In common with bacterial cholangitis the alkaline phosphatase may be elevated, but the presence of an eosinophilia should point to the possibility of a fluke infection.

Diagnosis

The diagnosis may be suggested by a history of watercress consumption and features of cholangitis and an eosinophilia. Praziquantel is the therapy of choice and surgical and endoscopic intervention may be required to deal with biliary tree obstruction.

Protozoal Infections

LEISHMANIASIS (SEE ALSO CHAPTER 117)

Visceral leishmaniasis or kala-azar can lead to massive hepatosplenomegaly.

Epidemiology

Leishmanial infection is transmitted by sandflies and is reported particularly around the Mediterranean basin, in South America and Asia.

Pathology

Host factors are thought to be important in determining the disease outcome following leishmanial infection. It is not known why some patients develop only localized lesions and others develop more serious systemic disease. Underlying HIV infection is associated with multisystem disease and reactivation of previous infections.[26]

Clinical features

The patient may present with fever or anemia. Massive hepatosplenomegaly may be present.

Diagnosis

The presence of organisms may be detected by bone marrow examination, liver biopsy or splenic aspiration. Hypergammaglobulinemia is often present. Serologic tests are often useful, but antibody tests may be negative in patients with HIV infection or other types of immunodeficiency.

Management

Therapy of leishmaniasis is somewhat limited by the toxicity of many of the antimicrobial agents. Antimonial compounds, for example, can cause pancreatitis. Liposomal and other preparations of amphotericin are being increasingly used with success. In the setting of immunosuppression maintenance regimens are often required with regular administration of amphotericin B or intravenous pentamidine.

MALARIA

During acute malaria the parasitic load within the reticuloendothelial system and particularly the liver may be large and this may result in hepatic dysfunction. This is thought to predispose the patient with malaria to bacteremia. Mild elevation of the transaminase values may occur, but hyperbilirubinemia is mainly associated with the hemolysis of malaria rather than hepatic dysfunction.

TOXOPLASMA

Mild hepatitis or granulomatous liver disease has been reported with both primary and reactivation forms of toxoplasmosis infection.

Fungal Infections

The liver may be involved as part of a systemic fungal infection in a patient with candidemia.[27] Cryptococcal, histoplasmosis and pneumocystis infection of the liver are mainly seen in patients with HIV infection.

Aspergillus infection of the liver with abscess formation is mainly seen in patients with neutropenia as a result of chemotherapy.

Biliary Tree Infections

ACUTE CHOLECYSTITIS

Pathology

Gallbladder infections are usually the results of gallstone formation and impaction within the cystic duct[28] with impaired biliary drainage leading to infection, edema and compressive effects on the local blood supply, which can cause gangrene of the gallbladder. Suppuration within the gallbladder can lead to bacteremia, septicemia, cholangitis and liver abscess formation. Acalculous cholecystitis can follow infection with *Salmonella* or *Campylobacter* spp. or can occur in acutely ill patients following major surgery or burns. In the setting of HIV infection, infection with *Salmonella* or *Campylobacter* spp. may be implicated or the gallbladder disease may be a feature of HIV cholangiopathy,[29] which is often associated with cytomegalovirus infection, cryptosporidiosis, microsporidiosis or lymphoma.

Clinical features

The patient may describe right hypochondrial discomfort, which can occur in waves. Radiation to the right shoulder is common. Feverishness or rigors can occur and the patient may develop bacteremia and septicemia. Right hypochondrial tenderness is usually present and the gallbladder may be palpable in one-third of cases. A degree of jaundice may be present depending on the extent of biliary tree obstruction.

Diagnosis

The diagnosis is usually made clinically, but ultrasound of the liver and gallbladder may demonstrate gallstones with thickening of the gallbladder wall or dilatation of the biliary tree in the presence of obstruction. Laboratory findings include an elevated white cell count, hyperbilirubinemia and elevated alkaline phosphatase. There may be modest elevations of the transaminase values. Impaired biliary drainage because of pancreatic carcinoma can also cause dilatation of the biliary tree and ERCP may be required to delineate the anatomy and to facilitate drainage if required. Magnetic resonance cholangiopancreatography (MRCP) is a helpful, noninvasive imaging technique useful in visualizing the biliary tract.[30]

Management

The priorities are to facilitate drainage of the biliary tree and to treat infection. Cholecystectomy, when performed by the open technique, has a high mortality and morbidity rate in patients with acute cholecystitis and the usual practice was for conservative management of the acute illness and elective cholecystectomy some weeks later. This,

however, required two hospital admissions and the emergency readmission rate was high for these patients.[31] Laparoscopic cholecystectomy is increasingly performed early in patients with acute cholecystitis[32] and appears successful, even when gangrenous cholecystitis[33] is present. A meta-analysis of four studies (375 patients)[34] concluded that early laparoscopic surgery resulted in a shorter total hospital stay but with significantly longer operation time. For frail patients who are unfit for surgery ERCP can be both life-saving and diagnostic, with endoscopic removal of stones by sphincterotomy, basket or balloon removal and stent insertion. Where ERCP is not available or not technically feasible, percutaneous biliary drainage can be performed.

Elective cholecystectomy can generally be performed subsequently, but emergency surgery may be required if the situation is complicated by a gangrenous gallbladder or poor response to antimicrobial therapy.[35]

Antimicrobial therapy is generally prescribed to cover Gram-negative bacilli, enterococci and anaerobes, although the importance of enterococcal infection is debated in this setting.[36] Piperacillin–tazobactam or ticarcillin–clavulanic acid is therefore useful. Carbapenems are increasingly used, particularly if the patient has had a prolonged inpatient stay or has undergone a number of invasive procedures. Aminoglycosides must be used carefully in this setting, particularly in the elderly because there is a high incidence of renal impairment in patients with biliary tree sepsis. Cephalosporins and quinolones do not adequately cover enterococcal infection. Antimicrobial prophylaxis is advised for procedures involving an obstructed biliary system.

CHOLANGITIS

Pathology

Bacterial cholangitis generally results from infection of an obstructed biliary tree and is most commonly caused by gallstones obstructing the common bile duct.[37] Other predisposing causes include congenital biliary tract disorders, sclerosing cholangitis, HIV cholangiopathy and bile duct strictures.

Clinical features

The symptoms and signs are generally similar to acute cholecystitis, but the patient may have no history of abdominal pain and present with septicemia.

Diagnosis

Bacteremia has been reported in half the cases of cholangitis. Blood cultures are important investigations. The alkaline phosphatase and bilirubin are usually elevated. Ultrasound may show dilatation of the biliary tree with stones, but the bile duct is often difficult to visualize and other imaging techniques, such as endoscopic ultrasound and MRCP[38] may be required. ERCP is useful for diagnosis when the patient has been stabilized.

Management

As with cholecystitis the priorities are supportive care for the patient with the appropriate antimicrobial chemotherapy and drainage of the obstructed biliary system.

CHRONIC CHOLECYSTITIS

Chronic cholecystitis is an unusual condition. Again gallstones are commonly seen. Chronic cholecystitis may be seen following infection with *Salmonella* or *Campylobacter* spp.

Management

Elective cholecystectomy is the treatment of choice. Laparoscopic cholecystectomy is increasingly used for gallstone disease and acalculous cholecystitis and is associated with lower morbidity and mortality rates.

SPLENIC INFECTION

Pathogenesis and pathology

Splenomegaly is present in many infections and may be a clue to the diagnosis. However, a large spleen is also evident in many inflammatory, infiltrative and malignant processes. Bacterial pathogens generally reach the spleen via the systemic circulation as part of a bacteremia but spleen infection can also occur contiguously from intra-abdominal sepsis or, more rarely, following percutaneous trauma. This may be obvious if there is a history of a percutaneous procedure or injury but blunt trauma may lead to hematoma formation with subsequent secondary infection and the diagnosis in this setting is often delayed. Splenic infarcts can be seen following septic emboli but can also occur with underlying hematologic conditions such as sickle cell disease and polycythemia. Vasculitides can also lead to splenic infarcts with risks of secondary bacterial infection and abscess formation. Rupture of an abscess can occur. Without appropriate intervention the abscess can rupture within the peritoneal cavity, with the development of peritonitis and often associated hemorrhage. More rarely, splenic abscesses rupture into the stomach, bowel, lung, kidney or, very rarely, externally.

Spleen involvement is common in viral infection such as Epstein–Barr virus infection and HIV. Protozoal infection, particularly leishmaniasis, can be associated with splenic enlargement. Splenic pneumocystis infection has been reported in patients with advanced HIV infection.

Clinical features of a splenic abscess

Only a minority of patients exhibit the classic features of left hypochondrial pain, fever and splenomegaly. Patients may complain of left shoulder pain or pleuritic pain. Left hypochondrial tenderness or, more rarely, a rub may be evident. More rarely there may be local swelling, erythema or tenderness. Splinter hemorrhages and a heart murmur suggest underlying endocarditis.

Diagnosis

The white blood cell count is usually elevated. A chest X-ray may demonstrate a left pleural effusion or elevation of the left hemidiaphragm. An ultrasound examination may be diagnostic but the most sensitive test is a CT scan which may also be useful in excluding underlying intra-abdominal sepsis. Blood cultures should be obtained and urine microscopy and an echocardiogram performed if there is suspicion of endocarditis.

Management

Blood cultures should help direct appropriate antimicrobial therapy. The presence of streptococci or staphylococci suggests seeding from bacteremia – particularly infective endocarditis – whereas polymicrobial infection is more usually seen when an abscess is secondary to local intra-abdominal infection as a result of a perforated viscus. Patients with splenic abscess are often elderly with underlying co-morbidities such as diabetes mellitus. Drainage of the abscess may be required but the spleen is highly vascular and the risks versus benefits of this approach, whether percutaneous[39] or open, have to be carefully considered for the individual patient. There should be close liaison with the radiologic and surgical teams and often splenectomy is required.

REFERENCES

References for this chapter can be found online at http://www.expertconsult.com

Barbara Doudier
Jean Delmont
Philippe Parola

Practice point | **17** |

Travelers' diarrhea

INTRODUCTION

Travel-related diarrhea is the first cause of morbidity in travelers returning from Caribbean areas, Central and South America, South Central Asia and Africa. Ignorance about this risk appears to be the most crucial factor determining travel-related morbidity rates. Episodes of travelers' diarrhea are mostly benign. Nevertheless, associated dehydration can be severe. Prior education and simple advice are key to prevention of travelers' diarrhea.

DEFINITION, EPIDEMIOLOGY AND CLINICAL FEATURES

The definition of acute travelers' diarrhea (TD) is an abnormally increased frequency or decreased consistency of stools for less than 3 weeks. There are three different types of TD – classic, moderate and mild – defined as follows:

- Classic TD consists of three or more unformed stools in 24 hours with one of the following symptoms: nausea, vomiting, abdominal pain, fever or blood in the stools.
- Moderate TD consists of one or two unformed stools in 24 hours and one of the above symptoms, or more than two unformed stools in 24 hours.
- Mild TD consists of one or two unformed stools in 24 hours without any other sign.

Risk factors for developing TD are well known. The number of ingested organisms that reach the intestine alive will indicate the type of TD. People with a previous history of gastric surgery or abnormal digestive motility, or those treated for gastric ulcer with antihistaminic drugs (bacteria can reach the small bowel because of reduction of gastric acid), have an increased risk of developing TD. 'Adventure' trips, consumption of unclean food or water or travel in countries with poor hygiene standards are other risk factors for TD.

The etiology of TD is wide ranging (Table PP17.1). Bacteria, viruses, parasites and occasionally biologic toxins or fungal agents are responsible for TD. Up to 50% of TD is caused by bacteria. The most common agent identified in TD is enterotoxigenic *Escherichia coli* (ETEC). Other pathogens are reported in Table PP17.1. Although travelers with doxycycline malaria prophylaxis or treated by antibiotics can develop *Clostridium difficile*-associated diarrhea, it is a rare cause of TD. *Vibrio cholerae* O1 or O139 is an important cause of diarrhea in developing countries but not a common cause of TD. In a large study of 17 353 ill returned travelers, patients with bacterial TD came most commonly from South East Asia. *Campylobacter* spp. are the principal cause of TD.

Viruses are a less common cause of TD. Rotavirus is predominant (10–25% of TD). Norovirus as Norwalk agent is inconsistently reported.

Table PP17.1 Usual pathogens causing travelers' diarrhea and their clinical characteristics

Pathogen	Clinical features
Bacteria	
Enterotoxigenic *Escherichia coli*	'Turista': short incubation, fecal diarrhea without blood or pus (enterotoxin) Cholera-like diarrhea
Enteroaggregative *E. coli*	'Turista'
Campylobacter jejuni	Dysentery: bloody diarrhea, abdominal pain, tenesmus, fever (enteroinvasion) Fecal diarrhea
Salmonella spp.	Dysentery (enteroinvasion) Fecal diarrhea
Shigella spp.	Dysentery (enteroinvasion) Aqueous diarrhea (enterotoxin) Fecal diarrhea
Vibrio parahaemolyticus	Dysentery (enteroinvasion) or aqueous diarrhea (enterotoxin)
Aeromonas hydrophila	Aqueous diarrhea (enterotoxin) or dysentery (enteroinvasion)
Plesiomonas shigelloides	Cholera-like diarrhea
Yersinia enterocolitica	Dysentery (enteroinvasion)
Viruses	
Rotavirus	Vomiting, aqueous diarrhea
Enteric adenovirus	Vomiting, aqueous diarrhea
Parasites	
Giardia lamblia	Chronic diarrhea, predominant upper gastrointestinal signs
Cryptosporidium parvum	Children, chronic diarrhea
Cyclospora cayetanensis	Chronic diarrhea, predominant upper gastrointestinal signs
Microsporidium spp.	Frequent with AIDS, chronic diarrhea
Isospora belli	Frequent with AIDS, chronic diarrhea
Entamoeba histolytica	Chronic diarrhea or acute bloody diarrhea

Parasites are rarely implicated in TD. However, *Giardia lamblia*, *Cryptosporidium parvum*, *Cyclospora cayetanensis*, *Microsporidium* spp. and *Isospora belli* have been reported as causes of prolonged TD. Giardiasis was frequently reported among returned travelers from South Central Asia (proportional morbidity: 150 per 1000 returned travelers).

Contamination of seafood by toxins (e.g. ciguatera toxin from contaminated reefs in tropical areas) is occasionally responsible for TD.

Most episodes of TD begin between 4 and 14 days after people's arrival at their destination but the incubation period can be shorter if the inoculum is particularly prevalent or in cases of *Staphylococcus aureus* food poisoning (incubation period: 2–6 hours). The illness is frequently self-limiting and short. Only 20% of people suffering TD report needing bed rest for 1–2 days. Clinical characteristics depend on the cause (see Table PP17.1), the patient's age and their immune status. Location helps to focus on possible implicating agents.

DIAGNOSIS

For most cases of mild TD, laboratory tests on feces are unrewarding. Laboratory tests on freshly collected stools are necessary for identifying the etiologic agent in four conditions:

- persistent or severe diarrhea;
- dysentery (blood in feces);
- fever;
- severe abdominal pain.

A stool culture is nearly always necessary in a patient with fever and colitis. Clinical features suggest specific causes and help in the selection of biologic investigations. If upper gastrointestinal signs are predominant, stool examination for *G. lamblia* and *Cyclospora* must be undertaken. *C. arvum* or *Microsporidium* must be looked for if the symptoms persist for more than 14 days. Generally, three freshly passed stools must be collected on different days. Laboratories should be able to examine stools for *G. lamblia*, *Entamoeba histolytica*, *Dientamoeba fragilis*, *Blastocystis hominis*, *Cryptosporidium* spp., *C. cayetanensis* and *Isospora belli*. *Salmonella*, *Shigella* and *Vibrio* should be sought using routine enriched and selective media. For viral causes, latex tests for rotavirus are available.

MANAGEMENT

Most episodes of TD are self-limiting and require no specific treatment. Necessity to treat depends of the severity of the illness and the traveler's inconvenience. The three important points in TD treatment are fluid replacement, antibiotics and antimotility agents. Oral or intravenous fluid replacement is essential in moderate to severe TD. Fluids with sugar and salt are recommended for mild TD. Children must receive oral rehydration solution. Extreme ages of life (the very old and the very young), pregnant travelers or people treated by diuretics should be monitored carefully.

The issue of diet is controversial. It would appear that if the duration of TD is less than 3 days, no benefit is obtained with diet.

Antibiotics are indicated if TD consists of more than four stools in 24 hours, associated with fever, blood, mucus or pus in the stool. Travelers may have a prescription for antibiotics that can be taken over

Table PP17.2 Infectious Diseases Society of America treatment recommendations for travelers' diarrhea

Drug	Dosage	Specific indications
Norfloxacin	400 mg q12 h	
Ciprofloxacin	500 mg q12 h	
Ofloxacin	200 mg q12 h	
Levofloxacin	500 mg q24 h	
Azithromycin	1000 mg q24 h	Children and pregnant women Fluoroquinolone resistance
Rifaximin	200 mg q8 h	

3 days if such symptoms occur during the trip. In cases of severe TD (fever, more than eight stools per day), persistent diarrhea for more than 2 days and fragile status, or if antibiotic therapy fails after 2 days, medical consultation is required.

When the indication for treatment is confirmed, quinolone therapy should be started as soon as possible. Ciprofloxacin (500 mg twice daily) for 3 days is the treatment of choice. Azithromycin is safe to use in children and pregnant women. Quinolones are active against most of the strains of ETEC, *Campylobacter* spp., *Salmonella* spp., *V. parahaemolyticus* and *V. cholerae*. If there is resistance to quinolones (e.g. *Campylobacter jejuni* in South East Asia), azithromycin is helpful (single dose 1 g or 500 mg/day for 3 days). The Infectious Diseases Society of America treatment recommendations are summarized in Table PP17.2.

Antimotility agents are forbidden in cases of fever and bloody diarrhea. They must be stopped if abdominal pain increases or diarrhea persists for more than 2 days.

PREVENTION

Prevention consists of improving food and water selection, water purification and prior hygiene education. Specific vaccination against typhoid and hepatitis A must be carried out before traveling. Chemoprophylaxis for a short period (7 days) must be limited to high-risk travelers (e.g. AIDS, gastric surgery, chronic intestinal disease) or if digestive discomfort would cause considerable inconvenience (e.g. business, competitive sport).

FURTHER READING

Further reading for this chapter can be found online at http://www.expertconsult.com

Management of persistent postinfectious diarrhea in adults

INTRODUCTION

The presence of diarrhea beyond 2 weeks of a confirmed or presumed infectious exposure is a useful working definition of persistent diarrhea as this helps to exclude most common acute bacterial and viral infections, although protozoal infections may persist for longer. Patients with persistent diarrhea after recent travel to a tropical or developing country can also be considered as having postinfectious diarrhea.

PATHOGENESIS AND CLINICAL FEATURES

Postinfectious irritable bowel syndrome

In a prospective study, we found that 25% of previously healthy patients developed a diarrhea-predominant type of irritable bowel syndrome (IBS) (Table PP18.1) after an episode of acute infectious diarrhea. Psychologic disturbances such as anxiety and stressful recent life events were important predictors for the development of IBS. Further studies support the presence of subcolitic inflammatory changes in this subset of IBS. Other potential pathogenic factors are small intestinal bacterial overgrowth, changes in the colonic microflora, lactose malabsorption, alterations in colonic motility and sensitivity, and bile acid malabsorption. Latent or potential celiac disease may also be present in a subset of patients with IBS as evidenced by the presence of serologic markers.

Table PP18.1 Points to note in the history and physical examination of patients who have persistent diarrhea

- Onset of diarrhea in relation to confirmed or presumed infectious illness
- Travel to or residence in tropics or developing countries
- Weight loss
- Nature of the stools: frequency, consistency, estimated volume, steatorrhea
- Bowel symptoms suggesting irritable bowel syndrome: abdominal pain relieved by defecation, constipation, passage of mucus, feeling of incomplete evacuation, bloating
- Other abdominal symptoms: flatulence (suggesting giardiasis, lactose malabsorption), blood in the stool (suggesting colitis, dysentery)
- Risk factors for HIV if appropriate
- Examination for evidence of weight loss, anemia, malabsorption, abdominal masses, lymph nodes

---

Inflammatory bowel disease

Some patients who have inflammatory bowel disease (IBD) in their initial presentation have a positive microbial finding. However, symptoms may persist or recur despite the eradication of the inciting organism. Commonly implicated pathogens are *Entamoeba histolytica, Shigella* spp., *Salmonella* spp., *Aeromonas* spp. and *Clostridium difficile*. Possible explanations for this association include bacterial infection added on to previously unrecognized IBD, and the precipitation of IBD by an altered intestinal microflora or by an immunopathogenic effect of bacterial products of inflammation.

Human immunodeficiency virus-associated enteropathy

HIV-associated enteropathy may present with chronic diarrhea and significant weight loss or malabsorption. It is believed that in the majority of HIV-infected patients who have chronic diarrhea, a potential pathogen can be detected.

Postinfective malabsorption

Tropical sprue presents with chronic gastrointestinal symptoms and malabsorption following an acute diarrheal episode that is usually contracted in a tropical country (although it has also been described in travelers to the Mediterranean area). Although a specific microbial agent has not been identified, the typical response to broad-spectrum antibiotics suggests an infectious pathogenesis. Intestinal infections with parasites, especially *Giardia lamblia*, may also present similarly.

Persistent intestinal infections

Occasionally infective colitis associated with *E. histolytica, Cryptosporidium* spp., *Campylobacter jejuni* or *Salmonella* spp. may persist beyond 6 weeks (Table PP18.2). The clinical spectrum of *G. lamblia* infection ranges from asymptomatic cyst excretion through chronic diarrhea with marked flatulence to intestinal malabsorption. *Cyclospora cayetanensis* is a newly recognized protozoal parasite that has been reported in many countries, but is most common in tropical and subtropical areas. It causes prolonged watery diarrhea in a characteristic relapsing cyclic pattern even in immunocompetent patients. Although cases of chronic diarrhea associated with *Blastocystis hominis, Aeromonas* spp. and *Plesiomonas shigelloides* have been reported, their pathogenic potential remains uncertain. In a middle-aged white man presenting with diarrhea, abdominal pain, weight loss and joint pains, Whipple's disease should be considered. Recently *Tropheryma whipplei*, the bacterium implicated in Whipple's disease, has been cultivated and its genome sequenced and analyzed.

Table PP18.2 Organisms that may be involved in chronic diarrhea and their antibiotic treatment

Organism		Antibiotic	Suggested dosage
Bacteria	*Shigella* spp.	Quinolones, e.g. ciprofloxacin,	500 mg q12h for 5 days
	Salmonella spp.	norfloxacin	400 mg q12h for 5 days
	Campylobacter spp.		
	Aeromonas spp.		
	Plesiomonas shigelloides		
	Spirochetes	Metronidazole	400 mg q8h for 10 days
	Clostridium difficile toxin-positive colitis	Metronidazole	400 mg q8h for 10–14 days
		Vancomycin (oral)	125 mg q6h for 10–14 days
		Colestyramine	4 g q8h for 10–14 days
Protozoa	*Giarida lamblia*	Metronidazole	2 g q24h for 3 days
		Tinidazole	2 g q24h for 1 day
		Albendazole	400 mg q24h for 5 days
	Entamoeba histolytica	Metronidazole	800 mg q8h for 5 days
		Tinidazole	1 g q12h for 3 days
	Cyclospora cayetanensis	Trimethoprim–sulfamethoxazole	2 tablets q12h for 7 days
	Isospora belii	Trimethoprim–sulfamethoxazole	2 tablets q6h for 14 days
	Blastocystis hominis	Metronidazole	800 mg q8h for 10 days
Helminths	*Strongyloides stercoralis*	Thiabendazole	25 mg/kg (maximum 1.5 g) q12h for 3 days
		Albendazole	400 mg q12h for 3 days (repeat at 3 weeks if required)
	Trichuris trichiura	Mebendazole	100 mg q12h for 3 days
	Capillaria philippinensis	Mebendazole	100 mg q6h for 20–30 days
	Mixed infection	Mebendazole	200 mg q12h for 5 days
		Albendazole	400 mg q24h for 3 days
Tropical sprue		Tetracycline plus	250 mg q6h for 30 days (minimum)
		Folic acid	5 mg q12h for 90 days

DIAGNOSIS

Patients can be stratified to an appropriate level of testing on the basis of the points listed in Table PP18.1.

Level 1 tests are:
- stool studies – microscopy, culture, ova, cysts and parasites, and tests for *C. difficile* toxin;
- blood studies – full blood count, erythrocyte sedimentation rate, C-reactive protein, biochemistry (electrolytes, protein, albumin) and studies for the detection of HIV antibodies; and
- sigmoidoscopy.

In a patient who has no history of travel to or residence in a tropical or developing country and no significant weight loss or blood in the stools, level 1 tests would usually be sufficient. To optimize the yield from stool examinations, three specimens, preferably when stools are loose, should be collected on separate days and processed rapidly. In places where facilities are readily available, sigmoidoscopy is the most expedient way to detect colitis and determine its cause through the biopsy of endoscopically visible lesions. Biopsies taken late in an infective colitis often show changes that are difficult to distinguish from IBD. When there is doubt about the diagnosis, a follow-up biopsy 6–8 weeks later is helpful, as infective colitis usually reverts spontaneously to normal. The decision to test further should be based on clinical indications and the results of the level 1 tests. For instance, in the presence of relevant exposure, or the finding of lymphopenia, the issue of testing for HIV should be addressed.

Level 2a tests are:
- lactose and fructose tolerance tests or a 2-week trial of dietary exclusion; and
- serology for IgA antigliadin, antiendomysium and anti-tissue transglutaminase.

For patients whose presentation is consistent with IBS (see Table PP18.1), level 2a tests can be considered, depending on the clinical circumstances and the facilities available.

Level 2b tests are:
- serum folate, vitamin B12, ferritin;
- gastroscopy with duodenal biopsy.

If there is a suspicion of malabsorption, evidence for this should be obtained as indicated for level 2b tests. Where there is positive evidence, and if stools are negative, endoscopy with duodenal biopsy is the next test of choice. Histologic examination contributes to the diagnosis of conditions such as tropical and celiac sprue through the diagnosis of villous atrophy, as well as helping to isolate *Giardia* spp., trophozoites and other infectious and parasitic agents that reside on enterocytes. Duodenal biopsy is also the first test of choice for the diagnosis of Whipple's disease which is characterized by the presence of foamy macrophages that stain positively to periodic acid–Schiff.

Level 3 tests are:
- colonoscopy;
- multislice CT scan;
- capsule endoscopy; and
- enteroscopy.

If the diagnosis remains uncertain, level 3 tests help to exclude Crohn's disease, colonic tumors, small intestinal diverticula (which may give rise to bacterial overgrowth) and intestinal lymphoma. Where the facilities are available, multislice CT scan has largely superseded barium studies for radiologic imaging of the small intestine. Capsule endoscopy may be helpful to identify lesions in the jejunum or ileum beyond the reach of the standard endoscope. Tissue diagnosis may be obtained subsequently by means of an enteroscopic technique.

MANAGEMENT

If malabsorption or weight loss is present and a specific infective diagnosis can be made, the indication for antimicrobial therapy is clear. If the diagnosis remains uncertain after thorough investigation, a chemotherapeutic trial of metronidazole or tetracycline appears justified. In the presence of HIV, a persistent search for an enteric pathogen is important because it is recognized that a potentially treatable pathogen can often be detected. Nutritional supplements may occasionally be required.

Patients who have a positive stool isolate but no malabsorption, weight loss or dysenteric stools pose a therapeutic dilemma. Many of these patients are persistent excretors or carriers of the organism and are suffering from postinfectious IBS; antibiotic treatment will either not improve the diarrhea or will produce a temporary improvement, possibly as a nonspecific effect of antibiotics on colonic flora. However, occasionally bacterial pathogens may give rise to protracted diarrhea and, as long as the pathogenic potential of an organism remains uncertain, a trial of antimicrobial chemotherapy can be justified. Repeated courses of antibiotics should not be pursued if the patient shows no improvement.

In patients who have postinfectious IBS, symptomatic treatment with loperamide, colestyramine and low-dose tricyclic antidepressant agents may be helpful. Clinical evidence of efficacy is now beginning to emerge for treatment with probiotic bacteria such as lactobacilli and bifidobacteria. Patients who have positive serology for celiac-associated antibodies should undertake a gluten-free diet with repeat serology after 3 months. IBS patients with lactose or fructose intolerance should modify their diet as appropriate.

FURTHER READING

Further reading for this chapter can be found online at http://www.expertconsult.com

Barbara Doudier
Geraldine Placko-Parola
Jean Delmont

Practice point | **19** |

Approach to liver abscesses

INTRODUCTION

Liver abscess is an important, potentially life-threatening disorder. The two most frequent varieties of liver abscess are pyogenic abscess and amebic abscess. Etiology, epidemiology and treatment have changed over time. Historically, pyogenic liver abscess (PLA) was described as primarily affecting young men secondary to suppurative appendicitis and pylephlebitis; surgery was rarely recommended. At present, source and treatment differ radically.

EPIDEMIOLOGY

In recent studies, the incidence of liver abscess (LA) in Europe was estimated at 18 cases per 100 000 hospital admissions and 2–3 cases per 100 000 population. This differs from countries such as Taiwan where the incidence of LA is 446 per 100 000 hospital admissions. Recent reports have noted that the average age of patients has increased substantially. Nowadays, the mean age is 56.4 years. A recent study showed that diabetes mellitus is a strong independent risk factor for PLA but is not a factor for a worse prognosis.

SOURCE

The prevailing causes of PLA have changed over the past few years. Recent studies have shown an increase in the proportion of cases with underlying biliary disease which is often the most common identifiable cause of PLA. Other underlying conditions include intra-abdominal infections, malignancy, cardiovascular disease, alcohol abuse, cirrhosis, diverticulitis and inflammatory disease.

Hematogenous seeding is not the most usual pathway for the development of LA but if a single micro-organism (typically *Streptococcus* or *Staphylococcus* spp.) is isolated from an LA, a distant source must be sought. The usual pathways for the development of LA include contiguous spread from the gallbladder, ascending biliary obstruction with gallstones, or surgical or traumatic wounds (notably perforation of the gastrointestinal tract by a foreign body). Almost 80% of abscesses are solitary. Most liver abscesses are right sided.

Amebic LA is prevalent in tropical countries; in temperate areas, it is usually observed in patients who have been staying in endemic countries.

MICROBIOLOGY

Most liver abscesses are polymicrobial. Gram-negative bacilli and anaerobes are predominantly isolated in culture. Some streptococcal species are specific for LA with simultaneous metastatic infections at others sites. *Klebsiella pneumoniae* has been described in some studies as an emergent organism that can cause primary and secondary LA. In New York in 2004, *K. pneumoniae* became the predominant etiology of PLA (23%). In Taiwan, *K. pneumonia* is recovered in 82% of cases. Moreover, *K. pneumoniae* isolates from primary LA have an increased number of virulence factors (especially *K. pneumoniae* genotype K1) which confer a risk of metastatic infections with ocular and neurologic complications.

Other organisms can be recovered from patients with LA. *Candida* species represent 22% of LA in some series. It usually occurs in immunocompromised patients with neutropenia. Gram-positive pathogens have been reported in patients who underwent embolization for hepatocellular carcinoma. Tuberculous LA is rare but must be considered if no other organism is recovered. Amebic LA should be considered in patients who traveled in endemic areas. Useful features in distinguishing pyogenic from amebic LA are outlined in Table PP19.1.

CLINICAL MANIFESTATIONS

Fever is the most common finding at presentation, occurring in almost 90% of cases. Other frequent symptoms are right upper quadrant pain (72%), chills (69%) and nausea (43%). The absence of right upper quadrant pain or hepatomegaly does not exclude the diagnosis of LA. Isolated fever can be the only complaint in elderly patients. Other manifestations include vomiting, weight loss, jaundice and diarrhea.

A recent study showed that the mean duration of fever was 4.6 days and the mean duration of hospitalization was 19.6 days, with no significant difference in length of stay between patients undergoing different treatments.

IMAGING STUDIES

Chest X-ray may show elevation of the right hemidiaphragm, right basilar infiltrate, pleural effusion, atelectasis or consolidation of the right base. A recent study showed that chest X-ray was abnormal in 33% of cases. Rarely, abdominal X-ray may show gas within a liver abscess.

Table PP19.1 Useful features in distinguishing pyogenic from amebic liver abscess

	Pyogenic liver abscess	Amebic liver abscess
Age >50 years	x	
Diabetes mellitus	x	
Chest pain	x	x
Rale/ronchi/ cough	x	
Jaundice	x	x
Low albumin	x	
Elevated bilirubin	x	x
Elevated alkaline phosphatase	x	x
Male predominance		x
Abdominal pain	x	x
Diarrhoea		x
Hepatomegaly		x
Abdominal tenderness	x	x
High indirect hemagglutination assay titers		x
Solitary abscess		x
Right lobe abscess		x

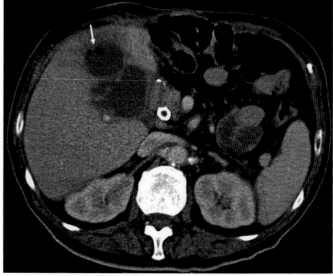

Fig. PP19.2 CT of a large, round, low-attenuation liver lesion with a smooth edge. The wall is thick and enhanced and localization is subcapsular. The appearance is evocative of amebic abscess.

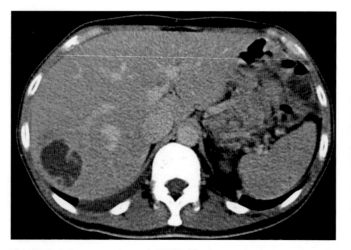

Fig. PP19.1 Contrast-enhanced CT of a low-attenuation lesion in the right liver lobe: shape is regular, septa appear inside.

Fig. PP19.3 Contrast-enhanced CT of two low-attenuation lesions. Gas-containing sign (arrow) is specific for pyogenic abscess.

Ultrasonography and CT are the imaging methods of choice. CT shows that abscesses typically appear with low attenuation. Shape is regular or irregular, with or without septa inside (Figs PP19.1, PP19.2). A wall is sometimes present. A gas-containing sign is specific for pyogenic abscess although it is uncommon (Fig. PP19.3). There is no differential diagnosis for a typical simple cyst. However, the differential diagnosis of atypical cysts includes benign tumors and malignancy. Both imaging studies and clinical features may help to distinguish an atypical cyst from a liver abscess.

NONSPECIFIC LABORATORY FINDINGS

The most common laboratory nonspecific abnormalities are increased polymorphonuclear cell count, elevated erythrocyte sedimentation rate, decreased albumin level and elevated alkaline phosphatase levels. Serum bilirubin and aspartate aminotransferase are elevated in 50% of patients.

MICROBIOLOGIC DIAGNOSIS

Diagnostic aspiration of the lesion is required to confirm a pyogenic abscess. Samples should be sent for Gram stain and aerobic and anaerobic culture. Blood cultures are necessary because 24% of patients with PLA have bacteremia. Amebic serology is necessary because amebic LA cannot be distinguished from PLA by imaging studies alone. Moreover, amebic serology is positive in 95% of cases of amebic abscess. High indirect hemagglutination assay (IHA) titers are observed with or without amebic cysts in stools.

Identifying the underlying source of a liver abscess is the second approach to diagnosis. In a recent study, a primary abnormality was present in 92% of cases. Possibilities include a contiguous biliary tract infection, peritonitis, pylephlebitis, colon cancer or hematogenous seeding of the liver.

Foreign body ingestion may lead to gastrointestinal perforation and subsequent migration of the foreign body in the liver, causing a migrated foreign body left-sided liver abscess.

TREATMENT

Successful treatment usually requires both antibiotic therapy and drainage. In contrast to PLA, drainage of amebic LA is not usually necessary. Three drainage methods exist. Percutaneous drainage guided by imaging is most often used as compared to surgical drainage. Efficacy of repeated percutaneous needle aspiration versus percutaneous drainage is always controversial. There is no significant difference in morbidity, mortality or time to resolution between percutaneous versus surgical drainage. Complications after one or the other technique differ: patients who underwent surgical drainage have complications of bleeding, wound infection and intra-abdominal abscess; patients who underwent percutaneous drainage have complications of peritonitis, catheter blockage and catheter dislodgement.

Nevertheless, surgical drainage must be used when there is no positive clinical outcome after 4–7 days of percutaneous drainage and when there are multiple, large or loculated abscesses, there is a risk of the catheter being plugged by viscous pus and if there is an underlying condition which requires surgical intervention (e.g. biliary tract lesion). For this last eventuality, some authors propose endoscopic retrograde cholangiopancreatography.

Antibiotic therapy includes initial parenteral treatment with one of the regimens outlined in Table PP19.2. There is no randomized study describing the optimal duration of therapy. Parenteral antibiotics are often prescribed for the first 2–3 weeks or until there is a favorable

Table PP19.2 Antibiotic therapy of pyogenic liver abscess

	First-intention therapy	Alternative therapy
Monotherapy		
β-Lactam/β-lactamase inhibitor	Ampicillin–sulbactam 3 g q6h	Piperacillin–tazobactam 3 g q4h
Carbapenem	Imipenem 1 g q8h	Ertapenem 1 g q24h
Bitherapy		
Metronidazole plus cephalosporin/fluoroquinolone	Metronidazole 500 mg q8h plus ceftriaxone 1 g q24h	Metronidazole 500 mg q8h plus ciprofloxacin 500 mg q12h

clinical outcome. The remainder of the course is completed with oral drugs such as metronidazole and a fluoroquinolone.

Specific therapy for amebic liver abscess is oral metronidazole 500–750 mg, three times a day for 7–10 days.

FURTHER READING

Further reading for this chapter can be found online at http://www.expertconsult.com

Infective and reactive arthritis

INTRODUCTION

Infective arthritis is an inflammation of the joint space caused by invasion of different micro-organisms. Hematogenous seeding of the joint is the most common mechanism of infection in native joints. The incidence of infective arthritis in adults caused by bacteria other than *Neisseria gonorrhoeae* is relatively low, but these infections can cause major morbidity as a result of pain, immobility and loss of joint function. Successful treatment requires prompt drainage of the joint, using multiple arthrocenteses or open arthrotomy, and prolonged antimicrobial therapy to achieve sterilization of the joint space as well as a satisfactory functional result. This chapter discusses infective arthritis in adults, with the major emphasis on bacterial infective arthritis. Viral and reactive arthritis are discussed briefly. Infective arthritis caused by *Borrelia burgdorferi* is discussed in Chapter 43 and mycobacterial arthritis in Chapter 30.

Bacterial Arthritis

EPIDEMIOLOGY

In 2005, according to the Centers for Disease Control and Prevention (CDC), there were an estimated 24 000 cases of pyogenic arthritis that were hospitalized in the USA; 58% of the patients were male, and 33% were 65 years of age or older.[1] The mean duration of hospitalization of patients who had a primary diagnosis of pyogenic arthritis was 7.8 days. These data are in agreement with other published incidence rates of bacterial arthritis in the general population.[2,3] Disseminated gonococcal infection with associated gonococcal infective arthritis is the leading cause of hospital admission due to infective arthritis in the USA, with an estimated incidence rate of 2.8 per 100 000 person years (Chapter 168).[4]

RISK FACTORS

Rheumatoid arthritis, diabetes mellitus, malignancy, old age, the use of systemic steroids and prior surgery on the joint suppress the immune system and, as such, are risk factors for acquiring bacterial arthritis.[5–8] Novel therapies such as etanercept and infliximab, and targeting tumor necrosis factor for the treatment of rheumatoid arthritis have come into widespread clinical use. These agents have been shown to be implicated as a possible risk factor for severe polyarticular infectious complications in this patient population.[9] Situations that increase the risk of bacteremia, such as injection drug use, indwelling intravenous catheters and skin infection, and situations that allow direct inoculation of

micro-organisms, such as intra-articular injection or arthroscopy, also predispose the joint to infection. Several cases of infective arthritis due to *Clostridium* spp. were reported to the CDC. All these cases underwent tissue allograft reconstruction surgery. Anaerobic cultures of the nonimplanted donor tissue yielded *Clostridium* spp. in selected cases. It is believed that the donor tissue was hematogenously seeded by bowel flora and that the aseptic processing techniques used for the implicated donor tissues did not eliminate spores of *Clostridium* spp.[10] Individuals with rheumatoid arthritis and/or receiving disease-modifying antirheumatic drugs are at increased risk of *Staphylococcus aureus* arthritis.[11] Emerging cases of methicillin-resistant *Staphylococcus aureus* arthritis are being reported from the community and the health-care setting.[12]

Disseminated gonococcal infection is more common among sexually active, menstruating women, although it can also occur during pregnancy and the peripartum period.[4] The male:female ratio is approximately 1:4. Often the microbiologic etiology of infective arthritis can be predicted based on the specific risk factor predisposing to infection (Table 40.1).[13]

PATHOGENESIS

Nongonococcal bacterial arthritis most often results from hematogenous seeding of the joint space as a result of bacteremia. Synovial tissue has a rich vascular supply but no basement membrane, factors that favor ingress of blood-borne organisms.[8,13] The bacteremia can be primary or secondary to an infection elsewhere in the body (e.g. pneumonia, cellulitis) or to injection drug use.[5] An identifiable focus of infection can be found in approximately 50% of cases.[8,14]

Direct inoculation of micro-organisms into the joint space due of trauma, arthrotomy, arthroscopy or diagnostic and therapeutic arthrocenteses is another mechanism of infection. The risk of septic arthritis after arthrocentesis has been reported to be 0.002–0.007%; after arthroscopy it is reported to be 0.04–0.4%.[15] Infection of the joint space as a result of contiguous soft tissue infection or periarticular osteomyelitis is much less common.

Once bacteria have entered the joint space there is ingress of polymorphonuclear leukocytes, which results in hydrolysis of proteoglycans and collagen through stimulation of locally synthesized cytokines and release of enzymes such as gelatinases.[1,16] If left untreated, destruction of the articular cartilage eventually occurs, leading to irreversible joint damage.[17–19]

Staphylococcus aureus is the most common etiologic agent of infective arthritis in adults (Table 40.2).[8,20–23] In young sexually active persons, *N. gonorrhoeae* is the predominant pathogen. Infection in patients who have rheumatoid arthritis is due to *S. aureus* in as many as 80% of patients. Group B streptococcal infection is more likely to occur in patients who have diabetes mellitus. Coagulase-negative staphylococci

Table 40.1 Epidemiologic and clinical features associated with specific etiologic agents of infective arthritis

Likely etiologic agent	Clinical or epidemiologic setting
Bacteria	
Staphylococcus aureus	Rheumatoid arthritis, injection drug use, arthroscopy, arthrotomy, polyarticular arthritis
Coagulase-negative staphylococci	Arthroscopy, arthrotomy, foreign material
Neisseria gonorrhoeae	Young, sexually active, history of sexually transmitted disease or unsafe sex, menstruation, pregnancy, multiple skin lesions
Pseudomonas aeruginosa and other aerobic Gram-negative bacteria	Injection drug use, elderly
Anaerobes	Human and animal bites, orthopedic allograft infection with allograft without sporicidal sterilization, anaerobic infection elsewhere in body
Usual oral flora	Human and animal bites
Eikenella corrodens	Human bite
Pasteurella multocida	Cat or dog bite
Streptobacillus moniliformis	Rat bite
Neisseria meningitidis	Multiple purpuric lesions
Other	
Mycoplasma spp.	Common variable hypogammaglobulinemia
Borrelia burgdorferi	Resident in endemic area, known or suspected tick exposure, history of erythema chronicum migrans
Troypheryma whipplei	Other manifestations of Whipple's disease
Mycobacteria	
Mycobacterium tuberculosis	Positive tuberculin skin test, resident in country where disease is endemic, known exposure history
Mycobacterium marinum	Exposure to aquatic environment
Mycobacterium avium intracelulare	HIV, T-cell suppression
Mycobacterium leprae	Resident in country where disease is endemic
Fungi	
Sporothrix schenckii	History of trauma with exposure to colonized soil (e.g. sphagnum moss)
Candida	Prior known or suspected candidemia or culture-negative central infection, neutropenia
Aspergillus	Prior known or suspected invasive aspergillus infection, prolonged neutropenia
Blastomyces dermatididis	Resident in area where disease is endemic, exposure to beaver dams
Coccidiomyces immitis	Resident in area where disease is endemic

Data from Smith & Piercy.[13]

Table 40.2 Etiologic agents of nongonococcal bacterial arthritis in adults

Micro-organisms	Cases (%)
Staphylococcus aureus	68
Streptococci (including β-hemolytic streptococci, viridans group streptococci and *Streptococcus pneumoniae*)	20
Haemophilus influenzae	1
Aerobic Gram-negative bacilli	10
Polymicrobial and miscellaneous	1
Unknown	<1

Data from Roberts & Mock.[23]

may cause infection following arthroscopy and other medical procedures, including intra-articular injections. Infective arthritis due to Gram-negative bacilli is more common in the elderly and in patients who have co-morbid illnesses.[24]

Anaerobic infection is uncommon except in the setting of septic arthritis occurring after human or animal bite injuries or diabetic foot infections. Among injection drug users, *Pseudomonas aeruginosa* and *S. aureus* are common pathogens.[25,26] Hypogammaglobulinemia is a risk factor for infective arthritis due to *Mycoplasma* spp.[27]

PREVENTION

Prevention of infective arthritis is obviously preferable to treatment of established infection. Examples of efforts to decrease the incidence of infective arthritis include the promotion of public health measures to prevent the acquisition of *N. gonorrhoeae*, measures to decrease the incidence of animal bites, prophylactic foot care in patients who have diabetes mellitus and eradication of injection drug use. Rapid and effective treatment of antecedent infections that may cause joint infections, such as catheter-associated bacteremia due to *S. aureus* or skin and soft tissue infection in patients who have rheumatoid arthritis and diabetes mellitus, as well as the administration of vaccines against *Haemophilus influenzae* and *Streptococcus pneumoniae*, are also effective preventive measures.[28] Eradication of the *S. aureus* carrier state with the use of topical mupirocin and chlorhexidine body washes in patients at risk for infective arthritis might play a role in reducing the risk of infection prior to joint surgery.[29]

CLINICAL FEATURES

Nongonococcal infective arthritis

Nongonococcal infective arthritis is typically monoarticular and has an acute presentation. Patients complain of pain and limitation of motion in over 90% of cases.[13] In one study, fever was present in 78% of patients within 24 hours of hospitalization, although it was rarely above 102°F (39°C).[19] Chills were uncommon. Physical examination usually reveals a large effusion and a marked decrease in active and passive range of motion of the joint. However, these findings may be minimal or absent in those patients who have rheumatoid arthritis, and they may be difficult to discern in infections of the hip or shoulder.

The knee is the most commonly involved native joint in adults. In a case series from the Netherlands, the percentage of cases involving a particular joint was: knee 55%, ankle 10%, wrist 9%, shoulder 7%, hip 5%, elbow 5%, sternoclavicular joint 5%, sacroiliac joint 2% and foot joint 2%.[3] Sacroiliac or sternoclavicular joint infection is more common among injection drug users and may be difficult to diagnose. Polyarticular infection occurs in approximately 15% of patients and is often due to *S. aureus*.[30] Thus, a polyarticular presentation does not always imply the presence of gonococcal, viral, reactive or noninfectious arthritis. It is more common among patients with rheumatoid arthritis and patients who have other co-morbid illnesses.

The case fatality rate for patients with nongonococcal bacterial arthritis is estimated to be between 10% and 16%, and as many as 50% of patients who survive their infection will have some degree of permanent loss of joint function.[8,20–22] Morbidity and mortality are dependent on a number of factors, including age, presence of rheumatoid arthritis, infection in the hip or shoulder, duration of symptoms before treatment, the presence of polyarticular arthritis, persistently positive joint fluid cultures after appropriate therapy, the presence of bacteremia and the virulence of the infecting organism.[2,8,31,32]

Gonococcal arthritis

Disseminated gonococcal infection presents with two distinct clinical entities.[4] Early after dissemination from mucosal surfaces such as the cervix or urethra the patient presents with bacteremia, fever, polyarthralgia, tenosynovitis (typically of the hands and fingers) and multiple maculopapular, pustular, vesicular or necrotic skin lesions. Asymmetric joint involvement is common. The knee, elbow, wrist, metacarpophalangeal and ankle joints are the most commonly involved. This presentation accounts for 60% of patients who present with disseminated gonococcal disease, and it has been described as the dermatitis–arthritis syndrome. If left untreated, the patient will present later with monoarticular arthritis, usually without tenosynovitis or skin lesions. Co-infection with HIV often leads to infection of unusual joints and an aggressive course.[33]

The outcome of disseminated gonococcal infection is almost always excellent (see Practice Point 29).

DIAGNOSIS

Although the history and physical examination can lead to a high index of suspicion for infection, a synovial fluid culture that yields a causative micro-organism is the only definitive method for diagnosing bacterial arthritis. Fever and rigors in the setting of an inflammatory arthritis have a low positive predictive value for bacterial arthritis and have been reported in crystal-induced arthropathy.[15] The erythrocyte sedimentation rate (ESR), C-reactive protein and leukocyte counts are elevated in the majority of cases, although again the positive predictive value of these tests in the setting of a monoarticular inflammatory arthritis is low. A rise in the ESR may help in the differential diagnosis of new joint pain and effusion in those patients who have rheumatoid arthritis.[13,34] Blood cultures are positive in up to 70% of all patients, and more often than this in patients who have polyarticular involvement.[22,30]

In disseminated gonococcal infection the majority of patients have an elevated ESR, and only 50% will have an abnormal leukocyte count. Anemia and abnormal liver function tests also may occur but these findings are usually transient.[4]

In approximately 80% of patients who have disseminated gonococcal arthritis there is a positive culture or *N. gonorrhoeae* DNA can be identified by polymerase chain reaction (PCR) or ligase chain reaction in samples from the cervix, urethra, rectum, pharynx or urine. Skin lesions yield *N. gonorrhoeae* in 30% of cases and blood cultures in 5%.

The diagnostic procedure of choice for bacterial arthritis is an arthrocentesis. This should be done immediately once the diagnosis of joint infection is suspected so as not to delay appropriate medical or surgical therapy. If synovial fluid cannot be obtained by blind needle aspiration (e.g. in the case hip joint infection), then aspiration should be done with the help of a radiologist. If necessary, an open arthrotomy should be performed to make a definitive diagnosis.

Synovial fluid is often cloudy or purulent in appearance. The synovial fluid should be routinely examined for uric acid and calcium pyrophosphate crystals, and a leukocyte count and differential should be obtained on each specimen. The leukocyte count is usually greater than 50 000/mm³ and often greater than 100 000/mm³, with more than 75% polymorphonuclear leukocytes. These findings can also be seen in patients who have inflammatory arthritis and crystal deposition arthritis. The sensitivity and specificity of a synovial fluid leukocyte count of >2 × 10⁹ for the presence of inflammatory arthritis have been estimated to be 84% and 84%.[35] For a differential count of >75% polymorphonuclear leukocytes, the sensitivity and specificity are 75% and 92%. Although many clinicians order synovial fluid glucose and protein levels, the results of these tests have been shown to be less informative than the leukocyte count and differential.[35] The synovial fluid lactic acid and lactate dehydrogenase levels are often elevated in patients who have infective arthritis, but elevation of these tests can be seen in other inflammatory joint disorders as well.[8]

Synovial fluid should be cultured for both aerobes and anaerobes and other organisms, depending on the clinical circumstances. A recent study performed at the Mayo Clinic showed superior performance of the BACTEC Peds Plus/F bottle over the conventional agar plate method for the detection of clinically significant micro-organisms from synovial fluid specimens.[36]

The synovial fluid culture will be positive in 90% of cases of nongonococcal arthritis, assuming that antibiotic therapy has not been started before the sample has been collected.[19] The Gram stain is positive in 50% of patients.[8]

In patients who have disseminated gonococcal infection, the synovial fluid cultures are positive in 25–30% of all patients and 50% of patients who present with monoarticular arthritis. The role of PCR in detecting bacterial pathogens in patients who have infective arthritis has not yet been well defined, although the technique seems a promising tool for the detection of infectious arthritis due to *N. gonorrhoeae*,

Borrelia burgdorferi and *Tropheryma whipplei*.[37] PCR can help to distinguish disseminated gonococcal infection from other inflammatory arthropathies such as Reiter's syndrome.[38]

Synovial tissue cultures are indicated only for chronic infective arthritis when mycobacterial or fungal arthritis is suspected or when synovial fluid cultures cannot be obtained by less invasive techniques.

Periarticular soft tissue swelling is the most common abnormality seen on plain radiography in patients who have bacterial arthritis. Periarticular erosions and osteoporosis as well as joint space narrowing due to cartilage destruction do not occur for several weeks. Thus, plain radiographs are not usually helpful in making a diagnosis of bacterial arthritis. Occasionally, in longstanding infection, periarticular osteomyelitis will be visible on plain radiograph (Fig. 40.1). It is often difficult to distinguish infection from inflammatory arthritis using radiographic methods in the setting of rheumatoid arthritis, but the development of a rapid destructive arthritis in one or two joints suggests infection. CT scans and MRI are more useful than plain radiographs for identifying concomitant periarticular osteomyelitis, soft tissue abscesses and joint effusions, but they are expensive and most often are not necessary (Fig. 40.2). Sacroiliac or sternoclavicular joint disease is optimally evaluated with these modalities, as well as with radionuclide studies. [111]Indium scans may be useful for identifying relatively asymptomatic septic arthritis in immunocompromised patients who have one or more known septic joints in whom there is a high index of suspicion for polyarticular infection.

In adults, the differential diagnosis for patients with an acute onset of fever, chills and an inflammatory arthritis of one or more joints includes bacterial arthritis, gout, pseudogout, rheumatic fever, reactive arthritis and rheumatic illnesses such as rheumatoid arthritis and psoriatic arthritis. Gout and pseudogout are the most common noninfectious inflammatory arthritides that need to be differentiated from bacterial arthritis.[8] They should be suspected when there is a history of previous episodes or there is chondrocalcinosis on plain film. Synovial fluid analysis using polarized light microscopy is the most useful diagnostic test for gout or pseudogout.

The articular manifestations of rheumatic fever occur in approximately 75% of first episodes, last for several weeks and do not cause permanent joint damage. Typically there is development of a migratory polyarthritis involving the knees, elbows, ankles and wrists that occurs within 1–5 weeks of the antecedent streptococcal pharyngitis. Joint symptoms can range from arthralgia without obvious physical findings to inflammatory arthritis that is indistinguishable from infective polyarthritis. Often more than six joints are affected. The diagnosis of rheumatic fever is dependent on satisfying the updated Jones criteria (see Chapter 166).[39]

Bacterial arthritis should be suspected in those patients at increased risk of infection. Fungal and mycobacterial infection is usually monoarticular but their presentation is usually over weeks to months instead of hours to days. Diseases that must be distinguished from disseminated gonococcal infection include viral and reactive arthritis, rheumatic fever and secondary syphilis.

MANAGEMENT

The keys to the management of infective arthritis are:
- drainage of the purulent synovial fluid;
- debridement of any concomitant periarticular osteomyelitis; and
- administration of appropriate parenteral antimicrobial therapy.

Experimental models of septic arthritis suggest that early drainage and antimicrobial therapy prevent cartilage destruction.[40] Local antimicrobial therapy is unnecessary and may cause a chemical synovitis.[8] Joint immobilization and elevation is useful for symptomatic relief of pain early in the course of the disease, but early active range of motion exercises are beneficial for ultimate functional outcome.

Synovial fluid drainage

The optimal method of drainage of an infected joint remains controversial, in part because no well-controlled randomized trials exist to guide therapy and because the therapy of each patient should be individualized.[41] Most adults who have septic arthritis have been managed with repeated joint aspirations instead of surgical debridement.[19] Patients who have disseminated gonococcal infection rarely require repeat joint aspirations, arthroscopy or arthrotomy.[4]

The use of arthroscopy has expanded in recent years because of the minimal morbidity of the procedure and the improved ability of arthroscopy to adequately drain purulent material from the joint compared with joint aspiration.[42–47] Large multicenter, randomized trials are needed to evaluate the comparative efficacy of these modalities.

Debridement

Recommended indications for surgical debridement have included effusions that fail to resolve with 7 days of conservative therapy and inability to adequately drain the infected joint by aspiration or arthroscopy, either because of location (hip and shoulder) or loculations of pus[8,13] (Fig. 40.3).

Antimicrobial therapy

Antimicrobial therapy should be administered as soon as the diagnosis is suspected and synovial fluid cultures obtained. Any delay in the administration of antimicrobial therapy may result in significant

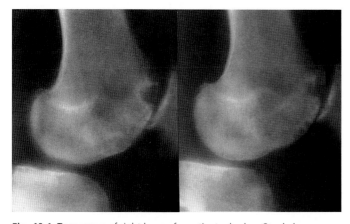

Fig. 40.1 Tomogram of right knee of a patient who has *Staphylococcus aureus* septic arthritis and periarticular osteomyelitis. Note the mixed sclerosis and lytic changes suggestive of osteomyelitis.

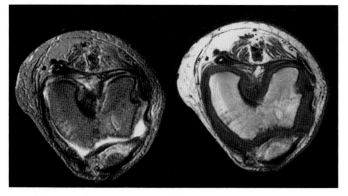

Fig. 40.2 MRI scan of right knee of a patient who has *Staphylococcus aureus* septic arthritis. Note the soft tissue inflammation and a joint effusion.

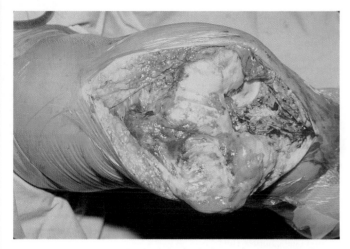

Fig. 40.3 Intraoperative photograph of right knee of a patient who has *Staphylococcus aureus* septic arthritis. Note the damaged joint and dark brown, boggy and hyperemic synovium.

cartilage loss and functional limitation of the affected joint. To date there are no randomized studies to help guide the clinician in the antimicrobial therapy of septic arthritis. Initial antimicrobial therapy should be based on the results of the Gram stain and the specific clinical and epidemiologic setting. If no micro-organisms are seen on the Gram stain, then empiric therapy for *S. aureus*, streptococci and gonococci (in young sexually active adults) should be given. Antimicrobials with anaerobic activity should be added to this regimen if septic arthritis occurs after the use of an allograft.[10] Administration of vancomycin or an antimicrobial with MRSA activity should be considered empirically in patients at risk for MRSA or when methicillin resistance is high in the community. Most experts administer 2–4 weeks of intravenous antimicrobial therapy for the treatment of nongonococcal septic arthritis.[8,13,48] In most cases this therapy can be administered on an outpatient basis after an initial period of hospitalization.

Suggested antimicrobials for specific pathogens causing infective arthritis are shown in Table 40.3.

Oral antimicrobial therapy with an effective agent with excellent bioavailability, such as ciprofloxacin or linezolid, is also acceptable, particularly if compliance with oral therapy can be assured.

Table 40.3 Antibiotic therapy of infective arthritis in adults for selected bacterial micro-organisms

Micro-organisms	Antibiotic therapy	Alternative therapy	
Staphylococcus aureus	Methicillin-sensitive strains	Nafcillin *or* oxacillin 1.5–2.0 g iv q4h *or* Cefazolin (or other first-generation cephalosporins in equivalent dosages) 1 g iv q8h	Vancomycin 15 mg/kg iv q12h, not to exceed 2 g in 24h unless serum levels are monitored
	Methicillin-resistant strains	Vancomycin 15 mg/kg iv q12h, not to exceed 2 g in 24h unless serum levels are monitored	Consult a specialist in infectious diseases Linezolid 600 mg iv/po q12h
Penicillin-sensitive streptococci *or* pneumococci with an MIC ≤0.1 μg/ml		Aqueous crystalline penicillin G 20 × 10⁶ U iv q24h either continuously *or* in six equally divided doses *or* Ceftriaxone 2 g iv or im q24h *or* Cefazolin 1 g iv q8h	Vancomycin 15 mg/kg iv q12h, not to exceed 2 g in 24h unless serum levels are monitored
Enterococci *or* streptococci with an MIC ≥0.5 μg/ml *or* nutritionally variant streptococci (all enterococci causing infection must be tested for antimicrobial susceptibility in order to select optimal therapy)		Aqueous crystalline penicillin G 20 × 10⁶ U iv q24h either continuously *or* in six equally divided doses, plus gentamicin sulfate 1 mg/kg iv or im q8h *or* Ampicillin sodium 12 g iv q24h either continuously or in six equally divided doses	Vancomycin 15 mg/kg iv q12h, not to exceed 2 g in 24h unless serum levels are monitored
Neisseria gonorrhoeae		Ceftriaxone 1 g im *or* iv q24h for 24–48h after clinical improvement *followed by* Cefixime 400 mg po q12h for 1 week *or* Ciprofloxacin 500 mg po q12h for 1 week *or* Ofloxacin 400 mg po q12h for 1 week	Ciprofloxacin 400 mg iv q12h for 24–48h after clinical improvement *or* Ofloxacin 400 mg iv q12h for 24–48h after clinical improvement *or* Spectinomycin 2 g im q12h for 24–48h after clinical improvement *followed by* Ciprofloxacin 500 mg po q12h for 1 week *or* Ofloxacin 400 mg po q12h for 1 week
Enterobacteriaceae *Pseudomonas aeruginosa, Enterobacter* spp.		Ceftriaxone 2 g iv q24h *or* Ciprofloxacin 750 mg po q12h (based on *in-vitro* susceptibility)	Levofloxacin 500 mg po q24h
Dosages recommended are for patients who have normal renal function.			

The therapy of gonococcal septic arthritis would require the use of ceftriaxone as the initial drug of choice, followed by oral therapy with a cephalosporin or a quinolone after initial clinical improvement (see Table 40.3). Given the increasing incidence of quinolone-resistant *N. gonorrhea*, however, we would advocate avoidance of empiric use of a quinolone pending the results of the *in-vitro* sensitivities.[49]

Viral Arthritis

Arthritis is a common complication of infections with hepatitis B virus, erythrovirus B19 (formerly paravovirus B19), rubella and alphaviruses, and is relatively rare with mumps virus, enteroviruses, adenoviruses and herpesviruses. The most common mechanism by which viruses cause arthritis is by invasion of the joint during the period of viremia. Other postulated mechanisms include immune complex deposition, insertion of the viral genome into the host DNA, thus promoting autoimmunity through an 'altered self', and direct viral infection of the immune system, thus altering the immune response.[50–53]

Typically, viral arthritis occurs during the prodromal stages of viral infection and is associated with a rash. Polyarticular involvement, including the small joints of the hands, is typical. There is no specific pattern of joint involvement that is unique to a given viral etiology. Diagnosis is based on historic and clinical clues (Table 40.4) and diagnostic testing specific for each individual virus, the details of which are discussed in the relevant chapters. Recently, an emerging form of acute and chronic distal joint arthritis related to chikungunya virus has been reported in the Far East.[54] Viral arthritis is usually self-limiting but may progress to a chronic arthropathy in certain instances. It is important that viral arthritis is distinguished from rheumatic fever and the initial presentation of autoimmune disorders, including rheumatoid arthritis.

Treatment is discussed in the chapters devoted to specific viruses. Prevention of viral arthritis is dependent on vaccination against the specific pathogen causing arthritis (e.g. mumps virus, rubella, hepatitis A virus, hepatitis B virus and varicella-zoster virus) (see Chapters 152, 154, 161 and 163).

Reactive Arthritis

Reactive arthritis describes the acute onset of an inflammatory arthritis soon after an infection elsewhere in the body in which micro-organisms cannot be cultured from the synovial fluid. In some

Table 40.4 Clinical or epidemiologic features of infective arthritis caused by selected viruses

Viral agent	Epidemiologic features	Clinical characteristics	Outcome
Rubella (including rubella vaccine)	No prior vaccination; 51–61% of rubella cases; 0–14% of patients receiving vaccination. Less common with new vaccine. Ratio of women:men – 9:1.	Symmetric arthritis of the metacarpal and proximal phalangeal joints, wrist, elbow, ankle, knee; onset variable in relationship to rash. May mimic rheumatoid arthritis. Post vaccination disease less symptomatic	Spontaneous resolution in days to weeks but may be chronic or recur.
Erythrovirus B19	60% of adult cases, females > males. Child care providers or school teachers; unusual in children	Sudden severe polyarticular arthritis in small joints. May mimic rheumatoid arthritis	Spontaneous resolution most common. Chronic arthritis can occur
Hepatitis A	10–14% of cases of hepatitis A; typical risk factors for acquisition of hepatitis A	Often associated with rash	Resolves spontaneously
Hepatitis B	10–25% of cases of hepatitis B; typical risk factors for acquisition of hepatitis B	Severe arthritis of sudden onset, symmetric, polyarthritis involving hand and knee; morning stiffness is considerable; skin rash may be present including urticaria	May last 1–3 weeks. Typically resolves during the preicteric phase. Chronic arthritis may occur with chronic hepatitis B infection
Hepatitis C	Typical risk factors for acquisition of hepatitis C	Can occur with acute or chronic infection. Sudden onset; joint pain in hands, wrists and shoulders often greater than physical findings. May mimic rheumatoid arthritis. Distinct from cryoglobulinemia with hepatitis C	May resolve spontaneously. Has been reported to persist for months and recur
HIV	Typical HIV-associated risk factors. Approximately 8% of HIV infected patients affected	Most cases are monoarticular but monoarticular and polyarticular presentations occur. Distinct from Reiter's syndrome or psoriatic arthritis which also occur in HIV-infected individuals. Occurs in multiple stages of HIV infection	Usually resolves in several weeks. May persist for months
Arthropod-borne Chikungunya O'nyong-nyong Sindbis virus Ross River agent Barmah Forest virus	East Africa, India, South East Asia, Philippines East Africa Sweden, Finland, Russia Australia, New Zealand, New Guinea Australia	May occur in epidemics. May be associated with rash. Constitutional symptoms may be present	Spontaneous resolution is typical. Chronic arthritis is unusual except with Sindbis virus

Data from Smith & Piercy,[13] Siegel & Gall,[50] Veno *et al.*,[58] Espinosa,[59] Naides.[60]

instances genetic material may be found in the joint using molecular diagnostic techniques. Reiter's syndrome (the classic triad of arthritis, urethritis and conjunctivitis) is a common example of reactive arthritis. Many patients who develop reactive arthritis are HLA-B27-positive. The micro-organisms that have been associated with reactive arthritis are detailed in Table 40.5.[55] A recent study that evaluated the risk of reactive arthritis following a large outbreak of O157:H7 and *Campylobacter* species found an incidence of arthritis of 17.6% and 21.7% respectively in patients who developed moderate or severe gastroenteritis symptoms.[56]

Typically, reactive arthritis begins several weeks after an antecedent infection. The initial clinical presentation is usually asymmetric oligoarticular arthritis without prominent constitutional symptoms. The syndrome also occurs without any identifiable symptoms of infection, however, particularly in the case of *Chlamydia trachomatis*. In the case of Reiter's syndrome, extra-articular manifestations are also present.

Laboratory abnormalities are nonspecific and include mild elevations in the leukocyte count, ESR and C-reactive protein. Radiographs usually show only soft tissue swelling in early disease, but juxta-articular osteoporosis and erosion may also be seen.

Reactive arthritis is normally a self-limited disease, but chronic arthritis and sacroiliitis can occur in up to 15–30% of patients. Treatment is with anti-inflammatory agents. The role of antibacterial therapy is controversial. Randomized trials evaluating the efficacy of antimicrobials in patients with reactive arthritis have been limited by small numbers of patients. In one study there was a trend towards efficacy for acute reactive arthritis due to *Chlamydia* spp.[57] Prevention of infection is reliant on effective prevention and treatment of precipitating antecedent infections.

Table 40.5 Micro-organisms associated with reactive arthritis

Definite association
• *Chlamydia trachomatis*
• *Shigella flexneri*
• *Salmonella enteritidis*
• *Salmonella typhimurium*
• *Yersinia enterocolitica*
• *Yersinia pseudotuberculosis*
• *Campylobacter jejuni*

Data from Hughes & Keat.[55]

REFERENCES

References for this chapter can be found online at http://www.expertconsult.com

Chapter | **41** | *Anthony R Berendt*

Acute and chronic osteomyelitis

INTRODUCTION AND EPIDEMIOLOGY

The osteomyelitic left fibula of the largest articulated fossil specimen of *Tyrannosaurus rex*, 'Sue', on display in the Field Museum of Natural History in Chicago,[1] vividly illustrates the ancient relationship between vertebrate bones and microbial pathogens, and the highly conserved biologic responses that have evolved to protect the host from this interaction. These responses, at their most successful, will prevent septicemic death and contain infection within a small part of the bone, either arresting and eradicating the infection, or creating a situation in which the infected portion of bone can be expelled from the body. It is common, however, for the eradicative responses to be incomplete, leading to chronic suppurative infection associated with pain, poor function and ill-health, and sometimes with progressive disability. This morbidity is as debilitating for the survivor of modern trauma, military conflict or sepsis developing osteomyelitis today, as it will have been for 'Sue' over 65 million years ago.

The formidable clinical reputation of osteomyelitis is perhaps well earned[2] but not inevitable with currently available treatments. Indeed, one way to make a poor outcome much more certain is to succumb to a nihilistic view that this is a condition characterized by intractability, recurrence and failure. Experiences from well-organized and skilled multidisciplinary teams suggest that with a positive approach, high rates of arrested infection and restored function can be achieved.[3] Difficulties in delivering success for all patients are partly due to variation; in the interplay of microbial virulence and host biology in each patient, in the extent of pre-treatment damage to bone stock and soft tissues, and in the clinical team's judgments and technical skill. The latter is unsurprising given the relative lack of good evidence to direct treatment, as a result of which most recommended management strategies are based on expert experience and opinion, not on randomized controlled trials.

The epidemiology of acute osteomyelitis has been studied in the northern and southern hemispheres[4–6] (Fig. 41.1). In all locations hematogenous osteomyelitis is a disease of children and adolescents and is much less common in adulthood. Incidences have been shown to be greater in the southern hemisphere. High rates are seen in Polynesians and in New Zealand, in Maori children compared to Caucasians,[4,5] but the relative importance of microbial, genetic, socioeconomic and cultural factors is unknown. In the northern hemisphere, rates of acute and subacute hematogenous osteomyelitis in children have been declining over decades,[6] compounded by the elimination of *Haemophilus influenzae* osteomyelitis[7,8] through immunization. A second peak in incidence occurs in older adults[9] and this includes vertebral osteomyelitis with an incidence of approximately 2 per 100 000 in both France and Sweden.[10,11]

Recent studies have stressed a growing role for community-acquired strains of methicillin-resistant *Staphylococcus aureus* (CA-MRSA) in acute hematogenous osteomyelitis,[8,12] the incidence of which may therefore rise once more.

The epidemiology of chronic osteomyelitis is less well documented, due as it is to a variety of different insults and manifesting in a variety of sites and ways. Cases are more frequently due to old trauma or instrumentation than to prior hematogenous infection. The enormous burden of war and civil unrest, the expansion and aging of human populations, and the rapid increases in automobile transport (and associated trauma) are all likely to have increased the prevalence of chronic osteomyelitis. A single example is the pandemic of type 2 diabetes. It is estimated that up to 25% of persons with diabetes will have a foot ulcer at some time during their life[13] and approximately 20% of patients attending foot ulcer clinics have osteomyelitis complicating the ulceration.[14] With global numbers of persons with diabetes at some 250 million, this suggests that around 12.5 million of today's current diabetics will have had, or will develop, osteomyelitis of one or more foot bones. The health-care burden of this is very substantial.

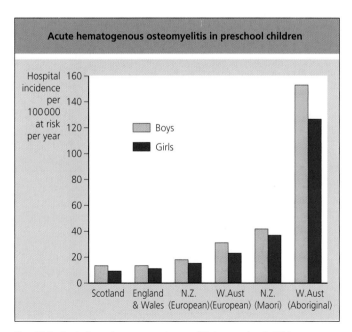

Fig. 41.1 Acute hematogenous osteomyelitis in preschool children. Data from Gillespie.[4]

PATHOGENESIS, PATHOLOGY AND CLASSIFICATION

Microbial factors

The pathogenesis of osteomyelitis begins with access and attachment[15] of organisms to bone either via hematogenous spread or from a contiguous focus of infection. Hematogenous spread may be from an obvious or an inapparent focus of infection or bacteremia. The contiguous focus may be infected soft tissue, a joint, orthopedic instrumentation or an area of chronic ulceration overlying bone.[16]

Staphylococci are the most common agents of bone infection. *Staphylococcus aureus* possesses numerous cell-wall-associated adhesins mediating specific attachment to a wide variety of extracellular matrix proteins found in bone[17] (Figs 41.2, 41.3). These include fibronectin, laminin, osteopontin, bone matrix sialoprotein and collagen. Yet other adhesins mediate attachment to components of thrombus such as fibrinogen and thrombospondin. Patients with hematogenous osteomyelitis commonly report some form of antecedent blunt injury to the affected part. This could expose bone matrix proteins (by microfracture of their mineral covering) and produce local thrombus to which staphylococci can attach. Where bone is directly exposed, necrosis of the outer surface provides an ideal substrate for bacterial attachment and subsequent invasion.

Post-attachment events include the elaboration of toxins that directly contribute to necrosis of tissues. In *S. aureus* the synthesis of these is controlled by quorum sensing mechanisms[18] and global virulence regulators.[19] Adherent bacterial growth leads to the formation of a biofilm, an adherent consortium of micro-organisms enmeshed in an exocellular polysaccharide. Biofilmed organisms manifest different phenotypes from planktonic ones, being much less susceptible to antimicrobial agents and to host defenses, and hence capable of prolonged survival.[20]

Small colony variants are another potential mechanism for persistence.[21] Altered gene expression affects metabolic pathways, growth rates, expression of virulence factors and antibiotic susceptibility. Small colony variants have been shown capable of persisting intracellularly including in endothelial cells, fibroblasts and osteoblasts, and have been recovered from clinical cases of chronic osteomyelitis.[22]

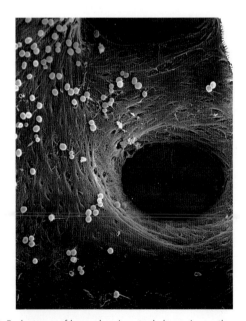

Fig. 41.2 Endosteum of bone showing staphylococci near the endosteal Haversian canal. *In-vitro* incubation of bone chips with *Staphylococcus aureus* interrupted at 48 hours (scanning electromicrograph). From Norden CW, Gillespie WJ, Nade S. Infections in bones and joints. Blackwell Scientific Publications; 1994, with permission.

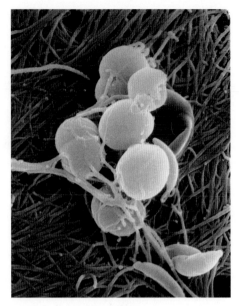

Fig. 41.3 Staphylococci enmeshed in glycocalyx near the Haversian osteum. *In-vitro* incubation of bone chips with *Staphylococcus aureus* interrupted at 48 hours (scanning electromicrograph). From Norden CW, Gillespie WJ, Nade S. Infections in bones and joints. Blackwell Scientific Publications; 1994, with permission.

Host factors

In hematogenous infection the pathogen most commonly localizes to the metaphysis of a large long bone just beneath the growth plate. The commonest sites are therefore femur, tibia, humerus, radius and ulna, but any bone can be involved and periosteal or epiphyseal seeding can occur. Extension across the growth plate is impeded in children; following epiphyseal fusion this route becomes possible and the joint can be involved. This is also the case in neonates since the joint capsule extends past the growth plate and encompasses some of the metaphysis as well as the epiphysis.

Infection triggers an acute inflammatory response, which in the rigid mechanical microenvironment of bone causes raised intraosseous pressures contributing to vascular thrombosis. Infection may be contained, in the resulting region of bone death, by the surrounding inflammation.

If infection is arrested at an early stage the effects on bone may be minimal. If infection progresses, pus may track to other areas of the bone along the medullary canal or through the Haversian systems in cortical bone from the medulla to the outer surface of the cortex. Here it may strip the periosteum (especially in the young where it is less adherent) and form a subperiosteal abscess. This may contribute to a bacteremia and major septicemic illness, or it may track out into the soft tissues and eventually form abscesses or a sinus, draining to the outside world.

Establishment of chronicity

Dead bone acts as an inert surface for biofilm formation and is surrounded by acute inflammation and suppuration. Both the inflammatory cytokines and mediators released during infection, and in some cases bacterial products themselves, can trigger bone resorption either by osteoclast activation or by stimulating phagocytic cells to take on a bone-resorbing phenotype.[23,24] Hence bone is lost from around the dead area, potentially ultimately separating it from the surrounding living bone to form the sequestrum. At the same time, where periosteal stripping has occurred, the resulting periosteal reaction produces a shell of new bone, the involucrum, around the dead bone. This will not be seen where the periosteal tissues themselves have been destroyed by infection or by pre-existing ulceration. Pus drains via one or more cloacae in the involucrum or from cortical breaches. This situation is compatible with life and function since the draining infection assumes a less aggressive nature and the mechanics of the bone can be preserved by a well-developed involucrum. The patient does, however, suffer ongoing bone pain, drainage, chronic debility and ill-health, and potential flares in infection that can affect the soft tissues, the bone or a neighboring joint, or lead to abscess formation or bacteremia.

Microbiology

The earliest descriptions established the primacy of *S. aureus* as a cause of osteomyelitis[25] and this remains the case today, accounting for over 50% of cases in pure or mixed growth.[26,27] In recent years there has been an increased importance of MRSA strains,[12] with community-acquired strains (CA-MRSA) of increasing importance in many locations worldwide. Where environmental contamination has been prominent, as in open fractures or blast injuries, or where infection arises from chronic wounds with their attendant complex polymicrobial flora, a wider variety of pathogens is seen with a rise in the importance of the Enterobacteriaceae[28] and of *Pseudomonas aeruginosa*. The latter is also associated with specific situations and risk factors, often involving initial interaction with a cartilaginous area adjoining bone, such as:

- puncture injuries to the foot through the soles of sneakers (training shoes) causing osteochondritis of the metatarsophalangeal joint;[29]
- malignant otitis externa involving the junction of the external auditory meatus and the skull base;[30]
- hematogenous seeding to vertebral end-plates in intravenous drug users and renal dialysis patients; and
- as a cause of chronic long bone osteomyelitis after open fracture and multiple procedures.

Anaerobes can play primary or synergistic roles and there is some evidence that their prevalence rises with increased efforts to isolate them.[31] Low-virulence organisms such as coagulase-negative staphylococci or enterococci are common in mixed infections, especially in diabetic foot osteomyelitis[32] or where infection arose in association with orthopedic instrumentation (even if metalware has subsequently been removed). In these situations they sometimes appear to be capable of acting as pathogens in their own right, being isolated in pure growth from reliable specimens.

Worldwide, infection with *Mycobacterium tuberculosis* remains important[33,34] and in appropriate geographic areas, *Brucella* spp. are important causes of spondylodiscitis.[35] *Salmonella typhi* and non-typhoidal *Salmonella* spp. have been identified as important in Africa, both in and outwith the context of sickle cell anemia or coincident HIV infection; various unusual *Salmonella* spp. have also been described in temperate zones from animal contact, such as with pet reptiles. Also of geographic importance are endemic fungal diseases including coccidioidomycosis, histoplasmosis and blastomycosis, all of which can produce bone lesions, as can late stage mycetomas. *Kingella kingae* has been shown to play an important role in childhood infections in Israel and France; for unclear reasons, this is not the case worldwide.[27] It would not be wrong to say that there are few surprises in the microbial 'small print' of causative pathogens, including atypical mycobacteria, *Nocardia*, melioidosis, yeasts, actinomycetes and even classic pathogens such as *Treponema pallidum*. Where chronic bone infection has been associated with multiple treatment attempts, multidrug-resistant organisms (MDROs) are common.

Pathology

The histologic appearances of osteomyelitis mirror the physiologic processes. The hallmarks are acute inflammatory cells within bone, and bone death, which may be associated with acute inflammation in the adjoining soft tissues, ulceration or purulence. Bacteria or fungi may rarely be demonstrable on special staining. As chronic infection develops, chronic inflammatory cells are admixed to the acute picture, and enhanced osteoclastic activity can be seen alongside new bone formation. In the case of a number of infections, including tuberculosis, granuloma formation occurs.

Classification

Osteomyelitis can be classified in several ways. *Temporal classifications*, namely acute, subacute and chronic, help to articulate the urgency and priorities of treatment and the prospects of cure. *Pathogenetic classifications*, namely hematogenous and contiguous focus, can help to direct attention to the likely spectrum of causative pathogens. Furthermore, this scheme also indicates whether the disease is 'inside-to-out' (hematogenous) and so effectively chronic in the bone by the time infection drains to the soft tissues, or 'outside-to-in' (contiguous focus), where there is often a substantial soft tissue problem to manage at the earliest point that bone is involved. *Anatomic schemes* can helpfully draw attention to specific challenges linked to regional anatomy; certainly the epidemiologies and treatments of skull base, long bone, diabetic foot and spinal osteomyelitis are different.

Most helpful of all, however, is the eponymous *anatomic-physiologic staging system* developed by Cierny & Mader[36] (Fig. 41.4). This details both the extent of bony involvement and key local and systemic factors that may affect prognosis. The staging system also inherently suggests

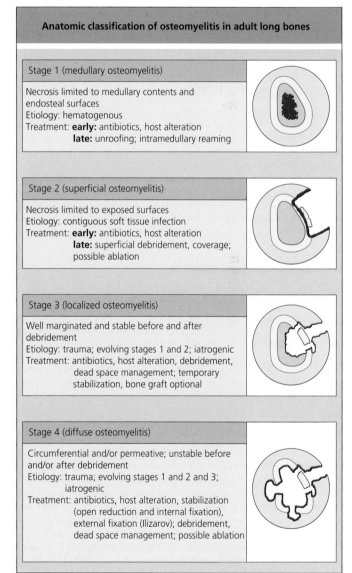

Fig. 41.4 Anatomic classification of osteomyelitis in adult long bones. Adapted with permission from Mader JT, Calhoun J. Osteomyelitis. In: Mandel G, Bennet J, Dolin R, eds. Infectious diseases. New York: Churchill Livingstone; 1995:1039–52.

different surgical strategies to precede antibiotic therapy and in some cases also predicts the reconstructive approach likely to be required.

PREVENTION

Since bone infection is relatively rare, an extensive literature on its prevention is lacking. Effective treatment of soft tissue infection, and careful attention to the prevention of health-care-associated infections (including orthopedic surgical site infections), may prevent a handful of cases of osteomyelitis but the data may never be forthcoming to prove this. Appropriate treatment of open fractures with debridement, antibiotics, stabilization and where needed, plastic surgery for soft tissue cover does have a demonstrated role in reducing infection and the subsequent risk of chronic osteomyelitis.[37] Finally it is clear that careful attention to pressure offloading can lead to primary healing and the secondary prevention of ulceration in the diabetic foot and other pressure situations.[38] It is highly likely that the systematic application of, and adherence to, these measures will prevent a substantial burden of diabetic foot osteomyelitis. Similarly, pressure sore risk assessment and care is essential in the prevention of decubitus ulcers and the osteomyelitis that sometimes complicates them.

CLINICAL FEATURES

Acute osteomyelitis

The classic descriptions are of an acute septic illness associated with agonizing pain localized to a bone.[2] Small children unable to localize or verbalize their pain may instead refuse to move a whole limb. There is high fever, prostration and systemic upset. Bacteremia complicates up to 50% of cases.

As the infection progresses, worsening sepsis is accompanied by increasing pain and bony tenderness together with soft tissue edema. Intra- or extraosseous abscesses may form. Without treatment, the outcome is either septicemic death or a prolonged febrile illness that resolves when pus drains spontaneously via a sinus.

Subacute osteomyelitis

The decline in acute hematogenous osteomyelitis of childhood appears to have been accompanied by a greater proportion of cases presenting with longer and more insidious histories, and with less systemic or local upset.[39] Often the major findings are that early radiologic changes are visible at presentation, not the case for classic acute osteomyelitis (see below). These painful bone lesions may mimic tumors[40] and hence are usually managed with biopsy or complete excision, often before they are recognized as being infective, and sometimes therefore without cultures being sent. Prognosis is, however, usually good.[41]

Chronic osteomyelitis

There is rarely a fever unless the infection is undergoing an acute flare. A degree of insidious ill-health is common, often noticed by the patient only after successful treatment. The most consistent features are bone pain, continuous or intermittent wound drainage, and impaired function; this may be profound (Figs 41.5, 41.6). Draining sinuses may alter in location and number over time through spontaneous remissions and relapses, healing and reopening via old or new routes. Where soft tissue loss preceded bone infection, continuous drainage or exposure of bone leads to persistent wounds. The abnormal soft tissue envelope is often confounded by scars from previous surgery, which can form preferential routes for sinus formation.

Progressive bony changes can include the expulsion of fragments or the whole of a sequestrum leading to self-arrest of infection. Relapse can occur decades after initial injury and infection.

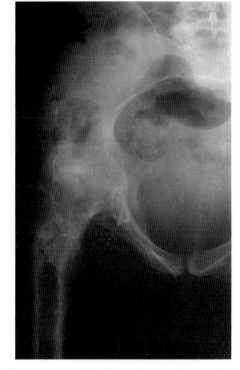

Fig. 41.5 Chronic osteomyelitis. The patient is a 30-year-old man who was born in Pakistan and who, as a child, had chronic osteomyelitis caused by *Staphylococcus aureus*. He is asymptomatic now except for occasional pain in the hip and a limp. The radiograph shows destruction of the femoral head and acetabulum, chronic changes in the femoral shaft and fusion of the right hip joint. Courtesy of Dr Joseph Mammone.

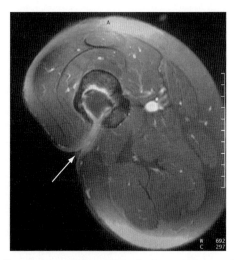

Fig. 41.6 Chronic active osteomyelitis in the femur. This case of osteomyelitis was secondary to a fracture and open reduction and internal fixation 30 years before. This axial, contrast-enhanced, fat-suppressed T1-weighted MRI scan shows cortical thickening and a focal intraosseous fluid collection with an enhancing rim, communicating via a sinus tract to the surface of the thigh (arrow).

Pathologic fracture of the osteomyelitic bone may occur, especially if a mechanically sound involucrum has failed to form. Rarely, after decades of continuous drainage, chronic osteomyelitis can be complicated by the development of squamous cell carcinoma or sarcoma in the soft tissue or bone. This may be presaged by increased pain, swelling, drainage or changes in the character of the ulcer tissue.

Osteomyelitis in specific anatomic situations

The accounts above relate particularly to long bone osteomyelitis but other important manifestations exist that are worthy of comment.

Vertebral osteomyelitis

The entity of infective discitis is recognized in childhood but is of particular significance in adults, especially the elderly.[42] Disc space and spinal infections may be postsurgical, in which case there is a greater likelihood of coagulase-negative staphylococci or other low virulence organisms being responsible; the majority of infections are, however, of hematogenous origin and due to *S. aureus* or the Enterobacteriaceae. It is suggested that the latter find a route, via the venous system, from sites of infection in bowel or urinary tract via retrograde flow into Batson's venous plexus which envelops the vertebrae. Seeding just beneath the vertebral end-plate is rapidly followed by involvement of the disc and the other adjoining vertebrae, setting up a pattern of a disc-space-centered infection. This process may occur at multiple separate or contiguous levels and is often accompanied by paraspinal or psoas abscess formation. Infection may track to form anterior or posterior epidural abscesses. These, retropulsion of disc space contents or mechanical instability of the spine from bone destruction, can cause cord compression or cord infarction, and paraplegia that may be irreversible (Figs 41.7–41.9). Nerve root irritation or compression at the lateral foraminae can lead to radicular symptoms and hence presentations with chest or abdominal pain rather than back pain. Tuberculosis of the spine manifests in similar ways.

In addition to the classic picture described above, isolated infections involving facet joints, posterior spinal elements and even the odontoid peg are well recognized. Severe back pain is an almost universal feature and with or without fever, should always raise the possibility of spinal infection.

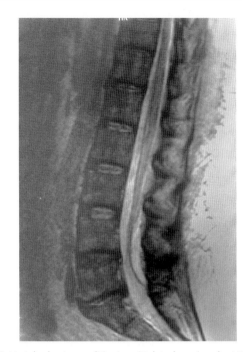

Fig. 41.8 Vertebral osteomyelitis. A sagittal, turbo spin echo MRI scan (T2-weighted) from the same patient as the scan in Fig. 41.7. Courtesy of Dr Joseph Mammone.

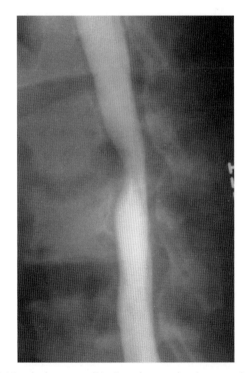

Fig. 41.9 Vertebral osteomyelitis. A myelogram showing posterior compression of the spinal cord by an inflammatory mass. Note the involvement of adjacent vertebral end-plates and the intervertebral disc. Courtesy of Dr Joseph Mammone.

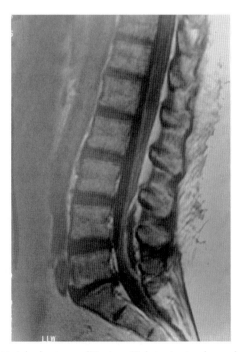

Fig. 41.7 Vertebral osteomyelitis. A sagittal, contrast-enhanced conventional spin echo MRI scan (T1-weighted) demonstrates a posteriorly located epidural abscess at the L4–L5 vertebral level with an enhancing rim and displacement of the nerve roots anteriorly. Courtesy of Dr Joseph Mammone.

Diabetic foot osteomyelitis

The peripheral neuropathy of diabetes has sensory, autonomic and motor components. Motor neuropathy causes differential loss of function of the distally innervated intrinsic foot musculature, resulting in changes to the biomechanics of the foot with clawing of toes and an equinus deformity. This leads to sites of excessive pressure, notably under the metatarsal heads, the heel, on the dorsal aspects of the interphalangeal joints and on the ends of the toes. In the context of loss of protective sensation and reduced skin compliance due to disordered sweating and lubrication, together with changes in collagen cross linking from excessive nonenyzmatic glycosylation, the result is ulceration. Alternatively, in dense neuropathy, sensation may be so impaired that foreign objects can accidentally fall inside footwear and be unnoticed, or be trodden on barefoot, and cause injury.

Ulceration may involve the periosteum or a joint capsule and hence allow infection to gain access to bone directly or via a chronic septic arthritis. Diabetic foot osteomyelitis therefore most commonly involves a metatarsal head (extending variably into the shaft and metatarsophalangeal joint), the phalanges at the interphalangeal joints or the terminal tuft, or the calcaneum. Infections of the bones of the midfoot may arise from soft tissue spread or because Charcot neuro-osteoarthropathy has led to collapse of the plantar arch and a 'rocker bottom' foot with plantar ulceration. Subsequent progression of infection is as for other sites, with the frequent development of spreading cellulitis, abscesses (that may be in the deep compartments of the foot) and necrosis. Fever is by no means universal, even with significant deep infection, and when present indicates severe disease with possible accompanying bacteremia or necrotizing fasciitis. Pain is substantially less than would normally be expected because of neuropathy; as a result presentation is delayed, especially in patients who are poorly educated, unmotivated or inadequately resourced to access health care promptly for foot problems (Fig. 41.10).

Osteomyelitis complicating decubitus ulcers

Decubitus ulcers occur where prolonged loading due to immobility interacts with poor quality soft tissue due to debility, especially if also complicated by neuropathy or cognitive impairment. Bone pain is a variable complaint; bone is often visible or palpable in large pressure ulcers,

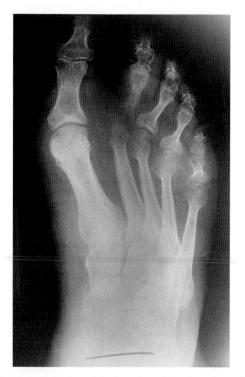

Fig. 41.10 Osteomyelitis in a diabetic patient. Diabetic patient with osteomyelitis and destruction of proximal second phalanx and metatarsal as well as second metatarsal-phalangeal joint. Courtesy of Dr Joseph Mammone.

and fragments may regularly be exfoliated into the drainage or dressings. The most common sites are the calcaneum, the femoral greater trochanter, the sacrum or the ischial tuberosity, depending on the areas of maximal pressure ulceration. Lesions may be bilateral. The soft tissue component is a dominant feature of the clinical problem; where the patient becomes systemically unwell this often reflects the development of abscesses, spreading soft tissue infection and/or bacteremia, rather than being directly due to the osteomyelitis. However, extensive involvement of bone is possible, particularly in the pelvis, and possible involvement of the hip joint should be borne in mind in patients with very advanced ulceration involving the structures around the hip.

Skull-base osteomyelitis

This condition is most common in elderly diabetic males and commences as a malignant otitis externa that then involves the petrous temporal bone.[43] It is also recognized in some postneurosurgical situations when midline involvement of the skull base is possible. Causative agents include *P. aeruginosa*, staphylococci or Enterobacteriaceae, though it may be hard to persuade surgeons to take biopsies for culture because of the complex anatomic relationships of the bones of the skull base to major neurovascular structures. Severe headache with referred ear and facial pain can occur, as can cranial nerve palsies. These are caused when nerves are compromised by inflammatory tissue in their anatomic course through the involved bone. Overall, significant morbidity and mortality still results and prolonged treatment is required.[44]

Mandibular osteomyelitis

Infections of mandibular reconstructions manifest as swelling and drainage from surgical wounds that resolve only with surgical debridement and targeted antibiotics. Infection of the native mandible is uncommon and is largely dealt with in dental practice. Localized infections associated with carious teeth manifest as pain, loosening of the tooth, and possibly a dental sinus draining beneath or lateral to the jaw. More challenging are cases with pain and diffuse sclerosis of the mandible without a realistic target for the dental or maxillofacial surgeon to resect; these are frequently culture negative but anaerobes may play an important role.

Chronic relapsing multifocal osteomyelitis (CRMO)

Another uncommon but important condition, CRMO is a term given to a culture-negative form of chronic bone inflammation (as seen histologically on bone biopsy) that does not produce the bone destruction typical of pyogenic osteomyelitis, and that arises apparently hematogenously.[45] Classically lesions are self-limiting, with different sites being involved at different times; there is a greater tendency for involvement of the sacrum, pelvis, spinal column and clavicle than is common in pyogenic hematogenous osteomyelitis. Pain is the dominant symptom, of insidious onset and therefore chronic at the time of presentation; wound drainage is not a feature. Some patients have other clinical manifestations making up the SAPHO syndrome (*s*ynovitis, *a*cne, *p*almoplantar pustulosis, *h*yperostosis, *o*steitis);[46] others have some but not all of these features, or other conditions such as sacroiliitis or inflammatory bowel disease; and yet other patients have nondestructive, culture-negative chronic osteomyelitis of similar appearances in single bones. Many accounts have emphasized a resolution of symptoms as the patient reaches adulthood, but a proportion of patients definitely have persistent pain and evidence of ongoing inflammation.[47] It is not clear whether this entity is a single condition that varies in extent and number of bones involved, or whether multiple conditions are being categorized as one. A genetic basis has been identified for a related condition, Majeed syndrome,[48] in which CRMO is accompanied by a dyserythropoietic anemia; a mutation in the LPIN2 gene (of unknown function) is strongly associated.[49] In the mouse, a chronic multifocal osteomyelitis condition is known to be due to an autosomal recessive gene mapping to chromosome 18[50] and since identified as likely to be a missense mutation in the *pstpip2* gene;[51] again, the human homologue PSTPIP2 is of unknown function.

The particular importance of this condition lies in its combination of diffuse bone involvement (offering no defined target for curative surgery) with unpredictable responses to medical therapies. These have included anti-inflammatory antibiotics such as tetracyclines and macrolides, nonsteroidal anti-inflammatories and bisphosphonates. Because there is no surgical solution for most cases and no clear medical therapy to offer, the prognosis can sometimes be worse than that predicted for a pyogenic chronic osteomyelitis.

DIAGNOSIS

Clinical features

Osteomyelitis should be suspected whenever a patient presents with bone or limb pain and fever. Differentials include soft tissue abscess (which does not rule out osteomyelitis), necrotizing fasciitis, pyomyositis and occasionally tumor. Pointers to chronic osteomyelitis include draining sinuses or chronic wounds that will not heal despite appropriate wound care, especially if in the context of risk factors for pressure ulceration. Visible or palpable bone is virtually pathognomonic of bone involvement, as is the expulsion of bony sequestra; a sterile metal probe has been shown to be useful for palpating bone in the diabetic foot, with a high specificity for underlying osteomyelitis.[52–54]

Blood tests

Elevations of inflammatory markers such as C-reactive protein (CRP) and erythrocyte sedimentation rate (ESR) are common, and in the absence of other causes have good specificity;[55,56] however, in a proportion of cases, levels will be falsely normal.[57] Biochemical and serologic tests are of limited value.

Radiology

Plain radiographs

Plain radiologic appearances are normal in early acute osteomyelitis,[58] becoming abnormal after 10–14 days when sufficient bone resorption has taken place to be visible on radiographs, and when periosteal reaction has laid down enough new mineral to be opacified.[59] Subcortical lucency is often seen when chronic septic arthritis leads to osteomyelitis of the subarticular bone. Areas of bone death are visible as denser parts of bone once the osteopenia of disuse and inflammation has reduced the mineral density of the surrounding viable bone. Over time, sclerotic areas and mature involucrum develop through the laying down of new bone. Fragmentation of sequestrum or of the infected segment of bone, including cortical breaches and pathologic fracture, occurs later in the disease.

As a diagnostic tool plain radiology is limited by its time dependence for the development of typical changes. Although the combination of destructive and reparative responses with evidence of bone death is relatively pathognomonic, particularly when serial films allow assessment of the timescale of changes (infection leads to rapid change compared to tumor), in some locations plain films are relatively unhelpful due to poor anatomic definition (e.g. in the spine) or because neuro-osteoarthropathy leads to abnormal appearances that can be confused with infection (as in the diabetic foot).[60]

Ultrasound

Ultrasound can be useful for the detection of soft tissue collections and also for examining the periosteum. It can show periosteal edema and elevation with subperiosteal pus, which can be aspirated under image guidance.[61] It can demonstrate sinus tracts and cortical breaches. In all these respects it is limited by the specification of the machine, the build of the patient and the skill of the operator.

Isotope scanning

Isotope scanning consists of several different modalities of different value. Triple phase bone scans are sensitive but nonspecific and while a negative scan largely rules out infection, the need to use other tests as well limits cost-effectiveness (Table 41.1, Figs 41.11, 41.12). White cell scans, despite being much more complex to perform and having inherent risks (including the rare but catastrophic injection of heterologous labeled white cells from another patient due to laboratory error), have a greater specificity and so can be useful. Fluorodeoxyglucose-positron emission tomography (FDG-PET) appears to be promising in studies to date.[63]

Computed tomography

CT has a place in surgical planning for the assessment of non-unions and complex bony architecture, and is well suited for identifying sequestra and soft tissue abscesses. It is easily affected by the presence of metalware, involves a significant radiation dose, and does not provide physiologic information about the intraosseous environment though it will identify cavities within bone. Other than for assessment of union and when MRI is contraindicated or unavailable, MRI scanning is preferred to CT.[64]

Magnetic resonance imaging

This provides information on soft tissues including sinus tracts, bone anatomy, and intraosseous edema and abscess formation. It is the most valuable of the imaging modalities in osteomyelitis,[64] including in diabetic foot osteomyelitis where this is required,[65–68] with high

Table 41.1 Tests for osteomyelitis.

Sensitivity, specificity, positive predictive values and negative predictive values of tests used to diagnose infection of bone

	Sensitivity (%)	Specificity (%)	Positive predictive value (%)	Negative predictive value (%)
Three-phase bone scan	95	33	53	90
Gallium scan	81	69	71	80
Indium-labeled white blood cell scan	88	85	86	87
MRI	95	88	93	92
Adapted from White et al.[62]				

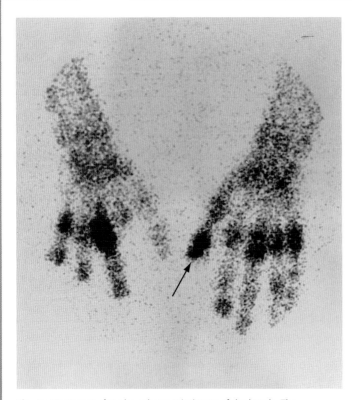

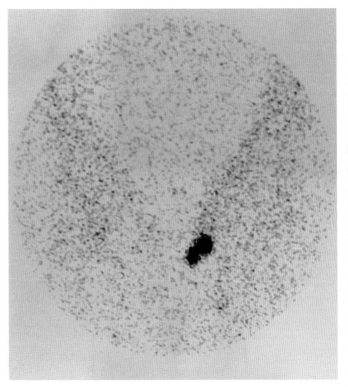

Fig. 41.11 Twenty-four-hour bone scintigram of the hands. The patient is a 50-year-old diabetic with a draining ulcer at the top of the right thumb (arrow). A biopsy grew *Staphylococcus aureus*. There is intense uptake in distal first phalanx and in multiple neuropathic joints. With permission from Jacobson AF, Harley J, Kipsky B, Pecoraro R. Diagnosis of osteomyelitis in the presence of soft tissue infection and radiologic evidence of osseous abnormalities. AJR Am J Roentgenol 1991;157:807–12.

Fig. 41.12 Leukocyte scintigram of the hands. This scan is from the same patient as the scan in Fig. 41.11. Again there is intense uptake in the distal first phalanx, but there is no accumulation of leukocytes in the multiple neuropathic joints. With permission from Jacobson AF, Harley J, Kipsky B, Pecoraro R. Diagnosis of osteomyelitis in the presence of soft tissue infection and radiologic evidence of osseous abnormalities. AJR Am J Roentgenol 1991;157:807–12.

sensitivity and if reported by an expert, specificity (Fig. 41.13). It is prone to postsurgical and postinstrumentation artifacts, with signal voids being created by metalware and by microscopic metallosis persisting even after metalware removal. Slow resolution of changes makes MRI of uncertain value in monitoring response to treatment, but it has proved very valuable in primary diagnosis and in surgical planning.

Bone biopsy

The criterion standard for diagnosing osteomyelitis is the culture of microbes from reliably obtained samples of bone, accompanied by inflammation in histologic samples. Bone biopsy may be performed safely either surgically or as a percutaneous procedure[69-71] under CT or fluoroscopic guidance. This is particularly useful in situations where there is a desire to avoid surgery, or when surgery is not always required for success (e.g. in the spine[72] and diabetic foot[70]). Bone samples or those of adjoining soft tissue are recommended in preference to superficial swabs or biopsies of sinus tracts, which have a greater range of organisms present that usually do not reliably represent the deep flora.[70,73] Obtaining multiple deep samples, and using separate instruments to avoid cross-contamination, increases sensitivity and specificity of culture in revision arthroplasty[74] and by extrapolation, in chronic osteomyelitis too. A range of conditions including use of broth enrichment culture is advised to maximize the chance of isolating the causative pathogens, despite which some 15–20% of chronic cases are culture-negative. Molecular diagnostic methods[75,76] are still not in routine use as a solution to this problem.

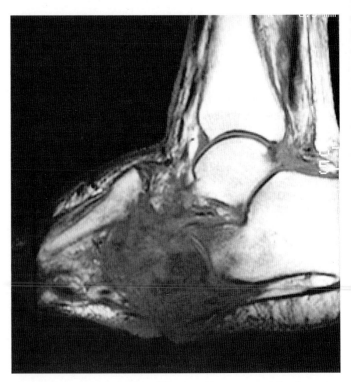

Fig. 41.13 T1-weighted image of the foot. The scan reveals forefoot amputation and a normal signal in distal tibia, talus and posterior calcaneus. The interior portion of the calcaneus has edema. The remainder of the tarsal bones have been destroyed and replaced by a low signal inflammatory mass.

MANAGEMENT

Acute osteomyelitis

Initial actions

The priority is to start antibiotics promptly in order to reduce the risks of bacteremia and of progressive bone death and destruction. Acute osteomyelitis should therefore be diagnosed clinically, prompting blood cultures and any other rapid cultures (e.g. aspiration of a collection) and initiation of empiric treatment without undue delay.

Immediately following on from this, a more full clinical and laboratory assessment can be carried out. Hematologic and biochemical testing provide a broader picture of the degree of systemic upset, plain radiology helps to rule out fracture and define pre-existing disease and a definitive confirmatory test such as MRI or white cell scanning can be organized.

Antibiotic therapy

Intravenous antibiotics should be commenced empirically and must include an agent active against *S. aureus*; the need to include activity against MRSA should be considered carefully based on risk factors and local prevalence. Once culture results are available, therapy can be rationalized (Table 41.2). There is very extensive experience, especially in children, of treating for 48–72 hours with intravenous antibiotics and then switching to oral therapy provided the clinical response has been prompt, the organism is susceptible to highly bioavailable oral therapy and adherence to the agreed regimen can be assured.[77–79] In acute osteomyelitis without complications, 4 weeks of therapy is generally adequate; this may need to be extended for longer periods if bone has already been killed but not yet removed.

The role of surgery

Surgery is not necessary in every case but orthopedic review is essential if available. Most surgeons no longer favor routine drilling of the bone.[80] Surgery should be reserved for clinical or imaging evidence of abscess formation, necrosis, or if infection fails to respond to appropriate antibiotics.

Prognosis

Acute osteomyelitis, diagnosed and treated promptly with appropriate antibiotics, carries a good prognosis with several studies showing cure rates of over 90% without major sequelae.[79] However, when diagnosis or treatment is delayed, and in a minority of cases despite appropriate therapy, serious sequelae can occur. Secondary septic arthritis can have a serious impact on longer term function in neonates or adults, and growth plate disturbance adjacent to a metaphyseal focus can lead to limb length discrepancy or angular deformity.[81] Chronic infection is highly likely if significant bone death occurs.

Chronic osteomyelitis

Initial actions

Whereas time is of the essence in acute osteomyelitis, this is not generally the case in chronic infection. Here, a process of patient-centered goal setting is required to ensure that realistic treatment aims are defined. As long as the patient remains medically stable, imaging and other diagnostics should usually be undertaken before antibiotics are commenced, planning for the surgery that will be necessary in most situations. While there is evidence that diabetic foot osteomyelitis may respond to antibiotics (and podiatry) alone,[82] and whilst most spinal infection can be treated with prolonged antibiotics without surgery,

Table 41.2 Antimicrobial therapy for infections of bone

Organism	ANTIMICROBIAL AGENT OF CHOICE	
	Agent	Alternative agents
Staphylococcus aureus (methicillin-sensitive)	Nafcillin or oxacillin 2 g q6h iv	Cefazolin, vancomycin, clindamycin
Staphylococcus aureus (methicillin-resistant)	Vancomycin 1 g q12h iv	Trimethoprim-sulfamethoxazole plus rifampin
Streptococcus pneumoniae	Penicillin G 5 × 10^6 U q6h iv*	Cefazolin, vancomycin, clindamycin
Group A β-hemolytic streptococci	Penicillin G 5 × 10^6 U q8h iv	Cefazolin, vancomycin, clindamycin
Enterococci	Ampicillin 2 g q4h iv†	Vancomycin
Haemophilus influenzae (β-lactamase-negative)	Ampicillin 2 g q4h iv	Trimethoprim-sulfamethoxazole, ceftriaxone
Haemophilus influenzae (β-lactamase-positive)	Ceftriaxone 1 g q12h iv	Trimethoprim-sulfamethoxazole
Klebsiella pneumoniae	Ceftriaxone 1 g q12h iv	Ciprofloxacin, piperacillin, imipenem
Escherichia coli	Cefazolin 1g q8h iv	Ciprofloxacin, ceftriaxone, imipenem
Pseudomonas aeruginosa	Ciprofloxacin 400 mg q12h iv or ceftazidime 1 g q8h iv	Pipercillin plus aminoglycoside, aztreonam
Serratia marcescens	Ceftriaxone 1 g q12h iv	Imipenem, trimethoprim-sulfamethoxazole, ciprofloxacin
Salmonella spp.	Depends on sensitivity test; choose between ampicillin, ceftriaxone, imipenem, ciprofloxacin	
Bacteroides spp.	Clindamycin 600 mg q8h iv	Imipenem, metronidazole

*If susceptible or intermediate resistance. If high level resistance, use ceftriaxone 1 g q24h or vancomycin 1 g q12h.
†If susceptible. If ampicillin resistant but vancomycin susceptible, use vancomycin. If resistant to both, check susceptibility to tetracyclines, chloramphenicol or experimental agents.

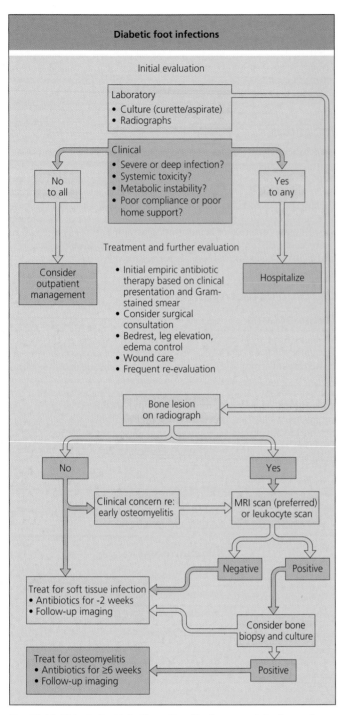

Fig. 41.14 Diabetic foot infections. Algorithmic approach to diagnosis and management. Adapted with permission from Lipsky BA, Pecoraro RE, Wheat LJ. The diabetic foot. Soft tissue and bone infection. Infect Dis Clin North Am 1990;4:409–32.

achieving reliable arrest of infection in the pelvis or long bones generally requires an operation (Figs 41.14, 41.15).

The role of surgery

There is a range of surgical debridement methods and reconstructive techniques, all geared towards control of infection, removal of the sequestra, skeletal stabilization and healing, and restoration of healthy soft tissue cover. Procedures include intramedullary reaming, limited cortical debridement, cortical windowing to access large and complex sequestra and endomedullary cavities, and segmental resection

for extensive disease.[83] In some cases conservative and reconstructive techniques are inappropriate and amputation provides the quickest and most acceptable route back to health. Plastic surgical techniques have proved exceedingly important in permitting postoperative soft tissue closure without excessive tension, largely through free muscle flaps with microvascular anastomosis. Advanced orthopedic methods, such as the Ilizarov circular frame,[84] allow the management of segmental defects and their reconstruction, using distraction osteogenesis to regenerate bone, or stabilizing the defect to accept a vascularized bone transfer such as a free fibula graft.[85] These technologies allow the surgeon to be much more radical in removing dead and infected tissue, thereby reducing the likelihood of recurrence.

While the role of surgery has been stressed here, it must be recognized that for some patients there are no surgical options that leave the patient with a better quality of life than the disease itself imposes. This group where 'cure is worse than disease' is joined by those who decline technically possible but high-risk or high-morbidity treatment, even if a successful outcome would be predicted to give good results. Finally, some conditions respond well enough to prolonged culture-directed antibiotic therapy and conservative wound care, with optimization of co-morbidities, that surgery can be deferred until the results of this strategy are clear. Many infections of spine, skull base and the diabetic foot fall into this category and a patient-centered approach is always important. In the case of diabetic foot osteomyelitis, it is not clear in which circumstances surgery is essential;[82] many cases can be managed successfully with antibiotics alone.[86]

Antibiotic therapy

Given the wide range of potential pathogens and the increasing prevalence of multidrug-resistant organisms (MDROs), empiric therapy should, whenever possible, be avoided until reliable deep samples have been obtained for culture. It is safe in the vast majority of patients to stop antibiotics at least 2 weeks before planned surgery or biopsy, provided the patient's prior history of infection and antibiotic response is considered carefully and mechanisms for urgent review are put in place. Patients must understand the rationale for the antibiotic-free period and know what to do if infection is flaring in advance of planned definitive diagnosis or treatment.

Once samples are obtained, empiric therapy can begin. As for acute osteomyelitis the choice of regimen must include activity against staphylococci, but given the higher prevalence of methicillin-resistant *S. aureus* and coagulase-negative staphylococci, and the increased likelihood of isolating Gram-negative pathogens, initial cover is frequently broader in spectrum. Regimens will need to balance the benefits of early appropriate therapy for all likely pathogens (favoring a broader spectrum) against risks of *Clostridium difficile* diarrhea and selection of MDROs in the patient flora and hospital environment (favoring a narrower spectrum).

Definitive antimicrobial regimens should, when possible, be based on culture and sensitivity results. There is experience in using prolonged intravenous therapy for up to 6 weeks including via outpatient parenteral antibiotic therapy (OPAT) programs,[87] in using switch regimens to move much earlier to oral therapy,[88] in relying largely on locally delivered treatment using antibiotic-loaded bone cement[89,90] or even calcium sulfate (plaster of Paris),[91,92] and in some situations (especially when surgical treatment is not undertaken) in using entirely oral regimens. A systematic review of available literature found no evidence of superior outcomes with any particular antibiotic choice or route of administration in all types of bone and joint infection;[93] more recently, a systematic review specifically of diabetic foot osteomyelitis reached similar conclusions.[82] However, adequately powered, randomized studies to answer these important questions directly are still lacking.

Duration of antibiotic therapy in chronic osteomyelitis varies substantially between and within centers. Where it is possible to have confidence in the judgment of the surgeon regarding the completeness of resection of dead bone, a logical scheme is to give 4–6 weeks of therapy following complete resection (and potentially less for more localized disease), and much more prolonged therapy when

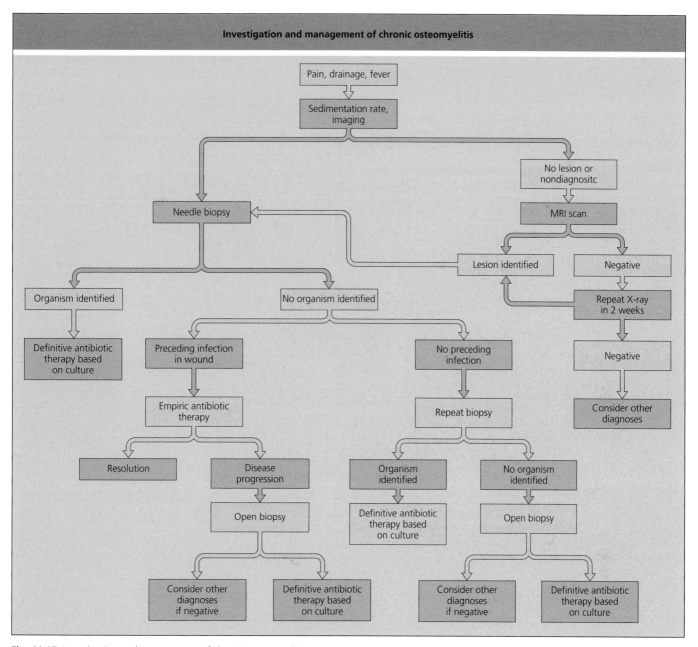

Investigation and management of chronic osteomyelitis

Pain, drainage, fever

Sedimentation rate, imaging

No lesion or nondiagnositc

MRI scan

Needle biopsy

Lesion identified

Negative

Repeat X-ray in 2 weeks

Organism identified

No organism identified

Definitive antibiotic therapy based on culture

Preceding infection in wound

No preceding infection

Negative

Empiric antibiotic therapy

Repeat biopsy

Consider other diagnoses

Resolution

Disease progression

Organism identified

No organism identified

Open biopsy

Definitive antibiotic therapy based on culture

Open biopsy

Consider other diagnoses if negative

Definitive antibiotic therapy based on culture

Consider other diagnoses if negative

Definitive antibiotic therapy based on culture

Fig. 41.15 Investigation and management of chronic osteomyelitis.

dead bone is known to persist.[14] The precise duration of this can be tailored to the specific circumstances of the patient, recognizing that relapse is much more likely in this situation. The goal therefore becomes to deliver a disease-free period while on therapy, during which important biologic events may occur (expulsion of a sequestrum, consolidation of an involucrum, healing of a fracture or nonunion) or even key personal milestones important to the patient's quality of life. If amputation has been necessary then the duration of postoperative antibiotic treatment can be based on the degree of infection in the remaining soft tissue and bone.

Soft tissue management

The soft tissues are critical as barriers to re-infection and as a delivery vehicle for host defenses and antibiotics. Their importance is often underestimated. Effort must be made to ensure the removal of chronically scarred and indurated soft tissues, surgical wound

closure without dead spaces or excessive tension, coverage of debrided bone with healthy tissue, and for chronic wounds not appropriate for surgery, an optimized wound-healing environment. This includes fastidious pressure offloading in decubiti and diabetic foot ulcers,[38] assessment and optimization of local vascularity (arterial and venous) and of systemic factors (hematocrit, oxygenation, nutrition and the minimizing of drugs that affect healing).

Adjunctive factors

Careful attention to co-morbidities as listed above is important for bone as well as for soft tissue healing. Of other specific adjunctive therapies used, virtually none has an established evidence base. A systematic review of diabetic foot osteomyelitis found no evidence to support any specific adjunctive therapies in diabetic foot osteomyelitis.[82] In particular, the use of hyperbaric oxygen, in widespread use in many centers, has not yet been validated for

455

osteomyelitis in large-scale, appropriately blinded, randomized controlled trials. The topic remains a controversial one with advocates on both sides.[94,95]

CONCLUSIONS

Osteomyelitis remains a fascinating and challenging condition requiring more basic and translational research. The development of consensus definitions and the widespread adoption of standardized classification and staging systems is an essential step in enabling multicenter studies to develop the most cost-effective diagnostic and therapeutic protocols. These will need to be developed and implemented by multidisciplinary teams that together can provide the surgical, medical and psychological expertise that patients with osteomyelitis so frequently need if they are to achieve the best possible outcomes. Development of competencies in these teams is perhaps the greatest priority of all so that more patients can experience, now, the best of what current treatments can offer.

REFERENCES

References for this chapter can be found online at http://www.expertconsult.com

Chapter | **42** | *Anthony R Berendt*

Infections of prosthetic joints and related problems

INTRODUCTION

Implant technology is one of the cornerstones of modern orthopedics. Of the few clouds on the extensive horizons that orthopedic instrumentation has opened up, infection is without doubt one of the darkest. Thus while hip replacement is one of the most cost-effective health-care interventions ever developed,[1] the chronically infected hip replacement is one of the most challenging and costly conditions for an orthopedic surgeon to treat.[2] Similarly, modern technology now permits a much greater likelihood of salvaging a functional limb after severe trauma, but if infection develops the limb may ultimately be lost after all, with much greater suffering and cost in the interim.

While both serious systemic sepsis leading to mortality and necrotizing soft tissue infections are relatively uncommon following orthopedic instrumentation, infection nonetheless causes significant morbidity. This may take the form of continuous wound drainage, implant failure from loss of mechanical fixation to the bone, progressively worsening pain and resultant disability, and chronic morbidity affecting physical and mental health parameters. Patients with chronic orthopedic implant infections have multiple dimensions to their problems, many of which lie outside the traditional 'comfort zone' of many orthopedic surgeons.

Perhaps for this reason, allied to the relative scarcity of these problems, the field remains bedeviled by a paucity of high-quality evidence. This has not prevented the establishment of the principles of good practice that form the basis of much of this chapter, nor a considerable degree of consensus among many different expert centers. Such expert consensus is the basis of forthcoming clinical practice guidelines for prosthetic joint infection that are expected to be produced by the Infectious Diseases Society of America in 2010. One key principle on which all are agreed is the necessity for these problems to be treated by a multidisciplinary team or via a co-ordinated multidisciplinary care pathway, with expertise in the whole range of skills required to treat and rehabilitate these patients optimally.

EPIDEMIOLOGY

Rates of infection following hip and knee replacement are cited as between 0.5% and 2% in large series from the Scandinavian joint replacement registries or specialist centers.[3,4] Rates of infection of less common arthroplasties such as shoulder, elbow and ankle are less well defined. Substantial datasets from large-scale surveillance schemes as in the UK suggest infection currently complicates 0.5% of hip replacements, 0.25% of knee replacements, 2.5% of hemiarthroplasties for fractured neck of femur and 1% of fixations for long bone fracture.[5] Ascertainment is a particular issue given the increasing trend for early

discharge after surgery. There are also issues of definition: while the Centers for Disease Control and Prevention (CDC) definitions for organ/space infection are clear in the event of a prosthesis being present,[6] diagnostic difficulties (see below) and the very slow evolution of infections with low-grade pathogens in some cases may reduce early recognition; so too may the effect of denial or a lack of diagnostic rigor from the surgical team. Finally, different approaches are required to diagnose a superficial compared to a deep infection; it remains to be seen whether the trend for health-care commissioners not to reimburse complications such as infection constitutes a perverse incentive that drives clinicians to avoid diagnosing infection in the early postoperative period.

PATHOGENESIS AND PATHOLOGY

Pathogenesis

Prosthetic joint infection is a paradigm of device-related infection and of the issues involved in treating complex surgical infection. There are three elements which come together:

- the effect of implants on host biology (affecting susceptibility and response to infection);
- the effect of implants on microbial biology (including susceptibility to host defenses and antimicrobials); and
- the effect of chronic infection on the biology of bone and soft tissue.

All foreign implants increase susceptibility to infection, as the work of Elek and Conen demonstrated, using human volunteers to assess the inoculum of *Staphylococcus pyogenes* required to cause a wound infection in the presence or absence of a piece of suture material.[7] Complement is depleted in the vicinity of an implant and white cell function is abnormal. The effect of these changes is to permit relatively low-virulence organisms to survive in the microenvironment of the prosthesis, as well as making infection with a higher-grade pathogen more likely. Finally, the act of implanting orthopedic instrumentation causes a degree of direct injury not only to the soft tissues but also to the bone. In addition to the sawing and drilling that is commonly necessary to prepare and anchor some implants, the use of polymethylmethacrylate bone cement leads to the death of bone at the cement–bone interface, since the cement generates considerable local heat as it cures.

Implants also profoundly affect the biology of microbes, in the first instance by providing substrates to support adhesion. This is mediated by a number of different mechanisms, including hydrophobic interactions between implant and microbial cell surface, and specific receptor–ligand interactions between implant surfaces conditioned with host proteins such as fibronectin and their cognate ligands on the bacterial cell surface.[8]

457

There is a substantial body of evidence that many micro-organisms will establish very large communities of adherent cells, involving one or more species, usually linked together with an exocellular polysaccharide that may be sufficiently abundant to be visible experimentally as 'slime'. This structure, known as a biofilm, can be demonstrated to have a complex internal structure, the nature of which will depend upon environmental factors including rates of flow of fluid across the biofilm and availability of key nutrients to the enormous numbers of microbes constituting the biofilm[9] (Fig. 42.1). The molecular basis for biofilm formation and the intercellular signaling events that occur are increasingly well understood[10] and are described in detail elsewhere.

Biofilms appear to be important in the persistent nature of implant-related infections. The mechanisms for this are not fully understood; while there is some evidence that local immune function is impaired,[11] there is also evidence that white cells can penetrate biofilms and kill at least some of the microbes present within them.[12] In the same way, the notion that antibiotics cannot penetrate biofilms now has little sway, but what is clear is that within a biofilm is a population of cells that do indeed phenotypically resist antibiotic action and will recover rapidly once antibiotic pressure is lifted.[13] These 'persisters' are of considerable interest, but still poorly understood. They may relate to small-colony variants, which have been shown to exist in the context of the gentamicin-loaded bone cement commonly used in joint replacement, and to constitute a mechanism for intracellular persistence and phenotypic antimicrobial resistance.[14,15]

The host mobilizes acute inflammatory responses to combat infection, even though these are not usually curative (Fig. 42.2). The result is a continuous process of acute inflammation which frequently leads to the formation of pus around the implant. The development of a sinus is a common response to this: by allowing pus to drain, it has the effect of decompressing the infection and, as a result, of averting the most harmful aspects of an infected collection. Patients with drain-

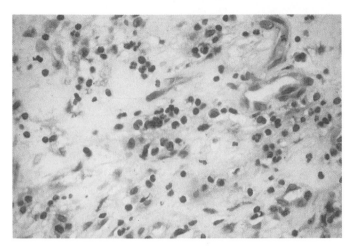

Fig. 42.2 Histologic features of infection. Periprosthetic tissue from a clinically infected total hip replacement from which multiple specimens grew an indistinguishable organism. Numerous neutrophils are present in the tissue.

ing sinuses may remain in relative health, and relative comfort, for considerable periods of time. Sinus blockage may trigger acute flares of soft tissue or systemic infection as the pathogens switch to more invasive phenotypes through quorum sensing mechanisms. Chronic sinuses may produce such extensive effects, in particular loss of soft tissue, so that primary closure of subsequent surgical incisions cannot be achieved.

Continuous inflammation does, however, have undesirable effects on bone biology in that it leads to the activation of osteoclasts and the recruitment of other cells that take on a bone-resorbing phenotype.[16] This activity is cytokine–directed and so is focused in the immediate vicinity of the implant, the effect being that bone is lost at the bone–cement or bone–metal interfaces. This ultimately leads to implant loosening; in the context of joint replacement the result is a progressively more painful, ultimately failing joint; in a fracture fixation or fusion construct, the result is mechanical instability that jeopardizes union and appears to make infection harder to control. The ultimate effects are hence a mechanically failed, infected arthroplasty or an infected non-union (Fig. 42.3).

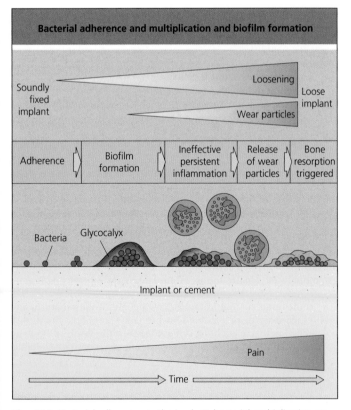

Fig. 42.1 Bacterial adherence to the implant, bacterial multiplication on the surface and biofilm formation. An ineffective host response triggers bone resorption, contributing to loosening, which is accelerated by wear particles and the host response to them.

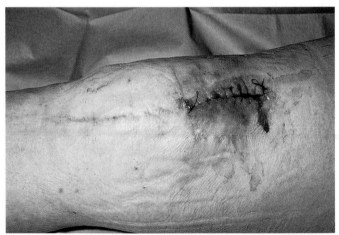

Fig. 42.3 An acutely infected knee replacement. The site was washed out but the infection failed to resolve. At reoperation the implant was found to be loose and it needed to be removed. *Staphylococcus aureus* was grown from deep specimens.

An additional feature that is not unique to infection is that once the loosening process begins, wear particles – from metal, high-density polyethylene used for some bearing surfaces or bone cement – accumulate at an increased rate. These particles trigger chronic inflammation that also contributes to bone loss;[17] the effects on immune function are unclear.

Pathology

The pathologic hallmark of infection is the presence of acute inflammatory cells in periprosthetic tissues[18,19] (see Fig. 42.2). By contrast, chronic inflammation is associated with aseptic loosening and uninfected non-union. The only situation in which a neutrophil infiltrate is not pathognomonic of infection is when an inflammatory arthritis is present. In addition, mycobacterial infections generally cause typical appearances of granuloma formation in the context of chronic inflammation.

Microbiology

The majority of orthopedic device-related infections are caused by skin commensals gaining access to the implant or to periprosthetic tissue at the time of surgery (Table 42.1). For this reason the majority of infections are due to aerobic Gram-positive cocci, with staphylococci pre-eminent.[5,20,21] Some infections are produced via hematogenous spread, mostly with *Staphylococcus aureus* and β-hemolytic streptococci, but rarely from oropharyngeal, bowel or urinary tract, or other causes of bacteremia.

The preponderance of staphylococci, including coagulase-negative staphylococci in equal numbers to *S. aureus*, also includes an important role for methicillin-resistant *S. aureus* (MRSA) in some centers (Fig. 42.4). This has also included infections with community-associated strains (CA-MRSA) increasingly prevalent in many urban environments in the USA, which on some occasions have been demonstrated to be introduced into, and transmitted within, the hospital environment.[22]

The very wide range of different pathogens described in the literature includes not only the full gamut of skin commensals but also less common pathogens including *Mycobacterium tuberculosis*, *Campylobacter* spp. and even *Clostridium difficile*, all in prosthetic joints. It is sensible for the infectious diseases physician to remember, and to remind orthopedic colleagues, that the range of possible pathogens and antimicrobial resistance patterns is significant, so that microbial diagnosis is a key element of successful treatment in many situations.

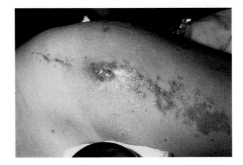

Fig. 42.4 A sinus tract discharging from an infected total hip replacement. *Staphylococcus aureus* was grown from deep specimens. Note the Koebner phenomenon; this patient's psoriasis was probably a significant risk factor for infection.

PREVENTION

The great difficulties and costs currently associated with the diagnosis and treatment of orthopedic implant infections fully justify increased attention to preventive measures. These can be considered in the pre- and perioperative, the immediate postoperative and the late postoperative stages.

Pre- and perioperative

At a system level, there is some evidence that separation of elective from emergency workstreams, including introducing 'ring-fenced' beds for orthopedic surgery, reduces infection rates.[23] Furthermore, the advent of care bundles has been a significant advance, and the systematic implementation of surgical site infection (SSI) care bundles has been highly successful in some institutions. Several guidelines for prevention of SSIs have been produced based on systematic reviews of the literature.[24,25]

Studies have demonstrated that certain patients are at greater risk of prosthetic joint infection, namely those who are obese, diabetic, taking steroids or of advanced age,[26,27] and in a multivariate analysis of a case-control group, with histories of malignant disease, prior surgery on the joint, or one or more factors from the National Nosocomial Infections Surveillance Score (NNISS) which integrates wound status, duration of surgery and American Society of Anesthesiology score as a simple indicator of co-morbidity.[28] While the possession of such risk factors is not an acceptable reason to withhold joint replacement from a deserving patient, it makes sense to identify patients at higher risk both to ensure preventive measures are reliably implemented and to trigger a heightened index of suspicion for infection if there are postoperative concerns.

It is standard orthopedic practice to attempt to identify and remove all sources of actual and potential sepsis, both local and distant, such as poor dentition, leg ulcers or exfoliative skin conditions, prior to arthroplasty. It is also sensible to ensure that treatable co-morbidities like diabetes are optimally controlled. In keeping with SSI prevention bundles and guidelines, preoperative shaving of the surgical site should be avoided if possible; if unavoidable, it should only be undertaken with an electrical clipper on the day of surgery.[24,25] There are no real options to undertake these measures in acute trauma where, instead, thorough wound toilet and debridement of devitalized tissues around the fracture are critical actions in reducing the infection rate.[29]

Good sterile technique remains of paramount importance and failings in this cannot readily be compensated for by other measures including prophylactic antibiotics. Surgical teams should maintain sterile technique at a high standard; however, if infection rates rise, all elements of practice should be observed for breaches of best practice. This also applies to theater discipline and the avoidance of unnecessary interruptions and human traffic in the operating room.

Table 42.1 Bacteria associated with infected implants presenting at different stages

Early infection (up to 3 months)	*Staphylococcus aureus* Coagulase-negative staphylococci Aerobic Gram-negative rods β-Hemolytic streptococci
Delayed infection (4–12 months)	Coagulase-negative staphylococci Other skin commensals *Staphylococcus aureus*
Late infection, including hematogenous seeding (more than 12 months)	Coagulase-negative staphylococci Other skin commensals *Staphylococcus aureus* Aerobic Gram-negative rods Anaerobes *Mycobacterium tuberculosis*

Historical data indicate that excessive use of diathermy for the control of bleeding or for incising tissue may increase risk of infection by creating a substantial volume of devitalized tissue. This risk must be balanced against the risk from hematoma formation, which has itself led to a long-running controversy over the use of suction drains, seen either as reducing the risk of infected hematoma or as increasing risk of infection by providing a portal of entry into the deep tissues. Good tissue handling, dead space management and effective wound closure are all important factors in preventing the access of pathogens to the deeper tissues in the postoperative period. In lower limb trauma (particularly tibial fractures) this attention to the soft tissues includes early plastic surgical intervention to ensure early wound closure with healthy tissue.[30]

The theater environment is also important, with a high level of cleanliness desirable. The use of ultraclean air was pioneered by Charnley when he developed hip replacement and it continues to be a mechanism that can greatly reduce the number of bacteria able to access the wound from the air.[31] Despite this the limitations of ultraclean air must be understood, including the turbulent airflows that can be induced by the presence of theater personnel and the entrainment of air, contaminated with skin scales shed by them, into the operative field or over exposed trays of surgical instruments.

The landmark Medical Research Council trials conducted by Lidwell demonstrated the importance of antibiotic prophylaxis though this was of equal (and independent) value to that conferred by ultraclean air.[32] A single dose of antibiotic may be sufficient, though it is considered good practice to redose if short half-life antibiotics are used and the wound remains open for over 2 hours. However, the data from Scandinavian arthroplasty registers suggest, based on historical controls, that infection rates may be reduced if 24 hours of prophylaxis is given. This is reflected in guidelines,[24,25] leading to obvious tension with the efforts to reduce to a minimum the selection pressures for MRSA and *C. difficile*. Prophylactic regimens must take into account local sensitivity patterns among key pathogens and there should be a process of periodic review and local guideline updating.

Early postoperative

In the early postoperative period the implant is surrounded by hematoma and lies at the bottom of a substantial soft tissue wound, albeit one that has usually been closed in layers to reconstitute anatomic barriers to externally derived infection. While it is too late to influence the events that have taken place in the operating room, efforts can still be made to minimize infection from external sources. Care should therefore be taken to comply with all other infection control care bundles in the postoperative period and to optimize wound care with strict non-touch, aseptic techniques. The infection specialist has an important leadership role in emphasizing the importance of all these measures.

Late postoperative

It seems self-evident that infections that might constitute sources of bacteremia should be treated particularly promptly in individuals with orthopedic instrumentation. However, it is important to understand that the microbiologic data suggest that the vast majority of cases of orthopedic device-related infection do not originate from distant sources but are acquired during the initial surgery.[20] Nonetheless hematogenous seeding of prosthetic joints (perhaps more so than static implants for fracture fixation or fusion) does without doubt occur, and it therefore makes sense to act as if it is a real possibility, ensuring timely, appropriate management of suspected or proven distant infection.

If the role of distant infection is uncertain, the need for prophylaxis associated with dental treatment is yet more problematic. Very small numbers of infections are demonstrably due to the kinds of organism typical of the orogingival flora. Most large centers will have anecdotal experience of such infections band in some such cases patients recall recent dental work. Theoretical considerations remind us that large numbers of oropharyngeal bacteria are released into the circulation not only during dental treatment but also during much more regular activities such as dental brushing or flossing. Thus, while much expert and pragmatic guidance currently favors the administration of prophylaxis within 2 years of implantation of a joint replacement or for any high-risk patient,[33] the evidence base for this remains scanty and the guidance therefore controversial.[34] There is consensus that prophylaxis for dental treatment is not indicated for fixed metalware, i.e. pins, plates and screws.[33]

CLINICAL FEATURES

Time to presentation

The clinical features of infection are often related to the time after implantation on the assumption that infections with high-grade pathogens present early, while lower virulence pathogens take correspondingly longer to achieve a sufficient burden to trigger a clinically evident inflammatory response. Thus early infections are defined as within 3 months of implantation, delayed as 4–12 months, and late infections, often thought to be hematogenous in origin, occur over a year after implantation. As originally described, early infections were thought to have a preponderance of virulent Gram-positive pathogens, delayed as being dominated by coagulase-negative staphylococci, and late being once again due to virulent causes of bacteremia and hematogenous seeding. At least one large study of cases of infection treated with debridement and implant retention at a range of times after implantation found no such relationships between pathogens and time after surgery.[20] It is possible that the dogma in the existing literature is biased by clinical management behaviors in some centers, lower grade infections taking longer to diagnose in the absence of a highly standardized clinical protocol for dealing with persistently draining wounds or those displaying signs of mild, apparently superficial, infection.

Acuity of presentation

Another commonly employed scheme is to describe the acuity of presentation. Acute infections are those with typical features of wound purulence and drainage, spreading soft tissue erythema and tenderness, systemic features such as fever, and short histories. In the context of a healed wound, acute infections also have the appearances of a septic arthritis or of a soft-tissue abscess associated with the implant. In the case of spinal instrumentation this can even, rarely, take the form of an epidural abscess.

These features would be contrasted with those typical in chronic infections where progressive pain, intermittent or continuous sinus drainage, and implant failure are much more likely to be present. In a small minority of cases a chronic infection is so indolent that it is an incidental finding at revision arthroplasty or implant removal for painful loosening (provided, that is, there is a routine of performing culture and histology on all cases of revision joint surgery or metalware removal). Very late-diagnosed infections of posterior spinal instrumentation, caused by coagulase-negative staphylococci or propionibacteria, have been recognized by the use of this rigorous diagnostic approach.[35]

Both the temporal and the acuity-based schemes for describing infections have their limitations if used alone. In combination, the two describe the timing of onset of symptoms in a way that is of some value even though it appears less effective at predicting the microbiology than was earlier supposed.

DIAGNOSIS

The particular difficulty surrounding the diagnosis of infection is the variability in the clinical presentation, in the ability to culture the causative pathogens, and in the density of neutrophils within periprosthetic tissues (as measured by the numbers seen per high power field in histologic analysis). In addition, the fact that most infections are caused by skin commensals raises significant issues of culture contamination and diagnostic specificity. As a result, no consensus criteria for defining infection have yet been established, and most diagnostic tests or protocols have been assessed against criteria variably defined by the investigator.

Crucial in making the diagnosis of infection is the maintenance of clinical vigilance. In the early postoperative period, persistent wound problems or complaints of pain should raise suspicions, even if typical features of wound infection are lacking. After the first few months, patients who complain that the implant was 'never right' should receive careful attention, especially if this is their first joint replacement or other orthopedic metalware. Patients who have known an uninfected implant and then receive an infected one are likely to be much more demanding since they know what to expect (an inapparent, normal-feeling joint after a few months). The danger with the 'first-timer' who develops infection is that they do not realize just how asymptomatic a good joint replacement or fracture fixation should be.

In the context of an acute infection, investigations are undertaken both to assess the degree of systemic upset and to evaluate the implant. Blood cultures may demonstrate an ongoing bacteremia; measurement of inflammatory markers provides a useful baseline for the assessment of clinical response to treatment; plain radiography demonstrates if the implant is soundly fixed, assesses the bone stock and any bony reactions, and excludes fracture or mechanical failure. If the patient is acutely unwell, ultrasound may help in assessing the presence of joint fluid or peri-implant collections for aspiration, with Gram stain and culture of the material obtained. Ultimately, the diagnosis can be made through surgical exploration, in part visually (though if explored promptly, an acute early infection may show only hematoma and tissue edema, and not frank pus), but in particular through the ability to obtain multiple specimens for culture and histology.[36]

In chronic infection, certain clinical features, such as sinus tract formation, are to all intents and purposes pathognomonic; however, the diagnostic problem is much greater with loose implants and with well-fixed but chronically painful implants (see Fig. 42.4). Plain radiographs are a standard part of assessment, allowing planning of further surgical options, examination for progressive loosening or implant failure, and assessment of the bone for chronic responses that may be due to infection (Fig. 42.5). However, features linked to infection, such as periosteal reaction, endosteal scalloping or extensive bone resorption, may in fact be caused by noninfective processes such as large diameter cementless implants, giant cell granulomas and stress shielding, respectively.

In the chronic situation, inflammatory markers are less helpful than in acute disease. When elevated in the absence of other causes of inflammation they may be of value;[37] however, it is well recognized that patients may have normal markers despite an unequivocal diagnosis of infection.

Aspiration of joint fluid for culture has been shown to have high sensitivity and specificity compared to cultures and histology obtained at revision, particularly if selectively performed in patients with an elevated erythrocyte sedimentation rate and/or C-reactive protein.[38-40] However, for those infections associated with lower numbers of neutrophils in periprosthetic tissue and with organisms isolated only on enrichment cultures, aspirates perform less well. The use of needle biopsy may enhance recovery of pathogens by providing a tissue sample and by allowing histologic analysis as well as culture, especially if multiple passes are made.

Exploration permits visual inspection of the prosthesis and the periprosthetic tissues. Purulence around the implant is diagnostic of infection and periprosthetic tissue samples are readily obtained, especially if the implant is being removed. Taking multiple independent samples increases the sensitivity of microbiologic diagnosis, which is also rendered more specific by requiring two or more samples to yield an indistinguishable organism and by histologic examination of periprosthetic tissue.[19,36]

Tissue samples should be sent in preference to swabs, but an increasing body of evidence suggests that bacteria adherent to the prosthesis can be dislodged with sonication,[41] allowing culture or other examinations and producing a test that may be at least as sensitive as the multiple sampling method and possibly of more value if there has been recent antibiotic therapy.[42] This, with molecular methods, may increase our understanding of the range of organisms that can infect orthopedic instrumentation. Despite some concerns,[43] an increasing number of reports suggest that polymerase chain reaction can yield causative pathogens,[41,44-46] though information on a full panel of antimicrobial sensitivities may require further work in contrast to what can be obtained with a cultured isolate. It may even be that gene expression profiling can help make the diagnosis of infection by characterizing distinctive patterns of gene expression in infected individuals.[47]

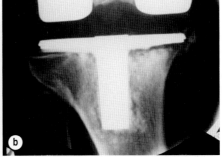

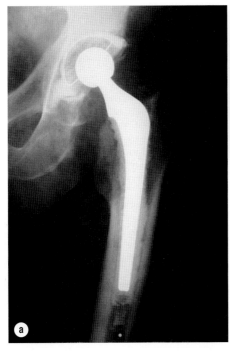

Fig. 42.5 Implant loosening in late infection. (a) Radiograph of the infected hip shown in Figure 42.4. There is an obvious radiolucent line at the bone–cement interface. This implant required revision. (b) Radiograph of a loose knee replacement, showing resorption of bone beneath the tibial component, a cause of instability. Coagulase-negative staphylococci were grown from multiple deep specimens.

MANAGEMENT

The cornerstone of successful management is the setting of realistic, patient-centered goals that take into account the specific symptoms and the options for reconstruction. The paramount aim is usually to control infection or sinus tract drainage, but for some it is the relief of intractable pain. In acute presentations there is a significant risk of serious sepsis and decision-making needs to be urgent; in chronic situations there is rarely this urgency and careful planning is important for best outcomes.

Assessment

At presentation, patients should initially be assessed for their systemic state as for any acute infection, with urgent treatment indicated for any sepsis syndrome. It is then appropriate to assess implant function and stability in order to establish whether an attempt should be made to salvage the existing implant or to revise it. This decision will also be related in part to the bone stock, which may set technical limits on possible reconstruction if the implant is indeed removed. Also of importance is the quality of the soft tissue envelope, defects or extensive scarring, which may point to the need for a plastic surgeon to be part of the treating team. It is likely that one or more co-morbidities will need to be addressed (given that medical co-morbidities are risk factors for infection); these can also include significant anxiety, depression or anger from chronic pain and disability, altered body image (from chronic wounds), social isolation, the iatrogenic nature of many infections, and the threat of permanent disability including the possibility of limb loss.

Treatment options

As stated above, a key decision to make is whether or not to attempt to salvage the implant. The rationale for attempting this is when the implant is soundly fixed and functioning well. Implant retention may be attempted with curative intent when there is a short history (within 2 weeks of onset of symptoms) and the pathogens are susceptible to both a fluoroquinolone and rifampin (rifampicin). Using this combination for 3–6 months, following a formal debridement and retention procedure in which all infected and necrotic soft tissues are removed and all modular components exchanged, leaving a stable implant covered by healthy soft tissue, cure rates of around 80% or more have been described.[48,49] Where antibiotic regimens are required that do not make use of this combination, there may be some grounds for optimism[50] (e.g. with β-lactam-sensitive streptococci other than enterococci),[51] but there is less published experience.

The alternative is to give longer term antibiotic therapy without necessarily expecting cure.[52] In this situation infection might be expected to recur if antibiotics were stopped because of the length of time it had been established, or because of significant biologic factors that are likely to favor recurrent infection such as cancellous bone graft or a large revision implant. Suppression is also appropriate when the implant is not required in the long term but has a temporary function to stabilize a healing fracture or a fusion procedure. In that situation the infection should be suppressed until bony union, followed by removal, bone and soft tissue debridement, and further antibiotic therapy. If implant removal is expected to carry significant risk, it may be reasonable to treat for 3–6 months after union and then discontinue antibiotics, or to decide to treat indefinitely.

Implant removal (without reimplantation) is an option when a temporary implant has fulfilled its role; however, in the case of prosthetic joints it can only be considered in certain locations, notably the hip where a Girdlestone's pseudarthrosis forms over time after excision arthroplasty. In most joints there is an unacceptable level of pain from the lack of an articular surface, and in fusions and fractures metalware removal prior to union results in considerable pain from

instability. Excision arthroplasty delivers cure rates in excess of 90% but just as when reimplantation is planned, it is essential that all foreign material including any bone cement has been removed.[53]

It is therefore much more common to remove prosthetic joints in the context of revision surgery, aimed at restoring function through reimplanting a prosthesis in the future. There is uncertainty as to whether an immediate reimplantation (a one-stage revision) is as effective as a delayed reimplantation (two-stage revision) which theoretically gives an opportunity to treat the infection without the presence of a prosthesis.[54–58] In many joints the bones are kept apart using some form of spacer, which may be fashioned from antibiotic-loaded bone cement to allow passive joint motion. Spacer devices have the additional advantages of allowing maintenance of limb and muscle length, management of any dead space and can act as a vehicle for the delivery of antibiotics impregnated into the cement. Special forms of spacer have been designed to cope with massive bone loss and allow for subsequent reconstruction with tumor-type endoprostheses.[59] Selected results of one- and two-stage revision with the use of bone cement are broadly similar, but a randomized controlled trial has not been carried out to test the question fully.

As described in relation to excision arthroplasty, it is not always possible to offer revision surgery and joint reconstruction. In some situations as at the knee joint, surgery to carry out fusion may be a limb-sparing technique that a patient will opt for. There are technical difficulties, however, because by the time fusion is carried out, there have often been several revision attempts and bone stock may be poor. A range of techniques is possible and it may be desirable to cover such a treatment plan with antibiotics, especially if infection is active when the fusion is undertaken. Amputation lies at the extreme end of treatment but has to be considered in cases of intractable infection with unreconstructable soft tissues and poor bone stock.[60]

Antibiotic duration and route of administration

It is essential that antibiotics achieve high levels at the site of infection. Three routes of administration are possible, with little good evidence to inform choices between them.[61]

Locally, antibiotics can be delivered via antibiotic loaded acrylic (bone) cement (ALAC). The bulk of the data and published experience relate to the use of aminoglycosides but other antibiotics that are heat stable (e.g. vancomycin) can be incorporated. Elution of antibiotic occurs over at least 1–2 weeks during which time there are very high local, but negligible systemic, levels. ALAC can be fashioned into beads on chains, spacers, cylinders or poured into molds to generate controlled shapes. In some studies it seems to play an important role in success.[59]

Systemic antibiotics can be delivered in two ways, either orally provided highly bioavailable drugs are used, or parenterally mainly via the intravenous route. Cost and convenience favor oral therapy with a somewhat greater risk of gastrointestinal intolerance, poor adherence to the treatment protocol and poor absorption if there are co-morbidities. Intravenous therapy ensures delivery but at the risk of vascular catheter infection and this is only sustainable for prolonged treatment if there are well-supervised outpatient parenteral therapy (OPAT) programs.[62] This can include self-administered outpatient parenteral antibiotic therapy (S-OPAT) which has advantages over health-care-worker administered therapy (H-OPAT).[62]

There are no proven advantages for durations of intravenous therapy beyond 6 weeks except on an exceptional basis for the treatment of a multidrug-resistant organism (MDRO). Total durations of therapy of 3–6 months have been associated with good outcomes,[49] though where there is doubt about the likelihood of cure, much longer periods of treatment are used.[52] Choices of antibiotic must take into account convenience (if OPAT is undertaken), side-effects and interactions, bioavailability and the antimicrobial resistance profile of the organism(s).

CONCLUSIONS

We have seen how prosthetic joint infection constitutes a major challenge to clinicians, scientists and indeed, to managers responsible for the organization of care. Prevention is of great importance, but equally we must stress that good outcomes are often possible with teamwork, skill and knowledge. There are still key questions to resolve, but the future of care will likely continue to include a specialist multidisciplinary team approach, with attention to careful patient assessment regarding goals, meticulous diagnostic and surgical debridement techniques, careful selection of antibiotics including duration, choice and route, and an understanding that in many circumstances, cure of infection, together with re-establishment of pain-free mechanical function, is often achievable.

REFERENCES

References for this chapter can be found online at http://www.expertconsult.com

Sammy Nakhla
Daniel W Rahn
Benjamin J Luft

Chapter | **43** |

Lyme disease

HISTORY

Lyme borreliosis is caused by the tick-borne spirochete, *Borrelia burgdorferi*, which is distributed throughout the Northern Hemisphere. The cutaneous manifestation, acrodermatitis chronica atrophicans (ACA) was first described in Germany by Buchwald in 1883. Afzelius subsequently described erythema migrans (EM) in Sweden and speculated that the rash was associated with tick bites. French physicians Garin and Bujadoux reported the first case of a neurologic manifestation, meningoradiculo-neuritis.[1-3] The disease was first treated with antibiotics in 1949 by Thyresson. In 1975, Steere and colleagues delineated the disease in the USA, while Burgdorfer and colleagues isolated and cultivated the causative agent.[1,2]

EPIDEMIOLOGY

Lyme disease is the most common vector-borne disease in the USA[4] and occurs widely throughout Europe and Asia.[5] The infecting organism, *B. burgdorferi*, is maintained in and transmitted by ticks of the *Ixodes ricinus* complex, including *Ixodes scapularis* in north-east and central USA, *Ixodes pacificus* on the west coast of the USA, *Ixodes ricinus* in Europe and *Ixodes persulcatus* in Asia (see Chapter 11).

In Europe, three species of the *B. burgdorferi* sensu lato complex are pathogenic, including *B. burgdorferi* sensu stricto, *Borrelia garinii* and *Borrelia afzelii*. *Borrelia burgdorferi* is the only pathogenic species in North America. The relative distribution of these species from region to region throughout Europe and Asia may account for the relative variability of disease syndromes associated with Lyme disease. Additional borrelial species *B. valaisiana* and *B. lusitaniae* have been identified by polymerase chain reaction (PCR) in skin biopsies or blood from a few patients with EM, ACA and with flu-like illnesses. However, these organisms have not yet been cultured from these lesions and their role in human illness remains unclear.[1,5,6]

Lyme disease is increasing in both incidence and recognition. The known endemic range is expanding, but the precise incidence and geographic spread are uncertain due to difficulties in establishing widely accepted diagnostic criteria. A National Surveillance Case Definition was adopted in the USA in 1990 to establish uniform diagnostic criteria for surveillance (Table 43.1). Over 90% of cases in the USA have been reported by 10 states in the north-east, upper midwest and Pacific coastal regions.[3] Even within these regions local distribution is highly variable. The recent upsurge in cases in the USA is a result of reforestation of land used for farming a generation ago, creating environments suitable for the deer reservoir,[7] and the outward migration of people from cities to rural areas.

Individuals who are exposed to natural outdoor habitats in the spring and early summer months are at greatest risk as this is the time when the tick vector is most active.[7,8] Erythema migrans is the sentinel clinical feature for most patients with Lyme disease. Those who do not manifest this skin lesion may come to medical attention months later with one or more symptoms of disseminated disease.

The seasonal variation of onset in temperate climatic zones follows the ecology of the predominant tick vectors. The life cycle and feeding habits of *I. scapularis* are best understood (Figs 43.1, 43.2). This tick has a three-stage life cycle (larva, nymph and adult) that spans 2 years. Larvae hatch from fertilized eggs in late spring and feed once for 2 or more days in midsummer. Preferred hosts are rodents and other small mammals. The next spring they molt into nymphs, and feed again for 3 or 4 days, with the same host range. Humans usually acquire Lyme disease from infected nymphs. After this second blood meal, the nymphs molt into adults. Adult *I. scapularis* has a narrower host range, with a preference for deer. Mating occurs on deer, and the female deposits her eggs and the cycle begins anew.[9]

In endemic areas, 30% or more of nymphs may be infected with *B. burgdorferi*; the rate of infection in adult ticks may be even higher, but infection rates in unfed larvae are less than 1%.[10] This pattern suggests that ticks acquire *B. burgdorferi* from reservoir hosts rather than transovarial transmission. The white-footed mouse, *Peromyscus leucopus*, is the primary reservoir host for *I. scapularis*.[11] As long as the organism, ticks, mice and deer are all present in the environment, the enzootic cycle will continue.

Variation in vector–host relationships provide the primary explanation for wide regional variation in the incidence of Lyme disease in California,[12] south-east USA[13] and elsewhere in North America. A primary determinant of transmission risk after a known tick bite is the duration of tick attachment before removal.[14,15] A tick attached for less than 24 hours has a low likelihood of transmitting *B. burgdorferi*.

Other modes of transmission have been postulated including transfusion of infected blood products[16] and biting flies,[17,18] but evidence strongly favors ixodid ticks as the primary and, most likely, exclusive vector of Lyme disease. Congenital transmission has been reported,[19,20] but the evidence regarding clinical disease resulting from transplacental transfer is inconclusive.

Borrelia burgdorferi sensu stricto strains likely differ in their host specificity and the degree of human pathogenicity.[9] A specific restriction fragment length polymorphism type of intergenic spacer (IGS) sequence and genotypic variants of the *OspC* gene are associated with hematogenous dissemination in patients with early stage Lyme disease.[20,21] Variations in *OspC* clonal types and risk of invasive disease are found in other pathogenic genospecies such as *B. afzelii* and *B. garinii*.[22,23]

Molecular analysis found a close relationship and overlapping genotypes between the European and North American populations.[24-26] A phylogeographic approach to the population history of Lyme disease

Table 43.1 Lyme disease: a summary of the US National Surveillance Case Definition

Definition	A systemic, tick-borne disease with protean manifestations: dermatologic, rheumatologic, neurologic and cardiac abnormalities. The initial skin lesion, erythema migrans, is the best clinical marker (occurs in 60–80% of patients)
Case definition	1. Erythema migrans present *or* 2. At least one late manifestation and laboratory confirmation of infection
General definitions	
1. Erythema migrans (EM)	• Skin lesion typically beginning as a red macute/papule and expanding over days or weeks to form a large round lesion, often with partial central clearing • A solitary lesion must measure at least 5 cm; secondary lesions may also occur • An annular erythematous lesion developing within several hours of a tick bite represents a hypersensitivity reaction and does not qualify as erythema migrans • The expanding EM lesion is usually accompanied by other acute symptoms, particularly fatigue, fever, headache, mildly stiff neck, arthralgias and myalgias, which are typically intermittent • Diagnosis of EM must be made by a physician • Laboratory confirmation is recommended for patients with no known exposure
2. Late manifestations These include any of the opposite *when an alternative explanation is not found*	Musculoskeletal system • Recurrent, brief attacks (lasting weeks or months) of objective joint swelling in one or a few joints, sometimes followed by chronic arthritis in one or a few joints • Manifestations not considered to be criteria for diagnosis include chronic progressive arthritis not preceded by brief attacks, chronic symmetric polyarthritis, or arthralgias, myalgias or fibromyalgia syndromes alone Nervous system • Lymphocytic meningitis, cranial neuritis, particularly facial palsy (may be bilateral), radiculoneuropathy or, rarely, encephalomyelitis alone or in combination • Encephalomyelitis must be confirmed by evidence of antibody production against *Borrelia burgdorferi* in CSF, shown by a higher titer of antibody in the CSF than in serum • Headache, fatigue, paresthesia or mildly stiff neck alone are not accepted as criteria for neurologic involvement Cardiovascular system • Acute-onset, high-grade (2nd or 3rd degree) atrioventricular conduction defects that resolve in days to weeks and are sometimes associated with myocarditis • Palpitations, bradycardia, bundle-branch block or myocarditis alone are not accepted as criteria for cardiovascular involvement
3. Exposure	• Exposure to wooded, brushy or grassy areas (potential tick habitats) in an endemic county no more than 30 days before the onset of EM • A history of tick bite is not required
4. Endemic county	• A county in which at least two definite cases have been previously acquired or in which a tick vector has been shown to be infected with *B. burgdorferi*
5. Laboratory confirmation	• Isolation of the spirochete from tissue or body fluid *or* • Detection of diagnostic levels of IgM or IgG antibodies to the spirochete in the serum or the CSF *or* • Detection of an important change in antibody levels in paired acute and convalescent serum samples • States may separately determine the criteria for laboratory confirmation and diagnostic levels of antibody • Syphilis and other known biologic causes of false-positive serologic test results should be excluded, when laboratory confirmation is based on serologic testing alone

reveals recent migration events and recombinant genomic types. In fact, a highly pathogenic clone seems to have spread rapidly in recent years to infect a broad range of host species in both continents.[27]

CLINICAL FEATURES

Although the most recognizable feature of Lyme disease is EM, it is a complex systemic illness with protean clinical manifestations. Like syphilis, Lyme borreliosis is a 'great imitator'; its symptoms range from cutaneous to musculoskeletal, cardiac to neurologic. It is interesting to note the differences in manifestations between North American and European disease arising from the endemicity of particular genomospecies in those regions.[5] Species and strain differences induce differing immunologic responses, rendering clinical and serologic diagnosis a formidable challenge.[21] Reported seropositivity depends upon the borrelial strain employed as antigen. Further confounding this diagnostic dilemma is the issue of co-infection with other tick-borne illnesses (i.e. ehrlichiosis, flaviviruses and babesiosis).

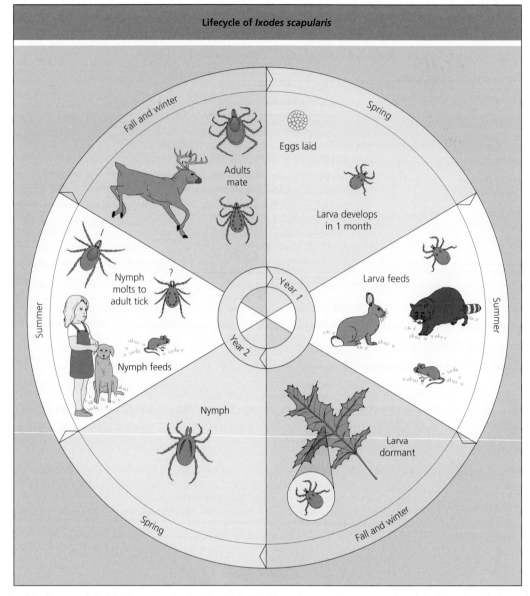

Fig. 43.1 Life cycle of *Ixodes scapularis* (also known as *Ixodes dammini*). The life cycle spans 2 years. Eggs hatch in the spring; six-legged larvae develop and feed once in the summer, acquiring *Borrelia burgdorferi* from their preferred host, the white-footed mouse. Next spring, the larvae molt into eight-legged nymphs, which feed once; mice are the preferred host, humans not being necessary for the ticks' life cycle. The nymphs molt into adult male and female ticks; mating often occurs while the female feeds on a deer, and the male may remain on the deer, the female falling off and then laying eggs. Adapted, with permission, from an illustration by Nancy Lou Makris in Rahn & Malawista.[101]

Lyme disease, human granulocytic ehrlichiosis and babesiosis not only share a common tick vector (*I. scapularis*), but also exhibit overlapping clinical features.[28] Despite these similarities recognition of co-infection is crucial to guide choice of antibiotic therapy.

Localized early disease

Lyme disease begins with EM at the site of a tick bite (Figs 43.3–43.6). In approximately one-third of cases, this skin lesion is missed or absent and patients present with symptoms of flu-like illness or disseminated disease. The interval between tick bite and appearance of EM varies from a few days to a month (median 7 days). The lesion begins as an erythematous papule and expands over several days to achieve a median diameter of 15 cm; favored sites are the groin, buttock, popliteal fossa and axilla. The Centers for Disease Control and Prevention (CDC) has determined 5 cm (in largest diameter) as the minimum diagnostic criterion for EM to distinguish this lesion from other diagnoses.[29] Transient and localized inflammatory reaction at the bite site after tick attachment is common; this resolves spontaneously and is not associated with an infection. Another useful differential point is that EM lesions tend to occur at sites not commonly seen in community-acquired cellulitis such as the axilla, popliteal fossa, back, abdomen and groin. Cellulitis lesions are typically tender to palpation and pruritic while EM lesions can be remarkably asymptomatic, despite their often striking appearance.[30] Although lesion size more than 5 cm is a useful diagnostic criterion, it should not be used to exclude EM when clinical and epidemiologic characteristics are suggestive of Lyme disease as early treatment is correlated with clinical response.[30–32]

The lesions of EM are generally annular with a sharply demarcated outer border and an erythematous or bluish hue. They are warm to the touch, flat and minimally or non-tender. Lesions may show partial central clearing, but can be indurated or even necrotic. This cutaneous lesion is the best clinical marker of Lyme disease, yet an

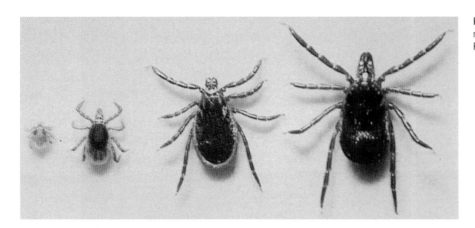

Fig. 43.2 *Ixodes scapularis*. Larva, nymph, adult male and adult female. Courtesy of Pfizer Central Research.

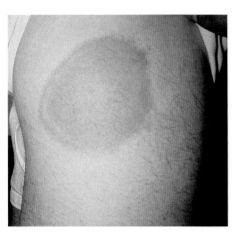

Fig. 43.3 Erythema migrans. A typical annular, flat, erythematous lesion with a sharply demarcated border and partial central healing. Courtesy of Dr Steven Luger, Old Lyme, Connecticut, USA.

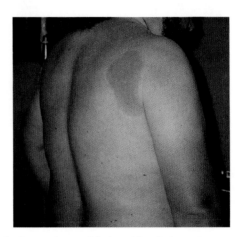

Fig. 43.5 Erythema migrans. A lesion with a dusky center, a common variant. Courtesy of Dr Steven Luger, Old Lyme, Connecticut, USA.

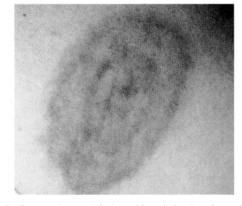

Fig. 43.4 Erythema migrans. A lesion with variation in color and a target-like appearance. The bite site is visible in the center. Courtesy of Dr Steven Luger, Old Lyme, Connecticut, USA.

annular erythematous lesion following a tick bite is not sufficient evidence for a definitive diagnosis of Lyme disease, especially in nonendemic areas.[8]

A lesion that may be mistaken for Lyme disease is known as southern tick-associated rash illness (STARI) which results from a bite of the *Amblyomma americanum* tick (also known as the lone star tick), not known to be able to transmit *B. burgdorferi*.[31] STARI can occur concomitantly with

human monocytic ehrlichiosis (HME) which is transmitted by the same tick vector. *Amblyomma americanum* ticks were originally thought to be restricted to southern states of the USA but have expanded northward over the past 30 years to as far north as Maine.[31,33]

Early disseminated disease

Within several days of the appearance of EM, many patients develop disseminated infection with the appearance of prominent systemic symptoms, the occurrence of multiple secondary skin lesions, or both. Malaise, fatigue, lethargy, headache, fever and chills, arthralgia and myalgia are particularly common, each occurring in one-half or more of patients. Symptoms may fluctuate rapidly and vary from a flu-like syndrome to a meningitis-like illness.

Secondary skin lesions may occur anywhere on the body and resemble primary lesions but are usually smaller, show less expansion with time and lack indurated centers. These manifestations of early disseminated infection appear to be more common in the USA than in Europe and may reflect biologic differences in infecting organisms. Erythema migrans, secondary skin lesions and associated symptoms resolve, even without antibiotic therapy, a median of 28 days after onset. Recurrent crops of evanescent lesions may occur, and fatigue, intermittent musculoskeletal pain and headaches may persist for months.

Late disseminated disease

After resolution of the signs and symptoms of early disease, most untreated patients (>50%) will develop some form of long-term sequelae from Lyme disease.[22] Predominant complications are involvement

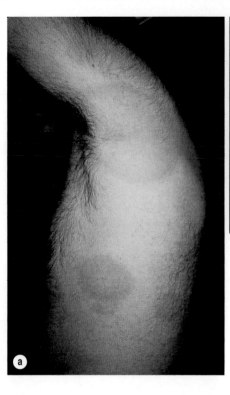

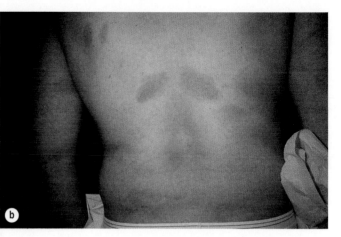

Fig. 43.6 Multiple erythema migrans lesions. Lateral (a) and posterior (b) views of the same patient with multiple erythematous macules of EM. Secondary lesions result from hematogenous spread. They may occur anywhere in the body. Secondary lesions are usually of uniform color and lack induration. Courtesy of Dr Steven Luger, Old Lyme, Connecticut, USA.

of the heart, nervous system and joints, but case reports have described involvement of multiple organs, including the liver,[23] subcutaneous tissue,[24] muscle,[25] eye structures[25] and spleen.[27] More than one organ system can be affected simultaneously or sequentially in an individual patient.

Carditis

Less than 10% of patients with untreated early Lyme disease develop carditis, generally a few weeks to a few months after EM. However, palpitations from an arrhythmia or unexplained syncope from high-degree atrioventricular block may be the presenting manifestation of Lyme disease.[34] The primary clinical manifestation of Lyme carditis is heart block, which may fluctuate from first-degree to complete heart block over minutes to hours and generally resolves spontaneously within a few weeks, even in untreated patients.[35] Although temporary pacing is frequently required, permanent pacing is rarely needed in the treated patient.[34]

Rarely, congestive heart failure has been linked to Lyme disease. A case report suggested that Lyme carditis might be a cause of chronic dilated cardiomyopathy.[36] Endomyocardial biopsy and electrophysiologic testing have revealed direct spirochetal invasion of cardiac muscle and widespread abnormalities of cardiac conduction.[37]

Neurologic manifestations

Frank neurologic abnormalities, including cranial neuropathy (particularly Bell's palsy), meningitis, radiculoneuropathy, myelopathy and encephalopathy occur in about 15% of patients. Neurologic symptoms generally begin a few weeks after EM (median 4 weeks), although some patients can initially present with neurologic manifestations alone.[8,38]

Subtle neurologic complaints without objective deficits (headache, irritability, paresthesias, photophobia and lethargy) may accompany early disease dissemination and represent the mildest end of the spectrum of neurologic Lyme disease. Multiple neurologic abnormalities may coexist or occur sequentially. The most common neurologic complication of Lyme disease is seventh nerve palsy and bilateral involvement may occur.[8] Occurrence of Bell's palsy in young people in the summer months in Lyme-endemic areas is highly suggestive of Lyme disease. Peripheral nerve abnormalities may involve sensory and motor nerve roots, plexi and motor and sensory nerve fibers.[39,40] Meningitis and radiculoneuropathy often wax and wane for weeks to months but ultimately resolve spontaneously.

Borrelia burgdorferi has been isolated from the cerebrospinal fluid (CSF) of a patient whose only complaint was tinnitus,[41] and has been demonstrated by PCR in patients with symptoms limited to headache, Bell's palsy or paresthesias, indicating that the symptoms associated with central nervous system (CNS) infection may be minimal.[42] The emergence of subtle neurologic manifestations years after onset of Lyme disease also supports the possibility of latent persistent infection in the CNS (see Late neurologic syndromes, below). Rarely, cases of demyelinating encephalopathy mimicking multiple sclerosis have been reported.[43,44]

Arthritis

Most people who have untreated Lyme disease develop arthritis. Brief, intermittent attacks of migratory musculoskeletal pain commonly begin early in Lyme disease and may persist for months before the appearance of overt arthritis. Frank arthritis occurs in 60% of patients in the USA, at a median of 6 months after EM, but, as with other symptoms of disseminated disease, arthritis may be among the presenting manifestation of Lyme disease.[45] Although the clinical expression varies, patients most often experience brief recurrent attacks of monoarticular or oligoarticular inflammatory arthritis involving large joints, particularly the knee.[46,47] Effusions may be massive (100 ml or more), causing popliteal cysts, which may rupture and result in a pseudothrombophlebitis syndrome.

Attacks last a few days to a few weeks and over time (months to years) decrease in severity, frequency and duration.[47] Arthritis has been reported to be milder in children than in adults.[48,49] Polyarthritis is decidedly uncommon. Synovitis becomes chronic in 20% of cases (see Chronic arthritis, below).

Late (persistent) disease

After the disseminated stage of Lyme disease, symptoms can vary substantially from self-limited inflammation that resolves spontaneously, only to recur years later and give rise to the chronic manifestations of disease. This has been called 'late Lyme disease'. Late Lyme disease may involve the CNS, the joints and the skin (particularly in Europe). Information is still emerging on this patient group. It is as yet unclear whether the clinical manifestations of late Lyme disease result from persistent sterile inflammation or persistent infection.

Late neurologic syndromes

In Europe, radiculoneuritis is the predominant late neurologic manifestation of B. burgdorferi infections in adults, with more frequent occurrence of meningitis in children.[2] Other reported CNS abnormalities include lymphocytic meningitis, peripheral neuropathy and cranial neuritis, collectively known as Garin–Bujadoux–Bannwarth (MPN–GBB) or Bannwarth's syndrome.[50] Bannwarth's series of 26 patients led to the discovery of the link between these neurologic syndromes and tick bite/EM.[2] Pfister and colleagues found 73% with radicular pain within the dermatomal distribution of the prior arthropod bite or EM.[50]

Both a mild, predominantly sensory, peripheral neuropathy and subtle encephalopathy may occur months to years after the onset of Lyme disease.[51,52] The diagnosis of Lyme encephalopathy hinges on the presence of cognitive deficits involving primarily short-term memory and concentration, and serologic or PCR evidence of antecedent infection with B. burgdorferi. Chronic fatigue, headaches and sleep disturbance frequently accompany these abnormalities and can be very problematic. Rarely, severe encephalomyelopathy has occurred with impairment of higher cortical function, seizures and spinal cord lesions. Chronic neuropathy in patients with ACA has been described. The most common manifestations include peripheral neuropathy with sensory deficits in a patchy distribution.[53]

Despite extensive study, the post-Lyme disease or chronic Lyme disease syndrome remains an enigmatic process. Its pathogenesis is not understood and even its clinical validity as an infectious disease has been questioned. The diagnosis is often based solely on clinical judgment rather than on well-defined clinical criteria. Four randomized placebo-controlled studies[54–57] have been performed, each with different entry criteria and with varying results. The results have varied from some improvement in fatigue and neurocognitive function to others that have shown no effect. In all of these studies, antibiotic therapy offers no sustained benefit to patients who have post-Lyme disease syndrome. These studies also showed a substantial placebo effect and a significant risk of treatment-related adverse events. To complicate our understanding of post-antibiotic Lyme disease, recent animal studies have demonstrated persistent infection in mice treated with a prolonged course of antibiotics.[58,59] Further research to elucidate the mechanisms underlying persistent symptoms after Lyme disease and controlled trials of new approaches to the treatment and management of these patients are needed.

Chronic arthritis

Arthritis becomes chronic in 20% of patients who have untreated Lyme disease, resulting in a syndrome that is clinically indistinguishable from other forms of monoarticular or oligoarticular inflammatory arthritis. Chronic Lyme arthritis is preceded by recurrent brief attacks of joint inflammation. The knee is by far the most commonly affected joint. Immunogenetic factors, particularly human leukocyte antigens (HLA-DR2 and DR4), may predict which people are at highest risk of developing chronic Lyme arthritis.[60] Even chronic Lyme arthritis may eventually remit spontaneously. Only a minority of patients develop radiographic evidence of erosions of cartilage or bone.[61] There have been no unequivocal cases of symmetric, peripheral, polyarticular, inflammatory arthritis with joint destruction resulting from Lyme disease. Differentiation from rheumatoid arthritis is rarely a problem.

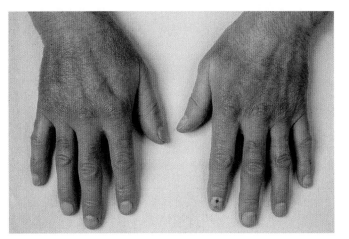

Fig. 43.7 Acrodermatitis chronicum atrophicans. Typical inflammatory bluish-red lesions of acrodermatitis chronicum atrophicans. Lesions usually occur on acral portions of extremities. Courtesy of Dr. Eva Asbrink.

In the diagnosis of persistent Lyme arthritis, culture from synovial fluid has generally been unsuccessful. PCR of synovial fluid has been shown to successfully detect B. burgdorferi DNA with an estimated sensitivity of approximately 80–85%.[62] There is concern that PCR positivity due to dead spirochetes may prevent its use as a means of determining whether infection is persistent, and reports of positive PCR in patients after antibiotic therapy exist.[58,59] However, as most studies have found that PCR is negative in patients receiving more than 1–2 months of antibiotic therapy,[63] B. burgdorferi is likely no longer present in the joints of most patients who have chronic antibiotic-refractory arthritis. Many clinicians now use PCR positivity from synovial fluid as a prerequisite before additional courses of antibiotics are given for persistent arthritis after a standard course of antibiotics.

Chronic skin involvement

Chronic skin involvement (acrodermatitis chronicum atrophicans) as a late manifestation of Lyme disease occurs primarily in Europe.[64] It usually occurs in an acral distribution and is characterized by violaceous discoloration and swelling at a site where EM occurred years earlier. The lesion eventually becomes atrophic (Fig. 43.7). Other clinical manifestations include fibrotic nodules, ulnar bands, sensory disturbances, muscular weakness, myalgias, arthralgias and tenderness on impact over bony prominences. In a study of 50 consecutive patients with ACA in Sweden, elevated antispirochetal antibody titers were found at indirect immunofluorescence and enzyme-linked immunosorbent assay (ELISA), and histologic biopsies demonstrated dermal lymphocytic infiltrates with plasma cells and telangiectasia.[64,65] Acrodermatitis chronicum atrophicans is thought to result from local persistence of B. burgdorferi, which has been isolated from a lesion 10 years after onset.[65] Lichen sclerosis et atrophicus or morphea-like lesions have also been described.

DIAGNOSTIC INVESTIGATIONS

Lyme disease is a diagnostic challenge by the clinician and the laboratory alike. The clinical presentation is highly variable with a myriad of possible outcomes depending on host factors and pathogen characteristics. Currently available diagnostic assays are not always precise and are subject to bias in their interpretation. The National Surveillance Case Definition of Lyme disease developed in the USA (see Table 43.1) requires either the presence of EM or a definite late manifestation of Lyme disease combined with laboratory confirmation of infection in a person who has had opportunity to be exposed to the causative agent. Definitive laboratory confirmation requires isolation of the causative organism from clinically involved tissue, but this is rarely achievable in clinical practice. Demonstration of specific serologic immune responsiveness against *B. burgdorferi* has been accepted as a substitute for bacteriologic isolation. Unfortunately the sensitivity and specificity of many tests has been poor.[66–68] For 75% of patients, a serum sample obtained 2 weeks after the initial sample will be positive, but prompt antibiotic treatment may prevent seroconversion.

Western blot confirmation of all positive and equivocal screening results is recommended.[69] The predictive value of laboratory tests used for the diagnosis of Lyme disease improves dramatically when used in patients with characteristic clinical features of the illness. Laboratory testing should only be used for confirmation; it should not be used for screening asymptomatic patients.

Detection of a specific immune response to *B. burgdorferi* remains the best means of confirming the diagnosis of Lyme disease. The first immune response in Lyme disease is mediated by T cells and is directed against a variety of epitopes.[70,71] This T-cell response subsequently localizes preferentially to involved tissues.[70,72] Unfortunately, tests to measure this response are not standardized, are technically demanding, require live cells and have varied in sensitivity and specificity.[73] For these reasons, measurement of the T-cell response cannot be recommended routinely for diagnosis.

The serologic response to *B. burgdorferi* has been well characterized (Fig. 43.8).[74] Specific IgM antibody, directed initially primarily against the flagellae of the organism, is detectable a few weeks after disease onset. The response broadens to include additional antigens over time and peaks by 3–6 weeks. Generally IgM antibody falls to within the normal range by 6 months, but occasionally it may remain elevated for much longer. Specific IgG antibody is detectable a few weeks after IgM and is directed against the same antigen, but IgG antibodies may not peak until many months after disease onset.

Both immunofluorescence assay (IFA) and ELISA have been used to detect this antibody response; in general, ELISA is preferable because of better sensitivity, objectivity and reproducibility, and because of its adaptability to automated systems. Regrettably, serologies for Lyme disease may be falsely positive or negative for various reasons.

Both IFA and ELISA may yield false-positive results because of epitopes in the test antigen preparations that cross-react with other bacteria.[68] False-positive results may also occur in conditions associated with polyclonal B-cell activation. Specificity is increased by a two-step approach in which all positive or equivocal results are confirmed by Western immunoblotting. This two-step approach was recommended by participants in a national conference on serologic diagnosis of Lyme disease held in 1994 under the sponsorship of the CDC.[69] A true positive ELISA is associated with immunoreactivity against

Table 43.2 Western blot criteria. Centers for Disease Control and Prevention Working Group recommendations for Western blot positivity

- All serum specimens found to be positive or equivocal by a sensitive enzyme immunoassay or immunofluorescent assay should be tested by a standardized Western blot procedure
- When Western immunoblot is used in the first 4 weeks of illness, both IgM and IgG procedures should be performed
- After the first 4 weeks of illness, IgG alone should be performed
- An IgM blot is considered positive if two of the following three bands are present: 24 kDa (OspC), 39 kDa (BmpA) and 41 kDa (Fla)
- An IgG blot is considered positive if five of the following 10 bands are present: 18, 21 (OspC), 28, 30, 39 (BmpA), 41 (Fla), 45, 58, 66 and 93 kDa

Recommendations of the Second National Conference on Serologic Diagnosis of Lyme Disease sponsored by the Centers for Disease Control and Prevention, the Association of State and Territorial Public Health Laboratory Directors and the Michigan Department of Health.

Osp, outer surface protein; Fla, flagella.

polypeptides specific for *B. burgdorferi*, reactivity that is absent in the various conditions associated with false-positive ELISA results. The currently recommended criteria for a positive Western blot are given in Table 43.2.

One special circumstance deserves mention. Antibiotic therapy administered early in the course of Lyme disease may result in a negative serology by curing the infection and eliminating antigen before systemic immune challenge.[68] One series indicated, however, that infection may persist after early antibiotic therapy despite persistently negative serologies.[71]

In a study of 17 patients with acute Lyme disease who received prompt treatment with oral antibiotics and subsequently developed 'chronic' illness, it was shown that none of them had diagnostic levels of antibodies to *B. burgdorferi* on either a standard ELISA or IFA.[71] On Western blot analysis, the level of immunoglobulin reactivity against *B. burgdorferi* was no greater than that of normal controls. These patients had a vigorous T-cell proliferative response to whole *B. burgdorferi* at levels similar to that of 18 patients with chronic Lyme disease with detectable antibodies. The T-cell response of both groups was greater than that of a control group. The investigators concluded that the presence of chronic Lyme disease cannot be excluded by the absence of antibodies against *B. burgdorferi* and that a specific T-cell response to *B. burgdorferi* is evidence of infection in seronegative patients with suggestive clinical parameters.[71]

This apparent dissociation between T- and B-cell immune responses may be attributed to the administration of antibiotics for EM and, therefore, the presence of low or undetectable levels of anti-*Borrelia* antibodies. Antibiotic therapy may have resulted in the elimination of most spirochetes at a critical early stage of the immune response, thereby hindering the development of a sustained B-cell response.[71] Persistent disease activity may result from harboring of *B. burgdorferi* in sites such as the CNS, which may not receive adequate concentrations of antibiotics to reach the minimum inhibitory concentrations (MICs) required against the majority of strains of *B. burgdorferi*. In support of this observation is the discovery of local production of anti-*Borrelia* antibody in the CNS in those suffering from neurologic symptoms of Lyme borreliosis in the absence of diagnostic serum antibodies levels.[75,76]

The concept of antigenic variation displayed by other borrelial species may represent an alternative explanation for the apparent absence of a specific antibody response in seronegative Lyme disease.[77] Classically, immunodominant 'variable major proteins' are replaced periodically by variant forms, enabling the organism to elude the host's antibody. Although *B. burgdorferi* does not precisely exhibit marked antigenic variation, antigenic diversity has been noted among strains found in humans, animals and ticks.[77]

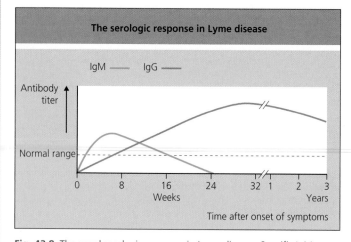

Fig. 43.8 The usual serologic response in Lyme disease. Specific IgM becomes detectable 1–2 weeks after symptom onset and the appearance of erythema migrans. The later appearance of IgG is frequently concurrent with systemic manifestations. IgG is nearly always elevated with late disease. Typically, and even in untreated patients, IgM falls over 4–6 months; persistence for longer than this predicts later manifestations.

Other laboratory findings

Lyme meningitis is characterized by lymphocytic pleocytosis (<300wbc) with elevated protein and usually normal CSF glucose (although hypoglycorrhachia is found on occasion). In protracted cases the IgG:albumin ratio can be found with oligoclonal banding of CSF proteins.[43,44]

Attacks of arthritis are accompanied by an inflammatory joint fluid containing a few hundred to 50 000 white blood cells, mostly polymorphonuclear, elevation in protein and normal glucose.[45] Radiographs of affected joints most often show only soft tissue swelling, but when joint inflammation has persisted for many months, there may be pannus formation and erosions of underlying cartilage and bone.[47] Some patients develop enthesopathy with calcifications of tendon and ligament attachment sites.

Cognitive deficits associated with late neurologic involvement may be quantified by neuropsychologic testing, a very helpful modality in the formal assessment of cognitive complaints.[51,52] A depressive overlay is often present, but findings should also reveal an organic encephalopathy primarily affecting short-term memory. Peripheral neuropathy and radiculoneuropathy cause abnormalities on electromyography and, less often, abnormalities of peripheral nerve conduction;[52] sensory fibers are more frequently affected than motor fibers. Although these findings on tests of CNS and peripheral nervous system function are not specific for Lyme disease, abnormal findings indicate a definite disorder of the nervous system, and the combination of central and peripheral nerve abnormalities characteristic of Lyme disease is uncommon in other diseases.

Specific laboratory confirmation of *B. burgdorferi* infection is possible with culture of affected tissue, or by PCR on skin, urine, joint fluid, blood or CSF. Although the causative organism has been cultured from a variety of affected tissues[78] and joint fluid,[79] this technique is not readily available in routine clinical laboratories. The PCR assay is a valuable adjunctive study[80,81] but is not considered a routine diagnostic test for Lyme disease.

Despite all the problems with diagnostic assays, most patients, even those with longstanding symptoms, can be adequately managed and effectively treated. At present, the diagnosis of chronic Lyme disease is loosely applied to a constellation of symptoms including fatigue, arthralgias, aches, pains, memory disturbances and impairment in concentration. Referring to these patients as having chronic Lyme disease when there is no clinical or laboratory evidence of *B. burgdorferi* infection is misleading and does a disservice to the patients and other physicians alike. Confusion over this designation has created misunderstanding and promotes phobias regarding the stigma of 'chronic' or lifelong disease.

An accurate diagnosis is usually readily achievable by a careful history of exposure and a history of EM with suggestive clinical features. Serologic assays interpreted under these circumstances remain the best screening methods for exposure followed by confirmation with immunoblotting techniques. A lack of response to antibiotic therapy in presumed Lyme disease is most likely due to incorrect diagnosis, thereby warranting a continued search for the cause of illness.[82,83]

Measurement of immunoreactivity in CSF is a useful adjunct in the diagnosis of CNS Lyme disease.[84] To have diagnostic value, a CSF index should be calculated comparing the ratios of specific antibody to total immunoglobulin in CSF and serum. A specific antibody response in CSF is not always detectable with CSF Lyme disease, but is helpful when positive.

DIAGNIOSTIC PITFALLS IN THE DIFFERENTIAL DIAGNOSIS

Erythema migrans is the classic skin lesion of Lyme disease and, in its typical appearance, can be confused with little else. However, atypical presentations may lead to confusion[85] and caution must be exercised when making this diagnosis in nonendemic areas.[86,87]

In later stages, Lyme disease may mimic a variety of cardiac, neurologic and arthritic disorders. Carditis can be confused with subacute bacterial endocarditis or acute rheumatic fever, but valvular lesions do not occur in Lyme disease. Blood cultures are negative.[88]

Bell's palsy caused by Lyme disease is indistinguishable from idiopathic Bell's palsy, but Lyme disease is one of very few causes of bilateral Bell's palsy (a helpful clue if present) and, by this stage of disease, patients are typically seropositive. Lyme meningitis presents a clinical picture similar to that of viral meningitis, but there is often an antecedent history of EM, the course is more protracted and Lyme meningitis is characterized by relapses and remissions. The peripheral neuropathy associated with the late neurologic manifestations of Lyme disease mimics other sensory neuropathies; however, a history of previous non-neurologic involvement is usually present and serologies can be helpful in the differential diagnosis. The rare patients who have demyelinating encephalopathy must be distinguished from patients who have multiple sclerosis; positive serology (particularly if present in CSF) or CSF PCR, combined with an exposure history, is very helpful in this circumstance.[88]

The typical patient with Lyme arthritis who has monoarticular inflammatory arthritis of a knee can be confused with reactive arthritis, crystal-induced arthritis or septic arthritis. At initial presentation, bacterial infection must always be excluded. The pattern of brief, recurrent attacks is more common in Lyme disease than other common forms of acute arthritis. Furthermore, patients who have Lyme arthritis are virtually always seropositive.

It is particularly important to differentiate fibromyalgia from 'chronic' Lyme disease because the prognosis and response to therapy are quite different.[83,88]

PATHOGENESIS AND PATHOLOGY

Borrelia burgdorferi has been unequivocally established as being the cause of Lyme disease. Clinical isolates differ in their outer surface protein expression[89] and genetic composition.[90] All three genospecies – *B. burgdorferi*, *B. garinii* and *B. afzelii* – have been isolated from patients who have Lyme disease and it is likely that disease expression in humans may vary depending upon the genospecies.[91]

Unlike *Treponema pallidum*, *B. burgdorferi* can be grown in culture although a specialized medium is required. Serial passage in culture alters surface protein expression with loss of pathogenicity in mice,[92] but the specific factors conferring pathogenicity have not yet been identified. *Borrelia burgdorferi* can penetrate endothelial monolayers and survive intracellularly in cultured fibroblasts.[93] Work is in progress to understand the mechanisms by which this organism can cause persistent infection despite a vigorous immune response.

The organism may evade eradication through an initially delayed and ineffective immune response. It disseminates preferentially to certain target organs where it engenders an immunologically mediated host response, with tissue injury occurring as a result of the inflammatory response. Why this lesion becomes persistent in some people and whether live organisms persist in all cases of chronic disease remain to be elucidated. An important question is how *B. burgdorferi* avoids destruction in the presence of the vigorous specific T- and B-cell responses that are usually apparent within a few weeks of onset of disease. In humans, the early immune response is directed primarily against a flagellar antigen. Vaccine studies in mice have shown that specific antibodies against this antigen do not protect against subsequent infection. Vaccination with outer surface protein (Osp) A, an immunodominant surface antigen to which antibodies appear much later in human disease, is protective.[94] It may be that, in human Lyme disease, *B. burgdorferi* is able to establish infection because of an ineffective initial immune response focused primarily against flagellae. Later, when the immune response broadens, infection may already be established and disease may be perpetuated through other mechanisms such as survival in sequestered, intracellular sites.[95]

HLA-DR4 predisposes to the development of persistent Lyme arthritis and DR4 is associated with a lack of response to antibiotics.[60] Patients who are HLA-DR4 positive and who have treatment-resistant Lyme arthritis have also been shown to have a strong immune response to an epitope on OspA that cross-reacts with human lymphocyte function antigen 1 (LFA-1), which may serve as an autoantigen.[96] This evidence suggests a possible autoimmune mechanism for chronic Lyme arthritis through a mechanism involving molecular mimicry between OspA and LFA-1 in HLA-DR4-positive individuals. No predictors of chronic neurologic disease have been described as yet. Histologic studies of affected tissues have provided evidence for immunologically mediated inflammation. Stains of EM lesions reveal a perivascular mononuclear infiltrate and fibrin deposition in the dermis, without epidermal changes except at the site of the bite.[8] Endomyocardial biopsies have revealed similar changes in the heart, with a focal perivascular infiltrate of mononuclear cells and fibrin deposition in both the endocardium and myocardium.[36] Biopsies of affected nerves show inflammatory infiltrates around endoneurial and perineurial vessels without vessel necrosis.[97] Both myelinated and unmyelinated fibers may be affected. Synovial biopsies from involved joints have revealed synovial lining cell hyperplasia and hypertrophy, vascular proliferation and lymphocytic infiltration of the subsynovial areas. The intensity of the infiltrate varies, and fibrin deposition may be pronounced. Aggregates of T and B cells, often with lymphoid follicle formation, are common and may be concentrated in perivascular areas with obliteration of vessels but without vessel necrosis.[47] Levels of interleukin (IL)-1,[98] prostaglandin E_2 and collagenase[99] in joint fluid are elevated, similar to the situation in rheumatoid arthritis. Spirochetes have been visualized in skin lesions,[63] heart tissue[36] and synovium,[95] but not in peripheral nerves, where it has been postulated that an autoimmune mechanism accounts for the inflammatory lesions.[100]

MANAGEMENT

The primary goals of therapy for Lyme disease are the control of inflammation and the eradication of the infection. Lyme disease is most responsive to antibiotic therapy early in the course of the disease. As with syphilis, some later disease manifestations do not seem to improve after administration of antibiotics.

Treatment regimens are based in part on data from controlled clinical trials and in part on clinical experience.[101] *In-vitro* antibiotic sensitivity testing does not reliably predict clinical response. Loose criteria for diagnosis accepted without critical review have led to widespread antibiotic use for presumptive Lyme disease in patients who almost certainly have other explanations for their symptoms. In one report, the leading reason for failure to respond to antibiotic therapy for Lyme disease was incorrect diagnosis.[102] In addition, the appropriate end point of antibiotic therapy is often not clear because of the difficulty of proving when the infection has been eradicated and because of the common persistence of symptoms long after treatment. Current treatment recommendations (Table 43.3) represent a distillation of available evidence and will no doubt be refined in time.[83]

Early localized or early disseminated disease

If antibiotic therapy is initiated early in the course of Lyme disease, EM typically resolves promptly and later stage disease is prevented.[83,103] Early localized infection, limited to a single skin lesion, with mild or no systemic symptoms, is uniformly responsive to short-course oral antibiotic therapy with a number of agents. Of the antibiotics studied to date, amoxicillin (500 mg q8h), doxycycline (100 mg q12h) and cefuroxime axetil (500 mg q12h) have been the most effective for this stage of disease.[104,105] Although the optimal duration of therapy is unknown, most clinicians currently recommend 2–3 weeks for both early localized and early disseminated disease.

The appearance of systemic symptoms (fever, arthralgias, fatigue) and secondary skin lesions reflects dissemination of the organism beyond the site of inoculation. As long as no neurologic symptoms are present, 3 weeks of oral therapy is sufficient for this group of patients. In a carefully performed prospective study, 10% of patients with a single EM lesion and no systemic symptoms had a positive PCR on blood. This was interpreted as demonstrating that clinically silent bloodstream invasion may be relatively common early in the course of infection.[80]

Some experts have recommended the addition of probenecid to amoxicillin, but this combination has been associated with a relatively high frequency of rashes and is not known to be superior to amoxicillin alone. The pediatric dose range of amoxicillin is 30–40 mg/kg per day in three divided doses. Herxheimer-like reactions, with intensification of fever and arthralgias, may occur shortly after initiation of therapy. If possible, doxycycline should be avoided in children under the age of 9 years and during pregnancy because of the possibility of staining of the teeth. Tetracyclines must be used with caution during summer in all patients because they may predispose the patient to sun-sensitive rashes or severe sunburn. Penicillin-allergic young children can be treated with cefuroxime or erythromycin, but results with macrolide antibiotics have been less satisfactory than those with penicillin, amoxicillin or tetracyclines.[83] Azithromycin has been studied systematically and found to be less effective than amoxicillin.[105]

Regardless of which agent is chosen, some patients experience a delayed resolution of systemic symptoms (headache, musculoskeletal pain, fatigue) which may persist as long as 3 months after completion of therapy. These symptoms usually resolve spontaneously and do not indicate continued infection requiring further antibiotic therapy.[103] A seemingly self-perpetuating fibromyalgia syndrome may develop in response to Lyme disease; this too is unresponsive to antibiotic therapy.[106] The likelihood of delayed resolution of symptoms is greatest in patients who have prominent systemic symptoms or a delay in diagnosis before institution of antibiotics.[83]

Disseminated disease

With the possible exception of arthritis, which usually responds to oral therapy, disseminated infection with target organ involvement should generally be treated with intravenous antibiotics. Carditis, meningitis, cranial neuropathy, radiculoneuropathy and arthritis are discussed separately.

Carditis

Although carditis resolves spontaneously, observational data suggest that resolution of heart block may be hastened by treatment with salicylates, corticosteroids, oral penicillin, oral tetracyclines and intravenous ceftriaxone and penicillin.[37,83] This response to either anti-inflammatory therapy or antibiotics suggests that the proximate cause of the heart block is the inflammatory reaction engendered by the Lyme spirochete rather than direct tissue destruction resulting from the infection. Control of the inflammatory response leads to resolution of clinical manifestations.

Heart block caused by carditis may progress suddenly, necessitating a temporary pacemaker, but permanent pacing is rarely necessary. Hospitalization with cardiac monitoring is prudent while antibiotic therapy is instituted. Although no comparative trials have been conducted, treatment with intravenous penicillin or a third-generation cephalosporin for a minimum of 2 weeks to eradicate systemic spirochetal infection is recommended. Salicylates or nonsteroidal anti-inflammatory agents may hasten symptom resolution. Systemic corticosteroids may be dramatically effective in reversing heart block, but they are rarely needed during antibiotic therapy for Lyme carditis.[83]

Table 43.3 Suggested antibiotic regimens for Lyme disease

Early disease	• Doxycycline, 100 mg po, q12h for 21 days, or • Amoxicillin (with or without probenecid) 500 mg, q8h for 21 days, or • Erythromycin, 250–500 mg po, q6h for 21 days, or • Azithromycin 500 mg daily for 7 days, or • Cefuroxime axetil, 500 mg po, q12h for 21 days Shorter courses (14 days) may suffice for localized early disease. Erythromycin and azithromycin less effective than other choices
Lyme arthritis	Initial treatment: • Doxycycline, 100 mg po, q12h for 30 days, or • Amoxicillin and probenecid, 500 mg each po, q6h for 30 days If initial treatment fails: • Penicillin G, 20 × 10⁶ IU iv, daily in divided doses for 14 days, or • Ceftriaxone sodium, 2 g iv, daily for 14 days
Neurologic manifestations	For facial nerve paralysis alone: • Doxycycline, 100 mg po, q12h for 21–30 days, or • Amoxicillin, 500 mg po, q8h for 21–30 days
Additional signs (e.g. Lyme meningitis, radiculopathy, encephalitis)	• Ceftriaxone, 2 g iv, daily for 30 days, or • Penicillin G, 20 × 10⁶ IU iv, daily in divided doses for 30 days Possible alternatives: • Cefotaxime sodium, 2 g iv, q8h for 30 days, or • Doxycycline, 100 mg po, q12h for 14–30 days, or • Chloramphenicol, 1 g iv, q6h for 14–30 days
Lyme carditis	• Ceftriaxone, 2 g iv, daily for 14 days, or • Penicillin G, 20 × 10⁶ IU iv, daily in divided doses for 14 days Possible alternatives: • Doxycycline, 100 mg po, q12h for 21 days, or • Amoxicillin, 500 mg po, q8h for 21 days
During pregnancy	Localized, early disease: • Amoxicillin, 500 mg po, q8h for 21 days Other manifestations: • Penicillin G, 20 × 10⁶ IU iv, daily in divided doses for 14–30 days, or • Ceftriaxone, 2 g, daily for 14–30 days

Neurologic manifestations

Data on the treatment of neurologic manifestations are derived primarily from clinical experience. The tendency for spontaneous resolution of Bell's palsy, the fluctuating course of meningitis, the clinical variation of neurologic syndromes and the delayed emergence of the subtle deficits associated with late neurologic Lyme disease must all be considered in evaluating the clinical response to antibiotic therapy.[38,50,104] The emergence of chronic neurologic impairment years after remission of acute neurologic symptoms highlights the danger of complacency about the potential consequences of incomplete eradication of CNS infection.

Bell's palsy

Historically, Lyme-associated facial palsy has been treated with oral antibiotics, whereas other neurologic syndromes have been treated intravenously. It is unclear whether this distinction is warranted. Facial palsy itself resolves completely or almost completely in nearly all patients (121 of 122 patients in one series).[107] Patients who have facial palsy should undergo a careful neurologic evaluation, including a CSF examination. Cerebrospinal fluid invasion has been demonstrated by PCR in patients who have minimal CNS complaints and facial palsy, most of whom have clinically silent CSF pleocytosis.[40] If facial palsy is the only clinical abnormality and CSF is normal, current practice is to administer oral antibiotics for 21–30 days, a practice that has resulted in favorable outcomes. Long-term follow-up of this group is impor-

tant and, if CSF examination is not possible, the preferred course at present is to administer intravenous antibiotics.

Meningitis

Intravenous penicillin for 10 days has been shown in clinical trials to be effective treatment of meningitis. In one small series, intravenous ceftriaxone for 14 days was superior to a 10-day course of penicillin.[108] Most experts prefer a 30-day course of treatment, however, because of the occasional occurrence of late neurologic relapses after shorter courses of therapy. It is not necessary to document clearing of all CSF abnormalities before discontinuation of therapy because clearing of inflammation may lag behind bacteriologic cure.[83] The co-occurrence of encephalopathy or encephalomyelopathy does not change this approach.

Radiculoneuropathy

Radiculoneuropathy is less clearly responsive to antibiotic therapy. Intravenous penicillin has not been shown to hasten resolution, and the response to ceftriaxone is unpredictable.[40,41] Current practice, however, is to administer intravenous antibiotic therapy based on favorable long-term outcome with this approach and the belief that radiculoneuropathy is driven by systemic infection. Resolution of neuropathy may be very gradual (taking place over months) and, with chronic involvement, this response may be incomplete. Doxycycline has been used orally and intravenously as an alternative to ceftriaxone or penicillin, but experience with this agent is limited.[109] One patient who had severe neurologic involvement, unresponsive to penicillin, responded favorably to chloramphenicol.[110]

Arthritis

Arthritis may respond to either oral[111] or parenteral[112] antibiotic therapy, but antibiotic failures occur with either approach. Amoxicillin plus probenecid given orally for 4 weeks cures the majority of patients and those who fail oral therapy do not appear to respond to intravenous therapy. In a carefully carried out PCR study, no joint fluids were PCR positive in patients who had received at least 8 weeks of antibiotic therapy. The optimal duration of therapy is unknown but an initial course for 4 weeks is recommended.

The role for parenteral therapy for Lyme arthritis is unclear. Patients who have concurrent neurologic involvement should receive intravenous treatment. In one randomized study, intramuscular benzathine penicillin given weekly for 3 weeks cured less than one-half of patients, but intravenous penicillin for 10 days cured a higher percentage.[112] Ceftriaxone given for 14 days has been found to be more effective than 10 days of penicillin.[83] The primary reason for selection of intravenous therapy is concurrent neurologic involvement, in which case ceftriaxone or cefotaxime for 2–4 weeks are probably the agents of choice.

Resolution is commonly delayed, with synovitis persisting for months after completion of antibiotic therapy before eventually resolving. It has been suspected that administration of intra-articular corticosteroids during or before antibiotic therapy increases the risk of antibiotic failure, but a single intra-articular injection after completion of antibiotic therapy may hasten resolution. Patients who do not respond to a first course of therapy may respond to a repeat course, but there is no known rationale for a course of longer than 8 weeks. Adjunctive treatment measures should include evacuation of large effusions and limitation of weightbearing during acute attacks. Chronic inflammatory arthritis may occur through an autoimmune mechanism rather than as a result of persistent infection.

Late Lyme disease

Late Lyme disease, a designation reserved for those patients who have symptoms that persist for longer than 1 year, generally involves persistent inflammation in the CNS, joints or skin (ACA). Generally, patients who have ACA respond to oral penicillin. Late neurologic and arthritic involvement, however, are less predictably responsive. In one report, only one-half of patients who had late neurologic symptoms showed either resolution or sustained improvement after 6 months of follow-up after a 2-week course of ceftriaxone.[52] Those who did not respond, however, did not show progressive worsening. Long-term follow-up of this patient group is essential. In a European trial ceftriaxone and penicillin for 2 weeks were both effective for late neurologic involvement.[113]

Persistent arthritis after antibiotic therapy occurs most often in people who have HLA-DR4.[60] They are usually PCR negative and may be treated satisfactorily with arthroscopic synovectomy after failing to respond to either oral or intravenous antibiotics, suggesting that the pathogenesis of antibiotic-resistant arthritis may involve mechanisms other than persistent infection.[114] A recent study has provided strong evidence of an autoimmune mechanism for chronic Lyme arthritis.[96] Comparative trials of different antibiotics and varying durations of therapy are currently in progress for the treatment of late manifestations of Lyme disease, but there are no controlled data involving treatment periods longer than 4 weeks.

Pregnancy

Lyme disease acquired during pregnancy represents a special category because the health of the fetus must also be considered. Case reports have provided convincing evidence that *B. burgdorferi* can cross the placenta. Stillbirth[115,116] and neonatal death[19,20] have been attributed to *B. burgdorferi* transmitted from mother to fetus in utero, but the evidence to support this conclusion is still incomplete. The vast majority of pregnancies complicated by maternal Lyme disease have normal outcomes. *Borrelia burgdorferi* has not been linked statistically to congenital anomalies,[103] and no increased risk of an adverse outcome of pregnancy has been associated with asymptomatic seropositivity[117] or history of previous Lyme disease. It is appropriate to maintain a lower threshold for institution of aggressive antibiotic therapy for suspected Lyme disease during pregnancy, but women should be reassured that no cases of fetal Lyme disease have occurred with currently recommended antibiotic regimens. Doxycycline and other tetracyclines should be avoided during pregnancy.

Previous controlled clinical trials indicate that antibiotic therapy offers no sustained benefit to patients who have post-Lyme disease syndrome. Further research to elucidate the mechanisms underlying persistent symptoms after Lyme disease and controlled trials of new approaches to the treatment and management of these patients are needed.[115,118]

PREVENTION

If possible, it is preferable to prevent Lyme disease by personal protection and avoidance of prolonged tick attachment if a tick bite occurs. One obvious issue with regard to prevention is whether an individual with a known ixodid tick bite in a Lyme disease endemic area should be treated prophylactically with antibiotics. This question has been studied in a Lyme disease endemic area in Connecticut. A randomized, double-blind trial of amoxicillin therapy for tick bites[15] showed that, although the tick infection rate approached 15%, the risk of Lyme disease in untreated people was so low – 1.2% (95% CI 0.1–4.1%) – that prophylactic therapy (although probably effective) was not warranted. In a recent survey of pediatricians in an endemic area, 26% (70/267) routinely administered prophylactic antibiotics after tick bites.[119]

Nadelman *et al.*[120] advocated a single dose of oral doxycycline (200 mg) within 72 hours after removal of an *I. scapularis* tick. They found this to significantly reduce the incidence of Lyme disease (1/235 in the doxycycline group vs 8/247 in the placebo group). Many clinicians argue that this practice is unwarranted and may promote the development of antibiotic resistance.[121,122] Prophylactic antibiotics may be cost-effective in endemic regions if the risk of transmission following tick bites is greater than 0.01.[122] Personal protection including protective clothing measures such as wearing light-colored clothing to provide a background that contrasts with the ticks is often recommended.[83] The use of insect repellent containing N,N-diethyl-M-toluamide (DEET) and the prompt removal of ticks reduce the risk of Lyme disease.

Another area of active research involves efforts to develop a Lyme disease vaccine. A recombinant vaccine based on OspA, Lymerix, was approved for use in the past but was subsequently withdrawn from the market.[123] Efficacy was reported to be 79%[124] after three doses. New recombinant-based vaccines currently under development are expected to have a broad range of specificity against the variants of *B. burgdorferi* distributed throughout the world.[125,126]

REFERENCES

References for this chapter can be found online at http://www.expertconsult.com

Postoperative infections in a patient with a prosthetic joint

INTRODUCTION

The major clinical issues involved in caring for an infected patient with an indwelling joint prosthesis are difficulties encountered in establishing the anatomic extent of involvement (i.e. is the prosthetic joint involved in the infection?), difficulties in selecting an appropriate therapeutic option once prosthetic joint infection has been diagnosed and difficulties in confirming the adequacy of the therapeutic approach chosen. Many of these clinical problems can be resolved by employing both evidenced-based judgments and clinical observations to select an appropriate option to satisfy the patient's orthopedic and infectious disease needs.

EXTRA-ARTICULAR INFECTIONS (AFTER IMPLANTATION OF A JOINT PROSTHESIS)

Postoperative suprafascial wound infections (such as suture abscesses, cellulitis and infected extra-articular hematomas) should be treated promptly by debridement (if needed) and antibiotic therapy, often intravenously, at least in part, for up to 2 weeks.

Urinary tract infections and pneumonia should also be treated promptly and for durations appropriate for the rapidity of the patient's clinical response. If the patient has blood culture evidence of bacteremia, then a course of intravenous antibiotic therapy for a minimum of 2 weeks should be administered. If the patient appears to have had a bacteremia (such as the presence of true rigors with fever or the presence of an intravenous site infection), this should be treated with at least a 2-week course of intravenous antibiotics.

PROSTHETIC JOINT INFECTIONS

Diagnosis

Prosthetic joint infection produces the cardinal symptoms of inflammation with a wide spectrum of severity. The frequencies of these presenting symptoms are listed in Table PP20.1. If a painful prosthesis is accompanied by a fever or purulent drainage from overlying cutaneous sinuses, infection may be presumed, pending further confirmatory tests. However, in most cases, infection must be differentiated from aseptic and mechanical problems (such as hemarthrosis, gout, bland loosening, dislocation, metallic debris-induced synovitis, osteolysis) which are more common causes of pain and inflammatory symptoms in these patients. Joint pain is nearly universally present. Constant joint pain is suggestive of infection, whereas mechanical loosening commonly causes pain only with motion and weight-bearing.

Table PP20.1 Presenting symptoms of prosthetic joint infection	
Symptom	**Frequency (%)**
Joint pain	95
Fever	43
Periarticular swelling	38
Wound or cutaneous sinus drainage	32

Radiologic abnormalities are found in 50% of septic prostheses. They are generally related to the duration of infection because it may take 3–6 months for such changes to appear. If both distal and proximal components of a prosthetic joint demonstrate radiographic pathology, sepsis is more likely than simple mechanical loosening. However, all of these radiographic changes are nonspecific for infection as they are also seen frequently with aseptic processes.

Abnormal uptakes on radioisotopic scans (technetium bone scan, sequential technetium–gallium bone scanning, indium-labeled leukocyte scanning) are also too nonspecific or too variably sensitive to be able to carry the burden of establishing the diagnosis of prosthetic joint infection. Increased technetium diphosphonate uptake on bone scans is seen routinely around normal prostheses for 6 months after arthroplasty. A normal or negative technetium scan can be considered evidence against the presence of infection, but a positive radioisotopic scan, of any type, is not definitive in establishing the diagnosis of arthroplasty infection. Elevated peripheral or joint space leukocyte counts, erythrocyte sedimentation rates and C-reactive protein levels, although suggestive, also are inadequate to diagnose prosthetic joint sepsis.

The single observation that delineates the presence of implant infection is isolation of the pathogen by aspiration of joint fluid or by surgical debridement. Arthrocentesis demonstrates the pathogen with a sensitivity of 86–92% and a specificity of 82–97% in the larger surveys. Gram staining is positive in only 32% of cases. Fluoroscopic guidance and arthrography are useful to document accurate needle placement for prosthetic joint aspiration. If difficulty is encountered in obtaining intra-articular fluid, irrigation with sterile normal saline solution, without antiseptic preservative additives, can be used to provide the necessary fluid for culture. Since fastidious micro-organisms, including anaerobes, may be causative agents in prosthetic arthroplasty infections, multiple specimens should be obtained and rapidly cultured in appropriately supportive media. If initial cultures reveal a relatively avirulent organism (such as coagulase-negative staphylococci, corynebacteria, propionibacteria or *Bacillus* species), a second aspirate should be considered to re-confirm the bacteriologic diagnosis and to substantially reduce the possibility that the isolate is artifactual.

Table PP20.2 Diagnostic value of the number of positive operative cultures (for the same organism) when three to six specimens are examined

Number positive	Probability of infection (%)
3 or more	94.8
2	20.4
1	13.3
0	3.4

From Atkins BL, Athanasou N, Deeks JJ, et al. Prospective evaluation of criteria for microbiologic diagnosis of prosthetic joint infection at revision arthroplasty. J Clin Microbiol 1998;36:2932–9.

As operative debridement cultures are also used to definitively diagnose prosthetic joint infection, the patient should not receive antimicrobial therapy for several weeks prior to surgery and no antibiotic therapy should be given preoperatively. Optimally several (between five and seven) specimens of tissue, purulence and fluid should be submitted for culture. The diagnostic value of the number of positive operative cultures for the same organism has been calculated (Table PP20.2). If at least three specimens are submitted to the microbiology laboratory, then a finding of one positive culture represents a 13.3% probability of a prosthetic joint infection, two positive cultures represent a 20.4% probability and three positive cultures a 94.8% probability. The results of these microbiologic techniques should confirm the presence and nature of the infection and allow for optimal treatment.

In the uncommon circumstance in which the clinical suggestion of sepsis is strong but the cultures are sterile, fastidious micro-organisms, particularly anaerobes, should be suspected. Mycobacteria and fungi should also be considered as possible etiologic pathogens in appropriate clinical circumstances and specific cultures for them should be obtained. To design the most efficacious and least toxic antimicrobial therapy, the patient's infecting strain of bacteria must first be available for *in-vitro* evaluation.

Therapeutic options

The most predictably effective treatment for prosthetic joint infection involves complete removal of all foreign materials (metallic prosthesis, cement and any accompanying biofilm). Explantation and re-implantation can be accomplished in a single stage (exchange procedure) or in a two-stage approach. The most successful protocol incorporates standardized antimicrobial therapy with a two-stage surgical method:

1. Removal of the prosthesis and cement followed by a 6-week course of bactericidal antibiotic therapy chosen on the basis of quantitative *in-vitro* susceptibility studies.
2. Re-implantation at the conclusion of the 6-week antibiotic course.

Use of methylmethacrylate cement impregnated with an antimicrobial agent (usually tobramycin or gentamicin with or without vancomycin) has not been subjected to controlled trials but is commonly practiced during re-implantation if a cemented prosthesis is employed. The antimicrobial agents leach from the hardened plastic (cement) to produce variable but high initial release and protracted diffusion of antibiotic into surrounding tissues at the bone–cement interface (at high levels for approximately 2 weeks). Antibiotic-loaded polymethylmethacrylate is also commonly used in cement spacers inserted after prosthesis removal to maintain the structural anatomy and to facilitate subsequent re-implantation. With this protocol, a 90–96% success rate has been achieved in total hip replacement infections and a 97% success rate in total knee replacement infections. The success of this regimen relies on thorough debridement techniques and effective antimicrobial therapy.

Systemic antibiotic potency against the infecting pathogen is standardized by using the serum bactericidal test. Blood is drawn at a time representing 25% of the interval between doses:

- at 1 hour post-dose for drugs given every 4 hours;
- at 1.5 hours post-dose for drugs given every 6 hours;
- at 2 hours post-dose for drugs given every 8 hours;
- at 3 hours post-dose for drugs given every 12 hours; and
- at 6 hours post-dose for drugs given every 24 hours.

The serum bactericidal test is performed with a goal of producing a minimum 1:8 titer against all infecting pathogens. In this manner, both Gram-positive bacteria (including methicillin-resistant *Staphylococcus aureus* and enterococci) and Gram-negative bacilli (including *Pseudomonas aeruginosa*) can be eliminated if the specific sensitivity of each isolate allows eradication. The empirical selection of a 6-week duration of antibiotic therapy may be critical for efficacy. Others have employed a similar approach to therapy but with only a 2-week course of antibiotic treatment before implantation of the new prosthesis. With this shorter protocol, the pathogen was eradicated in only 79% of cases with only 35% of the patients obtaining good function with the new prosthesis.

The single-stage (exchange procedure) treatment involves extraction of the metallic joint and cement with immediate implantation of a new prosthesis. Antibiotic-loaded methylmethacrylate cement is used during this implantation. The protocol is effective in 70–83% of cases. If the exchange operation is repeated (in those for whom the first replacement failed), and antibiotic-loaded cement is used, the success rate can be increased to 90%. It has been suggested that this mode of therapy is applicable only to infections with the less virulent micro-organisms, because high failure rates are observed when the pathogen is *Staphylococcus aureus* or a Gram-negative bacillus. Systemic antibiotics are administered rarely and without standardization in this regimen. Moreover, the customary selection of an aminoglycoside as a component in the re-cementing phase of these operations may not reflect the susceptibility of the pathogen being treated. Currently, surgeons have the additional option of including vancomycin with the aminoglycoside in loading the cement. This should increase the effectiveness of this local, depot administration of antibiotic therapy.

Although the two-stage removal and re-implantation approach is more effective, the single-stage procedure is often used for elderly or infirm patients who might not tolerate protracted bed rest and a second major operation. Patients chosen for the single-stage approach should also have infecting organisms which are very sensitive to aminoglycosides with or without vancomycin since these are the antibiotics that can be used most successfully when incorporated into the polymethylmethacrylate cement used in this procedure.

In contradistinction to the previously described therapeutic approaches, treatment with retention of the infected prosthesis can be a consideration in specific clinical circumstances. In patients with prosthetic joints infected with penicillin-susceptible streptococci, with symptoms for 10 days or less, 89.5% were successfully treated without implant removal. Early postoperative infections (<1 month after implantation) and early hematogenous infections (<1 month of symptoms) treated without prosthesis removal have had reported success rates of approximately 71% in small numbers of patients receiving a single debridement followed by 4–6 weeks of antibiotic therapy. Some of these cases may have had false-positive cultures in this setting, which could inflate the success rate. Other studies of similar patient populations have had very low success rates, such as 23% of those who had symptoms for <2 weeks (100% failure rate in those with symptoms for >2 weeks) and 38% and 36% success rates in two additional studies. When the pathogen is *S. aureus*, the success rate was 50% if symptoms were present for 2 days or less; the success rate was 10% if symptoms were present for >2 days.

Success with long courses (3–6 months) of antibiotic therapy using rifampin (rifampicin) in combination with other antimicrobial agents has been reported in selected patients with retained orthopedic implants. Most of these infected implants were fracture-fixation devices and not septic total joint prostheses; infections of the latter appear to be more difficult to cure. Nonetheless, rifampin appears to have an enhanced capacity to penetrate membranes and biofilms and therefore may be a critically important antibiotic in the treatment of infected prosthetic articulations without removal of the implant.

Deciding which therapeutic approach is appropriate in individual patients is highly dependent on isolating the pathogen. Knowledge about the infecting micro-organism is important in systemic antibiotic selection, in selecting antibiotics to be incorporated into polymethyl-methacrylate spacers (or deciding not to use a spacer if the pathogen is resistant to incorporated antibiotics) and in deciding whether to use a single-stage or a two-stage therapeutic approach. The etiologic bacteria also must be available to measure the bactericidal potency of designed therapy (using the serum bactericidal test).

In those circumstances in which the clinical suggestion of sepsis is strong but the prosthetic joint cultures are sterile, anaerobic bacteria (such as *Peptostreptococcus, Bacteroides, Propionibacterium acnes*) should be suspected and empiric antibiotic regimens should be designed to include anaerobic coverage. Consideration should also be given to the presence of other fastidious pathogens such as mycobacteria and fungi. In addition, the possible masking effect of any prior antibiotic therapy (particularly within 6 weeks of the diagnostic cultures) should be borne in mind when designing the necessarily empiric antimicrobial therapies in these circumstances.

Suppressive antibiotic therapy

Suppressive oral antimicrobial therapy may be of value in selected cases in which:

- prosthesis removal is not possible;
- the prosthesis is not loose;
- the pathogen is relatively avirulent
- the pathogen is exquisitely sensitive to an orally absorbed antibiotic; and
- the patient can tolerate an appropriate oral antibiotic.

Successful retention of a functioning hip arthroplasty was observed in 63% of patients when all of the above five criteria were fulfilled. When similar therapy was employed in total knee replacements infected with a variety of micro-organisms (both virulent and avirulent), successful joint function was only variably maintained in 26–82% of patients. The suppressive approach is not without risk.

Serial radiographs are needed over the course of treatment to monitor for progressive bone resorption at the bone–cement interface, which could reduce the success of any future revision surgery. Secondary resistance can emerge and, despite continual antibiotic therapy, the localized septic process can extend into adjacent tissue compartments or become a systemic infection. Moreover, the patient is subjected to the potential side-effects of chronic antibiotic administration.

Prevention

In view of the catastrophic effects of prosthetic arthroplasty infection, prevention of these septic processes is of prime importance. In anticipation of elective total joint replacement surgery, the patient should be evaluated for the presence of pyogenic dentogingival pathology, obstructive uropathy and dermatologic conditions that might predispose to infection and bacteremia. The use of prophylactic antibiotics in anticipation of bacteremic events (i.e. dental surgery, cystoscopy, surgical procedures on infected or contaminated tissues) has been suggested on the same empirical basis on which endocarditis prophylaxis is recommended. This approach to prevention is controversial, and no data are available with which to determine the adequacy or the cost-effectiveness of such measures. The American Dental Association and the American Academy of Orthopedic Surgeons have jointly advised that a single dose of prophylactic antibiotic be given to selected patients undergoing dental procedures associated with significant bleeding. Similarly the American Urologic Association and the American Academy of Orthopedic Surgeons have jointly advised that prophylactic antibiotics be considered in patients undergoing urologic procedures with higher bacteremia risk. Clinical decisions regarding prophylactic antibiotics for expected bacteremias in patients with prosthetic joints should be made on an individual basis.

FURTHER READING

Further reading for this chapter can be found online at http://www.expertconsult.com

Sepsis

This chapter examines the consequences of the systemic effects of infection, broadly referred to as sepsis.

EPIDEMIOLOGY

Definition and nomenclature

Physicians have long recognized that infection can lead to generalized circulatory collapse and death. In the 1990s Bone initiated a debate on the terminology of sepsis, identifying key clinical criteria and definitions.[1] Bone recognized that similar physiologic changes could occur in noninfective inflammatory processes, such as pancreatitis, and introduced the term the systemic inflammatory response syndrome (SIRS) to define a common set of diagnostic criteria for infected (sepsis) and noninfected patients.[1] The term SIRS has been criticized for being too imprecise[2] but the concept and definition of sepsis has remained.[3] It is important to remember that sepsis is a heterogeneous condition resulting from the interaction of host, pathogen and environmental factors. Some authors have questioned the validity of grouping all such patients together, particularly in research studies of new therapeutic agents.[4]

Severe sepsis (Table 44.1) may be defined simply as 'sepsis plus sepsis-induced organ dysfunction or tissue hypoperfusion'.[5] The challenge for clinicians is to recognize the presentation of sepsis/severe sepsis (Table 44.2) and intervene early.

Incidence and prevalence of sepsis

Host and environmental factors interact in the development of sepsis with varying rates in different patient populations. Furthermore, variation in the organization of health care in different medical systems makes comparisons between countries difficult. Angus and co-workers examined the epidemiology of sepsis in the USA.[6] Using existing databases they analyzed discharge records of over 6 million patients from seven US states during 1995 and extrapolated the results for the

Table 44.1 Definitions of infection-related syndromes

- *Bacteremia*: viable bacteria cultured from bloodstream – patient may or may not have evidence of sepsis/severe sepsis
- *Sepsis*: infection, documented or suspected, plus systemic manifestations (see Table 44.2)
- *Severe sepsis*: sepsis-induced organ dysfunction or tissue hypoperfusion (see Table 44.2)
- *Septic shock*: sepsis-induced hypotension not responding to fluid resuscitation

Table 44.2 Clinical signs and laboratory parameters in the diagnosis of sepsis

Infection – documented or suspected, plus some of the following:	
Clinical signs	Fever temperature >110.4° F (38.3° C) or Hypothermia temperature <96.8° (36° C) Heart rate >90 beats/min Hypotension SBP <90 mmHg, MAP <70 mmHg, SBP fall of >40 mmHg from baseline Prolonged capillary refill time or tissue mottling – indicates poor tissue perfusion Tachypnoea: respiratory rate >20 breaths/min or arterial CO_2 tension <32 mmHg (4.3 kPa) Altered mental state from baseline
Inflammatory markers	WBC >12 000 cells/mm³, <4000 cells/mm³ or >10% immature forms (bands) Plasma C-reactive protein >2× normal range Procalcitonin >2× normal range
Organ dysfunction	Metabolic acidosis: elevated base deficit ≥5, increased blood lactate Hypoxia: Pao_2/Fio_2 <300 Oliguria: urine output <0.5 ml/kg for >2 h despite fluid resuscitation Creatinine rise from baseline >40 μmol/l Coagulopathy: INR >1.5 in absence of anticoagulation, platelet count <100 × 10⁹/l Hyperbilirubinemia: bilirubin >4 mg/dl or 70 μmol/l Hyperglycemia or hypoglycemia in nondiabetic

INR; international normalized ratio; MAP, mean arterial pressure; SBP; systolic blood pressure; WBC, white blood count.
Adapted from Dellinger *et al*.[5]

whole US population. Data collected in this way should be viewed with some caution but the size of this study demands attention. They estimated an annual incidence for severe sepsis of 3 cases per 1000 (2.26 cases/100 hospital discharges), equivalent to 751 000 cases each year. Incidence rose from 0.2/1000 in childhood to 26/1000 over the age of 85. Severe sepsis was estimated to cost around $16 billion per year. In a separate study, Martin *et al.* reported similar figures and also that the incidence of sepsis in the USA was rising at around 9% per year, reaching 240/100 000 in 2000.[7] A review of 330 million emergency department attendances in the USA showed that 0.69% were for severe sepsis.[8]

In Europe Van Gestel *et al.* performed a point prevalence study in 47 intensive care units (ICU) across the Netherlands, showing that 29.5% of patients fulfilled severe sepsis criteria.[9] Extrapolating from these data indicated that severe sepsis was responsible for 0.61% of all hospital admissions but 11% of admissions to intensive care in The Netherlands. Similar data showed a point prevalence for severe sepsis in ICU admissions of 28.7% in the UK[10] and 27% in France.[11] In Australia and New Zealand severe sepsis has been estimated in 0.77 per 1000 of the population and is responsible for 11.8/100 ICU admissions.[12]

Morbidity and mortality rates

The mortality of sepsis varies because of variations in infection prevalence, case definition, ICU facilities and patient populations. In an analysis of four large sepsis trials, 14-day mortality averaged 26% and 28-day mortality 42%.[1] In the Angus study cited above overall mortality was 28.6%, equivalent to 215 000 deaths per annum in the USA.[6] In this study mortality in childhood was around 10%, rising to 38.4% in those over age 85.[6]

Factors associated with early death include the number of organ systems involved,[13] acidosis, and shock.[14] Late deaths are associated with medical co-morbidities, underlying illness and multiple sources of infection. *Pseudomonas aeruginosa*, *Candida* spp. and mixed infections have a higher attributable mortality than other agents. Patients

with sepsis often have serious co-morbidity, but even when this is taken into account the attributable mortality from severe sepsis is still 25%,[15] increasing to over 60% if four or more organs are failing.[13] Long-term mortality is high after an episode of severe sepsis.[16] Some studies have suggested that while the incidence of severe sepsis continues to increase, there has been a recent improvement in mortality, possibly due to the introduction of a more systematic approach to recognition and therapy.[10,17]

Risk factors for sepsis

Broadly speaking, risk factors for sepsis are those factors that weaken/breach host defenses, increasing the likelihood of bacterial invasion of otherwise sterile tissue as summarized in Figure 44.1.

PATHOGENESIS AND PATHOLOGY

Etiologic agents of sepsis

Bacteria are the commonest underlying pathogens in patients with community and hospital-acquired sepsis. Nonbacterial pathogens may also induce the pathologic responses leading to sepsis, including fungi, rickettsiae, protozoa and certain viruses. The epidemiology of community-acquired sepsis varies considerably between tropical and nontropical zones. Alterations in host immunity also influence the nature of the underlying organisms in sepsis.

Historically, Gram-negative bacteria were most commonly associated with septic shock but a shift in etiology occurred during the 1990s, with increasing infection due to Gram-positive bacteria and

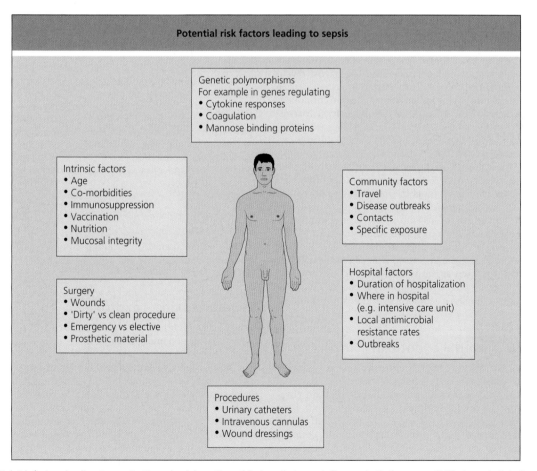

Potential risk factors leading to sepsis

Genetic polymorphisms
For example in genes regulating
• Cytokine responses
• Coagulation
• Mannose binding proteins

Intrinsic factors
• Age
• Co-morbidities
• Immunosuppression
• Vaccination
• Nutrition
• Mucosal integrity

Surgery
• Wounds
• 'Dirty' vs clean procedure
• Emergency vs elective
• Prosthetic material

Community factors
• Travel
• Disease outbreaks
• Contacts
• Specific exposure

Hospital factors
• Duration of hospitalization
• Where in hospital
  (e.g. intensive care unit)
• Local antimicrobial
  resistance rates
• Outbreaks

Procedures
• Urinary catheters
• Intravenous cannulas
• Wound dressings

Fig. 44.1 Potential risk factors leading to sepsis. Complex interaction of factors that may influence both the susceptibility to and clinical outcome of severe sepsis.

479

fungal pathogens particularly within the ICU.[13,18] Vincent *et al.* surveyed over 3000 ICU patients across Europe in the SOAP study. A microbiologic cause was only identified in 60% of patients with severe sepsis which is comparable to other studies and indicates the need for better diagnostic tests. Gram-positive bacteria were responsible for 40%, Gram-negative bacteria 38% and fungi (mainly *Candida* spp.) in 17% of cases. Twenty percent of patients were bacteremic, with pulmonary, abdominal, skin and urinary tract the most common local sites of infection.[13]

The epidemiology of severe bacterial sepsis continually changes in response to the emergence of new bacterial strains and alterations in host or environmental factors. Recent years have seen the emergence of community-acquired methicillin-resistant *Staphylococcus aureus* (MRSA)[19] and more virulent strains of *Clostridium difficile*[20] as causative agents of severe sepsis in the USA with subsequent spread to other parts of the world.

Bacterial products involved in sepsis

Bacteria produce a variety of exotoxins and endogenous cell wall products that induce proinflammatory responses *in vitro* that may culminate in sepsis *in vivo*. Such products are released by bacteria during local or systemic infection and, in turn, may have local or distant proinflammatory effects.[21] The innate immune system is our first line of defense against invading micro-organisms and immune activation through this route is central to the pathogenesis of sepsis.

Innate immune recognition of microbial products

In recent years the concept of pathogen recognition systems triggering an initial, and very rapid, innate immune response to pathogens has emerged.[21] Pathogen-associated molecular patterns (PAMPs) are the microbial products that trigger these receptor recognition systems that are found in almost all higher eukaryotes.[22] The same receptor systems may be triggered by other harmful stimuli known as damage-associated molecular patterns (DAMPs). The relevance of this to severe sepsis is that innate immunity is, in most cases, the first defense mechanism against invading organisms and this activation system plays a pivotal role in setting in motion the inflammatory and anti-inflammatory processes that determine whether the infection resolves, disseminates or leads to sepsis (Fig. 44.2).

Identification of the Toll-like receptor (TLR) family and the recognition of the central role of TLR in the innate response to infection is one of the most important discoveries in understanding the molecular basis for severe sepsis.[23] Toll receptors were first identified as important in the recognition of fungi in *Drosophila* and have been recognized in widely diverse organisms including plants, animals and insects. To date, 10 functional Toll receptors have been identified in humans; they are involved in the recognition and response to PAMPs and DAMPs (Table 44.3).[24] Further elucidation of the Toll receptor pathway and signaling in sepsis may lead to a greater understanding of the molecular basis for severe sepsis in different infections and lead to new therapeutic targets.[25] Endotoxin (lipopolysaccharide) is one of the most potent PAMPs and cellular activation by endotoxin is examined in more detail below.

Gram-negative bacterial endotoxin

Endotoxin (lipopolysaccharide, LPS) is found only in Gram-negative bacteria, where it forms part of the outer leaflet of the bacterial cell wall (Fig. 44.3). It consists of a polysaccharide domain covalently bound to a unique di-glucosamine-based phospholipid, lipid A (Fig. 44.3), which is the key toxic moiety of LPS. Lipid A and LPS induce a wide range of both proinflammatory and counterregulatory responses *in vitro* and *in vivo*. In human volunteers, administration of small amounts of endotoxin induce fever and release of cytokines including tumor necrosis factor (TNF), interleukin (IL)-1 and IL-6.[26]

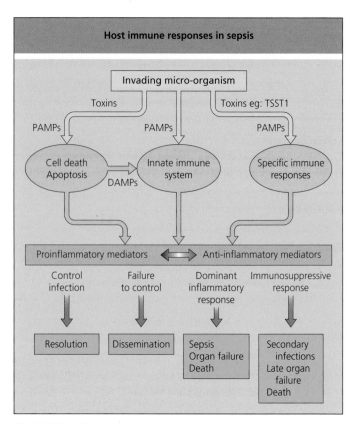

Fig. 44.2 Host immune responses in sepsis. Invading pathogens may activate the immune system by release of soluble toxins or by interaction of structural components (pathogen-associated molecular patterns, PAMPs) with the Toll-like receptor pathway. Immune activation releases a variety of inflammatory mediators that may have local or distant actions. Cell death and tissue damage may result from the direct effect of bacterial toxins or as a result of the inflammatory cascade initiated by the infection. Some host products released following cell damage are damage-associated molecular patterns (DAMPs) and may lead to further immune activation. Anti-inflammatory mediators are also released as part of a feedback loop to limit inflammatory damage. If the balance between proinflammatory and anti-inflammatory mechanisms is correct then localization and resolution of infection will occur. If there is a hyperinflammatory response then there is a risk of sepsis, organ damage and death. If an anti-inflammatory pathway predominates then there is an increased risk of secondary infection leading to further episodes of sepsis and death.

The cellular interaction of LPS is complex, involving both serum LPS-binding proteins and cell-bound and soluble LPS receptors[27] (Fig. 44.4).

Secreted toxins – exotoxins

Exotoxins are released by bacteria and other pathogens, and can cause substantial damage through direct toxic effects or by provoking inflammatory responses (Table 44.4). Type 1 toxins, such as superantigens, do not directly enter cells but bind to surface receptors, triggering specific responses. Type 2 toxins cause direct cell damage and there are many examples of these that are linked to bacterial pathogenesis (e.g. DNAse or protease enzymes). A good example discussed earlier is the emergence of a highly virulent strain of community-acquired MRSA associated with skin and soft tissue infections, necrotizing pneumonia and severe sepsis.[19] Pathogenicity is linked to the Panton–Valentine leukocidin (PVL) gene. PVL is directly toxic to neutrophils and the purified toxin can cause necrotizing pneumonia and sepsis in experimental models.

Table 44.3 Toll-like receptor binding ligands relevant to sepsis

Source	Stimulus	Released by	Receptor
Bacteria	Lipopolysaccharide, endotoxin, LPS	Gram-negative bacteria	TLR4
	Peptidoglycan	Gram-positive bacteria	TLR2
	Lipoteichoic acid	Almost all bacteria	TLR2
	Triacyl lipopeptides	Almost all bacteria	TLR1, TLR2
	Porins	*Neisseria* spp.	TLR2
	Flagellin	Flagellated bacteria	TLR5
	CpG DNA	All bacteria	TLR 9
Fungi	Zymosan	*Saccharomyces*	TLR2, TLR6
	Phospholipomannan	*Candida albicans*	TLR2
	Mannan	*Candida albicans*	TLR4
	O-linked mannosyl residues	*Candida albicans*	TLR4
	Glucans	*Candida albicans*	TLR2
Parasites	Glycosylphosphatidylinositol	*Plasmodium falciparum*	TLR2
Human cells	Heat shock proteins	Tissue damage	TLR4
	Fibronectin	Tissue damage	TLR4
	Hyaluronic acid	Tissue damage	TLR4
	Biglycans	Tissue damage	TLR4
	HMGB1	Tissue damage	TLR2, TLR4

HMGB1, high-mobility group box 1 protein; TLR; Toll-like receptor.
Adapted from van der Poll & Opal.[21]

A third type of bacterial exotoxin is formed of A and B subunits; the A subunit mediates cell entry and the B component is cytotoxic. A good example of the relevance to severe sepsis has come with the emergence of a hypervirulent strain of *C. difficile* known as NAP1/027.[20] Virulence of *C. difficile* NAP1/027 is linked to mutation of a toxin suppressor gene leading to increased production of both A and B toxins. Patients with infection due to NAP1/027 have more symptomatic disease and higher rates of toxic megacolon, severe sepsis and death.

Superantigenic toxins

Superantigenic bacterial toxins can cause profound hypotension, inflammation and organ failure.[28] Strains of *Staph. aureus* and *Streptococcus pyogenes* that are able to express these toxins are implicated in the pathogenesis of staphylococcal and streptococcal toxic shock. The principle behind immune activation by superantigens is outlined in Figure 44.5. Essentially, the bacterial toxin is capable of bypassing the normal highly antigen-specific mechanisms of T-lymphocyte activation by directly linking major histocompatibility complex (MHC) II on antigen-presenting cells to the Vβ subunit of the T-lymphocyte receptor. This triggers cell activation and massive cytokine release which, in turn, can lead to severe sepsis and organ failure.[29] Whether an individual infected with a superantigen-producing organism develops toxic shock is complex depending on the quantity of toxin produced, the presence or absence of pre-existing neutralizing antitoxin antibodies and on the composition of an individual's MHC molecules and T-lymphocyte repertoire of Vβ subunits.[30] An epidemic of menstruation-associated staphylococcal toxic shock syndrome occurred in the 1970s linked to use of a particular type of superabsorbent tampon that enhanced proliferation and increased toxin production by staphylococci in the vagina.[31]

Host genetic factors in susceptibility to sepsis

One of the most intriguing aspects of severe sepsis is why one individual will respond to a particular infection with devastating consequences of septic shock whilst another resolves a similar infection.

A full discussion is beyond the scope of this chapter but it is clear that genetic variation explains aspects of the human response to infection. Animal models and some human studies have linked polymorphisms in key bacterial response genes, including cytokine, mannose-binding protein, CD14 and Toll-receptor genes, to outcome in severe sepsis.[30,32] Human leukocyte antigen (HLA) type II polymorphisms have been linked to responses to superantigens.[33] Further understanding of the genetic basis for response to infection may lead to targeted therapies for patients with sepsis.

Host responses in severe sepsis

Some of the central pathways leading to tissue damage in severe sepsis are shown in Figure 44.5 and key mediators are listed in Table 44.5. Selected pathogenetic mechanisms are discussed in more detail below.

Inflammatory and anti-inflammatory cytokines

Historically much attention was given to the search for the 'key mediator' of sepsis and the focus has at various times settled on complement, arachidonic metabolites, kinins, lipid mediators and cytokines. Rather than being due to one mediator, severe sepsis is the result of a complex interaction of inflammatory and anti-inflammatory processes as depicted in Figure 44.5.

Throughout the 1990s attention focused on the cytokines TNF, IL-1 and interferon gamma (IFN-γ). The evidence that proinflammatory cytokines, such as TNF and IL-1, play a causative role in sepsis stems from several lines of research. First, IL-1 and TNF can induce septic shock in animals and inhibitors of these cytokines can prevent the onset of sepsis in these models.[34] Secondly, mice deficient in the genes encoding receptors for TNF are resistant to septic shock induced by endotoxin. Finally, these cytokines are elevated in human sepsis, and high levels of cytokines correlate with a poor outcome in some but not all studies. TNF is released early in response to LPS challenge,[26] and the cooperative effects of TNF, IL-1 and IFN-γ in producing inflammatory responses made these three cytokines prime targets for experimental intervention in sepsis.

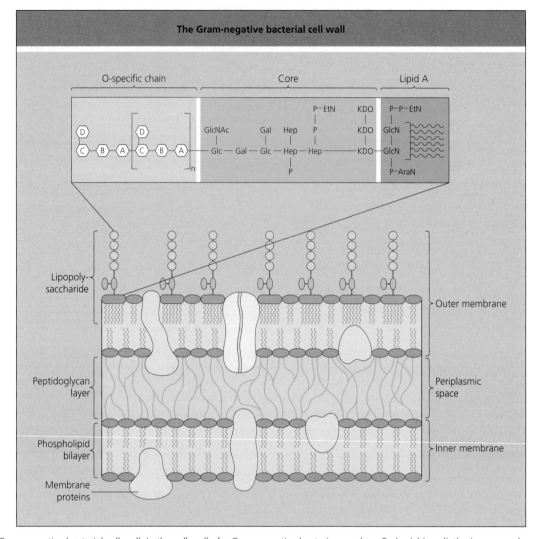

The Gram-negative bacterial cell wall

Fig. 44.3 The Gram-negative bacterial cell wall. In the cell wall of a Gram-negative bacterium such as *Escherichia coli*, the inner membrane is composed of phospholipids and membrane proteins and is separated from the outer membrane by the periplasmic space and peptidoglycan. Lipopolysaccharide (expanded box) is found only in the outermost leaflet of the outer membrane with the lipid A moiety in the membrane and the polysaccharide (O) side chain directed outwards. Lipid A is highly conserved across Gram-negative bacteria and consists of a phosphorylated diglucosamine backbone decorated with six or seven acyl side chains. Dephosphorylation or deacylation of lipid A abrogates its toxicity. Lipid A is covalently linked to an inner core of sugar residues that is relatively well conserved across species and antibodies directed against the core may protect against challenge with heterologous Gram-negative bacilli. The core is followed by an outer polysaccharide chain, of repeating sugar residues, that varies between different bacterial strains (O antigen). Antibodies directed against the O antigen will only protect against challenge with that individual bacterial strain. Gal, D-galactose; Glc, D-glucose; GlcNAc, *N*-acetyl-D-glucosamine; Hep, L-glycero-D-manno-heptose; KDO, 3-deoxy-D-manno-octulosonic acid.

High-mobility group box 1 protein (HMGB1) has attracted attention as a late mediator of inflammatory responses in sepsis.[35] HMGB1 does not appear until more than 8 hours after the onset of sepsis. It is a nuclear protein found in all human cells and is released from macrophages and natural killer cells following infectious challenge. Many cell types following cell injury also release it. HMGB1 is released following apoptosis and anti-HMGB1 monoclonal antibodies improve outcome in animal models of sepsis.[36]

Macrophage migration inhibitory factor (MIF) is released by a variety of cells during sepsis and also in response to glucocorticoids. MIF appears to be important in sepsis pathogenesis as it enhances release of other proinflammatory cytokines, including TNF, and upregulates macrophage expression of TLR4 which increases responsiveness to LPS.[37] Furthermore, MIF prolongs macrophage life by delaying apoptosis. These actions will tend to sustain a proinflammatory profile, potentially worsening tissue damage, and blockade of MIF protects animals from lethal sepsis.

In addition to the large number of proinflammatory mediators induced during severe sepsis, there are many counter-regulatory mediators

(see Table 44.5). Counter-regulatory mediators have specific actions and may neutralize or detoxify bacterial products, block the synthesis or release of cytokines, neutralize circulating inflammatory mediators or downregulate cell responses to inflammatory stimuli. Thus, it is the balance between these opposing mechanisms that will determine whether inflammation is successful in eliminating infection and then 'shutting down', or progressing so that healthy tissues become victims of 'friendly fire' (see Fig. 44.5). In individual patients with severe sepsis it may be this balance between the proinflammatory and anti-inflammatory processes that determines whether infection resolves, disseminates or leads to severe sepsis.

Coagulopathy

Widespread activation of coagulation pathways is common in sepsis and disseminated intravascular coagulation (DIC) may occur as a result. Bacterial products and inflammatory mediators can activate coagulation, anticoagulation and fibrinolytic pathways with a net procoagulant profile. Activated monocytes and endothelial cells increase secretion of tissue factor, which initiates the coagulopathy

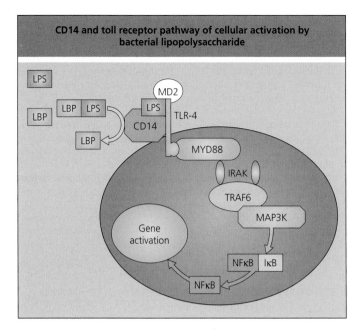

Fig. 44.4 CD14 and toll receptor pathway of cellular activation by bacterial lipopolysaccharide. Schematic representation of events at the inflammatory cell surface. Lipopolysaccharide (LPS), either free or as part of lipoprotein complexes, is bound by LPS-binding protein (LBP) in the fluid phase. The LPS–LBP complex binds to the cell surface receptor CD14 on neutrophils and macrophages. CD14 lacks an intracellular domain and acts as a co-receptor presenting LPS to toll-like receptor 4 (TLR-4), leading in turn to activation of intracellular signaling and gene activation. IκB, inhibitor of kappa B; IRAK, interleukin 1 receptor-associated kinase; MAP3K, mitogen-activated protein 3-kinase; MYD88, myeloid differentiation factor 88; NFκB, nuclear factor kappa B; TRAF6, tumor necrosis factor receptor-associated factor 6.

Table 44.4 Examples of bacterial exotoxins in sepsis

Category	Source	Examples
Pore-forming exotoxins	*Staphylococcus aureus*	α-Hemolysin Panton–Valentine leukocidin (PVL)
	Streptococcus pyogenes	Streptolysin-O
	Escherichia coli	*E. coli* hemolysin
	Aeromonas spp.	Aerolysin
Superantigens	*Staph. aureus*	Toxic shock syndrome toxin 1, enterotoxins A–F
	Strep. pyogenes	SPEA, SPEC, SMEZ
Enzymes	*Staph. aureus*	Coagulase, DNAse, proteases
	Strep. pyogenes	IL-1β convertase, proteases
	Clostridium perfringens	Phospholipase C

IL-1, interleukin-1; SPE, streptococcal pyrogenic exotoxin.

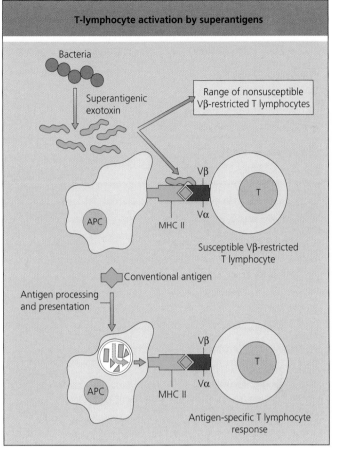

Fig. 44.5 T lymphocyte activation by superantigens. In the conventional response to bacterial antigens (bottom) the antigen is processed and presented by the antigen-presenting cell (APC) in association with MHC II. Only T lymphocytes with the correct antigen recognition site can then be activated (i.e. this is a highly antigen-specific process). Superantigens (top) are able to bypass this process by bridging between MHC II and the Vβ subunit of the T-lymphocyte receptor. Thus the entire population of T lymphocytes expressing that particular Vβ subunit can be activated; this can be up to 20% of the total T-lymphocyte population.

seen in sepsis.[38] Involvement of platelets and von Willebrand's factor may also stimulate coagulation.

Anticoagulant pathways involve antithrombin II, activated protein C and tissue-factor pathway inhibitor (TFPI) which are important in counteracting the procoagulant effect of inflammation.[38] Plasminogen activator inhibitor type 1 (PAI-1) is important in controlling fibrinolysis. Occlusion of small blood vessels during DIC leads to further tissue damage. There is a high risk of bleeding due to thrombocytopenia and exhaustion of clotting factors and activated protein C. This is seen in its most extreme in purpura fulminans in meningococcal bacteremia. Modulation of coagulation has been a therapeutic target in severe sepsis and recombinant human activated protein C is licensed for use in severe sepsis with a high risk of mortality.

Nitric oxide

Nitric oxide (NO) may be involved in the pathophysiology of sepsis through a number of mechanisms.[39] First, NO is a free radical and has the ability to kill phagocytosed organisms. Second, NO is a potent vasodilator and a basal level of NO is required for the maintenance of normal arteriolar tone. Synthesis of NO is increased by a number of bacterial products, including LPS and cytokines. In particular, TNF, IL-1 and IFN-γ appear to increase NO synthesis synergistically. Sepsis is characterized by widespread peripheral vasodilatation and loss of the normal regulation of tissue blood flow. There is considerable experimental evidence in animals to suggest that the vasodilatation in sepsis is mediated by increased NO levels. In humans, elevated urinary nitrite levels are found in sepsis, implying increased NO synthesis.

Table 44.5 Examples of important soluble mediators in sepsis

Target	Proinflammatory mediators	Inhibitory or counter regulatory mediators
Monocyte/ macrophage	TNF, IL-1, IL-8, IL-6, IL-12, IFN-γ, tissue factor, prostanoids, kinins, leukotrienes, PAF, NO, MIF, HMGB1	IL-1 Ra, sTNFr, TGF-β
Neutrophils	Integrin expression, superoxide production, kinins	BPI, CAP 57, defensins, acyloxyacylhydrolase
Lymphocytes	IFN-γ, IFN-β, IL-2	IL-4, IL-10, sIL-2r
Endothelia	Selectins, VCAM, ICAM, NO, tissue factor	Tissue factor pathway inhibitor
Platelets	Serotonin, prostanoids	PDGF
Coagulation pathway	Tissue factor, coagulation cascade leading to thrombin generation	TFPI, AT-III, PAI
Plasma components	Complement activation, bradykinin	Lipoprotein complexes, LBP, CRP

AT-III, antithrombin III; BPI, bacterial/permeability-increasing protein; CRP, C-reactive protein; HMGB1, high-mobility group box 1 protein; ICAM, intercellular adhesion molecule; IFN, interferon; IL, interleukin; LBP, lipopolysaccharide-binding protein; MIF, macrophage migration inhibitory factor; NO, nitric oxide; PAF, platelet-activating factor; PAI, plasminogen activator inhibitor; PDGF, platelet-derived growth factor; sIL-2r, soluble IL-2 receptor; sTNFr, soluble tumor necrosis factor receptor; TFPI, tissue factor pathway inhibitor; TGF-β transforming growth factor beta; TNF, tumor necrosis factor; VCAM, vascular cell adhesion molecule.

Complement

Activation of complement leads to a proteolytic cascade resulting in the liberation of molecules that can act as opsonins and chemoattractants, and can also mediate bacterial lysis. Lipopolysaccharide and other bacterial products activate complement by the alternative pathway. Massive local activation of complement during sepsis will fuel the inflammatory response by recruiting neutrophils, and through the activation of kinins and histamine will contribute to increased endothelial permeability and capillary leakage. C5a is increased during severe sepsis and C5a receptors are upregulated.[40] C5a recruits neutrophils and other inflammatory cells to sites of inflammation. C5a also activates neutrophils by increasing the release of neutrophil granule proteins and prolongs neutrophil lifespan by inhibiting apoptosis. Blockade of C5a improves outcome in models of severe sepsis.

Neutrophil–endothelial cell interactions

An early response to the local production of inflammatory mediators is the upregulation of adhesion molecules on endothelial cells and the release of chemokines that recruit neutrophils and other inflammatory cells to the site of infection. Exposure of neutrophils to LPS and some cytokines enhances the ability of neutrophils to release inflammatory molecules and primes neutrophils for the generation of oxygen radicals and proteolytic enzymes. These mechanisms enable neutrophils to survive longer in an inflammatory environment and to kill more bacteria, but excessive activation of endothelial adhesion may result in the migration of primed activated neutrophils into sites distant from infection. The ensuing tissue damage stimulates a vicious cycle of re-recruitment of inflammatory cells that may ultimately lead to organ damage and failure.

Immunosuppression as a result of sepsis

Sepsis is a dynamic condition and the dominant pathologic processes can change rapidly. After the initial inflammatory episode of sepsis patients may enter a phase of relative immunosuppression.[41] This can be followed by recovery but additional infectious or noninfectious insults may trigger further inflammatory responses, relapse of severe sepsis and worsening of tissue damage (see Fig. 44.5).

The mechanism underlying immunosuppression is multifactorial. The responses of immune cells may be blunted for a period of time with neutrophils, monocytes and lymphocytes releasing fewer inflammatory mediators for a given stimulus.[42] In part this is due to down-regulation of cellular receptors, anti-inflammatory cytokines such as IL-10 and transforming growth factor beta. In addition, evidence has accumulated that sepsis can trigger apoptosis and cell death of a variety of cell types including lymphoid cells.[43] The contribution of sepsis-related immunosuppression to mortality is not fully understood and experimental approaches to boost immunity after the initial phase of sepsis are under evaluation.

Pathophysiologic events leading to organ failure in sepsis

How do the complicated and often confusing inflammatory responses outlined above lead to tissue damage and eventually multiorgan failure? At the cellular level, the end result of the inflammatory process is apoptosis and cell death. In part this is mediated by local hypoxia but apoptosis may also be induced by some proinflammatory mediators. In the whole organism the key to organ damage lies in the breakdown of normal vascular homeostasis, oxygen delivery and oxygen utilization by tissues. This leads to hypoxia and lactic acidosis which further impair organ function (Fig. 44.6). All organs may be affected but clinically the most important are depressed myocardial function, alterations in the peripheral vasculature and failure of oxygen exchange in the lung.

Cardiac function

One of the features of severe sepsis is peripheral vasodilatation, which should lead to an increase in cardiac output to compensate. The rise in cardiac output is often less than that predicted and it is recognized that most patients who have severe sepsis have impaired myocardial function. Cumulative evidence suggests that the impairment of myocardial contractility seen in sepsis is a consequence of circulating cytokines. Tumor necrosis factor directly reduces myocyte contractility and induction of myocardial NO synthesis by cytokines also impairs myocardial function. IL-6 has also been shown to impair myocardial function.

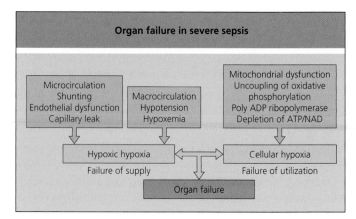

Fig. 44.6 Organ failure in severe sepsis. Organ dysfunction and finally organ failure is the result of cellular hypoxia and acidosis. Hypoxia and acidosis result both from a failure of oxygen delivery due to disturbances in circulation and limitation of the cellular ability to utilize oxygen as a result of mitochondrial dysfunction.

Peripheral vasculature

The hallmark of severe sepsis is widespread peripheral vasodilatation and, in refractory septic shock, it may resist all attempts at pharmacologic intervention. As mentioned earlier, this is largely the consequence of increased NO production in response to cytokines. The most serious consequence of the vasodilatation is the loss of homeostatic regulation of tissue blood flow. Thus, much of the circulating blood volume is shunted through capillary beds, bypassing deep tissues and reducing the opportunity for oxygen extraction. This in turn exacerbates tissue hypoxia and helps to drive the metabolic acidosis that is one of the prominent features of severe sepsis. Further local impairment of perfusion may occur as the result of aggregation of platelets and activation of coagulation in the microcirculation.

Renal failure

Renal impairment is common in severe sepsis and is related to impairment of the renal microvasculature reducing renal perfusion and glomerular filtration followed by the development of acute tubular necrosis.[44]

Respiratory failure

The lung is one of the most vulnerable organs in sepsis, and TNF, platelet-activating factor (PAF), C5a, IL-8 and thromboxane appear to play prominent roles in the development of the adult respiratory distress syndrome (ARDS). The passage of neutrophils across the endothelium and subsequent degranulation in the lung interstitium leads to impairment of endothelial integrity and the accumulation of fluid and inflammatory cells in the alveolar spaces. Impaired gas exchange inevitably produces hypoxia, which further worsens the situation. The combination of hypoxia and increased pulmonary thromboxane synthesis increases pulmonary vascular resistance, in contrast to the fall in systemic vascular resistance. Thus the end result of the pulmonary events in sepsis is the development of interstitial edema and pulmonary hypertension, the hallmarks of ARDS.[45]

PREVENTION

The morbidity, mortality and hospital costs associated with severe sepsis demand that strenuous efforts must be made to reduce the incidence of this serious disease. These can be divided as follows:
- vaccination strategies for at-risk populations;
- assiduous infection control for high-risk patients;
- use of prophylactic antibiotic therapies; and
- prompt recognition and treatment of infection and severe sepsis.

Vaccination strategies are discussed elsewhere under sections on specific pathogens but it is worth noting the success of meningococcal type C conjugate vaccine in reducing the incidence of fulminant meningococcal disease. Interestingly, a recent study from the USA detected a reduction in invasive pneumococcal disease in adults after their children had been immunized with the pneumococcal conjugate vaccine.[46] Unfortunately the majority of cases of severe sepsis are caused by organisms for which no vaccine is available.

CLINICAL FEATURES

A rigorous history, physical examination and directed investigations are essential to arrive at the correct diagnosis of any infectious disease. However, severe sepsis and shock is a medical emergency and therefore full assessment may have to be delayed until resuscitation and empiric antimicrobial therapy have been commenced. The aims of clinical evaluation are to establish the diagnosis of sepsis, estimate disease severity and prognosis, and elucidate the underlying cause. The exact presentation will depend on the site of infection, the nature of the infecting organism, the host response and coexistent illness.

History and symptomatology

Symptoms that suggest the onset of sepsis are often nonspecific and include sweats, chills or rigors, breathlessness, nausea and vomiting or diarrhea, and headache. Confusion may be found in 10–30% of patients, especially the elderly, and sepsis-related encephalopathy is associated with a poorer clinical outcome. There may be specific localizing symptoms or signs to suggest the underlying pathology, such as cough, dysuria or meningism, but in many cases there are no clues. Other important information to elicit includes recent travel, contact with animals, local infectious disease outbreaks, recent surgical procedures, indwelling prosthetic devices, hospitalization, prior antibiotics, underlying pathology and immunosuppressive illness or medication (see Fig. 44.1).

Physical signs on examination

With progression to severe sepsis and shock there is increasing evidence of organ dysfunction; the key physical signs and physiologic changes indicating this are encapsulated in Table 44.2 and Figure 44.7. Remember that sepsis is a dynamic evolving clinical picture and frequent re-evaluation of the patient is essential.

The characteristic patient is febrile, tachypneic, tachycardic with warm peripheries and a bounding arterial pulse, hypotensive, disoriented and oliguric. With impending circulatory collapse the patient

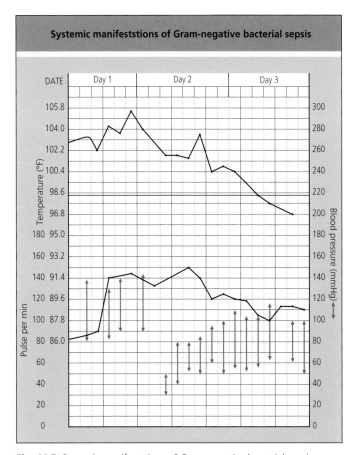

Fig. 44.7 Systemic manifestations of Gram-negative bacterial sepsis. Observation chart of a 49-year-old woman admitted to hospital with a suspected drug fever. For the first 24 hours she was observed without antimicrobial chemotherapy and demonstrated a persistent fever and tachycardia (sepsis). At this point she suddenly became confused, hypotensive and oliguric, indicating the development of severe sepsis. The underlying cause was an *Escherichia coli* bacteremia from an unsuspected urinary tract infection. She responded to fluid replacement and antibiotics and made a full recovery.

may develop peripheral vasoconstriction with cool peripheries and a prolonged capillary refill time. The observation chart of a patient with severe sepsis is shown in Figure 44.7 and the clinical course of a patient with streptococcal toxic shock in Figure 44.8. Some patients, particularly the elderly or immunocompromised, have a more subtle presentation necessitating a high index of suspicion to recognize early disease. Most patients are febrile but severe sepsis may present with hypothermia. A detailed physical examination is vital and it is important to examine the skin, all wounds and to perform full ear, nose and throat, rectal and vaginal examinations and fundoscopy as these sites

are often overlooked. In the hospitalized patient pay particular attention to indwelling intravenous/intra-arterial lines, insist on exposing and examining all wounds, and carefully review the pressure areas as these are frequently neglected sites.

Occasionally, the physical examination will directly establish the diagnosis; helpful signs include the purpuric rash or peripheral gangrene of meningococcemia (Fig. 44.9), peripheral emboli in endocarditis, the erythematous rash or desquamation in staphylococcal or streptococcal toxic shock (Fig. 44.10), ecthyma gangrenosum in patients who have neutropenia and *P. aeruginosa* bacteremia, or the

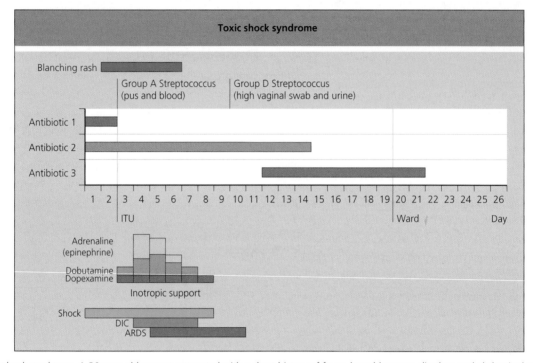

Fig. 44.8 Toxic shock syndrome. A 30-year-old woman presented with a short history of fever, breathlessness, diarrhea and abdominal pain. She was pyrexial and hypotensive with a blanching macular rash noted on day 2. Blood cultures grew a group A β-hemolytic streptococcus. Laparotomy revealed 800 ml of peritoneal pus with no intestinal perforation consistent with spontaneous bacterial peritonitis. She required ventilatory support plus inotropes to maintain blood pressure for 6 days and developed evidence of disseminated intravascular coagulation (DIC) and adult respiratory distress syndrome (ARDS). She made a gradual recovery complicated by an enterococcal urinary tract infection, finally leaving hospital 27 days after presentation. The group A streptococcal isolate from her blood was subsequently shown to release streptococcal mitogenic exotoxin Z (SMEZ), a potent superantigen. Courtesy of Dr P Gothard and Dr S Sriskanden, Hammersmith Hospital, London.

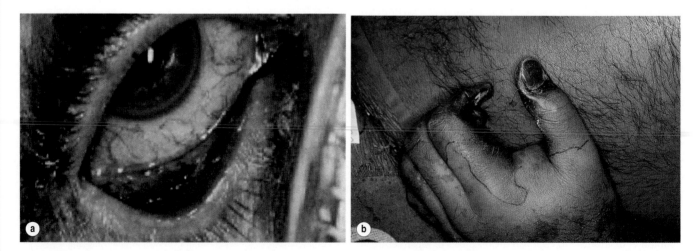

Fig. 44.9 Cutaneous changes in meningococcal infection. (a) Petechial hemorrhages are the hallmark of meningococcal infection and may be found on the periphery or, as in this case, the conjunctivae. (b) In severe disease the purpura may become confluent (purpura fulminans) and lead to severe digital gangrene. Courtesy of J Cohen, Brighton.

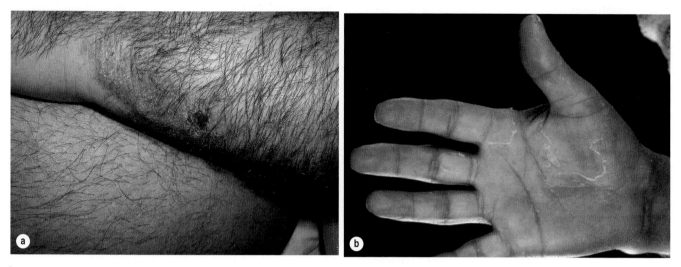

Fig. 44.10 Cutaneous changes in toxic shock. (a) Localized infection at the edge of a patch of eczema in a patient presenting with staphylococcal toxic shock syndrome. (b) Desquamation of the palm following an episode of staphylococcal toxic shock. Courtesy of Dr M Jacobs.

retinal lesions of *Candida* endophthalmitis. Focal physical signs may help to identify the site of infection, for example renal angle tenderness, pulmonary consolidation, new cardiac murmur or finding an intra-abdominal mass.

If the patient is hypotensive, other causes of shock such as cardiac dysfunction (including myocardial infarction and cardiac tamponade), hypovolemia and redistributive shock from pancreatitis and physical injuries need to be considered. Remember that hypotension in sepsis is often multifactorial and sepsis may complicate or coexist with other causes of shock.

DIAGNOSIS

Laboratory investigations

These can be broadly divided into those that help to confirm that the patient has sepsis and detect and follow complications such as organ failure, and those that establish the underlying cause.

Hematologic and biochemical evaluation in sepsis

Full blood count and blood film

Look for a neutrophil leukocytosis or leukopenia. The blood film may suggest bacterial infection with toxic granulation of neutrophils (increased band forms) even when the white cell count is normal. Leukopenia is a poor prognostic sign. Low platelet count suggests DIC and evidence of microangiopathic hemolysis may be visible. In patients who have traveled to an endemic area perform blood films for malaria parasites.

Coagulation screen

Look for evidence of DIC – prolonged prothrombin or activated partial thromboplastin time, low fibrinogen and elevated markers of fibrinolysis (fibrin degradation products or D-dimer levels).

Electrolytes and renal function

Monitor renal function closely; elevated potassium may indicate rhabdomyolysis, which may complicate severe sepsis.

Liver tests

Minor abnormalities are common in patients with sepsis and do not necessarily signify hepatic infection. Elevated bilirubin, alkaline phosphatase or transaminases of two to three times the normal level may be seen in up to 30–50% of patients. These are generally transient and not of prognostic importance. More markedly abnormal liver tests suggest underlying hepatic or biliary tract infection. Progressively deteriorating liver biochemistry in patients who have sepsis suggests hepatocellular damage or acalculous cholecystitis, which may complicate severe sepsis.

Plasma albumin

An acute fall in albumin, to as low as 1.5–2.0 g/dl over 24 hours, may occur as a result of widespread endothelial damage and capillary leakage of protein. In patients with chronic underlying illness or prolonged infection, the albumin may fall due to poor nutrition and a switch in hepatic metabolism towards acute-phase proteins.

Blood glucose

Hypoglycemia or hyperglycemia may occur in severe sepsis. In patients who are diabetic close monitoring and normalization of blood glucose are essential.

Arterial blood gases

Typically the patient has a metabolic acidosis with compensatory respiratory alkalosis. The degree of acidosis is a marker of the severity of illness. The onset of hypoxia indicates severe disease and a high risk of ARDS. Measurement of venous and arterial oxygen content allows calculation of oxygen delivery and consumption.

Plasma lactate

This is often increased three- to fivefold in severe sepsis (normal 1.0–2.5 mmol/l) and relates to the degree of tissue hypoxia. Lactate estimations are helpful in diagnosing severe sepsis, predicting mortality and monitoring the response to therapy.[5,47]

Other biochemical investigations

Amylase, creatinine phosphokinase, calcium and magnesium levels may be disturbed in patients with severe sepsis.

C-reactive protein

C-reactive protein (CRP) is an acute-phase reactant that rises within a few hours of bacterial infection. High levels are detectable in most patients who have severe sepsis although the level of CRP does not reliably distinguish infective from noninfective causes of shock or between sepsis and severe sepsis.[48] Patients with fulminant sepsis may have a normal CRP at presentation.

Procalcitonin

Procalcitonin has been suggested as a more sensitive and specific marker of bacterial infection than CRP and is preferred in some centers. Procalcitonin levels may be able to discriminate between sepsis and severe sepsis but this has not entered routine clinical practice.[48,49]

Endotoxin or cytokine levels

In some but not all studies plasma levels of endotoxin and cytokines such as TNF and IL-6 have correlated with outcome of Gram-negative sepsis. Variation in reported data along with technical difficulties in performing these assays in real time makes routine testing impractical in most settings.

Microbiologic investigations in sepsis

Establishing an accurate microbiologic diagnosis of the cause of sepsis is a crucial part of patient management. Microbiologic diagnosis is needed to confirm the diagnosis and to direct antimicrobial therapy, particularly with reports of increased antimicrobial resistance in patients with severe sepsis. Despite modern laboratory techniques microbiologic confirmation can only be achieved in around 60% of cases and there is a clear need for improved diagnostic methods.[50] Ideally, all relevant cultures should be taken before initiating antibiotic therapy, but treatment is urgent and should not be unduly delayed.

Blood cultures are the most important microbiologic investigation. Two or three separate blood cultures (total 20–30 ml of blood) should be inoculated into one of the standard commercial blood culture media.[5] Culturing an inadequate volume of blood is the most common reason for not detecting bacteremia.[51] The bottles should be incubated aerobically and anaerobically at 98°F (37°C), preferably agitated, for 7 days. The development of automated blood culture analysis allows for more rapid identification of positive cultures. Where there is a high risk of underlying fungal infection then specific fungal media may be helpful.

Sputum and urine microscopy and culture should be performed in all cases. All wounds should be swabbed and sterile body sites such as cerebrospinal fluid (CSF), joint or pleural fluid sampled as indicated. In cases in which toxic shock syndrome is suspected, wound, nose, throat and vaginal swabs should be taken. If staphylococci or streptococci are isolated in cases of toxic shock then the appropriate reference laboratories can assay the isolate for toxin production. Cultures should be repeated as directed by previous results and the condition of the patient.

Histopathologic changes in sepsis

Organ pathology in sepsis is due to the combined effects of hypoxia, impairment in tissue perfusion and severe acidosis. In the lung the changes are those of ARDS, with early findings of interstitial and alveolar edema, fibrosis developing at a later stage. The kidneys may show acute tubular necrosis that is generally reversible (Fig. 44.11). Hepatic changes are of an ischemic zonal necrosis and some cases may develop an acalculous cholecystitis. In the brain there may be areas of focal ischemia or hemorrhage. In severe cases of septic shock associated with *Neisseria meningitidis* or *Capnocytophaga canimorsus* there may be peripheral gangrene due to severe impairment of perfusion (see Fig. 44.9 and also Fig. 12.6) and hemorrhage into the adrenal glands (Fig. 44.12). The gut is also affected by ischemia and may show mucosal ulcerations and areas of infarction.

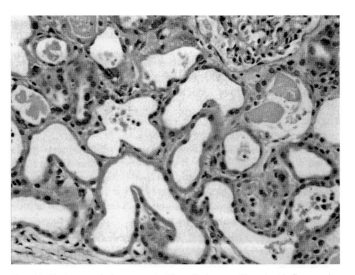

Fig. 44.11 Acute tubular necrosis. The tubules are dilated with flattened epithelial cells, and contain debris; the glomerulus is not greatly affected. Hematoxylin and eosin. With permission from Williams JD et al., Clinical Atlas of the Kidney. London: Mosby; 1991.

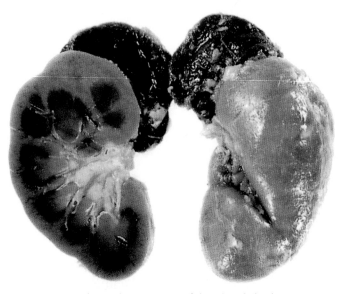

Fig. 44.12 Acute hemorrhagic necrosis of the adrenal glands (Waterhouse–Friderichsen syndrome). Both adrenal glands of a child with meningococcal septicemia show hemorrhagic necrosis leading to acute adrenal failure. With permission from Stevens A, Lowe J. Pathology. London: Mosby; 1995.

Radiologic investigations

Chest radiography is necessary in all cases and may show signs of ARDS. Other studies may also be indicated. Radiologic investigations can be of great help in identifying occult sites of infection (Fig. 44.13) and close liaison with the diagnostic radiology department is vital. Ultrasound and CT are particularly useful when trying to detect deep abscesses; in selected cases nuclear medicine techniques may pinpoint the site of infection. Access to an interventional radiologist who can perform percutaneous sampling/drainage of sites of infection is invaluable.

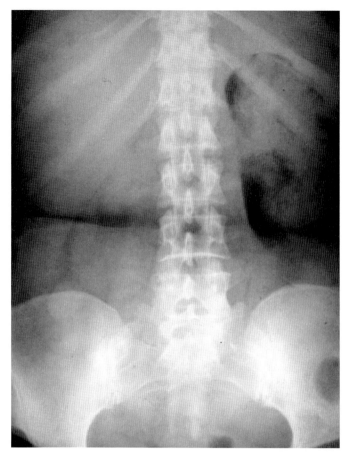

Fig. 44.13 Radiologic detection of occult foci of infection in severe sepsis. Plain abdominal X-ray in a diabetic with an *Escherichia coli* urinary tract infection and pyelonephritis who had developed hypotension and oliguria. X-ray reveals gas around the kidney due to a perinephric abscess requiring urgent drainage.

MANAGEMENT

Mortality from sepsis and multiorgan failure remains high but by early recognition and prompt therapeutic intervention patients can be prevented from progressing down this path. There is no complete consensus on how best to manage severe sepsis and few randomized trial data dealing with optimal treatment. An approach to therapy is encapsulated in the Surviving Sepsis Campaign guidelines first produced in 2004 and updated in 2008.[5,52] These guidelines have not met with universal approval, mainly because severe sepsis is not a homogeneous condition and a generalized approach to treatment can be criticized. However, they do provide a logical and structured approach to the septic patient.

The key principles in the management of severe sepsis are:

- treat infection with prompt and effective antimicrobial therapy and, where indicated, source control;
- maintain tissue perfusion/oxygenation and preserve organ function; and
- prevent complications during/following the episode of severe sepsis.

Antibiotic chemotherapy

Incorrect empiric antibiotic choice is strongly associated with a higher mortality in severe sepsis.[18,53] Furthermore, delay in administration of antibiotics worsens survival. Kumar *et al.* reviewed 2154 patients with

Table 44.6 Principles of antibiotic administration and selection of antimicrobial agents in severe sepsis

Antibiotic administration
Intravenous high dose therapy within 1 h of the recognition of severe sepsis
Broad-spectrum choice to include one or more drugs active against the likely infecting pathogen
Chosen antibiotic should penetrate the likely site of infection
Review antibiotic choice every 24 h in the light of clinical response and microbiology results
Consider combination therapy for known or suspected *Pseudomonas* infection or in neutropenic sepsis

Selection of antimicrobial agent
Clinical syndrome/likely microbiology
Site of infection
Risk of resistance based on local and national data
Host factors including immunocompromised state
Co-morbidities including organ function and drug allergy
Risk of *Clostridium difficile* and other hospital-acquired infections based on local epidemiology

septic shock and found that only 50% had received antibiotics within 1 hour of the onset of shock.[14] In this study the mortality rate was 20.1% if antibiotics were administered within the first hour after the onset of hypotension and rose by 7.6% per hour of delay, becoming statistically significant if antibiotics were delayed more than 2 hours.

It is not possible to provide specific antimicrobial guidelines for severe sepsis as there are many local variables that must be taken into consideration such as local resistance patterns and risks of *C. difficile*. An overview of the principles underpinning antibiotic choice in severe sepsis is provided in Table 44.6. There are few outcome data on duration of antibiotic therapy in severe sepsis and a course of 7–10 days is frequently recommended, although shorter courses may be given to selected patients and helps to reduce resistance.

Antibiotic-induced endotoxin release

In experimental models, and some limited situations in humans, release of endotoxin from bacteria has been shown to increase the inflammatory response.[54] Thus, a school of thought has developed that antibiotics should be chosen on the basis of their potential to cause endotoxin release.[55] However, beyond a handful of small studies there are few clinical data to support a major role for this hypothesis in severe sepsis. Antibiotics should be selected on the basis of efficacy for the specific clinical picture, rather than on the risk of endotoxin release.

Source control – detection and removal of infected material

It is essential to drain/remove all possible infective foci as these are often the cause for treatment failure (see Fig. 44.13). Thus, abscesses should be drained, dead tissue resected and infected foreign material, such as an infected central venous catheter, removed. Guidance suggests that source control should occur as early as possible after initial resuscitation and is ideally performed within 6 hours of the onset of severe sepsis.[5] One exception to early intervention is severe necrotic pancreatitis where current practice is to defer percutaneous drainage due to the high complication rate and secondary infective risk.[56] The critically ill patient on intensive care may have repeated episodes of sepsis; locating the underlying focus often requires considerable determination, repeated radiologic investigation and sometimes persistent discussions with surgical colleagues.

Supportive therapy

The goal of supportive therapy is to try to maintain tissue oxygen delivery, a concept advanced by Shoemaker and others throughout the 1970s.[57] The potential benefit of early aggressive supportive therapy is shown in a study by Rivers et al.[58] in which 263 patients with severe sepsis were randomized to receive standard therapy or 'goal-directed' therapy where cardiac preload, afterload and contractility were actively managed to try to balance oxygen delivery with demand prior to admission to the ICU. In-hospital mortality was reduced from 46.5% in the standard group to 30.5% in the goal-directed group (p <0.009). Goal-directed therapy appears to improve outcome during initial resuscitation when patients first develop severe sepsis and the applicability of this approach to all comers with sepsis has been questioned. However, the Rivers study establishes the importance of paying attention to prompt and effective resuscitation in severe sepsis.

Ideally, patients who have sepsis should be closely monitored in an intensive therapy or high-dependency unit. Indeed a review of 41 patients who had septic shock revealed increased mortality when patients were managed outside of the intensive therapy unit, 70% versus 39%, even though the patients had less severe illness.[59] Minimal requirements for safe management include facilities for measurement of blood pressure, cardiac monitoring, central venous pressure recording, arterial blood gas analysis, oxygen and facilities for assisted/mechanical ventilation or dialysis when required. Invasive monitoring is useful in excluding other causes of shock and in directing therapy. However, invasive monitoring is not a substitute for repeated examination and clinical assessment of the patient. Many factors such as cardiovascular disease, hypovolemia or inotropic drugs can confound such data; results must be interpreted in the context of the clinical situation. Normal values and the typical ranges for hemodynamic parameters in severe sepsis are given in Table 44.7.

Severe sepsis is a heterogeneous condition and it is not possible to be didactic about the management of individual patients. Patients should be monitored closely during resuscitation and interventions tailored to physiologic measurements of organ function/perfusion. Improvement in acidosis and reduction in serum lactate is a reliable guide to improved tissue perfusion and oxygenation. A stepwise approach to initial resuscitation is provided by the Surviving Sepsis Campaign guidelines:[5]

- Begin resuscitation immediately in patients with hypotension or serum lactate >4.0 mmol/l.

- Do not delay pending ICU admission.
- Resuscitation goals:
  - CVP 8–12 mmHg
  - Mean arterial pressure >65 mmHg
  - Urine output >0.5 ml/kg/h
  - Central venous oxygen saturation >70%.

Intravenous fluid therapy

Fluid resuscitation is critical and should precede any pharmacologic agents. Crystalloid or colloids can be used as there are no clear data supporting one over the other.[5] Concerns over the safety of human albumin have been decreased by the SAFE study which showed equal efficacy and safety when albumin was used in comparison to saline in ICU patients.[60] One recent study has found an unexplained increase in adverse events in patients who were resuscitated with pentastarch compared to Ringer's lactate.[61] This finding requires further investigation before a definitive recommendation can be made about colloid solutions based on starch derivatives. In hypotensive or hypovolemic adults, an initial fluid challenge of 1000 ml crystalloid or 300–500 ml colloid should be administered over 30 minutes. Fluid filling should be continued as long as patients have evidence of hypovolemia and impaired organ perfusion. Patients must be monitored closely as cardiac filling pressures increase to avoid cardiac failure.

Vasopressors

Pharmacologic intervention is indicated if evidence of hypoperfusion – persistent hypotension or acidosis – persists despite fluid filling. Initial treatment is with noradrenaline (norepinephrine) or dopamine. There is no evidence that one agent is superior to the other. In refractory cases vasopressin or terlipressin may also be considered but large trial data on these agents are lacking.[62] The dose of pressor agents is titrated to maintain an arterial pressure of 65 mmHg or greater with improved organ perfusion. Patients receiving pressor agents require continuous arterial pressure monitoring and close attention to peripheral perfusion as ischemia of the extremities may complicate their use. There is no role for 'renal dose' dopamine in the management of severe sepsis.

Inotropes

Substantial experimental and clinical data indicate that myocardial function is impaired in severe sepsis. Inotropes increase cardiac contractility and can increase cardiac output and tissue perfusion in severe sepsis. Adrenaline (epinephrine) or dobutamine can fulfill this role and there is no evidence that either agent is superior. Inotropes are indicated where there is evidence of a persistent low cardiac output despite fluid resuscitation and treatment with pressor agents. Inotropes should not be given to patients who are still hypovolemic. Some researchers have used inotropes to try to achieve supranormal oxygen delivery in severe sepsis but there is no evidence that this strategy improves clinical outcome and it is potentially deleterious.[63]

Insulin therapy in severe sepsis

Assiduous control of the blood glucose level is essential in diabetic patients with severe sepsis. Several studies had previously indicated a benefit from tight glycemic control with intensive insulin therapy in nondiabetic patients with critical illness, including those with severe sepsis.[64] However, a large multicenter randomized study reported in 2008 has shown no overall benefit from insulin therapy in sepsis and a significant increase in hypoglycemic events.[61] Therefore, at this time, insulin should only be used in septic patients with hyperglycemia until more data are available.

Table 44.7 Hemodynamic changes in severe sepsis

Parameter	Normal range	Changes in severe sepsis
Heart rate (HR)	72–88 beats/min	Sinus tachycardia
Mean arterial pressure (MAP)	70–105 mmHg	Hypotension <60 mmHg
Cardiac output (CO)	4–8 l/min	Increased but not enough to compensate for low SVR
Systemic vascular resistance (SVR)	800–1500 dyne/s/cm²	Reduced (<600 if no pressor agents)
Oxygen delivery (Do_2)	520–720 ml/min/m²	Decreased
Oxygen consumption (Vo_2)	100–180 ml/min/m²	Typically increased

CO = SV × HR; SVR = (MAP – CVP)/CO × 79.92
Do_2 = CI × arterial oxygen × 10; Vo_2 = CI × (arterial – venous oxygen) × 10
CI, cardiac index (CO/m² surface area); CVP, central venous pressure; SV, stroke volume.

Blood products in severe sepsis

There is some controversy around red cell transfusions in patients with severe sepsis. Early goal-directed therapy suggests transfusion of red cells to maintain a hematocrit >30% in patients with a superior vena cava oxygen saturation of <70% after fluid resuscitation. In contrast, the Transfusion Requirements in Critical Care trial suggests that there is no benefit in transfusing above a threshold hemoglobin of 7 g/dl in patients in ICU.[65]

Thrombocytopenia is common in severe sepsis. Platelet transfusion should be considered if the absolute platelet count is less than $5 \times 10^9/l$ in the absence of bleeding or less than $30 \times 10^9/l$ in the presence of bleeding. Replacement of coagulation factors with fresh frozen plasma or cryoprecipitate may be required to combat bleeding. Plasma also contains potentially proinflammatory components such as complement and replacing these may increase inflammation.

Other supportive treatments

Patients with severe sepsis should receive thromboprophylaxis unless there is a specific contraindication. Stress ulcer prophylaxis is indicated with an H_2 blocker or a proton pump inhibitor. Nutrition should be maintained, preferably by the enteral route. In renal impairment or severe acidosis early consideration should be given to hemofiltration. In the intubated and ventilated patient a reduced risk of ARDS and improved clinical outcome can be achieved using a volume and pressure limited strategy and, where necessary, permissive hypercapnia.[5]

IMMUNOMODULATION AND ADJUNCTIVE THERAPIES IN SEVERE SEPSIS

The concept that organ damage in sepsis is the result of the host inflammatory response has led to an enormous research effort to understand and intervene in this process. Many therapeutic strategies have been investigated in the laboratory setting and within large randomized clinical trials. This has highlighted the difficulties inherent in performing interventional studies in sepsis and initial results have often been conflicting and disappointing with the notable failure of antiendotoxin and anticytokine treatments. In the past decade a number of adjunctive treatments – namely low-dose corticosteroids, intravenous immunoglobulins and recombinant human activated protein C – have entered clinical practice for selected groups of patients with severe sepsis and these are discussed in more detail below.

Corticosteroids

There has been considerable controversy surrounding the use of corticosteroids in severe sepsis. In animal models pretreatment with corticosteroids protected against endotoxemia, and initial promising reports in humans led to the widespread use of high-dose corticosteroids in sepsis. Subsequently, two large multicenter trials failed to show benefit and meta-analyses of suitable trials confirmed that the use of high-dose corticosteroids in sepsis is not of benefit and may potentially be deleterious by increasing rates of secondary infection.[66] However, impairment of the hypothalamic–pituitary–adrenal axis is seen in some patients with sepsis and is associated with a poor outcome. This led to a re-evaluation of the role of lower dose corticosteroid replacement therapy.

In 2002 Annane et al. reported a significant increase in survival of patients with severe sepsis, who had catecholamine-refractory shock and a poor response to synacthen, indicating adrenal failure, when treated with a combination of hydrocortisone and fludrocortisone.[67] As a result of this, corticosteroid replacement has been recommended for patients with severe sepsis and a poor response to

fluids and vasopressors.[5] Hydrocortisone is usually given at a dose of 200–400 mg/day in divided doses with or without fludrocortisone 50 µg/day.

In 2008 a large multicenter study, CORTICUS, was reported which failed to confirm the mortality benefit seen in earlier studies.[68] However, in this study, shock resolution was significantly faster in patients receiving hydrocortisone therapy, supporting a rationale for steroid replacement therapy in severe sepsis. Further work will be required to define the precise role of corticosteroid therapy for patients with severe sepsis.

Intravenous immunoglobulin therapy

Intravenous immunoglobulin therapy (IVIG) administration has been examined in bacterial sepsis with variable data.[69] At present it is not possible, on the basis of the available evidence, to recommend IVIG for unselected patients with severe sepsis. In severe sepsis associated with toxin-producing bacteria, for example staphylococcal or streptococcal toxic shock syndrome, there is a stronger rationale for the use of high-dose IVIG. Toxic shock is seen in persons with low levels of antitoxin antibodies and pooled IVIG contains neutralizing antibodies against a variety of superantigenic toxins. Experimental data and anecdotal reports would support the use of IVIG in this setting but there are as yet no substantial clinical trials. More recently IVIG has been suggested for use in patients with severe infections due to *Staph. aureus* strains producing the Panton–Valentine leukocidin toxin[70] and for severe *C. difficile* infection.[71]

Recombinant human activated protein C

Modulators of coagulation are protective in animal models of severe sepsis and have entered human trials. Of these, recombinant human activated protein C (rhAPC) is most promising. In a phase III multicenter trial of rhAPC versus placebo (PROWESS) in 1690 patients with severe sepsis, 28-day mortality was reduced from 30.8 to 24.7% ($p <0.005$), a relative reduction in risk of death of 19.4%.[72] There was a small but significant increase in serious bleeding in the active therapy group. On the basis of these results rhAPC (drotrecogin alpha) was granted a product license for the treatment of severe sepsis and organ failure in adults in 2002. rhAPC has been recommended in adult patients with sepsis-induced organ dysfunction and a high risk of death (i.e. APACHE II score >25) and who have no contraindications that would increase the risk of bleeding.

PROWESS was followed by the ADDRESS trial which looked at the use of rhAPC in patients with sepsis at a lower risk of death.[73] In this study, involving 2613 patients, no mortality benefit from rhAPC could be detected over placebo but there was a significant increase in 28-day mortality rate if they received rhAPC rather than placebo. Furthermore, in subgroup analysis of patients enrolled into ADDRESS but at high risk of death (similar criteria to the PROWESS study) no benefit from rhAPC could be detected.

So where does this leave rhAPC in the treatment of severe sepsis? On the basis of a well-randomized and performed clinical trial rhAPC has a product license and has entered treatment guidelines in many countries. On the available evidence it is reasonable to continue to prescribe rhAPC for patients with severe sepsis who fulfill the original PROWESS entry criteria and who do not have a high risk of bleeding complications. rhAPC should not be given to patients with single organ failure or a low risk of death due to the risk of bleeding. Further randomized trials of rhAPC are planned which may answer these questions.

REFERENCES

References for this chapter can be found online at http://www.expertconsult.com

Infections associated with intravascular lines, grafts and devices

Infections of Intravascular Lines and Devices

INTRODUCTION

Intravascular lines and devices are used increasingly in health care for the administration of fluids, medication, blood products and nutrition, for hemodynamic monitoring and for hemodialysis. However, catheter-related bloodstream infection (CRBSI) has become a leading cause of nosocomial bacteremia, and carries an associated morbidity, mortality, increased length of hospital stay, and cost of care.[1,2] Approximately 3 in every 1000 patients admitted to hospital in the UK will acquire bacteremia, and almost one-third of these are secondary to intravascular catheter infection.[3]

EPIDEMIOLOGY

All kinds of intravascular catheters and devices carry a risk of infection, but the risk varies considerably with the device used. Peripheral cannulae, usually only in place for up to 72 hours, are associated with a low risk of bloodstream infection, although the frequency of their use means they still cause significant morbidity. The majority of serious catheter-related infections are associated with central venous catheters (CVCs). Tunneled and cuffed or surgically implanted catheters carry much lower rates of infection than standard non-tunneled CVCs, with totally implantable ports having the lowest rates per 1000 catheter days (Table 45.1).

In addition to the type of catheter used, a number of factors during insertion, as well as patient factors, may predispose to catheter-related infection (Table 45.2).

PATHOGENESIS

Colonization of intravascular catheters may occur by either of two main routes. Extraluminal colonization, originating from the skin insertion site and migrating along the extraluminal surface, is the predominant mechanism in short-term catheters such as the non-tunneled central venous catheters used most frequently in intensive care units. Intraluminal colonization, originating from colonization of the catheter hub, or less commonly from contaminated infusate, is the predominant mechanism in longer-term lines including tunneled CVCs used for chemotherapy or parenteral nutrition. Less commonly, catheters may become colonized hematogenously, secondary to a distant site of infection (Fig. 45.1). The relative likelihood of each of the two main routes of colonization is important when considering methods for the prevention and diagnosis of catheter-related infection in a particular clinical setting.[1,2]

The commonest micro-organisms implicated in catheter-related infection include skin flora, particularly the staphylococci (most commonly coagulase-negative staphylococci but also *Staphylococcus aureus*), yeasts and aerobic Gram-negative bacilli (Fig. 45.2).

The ability of micro-organisms to form a biofilm on the surface of an intravascular catheter is important in explaining the persistence of catheter infection. A biofilm comprising host proteins, microcolonies of the infecting organisms and the extracellular polysaccharide matrix (slime) they produce, allows persistence of organisms in a relatively protected environment. Antibiotics at doses much higher than those needed to kill organisms in planktonic state may still be insufficient to kill sessile bacteria within a biofilm.[8] This explains why systemic antibiotics alone often do not succeed in eliminating infection until the line is removed.

CLINICAL FEATURES

Catheter-related infection may be local or systemic or the two may coexist.

Local infection

Localized catheter infections include exit site infection, tunnel infection and pocket infection (Fig. 45.3). They may present with signs of inflammation, purulence or frank cellulitis. Local infection may coexist with systemic infection (frank purulence may be predictive of CRBSI[9]), but may also exist independently. The vast majority of CRBSI occur without local signs[9] and as such the absence of such signs should not reassure against a diagnosis of CRBSI in a patient with unexplained fever.

Systemic infection

Catheter-related BSI may present nonspecifically with fever and chills, with or without septic shock, and should be considered when these features are present in a patient without an obvious alternative source of infection. Blood cultures growing *S. aureus*, coagulase-negative staphylococci or *Candida* species should particularly suggest the diagnosis.

Definitions of catheter colonization, local infection and CRBSI are outlined in Table 45.3.

Table 45.1 Rates of bloodstream infection (BSI) caused by the various types of devices used for vascular access

Catheter type	RATES OF DEVICE-RELATED BSIs PER 100 CATHETERS		RATES OF DEVICE-RELATED BSIs PER 1000 CATHETER DAYS	
	Pooled mean	95% CI	Pooled mean	95% CI
Peripheral venous cannulas				
Plastic catheters	0.2	0.1–0.3	0.6	0.3–1.2
Steel needles	0.4	0.0–2.3	1.6	0.0–9.1
Cutdowns	3.7	0.1–20.6	8.8	0.2–49.3
Arterial catheters used for hemodynamic monitoring	1.5	0.9–2.4	2.9	1.8–4.5
Central venous catheters				
Standard noncuffed, nonmedicated	3.3	3.3–4.0	2.3	2.0–2.4
Antibiotic coated	0.2	0.0–1.0	0.2	0.1–1.4
Control nonmedicated	4.4	3.5–5.5	—	—
Antiseptic-impregnated	3.1	2.4–3.9	2.9	2.3–3.7
Control nonmedicated	3.8	1.5–7.8	—	—
Peripherally inserted central catheters (PICCs)	1.2	0.5–2.2	0.4	0.2–0.7
Silver-impregnated cuffs	3.3	1.9–5.4	3.2	1.9–5.3
Tunneled but noncuffed	12.4	10.7–16.6	1.8	1.4–2.0
Pulmonary artery catheters	1.9	1.1–2.5	5.5	3.2–12.4
Heparin-bonded	0.4	0.2–0.9	2.6	1.1–5.2
Hemodialysis catheters				
Noncuffed	16.2	13.5–18.3	2.8	2.3–3.1
Cuffed	6.3	4.2–9.2	1.1	0.7–1.6
Tunneled and cuffed central venous catheters	20.9	18.2–21.9	1.2	1.0–1.3
Subcutaneous central venous ports	5.1	4.0–6.3	0.2	0.1–0.2
Peripherally inserted central ports	0.0	0.0–2.8	0.0	0.0–0.1
Intra-aortic balloon counter-pulsation devices	1.9	0.9–3.6	5.5	2.5–10.5
Left ventricular assist devices	22.5	17.5–28.5	4.5	3.6–5.7

Based on 206 published prospective studies in which every device was evaluated for infection. From Kluger & Maki.[4] Copyright The University of Chicago Press.

PREVENTION

Catheter-related infections are highly preventable. Considerable evidence now exists confirming the efficacy of specific interventions, and these measures have been incorporated into several national guidelines for prevention, such as those of the US Centers for Disease Control and Prevention (CDC) Healthcare Infection Control Practices Advisory Committee (HICPAC)[2] (Table 45.4), the English epic2 (evidence-based practice in infection control) guidelines[3] and the French Intensive Care Society (SRLF) consensus guidelines.[11]

As catheter-related infection may follow either extraluminal or intraluminal colonization, prevention strategies should focus on these two potential routes of acquisition.

Prevention of colonization of the external surface of the line

Measures to prevent extraluminal colonization are of primary importance with short-term lines, where the role of microbial colonization of the insertion site is so important in the pathogenesis of infection. The aim is to reduce the populations of skin micro-organisms at the time of insertion and during subsequent manipulations, dressings and care.

Maximum sterile barrier

The use of maximum sterile precautions, similar to those used in the operating theater (including sterile gown, gloves and cap, and a large sterile drape) has been shown to significantly reduce infection when compared with standard precautions (sterile gloves, small sterile drape).[2] In a randomized controlled trial, use of maximum sterile precautions led to a reduction in catheter colonization, bacteremia and cost.[12] This approach has also been found to reduce catheter-related infection associated with pulmonary artery catheters.[13]

Choice of cutaneous antiseptic

The impact of the choice of antiseptic solution is the subject of a meta-analysis of eight randomized controlled trials of chlorhexidine gluconate versus povidone-iodine.[14] The use of chlorhexidine gluconate rather than povidone-iodine was associated with a 50% reduction in the risk of catheter-related bloodstream infection. The efficacy of chlorhexidine may be concentration related, and a study comparing 0.5% chlorhexidine with 10% povidone-iodine failed to show a significant difference in catheter colonization or bacteremia,[15] whereas a study by Maki et al. showed a trend to less bloodstream infection with 2% aqueous chlorhexidine compared with 10% povidone-iodine or 70% alcohol.[16] Finally, povidone-iodine in ethanol is more effective than povidone-iodine alone.[17] The HICPAC guidelines strongly recommend cutaneous antisepsis with a 2% chlorhexidine-based preparation.[2]

Table 45.2 Risk factors for intravascular device-related bloodstream infection

Risk factors (number of studies)		Relative risk or odds ratio
Patient characteristics	Underlying disease:	
	AIDS (2)	4.8
	Neutropenia (2)	1.0–15.1
	Gastrointestinal disease (1)	2.4
	Surgical service (1)	4.4
	Placement in intensive care unit or coronary care unit (3)	0.4–6.7
	Extended hospitalization (3)	1.0–6.7
	Other intravascular devices (2)	1.0–3.8
	Systemic antibiotics (3)	0.1–0.5
	Active infection at another site (2)	8.7–9.2
	High APACHE III score (1)	4.2
	Mechanical ventilation (1)	2.0–2.5
	Transplant patient (1)	2.6
Features of insertion	Difficult insertion (1)	5.4
	Maximal sterile barriers (1)	0.2
	Tunneling (2)	0.3–1.0
	Insertion over a guidewire (8)	1.0–3.3
	Insertion site:	
	Internal jugular vein (6)	1.0–3.3
	Subclavian vein (5)	0.4–1.0
	Femoral vein (2)	3.3–4.8
	Defatting insertion site (1)	1.0
	Use of multilumen catheter (8)	6.5
Catheter management	Routine change of iv set (2)	1.0
	Nurse: patient ratio	
	1:2.0	61.5
	1:1.5	15.6
	1:1.2	4.0
	1:1	1.0
	Inappropriate catheter usage (1)	5.3
	Duration of catheterization >7 days (5)	1.0–8.7
	Colonization of catheter hub (3)	17.9–44.1
	Parenteral nutrition (2)	4.8

Adapted from Safdar et al.[5]

Site of catheter

The subclavian site is associated with less risk of infection than either the femoral or internal jugular site.[2,3] The commonly used internal jugular site is at risk of infection for several reasons, including its proximity to oropharyngeal secretions, the difficulty of applying an occlusive dressing and the presence of hair.[18] Peripherally inserted central catheters (PICC lines) are inserted in the superior vena cava via the veins of the upper arm. The HICPAC guidelines suggest that they are associated with lower rates of infection than other non-tunneled central venous catheters, and that this may be due to being distant from the oropharyngeal secretions and less heavy colonization of the antecubital site.[2] However, a prospective cohort study using data from two randomized trials found rates of infection in hospitalized patients with PICC lines to be similar to that of other non-tunneled lines, and much greater than when PICCs are used exclusively in the outpatient setting.[19]

Dressings

Appropriate adhesive dressings are crucial in the prevention of extra-luminal colonization. Transparent, semipermeable dressings have gained favor, allowing regular observation of the line site, permitting showering and requiring less frequent replacement. Although initial reports described a high rate of colonization of the exit site with these dressings, a meta-analysis comparing transparent with gauze dressings found no significant difference in rates of CRBSI.[20]

Chlorhexidine-impregnated sponges, which can be placed over the line insertion site and fixed with a transparent dressing, have been the subject of a meta-analysis of eight randomized controlled trials.[21] Although their use was associated with a trend towards reduction of vascular catheter infection, the number of sponges needed to prevent one infection was high and their use has not been widely recommended. A recent large randomized controlled trial, however, confirms the preventive efficacy of this method, showing a 70% decreased rate of CRBSI.[22]

Prevention of endoluminal contamination

Number of lumens

Despite a perception that the greater the number of lumens, the higher the risk of catheter infection, this has not been shown conclusively in either randomized controlled trials or meta-analysis, with two meta-analyses reaching differing conclusions.[23,24] The English epic guidelines suggest using a single-lumen catheter unless multiple lumens are essential for patient management.[3]

Heparin

Catheter-related thrombosis may be associated with catheter-related sepsis. A meta-analysis of 14 clinical trials indicates that the risk of catheter-related thrombosis is significantly reduced by prophylactic-dose heparin.[25] The risk of microbial colonization of the CVC was also significantly reduced, but not that of CRBSI. The epic guidelines conclude that there is insufficient evidence to recommend the routine use of heparin to reduce CRBSI, but make the point that patients with intravascular catheters are often receiving prophylactic heparin for deep vein thrombosis prophylaxis, and that heparin flushes may be useful for maintaining line patency in infrequently accessed lines or in accordance with manufacturers' recommendations for hemodialysis lines or implanted ports.[3]

Antibiotic locks in prevention

Routine use of antibiotic locks for prevention of CRBSI has not been shown to be beneficial and may promote resistance. Their use may be appropriate in selected cases, for example for the prevention of recurrent infection in patients with long-term tunneled or implanted lines (e.g. patients on hemodialysis) who experience multiple episodes of confirmed infection despite optimum antiseptic practice.[2,3]

Replacement of administration sets

Studies have shown that replacement of intravenous administration sets no more frequently than every 72 hours is safe and cost-effective. Administration sets for total parenteral nutrition should be changed every 24 hours, and those for blood products should be disposed of after the infusion or after 12 hours, whichever is sooner.[3]

Other strategies for prevention

Tunneled or totally implanted devices

Long-term tunneled or totally implanted venous access devices are associated with lower rates of infection than non-tunneled long-term lines, with totally implanted systems having the lowest rates.

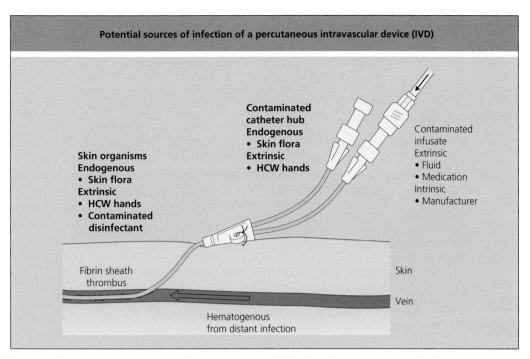

Fig. 45.1 Potential sources of infection of a percutaneous intravascular device (IVD). These include contiguous skin flora, contamination of the catheter hub and lumen, contamination of infusate and hematogenous colonization of the IVD from distant, unrelated sites of infection. HCW, health-care worker. From Crnich & Maki.[6] Copyright The University of Chicago Press.

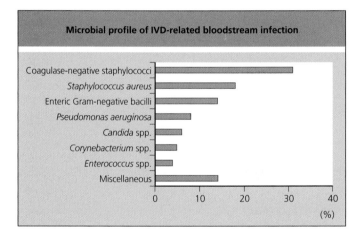

Fig. 45.2 Microbial profile of intravascular device-related bloodstream infection. Based on an analysis of 159 published prospective studies. From: Maki et al.[7]

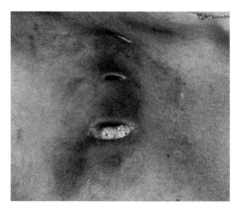

Fig. 45.3 Drained infusion port pocket abscess with evidence of intravascular device-related inflammation. From Raad et al.[34]

For patients requiring long-term intermittent access, totally implanted devices are preferred. For situations where frequent or regular access is needed, a tunneled line is preferable.[2,3]

Tunneling of short-term internal jugular or femoral lines reduces infection rates;[26] no such difference is seen with subclavian lines.[27] However, the apparent risk reduction associated with the tunneling of nutrition catheters disappeared completely with the introduction of a specialist nutrition nurse in one study,[28] suggesting that rigorous aseptic nursing care may be the more significant factor.

Antimicrobial catheters

Antiseptic catheters

Catheters coated with chlorhexidine and sulfadiazine silver on their outer surface were associated with reduced rates of colonization and catheter-related bloodstream infection in a meta-analysis,[29] and have been shown to be cost-effective in high-incidence settings.[30] The antimicrobial activity decreases over time and benefit is likely to be realized in the first 15 days.[31] A second-generation catheter impregnated on both the external and internal surfaces, and with three times the concentration of chlorhexidine, was associated with reduced rates of colonization but without significant reduction in bacteremia.[32] However a possible explanation for this may be underpowering of the studies, given a low baseline infection rate. Rare cases of anaphylaxis have been reported to these catheters in Japan and the UK.[33]

Antibiotic-coated catheters

Catheters impregnated with minocycline and rifampicin on both the external and internal surfaces have been shown to significantly reduce rates of CRBSI in randomized controlled trials.[34,35] A prospective randomized study comparing first-generation chlorhexidine/sulfadiazine catheters with minocycline/rifampicin showed the latter to be associated with significantly lower rates of CRBSI;[36] this has subsequently been confirmed in a meta-analysis.[33] The duration of antimicrobial activity is greater than that of first-generation chlorhexidine/sulfadiazine catheters and may extend beyond 4 weeks.[33]

Table 45.3 Proposed definitions for intravascular device (IVD)-related colonization, local infection and bloodstream infection, based on microbiologic confirmation of the IVD as the source

IVD colonization	• Positive semiquantitative* (or quantitative†) culture of the implanted portion or portions of the IVD
	• Absence of signs of local or systemic infection
Local IVD infection	• Positive semiquantitative* (or quantitative†) culture of the removed IVD or a positive microscopic examination or culture of pus or thrombus from the cannulated vessel
	• Clinical evidence of infection of the insertion site (i.e. erythema, induration or purulence), *but*
	• Absence of systemic signs of infection and negative blood cultures, if done
IVD-related bloodstream infection (BSI)	If the IVD is removed:
	• Positive semiquantitative* (or quantitative†) culture of the IVD or a positive culture of the catheter hub or infusate (or positive microscopic examination or culture of pus or thrombus from the cannulated vessel) *and* one or more positive blood cultures, ideally percutaneously drawn, concordant for the same species, ideally by molecular subtyping methods
	• Clinical and microbiologic data disclose no other clear-cut source for the BSI
	If the IVD is retained:
	• If quantitative blood cultures are available, cultures drawn both from the IVD and a peripheral vein (or another IVD) are both positive and show a marked step-up in quantitative positivity (fivefold or greater) in the IVD-drawn culture
	• Clinical and microbiologic data disclose no other clear-cut source for the BSI
	or
	• If automated monitoring of incubating blood cultures is available, blood cultures drawn concomitantly from the IVD and a peripheral vein (or another IVD) show both are positive, but the IVD-drawn blood culture turns positive more than 2 hours before the peripherally drawn culture
	• Clinical and microbiologic data disclose no other clear-cut source for the BSI

*Roll plate of cannula segment(s) >15 cfu
†Sonication culture of cannula segment(s) ≥10^3 cfu.
Adapted from Crnich & Maki.[10]

Table 45.4 Guideline for the prevention of intravascular device-related bloodstream infection

Recommendation		Strength of evidence*
General measures	Educate all health-care workers involved with IVD care and maintenance	IA
	Ensure adequate nursing staffing levels in intensive care units	IB
Surveillance	Monitor institutional IVD infection rates of IVD-related BSI	IA
	Express rates of CVC-related BSI per 1000 CVC-days	IB
At catheter insertion	Aseptic technique:	
	Hygienic hand care before insertion or manipulation of any IVD	IA
	Clean or sterile gloves during insertion and manipulation of noncentral IVDs	IC
	Maximal barrier precautions during insertion of CVCs: mask, cap, sterile gown, gloves, drapes	IA
	Dedicated IVD team strongly recommended	IA
	Cutaneous antisepsis: first choice, 2% chlorhexidine; however, tincture of iodine, an iodophor or 70% alcohol are acceptable (no recommendations for use of chlorhexidine in infants less than 2 months, unresolved issue)	IA
	In adults, other than hemodialysis catheters (jugular site preference), use a subclavian site rather than a jugular or femoral site for CVC access (in pediatric patients, no recommendations for preferred site, unresolved issue)	IA
	Use of sutureless securement device	NR
	Sterile gauze or a semipermeable polyurethane dressing to cover site	IA
	No systemic or topical antibiotics at insertion	IA
Maintenance	Remove IVD as soon as no longer required	IA
	Monitor IVD site daily	IB
	Change dressing of CVC insertion site at least weekly	II
	Do not use topical antibiotic ointments	IA
	Change needleless iv systems at least as frequently as the administration set; replace caps no more frequently than every 3 days or per manufacturers' recommendations	II
	Complete lipid infusions within 12 hours	IB

Table 45.4 Guideline for the prevention of intravascular device-related bloodstream infection—cont'd

Recommendation		Strength of evidence*
	Replace administration sets no more frequently than every 72 hours. When lipid-containing admixtures or blood products are given, sets should be replaced every 24 hours; with propofol, every 6–12 hours	IA
	Replace peripheral IVs every 72–96 hours	IB
	Do not routinely replace CVCs or PICCs solely for prevention of infection	IB
	Do not remove CVCs or PICCs solely because of fever unless IVD infection is suspected but replace catheter if there is purulence at the exit site, especially if the patient is hemodynamically unstable and IVD-related BSI is suspected	II
Technology	Use antimicrobial-coated or antiseptic-impregnated CVC in adult patients if institutional rate of BSI is high despite consistent application of preventive measures and catheter likely to remain in place >5 days (no data or recommendations for pediatric patients)	IB
	Use of chlorhexidine-impregnated sponge dressings (no recommendation for adults or children – unresolved issue; do not use in neonates <7 days old or of gestational age <26 weeks)	NR
	Use prophylactic antibiotic lock solution only in patients with long-term IVDs who have continued to experience IVD-related BSIs despite consistent application of infection control practices	II

BSI, bloodstream infection; CVC, central venous catheter; IVD, intravascular device; PICC, peripherally inserted central catheter.
*IA, strongly recommended for implementation and supported by well-designed experimental, clinical or epidemiologic studies; IB, strongly recommended for implementation and supported by some experimental, clinical or epidemiologic studies and a strong theoretical rationale; IC, required by state or federal regulations, rules or standards; II, suggested for implementation and supported by suggestive clinical or epidemiologic trials or a theoretical rationale – unresolved issue, an unresolved issue for which evidence is insufficient or no consensus regarding efficacy exists; NR, no recommendation for or against at this time.
Adapted from O'Grady et al.[2]

Clinical studies have shown conflicting results regarding emergence of resistance to either of the antibiotics concerned, although *in-vitro* studies have indicated that resistance may develop, particularly among staphylococci.[2,33] Some studies have reported an increased risk of colonization with *Candida* species in patients with these catheters.[33]

Silver-impregnated catheters

Silver has broad-spectrum antimicrobial activity; however activity is greater against Gram-negative than Gram-positive organisms. A meta-analysis failed to show any benefit in terms of catheter colonization or CRBSI with any of the available silver-impregnated vascular catheters.[33]

The CDC's Hospital Infection Control Practices Advisory Committee guidelines[2] suggest that antimicrobial catheters (chlorhexidine/sulfadiazine or minocycline/rifampicin) be considered in settings where a high rate of CRBSI persists despite the implementation of other measures (education, training, optimal skin antisepsis, maximum sterile barrier) for patients who are expected to need the catheter for more than 5 days. The English epic guidelines[3] suggest the use of antimicrobial catheters for patients who are at high risk of infection and likely to need central venous access for 1–3 weeks.

Results of a meta-analysis of antimicrobial catheters are shown in Figure 45.4.

Antiseptic cuffs

Silver-impregnated cuffs failed to reduce the incidence of CRBSI, in either short-term or long-term catheterization.[2,3]

Catheter replacement

Short-term peripheral cannulae should be replaced every 48–72 hours to prevent thrombophlebitis and infection.[2] However, routine replacement has not been shown to reduce the infection risk associated with central venous catheters, dialysis catheters or peripheral arterial lines[24] and is not recommended.[2,3] The use of guidewire exchange should not be used in cases of confirmed catheter-related infection. However, exchange over a guidewire may be used in cases of suspected line infection where there is no evidence of local infection of the line site. The tip should be sent for culture and if infection is confirmed, the new catheter should be removed and access established at an alternative site.[3]

Multifaceted approach

The very nature of the prevention measures outlined above necessitates a multifaceted approach to their implementation. A number of studies have demonstrated that the combination of several simple measures (the 'prevention bundle' approach)[37] may dramatically reduce the incidence of CRBSI. A multicenter study across 103 intensive care units in Michigan evaluated the implementation of five prevention measures (hand hygiene, maximum sterile barrier, chlorhexidine skin antisepsis, avoidance of the femoral site where possible and prompt removal of unnecessary lines).[38] A dramatic reduction in the incidence of CRBSI, with median rates lowered to zero, was seen at 3 months and maintained at 18. Several authors have demonstrated the importance of staff education programs, standardization of aseptic care and adequate staffing levels. Surveillance and feedback of infection rates can reduce the incidence of CRBSI without any additional intervention.[39] Rates of infection go up when inexperienced staff are responsible for line care, and specialist 'IV teams' have been shown unequivocally to reduce rates of CRBSI.[2]

DIAGNOSIS

Clinical diagnosis

Clinical features are unreliable for the diagnosis of catheter-related infection. Fever and chills have poor specificity, whereas local inflammation of the line site is associated with greater specificity but a

CRBSI in trials comparing antimicrobial CVCs with standard CVCs

	CVCs (n/N)		OR	OR (95% CI)	NNT
	Standard	Comparator			
Silver alloy coated					
Bach et al (1999)[45]	2/33	2/34		0·97 (0·13–7·21)	561
Harter et al (2002)[57]	8/93	5/107		0·53 (0·17–1·62)	25
Goldschmidt et al (1995)[54]	10/113	6/120		0·56 (0·20–1·51)	26
Total (FEM)	20/239	13/261		0·58 (0·29–1·17)	30
Test for heterogeneity: Q=0.29 (2df), p=0.86; I^2=0%					
Silver iontophoretic					
Moretti et al (2005)[66]	1/262	0/252		0·14 (0·00–7·09)	262
Corral et al (2003)[50]	1/103	4/103		3·40 (0·58–19·97)	NA
Total (FEM)	2/365	4/355		1·98 (0·40–9·95)	NA
Test for heterogeneity: Q=2.11 (1 df), p=0.15; I^2=0%					
Silver impregnated					
Kalfon et al (2007)[61]	8/297	8/320		0·93 (0·34–2·50)	517
First-generation CSS					
Tennenberg et al (1997)[75]	9/145	5/137		0·58 (0·20–1·70)	39
Maki et al (1997)[64]	9/195	2/208		0·25 (0·08–0·84)	27
Marik et al (1999)[65]	2/39	1/36		0·56 (0·06–5·43)	43
Hannan et al (1999)[56]	3/177	1/174		0·37 (0·05–2·66)	89
Bach et al (1996)[44]	3/117	0/116		0·13 (0·01–1·30)	39
Collin et al (1999)[49]	4/139	1/98		0·41 (0·07–2·46)	54
Sheng et al (2000)[73]	2/122	1/113		0·55 (0·06–5·36)	133
Heard et al (1998)[58]	6/157	5/151		0·86 (0·26–2·87)	196
Osma et al (2006)[67]	1/69	4/64		3·73 (0·63–22·16)	NA
Pemberton et al (1996)[69]	3/40	2/32		0·83 (0·13–5·06)	80
Ciresi et al (1996)[47]	8/127	8/124		1·03 (0·37–2·82)	NA
Jaeger et al (2005)[60]	8/55	1/51		0·20 (0·05–0·78)	8
Logghe et al (1997)[63]	15/342	17/338		1·15 (0·57–2·35)	NA
Total (FEM)	73/1724	48/1642		0·68 (0·47–0·98)	72
Test for heterogeneity: Q=14.95 (12 df), p=1.00; I^2=26.4%					
Second-generation CSS					
Rupp et al (2005)[72]	3/393	1/384		0·38 (0·05–2·87)	199
Ostendorf et al (2005)[68]	7/94	3/90		0·45 (0·13–1·61)	24
Brun-Buisson et al (2004)[46]	5/175	3/188		0·56 (0·14–2·26)	79
Total (FEM)	15/662	7/662		0·47 (0·20–1·10)	154
Test for heterogeneity: Q=0.11 (2 df), p=0.95; I^2=0%					
Benzalkonium chloride					
Jaeger et al (2001)[59]	1/25	1/25		1·00 (0·06–16·45)	NA
Minocycline–rifampicin					
Raad et al (1997)[70]	7/136	7/136		0·14 (0·03–0·61)	19
Marik et al (1999)[65]	2/39	0/38		0·14 (0·01–2·20)	20
Chatzinikolaou et al (2003)[48]	1/64	0/66		0·13 (0·00–6·61)	64
Leon et al (2004)[62]	11/180	6/187		0·52 (0·20–1·37)	34
Hanna et al (2004)[55]	14/174	3/182		0·25 (0·09–0·65)	16
Total (FEM)	35/593	9/603		0·29 (0·16–0·52)	21
Test for heterogeneity: Q=2.93 (4 df), p=1.00; I^2=0%					
Total antimicrobial CVCs (FEM)	154/3905	90/3868		0·58 (0·45–0·75)	77
Test for heterogeneity: Q=29.94 (28 df), p=0.32; I^2=13.2%					

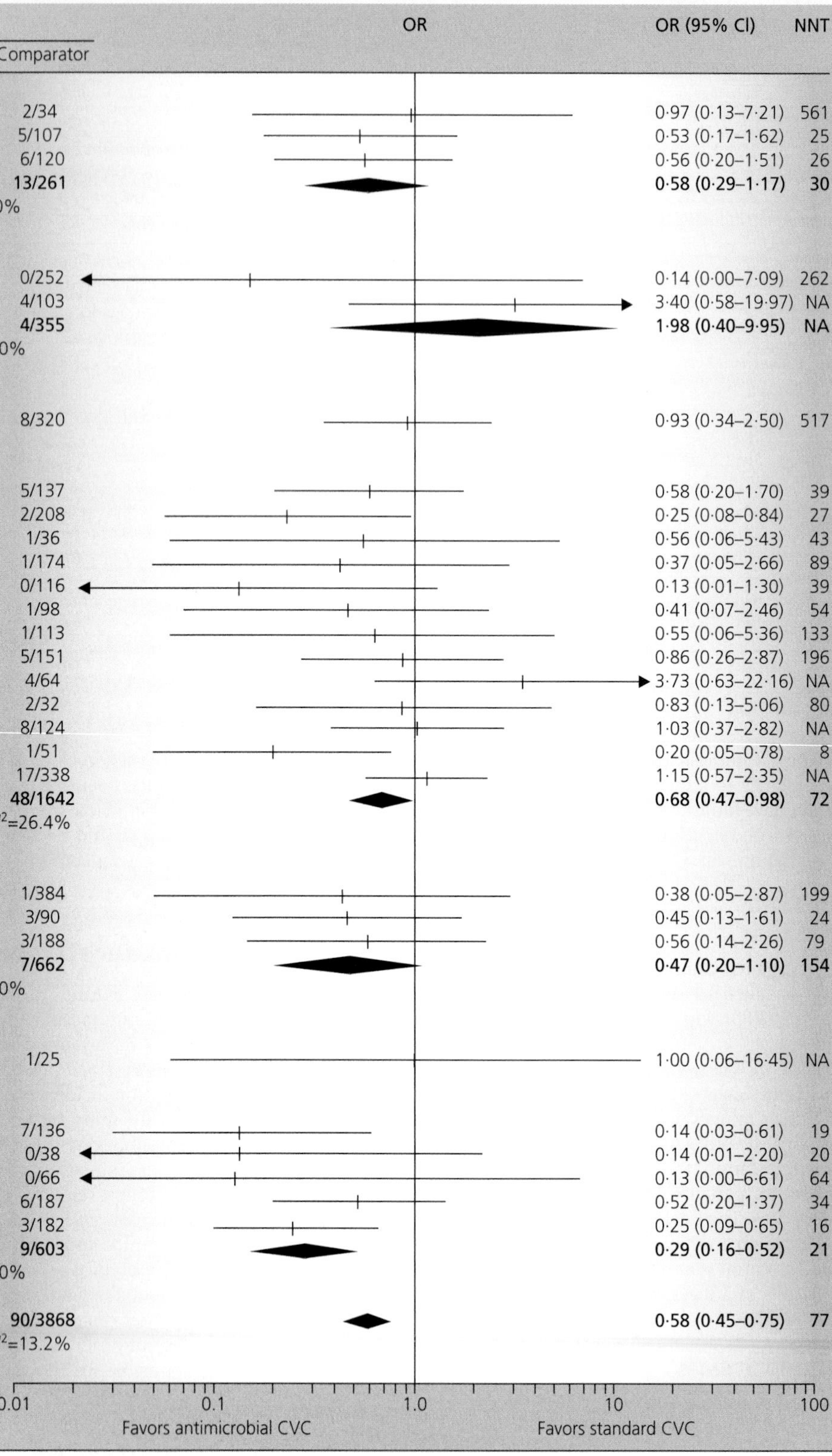

0.01   0.1   1.0   10   100

Favors antimicrobial CVC   Favors standard CVC

Fig. 45.4 Catheter-related bloodstream infection in trials comparing antimicrobial central venous catheters (CVCs) with standard CVCs. From Casey et al.[33] Reprinted from the Lancet Infectious Diseases. Copyright Elsevier 2008.

sensitivity of 3% or less.[9] Removal of a catheter in response to a clinical suspicion alone in a febrile patient results in unnecessary removal in 70–80% of cases.[26] It is therefore preferable to make a diagnosis of catheter-related infection microbiologically, ideally while the catheter remains in place.

Diagnostic methods with the catheter *in situ*

In the absence of septic shock, a 'watchful waiting' approach has been shown in a randomized trial to be a safe alternative to immediate catheter removal in patients in intensive care.[40] The notable exception to this approach might be those patients where the consequences of missing a catheter-related infection are potentially more serious, such as in the presence of an intravascular foreign body.

In order to rule out the line as the source of an unexplained fever, diagnostic techniques with a high negative predictive value are required.

Culture of the skin insertion site or hub

Several studies have evaluated the role of culturing swabs taken from the skin around the catheter insertion site, and swabs of the catheter hub.[41–44] Routine surveillance cultures of these sites have failed to predict line sepsis and therefore, in the absence of clinical suspicion, these methods are unhelpful. However, several authors have noted that catheter-related bacteremia is uncommon when these cultures are negative (negative predictive value >90%[41,42,44]), and as such these samples may be useful in eliminating the line as a source in cases of unexplained fever.

Paired quantitative blood cultures

This method involves taking paired blood cultures simultaneously from the line and peripherally, and culturing each using a quantitative technique. If the blood culture taken from the line is positive with a colony count several times higher than that of the peripheral culture, it is predictive of catheter-related bloodstream infection.[1,45] When sepsis is not related to the catheter, the colony counts are similar from the two sites. Studies have reported different cut-off points of between 4- to 10-fold as being highly predictive of CRBSI; both the Infectious Diseases Society of America (IDSA) and the French Society of Intensive Care (SRLF)[11] have chosen a ratio of 5:1 for a positive diagnosis. A meta-analysis found paired quantitative cultures to be the most accurate test for diagnosis of catheter-related bloodstream infection, with sensitivity and specificity of 75% and 97%, respectively, for short-term lines and 93% and 100%, respectively, for long-term lines.[46] However, as this technique is labor intensive and expensive, it has not been widely adopted.

A single catheter-drawn quantitative blood culture yielding more than 100 colony forming units (cfu)/ml may be diagnostic without a paired peripheral culture, particularly when taken from tunneled catheters.[1] However, this method cannot distinguish between catheter-associated bacteremia and high-grade bacteremia from another source, and is associated with low sensitivity in short-term catheters.

Differential time to positivity of paired blood cultures

This technique is derived from the same concept as paired quantitative blood cultures as described above, but takes advantage of the fact that most diagnostic laboratories use automatic blood culture machines which detect 'time to positivity' on a continuous basis. The 'time to positivity' is inversely proportional to the initial inoculum[47] and can therefore be used as a less labor-intensive method of estimating differences in bacterial load between the two samples. When a blood culture taken from the CVC becomes positive at least 2 hours earlier than that taken peripherally, it is highly predictive of CRBSI. This method has been validated in oncology, hematology and

pediatrics.[47–51] Although paired culture techniques are more sensitive for long-term catheters, evidence exists to support their use in short-term lines also.[51] A meta-analysis found this technique to have a sensitivity and specificity of 89% and 87%, respectively, for short-term catheters and of 90% and 72%, respectively, for long-term catheters. Differential time to positivity is a relatively easy technique with minimal added costs. Difficulties may arise when insufficient blood can be aspirated via the line in order to carry out the culture, which may occur in up to a quarter of cases.[52]

Acridine orange leukocyte cytospin, endoluminal brush

Aspiration of a small (50–100 microliter) sample of blood from the catheter and direct examination using acridine orange leukocyte cytospin (AOLC) is a rapid diagnostic method, giving a result in 30–60 minutes. The sample is spun, stained with acridine orange and examined for the presence of bacteria using ultraviolet microscopy (Fig. 45.5). First evaluated favorably in neonates, in adults the sensitivity of this method has been very variable between studies.[53] The use of endoluminal brushing of the catheter prior to sampling has been proposed to increase sensitivity.[54] However, theoretical risks of embolization or induced bacteremia cannot be excluded. A study using AOLC followed by Gram staining reported a sensitivity of 96% and sensitivity of 92%.[55] Currently these techniques have not been widely adopted and require further investigation.

Diagnostic methods requiring line removal

Qualitative culture of catheter tip

Older methods of qualitative culture of the catheter tip in liquid broth were oversensitive and did not distinguish infection from colonization or contamination, and have been abandoned.

Semiquantitative culture of catheter tip

Semiquantitative culture (roll plate) of the catheter tip, described by Maki *et al.* in 1977,[56] is one of the most widely used methods of

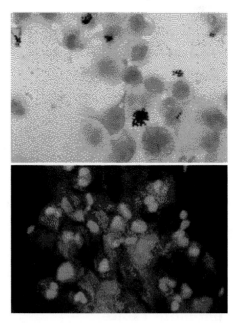

Fig. 45.5 Examples of Gram stain and acridine orange leukocyte cytospin (AOLC) tests positive for septicemia. Top: Gram-positive staphylococci (*Staphylococcus aureus*); bottom: stained with acridine orange (*Candida albicans*). Red and green cells are leukocytes. From Kite *et al.*[55] Copyright Elsevier 1999.

catheter culture. The distal catheter segment is rolled across the surface of an agar plate and incubated for 24–48 hours; the presence of more than 15 cfu was found to correlate with local signs of inflammation in the patients studied, most of whom had short-term peripheral catheters rather than CVCs. A meta-analysis examined 14 trials of this method in short-term central venous catheters and found pooled sensitivities and specificities of 84% and 85%, respectively.[46] A significant limitation of this method is that it only analyses the extraluminal portion of the catheter. The accuracy of this technique in diagnosing CRBSI in long-term CVCs, for which the intraluminal route of colonization is more important, is of concern, with sensitivity reportedly as low as 45%.[34]

Quantitative culture of catheter tip

Several quantitative methods have been described. Flushing of the catheter tip with broth examines only the internal surface. Vortexing the catheter tip in 1 ml sterile water as described by Brun-Buisson et al.[57] allows the release of organisms from both the internal and external surfaces of the catheter. A threshold of 10^3 cfu/ml correlated with systemic signs of infection, with or without catheter-associated bacteremia, and exhibited high specificity (88%) and sensitivity (97%) in critically ill patients. An alternative method using sonication of the catheter tip in broth gave similar results.[58] Quantitative culture of catheter segments was more accurate than roll plate and qualitative methods in a receiver operating characteristic (ROC) curve analysis.[59] Pooled sensitivity and specificity of quantitative segment culture for short-term catheters was 82% and 89%, respectively, and 83% and 97%, respectively, for long-term catheters in a meta-analysis.[46]

Direct examination of catheter tip

Gram staining or acridine orange staining of the catheter tip appears to offer good sensitivity and specificity but is labor intensive and time consuming and has not been widely adopted.

MANAGEMENT

Line removal

In the presence of septic shock, without an alternative source, the line should be removed and empiric antibiotics commenced. Other indications for early line removal include deep localized infection such as tunnel infection, frank cellulitis, pocket infection or port abscess. Catheter-related infections caused by S. aureus or Candida spp. are associated with high failure rates if treatment is attempted with the line still in place, and therefore line removal is recommended when these organisms are implicated.[1] The same is probably true of Pseudomonas and possibly other aerobic Gram-negative bacteria. Catheter infections complicated by septic thrombosis, endocarditis or osteomyelitis also require line removal. When dealing with tunneled or surgically implanted lines, it is clearly particularly important to make every attempt to confirm the diagnosis of catheter-related infection in order to avoid unnecessary line removal. In the case of coagulase-negative staphylococci, treatment with prolonged antibiotics plus lock therapy may be successful without line removal. Some authors have also reported the success of this approach with other organisms, provided no complications are present, in cases where line salvage is required.[1]

Empiric antibiotic choice

Antibiotics for suspected catheter-related infection are often started empirically. The choice of antibiotic will depend on clinical severity and risk factors in an individual patient. Direct staining of a catheter insertion site swab, or of the catheter itself, may help guide therapy.[60]

Although evidence is lacking to support a particular choice of antibiotic combination for empiric treatment, usually a glycopeptide is chosen, due to the high prevalence of resistant Gram-positive organisms in these infections. The addition of broad spectrum Gram-negative (including pseudomonal) cover is appropriate in cases of severe sepsis or immunocompromise.[1] Antibiotics can then be rationalized when culture results become available.

Antibiotic choice and duration

Limited evidence exists regarding optimal duration of antibiotic treatment for CRBSI; suggestions below are based on consensus opinion as outlined in the guidelines of the IDSA.[1]

Coagulase-negative staphylococci

Coagulase-negative staphylococci, being skin commensals, are the commonest cause of catheter-related infection but also the commonest contaminants. In order to confirm the diagnosis of coagulase-negative staphylococcal CRBSI, at least two positive blood cultures, of which one should be from a peripheral sample, are needed.[34] If the line has been removed, and the patient lacks risk factors for complicated disease (such as a prosthetic graft), a short course of 5–7 days of antibiotic is likely to be sufficient.

If it is preferable that the line be retained, and the patient lacks risk factors for complicated disease, it is reasonable to try treatment with the line in situ. Eighty percent of CRBSI caused by coagulase-negative staphylococci may be successfully treated without catheter removal, with a 20% chance that bacteremia will recur.[61] The IDSA guidelines recommend a 10–14-day course of systemic antibiotic and antibiotic lock therapy for non-tunneled lines or 7 days of systemic antibiotic followed by 14 days of lock therapy for tunneled lines.

Staphylococcus aureus

Staphylococcus aureus is associated with a higher rate of complicated or metastatic infection, such as septic thrombosis or endocarditis. The duration of treatment will depend on the likelihood of such complications. Persistence of fever and/or bacteremia at 72 hours after catheter removal and antibiotic initiation is predictive of complicated disease.[34] A study examining the use of transesophageal echocardiography in patients with S. aureus bacteremia made a diagnosis of endocarditis by Duke Criteria in 23% of patients.[62] The use of transthoracic echocardiography was associated with a sensitivity of just 32%. The authors, and the IDSA guidelines, recommend transesophageal echocardiogram in all patients with S. aureus bacteremia, and the extension of treatment to 4–6 weeks when this complication is present.[1] For treatment of seemingly uncomplicated S. aureus bacteremia, not less than 14 days of treatment following catheter removal is recommended.[1,63] In selected cases where salvage of a tunneled line is required, in the absence of complications and with a negative transesophageal echo, the IDSA guidelines suggest 14 days of systemic antibiotics plus lock therapy.

Gram-negative bacilli

The incidence of Gram-negative intravascular catheter infections may be increasing. They are a relatively common cause of CRBSI in immunocompromised patients with long-term tunneled catheters and of infections associated with contaminated infusate.[1] Retrospective studies have shown high rates of relapse if the catheter is not removed;[64,65] however, anecdotal success has been reported with systemic antibiotics plus antibiotic lock therapy for salvage of tunneled catheters.

Candida species

All cases of catheter-related candidemia should be treated with systemic antifungals to avoid the complication of sight-threatening candidal endophthalmitis.[1] Several prospective studies have identified catheter retention as a risk factor for persistent candidemia or increased mortality.[34] Failure to remove the catheter was associated with poorer response to antifungals in a large retrospective study of patients with cancer, provided the candidemia was catheter related.[66] However, in cases of noncatheter related candidemia, catheter removal had no effect on outcome. Clinical characteristics that suggested a noncatheter source for the candidemia included disseminated infection at diagnosis, recent chemotherapy and neutropenia; characteristics that implicated the catheter included isolation of *Candida parapsilosis*, paired blood culture techniques supportive of a catheter source of candidemia, and parenteral nutrition.

Fluconazole at a dose of 400 mg/day has been shown to be as effective as amphotericin in non-neutropenic patients with candidemia, with less associated toxicity.[67] Fluconazole may therefore be used for susceptible isolates.[1] For empiric treatment before speciation and sensitivity results are available, amphotericin B is recommended in hemodynamically unstable patients or those who have received prolonged fluconazole therapy. Otherwise, empiric treatment with fluconazole is recommended.[1] Catheter-related *Candida krusei* infections should be treated with amphotericin B.[1] Non-tunneled CVCs should be removed; in the case of a tunneled line it is important to determine if the candidemia is catheter related or secondary to another source such as the gastrointestinal tract. If the catheter is confirmed as the source, it should be removed. Duration of treatment should be for 14 days after the last positive blood culture and when signs and symptoms of infection have resolved.[1]

Treatment of a positive catheter tip culture without bacteremia

There is a lack of evidence to guide the management of positive catheter tip cultures without definite evidence of bacteremia. IDSA guidelines suggest that it is not usually necessary to treat; however, if *S. aureus* or *Candida* spp. are isolated, particularly in the context of risk factors such as valvular heart disease or prosthetic graft, patients should be watched closely for evidence of persistent infection and blood cultures should be taken. Some experts would advocate a short course (5–7 days) of antimicrobial treatment.

Complications

Persistence of fever and/or bacteremia 72 hours after catheter removal and initiation of appropriate antibiotics should prompt a thorough search for complicated or secondary infection including septic thrombosis, endocarditis and osteomyelitis. This is particularly important in the case of *S. aureus* infection. If a secondary source of infection is found, antibiotic treatment will need to be prolonged, usually to a minimum of 4–6 weeks. Superficial septic thrombosis may also necessitate excision of the vein; septic thrombosis of the great central veins and arteries requires anticoagulation in addition to antibiotic treatment.[1]

Antibiotic line locks

The technique of line locking involves instilling antibiotics at high concentration (>100 times the minimum inhibitory concentration of the organism) at sufficient volume to fill the lumen of the catheter, and leaving them in place for a period of several hours or even days while the catheter is not in use (such as overnight). *In-vitro* studies have demonstrated that these higher concentrations of antibiotics are needed to kill sessile bacteria growing in a biofilm,[8] and *in-vivo* studies have shown higher rates of successful catheter salvage using antibiotic locks in addition to systemic treatment when compared with systemic antibiotics alone.[1] Antibiotics that can be used in this way include vancomycin, teicoplanin, gentamicin or amikacin, usually for a duration of 2 weeks. Attempts to use antifungals in this way have been less successful and are not recommended. Lock therapy is unlikely to be successful if extraluminal infection is present and as such the role of this approach with short-term or recently inserted lines is uncertain.

Infections of Arterial Grafts

INTRODUCTION

Reconstructive surgery of occluded or aneurysmal arteries may involve the implantation of either an autologous vein graft or a prosthetic graft. Graft infection, more common with prosthetic grafts, is a much feared complication which may lead to limb loss or death.

EPIDEMIOLOGY

The risk of arterial graft infection varies with the site of the graft, with higher rates associated with lower limb revascularization and lower rates in aortic graft replacement (Table 45.5). Many patient or operative factors may influence the risk of infection, including diabetes, prolonged operating time, malnutrition and lower limb infection at the time of surgery (Table 45.6).

PATHOGENESIS

Early graft infection (during the first 30 days) is relatively uncommon and usually secondary to early groin or lower limb wound infection. Lower limb graft infection more commonly presents beyond 4 months, and aortic graft infection may present years later.[69] Intraoperative contamination of the graft with skin flora may occur in as many as 56% of arterial grafts,[70] implying this as the likely route of acquisition for the majority of graft infections. Contiguous spread from local wound infection or hematogenous spread from a distant site (such as an infected intravascular catheter) may also occur. Once present, micro-organisms can adhere to the graft and form biofilms similar to those seen in catheter-related infection. In this way they can evade the immune system and antibiotic activity, making treatment without graft removal extremely difficult.

Staphylococci, predominantly *S. aureus*, are the most commonly implicated pathogens, with *S. aureus* being responsible for up to 55% of all deep wound and graft infections in the UK.[71] Around 70% of *S. aureus* isolated from vascular surgical-site infections are methicillin resistant.[71] Gram-negative bacteria account for to up to one-third of such infections and anaerobes may be implicated in patients with ischemic tissue. Early infection is more likely to be caused by *S. aureus* or Gram-negative organisms, with less virulent organisms such as coagulase-negative staphylococci, enterococci and streptococci being implicated in late infection.

Table 45.5 Rates of infection by location of arterial graft	
Location of arterial graft	**Rates of infection (%)**
Thoracic aorta	1.2–3.0
Aortoiliac	0.0–1.3
Aortofemoral	0.5–3.0
Femorofemoral	3.6–5.0
Femoropopliteal	2.0–4.6
Axillofemoral	5.3–6.0
Cervical	0.0–0.2
Adapted from Goëau-Brissonnière & Coggia.[68]	

Table 45.6 Patient, procedure and environmental risk factors for surgical site infection

Patient-related risk factors	Nasal carriage of *Staphylococcus aureus* Prolonged preoperative length of stay Postoperative bacteremia End-stage renal disease Obesity Malnutrition/low serum albumin Older age Smoking, nicotine use Diabetes mellitus Prior incision site irradiation Malnutrition/low serum albumin Autoimmune disease/corticosteroid therapy Malignancy and chemotherapy
Procedure-related risk factors	Femoral/groin incision Remote infection Biomaterial implant Emergency/preoperative procedure American Society of Anesthesiology score >2 Extended operative time Hypothermia Shock Hyperglycemia
Environmental risk factors	Operating suite ventilation – environmental surface cleaning Instrument and vascular implant sterility Surgical attire and sterile operative technique

From Bandyk.[69] Copyright Elsevier 2008.

PREVENTION

Prior to elective vascular surgery, every attempt should be made to reduce a patient's individual risk factors for infection. Diabetic control and nutritional state should be optimized, and local or distant sites of infection eradicated or minimized.

Despite being classified as clean procedures, the additional risk associated with the implantation of prosthetic material justifies the use of prophylactic antibiotics in vascular surgery. A meta-analysis has examined 35 randomized controlled trials of preventive measures in arterial surgery.[72] Prophylactic systemic antibiotics reduced the risk of wound infection and early graft infection by between three-quarters and two-thirds (RR 0.25 and 0.31, respectively). Prophylaxis continued beyond 24 hours was not associated with any additional benefit. Other interventions including preoperative bathing or showering with antiseptic agents or suction groin-wound drainage lacked evidence of effectiveness. No benefit was demonstrated from the use of rifampin (rifampicin)-impregnated grafts in preventing either early or late graft infection.

First- or second-generation cephalosporins or co-amoxiclav are commonly used for prophylaxis in vascular surgery. The increasing prevalence of methicillin-resistant *S. aureus* (MRSA) and high rates of methicillin resistance among coagulase-negative staphylococci has raised the question as to whether glycopeptides should be added to prophylaxis regimens. Routine use of glycopeptides has not generally been adopted, in part due to concern that this would promote the emergence of glycopeptide resistance among enterococci and staphylococci. However, their use in high-risk patients has been advocated, for example in patients with a history of MRSA colonization or infection, or in settings with a high prevalence of methicillin-resistant staphylococci.[63,73,74] However, a threshold defining 'high prevalence' has not been well established. Wide use of MRSA screening and subsequent decontamination has been recommended in the UK, including preoperatively for all elective surgery.

CLINICAL FEATURES

Early infection will often present with local signs of cellulitis, purulent drainage or wound dehiscence in combination with systemic signs of sepsis. Early infection with virulent organisms may quickly progress to pseudoaneurysm formation and hemorrhage, whereas more indolent infection may present with cutaneous sinus tracts or graft thrombosis. Late infection of aortic grafts will more typically present with unexplained fever or bacteremia, but may present with catastrophic gastrointestinal hemorrhage from aortoenteric fistula formation.

DIAGNOSIS

Before empiric antibiotics are started, at least two blood cultures should be taken. The presence of fluid collections around the graft is highly suggestive of graft infection, although it may be a normal finding in the early postoperative period. Deep fluid collections should be aspirated for culture, preferably prior to antibiotic treatment in a hemodynamically stable patient. Fluid cultures may, however, be negative in cases of infection caused by less virulent organisms such as coagulase-negative staphylococci. Imaging with contrast CT may show failure of the graft to become incorporated into adjacent tissues, perigraft fluid or gas, pseudoaneurysm formation, focal bowel wall thickening or intragraft thrombus[75] (Fig. 45.6). Nuclear medicine scans are unhelpful in the early postoperative period when they are likely to be falsely positive, but may be useful in difficult late cases. Sinography, in which contrast is injected into a cutaneous sinus, may show tracking of dye along a non-incorporated infected graft.[75] Ultrasound may be used to identify infrainguinal pseudoaneurysm formation or graft thrombus.

MANAGEMENT

With few exceptions, the management of arterial graft infection is surgical. Intravenous antibiotic therapy is initiated preoperatively and usually continued for a minimum of 4–6 weeks postoperatively.

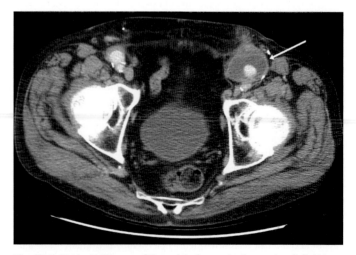

Fig. 45.6 Contrast CT scan of the pelvis demonstrating perigraft fluid in a patient with an infected left-sided aortoiliac graft (arrow).

In patients who are profoundly septic on presentation, empiric antibiotics should cover the range of nosocomial pathogens, for example combining a glycopeptide with an antipseudomonal penicillin, to be rationalized in the light of positive culture results.

Options for surgical intervention

Choice of surgical intervention must consider the location of the graft, extent of infection, virulence of the organism, options for preserving distal perfusion and a patient's likely ability to tolerate the proposed procedure.

For infrarenal aortic grafts, the gold standard approach has been total excision of the graft with bypass through a noninfected (extra-anatomic) site, most often axillobifemoral, to restore distal perfusion. Risks of this approach include stump blowout, bypass thrombosis and graft re-infection.[75] Graft excision and *in-situ* replacement with a prosthetic graft has greater patency but, as would be expected, higher rates of re-infection, and is generally only recommended as a holding procedure in low-virulence infections. Attempts at replacement with fresh or cryopreserved aortic allograft have been disappointing. *In-situ* replacement with an autogenous vein graft carries a lower risk of re-infection (although this may still occur in the context of virulent Gram-negative pathogens), but disadvantages include longer operative time,

and risks of deep vein thrombosis, lower limb paresis and edema, and the need for fasciotomy. A meta-analysis of surgical options for low-virulence infections of aortic grafts[76] questioned whether extra-anatomic bypass should remain the gold standard, as *in-situ* replacements were associated with fewer adverse events. However, the authors comment that drawing such conclusions may be misleading, given the broad clinical spectrum of graft infection and individual patient subgroups that may benefit from one approach over another.

For infrainguinal graft infection, complete excision is usually required, with either *in-situ* replacement with autogenous vein graft or extra-anatomic prosthesis. Successful management without graft removal has been described in selected patients, using surgical debridement of the graft bed followed by the placement of a muscle flap.[77]

REFERENCES

References for this chapter can be found online at http://www.expertconsult.com

Myocarditis and pericarditis

Myocarditis

EPIDEMIOLOGY

The term myocarditis applies to a variety of disease states that produce inflammation of the myocardium. In its acute form, myocarditis ranges from an asymptomatic illness with reversible changes to fulminant myocardial necrosis and death. In its chronic form, lymphocytic infiltration of the myocardium may cause subacute deterioration of cardiac function; indeed, chronic myocarditis may predate the development of 'idiopathic' dilated cardiomyopathy (IDC). The possible association between viral myocarditis and IDC is intriguing and potentially important. Although frequently ascribed to inflammation caused by an infectious agent, myocarditis may also be seen in allergic reactions, drug reactions and in association with systemic inflammatory disease. A diagnosis of acute infectious myocarditis is suggested when unexplained heart failure or malignant arrhythmias occur in the setting of a systemic febrile illness or after symptoms of an upper respiratory tract infection.

The incidence of infectious myocarditis in the general population is unknown. In a prospective study of Finnish military recruits conducted over several years, a mean annual incidence of 0.02% was found.[1] The prevalence of clinically significant myocarditis is higher in children and young adults than in older adults, and is thought to be a major cause of sudden cardiac death in adults under the age of 40 years.[2-4] Within immunosuppressed patients, myocarditis is more prevalent, affecting approximately 50% of AIDS patients at autopsy.[5]

PATHOGENESIS AND PATHOLOGY

In myocarditis, damage to cardiac myocytes appears to involve one or more of four possible mechanisms:
- direct cytopathic effects of an infectious agent;
- cellular injury secondary to circulating exogenous or bacterial toxins;
- specific cell-mediated or humoral immunologic response to the inciting agent or induced neoantigens; and
- nonspecific cellular injury caused by generalized inflammation.
Histologically, both myocyte necrosis and infiltration by inflammatory cells in the absence of ischemia are pathognomonic of the disease. The infiltrate may be composed of a variety of cell types, including neutrophils, lymphocytes, macrophages, plasma cells, eosinophils and/or giant cells (Fig. 46.1).

The pathologic abnormalities associated with myocarditis vary considerably depending on the etiologic agent and individual host response. Coxsackie virus, for example, appears to infect cardiac myocytes directly

while infection with parvovirus B19 appears to involve the vascular endothelium. The time after infection when tissue is obtained for analysis also greatly influences the histologic appearance. In acute enteroviral myocarditis, for example, few inflammatory cells may be seen, whereas cellular infiltrates are the hallmark of chronic enteroviral myocarditis. Analysis of endomyocardial biopsy specimens obtained during infection with different agents shows considerable overlap, however. Thus, a histologic diagnosis of myocarditis usually does not indicate the agent responsible.

Bacteria

Bacteria may cause myocarditis by a variety of mechanisms. Bacteremia caused by a wide variety of species may result in metastatic foci within the myocardium. Myocarditis has been noted in association with streptococcal and staphylococcal bacteremia, meningococcemia, bartonellosis, brucellosis, leptospirosis and Whipple's disease. However, the resulting myocardial dysfunction is only clinically significant in a subset of patients with overwhelming infections. In contrast, myocardial involvement in bacterial endocarditis is more common and is often clinically significant. Bacteria (especially *Staphylococcus aureus*) may directly invade the myocardium from infected valves to cause abscesses, valvular failure and conduction abnormalities, or may embolize throughout the myocardium to cause global ventricular dysfunction. Cardiac infections caused by salmonellae are particularly serious; mural involvement responds poorly to antimicrobial agents and, without surgical therapy, mortality is 100%.

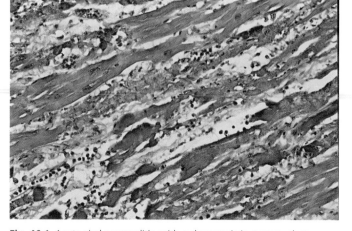

Fig. 46.1 Acute viral myocarditis, with a characteristic mononuclear infiltrate.

Bacterial toxin production can also be clinically significant. Subtle evidence of toxin mediated myocarditis can be detected in as many as two-thirds of patients who have diphtheria, occurring 1–2 weeks after the onset of illness, often when the oropharyngeal manifestations are improving.[6] Patients who have electrocardiogram (ECG) changes of myocarditis have a mortality rate three to four times that of patients who have normal tracings, with atrioventricular nodal and left bundle branch block carrying a mortality rate of 60–90%.[7]

Finally, cardiac involvement (including myocarditis) occurs in up to 50% of cases of acute rheumatic fever (ARF). Pancarditis (e.g. endocarditis, myocarditis and pericarditis) in cases of ARF is likely the result of an overexuberant host immune reaction to upper respiratory tract infection with rheumatogenic strains of group A streptococci. 'Molecular mimicry' (e.g. immunologic cross-reactivity to cardiac antigens elicited by streptococcal products) underlies the postulated pathogenesis of this disease, as investigators have failed to demonstrate the presence of streptococci within inflammatory cardiac lesions.

Spirochetes

Spirochetes such as *Borrelia burgdorferi*, the etiologic agent of Lyme disease, are important causes of myocarditis with cardiac manifestations occurring in approximately 8% of patients.[8] The cardiac manifestations of Lyme disease may occur in an isolated manner, or coincident with other features such as erythema chronicum migrans or neurologic abnormalities. The most prevalent abnormality is fluctuating atrioventricular block, but some patients have evidence of more diffuse myopericardial involvement. Indeed, organisms have occasionally been demonstrated in endomyocardial biopsy tissue both pre-mortem[9] and at autopsy,[10] providing supportive evidence for direct spirochetal invasion. Myocardial involvement is common in cases of fatal leptospirosis (Weil's disease), where arrhythmias or acute circulatory collapse may occur in conjunction with hepatorenal or central nervous system syndromes. At autopsy, myocardial inflammation, coronary arteritis and aortitis are common findings.

Gummatous involvement of the myocardium during late syphilis is an exceedingly rare cause of myocarditis. Cardiac manifestations reported in the literature include conduction abnormalities and myocardial infarction usually involving the left ventricle at the base of the interventricular septum with destruction of myocytes and replacement with fibrous tissue.[11]

Rickettsiae

Rickettsiae produce systemic vasculitis by endothelial invasion, which not infrequently involves the myocardium. Rocky Mountain spotted fever (caused by *Rickettsia rickettsii*) and scrub typhus (caused by *R. tsutsugamushi*) infections may cause transient cardiac dysfunction in severe illness, which invariably clears with disease resolution. *Coxiella burnetii* (the agent of Q fever) is a rare cause of myocarditis, but this may progress to heart failure and death.[12]

Parasites

Several parasites are known to cause chronic myocarditis and sustained myocardial dysfunction, primarily in the developing world. Chagas disease (American trypanosomiasis), widely distributed in Central and South America, is caused by the protozoan *Trypanosoma cruzi*. The organism enters the human host via the bite of the reduviid bug. Rarely, patients develop fever, myalgias, hepatosplenomegaly and myocarditis during acute infection, when myocardial parasites are abundant. Far more common is the development of biventricular failure from chronic myocarditis, which occurs in 30% of infected individuals. In chronic Chagas disease the heart is enlarged and microscopic evidence of focal mononuclear cell infiltrates is commonly found, despite the fact that parasites may be demonstrated in only a minority of patients. A history of residence in Central or South America should increase clinical suspicion for this pathogen.

Assessment of epidemiologic exposure is also essential for the diagnosis of *Trichinella spiralis*, an important parasite with worldwide distribution that has been linked to fatal myocarditis. Myocarditis generally develops in severe infections, in which the cardinal features of periorbital edema, myositis, fever and eosinophilia are present. Recent consumption of poorly cooked pork enhances the likelihood of this diagnosis. Other parasites and/or their ova, including *Ascaris*, *Schistosoma* and *Taenia solium*, may lodge in the myocardium during their systemic phase. The presence of eosinophilia in the context of acute heart failure should prompt a search for their presence, although eosinophilia is an important distinguishing factor for patients who have hypersensitivity myocarditis and hypereosinophilic syndrome as well.

Viruses

Viral infections are the most common cause of myocarditis in the Western world (Table 46.1). The enteroviruses (Coxsackie A and B, echovirus) have historically been regarded as the most common cause of viral myocarditis. However, the increasing use of molecular techniques such as polymerase chain reaction (PCR) have implicated other viral pathogens such as parvovirus B19 and human herpesvirus 6 (HHV-6). In a recent study from Germany, parvovirus B19 and HHV-6 were the most frequently isolated viruses in a cohort of 87 patients with viral myocarditis, accounting for 56% and 18% of infections, respectively.[13] In addition, the persistence of these viral genomes within the myocardium may play a role in the progression of acute viral myocarditis to dilated cardiomyopathy.[14–16] Earlier studies using molecular techniques suggest that 18–53% of patients who have myocarditis or IDC may have persistent enteroviral infection.[17]

Until recently, evidence of a causal link between enterovirus infection and myocarditis was primarily circumstantial, since many patients report an antecedent viral syndrome.[18,19] Observations of increased enteroviral antibody titers or a fall in convalescent titers have been offered as further evidence that enteroviruses are the causative agents. Unfortunately, these infections are common in the general population and it has been difficult temporally to associate serologic changes with changes in cardiac function. In one study it was found that 34% of patients who had IDC had Coxsackie virus B titers of 1:40, but the same incidence was found in control individuals.[20] However, if a cutoff antiviral titer of 1:1024 was used, 30% of patients who had IDC were abnormal as compared with 2% of control individuals.[21] Viral culture from myocardial biopsies has not been revealing.

Given the lack of confirmatory culture or serologic data, animal models of viral myocarditis have been constructed to demonstrate the pathogenicity of the enteroviruses. Murine models of acute Coxsackie B viral myocarditis demonstrate viral attachment, myocyte penetration and subsequent viral replication, with resulting scattered foci of cellular necrosis. This initial phase terminates with viral clearance by mononuclear cells and the expression of proinflammatory cytokines, including tumor necrosis factor and interferon gamma (IFN-γ).[22–24] The chronic phase of infection is characterized by the presence of macrophages and T cells, not replicating virus, within myocardial tissue.[25–27] Interestingly, depletion of T cells prevents the later stages of myocardial injury although replicating virus persists within the myocardium after T-cell depletion.[28] These experiments highlight the importance of T cells in the perpetuation of myocardial injury although the antigens to which they are directed remains unknown.

Immunocompromised patients

Immunocompromised patients are subject to the same infections as the immunocompetent; however, their risk for clinically significant myocarditis is higher than in the general population, and they are uniquely at risk for opportunistic pathogens. In end-stage AIDS, as many as 10% of patients will have clinically significant cardiomyopathy.[29] The increasing use of highly active antiretroviral therapy has led to a significant decrease in the incidence of this type of cardiac

Table 46.1 Infectious causes of myocarditis

Region	Normal host		Immunocompromised host
Developed world	Common and/or important	Viruses: Coxsackie viruses (A and B), human herpes virus 6, influenza echovirus, cytomegalovirus (CMV), Epstein–Barr virus (EBV), influenza viruses (A and B), adenovirus, parvovirus B19, hepatitis B virus, hepatitis C virus Bacteria: *Corynebacterium diphtheriae*, *Borrelia* spp., any organism associated with infective endocarditis Parasites: *Trichinella spiralis*, *Trypanosoma cruzi*	Viruses: HIV, CMV, EBV, varicella-zoster virus (VZV), adenovirus, parvovirus Fungi: *Candida, Aspergillus, Cryptococcus* Parasites: *Toxoplasma gondii, Trypanosoma cruzi*
	Uncommon	Viruses: adenovirus, parvovirus, respiratory syncytial virus, hepatitis B virus, ?hepatitis C virus Bacteria: staphylococci, streptococci, meningococci, *Salmonella, Listeria, Clostridium, Rickettsia, Bartonella, Ehrlichia, Campylobacter jejunii*	Fungi: *Histoplasma, Blastomyces, Coccidioides imitis*, zygomyces
Developing world		Viruses: poliovirus, mumps virus, rubella virus, arenaviruses, dengue virus, rabies virus, chikungunya virus, Ebola virus, yellow fever virus Bacteria: *Leptospira* spp. Parasites: *Trypanosoma cruzi, Trypanosoma gambiense*	

involvement in patients with HIV.[30] In a study of 33 patients infected with HIV who underwent cardiac biopsy, specific DNA hybridization demonstrated HIV in five out of 33 patients and cytomegalovirus (CMV) in 16, suggesting that cardiotropic viral infections may be important in pathogenesis.[31] Although HIV itself has been cultured from heart tissue[32] and shown to be present by *in-situ* hybridization,[33] it is only rarely present in cardiac myocytes in patients with demonstrable pathology. Thus, whether the virus itself causes heart failure, sets the stage for other cardiotropic pathogens, or is a correlate for the causative nutritional wasting present in late stage AIDS is unknown. In children with AIDS, myocarditis is perhaps even more common postmortem than in adults, and may be associated with different pathogens; in one study, adenoviruses were detected in over 30% of hearts with histologic evidence of myocarditis.[34] Both *Cryptococcus neoformans*[35] and *Toxoplasma gondii*[36] are also important opportunistic causes of myocarditis in the setting of advanced HIV disease.

Other disseminated fungal infections (such as disseminated candidiasis, aspergillosis and histoplasmosis) or viral infections such as herpes simplex virus or varicella-zoster virus may also present with myocarditis in the immunocompromised patient, but can usually be identified by associated findings. Cytomegalovirus is an important pathogen in solid organ and hematopoietic stem cell transplant recipients with myocarditis. In heart transplant recipients, CMV infection is a risk factor for a form of immune-mediated cardiac rejection that presents as accelerated coronary atherosclerosis; importantly, prophylactic ganciclovir significantly reduces the incidence of this complication.[37] Finally, the role of CMV in myocarditis of immunocompetent patients is also intriguing; a recent study found intramyocyte CMV DNA in 14% of patients who had myocarditis but none was found in control individuals.[38]

A wide variety of other diseases may cause myocardial inflammation. Important noninfectious causes of myocarditis are listed in Table 46.2.

CLINICAL FEATURES

The clinical expression of acute myocarditis ranges from an asymptomatic state to rapidly progressive myocardial dysfunction and death. Complaints on presentation may include fever, fatigue, malaise, chest pain, dyspnea and palpitations; arthralgias and upper respiratory tract

Table 46.2 Noninfectious causes of myocarditis

Connective tissue disorders	Systemic lupus erythematosus, rheumatoid arthritis, systemic sclerosis, dermatomyositis, polymyositis,
Idiopathic inflammatory/ infiltrative disorders	Kawasaki disease, sarcoidosis, giant cell myocarditis
Insect and arachnid stings	Wasp, scorpion, spider stings
Medications	Cocaine, ethanol, arsenic, cyclophosphamide, daunorubicin, adriamycin, sulfonamides, tetracycline, methyldopa
Post-irradiation myocarditis	
Peripartum myocarditis	
Pheochromocytoma	
Thrombotic thrombocytopenic purpura	
Thyrotoxicosis	

symptoms may be associated with viral myocarditis, but are nonspecific. Chest pain may be vague, pleuritic (suggesting pericardial involvement) or angina-like. The majority of patients, however, have no precordial discomfort.

Physical examination may reveal tachycardia out of proportion to the height of fever or degree of heart failure. Cardiac auscultation may be unrevealing, or may demonstrate muffled heart sounds, extra beats, transient murmurs or loud ventricular gallops; friction rubs are uncommon and indicate pericardial involvement. In severe cases, signs of congestive heart failure (CHF) are present, and pansystolic apical pulses may be palpated.

The electrocardiographic manifestations of myocarditis are usually transient and occur far more frequently than clinical myocardial involvement. Indeed, mild asymptomatic myocardial involvement diagnosed by serial electrocardiographic changes was present in over

1% of military conscripts with acute viral syndromes. ST segment elevation and T wave inversions may be seen acutely, and reflect the focal nature of the myocardial inflammation. These changes usually return to normal within 2 months. Atrial and ventricular arrhythmias are common in severe cases. Atrioventricular nodal or intraventricular conduction defects denote involvement of the conduction system and suggest more widespread disease or specific etiologies (e.g. Lyme carditis). Although usually transient and without sequelae, complete heart block may cause sudden death in these patients. Routine radiologic examination demonstrates cardiomegaly and pulmonary vascular congestion in severe cases.

DIAGNOSIS

The clinical diagnosis of myocarditis is often difficult and requires a high index of suspicion. When unexplained heart failure or malignant arrhythmias occur in the setting of an acute febrile illness, the clinical diagnosis of infectious myocarditis is suggested. Heart failure of recent onset mandates that the physician first consider ischemic, valvular, primary pulmonary or congenital disease in the differential diagnosis. Other causes of acute myocardial dysfunction, such as rheumatologic disease, endocrinopathies, electrolyte disturbances and toxin exposure (e.g. ethanol, cocaine and heavy metals), must also be ruled out.

Electrocardiogram changes are important ancillary findings but, given the high incidence of nonspecific ST segment and T wave changes seen in acute viral syndromes, they alone are often non-diagnostic. Similarly, laboratory abnormalities such as leukocytosis and an elevated erythrocyte sedimentation rate are also nonspecific. Serum creatinine phosphokinase (CPK) elevations, on the other hand, do signify acute myocardial injury and thus are very important. Unfortunately, these elevations do not differentiate the cause of that injury (i.e. ischemic versus inflammatory). Myocardial enzyme release parallels myocyte necrosis, as in small-to-moderate myocardial infarctions. However, in contrast to ischemic necrosis, in which CPK levels return to normal within 72 hours, elevated CPK levels may persist for 6 days in myocarditis.[39] The CPK-MB is elevated in 70% of patients who have myocarditis and ST segment elevation on ECG, but is usually normal if only T wave changes are present. Although serum assays for troponin T (a cardiac contractile protein) offer greater specificity for myocardial damage and persist for 2–3 days longer than CPK-MB determinations, they also are not specific for myocarditis.

Echocardiography is a valuable tool in the initial evaluation of the patient and in follow-up. Echocardiograms in myocarditis commonly show variable degrees of cardiac dysfunction, often with striking focal wall motion abnormalities. Dyskinesia or akinesia is most often biventricular. Furthermore, the test may eliminate other anatomic causes of CHF and may demonstrate the presence of ventricular thrombi or pericardial effusions. Echocardiographic changes generally resolve within a few days in parallel with the clinical course; if progressive ventricular dysfunction is demonstrated, chronic myocarditis may be suggested.

Many other imaging modalities for diagnosing acute myocarditis have been studied. However, validation of these diagnostic tools has been challenging in the absence of a reliable gold standard. Cardiovascular magnetic resonance (CMR) is able to distinguish between the different etiologies of myocardial damage, including myocarditis, ischemic heart disease and other cardiomyopathies, as well as assessing ventricular volume and function.[40] The high spatial resolution and contrast used in CMR allows for small areas of myocardial injury to be identified, which is useful for diagnosis of myocarditis since it usually presents as focal or patchy inflammation of the ventricles. Though safe and non-invasive, CMR cannot be used in patients with pacemakers or defibrillators. In addition, cost, availability and expertise continue to limit its widespread use in the clinical setting.

Despite advances in imaging techniques, endomyocardial biopsy is still considered the reference technique for diagnosis of myocarditis. However, it remains limited by the lack of sensitivity and specificity along with its invasive nature. Even in post-mortem specimens with proven myocarditis, the probability of diagnosing myocarditis based on the Dallas criteria (see below) with one biopsy was only 17–28%, which increased to approximately 67% with more than five biopsies.[41-43] Because the inflammation involves both ventricles, a transvenous approach is generally employed in order to obtain a biopsy of the right ventricular septum. In experienced hands the procedure is relatively safe, although deaths have occurred. Biopsy studies in acute disease have generally been carried out in cases of fulminant myocarditis. Studies using serial biopsies have demonstrated findings similar to those seen in the murine model. In the majority of cases, histologic evidence of myocarditis has resolved 3–4 weeks after the onset of symptoms and late biopsy is therefore unhelpful.[44] Because of the focal nature of the disease, many practitioners have recommended obtaining four or five biopsies from different sites at initial catheterization. Repeat biopsies and/or left heart catheterization with biopsy have sometimes been necessary to establish the diagnosis firmly but increase the risk of complications such as ventricular wall rupture. In addition, the use of quantitative (qPCR) and qualitative (nested PCR) molecular techniques in conjunction with endomyocardial biopsies has increased the ability to detect viral genomes. However, due to the uncertainty regarding the number of biopsy specimens required to attain clinical sensitivity, a positive PCR result is diagnostic while a negative PCR does not exclude viral disease.[45]

Disagreement among pathologists regarding histopathologic interpretation of specimens has also been problematic. A working standard, termed the Dallas criteria, is now used by the majority of investigators to define the disease.[44]

- Active myocarditis is defined as 'an inflammatory infiltrate of the myocardium with necrosis and/or degeneration of adjacent myocytes not typical of the ischemic damage associated with coronary heart disease'.
- Borderline myocarditis is present when infiltration is sparse, or when cardiac myocytes are infiltrated with leukocytes, but associated myocyte necrosis is not present; myocarditis cannot be diagnosed in the absence of inflammation.
- The absence of myocarditis indicates normal myocardium or pathologic changes of a noninflammatory nature (fibrosis, atrophy, hypertrophy).

The adoption of the Dallas criteria has led to 90% concordance among experienced pathologists. Application of the criteria in the Multicenter Treatment Trial for Myocarditis (MTT) suggests that the prevalence of 'active myocarditis' in patients who have recent onset (<12 months) CHF is approximately 10%;[46] a recent study demonstrated identical findings.[47] However, these patients are qualitatively different from those who have acute infectious myocarditis in which fever and acute ECG changes are present. They are best characterized as having IDC with myocardial inflammation.

The rationale for the development of the Dallas criteria was to identify patients prospectively who were likely or unlikely to benefit from immunosuppressive therapy. Given the results of the MTT (see below), many physicians have called into question the utility of the endomyocardial biopsy. In selected cases, however, the biopsy can provide valuable clinical data. Rarely, a biopsy will identify specific disease processes (i.e. toxoplasmosis, CMV, giant cell myocarditis, trichinosis, sarcoidosis) for which specific therapy is available or for which a prognosis can be given (i.e. Pompe's disease, amyloidosis). Because the prognosis in most cases of acute myocarditis is favorable (and an etiology is rarely discovered in cases of cardiomyopathy of gradual onset), we believe that the endomyocardial biopsy is unnecessary for the majority of patients with suspected myocarditis. Notable exceptions include transplant recipients and patients who have AIDS, for whom the discovery of a treatable etiology is more likely. In the setting of progressive clinical deterioration (such as arrhythmias or heart failure refractory to standard therapy) in which the diagnosis is unknown, endomyocardial biopsy should also be considered.

Thus, the approach for the immunocompetent patient who has acute myocarditis should focus on the management of CHF and its complications (see below). A thorough history (with attention to epidemiologic detail) and physical examination will unearth the majority of nonviral etiologies, in which signs and symptoms other than CHF frequently dominate the clinical picture. In the febrile patient, blood cultures should be obtained. Serologic testing for HIV should always be performed given the high prevalence of myocarditis in patients with AIDS; testing for Lyme disease, Chagas disease and autoimmune diseases should be performed in the appropriate clinical context. A complete blood count with differential should be performed to rule out eosinophilia (which may suggest parasitic infection or hypersensitivity myocarditis). Testing for CMV in blood is unlikely to be helpful because CMV reactivation in the presence of unrelated acute febrile illnesses is relatively common. Although enteroviruses are prominent pathogens, routine use of acute and convalescent enteroviral titers adds little to clinical management. Noninvasive testing for enteroviruses and adenoviruses by serum PCR is possible (although not widely available), but studies have not been performed to demonstrate that this information affects outcome. Perhaps future advances in virology and molecular biology coupled with targeted antiviral therapy will provide more options for the diagnosis and treatment of myocarditis; for now, however, the majority of cases remain classified as 'idiopathic' and are treated expectantly.

MANAGEMENT

The natural history of acute infectious myocarditis is quite variable, although the majority of cases run a benign, self-limited course. Acute cardiac dysfunction does not predict chronic impairment, as most of these individuals demonstrate normalization of laboratory, echocardiographic and histologic parameters within 1 month of symptom onset. For this reason, supportive care in lieu of aggressive, invasive procedures is of primary importance.

General measures target CHF, arrhythmias and other derangements associated with myocarditis. Animal models have demonstrated that exercise during viral myocarditis is associated with higher mortality and more extensive histologic damage; thus, bed rest may be important. Conventional therapy has included oxygen, diuretics, angiotensin-converting enzyme (ACE) inhibitors and beta-blockade, as for any patient who has CHF. Anticoagulation for patients who have intracardiac thrombi and/or severely depressed myocardial function is also important. In the murine model, early treatment with the ACE inhibitor captopril decreased left ventricular mass and myocardial necrosis, suggesting benefits above and beyond afterload reduction.[48] Randomized trials in humans have yet to be conducted, although afterload reduction appears safe and effective in other settings. Rarely, fulminant heart failure requires the use of inotropic support, intra-aortic balloon pumps or ventricular assist devices as a bridge to the resumption of cardiac function.[49] Unfortunately, there are no clinical or laboratory indicators to identify those patients who will spontaneously recover; indeed, patients who have fulminant myocarditis may have a better prognosis than those with acute, nonfulminant myocarditis.[50] For those who do not respond, cardiac transplantation is an option; however, patients who have myocarditis before transplantation have a significantly higher incidence of rejection and death in the first year.

As significant arrhythmias are probably associated with the majority of deaths in acute myocarditis, all hospitalized patients should be monitored on telemetry. Premature beats are common and do not require therapy. Supraventricular tachycardia, however, worsens heart failure and should be electrically converted. The use of anti-arrhythmic agents for high-grade ventricular ectopy has not been studied. Care should be exercised with any antiarrhythmic agent (including digoxin, which has a low threshold for toxicity in these patients) but sustained ventricular arrhythmias should be treated aggressively. Complete heart block is an indication for temporary venous pacing. The condition often resolves without a need for permanent pacemaker placement.

If a specific infection is identified (such as Lyme or staphylococcal carditis), antimicrobial therapy should be directed at the causative

pathogen. As noted above, viruses are the likely cause of most cases of myocarditis, but patients who have putative viral myocarditis most commonly present after viral replication has ceased. Murine models of CMV-induced myocarditis confirm that ganciclovir or cidofovir improves outcomes in the acute (<24 hours) phase of infection, but are ineffective later.[51] Pleconaril is a novel compound that has antiviral activity against the enteroviruses (including Coxsackie viruses A and B) and thus has potential for treating the most common etiology of myocarditis. Clinical response was favorable in three-quarters of patients treated in one report,[52] but high rates of spontaneous recovery make conclusions speculative. Antiviral therapy with interferon-α for patients with enterovirus-induced myocarditis has also been studied.[53]

Contrary to expectations, most studies of immunosuppressive therapy such as prednisone, azathioprine and ciclosporin have not favorably influenced outcome. A meta-analysis evaluating 316 patients enrolled in five trials demonstrated no benefit of immunosuppressive therapy as compared to placebo or conventional therapy in terms of the pooled outcome of all-cause death and heart transplantation (odds ratio 1.03; 95% confidence interval 0.58–1.80).[54] Similarly, although multiple case reports and case series have documented successful treatment of acute myocarditis with intravenous immunoglobulin (IVIG), this difference was not observed in the only randomized controlled trial comparing IVIG to placebo for treatment of acute myocarditis in 62 patients. Treatment with IVIG showed no benefit in terms of improvement in cardiac function, survival, or need for a left ventricular assist device or transplant.[55] Trials evaluating the use of immunosuppression and other treatment strategies are needed, but are inherently difficult to perform given the low incidence of acute myocarditis, difficulty in diagnosis and the low rate of events such as death or need for cardiac transplant.

Pericarditis

EPIDEMIOLOGY

Interest in the pericardium dates to antiquity. The writings of Homer and Maximus relate the history of the 'hairy hearts of heroes' such as Aristomenes, the legendary Messinian warrior; his heart was cut out in battle and found to be 'stuffed with hair', probably the first recorded case of fibrinous pericarditis. Significant understanding of the etiology and pathophysiology followed, from Galen's first pericardial resection in the 2nd century AD to Lower's classic description of tamponade, constrictive pericarditis and pulsus paradoxus in the 17th century. Medical advances in antibiotic therapy, surgical technique, antineoplastic therapy and hemodialysis have substantially altered the spectrum and prognosis of pericardial disease in the 21st century. Imaging modalities have also made a significant impact; since the advent of echocardiography in 1955, pericardial effusions are now readily diagnosed. The etiologic determination of pericardial disease, however, remains difficult. Timely, directed therapy depends in large part on the diligence of the clinician.

The incidence of pericardial inflammation detected in several autopsy series ranges from 2% to 6%, whereas pericarditis is diagnosed clinically in only about 1 out of 1000 hospital admissions. The relative frequency of each etiologic process depends upon the clinical setting. Thus, viral or idiopathic pericarditis often presents in the outpatient clinic, whereas malignant or uremic effusions are more frequently seen in referral centers.

PATHOGENESIS AND PATHOLOGY

The human pericardium forms a strong, flask-shaped sac that encloses the heart and the origins of the great vessels. It is composed of a fibrous outer layer and an inner serous membrane formed by a single layer of mesothelial cells. This membrane is attached to the surface of the heart to form the visceral pericardium; it reflects upon itself, lining the inside of the collagen-based fibrous layer to form the parietal pericardium. The visceral pericardium continuously produces a clear pericardial fluid, which serves as a lubricant; it is also the source of excess fluid in disease states. The human pericardium normally contains up to 50 ml of this fluid, which drains via the thoracic and right lymphatic duct into the central circulation. Pericardial effusion may develop in response to pericardial injury (as in pericarditis) or may be secondary to other processes that alter the secretion and drainage of pericardial fluid. The pathologic changes seen in acute pericarditis are those of nonspecific inflammation with cellular infiltration, fibrin deposition and the outpouring of pericardial fluid. These changes may resolve spontaneously over time, or may organize with fibrous adhesions between the epicardium and visceral pericardium, the visceral and parietal pericardium, or the pericardium and adjacent sternum and pleura (Fig. 46.2). Thus, inflammation, fluid exudation and fibrin organization account for the cardinal manifestations of pericarditis: chest pain, pericardial effusion and constriction.

The causes of this pericardial inflammation are numerous, including both infectious (Table 46.3) and noninfectious (Table 46.4) etiologies.

Noninfectious agents

The three most prevalent noninfectious causes of pericardial disease are malignancies, uremia and connective tissue disorders.

- Neoplasms may cause pericarditis or effusions by direct involvement of the pericardium (in which malignant cells are usually demonstrated within pericardial fluid) or by obstruction of the pericardial lymphatic drainage (with resulting 'benign' effusions).
- Uremic pericarditis, which affects up to 20% of patients on chronic hemodialysis, is characterized by the appearance of a shaggy, fibrinous exudate without cellular infiltration.
- Collagen vascular diseases (most commonly systemic lupus erythematosus and rheumatoid arthritis) are notable for their propensity to involve the pericardium; immune complex deposition is thought to be primary in the pathogenesis of pericardial disease.

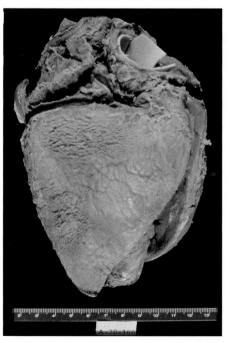

Fig. 46.2 Heart at autopsy of a patient who had acute suppurative pericarditis. The parietal pericardium has been stripped from the specimen, revealing a 'bread and butter' appearance.

Table 46.3 Infectious causes of pericarditis

Viruses	Mycobacteria
Cytomegalovirus Herpes simplex virus Coxsackie A virus Coxsackie B virus Echovirus Adenovirus Influenzavirus Mumpsvirus Varicella-zoster virus Epstein–Barr virus HIV	*Mycobacterium tuberculosis* *Mycobacterium chelonae* *Mycobacterium avium* complex
	Spirochetes *Borrelia burgdorferi*
Bacteria *Streptococcus pneumoniae* *Streptococcus* spp. *Staphylococcus aureus* *Neisseria meningitidis* *Listeria monocytogenes* *Haemophilus influenzae* *Francisella tularensis* *Brucella melitensis* Enteric Gram-negative rods *Actinomyces* spp. *Nocardia asteroides* *Legionella pneumophila* *Tropheryma whipplei* *Salmonella* spp. *Campylobacter* spp. *Rickettsia/Coxiella burnetii*	Mycoplasma *Mycoplasma pneumoniae* *Ureaplasma urealyticum* *Mycoplasma hominis*
	Fungi *Histoplasma capsulatum* *Coccidioides immitis* *Cryptococcus neoformans* *Blastomyces dermatiditis* *Candida* spp. *Aspergillus fumigatus*
	Parasites *Toxoplasma gondii* *Entamoeba histolytica* *Echinococcus granulosus* *Schistosoma* spp.

Table 46.4 Noninfectious causes of pericarditis

Idiopathic
Connective tissue disorders
Acute rheumatic fever, systemic lupus erythematosus, rheumatoid arthritis, scleroderma, mixed connective tissue disease, Wegener's granulomatosis, polyarteritis nodosa, temporal arteritis
Metabolic
Uremia, hypothyroidism
Malignancies
Lung cancer, breast cancer, leukemia, lymphoma, melanoma, others
Acute myocardial infarction
Post-myocardial infarction syndrome (Dressler syndrome)
Dissecting aortic aneurysm
Traumatic
Chest trauma, postsurgical hemopericardium, pacemaker insertion, cardiac catheterization, esophageal rupture, pancreatic–pericardial fistula
Post-irradiation
Idiopathic infiltrative/inflammatory disorders
Sarcoidosis, amyloidosis, inflammatory bowel disease, Behçet's disease, familial Mediterranean fever
Medications
Procainamide, hydralazine, isoniazid, phenylbutazone, dantrolene, doxorubicin, dilantin, methysergide, minoxidil

Infectious agents

A variety of microbes have been reported to cause pericarditis. Chief among these are viruses, which can produce a clinical syndrome of myopericarditis, but often other infectious agents are also implicated.

Viruses

The most common etiologies of viral pericarditis include Coxsackie A and B, echovirus type 8, adenovirus and HIV (see Table 46.3). As is the case for myocarditis, these viruses have only rarely been isolated from pericardial fluid or tissue; as such, evidence for viral causation of pericardial inflammation is primarily based upon isolation of virus from other sites, such as stool, and by demonstration of a fourfold rise in serum antibody titers. Most recently, PCR testing has found evidence of adenovirus, enterovirus and CMV in pericardial fluid and tissue from patients with acute pericarditis.[56]

Bacteria and other infectious agents

Bacteria may cause pericarditis by a number of different mechanisms. Hematogenous seeding of the pericardium may occur during the course of bacteremia caused by a variety of organisms. In the pre-antibiotic era, most cases of purulent pericarditis were seen as complications of bacteremia or pneumonia. Today, extension of infection from a contiguous focus within the chest is seen as a postoperative or post-traumatic complication. Subdiaphragmatic abscesses may also cause pericardial infection by direct extension. Highly invasive bacterial infections within the heart, such as acute staphylococcal endocarditis, may erode into the pericardium from a perivalvular abscess to cause purulent pericarditis. Pericardial effusions in patients who have subacute infective endocarditis provide another mechanism by which bacterial infection can lead to pericardial disease. Pathologic changes in the pericardium are caused by immune complex deposition, resulting in sterile exudates. Although common, these effusions are not correlated with prognosis, and most resolve without specific therapy.

The microbiology of bacterial pericarditis continues to evolve (see Table 46.3). Before antibiotics, uncontrolled pneumococcal, streptococcal or staphylococcal pulmonary infections were most frequently implicated. Streptococci and staphylococci remain important pathogens today (particularly in traumatic and post-thoracotomy pericarditis), with Gram-negative bacilli, atypical bacteria and *Candida* also assuming important roles. Pericardial involvement has also been documented in the course of such illnesses as tularemia, brucellosis, salmonellosis, legionellosis, meningococcal disease and Q fever.[57] In children, bacteria cause proportionately more cases of pericarditis than is the case in adults; *Staph. aureus* and *Haemophilus influenzae* are the most common etiologic agents.

Pericarditis caused by *Mycoplasma* spp. deserves special mention. Although pericarditis has been recognized in the course of *Mycoplasma* disease since 1944, culture of the organism has proved difficult. Therefore, autoimmune phenomena have been invoked to explain the association. In one report, *Mycoplasma pneumoniae*, *M. hominis* and *Ureaplasma urealyticum* were isolated from pericardial fluid and/or tissue cultures in five patients with large pericardial effusions.[58] Treatment with doxycycline after drainage of the effusions resulted in complete resolution in all five cases. Pericarditis caused by *Mycoplasma* spp. is thus more common than previously recognized, and fluid obtained for culture should always be analyzed for the presence of these organisms.

Mycobacteria continue to be important causes of acute pericarditis, pericardial effusion and constrictive pericarditis, particularly in developing countries. The incidence of tuberculous pericarditis among patients who have pulmonary tuberculosis ranges from 1% to 8%.[59] While the overall incidence of tuberculous pericarditis has significantly declined in the United States, countries with a high prevalence of tuberculosis and HIV such as South Africa continue to have a higher burden of disease. In a study from the Western Cape province of South Africa, tuberculous pericarditis was the most common cause of pericardial effusions and accounted for 69.5% of the 233 cases of pericardial effusion. Of note, 50% of patients in this study were HIV positive.[60]

Histoplasma capsulatum is the most common cause of fungal pericarditis; in large outbreaks, pericarditis was noted in 6% of patients who had symptomatic histoplasmosis. It most commonly develops as a noninfectious inflammatory response that resolves spontaneously without therapy. Occasionally, seeding of the pericardium occurs in the course of disseminated infection. In contrast, pericarditis has only rarely been reported in cases of severe coccidioidomycosis.

In the severely immunosuppressed or post-thoracotomy patient, infection caused by *Candida* spp., *Aspergillus fumigatus* or *Cryptococcus neoformans* has occasionally resulted from either fungemia or direct inoculation.

Pericarditis in AIDS

In contrast to other immunocompromised states, pericardial disease in patients who have AIDS is quite common. Effusions are frequently noted in end-stage AIDS (occurring in 16–40% of patients) and are associated with a poor prognosis. Etiologies include a variety of pathogens (including viruses, bacteria, fungi and mycobacteria), although in the majority of cases no causative agent can be defined. Malignant effusions secondary to lymphomatous involvement of the pericardium have also been noted. Furthermore, although extrapericardial disease suggested specific infectious or malignant etiologies in 55% of patients who had pericardial effusions in one trial, these assumptions proved incorrect for all those in whom pericardiocentesis was performed.[61]

CLINICAL FEATURES

Acute pericarditis is most often recognized by its chief presenting manifestation: chest pain. The pain is usually precordial or retrosternal, often with radiation to the trapezius ridge or neck; it is exacerbated by lying supine, coughing or deep inspiration, with relief upon sitting upright or forward. The patient's discomfort may be caused by inflammation of the adjacent pleura, accounting for the pleuritic component that often accompanies the pain. This pain is distinguished from the pain of myocardial ischemia by its quality, its duration (pain may last for days without therapy) and the absence of associated factors (i.e. pain is unchanged with exertion or rest). Patients may also report that splinting reduces the pleuritic discomfort.

A pericardial friction rub is the pathognomonic physical finding of acute pericarditis. Characterized as scratchy or grating, it is best appreciated along the left sternal border with respirations suspended and the patient leaning forward. The classic friction rub has three components, corresponding to atrial systole, ventricular systole and the rapid ventricular filling phase of early diastole, although one or more of these phases are usually absent. Of note, the friction rub frequently waxes and wanes in intensity and may disappear altogether with the accumulation of fluid within the pericardial sac. The pericardial rub may again become prominent in tamponade, in which the pericardium rubs against the adjacent pleura.

Pericardial effusions range from the asymptomatic to those causing cardiac tamponade. The rate of fluid accumulation is a major determinant in physiologic manifestations. When the effusion develops slowly, the pericardium may stretch to accumulate as much as 2 liters of fluid. The normal pericardium, however, can accommodate the rapid accumulation of only 100–200 ml of fluid before signs and symptoms of tamponade develop. Patients may then complain of dyspnea or a dull retrosternal ache, and examination will reveal jugular venous distension, the most common physical finding in acute tamponade. A fall of 10 mmHg or more in systolic blood pressure during inspiration (the pulsus paradoxus) is recognized as a hallmark of critical cardiac tamponade, although it may be absent if hypotension is already present.

effusions, characteristic ECG changes are often absent. Cardiac arrhythmias are uncharacteristic in isolated pericardial disease; their presence implies myocardial involvement. The ECG typically evolves through four stages during acute pericarditis.

- Diffuse ST-segment elevation (usually concave up) with reciprocal ST depression in aVR and V1 accompanies the onset of chest pain and is virtually diagnostic of pericarditis; these findings are present in 50% of patients who have acute pericarditis.[62] PR depression in the inferolateral leads is frequently seen in this stage (Fig. 46.4).
- ST and PR segments normalize, typically several days later.
- Diffuse T wave inversions develop, generally after ST segments become isoelectric.
- Electrocardiograph changes normalize; long-term inversion of T waves suggests 'chronic' pericarditis.

Elevated CPK and troponin I levels are common in cases of acute pericarditis. Whether this signifies clinically relevant myocardial changes has not been adequately evaluated.

DIAGNOSIS

A number of studies have established the utility of using a stepped approach.[63] One study prospectively evaluated 231 consecutive patients who had acute pericardial disease of unknown cause.[64] Pericardiocentesis was performed in patients who had tamponade, suspicion of purulent pericarditis or symptoms and/or effusion persisting for more than 1 week after initiation of nonsteroidal anti-inflammatory drug (NSAID) therapy. Pericardial biopsy was undertaken if clinical activity persisted at 3 weeks and the etiology was unknown. Despite this extensive evaluation, a specific diagnosis was confirmed in only 32 patients: neoplasia in 13, tuberculosis in nine, rheumatic disease in four, purulent pericarditis in two, toxoplasmosis in two and viral pericarditis in two. Diagnostic yield was substantial when pericardiocentesis or biopsy was performed to relieve tamponade, but poor when used solely for diagnostic purposes. Over a mean follow-up of 31

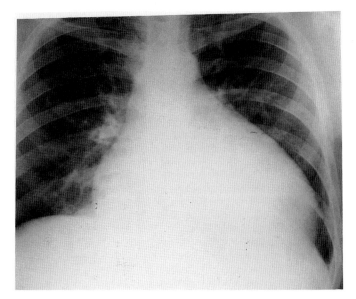

Fig. 46.3 Cardiomegaly in a patient who has pericarditis. The presence of a 'water-bottle' heart on this plain film suggests a large pericardial effusion.

Enlargement of the cardiac silhouette on routine radiography does not usually occur until at least 250 ml of fluid have accumulated in the pericardial space. Other findings on chest radiogram, such as a 'water bottle' heart (Fig. 46.3) or a prominent fat stripe sign, are found only in large pericardial effusions; their absence does not rule out the presence of a hemodynamically significant effusion. Chest radiograms may also provide etiologic clues for pericardial disease, such as pneumonic infiltrates or mediastinal adenopathy.

Electrocardiographic changes in acute pericarditis imply inflammation of the pericardium. Thus, in uremic or neoplastic pericardial

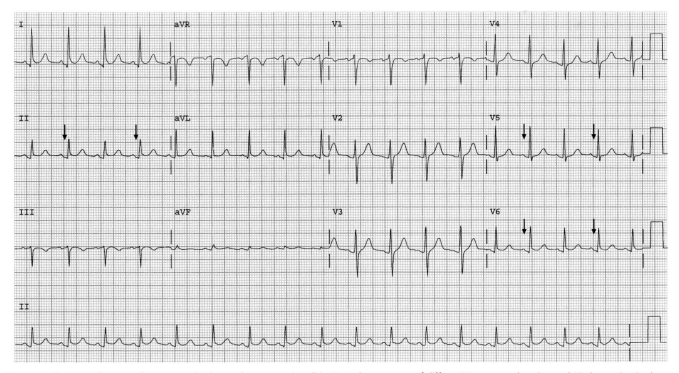

Fig. 46.4 Electrocardiogram of a patient who has early acute pericarditis. Note the presence of diffuse ST segment elevation and PR depression in the inferolateral leads (arrows). 25 mm/s; 10.0 mm/mV; F–W 0.05–100.

months, no patient diagnosed with idiopathic pericarditis and treated with NSAIDs showed signs of recurrent or chronic pericardial disease.

Because of the recent interest in subxiphoid pericardial biopsy and drainage of pericardial effusions, we recently undertook a prospective nonrandomized trial of all patients who had large pericardial effusions hospitalized at our institution. These patients underwent a similar stepped preoperative approach, with subsequent subxiphoid pericardial biopsy and drainage of their effusions.[65] Diligent handling and extensive microbiologic analysis (including cultures for aerobic and anaerobic bacteria, viruses, chlamydiae, mycoplasmas, fungi and mycobacteria) of pericardial fluid and tissue allowed specific diagnoses to be established in 53 out of 57 patients, confirming prior reports of high diagnostic yield when stepped algorithms are used for large effusions. More than one-third of the patients had malignancy or a history of irradiation to the thorax for malignancy. Infections (mostly viral), collagen–vascular disease and uremia were also frequently implicated (Table 46.5). Unexpected pathogens included CMV in three patients, herpes simplex virus 1 in one, *M. pneumoniae* in two, *Mycobacterium avium* complex in one and *Mycobacterium chelonei* (see Table 46.3) in one patient. No patient showed evidence of Coxsackie A or B viral infection. Comparison of this study with two other important series shows a significant variation in etiologies as a result of different populations, diagnostic strategies and investigator interests (i.e. infectious disease specialist versus cardiologist).

A comparison of diagnostic yield between pericardial fluid and biopsy demonstrated that fluid analysis was far more sensitive for malignancy; tissue provided additional information only in infected patients in whom fluid was not available for analysis. Previous studies demonstrated similar utility of pericardial fluid analysis; in a retrospective study of 93 cases of malignant effusion with both pericardial fluid and tissue analysis, cytology was correct in 87 cases (diagnostic accuracy 94%) with 100% specificity.[67]

In summary, acute pericarditis is most often viral or idiopathic in etiology; as such, invasive workups are usually not necessary. For the patient who has large effusions, tamponade or presentation suggestive of purulent pericarditis, early and aggressive intervention will often yield diagnostic and therapeutic rewards.

As noted previously, a wide variety of infectious and noninfectious agents can cause acute pericarditis and/or pericardial effusions (see Tables 46.1 and 46.2). For the patient presenting with acute chest pain, initial evaluation should focus on identifying conditions that may be rapidly fatal. Thus, myocardial infarction, aortic dissection, purulent pericarditis and cardiac tamponade should be systematically ruled out. An appropriate workup includes a thorough history and physical examination, ECG and chest X-ray (to rule out intrathoracic malignancy, tuberculosis or a widened mediastinum suggestive of aortic dissection) and routine laboratory studies including complete blood counts, serum chemistries, serial CPK with MB fraction determination, thyroid function tests, rheumatoid factor and antinuclear antibodies; blood cultures should be obtained for the febrile patient. Due to the serious consequences of untreated tuberculous pericarditis, a tuberculin skin test should be placed as well.

For the majority of individuals, a specific etiology will not be apparent, and a diagnosis of acute viral or idiopathic pericarditis will be made. Because either entity typically follows a brief and benign course, a full diagnostic evaluation is not appropriate. The confirmation of a particular viral agent is not necessary, as serologic titers and/or viral cultures are quite nonspecific, the workup is costly and a retrospective diagnosis is usually not helpful in management. Because significant pericardial effusion may accumulate even in idiopathic disease, however, all patients should be carefully evaluated for its presence; hemodynamic compromise on physical examination, cardiac enlargement on chest radiography or significant effusions on echocardiography necessitates rapid intervention. For patients who have large effusions, and for those in whom another diagnosis is suggested, a more thorough workup often includes pericardial drainage with or without pericardial biopsy.

As noted above, noninvasive diagnosis of pericardial disease in patients who have AIDS is extremely difficult. Because specific etiologic diagnosis often has important treatment ramifications, pericardial effusions in these patients should be managed on an individualized basis, with invasive diagnostic testing employed in those whose baseline health would benefit from aggressive therapeutic measures.

Echocardiography has largely replaced other methods for the detection of pericardial fluid. With experience, operators can detect as little as 20 ml of excess fluid posterior to the left ventricle. Echocardiography can also provide ancillary data in assessing the patient who has an effusion. Increased respiratory flow variation across the mitral valve with Doppler echocardiography is characteristic of cardiac tamponade. In addition, other etiologies of myocardial dysfunction such as left and right ventricular infarction can be ruled out. Finally, the echocardiogram can direct attempts at pericardiocentesis by identifying the location of pericardial fluid.

CT scans of the chest are primarily helpful in the diagnosis of pericardial thickening. Significant effusions are also readily demonstrated (Fig. 46.5). In addition, CT scans are more sensitive for the demonstration of small parenchymal nodules and mediastinal lymphadenopathy than is conventional radiography, and thus have clinical utility in the diagnosis of malignant pericarditis. Similarly, MRI may be useful in the non-invasive characterization of pericardial fluid as well as pericardial thickness.

Table 46.5 Etiology of large pericardial effusions[65]	
Etiology	**% of 75 diagnoses**
Malignancy	27
Viral	16
Collagen vascular disease	14
Radiation	11
Uremia	11
Mycobacterial	5
Mycoplasma	3
Bacterial	1
Idiopathic	5
Other	8

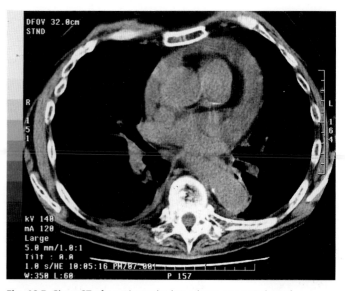

Fig. 46.5 Chest CT of a patient who has a large crescent-shaped pericardial effusion.

Cardiac catheterization is reserved for patients in whom pericardial constriction is believed to play a role in symptomatology. In those who have chest pain of undetermined etiology, catheterization is also useful for ruling out myocardial ischemia as a confounding diagnosis.

MANAGEMENT

Nearly all patients who have acute pericarditis should be hospitalized for relief of symptoms, diagnostic evaluation and observation for complications. Specific medical therapy is tailored to the cause of pericarditis. Aspirin, at doses of 2–6 g/day, or other NSAIDs are effective in reducing symptoms of pericarditis and are the agents of choice for idiopathic or viral pericarditis. Corticosteroids should be reserved for symptomatic nonresponders. Prednisone, however, is the drug of choice in pericarditis associated with connective tissue disease.

Idiopathic or viral pericarditis generally follows a benign, self-limited course but the occasional patient will present with recurrent pericardial pain. Treatment for recurrences generally begins with NSAIDs; corticosteroids have been used successfully for NSAID-resistant cases. Colchicine has shown promise as a steroid-sparing agent in a number of small trials.[70] Pericardiectomy for recurrent pericarditis should be reserved for those who fail medical therapy.[71]

Targeted intravenous antibiotics and surgical drainage of the pericardium remain the mainstays of therapy for purulent pericarditis. Pericardiocentesis urgently performed for the critically ill patient does not obviate the need for complete drainage and irrigation; fluid may reaccumulate rapidly and sequelae such as constriction may develop in hours. There is no rationale for intrapericardial antibiotic administration, as pericardial penetration of antibiotic is excellent.

Tuberculous pericarditis remains a diagnostic and therapeutic challenge. Clinical features are nonspecific, the disease course is confusing and laboratory evaluation is often nondiagnostic, particularly in low prevalence settings and in patients who have localized disease. For example, although large effusions are more likely to be tuberculous, up to 50% of tuberculous effusions resolve spontaneously despite ongoing tissue infection. The tuberculin skin test may be negative in up to 30% of patients as a result of cutaneous anergy yet may be positive in the patient who has acute idiopathic pericarditis and benign natural history. Suggestive, but not diagnostic, findings include a recent history of pulmonary tuberculosis, a positive sputum smear or culture or a high pericardial fluid adenosine deaminase level (>45 units/l).[72] Even granulomatous inflammation of the pericardium is not diagnostic, as this may be demonstrated in pericardial disease from other causes, such as histoplasmosis, sarcoidosis and rheumatoid arthritis. Additionally, a negative biopsy of the pericardium does not rule out tuberculous pericarditis, as removal of the entire pericardium may be necessary to demonstrate clear-cut evidence of tuberculosis.[73]

Definitive diagnosis rests upon the demonstration of the tubercle bacillus in pericardial fluid and/or tissue. However, the need for early therapy demands that treatment often be undertaken based upon a presumptive diagnosis. Initial treatment should consist of four drugs including isoniazid and rifampin (rifampicin) until sensitivities are known. The use of concomitant prednisone (at doses of 60 mg/day initially) to reduce pericardial inflammation is supported by two large controlled trials in Transkei, South Africa. Clinical improvement occurred more rapidly, 2-year mortality was lower (4 versus 11) and pericardiectomy was required less often (21% versus 30%) compared with those treated with four-drug therapy alone.[74] These data also highlight the incidence of constrictive complications in this disease. Complete pericardiectomy is advocated for those who have recurrent effusions or cardiac compression with constrictive physiology after 4–6 weeks of oral therapy. Such early pericardiectomy is associated with a good outcome; mortality is substantially higher in patients who undergo pericardiectomy at the late stage of calcific pericardial constriction.[75,76]

REFERENCES

References for this chapter can be found online at http://www.expertconsult.com

Endocarditis and endarteritis

INTRODUCTION

This chapter reviews infective endocarditis (IE) and other endovascular infections in the context of their evolving epidemiology, diagnostic tools and therapeutic strategies. These diseases are invariably lethal if not aggressively treated with antibiotics associated or not to surgery. Continuous developments in diagnostic criteria, including the use of echocardiography and molecular microbiology, have led to prompter disease recognition and therapy.[1] In spite of global improvements in health care, the incidence of IE has not decreased. Rheumatic heart disease, which was a primary risk factor for IE, has almost vanished from industrialized countries, but remains the primary risk factor in developing countries, where it is associated with poverty, crowding and poor health-care conditions[2] (see Chapter 48). In industrialized countries it is being replaced with new at-risk groups, including intravenous drug users (IVDU), elderly people with degenerative valves lesions, patients with health-care-associated conditions such as chronic dialysis, and patients who have intravascular prostheses.[3–5]

Whenever appropriate, the text and the figures in the chapter indicate the levels of recommendations and the levels of evidence for treatment suggestions, as summarized in Table 47.1.

Table 47.1 Levels of recommendations and levels of evidence for treatment suggestions

Classification of recommendations

Class I: Conditions for which there is evidence and/or general agreement that a given treatment is effective
Class II: Conditions for which there is conflicting evidence and/or divergence of opinion about the efficacy of a given treatment
- *Class IIa*: Evidence in favor of efficacy
- *Class IIb*: Efficacy not well established by opinion or evidence
Class III: Conditions for which there is evidence and/or general agreement that a given treatment is not effective and in some cases may be harmful

Level of evidence

Level of evidence A: Data derived from multiple randomized clinical trials or meta-analyses
Level of evidence B: Data derived from a single randomized trial or nonrandomized studies
Level of evidence C: Only consensus opinion of experts, case studies or standard of care

---

Adapted from European Society of Cardiology[24] and American Heart Association[38] guidelines.

EPIDEMIOLOGY

The overall incidence of IE has remained between 2 and 6 per 100 000 population per year over the last 30 years.[3–5] There is a persisting predominance in males, with a 1.5:1 to 2:1 male:female ratio. Mortality remains high, and ranges from 10% to more than 30%, depending on multiple factors including the type of organism (e.g. oral streptococci are less aggressive than *Staphylococcus aureus*), underlying conditions and whether the infection occurs on a native or a prosthetic valve. In one study, mortality of *S. aureus* prosthetic valve IE was reported to be as high as 47%.[6]

In parallel, risk factors and infecting micro-organisms are evolving. Chronic rheumatic heart disease is now rare in industrialized countries[5] (see Chapter 48), and formerly classic pathogens such as pneumococci and gonococci have become uncommon. Oral streptococci tend to remain predominant in the general population,[2,4,5] but *S. aureus* and coagulase-negative staphylococci (mainly *S. epidermidis*) have become predominant in IVDU, in prosthetic valve IE and in patients with health-care-related conditions,[3,7–9] and group D streptococci (mainly *Streptococcus bovis*, recently renamed *S. gallolyticus*) are increasingly prevalent in elderly patients and often related to colon tumors.[3–5]

Intravenous drug users involve mostly young individuals (mean age 30–40 years).[10] However, the other risk factors are more frequent in the elderly, and the mean age of patients with IE has progressively increased from 30 years in the 1950s, to 50 years in the 1980s and 55 to >60 years since the 1990s.[3,4,11,12] In one review totalizing 3784 episodes of IE between 1993 and 2003, the incidence of IE varied from <5 to >15 per 100 000 patients per year in individuals younger and older than 65 years, respectively.[3] The clustering of risk factors in elderly patients correlated with a more than three times increased incidence of IE in this group. Therefore, the results of different epidemiologic studies may vary according to the population analyzed.[5,9]

Infective endocarditis is commonly classified in four categories, which are discussed below:
- native valve IE (NVE);
- prosthetic valve IE (PVE);
- IE in intravenous drug users; and
- nosocomial (or health-care-related) IE.

Native valve infective endocarditis

Risk factors for NVE include congenital heart disease and acquired abnormalities such as chronic rheumatic heart disease and degenerative heart disease. People who have cardiac abnormalities that result in high-to-low pressure gradients are at greater risk of infection. Turbulent blood flow may provoke damage or peeling of the endothelium and formation of nonbacterial thrombotic vegetations. Circulating bacteria tend to adhere on the low-pressure side of such Venturi-like systems.

These observations explain why left-sided valves and left-to-right ventricular or arterial shunts are the most common sites of IE.

Congenital heart disease

Congenital heart disease is a lifelong risk factor. It is a major risk factor in children, in whom it accounts for 30–40% of IE.[13] Although a less frequent risk factor in adults, it still represents about 5% of IE cases.[14] This includes all of the cardiac abnormalities associated with turbulent blood flow. Tetralogy of Fallot carries the highest risk for IE, followed by bicuspid aortic valve, coarctation of the aorta and ventricular septal defect. In contrast, secundum atrial septum defects rarely put the patient at risk, probably because they result in a low-pressure shunt.

Surgical or medical closure of a patent ductus arteriosus usually eliminates the risk of endovascular infection. However, surgical correction does not exclude the risk of IE in patients suffering major congenital heart disease, such as tetralogy of Fallot.[14] The type of surgical correction may influence the risk of subsequent infection in this situation. In the largest long-term survey, involving 1142 patient years of observation, IE occurred in 23% of patients treated with anastomotic operations but in only 9% of patients treated with pulmonary valvulotomy or infundibular resection or both.[15] Vascular anastomoses are likely to generate turbulent blood flow, which might explain the greater risk of IE following anastomotic rather than plastic repair.

Rheumatic heart disease

Rheumatic heart disease was the most frequent acquired cardiac anomaly leading to IE in the pre-antibiotic era. In one series, the frequency of chronic rheumatic heart disease in patients who had developed IE decreased from approximately 22% between 1933 and 1952 to less than 1% between 1963 and 1972.[16] Although the prevalence of the disease has decreased to less than 10 per 100 000 population per year in industrialized countries, it remains the predisposing factor of IE in up to 50% of cases in certain developing countries.[2] Moreover, occasional clusters of rheumatic fever were recently described in the USA, and were linked to peculiar clones of group A streptococci.[17] Thus, rheumatic heart disease remains an important risk factor for IE.

Mitral valve prolapse

Mitral valve prolapse is a relatively common condition affecting 2–3% of the population. It has been associated with at least three autosomal-dominant inherited loci, located on chromosomes 11, 13, and 16.[18] Patients with valve regurgitation have a 10- to 100-fold increased risk of IE, and the risk of IE may be especially important in children and in patients over the age or 50 years.[19] Interestingly, mitral valve prolapse is associated with body leanness, lower blood pressure and lower prevalence of diabetes in American Indians. Thus, the inherited valve alteration is ironically associated with cardiovascular protective parameters, referring to as a Darwinian paradox.

Degenerative valve lesions

Degenerative valve lesions are present in up to 25% of patients aged over 40 years and in 50% of patients aged over 60 years with IE.[20] They involve local inflammation, micro-ulcers and microthrombi of the endothelium, which are quite similar to atherosclerosis. A recent echocardiography study identified degenerative valve lesions that might increase the risk of IE in up to 50% of patients aged more than 60 years.[21] This may explain, at least in part, the increased risk of IE in elderly individuals.

Prosthetic valve infective endocarditis

PVE occurs in 1–5% of cases, or 0.3–0.6% per patient years.[22,23] The issue of whether mechanical or bioprosthetic valves are more prone to infection remains unresolved.[22] PVE is usually classified as either early infection or late infection, depending on whether the symptoms of infection occur within 12 months after surgery or later.[24,25] This stratification is based on differences in the types of pathogen responsible for PVE during the two periods:

- early PVE implicates more often surgically related and drug-resistant microbes (e.g. methicillin-resistant staphylococci);
- late PVE implicates more often oral streptococci and sometimes Gram-negative bacteria of the so-called HACEK group (including *Haemophilus* spp., *Actinobacillus actinomycetemcomitans*, *Cardiobacterium hominis*, *Eikenella corrodens* and *Kingella kingae*).

The switch between these two periods is somewhat empiric and was formerly considered to be 2 months post-surgery. However, it was recently shown that the major shift from one type of organisms to the other occurred earlier than 12 months post-surgery.[25] Patients with a prosthetic valve implanted during active IE have a greater risk (up to seven times) of subsequent PVE than patients undergoing elective valve replacement, although the infection may be due to a different organism.

Infective endocarditis in intravenous drug users

Intravenous drug users and HIV patients constitute a special risk group of relatively young people, with a median age varying between 30 and 40 years.[10] However, they may progressively increase in elderly patients in coming years. Men are more often affected than women. The tricuspid valve is infected in more that 50% of cases, followed by the aortic valve in 25% and the mitral valve in 20%, with mixed right-sided and left-sided IE in a few cases. It has been suggested that repeated injections of impure drugs and particulate material might produce microtrauma to the tricuspid leaflets, thus facilitating microbial colonization and infection. However, 20–40% of intravenous drug users suffering IE have pre-existing cardiac lesions, often caused by previous valve infection. The responsible bacteria often originate from the skin, which explains the predominance of *S. aureus* infections (Table 47.2), but streptococci and other micro-organisms are also encountered; some pathogens, such as *Pseudomonas aeruginosa* and fungi, may produce severe forms of IE.

Immune deficiency related to HIV is a risk factor, as well behaviors associated with this particular at-risk group (e.g. alcohol intake and intravenous injections).[10] In one study, the risk of IE was unaffected in patients with >500 CD4 cells/mm³, but increased approximately fourfold in those with <200 CD4 counts. The mortality of IE was also higher in patients with AIDS, especially in advanced cases, than in other patients.[26]

Nosocomial (or health-care-related) infective endocarditis

Nosocomial IE is another growing category of patients. In a recent series it accounted for 22% of 109 cases overall, and 16% of cases excluding early PVE in cardiac surgery patients.[27] Many patients had debilitating underlying conditions, but less than 50% had obvious cardiac predisposing factors. In most circumstances a potential source of bacteremia could be identified, such as the presence of intravenous lines or invasive procedures. Pathogens usually originated from the skin or the urinary tract, staphylococci and enterococci being the most common. In one study, up to 13% of nosocomial *S. aureus* bacteremias were responsible for subsequent IE.[28] Moreover, possible right-sided IE was reported in 5% of bone marrow transplant recipients who had central venous catheters. Overall, mortality was up to 50%.

The general increase in health-care-associated IE was confirmed in recent surveys, where it represented more than 30% of all IE due to *S. aureus*, and in which chronic hemodialysis – which increased fourfold between 1993 and 1999 – was an independent risk factor.[8] As a result, it was recently proposed that a fifth category of 'hemodialysis-related IE' be added to the four categories of IE listed above.[29]

Table 47.2 Microbiology of IE in the general population and in specific at-risk groups

Pathogens	NO. OF EPISODES (% OF TOTAL)			
	Native valve	Intravenous drug abusers	Prosthetic valve	
			Early	Late
Staphylococci:	124 (44)	60 (69)	10 (66)	33 (45)
Staphylococcus aureus	106 (38)	60 (69)	3 (21)	15 (20)
Coagulase negative	18 (6)	0 (0)	7 (45)	18 (25)
Streptococci:	86 (31)	7 (8)	0 (0)	25 (35)
Oral streptococci	59 (21)	3 (3)		19 (26)
Others (non-enterococcal)	27 (10)*	4 (5)		6 (9)
Enterococcus spp†	21 (8)	2 (2)	1 (7)	5 (7)
HACEK group	12 (4)‡	0 (0)	0 (0)	1 (1.5)
Polymicrobial	6 (2)	8 (9)	0 (0)	1 (1.5)
Other bacteria	12 (4)§	4 (5)	0 (0)	2 (3)
Fungi	3 (1)	2 (2)	0 (0)	0 (0)
Negative blood culture	16 (6)	4 (5)	4 (27)	5 (7)
Total episodes	280 (100)	87 (100)	15 (100)	72 (100)

*Including 9 *S. agalactiae*, 6 *S. bovis* (renamed *S. gallolyticus*), 3 *S. pneumoniae*, 2 *S. pyogenes*, 1 group G streptococcus, and 1 *Abiotrophia* spp.
†Mostly (>80%) represented by *S. faecalis*.
‡Includes *Haemophilus* spp., *Actinobacillus actinomycetemcomitans*, *Cardiobacterium hominis*, *Eikenella corrodens* and *Kingella kingae*.
§Includes 4 *Escherichia coli*, 2 *Corynebacterium* spp., 2 *Proteus mirabilis*, 1 *Mycobacterium tuberculosis* and 1 *Bacteroides fragilis*.
Adapted from Moreillon & Que.[3]

PATHOGENESIS, PATHOLOGY AND INFECTING MICRO-ORGANISMS

The key issues in the pathogenesis of IE, discussed below, are:
- the predisposing host factors;
- the characteristics of the infecting micro-organisms;
- the role of transient bacteremia; and
- the inability of the immune system to eradicate micro-organisms once they are located on the endocardium.

Predisposing host factors

The normal valve endothelium is very resistant to colonization and infection by circulating bacteria. On the other hand, mechanical lesions of this endothelium result in exposure of the underlying extracellular matrix proteins, the production of tissue factor, and the deposition of fibrin and platelets as a normal healing process. Such nonbacterial thrombotic endocarditis is an ideal nidus for bacterial adherence and infection (Fig. 47.1) (reviewed in Moreillon *et al.*[30]).

Endothelial damage may result from mechanical aggression due to turbulent blood flow in cases of congenital cardiac abnormalities or prosthetic valves, or lesions provoked by electrodes or catheters. Alternatively, endothelial damage can result from inflammation, as rheumatic carditis or in elderly individuals with degenerative valve lesions, which involve inflammation, micro-ulcers and micro-thrombi.[20,21] It was suggested that the presence of *Chlamydia pneumoniae* or cytomegalovirus in endovascular locations could be linked to arteriosclerosis. Whether these organisms also promote degenerative valve lesions promoting IE remains to be demonstrated.

Characteristics of the micro-organisms

The organisms most frequently responsible for IE are also those that have the greatest ability to adhere to and colonize damaged valves.[30] Together, *S. aureus*, *Streptococcus* spp. and enterococci are responsible

for over 80% of all cases of IE (see Table 47.2). IE pathogens possess several surface adhesins that mediate attachment to extracellular matrix proteins of the host. These adhesins are collectively referred to as MSCRAMMs, for microbial surface component reacting with adhesive matrix molecules. They include both proteins and polysaccharides.

In *S. aureus*, fibrinogen-binding protein A (also called clumping factor A or ClfA) and fibronectin-binding protein A (FnBPA) are involved in valve colonization and invasion, whereas other MSCRAMMs seem less implicated.[31] Figure 47.2 presents a likely scenario in the case of IE due to this organism. In streptococci, several surface proteins as well as platelet-activating factors and exopolysaccharides are involved in bacterial adherence to damaged valves. This abundance of surface adhesins makes IE pathogens particularly prone to colonize susceptible valve tissues.

Aside from bacterial colonization of pre-existing valve lesions, invasion of endothelial cells may also occur in certain circumstances. Direct invasion of the valve endothelium was demonstrated in experimental endocarditis with *S. aureus*.[31] During inflammation, endothelial cells express a variety of molecules, including integrins of the β_1 family (very late antigen, VLA), which bind fibronectin. Fibronectin bound to endothelia is a privileged ligand for pathogens expressing fibronectin-binding proteins, including *S. aureus*. Bridging *S. aureus* and endothelial cells via fibronectin triggers internalization of the attached microbes by the host cell. Thus, local inflammation due to degenerative lesions, e.g. arteriosclerosis, or as yet undetermined conditions may promote direct endothelial infection. These events may also be important in the pathogenesis of IE due to intracellular pathogens such as *Coxiella burnetii* (the agent of Q fever), *Chlamydia* spp., *Legionella* spp. and *Bartonella* spp.[32]

The role of transient bacteremia

The role of transient bacteremia was demonstrated in animals with catheter-induced aortic valve vegetations and dental manipulation.[33] Both the magnitude of bacteremia during dental procedures and the ability of the pathogen to attach to damaged valves were important. Out of a great variety of gingival micro-organisms circulating in the blood after the procedure, only those able to attach to damaged valves (i.e. streptococci and *S. aureus*) produced IE.

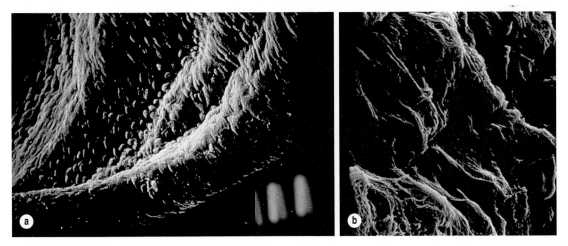

Fig. 47.1 Scanning electron microscopy of a rabbit aortic valve leaflet. (a) A normal valve, covered by a monolayer of endothelial cells. (b) The meshwork of fibrin and platelets covering a damaged valve. Mechanical lesions of the valve were created by inserting a catheter through the right aortic carotid and across the aortic valve.

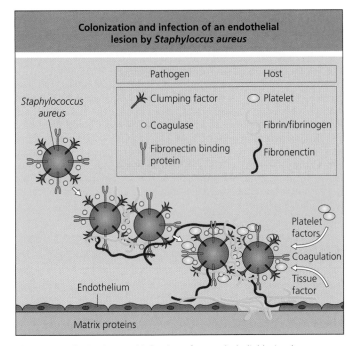

Fig. 47.2 Colonization and infection of an endothelial lesion by *Staphylococcus aureus*. Exposure of the subendothelial matrix triggers the deposition of platelet–fibrin clots and other plasma-soluble and matrix proteins, including fibrinogen, fibrin, fibronectin and thrombospondin. Triggering of the coagulation cascade is also mediated by tissue factor, which contributes to platelet activation and the constitution of a nonbacterial thrombotic vegetation. *S. aureus* is equipped with a wealth of surface determinants that may promote binding and colonization of nonbacterial thrombotic vegetations. The main players are fibrinogen-binding protein A (clumping factor A, or ClfA) and fibronectin-binding protein A (FnBPA), which synergize for valve adhesion and invasion of endothelial cells.[31] Coagulase might also help trigger platelet aggregation.

Bouts of transient bacteremia occur not only during medicosurgical procedures, but also during normal activities such as chewing and tooth-brushing. Such spontaneous bacteremias are usually of low grade and short duration (1–100 CFU/ml of blood for less than 10 minutes),[34] but their high frequency may explain why most IE cases occur outside medicosurgical procedures.[12,35] Also of increasing concern are health-care-associated bacteremias, such as in chronic hemodialysis patients who represent a quasi new at-risk group for IE.[8,29]

The role of host defenses

IE is most often due to Gram-positive organisms, and rarely to Gram-negative bacteria (see Table 47.2). The reason for this is probably multifactorial. Differences in bacterial adherence to damaged valves may be one explanation. However, differences in the susceptibility of Gram-positive and Gram-negative bacteria to serum-induced killing may also account for these variations. The C5b–C9 membrane-attack complex of complement kills Gram-negative bacteria by perforating their outer membrane. In contrast, complement does not kill Gram-positive bacteria because they lack an outer membrane, and their plasma membrane is protected from the membrane-attack complex by the thick surrounding peptidoglycan.

The importance of serum was demonstrated in experimental IE induced by serum-susceptible *Escherichia coli*. These organisms were spontaneously cleared from the valves. Yet, some Gram-negative bacteria may carry thick capsules or other modifications of their surface that help them resist complement-induced killing. Important Gram-negative bacteria that provoke IE include bacteria of the HACEK group, as well as *P. aeruginosa*.

Although Gram-positive bacteria are resistant to complement, they may be the targets of other nonspecific immune factors such as platelet microbicidal proteins (PMPs). PMPs are peptides produced by activated thrombocytes that kill bacteria by damaging their plasma membrane. The protective role of PMPs was suggested by experimental endocarditis, where thrombocytopenic rabbits demonstrated greater bacterial densities in their vegetations than rabbits with normal platelet counts. Likewise, micro-organisms recovered from patients with IE were consistently resistant to PMP-induced killing, whereas similar bacteria recovered from patients with other types of infection were susceptible to PMPs.[36] Therefore platelets, which are a major component of the vegetations, are key players in the nonspecific defense against IE.

Humoral and cellular immunity seem to play only a limited role in defense against IE. Immunization studies in experimental endocarditis gave contradictory results. Immunization of rats against the streptococcal MSCRAMM FimA conferred cross-protection against IE due to several viridans group streptococci.[37] In contrast, immunization of rabbits against the enterococcal aggregation substance failed to protect

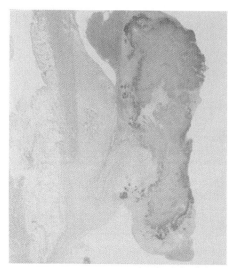

Fig. 47.3
Microscopic appearance of a vegetation from a patient suffering mitral valve infective endocarditis due to *Streptococcus sanguis*. The purple area represents clusters of streptococci packed within a fibrin-platelet meshwork. Professional phagocytes are essentially absent from the lesion.

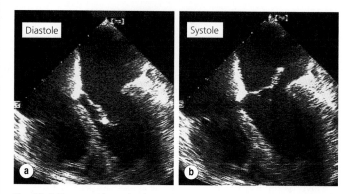

Fig. 47.4 Transesophageal echocardiography of a mitral valve infective endocarditis. The echocardiogram is from the patient described in Figure 47.3. Arrows indicate a large pediculated vegetation, which oscillates from the left ventricle to the left atrium during the systole. Courtesy of Dr X Jeanrenaud.

the animals against experimental IE. In this case, specific antibodies arising from vaccination could not appropriately penetrate inside the vegetation *in vivo*. Administration of granulocyte colony-stimulating factor did not influence the course of infection either. IE is not noticeably more frequent in immunocompromised patients than in those without immune defects, except for HIV patients who may have additional risk factors and risk components.[10] In established infection, bacteria are clustered in amorphous platelet–fibrin clots (the vegetations), permitting little access to professional phagocytes to remove the bacteria (Fig. 47.3). Figure 47.4 presents an echocardiographic picture of a large oscillating vegetation, which occurred in the context of a mitral valve streptococcal IE. Such a 'therapeutic sanctuary' explains why successful treatment of IE relies primarily on antibiotic-induced killing of bacteria rather than on host defenses.

PREVENTION

Because of its severity, it is generally agreed that IE should be prevented whenever possible. Choice of appropriate prophylactic measures requires:
- identification of patients at risk;
- determination of the procedures or circumstances that may result in bacteremia;
- choice of an appropriate antimicrobial regimen; and
- balancing of the known risks against the possible benefits of intervention.

Because prospective studies of IE prophylaxis in humans raise ethical issues and would require too many patients, the practice of IE prophylaxis is still based on its proven efficacy in experimental animal models. Recently, a working group of the American Heart Association revisited the guidelines for prophylaxis based on a risk assessment of both underlying cardiac conditions and medicosurgical practices most likely to promote IE.[38] The group reviewed the English language literature on the subject from 1950 to 2006 and concluded the following:
- Only an extremely small number of cases of IE might be prevented by antibiotic prophylaxis for dental procedures, even if such prophylactic therapy were 100% effective.
- IE prophylaxis for dental procedures is reasonable only for patients with underlying cardiac conditions associated with the highest risk of adverse outcome from IE.
- For patients with these underlying cardiac conditions, prophylaxis is reasonable for all dental procedures that involve manipulation of gingival tissue or the periapical region of teeth or perforation of the oral mucosa.
- Prophylaxis is not recommended based solely on an increased lifetime risk of acquisition of IE.
- Administration of antibiotics solely to prevent IE is not recommended for patients who are to undergo a genitourinary or gastrointestinal tract procedure.

The content of the new guidelines is summarized in Tables 47.3 and 47.4. The critical review by the working group helps settle unproven assumptions and potential medicolegal issues on the topic. Moreover, the new guidelines greatly simplify the choice of prophylactic drugs and thus may improve compliance. Due to the lack of controlled prospective studies, the level of evidence of most of these propositions is II-B, except for prophylaxis before cardiac surgery, which is I-A.

Since the working group gathered international experts, the new guidelines will most likely be adopted by most European countries, with possible minor modifications.[24] For example, the 2008 guidelines from the British National Institute for Health and Clinical Excellence (NICE) are even more restrictive, as they propose to completely abandon IE prophylaxis (www.nice.org.uk/CG064). Patients with healthy gums are at lower risk of bacteremia than those with severe gingivitis, hence the importance of primary prevention by general hygiene of the dental sphere and other body sites that might be susceptible to release pathogens into the blood.

CLINICAL FEATURES

IE may follow an acute or subacute course. The general clinical features (Table 47.5) are not usually specific. Figure 47.5 depicts the dynamics of infection-related events (critical phase) and infection-unrelated events (continuation phase) that may occur during antibiotic treatment.

Acute infective endocarditis

Acute IE can be devastating. It is most frequently caused by *S. aureus* (and sometimes by *Staphylococcus lugdunensis* and *Staphylococcus capitis*) followed by certain streptococci of the *Streptococcus milleri* group (*Streptococcus constellatus*, *Streptococcus anginosus* and *Streptococcus intermedius*) and enterococci. Bacterial production of proteases and other exoproteins contributes to rapid destruction of valve leaflets and the development of abscesses located in the valve ring and the myocardium. Myocarditis and pericardial effusions are frequent. Patients are prostrate and have a high fever. Hypotension and shock may occur, caused both by the septic state and by cardiac failure. Valve vegetations may vary from a few millimeters in diameter to more than 1 cm. Large vegetations are frequent in acute *S. aureus* and fungal IE (Fig. 47.6) and are more likely to detach and give rise to septic emboli. Complications in peripheral organs mainly result from embolic lesions; these may include skin abscesses and retinal emboli (Fig. 47.7), as well as abscesses in the brain and the spleen (Fig. 47.8).

Table 47.3 Cardiac conditions associated with the highest risk of adverse outcome from infective endocarditis (IE), and procedures for which antibiotic prophylaxis is recommended or not recommended

Underlying cardiac conditions where antibiotic prophylaxis is recommended

Prosthetic cardiac valve
Previous IE
Congenital heart disease (CHD)*
- Non-repaired cyanotic CHD, including palliative shunts and conduits
- Repaired congenital heart defect with prosthetic material or device, either by surgically or by catheter intervention, during the first 6 months after the procedure†
- Repaired CHD with residual defects at the site or adjacent to the site of a prosthetic patch or device (a situation that inhibits endothelialization)
Cardiac transplantation recipients who develop cardiac valvulopathy

Procedures where antibiotic prophylaxis is recommended for the above conditions

All dental procedures that involve manipulation of gingival tissues or periapical region of teeth, or perforation of oral mucosa
Procedures on respiratory tract or infected skin, skin structures or musculoskeletal tissues only if they imply overt incision of the skin or mucosa

Procedures where antibiotic prophylaxis is not recommended

Procedures on the genitourinary or gastrointestinal tracts, if indication for prophylaxis implicates only endocarditis prevention

*Antibiotic prophylaxis is not recommended for any CHD other than those listed above.
†Endothelialization occurs during the first 6 months after implantation.
Adapted from European Society of Cardiology[24] and American Heart Association[38] guidelines.

Major indications for urgent valve replacement include refractory cardiac failure due to valve destruction and persistent sepsis related to myocardial abscesses. A defect in atrioventricular conduction is often an early sign of septal invasion by a contiguous valve ring abscess, which usually requires urgent surgery.

Subacute infective endocarditis

Subacute IE is not usually due to *S. aureus*, but it may be due to any of the organisms listed in Table 47.2. It can mimic chronic wasting diseases. The duration between initiation and diagnosis can vary from a few days to more than 5 weeks. Fever is almost always present (see Table 47.5). Physical signs reflect the existence of cardiac or peripheral complications. These include a new or changing heart murmur, evidence of embolic events and immunologic signs of chronic inflammation. Immune complexes (or rheumatoid factor) are present in up to 50% of patients after 6 weeks of subacute infection. Their level decreases during effective treatment. Immune phenomena may be the cause of petechiae, splinter hemorrhages, Osler nodes and Roth spots, arthritis and glomerulonephritis. Osler nodes are small and painful nodular lesions on the pads of the fingers or toes or on the thenar or hypothenar eminences (Fig. 47.9). They are caused by an allergic vasculitis. Although classic, they are not pathognomonic of subacute IE. Roth spots are rounded retinal hemorrhages with a white center. Focal or diffuse glomerulonephritis is present in most cases.

Vascular complications

Peripheral septic emboli are due to fragmentation of the vegetations and often bring the patient to consultation. Therefore they peak at the time of diagnosis and decrease rapidly during the first week of effective antibiotic therapy (see Fig. 47.5).[39] They are more frequent with *S. aureus* than with oral streptococci, when the size of vegetation is >10 mm, and when the mitral valve is involved.[40] Other types of vascular manifestation are the consequence of immune-related vasculitis. Mycotic aneurysms are found in up to 15% of cases, and are especially common in *S. aureus* IE. They may arise from direct

Table 47.4 Recommended antibiotic regimens for endocarditis prophylaxis for risk factors and procedures listed in Table 47.3

		REGIMEN: SINGLE DOSE 30–60 MIN BEFORE PROCEDURE	
For dental procedures*	**Agent**	**Adults**	**Children**
Oral route	Amoxicillin	2 g	50 mg/kg
Unable to take oral antibiotics	Ampicillin	2 g iv or im	50 mg/kg iv or im
	or		
	cefazolin or ceftriaxone	1 g iv or im	50 mg/kg iv or im
Allergic to penicillin – oral route	Cephalexin†,‡	2 g	50 mg/kg
	or		
	clindamycin	600 mg	20 mg/kg
	or		
	clarithromycin	500 mg	15 mg/kg
Allergic to penicillin – unable to take oral antibiotics	Cefazolin or ceftriaxone	1 g iv or im	50 mg/kg iv or im
	or		
	clindamycin	600 mg iv or im	20 mg/kg iv or im

*Regimens for other procedures should be targeted at the most probable pathogen implicated. For streptococci, antibiotics are the same as above. For staphylococci, anti-staphylococcal β-lactams or vancomycin should be considered. For enterococci, amoxicillin or ampicillin, as above, or vancomycin should be considered. The risk of methicillin-resistant staphylococci (preferred vancomycin) and vancomycin-resistant enterococci (preferred amoxicillin or ampicillin) should be taken into account.
†Or other first- or second-generation cephalosporin.
‡Cephalosporins should not be used patients with type 1 allergy to β-lactams.
Adapted from European Society of Cardiology[24] and American Heart Association[38] guidelines.

Table 47.5 Clinical features of IE in the general population and in specific at-risk groups

Clinical features	NO. OF EPISODES (% OF TOTAL)			
	Native valve	Intravenous drug abusers	Prosthetic valve	
			Early	Late
Symptoms				
Fever	170 (75)	42 (87)	7 (77)	47 (78)
Chills	104 (46)	(73)	5 (55)	32 (53)
Arthralgias/myalgias	44 (19)	(27)	–	10 (17)
Back pain	22 (10)	5 (10)	–	2 (2)
Pleuritic chest pain	10 (4)	17 (45)	–	3 (5)
Clinical signs				
Cardiac murmur	196 (86)	45 (93)	8 (88)	58 (96)
Petechiae, emboli	80 (35)	3 (6)	3 (33)	30 (50)
Osler nodes, Janeway lesions, Roth spots	26 (11)	3 (6)	0 (0)	6 (10)
Splinter hemorrhages*	28/80 (35)	3/15 (30)	5/7 (71)	17/33 (51)
Palpable spleen*	15/80 (19)	3/15 (30)	2/7 (28)	2/33 (6)
Central nervous system manifestations[†]	38/148 (25)	4/33 (12)	0/2 (0)	5/27 (18)
Renal insufficiency[†]	45/148 (30)	5/33 (15)	1/2 (50)	8/27 (30)
Temperature (°C)				
<37.8	64 (28)	15 (31)	3 (34)	21 (35)
37.8–38.9	82 (36)	12 (25)	6 (66)	22 (37)
≥39	81 (36)	21 (44)	0 (0)	17 (28)
Total episodes	228	48	9	60

*As reported by Sandre & Shafran.[58]
[†]As reported by Watanakunakorn & Burkert.[57]

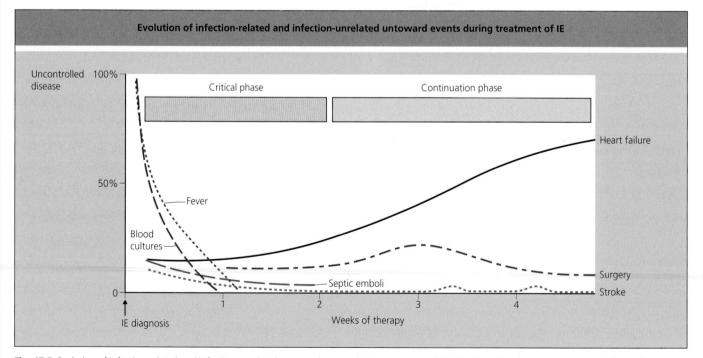

Evolution of infection-related and infection-unrelated untoward events during treatment of IE

Uncontrolled disease 100%

Critical phase   Continuation phase

Heart failure

50%

Fever

Blood cultures

Surgery

Septic emboli

Stroke

0

IE diagnosis   1   2   3   4   Weeks of therapy

Fig. 47.5 Evolution of infection-related and infection-unrelated untoward events during treatment of IE. Infection-related events occur mostly during the first 2 weeks of therapy. These include persistent fever, positive blood cultures, acute heart failure and septic emboli, which if persistent may require therapy readjustment and/or adjunctive surgery. These first 2 weeks represent a critical phase during which initiation of outpatient parenteral antibiotic therapy (OPAT) has to be carefully weighed. OPAT should not be initiated if all these parameters are not under control. Later events (continuation phase) are not related to inappropriate antibiotic treatment and may occur irrespective of hospital stay, i.e. hospital stay does not prevent and OPAT does not provoke such complications. OPAT is feasible during this phase, provided that logistics and medical follow-up (once or twice weekly) are organized. (For details, see Andrews & von Reyn.[54])

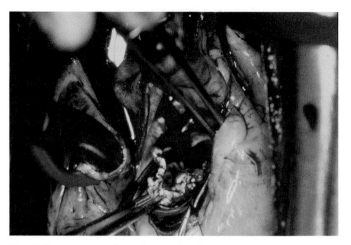

Fig. 47.6 Aortic valve of a patient undergoing emergency valve replacement for acute endocarditis caused by *Staphylococcus aureus*. In this patient, emergency valve replacement was mandatory because of multiple embolizations and acute heart failure. Here, the aorta has been opened and the valve is viewed from its upper side. The lower tweezers are holding a valve leaflet covered with vegetations. Next to the upper tweezers, a portion of a cuspid with a normal appearance can be distinguished.

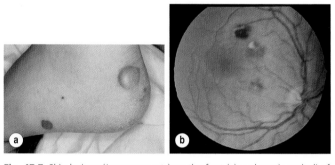

Fig. 47.7 Skin lesions (Janeway spots) on the foot (a) and septic emboli of the retina (b), the results of peripheral emboli in acute endocarditis caused by *Staphylococcus aureus*. These occurred in the patient described in Figure 47.6 and were present on admission to hospital.

invasion of the arterial wall by the infecting organisms, from septic embolization of the vasa vasorum or from the deposition of immune complexes with ensuing inflammation and weakening of the arterial wall. Mycotic aneurysms tend to be located at the bifurcation points of vessels. They may heal during antibiotic therapy or become clinically evident later, even months after the clinical cure of the disease. As such, the true incidence of mycotic aneurysms during IE is probably underestimated. In right-sided IE, embolization occurs in the pulmonary circulation and gives raise to pulmonary infiltrates and lung abscesses.

Neurologic complications

Neurologic manifestations occur in up to 40% of cases.[27] Anatomic alterations include cerebral infarction, arteritis, abscesses, mycotic aneurysms, intracerebral or subarachnoid hemorrhage, encephalomalacia, cerebritis and meningitis. Like peripheral emboli, embolic strokes peak at the time of diagnosis and decrease rapidly during efficacious antibiotic therapy.[40] The frequency of stroke is similar between NVE and PVE.

Neurologic events may be considered as a contraindication for cardiac surgery, due to the risk of anticoagulation-related cerebral hemorrhage. Nevertheless, recent studies indicate that surgery may be performed with a minimum risk of neurologic complications (3–6%), which offsets the risk of postponing valve surgery for uncontrolled infection and/or acute heart failure.[41] Such difficult situations should be handled via an interdisciplinary approach.

DIAGNOSIS

Precise clinical and microbiologic diagnosis is mandatory in order to guide therapy. In theory, IE combines persistent bacteremia and anatomic lesions of the valves. However, blood cultures may remain negative in up to 10% of cases (Tables 47.2, 47.6). Diagnosis of IE is difficult in blood culture-negative IE, or when changes in the valve status cannot be assessed owing to lack of information on pre-existing cardiac lesions. Therefore, criteria taking into account microbiology, valve status (as determined by echocardiography or pathology), serology and clinical features were recently assessed and validated to improve the diagnosis of IE in difficult cases (Table 47.7).[1]

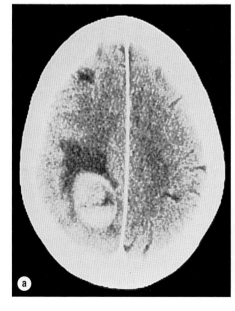

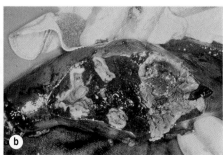

Fig. 47.8 A cerebral abscess (a) and multiple abscesses and ischemic necroses of the spleen (b), the results of peripheral emboli in acute endocarditis caused by *Staphylococcus aureus*. Again these occurred in the patient described in Figure 47.6; they developed after admission to hospital.

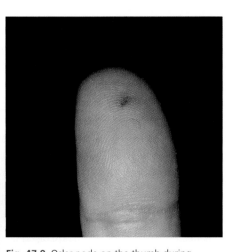

Fig. 47.9 Osler node on the thumb during subacute endocarditis. This was a rounded, tender, inflamed mass about 5 mm in diameter.

Table 47.6 Rare causes of IE associated with negative blood cultures

Pathogen	Diagnostic procedure	Proposed therapy and criteria for cure*
Brucella spp.	Blood cultures Serology Culture, immunohistology and PCR of surgical material	Doxycycline plus rifampin (rifampicin) or co-trimoxazole Treatment for >3 months Cure is considered when antibody titers are <1:160
Coxiella burnetii (agent of Q fever)	Serology: IgG phase I >1:800 Tissue culture, immunohistology and PCR of surgical material	Doxycycline plus hydroxychloroquine Doxycycline plus quinolone Treatment >18 months Cure is considered when IgG phase I titers are <1:800, and IgA and IgM titers are <1:50
Bartonella spp.[†]	Blood cultures Serology Culture, immunohistology and PCR of surgical material	β-lactams or doxycycline plus aminoglycoside Treatment >6 weeks Surgery required in up to 90% of cases
Chlamydia spp.[‡,§]	Serology Culture, immunohistology and PCR of surgical material	Doxycycline Newer fluoroquinolones Long-term treatment, optimal duration unknown
Mycoplasma spp.[§]	Serology Culture, immunohistology and PCR of surgical material	Doxycycline Newer fluoroquinolones Treatment >12 weeks
Legionella spp.[§]	Blood cultures Serology Culture, immunohistology and PCR of surgical material	Macrolides plus rifampin Newer fluoroquinolones Treatment >6 months
Tropheryma whipplei[¶] (agent of Whipple's disease)	Histology and PCR of surgical material	Co-trimoxazole β-lactam plus aminoglycoside (long-term treatment, optimal duration unknown)

*Because of the lack of large series on IE due to these pathogens, optimal treatment duration is mostly unknown (evidence level II-B). Treatment durations in the table are indicative and are based on selected case reports.
[†]Several therapeutic regimens were reported, including amino-penicillins and cephalosporins combined with aminoglycosides, doxycycline, vancomycin and quinolones.
[‡]Beware of serologic cross-reaction with the more common IE pathogen *Bartonella* spp.
[§]Newer fluoroquinolones are more potent than ciprofloxacin against intracellular pathogens such as *Mycoplasma* spp., *Legionella* spp. and *Chlamydia* spp.
[¶]Treatment of Whipple IE remains highly empiric. Successes were reported with long-term (>1 year) co-trimoxazole therapy.
Adapted from Brouqui & Raoult (2001)[32] and (2006).[44]

Blood cultures

Blood cultures are of primary importance because they reveal the infecting organism and guide antibiotic therapy. The volume of blood cultured is critical because bacteremia is often of low grade, representing only 1–100 bacteria/ml of blood. A minimum of two (ideally three) sets of blood cultures consisting of 20 ml of blood should be taken at 60 min intervals before any antibiotic administration, and distributed into a two-bottle system for incubation. For the most frequent pathogens, two sets will reveal the organism in *c.* 90% and three sets in up to 98% of cases.[42] Some centers have developed special IE culture protocols to optimize the detection of fastidious organisms, including blood collection in lysis-centrifugation tubes and subcultures on specific media. Whenever possible, the laboratory should be made aware of the possibility of IE.

Culture-negative infective endocarditis

Blood culture-negative IE falls into two categories that are important for diagnosis and treatment. In the first category are patients who have received antibiotics prior to blood cultures. These represent *c.* 50% of culture-negative cases.[43] In the second category are patients with IE due to fastidious or as yet noncultivable organisms, represented mostly by *Coxiella burnetii* and *Bartonella* spp. (in *c.* 70% of cases), *Brucella* spp. (in endemic areas) and rarely (in *c.* 1% of cases) *Tropheryma whipplei*, maybe *Legionella* spp. and sometimes fungi (especially *Aspergillus*).[43] The laboratory must be made aware of these possibilities. Table 47.6 lists the principal organisms of this group, and proposed diagnostic procedures

and therapies.[32] Since these cases of IE are rare, most therapeutic recommendations are based on limited experience including case reports and small series. Therefore, any of these conditions require a special case-by-case attention by the caregiver (evidence level II-A to II-B).

Microbiologic cultures

Bacteria of the HACEK group are usually detected after prolonged (>1 week) incubation of the blood cultures. In contrast, *Abiotrophia* spp. grow well in blood, but fail to grow when subcultured on conventional agar media. These so-called deficient bacteria do grow as satellite colonies if the plates are streaked with *S. aureus*, or if the growth medium is enriched with vitamin B6. These methods should be applied when bacteria are observed microscopically in blood cultures, but fail to grow on the subculture plates.

Brucella spp., *Bartonella* spp., *Legionella* spp. and *Mycobacteria* spp. are rare causes of IE that require special culture techniques.[44] The precise description of these techniques is beyond the scope of this chapter. Serologic tests may help define both culture strategies and other diagnostic procedures. Tissue cell cultures may be performed in specialized laboratories for the detection of strict or facultative intracellular bacteria. These include *C. burnetii*, *Chlamydia* spp., *Legionella* spp. and *Bartonella* spp.

If the patient undergoes surgery, it is of the utmost importance to obtain valve samples for cultures and other microbiologic tests. The importance of cultures cannot be emphasized enough, because it fulfills both diagnostic and therapeutic purposes. Indeed, cultures allow testing for antimicrobial susceptibility.

Table 47.7 Modified Duke criteria for diagnosis of infective endocarditis

Definition terminology used in the criteria	
Major criteria 1. Blood culture	Positive blood cultures (≥2/2) with typical IE micro-organisms (viridans streptococci, *S. bovis* (renamed *S. gallolyticus*), HACEK* group, or community-acquired *S. aureus* or enterococci in the absence of primary focus) Persistently positive blood cultures defined as two culture sets drawn >12 h apart, or three or the majority of four culture sets with the first and last separated at least by 1 h
2. Endocardial involvement	Single positive culture for *Coxiella burnetii* or anti-phase I antibody titer >1:800 New valve regurgitation Positive echocardiogram for IE (transesophageal echo recommended in patients with prosthetic valves and patients rated as 'possible' IE by clinical criteria) defined as: (i) oscillating intracardiac mass in the valve or supporting structure, *or* in the path of regurgitant jets, *or* on implanted material, in the absence of an alternative anatomic explanation, *or* (ii) abscess, *or* (iii) new partial dehiscence of prosthetic valve
Minor criteria 1. Predisposing cardiac condition or intravenous drug use 2. Fever: >38°C (100.4°F) 3. Vascular phenomena: arterial emboli, mycotic aneurysms, petechiae, Janeway lesions 4. Immunologic phenomena: glomerulonephritis, Osler nodes. Roth spots, rheumatoid factor 5. Microbiology: positive blood cultures, but not meeting major criteria, serologic evidence of active infection with plausible micro-organisms	

Diagnosis	
Definite • Pathology or bacteriology of vegetations, *or* • 2 major criteria, *or* • 1 major and 3 minor criteria, *or* • 5 minor criteria **Possible** • 1 major and 1 minor criterion, *or* • 3 minor criteria	**Rejected** • Firm alternative diagnosis, *or* • Resolution of IE syndrome after <4 days of antibiotic therapy, *or* • No pathologic evidence at surgery or autopsy after <4 days of antibiotic therapy • Does not meet criteria mentioned above

*Includes *Haemophilus* spp., *Actinobacillus actinomycetemcomitans*, *Cardiobacterium hominis*, *Eikenella corrodens* and *Kingella kingae*.
Adapted with modifications from Li *et al*.[1]

Histology

A number of special stains may help guide the etiologic diagnosis. Important techniques include Gram stain, periodic acid–Schiff (PAS) stain for Whipple's disease, Giemsa and Warthin–Starry stains for numerous bacteria including *Bartonella* spp., Ziehl-Neelsen stain for *Mycobacteria* spp. and Gimenez stain for *C. burnetii* and *Legionella* spp. While not strictly diagnostic, these techniques help delineate more specific etiologic procedures.

Polymerase chain reaction amplification

Polymerase chain reaction (PCR) amplification of the 16S or 23S ribosomal RNA genes (and sometimes other loci) has become a critical method for bacterial identification from culture and tissue samples. It has been successfully applied to IE surgical material,[45] including cutaneous biopsies of peripheral septic emboli. PCR is invaluable to detect poorly or noncultivable bacteria such as *Tropheryma whipplei*.[44] Figure 47.10 depicts a case of culture-negative aortic valve IE necessitating valve replacement. *T. whipplei* was identified by histology and PCR amplification of the surgical material.

Serology

Serologic tests are included in the Duke diagnostic criteria (see Table 47.7).[1] Common tests include the agglutination test for *Brucella melitensis*, indirect fluorescence for *Legionella pneumoniae*, ELISA for *Mycoplasma pneumoniae*, and complement fixation, ELISA and indi-

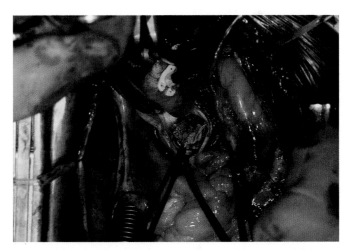

Fig. 47.10 Blood culture-negative aortic valve endocarditis caused by *Tropheryma whipplei* in a 48-year-old patient. The patient was admitted to hospital for acute abdominal pain. Abdominal surgery revealed an ischemic necrosis of the transverse colon, presumably due to arterial embolization. An echocardiogram revealed exuberant vegetations on the aortic valve. All blood cultures were negative. Emergency valve replacement was performed for cardiac insufficiency. *T. whipplei* infection was identified by histology and by using broad-spectrum polymerase chain reaction amplification of the surgical material. The patient was treated with long-term (>1 year) co-trimoxazole (see Table. 47.6). Courtesy of Dr F Bally.

rect immunofluorescence for *Chlamydia* spp. Of note, cross-reaction may occur between *Bartonella* spp. and *Chlamydia* spp. Since culture-proven IE due to *Chlamydia* spp. is notoriously rare, *Bartonella* should be suspected in the case of a positive *Chlamydia* serology. It is important because antimicrobial therapy differs (see Table 47.6). Serology is also critical in the diagnosis of *C. burnetii* IE, as an elevated IgG phase I antibody titer is pathognomonic of the disease.

Other tests

Although many laboratory findings may be abnormal, most of them are nonspecific. The erythrocyte sedimentation rate and the C-reactive protein are elevated in 90–100% of cases. Acute IE may be accompanied by high or low leukocyte counts with increased polymorphonuclear cells and immature forms, as well as other blood and chemistry abnormalities related to active infection. In subacute IE, nonspecific abnormalities accompanying chronic infection are common but not universal, including anemia with low serum iron concentration, low iron-binding capacity and thrombocytosis, leukocytosis, hypergammaglobulinemia and circulating immune complexes. Urinalysis often reveals proteinuria and microhematuria. Although these tests are not specific of IE, their return to normal values during treatment is an indirect marker of treatment efficacy.

MANAGEMENT

General principles

Successful treatment of IE relies on microbial eradication by antimicrobial drugs. Combined medical and surgical treatment is needed in more than 30% of cases, but the timing of surgery may vary along the duration of therapy (see Fig. 47.5). Both experimental and clinical studies have indicated the importance of using bactericidal drugs. For instance, 2 weeks of penicillin treatment for streptococcal IE was insufficient to prevent relapses, whereas 2 weeks of the bactericidal combination of penicillin plus an aminoglycoside successfully cured patients. Synergistic drug combinations are even more important against enterococcal IE, where combining β-lactams with aminoglycosides is mandatory to ensure treatment success.

Therapeutic schemes recommended for the most common pathogens are presented in Tables 47.8–47.11. High concentrations of antibiotics in the serum are desirable to ensure penetration into vegetations. Moreover, prolonged (4–6 weeks) treatment is mandatory to kill dormant bacteria clustered in the infected foci (see Fig. 47.3). Antibiotic choice is based on the minimal inhibitory concentration (MIC) of the drug for the pathogen. More sophisticated tests, such as inhibitory or bactericidal concentrations of the serum, have been proposed, but their utility for conducting therapy is not validated.

Drug treatment of PVE is longer (at least 6 weeks) than that of NVE (2–6 weeks), but qualitatively similar, except for staphylococcal PVE that should include rifampin (rifampicin) whenever the strain is susceptible to this agent. Treatment failure may be due to inadequate antibiotic administration, the presence of a surgically removable focus or antibiotic resistance. The three most problematic microbes with respect to antibiotic resistance are penicillin-resistant streptococci, methicillin-resistant and vancomycin-resistant staphylococci and multidrug-resistant enterococci. Culture-negative IE due to intracellular pathogens may also fail to respond to standard therapy (see Table 47.6).

Penicillin-resistant streptococci

The most common streptococci responsible for IE are oral streptococci of the viridans group, followed by enteric *S. bovis* (recently renamed *S. gallolyticus*), and more rarely group A, B, C and G

streptococci, pneumococci and nutritionally variant streptococci (*Abiotrophia defectiva*, *Granulicatella adiacens* and *Gemella*). Except for *S. gallolyticus* and group A streptococci, which are still uniformly susceptible to penicillin, all streptococci may demonstrate intermediate penicillin resistance (MIC of 0.1–1 mg/l) or full penicillin resistance (MIC >1 mg/l). Treatment of IE due penicillin-susceptible and penicillin-resistant streptococci is qualitatively similar, except that short-course (2 weeks) therapy should not be used in case of resistance, and combinations of β-lactams with aminoglycosides are preferred in these cases (Table 47.8).[46] Little experience exists with highly resistant isolates (MIC >4 mg/l). Vancomycin might be preferred in such circumstances.

Methicillin-resistant and vancomycin-resistant staphylococci

Methicillin-resistant *Staphylococcus aureus* (MRSA) produces low-affinity penicillin-binding protein 2A (PBP2A), which confers cross-resistance to most β-lactams. They are usually resistant to multiple antibiotics, leaving only vancomycin to treat severe infections (Table. 47.9). Treatment for health-care-associated MRSA (HC-MRSA) and community-acquired MRSA (CA-MRSA) is similar.

However, vancomycin-intermediate *S. aureus* (VISA) (MIC 4–16 mg/l) and hetero-VISA (MIC <2 mg/l, but with subpopulations growing at higher concentrations) have emerged worldwide, and were associated with IE treatment failures.[47] Moreover, few highly vancomycin-resistant *S. aureus* (MIC >32 mg/l) carrying a vancomycin-resistance cassette acquired from enterococci were isolated from infected patients in recent years. Treating IE caused by vancomycin-resistant staphylococci requires new approaches. New lipopeptide daptomycin (6 mg/kg/day intravenously) was recently approved for *S. aureus* bacteremia and right-sided IE.[48] Compassionate studies suggest that daptomycin might also overcome methicillin-resistance and vancomycin-resistance in left-sided IE, but definitive studies are missing. Importantly, daptomycin needs to be administered in appropriated doses to avoid resistance selection.[48] Other alternatives include newer β-lactams with relatively good PBP2A affinity,[49] tigecycline, quinupristin–dalfopristin combined or not with β-lactams, β-lactams plus oxazolidinones, and β-lactams plus vancomycin. Such cases warrant consultation of infectious disease specialists.

Multidrug-resistant enterococci

Most (>80%) enterococcal IE cases are due to *Enterococcus faecalis*, followed by *Enterococcus faecium* and rarely other enterococci. *E. faecalis* and *E. faecium* are frequently resistant to gentamicin.[50] An aminoglycoside MIC >500 mg/l is synonymous with loss of bactericidal synergism with cell wall inhibitors. Streptomycin may remain active in such cases, and thus be used instead. A recently described alternative against gentamicin-resistant *E. faecalis* suggests combining ampicillin with ceftriaxone,[51] which synergize by inhibiting complementary PBPs. Otherwise, more prolonged courses of β-lactams or vancomycin must be envisioned (Table 47.10).

β-lactam resistance and vancomycin resistance are mainly observed in *E. faecium*. However, dual resistance is rare and β-lactams might be used against vancomycin-resistant strains and vice-versa. Various results were reported with quinupristin–dalfopristin, linezolid, daptomycin and tigecycline. Such situations require the expertise of an infectious disease specialist.

Gram-negative bacteria

HACEK-related species

Haemophilus, *Actinobacillus*, *Cardiobacterium*, *Eikenella* and *Kingella* species are fastidious organisms that represent less than 5% of all IE cases (Tables 47.2, 47.11). Because they grow slowly, MIC tests may be

Table 47.8 Suggested treatment for native valve endocarditis due to streptococci

Antibiotic	Dosage and route	Duration (weeks)	Level of evidence	Comments
Penicillin-susceptible (MIC <0.1 mg/l) viridans streptococci and *S. bovis* **(renamed** *S. gallolyticus*)*				
Standard treatment Penicillin G	6 × 2–3 million U iv q24h	4	I-A	Preferred in patients older than 65 years or with impaired renal function
Ceftriaxone[†]	1 × 2 g iv or im q24h *Pediatric doses:*[‡] Penicillin G 200 000 U/kg q24h in four to six equally divided doses. Ceftriaxone 100 mg/kg iv or im q24h in one dose	4	I-A	
Short-term treatment Penicillin G with gentamicin[§]	6 × 2–3 million U iv q24h 1 × 3 mg/kg iv or im q24h in one daily dose *Pediatric doses:*[‡] Penicillin and ceftriaxone as above. Gentamicin 3 mg/kg iv or im q24h in one dose or in three equally divided doses	2 2	I-B	
Ceftriaxone[†] with netilmicin	1 × 2 g iv or im q24h 1 × 4 mg/kg iv q24h	2 2	I-B	
In β-lactam allergic patients				
Vancomycin[¶]	2 × 15 mg/kg iv q24h *Pediatric doses:*[‡] 40 mg/kg iv q24h in two to three equally divided doses	4	I-B	
Penicillin-resistant (MIC >1 mg/l) strains (some guidelines consider a limit at 0.5 mg/l for full resistance)				
Penicillin G with gentamicin[§] Vancomycin[¶]	6 × 3 million U iv q24h 3 mg/kg iv or im q24h in one daily dose 2 × 15 mg/kg iv q24h *Pediatric doses:*[‡] As above	4 2 4	I-B I-B	Recommended against highly resistant strains or for β-lactam allergic patients

*Notes for other streptococcal species: (i) short-term 2 weeks' therapy should not be used due to the lack of experience; (ii) IE due to *S. pneumoniae* is often accompanied by meningitis. Ceftriaxone (not penicillin) and perhaps vancomycin should be used in this case; (iii) IE due to nutritionally variant streptococci (e.g. *Abiotrophia*) should include aminoglycosides for at least 4 weeks.
[†]Preferred for outpatient therapy.
[‡]Pediatric doses should not exceed adult doses.
[§]Renal function and gentamicin concentrations in the serum should be monitored once a week. When given in a single daily dose, pre-dose (trough) concentrations should be <1 mg/l and post-dose (peak; 1 h after injection) concentrations should be c. 10–12 mg/l.
[¶]Vancomycin concentrations in the serum should achieve 10–15 mg/l at pre-dose (trough) level and 30–45 mg/l at post-dose level (peak; 1 h after infusion is completed).
Adapted with modifications from Moreillon & Que,[3] and from European Society of Cardiology[24] and Infectious Diseases Society of America[59] guidelines.

difficult to interpret. Some HACEK bacilli now produce β-lactamases, thus ampicillin is no longer the first-line option. Conversely, they are susceptible to ceftriaxone, other third- and fourth-generation cephalosporins, and quinolones. β-lactam based treatments are presented in Table 47.11. Ciprofloxacin (2 × 400 mg/day intravenously or 1000 mg/day orally) is a less well-demonstrated alternative (II-C).

Non-HACEK species

The International Collaboration on Endocarditis (ICE) reported non-HACEK Gram-negative bacteria in 49/2761 (1.8%) of IE cases.[52] Most (59%) were PVE, and only 4% occurred in intravenous drug users. *Escherichia coli* (29%) and *Pseudomonas aeruginosa* (14%) were most frequently reported, followed by *Salmonella* spp., *Klebsiella* spp.,

Serratia marcescens and *Neisseria gonorrhea*. Early surgery was frequent (51%) and intrahospital mortality was 24%. The treatment paradigm of such cases is early surgery plus long-term (>6 weeks) antibiotics with bactericidal combinations of β-lactams with aminoglycosides, and sometimes with quinolones or co-trimoxazole (II-B).

Culture-negative endocarditis

Treatments of IE due to rare pathogens and outcome criteria are summarized in Table. 47.6. Treatment durations in the table are indicative, and based on selected case reports. IE due to *Brucella* spp. responds to prolonged (>3 months) treatment with doxycycline plus co-trimoxazole or rifampin combined or not with streptomycin and surgery.[32]

Table 47.9 Suggested treatment for native valve and prosthetic valve endocarditis due to staphylococci (see suggestions for right-sided IE in footnotes)

Antibiotic	Dosage and route	Duration (weeks)	Level of evidence	Comments
Native valves				
Methicillin-susceptible staphylococci				
Oxacillin or (flu)cloxacillin with gentamicin*	6 × 2 g iv q24h 3 mg/kg iv or im q24h in two to three equally divided doses *Pediatric doses:*§ Oxacillin or (flu)cloxacillin 200 mg/kg iv q24h in four to six equally divided doses. Gentamicin 3 mg/kg iv or im q24h in three equally divided doses	4–6 3–5 days	I-A	The clinical benefit of gentamicin addition has not been formally demonstrated. Its use is optional
Alternative for patients allergic to penicillins (except for immediate-type penicillin hypersensitivity)				
Cefazolin (or other first generation cephalosporins) with gentamicin*	3 × 2 g iv q24h 3 mg/kg iv or im q24h in two to three equally divided doses *Pediatric doses:*§ Cefazolin 100 mg/kg iv q24h in three equally divided doses. Gentamicin as above	4–6 3–5 days	I-B	The clinical benefit of gentamicin addition has not been formally demonstrated. Its use is optional
Vancomycin†	2 × 15 mg/kg iv q24h *Pediatric doses:*§ 40 mg/kg iv q24h in two to three equally divided doses	4–6	I-B	Recommended only for β-lactam allergic patients
Methicillin-resistant staphylococci				
Vancomycin†	2 × 15 mg/kg iv q24h *Pediatric doses:*§ As above	4–6	I-B	
Prosthetic valves				
Methicillin-susceptible staphylococci				
Oxacillin or (flu)cloxacillin, with rifampin‡ and gentamicin*	6 × 2 g iv q24h 3 × 300 mg po q24h 3 mg/kg iv or im q24h in two to three equally divided doses *Pediatric doses:*§ Oxacillin and (flu)cloxacillin as above. Rifampin 20 mg/kg iv or po q24h in three equally divided doses	≥6 ≥6 2	I-B	Rifampin increases the hepatic metabolism of warfarin and other drugs Although the clinical benefit of gentamicin has not been demonstrated, it is recommended for PVE
Vancomycin† with rifampin‡ and gentamicin*	2 × 15 mg/kg iv q24h 3 × 300 mg po q24h 3 mg/kg iv or im q24h *Pediatric doses:*§ As above	≥6 ≥6 2	I-B	Recommended only for β-lactam allergic patients Monitor renal function and serum levels of gentamicin
Methicillin-resistant staphylococci				
Vancomycin† with rifampin‡ and gentamicin*	2 × 15 mg/kg iv q24h 3 × 300 mg po q24h 3 mg/kg iv or im q24h in two to three equally divided doses *Pediatric doses:*§ As above	≥6 ≥6 2	I-B	Monitor renal function and serum levels of gentamicin

Right-sided IE: Uncomplicated staphylococcal right-sided IE (i.e. with fully susceptible organisms and no cardiac failure or peripheral complications) has been successfully treated with short-course (2 weeks) treatment of cloxacillin alone or combined with gentamicin,[60] and with 4 weeks' oral therapy combining ciprofloxacin (2 × 750 mg q24h), or preferentially a more recent quinolone with rifampin (2 × 300 mg q24h). Recently, daptomycin (6 mg/kg q24h for 4 weeks) was accepted against both methicillin-susceptible *S. aureus* and MRSA.

*Renal function and gentamicin concentrations in the serum should be monitored once a week (twice in case of renal failure). When given in three divided doses, pre-dose (trough) concentrations should be <1 mg/l and post-dose (peak; 1 h after injection) concentrations should be between 3 and 4 mg/l.

†Monitor vancomycin concentrations in the serum as indicated in Table 47.8.

‡Rifampin (rifampicin) is believed to play a special role in prosthetic device infective endocarditis (PVE), because it helps eradicate bacteria attached to foreign material. Rifampin should never be used alone, because it selects for resistance at a high frequency (c. 10^{-6}).

§Pediatric doses should not exceed adult doses.

Adapted with modifications from Moreillon & Que,[3] and from European Society of Cardiology[24] and Infectious Diseases Society of America[59] guidelines.

Table 47.10 Antibiotic treatment of endocarditis due to *Enterococcus* spp.

Antibiotic	Dosage and route	Duration (weeks)	Level of evidence	Comments
β-lactam and gentamicin-susceptible strains (for resistant isolates, see footnotes)				
Penicillin G with gentamicin*	6 × 3–5 million U iv q24h 3 mg/kg iv or im q24h in two to three equally divided doses *Pediatric doses:*[‡] Penicillin G 200 000 U/kg iv q24h in four to six equally divided doses. Gentamicin 3 mg/kg iv or im q24h in three equally divided doses	4–6 4–6	I-A	6 weeks of therapy recommended for patients with symptoms of >3 months' duration
Ampicillin or amoxicillin with gentamicin*	6 × 2 g iv q24h 3 mg/kg iv or im q24h in two to three equally divided doses *Pediatric doses:*[‡] Ampicillin or amoxicillin 300 mg/kg iv q24h in four to six equally divided doses. Gentamicin as above	4–6 4–6	I-A	
Vancomycin[†] with gentamicin*	2 × 15 mg/kg iv q24h 3 mg/kg iv or im q24h in two to three equally divided doses *Pediatric doses:*[‡] 40 mg/kg iv q24h in two to three equally divided doses. Gentamicin as above	6 6	I-A	

In cases of high-level resistance to gentamicin (MIC >500 mg/l): if susceptible to streptomycin, replace gentamicin with streptomycin 15 mg/kg q24h in two equally divided doses (I-A); otherwise, use a more prolonged course of β-lactam therapy. Combining ampicillin with ceftriaxone was recently suggested against gentamicin-resistant *E. faecalis*[51] (II-A, II-B).
In cases of β-lactam resistance: (i) if due to β-lactamase production, replace ampicillin with ampicillin–sulbactam or amoxicillin with amoxicillin–clavulanate (I-C); (ii) if due to PBP5 alteration, use vancomycin-based regimens.
In cases of multidrug resistance to aminoglycosides, β-lactams and vancomycin: some suggested alternatives are: (i) linezolid 2 × 600 mg iv or po q24h foo 8 weeks (II-A, II-C) (control hematologic toxicity); (ii) quinupristin–dalfopristin 3 × 7.5 mg/kg q24h for ≥8 weeks (II-A, II-C); (iii) β-lactam combinations including imipenem plus ampicillin or ceftriaxone plus ampicillin for ≥8 weeks (II-B, II-C).
*Monitor renal function and gentamicin concentrations in the serum as indicated in Table 47.9.
[†]Monitor vancomycin concentrations in the serum as indicated in Table 47.8.
[‡]Pediatric doses should not exceed adult doses.
Adapted with modifications from Moreillon & Que,[3] and from European Society of Cardiology[24] and Infectious Diseases Society of America[59] guidelines.

Table 47.11 Antibiotic treatment of endocarditis due to fastidious Gram-negative bacteria of the HACEK group*

Antibiotic	Dosage and route	Duration (weeks)	Level of evidence	Comments
Ceftriaxone[†]	1 × 2 g iv or im q24h	4	I-B	
Ampicillin[‡] with gentamicin[§]	6 × 2 g iv q24h 3 × 1 mg/kg iv or im q24h *Pediatric doses:*[¶] Ceftriaxone 100 mg/kg iv or im q24h in one dose. Ampicillin 300 mg/kg iv q24h in four to six equally divided doses. Gentamicin 3 mg/kg iv or im q24h in one dose or in three equally divided doses	4 4	II-A, II-B	Studies suggest that gentamicin once a day might be adequate

*Includes *Haemophilus* spp., *Actinobacillus actinomycetemcomitans*, *Cardiobacterium hominis*, *Eikenella corrodens* and *Kingella kingae*.
[†]Preferred for outpatient treatment.
[‡]Ampicillin should not be used if microbes produce β-lactamases.
[§]Monitor renal function and gentamicin concentrations in the serum as indicated in Table 47.9.
[¶]Pediatric doses should not exceed adult doses.
Adapted with modifications from Moreillon & Que,[3] and from European Society of Cardiology[24] and Infectious Diseases Society of America[59] guidelines.

IE due to *C. burnetii* is often treated with a combination of doxycycline plus a fluoroquinolone given for up to 3 years, but recurrences are common. Recently, doxycycline combined with hydroxychloroquine appeared more effective. Hydroxychloroquine increases the phagolysosome pH (from 4.7 to 5.8) and improves tetracycline-induced bacterial killing.

IE due to *Bartonella* spp. should be suspected in homeless at-risk patients. Treatment includes primarily β-lactams (amoxicillin and ceftriaxone) combined with aminoglycosides (netilmicin or gentamicin) for at least 2 weeks, or β-lactams combined with other drugs (e.g. doxycycline) for a total of over 6 weeks. Up to 90% of patients may undergo surgical valve replacement.

Treatment of IE due to *Chlamydia* spp., *Mycoplasma* spp. and *Legionella* spp. is unknown. Since these organisms are highly susceptible to newer fluoroquinolones *in vitro*, these drugs should be part of the therapeutic regimen.

IE due to *T. whipplei* is very rare. A review of 35 cases proposes sequential administration of penicillin or ceftriaxone plus gentamicin for 2–6 weeks, followed by long-term (>1 year) co-trimoxazole.[53] Surgical valve replacement may be required for successful therapy (see Table 47.6).

Outpatient parenteral antibiotic therapy for infective endocarditis

Outpatient parenteral antibiotic therapy (OPAT) for IE should be envisioned to consolidate antimicrobial therapy once infection-related complications are under control. These occur during the first 2 weeks of treatment (critical phase; see Fig. 47.5) and include persistent fever or positive blood cultures, perivalvular abscesses, acute heart failure necessitating emergency surgery, septic emboli and stroke.[54] The critical phase is followed by a continuation phase, during which noninfection complications may occur (see Fig. 47.5). These are not related to antibiotic failure and may occur independently of the hospital stay. OPAT may be envisioned at this stage provided that feasibility and logistics are ensured. Critical issues are medical and social staff support, enforcing drug administration and monitoring drug efficacy. In case of problems, the patient should have direct access to the medical staff in charge. In such appropriate conditions OPAT performs equally well independently of the pathogen and NVE or PVE.[54]

Surgery

The leading indications for surgery are:
- refractory cardiac failure caused by valvular insufficiency;
- persistent sepsis caused by a surgically removable focus or a valvular ring or myocardial abscess; and
- persistent life-threatening embolization.

The decision when to operate on an unstable patient requires a multidisciplinary approach.

Endarteritis and Mycotic Aneurysms

Endarteritis is the inflammation of the arterial wall. The term mycotic aneurysm was coined by Osler to define a nonsyphilitic aneurysm resulting from infective endarteritis. Arterial infection may result from:
- microembolization of bacteria in the vasa vasorum;
- hematogenous seeding of the arterial intima or of thrombi lining atherosclerotic plaques during bacteremia;
- extension from contiguous infected foci; or
- arterial trauma with direct bacterial contamination.

The first two mechanisms are most important during IE. Other risk factors include pre-existing endarterial lesions (e.g. congenital malformations such as patent ductus arteriosus and aortic coarctation, atherosclerosis of large vessels, vascular prosthesis and sometimes depressed host immunity due to diabetes, cirrhosis or corticosteroid therapy). Infected aneurysms represent 2.6% of all aneurysms, with a male:female ratio of about 3:1.[55]

MICROBIAL PATHOGENS AND CLINICAL MANIFESTATIONS

In the context of IE, the pathogens of endarteritis follow the pattern shown in Table 47.2. In the absence of IE, on the other hand, Gram-negative bacteria are found more frequently. *Salmonella* spp., *E. coli* and other enterobacteria are isolated in more than 50% of cases of abdominal aortitis.[55] *Salmonella choleraesuis* and *Salmonella typhimurium* seem to have a particular tropism for atherosclerotic arteries. It was proposed that all patients over 50 years of age who develop *Salmonella* bacteremia should undergo abdominal imaging to detect possible aortic lesions. *S. aureus* is the organism most often associated with extra-abdominal lesions and infections of vascular prostheses, and it has been reported in about 30% of endarteritis overall. Other pathogens, including fungi, are occasionally reported.

Signs and symptoms depend on the anatomic site of the disease. Local signs include pain, erythema and manifestations due to compression of contiguous organs and distal ischemia or embolization. Fever and leukocytosis are almost always present.

DIAGNOSIS AND MANAGEMENT

Diagnosis requires a high degree of clinical suspicion. Microbiologic documentation is essential. Blood cultures and cultures of surgical specimens should be performed, if possible before starting antibiotic treatment. All laboratory techniques described for IE etiology diagnosis apply to endarteritis. Ultrasonography, CT, MRI and gallium- or indium-labeled leukocyte scans and especially fluorodeoxyglucose–positron emission tomography (FDG-PET) scanning (see Practice Point 21) are helpful to delineate the lesions. Although none of these techniques will distinguish between sterile and infected fluids, they may guide more invasive diagnostic procedures such as percutaneous needle aspiration of the affected area.

Appropriate antibiotic therapy and surgical resection of the infected vessel with extensive local debridement is mandatory. The material should be carefully examined both by the pathologist and by the microbiologist. Whenever possible, autologous vascular graft and bypass in uninfected tissue should be performed in order to decrease the risk of re-infection. Implantation of rifampin-bond prostheses was also shown to decrease re-infection.[56] Antibiotics should be given for at least 4–6 weeks. Certain situations are so complicated that therapeutic strategies must be adapted for each particular case. Sometimes patients are kept on antibiotics for much longer periods of time, even for life. Despite antibiotic treatment, the morbidity of vascular infections remains high. Infections of lower extremity arteries result in amputation in as many as 20% of cases. Moreover, the mortality rate of patients who have infected aneurysms that are diagnosed late may exceed 70%.

REFERENCES

References for this chapter can be found online at http://www.expertconsult.com

Cameron Wolfe
Kumar Visvanathan

Chapter | 48 |

Rheumatic fever

Acute rheumatic fever (ARF) is an autoimmune condition arising from group A *Streptococcus* infection, characterized by nonsuppurative, inflammatory lesions of heart valves, brain, joints and skin. Less commonly, cardiac muscle, pericardium or lungs are involved. In its classically described form, ARF presents as a febrile and essentially self-limited illness. However, inflammation of the heart valves has the potential for chronic progressive damage, known as rheumatic heart disease (RHD). Globally RHD remains the most common cause of acquired heart disease and cardiac morbidity in childhood.

EPIDEMIOLOGY AND HISTORY

Original descriptions of the disease date to Thomas Sydenham (1624–1689), but it was not until 1812 that William Charles Wells made the association of rheumatism and carditis. Associations with sore throat became evident in the 1880s and by the turn of the 19th century histopathologic descriptions were available through the work of Ludwig Aschoff.

Rheumatic fever is a disease of poverty and social injustice. It is borne of, and indicative of, community disadvantage. During the 1900s it became progressively uncommon in industrialized countries, and was consigned to the realms of the medically esoteric. Conversely, it became increasingly recognized in resource-poor countries.

In the West, the incidence of ARF and rheumatic heart disease began to decline before the availability of antibiotics, and dropped in earnest through the early 1960s and 1970s. Human factors such as improvements in living, sanitation and medical care, as well as reduction in household crowding, are proposed to have made the greatest impact in reducing the incidence of group A streptococcal infections. Current reliable data on the incidence of ARF are rare; however, estimates of the developed world suggest an annual incidence of 1 per 100 000; this compares to 100 and 150 per 100 000 in the Sudan and China, respectively.[1] The highest reported incidence was 508 per 100 000 children aged 5–14 years, between 1987 and 1996, in the Aboriginal population of northern Australia[2] – extraordinary for a country so developed in other respects. Recent estimates put the global burden at a minimum of 18.1 million people affected, with clear regional differences as seen in Figure 48.1.[3] Yearly mortality has been put at approximately 376 000 deaths. It is not clear if the increase in developing countries represents a higher disease burden or better diagnostic efforts.

In the indigenous Australian population residing in northern Australian communities, rheumatic heart disease affects over 2% of the community, leading to hospitalization rates eight times as great in this group as in the nonindigenous.[4] Acute rheumatic fever is common in other Pacific Island nations with very high rates. Much of sub-Saharan Africa, the Indian subcontinent, poorer sections of Latin America and large parts of Asia also have prevalence rates of rheumatic heart disease of greater than 2 per 1000.

Whilst the incidence has fallen in most areas of the developed world, there have been sporadic outbreaks in the United States, for example in Salt Lake City, Utah.[5] It would seem that emergence of more virulent group A streptococci are to blame in these instances.

First episodes of ARF occur most commonly in children between the ages of 5 and 15 years. It is most uncommon to present in the first 2 years of life. (Whether this is because of a need for multiple 'primary' infections or simply reflective of a more immature immune response is not known.) Conversely, first initial episodes become rare beyond the age of 35. Incidence is equal in both males and females, although females appear more likely to suffer Sydenham's chorea and mitral stenosis. The attack rate of rheumatic fever after untreated streptococcal exudative tonsillitis in military recruitment camps has been carefully studied; it is consistently around 3%.

PATHOGENESIS

Acute rheumatic fever requires infection of a susceptible host with a 'rheumatogenic' group A streptococcus. An abnormally vigorous, tissue-specific immune response then ensues. Several theories exist as to the cause of the pathogenicity:

- that streptococcal products (e.g. streptolysins) are directly toxic;
- that a serum sickness develops; or
- that molecular mimicry occurs.

Whilst not proven beyond doubt, mimicry appears likely given the presence of epitopes in human tissue that are immunologically similar to group A streptococcal antigens. This leads to both humoral and cellular responses. Cross-reacting antibodies bind epitopes in human myosin, sarcolemmal membrane proteins, keratin, actin and proteins in synovium and articular cartilage. For example, similarities exist between the α-helical coiled region of the M protein and the rod region of the cardiac myosin.[6] In patients who suffer from Sydenham's chorea, antibodies cross-reacting with neurons of the caudate and subthalamic nuclei, as well as the streptococci, have been found.[7]

Cell-mediated immune responses are also elevated early in ARF, suggesting early T-cell activation may be critical in pathogenesis, with humoral responses simply secondary to antigens released from already damaged tissues. CD4 and CD8 lymphocytes in rheumatic fever patients are found in increased numbers in the blood, as well as in human heart valve tissue. The M protein contains both T- and B-cell epitopes. The M protein (as well as streptococcal pyogenic exotoxins) can also act as a superantigen to further augment the immune response.

Recent interest has also focused on the innate immune system. Toll-like receptors (TLRs) form a component of microbial recognition and innate response. As an indicator of host factors being capable of affecting the pathogenesis of ARF, polymorphisms in TLR-2 (in particular Arg 753 Gln) have been shown to have a strong association

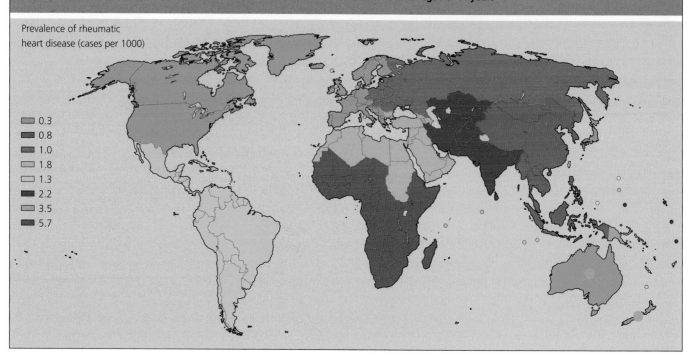

Prevalence of rheumatic heart disease in children aged 5–14 years

Prevalence of rheumatic heart disease (cases per 1000)

- 0.3
- 0.8
- 1.0
- 1.8
- 1.3
- 2.2
- 3.5
- 5.7

Fig. 48.1 Prevalence of rheumatic heart disease in children aged 5–14 years. The circles within Australia and New Zealand represent indigenous populations. Courtesy of JR Carapetis

with risk of ARF.[8,9] There has also been much interest in detecting an HLA association, although this has been difficult to prove and studies have given conflicting and varied reports depending on the population studied. The HLA-DR7 allele is frequently associated with the disease, especially with chronic multivalvular lesions.[10] HLA-DRB1*07 has been strongly associated in populations from Pakistan whilst HLA-DRB1*0701 and DQA1*0201 are associated in Egyptian groups. In addition, different associations have been found in Turkish, Taiwanese and Brazilian populations.[11,12]

There are variations in the organism that also affect the probability of rheumatic fever development. Variations in the M protein serotype affect 'rheumatogenicity'. Table 48.1 outlines the serotypes associated with nonsuppurative sequelae of group A streptococci. The serotypes can be divided into class I or class II M proteins. Outbreaks of ARF have almost exclusively occurred with class I M proteins. Streptococci from this class typically express more M protein and possess a larger capsule. They also lack the production of serum opacity factor. The effect of the M protein in this regard was confirmed when comparisons of the two outbreaks in Salt Lake City revealed similar M protein structure and capsular size in >80% of isolates, even though they were 12 years apart. They both possessed the *emm*18 gene which encodes for M subtype 18. The waning of the outbreak corresponded to the absence of the *emm*18 strain. There have also been interesting changes in the serotypes in circulation. At least in the USA there appears to

have been a virtual disappearance of types 14, 18, 19 and 29 when comparing isolates from the 1960s to those found in the early part of this decade.[13] Whether this is the cause of, or is unrelated to the decline in incidence in the USA has not been elucidated.

Previously it was assumed that pharyngeal infection with group A streptococci was required in order to precipitate ARF. This was challenged recently by an Australian group looking at strains causing pyoderma where ARF was postulated in the absence of recent pharyngitis. This theory has yet to be proved.[14]

Patients who have suffered an initial attack of rheumatic fever continue to have a significant predilection for recurrence of ARF following subsequent episodes. This risk appears greatest in the first 2 years after primary presentation and certainly wanes considerably after 5 years.

CLINICAL FEATURES

The onset of ARF always follows a latent period after a streptococcal sore throat. The average duration of this is 19 days, although it can last between 1 and 5 weeks. There is no difference in latency between first and recurrent episodes. Acute illness may present with a variety of signs and symptoms. The most important of these are described by the 'major manifestations' contained within the modified Jones criteria currently used for diagnosis. They include carditis, polyarthritis, chorea, subcutaneous nodules and erythema marginatum. A number of other additional features have been associated with ARF but are less specific, and are hence termed 'minor manifestations'.

Most manifestations of ARF are accompanied by fever (chorea may occur in isolation). Temperatures rarely exceed 102.2°F (39°C) and are very responsive to salicylate therapy.

Arthritis is the most common feature, occurring in 75% of first attacks, and is usually one of the first symptoms. Carditis occurs in a little under half of all cases, whereas chorea (15%), nodules and erythema marginatum (10%) are less common. The most common presentation is fever and polyarthralgia, with or without the murmur of mitral regurgitation.

Table 48.1 M protein serotypes

Condition	Serotypes
Acute rheumatic fever	1, 3, 5, 6, 14, 18, 19, 24, 27, 29
Acute glomerulonephritis – pharyngitis associated	1, 4, 12, 25
Acute glomerulonephritis – pyoderma associated	2, 49, 55, 59–61

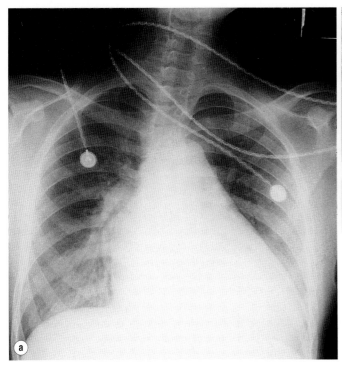

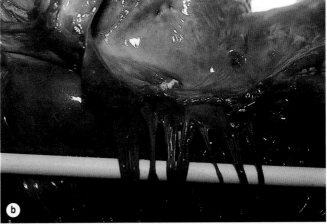

Fig. 48.2 (a) Chest radiograph of a 15-year-old boy who had multiple recurrences of acute rheumatic fever, showing gross cardiac enlargement and failure. He had mitral regurgitation and stenosis, and aortic regurgitation and stenosis. He died 2 days after this radiograph was taken, of intractable cardiac failure. (b) Post-mortem cardiac examination of the same boy, showing thickened, shortened mitral valve cusps with calcific vegetation and thickened chordae tendinae. (Photographs kindly provided by Professor Bart Currie, Darwin, NT, Australia.)

Carditis is more common in younger patients. Acute rheumatic fever can affect the pericardium (usually asymptomatic, present only with a subtle pericardial rub or effusion), the myocardium (hard to detect without the assistance of echocardiography, and rarely a cause of cardiac failure) or the endocardium (the most common and important). Initially valves become inflamed, friable and often have regurgitation. With time, and especially with repeated infections, the valves stiffen, become thickened and shortened, and eventually stenotic. Occasionally the valvular chordae can also shorten. The mitral valve is by far the most commonly affected. The aortic valve is also commonly affected, whereas disease of the pulmonary or tricuspid valve is rare (Fig. 48.2).

Clinically, a pansystolic murmur, consistent with mitral regurgitation, is the most common sign, sometimes associated with the low-pitched mid-diastolic (Carey Coombs) murmur. This is heard over the left ventricular impulse and is associated with acute valvulitis. It may be a feature of primary heart block, leading to early atrial systole and therefore increased flow at the time of the rapid filing phase.

Cardiac failure is possible in the acute phase of rheumatic fever. Rarely, it can even be life-threatening. Using echocardiography it is evident that the congestive heart failure is due to acute valvular dilatation, rather than myocarditis. Accordingly, troponin levels are usually not elevated. First-degree or greater degrees of heart block are also possible, although not specific enough to be diagnostic alone (Fig. 48.3).

Histopathology classically reveals 'Aschoff bodies' within the myocardium; these are perivascular foci of inflammation, consisting of areas of central necrosis surrounded by a rosette of large mononuclear and multinuclear giant cells (macrophage/histiocyte in origin).[15]

Examination reveals erythematous, painful, hot and swollen joints, which may contain sterile purulent effusions. The arthritis tends to be migratory, asymmetric, polyarticular and affects large joints. Each joint is most severely affected from a few days to a week, and returns to normal within 2–3 days. There are atypical cases of only monoarticular involvement, or persistent and additive disease.[16] The hallmark of rheumatic fever arthropathy is that it is exquisitely responsive to non-steroidal anti-inflammatory medication.

Perhaps the most intriguing manifestation of ARF was named by the English physician Thomas Sydenham. He described a classic chorea in 1686, also known as St Vitus' dance. It occurs in between 1%

and 30% of cases of rheumatic fever, and may follow a latent period of up to 6 months after the primary infection. It commonly occurs in isolation from other symptoms, and is far more common in females. Choreiform movements most frequently involve the face, arms and hands. It is generalized in almost 80% of patients and is unilateral in the remainder. The patient's tongue may dart erratically when protruded. Classic patterns of the chorea also include the 'mild-maid's grip' (the rhythmic squeezing when grasping the examiner's fingers), the 'spooning' position (a flexion of the wrists and extension of the fingers when the hands are extended) and the 'pronator sign' (when the arms and palms are outturned when held above the head). All movements worsen upon purposeful action or with anxiety and disappear during sleep. The chorea typically lasts for 1–2 months, and is almost always gone within 6.

Recent work looking at the EEG patterns of patients with Sydenham's chorea shows a parieto-occipital localization in almost 90% with lateralization in a little over 50%. Almost a third had abnormalities seen even after clinical symptoms had resolved. MRI scanning rarely if ever reveals pathology; positron emission tomography (PET) imaging can reveal abnormalities, especially in the basal ganglia, but is rarely used in clinical settings.[17,18]

Erythema marginatum and subcutaneous nodules are both rare manifestations of acute rheumatic fever (2%). The rash is pink and serpiginous, beginning as a macule which then clears centrally (Fig. 48.4). Multiple lesions affect the trunk and limbs, but rarely the face, and can move in front of the examiner, appearing more vasomotor than truly cutaneous. Although they can be present for weeks to months, this does not correlate with ongoing rheumatic inflammation. Nodules in ARF usually appear some weeks after the onset of fever and arthralgia. They are most common over bony surfaces and tendons, for example at the elbows, knees or Achilles tendon, even the spinous processes. Typically they are painless. Their clinical relevance is tied to their strong association with severe carditis.

Less common clinical symptoms seen in acute rheumatic fever include 'rheumatic pneumonia', referring to pulmonary infiltrates seen in some patients with acute carditis. Mild elevations in liver transaminases, microscopic hematuria, pyuria and proteinuria are occasionally found. Blood C-reactive protein (CRP) and erythrocyte sedimentation rate (ESR) are usually impressively elevated in the acute phase of disease.

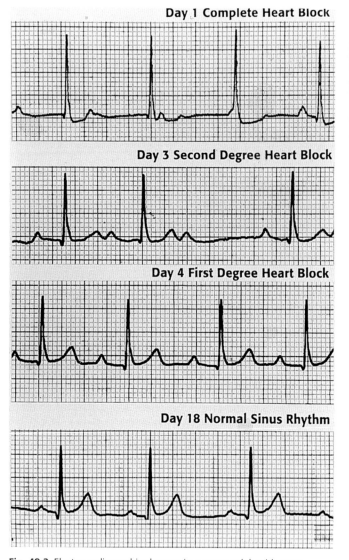

Fig. 48.3 Electrocardiographic changes in a young adult with acute rheumatic fever, showing evolution over 18 days from complete heart block to second-degree (Wenckebach) block to first-degree block and then to normal sinus rhythm. (Reproduced with permission from Bishop W, Currie B, Carapetis J, Kilburn C. A subtle presentation of acute rheumatic fever in remote northern Australia. *Aust N Z J Med* 1996;26:241–2.)

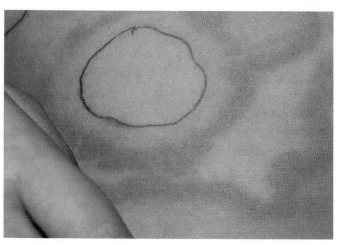

Fig. 48.4 Erythema marginatum on the trunk of an 8-year-old Caucasian boy. The pen mark shows the location of the rash approximately 60 minutes previously. (Photograph kindly provided by Professor Mike South, Royal Children's Hospital, Adelaide, Australia.)

highly prevalent, it may be very difficult to differentiate PANDAS, hence some regional boards recommend rarely, if ever, diagnosing the syndrome.[4]

DIAGNOSIS

There remains no definitive diagnostic test for ARF. In 1944, Jones developed the first set of diagnostic criteria, which were later revised in 1992. The 'updated' Jones criteria (Table 48.2) apply to the initial diagnosis of rheumatic fever. Their careful application is critical to arrive at the correct diagnosis, given the ongoing implications for secondary prophylaxis and cardiac follow-up. At least two major manifestations, or one major and two minor manifestations are required, in addition to evidence of recent streptococcal infection. Exceptions to the criteria exist, allowing a 'presumptive diagnosis': rheumatic chorea may be diagnosed in the absence of other manifestations or preceding streptococcal infection. Low-grade carditis may also occur as a delayed presentation, after streptococcal titers have fallen.

The modified Jones criteria are not beyond reproach. When one considers that merely fever and arthralgia, along with an elevated CRP would be diagnostic, the necessity to include recent streptococcal disease becomes evident. Because the presentation can be varied between individuals, careful exclusion of differential diagnoses is important. A number of differentials are listed in Table 48.3.

There is a separate clinical entity, known as poststreptococcal reactive arthritis. It has a shorter incubation period after bacterial infection, can follow non-group A streptococci and does not have the same dramatic responsiveness to salicylates. It carries no long-term risk of carditis, and therefore needs no long-term secondary prophylaxis. That said, only a very careful clinician would make this diagnosis in an area with highly endemic rheumatic fever. Hence some authorities recommend treating this for a year, and discontinuing if no evidence of carditis is found.

A group of disorders known as pediatric autoimmune neuropsychiatric disorders associated with streptococci (PANDAS) warrant attention; they include some of the tic disorders, some patients with Tourette's syndrome and obsessive–compulsive symptoms. They all have a temporal association with group A streptococcal infections. Some studies have associated antineuronal antibodies with the development of these conditions, but this remains inconclusive. The majority seem to have concurrent cardiac complaints. Currently there are insufficient data to support secondary prophylaxis in this group of patients.[19] In populations where acute rheumatic fever remains

Table 48.2 Guidelines for the diagnosis of initial attack of rheumatic fever*

Major manifestations	Minor manifestations	Supporting evidence of group A streptococcal throat infection
Carditis Polyarthritis Chorea Erythema marginatum Subcutaneous nodules	Clinical findings: • Arthralgia, fever Laboratory findings: • Elevated acute phase reactants (CRP, ESR) Prolonged PR interval	Positive throat culture Rapid streptococcal Ag test Elevated or rising Ab titer: • antistreptolysin, anti-DNaseB, antihyaluronidase

CRP, C-reactive protein; ESR, erythrocyte sedimentation rate.
*Jones criteria, updated 1992.[20]

Table 48.3 Differential diagnoses of the three most common major manifestations of acute rheumatic fever

	Polyarthritis	Carditis	Chorea
Differential diagnoses	Connective tissue disease Immune complex disease Septic arthritis (including gonococcal) Viral arthropathy Henoch–Schönlein purpura Reactive arthropathy Sickle cell anemia Infective endocarditis Leukemia or lymphoma	Innocent murmur Mitral valve prolapse Congenital heart disease Infective endocarditis Hypertrophic cardiomyopathy Myocarditis (viral or idiopathic) Pericarditis (viral or idiopathic)	Systemic lupus erythematosus Drug reaction Wilson's disease Tic disorder Choreo-athetoid cerebral palsy Encephalitis Huntington's chorea Intracranial malignancy Chorea gravidarum

What constitutes evidence of recent streptococcal infection is important to define. It may be demonstrated by a positive throat swab and culture, rapid antigen test or positive antistreptococcal serology. Within 2 months of onset, approximately 80% of patients with ARF will have an ASO titer greater than 200 Todd units/ml. If one of the other serologic tests (anti-DNase B, antihyaluronidase) is also performed, the sensitivity exceeds 90%. Serology, in the absence of culture, is clearly limited in areas with high prevalence of streptococcal impetigo, as children will have continually positive serology. Testing for class I antibodies as an indicator of rheumatic fever has poor specificity and is not presently recommended given the high likelihood of having class I antibodies in any endemic population.[21]

The B cell antigen D8/17 is expressed in a high percentage of those affected by ARF, a moderate amount in close family members, and yet sparsely in the general community. It appears to be inherited in a non-HLA-associated and autosomally recessive manner.[22,23] Although its availability is not extensive, this test has potential for aiding diagnosis; however, laboratories with flow cytometry facilities are required to undertake testing.[24,25]

The increasing specificity of the Jones criteria is appropriate for Western communities where the incidence is low and overdiagnosing rheumatic fever leads to unnecessary prescribing of long-term antibiotics. However, in developing countries where the incidence remains high, a greater sensitivity is desirable, given the profound morbidity of undertreated cardiac disease.

Echocardiographic recognition of clinically silent carditis is not included in the modified Jones criteria. However, it is increasingly recognized that these lesions may progress and warrant attention. The World Health Organization therefore incorporated echocardiographically diagnosed, clinically silent rheumatic valve involvement into recent guidelines, stating they should be treated as rheumatic heart disease until proven otherwise. To support this, recent studies in the developing world screening schoolchildren with echocardiography detected 2.2–3% prevalence of rheumatic heart disease. Only 2.2 per 1000 cases were detected in corresponding groups based on clinical grounds.[26] The use of echocardiography to screen was also supported by Brazilian work showing that, despite 34% of carditis patients normalizing their clinical examination after acute phase resolution, echocardiography showed progression to chronic subclinical valvular disease in over 80%. The financial costs in providing accurate echocardiography to the Third World, as well as suitable training of technicians, remain sizable stumbling blocks.

PREVENTION

Primary prophylaxis (antibiotic therapy of group A streptococcal upper respiratory tract infection) has been the cornerstone of primary prevention since the widespread availability of antibiotics. As treatment initiated within 8 days of the onset of symptoms, oral or intramuscular penicillin is effective at preventing subsequent development of rheumatic fever (for suggested dosing of antibiotics, see Table 48.4). Whilst courses of macrolides, cephalosporins and even later generation quinolones are effective against group A steptococci, they have not been studied in the context of prevention. Their added expense and broader antimicrobial spectrum argue against their use as first-line agents. Recent New Zealand data suggest daily amoxicillin is noninferior to twice-daily penicillin V for the treatment and eradication of streptococci.[27]

Table 48.4 Recommended doses* of antibiotics to prevent rheumatic fever

Indication and antibiotic	Route	Dose in children (<27 kg)	Dose in adult	Frequency	Duration
Options for treatment of group A streptococcal infection ('primary prophylaxis')					
Penicillin V (phenoxymethyl penicillin)	po	250 mg	500 mg	q12h	10 days
Benzathine penicillin G	im	450 mg (600 000 U)	900 mg (1.2 million U)	–	Single dose
Erythromycin (allergy to pen)	po	20 mg/kg (max 250 mg)	250 mg	q12h	10 days
Options for prevention of rheumatic fever recurrences ('secondary prophylaxis')					
Benzathine penicillin G	im	900 mg (1.2 million U)	900 mg (1.2 million U)	Every 3–4 weeks	Depending on severity of carditis
Penicillin V (phenoxymethyl penicillin)	po	250 mg	250 mg	q12h	
Erythromycin (allergy to pen)	po	250 mg	250 mg	q12h	

*Doses as recommended by the American Heart Association.[28]

In regions where acute rheumatic fever remains prevalent, primary antibiotic prophylaxis is important. In settings where the disease is now rare, however, the benefits of antibiotics in the treatment of group A streptococcal pharyngitis (prevention of rheumatic fever, suppurative sequelae and attenuating symptoms) do not outweigh cost, adverse drug reactions and potential for induction of resistance in other organisms.[29] Protecting sore throat sufferers against suppurative and nonsuppurative complications in modern Western society can be achieved only by treating with antibiotics many who will derive no benefit. In emerging economies where rates of, for example, acute rheumatic fever are high, the number needed to treat may be much lower.

Unfortunately there are few data showing conclusive reduction in the incidence of ARF in developing countries. Additionally, not all cases of ARF are preceded by an obviously sore throat, making prevention difficult. Diagnosing and treating acute pharyngitis remains imperative, although countries also require aggressive measures to improve housing, control skin disease, advance education of health staff and the wider community and attempt to close social and health disparities.[30,31]

There have been no controlled studies showing tonsillectomy to be effective. It is not currently recommended for primary prevention of ARF.[1]

Use of vaccines in primary prevention

A number of different M-protein based subunit vaccines are in varying stages of development. The M protein contains both a hypervariable region and a conserved C terminal region. The hypervariable N region has been shown to be highly immunogenic and can induce strain-specific immunity. A 26-valent vaccine candidate (recombinant protein vaccine) that has been successful in both phase I and phase II human clinical trials has been shown to induce antibodies capable of opsonization of not only the specific M types represented in the vaccine, but also subtype variants. There can be very small differences in amino acid sequences of subtype variants, indicating potential for broad coverage even in highly immunized populations where variant strains may develop under selective pressure.[32]

The C terminal has also been incorporated into a number of vaccine studies, showing reduced colonization of pharyngeal tissues in mice. Given this is the primary route of infection with group A streptococci in humans, it raises hope for ARF prevention. Conjugating N terminal proteins to either tetanus or diphtheria toxoid has also been an avenue of investigation successful in mouse models. Alternatively, a number of different peptides derived from the N terminus have been combined into a larger 'heteropolymer' for subcutaneous injection, showing protective effects in proof-of-concept animal models. Lipopeptide molecules and even protein vesicles ('proteosomes') have also been explored.[33] A novel approach taking shape in vaccine research includes using a nonpathogenic *Lactococcus lactis* strain that expresses a protein derived from the conserved region of the M protein as an intranasal vector for immune stimulation.[34]

Unfortunately, widespread rollout of a tested, cost-effective and efficacious human vaccine remains some years away. An excellent review of current development is included.[35]

Secondary prophylaxis

After an initial attack of ARF, patients are at higher risk of recurrence after subsequent episodes of streptococcal upper respiratory infections. This risk is highest in the first few years after the initial attack and fades thereafter. With each relapse, the likelihood of more significant rheumatic heart disease increases. Secondary prophylaxis (see Table 48.4) therefore becomes crucial to reduce long-term morbidity and mortality. Best preventive responses have been achieved with 3-weekly benzathine penicillin G injections, although 4-weekly injections are often given to improve compliance and decrease cost.[36,37] Daily oral penicillin is an alternative, although compliance is problematic; the same is true for daily oral sulfadiazine. Penicillin-allergic patients should be offered erythromycin.

The duration of secondary prophylaxis is determined by risk of recurrent disease. Certainly in the first 5 years it appears significant. It is also judged on the degree of pre-existing heart disease and the likelihood of ongoing streptococcal exposure. In New Zealand experience, data collected in the 1990s suggest antibiotic cessation may be considered at 21 years of age, or at least 10 years after the last attack.[38] For those with more severe carditis (based on at least moderate clinical or echocardiographic valvular dysfunction) some groups would consider cessation of prophylaxis only after age 30 years and more than 10 years after the last clinical relapse. Others would argue that continued prophylaxis for life is warranted.[28]

On a regional and national level, the establishment of formal control programs is highly desirable.[1,4,30] Such a program requires national commitment (including budgetary), a centralized registry of patients and ideally a multidisciplinary steering committee for appropriate oversight. Priorities include education and advocacy, case finding through surveillance, coordinating secondary prophylaxis and follow-up. The more complex primary preventive strategies that address health and social inequalities must follow.

MANAGEMENT

The main initial aims of management in ARF are to confirm the diagnosis, treat any cardiac failure and quiet inflammation. Ensuring ongoing secondary prophylaxis and clinical follow-up are subsequently important. While there is no evidence that acute treatment reduces the likelihood or severity of long-term valvular damage, there is considerable potential symptomatic benefit for the patient. Hospital admission is still recommended so as to ensure relevant investigations are performed in a timely manner, medical treatment is conducted, and education for patient and family takes place.

Initial investigations should include attempts at proving recent streptococcal infection through throat cultures and at least two of the serologic tests. Additionally, an ESR, CRP, white blood count, chest X-ray and, if possible, an echocardiogram should be considered in every patient. Other investigations may be required to exclude alternate diagnoses, including blood cultures for infective endocarditis, viral serology and autoimmune markers.

Previously bed rest was recommended. This is no longer the case, provided heart failure is adequately controlled. Ongoing active streptococcal infection warrants treatment with antibiotics. Oral penicillin V or amoxicillin is reasonable, or erythromycin if allergic. Intravenous administration is not required unless the patient is unable to take oral medication.

Anti-inflammatory medications are useful for a number of reasons. They result in rapid symptomatic improvement for patients, with fevers and arthralgias resolving within 1–2 days. Occasionally they are withheld to allow characteristic clinical features (e.g. migratory polyarthritis) to appear. Pain in these cases can be controlled by codeine until the diagnosis is made. Unfortunately, meta-analysis has shown no long-term benefits in those using anti-inflammatory agents (either steroidal or nonsteroidal) but this does enable clinicians to choose to withhold them for diagnostic purposes with reassurance; for example, aspirin at a dose of 80–100 mg/kg/day (4–6 g/day in adults) in four or five divided doses for 2 weeks, then reducing to 60–70 mg/kg/day for a further 2–4 weeks.

The more potent anti-inflammatory action of corticosteroids should be brought to bear when salicylates fail or when carditis with heart failure is severe. For example, 40–60 mg/day of oral prednisolone or even intravenous methyl prednisone in fulminant cases can be considered. All anti-inflammatory agents should be tapered as there is a risk of rebound if stopped abruptly. Intravenous immunoglobulin was ineffective in a randomized, placebo-controlled trial.[39]

The management of cardiac failure includes use of diuretics, angiotensin-converting enzyme inhibitors and fluid restriction. Digoxin may be used for atrial fibrillation, although it also has the potential to induce arrhythmias in the rare patient with concurrent active myocarditis. It is now a rare situation to require valve surgery for life-threatening cardiac failure in the acute setting.

Valve surgery is more often required for chronic disease. In recent years there has also been a trend to offer valve repair rather than replacement or to use homografts or xenograft valves rather than mechanical prostheses (to avoid the need for anticoagulation). This trend further enhances the need for regular monitoring of chronic valvular disease, as late surgical repair is technically difficult with an extensively damaged valve.

Mild cases of chorea do not usually require treatment. If chorea impairs normal daily activities, or leads to considerable embarrassment or discomfort to the patient, intervention is reasonable. Haloperidol, carbamazepine and diazepam have been traditionally used, although valproate, pimozide and chlorpromazine are equally effective. Associated anxiety can respond to behavioral therapy. Plasmapheresis and intravenous immunoglobulin have been shown to have benefit in a small trial, but cannot yet be recommended as mainstream treatment.[40] Salicylates and steroids have no role in chorea therapy.

PROGNOSIS AND FOLLOW-UP

Acute rheumatic fever resolves spontaneously, usually within 12 weeks, even if left untreated. With treatment most patients will be able to leave hospital in less than 2 weeks. The likelihood of developing rheumatic heart disease relates to the severity of the acute carditis and the number of episodes of subsequent recurrent ARF. Some 30–50% of all people with ARF will eventually develop rheumatic heart disease, increasing to 70% in patients with severe carditis on initial presentation. All patients should be added to a local registry, where available, to facilitate accurate follow-up.

Mortality in chronic rheumatic heart disease can result from progressive cardiac failure, infective endocarditis or thromboembolic stroke. Estimates of stroke-related deaths range from 100 000 per year to almost 270 000 per year in less developed countries.[3]

Depending on the population studied, 75% of recurrences occur in the first 2 years, and 90% in the first 5 years. This is likely related to immune sensitization that wanes with time. Unfortunately, a lack of carditis initially does not ensure subsequent episodes are free. As a result, regardless of the clinical features of the initial episode, the priorities of long-term management are to ensure adherence to secondary prophylaxis, treat cardiac failure and educate about the need to treat streptococcal upper respiratory or skin infections early.

Those patients who have proven rheumatic heart disease should be stratified according to the severity of disease. Mild cases should undergo echocardiography every 1–2 years where possible. Severe cases should be followed every 3–6 months, depending on progression. Patients should be given endocarditis prophylaxis during dental procedures, and should have yearly dental reviews. In those who take oral daily penicillin for ARF secondary prevention, their oral cavity may contain viridans streptococci relatively resistant to penicillin, and hence should be offered clindamycin, azithromycin or clarithromycin for endocarditis prophylaxis.[41] (See Chapter 47 for further information on endocarditis prophylaxis.) Some national guidelines also suggest vaccination with the influenza vaccine (yearly) and a locally available pneumococcal vaccine (5-yearly) could be considered.[4] This is in addition to penicillin, and is solely based on expert opinion.

REFERENCES

References for this chapter can be found online at http://www.expertconsult.com

Nuclear medicine scanning

INTRODUCTION

Nuclear medicine techniques have a lot to offer in visualization of infectious foci. They point to the localization of a particular metabolic process, leading to elevated uptake of a radiopharmaceutical. Furthermore, with these techniques it is possible to monitor the effect of therapy.

TECHNIQUES

A wide variety of approaches to scintigraphic imaging of infectious disorders, depicting the different stages of the inflammatory response, have been developed (Table PP21.1). Table PP21.2 shows the advantages and disadvantages of the scintigraphic techniques that are currently used in clinical practice.

PROSTHETIC JOINT INFECTION

A negative bone scintigraph effectively rules out infection. However, the majority of infections occur within 1 year after implantation, and at that time enhanced periprosthetic uptake is observed on the bone scan in most patients. Therefore, an abnormal bone scan will require additional studies to determine the cause of the abnormality.

Although not the ideal agent in these patients, ^{67}Ga-citrate can be used to delineate infected prostheses, with a moderate overall accuracy

of 70–80%. Radiolabeled leukocytes can accurately delineate infections in this patient population. However, in many cases the physiologic uptake of the labeled leukocytes in the bone marrow complicates the interpretation of the images.

In combination with sulfur colloid that accumulates in active marrow but not in infection, accuracy in diagnosing painful prostheses exceeds 90%. Furthermore, infected prostheses can be diagnosed very accurately using radiolabeled antigranulocyte antibody preparations. ^{18}F-fluorodeoxyglucose positron emission tomography (FDG-PET) also has a high sensitivity in diagnosing infected joint prostheses. Specificity, however, is lower than specificity of combined leukocyte scintigraphy and bone scanning.

OSTEOMYELITIS

A three-phase bone scan in otherwise normal bone is able to diagnose osteomyelitis with high sensitivity and specificity. In patients with other osseous abnormalities, ^{67}Ga-citrate or radiolabeled leukocytes can be applied to increase specificity; however, radiolabeled leukocytes are less suitable for diagnosing chronic low-grade osteomyelitis or suspected vertebral osteomyelitis. FDG-PET proved to be superior to MRI, ^{67}Ga-citrate scintigraphy and three-phase bone scan in patients suspected of vertebral osteomyelitis (Fig. PP21.1). In addition, FDG-PET is a very sensitive tool even for chronic and low-grade osteomyelitis.

Case study (Fig. PP21.1)

A 56-year-old woman experienced persisting fever despite adequate antibiotic treatment of her *Staphylococcus aureus* sepsis and endocarditis. PET showed increased FDG uptake in both shoulders, the left sternoclavicular joint, and the thoracic and lumbar spine. Septic arthritis of both shoulders was confirmed by puncture and culture and surgical treatment was needed several times. MRI confirmed spondylodiscitis of the sixth and seventh thoracic vertebrae and the third and fourth lumbar vertebrae, for which prolonged antibiotic treatment was prescribed.

VASCULAR INFECTIONS

CT is most often used for the assessment of vascular graft infection. However, hematomas and seromas in the vicinity of a vascular graft appear anatomically similar to an abscess, thus making it difficult to distinguish between noninfected and infected prosthetic grafts on CT images. The background activity of the images obtained with ^{67}Ga and radiolabeled immunoglobulins in many cases is too high for accurate visualization of vascular lesions.

Table PP21.1 Approaches to scintigraphic imaging of infectious disorders		
Physiologic characteristics	**Targeting mechanism**	**Radiolabeled compound**
Enhanced vascular permeability	Nonspecific uptake	[67]Gallium-citrate
Enhanced influx of granulocytes	Granulocyte influx	[111]Indium-leukocytes [99m]Technetium-leukocytes
	Antigen binding	Radiolabeled antigranulocyte monoclonal antibodies (e.g. LeuTech®, LeukoScan®)
Increased metabolic activity	Enhanced glucose uptake	^{18}F-fluorodeoxyglucose (FDG)

Table PP21.2 Advantages and disadvantages of currently available scintigraphic techniques

⁶⁷Gallium-citrate

Mechanism

- Accumulates as an iron analogue through binding to circulating transferrin
- This complex extravasates at the site of inflammation due to locally enhanced vascular permeability
- ^{67}Ga is transferred to lactoferrin that is locally excreted by leukocytes or to siderophores produced by micro-organisms

Advantages

- High sensitivity for both acute and chronic infection and noninfectious inflammation
- Inexpensive, easy labeling technique

Disadvantages

- Poor specificity (bowel excretion, accumulation in malignant tissues and areas of bone modeling)
- High-energy gamma radiation, causing high radiation absorbed doses
- Optimal imaging often requires delay of up to 72 h after the injection

¹¹¹Indium- or ^{99m}Technetium-leukocyte scintigraphy

Mechanism

- A blood sample (50 ml) is collected
- Leukocytes are separated *in vitro* from red blood cells
- Leukocytes are labeled with radioactive isotopes (^{111}In or ^{99m}Tc) and re-injected

Advantages

- Good diagnostic accuracy

Disadvantages

- Laborious procedure
- Handling of potentially contaminated blood, risk of transmission of infection
- Less sensitive in chronic low-grade infections and infections of the central skeleton

Antigranulocyte monoclonal antibodies and antibody fragments

Mechanism

- *In-vitro* labeling of monoclonal antibodies against surface antigens present on granulocytes
- Injection of radiolabeled antibodies and *in-vivo* binding to leukocytes

Advantages

- Easier labeling procedure
- No need for handling of potentially contaminated blood

Disadvantages

- Long time interval between injection and imaging
- Monoclonal antibodies: induction of human anti-mouse antibodies

¹⁸F-fluorodeoxyglucose positron emission tomography (FDG-PET)

Mechanism

- Accumulation in tissues with high rate of glycolysis (malignant cells, activated leukocytes)

Table PP21.2 Advantages and disadvantages of currently available scintigraphic techniques—cont'd

Advantages

- High resolution resulting in superior images
- Sensitivity in chronic low-grade infections and in infections of the central skeleton
- Early imaging (1 h after injection)

Disadvantages

- No differentiation between infection and malignancy (an advantage in fever of unknown origin)
- Relatively expensive
- More limited availability

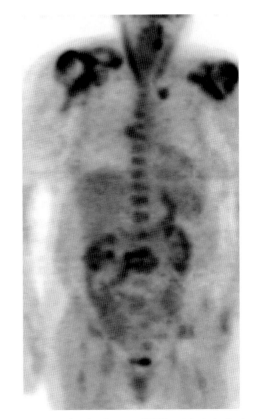

Fig. PP21.1 PET scan showing increased FDG uptake in both shoulders, the left sternoclavicular joint, and the thoracic and lumbar spine.

Vascular infections can be detected accurately with radiolabeled white blood cells; the overall sensitivity, specificity and accuracy of ^{111}In-labeled leukocytes is >90%. More recently, FDG-PET has been shown valuable in diagnosing vascular infections (Fig. PP21.2). In a systematic comparison between CT and FDG-PET in patients suspected of vascular graft infection, the sensitivity of FDG-PET (91%) was significantly higher than that of CT (64%). When the PET criterion for infection was defined as focal abnormal uptake, the specificities of FDG-PET and CT were comparable. It is to be expected that specificity and positive predictive value are even better after a certain period following surgery.

Case study (Fig. PP21.2)

A 69-year-old woman was admitted because of fever and chills. She also complained of pain in the upper abdomen radiating to her left leg. Her medical history was remarkable for severe arterial insufficiency

Fig. PP21.2 PET scan showing increased FDG uptake at the aortomesenteric bypass: (a) coronal view; (b) sagittal view, upper panels. Lower panels: FDG-PET-CT scan.

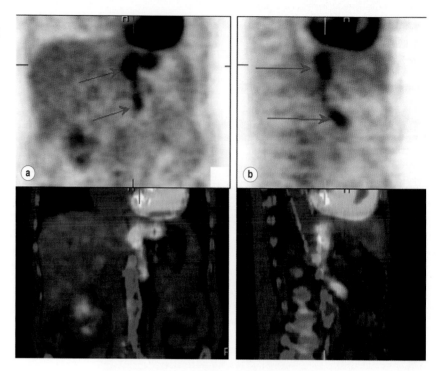

with mesenterial ischemia for which a bypass from the aorta to the superior mesenteric artery was performed 2 years earlier. She had also undergone an aorto-iliacal bypass some 15 years previously.

Blood cultures grew *Escherichia coli*. The first abdominal CT scan showed no signs of infection. PET, however, showed increased FDG uptake at the aortomesenteric bypass. An infection of the vascular prosthesis was diagnosed. The prosthesis could not be removed, so suppressive therapy with ciprofloxacin was started.

METASTATIC INFECTIOUS FOCI

Timely identification of metastatic complications of bloodstream infections, although critical, is often difficult. In a retrospective study in 40 patients with a high suspicion of metastatic complications after bloodstream infection, FDG-PET diagnosed a clinically relevant new focus in 45% of cases while, on average, four conventional diagnostic tests had been performed before FDG-PET. FDG-PET is very promising in detecting metastatic infectious foci in patients with a high level of clinical suspicion (see Fig. PP21.1).

ABDOMINAL INFECTIONS

For this purpose, ultrasonography, CT and MRI are currently considered the modalities of choice. However, in early stages of infection or in postoperative patients with equivocal anatomic changes, scintigraphic imaging can be very useful.

Although ^{67}Ga-citrate has a reasonable diagnostic accuracy for diagnosing abdominal infection, the physiologic gastrointestinal uptake of ^{67}Ga-citrate limits the interpretation of the images. Radiolabeled white blood cells are more suitable in these patients. Because ^{111}In-labeled leukocytes normally do not localize in the gastrointestinal tract, they have an advantage over ^{99m}Tc-labeled leukocytes. In patients with polycystic kidney disease, FDG-PET proved to be very helpful in suspected renal or hepatic cyst infection by correctly pointing to the infected cysts. In addition, FDG-PET appears to be a sensitive and specific adjunct in the diagnosis of suspected alveolar echinococcosis and can help in differentiating alveolar from cystic echinococcosis in the liver. FDG-PET also appears to be valuable in assessing the efficacy of chemotherapy in these patients.

FEVER OF UNKNOWN ORIGIN

The value of FDG-PET has been studied in 292 patients with fever of unknown origin (FUO) showing an overall helpfulness of FDG-PET of 36%. FDG-PET appears to be superior to ^{67}Ga-citrate scintigraphy because the diagnostic yield is at least similar to that of ^{67}Ga-citrate scintigraphy and the results are available within hours instead of days.

Based on the results of these studies and resulting from the favorable characteristics of FDG-PET, conventional scintigraphic techniques may in the future be replaced by FDG-PET in the investigation of patients with FUO in institutions where this technique is available.

DISCUSSION

Leukocyte scintigraphy is still considered the 'gold standard' nuclear medicine technique for the imaging of infection and inflammation by many clinicians, but a gradual shift from cumbersome and even hazardous techniques to approaches, based on small agents binding to their targets with high affinity, is ongoing. The ideal agent will be determined by the clinical situation and local availability.

FDG-PET has a lot to offer in visualization of various infectious foci in many organ systems. It is shown to be superior to other scintigraphic techniques in FUO, chronic low-grade osteomyelitis and vertebral osteomyelitis. FDG-PET has also shown promising results in vascular graft infections and the evaluation of metastatic infectious foci in patients with bloodstream infections. FDG-PET may prove to be as useful in the rapid detection and management of infectious diseases as it is in the management of malignant diseases. In addition, combined PET-CT scans are suspected to further increase the usefulness of this imaging modality.

FURTHER READING

Further reading for this chapter can be found online at http://www.expertconsult.com

Approach to the patient with persistent bacteremia

INTRODUCTION

Persistent bacteremia, generally defined as continuous bacteremia for at least 3 days, is a common clinical problem and presents a unique therapeutic challenge. The frequency of persistent bacteremia has been rising over the past 10 years, reflecting an increase in resistant organisms such as meticillin-resistant *Staphylococcus aureus* (MRSA) and the upsurge of implantable intravascular devices. This trend is particularly concerning as persistent bacteremia is associated with longer hospitalizations and higher morbidity and mortality compared with shorter duration bacteremia. Effective management entails a comprehensive approach including a diligent search for metastatic foci of infection coupled with optimal antibiotic therapy. The differential diagnosis of persistent bacteremia is usually quite straightforward:

- inappropriate or inadequate antibiotics;
- an extravascular focus of infection; or
- endocarditis or intravascular infection.

INAPPROPRIATE OR INADEQUATE ANTIBIOTICS

Persistent bacteremia is often related to inappropriate antibiotic therapy through either inadequate empiric coverage or subtherapeutic dosing. Careful reassessment of initial empiric antibiotic choices based on culture and susceptibility results is the critical element in the management of persistent bacteremia.

The choice for empiric coverage of antibiotics should be dictated by the clinical presentation. In patients with endocarditis, adequate antistaphylococcal coverage, including MRSA, and antistreptococcal coverage in conjunction with a synergistic aminoglycoside should be considered (see Chapter 47). Those patients with foreign bodies (e.g. prostheses or implantable intravascular devices) should be administered antibiotics that cover nosocomial pathogens including MRSA and resistant gram-negative bacteria such as *Klebsiella*, *Serratia*, and *Pseudomonas* species.

Suboptimal dosing represents a selective pressure that is imposed on the bacteria which in turn facilitates the emergence of resistance. MRSA is being reported with increasing frequency as a cause of persistent bacteremia and infective endocarditis.

Recommendations of maintaining higher vancomycin trough levels of 15–20 µg/ml in MRSA pneumonia have now been extrapolated to MRSA bacteremias. MRSA infections with strains expressing higher vancomycin minimum inhibitory concentrations (MICs) of 2–4 µg/ml are associated with vancomycin-treatment failure and poor outcomes. As such, recent guidelines suggest lowering the breakpoint of the MIC for susceptibility for MRSA from 4 µg/ml to 2 µg/ml and consider increasing vancomycin dosing or use alternative antibiotics when the vancomycin MIC is ≥2 µg/ml.

For infections with *Pseudomonas* spp. and other resistant gram-negative pathogens such as *Acinetobacter* spp., successful eradication necessitates higher doses of broad-spectrum β-lactams at shorter intervals to maintain levels above the MIC. Likewise, higher doses of fluoroquinolones and aminoglycosides emphasize the concentration-dependent activity of these antimicrobials while taking advantage of their sustained postantibiotic effect. Studies are underway with continuous infusions of anti-pseudomonal β-lactams to facilitate consistent levels of the antimicrobial above the MIC, especially in the critically ill patient. Such continuous infusions have been shown to be effective in animal experiments.

FOCUS OF INFECTION

The identification of a metastatic focus of infection, particularly a removable or drainable focus, is a key component in the evaluation of a patient with persistent bacteremia (Table PP22.1). Even optimal antibiotic therapy is unlikely to be curative unless source control is achieved.

The growing use of devices such as central venous catheters, automatic implantable cardioverter defibrillators (AICDs), cardiac pacemakers and central implantable spinal pumps in the medical community has resulted in increased incidence of bloodstream infections. The presence of a central vascular catheter is an independent risk factor for persistent bacteremia even if another source of infection is identified. Patients with persistently positive blood cultures should

---

Table PP22.1 Potential foci of infection in persistent bacteremia

- Implanted devices
  - Central venous catheters
  - Automatic implantable cardioverter defibrillator (AICD) or cardiac pacemaker
  - Implantable spinal pump
- Intra-abdominal process
- Osteomyelitis (particularly vertebral)
- Epidural abscess
- Intravascular infection
  - Endocarditis with or without valvular ring abscess
  - Mycotic aneurysm
  - Thrombophlebitis
  - Pylephlebitis

be examined carefully for evidence of local inflammation at the site of implanted devices. If present, the device should be removed and cultured. Even if there is no local inflammation, in the absence of another identifiable source, persistent bloodstream contamination necessitates the removal of the device. Empiric antibiotic regimens that cover nosocomial pathogens such as MRSA and *Pseudomonas* spp. should be initiated while awaiting definitive diagnostics and procedures.

In those patients without implanted devices, other foci of infection should be explored. Certain pathogens such as *Salmonella* spp. and *Staphylococcus aureus* are more likely to result in metastatic infectious lesions and their presence should trigger an investigation for metastatic disease. Some studies indicate that intermittent bacteremia often denotes an occult abscess whereas persistent bacteremia is more suggestive of an endovascular source. However, in a review of patients with persistent bacteremia, a non-endovascular source was implicated in 23% of cases. Patients with burns, cirrhosis or baseline intra-abdominal pathology are at particular risk of persistent bacteremia, perhaps related to mucosal barrier dysfunction and/or diminished bacterial clearance capacity. In these patients, an aggressive search for an intra-abdominal process should be undertaken.

Infections in areas with poor blood supply, such as bone or the peripheral extremities of patients with severe neuropathy, may contribute to persistent bacteremia without an apparent endovascular focus. Persistent bacteremia in a patient with bone pain, back pain and/or neurologic symptoms should trigger a workup for osteomyelitis (particularly vertebral) or an epidural abscess with MRI of the involved area.

ENDOCARDITIS OR INTRAVASCULAR INFECTION

Endovascular infections account for most cases of persistent bacteremia. Factors supporting a diagnosis of endocarditis include:

- a new or changing heart murmur;
- valvular vegetations on echocardiogram;
- peripheral stigmata of endocarditis, including septic emboli or glomerulonephritis; and
- persistent bacteremia with a typical pathogen such as *Streptococcus* spp., *Staphylococcus aureus*, enterococci or the HACEK organisms.

In patients with prosthetic heart valves, persistently positive blood cultures without another identifiable source of infection are virtually pathognomonic for prosthetic valve endocarditis and should immediately be assessed with a transesophageal echocardiogram to assess for valve function and possible leakage.

Persistently positive blood cultures while on optimal antibiotic therapy, in the absence of an intravascular device and without other identifiable foci of infection, most commonly result from intravascular suppuration. Possible intravascular infections are native valve endocarditis with or without associated valvular ring abscess, mycotic aneurysm, thrombophlebitis or pylephlebitis (Fig. PP22.1) and should be explored with appropriate diagnostic studies such as transesophageal echocardiogram or nuclear medicine studies (for more details on imaging studies, see Practice Point 21).

While diagnostic tests are pending, optimal empiric antibiotic therapy should be initiated in all patients where the clinical scenario supports this diagnosis. In addition, when the diagnosis of suppurative intravascular infection has been established, a low threshold for surgical exploration should be maintained because this often subtle and

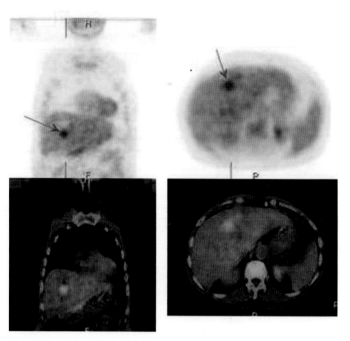

Fig. PP22.1 Pylephlibitis. This previously healthy 68-year-old man was admitted with fever that had been present for 2 weeks and diffuse abdominal pain. Physical examination was normal except for a temperature of 102.4°F (39.1°C) and a heart rate of 98 bpm. Blood cultures grew *Escherichia coli*, *Pseudomonas aeruginosa* and coagulase-negative staphylococci. Because of persisting fever despite treatment with piperacillin–tazobactam, an FDG-PET CT scan was performed, which showed increased FDG-uptake in the portal vein (arrow) and several smaller areas in the liver. CT confirmed the presence of a portal vein thrombosis and small liver abscesses, so a diagnosis of pylephlebitis was made. The patient was treated with amoxicillin–clavulanic acid and ciprofloxacin for 6 more weeks and low-molecular-weight heparin for 6 months, with a complete resolution of his symptoms. Courtesy of Chantal Bleeker-Rovers, MD.

highly lethal process is unlikely to be eradicated unless the lesion is excised, even in the presence of optimal antibiotic therapy.

CONCLUSION

Many hospitalized individuals with bacteremia are at risk for persistent bacteremia, particularly those with resistant organisms, intravascular infections and foreign bodies. Rates of persistent bacteremia are expected to rise as populations at risk expand with the increase of implantable devices.

Table PP22.2 outlines the approach to the patient with a persistent bacteremia. The key points in the diagnostic approach remain a careful history and physical examination, thorough consideration of likely pathogens and further diagnostic workup with imaging studies as indicated by the clinical scenario, judicious assessment of antimicrobials, and pursuit of definitive treatment through source control. Aggressive attempts to minimize the risk of complications associated with persistent bacteremia are vital in view of the higher rates of morbidity and mortality associated with this clinical entity.

Table PP22.2 Evaluation of a patient with persistent bacteremia (≥3 days)

- Obtain full history and physical, examining the patient thoroughly for any identifiable sources of infection, visible or implanted
- Assess antibiotic coverage and dosing to ensure optimal levels based on culture and susceptibility results and/or on clinical scenario
- Obtain diagnostic imaging based on organisms isolated and clinical scenario:
  - if organism isolated is consistent with a diagnosis of endocarditis, obtain transthoracic or transesophageal echocardiogram
  - if organism(s) is gram-negative, fungal pathogen or polymicrobial, or patient is at risk of bacterial translocation via the gut, obtain abdominal imaging to rule out occult abdominal process
  - if patient has back pain or neurologic symptoms, obtain MRI of head/spine to evaluate for epidural abscess or vertebral osteomyelitis
- For patients with intravascular devices and/or catheters:
  - identify and remove any temporary peripheral catheters and send for culture
  - if there is expressible purulence, culture and consider surgical intervention
  - if intravascular device such as AICD or tunneled catheter is present and no other source of infection is identified, remove and send for semiquantitative culture
- For patients who remain persistently bacteremic on optimal antibiotic therapy despite removal of all foreign bodies:
  - consider radiolabeled white blood cell scan or positron emission tomography to evaluate for evidence of intravascular suppuration
  - if suggestive of a suppurative process, obtain surgical consult for definitive evaluation and treatment

FURTHER READING

Further reading for this chapter can be found online at http://www.expertconsult.com

Vaginitis, vulvitis, cervicitis and cutaneous vulval lesions

Vaginitis

Vaginal symptoms are extremely common, and vaginal discharge is among the 25 most common reasons for consulting physicians in private office practice in the USA. Vaginitis is found in more than one-quarter of women attending sexually transmitted disease (STD) clinics. Not all women with vaginal symptoms have vaginitis; approximately 40% of women with vaginal symptoms will have some type of vaginitis (Table 49.1).

Bacterial Vaginosis

EPIDEMIOLOGY

Bacterial vaginosis is the most common cause of vaginitis in women of child-bearing age. It has been diagnosed in 17–19% of women seeking gynecologic care in family practice or student health-care settings.[1]

Table 49.1 Causes of vaginitis in adult women

Common infectious vaginitis	Bacterial vaginosis (40–50%)
	Vulvovaginal candidiasis (20–25%)
	Trichomonal vaginitis (15–20%)
Uncommon infectious vaginitis	Foreign body with secondary infection
	Desquamative inflammatory vaginitis (clindamycin responsive)
	Streptococcal vaginitis (group A)
	Ulcerative vaginitis associated with *Staphylococcus aureus* and toxic shock syndrome
	Idiopathic vulvovaginal ulceration associated with HIV
Noninfectious vaginitis	Chemical/irritant
	Allergic, hypersensitivity and contact dermatitis (lichen simplex)
	Traumatic
	Atrophic vaginitis
	Postpuerperal atrophic vaginitis
	Desquamative inflammatory vaginitis (corticosteroid responsive)
	Erosive lichen planus
	Collagen vascular disease, Behçet's syndrome, pemphigus syndromes
	Idiopathic

The worldwide prevalence ranges from 11% to 48% of women of reproductive age, with variation according to population studied.[2] The prevalence increases considerably in symptomatic women attending STD clinics, reaching 24–37%. Bacterial vaginosis has been observed in 16–29% of pregnant women. *Gardnerella vaginalis* has been found in 10–31% of virgin adolescent girls, but is found significantly more frequently among sexually active women, reaching a prevalence of 50–60% in some at-risk populations.

Evaluation of epidemiologic factors has revealed few clues as to the cause of bacterial vaginosis. Use of the intrauterine device and douching was found to be more common in women with bacterial vaginosis. Bacterial vaginosis is significantly more common among black and sexually active women, including lesbians.

PATHOGENESIS AND PATHOLOGY

Bacterial vaginosis is not due to a single organism and is the result of massive overgrowth of mixed complex flora or microbiota, including peptostreptococci, *Bacteroides* spp., *G. vaginalis*, *Mobiluncus* spp. and genital mycoplasma.[1] There is little inflammation, and the disorder represents a disturbance of the vaginal microbial ecosystem rather than a true infection of tissues. The overgrowth of mixed flora is associated with a loss of the normal *Lactobacillus* spp. dominated vaginal flora. No single bacterial species is responsible for bacterial vaginosis. Experimental studies in human volunteers and studies in animals indicate that inoculation of the vagina with individual species of bacteria associated with bacterial vaginosis (e.g. *G. vaginalis*), rarely results in bacterial vaginosis. In support of the role of sexual transmission is the higher prevalence of bacterial vaginosis among sexually active young women than among sexually inexperienced women, and the observation that bacterial vaginosis-associated micro-organisms are more frequently isolated from the urethras of male partners of females with bacterial vaginosis.[1]

The cause of the overgrowth of anaerobes, *Gardnerella*, *Mycoplasma* and *Mobiluncus* spp. is unknown. Theories include increased substrate availability, increased pH and loss of the restraining effects of the predominant *Lactobacillus* spp. flora. It has been reported that normal women are predominantly colonized by hydrogen peroxide-producing strains of lactobacilli, whereas women with bacterial vaginosis have reduced population numbers of lactobacilli, and the species present lack the ability to produce hydrogen peroxide.[3] The hydrogen peroxide produced by lactobacilli may inhibit the pathogens associated with bacterial vaginosis, either directly by the toxicity of hydrogen peroxide, or as a result of the production of a hydrogen peroxide–halide complex in the presence of natural cervical peroxidase.

Accompanying the bacterial overgrowth in bacterial vaginosis is the increased production of amines by anaerobes, facilitated by microbial decarboxylases. Volatile amines in the presence of increased vaginal pH produce the typical fishy odor, which is also produced when 10%

potassium hydroxide is added to vaginal secretions. Trimethylamine is the dominant abnormal amine in bacterial vaginosis. It is likely that bacterial polyamines together with the organic acids found in the vagina in bacterial vaginosis (acetic and succinic acid) are cytotoxic, resulting in exfoliation of vaginal epithelial cells and creating the vaginal discharge. *Gardnerella vaginalis* attaches avidly to exfoliated epithelial cells, especially at the alkaline pH found in bacterial vaginosis. The adherence of *Gardnerella* organisms results in the formation of the pathognomonic clue cells. Using broad-range DNA probes, new molecular methods have identified at least 35 new bacterial phylotypes (species) previously noncultivable in women with bacterial vaginosis, including *Atopobium vaginae* and clostridial species BVAB I, II and III, offering new insights into pathogenesis.[4]

PREVENTION

Because the pathogenesis of bacterial vaginosis is obscure, preventive measures have not been forthcoming. Although not proven to be sexually transmitted, barrier contraception may reduce occurrence and avoiding douching is recommended.

CLINICAL FEATURES

As many as 50% of women with bacterial vaginosis may be asymptomatic. An abnormal malodorous vaginal discharge, often described as fishy, that is infrequently profuse and often appears after unprotected coitus, is usually described. Pruritus, dysuria and dyspareunia are rare. Examination reveals a nonviscous, grayish-white adherent discharge.

Bacterial vaginosis has been incorrectly considered to be largely of nuisance value only. There is now considerable evidence of serious obstetric and gynecologic complications of bacterial vaginosis, including asymptomatic bacterial vaginosis diagnosed by Gram stain. Obstetric complications include chorioamnionitis, pre-term labor, prematurity and postpartum fever.[5] Gynecologic sequelae are postabortion fever, posthysterectomy fever, cuff infection and chronic mast cell endometritis. A more recent association is reported between untreated bacterial vaginosis and cervical inflammation and low-grade dysplasia.[6] Bacterial vaginosis is a risk factor for HIV acquisition and transmission.[7] Bacterial vaginosis is also a risk factor for acquisition of herpes simplex virus 2, gonorrhea and chlamydial infection.[8]

DIAGNOSIS

Signs and symptoms are unreliable in the diagnosis of bacterial vaginosis (Table 49.2). The clinical diagnosis can reliably be made in the presence of at least three of the following objective criteria:
- adherent, white, nonfloccular homogeneous discharge;
- positive amine test, with release of fishy odor on addition of 10% potassium hydroxide to vaginal secretions;
- vaginal pH >4.5; and
- presence of clue cells on light microscopy.

These features are simple and reliable, and tests for them are easy to perform. The presence of clue cells is the single most reliable predictor of bacterial vaginosis. Clue cells are exfoliated vaginal squamous epithelial cells covered with *G. vaginalis*, giving the cells a granular or stippled appearance with characteristic loss of clear cell borders. Of observed epithelial cells, diagnostic significance is indicated by 20% clue cells. Occasionally, clue cells covered exclusively by curved

Table 49.2 Diagnostic features of infectious vaginitis

		Normal	*Candida* **vaginitis**	**Bacterial vaginosis**	*Trichomonas* **vaginitis**
Symptoms		None or physiologic leukorrhea	Vulvar pruritus, soreness, increased discharge, dysuria, dyspareunia	Malodorous moderate discharge	Profuse purulent discharge, offensive odor, pruritus, and dyspareunia
Discharge	Amount	Variable, scant to moderate	Scant to moderate	Moderate	Profuse
	Color	Clear or white	White	White/gray	Yellow
	Consistency	Floccular nonhomogeneous	Clumped but variable	Homogeneous, uniformly coating walls	Homogeneous
	'Bubbles'	Absent	Absent	Present	Present
	Appearance of vulva and vagina	Normal	Introital and vulvar erythema, edema and occasional pustules, vaginal erythema	No inflammation	Erythema and swelling of vulvar and vaginal epithelium (strawberry cervix)
	pH of vaginal fluid	<4.5	<4.5	>4.7	5.0–6.0
	Amine test (10% potassium hydroxide)	Negative	Negative	Positive	Occasionally present
	Saline microscopy	Normal epithelial cell, lactobacilli predominate	Normal flora, blastospores (yeast) 40–50% pseudohyphae	Clue cells, coccobacillary flora predominate, absence of leukocytes, motile curved rods	PMNS +++, motile trichomonads (80–90%), no clue cells, abnormal flora
10% potassium hydroxide microscopy		Negative	Positive (60–90%)	Negative (except in mixed infections)	Negative

Gram-negative rods belonging to *Mobiluncus* spp. can be demonstrated. The offensive fishy odor may be apparent during the physical examination or may become apparent only during the amine test. Gram strain of vaginal secretions is extremely valuable in diagnosis, with a sensitivity of 93% and specificity of 70%.

Although cultures for *G. vaginalis* are positive in almost all cases of bacterial vaginosis, *G. vaginalis* may be detected in 50–60% of women who do not meet the diagnostic criteria for bacterial vaginosis. Accordingly, vaginal culture has no part in the diagnosis of bacterial vaginosis. DNA probes for *G. vaginalis* are both sensitive (95%) and specific (99%), but are not widely used by practitioners because of costs and lack of insurance reimbursement. Diagnostic cards are now available for rapid diagnosis, measuring pH, amines or sialidase.

MANAGEMENT

Poor efficacy has been observed with triple sulfa creams, ampicillin, quinolones, erythromycin, tetracycline, acetic acid gel and povidone–iodine vaginal douches.[9]

The most widely used oral therapy remains metronidazole or tinidazole. Most studies using multiple divided dose metronidazole regimens of 800–1200 mg/day for 1 week achieved clinical cure rates in excess of 90% immediately, and of approximately 80% at 4 weeks. Although single-dose therapy with 2 g metronidazole achieves comparable immediate clinical response rates, higher recurrence rates have been reported. The CDC recommended regimen is metronidazole 500 mg twice daily for 7 days.[9] The beneficial effect of metronidazole results predominantly from its anti-anaerobic activity and because *G. vaginalis* is susceptible to the hydroxymetabolites of metronidazole. Although *Mycoplasma hominis* and *Mobiluncus curtisii* are resistant to metronidazole, the organisms are usually not detected at follow-up visits of successfully treated patients. Similarly, metronidazole and tinidazole are considered therapeutic equivalents although tinidazole has fewer of the commonly experienced side-effects.

Topical therapy with 2% clindamycin cream once daily for 7 days, clindamycin ovules for 3 days or metronidazole gel 0.75% administered daily for 5 days have been shown to be as effective as oral metronidazole, without any of the side-effects of the latter.[9]

In the past, asymptomatic bacterial vaginosis was not treated, especially because patients often improve spontaneously over several months. However, the growing evidence linking asymptomatic bacterial vaginosis with numerous obstetric and gynecologic upper tract complications has caused reassessment of this policy, especially with additional convenient topical therapies.[5,10] Asymptomatic bacterial vaginosis should be treated before pregnancy, in women with cervical abnormalities and before elective gynecologic surgery. Routine screening for and treatment of asymptomatic bacterial vaginosis in pregnancy remains controversial, pending the outcome of studies proving that therapy of bacterial vaginosis reduces pre-term delivery and prematurity.[11]

Despite indirect evidence of sexual transmission, no study has documented reduced recurrent rates of bacterial vaginosis in women whose partners have been treated with a variety of regimens, including metronidazole. Accordingly, most clinicians do not routinely treat male partners.

After therapy with oral metronidazole, approximately 30% of patients initially responding experience recurrence of symptoms within 3 months.[1] Reasons for recurrence are unclear, including the possibility of re-infection, but recurrence more likely reflects vaginal relapse, with failure to eradicate the offending organisms and re-establish the normal protective *Lactobacillus* spp. dominant vaginal flora. Management of bacterial vaginosis relapse includes oral or vaginal metronidazole, or topical clindamycin, usually prescribed for 14 days. New experimental approaches including exogenous *Lactobacillus* spp. recolonization using selected bacteria-containing suppositories have been encouraging. Maintenance antimicrobial agents administered twice weekly for 4–6 months have been reasonably effective but results are less than desirable.[12]

Trichomoniasis

EPIDEMIOLOGY

Studies estimate that 3–5 million American women contract trichomoniasis annually, with a worldwide distribution of approximately 180 million annual cases.[1,13] The prevalence of trichomoniasis correlates with the overall level of sexual activity of the specific group of women under study, being diagnosed in about 5% of women in family planning clinics, in 13–25% of women attending gynecology clinics, in 50–75% of prostitutes and in 7–35% of women in STD clinics. In many industrialized countries, recent surveys indicate a decline in the incidence of trichomoniasis.[13]

PATHOGENESIS AND PATHOLOGY

Sexual transmission is the dominant method of introduction of *Trichomonas vaginalis* into the vagina.[1] *Trichomonas vaginalis* was identified in the urethra of 70% of men who had had sexual contact with infected women within the previous 48 hours. There is also a high prevalence of gonorrhea in women with trichomoniasis, and both of these are significantly associated with use of nonbarrier methods of contraception.

Recurrent trichomoniasis is common and is indicative of a lack of significant protective immunity. Nevertheless, an immune response to *Trichomonas* spp. does develop, as indicated by low titers of serum antibody, but this is insufficient for diagnostic serology. Antitrichomonal IgA has been detected in vaginal secretions, but a protective role is not defined.

Delayed hypersensitivity in natural infection can also be demonstrated. The predominant host defense response is provided by the numerous polymorphonuclear leukocytes (PMNs), which respond to chemotactic substances released by trichomonads and are capable of killing *T. vaginalis* without ingesting trichomonads. *Trichomonas vaginalis* destroys epithelial cells by direct cell contact and cytotoxicity. The urethra, paraurethral, Bartholin's and Skene's glands are infected in the majority of patients, and organisms are occasionally isolated from urine.

PREVENTION

Sexual transmission of trichomonads is efficiently prevented by use of barrier contraception. Spermicidal agents such as nonoxynol-9 also reduce transmission. Re-infection of women is common, hence the mandatory requirement of treatment, preferably simultaneously, of all sexual partners with metronidazole. Women can acquire the disease from other women, but men do not usually transmit infection to other men.

CLINICAL FEATURES

Infection with *Trichomonas* spp. in women ranges from an asymptomatic carrier state to severe acute inflammatory disease.[14,15] Vaginal discharge is reported by 50–75% of women diagnosed with trichomoniasis; however, the discharge is not always described as malodorous. Pruritus occurs in 25–50% of patients and is often severe. Other infrequent symptoms include dyspareunia, dysuria and, rarely, frequency of micturition. Lower abdominal pain occurs in fewer than 10% of patients and should alert the physician to the possibility of concomitant salpingitis caused by other organisms. Symptoms of acute trichomoniasis often appear during or immediately after menstruation. Although controversial, the incubation period has been estimated to range from 3 to 28 days.

Physical findings represent a spectrum depending on the severity of disease. Vulvar findings may be absent, but are typically characterized in severe cases by diffuse vulvar erythema (10–33%), edema and a copious, profuse and malodorous vaginal discharge, which is often described as being yellow-green and frothy, but is frequently grayish-white.[11] Frothiness is seen in a minority of patients and is more commonly seen in bacterial vaginosis.

The vaginal walls are erythematous and in severe cases may be granular in appearance. Punctate hemorrhages (colpitis macularis) of the cervix may result in a strawberry-like appearance that, although apparent to the naked eye in only 1–2% of patients, is present in 45% of cases on colposcopy.[11]

The clinical course of trichomoniasis in pregnancy is identical to that seen in the nonpregnant state, and when untreated it is associated with premature rupture of membranes and prematurity. Trichomoniasis is reported to facilitate HIV transmission. Trichomoniasis is a risk factor for development of posthysterectomy cellulitis, tubal infertility, cervical neoplasia and pelvic inflammatory disease.[16]

DIAGNOSIS

None of the clinical features of vaginitis caused by *Trichomonas* spp. are sufficiently specific to allow a diagnosis of trichomonal infection based on signs and symptoms alone (see Table 49.2).[10] Definitive diagnosis requires the demonstration of the organism. Vaginal pH is markedly elevated, almost always above 5.0, and not infrequently 6.0. On saline microscopy, an increase in the number of PMNs is almost invariably present. The ovoid parasites are slightly larger than PMNs and are best recognized by their motility. The wet mount is positive in only 40–80% of cases (low sensitivity). Gram stain is of little value because of its inability to differentiate PMNs from nonmotile trichomonads, and use of Giemsa, acridine orange and other stains has no advantage over saline preparations. Although trichomonads are often seen on Papanicolaou smears, this method has a sensitivity of only 60–70% when compared with saline preparation microscopy, and false-positive results are not infrequently reported.

Several equivalent culture medium methods are available, and growth is usually detected within 48 hours. Culture including 'In-Pouch' is now recognized as the most sensitive method for detecting the presence of trichomonads (95% sensitivity) and should be considered in patients with vaginitis in whom an elevated pH is found together with PMN excess and absence of motile trichomonads. Several new diagnostic kits using DNA probes or rapid antigen detection are now available commercially and are replacing culture because of rapid confirmation[17] (e.g. Affirm VP, BectonDickenson; OSOM Trichomonas Rapid Test, Genzyme).

MANAGEMENT

Therapy is indicated in all nonpregnant women diagnosed with *Trichomonas* vaginitis, even if asymptomatic, and consists of administering the 5-nitroimidazole group of drugs – metronidazole, tinidazole and ornidazole – which are all of similar efficacy.[9] Oral therapy as opposed to topical vaginal therapy is preferred because of the frequency of infection of the urethra and periurethral glands, which provide sources for endogenous recurrence. Treatment of all sexual partners is mandatory.

Treatment consists of oral metronidazole, 500 mg every 12 hours for 7 days, which has a cure rate of 95%. Comparable results have been obtained with a single oral dose of 2 g metronidazole, achieving cure rates of 82–88%. The latter cure rate increases to greater than 90% when sexual partners are treated simultaneously. The advantages of single-dose therapy include better patient compliance, lower total dose, shorter period of alcohol avoidance and possibly decreased incidence of subsequent vaginitis caused by *Candida* spp. A disadvantage of single-dose therapy is the need to insist on simultaneous treatment of sexual partners.

The 5-nitroimidazoles are not in themselves trichomonacidal, but low-redox proteins reduce the nitro group, resulting in the formation of highly cytotoxic products within the organisms. Aerobic conditions interfere with this reduction process and decrease the antianaerobic activity of the 5-nitroimidazoles. Most strains of *T. vaginalis* are highly susceptible to metronidazole, with minimum inhibitory concentrations (MICs) of 1 mg/l. Similar efficacy results are reported with tinidazole but the latter has a superior tolerance profile.

Patients not responding to an initial course often respond to an additional standard course of 7-day therapy. Some patients are refractory to repeated courses of therapy, even when compliance is assured and sexual partners are known to have been treated. If re-infection is excluded, these rare patients may have strains of *T. vaginalis* that are resistant to metronidazole, which can be confirmed *in vitro*. Increased doses of metronidazole and longer duration of therapy are necessary to cure these refractory patients. The patients should be given maximal tolerated dosages of oral metronidazole of 2–4 g/day for 10–14 days. Rarely, intravenous metronidazole, in dosages as high as 2–4 g/day, may be necessary, with careful monitoring for drug toxicity. Considerable success has been observed in treating resistant infections with oral tinidazole; however, the drug is not readily available and the optimal dose to be used is unknown.[18] Most investigators use high-dose tinidazole 1–4 g/day for 14 days.[18] Rare patients not responding to nitroimidazoles can be treated with topical paramomycin.

Side-effects of metronidazole include an unpleasant or metallic taste. Other common side-effects include nausea (10%), transient neutropenia (7.5%) and a disulfiram-like effect when alcohol is ingested. Caution should be taken when 5-nitroimidazoles are used in patients taking warfarin. Long-term and high-dose therapy increase the risk of neutropenia and peripheral neuropathy. In experimental studies, metronidazole has been shown to be mutagenic for certain bacteria, indicating a carcinogenic potential, although cohort studies have not established an increase in cancer morbidity. Thus, the risk to humans of short-term low-dose metronidazole treatment is extremely small. Superinfection with *Candida* spp. is by no means uncommon.

Treatment of symptomatic trichomoniasis in pregnancy is identical.[9] Metronidazole readily crosses the placenta and, because of concern for teratogenicity, some consider it prudent to avoid its use in the first trimester of pregnancy. More recently investigators have become more comfortable with the use of metronidazole throughout pregnancy. Topical clotrimazole and povidone–iodine jelly offer minimal benefit. Some concern exists about treating asymptomatic trichomoniasis in pregnancy because one trial found a higher rate of pre-term birth (RR 1.8) compared to control women.[19]

Vulvovaginal Candidiasis

EPIDEMIOLOGY

Vulvovaginal candidiasis (VVC) accounts for approximately one-third of vaginitis cases. In the USA, *Candida* spp. are now the second commonest cause of vaginal infections.[20,21]

It is estimated that 75% of women experience at least one episode of VVC during their child-bearing years, and approximately 40–50% experience a second attack. A small subpopulation of women of undetermined magnitude, probably 5–8% of adult females, suffers from repeated, recurrent, often intractable episodes of *Candida* vaginitis.[22]

Point-prevalence studies indicate that *Candida* spp. may be isolated from the genital tract of approximately 20% of asymptomatic, healthy women of child-bearing age. The natural history of asymptomatic colonization is unknown, although animal and human studies suggest that vaginal carriage continues for several months and perhaps years. Several factors are associated with increased rates of asymptomatic vaginal colonization with *Candida* spp., including pregnancy (30–40%), use of oral contraceptives, uncontrolled diabetes mellitus and frequency of visits to STD clinics. The rarity of isolation of

Candida spp. in premenarchal girls, the lower prevalence of *Candida* vaginitis after menopause and the possible association with hormone replacement therapy emphasize the hormonal dependence of VVC.

PATHOGENESIS AND PATHOLOGY

The organism

Between 85% and 90% of yeast isolated from the vagina are *Candida albicans* strains. The remainder are other species, the commonest of which are *Candida glabrata* and *Candida tropicalis*. Non-*albicans Candida* spp., although less virulent, are capable of inducing vaginitis and are often more resistant to conventional therapy. Some, but not all, recent surveys indicate an increase in VVC caused by non-*albicans Candida* spp., particularly *C. glabrata*.[21,23]

Germination of *Candida* spp. enhances colonization and facilitates tissue invasion. Factors that enhance or facilitate germination (e.g. estrogen therapy and pregnancy) tend to precipitate symptomatic vaginitis, whereas measures that inhibit germination (e.g. bacterial flora and local mucosal cell-mediated immunity) may prevent acute vaginitis in women who are asymptomatic carriers of yeast.

Candida organisms gain access to the vaginal lumen and secretions predominantly from the adjacent perianal area. This finding is borne out by epidemiologic typing studies. *Candida* vaginitis is seen predominantly in women of child-bearing age, and only in the minority of cases can a precipitating factor be identified to explain the transformation from asymptomatic carriage to symptomatic vaginitis in individual patients.

Host factors

A number of host factors are associated with increased asymptomatic vaginal colonization by *Candida* spp. and with *Candida* vaginitis. During pregnancy, the vagina is more susceptible to vaginal infection, resulting in higher incidences of vaginal colonization, vaginitis and lower cure rates. The clinical attack rate is maximal in the third trimester, and symptomatic recurrences are also more common throughout pregnancy. The high levels of reproductive hormones result in a higher glycogen content in the vaginal environment, which provides an excellent carbon source for growth and germination of *Candida* spp. A more common mechanism is where estrogens enhance vaginal epithelial cell avidity for *Candida* spp. adherence, and a yeast cytosol receptor or binding system for female reproductive hormones has been documented. These hormones also enhance yeast mycelial formation. Several studies have shown increased VVC associated with oral contraceptive use[24] and uncontrolled diabetes mellitus. Glucose tolerance tests have been recommended for women with recurrent VVC; however, the yield is low, and testing is not justified in otherwise healthy premenopausal women.

Symptomatic VVC is frequently observed during or after courses of systemic antibiotics. Although no antimicrobial agent is free of this complication, broad-spectrum antibiotics, such as tetracycline, and β-lactams are mainly responsible, and are thought to act by eliminating the normal protective vaginal bacterial flora. The natural flora provides a colonization resistance mechanism and prevents germination of *Candida* spp. The provider of this protective function has been singled out to be *Lactobacillus* spp.[25] *Lactobacillus–Candida* interaction includes competition for nutrients, steric interference with adherence of *Candida* spp. and elaboration of bacteriocins that inhibit yeast proliferation and germination.

Other factors that contribute to an increased incidence of *Candida* vaginitis include the use of tight, poorly ventilated clothing and nylon underclothing, which increase perineal moisture and temperature.

Candida spp. may cause cell damage and resulting inflammation by direct hyphal invasion of epithelial tissue. It is possible that proteases and other hydrolytic enzymes facilitate cell penetration with resultant inflammation, mucosal swelling, erythema and exfoliation

of vaginal epithelial cells. The characteristic nonhomogeneous vaginal discharge consists of a conglomerate of hyphal elements and exfoliated nonviable epithelial cells with few PMNs. *Candida* spp. may also induce symptoms by hypersensitivity or allergic reactions, particularly in women with idiopathic recurrent VVC (see Noninfectious vaginitis and vulvitis, below).[18,26]

Oral and vaginal thrush correlate well with depressed cell-mediated immunity in debilitated or immunosuppressed patients.[26] This is particularly evident in patients who have chronic mucocutaneous candidiasis and AIDS.

Pathogenesis of recurrent and chronic *Candida* vaginitis

Careful evaluation (Fig. 49.1) of women with recurrent vaginitis usually fails to reveal any precipitating or causal mechanism.[22] In the past, investigators attributed frequent episodes to repeated fungal re-inoculation of the vagina from a persistent intestinal source or to sexual transmission.[22]

The intestinal theory is based on the report of recovery of *Candida* spp. on rectal culture in almost 100% of women with VVC. Typing of simultaneously obtained vaginal and rectal isolates almost invariably reveals identical strains. This theory has been criticized in the past few years because of lower concordance between rectal and vaginal cultures in patients with recurrent VVC. Moreover, long-term therapy with oral nonabsorbable nystatin is not effective in preventing recurrences. It is likely that frequent relapses of VVC originate from a vaginal and not an intestinal reservoir. Vaginal persistence of *Candida* spp. is a consequence of use of fungistatic and not fungicidal drug therapy.

Although sexual transmission of *Candida* organisms occurs via vaginal intercourse and orogenital contact, the role of sexual re-introduction of yeast as a cause for recurrent VVC is doubtful. Recurrent VVC frequently occurs in celibate women and only a minority of male partners of women who have recurrent VVC are colonized with *Candida* spp. Although most studies aimed at treating male partners have not reduced the frequency of recurrent episodes of vaginitis, in one study reduction was achieved in recurrent VVC by treating colonized male partners.[27]

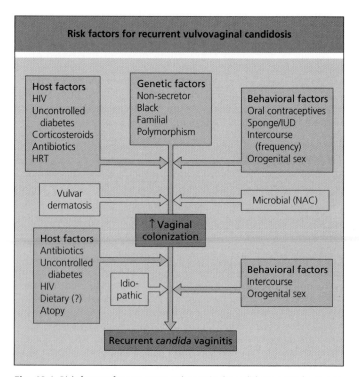

Fig. 49.1 Risk factors for recurrent vulvovaginal candidosis. HRT, hormone replacement therapy; NAC, non-*albicans Candida* spp., IUD, intrauterine device.

Vaginal relapse implies that incomplete eradication or clearance of *Candida* spp. from the vagina occurs after antimycotic therapy. Organisms persist in small numbers in the vagina and result in continued carriage of the organisms, and when host environmental conditions permit, the colonizing organisms increase in number and undergo mycelial transformation, resulting in a new clinical episode.

Whether recurrence is caused by vaginal re-infection or relapse, women with recurrent VVC differ from those with infrequent episodes in their inability to tolerate small numbers of *Candida* organisms re-introduced or persisting in the vagina. On the basis of typing of organisms, women with recurrent and infrequent infection have the same distribution frequency of *Candida* strains as women without symptoms.

Host factors responsible for frequent episodes are not clearly delineated, and more than one mechanism may be operative. There is no evidence of complement, phagocytic cells or immunoglobulin deficiency in these patients. Recurrent VVC is rarely caused by drug resistance.[28]

Current theories about the pathogenesis of recurrent VVC include qualitative and quantitative deficiency in the normal protective vaginal bacterial flora and an acquired, often transient antigen-specific deficiency in T-cell function that similarly permits unchecked yeast proliferation.[26,29] Another theory is that of an acquired acute hypersensitivity reaction to *Candida* antigen, which is accompanied by elevated vaginal titers of *Candida* antigen-specific IgE. This theory has a clinical basis in that patients with recurrent VVC often present with severe vulvar manifestations (rash, erythema, swelling and pruritus) with minimal exudative vaginal changes, little discharge and lower numbers of organisms. Allergic responses to *Candida* spp. have been reported to involve the male genitalia immediately after coitus with a woman infected with *Candida* spp. and are characterized by the acute onset of erythema, edema, severe pruritus and irritation of the penis. As yet, only a minority of women with recurrent VVC have been shown to have elevated *Candida*-specific vaginal IgE. Limited studies using *Candida* antigen desensitization have been found to be helpful in reducing the frequency of recurrent episodes of vaginitis.

Women who are HIV seropositive have higher vaginal colonization rates than seronegative women, but the attack rate of symptomatic VVC appears similar. Reports of chronic, severe recurrent VVC are largely unsubstantiated. Recurrent VVC in the absence of other risk factors for HIV is not an indication for HIV testing.[22]

Recent reports indicate an important role for host genetic factors that explain racial blood group and family predilections to VVC. Genetic factors include quantity of vaginal mannose-binding lectin (MBL) which is reduced in vaginal secretions of women with recurrent VVC. Other genetic factors influence host immune reactivity in response to *Candida* antigen.[30]

PREVENTION

In women with confirmed recurrent VVC linked to frequent courses of systemic antibiotics, prophylactic antimycotics are justified. A useful regimen is fluconazole 150 mg once weekly for the duration of antibiotic therapy. No other dietary or alternative method such as the use of probiotic preparations of lactobacilli has stood the test of time in preventing VVC.[31] In women prone to VVC, avoiding the use of oral contraceptives, intrauterine devices and the contraceptive sponge is prudent.

CLINICAL FEATURES

The most frequent symptom of VVC is vulvar pruritus because vaginal discharge is not invariably present and is frequently minimal.[21] Although described as typically cottage cheese-like in character, the discharge may vary from watery to homogeneously thick. Vaginal soreness, irritation, vulvar burning, dyspareunia and external dysuria are commonly present. Odor, if present, is minimal and nonoffensive. Examination frequently reveals erythema and swelling of the labia and vulva (Fig. 49.2), often with discrete pustulopapular peripheral lesions

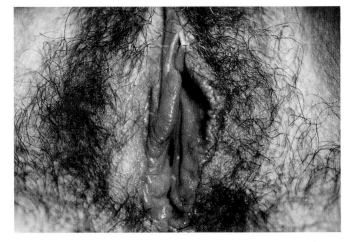

Fig. 49.2 Typical *Candida* vulvovaginitis with bilateral symmetric erythema and edema of vestibule and labia.

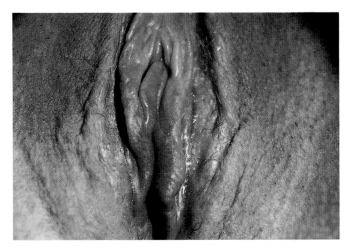

Fig. 49.3 Severe *Candida* vulvovaginitis with bilateral painful fissure formation in the vulva.

and linear fissures (Fig. 49.3). The cervix is normal and vaginal mucosal erythema with adherent whitish discharge is present. Characteristically, symptoms are exacerbated in the week before the onset of menses, with some relief with the onset of menstrual flow.

DIAGNOSIS

The relative lack of specificity of symptoms and signs precludes a diagnosis that is based only on history and physical examination. Most patients with symptomatic VVC may be readily diagnosed on the basis of simple microscopic examination of vaginal secretions and finding of a normal pH. A wet mount or saline preparation has a sensitivity of 40–60%. The 10% potassium hydroxide preparation is more sensitive in diagnosing the presence of germinated yeast. A normal vaginal pH (4.0–4.5) is found in *Candida* vaginitis, and the finding of a pH in excess of 4.5 should suggest the possibility of bacterial vaginosis, trichomoniasis or a mixed infection.[21]

Although routine fungal cultures are unnecessary, vaginal culture should be performed in the presence of negative microscopy in a symptomatic patient. The Papanicolaou smear is unreliable, being insensitive and positive in only about 25% of cases. There is no reliable serologic technique for the diagnosis of *Candida* vaginitis. Unfortunately, no reliable laboratory test based upon rapid antigen detection is available commercially. DNA probes are useful and reliable but not widely available.

MANAGEMENT

Topical agents for acute *Candida* vaginitis

Antimycotics are available for local use as creams, vaginal tablets, suppositories and coated tampons (Table 49.3). There is little to suggest that the formulation of the topical antimycotic influences clinical efficacy.[22] Extensive vulvar inflammation dictates local vulvar application of antimycotic cream and, if severe, in combination with a topical steroid.[32]

The average mycologic cure rate of 7- and 14-day courses of nystatin is 75–80%. Azoles appear to achieve slightly higher clinical mycologic cure rates than the polyenes (nystatin): 85–90%. Although many studies have compared the clinical efficacies of the various azoles, there is little evidence that any one azole agent is superior to others.[33] Topical azoles are remarkably free of local and systemic side-effects; nevertheless, the initial application of topical agents is not infrequently accompanied by local burning and discomfort.

Systemic agents for acute *Candida* vaginitis

There has been a major trend toward shorter treatment courses with progressively higher antifungal doses, culminating in highly effective single-dose topical regimens. Although short-course regimens are effective for mild and moderate vaginitis, cure rates for severe and complicated vaginitis are lower.

Oral systemic azoles available for the treatment of VVC include ketoconazole 400 mg every 12 hours for 5 days, itraconazole 200 mg/day for 3 days (or every 12 hours single-day regimen) and, finally,

Table 49.4 Classification of vulvovaginal candidiasis

Uncomplicated	Complicated
Candida albicans + Infrequent episodes + Mild-to-moderate vaginitis + Normal host	Non-*albicans Candida* spp. Resistant *Candida albicans* (rare) *or* History of recurrent vulvovaginal candidiasis *or* Severe vulvovaginal candidiasis *or* Abnormal host, for example, uncontrolled diabetes, pregnancy, immunocompromised

fluconazole 150 mg single dose.[34] All the oral regimens achieve clinical cure rates in excess of 80%. Oral regimens are generally preferred by women because of convenience and lack of local side-effects. None of the systemic regimens is approved for use during pregnancy. Hepatotoxicity with ketoconazole precludes its widespread use in VVC.[33]

Vulvovaginal candidiasis is classified as uncomplicated or complicated on the basis of the likelihood of achieving clinical and mycologic cure with short-course therapy (Table 49.4). Uncomplicated VVC represents by far the most common form of vaginitis seen, is caused by highly sensitive *C. albicans* and, provided that the severity is mild to moderate, patients respond well to all topical or oral antimycotics, including single-dose therapy. In contrast, patients who have complicated VVC have a relatively resistant organism, a host factor or a severity of infection that dictates more intensive and prolonged therapy lasting 7–14 days. Most non-*albicans Candida* infections respond to conventional topical or oral antifungals provided they are administered for sufficient duration. However, vaginitis caused by *C. glabrata* often fails to respond to azoles and may require treatment with vaginal capsules of boric acid 600 mg/day for 14 days.[35] Patients with severe vulvovaginitis require more prolonged systemic or topical therapy. The former can be provided by a second dose of fluconazole 150 mg, 72 hours after the first dose.[36]

Treatment of recurrent vulvovaginal candidiasis

The management of women who have recurrent VVC aims at control rather than cure. The clinician should first confirm the diagnosis of recurrent VVC. Uncontrolled diabetes mellitus must be controlled and use of corticosteroids or other immunosuppressive agents should be discontinued where possible. Unfortunately, in the majority of women with recurrent VVC, no underlying or predisposing factor can be identified. Recurrent VVC requires long-term maintenance with a suppressive prophylactic regimen. Because of the chronicity of therapy, the convenience of oral treatment is apparent, and the best suppressive prophylaxis has been achieved with weekly oral fluconazole at a dosage of 150 mg.[37] An effective topical prophylactic regimen consists of weekly vaginal suppositories of clotrimazole 500 mg.[21,22]

Atrophic Vaginitis

Clinically significant atrophic vaginitis is quite rare, and the majority of women with mild-to-moderate atrophy are asymptomatic. Because of reduced endogenous estrogen, the epithelium becomes thin and lacking in glycogen, which contributes to a reduction in lactic acid production and an increase in vaginal pH. This change in the environment encourages the overgrowth of nonacidophilic coliform organisms and the disappearance of *Lactobacillus* spp. Despite these major but usually gradual changes, symptoms are mostly absent, especially in the absence of coitus.

Table 49.3 Therapy for vaginal candidiasis – topical agents

TOPICAL AGENTS		
Drug	**Formulation**	**Dosage regimen**
*Butoconazole	2% cream	5 g q24h for 3 days
*Clotrimazole	1% cream 100 mg vaginal tablets 100 mg vaginal tablets 500 mg vaginal tablets	5 g q24h for 7–14 days 1 tablet q24h for 7 days 2 tablets q24h for 3 days 1 tablet, single dose
*Miconazole	2% cream 100 mg vaginal suppository 200 mg vaginal suppository 1200 mg vaginal suppository	5 g q24h for 7 days 1 suppository q24h for 7 days 1 suppository q24h for 3 days 1 suppository, single dose
Econazole	150 mg vaginal tablet	1 tablet q24h for 3 days
Fenticonazole	2% cream	5 g q24h for 7 days
*Tioconazole	2% cream 6.5% cream	5 g q24h for 3 days 5 g, single dose
Terconazole	0.4% cream 0.8% cream 80 mg vaginal suppository	5 g q24h for 7 days 5 g q24h for 3 days 80 mg q24h for 3 days
Nystatin	100 000 U vaginal tablets	1 tablet q24h for 14 days

*Drugs available over the counter, without prescription.

With advanced atrophy, symptoms include vaginal soreness, dyspareunia and occasional spotting or discharge. Burning is a frequent complaint and is often precipitated by intercourse. The vaginal mucosa is thin, with diffuse redness, occasional petechiae or ecchymoses with few or no vaginal folds. Vestibular atrophy may also be apparent and discharge may be serosanguinous, thick or watery, and the pH of the vaginal secretions ranges from 5.5 to 7.0. The wet smear frequently shows small, round epithelial or parabasal cells which represent immature squamous cells that have not been exposed to sufficient estrogen. The *Lactobacillus* spp. dominated flora is replaced by mixed flora of Gram-negative rods. Bacteriologic cultures in these patients are unnecessary, and can be misleading.

The treatment of atrophic vaginitis consists primarily of topical vaginal estrogen. Nightly use of half or all the contents of an applicator for 1–2 weeks is usually sufficient to alleviate the atrophic vaginitis.

Noninfectious Vaginitis and Vulvitis

Women frequently present with acute or chronic vulvovaginal symptoms caused by noninfectious etiologies. Symptoms are indistinguishable from those of infectious syndromes, but are most commonly confused with those of acute *Candida* vaginitis, including pruritus, irritation, burning, soreness and variable discharge.

Noninfectious causes include irritants [physical (e.g. minipads) or chemical (e.g. spermicides, povidone–iodine, topical antimycotics, soaps and perfumes, topical 5-fluorouracil)] and allergens, which are responsible for immunologic acute and chronic hypersensitivity reactions, including contact dermatitis (e.g. latex condoms, antimycotic creams). An enormous list of topical factors responsible for local inflammatory reactions and symptoms exists and many more have yet to be defined. Depending on the site of contact, symptoms may be vaginal or vulvar. Included in this category are systemic dermatoses that may present in the vulva (e.g. psoriasis, Fig. 49.4) or vulva-specific dermatosis (e.g. lichen sclerosus).

A noninfectious mechanism may coexist with or follow an infectious process, and should be considered when the three common infectious causes and hormone deficiency are excluded and in the presence of a normal vaginal pH, normal saline and potassium hydroxide microscopy, and, ultimately, a negative yeast culture. Unfortunately, given the anticipated 20% colonization rates in normal asymptomatic women, occasionally a positive yeast culture in a symptomatic patient reflects the presence of an innocent bystander and not the cause of the vulvovaginal symptoms. The only logical way of establishing the role of *Candida* spp. in this context is to treat with an oral antifungal agent and assess the clinical response.

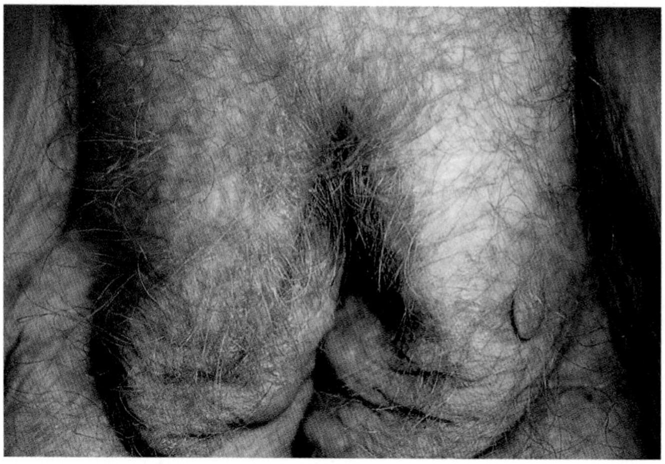

Fig. 49.4 Vulvar psoriasis resulting in pruritus vulva and misdiagnosed as *Candida* vulvovaginitis.

Once a local chemical irritant or allergic reaction is suspected, a detailed inquiry into possible causal factors is essential. Offending agents or behaviors should be eliminated wherever possible, including avoiding chemical irritants and allergens (e.g. soaps, detergents). The immediate management of severe vulvovaginal symptoms of noninfectious etiology should not rely on topical corticosteroids, which are rarely the solution and frequently high-potency corticosteroid creams cause intense burning. Local relief measures include sodium bicarbonate sitz baths and oral antihistamines.

A syndrome of hyperacidity of the vagina causing overgrowth of lactobacilli has been described but not confirmed. A rebound increase in population numbers of lactobacilli is thought to occur after completion of topical antimycotics and is alleged to suppress population numbers of healthy resident flora. The proposed syndrome of cytolytic vaginosis is characterized by vulvovaginal burning, irritation, soreness and dyspareunia, and is usually incorrectly diagnosed as VVC. The finding of large numbers of lactobacilli on wet count and a low pH, together with extensive squamous epithelial cell cytolysis is said to confirm the diagnosis. Recommended therapy for cytolytic vaginosis is daily alkaline douching using sodium bicarbonate to elevate the low vaginal pH and suppress growth of lactobacilli.

Vulvitis

Most of the important infectious and noninfectious causes of vulvitis have been described in the section on vaginitis. Human papillomavirus and genital herpes are described in Chapters 59 and 58, respectively. Bacterial vulvitis due to streptococci, anaerobes and Gram-negative rods occurs infrequently and should be diagnosed by clinical features and bacterial culture. Specific antimicrobial treatment is indicated for patients with the diagnosis of bacterial vulvitis. Occasionally a Bartholin's abscess creates a painful swelling in the vulva. This can be due to *N. gonorrhoeae* or to a variety of pathogens, particularly Grampositive organisms. A Bartholin's cyst infection should be treated with appropriate antibiotics and occasionally may require drainage. Other causes of vestibulitis or vulvitis include lichen sclerosus, erosive lichen planus and theoretically any cause of dermatosis or dermatitis such as psoriasis (see Fig. 49.4), eczema and pemphigus.

Cervicitis

EPIDEMIOLOGY

The presence of a purulent exudate in the cervical os has been highly associated with cervical infection with *Chlamydia trachomatis*, *N. gonorrhoeae*, herpes simplex virus and cytomegalovirus. Infection with *T. vaginalis* correlates with colpitis macularis and inflammatory changes of the ectocervix.[38,39] Not infrequently, mucopurulent endocervicitis or ectocervicitis is seen in the absence of these pathogens, indicating that additional, as yet unrecognized causes exist. A role for disruption of vaginal flora, specifically overgrowth of anaerobes as typified in bacterial vaginosis in causing cervical inflammation has been proposed. Rare causes of cervicitis include *Mycobacterium tuberculosis* and *Actinomyces israelii*, the latter almost invariably in the presence of intrauterine devices. Although the most important and prevalent infection of the cervix is undoubtedly human papillomavirus, this virus does not cause cervicitis and is discussed in Chapter 156. To the growing number of etiologic agents implicated in cervicitis, must be added *Mycoplasma genitalium*.[40]

The prevalence of genital chlamydial infection ranges from 8 to 40%.[41] Risk factors include young age, unmarried status, lower socioeconomic conditions, number and recent change of sexual partner, ectopy, oral contraceptive use and concurrent gonococcal infection; the last may reactivate latent chlamydial infection and increases shedding of chlamydia from the endocervix.[42] Risk factors for gonococcal mucopurulent cervicitis are identical to those of *Chlamydia* spp. but also include urban dwelling, prostitution, illicit drug use and minority racial status. Up to 60% of women with *N. gonorrhoeae* have co-infection with chlamydia.[41] Herpetic cervicitis is rare in the absence of genital lesions and is most commonly associated with first episode, primary disease with an 80% viral isolation rate.[39] Cytomegalovirus is thought to be responsible for approximately 5% of cases of cervicitis and is usually asymptomatic. When it is isolated from cervical secretions, the detection may not imply a causal relationship with present pathology.

CLINICAL FEATURES

Cervicitis is frequently asymptomatic and is detected on routine pelvic examination. Alternatively, cervical inflammation is recognized because of signs and symptoms of concomitant infection (e.g. vaginal trichomoniasis, genital herpes or salpingitis). Mucopurulent cervicitis may result in a purulent vaginal discharge in its own right. Accordingly, cervical speculum evaluation should be an essential part of vaginal examination in women with an abnormal discharge. Mucopurulent endocervicitis results in swelling and erythema of the zone of ectopy, associated with friability, contact bleeding, spotting and a yellow or green endocervical exudate. The purulent discharge is best appreciated by obtaining an endocervical swab specimen and observing the latter against a white background.

Trichomoniasis is associated with ectocervical squamous epithelial mucosal inflammation, giving the cervix a 'strawberry' appearance due to microscopic focal patchy petechiae (colpitis macularis) in 5–20% of patients.[15] Primary herpes cervicitis may be associated with severe necrosis that is reminiscent of cervical cancer. Most commonly, primary herpetic cervicitis is characterized by increased surface vascularity, and micro- and macro-ulcerations with and without necrotic areas. Asymptomatic shedding of herpesvirus occurs in the absence of cervical lesions.

DIAGNOSIS

Mucopurulent cervicitis is confirmed when a Gram-stained specimen of green or yellow endocervical exudate reveals more than 30 PMNs per high power field.[1] Microscopic examination of cervical mucus from a patient with mucopurulent endocervicitis reveals an overabundance of inflammatory cells, obliterating the background ferning pattern. A similar excess of inflammatory cells can be found in a Papanicolaou smear. These two microscopic studies are not reliable in identifying the underlying cause of mucopurulent cervicitis. For a diagnosis of *C. trachomatis* cervicitis, culture techniques to identify the obligate intra-parasites served as the gold standard in the past. Now the development of the more widely available enzyme-linked immunosorbent assay antigen detection tests has been replaced by highly sensitive DNA amplification techniques, particularly ligase chain reaction, allowing diagnosis not only from cervical specimens, but also by screening

urine specimens. Gram stain of cervical mucus may reveal intracellular Gram-negative diplococci, but has low sensitivity and specificity in the diagnosis of gonococcal cervicitis. Diagnosis relies mainly upon culture of the endocervix using a modified Thayer–Martin medium; however, diagnostic methodologies now include use of DNA probes, especially for screening purposes, given the high sensitivity of these newer techniques.

Although Papanicolaou smears in herpetic cervicitis are useful in revealing multinucleated giant cells, viral culture and fluorescein-conjugated monoclonal antibodies are the mainstay of clinical diagnosis; polymerase chain reaction is used for monitoring asymptomatic viral shedding in a research context.

The clinical differentiation of the various causes of cervicitis is not possible, but requires the aforementioned diagnostic tests, recognizing that frequently more than one etiologic agent may be present simultaneously because many of the pathogens share risk factors and behavior. The most important diagnostic problem is that of overdiagnosis of cervicitis. All too frequently physiologic changes in the appearance of the cervix, in spite of the use of colposcopy, are interpreted as reflecting pathologic cervicitis. Regrettably, after failed attempts to identify pathogenic micro-organisms, patients are needlessly treated with cervical ablative techniques. Cervical ectopy is often mistaken for cervicitis with eversion of endocervical columnar cells, and is commonly seen in women on oral contraceptives.[42] Other physiologic changes related to childbirth and dilatation of the cervical canal are mistakenly diagnosed as cervicitis.

Equally important is the failure to recognize that a friable, abnormal cervix may reflect dysplasia and neoplasia. If the Papanicolaou smear reports inflammatory cells with or without atypia, the presence of atypical squamous cells of undetermined significance (ASCUS) should be considered in the differential diagnosis between a benign change in reaction to a stimulus and a low-grade squamous intraepithelial lesion. Accordingly, women with a Papanicolaou smear showing ASCUS should have their smears repeated. Persistence of an ASCUS smear should prompt colposcopy.

MANAGEMENT

Antimicrobial regimens for infectious cervicitis are provided in the chapters on pelvic inflammatory disease, gonorrhea and chlamydial infections (see Chapters 50 and 177; and Practice Point 29).

REFERENCES

References for this chapter can be found online at http://www.expertconsult.com

Infections of the female pelvis including septic abortion

Infections of the female pelvis constitute a diverse group. This chapter considers three groups of infections: pelvic inflammatory disease (PID), postpartum and postabortal infections (including postpartum endometritis and Caesarian section, episiotomy infections and postabortion sepsis) and postsurgical gynecologic infections.

Pelvic Inflammatory Disease

EPIDEMIOLOGY

Pelvic inflammatory disease (PID) refers to an acute clinical syndrome that results when vaginal or cervical organisms ascend into the upper structures of the female reproductive tract unrelated to pregnancy or surgery.[1] Depending on which areas are infected, PID may manifest itself as endometritis, parametritis, salpingitis, oophoritis, pelvic peritonitis, tubo-ovarian abscess, periappendicitis, perihepatitis (Fitz-Hugh–Curtis syndrome) and perisplenitis.

Pelvic inflammatory disease and sexually transmitted diseases (STDs) share many of the same risk factors and, in the USA, 40–80% of PID is attributed to STDs. Bacterial vaginosis (BV) is commonly found in women with PID.[2] Identified risk factors for PID include younger age, unmarried status, lower socioeconomic status, sexual behavior (number of sexual partners, age of sexual debut, rate of acquiring new partners), substance abuse, poor health-care behavior (treatment-seeking and compliance with treatment instructions), douching and intrauterine device insertion.[1,3] In studies from the USA and Europe, about three-quarters of women who had PID were under 25 years of age, and about one-half had never been pregnant.[1] Oral contraceptive users tend to have clinically and laparoscopically milder infection than do nonusers, and oral contraceptives appear to protect against chlamydial PID.[4]

PATHOGENESIS AND PATHOLOGY

The vast majority of PID cases result from a direct canalicular spread of organisms from the endocervix to the mucosa of the endometrium and fallopian tubes, although the precise mechanisms are poorly understood. Postinfectious scarring (e.g. intratubal adhesions, tubal occlusion, peritubal scarring and damaged fimbrial ostia) results in the long-term sequelae of PID.

Occurrence of PID is described only among sexually active women, and its risk is associated with the number of sexual partners and the frequency of sexual acts among women with only one sexual partner. Multiple organisms have been implicated as etiologic agents of PID (Table 50.1). The rates of isolation of these organisms are variable. They may vary with geographic region, duration

Table 50.1 Common etiologic agents of pelvic inflammatory disease

Aerobic bacteria	*Neisseria gonorrhoeae* *Chlamydia trachomatis* *Gardnerella vaginalis* *Escherichia coli* *Streptococcus* spp. *Haemophilus influenzae*
Anaerobic bacteria	*Bacteroides* spp. *Peptostreptococcus* spp. *Peptococcus* spp. *Prevotella* spp. *Porphyromonas* spp.
Mycoplasmas	*Mycoplasma hominis* *Mycoplasma genitalium*

Data from Westrom & Eschenbach.[1]

of infection and the site of sampling (i.e. cervix, fallopian tubes or endometrium). The most commonly recovered organisms are *Neisseria gonorrhoeae* and *Chlamydia trachomatis*, followed by other aerobic and anaerobic bacteria associated with BV (e.g. *Gardnerella vaginalis*, *Mycoplasma hominis*, *Prevotella bivia* and *Porphyromonas*, *Prevotella* and *Peptostreptococcus* spp.). *Mycoplasma genitalium* may also be an etiologic agent of PID. Rates of isolation of 10–20% in the upper genital tract, and as high as 85% (5–27% in studies from Europe versus 44–70% in those from North America) in the lower genital tract, have been reported for *N. gonorrhoeae*. For *C. trachomatis*, rates of 1.2–31% in the upper genital tract and 31% in the lower genital tract have been reported.[1,2,5] It is estimated that between 10% and 40% of women who have untreated gonococcal or chlamydial cervical infection will develop acute upper tract infection. Finally, *M. genitalium* can be found in up to 14% of women with PID.[6] However, PID is a polymicrobial infection, even in the setting of gonococcal or chlamydial cervicitis. It has been suggested that, in many cases of PID, STD organisms initiate the inflammation of the tubal mucosa and this process facilitates the invasion of the mucosa by organisms endogenous to the lower genital tract.[1]

PREVENTION

Prevention is directed at reducing a woman's risk of acquiring an STD, and the detection and treatment of lower genital tract infections. Women screened and treated for asymptomatic chlamydial infection

551

were nearly 60% less likely than unscreened women to develop PID.[7] Prompt and correct treatment of upper tract infections will ameliorate some of the long-term sequelae.

CLINICAL FEATURES

The most common clinical complaint in a woman who has PID is bilateral lower abdominal or pelvic pain. Other complaints include an abnormal vaginal discharge, dyspareunia, dysmenorrhea and abnormal uterine bleeding. In more severe cases, nausea, vomiting, fever and diffuse abdominal pain may occur. The hallmark findings of PID are cervical motion tenderness and uterine or adnexal tenderness in the absence of other potential cause of the illness. Whereas gonococcal PID tends to have an abrupt, fulminant presentation within 1 week of the onset of menses, chlamydial PID is characterized by a subacute course with mild symptoms, often described as just a dull pain, and mild findings. It is not unusual for a woman who has chlamydial PID to be unaware of her infection and to present as a relatively asymptomatic contact of a male with urethritis. The clinician should be alert to adnexal masses or fullness as the major signs of chlamydial infection. Women who have HIV infection and PID may present with more clinically severe disease.[8]

The common complications and sequelae of PID include ectopic pregnancy, tubal infertility, recurrent PID, chronic abdominal pain, tubo-ovarian abscesses and pelvic adhesions. A woman's risk of ectopic pregnancy increases seven- to 10-fold after an episode of PID. The number of episodes of PID, the woman's age and the severity of tubal inflammation determined at laparoscopy influence the fertility prognosis of PID.[1] It appears that PID caused by chlamydial infection may result in more infertility than PID caused by gonococcal infection. Recurrent pelvic infections will develop in up to one-third of women who have had PID. Chronic abdominal pain lasting more than 6 months occurs in 15–18% of women after PID. Pyosalpinx, tubo-ovarian abscesses and pelvic adhesions occur in 15–20% of women who have had PID and often require surgical intervention. Mortality from acute PID is rare. The most common cause of death from PID is a ruptured tubo-ovarian abscess with subsequent peritonitis. The mortality rate from this complication of PID is 6–8%.

DIAGNOSIS

The clinical diagnosis of PID is imprecise. The traditional clinical signs and symptoms of PID are neither sensitive nor specific for the syndrome. Laparoscopy confirms salpingitis in 45–89% of women who have clinically diagnosed PID. Of women who have acute clinical PID, 6–45% have normal fallopian tubes and 5–33% have other conditions, including ectopic pregnancy, appendicitis, hemorrhagic ovarian cysts, endometritis, pelvic adhesions and torsion of an adnexal structure.[5,9] False-negative clinical diagnoses for PID range from 16% to 47%.[9] The diagnoses prior to laparoscopy in women who have laparoscopically confirmed PID included ectopic pregnancy, ovarian cyst, hemorrhagic ovarian cyst, endometriosis, fibroids, ovarian tumor, appendicitis, pyelonephritis and uncertain diagnosis. Although laparoscopy can be used to obtain a more accurate diagnosis, it is neither readily available in most cases nor justifiable in clinically mild disease.

Women who have lower abdominal tenderness, adnexal tenderness or cervical motion tenderness – the Centers for Disease Control minimum criteria – should be treated for PID if there is no other diagnosis that should be considered.[10] One analysis on a large number of women enrolled in a clinical trial showed that lower abdominal tenderness alone was the most sensitive of the physical findings.[11] However, many clinicians may be uncomfortable treating for PID based on history and physical examination alone.

Tests to document an inflammatory and infectious process in the lower genital tract can be used to increase the sensitivity of the clinical signs. A pregnancy test should be done to make sure that the pain is not caused by an ectopic pregnancy. Within the setting of a patient with lower abdominal or pelvic tenderness, the presence of an increased number of leukocytes (a ratio of more than 1:1 white blood cells:vaginal epithelial cells) or findings consistent with BV on a wet mount are considered supportive of a diagnosis of PID. Similarly, an endocervical Gram stain, obtained after cleaning the ectocervix, showing Gram-negative intracellular diplococci, 30 or more polymorphonuclear leukocytes per high power field, or a positive test (culture or PCR) for either *N. gonorrhoeae* or *C. trachomatis* are also useful in establishing the diagnosis. Erythrocyte sedimentation rate, C-reactive protein and complete white blood cell count may also be useful. Pelvic and endovaginal ultrasound can detect findings consistent with severe PID, including tubo-ovarian abscesses, dilated fallopian tubes and cul-de-sac fluid. Ultrasound is less useful in mild or atypical clinical presentations. CT scanning has the same limitations as ultrasound. However, in severe cases of PID with atypical ultrasound findings CT can be useful.[12] For example, spiral CT scanning optimizes identification of small air bubbles that are specific for abscess.[13]

More invasive tests may also be considered in a woman where PID is suspected. Endometrial biopsy documenting endometrial neutrophils or plasma cells confirms the diagnosis but requires at least 24 hours for processing. Purulent material from the peritoneal cavity obtained by culdocentesis, a painful procedure, may support the diagnosis of PID but may also occur with other intra-abdominal infections such as appendicitis. Laparoscopy is the gold standard for the diagnosis and staging of acute PID. The minimum criteria for visual confirmation of PID include hyperemia of the tubal surface, edema of the tubal wall and a sticky exudate on the tubal surface and from the fimbriated end when patent.[14]

MANAGEMENT

Management of a patient who has PID includes therapy, education, careful follow-up and partner management. The goal is to cure the patient, prevent recurrences and, ultimately, to preserve fertility. Empiric treatment should be instituted as soon as the diagnosis is suspected. Based on the polymicrobial nature of PID, therapy must provide broad-spectrum coverage. Several antimicrobial regimens have proved to be highly effective in achieving clinical cure of PID.[10] Studies from the pre-antibiotic era documented infertility rates after PID of 60–70%, indicating that prompt institution of antimicrobial therapy does influence fertility outcome.[1]

Pelvic inflammatory disease should always be treated with a minimum of two antibiotics for at least 10–14 days (Table 50.2). The combination regimen of an extended-spectrum parenteral cephalosporin plus doxycycline provides good coverage for most potential pathogens, including β-lactamase-producing strains. An alternative parenteral inpatient regimen is the combination of clindamycin plus an aminoglycoside. Oral regimens listed in Table 50.2 also provide excellent coverage. However, with recent data suggesting that quinolone-resistant *N. gonorrheae* (QRNG) is becoming more common, quinolones are no longer recommended for first-line therapy unless QRNG is not suspected as being involved, based on either negative testing or low local prevalence of this organism.[15]

Recent data from a large randomized clinical trial comparing inpatient and outpatient therapy indicate that outpatient therapy is associated with similar short- and long-term treatment outcomes in women with mild to moderate PID.[16] Hospitalization is recommended for women whose tolerance or compliance with outpatient regimens is uncertain, or who have factors that complicate treatment, severe illness or an uncertain diagnosis (Table 50.3).

Supportive therapy includes hydration, bed rest in the semi-Fowler position to localize the infection to the pelvis, pelvic rest and pain relief. The patient should abstain from sexual intercourse until test-of-cure studies and resolution of signs and symptoms. All sexual partners in the previous 30 days should be evaluated and presumptively treated for gonococcal and chlamydial infection. Explicit and clear patient education cannot be overemphasized in the treatment of PID, especially in the context of outpatient management.

Table 50.2 Recommended treatment of pelvic inflammatory disease

Oral treatment		
Regimen A	With or without	Ofloxacin 400 mg po q24h for 14 days, or Levofloxacin 500 mg po q24h for 14 days Metronidazole 500 mg po q12h for 14 days
Regimen B	Either	Ceftriaxone 250 mg im, or Cefoxitin 2 g im plus probenecid 1 g po in a single dose concurrently, or Other parenteral third-generation cephalosporin (e.g. ceftizoxime or cefotaxime)
	Plus	Doxycycline 100 mg po q12h for 14 days
	With or without	Metronidazole 500 mg po q12h for 7 days
Parenteral treatment		
Regimen A*	Either	Cefotetan 2 g iv q12h, or Cefoxitin 2 g iv q6h
	Plus	Doxycycline 100 mg iv or po q12h
Regimen B	Plus	Clindamycin 900 mg iv q8h Gentamicin loading dose iv or im (2 mg/kg body weight) followed by a maintenance dose of 1.5 mg/kg; single daily dosing may be substituted

Parenteral regimens should be continued for 48 hours after substantial clinical improvement. Doxycycline 100 mg po q12h or clindamycin 450 mg po q6h should then be administered for a total of 14 days.
*This regimen should not be used if quinolone-resistant *N. gonorrheae* is suspected.
Data from Centers for Disease Control and Prevention.[10]

Table 50.3 Recommendations for hospitalizing patients who have pelvic inflammatory disease

Uncertain tolerance or compliance with outpatient regimen	Substance abusers Nausea and vomiting Follow-up at 72 hours after starting antibiotic treatment is problematic
Complicating factors	Pregnancy Suspected pelvic or tubo-ovarian abscess
Severe illness	Temperature over 101°F (38.3°C) White blood cell count >15 000/ml Peritoneal signs Septic
Uncertain diagnosis	Failure to respond clinically to outpatient treatment Inability to exclude surgical emergencies (ectopic pregnancy, appendicitis)

The incidence of ascending infection among pregnant women who have intact membranes is unknown but is believed to be rare.[17] However, given the high-risk of miscarriage and pre-term delivery associated with PID, pregnant women who have PID must be hospitalized and given parenteral antibiotic therapy.[10]

Women who have tubo-ovarian abscesses should be hospitalized and begun on broad-spectrum antibiotics (aminoglycoside plus clindamycin or metronidazole). The vast majority of abscesses with a diameter of 4–6 cm respond to antibiotics alone, whereas only 40% of those that are 10 cm or larger respond to medical therapy alone.[18] Increasing abscess size or failure to defervesce 72 hours after administration of antibiotics suggests medical failure and requires surgical intervention (e.g. percutaneous or transvaginal drainage under sonographic guidance, laparoscopic drainage or laparotomy). Leaking or ruptured abscesses require immediate laparotomy after stabilization of the patient. Extensive surgery such as complete hysterectomy is rarely indicated except in life-threatening complications such as extensive necrotic myometrium.

Postpartum Endometritis and Caesarian Section

EPIDEMIOLOGY

Postpartum endometritis, an infection of the uterus, is the most common cause of maternal postpartum fever and includes the inflammatory conditions of endometritis, endomyometritis and endoparametritis. It can be categorized into early infection (i.e. onset within 48 hours of delivery) and late infection (i.e. onset 2 days to 2 weeks after delivery). The most significant risk factor for postpartum endometritis is Caesarian section; the incidence of postpartum endometritis after vaginal delivery is 2–5% whereas the rate after Caesarian section ranges from 20% to 55%.[19] Postpartum upper tract infections following vaginal delivery are about 10 times more common in developing countries than in developed countries as a result of unclean delivery practice, traditional birth practices and the high prevalence of STDs in some populations.[20]

PATHOGENESIS AND PATHOLOGY

Early postpartum endometritis usually is associated with nonelective Caesarian section and is probably the result of direct uterine contamination by organisms in the amniotic cavity. This is in direct contrast to women who develop late postpartum endometritis, which usually develops after vaginal delivery. The timing of these late infections suggests an ascending infection similar to the mechanisms for PID. Wound infections after Caesarian section appear to be the result of a direct contamination of the wound by organisms in the endometrium at the time of surgery.

Postpartum endometritis is a mixed aerobic–anaerobic infection (Table 50.4). *Ureaplasma urealyticum* and *Mycoplasma hominis* have also been isolated from the endometrium and blood of infected women, but their clinical significance is not clear.[21] *Chlamydia trachomatis* is associated with the late form of postpartum endometritis.[22] Group A β-hemolytic streptococcal endometritis is rare and clustered cases are probably related to a common source, often a caregiver. Herpes simplex endometritis has also been reported.[23] Bacteremia occurs in 10–20% of patients and most common blood isolates are group B streptococci, *Gardnerella vaginalis* and *Peptostreptococcus* spp.

PREVENTION

The timely diagnosis and treatment of lower tract syndromes during pregnancy, especially bacterial vaginosis, may prevent some postpartum endometritis. However, the only intervention which clearly reduces the risk of endometritis is the use of prophylactic antibiotics for patients

Table 50.4 Common endogenous micro-organisms identified as potential etiologic agents in postoperative pelvic infections

Aerobic bacteria	*Streptococcus* spp.
	Enterococcus spp.
	Staphylococcus aureus
	Staphylococcus epidermidis
	Escherichia coli
	Klebsiella pneumoniae
	Gardnerella vaginalis
Anaerobic bacteria	*Bacteroides* spp.
	Peptostreptococcus spp.
	Prevotella bivia
	Prevotella disiens
	Fusobacterium spp.
Mycoplasmas	*Mycoplasma hominis*
	Ureaplasma urealyticum

requiring a nonelective Caesarian section after labor or rupture of membranes, with a two-thirds to three-quarters reduction in infection.[19,24,25]

CLINICAL FEATURES

Risk factors for postpartum endometritis include duration of labor, length of time membranes remain ruptured, presence of STDs, presence of BV, the number of vaginal examinations, the use of internal fetal monitoring and socioeconomic status.[21,26,27]

Postpartum endometritis should be suspected in any woman who develops significant fever (oral temperature 101.3°F (38.5°C) or higher in the first 24 hours after delivery or 100.4°F (38°C) or higher for at least 4 consecutive hours, 24 hours or more after delivery). The diagnosis of postpartum endometritis can be made on the basis of clinical features of fever and when signs which suggest an endometrial inflammatory process, such as abdominal pain, uterine tenderness, foul lochia, increased uterine bleeding and uterine subinvolution, are present. Late-onset endometritis tends to have a mild, subacute clinical presentation.

Acute complications of postpartum endometritis include pelvic abscess and puerperal ovarian vein thrombophlebitis. Puerperal ovarian vein thrombophlebitis is an acute thrombosis of one or both ovarian veins postpartum, is usually associated with postpartum endometritis with an onset of 2–4 days after delivery, and can be associated with septic pulmonary emboli. The reported incidence is 1 in 2000 deliveries.[28] Chronic complications and sequelae result from postinfectious scarring.

DIAGNOSIS

Blood cultures should be obtained from all patients before starting therapy. Tests for the detection of cervical infection with *N. gonorrhoeae* and *C. trachomatis* should be obtained from all women at risk of STDs. Quantitative endometrial cultures obtained using a triple lumen catheter, which minimizes contamination, may provide useful information but is rarely used in clinical practice. A complete white blood cell count should be done. If an adnexal mass is felt on examination, then ultrasound or CT can be used to confirm the diagnosis.

MANAGEMENT

Postpartum endometritis is commonly treated parenterally with a broad-spectrum antibiotic regimen with activity against *Bacteroides fragilis* and other penicillin-resistant anaerobic bacteria, such as second-generation cephalosporins (cefoxitin or cefotetan) or the extended-spectrum penicillins (ticarcillin–clavulanate or sulbactam–ampicillin).[27] The combination of aminoglycoside plus clindamycin remains an appropriate regimen.[29] Once-daily administration of aminoglycosides appears to be effective and safe in the treatment of endometritis.[29]

Women should continue to receive parenteral therapy until fever has resolved, uterine tenderness and abdominal pain are gone, and white blood cell count has normalized. Subsequent oral antibiotic therapy with erythromycin or doxycycline is only indicated in women who require it for a documented chlamydial infection for a total of 10–14 days.

Reasons for failure to respond to antimicrobial therapy include inappropriate antibiotics (enterococcal infection or resistant anaerobic infection), pelvic or wound abscess, or ovarian vein thrombophlebitis. When postpartum septic pelvic thrombophlebitis is suspected, heparin should be given.[28] Late postpartum endometritis can be managed in the same way as PID (see Table 50.2).

Episiotomy Infections

EPIDEMIOLOGY

Episiotomy infections are rare. The rate of infection of episiotomies is 0.1% overall but increases to 1–2% of episiotomies complicated by third- or fourth-degree extensions. Episiotomy infections, however, can have severe and even fatal consequences.

PATHOGENESIS AND PATHOLOGY

Episiotomy infections have been classified into four categories based on the depth of infection in the soft tissue: simple infection, superficial fascial infection, superficial fascial necrosis and myonecrosis.[30] Bacteria implicated in episiotomy infections include skin pathogens, streptococci and staphylococci, and bacteria associated with vaginal flora, Enterobacteriaceae and anaerobic bacteria, including *B. fragilis*. *Clostridium perfringens* and *C. sordellii* are likely if myonecrosis is present. Methicillin-resistant *Staphylococcus aureus* has also been reported as a cause of episiotomy infection.[31]

PREVENTION

Treatment standards should be introduced that reduce the liberal or routine use of episiotomies, as they appear to increase the risk of third- and fourth-degree tears. In the USA from 1980 to 2005 there has been an overall decline in the use of episiotomy from 64% to 19%.[32]

CLINICAL FEATURES

The simple wound infection is a local infection limited to incision site in the skin and the superficial fascia. Clinically there is edema and erythema only along the incision. A superficial fascial infection involves two layers of the superficial fascia and resembles a cellulitis with erythema, edema and pain. Often, infection of the episiotomy site may be associated with dehiscence. The superficial infection may be indistinguishable on the basis of skin appearance from an early superficial fascial infection with necrosis (necrotizing fasciitis). Necrotizing fasciitis involves all layers of the superficial fascia (and may involve the deep fascia). Skin anesthesia may precede the skin breakdown, because of nerve involvement. As nutrient vessels are occluded, the skin may turn dusky and develop bullae and then frank necrosis. Subcutaneous gas may be present with the mixed infection. These patients often have evidence of marked toxicity out of proportion to the clinical findings. In myonecrosis, pain is often the dominant feature. Patients are extremely toxic, restless and confused or disoriented.

DIAGNOSIS

Prompt diagnosis is of paramount importance because necrotizing fasciitis and myonecrosis are rapidly progressive. Frozen section examination of full-depth biopsy specimens has been helpful in the diagnosis of necrotizing fasciitis.[33] However, surgical exploration is warranted if necrotizing fasciitis or myonecrosis is suspected.

MANAGEMENT

Management of a simple episiotomy wound infection includes opening of the incision and exploration to ensure that there is no accumulated blood or a rectovaginal opening. Any superficial fascial infection should be managed with broad-spectrum antibiotic coverage (e.g. ampicillin–gentamicin–metronidazole or ampicillin–gentamicin–clindamycin) and observed closely. After initial management and control of the infection, early repair in the immediate postpartum period can be considered in a patient with dehiscence secondary to infection.[34]

More extensive surgical exploration should be undertaken if erythema and edema extend beyond the incision site, there is no improvement in 24–48 hours after the start of antibiotics, if the patient deteriorates, or if the patient has severe systemic manifestations. In the case of necrotizing fasciitis, the superficial fascia will separate easily from the deep fascia with a probe or finger (this does not occur in healthy tissue), the incisions will be bloodless and the exudate will be serosanguinous rather than purulent. Surgical debridement of all necrotic and pale tissue should be performed promptly and broad-spectrum antibiotic therapy should be instituted. The wound should be left open after debridement. A second-look procedure is often necessary after 24 hours.

Myonecrosis is an extremely rare event that is usually caused by *C. perfringens* or *C. sordellii* but may result from an extension of necrotizing fasciitis through the deep fascia to the muscle. Therapy includes high-dose penicillin and urgent surgical debridement. Hyperbaric oxygen therapy remains controversial and should be considered only as adjunctive therapy.

Postabortion Sepsis

EPIDEMIOLOGY

Postabortion sepsis is an ascending infection of the female pelvis after spontaneous or induced abortion. Inflammatory conditions associated with infectious complications of abortion are similar to those for PID but can be complicated by retained, poorly perfused tissue and uterine or bowel trauma. The mortality from abortion in developed countries is low (an estimated 0.6 per 100 000 cases), and abortion accounts for only 5% of all maternal mortality in the USA. Infection is the major cause when mortality does result from abortion complications. In a review of 107 deaths caused by abortion in the USA between 1975 and 1977, 33% were caused by sepsis.[35] In developing countries the World Health Organization estimates that illegal abortion accounts for 25–50% of the 500 000 maternal deaths that occur each year.

PATHOGENESIS AND PATHOLOGY

The bacteria associated with postabortion sepsis are similar to those associated with PID. However, the potential of direct uterine or bowel injury and retention of the products of conception after an abortion may result in injured and poorly vascularized tissue and an enlarged spectrum of enteric organisms, including *C. perfringens*. In developing countries, tetanus is a cause of mortality after abortion. More recently,

C. sordellii has been associated with fulminant infections, secondary to lethal toxic shock-like syndrome, in women undergoing medical abortion with mifepristone.[36]

PREVENTION

Prevention measures include providing effective and acceptable contraception and appropriate medical management of abortion. Prophylaxis for cervical and vaginal infections, particularly for BV, before voluntary termination of pregnancy seems to decrease the risk of postabortal infection.[10] Prompt diagnosis and effective treatment of endometritis after the procedure is extremely important as delayed treatment is a common feature in cases of death from septic abortion.

CLINICAL FEATURES

The diagnosis of septic abortion should be considered in any woman who has a temperature of 100.4°F (38°C) or higher on two occasions more than 24 hours after an abortion and in any woman of reproductive age who presents with fever, abdominal pain and bleeding. Additionally, details of the procedure, including microbiologic studies and pathology of the aborted tissues, should be obtained. Physical examination findings typically include uterine tenderness, foul or purulent cervical discharge and products of conception at the cervical os. In more severe infections the patient may be hypotensive or in shock. The presence of cervical or vaginal lacerations should be assessed. Women who have clostridial infection may have severe disseminated intravascular hemolysis.

Fortunately rare, infection with *C. sordellii* may have atypical features, in that classic indicators of infection, such as fever, a purulent discharge, uterine tenderness and an elevated white blood cell count, are notably absent until the patient is in shock, and the only early warning may be excessive uterine bleeding.[36]

Acute complications of septic abortion are seen in advanced stages of the disease process and include the respiratory distress syndrome, septic shock, renal failure, abscess formation, septic pelvic vein thrombophlebitis and septic emboli, and disseminated intravascular coagulopathy; death may also occur. The chronic complications are similar to those of PID and include infertility, chronic pelvic pain and ectopic pregnancy.

DIAGNOSIS

Except for women who have mild, early, uncomplicated postabortion endometritis, all women should have blood and cervical cultures as well as a complete white blood cell count and urinalysis. Upright and flat abdominal and pelvic radiographs should be done to assess the presence of air in the abdominal cavity, dilated bowel and gas in the uterus. Pelvic ultrasound can determine the presence of retained tissue and other fluid collections, and the disruption of the myometrium by fluid or gas. CT is useful in assessing the entire abdomen. Laparoscopy can be used to examine the uterus for perforation but is suboptimal for a detailed examination of the bowel.[35]

MANAGEMENT

Any woman who has an incomplete or failed abortion or retained clotted or liquid blood (hematometra) should undergo immediate re-evacuation.[37] This tissue serves as a nidus for infection. The recommended treatment of PID (see Table 50.2) is appropriate for a woman who has early, uncomplicated postabortion infection limited to the endometrial cavity. The patient should be evaluated 48 hours after institution of therapy. If fever or pain persists, then the patient should be hospitalized and evaluated as above.

Women who have more severe illness should be hospitalized and begun on broad-spectrum antibiotics such as ampicillin, gentamicin and clindamycin. If clostridial infection is suspected, high-dose penicillin therapy should be used in place of ampicillin. These patients should be monitored closely and aggressively evaluated for uterine perforation and bowel injury. In the case of suspected *C. sordellii* infection, some experts recommend the combination of clindamycin and imipenem–cilastatin.[38] Laparotomy with possible hysterectomy should be performed if there is failure to respond to uterine evacuation and medical therapy, uterine perforation with necrotic myometrium or suspected bowel injury, pelvic and adnexal abscesses, or clostridial myometritis. Indications for a total hysterectomy with removal of adnexae include a discolored, woody appearance of the uterus and adnexae, clostridial sepsis, pelvic tissue crepitation and gas in the uterine wall on radiographs.

Postoperative Gynecologic Infections

EPIDEMIOLOGY

Hysterectomy is the most frequently performed elective surgical procedure among women of reproductive age in the USA.[32] The spectrum of postoperative infections after hysterectomy includes vaginal cuff cellulitis, pelvic cellulitis, vaginal cuff abscess, phlegmon, pelvic abscess and wound infections.[24] Rates of infection after abdominal hysterectomy ranged from 11% to 38% without antibiotic prophylaxis and from 4% to 8% with antibiotic prophylaxis. For vaginal hysterectomies, infection rates varied between 12% and 64% without antibiotic prophylaxis and between 0% and 10% with antibiotic prophylaxis.[39] Risk factors for postoperative infection include duration of surgery, younger age, lower socioeconomic status and the presence of BV.

PATHOGENESIS AND PATHOLOGY

Bacterial contamination of the operative site with flora of the lower reproductive tract occurs at the vaginal incision. The exposure in a vaginal hysterectomy occurs from the initial vaginal incision throughout the procedure and the exposure in an abdominal hysterectomy occurs near the end of the procedure. Hospitalization itself, regardless of whether antimicrobial prophylaxis is given, changes the vaginal flora, resulting in an increase in colony counts of *Escherichia coli*, *Enterococcus faecalis* and *Bacteroides* spp. and a decline in *Staphylococcus epidermidis* and *Streptococcus* and *Peptostreptococcus* spp.

Postoperative infections involve a mix of aerobic and anaerobic bacteria from the lower reproductive tract (see Table 50.4). *Bacteroides fragilis* and *Fusobacterium* spp. are more common in infections than when they are found in normal vaginal flora.

PREVENTION

Patients undergoing elective hysterectomy should be screened and, if necessary, treated for bacterial vaginosis several weeks before surgery. Preoperative single-dose antibiotic prophylaxis substantially reduces the rate of postoperative febrile morbidity in these procedures.[24,39]

CLINICAL FEATURES

Postoperative fever itself does not indicate infection but should prompt the clinician to evaluate the patient for one.

In pelvic cellulitis symptoms usually occur 2–3 days after surgery and include fever (temperature over 100.4°F (38°C)) and complaints of increasing abdominal and pelvic pain that may not be symmetric.[40] Parametrial tenderness without palpable mass is found on bimanual examination.

Histologic vaginal cuff cellulitis will develop in all women postoperatively as part of the normal healing process and most cases resolve without antibiotic therapy. Women who have more severe cellulitis will complain of increasing central or lower abdominal pain, increasing vaginal discharge or low-grade fever, usually within the first 2 weeks postoperatively. Bimanual pelvic examination may show only mild suprapubic tenderness to deep palpation without masses. Speculum examination will show a tender, indurated, hyperemic vaginal surgical margin.

In a vaginal cuff abscess patients typically have fever 2–3 days postoperatively and may report vaginal fullness. On examination a tender, palpable collection will be found above the vaginal surgical margin. A phlegmon would be diagnosed if a tender mass were felt in one or both parametrial areas and if no abscess could be identified on radiographic studies.

Pelvic abscesses are a late postoperative complication that present many weeks after surgery and most have a palpable mass in the pelvis. Wound infections are characterized by pain, marginal cellulitis and purulent exudate. Septic pelvic vein thrombophlebitis and osteomyelitis pubis are both rare complications of gynecologic surgery.

DIAGNOSIS

Microbiologic cultures obtained from drained abscesses are useful in guiding therapy. Cultures of the vaginal cuff are likely to be contaminated with vaginal flora. Abdominal and pelvic ultrasound and CT scans are useful to confirm the presence of a fluid collection when pelvic abscesses are suspected.

MANAGEMENT

Patients who have pelvic cellulitis should be treated with a broad-spectrum parenteral antibiotic regimen, such as a second-generation cephalosporin (cefoxitin or cefotetan), extended-spectrum penicillin (ticarcillin–clavulanate or sulbactam–ampicillin), or an aminoglycoside plus clindamycin, for 24–36 hours after the patient becomes afebrile. Cuff abscesses should be managed similarly, and the abscess should be drained. Vaginal cuff cellulitis can be managed on an outpatient basis with oral antibiotics such as amoxicillin–clavulanic acid, but patients should have a follow-up evaluation 72 hours after starting therapy. Medical therapy that covers Gram-negative aerobes and Gram-negative anaerobes (aminoglycoside–clindamycin or aminoglycoside–metronidazole) is often successful in treating postoperative pelvic abscesses that are inaccessible to drainage.

Patients who fail to respond to medical therapy alone (no defervescence in 72 hours or enlarging abscess) will require laparotomy and drainage, or excision. Abscesses accessible from a cutaneous surface should be drained. Patients should be treated with parenteral antibiotics until all signs and symptoms have resolved.

Some clinicians give postdischarge outpatient treatment with metronidazole and amoxicillin for 1 week after discharge in those patients who responded to medical management. All patients who have pelvic abscesses should be re-evaluated 2 weeks after discharge to ensure no recurrence of the abscess has occurred.

REFERENCES

References for this chapter can be found online at http://www.expertconsult.com

Marleen Temmerman
Hans Verstraelen

Chapter | **51** |

Complications of pregnancy: maternal perspectives

EPIDEMIOLOGY

Medical progress, such as effective antibiotics and vaccines, in combination with improved living conditions has modified the sequelae of infections, yet infectious morbidity in pregnancy remains a serious problem.

Any acute or chronic infection may occur before conception, during pregnancy or during the puerperium and may have serious consequences for the mother, the fetus and the neonate. Some microorganisms are known to cause congenital infections and are discussed in Chapter 52. Others primarily influence the health of pregnant women and are described below.

The problem of maternal infections during pregnancy is addressed with emphasis on organ systems, including genitourinary tract infections, respiratory tract infections, gastrointestinal infections, puerperal sepsis, wound infection, mastitis, thrombophlebitis, endocarditis and meningitis. The infectious etiology of pre-term birth, premature pre-term rupture of membranes (pPROM) and chorioamnionitis deserves special attention. In addition, the implications of specific infections, including malaria, listeriosis, Lyme disease, varicella-zoster, HIV and other sexually transmitted diseases (STDs), are summarized in Tables 51.1 and 51.2.

The topic of infections in pregnancy is too wide to summarize in a single chapter. The interested reader will find excellent reviews by Sweet and Gibbs, Ledger, Hurley and Lamont.[1–4]

Incidence and prevalence

The primary infectious risk factor to poor pregnancy outcome, including pre-term birth, pPROM, spontaneous abortion, perinatal morbidity and mortality and maternal infections, does not relate to a specific micro-organism, but rather to a perturbation of the vaginal ecosystem and to bacterial vaginosis in particular. Bacterial vaginosis is a particularly common, albeit often asymptomatic condition, characterized by a loss of the resident lactobacilli and the concomitant overgrowth with a wide variety of mostly anaerobic species associated with ascending genital tract infection.[5–10]

Group B streptococci (GBS) continue to be a leading cause of perinatal infections.[11] The reported rates of GBS colonization in the genital tract range from 5% to 40%, with an average transmission rate to the neonate of 60%. The rates of early-onset GBS infection in the neonate, especially in pre-term and low-birth-weight babies, can be as high as 3 in 1000; however, the role of GBS in the occurrence of pre-term birth remains unclear.

Sexually transmitted infections, including trichomoniasis, gonorrhea, *Chlamydia* infection and syphilis, have also been associated with adverse pregnancy outcome, including pre-term birth, pPROM, low birth weight and postpartum infection.[12,13]

Prevalence rates of HIV in pregnant women are increasing all over the world but have reached endemic proportions in developing countries. The impact of maternal HIV infection on pregnancy outcome is still debated but most data from large studies of pregnant women who do not use drugs show an increased risk of adverse obstetric outcome, including abortion, prematurity, low birth weight and stillbirth.[13,14] However, the main risk remains mother-to-child transmission, with perinatal HIV transmission rates reported to occur with 15–40% of births among HIV-infected women.

Urinary tract infections (UTIs) are the most common infections in pregnancy, with or without clinical signs or symptoms. Asymptomatic bacteriuria is found in 4–7% of pregnant women, of whom 25–30% will develop pyelonephritis later in pregnancy.

Upper respiratory tract infections are common but of limited consequence for mother and child. In contrast, pneumonia is a serious illness for a pregnant woman.

Gastrointestinal infections caused by viruses are usually mild with no harm to the pregnancy and no need for specific medication. Meningitis is rare except for areas in which HIV and cryptococcal meningitis are endemic. Bacterial endocarditis is also uncommon and incidence rates vary from 1 in 4000 to 1 in 16 000 deliveries.

Febrile illness at delivery is uncommon in uncomplicated term pregnancies. Common underlying causes are chorioamnionitis, pyelonephritis, influenza and listeriosis.

The overall incidence of postpartum infections varies between 1% and 10%, depending on the definitions used, particularly for mastitis and postpartum endometritis. Postpartum infections consist of genital tract infections, puerperal mastitis, pelvic thrombophlebitis, UTIs, wound infections, complications of anesthesia and other infectious complications.

Genital tract infections of the uterus are the most common cause of puerperal infection and are categorized as endometritis, endomyometritis or endoparametritis depending on the extent of the infection. Wound and episiotomy infections occur frequently. After Caesarian section, wound infection defined as erythema, positive discharge and/or positive wound cultures varies between 5% and 10%, with emergency cases at higher risk of infection.

Septic thrombophlebitis is a rare complication of pregnancy with reported incidence rates of 1 in 2000 deliveries. The incidence of puerperal mastitis is estimated at around 1% in lactating women. Most have a mild disease.

Burden of disease, morbidity and mortality

In the general population the attributable risk of infections for adverse pregnancy outcome depends on the prevalence rates of infections in the population as well as on the socioeconomic and cultural factors that influence health, health behavior and health-seeking behavior. All infections that manifest with fever increase the risk of pre-term birth because of the release of pyrogens that increase myometrial activity.

Table 51.1 Implications of specific infections on pregnancy

	Impact on mother and child	Prevention	Management
Malaria	More frequent, more severe in pregnancy, especially in nonimmune women; increased risk of hypoglycemia in the mother LBW, IUGR, pre-term birth, abortion and stillbirth increased Congenital malaria (fever, hepatosplenomegaly, jaundice, anemia)	Chemoprophylaxis in travelers to endemic areas If no *Plasmodium falciparum* resistance, chloroquine phosphate 500 mg/week po In case of resistance proguanil 200 mg po q24h plus chloroquine 500 mg po q24h Avoid exposure	Prompt treatment with chloroquine or quinine according to resistance patterns Similar treatment regimens to those in nonpregnant women
Listeriosis	Mild maternal infection, but increased susceptibility Serious impact on the fetus: amnionitis, pre-term birth, septic abortion, stillbirth, fatality rate 3–50%	Early diagnosis in any febrile illness in pregnancy, cervical and blood cultures for *Listeria monocytogenes* Avoid implicated foods (e.g. unpasteurized cheese)	Ampicillin 2 g iv q6h plus gentamicin 2 mg/kg q8h for 1 week
Lyme disease	Erythema migrans in the mother, risk of transmission unknown, probably low Pre-term birth, stillbirth, syndactyly, cortical blindness, rash	Protective clothes in tick-infected areas (rural forest); remove ticks	Early treatment with amoxicillin 500 mg po q6h for 10–30 days or ceftriaxone 2 g iv for 14 days
Varicella-zoster	Rare in adults, fever, malaise followed by rash, 20% risk of varicella pneumonia Risk of abortion, stillbirth Congenital varicella (limb hypoplasia, cortical atrophy, retardation, IUGR, cutaneous scars, microphthalmia)	IgG testing if exposed If no IgG: varicella-zoster immunoglobulin 125 units/10 kg, max 625 units im, <96h after exposure	In cases of pneumonia: admission, respiratory support, aciclovir 10–15 mg/kg for 7 days Ultrasound assessment of the fetus
Measles	Increased maternal mortality secondary to pneumonia Risk of prematurity Developmental abnormalities (e.g. congenital heart disease, cleft lip, cerebral leukodystrophy and cyclopia have been reported)	Passive immunization in susceptible exposed women with pooled immunoglobulins 0.25 ml/kg within 6 days of exposure Avoid measles vaccine in pregnancy	Symptomatic
Group B streptococci	Sepsis in 1–3/1000 neonates, high mortality rates	Non consensus Antenatal case detection and treatment, or intrapartum treatment of women at risk?	Penicillin G 5 million units iv followed by 2.5 million units q4h until delivery or ampicillin 2 g followed by 1 g q4h until delivery

LBW, low birth weight; IUGR, intrauterine growth retardation.

Intra-amniotic infection diagnosed on clinical criteria occurs in 1–5% of pregnancies, with or without ruptured membranes. Consequences are pre-term birth, pPROM and postpartum and neonatal infections. The mother and the fetus are put at risk with pPROM as it is associated with pre-term birth and frequent infectious morbidity. Ascending infections, either the cause or the result of pPROM, may lead to intra-amniotic infection, chorioamnionitis, placentitis and fetal infections, including pneumonia and bacteremia.

The impact of asymptomatic UTI on pregnancy complications such as hypertension, anemia and poor obstetric outcome remains controversial. In contrast, ascending UTIs clearly play a role in the etiology of pre-term delivery and neonatal death.

Lower respiratory tract infections, meningitis and bacterial endocarditis are all life-threatening conditions for the mother and should be treated without delay.

Although postpartum infections are seldom life-threatening, sepsis remains an important cause of maternal death worldwide. Maternal mortality rates of 1–5 per 100 000 live births are registered in the Western world, whereas 100–600 per 100 000 pregnant or child-bearing women in developing countries die as a consequence of reproduction. In addition, for every woman who dies in childbirth another 30 women suffer from injuries, infections and disabilities. Overall, 25% of maternal mortality is considered to be caused by infections and this number can be lowered substantially by better health services and prompt treatment.

A number of reports estimating the role of infections in maternal death are summarized in Table 51.3. Few etiologic studies have been carried out in developing countries but the role of infections is likely to be more important. Personal observations (MT) from Nairobi, Kenya indicate that infections play a role in up to 40% of mothers dying in childbirth. The silent tragedy of maternal death should receive more attention from the international community, and also from the research world, because a substantial proportion of maternal deaths as a result of infections, bleeding and eclampsia are avoidable and interventions have to be tested to lower this unacceptable consequence of giving birth.

Postpartum genital infections may lead to chronic pain and discomfort, bleeding irregularities and infertility caused by ascending infections. Wound infections may increase pain and discomfort and prolong hospital stay. Pelvic vein thrombophlebitis may lead to serious complications such as septic pulmonary emboli.

Table 51.2 Implications of some sexually transmitted diseases on pregnancy

	Impact on mother and child	Prevention	Management
Neisseria gonorrhoeae	Ophthalmia neonatorum, pre-term delivery, puerperal infections	Silver nitrate 1% or tetracycline eye ointment	Spectinomycin 2 g im, ceftriaxone 250 mg im, or standard antimicrobial treatment
Chlamydia trachomatis	Ophthalmia neonatorum, puerperal infections, pre-term delivery	Tetracycline eye ointment	Erythromycin 500 mg for 4–7 days
Bacterial vaginosis	Risk of pre-term birth	Case detection and treatment is still under study	Metronidazole 250 mg q8h for 3–7 days or erythromycin base 333 mg q8h for 3–14 days
Trichomonas vaginalis	Risk of pre-term birth	Case detection and treatment no proven effect	Metronidazole 2 g single dose
Condylomata acuminatum	Risk of respiratory papillomatoses 1/80–1/1500	Case detection and treatment	Topical trichloroacetic acid (85%)/ surgery
Herpex simplex	Neonatal herpes 50% in mother with primary herpes at delivery	History from pregnant woman, careful inspection of the genital tract on the day of delivery	In case of active lesions, Caesarian section or vaginal delivery under aciclovir 200–400 mg q8h (under study)
HIV	Transmission in 25–45% Risk of abortion, pre-term delivery, puerperal infections	Antiretroviral therapy according to the most recent guidelines Elective Caesarian section No breast-feeding	Avoid long labor, rupture of membranes <4 h Treat with antiretroviral therapy, according to the most recent guidelines

Table 51.3 Cases of maternal death from infections

	Date of study	%
Michigan	1950–1971	23
Iowa	1926–1980	56
	1950–1980	16
South Carolina	1970–1984	14
Oklahoma	1950–1979	7
Data from Sweet & Gibbs.[1]		

Risk factors

Poverty is the most important risk factor for maternal infections during pregnancy. Poor women are more susceptible to malnutrition, infections, including STDs, less adequate sanitary conditions and lower access to preventive and curative health care than those who are financially better off.

Risk factors for UTI in pregnancy include sexual activity, older age, history of UTIs, lower socioeconomic status, diabetes mellitus, sickle-cell disease and specific bacterial factors such as the serotype and the virulence determinants of the micro-organisms.

Risk factors for lower respiratory disease include low socioeconomic status and HIV infection, particularly for infections with *Streptococcus pneumoniae*. Bacterial endocarditis has been reported more often in urban settings and among drug users.

Risk factors for puerperal genital infections include socioeconomic variables, anemia, STD, obstetric factors such as length of rupture of membranes, pre-term delivery, Caesarian section and number of vaginal examinations. Puerperal fever caused by group A β-hemolytic streptococci, once one of the most striking examples of iatrogenic infections in the 19th century, is a rare event in modern obstetrics, although sporadic outbreaks have been reported. A toxic-shock-like syndrome can occur caused by the release of pyrogenic exotoxins from streptococcal isolates (see Chapter 44).

Factors known to increase the risk for wound infections are age, obesity, bacterial contamination, operating time and duration of preoperative hospitalization, emergency procedures, number of vaginal examinations, duration of internal fetal monitoring, length of labor and underlying maternal disease. Puerperal mastitis can be related to poor nursing techniques and lack of strict hygiene measures.

PATHOGENESIS AND PATHOLOGY

Pathogenesis

The pathogenesis of most infections is similar in pregnant and non-pregnant women except for possible alterations in the immune system as noted below. Of specific interest is the role of infectious agents in the onset of labor or, more importantly, of pre-term labor. Although the exact mechanism of the onset of labor is still part of the human parturition puzzle, there is convincing evidence for the role of prostaglandins in the initiation of parturition. Arachidonic acid, one of the precursors of prostaglandins, is made available for prostaglandin synthesis by the enzyme phospholipase A_2. This enzyme, produced by many micro-organisms but especially by anaerobes, might be one of the mechanisms of pre-term initiation of labor. Micro-organisms can stimulate the release of cytokines, such as interleukins and tumor necrosis factor, that stimulate prostaglandin precursors, thus leading to uterine contractions.

In theory, the amniotic cavity is sterile, protected by the placental membranes, with the cervical mucus serving as an effective barrier preventing micro-organisms from entering the uterine cavity. With the onset of labor and the rupture of membranes, bacteria may ascend and result in an amniotic infection. Pathogens may also gain access to the amniotic cavity through intact membranes or after invasive procedures such as amniocentesis, chorion villus sampling, umbilical blood sampling and cervical cerclage.

Urinary tract infections are caused by organisms that are part of the normal fecal flora, with *Escherichia coli* responsible for 80–90% of infections. Others are facultative Gram-negative bacteria, including *Klebsiella, Proteus, Enterobacter* and *Pseudomonas* spp., and Gram-positive bacteria such as staphylococci and GBS. Symptomatic UTIs are more frequent in pregnancy for several reasons, including decreased ureteric muscle tone and activity, dilatation of the ureter and renal pelvis because of the progesterone effect, and mechanical obstruction caused by an enlarging uterus, changes of the bladder and alterations in the properties of urine during pregnancy. Bacteriuria is of concern because of the increased risk of pyelonephritis associated with pre-term labor caused by pyrogens, ureteric contractions leading to reflex myometrial contractions, the release of bacterial enzymes that may weaken the membranes and bacterial products that stimulate prostaglandin synthesis.

The most common organisms causing pneumonia in pregnant women are *S. pneumoniae, Haemophilus influenzae*, group A β-hemolytic streptococci and coagulase-positive staphylococci.

Postpartum endometritis seems to be a mixed infection with aerobic and anaerobic bacteria from the genital tract. Sexually transmitted diseases, including *Chlamydia trachomatis* and *Neisseria gonorrhoeae*, are important risk factors for ascending infections. Caesarian section is the single most important predisposing factor for pelvic infection. Wound infections are determined by the surgical techniques used, the amount of bacterial contamination and the resistance of the patient. An adequate blood supply is necessary to avoid acidosis in the wound. Organisms involved are *Enterococcus faecalis, E. coli, Staphylococcus aureus, Strep. pyogenes, Proteus* spp. and anaerobes. Predisposing factors for septic pelvic thrombophlebitis include changes in coagulation factors, alterations in the vein wall and stasis of blood flow.

In most cases of mastitis, *Staph. aureus* is the responsible organism, although *Staph. epidermidis* and viridans streptococci may also be isolated and are of questionable significance. Sporadic mastitis, usually the result of poor nursing technique, manifests as a cellulitis of the breast, primarily involving the interlobular connective tissue, to which the pathogens gain entry via a cracked or fissured nipple. In epidemic mastitis, however, infection occurs via the ductal system and spreads throughout the entire breast, resulting in mammary adenitis. The role of *Candida albicans* in causing mastitis is controversial.

Immunity

The normal course of pregnancy is associated with a variety of changes in humoral and cellular immunity, such as a loss in CD4⁺ cells and other alterations in T-cell subsets.[15-19] Reports on T-cell subsets during pregnancy have been conflicting. Some studies have found a progressive fall in the CD4⁺ count throughout pregnancy, from a mean of 950 cells/ml before 18 weeks to 720 cells/ml at term. Others have either reported a U-shaped CD4⁺ cell count profile during pregnancy, with a minimum at approximately 32 weeks of gestation (CD4 of 30% and a CD4⁺ count of 876 cells/ml), or have found stable CD4 levels and CD4:CD8 ratios during pregnancy with a rise (rebound) afterwards. Such differences may be attributable to different methodology (manual fluorescence microscopy versus automated flow cytometry), to differences in study populations or to the fact that blood was taken at different times during pregnancy. The altered immune status of pregnant women may possibly alter the response of the host to infectious agents.

Despite conflicting laboratory data, most studies agree that the humoral immune response (polymorphonuclear cells, PMNs) in pregnancy is similar to that in nonpregnant women but that the cellular immune response is diminished. Mortality rates of, for example, pneumococcal pneumonia, malaria or influenza have been found to be higher in pregnant than in nonpregnant women.

PREVENTION

Elimination of poverty and improvement of antenatal and obstetric care in deprived groups of society are primary strategies to prevent adverse pregnancy outcome. The challenge of identifying women at risk of adverse obstetric outcome is still a subject of intensive research. Early markers of infection-related pre-term birth are needed to identify a subset of women at risk for pre-term delivery who could benefit from antimicrobial therapy. A vaginal pH ≥5.0 and the presence of vaginal neutrophils at a rate of more than 5 per oil-field on Gram stain were found to be strongly associated with early pre-term birth.[20] A modified scoring system applied to Gram-stained vaginal smears in early pregnancy differentiating normal smears from bacterial vaginosis-like smears, smears dominated by atypical Gram-positive rods and lactobacilli-dominated smears showing heavy leukorrhea of unknown cause yielded a sensitivity of 70% in predicting spontaneous pre-term birth.[21] A number of molecular markers have been scrutinized for their putative predictive value with regard to the occurrence of pre-term birth. Overall, at present the most potent factors found to be associated with early spontaneous pre-term birth are a positive cervical–vaginal fetal fibronectin test, and elevated alpha-fetoprotein, alkaline phosphatase and granulocyte colony-stimulating factor serum levels, along with a shortened cervical length.[21,22]

Case detection and treatment of genitourinary infections is recommended in pregnant women who note an abnormal discharge. Screening for genitourinary pathogens with a potential negative impact on pregnancy outcome, such as bacterial vaginosis, trichomoniasis, GBS, gonorrhea, *Chlamydia* and others, depends on the prevalence of infectious agents in the population, the expected outcome of the intervention and the available resources. Recent intervention studies have provided convincing evidence of the benefit of identifying and treating bacterial vaginosis in pregnancy but only in women at high risk for pre-term birth.[10,11] As a result, the practice of routine screening for bacterial vaginosis in asymptomatic women at low risk for pre-term delivery cannot be justified according to published studies.

Screening for GBS in pregnant women is still a subject of debate. Between 10% and 30% of pregnant women are colonized with GBS, an important source of perinatal morbidity and mortality. Recently, the Centers for Disease Control and Prevention issued recommendations for the active prevention of GBS, which have been adopted by the American College of Obstetricians and Gynecologists.[23] A strategy based on late prenatal cultures, followed by intrapartum treatment with penicillin or other broad-spectrum antibiotics is recommended. Others argue that routine antimicrobial treatment with a broad-spectrum antibiotic is optimal for pregnant women at high risk of adverse pregnancy outcome in order to reduce the incidence of infectious complications such as pre-term birth, neonatal infections and maternal infectious morbidity.[24] Risk may be based solely on laboratory findings or on clinical and obstetric factors (bad obstetric history, clinical signs and symptoms). However, many questions remain unanswered, especially the benefit of screening and treating low-risk groups and the ideal antimicrobial regimen. The existing evidence is hampered by methodologic weaknesses such as small numbers, use of combinations of antibiotics and differences in populations studied. Although practice guidelines have been established it is essential to prove that the costs and the benefits associated with screening and treating genital infections in pregnant women outweigh the potential risks and effects. Only prospective, randomized and blinded clinical trials with large study populations can determine the effect of antimicrobial therapy on infectious morbidity and mortality in pregnancy.

Intercourse during pregnancy has been implicated as a risk factor for pre-term birth. This could be because of the effect of STDs or because of increased myometrial activity and cervical ripening caused by the prostaglandins in sperm. After correcting for STDs, there is little evidence of a causal relation between sexual intercourse and pre-term birth.

Randomized trials of condom use versus unprotected sex in high-risk groups for poor pregnancy outcome have not been carried out to date.

Detection and treatment of maternal bacteriuria in early pregnancy, preferably around 16 weeks, can reduce the risk of pyelonephritis, pre-term delivery and neonatal mortality.

Routine examination of stools for pathogens is not useful in pregnant women, except in populations that have high rates of anemia and malnutrition.

Prevention of puerperal infections is a major concern in obstetrics. Antenatal detection and treatment of STDs and hygienic standards during delivery decrease the risk for puerperal infection. The indications for cervical cerclage have to be carefully weighed against the risks, and antibiotic prophylaxis should be given. Active management of labor – including shorter labor, fewer vaginal examinations and reduced Caesarian section rates – help to prevent genital infections. Antibiotic prophylaxis in cases of long, complicated or operative deliveries is effective, although resistance is a limiting factor.

Mastitis can be prevented through good nursing technique, including strict hygiene measures.

CLINICAL FEATURES

Infections in pregnancy can be asymptomatic but usually manifest with symptoms similar to those in nonpregnant individuals.[1-4] The course of the infection may be worse because of alterations in immune response and because of the potential hazards for the outcome of pregnancy and the well-being of the fetus.

The clinical diagnosis of intra-amniotic infection is based upon fever, uterine tenderness, fetal tachycardia, leukocytosis and elevated C-reactive protein, with or without ruptured membranes.

Urinary tract infections are the most common infectious complications of pregnancy and can be asymptomatic or manifest with signs of cystitis such as frequency, urgency and dysuria. Fever, flank pain and chills occur with ascending UTIs.

Lower respiratory tract infections manifest with cough, fever and chest pain.

Gastrointestinal infections appear as diarrhea and are usually self-limiting and without complications. If the diarrhea persists beyond 24 hours, a stool specimen should be obtained for culture. Acute appendicitis can be a diagnostic dilemma as the clinical presentations differ from those seen in nonpregnant women because of the large uterus and the altered immune response. Appendicitis may manifest as upper right quadrant pain with nausea and vomiting, without leukocytosis or fever, and should be differentiated from acute cholecystitis and amebic liver diseases.

Meningitis should be considered in every patient with headache, malaise, nausea, vomiting and fever. The diagnosis of bacterial endocarditis in pregnant women should be considered in any febrile, lethargic patient with no signs of localizing infection. Cutaneous lesions and heart murmurs should be sought. Blood cultures are required for diagnosis.

Diagnostic criteria for postpartum endometritis include fever, uterine and/or adnexal tenderness, purulent or foul lochia and leukocytosis in the absence of other signs of infection within the first 5 days after delivery. Late postpartum endometritis may occur weeks after delivery. Retention of placental products has to be excluded.

Early wound infection starts usually within 48 hours postpartum and manifests with fever and cellulitis or edema of the wound. Early wound infection is often caused by group A or group B streptococci, or *Clostridium perfringens*. In clostridial infection, wound cellulitis is associated with a watery discharge and a bronze appearance of the skin. Late-onset wound infections occur about 4–8 days after surgery, and manifest with fever and an erythematous, draining wound.

Early recognition of life-threatening complications such as necrotizing fasciitis is crucial. Cutaneous findings can be minimal and include cellulitis, edema and sometimes crepitations. However, the patient may be critically ill and require prompt treatment. A surgical exploration of the wound may be necessary to make the diagnosis.

Puerperal mastitis occurs with breast engorgement and milk stasis, often in the second or third week after delivery. The onset of sporadic mastitis is rather sudden, with breast tenderness, chills, fever, malaise and headache mimicking a flu-like syndrome. The breast may show foci of local infection characterized by erythema, tenderness and warmth. The development of a breast abscess is rare in lactating women.

Patients with ovarian vein thrombophlebitis, which is more frequently present on the right, usually have distinct clinical findings. They present with fever and lower abdominal pain, and on examination are acutely ill with tachycardia and tachypnea and may be in respiratory distress. Abdominal examination usually shows direct tenderness, guarding and a tender abdominal mass. Pelvic pain thrombophlebitis without pulmonary emboli manifests less dramatically and has a more rapid response to therapy. These patients are more often not as critically ill, and just have fever and tachycardia.

DIAGNOSIS

Most infections that manifest with clinical signs and symptoms do not give rise to diagnostic difficulties, as they are related to specific infections of the urinary or reproductive tract, or to common infections in the community. Outlining a complete scheme of investigations is beyond the scope of this chapter, but a summary of the most important diagnostic leads and laboratory tests is presented in Table 51.4 (see also Chapter 98).

Rapid and inexpensive tests for the early detection of intra-amniotic infection in patients in pre-term labor, including amniotic fluid Gram stain, leukocyte esterase, amniotic fluid glucose concentration and the Limulus amebocyte lysate assay for endotoxin, have been tested in women admitted with pPROM or pre-term birth. The greatest sensitivity for predicting infection was demonstrated by a low glucose level in amniotic fluid but none of the tests had sufficient accuracy to allow clinical decisions.[24,25] For women with cervical dilatation in the mid-trimester of pregnancy, amniocentesis to determine the microbiologic characteristics of the amniotic cavity should be considered before placing a cerclage because of the poor prognosis in women with microbial invasion of the amniotic cavity.

The diagnosis of UTI is based on quantitative cultures with more than 100 000 cfu/ml clear-voided urine (midstream) in asymptomatic patients, or more than 100 cfu/ml in symptomatic patients. Direct suprapubic bladder aspiration is a better technique for obtaining

Table 51.4 Clinical and laboratory criteria in the diagnosis of infection in pregnancy

History	Signs, symptoms, onset, specific localization, additional signs such as pain, rash, uterine tenderness, leakage of amniotic fluid, exposure to infections, pets, occupation, hobbies, travel, place of residence, history of infections
Clinical examination	Auscultation of heart and lungs, assessment of the uterus and cervix, examination of the breasts, detection of masses, enlargement of spleen, liver, lymph nodes, signs of thrombophlebitis
Laboratory tests	White blood cell count and differential, C-reactive protein, serum enzymes, blood smears, blood cultures, throat and vaginal swabs, specific antibodies, urine culture

uncontaminated urine but is less readily accepted by patients and/or physicians. To avoid screening all pregnant women with expensive and time-consuming urine cultures, rapid screening tests such as leukocyte esterase dipstick, microscopy for pyuria, nitrite tests and enzymatic screening tests have been developed. The rapid enzymatic test seems to be a reliable alternative to culture screening, with a sensitivity of 100%, a specificity of 81% and a negative predictive value of 100%.[26]

The key to the care of lower respiratory tract infections is an early diagnosis, with careful clinical evaluation and examination, if possible, of a sputum sample and a blood culture. One should not hesitate to take a chest radiograph, as well as an arterial Po_2 in pregnant women if a serious lower respiratory tract infection is suspected. In patients with meningitis, a spinal tap with Gram stain, culture and chemical analysis of the cerebrospinal fluid is indicated.

Postpartum endometritis is a clinical diagnosis supplemented by a cervical swab for aerobic culture to identify pathogens that may require additional measures besides the antibacterial therapy. Isolation of group A streptococci should lead to isolation of the patient whereas that of GBS should prompt further action in relation to the neonate. Culturing techniques of the endometrium with double- and triple-lumen devices have been hampered by vaginal and cervical contamination and are not used routinely.

The diagnosis of early wound infection is made clinically and confirmed by a Gram stain. Gram-positive rods are highly suggestive of clostridia, and Gram-positive cocci indicate the presence of group A streptococci or *Staph. aureus*.

The diagnosis of mastitis is a clinical diagnosis. Mammography and ultrasound can be useful in the early diagnosis of an abscess and to differentiate infection from a breast malignancy. However, this technique is rarely used because of pain and discomfort to the patient.

Pelvic vein thrombophlebitis is a difficult clinical diagnosis often confused with acute appendicitis, torsion of an adnexa, urolithiasis, pyelonephritis, leiomyoma and pelvic abscess. In case of clinical suspicion of a pelvic vein thrombophlebitis, additional examinations such as venography, CT scan and sonography have to be performed.

MANAGEMENT

A number of interventions with proven value in the management of morbidity related to infection during pregnancy are discussed. The serologic screening and subsequent management of viral infections, including rubella, toxoplasmosis, cytomegalovirus, HIV and others, is discussed in Chapter 52.

Although the initiating mechanism of pre-term labor is unknown, the potential role of ascending infection and intrauterine inflammation is clear. Consequently, attempts to prolong gestation and improve pregnancy outcome using antimicrobials have been made. A number of prospective, randomized clinical trials with antibiotics have been reviewed. Among women in pre-term labor with intact membranes the use of prophylactic antibiotics is associated with a reduction in maternal infection, though not with a clear benefit for length of gestation and neonatal outcome, and hence this treatment is not recommended for routine practice.[27] In contrast, among women with pre-term rupture of membranes, antibiotic administration is associated with a significant reduction in intrauterine infection, with delay in delivery and a reduction in major markers of neonatal morbidity. These data support the routine use of antibiotics in pPROM, such as erythromycin, while co-amoxiclav should be avoided.[28] In addition, routine antibiotic prophylaxis given during the second or third trimester of pregnancy reduces the risk of pre-labor rupture of membranes when given to unselected pregnant women and is associated with beneficial effects on birth weight and the risk of postpartum endometritis among women with a previous pre-term birth. However, as infection is the underlying cause of pre-term birth in only a fraction of women, improved diagnostic methods are needed to identify those patients who will most gain from routine antibiotic prophylaxis.[29]

As bacteriuria in pregnancy, if untreated, may lead to pyelonephritis in up to a third of women, with potential hazards for mother and fetus, screening and management in pregnancy is justified. Antibiotic treatment is effective in clearing asymptomatic bacteriuria and in reducing the risk of pyelonephritis in pregnancy.[30] There are, however, insufficient data to recommend any specific regimen. The choice of antibiotic should be guided by antimicrobial susceptibility testing, but this decision is becoming more difficult because of increasing rates of antimicrobial resistance to commonly prescribed antibiotics.[31] Also, the optimal duration of antimicrobial therapy for treatment of bacteriuria in pregnant women has not been determined.[32]

Similarly, antibiotic treatment has been shown to be highly effective for the cure of symptomatic cystourethritis; however, there are insufficient data to recommend any specific treatment regimen for symptomatic urinary tract infections during pregnancy. Accordingly, susceptibility tests should be obtained. Most antibiotics studied were shown to be very effective, while complications are rare.[33] Common antimicrobial treatment options include 3-day courses of trimethoprim–sulfamethoxazole (TMP–SMZ) 160/800 mg q12h or a 7-day course of nitrofurantoin 100 mg q6h, or cephalexin 500 mg q6h. TMP–SMZ should be avoided in the third trimester because sulfonamides cross the placenta and compete with bilirubin in the fetus. Trimethoprim is a folate antagonist and should be combined with folic acid if given in high doses. In view of the high rate of recurrence of bacteriuria in pregnancy, suppressive therapy is recommended until 2 weeks postpartum in women with recurrent bacteriuria. Pregnant women with acute pyelonephritis require admission for parenteral administration of antibiotics and careful monitoring.

Penicillin is the drug of choice in women with lower respiratory tract infections caused by pneumococci. The fever may cause premature contractions. Because of possible cardiopulmonary complications, β-mimetic tocolytic drugs should be avoided or, if necessary, administered with caution.

Treatment of gastrointestinal infections is usually not necessary during pregnancy except when the problems persist and interfere with the mother's health. Metronidazole should be prescribed for *Entamoeba histolytica* infection. Pregnant women with acute appendicitis should undergo surgical exploration by the obstetrician together with the surgeon, and antibiotics should be prescribed.

Treatment of postpartum genital infection includes appropriate antibiotics with good anaerobic coverage. After Caesarian section the desired results have been obtained with a combination of clindamycin and gentamicin.[34] Newer antibiotics such as the monobactams may replace gentamicin in combination with clindamycin, and the newer cephalosporins with a wide spectrum of activity are increasingly used. Intravenous antibiotics should be continued for 24–48 hours after the patient has become afebrile, and can be stopped without changing to oral antibiotics unless a staphylococcal infection is present. The reduction of endometritis by some two-thirds and the decrease in wound infections justifies a policy of routine prophylactic antibiotics to women undergoing elective or nonelective Caesarian section.[35]

The treatment of early wound infections may require excision of the necrotic tissue and aggressive antibiotic treatment with a cephalosporin or clindamycin. In late-onset (after 5 days) wound infection incision of the wound and drainage is required. If the patient does not become afebrile after 24 hours, antibiotics should be prescribed. Open wounds can be allowed to close spontaneously by granulation after wound debridement and packing. Surgical closure of Caesarian section has been shown to be successful and requires less healing time. The procedure may be carried out under general or local anesthesia, and antibiotic prophylaxis is generally used. Episiotomy incisions should not be re-sutured but given time to heal by granulation, unless the sphincter muscle or the rectal mucosa is involved. In rare complications such as necrotizing fasciitis or clostridial gas gangrene, treatment must be aggressive, including high doses of broad-spectrum antibiotics and extensive drainage and debridement.

Therapy of mastitis includes continuation of lactation and treatment with a penicillinase-resistant penicillin or a cephalosporin, given orally except in the case of a severely sick patient. Ice packs, breast support, analgesics and regular emptying of the infected breast may help to prevent abscesses. In case of abscess formation, surgical incision and drainage should be performed.

Table 51.5 Risk factor assignments for antibiotics in pregnancy[36]

Agent		Category	Potential toxicity
1	Penicillin	B	
2	Cephalosporin	B_M	
3	Monobactam	B_M	
4.1	Aminoglycoside/group 1	C*	Fetal ototoxicity, maternal oto- and nephrotoxicity
4.2	Aminoglycoside/group 2 (spectinomycin)	B	
5	Chloramphenicol	C	Gray syndrome (cardiovascular collapse in babies) when given near term
6	Tetracycline	D	Adverse effects on fetal teeth and bones, congenital defects, maternal liver toxicity
7.1	Macrolide: erythromycin	B	! Estolate salt form can induce maternal hepatotoxicity
7.2	Other macrolides	$C–C_M$	
8	Clindamycin	B	
9	Fluoroquinolone	C_M	
10.1	Sulfonamides	B*	No teratogenic effect, to be avoided near term because of potential toxicity to the newborn (kernicterus)
10.2	Trimethoprim–sulfamethoxazole	C_M	Megaloblastic anemia, folate activity

*Adapted from ref.[36]

Treatment of pelvic vein thrombophlebitis includes broad-spectrum antibiotics, heparin for 7–10 days intravenously, followed by long-term anticoagulation with oral anticoagulants. Surgery, including bilateral ovarian vein and inferior vena cava ligation, may be required for patients who do not respond to treatment. Hysterectomy is seldom required.

Antibiotics in pregnancy

Antibiotics are frequently used during pregnancy. Several studies have shown that 25–40% of pregnant women take antibiotics, mainly in the second trimester, while the incidence of antibiotic intake is around 5% in the first trimester. Administration of a drug to a pregnant woman presents a unique problem. The pharmacologic mechanisms must be well considered, and the fetus must always be kept in mind. Most drugs or chemical substances taken during pregnancy can cross the placenta to some extent throughout pregnancy, but the fetus is at highest risk during the first 3 months of gestation.

Risk factors have been assigned to all level of risk that a drug poses to the fetus (A, B, C, D and X). The definitions used for the risk factors, described by Briggs *et al.*,[36] are summarized below.

- Category A: Controlled studies in women fail to demonstrate a risk to the fetus in the first trimester (and there is no evidence of a risk in later trimesters), and the possibility of fetal harm appears remote.
- Category B: Either animal reproduction studies have failed to demonstrate a risk to the fetus and there are no adequate and well-controlled studies in pregnant women, or animal reproduction studies have shown an adverse effect, but adequate and well-controlled studies in pregnant women have failed to demonstrate a risk to the fetus in any trimester.
- Category C: Animal reproduction studies have shown an adverse effect on the fetus and there are no adequate and well-controlled studies in humans. However, potential benefits may warrant use of the drug in pregnant women despite potential risks.
- Category D: There is positive evidence of human fetal risk based on adverse reaction data from investigational or marketing experience or studies in humans, but potential benefits may warrant use of the drug in pregnant women despite potential risks.

- Category X: Studies in animals or humans have demonstrated fetal abnormalities or there is evidence of fetal risk based on human experience or both, and the risk of the use of the drug in pregnant women clearly outweighs any possible benefit. The drug is contraindicated in women who are or may become pregnant.

Many older drugs have not been given a letter by their manufacturers, and the risk factor assignments were made by Briggs *et al.*[36] In cases where the manufacturer has rated the product in its professional literature, the risk factor is shown with a subscript (e.g. C_M). Risk markers with an asterisk indicate that risks to the fetus depend on when or for how long the antibiotic is used. The classification of the most commonly used antibiotics is summarized in Table 51.5.[36]

CONCLUSIONS

Infectious diseases are important risk factors for maternal and neonatal morbidity and mortality and can be detected early with improved outcomes or prevented entirely. Maternal mortality due to infections is an unbearable tragedy and must be addressed by improved access to modern obstetric care for all pregnant women. This care must be affordable, even in resource-limited countries, and should be a priority for governments and international agencies.

Preventing pre-term birth is a global issue, including industrialized countries. A substantial portion of pre-term births can be prevented with improvements in the detection and management of infections during pregnancy. Further research is required to identify women and babies at risk, and to develop preventive, diagnostic and management strategies to enhance care with maximal benefits at minimal costs and adverse effects.

REFERENCES

References for this chapter can be found online at http://www.expertconsult.com

Ari Bitnun
Elizabeth Lee
Ford-Jones
Greg Ryan

Chapter | 52 |

Implications for the fetus of maternal infections in pregnancy

The number of pathogens capable of infecting the fetus, and the spectrum of disease in the fetus and newborn infant caused by various pathogens has expanded substantially. Advances in molecular technology (e.g. polymerase chain reaction, PCR) and wider availability of intrauterine diagnostic testing (e.g. maternal serum alpha-fetoprotein screening, ultrasound, amniocentesis, fetal blood sampling) have provided new opportunities to link pathogens to untoward events. Congenital infection in pregnancy may come to clinical attention through:

- a history of maternal risk factors;
- known exposure;
- documented acute maternal infection;
- laboratory screening;
- detection of fetal abnormalities on clinical examination or ultrasonography;
- suggestive findings in the neonate; and
- suggestive findings in the child.

Depending on the scenario, one or a range of infections must be considered in the differential diagnosis.

Fortunately, the vast majority of maternal infections have no deleterious effect on the fetus, either because there is no transmission to the intrauterine site or because the fetal infection is asymptomatic. Fear and poor understanding of risk on the part of the parents or physician can lead to unnecessary termination of pregnancy.

EPIDEMIOLOGY

Although many micro-organisms are known to cause congenital (intrauterine) infection (Table 52.1), only more common agents are discussed (see below). A brief summary of infections transmitted primarily at the time of delivery is given at the end of the chapter.

Because the use of appropriate diagnostic testing is highly variable and because many of these diseases are not reportable to public health departments, there are few data on incidence.

Geography

There is considerable geographic variation in the risk of exposure to pathogens associated with congenital and perinatal infections. This variation may be related directly to the biology of the pathogen (e.g. *Plasmodium* spp., *Trypanosoma cruzi*), culinary practices, including handling and ingestion of fresh raw meat (e.g. toxoplasmosis) or regional variation in breast-feeding rates. The geographic distribution of certain pathogens may change over time, particularly arthropod-borne or zoonotic infections; an example of this is the recent introduction of West Nile virus to North America.

Other factors associated with infection

Epidemiologic factors associated with maternal–fetal infection are summarized in Table 52.2. The risk of congenital infection often reflects maternal immunity rates as well as the risk of exposure to the pathogen. Cytomegalovirus (CMV) and *Treponema pallidum* are excellent examples of this. Annual seroconversion rates to CMV for healthcare workers, usually in the range of 2–4%, are generally lower than rates in day-care workers or susceptible parents of children in day care (12–45%).[3] Syphilis in pregnancy generally affects women who are young, unmarried, of low socioeconomic status and who receive inadequate prenatal care.

PATHOGENESIS AND PATHOLOGY

Infections occurring in the neonate may be acquired in the following ways:

- transplacentally in utero (congenital or intrauterine) by direct blood flow to the amniotic fluid or from the genital tract via the cervical amniotic route, during pregnancy or just before delivery. The placenta can be infected and even act as a repository for pathogen growth;
- at the time of birth (perinatal) through vaginal secretions and blood; and
- after birth but during the neonatal period (postnatal), from the mother, her breast milk or other sources.

Adverse outcomes from intrauterine infection include abortion, stillbirth, premature delivery, physical defects, intrauterine growth restriction (e.g. rubella, enterovirus, herpes simplex virus (HSV)) and postnatal persistence of infection (e.g. rubella, CMV, HSV, toxoplasmosis).

A general association between certain outcomes and timing and site of infection exists:

- embryo: malformations, spontaneous abortion;
- fetus: stillbirth, neurologic sequelae; and
- placenta: preterm birth, stillbirth and neonatal death.

Factors affecting fetal disease

The risk of transplacental transmission and disease manifestations are influenced by a multitude of factors, including the pathogen's propensity for causing fetal infection, the pregnant woman's immunologic status to the pathogen, placenta function and the timing of infection in regard to fetal development.

Table 52.1 Infectious agents known to cause congenital infection

Viruses	Herpesviruses
	Cytomegalovirus
	Herpes simplex virus
	Varicella zoster virus
	Human herpesvirus 6[2]
	Human herpesvirus 7[2]
	Parvovirus B19
	Rubella virus
	Measles virus
	Enteroviruses
	Coxsackie B
	Echoviruses
	Polioviruses
	Parechoviruses
	Human immunodeficiency viruses
	HIV-1
	HIV-2
	Lymphocytic choriomeningitis virus
	Hepatitis B virus
	Vaccinia
	Smallpox
	Adenovirus
	Western equine encephalitis virus
	Venezuelan encephalitis virus
	West Nile virus
Bacteria	*Treponema pallidum*
	Mycobacterium tuberculosis
	Listeria monocytogenes
	Brucella spp.
	Campylobacter fetus
	Salmonella typhi
	Borrelia burgdorferi
	Coxiella burnetti
Protozoa	*Toxoplasma gondii*
	Plasmodium spp.
	Trypanosoma cruzi
Fungi	*Coccidioides immitis*

Adapted with permission from Guerina.[1]

Table 52.2 Factors associated with maternal–fetal infection

Association	Pathogen
Seasonality (in North America)	Parvovirus B19 (winter, spring) Rubella (winter, spring) Enterovirus (summer, autumn) West Nile virus (summer, autumn)
Handling/ingestion of uncooked, previously unfrozen meat	*Toxoplasma gondii*
Children: Day care School Household	CMV, parvovirus Parvovirus CMV, parvovirus
Exposure in travel to certain geographic regions	*Toxoplasma gondii*, *Mycobacterium tuberculosis*, *Plasmodium* spp., *Trypanosoma cruzi*, *Borrelia burgdorferi*, hepatitis B virus, *Brucella* spp., West Nile virus
Kitten/cat feces within 21 days of primary infection (handling animals, kitty litter, gardening)	*Toxoplasma gondii*
Number of sexual partners, sex industry worker/partner, illicit drug use	*Treponema pallidum*, herpes simplex virus, hepatitis B virus, hepatitis C virus, HIV
Sexually active adolescents	CMV, herpes simplex virus, hepatitis B virus, hepatitis C virus, HIV
Unimmunized (e.g. immigrant from developing world; World Health Organization Expanded Program of Immunization does not include rubella)	Rubella
Other incompletely immunized	Measles, mumps, tetanus, diphtheria, poliomyelitis, hepatitis B, varicella-zoster virus

Pathogen

The explanation as to why certain pathogens have a propensity for causing congenital infections is incompletely understood. In part, this may reflect the tendency of certain infecting organisms to invade the mother's bloodstream, thereby coming in contact with the placenta and fetus. Inoculum size, as measured by quantity of pathogen in the blood, may also be an important factor (e.g. viral load in HIV).

The specific manifestations of different pathogens reflect their individual propensity for certain stages of organogenesis as well as specific organs and tissues. Rubella virus and varicella zoster virus (VZV) cause developmental anomalies through cell death, inhibition of cell growth or chromosomal damage. Inflammation, and the resulting tissue destruction, is thought to be responsible for the structural abnormalities characteristic of HSV, congenital syphilis and toxoplasmosis. Parvovirus B19, by binding to the P antigen on erythrocyte precursors and thereby inhibiting the required rapid increase in erythrocyte numbers during the second trimester, can cause profound anemia and nonimmune hydrops.

Postnatal persistence of CMV, HSV, *Toxoplasma gondii* and rubella can result in progressive tissue damage and onset or worsening of clinical disease later in life. Thus, hearing loss associated with congenital CMV can become manifest after 2 years of age, and the chorioretinitis of congenital toxoplasmosis can recur in later years despite prior therapy.[4,5] Progressive encephalitis may occur with congenital rubella, with onset typically in the teenage years.[6]

Maternal immunity

Before conception

Preconception immunity in the immunocompetent mother is usually protective to the fetus. Exceptions include viruses with known latency such as CMV and occasionally HSV, rubella when maternal immunity has waned, untreated *Treponema pallidum* and HIV. Immunosuppressive disorders and immunosuppressive therapy will also alter the risk of fetal disease (e.g. HIV-1 infection facilitates the transmission of *T. gondii*).

The length of time before conception during which infection may occur without causing later fetal damage is not known. In the immunocompetent mother, it is advisable to have an interval of 7–9 months between *T. gondii* acquisition and conception. Over 50% of infants born to mothers with primary or secondary syphilis will have congenital infection, decreasing to 40% with early latent syphilis and to 10% or less with late latent infection.[7]

During pregnancy and before delivery

The risk of transplacental transmission and severity of disease are increased with primary maternal infection during pregnancy. Thus, the rate of intrauterine transmission of CMV is about 40% with primary maternal infection, but only 1% among previously seropositive mothers. Neurologic sequelae are approximately three times higher in the context of primary infection.

In late gestational infections, the fetus is at high risk of severe disease when delivered before transplacental transfer of specific antibody has taken place. For example, the mortality from varicella-zoster virus infection acquired transplacentally from a mother who develops skin lesions from 5 days prior to delivery to 2 days after delivery is 30% in the absence of treatment.

Placenta

In early gestation, the small developing placenta effectively excludes most pathogens. As the placenta matures, with expansion of the maternal–fetal interface, this barrier becomes more porous, rendering transplacental transmission more likely. For a variety of pathogens, including CMV, rubella virus, *Treponema pallidum*, *Plasmodium* spp. and *Mycobacterium tuberculosis*, placental infection may occur without fetal infection. Thus, the placenta can prevent infections from reaching the fetus; in part, this is due to it serving as a physical barrier to the pathogen. In addition, placental macrophages and local production of antibodies and cytokines may be important.

Fetus

Fetal disease may result from many pathogens at any time during gestation. In general, transplacental transmission (via umbilical blood flow or direct spread to the amniotic fluid) is less likely early in gestation, but the results of infection, if it occurs, are more likely to be severe. The deficiencies in immune function of the young fetus in both humoral and in cellular function contribute to the increased risk of severe disease through unchecked tissue damage, organ dysfunction and teratogenicity. Detectable IgM is rarely produced before 20–24 weeks of gestation.

Certain pathogens are associated with particular effects at certain stages of cell development. For example, maternal rubella infection in pregnancy prior to 16 weeks, but not thereafter, is associated with the development of congenital defects.[8] Congenital varicella syndrome occurs almost exclusively before 20 weeks of gestation; the highest risk occurs if the mother had varicella infection between 13 and 20 weeks.[9] While transmission of *T. gondii* occurs in only about 15% of first trimester infections, severe disease occurs in about 40% of infected infants.[10] In the third trimester the reverse is true with 60% transmission, but the disease is generally milder or asymptomatic.

PREVENTION

Prevention of maternal infection in pregnancy should include education, immunization, laboratory screening, monitoring for evidence of infection and, where appropriate, intervention (Table 52.3).

Education and exposure avoidance

While exposure to potential pathogens during pregnancy cannot be completely eliminated, relatively simple interventions can offer significant protection (Table 52.3). All women who are planning pregnancy should be given advice pertinent to infection prevention:

- Wash hands thoroughly before eating and before and after food preparation (e.g. enteric pathogens, *Listeria* spp., *T. gondii*).

- Wash hands after coming in contact with saliva, stool, urine or other body secretions (e.g. enteric pathogens, *Listeria* spp., CMV, rubella).
- Avoid eating unpasteurized milk or cheese and undercooked meat (e.g. *Listeria* spp., *Brucella* spp., *T. gondii*).
- For those with high-risk behaviors such as intravenous drug use or multiple sexual partners, provide information on the risk posed by HIV, hepatitis B, hepatitis C, syphilis and other sexually transmitted infections.
- Inform physician following exposure to erythema infectiosum (fifth disease, parvovirus B19), chickenpox/shingles, pertussis (whooping cough) or other infection.
- For women with recurrent genital herpes, inform physician if they have recurrent lesions late in gestation or when in labor.
- Inform women that testing for rubella immunity and evidence of hepatitis B virus, HIV and syphilis infection is routinely sought in pregnancy.

Active and passive immunization

All women should be immune to measles, mumps, rubella, tetanus, diphtheria, poliomyelitis, hepatitis B and varicella, either by natural infection or by vaccination. Influenza and pneumococcal immunization are recommended for women who are at high risk of infection. Immune globulin products may be indicated on exposure to measles, hepatitis A or B virus, tetanus, varicella or rabies and, in the case of certain travel, to poliomyelitis, yellow fever, typhoid and hepatitis B virus. Although inactivated vaccines are generally considered safe, some physicians wait until after the first trimester to administer them. Live viral or bacterial vaccines should be avoided during pregnancy. However, the risk of congenital rubella syndrome after administration of vaccine to a pregnant woman is very low.[11]

Screening for infection during pregnancy

Rubella screening alerts the physician to which mothers require postpartum immunization. Also, if the susceptible woman has known exposure or disease, the physician can confirm acute infection through study of a second serum sample. Antenatal screening for syphilis allows for treatment of the mother as well as prevention of infection in the infant. Hepatitis B virus screening allows for preventive management of the infant of the hepatitis B surface antigen (HBsAg)-positive mother.

The interpretation of other serology in pregnancy in the absence of seroconversion is fraught with difficulty as the acuity of the infection often cannot be determined. A woman at high risk of CMV infection (e.g. a day-care worker) would therefore be advised to establish her immune status before pregnancy. However, the general value of routine antenatal screening for CMV, as is practiced in some European countries, is debatable, in part because of the difficulty in interpreting serology results. Thus, a positive IgM for CMV in the absence of suggestive symptoms may represent a false-positive test result. If confronted with this scenario, antibody avidity assays may be helpful in determining the timing of infection.[12]

Screening for toxoplasmosis is not universally recommended, but some have argued for its implementation.[13] *Toxoplasma gondii*-specific IgM antibody can persist for more than a year in about one-third of infections, making it difficult to establish the timing of maternal infection. If *T. gondii*-specific IgM is detected during pregnancy, additional serologic testing that includes the Sabin–Feldman dye test, IgM ELISA and avidity assays should be undertaken through a reference laboratory (e.g. Toxoplasma Serology Laboratory, Palo Alto Medical Foundation, Palo Alto, CA).[14] If serology is suggestive of acute infection, amniotic fluid sampling and testing by PCR can be used to confirm fetal infection.[14] Practitioner-based testing for acute toxoplasmosis in the absence of a community-based program should be discouraged in countries where screening and treatment are not routine.

Table 52.3 Summary of preventive antenatal strategies

Pathogen	Exposure avoidance	Infection screening	Potential maternal–fetal medical interventions
CMV	Hand washing after handling respiratory secretion and urine	Some jurisdictions support routine screening of day-care workers pre-pregnancy	CMV hyperimmune globulin and oral valganciclovir for pregnant women with confirmed acute infection may be of benefit
HIV	Avoid high-risk behaviors such as unprotected sex with multiple partners, intravenous drug use Condom use	Recommended for all women; testing strategies vary with jurisdiction (opt in vs. opt out) Repeat testing late in pregnancy for those at 'high risk' should be considered Exclude associated infections such as hepatitis B, hepatitis C, syphilis and other STIs	Antiretroviral therapy to mother and baby Elective Caesarian section if maternal viral load >1000 copies/ml
Parvovirus B19	Hand washing	Following exposure or during epidemic	Intrauterine transfusion may be of benefit in selected cases
Rubella	Hand washing	Routine and following exposure	If susceptible, immunize well before conception or postpartum
VZV	Avoid exposure to children with chickenpox if nonimmune	Following exposure or during outbreak	Immunization prior to or after pregnancy if nonimmune If susceptible, some experts recommend varicella zoster immune globulin within 96 hours of exposure Oral aciclovir in mother if develops chickenpox
Treponema pallidum	Avoid high-risk behaviors such as unprotected sex with multiple partners Condom use	Routine; if high risk, third trimester intrapartum testing Exclude associated infections such as HIV, hepatitis B, hepatitis C, gonorrhea and other STIs	Penicillin Monthly serologic follow-up
Toxoplasma gondii	Avoid eating undercooked meat and wash hands thoroughly after handling Wash fruits and vegetables before eating and after handling Avoid contact with materials potentially contaminated with cat excreta such as kitty litter boxes Wear gloves while gardening	Some jurisdictions recommend routine screening; if not, screen following suspected exposure	Spiramycin or pyrimethamine–sulfadiazine with folinic acid for documented maternal infection

Monitoring for evidence of infection (clinical manifestations and ultrasound findings)

Maternal illness

Rash in pregnancy requires exclusion of syphilis, rubella, parvovirus B19 and enterovirus infection. Arthritis occurs with parvovirus B19 infection as well as with rubella. In the presence of acute mononucleosis-like symptoms of fatigue and lymphadenopathy, Epstein–Barr virus, CMV, *T. gondii* and HIV infection must be considered.

Fetal ultrasonography

Ultrasound findings of in-utero infection are provided in the Clinical features section below and in Table 52.4.

Screening for congenital infections in newborns

Routine neonatal screening for congenital toxoplasmosis is practiced in several countries;[15,16] detection of *T. gondii*-specific IgM in newborn dried blood spots has been used for this purpose. Some have also advocated for routine neonatal CMV screening.[17] Potential strategies for detection of congenital CMV infection include shell vial culture of urine or saliva or PCR for CMV DNA in neonatal dried blood spots. The cost-effectiveness of screening neonates for congenital infections has not been established.[13]

Intervention

A variety of interventions are available to prevent congenital infections. These are detailed in the management section below and in Table 52.3.

Table 52.4 Clinical features of in-utero infection

General	Intrauterine growth retardation: all etiologies Hydrops fetalis: parvovirus B19, CMV, syphilis, toxoplasmosis, HSV, Coxsackie B3 Placentamegaly: CMV, syphilis
Head and neck	Hydrocephalus: toxoplasmosis, CMV, enterovirus Microcephaly: CMV, rubella, HSV, varicella, toxoplasmosis Intracranial calcification: CMV, toxoplasmosis, HSV, rubella, HIV, parvovirus B19, West Nile virus, lymphocytic choriomeningitis virus
Heart	Congestive heart failure: parvovirus B19, syphilis, CMV, toxoplasmosis Pericardial effusion: parvovirus B19, syphilis, CMV, toxoplasmosis Cardiac defects: rubella, parvovirus B19, mumps (not proven) Myocarditis: enterovirus
Lungs	Pleural effusion: parvovirus B19, syphilis, toxoplasmosis Pulmonary hypoplasia: CMV
Abdomen	Hepatosplenomegaly: CMV, rubella, toxoplasmosis, HSV, syphilis, enterovirus, parvovirus B19 Echogenic bowel: CMV, toxoplasmosis Hepatic calcifications: CMV, toxoplasmosis Meconium peritonitis: CMV, toxoplasmosis Ascites: parvovirus B19, CMV, toxoplasmosis, syphilis
Extremities	Limb reduction, limb restriction: varicella

CLINICAL FEATURES

Fetal

The features of in-utero infections are summarized in Table 52.4. Some fetal abnormalities detected on antenatal ultrasonography may be caused by infection. However, no ultrasonographic findings are pathognomonic for a particular agent.[18] Postnatal follow-up of infants, including ophthalmologic examination, cranial neuroimaging (i.e. CT and MRI), head growth and developmental progress over at least the first 2 years of life, is important in identifying affected infants.

Spontaneous abortion and stillbirth

Pregnancy loss has been associated with infection with CMV, enterovirus, HSV, HIV, parvovirus B19, rubella, *Treponema pallidum* and *T. gondii*. Fetal loss occurring with any maternal viral infection requires comprehensive pathologic and microbiologic evaluation to determine the role of the infection in pathogenesis.

Syndromes of congenital infection
General

The majority of infected infants have no symptoms at birth although some will develop sequelae later in childhood (Table 52.5). Routine investigation of premature or low birth weight infants for possible congenital infection only rarely yields positive results. Prematurity is typical of congenital syphilis and common in perinatal HSV infection. Intrauterine growth retardation occurs with rubella, CMV, toxoplasmosis and, occasionally, enteroviruses. The clinical findings in congenital infection are summarized in Table 52.6.

Table 52.5 Early onset and late onset manifestations of selected congenital infections

Micro-organism	Proportion infected with symptoms at birth	Selected early onset manifestations	Proportion with late onset manifestations	Late onset manifestations
CMV	10%	Low birth weight, petechial/purpuric rash, hepatosplenomegaly, thrombocytopenia, chorioretinitis, microcephaly, cerebral calcifications	5–15%	Sensorineural hearing loss, microcephaly, mental retardation, motor deficits, chorioretinitis
Rubella	First 16 weeks, decreasing from 90% to 24%	Low birth weight, blueberry muffin rash, hemolytic anemia, thrombocytopenia, hepatosplenomegaly, cardiac defects, cataract, bony lucencies	>20%	Sensorineural hearing loss, visual defects, multiple endocrinopathies, panencephalitis
Treponema pallidum	30% (30–40% stillborn)	Low birth weight, snuffles, diffuse rash, pseudoparalysis (perichondritis, osteitis), chorioretinitis, aseptic meningitis, hemolytic anemia	Unknown	Sensorineural hearing loss, visual defects, abnormal dentition, bone and joint abnormalities, CNS abnormalities
Toxoplasma gondii	Severe organ damage in 20% of infants of untreated mothers and 2% in treated mothers	Low birth weight, hepatosplenomegaly, macrocephaly with hydrocephalus, or microcephaly, intracranial calcifications	40% of infants of untreated mothers; 17% of infants of treated mothers	Chorioretinitis most common, sensorineural hearing loss

Table 52.6 Clinical findings in congenital infection[19,20]

Prematurity	Syphilis, HSV
Intrauterine growth retardation	All etiologies including tuberculosis
Anemia with hydrops	Parvovirus B19, syphilis, CMV, toxoplasmosis
Bone lesions	Syphilis, rubella
Cerebral calcification	Toxoplasmosis (widely distributed) CMV and HSV (usually periventricular) Parvovirus B19, rubella, HIV, West Nile virus, lymphocytic choriomeningitis virus
Congenital heart disease	Rubella, parvovirus B19, mumps (not proved)
Hepatosplenomegaly	CMV, rubella, toxoplasmosis, HSV, syphilis, enterovirus, parvovirus B19
Hydrocephalus	Toxoplasmosis, CMV, syphilis, possibly enterovirus
Hydrops, ascites, pleural effusions	Parvovirus B19, CMV, toxoplasmosis, syphilis
Jaundice	CMV, toxoplasmosis, rubella, HSV, syphilis, enterovirus
Limb paralysis with atrophy and cicatrices	Varicella
Maculopapular exanthem	Syphilis, measles, rubella, enterovirus
Microcephaly	CMV, toxoplasmosis, rubella, varicella, HSV
Ocular findings (see below)	CMV, toxoplasmosis, rubella, HSV, syphilis, enterovirus, parvovirus B19
Progressive hepatic failure and clotting abnormalities	Echovirus, Coxsackie B virus, enterovirus, HSV, toxoplasmosis
Pseudoparalysis	Syphilis
Purpura (usually appears on first day)	CMV, toxoplasmosis, syphilis, rubella, HSV, enterovirus, parvovirus B19
Vesicles	HSV, syphilis, varicella, CMV, parvovirus B19, enterovirus
Cataracts	Rubella, HSV, VZV, parvovirus B19, toxoplasmosis, syphilis
Chorioretinitis	HSV, VZV, rubella, CMV, toxoplasmosis, West Nile virus
Optic atrophy	HSV, VZV, rubella, CMV, toxoplasmosis, syphilis
Microphthalmia	Rubella, HSV, parvovirus B19, toxoplasmosis, CMV, varicella
Coloboma	CMV
Keratoconjunctivitis	HSV
Pigment retinopathy	Rubella
Glaucoma	Rubella, toxoplasmosis, syphilis
Iritis	HSV, rubella, syphilis
Anophthalmia	CMV
Peter's anomaly	CMV
Horner syndrome	VZV

Sepsis-like illness

HSV acquired just before delivery or intrapartum may present as a perinatal syndrome, often without skin lesions, and resemble neonatal sepsis or pneumonitis. An early laboratory clue is abnormal liver enzymes. Shock, coagulopathy, fulminant hepatitis and, often, skin lesions follow. Congenital tuberculosis and enteroviral infections can also present in this way.

Hepatitis

Enteroviruses, HSV and *T. gondii* can cause overwhelming acute neonatal liver failure in the first week of life. Other infections, including CMV and parvovirus B19, can also present with hepatic findings.

Central nervous system

Central nervous system (CNS) involvement may occur with all of the congenital infections (as well as with perinatally acquired HSV and enteroviral infections), although initial findings may be very subtle. Occult findings in congenital neurosyphilis have led to general recommendations that neurosyphilis be assumed with any cerebrospinal fluid (CSF) abnormality.[21] With newer molecular techniques, CNS involvement may be better recognized (i.e. PCR detection of CMV DNA in the CSF). Clinical symptoms and signs may be preceded by ophthalmologic and neuroimaging findings. Central nervous system calcifications can be observed in congenital CMV, toxoplasmosis, HSV, HIV, rubella, parvovirus B19 and lymphocytic chorioretinitis virus (LCM).

Cardiac

Rubella infection causes structural defects including patent ductus arteriosus; parvovirus B19 may cause intrauterine congestive heart failure with resulting prenatal closure of the foramen ovale and Epstein's anomaly, and occasionally acute and chronic lymphocytic myocarditis.[22] Viral myocarditis is characteristically caused by Coxsackie B virus or other enteroviruses.

Ophthalmologic

Ophthalmologic abnormalities are seen in a variety of congenital infections (see Table 52.9).[19]

Deafness

Sensorineural deafness is a common sequela of congenital CMV and rubella, as well as of untreated *T. gondii* and *Treponema pallidum* infections. One-third of sensorineural hearing loss in childhood is caused by congenital CMV infection. Of rubella-infected infants, 80% or more may have deafness, often as the only significant consequence. Given the progressive nature of impairment, serial hearing evaluations to age 6–9 years are recommended for CMV-infected infants.

Specific infections

Cytomegalovirus

Between 85% and 90% of children with congenital CMV infection are asymptomatic at birth. Common clinical manifestations in symptomatic newborns include small for gestational age growth parameters, petechiae, thrombocytopenia, jaundice and hepatosplenomegaly. More severely affected infants may also have microcephaly, CNS calcifications, chorioretinitis or sensorineural hearing loss.

Symptomatic infants are at high risk of significant neurologic and developmental dysfunction, particularly if abnormalities are noted on cranial CT or if chorioretinitis exists. Cerebral calcifications tend to be periventricular. Most children with an abnormal newborn CT scan (90%) develop at least one neurologic sequela as compared with 29% of those with normal study, making cranial CT scan a good predictor of an adverse neurodevelopmental outcome. Normal development at 12 months of age makes subsequent neurodevelopmental or intellectual impairment unlikely. Infants with asymptomatic infection have a 5–15% risk of sensorineural hearing loss, mental retardation, motor spasticity or microcephaly evolving in the early years. Hearing loss may be late in onset, fluctuating and progressive, necessitating long-term follow-up (see Deafness above).

Enteroviruses (coxsackieviruses, echovirus)

Although high rates of maternal infection in pregnancy (up to 25%) have been reported, disease is limited to case reports or series of infected infants with a variety of entities including growth retardation, CNS malformations, blueberry muffin rash, hepatic necrosis, myocarditis or pericarditis.

Herpes simplex virus

Intrauterine HSV infection is characterized by the triad of skin vesicles or scarring, eye lesions and microcephaly or hydranencephaly. It may follow primary or recurrent, symptomatic or asymptomatic, HSV-1 or HSV-2 maternal infection at any stage of gestation. Acquisition just before delivery can lead to disease identical to that acquired at delivery, except that it occurs within the first 48 hours of life. The presence of even a single vesicle should prompt ophthalmologic examination, lumbar puncture with CSF analysis and cranial imaging.

Parvovirus B19

Seroprevalence studies indicate that approximately half of women of childbearing age are susceptible to parvovirus B19 and that the annual seroconversion rate among such women is about 1.5%. The risk of transplacental transmission of the infection is approximately 30%.[23] The vast majority of such infections, both symptomatic and asymptomatic, are followed by delivery of a healthy term infant.

The most common clinical manifestations of congenital infection with parvovirus B19 are pregnancy loss and nonimmune hydrops fetalis. The rate of fetal loss has been estimated at 5–9%, though it remains unclear what proportion of these are specifically due to parvovirus B19 infection.[23] Nonimmune hydrops fetalis is uncommon, occurring in 0–1.6% of parvovirus B19 infections; on the other hand, this virus is responsible for 10–20% of all nonimmune hydrops fetalis cases.

Rubella

The clinical features of congenital rubella syndrome (CRS) can be divided into the categories of transient, in newborns and infants; permanent, at birth or during the first year of life; and delayed, occurring in 10–20% of patients, usually in the second decade of life.[11] In rare cases, maternal reinfection has resulted in CRS.

Varicella-zoster virus

The congenital varicella syndrome (or fetal varicella-zoster syndrome, better reflecting the pathogenesis), including cicatricial skin scars, eye abnormalities including microphthalmia, hypoplastic limbs, and autonomic nervous system damage causing gastroesophageal reflux with or without CNS abnormalities, occurs almost exclusively with maternal varicella infection acquired before 20 weeks of gestation. Generally, after 20 weeks, manifestations include skin scars, as with postnatal VZV infection, and childhood shingles. Only rarely has this syndrome been reported after gestational zoster.

Subclinical maternal VZV infection is now recognized as a cause of neurologic symptoms and signs in children without other manifestations of congenital varicella syndrome, including dermatologic findings, suggesting the damage done by intrauterine varicella is underestimated. If the CNS is relatively spared, a good long-term outcome can occur.

Treponema pallidum

Most commonly, physicians are required to investigate the asymptomatic infant whose mother had positive serologic testing for syphilis. Among such infants, bone lesions are the most frequently encountered abnormality, occurring in 20% of infected cases. Cerebrospinal fluid examination is required for all infants with possible congenital syphilis and some experts believe that minimal abnormalities in the CSF should be considered to indicate neurosyphilis. These include leukocyte counts of $5/mm^3$ or more and protein concentration of 100 mg/dl or greater.

Toxoplasma gondii

The diversity of findings may be classified according to timing of symptomatology as:

- symptomatic neonatal disease;
- disease in the first months of life, usually with neurologic and ophthalmologic findings;
- sequela of previously undiagnosed infection (i.e. chorioretinitis later in childhood); and
- subclinical disease.

Severely affected children may present with the classic triad of hydrocephalus, intracranial calcifications and chorioretinitis. Of asymptomatic infected infants, half will have abnormalities on cranial imaging or on ophthalmologic examination. Among 23 000 mothers and infants in the Collaborative Perinatal Project, infants of IgG *T. gondii* antibody-positive mothers had a twofold increase in hearing loss, a 60% increase in the incidence of microcephaly and a 30% increase in the occurrence of low intelligence quotient (IQ <70).

Other

Intrauterine adenovirus infection has been associated with fetal myocarditis, pneumonia and encephalitis. Measles infection in pregnancy increases the risk of prematurity in the first 2 weeks after rash. Congenital West Nile virus infection has been associated with chorioretinitis and significant brain injury.[24]

DIAGNOSIS

Diagnosis of fetal infection

Attribution of adverse outcome to a particular micro-organism in early fetal life is problematic and frequently requires molecular diagnostic testing (e.g. DNA detection by PCR). Detection of micro-organism-specific IgM is hampered not only by the testing method but also by the failure of the fetus to reliably produce IgM-specific antibody before 22–24 weeks. Fetal infection may follow maternal infection by at least 4–6 weeks, providing false reassurance if fetal diagnosis, through direct detection or antibody production, is attempted too soon after maternal infection.

Antenatal diagnosis of fetal infection requires a multidisciplinary approach to exclude noninfectious causes and to obtain maternal–fetal studies. In the absence of fetal disease, prenatal diagnosis of fetal infection is not warranted because the predictive values of positive and negative results cannot be used as a basis for management decisions.[25] For example, in contrast to genetic diseases for which the outcome is reasonably certain, most infants with congenital CMV infection are asymptomatic and do not suffer sequelae. Follow-up of infants with suspected congenital infections over the ensuing months is needed to determine the presence, extent and damage, if any, resulting from the infection.[26]

Maternal testing

Many maternal infections are asymptomatic and all infections, symptomatic or otherwise, can pose a risk to the fetus. Laboratory tests are listed in Table 52.7. Routine broad screening of a single serum is unlikely to be helpful and is rarely indicated. The diagnosis of a primary CMV infection can be made by demonstration of seroconversion of CMV-specific IgG antibodies from negative to positive, but not by boosting of a titer, as this may occur with recurrent infection. Differentiation of the serofast state from inadequately treated syphilis can be difficult. A serofast patient usually has a titer of ≤1:4; although titers can be as high as 1:8,[27] caution in interpretation is essential.

Maternal symptoms and their likelihood

Although fetal disease follows both symptomatic and asymptomatic maternal infection and maternal infections are frequently asymptomatic, the following symptoms should suggest a search for micro-organisms: a flu- or acute mononucleosis syndrome-like illness (CMV, *T. gondii*, HIV) and arthritis or rash (parvovirus B19, rubella, *Treponema pallidum*). Maternal history relevant to congenital infections is summarized in Table 52.8.

Fetal testing

Detection of the micro-organism by culture or its DNA by PCR in amniotic fluid or fetal blood is promising, but should generally not be undertaken in the absence of fetal abnormalities because of the uncertain sensitivity and specificity. After 18 weeks of gestation, and at least 4 weeks after maternal infection, PCR testing of the amniotic fluid will detect 97% of *T. gondii*-infected fetuses.[28] Fetuses infected with CMV are likely to have positive amniotic fluid cultures after 20–22 weeks of gestation because fetal kidney infection is common.

Neonatal testing

In evaluating the neonate with suspected congenital infection at birth, it is necessary to:
* review the maternal history including serologic screening (Tables 52.7 and 52.8);
* review ultrasonography undertaken in pregnancy (Table 52.4);

Table 52.7 Laboratory evidence of clinically significant maternal infection

Micro-organism	Detection by culture, PCR (site)	Serology
CMV	Infrequently (blood/serum)	• Seroconversion • Possibly CMV IgM capture ELISA • Possibly IgG avidity testing to determine timing of infection
Enterovirus	Yes (stool, throat, other)	• Seroconversion
HSV	Yes (vesicle)	• Seroconversion • Research lab required to differentiate between HSV-1 and HSV-2
Parvovirus B19	Yes (blood)	• Seroconversion, • Parvovirus B19-specific IgM
Rubella	Infrequent (nasopharynx, urine)	• Seroconversion • Rubella-specific IgM
VZV	Yes (vesicle)	• Seroconversion
Treponema pallidum	Yes (lesion, wet field)	• VDRL/RPR ≥1:8 and positive treponemal test
Toxoplasma gondii		• Seroconversion • Toxoplasmosis-specific IgM with confirmatory testing in reference laboratory to determine timing of infection

Table 52.8 Maternal history relevant to congenital infections

Woman's history

Underlying illness and medications

Previous history of sexually transmitted disease (HSV, syphilis, chlamydia, gonorrhea, HIV)

Drug or alcohol use, current and previous

Travel during pregnancy (consider culinary practices and other factors in region traveled)

Occupation
- Working with children wearing diapers or who have disabilities (CMV)
- Working with elementary school children (parvovirus, rubella)
- Working with animals or raw meat products (*Toxoplasma gondii*)
- Working in the sex trade industry (HIV, syphilis, tuberculosis, hepatitis B virus, hepatitis C virus)

Household exposure to young children (CMV)

During her pregnancy
- Has she eaten raw meat or tasted it while cooking? (toxoplasmosis)
- Has she consumed unwashed vegetables? (food-borne pathogens, toxoplasmosis)
- Has she changed kitty litter without wearing gloves? (toxoplasmosis)
- Has she worked in soil/garden without wearing gloves? (toxoplasmosis)
- Has she had any illness she might not have mentioned until now?
- Cold sore? (HSV)
- Dysuria, burning, itching? (HSV)
- Profound fatigue? (CMV, toxoplasmosis, HIV)
- Swollen glands? (CMV, toxoplasmosis, HIV)
- Arthritis? (rubella, parvovirus B19)
- Rash? (rubella, parvovirus B19, syphilis, enterovirus)

Has her husband/partner had any particular illness?
- Skin sores anywhere? (HSV, syphilis, HIV)

Routine serologic testing

HBsAg, rubella-specific antibody, syphilis serology (treponemal and/or non-treponemal tests)
- First trimester
- If high risk, repeat third trimester, delivery

Antenatal care

- If absent, see Table 52.9

Table 52.9 Evaluation of neonate with suspected congenital infection

Clinical	Physical examination (gestational age, height, weight, head circumference) to identify prematurity, intrauterine growth retardation, microcephaly Measure liver/spleen size Ophthalmologic examination (by pediatric expert)
Laboratory	Complete blood count and smear Platelet count Liver transaminase levels Bilirubin level, direct and indirect CSF examination (cells, protein, with pertinent antibody detection; see Table 52.10) Laboratory testing (detection of agent, maternal and infant (not cord) serology) Immunoglobulin determinations Hold pretransfusion blood for possible additional tests
Other	Cranial CT scan with enhancement Long-bone radiographs (if syphilis or rubella likely) Placental pathology Audiology assessment Multidisciplinary follow-up

- submit maternal serology for documentation of a source of infection;
- detect the organism in the infant through culture (or molecular detection techniques);
- sequentially test the infant serologically; and
- appreciate the enormous rate of false-positive and false-negative test results obtained through IgM-specific testing and use of cord blood.

False-negative IgM tests in infants are very common (e.g. only 25% of infants with clinical manifestations of intrauterine infection had VZV IgM).[29] An exception is the rubella-specific IgM test, which is highly sensitive and specific. Parvovirus-specific IgM is frequently negative when virus is detected by PCR.

Serologic documentation of maternal infection and acute and follow-up serology of the infant over the first months or year of life can be diagnostic, albeit not sufficiently quickly to facilitate decisions about therapy. Passively transferred antibody will disappear during the first 6–12 months, whereas antibody persists or rises in the infected infant. Follow-up serology is more complicated in the case of congenital CMV as infection may also be acquired at birth or postnatally through breast milk or other contact.

Cord blood is not acceptable for specific antibody testing for syphilis, *T. gondii* or CMV because of false-positive and false-negative results. Total cord IgM levels may be falsely elevated through contamination by maternal blood. Cases of congenital syphilis have been reported in which both mothers' and neonates' titers were negative at birth but the infants subsequently developed clinical syphilis at 3–14 weeks of age with strongly positive titers.

The futility of a single serologic (syphilis, toxoplasmosis, other agents, rubella, CMV, herpesvirus (STORCH)) screen is well known and a more directed approach is required. Every effort should be made to recover the organism from the neonate and follow-up maternal and infant blood (Table 52.11).

Definitions of selected congenital infections

Because of delayed onset and/or recognition of signs of infection as well as the varied availability of diagnostic tests, definitions have been developed that take into consideration the likelihood of infection (Table 52.12).

- evaluate the infant clinically (Tables 52.6 and 52.9);
- attempt detection of the pathogen in the neonate; and
- undertake judicious maternal and infant serologic testing pertinent to the most likely diagnoses.

Detection of the micro-organism in the neonate

The best evidence for infection with CMV, enterovirus, HSV, parvovirus B19, rubella, syphilis, and *T. gondii* comes from detection of the agent in culture or by molecular detection techniques in the neonate (see below).

Maternal and infant testing pertinent to the most likely diagnoses

Diagnostic tests are summarized in Table 52.10. Over- and underdiagnosis of congenital infection has arisen as a result of failure to:

Table 52.10 Laboratory investigation and follow-up of neonate with suspected congenital infection

Infection	Mother at birth	Neonatal (not cord blood)	Follow-up of infant
CMV	Antibody	Virus detection in urine, saliva, blood leukocytes, CSF IgM capture enzyme-linked immunosorbent assay (ELISA) and radioimmunoassay antibody	Repeated antibody testing to 6–12 months; passive maternal antibody disappears at 4–9 months; negative infant and maternal antibody rules out infection, although intrapartum cervical and postpartum breast milk transmission is common
Enterovirus	Virus detection in stool, throat, blood, of mother of infant with suspected congenital enteroviral infection Bank serum	Virus detection in stool, throat, CSF, nose, blood, other Bank birth and 2nd serum at 2–4 weeks	Selective testing of paired infant and maternal sera appropriate to infant, maternal or community isolates
HSV	Antibody	Virus detection in skin vesicles, throat, CSF, urine, nose, conjunctiva, rectal swab Antibody	Repeated antibody testing to 6–12 months (cannot differentiate between type 1 and type 2 viruses) Negative infant and maternal antibody rules out infection
Parvovirus B19	IgM and IgG antibody Detection of DNA (e.g. by PCR) in blood	Detection of DNA (e.g. by PCR) in blood, bone marrow Parvovirus-specific IgM	Repeated antibody testing to 6–12 months Infected infants and their mothers may lack IgM antibody
Rubella	Rubella-specific IgG and IgM antibody	Rubella-specific IgM antibody Virus detection in urine, nasopharynx, CSF, blood CSF rubella-specific IgM antibody	Repeated antibody testing to 6–12 months Negative infant antibody at 6–12 months usually rules out infection
VZV	Antibody	Virus detection in skin lesions Antibody	Antibody testing 6–12 months postnatally Intrauterine infection commonly manifest only as persistent antibody and childhood zoster
Toxoplasma gondii	Toxoplasma-specific IgM and IgG antibody To determine acuity of infection in IgM-positive mother, need reference laboratory testing Seroconversion or fourfold rise in *Toxoplasma*-specific IgG in pregnancy	Reference laboratory testing of *Toxoplasma gondii* specific: IgM-ISAGA, DS-IgM-ELISA. IgE-ELISA, IgA-ELISA and virus detection by PCR in CSF (screening *Toxoplasma gondii*-IgM can be falsely positive and negative) Culture, PCR and histopathology of the placenta	Repeated antibody testing to 6–12 months Negative infant antibody at 6–12 months usually rules out congenital infection
Treponema pallidum	Nontreponemal antibody tests (quantitative): VDRL, RPR Treponemal antibody tests: EIA, TPPA, FTA, ABS If positive, maternal HIV status	Detection of treponemes in nasal secretions, skin lesions, etc. by darkfield examination Quantitative VDRL, RPR Serum treponemal antibody (e.g. EIA, TPPA, FTA, ABS)	Repeated quantitative VDRL/RPR and treponemal antibody testing to 12–15 months No test at birth can differentiate between the asymptomatic infected and uninfected neonate Passively transferred antibody disappears at 6 months (VDRL, RPR) and 12–15 months (treponemal tests)

Table 52.11 Appropriate specimens to diagnose congenital infection[20]

Specimen	Tests	Interpretation
Urine	Viral culture/detection (CMV, HSV, rubella)	Urine for CMV must be obtained at ≤2 weeks of age Positive is diagnostic
Throat swab	Viral culture (CMV, HSV, rubella, enteroviruses)	Positive is diagnostic
Blood	Agent detection (CMV, parvovirus B19)	Positive is diagnostic
Neonatal serum (single specimen)	Rubella-specific IgM	Positive is diagnostic although determination of status at 10–12 months is confirmatory

(Continued)

Table 52.11 Appropriate specimens to diagnose congenital infection[20]—cont'd

Specimen	Tests	Interpretation
Sequential neonatal, infant sera over 6–12 months	All	Passive maternal antibody in uninfected infant disappears at 4–9 months for CMV (unless peri-, postnatal transmission); 8 months for *Toxoplasma. gondii*; 6 months VDRL, rapid plasma reagin; 12–15 months treponemal Positive specific antibody at 8–12 months suggests congenital toxoplasmosis, parvovirus B19, rubella, VZV infection
Single maternal serum at delivery	*Toxoplasma gondii*-specific IgM	If IgM -specific antibody positive, reference laboratory testing of maternal, infant sera and placenta
Serology of both mother and infant	All	Negative maternal serology rules out source of infection Serial infant serology identifies passive maternal antibody (titers fall) and active infection (titers remain the same, rise over months)
CSF culture, detection	Detection CMV, enteroviruses, HSV, *Toxoplasma gondii* (reference laboratory), parvovirus B19 Rubella-specific IgM antibody VDRL/RPR and/or treponemal tests (non-bloody tap)	Positive is diagnostic
Skin lesions culture, detection	If active/vesiculated at birth: herpes, enteroviruses VZV Syphilis darkfield microscopy	Positive is diagnostic
Nasopharyngeal secretions	Syphilis darkfield microscopy	Positive is diagnostic
Stool cultures	Enteroviruses	Positive is diagnostic
Placenta	Variable	May be supportive of specific pathogen

Table 52.12 Definitions of selected congenital infections

CMV	Confirmed	Detection of CMV in the first 2–3 weeks of life in urine, throat or other sources in newborn with one or more of: • Small for gestational age • Hematologic findings (petechiae, purpura, splenomegaly, jaundice at birth) • Neurologic findings (microcephaly, chorioretinitis, neurologic abnormality, intracranial calcifications, hearing impairment) • Laboratory findings: direct hyperbilirubinemia >3 mg/dl, thrombocytopenia (platelet count <75 000/ml), liver function abnormality (alanine aminotransferase >100 mg/dl)
	Possible	As for Confirmed, except viral detection only after 3 weeks of age and other diseases ruled out
HSV	Congenital	Detection of HSV within 24 hours of birth or stable positive titer over 3 months in infants with one or more of: skin, eye and brain lesions
	Perinatal	Detection of HSV after 24 hours and in first 6 weeks of life further characterized by clinical and laboratory findings as one of: • Disseminated • CNS • Skin, eye, mouth disease (with negative CSF PCR)
Rubella	Confirmed	Defects of congenital rubella syndrome present and one more of: • Virus detected • Positive rubella-specific IgM antibody • Positive infant serology after disappearance of passively transferred maternal antibodies at 3–12 months
	Compatible	Insufficient laboratory data for confirmation of diagnosis but any two complications from (a) or one from (a) and one from (b): (a) Cataracts or congenital glaucoma, congenital heart disease, hearing loss, pigmentary retinopathy (b) Purpura, splenomegaly, jaundice, radiolucent bone disease, meningoencephalitis, microcephaly, mental retardation
	Possible	Presence of some compatible clinical findings, but insufficient criteria for either the Confirmed or Compatible categories

Table 52.12 Definitions of selected congenital infections—cont'd

Syphilis	Confirmed	Identification of *Treponema pallidum* in nasal or skin lesions
	Presumptive	One or more of:
		• Infant born to mother with untreated or inadequately treated syphilis
		• Treated with drug other than penicillin and/or
		• <30 days to 3 months before delivery
		• Infant has reactive treponemal test with findings of one or more of abnormal physical examination, long bone radiographs, CSF (including reactive CSF-VDRL and/or a leukocyte count of 20 ml or greater or a protein concentration of 100 mg/dl or greater), fourfold higher VDRL than mother has
		• Infant has documented fourfold rise in titers and positive treponemal test
		• Infant has reactive treponemal test that does not revert by 12–15 months
Toxoplasma gondii	Confirmed	• *Toxoplasma gondii*-specific IgM (or if available, Sabin–Feldman dye test >300 IU) in maternal sera with infant findings of chorioretinitis, cerebral calcifications or hydrocephalus in the absence of CMV infection
		• Positive antibody in infant at 8–10 months (after disappearance of passively transferred maternal antibody) with or without clinical findings
	Compatible	• Chorioretinitis with positive *Toxoplasma gondii*-specific antibody after 8–10 months of age
		• Cerebral calcifications and/or hydrocephalus with positive *Toxoplasma gondii*-specific antibody after 8–10 months of age in the absence of CMV infection
Parvovirus B19		Detection of parvovirus B19 by:
		• Direct electron microscopy or nucleic acid in blood and/or tissue obtained within the first 3 weeks of life in the presence of fetal or neonatal findings of hydrops and anemia
		• Parvovirus B19-specific IgM in the first 3 weeks or persistent IgG beyond 3–12 months with either documented maternal infection or fetal/neonatal findings of hydrops/anemia or cranial calcification
Varicella		One or more of:
		• Anomalies of congenital varicella syndrome (skin, eye, limb, neurologic)
		• Acute varicella at birth with viral detection
		• Herpes zoster in the first year of life with viral detection
		• VZV-specific IgM at birth, persistent IgG to 12 months or detection of specific lymphocyte transformation in response to VZV virus antigen

MANAGEMENT

General

A thorough understanding of the consequences of infection in pregnancy is required to counsel parents regarding risks to the fetus and possible courses of action. Selected maternal infections should be followed by ultrasonography to identify adverse effects. Antenatal diagnosis is generally attempted if fetal abnormalities are present. After delivery, additional information about contagiousness, breast-feeding and risk of transmission in subsequent pregnancies should be conveyed. Comprehensive long-term pediatric follow-up is required to identify and manage the spectrum of cognitive, motor, visual, hearing and other impairments that may be imparted by some of these infections.

Specific infections

Cytomegalovirus

The management of a pregnant woman with serologic evidence of acute CMV infection is difficult, in part because it is not possible to predict the outcome of the fetus; most infants born to such women are normal. Termination of pregnancy is certainly an option when significant abnormalities are detected on fetal ultrasound. The potential role of antenatal treatment of the mother with CMV-immune globulin[30] or valganciclovir[31] in preventing congenital CMV infection or disease is intriguing, but requires further study.[32]

Neurologic outcome cannot be reliably predicted until the infant is 2 or 3 years of age, during which head growth is monitored and achievement of developmental milestones is documented. Infants with abnormal cranial imaging are more likely to have cognitive and other deficits on follow-up.[33] Progression of existing retinal lesions or delayed development of chorioretinitis during childhood has been reported in about 20% of children, whereas hearing loss will evolve in about 30% of children, as late as school age. Children with asymptomatic congenital CMV infection show no differences in IQ score or other neuropsychologic test performance as compared with uninfected children.[34]

The benefit of and indications for antiviral therapy remain controversial. In a phase III randomly controlled trial, ganciclovir therapy (6 mg/kg/dose twice daily for 6 weeks), given to infants with evidence of CNS disease, chorioretinitis or hearing loss at baseline, protected infants from further hearing deterioration.[35] Transient effects on growth and resolution of transaminase elevation were also seen. Approximately two-thirds developed neutropenia, with half requiring dose reduction. The study has been criticized because less than 50% of subjects had evaluable data at baseline and at 6 months. The potential role of oral valganciclovir,[36] and prolonged therapy with ganciclovir or valganciclovir remain to be defined.[37]

Several studies have suggested a link between the development of sequelae, such as hearing loss, and viral burden, as measured by CMV antigenemia, quantitative PCR in blood and quantitative urine culture.[38,39] It is plausible that these measures of viral burden could be useful in selecting subjects for whom antiviral therapy is likely to be beneficial. Prevention through vaccination is urgently needed.

Herpes simplex virus

As intrauterine infection is rare, infected women should be assured that maternal infection is common but that fetal infection is unusual.

Parvovirus B19

After maternal exposure and documented infection, serial ultrasonography for 1–14 weeks will identify the hydropic fetus. For the fetus with nonimmune hydrops fetalis and a low hematocrit and reticulocyte count, one or more intravascular fetal transfusions of packed erythrocytes, until marrow aplasia resolves, have been used with good results. Hydropic fetuses with an intermediate hemoglobin and a high reticulocyte count, in whom the process is resolving spontaneously, need not be transfused and show no sequelae. There is no medical indication for termination of the pregnancy complicated by parvovirus B19 infection.

Rubella

Infected infants should be considered infectious for the first year of life unless repeated nasopharyngeal and urine cultures are negative. Long-term follow-up will identify progressive hearing loss and visual deterioration, endocrinopathies and subacute sclerosing panencephalitis.

Treponema pallidum

All infected women should receive penicillin therapy appropriate to their stage of disease to minimize or eliminate the risk of transmission to the fetus. If serology has been positive for less than 1 year, the patient may be treated with intramuscular benzathine penicillin G 2.4 million units as a single dose (some experts recommend two doses 1 week apart). If the patient has been seropositive for 1 year or more, benzathine penicillin G 2.4 million units in a single dose weekly for 3 successive weeks is required. Maternal CSF examination (protein, cell count, CSF-VDRL) is required only if neurosyphilis is suspected; it is not routinely required in patients with infectious syphilis if the neurologic examination is negative. Retreatment during pregnancy is unnecessary if titers followed monthly continue to fall. In the presence of penicillin allergy, desensitization is the preferred management; any other therapy will necessitate treatment of the infant after birth. All women with positive serology require HIV testing and testing of their recent sexual contacts, as well as repeat testing in the third trimester and at birth.

All infants born to seropositive mothers should be evaluated for possible congenital syphilis. Quantitative nontreponemal serology (rapid plasma reagin (RPR)/VDRL) should be done for all cases. Cord blood should not be used for RPR/VDRL testing as it may be falsely negative or positive.[40] The extent of investigation of the infant is dependent on the adequacy of and response to therapy in the mother, placental pathology and initial evaluation of the infant.[41] A full evaluation including complete blood count, treponemal and nontreponemal serology, long bone X-rays and CSF analysis (including nontreponemal titers in the CSF) is indicated for those deemed at risk.

The decision to treat an infant as possible congenital syphilis should follow a thorough evaluation of the maternal history, as well as the infant's clinical manifestations, laboratory results and radiographic findings.[41] Aqueous crystalline penicillin G 100 000–150 000 IU/kg (given every 8–12 hours) intravenously for 10–14 days is the recommended standard regimen.[41] After the second week of life, or with confirmed neurosyphilis or severe disease, aqueous penicillin 200 000–250 000 IU/kg per day may be used.[21] A preliminary study suggests that selected asymptomatic infants may be treated with intramuscular benzathine penicillin 50 000 IU/kg once, provided that there are no signs of congenital syphilis on physical examination, CSF cell count is normal and CSF-VDRL is negative, and radiographic studies of the long bones of the lower extremities, platelet counts and liver function tests are normal. Follow-up of all infants is required up to 1 year or beyond to ensure that the appropriate falls in titers have occurred and that treatment or retreatment is not required.

Toxoplasma gondii

If acutely infected women can be identified and treated in pregnancy through organization of a regional system of screening, there is evidence that the outcome is improved. Maternal spiramycin therapy may reduce the rate of transmission to the fetus and is recommended prior to 18 weeks' gestation. Once congenital infection is established, the combination of pyrimethamine and sulfadiazine is required to improve fetal outcome. The regimen currently recommended for treatment in North America is given in Table 52.13 (see also Practice Point 25).

The outcome of congenitally infected infants with treatment started at birth has been shown to be substantially better than that of historic controls not treated or treated for 1 month only.[42] Normal cognitive, neurologic and auditory outcome was observed in all children who did not have neurologic disease at birth. Furthermore, more than 70% of those with moderate or severe neurologic disease at birth had normal cognitive and/or neurologic outcome and none had sensorineural hearing loss. In contrast, when infants are not treated, late sequelae after subclinical disease include active chorioretinitis in 85%, including some cases of blindness or impaired vision, developmental delay in 20–75% and moderate hearing loss in 10–30%.

Perinatal infections

These occur as a result of ascending infection and premature rupture of the membranes or through intrapartum transmission. Their management and prevention are summarized in Table 52.14.

Specific infections

Enterovirus

Enteroviruses are among the commonest pathogens encountered by the newborn in the first months of life. The most common symptoms are undifferentiated fever and aseptic meningitis. A sepsis-like syndrome with or without myocarditis and hepatitis is occasionally seen; this is commonly associated with a nonspecific late-gestational febrile illness in the mother. Pleconaril is a potential therapeutic agent,[43] but is not currently available outside of the research setting. A randomized, double-blind, placebo-controlled clinical trial sponsored by the US National Institutes of Health evaluating pleconaril in enteroviral-associated neonatal sepsis syndrome is currently underway. Given the likelihood that an infected infant has received no passive maternal antibody, high-dose intravenous immune globulin may be reasonable in the acutely ill infant, although efficacy has not been demonstrated.

Herpes simplex virus

Because it is the primary infection, rather than recurrent infection in pregnancy, that is a risk to the fetus, transmission cannot be eliminated despite the best obstetric care. Primary infection is characterized by more prolonged shedding (mean of 11 days) and a 33% risk of transmission to the newborn if shedding occurs at delivery. Conversely, in recurrent infection, shedding lasts 2–4 days, and if present at birth, is associated with a 2% risk of transmission.

Neither a positive nor a negative clinical history will predict the neonatal risk for HSV infection. Of women with no previous history of genital HSV, 0.2% will have positive genital cultures at delivery.[44] Because viral shedding at the time of delivery cannot be predicted by third trimester cultures, screening is not recommended.

Women with recurrent disease should be reassured; the risk of neonatal infection in this situation is at most 1 in 2000 births. For women with first episode genital herpes during pregnancy or those with multiple recurrences, oral aciclovir or valaciclovir has been utilized to reduce the risk of active lesions at delivery and the need for Caesarian section.[45,46] Caesarian section is generally recommended for women with active lesions at birth or a clinical primary infection during pregnancy, particularly in the last half of gestation; infection may occur in spite of Caesarian section. Fetal scalp monitors should be

Table 52.13 Treatment of toxoplasmosis in the fetus and infant

Manifestation of disease	Medication	Dosage	Duration of therapy
In pregnant women with acute toxoplasmosis (first 21 weeks of gestation or until term if fetus not infected)	Spiramycin	1 g q8h without food	Until fetal infection documented or excluded at 21 weeks; if documented, in alternate months with pyrimethamine, leukovorin, and sulfadiazine until term (France)
If fetal infection confirmed after week 17 of gestation or if maternal infection acquired in last few weeks of gestation	Pyrimethamine and Sulfadiazine Leukovorin (folinic acid)	Loading dose: 100 mg/day in two divided doses for 2 days then 50 mg/day Loading dose: 75 mg/kg per day in two divided doses (maximum 4 g/day) for 2 days then 100 mg/kg per day in two divided doses (maximum 4 g/day) 10–20 mg/day	Until term (leukovorin is continued 1 week after pyrimethamine is discontinued)
Congenital *Toxoplasma gondii* infection in the infant	Pyrimethamine and Sulfadiazine and Leukovorin Corticosteroids (prednisolone) have been used when CSF protein is ≥1 g/dl and when active chorioretinitis threatens vision	Loading dose: 2 mg/kg per day for 2 days, then 1 mg/kg per day for 2–6 months, then this dose every Monday, Wednesday and Friday 100 mg/kg per day in two divided doses 10 mg 3 times a week 1 mg/kg per day in two divided doses	1 year 1 year 1 year Until resolution of elevated (≥1 g/dl) CSF protein level or active chorioretinitis that threatens vision

Adapted with permission from Hohlfeld et al[28] and Remington et al.[10]

Table 52.14 Preventive strategies and intrapartum management for selected perinatally acquired infections

Micro-organism	Clinical situation	Preventive management	Comment
Enterovirus	Active maternal enteroviral infection (i.e. fever, abdominal pain) at delivery	Attempt to defer delivery	May allow transmission of antibody
Hepatitis B virus	Maternal HBsAg status unknown	Neonatal passive plus active immunization	Many experts recommend universal neonatal immunization
HSV	Maternal lesions at delivery	Active observation of neonate for signs of infection	See detailed guidelines Caesarian section for active lesions or primary infection in (late) pregnancy
HIV-1	HIV-positive mother	Maternal antiretroviral therapy* Single or combination antiviral therapy of infant*	Antenatal delivery screening and therapy is recommended
Rubella	High risk, no antenatal care, no serology at delivery	Postpartum immunization of susceptible mother before hospital discharge	Failure to immunize prior to discharge has resulted in subsequent infected neonates
VZV	Maternal lesion within 1 week before or after delivery	Varicella-zoster immune globulin ± aciclovir therapy of neonate	Postpartum immunization of mothers known to be susceptible
Treponema pallidum	High risk, no antenatal care, no serology at delivery	Evaluation and possible therapy with follow-up of neonate	In high-risk women repeat screen in third trimester, delivery

*Potential interventions vary depending on the timing of diagnosis; intrapartum iv zidovudine with or without other antiretroviral agents should be given to the mother; the infant should receive zidovudine; the addition of other antiretroviral agents for the infant may be considered in selected cases.

avoided. Viral cultures should be obtained from the maternal cervix at birth. Infant cultures (i.e. urine, mouth, nasopharynx, stool/rectum) should be obtained at 24 hours and the child carefully observed for symptoms of neonatal HSV requiring therapy. Initial evaluation of all infants with suspected or confirmed HSV infection must include CSF PCR to detect subclinical CNS disease.

Neonatal HSV disease may manifest as disseminated disease, involving multiple organs, most notably the lungs and liver, localized CNS disease and isolated skin/mucosal disease. Skin lesions may be absent in disseminated and CNS disease. Aciclovir therapy for presumed or confirmed HSV infection is prescribed at a dose of 60 mg/kg per day intravenously q8h for 14–21 days.[47] For isolated skin and mucosal surface involvement, 14 days is sufficient, whereas 21 days of therapy is required with disseminated disease, encephalitis, or in the presence of an abnormal CSF profile. While mortality is certainly reduced with therapy, morbidity remains significant. Contact isolation of the infant with lesions is required.

Relapses of neonatal HSV infection with cutaneous and neurologic involvement have been reported, in some cases with the development of neurologic damage.[48] Long-term suppressive oral aciclovir has been suggested as a strategy to prevent such recurrences. In one small prospective study, 81% of infants on long-term suppressive aciclovir therapy had no recurrences, though 46% developed neutropenia.[49] Recurrent HSV encephalitis with aciclovir-resistant virus, while on suppressive acyclovir therapy, has recently been reported.[50]

Varicella-zoster virus

A neonate whose mother has developed varicella 5 days before delivery to 48 hours after delivery should receive a dose of 125 U (1.25 ml or 1 vial) of zoster immune globulin as soon as possible. These infants carry a 30% risk of infection without the protection of passive maternal antibody and a 30% mortality rate without antiviral therapy. Aciclovir at a dose of 1500 mg/m^2 per day is used to treat symptomatic neonates,[51] with dose adjustments for liver and renal failure or prematurity. Isolation of the exposed hospitalized infant is required.

HIV

In the absence of intervention the risk of mother-to-child transmission of HIV is approximately 40% (5% in utero, 20% intrapartum and 15% breast-feeding). Both early and late in-utero transmission can occur, though the latter is much more common. Fetal diagnostic testing may result in iatrogenic infection of the fetus and is contraindicated.

Prevention of mother-to-child transmission of HIV is achievable through antiretroviral therapy of the mother and infant and, where appropriate, elective Caesarian section (viral load >1000 copies/ml). Optimal preventive therapy consists of highly active antiretroviral therapy to the mother throughout the pregnancy or beginning in the second trimester, intrapartum intravenous zidovudine, and 6 weeks of oral zidovudine in the babies (see Chapter 98). In resource-poor settings, single dose nevirapine to mother and child and short course dual antiretroviral therapy have led to reductions in transmission of 50% or more. The potential for resistance development in women receiving single dose nevirapine is of concern. Elective Caesarian section can reduce the risk of transmission by half among women who received no antiretroviral therapy or zidovudine monotherapy.

Hepatitis B virus

In four studies of over 33 000 pregnant women in North America, a prevalence of HBsAg carriage of 0.8% was documented; 52% of women acknowledged no known risk factors. The risk of perinatal infection is greater if the maternal infection was acquired in the third trimester (80–90% vs <10% in the first trimester). If HBsAg positivity is accompanied by e-antigen positivity, the neonate is both more likely to become infected (70–90% vs 20–25%) and more likely to become a chronic carrier (85% vs 5%). The strongest predictor of transmission may be maternal hepatitis B virus DNA load.

Infants of carrier mothers should receive 0.5 ml hepatitis B immune globulin within 12 hours of birth and either 5 µg of the Merck hepatitis B vaccine (Recombivax HB) or 10 µg of the Smith Klein Beecham hepatitis B vaccine (Engerix-B). The second dose of vaccine is given at 1–2 months of age and the third dose at 6 months of age. Infants born to mothers of unknown status should receive the first dose of hepatitis B vaccine within 12 hours of birth and complete the vaccination series as indicated above. The need for and timing of hepatitis B immune globulin depends on availability of maternal HBsAg results and the infant's gestational age.[52]

Hepatitis C virus

The vertical transmission rate of hepatitis C virus (HCV) is between 2.4% and 11.9%. The risk of transmission is almost three times higher from women who are co-infected with HIV. Transmission from mothers who are HCV RNA negative is uncommon.[53] Confirmation of HCV infection in infancy requires the detection of HCV RNA after 1 month of age or the presence of HCV antibodies after 18 months of age.[54] Among vertically infected infants followed for 10–15 years, 20% clear the infection, 50% have chronic asymptomatic infection and 30% have chronic active infection.[55]

Group B streptococcus

Of the 10–35% of women asymptomatically carrying group B streptococcus (GBS), 50% of their infants will be colonized on their skin and mucous membranes. Of those colonized, 1–2% will develop early-onset disease. Two alternative approaches (i.e. screening, risk factor identification) to the prevention of group B streptococcal disease have been developed in the USA with a 70% reduction in the incidence of early-onset disease.[56] According to the more effective screening-based approach, all pregnant women should be screened at 35–37 weeks' gestation for anogenital group B streptococcus colonization. Intrapartum antibiotics are offered to all culture-positive women, regardless of risk factors. If the results of cultures are not known at the time of labor, intrapartum antibiotics are used in the presence of prematurity (<37 weeks' gestation), prolonged rupture of membranes (≥18 hours) or intrapartum fever (≥100.4°F/38°C). Also, women with a previously infected infant and women with group B streptococcus bacteriuria during the current pregnancy or a history of postpartum GBS sepsis are treated with intrapartum antibiotics (see Practice Point 26). In geographic regions with differing epidemiologic data, this approach may not be appropriate.

Absence of antenatal care

For women in whom there has been inadequate antenatal care, detection of infection is required at delivery as summarized in Table 52.15.

Table 52.15 Evaluation of women presenting in labor with limited or no antenatal care

Mother	• Genital examination for findings suggestive of sexually transmitted disease • Cultures for *Chlamydia trachomatis*, *Neisseria gonorrhoeae* • Serologic testing for HBsAg,* hepatitis C virus, HIV,* syphilis (treponemal and nontreponemal testing) • Adequate follow-up
Infant	• Prophylactic eye care • Serologic testing for HBsAg, hepatitis C virus, HIV, syphilis (treponemal and nontreponemal testing) • First dose of hepatitis B vaccine • Adequate follow-up

*HBsAg and HIV serology should be done stat in order to allow for prompt initiation of preventive interventions if the mother tests positive.

Breast-feeding

Contraindications and precautions with breast-feeding

In North America and other developed countries breast-feeding is contraindicated if the mother is infected with HIV, human T-cell lymphotropic virus 1 (HTLV-1) or HTLV-2.[57] In resource-poor settings, the potential benefits and harms associated with breast-feeding versus formula feeding need to be carefully weighed. Breast-feeding is not contraindicated with hepatitis B or hepatitis C infection.

Viral contamination of milk with rubella, HSV and CMV has also been reported, but serious sequelae have not generally occurred. CMV acquired through breast milk can pose a risk to extremely premature infants. In this setting, the potential benefits and risk of breast-feeding need to be considered. Mothers with herpetic lesions on their breasts should refrain from breast-feeding from the affected side(s). They should cover active lesions and wash their hands before breast-feeding.

Contaminated milk has been implicated in neonatal infection with *Staphylococcus aureus*, group B streptococcus, *Mycobacterium* spp. and possibly *Salmonella* spp. In mothers who have active pulmonary tuberculosis, contact with the infant must be avoided until the mother has received adequate antituberculous therapy and is considered noninfectious. In the setting of mastitis, breast feeding can usually be continued; in the presence of a breast abscess or frank pus, temporary discontinuation of breast-feeding on the affected side is warranted.[57]

Breast-feeding and drug therapy

The American Academy of Pediatrics recommends that breast-feeding be discontinued while a nursing mother is being treated with metronidazole, and warns about the use of nitrofurantoin and sulfa drugs, which can cause hemolysis in glucose-6-phosphatase-deficient infants.[58] Although it would be unusual for an effective maternal medication to be contraindicated because of risks to the infant through breast milk, physicians should be aware of information specific to agents being used. Frequent feeding exposes the infant to more drug than feeding at 4-hour intervals. Mothers can be encouraged to avoid frequent feedings to reduce drug exposure and the consequent changes in the infant's gastrointestinal flora and risk of oropharyngeal candidiasis.

REFERENCES

References for this chapter can be found online at http://www.expertconsult.com

Management of an HIV-positive pregnant woman who has a positive VDRL test from an area endemic for *Treponema* infection

INTRODUCTION

The dual epidemics of venereal syphilis (*Treponema pallidum* subsp. *pallidum*) and HIV are responsible for increasing tolls of morbidity and mortality among pregnant women and their offspring. Syphilis and HIV infection are closely interrelated. As sexually transmitted diseases, each poses a risk for the other, and there is now substantial evidence that genital ulcerative diseases, including syphilitic chancres, facilitate the bidirectional transmission of HIV-1. Although a simple screening test for syphilis and effective antibiotics are available, the disease remains uncontrolled in resource-scarce regions where antenatal testing and treatment are not always accessible. Moreover, in many of these countries, the endemic (i.e. nonvenereal) treponematoses yaws, endemic syphilis and pinta, caused by *T. pallidum* subsp. *pertenue*, *T. pallidum* subsp. *endemicum* and *T. carateum*, respectively, have not only not been eliminated but are also resurging in some places because of the breakdown of once successful control programs.

In the pregnant female, regardless of HIV-infection status, untreated syphilis poses a grave risk to the fetus or neonate on top of whatever morbidity, acute or chronic, it may inflict upon the mother. The possibility of infection with a nonvenereal treponematosis in such individuals poses a further diagnostic challenge inasmuch as it is impossible to distinguish these infections from venereal syphilis using currently available serologic tests. Health-care professionals managing patients residing in or emigrating from areas endemic for the nonvenereal treponematoses need to be aware of the clinical and epidemiologic features that distinguish these diseases from venereal syphilis. They also need to know how HIV co-infection may influence the management and outcome of syphilis in pregnant women and their offspring (Table PP23.1).

CLINICAL FEATURES

A detailed discussion of the clinical features of the treponematoses is beyond the scope of this commentary (see Chapters 57, 104 and 171); the salient clinical features of these diseases, however, are summarized in Table PP23.1.

Treponema pallidum infections are divided into early (i.e. primary, secondary and early latent) and late (i.e. late latent and tertiary) stages. Early lesions, as well as blood and exudative body fluids, are infectious. Primary lesions of venereal syphilis (chancres) occur usually in the anogenital area of sexually active individuals; a substantially greater proportion of heterosexual men present with genital ulcers than women and gay men. By contrast, acquisition of nonvenereal treponematoses occurs earlier in life, usually in childhood, with pri-

mary lesions often occurring on an extremity. Although anecdotal reports indicate that syphilis manifestations in HIV-infected patients may be florid and/or predispose to central nervous system complications, the manifestations of syphilis in most HIV-infected patients appear to be essentially the same as in HIV-uninfected patients.

No studies are available on the impact of HIV infection on the course or severity of the nonvenereal treponematoses. With both venereal and nonvenereal treponematoses, mucocutaneous lesions are the most common form of secondary disease; extracutaneous manifestations, occasionally severe, can occur in secondary syphilis (nonvenereal as well as venereal) and yaws. The gummatous lesions of late yaws can be extremely destructive. Venereal syphilis is the only treponematosis that involves the central nervous system or that causes congenital infection.

SERODIAGNOSTIC TESTS

Visualization of spirochetes in lesion exudate by darkfield examination is the definitive method for diagnosing primary treponemal infection. A presumptive diagnosis is possible with the use of non-treponemal and treponemal serologic tests. The nontreponemal tests (NTTs), represented by the VDRL test and the rapid plasma reagin (RPR) test, detect antibodies to a defined mixture of cardiolipin, lecithin and cholesterol. These tests have traditionally been designated as 'nontreponemal' based upon the belief that lipoidal antigens of host origin induce the antibodies being detected. Nontreponemal tests are used to screen for syphilis because they are easy to perform and have reasonably high sensitivity. Because they are titratable and usually decline in parallel with disease activity, they are also used to monitor the response to therapy. Falsely reactive NTTs are usually of low titer (<1:8) and may occur in a variety of conditions (see Chapter 57). Although pregnancy is a recognized cause of a falsely reactive NTT, one must exercise great caution in labeling a reactive NTT in a pregnant patient as a false-positive result.

The second type of serodiagnostic test, represented by the fluorescent treponemal antibody-absorption test (FTA-ABS), the *T. pallidum* hemagglutination assay (TPHA) and the *T. pallidum* particle agglutination assay (TPPA), detects antibodies directed against *T. pallidum* antigens and hence is designated as 'treponemal'. Treponemal tests are used to confirm that reactivity in a NTT is indeed due to syphilitic infection. Because they are more difficult and expensive to perform than NTTs, treponemal tests may not always be available in underdeveloped countries. In resource-scarce settings, traditional treponemal tests have been replaced by rapid treponemal tests which detect by immunochromatography serum antibodies specific for a variety of recombinant treponemal antigens (e.g. Determine Syphilis Tp test). These tests require only a drop of blood obtained by finger stick, can

Table PP23.1 Overview of treponemal infections

Disease	Organism	Endemic areas	Primary lesion	Secondary lesions	Tertiary lesions	Congenital infection
Venereal syphilis	*Treponema pallidum* subsp. *pallidum*	Worldwide	Chancre, usually in anogenital region	Mucocutaneous lesions (condyloma lata, papules, macules or maculopapules) Visceral involvement Central nervous system (CNS) involvement (usually aseptic meningitis)	Gummas, including CNS Carditis/aortitis Neurosyphilis (meningovascular, tabes, paresis)	Yes
Yaws	*Treponema pallidum* subsp. *pertenue*	Rural areas of Africa, Central and South America, the Caribbean, equatorial islands of South East Asia and remote parts of India and Thailand	Papule Papilloma Ulcer, usually on an extremity	Diffuse papules, papillomas and ulcers Osteitis Dactylitis	Destructive gummas of skin and bone	No
Pinta	*Treponema carateum*	Underdeveloped rural areas of Mexico and northern South America	Erythematous papule, usually on an extremity	Scaly papules Areas of altered skin pigmentation	Areas of altered skin pigmentation Hyperkeratosis	No
Endemic bejel	*Treponema pallidum* subsp. *endemicum*	West Africa, small foci in Zimbabwe, Botswana, Arabian peninsula and central Australia	Oral mucosal ulcer	Oral and pharyngeal ulcers Mucous patches Condyloma lata Periostitis	Gummas of skin, bone and joints	No

be performed with minimal training and do not require expensive equipment or refrigeration. Rapid treponemal tests have been shown to have a high sensitivity (85–90%) and specificity (92–98%) when compared to the traditional treponemal tests. However, rapid tests have not been studied in the context of nonvenereal treponematoses. Molecularly based efforts to design serodiagnostic tests capable of distinguishing venereal syphilis from the nonvenereal treponematoses, principally yaws, have thus far been unsuccessful. It is hoped that the availability of the genomic sequence for *T. pallidum* and, eventually, those of other pathogenic treponemes may enable investigators to identify polymorphisms that can be exploited for developing disease-specific serodiagnostic or polymerase chain reaction (PCR)-based tests.

Both treponemal and nontreponemal serologic tests are generally reliable for the diagnosis and management of syphilis in patients co-infected with HIV. However, HIV-infected syphilis patients may on occasion show higher than expected NTT titers, false-negative treponemal or nontreponemal tests, or delayed seroreactivity. When serologic tests and clinical syndromes suggestive of early syphilis do not correspond, alternative tests such as biopsy of suspicious lesions should be performed. When available, lesions can also be analyzed by PCR for the presence of *T. pallidum* DNA. As with serologic tests, the PCR tests in widespread usage cannot distinguish between the pathogenic treponemes.

SYPHILIS TESTING DURING PREGNANCY

It is estimated that, of all pregnant women who have untreated syphilis, only 20% will both carry the fetus to term and deliver a normal child. Complications include stillbirth (30%), neonatal death (10%) and mental handicap (40%). Because of the seriousness of these complications, pregnant women should be screened serologically for

syphilis early in pregnancy. For communities and populations in which the prevalence of syphilis is high or for patients at high risk, serologic testing should be performed twice during the first trimester, at 28 weeks gestation and at delivery. Rapid tests are less useful in areas with high prevalence, since a high proportion of pregnant women could have antibodies as a result of past, treated infection. Nevertheless, pregnant women who are seropositive but who lack clinical manifestations should be considered to be infected unless an adequate treatment history is clearly documented and sequential serologic, nontreponemal (e.g. RPR) antibody titers have declined appropriately. Given the inability of serodiagnostic tests to distinguish between venereal and nonvenereal treponematoses, syphilis should be the presumed diagnosis in asymptomatic, seropositive patients unless a diagnosis of nonvenereal treponematosis can be established unequivocally (see Table PP23.1).

TREATMENT

Penicillin is the antimicrobial of choice in the treatment of syphilis during pregnancy (Table PP23.2). Treatment during pregnancy should consist of the penicillin regimen appropriate for the stage of syphilis. Some specialists recommend a second dose of benzathine penicillin 2.4 million units intramuscularly, 1 week after the initial dose. The present consensus is that alternative regimens are potentially too harmful to the fetus (e.g. tetracycline), lack efficacy because of the inability of the drug to cross the placenta (e.g. erythromycin), have documented evidence of antimicrobial resistance (e.g. azithromycin) or are insufficiently studied (e.g. ceftriaxone). The current Centers for Disease Control and Prevention guidelines remind the practitioner of the importance of evaluating the HIV-infected patient both clinically and serologically for treatment

Table PP23.2 Treatment of syphilis during pregnancy in HIV-infected women

Primary or secondary syphilis	Benzathine penicillin G 2.4 million units im (single dose)
Early latent syphilis	Benzathine penicillin G 2.4 million units im (single dose)
Late latent syphilis or latent syphilis of unknown duration	Benzathine penicillin G 7.2 million units in three doses each of 2.4 million units im at 1-week intervals
Tertiary syphilis	Benzathine penicillin G 7.2 million units in three doses each of 2.4 million units im at 1-week intervals
Neurosyphilis	Aqueous crystalline penicillin G 18–25 million units q24h administered as 3–4 million units iv q4h for 10–14 days

failure. This is accomplished by blood draws at 3, 6, 9, 12 and 24 months after the course of therapy has been completed. The guidelines go on to suggest considering cerebrospinal fluid examination approximately 6 months after treatment, emphasizing that this is of unproven benefit. The treatment regimens for nonvenereal treponematoses are the same as those used for the comparable stage of venereal syphilis.

Because penicillin is clearly the preferred treatment, penicillin skin testing is recommended for reportedly penicillin-allergic pregnant women who have syphilis. If the penicillin allergy is confirmed, desensitization can be accomplished using incremental doses of oral penicillin V over 4–6 hours. A Jarisch–Herxheimer reaction, which presents with fever, headache and myalgia, can occur within hours of initiation of penicillin therapy in early syphilis. Women treated for syphilis during the second half of pregnancy may also experience self-limiting uterine contractions, decreased fetal activity and fetal heart rate abnormalities after penicillin treatment, but premature labor or fetal distress is rare. Women should be warned of the symptoms of the Jarisch–Herxheimer reaction and be instructed to use acetaminophen (paracetamol) to control these symptoms and to self-monitor uterine and fetal activity during the first 48 hours after penicillin therapy. In the second half of pregnancy, management and counseling may be facilitated by a fetal ultrasound but this should not delay therapy. Ultrasound signs of fetal syphilis (hepatomegaly, hydrops fetalis) indicate a greater risk to fetal health; such cases should be managed in consultation with specialists in high-risk obstetrics.

FURTHER READING

Further reading for this chapter can be found online at http://www.expertconsult.com

Theodore Jones
William R Bowie

Practice point | **24** |

Treatment of a positive *Toxoplasma* titer in pregnancy

INTRODUCTION

Clinically recognized toxoplasmosis is infrequent, but serologic evidence of toxoplasmosis is common. In immunologically competent people, even symptomatic toxoplasmosis is usually of minimal clinical significance. This is not the case in pregnancy. When symptomatic or asymptomatic infection is acquired just before or during pregnancy, *Toxoplasma gondii* readily crosses the placenta to infect the fetus, often with immense clinical and financial implications. The number of individuals in this country infected with *Toxoplasma gondii* is nearly one in four. In fact, nearly 85% of women of child-bearing age have not been exposed to the organism in the past. It is estimated that in North America, approximately one pregnancy in 1000 is affected, with higher rates reported in Europe. Although definitive proof is lacking, because early treatment of the mother has been thought to decrease the risk of infection of the fetus and diminish the sequelae in infected fetuses, appropriate management of the mother is essential.

Since the majority of infected women are either asymptomatic or have nonspecific and transient symptoms, the diagnosis is rarely made clinically. Rather, the health-care provider and the woman are typically faced with a positive serologic test without clear information on when the infection was acquired. 'Positive' serology with routine tests does not reliably determine the acuteness of infection, which is what determines management. An inappropriate response may result in unwarranted psychologic distress, unnecessary evaluations and treatments, and even unnecessary termination of pregnancy. In the USA, a recent study of obstetricians and gynecologists revealed that few were aware that 'positive' IgM antibody did not necessarily indicate acute infection, or that the US Food and Drug Administration had sent out an advisory about this problem with serologic tests for toxoplasmosis.

PATHOGENESIS

The definitive hosts of *T. gondii* are felines, and people are infected by direct or indirect contact with oocysts excreted by cats. Oocysts, spread for example in cat litter or soil or sand contaminated by cat feces, are highly infective. When ingested by animals or humans, they ultimately result in cysts in tissues. These also infect humans when uncooked or inadequately cooked meat containing viable cysts are ingested. Rarely, humans can also be infected by blood transfusions (see Chapters 52 and 183).

During acute infection of humans, toxoplasmosis is disseminated widely. Infection acquired immediately before conception or during pregnancy carries with it the risk of spread to the fetus. Though the risk of transmission in the first trimester (10–15%) is the lowest, its impact on the fetus is greatest, resulting in severe sequelae or death. Infection in the second trimester has been associated with a 25–40% transmission and has been found to have nonfatal effects in most circumstances. The highest proportion of fetuses infected occurs in the third trimester (>60% transmission). However, nearly all affected fetuses have mild or asymptomatic manifestations.

The classic triad of clinical features in severely infected infants who survive includes hydrocephalus, intracranial calcifications and chorioretinitis. Asymptomatically infected infants are typically not recognized at birth, but many, if not most, are thought to be at risk of subsequently developing chorioretinitis, hearing loss or subtle neurologic manifestations.

The economic impact of congenital toxoplasmosis is substantial, and screening programs to detect infection in pregnancy or at birth have been considered. In the USA, routine screening for toxoplasmosis in pregnancy is rarely recommended, but in some other countries screening is repeated serially in pregnancy, particularly in France.

INVESTIGATION

The focus of this Practice Point is on immunocompetent pregnant women who have had a 'positive' test for antibody to *T. gondii*. This will usually have been performed as a screening test rather than a diagnostic one. Depending on the laboratory, this will be either a positive IgG titer, or possibly a positive titer for both IgG and IgM. Evaluation for falling or rising titers is standard, but unless timing is fortuitous, stable titers are usually found rather than a definitive change.

Difficulties in interpretation of serologic results

There are several substantial problems in the interpretation of results.

- First, there are problems with sensitivity and, more frequently, specificity of many of the commercially available tests.
- Second, potential markers for acute infection, such as IgM and IgA, may persist long after the risk of transmission to the fetus ends. This may diminish the ability of IgM and IgA results that may be true positives to establish acuteness of infection. For this reason, when the IgM is reported as being 'positive', the possibilities are that it can be a false-positive (with the rate of false-positives dependent on the test and the laboratory), a true-positive indicative of recent infection or a true positive but simply reflecting persistence of IgM antibody.
- Third, the history and physical examination rarely adds to the clinician's ability to determine the acuteness of infection.

Negative anti-*Toxoplasma gondii* IgG and IgM

Unless it is very early in infection, negative anti-*Toxoplasma gondii* IgG and IgM indicate absence of previous infection. Women with such results are susceptible to infection. Primary prevention messages should be strongly reinforced. Subsequent repeat testing is required if one wishes to exclude infection later on in the pregnancy.

IgG titer only available, and is positive

An IgM test should be requested on the same or a new serum specimen because a single positive IgG titer provides no information about acuteness of infection. The presence of IgG antibody with a negative IgM antibody excludes recent infection. If performed early in pregnancy, no further investigation is required for toxoplasmosis. If performed late in pregnancy, there is an outside possibility that acute infection may have arisen earlier in pregnancy, with subsequent disappearance of IgM. Because of long-term persistence of IgM this is unlikely, but if there is any clinical concern of toxoplasmosis then the infant should be screened at birth.

Initial negative IgG titer with positive or equivocal IgM titer

When the IgG titer is negative, it is highly likely that the IgM titer is falsely positive. However, because the woman could be in the process of seroconverting, testing should be repeated in parallel on a second sample that is collected approximately 3 weeks after the first. If the IgG titer remains negative, then the result is probably falsely positive. Unless there are other features suggesting active infection, no further investigation is needed. Recent acquisition of infection is strongly suggested if the IgG titer becomes positive or there is a significant increase in the IgM titer.

Initial or subsequent positive IgG titer, and IgM titer is positive

Unless there is seroconversion or a significant increase in titers, interpretation at this stage is much more difficult because this information by itself does not establish acuteness of infection. Though IgM antibody levels rise within days of the infection and remain present – in general, for 2–3 weeks – it has been reported to persist for as long as 2–3 years in as many as 27% of women when immunosorbent agglutination assays are used. Often, this will confound additional efforts at clinical assessment with serology and other studies in the mother and potentially in the fetus.

History and examination of the mother

Although symptoms are usually absent or so nonspecific in over 90% of women with primary toxoplasmosis infection in pregnancy, a careful history and examination might detect symptoms that provide a clue to the onset of the disease. Most helpful would be development of lymphadenopathy, typically involving one node or a few nodes. A physical examination should be performed, looking in particular for abnormal lymphadenopathy and ocular disease.

Serologic studies in the mother

Pregnant women are often screened for a variety of processes (e.g. rubella, HIV), and this serum might have been stored. If available, prior stored serum should be tested for antibody to *T. gondii*. The results may be very helpful in determining the chronicity of infection.

Additional testing is required on available or newly acquired serum. If repeat testing on specimens run in parallel (i.e. testing is performed on all specimens at the same time) shows or has shown seroconversion or a fourfold or greater rise, then infection is acute. Usually titers are stable, and further testing is required in specialized or reference laboratories. A battery of tests is usually performed to assess acuteness of infection. Results should be interpreted in consultation with the reference laboratory. The two tests most often employed to assess acuteness of infection are IgG avidity and differential agglutination testing, but numerous other tests may be used by reference laboratories. If these additional results are consistent with acute infection or if they do not exclude acute infection, the woman should be managed as below.

MANAGEMENT

Studies diagnostic of or consistent with acute infection in pregnancy or immediately before conception

Management is in part determined by the time when infection was acquired. If results are consistent with infection immediately before or just after conception, the risk of delivering an infected baby is low. Either the fetus is not infected or if the fetus is infected it is likely to abort. When infection occurs later, the risk of having a viable but affected infant is much greater.

The mother should immediately be started on treatment (see below) for the duration of pregnancy and the fetus should be assessed by ultrasound. Amniocentesis for polymerase chain reaction (PCR) should be strongly considered.

Fetal ultrasound may show features consistent with infection, especially increased size of the ventricles. Negative studies do not exclude fetal involvement and studies may need to be performed serially.

With or without fetal abnormalities, amniocentesis should be considered at 18 weeks or later. If performed, as a minimum the amniotic fluid should be tested by PCR. Reference laboratories may do additional testing on amniotic fluid, such as mouse or cell culture inoculation. Although PCR can be falsely positive or falsely negative, if it is positive treatment of the mother should be switched to pyrimethamine and sulfadiazine.

Some authorities also sample fetal blood to detect the parasite or a fetal immunologic response, but PCR on amniotic fluid is probably safer.

Treatment of the mother

Initial treatment is with spiramycin 1 g orally every 8 hours. Spiramycin reduces the incidence and severity of fetal infection; however, when the fetus is known to be infected, pyrimethamine and sulfonamides are more active than spiramycin. Hence, ultrasound or amniotic fluid findings suggestive of fetal involvement should prompt a change of treatment to pyrimethamine and a sulfonamide. A variety of dosage regimens have been used, but currently suggested is pyrimethamine 25 mg/day and sulfadiazine 2 g orally every 12 hours, with supplemental folinic acid 5 mg/day. When treatment of the mother is initiated, it should be continued for the duration of the pregnancy.

The reader is cautioned to consider the fact that, while treatment of the woman with primary toxoplasmosis is suggested by most references, the effectiveness of prenatal treatment is not clear. Conflicting results have been noted in controlled and uncontrolled cohort studies: controlled studies failed to demonstrate benefit in treated women compared to untreated women, while several uncontrolled studies found a higher risk for congenital toxoplasmosis in untreated neonates. A recent systematic review further demonstrated the problem, with five studies demonstrating benefit while four failed in this regard.

Spiramycin is a macrolide with possible adverse reactions including nausea, vomiting, anorexia and diarrhea. Sulfadiazine has typical adverse reactions associated with sulfonamides, including concerns of kernicterus. The major adverse reaction to pyrimethamine is dose-related bone marrow suppression. To assess hematologic abnormalities, testing is recommended at least once weekly to detect anemia, leukopenia and thrombocytopenia.

Although other drugs have been used to treat toxoplasmosis, there is minimal experience with them in the context of pregnancy and fetal infection.

Termination of pregnancy

Many women with 'positive' serology for toxoplasmosis have had inappropriate termination of pregnancy. Positive IgG and IgM serology is not of itself an indication for termination. Most of these women will not have infected fetuses, but even if the fetus is infected, with appropriate long-term treatment the infants often do well. Termination should only be considered when there is documented evidence of fetal involvement, especially if infection was acquired early in the first trimester. However, even most of these infants who survive have done well with treatment of the mother followed by treatment of the infant.

Initial management of the infant at birth

If there is any question about the possibility of fetal acquisition of toxoplasmosis, the infant should be evaluated, including by one or a series of serologic tests. If clinical, serologic or other testing suggests congenital toxoplasmosis, the infant should be treated for 1 year. On this treatment, even infants who have clinically apparent manifestations such as intracranial calcifications, meningitis or chorioretinitis are highly likely to have a favorable outcome.

HIV infection and toxoplasmosis in pregnancy

In contrast to immunocompetent women, women who have HIV infection whose antibody to *T. gondii* is IgG positive and IgM negative are at risk of transmitting HIV to the fetus. Appropriate management is unclear. Important variables probably include the degree of immunosuppression, concurrent *Pneumocystis jirovecii* prophylaxis with trimethoprim–sulfamethoxazole (co-trimoxazole), *Mycobacterium avium-intracellulare* treatment or prophylaxis with macrolides, *T. gondii* treatment or suppression, and infection acquired in pregnancy. Acute infection with *T. gondii* in pregnancy should be managed aggressively, probably with pyrimethamine and sulfadiazine, whether or not there is objective evidence of fetal involvement (see Chapter 91).

Other considerations

Pregnant women who have possible or proven toxoplasmosis are likely to feel guilty that they did something that put their fetus at risk. It is prudent for women who are or might be pregnant to avoid direct or indirect contact with cats or raw or inadequately cooked meat. However, most people with toxoplasmosis are totally unaware of when or how they became infected. Care should be taken to avoid adding guilt to the stress that women who have 'positive' serology undergo.

FURTHER READING

Further reading for this chapter can be found online at http://www.expertconsult.com

A pregnant patient with a previous pregnancy complicated by group B streptococcal disease in the infant

INTRODUCTION

The group B streptococcus (GBS, *Streptococcus agalactiae*) is recognized as an important cause of invasive disease in neonates and pregnant women. Among neonates, premature infants are at the greatest risk of adverse outcomes from GBS infection. These premature infants account for 25% of cases of GBS disease among neonates. The disease manifests itself as an early-onset form (<7 days after birth), a late-onset form (7 days to 3 months after birth) and a very late form (>3 months after birth). Disease among infants usually presents as bacteremia, pneumonia and meningitis. However, they may experience other syndromes, including soft tissue and bone infection. Initial reports of GBS disease in the 1970s indicated mortality rates as high as 50%. Current mortality rates are less than 5%, largely due to advances that have evolved in neonatal care since the 1990s.

EPIDEMIOLOGY

The organism colonizes the gastrointestinal tract of humans, with the genitourinary tract being the most common site for secondary spread. Colonization rates vary widely among different ethnic groups, geographic areas and age groups. These rates generally indicate that 10–30% of pregnant women have vaginal or rectal colonization with GBS. Data from the USA have suggested that prior to the implementation of recommendations for the prevention of early-onset GBS using maternal intrapartum antimicrobial prophylaxis (IAP), the incidence of GBS neonatal disease was 1–4 cases per 1000 live births. Among these cases, early-onset disease occurred in approximately 1 infant per 100–200 colonized women and was responsible for 75% of cases among infants. Since the widespread use of IAP, the incidence of early-onset GBS disease has decreased significantly (by approximately 80%), resulting in an incidence rate of less than 1 case per 1000 live births.

The incidence of early-onset disease is higher in babies born to women less than 20 years of age and in those who are of black race in the USA. Intrapartum risk factors include premature onset of labor (<37 weeks gestation), prolonged rupture of membranes (>18 hours) and intrapartum fever (>100.4°F/>38°C). Additional risk factors include heavy vaginal colonization with GBS, previous delivery of an infant who had GBS disease and the presence of low maternal levels of anti-GBS capsular antibody. Women who have GBS bacteriuria are at an increased risk of delivering an infected baby with early-onset disease. This is related in part to the fact that women who have GBS bacteriuria are usually heavily colonized with GBS. Bacteriuria caused by GBS is associated with an increased risk of preterm labor.

MICROBIOLOGY

Group B streptococci are represented by several serotypes, including Ia, Ib and II–VIII. While all serotypes may cause disease in humans, serotype III is the main cause of early-onset meningitis as well as of late-onset GBS disease among neonates.

In the determination of the GBS carrier status of a pregnant woman, culture techniques that maximize the recovery of GBS are essential. The optimal method for GBS screening involves collection of a single vaginal–anorectal swab or two separate swabs from the vagina and rectum. These swabs may be taken by the health-care provider of the patient with appropriate instructions. Swabs should be placed in a transport medium if the bacteriology laboratory is off-site and subcultured onto selective broth medium. After overnight incubation, the specimen is subcultured onto solid blood agar. Slide agglutination tests or other tests used to detect GBS antigen may be used to enable specific identification of GBS.

PREVENTION

Vaccination as a GBS disease-preventive strategy is currently the subject of research. Chemoprophylaxis has become established as a useful preventive strategy. Given that the majority of newborns who have GBS disease acquire infection in utero, the administration of antibiotics to neonates (postnatal prophylaxis) will not prevent the majority of GBS disease. Intrapartum chemoprophylaxis (administration of antibiotic during labor) has the potential of preventing neonatal as well as maternal GBS disease.

Guidelines on intrapartum chemoprophylaxis have been established by various countries. However, it should be noted that there are differences in the approach to antenatal screening for GBS and chemoprophylaxis between countries. Some countries do not have specific recommendations for routine antenatal screening based on the perceived risks versus benefits in their regions. Guidelines are based on collective evidence showing a beneficial effect of intrapartum prophylaxis in preventing early-onset GBS sepsis in specific jurisdictions. The most widely accepted recommendations are those proposed by the US Centers for Disease Control and Prevention (Fig. PP25.1). Based on these recommendations, the following summary points can be made.

Screening

All pregnant women (exceptions noted) should be screened at 35–37 weeks gestation for vaginorectal colonization. The exceptions are women who had previous infants with invasive GBS disease and women with GBS bacteriuria during the current pregnancy.

Culture techniques that maximize the likelihood of GBS recovery should be used. Because lower vaginal and rectal cultures are recommended, cultures should not be collected by speculum examination. Laboratories should report results to both the anticipated site of delivery and the health-care provider who ordered the test. Ideally, laboratories that perform GBS cultures will ensure that clinicians have continuous access to culture results.

IAP indicated

- *Women identified as GBS carriers during the current pregnancy.* At the time of labor or rupture of membranes, IAP should be offered to these women.
- *Women who have previously given birth to an infant who had GBS disease.* Prenatal screening is not necessary for these women.
- *Women with GBS bacteriuria.* These women are usually heavily colonized with GBS. Women who have symptomatic or asymptomatic GBS urinary tract infections in pregnancy should be managed according to current standards of care for urinary tract infections in pregnancy.
- *If the results of cultures are not known at the time of labor or rupture of membranes* and *any of the following risk factors is present.* Gestation less than 37 weeks, duration of membrane rupture of 18 hours or longer, or intrapartum temperature >100.4°F (>38°C). If these women are febrile due to chorioamnionitis, appropriate broad-spectrum antimicrobial therapy that includes an agent that is active against GBS should replace intrapartum chemoprophylaxis.

IAP not indicated

- *Women who are colonized and have a planned Caesarian section prior to rupture of membranes.* These women are felt to be at an extremely low risk of delivering an infant who has early-onset GBS.
- *Previous pregnancy with positive GBS screening culture* (unless a culture is also positive in the current pregnancy or GBS bacteriuria is present).
- *Negative vaginal and rectal GBS screening culture in late gestation* (regardless of risk factors).

INFECTION CONTROL IN THE NEONATAL NURSERY

Adequate hand hygiene is regarded as the most effective way to prevent the spread of GBS within a nursery. The routine culturing of babies to determine colonization status is not recommended. The treatment of asymptomatic carriers is not recommended. Cultures may be considered as part of an epidemiologic investigation of an outbreak of late-onset or very late-onset cases. In the event of an outbreak, cohorting of ill and colonized infants and the use of contact precautions should occur.

Newborn management following IAP

The recommendations for the prevention of GBS disease are accompanied by a suggested approach to the management of neonates born to mothers who have received intrapartum antimicrobial prophylaxis (Fig. PP25.1). This approach is based on the gestational age of the neonate, the presence or absence of symptoms and signs of sepsis and whether sufficient time has elapsed between IAP and delivery. Antibiotics must be administered at least 4 hours prior to delivery to allow for adequate antibiotic levels in the amniotic fluid.

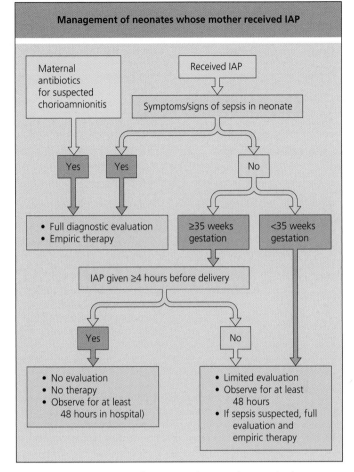

Fig. PP25.1 Management of neonates whose mothers received intrapartum antimicrobial prophylaxis (IAP).

MANAGEMENT OF A PREGNANT WOMAN WITH A PREVIOUS AFFECTED NEWBORN

Any woman who has lost an infant as a result of GBS disease needs the usual understanding and support given to any woman who has lost an infant during the neonatal period. Intrapartum prophylaxis is recommended regardless of screening cultures because of the previous delivery of a baby who had GBS disease. Routine vaginal–rectal screening for GBS is not necessary in this setting. However, it would be appropriate to obtain urine cultures at different antenatal visits to determine whether GBS bacteriuria is present, given that these women are at an increased risk of having GBS-affected infants.

Penicillin G (5 megaunits intravenously initially followed by 2.5 megaunits intravenously q4h) should be given intrapartum until delivery (Table PP25.1). Ampicillin (2 g intravenously initially and then 1 g intravenously q4h until delivery) is an acceptable alternative. Penicillin G is preferred because it has a narrow spectrum and is thus potentially less likely to select out resistant bacteria.

The use of IAP in women who are allergic to penicillin takes into account the risk of anaphylaxis and the background prevalence of GBS resistance to erythromycin and clindamycin. Given the relatively high rates of GBS resistance to these two latter agents, women who are allergic to penicillin but who are at low risk of anaphylaxis may receive cefazolin 2 g initially, then 1 g q8h. If the isolate has been shown to be susceptible to clindamycin, this agent may be used. Vancomycin should be reserved for women who are at high-risk of anaphylaxis in the setting where susceptibility testing of the GBS isolate has not been performed.

Table PP25.1 Alternative antibiotic regimens for intrapartum antimicrobial prophylaxis

Drugs	Doses	Comments
Penicillin	5 megaunits iv load, then 2.5 megaunits iv q4h	Preferred agent
Ampicillin	2 g iv load, then 1 g iv q4 h	Alternative agent
Cefazolin	2 g iv load, then 1 g iv q8 h	Use if risk of anaphylaxis is low in penicillin-allergic patient
Clindamycin	900 mg iv q8 h	Use if risk of anaphylaxis is high in penicillin allergic patient *and* the GBS isolate is known to be susceptible to clindamycin
Vancomycin	2 g iv load, then 1 g iv q12 h	Use if risk of anaphylaxis is high in penicillin allergic patient *and* the susceptibility of the GBS isolate is unknown or the isolate is known to be resistant to clindamycin

Group B streptococci are associated with various complications during pregnancy. These include septic abortion, urinary tract infections, chorioamnionitis, wound infection and endometritis. Although IAP may have a beneficial effect on endometritis, an assessment is necessary in the immediate postpartum period in order to guide further antibiotic therapy directed at the mother.

The newborn infant of a mother who has received intrapartum prophylaxis requires a special management approach. The approach outlined in Figure PP25.2 may be used as a guide to the management of the neonate. However, if the infant is believed to have invasive GBS disease, the following apply.

- Ampicillin plus an aminoglycoside is the initial treatment of presumed GBS disease.
- Penicillin G may be given alone when GBS is proved to be the etiologic agent and clinical and microbiologic responses have been documented.
- In cases of meningitis, a second lumbar puncture at 24–48 hours after the start of treatment is recommended by some experts; this may have prognostic significance.
- Bacteremia without a defined focus should be treated for a minimum of 10 days. Uncomplicated meningitis should be treated for 14–21 days (longer periods of treatment are needed in infants who have complicated courses).
- Osteomyelitis should be treated for a minimum of 4 weeks.
- There is a high incidence of co-infection among twins, and the twin of an index case should be observed or evaluated for sepsis as clinically indicated.

FURTHER READING

Further reading for this chapter can be found online at http://www.expertconsult.com

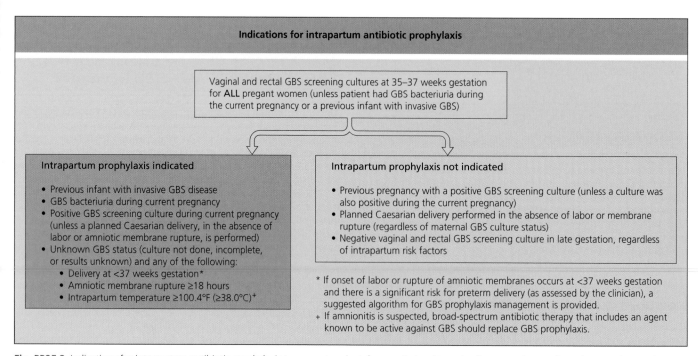

Fig. PP25.2 Indications for intrapartum antibiotic prophylaxis to prevent perinatal group B streptococcus disease under a universal prenatal screening strategy based on combined vaginal and rectal cultures collected at 35–37 weeks gestation from all pregnant women.

Cystitis and urethral syndromes

Urinary tract infections (UTIs) are the second most common infectious cause for consultation and prescription of antibiotics among family physicians and are a common cause of morbidity in institutional care. Most infections are limited to the lower urinary tract but may cause pyelonephritis and bacteremia. The global incidence is estimated to be 2–3%, or at least 150 million cases per annum, costing billions of dollars annually.[1] Most cases of cystitis are uncomplicated and respond readily to antimicrobial treatment and typically occur in otherwise healthy nonpregnant women. Complicated infections, associated with anatomic or functional abnormalities, have an increased risk of therapeutic failure.

Acute Cystitis

EPIDEMIOLOGY

In the first 3 months of life UTIs are about three times more common in males than females, but thereafter infections occur more frequently in females. The prevalence of bacteriuria in preschool- and school-aged girls is 30 times higher than that in boys; 5–6% of girls will have had at least one episode of bacteriuria during their school-age years.[2] Thereafter the prevalence increases with onset of sexual activity before falling during the thirties and then rising at about 1% per decade thereafter (Table 53.1). About 50% of adult women report at least one UTI during their life.[1]

Table 53.1 Prevalence of bacteriuria in different age groups

	Group	Prevalence (%)
Females	Schoolgirls	1.2
	Sexually active young women	2–4
	Women >60 years 70 years 80 years	6–8 5–10 20
	Institutionalized elderly	30–50
Males	Childhood to middle age	<1
	Men 60–65 >80 years	1–3 >10
	Institutionalized elderly	20–30

Among college women more that two-thirds of acute episodes may be attributable to intercourse.[3] Risk factors for symptomatic UTI include asymptomatic bacteriuria during childhood, previous UTI, and use of a diaphragm and spermicide. Sexual activity is not a risk factor for UTI in postmenopausal women

In pregnancy asymptomatic bacteriuria occurs in 4–7% of women, predisposing them to developing acute pyelonephritis (15–40% of cases) during the third trimester or in the puerperium. Up to 20% of such patients have significant abnormalities of the urinary tract. Bacteriuria of pregnancy has also been associated with increased risk of pre-eclampsia, lowered fetal birth weight, prematurity and increased perinatal mortality rates.[4]

Men have low rates of bacteriuria until advanced age when rates rise dramatically and UTI is associated with abnormalities of the urinary tract.[2] A lowered CD4 lymphocyte count from HIV infection is a risk factor for UTI.[5]

In the elderly, both concurrent disease of the urinary tract and other medical conditions contribute to the high prevalence of UTI (Table 53.2). Instrumentation is associated with an increased risk of infection of 1% of ambulatory patients and 5–10% of hospitalized patients.

PATHOGENESIS

Infecting organisms

In uncomplicated cystitis more than 95% of infections are caused by a single organism. The most common pathogen is *Escherichia coli* (80–90% of cases), and these usually possess fimbriae or pili that adhere to host receptors. *Staphylococcus saprophyticus* accounts for 10–20% of cases in young women during late summer and autumn (Table 53.3).[6] A small number of serotypes of *E. coli* account for most UTIs and some clones have become widespread.[7]

Complicated infections and infections among the institutionalized elderly may be polymicrobial (30% of cases), particularly when stones are present. There is an increased incidence of resistant Gram-negative, *Pseudomonas aeruginosa* and yeast infections in this group. Urease-producing organisms (*Proteus*, *Providencia* and *Morganella* spp.) are of concern because urease leads to the conversion of urea to ammonia, an increase in the pH of urine, precipitation of struvite crystals ($MgNH_4PO_4.6H_2O$), and stone formation.

Mechanisms

Cystitis is almost always caused by ascending infection, although *S. aureus* may infect the urine from the bloodstream. The increased susceptibility of women to UTI is probably related to the shorter distance between the anus and urethral orifice, shorter length of urethra and

Table 53.2 Risk factors for lower urinary tract infection

Young adults	Women	Past history of UTI Sexual intercourse Diaphragm use Spermicide	Parity Diabetes (women) Primary biliary cirrhosis Sickle cell anemia (pregnancy) Instrumentation Homosexual activity
	Men	Lack of circumcision AIDS	

Elderly people	Women	Loss of estrogen effect
		Incomplete emptying of bladder
			Abnormalities of urinary tract
			  Rectoceles
			  Urethroceles
			  Bladder diverticula

	Men	Strictures
		Instrumentation
			Prostatic disease
			  Benign enlargement
			  Calculi
			  Loss of bactericidal
			  secretions

	Both sexes	Neurologic disease
		  Alzheimer's disease
		  Parkinson's disease
			Cerebrovascular disease

Table 53.3 Organisms associated with urinary tract infections

Common organisms	Escherichia coli Staphylococcus saprophyticus	
Less common organisms	Klebsiella spp. Enterobacter spp. Proteus spp. Morganella spp. Citrobacter spp. Group B streptococcus Group D streptococcus Enterococci	Pseudomonas aeruginosa Acinetobacter spp. Serratia spp. Yeasts Corynebacterium urealyticum
Rare indications	Haemophilus influenzae Mycobacterium tuberculosis Anaerobes	Salmonella spp. Shigella spp. Adenovirus (type 11)
Unproven causes	Gardnerella vaginalis Ureaplasma urealyticum Mycoplasma hominis	

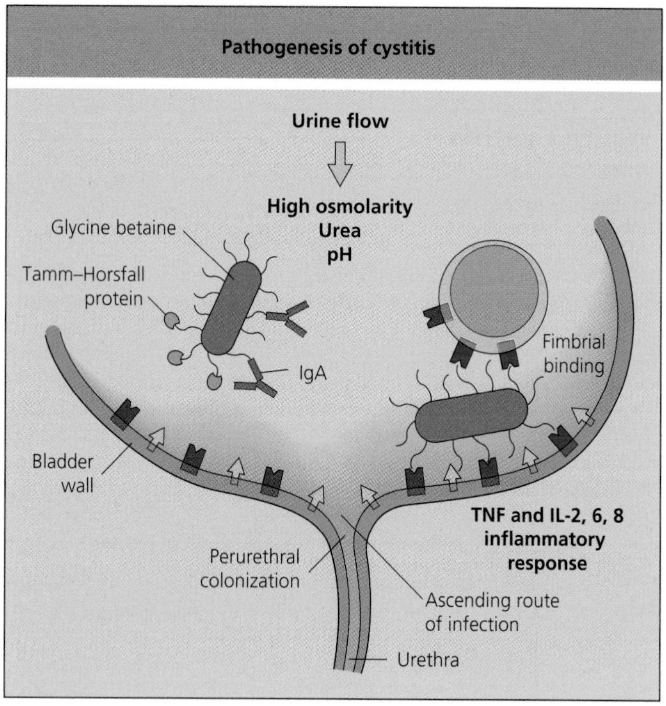

Pathogenesis of cystitis

Urine flow

High osmolarity
Urea
pH

Glycine betaine

Tamm–Horsfall protein

IgA

Fimbrial binding

Bladder wall

Perurethral colonization

TNF and IL-2, 6, 8 inflammatory response

Ascending route of infection

Urethra

Fig. 53.1 Pathogenesis of cystitis. Factors favoring bacterial persistence and infection include bacterial binding to bladder mucosa (fimbriae), and high bacterial growth rates despite high osmolarity and urea concentrations and low pH. Factors favoring bacterial elimination include high urine flow rate, high voiding frequency, bactericidal effects of bladder mucosa, secreted proteins that bind to fimbrial adhesins and the inflammatory response. IL, interleukin; TNF, tumor necrosis factor.

the absence of the antibacterial barrier provided by prostatic fluid in males. In other respects the pathogenesis is similar in men and women and depends on a series of complex, interdependent host–parasite interactions that enable colonization of the periurethral area from the bowel, ascent of organisms into the bladder, growth in urine, tissue invasion and evasion of immune response (Fig. 53.1) to occur.

Colonization

The region between the anus and urethra is normally colonized by specialized flora including lactobacilli that inhibit colonization with enteric organisms. Spermicides (nonoxynol-9), diaphragms, estrogen deficiency and antibiotics (particularly β-lactams) may cause a reduction in these organisms and increase colonization by enteric organisms including uropathogens.[8]

Some women with recurrent UTI have an increased susceptibility to persistent colonization of the periurethral zone and E. coli adheres more strongly to vaginal epithelial cells from these patients.[9] Nonsecretors of histo-blood group antigens (Lewis blood group [Le(a+b–)] and recessive [Le(a–b–)] phenotypes) are at greater risk of recurrent UTI.[10] Likewise, bowel carriage of *E. coli* possessing DNA sequences for P fimbriae, is more common among patients with the P blood group.[11]

Ascent

Bacteria normally enter the bladder by ascending along the mucosal sheath. This may result from mechanical instrumentation, sexual activity and motility of the organisms.

Fimbriae: role in mucosal adherence and inflammation

Symptomatic bacteriuria is highly correlated with the presence of bacteria that mediate attachment to uroepithelial cells. Type I (mannose-sensitive) fimbriae are important in initiating colonization of the bladder, but are not expressed subsequently following phase variation of the organisms. This may prevent binding to Tamm-Horsfall protein and IgA, and decrease recognition by phagocytic cells, which possess type I receptors.[12] Type II fimbrial attachment (mannose-resistant) is mediated by P fimbriae (Gal-Gal), which are associated with pyelonephritis, and attach to a variety of receptors associated with the globose series of glycolipids.[13] Attachment of bacteria

to the mucosa and cell wall components, such as lipid A, activate an inflammatory response, including production of tumor necrosis factor (TNF) and interleukin (IL)-2, IL-6 and IL-8, and attraction of inflammatory cells.[14]

In contrast, asymptomatic bacteriuria is usually caused by organisms that neither possess fimbriae nor excite an inflammatory response unless tissue invasion occurs. The pathogenesis of these infections is not known.

Biofilm formation

Uropathogenic *E. coli* readily form biofilms on the mucosal surfaces, epithelial cells and catheter surfaces. Bacteria within biofilms are characterized by a slow metabolic rate and localization within an exopolysaccharide coating, and are protected from opsonization and phagocytosis by host cells.[15] Sessile communities are maintained by quorum sensing molecules that may interact with the host's signaling systems. Recently intracellular bacterial communities have been found within facet cells which line the transitional epithelium in animal models and up to 20% of sexually active women with *E. coli* cystitis.[16] A larger number have filamentous organisms in the urine which is the hallmark of recent residence in sessile colonies (Fig. 53.2).

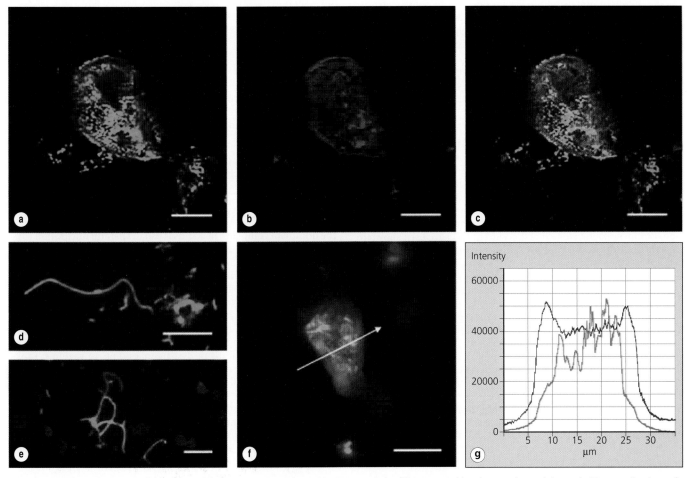

Fig. 53.2 Electron microscopy findings in urine from women with cystitis. TEM analysis of human cystitis urine specimens (a) revealed large collections of bacteria associated with nuclei and other cellular debris. These collections of bacteria from human urines (b) have similar morphology and organization as those recovered from intact murine intracellular bacterial communities (c). Bacteria and filaments were also observed intracellularly within exfoliated epithelial cells in a urine sample quickly fixed and analyzed from an *E. coli* cystitis patient (d). SEM analysis of cystitis urines deemed positive for intracellular bacterial communities and filaments captured large bacterial biofilm-like collections (e and f) composed of bacteria with a smaller, more coccoid morphology than typical *E. coli*. Long filaments were also captured by SEM (g). Scale bars: 2 μm (a and d); 1 μm (b and c); 5 μm (e–g). Courtesy of Rosen *et al.*[16]

Urodynamics

Normal structure and function of the urinary tract promotes elimination bacteria from the urinary tract because voiding eliminates free organisms and the bladder mucosa is bactericidal to many organisms on contact. Similarly, adequate urine flow promotes removal of bacteria from the upper urinary tracts. These defense mechanisms are potentially compromised by low urine flow rate, infrequent voiding, residual bladder urine and reflux of urine.[17] Neurologic disease, diabetes, debility and anatomic changes impair bacterial clearance by these mechanisms, particularly in the elderly. In postmenopausal women urinary incontinence, cystocele and postvoiding residual urine are the commonest risk factors for UTI.[18]

Growth in bladder urine

Growth in urine is essential for invasion of the urinary tract. Gonococci, anaerobes and urethral commensals are inhibited whereas uropathogens grow well in urine. Bacteria derive protection from the inhibitory effects of high osmotic forces, extremes of pH and high urea concentrations by the intracellular accumulation of osmolytes normally present in urine (e.g. glycine betaine) that stabilize macromolecular structures.[19]

Immune response

Locally produced urinary antibodies produced in response to febrile UTI (monomeric and dimeric IgA and IgG) decrease adherence by interference with adhesion receptors and agglutination of bacteria. Hyperimmunization can protect animals against experimental UTI.[20]

PREVENTION

Normal urinary tract

Recurrent or closely spaced symptomatic UTIs cause considerable morbidity and anxiety when no cause is found. Patients are often told to empty their bladder completely, maintain a high fluid intake and to void after intercourse, but there is little evidence to support these measures. Application of antiseptic cream (e.g. 0.5% cetrimide) to the urethral orifice may prevent infections. Women who use a diaphragm and spermicide should consider alternative methods of contraception. Postmenopausal women with recurrent UTI have been shown to benefit from the application of estriol vaginal cream (0.5 mg/day for 2 weeks then twice weekly).[21]

If these measures fail, chemoprophylaxis should be considered if there are two or more symptomatic UTIs within 6 months, or three or more over 12 months. A useful strategy is to give a 6-month trial of prophylaxis; if there is a reversion to the previous pattern, consider prophylaxis for 2 years. Postcoital prophylaxis is preferable, where applicable, as it results in administration of smaller amounts of antimicrobials than continuous prophylaxis and is equally effective. Continuous prophylaxis is highly effective but vaginal and oral candidiasis and gastrointestinal symptoms can be troublesome[22] (Table 53.4). Nitrofurantoin is an excellent agent because it does not alter the fecal flora, and resistance during treatment is rare. Use of trimethoprim–sulfamethoxazole (TMP–SMX) for as long as 5 years is effective and well tolerated.

Cranberry juice

Cranberry juice may decrease the number of symptomatic UTIs over a 12-month period but there are a large number of dropouts/withdrawals, indicating that cranberry juice may not be well tolerated and the optimum dosage and method of administration (e.g. juice, tablets or capsules) is uncertain.[23] Cranberry juice inhibits adherence of both type I fimbriated *E. coli* and P-fimbriated *E. coli* to uroepithelial cells.

Table 53.4 Drug regimens for prophylactic therapy administered as a single dose at night

Drug	Dose
Nitrofurantoin	50 mg
Trimethoprim	100 mg
Trimethoprim-sulfamethoxazole (co-trimoxazole)	480 mg
Norfloxacin	200 mg
Cephalexin	125 mg
Hexamine hippurate	1.0 g

Other prevention strategies

Competitive exclusion of uropathogens using probiotics (i.e. lactobacilli) or receptor analogues has been touted as a possible approach to reduce the risk of UTI by reducing colonization by uropathogens. While this approach holds promise, more research is needed.

Abnormal urinary tract

Any lesions in the urinary tract should be corrected if possible. Urologic referral is essential when abnormalities are found. Large residual volumes and high pressure may require intermittent self-catheterization. Low-dose chemoprophylaxis is often effective.

Vaccine

There is no vaccine currently available, although type I and type II pili and multiple heat-killed uropathogenic bacteria have been trialed. Anatomic and functional abnormalities may limit vaccine applicability.[24]

CLINICAL FEATURES

Symptomatic infection

The dominant complaint in cystitis is usually painful micturition (dysuria), which may be associated with frequency, urgency, strangury, initial and terminal hematuria, suprapubic discomfort and voiding small amounts of turbid urine. Low-grade fever may occur, but is usually absent. Pyuria or hematuria is almost always present. Elderly patients usually have similar symptoms but occasionally present with incontinence or smelly urine, or in men, epididymo-orchitis.[25]

Dysuria caused by bacterial cystitis should be distinguished from that caused by vaginitis, vulvitis and urethritis (see Chapter 49). Vaginal discharge, pruritus or dyspareunia points to vaginitis. Labial discomfort as the stream of urine is passed suggests vulvitis which is often caused by genital herpes and candidiasis. In urethritis there may be a history of a new sex partner, urethral discharge, mucopurulent cervicitis or bartholinitis. *Chlamydia trachomatis* and *Neisseria gonorrhoeae* are the usual causes.

Dysuria caused by chronic conditions such as interstitial cystitis and *Mycobacterium tuberculosis* infection may cause initial confusion but usually persists following attempts at treatment.

Asymptomatic bacteriuria

Asymptomatic bacteriuria is very common in elderly patients. It is poorly correlated with fatigue, poor appetite and urinary incontinence. Similarly, symptoms such as frequency, dysuria and hesitancy, which may be caused by infection, are common and nonspecific and often fail to respond to treatment of coexisting bacteriuria.[26] Asymptomatic UTIs have been shown to increase morbidity in pregnancy but not in the elderly.

DIAGNOSIS

The diagnosis of UTI can only be proven by culture of an adequately collected urine sample. This is essential in all suspected cases in males, infants and children. A presumptive diagnosis can be made in sexually active women in the presence of typical clinical features together with the presence of pyuria if sexually transmitted infections are unlikely.[27] A culture should be performed if a complicated infection is suspected or symptoms have relaped within a month of treatment.

Pyuria

The preferred method for assessment of pyuria is microscopic examination of uncentrifuged fresh urine using a hemocytometer, although counts per microscopic field are reasonably reliable in the clinical laboratory. Urine from adult patients who have symptomatic UTI almost always (>96%) contains more than 10 leukocytes/ml. Pyuria occurs less frequently in asymptomatic bacteriuria of pregnancy (50% positive) and the elderly (90% positive).

Pyuria alone is not a reliable predictor of infection. Specimens from women with vaginitis often contain white cells and there are many other causes of inflammation within the urinary tract (Table 53.5).

Urine dipsticks using esterase provide a simple inexpensive method for detecting pyuria. A positive test indicates a minimum of eight white blood cells per high power field and has a sensitivity of 88–95%

Table 53.5 Conditions associated with pyuria but without culturable bacteria using standard bacterial isolation techniques

Recent treatment of UTI	
Organism not culturable on usual bacterial media	Adenovirus Anaerobes *Chlamydia trachomatis* Fungal infections Herpes simplex Leptospirosis *Mycobacterium tuberculosis* *Neisseria gonorrhoeae*
Noninfectious causes	Cyclophosphamide therapy Foreign bodies Glomerulonephritis Interstitial cystitis Neoplasms Stones Transplant rejection Trauma Tubulointerstitial disease Vaginal contamination

and specificity of 94–98% compared with the counting chamber method.[28] The presence of blood, rifampin (rifampicin), nitrofurantoin, bilirubin and ascorbic acid may result in a false-negative test, whereas trichomonads, imipenem and amoxicillin-clavulanate may give a false-positive test.[29]

Detection of bacteria

The presence of bacteria on microscopy of urine correlates well with culture results. Experienced laboratories can reliably detect 10^8 organisms per liter in unstained specimens. The nitrite test is reliable for detecting Gram-negative bacilli in first morning urines but not other specimens because of inadequate time for reduction of nitrate to nitrite.

Midstream urine specimens

The simplest method for obtaining urine for quantitative culture is to collect a clean midstream specimen. This minimizes the confounding effects of contamination from the first few milliliters of urine.

The sensitivity and specificity of quantitative culture for diagnosis of UTI is dependent on the presence of symptoms and pyuria:

- in asymptomatic women, a single count of 10^4–10^5/ml has a 95% chance of representing contamination;[30]
- in symptomatic women with pyuria (>10 white blood cells/ml) a single count of more than 10^5/ml has a very high specificity (>99%) but a low sensitivity (51%) for UTI.[31]

Routine application of this criterion would fail to diagnose one-third of women with a UTI (Table 53.6).

Specimens from males are less likely to be contaminated and lower counts (>10^3/ml) are highly predictive of infection. Gram-positive bacteria and yeasts in urine tend to be associated with lower counts than Gram-negative bacilli.

In practice specimens are often poorly collected and delays in processing without refrigeration allow bacterial multiplication. In the presence of symptoms and pyuria, a bacterial count greater than 10^3/ml is a reasonable criterion for significant bacteriuria in routine laboratories, bearing in mind that this represents 10 organisms on a plate if a 0.01 ml loop is used. Others argue that over 10^4/ml is more realistic. Obstruction, antimicrobial agents and, possibly, diuresis can cause false-negative results.

Suprapubic aspiration

Suprapubic aspiration of urine from a distended bladder is an efficient means of diagnosis. Any bacteria identified can be regarded as significant because the technique avoids contamination. In most infected specimens bacteria can be seen microscopically and treatment started promptly. Provided the patient has a full bladder it is safe and acceptable.

Catheter specimens

Catheterization specifically for a urine culture may be justifiable if the patient is unable to co-operate to obtain an uncontaminated sample or to hold urine in the bladder for a suprapubic aspiration.

Table 53.6 Value of quantitative urine culture in diagnosis of urinary tract infection with Gram-negative bacilli in women

	Number of specimens	Organisms/ml of urine	Sensitivity (%)	Specificity (%)
Asymptomatic women	Two	>10^5	>95	>80
Symptomatic women with pyuria	One One One	>10^5 >10^3 >10^2	51 80 95	99 90 85

Catheterization rarely leads to false-positive results, but may introduce bacteria into the bladder. Straight plastic catheter or Alexa bag techniques are satisfactory.

Imaging of the urinary tract

All men, children and infants need investigations of the urinary tract if they have a UTI regardless of the clinical features at presentation. This is not cost-effective in women unless there is some evidence of an unusual clinical pattern, such as urinary infection in childhood, treatment failure, persistent microscopic hematuria or pyuria at follow-up. An ultrasound examination including postmicturition bladder volumes plus a plain abdominal radiograph, including the kidneys, ureters and bladder, are adequate in most instances. Cystoscopy rarely yields useful information in women with acute cystitis.

MANAGEMENT

The cornerstone of management is effective antimicrobial therapy (Table 53.7). Drinking large amounts of fluids and alkalinizing agents may decrease bacterial counts and improve symptoms, but add little to effective antimicrobial therapy.

Follow-up visits at 7–14 days after completion of therapy give the opportunity to obtain urine cultures and discuss the importance of the diagnosis. It is essential to relieve anxiety about sexual activity and perceived long-term consequences, and to discuss advice offered by the family and the media.

Acute uncomplicated bacterial cystitis

Short-course therapy has now become standard treatment because of improved compliance, lower cost, fewer side-effects and decreased likelihood of the emergence of resistant strains.[32] A treatment algorithm is given in Figure 53.3. Short-course therapy is contraindicated in complicated infections.

Three-day therapy

A 3-day regimen is recommended because it provides the advantages of short-course therapy and has a slightly higher success rate than single-dose therapy, particularly in older women. It is appreciated by patients because it may take several days for symptoms to abate. Three

Table 53.7 Drug treatment regimens for a 3-day course of oral therapy for bacterial cystitis

Drug	Dose
Trimethoprim	300 mg q24h
Trimethoprim-sulfamethoxazole (co-trimoxazole)	960 mg q12h
Ciprofloxacin	250 mg q12h
Fleroxacin	400 mg q24h
Levofloxacin	500 mg q24h
Lomefloxacin	400 mg q24h
Nalidixic acid	500 mg q8h
Norfloxacin	400 mg q12h
Amoxicillin	250 mg q8h
Amoxicillin-clavulanate	500/125 mg q12h
Cephalexin	250 mg q8h
Cephradine	250 mg q8h
Cefpodoxime proxetil	100 mg q12h
Pivmecillinam	200 mg q8h

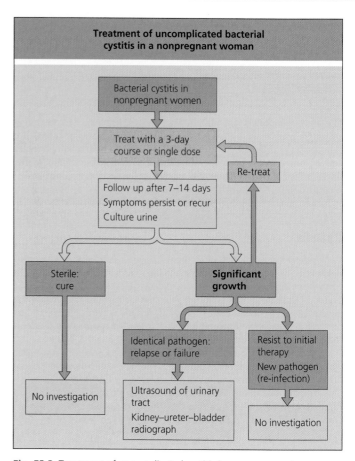

Fig. 53.3 Treatment of uncomplicated cystitis in a nonpregnant woman.

days of trimethoprim-sulfamethoxazole (TMP-SMX; co-trimoxazole), trimethoprim alone, the quinolones or pivmecillinam are as effective as longer courses with fewer side-effects. β-Lactams as a group are less effective than trimethoprim, TMP-SMX or the quinolones.[33] There is insufficient evidence to recommend nitrofurantoin for 3 days rather than 5 days.

Single-dose therapy

Single-dose therapy is essentially 1 day of treatment given in a single dose that produces inhibitory concentrations of antibiotic over a 12–24-hour period. It is most suitable for cystitis in sexually active women and for younger patients who have normal urinary tracts and a short history (<7 days) (Table 53.8).

Amoxicillin is less effective than either TMP–SMX or trimethoprim alone and is no longer recommended in single-dose regimens.

Table 53.8 Suggested drug treatment regimens for single-dose treatments

Drug	Dose
Trimethoprim	600 mg
Trimethoprim-sulfamethoxazole (co-trimoxazole)	1.92 g
Ciprofloxacin	500 mg
Fleroxacin	400 mg
Norfloxacin	800 mg
Fosfomycin trometamol	3 g

Fluoroquinolones are very effective, although they may be less effective against *S. saprophyticus* than Gram-negative bacilli. Fosfomycin trometamol is marketed specifically as single-dose therapy and is highly effective but is relatively expensive.

Those who fail to respond to single-dose therapy have an increased risk of abnormalities within the urinary tract.[34]

Therapeutic agents

Both TMP-SMX and trimethoprim (TMP) alone are highly effective, but as sulfonamides have occasional severe side-effects, especially in the elderly, TMP is preferred. There is no evidence that the combination with sulfamethoxazole prevents the emergence of resistance.

The fluoroquinolones have essentially superseded nalidixic acid and oxolinic acid. All these agents are extremely active and effective against most pathogens, including many hospital pathogens. Norfloxacin is usually the most inexpensive fluoroquinolone for the treatment of cystitis in some countries.

Nitrofurantoin is ineffective against *Proteus mirabilis.* The side-effects of nausea and vomiting can be minimized by treating with 50 mg q8h or 100 mg q18h without loss of efficacy, rather than 100 mg q6h.

Mecillinam has been widely used in Scandinavia without apparent resistance problems developing in Gram-negative organisms. *In-vitro* studies show resistance in Gram-positive organisms, but clinical studies show that there is a high cure rate for *S. saprophyticus*, presumably because of the very high concentrations achieved in the urine.

Amoxicillin is the treatment of choice for treating *Streptococcus faecalis*, but increasing resistance has limited its usefulness against other uropathogens. Combinations of β-lactams with β-lactamase inhibitors may be effective, but there is a high rate of diarrhea. Cephalosporins such as cephalexin, cephradine and cefaclor are useful, particularly in renal failure.

Fluoroquinolones have been shown to produce arthropathies in immature animals and are therefore contraindicated in pregnant women. Antibiotics, such as penicillins, may interfere with the effectiveness of oral contraceptives by altering the enterohepatic recycling of estrogen and reducing the contraceptive effect. Women who use oral contraceptives may need to use barrier methods of contraception while on treatment.

Choice of initial therapeutic agent

Trimethoprim and TMP-SMX have been regarded as the agents of first choice but there is pressure to use quinolones as resistance rates of *E. coli* and other Gram-negative organisms rise and exceed 10–20%. *In-vitro* resistance reduces the clinical success of TMP-SMX from 95% to 60% and bacterial eradication from 93% to 50%. Thus the expected clinical and bacterial success rates for a 10% resistance rate in Gram-negative infections will be 92% and 89%, and for a 20% resistance rate 88% and 84%, respectively.[35] The net effect on success on intention to treat will be smaller, because Gram-positive uropathogens remain susceptible to TMP or TMP-SMX.

The decision to change policy is made more difficult if reliable estimates of resistance rates in the local setting are lacking. Resistance rates reported by clinical laboratories are often misleading because isolates from patients who have failed therapy or are at a high risk of resistance are over-represented.[36] Using quinolones as a first choice may be a short-term solution because resistance to these agents is steadily rising worldwide and is reported to be more than 20% in several countries. There are now efforts to reverse quinolone use in some centers.[37]

Where resistance to TMP-SMX is a potential problem a reasonable approach is to use it unless the patient has risk factors for TMP-SMX resistance. These include previous infection with TMP-SMX-resistant organisms, recent use of TMP-SMX or another antimicrobial agent, recent hospitalization or recurrent UTI in the past year. Alternatives include fluoroquinolones (3 days), nitrofurantoin (5–7 days), pivampicillin (3 days) and fosfomycin (single dose).

Recurrent infections

The major problem with uncomplicated acute cystitis is recurrence. About one-half of adult women will have another infection within 1 year, many within 3 months. Recurrence rates vary (0.3–7.6 episodes per year) and may occur in clusters. With treatment of each episode, 20–30% will cease having recurrences. If episodes are closely spaced, self-administered therapy, preferably after obtaining a urine specimen, postcoital therapy or prophylaxis can be considered. Self-initiated therapy should be reserved for those who are not at risk of sexually transmitted infections or pregnancy, and who do not have significant co-morbid conditions.[38] A treatment algorithm is given in Figure 53.4.

Complicated infections

Complicated infections are more likely to be caused by unusual organisms and should be treated for 7–14 days. Quinolones are an appropriate initial choice but treatment should be altered in response to results from culture and sensitivity testing. Patients who fail short-course treatment often have abnormalities of the urinary tract (e.g. stones, diverticula, strictures, chronic bacterial prostatitis). These should be corrected where possible and infection treated with more prolonged courses of therapy of 7–14 days.

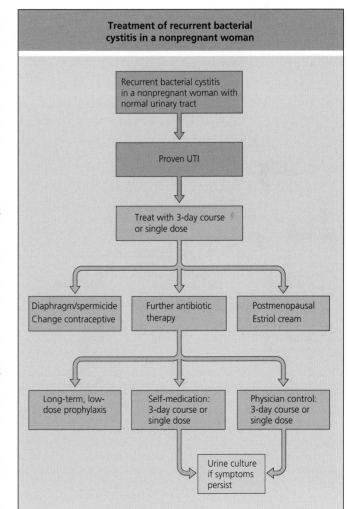

Fig. 53.4 Treatment of recurrent bacterial cystitis in a nonpregnant woman.

Urinary tract infections in pregnancy

The risks of symptomatic infection and pyelonephritis during the third trimester of pregnancy in mothers and prematurity in infants can be prevented by early detection and eradication of asymptomatic bacteriuria. In the first instance single-dose or a 3-day course of therapy is appropriate (Fig. 53.5). If relapse or re-infection occurs, then the patients should be re-treated. At that stage the simplest strategy is to institute prophylaxis (e.g. nitrofurantoin 50 mg at night), although some prefer close surveillance with repeated cultures and prompt treatment of each episode. All such patients need evaluation of the urinary tract with ultrasonography and a plain abdominal radiograph after delivery.

There is probably no absolute contraindication to any antimicrobial agent during pregnancy, but caution is urged with some agents. The β-lactams (e.g. amoxicillin, amoxicillin-clavulanate, cephalexin) are considered safe and the antifolate activity of trimethoprim and TMP-SMX is minimal in short courses and probably safe between 16 and 30 weeks of gestation (Table 53.9).

Males

Lower UTI in males may be complicated by infection of prostatic fluid, even if there is no clinical prostatitis. For this reason there is reluctance to treat men with short regimens and 7-day courses are recommended even for apparently uncomplicated cystitis. Long-term suppressive therapy may be helpful for frequent recurrences.

Asymptomatic bacteriuria

Asymptomatic bacteriuria is often best left untreated except in pregnancy. In elderly patients it is extremely common and there is no convincing evidence that treatment benefits the patient either in terms of recurrent symptomatic episodes or mortality rate. Antimicrobial therapy is associated with adverse effects, the potential for development of resistant strains and financial cost.

Invasive procedures

Asymptomatic bacteriuria should be treated if a patient is to undergo an invasive procedure of the genitourinary tract. Mucosal trauma may cause postprocedural bacteremia, and occasionally septic shock and death. The antimicrobial agent should be selected on the basis of the sensitivity of the infecting organism. Likewise, it is prudent to treat any urinary infections before the insertion of permanent indwelling devices, particularly prosthetic joints.

Treatment in the presence of renal failure

If treatment is truly indicated, drugs that achieve adequate urine concentrations in the presence of renal failure should be used. The best levels may be achieved with penicillins and cephalosporins. Trimethoprim and fluoroquinolones will probably achieve adequate concentrations, whereas nitrofurantoin, sulfamethoxazole and doxycycline are present in very low concentrations when creatinine clearance falls below about 0.16 ml/s.

Infections with *Candida* spp.

Infections with *Candida* spp. may occur either from hematogenous spread or via the ascending route. There is an increased risk in those with diabetes, prolonged antimicrobial therapy and instrumentation of the urinary tract. The natural history has not been well defined, but most infections are asymptomatic, limited to the lower urinary tract and may resolve in otherwise normal patients. Most trials in asymptomatic candiduria have failed to show a clinical benefit but candiduria in the presence of urinary manipulation should be treated. Symptomatic candiduria should always be treated. Oral fluconazole (200 mg/day, 14 days) is the treatment of choice, although some species such as *Candida krusei* may be resistant.[39] Intravenous amphotericin B (0.3 mg/kg/day, 1–7 days) is usually effective, presumably because of prolonged renal excretion. Oral flucytosine often fails with development of resistance. If a catheter is present, bladder washouts with amphotericin B may be used, but are of questionable efficacy. Casofungin may be effective despite minimal urinary excretion.

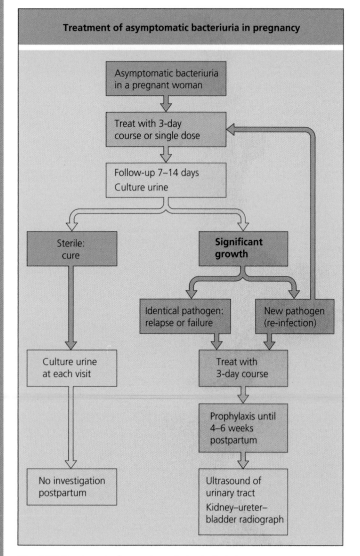

Treatment of asymptomatic bacteriuria in pregnancy

- Asymptomatic bacteriuria in a pregnant woman
- Treat with 3-day course or single dose
- Follow-up 7–14 days Culture urine
- Sterile: cure
- **Significant growth**
- Culture urine at each visit
- Identical pathogen: relapse or failure
- New pathogen (re-infection)
- Treat with 3-day course
- Prophylaxis until 4–6 weeks postpartum
- No investigation postpartum
- Ultrasound of urinary tract Kidney–ureter–bladder radiograph

Fig. 53.5 Treatment of asymptomatic bacteriuria in pregnancy.

Table 53.9 Possible toxicities of antimicrobial agents in pregnancy

Agent	Toxicity
Trimethoprim sulfonamides	Antifolate activity and megaloblastic anemia
Sulfonamides (protein bound)	Kernicterus of newborn
Sulfonamides/nitrofurantoin	Hemolytic anemia in glucose-6-phosphate dehydrogenase deficiency
Tetracycline	Fatty liver/hepatic necrosis in mother, stained teeth in baby
Fluoroquinolones	Not approved

Urethral Syndromes

PATHOGENESIS AND CLINICAL FEATURES

Following the introduction of quantitative bacterial counts, about half of women with acute symptoms of cystitis did not have significant – >10^5 colony forming units (cfu)/ml – bacteriuria. These women were said to have acute urethral syndrome or dysuria-pyuria syndrome. Many women with acute urethral syndrome have periurethral colonization with uropathogenic organisms and low numbers of E. coli, S. saprophyticus and enteric Gram-negative organisms present in their urine. Furthermore, many such patients responded to antibiotic therapy, suggesting that this was essentially a UTI. These patients probably have bacterial urethritis with little infection of the bladder and the diagnosis may be missed because of the low numbers of organisms present.

There remains a group with similar symptoms who do not have a low-count bacteriuria. It is possible that symptoms are caused by infection confined to the proximal urethra, especially if there is pyuria. A recent randomized controlled trial found that trimethoprim (300 mg daily) was superior to placebo in women with dipstick-negative acute dysuria, suggesting that infection is one cause of this syndrome.[40] Ureaplasma urealyticum and Chlamydia trachomatis are possible pathogens but trials with tetracycline have not been helpful. Multiple other causes have been suggested, including chemicals (e.g. bubble baths and deodorants), trauma, atrophic vaginitis in postmenopausal women and psychologic factors, but are mostly unproven.

MANAGEMENT

Management of the urethral syndrome is difficult. A pelvic examination should be carried out to exclude herpes simplex, gonorrhea and vaginitis. The symptoms usually settle in a few days, although some patients appear to benefit from a high fluid intake. Antimicrobial therapy may be helpful, particularly if pyuria is present, presumably reflecting bacterial urethritis or chlamydial infection. Antibiotics useful for treatment of UTI are often prescribed in the first instance. Tricyclic antidepressants are sometimes used in chronic dysuria but the benefit is unproven.

REFERENCES

References for this chapter can be found online at http://www.expertconsult.com

Prostatitis, epididymitis and orchitis

Prostatitis

The diagnosis of prostatitis syndrome refers to a variety of inflammatory and noninflammatory conditions probably not always affecting the prostatic gland itself. In 1978 a classification system[1] was developed to differentiate inflammatory from noninflammatory entities and was much used in the past. However, many aspects of chronic prostatic symptoms remained enigmatic. In 1999 a consensus conference at the National Institute of Diabetes, Digestive and Kidney Diseases (NIDDK) of the National Institutes of Health (NIH) developed a new classification system[2,3] based on the clinical presentation of the patients, the presence or absence of leukocytes in the expressed prostatic secretion (EPS) or voided bladder urine after prostatic massage (VB$_3$), and the presence or absence of bacteria in the EPS or VB$_3$. In addition, the inflammatory conditions are categorized into symptomatic and asymptomatic presentations, identifying patients who are incidentally diagnosed from biopsies, evaluations for fertility disorders or routine examinations. The term chronic pelvic pain syndrome (CPPS) was chosen, because it has not been scientifically demonstrated either that CPPS is primarily a disease of the prostate or that it is an inflammatory process.[2,3] Table 54.1 illustrates the NIH consensus.

EPIDEMIOLOGY

Definition and nomenclature

Acute bacterial prostatitis (ABP, NIH I) is an acute febrile illness that may be characterized by intense pain in the perineum and rectum, fever, voiding difficulties, systemic symptoms of sepsis and a tender, swollen prostate on rectal examination. The chronic prostatitis syndromes – chronic bacterial prostatitis (CBP) or chronic prostatitis/chronic pelvic pain syndrome (CP/CPPS) – cause symptoms that in the majority of cases cannot be differentiated from each other (Table 54.2). Patients with CBP (NIH II), however, often present with recurrent urinary tract infections. Pathogens must be present in EPS or VB$_3$ for a conclusive diagnosis of CBP.[4] In patients who have signs of inflammation (CP/CPPS, NIH IIIA), leukocytes (neutrophils, macrophages) are present in EPS or VB$_3$ or in ejaculate. In noninflammatory CP/CPPS (NIH IIIB) no signs of inflammation are detectable. In asymptomatic inflammatory prostatitis (NIH IV), detected either by prostatic histology or by the presence of leukocytes in seminal fluid or in prostate secretion during evaluation for other disorders, the patients have no subjective symptoms (see Table 54.1).

Incidence and prevalence

Because of classification difficulties, few data are available to determine the incidences of all the prostatic entities. Acute prostatitis is infrequent, with a probable incidence of fewer than 1 in 1000 adult men per year. However, prostatic symptoms are common. In the USA approximately 30% of men between 20 and 50 years of age experience 'prostatitis-like' symptoms[5] and these symptoms are responsible for about 25% of physician office visits by men for genitourinary complaints.[5–7] Prostatitis is the most common urologic diagnosis in men under 50 years of age and the third most common urologic diagnosis in men over 50 years of age.[8] It has been demonstrated that a diagnosis of chronic prostatitis can have a quality of life impact similar to a diagnosis of angina or Crohn's disease.[9] Thus, prostatitis is a major health-care issue, perhaps as important as the other two major prostatic diseases, namely benign hyperplasia and carcinoma.[10]

The term prostatitis implies inflammation, but only 5–10% of patients who have this diagnosis actually have a proven bacterial infection;[5,11] the remainder do not have 'significant' prostatic fluid bacterial counts. About half of these men have inflammatory CP/CPPS (NIH IIIA) with an elevated leukocyte count in prostatic fluid;[4,5,11–16] the remainder are categorized as having noninflammatory CP/CPPS (NIH IIIB). This is a diagnosis of exclusion and, in most cases, it cannot be proven that the symptoms arise from the prostate itself.

The most frequent form of prostatitis is asymptomatic inflammatory prostatitis (NIH IV). Significant scientific interest in this entity has evolved because of probable involvement in the initiation of prostate cancer.[17,18]

Risk factors

Urinary tract infections (UTIs) are the major underlying determinant of both ABP and CBP. Strains of *Escherichia coli* responsible for both ABP and CBP appear to have at least similar or even more urovirulence determinants to the *E. coli* strains that cause pyelonephritis.[19,20] Prostatic calculi can account for recurrences of CBP.[4] Bacterial microcolonies enclosed within biofilms inside prostatic acini and ducts can be a focus for bacterial persistence.[14] Inflammatory CP/CPPS may be due to intraprostatic reflux of urine causing inflammation.[21] Other presumed and unproven causes of inflammatory CP/CPPS are immunologic reactions to spermatozoa and migration of sexually transmitted organisms from the urethra.

CLINICAL FEATURES

Diagnosis

ABP is diagnosed by its clinical presentation.[6,16,22] It presents as an acute febrile illness with irritative and obstructive voiding symptoms. Prostatic massage is contraindicated and the diagnosis depends upon:
- urine and blood cultures;
- a gentle examination of the prostate that demonstrates acute inflammation; and
- urinalysis, which usually demonstrates pyuria.

Table 54.1 The National Institutes of Health consensus classification of prostatitis syndromes[2]

Category	Characteristic clinical features	Bacteriuria*	Inflammation†
I. Acute bacterial	Acute urinary tract infection (UTI)	+	+
II. Chronic bacterial	Recurrent UTI caused by the same organism	+	+
III. Chronic prostatitis/chronic pelvic pain syndrome (CP/CPPS) A. Inflammatory subtype‡ B. Noninflammatory subtype§	Primarily pain complaints, but also voiding complaints and sexual dysfunction	− −	+ −
IV. Asymptomatic	Diagnosed during evaluation of other genitourinary diseases	−	+

*In chronic bacterial prostatitis VB$_2$ can be sterile and bacteriuria can only be detected in expressed prostatic secretion (EPS) or VB$_3$.
†Objective evidence of an inflammatory response in EPS, postprostate massage urine or semen or by histology.
‡Formerly termed 'nonbacterial prostatitis'.
§Formerly termed 'prostatodynia'.

Table 54.2 Symptoms in patients with the chronic prostatitis syndromes

Urethral symptoms	• Burning in the urethra during voiding • Discharge • Difficult urination • Stranguria • Frequency • Nocturia
Prostatic symptoms	• Pressure behind pubic bone • Perineal pressure tension in testes and epididymes • Inguinal pain • Anorectal dysesthesia • Diffuse anogenital syndromes • Lower abdominal discomfort
Sexual dysfunction	• Loss of libido • Erectile dysfunction • Ejaculatory dysfunction • Pain during or after orgasm
Other symptoms	• Myalgia • Headache • Fatigue

Depending on the patient's history, two different types of acute bacterial prostatitis – spontaneous and manipulated – have been described.[23] Approximately 10% of acute prostatitis cases might be elicited by previous manipulation of the lower urinary tract (e.g. prostatic biopsies, transurethral manipulation). Patients with acute bacterial prostatitis secondary to manipulation are older and appear to have a higher risk of prostate abscess formation.

Prostatic abscesses may occur in patients who have acute prostatitis. This diagnosis is made by clinical examination and transrectal ultrasonography. Focal hypoechoic zones with irregular internal echoes, septations and indirect borders with the surrounding parenchyma are typical patterns. The abscess may be distinct or more diffuse. Prostatic abscesses are usually due to the same uropathogens that are responsible for ABP, although a variety of anaerobes and fungi are implicated sporadically. Systemic mycoses, particularly *Cryptococcus neoformans*, *Blastomyces dermatitidis*, *Coccidioides immitis* or *Histoplasma capsulatum*, can rarely involve the prostate gland and produce prostatic abscesses. *Candida albicans* can also cause prostatic abscesses.

Chronic bacterial prostatitis is a rather precise diagnosis. It often presents as the source of acute recurrent UTI and/or recurrent ABP. Patients presenting with prostatic complaints should have a prostatic massage to localize the infection. The method of choice is the Meares and Stamey localization technique (Fig. 54.1).[24] Increased numbers of neutrophils and fat-laden macrophages are typical cytologic signs in the EPS. Although increased numbers of leukocytes may be found in the EPS, it is generally accepted that over 10 neutrophils per high-power field indicates prostatitis.[16,20] In patients for whom an EPS cannot be obtained, increased numbers of neutrophils in the urine after prostatic massage (VB$_3$) is an indication of prostatitis if first voided urine (VB$_1$) and midstream urine (VB$_2$) do not contain these cells. In patients who have CBP, bacterial pathogens will be present in the EPS or VB$_3$ in larger numbers, usually a 10-fold higher concentration than in the VB$_1$ and VB$_2$.[16,20] The exact technique for localizing infection with the Meares and Stamey technique is outlined in Figure 54.1 and should be followed carefully.[24]

A simpler screening test to assess inflammation/infection is the two-glass pre- and post-massage test (PPMT). Compared with the four-glass test, the PPMT has a rather good concordance with the four-glass test for the initial evaluation.[25] The PPMT is therefore a reasonable alternative when EPS cannot be obtained or when microbiologic assistance is not available (EPS, due to its usually small volume, has to be processed and plated immediately).

The role of *Chlamydia trachomatis* and *Ureaplasma urealyticum* in bacterial prostatitis is uncertain and there are no widely accepted criteria for defining prostatitis due to these or other infrequently isolated pathogens (Table 54.3).[26–28]

Ejaculate analysis is sometimes recommended in men who have CBP to obtain further information but studies of seminal fluid are mostly unhelpful. A proportion of men who have CBP have bacteriospermia (>10^3 cfu/ml) and the organisms present are usually identical to those in the EPS.[29] As semen cultures identify significant bacteriospermia in only about 50% of semen specimens from men with CBP,[30] culture of the ejaculate alone is not sufficient to diagnose CBP.[22,30]

Biochemical analysis of EPS has been used as an additional diagnostic criterion for CBP but these observations have not been shown to be sufficiently sensitive or specific to add to the diagnosis (Fig. 54.2).[16,20] The pH is usually increased (>7.8) in the EPS from patients who have CBP.

Biopsy under ultrasonographic guidance, particularly if nodules are present, is used for histology and culture.[4,12,31] Inflammatory findings in the prostate are usually nonspecific and the primary indication for biopsy is to exclude prostatic cancer.

Evaluation of bladder emptying by flow rate measurements and ultrasonography can be useful in patients who have voiding disturbances.[31] On occasion this diagnostic workup should include a voiding

Meares and Stamey localization technique

1. Approximately 30 minutes before taking the specimen, the patient should drink 400 ml of liquid (two glasses). The test starts when the patient wants to void
2. The lids of four sterile specimen containers, which are marked VB_1, VB_2, EPS and VB_3, should be removed. Place the uncovered specimen containers on a flat surface and maintain sterility
3. Hands are washed
4. Expose the penis and retract the foreskin so that the glans is exposed. The foreskin should be retracted throughout
5. Cleanse the glans with a soap solution, remove the soap with sterile gauze or cotton and dry the glans
6. Urinate 10–15 ml into the first container marked VB_1
7. Urinate 100–200 ml into the toilet bowl or vessel and without interrupting the urine stream, urinate 10–15 ml into the second container marked VB_2
8. The patient bends forward and holds the sterile specimen container (EPS) to catch the prostate secretion
9. The physician massages the prostate until several drops of prostate secretion (EPS) are obtained
10. If no EPS can be collected during massage, a drop may be present at the orifice of the urethra and this drop should be taken with a 10 ml calibrated loop and cultured
11. Immediately after prostatic massage, the patient urinates 10–15 ml of urine into the container marked VB_3.

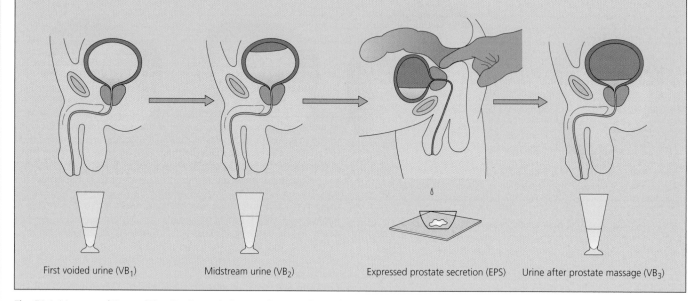

First voided urine (VB_1)   Midstream urine (VB_2)   Expressed prostate secretion (EPS)   Urine after prostate massage (VB_3)

Fig. 54.1 Meares and Stamey[24] localization technique to diagnose chronic bacterial prostatitis. Prostate secretion can be more readily obtained if the patient has not ejaculated for approximately 3–5 days before the examination.

cystourethrogram. Urodynamic changes are present in about one-third of patients who have CBP. In the presence of abnormal flow rate measurements, further studies should be performed to differentiate between functional and anatomic changes.

Urethrocystoscopy may reveal visible inflammatory changes in the posterior urethra. Prostatic sonography may demonstrate prostatic calculi (Fig. 54.3). Prostatic calculi may serve as nidi for pathogens and lead to CBP; however, as they are common and increase with age, their role remains controversial. Figure 54.4 outlines the diagnostic investigation of patients who present with possible CBP.[22]

Chronic prostatitis/chronic pelvic pain syndrome is a less specific diagnosis. In CP/CPPS (NIH IIIA) inflammatory cells in the EPS with negative cultures from both the EPS and VB_3 are found. Although numerous investigators have attempted to demonstrate that CP/CPPS (NIH IIIA) is due to difficult-to-culture pathogens such as *C. trachomatis* or genital mycoplasmas, there is no consensus that these organisms cause CP/CPPS (NIH IIIA).[26,32,33] As a result, this diagnosis is currently poorly defined and is presumed to be caused by largely unknown etiologic and pathogenetic processes.

In CP/CPPS (NIH IIIB) neither inflammatory cells nor positive cultures are found in EPS and VB_3. For a better discrimination of NIH IIIA from NIH IIIB, novel parameters, such as interleukin-8, have been investigated.[34,35] The exact limits of these parameters, however, are currently under discussion.

MANAGEMENT

Treatment varies according to the severity of the patient's presenting symptoms and the probable etiologic agent. Antimicrobial treatment should be initiated immediately in patients who have acute bacterial prostatitis after blood and urine cultures have been obtained. Prostatic massage is contraindicated. Parenteral treatment with a fluoroquinolone or a β-lactam with an aminoglycoside are appropriate initial regimens. After initial improvement, a switch to an oral regimen is appropriate and should be prescribed for about 2–4 weeks. Optimal antibiotics would be fluoroquinolones, if tested susceptible.

Patients who have possible CBP require investigation for evidence of inflammation and an etiologic agent. Selection of an appropriate antimicrobial agent that has optimal pharmacokinetics for prostatic secretion and tissue is important.[36] Antibacterial diffusion into prostate secretion depends upon the lipid solubility, molecular size and pKa of the agent.[36] For example, trimethoprim, a weak base with a pKa of 7.4, penetrates well into the acid prostatic secretion. However, because the pH of prostatic fluid in patients who have CBP is often alkaline, concentrations in prostatic secretion may be inadequate.[37,38] In contrast, the fluoroquinolones exist as zwitterions with a pKa in acid and alkaline milieus[39] (Table 54.4). Due to the relatively large

Table 54.3 Prostatitis infections by unconventional fastidious pathogens

Species	Clinical features	Comment
Haemophilus influenzae		Single case reports
Neisseria gonorrhoeae	Associated with history of gonococcal urethritis	Decreasing due to effective antibiotic treatment
Mycobacterium tuberculosis	Urogenital manifestation	Associated with HIV infection
Anaerobes	Prostatic abscesses	
Brucella spp.	Disseminated disease	Consumption of unpasteurized diary products and occupational contact
Candida spp.	In immuno-compromised patients with indwelling urinary catheters	
Coccidioides immitis, Blastomyces dermatitidis, Histoplasma capsulatum	Disseminated disease	Associated with HIV infection
Trichomonas vaginalis	Chronic inflammation	May be associated with urethritis

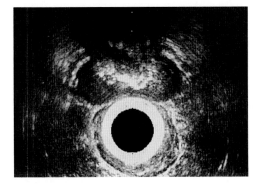

Fig. 54.3 Transrectal ultrasonography of the prostate with diffuse calcifications (prostatitis calcarea).

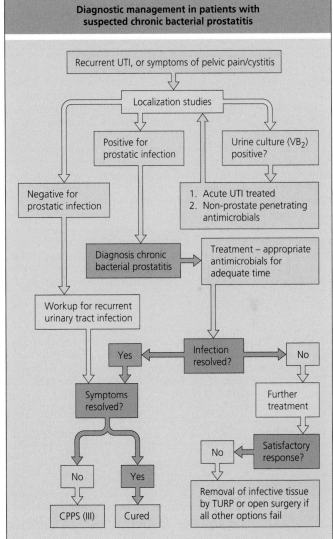

Fig. 54.4 Diagnostic management in patients with suspected chronic bacterial prostatitis. TURP, transurethral resection of prostate; UTI, urinary tract infection. Modified from Schaeffer et al.[22]

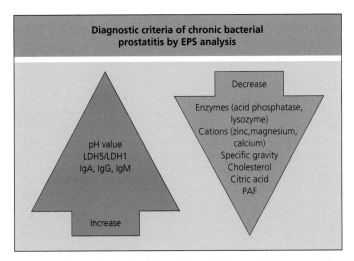

Fig. 54.2 Diagnostic criteria of chronic bacterial prostatitis by expressed prostatic secretion analysis. LDH, lactate dehydrogenase; PAF, prostatic antibacterial factor.

differences in pKa values of the different fluoroquinolones (Table 54.4), the prostatic fluid:plasma concentration ratios range from 0.10 to 1.57 (Table 54.5).[40–46] The concentration of some fluoroquinolones in the alkaline seminal fluid may even exceed that in plasma (Table 54.5).[42,44] There exists a positive correlation of the isoelectric points of the fluoroquinolones and the prostatic secretion to plasma concentration ratios, investigated in volunteers (Fig. 54.5).

Other studies have examined fluoroquinolone concentrations in prostatic tissue obtained at transurethral resection and they appear to be consistently at or above corresponding plasma concentrations.[47] These investigations, however, resemble a mixture of different pharmacokinetic compartments (e.g. intracellular, extracellular, interstitial

Table 54.4 Dissociation constants of fluoroquinolones[39]

Quinolone	Pk_{a1}	Pk_{a2}
Ciprofloxacin	6.1	8.7
Enoxacin	6.3	8.7
Fleroxacin	5.5	8.1
Gatifloxacin	6.0	9.2
Levofloxacin	6.1	8.2
Lomefloxacin	5.8	9.3
Moxifloxacin	6.4	9.5
Norfloxacin	6.3	8.4
Ofloxacin	6.0	8.2
Pefloxacin	6.3	7.6
Sparfloxacin	6.3	8.8

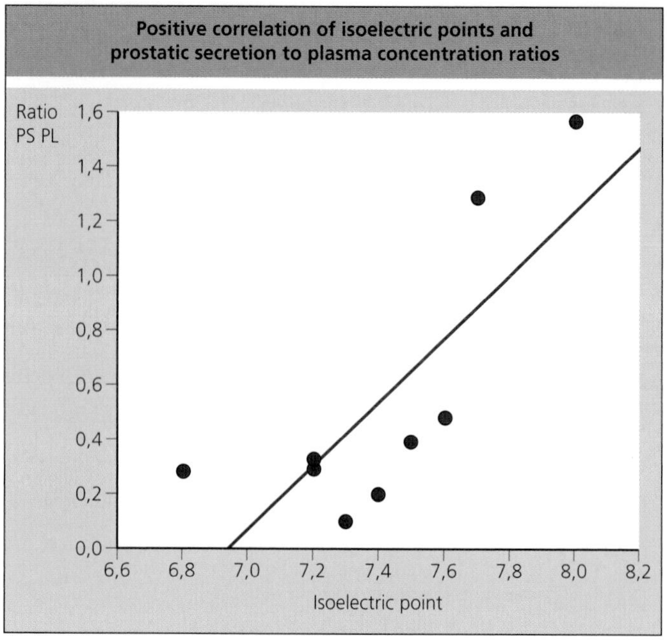

Fig. 54.5 Positive correlation of the isoelectric points and the prostatic secretion to plasma concentration ratios (PS/PL) of nine quinolones (see Table 54.5) (Pearson correlation, $P = 0.013$). Modified from Wagenlehner et al.[42]

compartment). Therefore assessment of concentrations in the prostatic fluid is the more precise method. Macrolides also penetrate into prostatic and seminal fluids very well; however, due to their restricted Gram-positive activity, they play only a limited role in the monotherapy treatment of CBP.[36,48]

Although it remains unproven, considerable evidence suggests that bacteria in prostatic tissue survive in a milieu protected by biofilms. Antimicrobial agents (particularly the fluoroquinolones and the macrolides) that are active in biofilm infection may be preferred drugs. Theoretically a combination therapy of fluoroquinolones and macrolides might be beneficial because of the anti-biofilm activity of the macrolides; however, no such data from studies in CBP patients are available. Most studies in patients who have CBP have not been well controlled and have been variably designed.[47,49] As a result, comparison is difficult. Duration of therapy has ranged from 14 to 150 days and follow-up investigation has not been standardized. An EPS should

be obtained from all patients at 4–8 weeks and at 6 months after treatment to ensure that the pathogens have been eradicated.[49]

Overall, it appears that 60–80% of patients who have *Escherichia coli* and other Enterobacteriaceae can be cured with a 4- to 6-week course of therapy (Table 54.6).[50-56] However, prostatitis due to *Pseudomonas aeruginosa* or enterococci often fails to respond to treatment and the increasing fluoroquinolone resistance among Enterobacteriaceae leads to increasing treatment failures in those species as well. In the case of CBP due to fluoroquinolone-resistant strains, prolonged treatment with co-trimoxazole for 2–3 months is recommended.

Table 54.5 Median concentrations of fluoroquinolones in prostatic and seminal fluid and fluid to plasma concentration ratios (normalized to a dose of 400 mg)

Quinolone	Dose (400 mg)	Time (h)	Subjects (n)	Prostatic fluid (mg/l)	Ratio of prostatic:plasma concentration*	Seminal fluid (mg/l)	Ratio of seminal:plasma concentration	Reference
Norfloxacin	po	1–4	7	0.08	0.10	n.d.	–	Naber & Sorgel[41]
Ciprofloxacin	iv	4	8	0.18	0.20	5.06	7.1	Naber et al.[45]
Fleroxacin	po	2–4	8	1.00	0.28	5.80	1.7	Naber & Sorgel[41]
Levofloxacin	po	3	8	1.42	0.29	5.14	1.0	Bulitta et al.[40]
Ofloxacin	iv	4	5	0.66	0.33	2.05	4.0	Naber et al.[46]
Enoxacin	po	2–4	10	0.29	0.39	2.19	2.2	Naber & Sorgel[41]
Lomefloxacin	po	4	7	1.38	0.48	2.03	1.2	Naber & Sorgel[41]
Gatifloxacin	po	4	7	1.03	1.29	1.75	1.0	Farker et al.[43] Naber et al.[44]
Moxifloxacin	po	3–4	8	3.99	1.57	2.43	1.0	Wagenlehner et al.[42]

n.d., no data.
*Ordered according to prostatic fluid to plasma ratios.

Table 54.6 Eradication of pathogens (bacteriologic cure) in patients with chronic bacterial prostatitis treated with fluoroquinolones

Quinolone	Daily dosage (mg)	Duration of therapy (days)	Number of evaluable patients	Bacteriologic cure (%)	Duration of follow-up (months)	Year of study	References*
Norfloxacin	800	28	14	64	6	1990	Schaeffer & Darras[50]
Ofloxacin	400	14	21	67	12	1989	Pust et al.[51]
Ciprofloxacin	1000	14	15	60	12	1987	Weidner et al.[52]
Ciprofloxacin	1000	28	16	63	21–36	1991	Weidner et al.[53]
Ciprofloxacin	1000	60–150	7	86	12	1991	Pfau[54]
Ciprofloxacin	1000	28	34	76	6	2000	Naber et al.[55]
Ciprofloxacin	1000	28	78	72	6	2001	Naber[56]
Lomefloxacin	400	28	75	63	6	2001	Naber[56]

Only studies are listed in which the diagnosis was derived from application of the Meares and Stamey technique and a follow-up of at least 6 months was available.

Chronic bacterial prostatitis can be a relapsing illness and recurrent episodes are best managed by continuous low-dose suppressive therapy with an effective regimen such as a fluoroquinolone, intermittent treatment whenever symptoms recur, or efforts to resect infected prostatic tissue, particularly prostatic calculi, in order to effect a surgical cure.[5] The last is rarely successful and should only be carried out with very specific indications.

A prostatic abscess may require drainage in addition to antimicrobial treatment. Occasionally, anaerobes or mixed infections may be responsible for the abscess. Cultures should always be obtained and, if fungal infection is suspected, the laboratory should be informed. Most treatment regimens should include an agent effective against anaerobes. Prostatic abscesses can be drained through the urethra, the perineum or the rectum.

Inflammatory CP/CPPS (NIH IIIA) is managed with α-blockers for 3–6 months, although a recent study has not shown any improved effect compared to placebo.[56A] A pollen extract (Cernilton) has recently been shown to significantly improve pain and total symptoms, specifically in patients with CP/CPPS (NIH IIIA).[56B] Occasionally, patients appear to have a very specific response to antimicrobial therapy and, whenever this occurs, a prolongation of therapy is indicated. However, most patients who have inflammatory CP/CPPS do not experience any change in symptoms with antibacterial therapy. Other treatment regimens include anti-inflammatory agents, phytotherapeutics and pain medications. However, all regimens are empiric and treatment is often unsatisfactory.

Noninflammatory CP/CPPS (NIH IIIB) is an imprecise diagnosis for which therapy is controversial. Although the symptoms can mimic those of CBP, the absence of inflammation or any signs of infection are presumed to mean that no microbial agent is involved.[2,3] Noninflammatory CP/CPPS is probably the most frequent entity when patients are presenting with symptoms of prostatitis. Treatment regimens are similar to those used for inflammatory CP/CPPS, with the exception that antibiotics do not have any role in this entity.

Epididymitis and orchitis

Epididymitis is an acute painful swelling in the scrotum, which is usually unilateral.[57] The testes may be involved in the inflammatory process as 'epididymo-orchitis'. Inflammatory processes of the testes, especially viral orchitis, less often involve the epididymis.

EPIDEMIOLOGY

Orchitis and epididymitis are classified as acute or chronic processes according to their cause (Table 54.7). Chronic inflammation with induration develops in about 15% of patients following an episode of acute epididymitis. Viral and bacterial inflammation of the testes can lead to testicular atrophy and destruction of spermatogenesis.[58]

Epididymitis is common among individuals who have high-risk sexual behaviors (frequent change of sexual partners) and is one of the leading causes of acute admission to hospital among military personnel. It occurs in 1–2% of patients who have gonococcal and chlamydial urethritis, with an equal risk from each. It is usually unilateral and is due to an extension of the urethral infection via the vas deferens to the epididymis.

In middle-aged and older men, epididymitis is usually due to the same organisms as those that cause UTI and is presumably a direct extension from the urinary tract. Epididymitis is more common in patients who have indwelling catheters. Bladder outlet obstruction and urogenital abnormalities are also risk factors for acute and chronic epididymo-orchitis.

Mumps orchitis was common before widespread vaccination but became rare in the 1990s. However, due to decreasing vaccination coverage in western populations, mumps notifications and orchitis cases

Table 54.7 Classification of epididymitis and orchitis

Acute epididymitis or epididymo-orchitis	Granulomatous epididymitis or orchitis	Viral orchitis
Neisseria gonorrhoeae	Mycobacterium tuberculosis	Mumps
Chlamydia trachomatis	Treponema pallidum	Enteroviruses
Escherichia coli	Brucella spp.	
Streptococcus pneumoniae	Sarcoid	
Klebsiella spp.	Fungal	
Salmonella spp.	Parasitic	
Other urinary tract pathogens	Idiopathic	
Idiopathic		

have increased rapidly in the past few years. Mumps orchitis occurs in 20–30% of postpubertal men who have mumps. Other viral infections can also cause orchitis, particularly enteroviruses. The testes can also be involved as a continuation of epididymitis, particularly when suppurative UTI pathogens are involved. Granulomatous orchitis is a rare condition of uncertain etiology.[59] With regard to chronic inflammatory conditions, a so-called 'low-grade autoimmune orchitis'[60] has been described.

Epididymo-orchitis can lead to abscess formation, testicular infarction, testicular atrophy, chronic epididymitis and infertility.[57] In men who have azoospermia, postinflammatory epididymal obstruction can sometimes be cured by reconstructive surgery.[61]

CLINICAL FEATURES

Inflammation, pain and scrotal swelling characterize acute epididymitis.[57] Frequently the tail of the epididymis is involved first. The spermatic cord is usually tender and enlarged. The testes may be spared or may be involved to produce a contiguous large painful mass. Acute epididymitis always requires immediate evaluation by Doppler duplex scanning to differentiate between acute epididymitis and spermatic cord torsion. The latter requires urgent surgical intervention to prevent testicular infarction.[62]

The microbiologic diagnosis of acute epididymitis must be made as specifically as possible. A urethral Gram stain, urine culture and other studies (e.g. amplification techniques) for identification of *Neisseria gonorrhoeae* and *C. trachomatis* should be obtained for all patients. Blood cultures are valuable if the patient is febrile or has systemic signs of toxicity. Ejaculate analysis according to World Health Organization (WHO) criteria, including leukocyte analysis, may be of value. A transiently decreased sperm count or azoospermia is common. Infertility is a rare complication unless there is bilateral involvement.

Chronic epididymitis is characterized by thickening and induration of the epididymis. Especially in patients who are infertile, ejaculate analysis concerning semen quality is a necessary investigation to exclude azoospermia[60] and changes of sperm maturation.[63]

Orchitis, an isolated inflammation of the testis, is a rare event. Most frequently it occurs in association with epididymitis, as epididymo-orchitis (see Table 54.7). Testicular swelling, frequently accompanied by fever, is typical. Antibody and other specific serum investigations should be carried out to identify mumps, enteroviruses and other potential viral pathogens. In chronic infections, ejaculate analysis may demonstrate structural sperm defects providing reduced sperm motility and number.[60] Testicular biopsy in these cases may demonstrate focal inflammation, mixed atrophy and complete Sertoli-cell-only syndrome in the follow-up.[58]

MANAGEMENT

In acute epididymitis (epididymo-orchitis), antimicrobial agents should be chosen for initial empiric treatment based on the probability of the etiologic agent. In sexually active men who are at risk of *C. trachomatis* or *N. gonorrhoeae*, a therapeutic regimen that covers both these pathogens is mandatory.

Antibiotic resistance in *N. gonorrhoeae* has increased dramatically over the past few years. The WHO surveillance of antibiotic resistance in *N. gonorrhoeae* in the Western Pacific Region, carried out in 2005, revealed resistance rates of penicillins and quinolones up to 100%, and of tetracyclines up to 80% in some countries.[64] Penicillin- and fluoroquinolone-resistant strains have already reached western countries. The Centers for Disease Control and Prevention (CDC) therefore adapted to this resistance trend and now recommend ceftriaxone as first-line agent for the treatment of acute epididymitis caused by *N. gonorrhoeae* in a rather low single dose of 250 mg intramuscularly.[65] Additional treatment of nongonococcal agents with a tetracycline is also recommended.[65]

Additional therapy includes scrotal support. Abscesses may require surgical drainage. If urinary tract pathogens are considered to be the probable etiologic agent, fluoroquinolones or trimethoprim–sulfamethoxazole are appropriate choices. Experimental[66] and clinical[67] studies suggest that the fluoroquinolones are very effective, if the pathogens test susceptible.

Interferon alpha (IFN-α) has been prescribed for the treatment of acute mumps orchitis.[60,68] However, further studies in which testicular biopsies were performed after treatment have shown that systemic treatment with IFN-α is not completely effective in preventing testicular atrophy after mumps orchitis.[69] Therapy with nonsteroidal anti-inflammatory agents has also been recommended,[70] as has treatment with long-acting gonadotrophin-releasing hormone agonists.[71] Use of steroids should be avoided, because concentrations of testosterone could be decreased and concentrations of follicle-stimulating and luteinizing hormones could be increased, facilitating testicular atrophy.[72]

REFERENCES

References for this chapter can be found online at http://www.expertconsult.com

Chapter | **55** | *Dimitri M Drekonja*
James R Johnson

Pyelonephritis and abscesses of the kidney

INTRODUCTION

Acute pyelonephritis, an acute infection (usually bacterial) of the kidney and renal pelvis, is one of the most common serious infectious diseases of otherwise healthy individuals, and is an even greater problem for compromised hosts. New approaches to the diagnosis and management of this disorder and its sequelae, including intrarenal and perinephric abscess, have resulted in improved outcomes for patients.

EPIDEMIOLOGY

Annually in the USA, approximately 200 000 adults are admitted to hospital for renal infection;[1,2] many others are managed as outpatients. In Seattle, Washington, the annual risk of pyelonephritis is approximately 12–13/10 000 for women and 3–4/10 000 for men.[3]

Complicated versus uncomplicated pyelonephritis

Pyelonephritis can be stratified as 'complicated' or 'uncomplicated', depending on the presence of underlying urologic or medical conditions that predispose to kidney infection or that aggravate the severity or intransigence of such infections once they occur.[1] Uncomplicated and complicated pyelonephritis have distinctive host substrates, microbial flora, pathogenetic mechanisms, clinical presentations and requirements for and response to therapy.

Risk factors

Although little is known about the specific risk factors for uncomplicated pyelonephritis, recognized risk factors for uncomplicated cystitis would be predicted to predispose to pyelonephritis also. Such associations include female sex and, among adolescent or adult women, sexual intercourse, a history of previous urinary tract infections (UTIs), use of spermicide-diaphragm contraception and being a nonsecretor of blood group substances (see Chapter 42). The postmenopausal state has also been associated with increased rates of UTI.[4,5] Among children, the P_1 blood group phenotype is associated with an increased pyelonephritis risk.[6] Further evidence for an inherited cause of pyelonephritis comes from a study involving a cohort of children predisposed to acute pyelonephritis. Investigators found increased rates of pyelonephritis in relatives of these children when compared to relatives of matched controls, despite similar rates of cystitis in the two groups. Expression of CXCR1 on peripheral blood neutrophils was

significantly decreased in the families with a history of pyelonephritis, suggesting this receptor may play a role in the pathogenesis of the disease.[7]

Pyelonephritis in compromised hosts, which by definition is 'complicated', is promoted by almost any anatomic or functional abnormality of the urinary tract, urinary tract instrumentation, diabetes mellitus, pregnancy (during which the risk of pyelonephritis is 1–2%) and conditions associated with sensory impairment (such as diabetic or alcoholic neuropathies and spinal cord injury).[1] Among the commonly implicated urologic conditions are posterior urethral valves (in infant boys), congenital vesicoureteral reflux (in girls), indwelling or intermittent urinary catheterization, other instrumentation of the urinary tract, neurogenic bladder, urolithiasis, ureteral diversions, any obstruction to normal urinary flow and kidney transplantation. Pyelonephritis in an immunosuppressed host does not imply that the infection is complicated per se, as the spectrum of expected infectious agents is similar to that seen in immune competent hosts, as is the response to and duration of therapy.

Renal abscess, which can be intrarenal, intrarenal with perirenal extension or entirely perirenal, typically develops as a consequence of acute pyelonephritis and is among the most serious local complications of this illness. It occurs predominantly in compromised hosts, notably patients who have diabetes mellitus or have undergone recent surgery or instrumentation of the urinary tract. Urinary reflux and obstruction are prominent risk factors for renal abscess. Rarely, a renal abscess may develop during a severe episode of otherwise uncomplicated pyelonephritis in an intact host.

PATHOGENESIS

Route of infection

Irrespective of the presence of predisposing host conditions, in almost all patients acute pyelonephritis arises via an ascending route of infection.[1] The causative micro-organisms enter the urethra, colonize the bladder, then ascend the ureters to the renal pelvis and subsequently invade the renal parenchyma. In most cases, the pathogens arise from the host's own intestinal (and, in women, vaginal) flora,[8] although in patients who have indwelling catheters or nephrostomy tubes organisms may be transferred on the hands of health-care workers and thus bypass the intestinal, vaginal and/or bladder colonization steps.

Microbial flora

Organisms must have substantial intrinsic virulence to overcome the many defense mechanisms of a healthy urinary tract and cause pyelonephritis in an intact host. In contrast, organisms of lesser intrinsic virulence can infect the kidney in patients who have impaired urinary tract defenses. Paradoxically, the less virulent organisms associated with complicated pyelonephritis are more often resistant to antimicrobial agents than are the more virulent ones that cause uncomplicated pyelonephritis. This, together with the impaired defense mechanisms of compromised hosts, makes such infections more difficult to treat and cure than uncomplicated pyelonephritis.

In uncomplicated pyelonephritis the distribution of microorganisms is similar to that in uncomplicated cystitis, with approximately 80% of isolates being *Escherichia coli* and the remainder other Gram-negative bacilli (predominantly *Klebsiella* and *Proteus* spp.), *Staphylococcus saprophyticus* (especially in young women), *Enterococcus* spp. (especially in older men) and occasionally group B or other streptococci.[1] The *E. coli* strains that cause uncomplicated pyelonephritis exhibit multiple virulence properties that contribute to their ability to invade the urinary tract and stimulate inflammation and tissue damage (Fig. 55.1).[9]

Among the various adhesins expressed by these strains, the most prevalent and pathogenetically important are type 1 fimbriae and P fimbriae. P fimbriae are strongly epidemiologically associated with pyelonephritis[9] and contribute to kidney infection in a monkey model.[10] They recognize Galα(1–4)Gal-containing receptors on host epithelial surfaces, including the mucosal lining of the colon, vagina and urinary tract. The P fimbrial adhesin molecule PapG is situated at the tip of the fimbrial stalk and mediates attachment to receptors on the host cell. PapG occurs in three known variants, of which the class II variant is the most common among strains that cause uncomplicated pyelonephritis and bacteremic UTIs, whereas the class III variant is associated with cystitis and with complicated UTIs.

Type 1 fimbriae are structurally similar to P fimbriae but have a binding specificity for mannose-containing receptors on host cells. Since type 1 fimbriae are produced by almost all *E. coli*, epidemiologic associations of type 1 fimbriae with UTI or pyelonephritis are difficult to demonstrate. However, in the mouse model of UTI, deletion of the type 1 fimbrial adhesin gene or immunization against the corresponding FimH adhesin molecule reduces both bladder and kidney infection. Other important virulence factors of pyelonephritogenic *E. coli*

include cytotoxins such as α-hemolysin (which destroys or impairs the function of host epithelial cells, phagocytes and lymphocytes), iron sequestration systems such as the aerobactin system, polysaccharide capsules, lipopolysaccharide and serum resistance proteins (which protect the organism against phagocytosis and/or complement-mediated lysis).[9,11]

In complicated pyelonephritis, although *E. coli* still is the single most common pathogen, it is less prevalent than in uncomplicated pyelonephritis and is represented by less virulent strains. Other Gram-negative bacilli are more commonly encountered, including *Pseudomonas aeruginosa*, *Enterobacter* spp. and other Enterobacteriaciae.[1]

Factors promoting ascending infection

Vaginal colonization with urovirulent organisms is promoted by sexual intercourse, particularly with the use of a spermicide, which kills normal lactobacillus-based vaginal flora and permits overgrowth with *E. coli* and other coliform bacteria.[8] Similar changes in the vaginal flora occur after the menopause as a result of estrogen depletion, and are induced by the use of certain antimicrobial agents, notably β-lactams.

In women, sexual intercourse promotes the entry of periurethral bacteria into the bladder on a mechanical basis. In catheterized patients, bacteria can be introduced into the bladder at the time of catheter insertion, or can migrate into the bladder along the external or luminal surfaces of catheters.[12] With improper catheter care, infected urine from the collecting bag and drainage tubing can reflux into the bladder. Antireflux valves are standard on most indwelling catheters; however, there is little evidence that they prevent bacteriuria or catheter-associated UTI. Catheter-associated organisms persist within the urinary tract in part by cementing themselves to the catheter within glycocalyx matrices that protect them against natural host defense mechanisms and antimicrobial agents. Uropathogenic *E. coli* have been demonstrated to invade the bladder epithelium in a mouse UTI model, suggesting a possible method for evading host defenses and establishing a persisting intracellular reservoir from which organisms could re-emerge to cause recurrent UTI. Whether this phenomenon

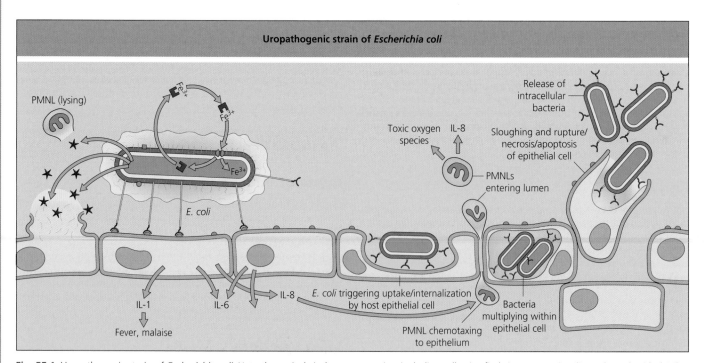

Fig. 55.1 Uropathogenic strain of *Escherichia coli*. Note the typical virulence properties, including adhesive fimbriae, cytotoxins, lipopolysaccharide (LPS), capsular polysaccharide, the aerobactin iron sequestration system and outer membrane proteins important in serum resistance. Bacterial interactions with host cells trigger cytokine production, inflammatory cell infiltration and bacterial internalization within epithelial cells. Internalized bacteria can multiply intracellularly and stimulate sloughing, rupture, necrosis or apoptosis of host cells. IL, interleukin; PMNLs, polymorphonuclear leukocytes.

contributes to the pathogenesis of UTI, and specifically pyelonephritis, in humans is undefined.

Ascent of pathogens from the bladder up the ureters is facilitated by vesicoureteral reflux, which may be pre-existing or which in the intact host can result from a reversible ureteral aperistalsis induced by exposure of the ureteral wall to lipopolysaccharide from adherent bacteria.[13] Bacterial flagellae also likely contribute to ureteral ascent against urine flow.[14] Among several UTI-promoting physiologic alterations of pregnancy, ureteral hypotonia and some degree of ureteral obstruction may contribute to bacterial entry into the upper urinary tract in pregnant women and its persistence once there.[10] Once within the renal pelvis, micro-organisms migrate up the collecting ducts into the tubules, a process promoted by intrarenal reflux (if present in the particular host) and by bacterial adhesins that recognize receptors along this epithelial surface or in subjacent tissues.[9,13]

PATHOLOGY

Within the urinary tract, pathogenic bacteria adhere to the mucosa and trigger a local cytokine/chemokine network, with production of interleukin (IL)-1, IL-6, IL-8 and tumor necrosis factor, and recruitment of polymorphonuclear leukocytes (PMNLs) and lymphocytes. Triggers include the interaction of bacterial lipopolysaccharide with host cell Toll-like receptor 4 (TLR4), P fimbrial binding to host membrane glycolipids, which activates an intracellular ceramide signaling pathway, and type-1-fimbria-mediated bacterial internalization. The influx of inflammatory cells leads to the generation of reactive oxygen species, leukotrienes, prostaglandins and other mediators of inflammation, which together with bacterial cytotoxins produce tissue damage, edema and, in the kidney, intense local vasoconstriction (see Fig. 55.1).[1,13] These phenomena presumably are responsible for the characteristic signs and symptoms of pyelonephritis, including dysuria and suprapubic pain from bladder involvement, flank pain and costovertebral angle tenderness from kidney involvement, and fever and malaise from inflammatory cytokines that enter the systemic circulation.

Histologically, in acute pyelonephritis the mucosa and submucosa of the collecting system, the tubules and the interstitium are edematous and infiltrated with PMNLs (Fig. 55.2). Tubules may necrose. Microabscesses form within the mucosa and interstitium, and can coalesce to form macroscopic abscesses.[1]

Grossly, the kidneys are diffusely or focally swollen and edematous. On sectioning, streaks of yellowish inflammatory infiltrate extend from the papillae and medulla toward the cortex, sometimes reaching the capsule and rupturing it.[1] When macroscopic abscesses do form, typically they localize at the corticomedullary junction but can be subcapsular or extend into the perirenal space.[7] In hyperglycemic diabetic patients, rapid fermentation of glucose by Gram-negative bacilli (or, rarely, yeasts) can produce gas within the renal parenchyma (emphysematous pyelonephritis; Fig. 55.3), within an abscess (gas abscess) or within the renal pelvis and collecting system (emphysematous pyelitis).[15] Papillary necrosis, which occasionally complicates acute pyelonephritis among diabetic patients, may make the infection worse because of the obstruction caused by sloughed tissue (Fig. 55.4).[1]

Functionally, the intense interstitial inflammatory process leads to a reduction in urinary concentrating capacity. Decreased renal blood flow, functional tubular obstruction from inflammatory cells and necrotic debris, and inflammation-induced tubular dysfunction result in delayed excretion of radiographic contrast dye[1] but only rarely manifest as clinically apparent renal dysfunction.[16]

Bacteremia develops in between 10% and 65% of patients who have acute pyelonephritis, depending on the severity of infection and increasing in proportion to the age of the host. Bacterial entry into the bloodstream may be promoted by P fimbriae and by tissue destruction mediated by microbial cytotoxins. Systemic complications of pyelonephritis, which are more common among patients who have Gram-negative bacteremia, include septic shock, disseminated intravascular coagulation and

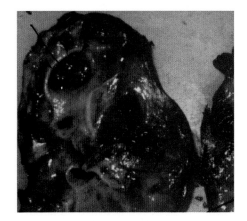

Fig. 55.3 Emphysematous pyelonephritis. Cortical necrosis (solid arrow), diffuse cortical hemorrhage (open arrow) and dilatation of the collecting system (arrowheads) in a nephrectomy specimen from a diabetic patient who received combined medical/surgical therapy and survived emphysematous pyelonephritis due to an unusual pathogen, namely *Candida albicans*.

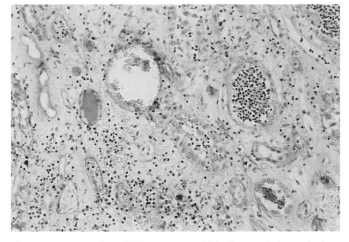

Fig. 55.2 Acute pyelonephritis. Note interstitial edema, tubules packed with PMNLs and a diffuse interstitial acute inflammatory infiltrate in this autopsy specimen from a diabetic patient who had refractory *Escherichia coli* urosepsis.

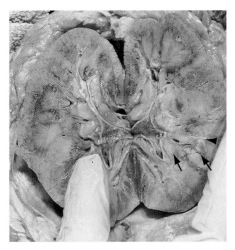

Fig. 55.4 Acute papillary necrosis (arrows) in an autopsy specimen from a diabetic patient who died from refractory *Escherichia coli* urosepsis. Necrotic papillae (arrows) failed to take up formalin, so appear pink, in contrast to the grayish-tan formalinized tissue.

the acute respiratory distress syndrome (ARDS). Pregnant women who have pyelonephritis are particularly prone to these complications, and also may develop premature labor as a result of the irritative effect of lipopolysaccharide on the uterus.[17]

Hematogenous renal abscesses

Intrarenal abscesses can also be caused by certain hematogenously borne pathogens, most commonly *Staphylococcus aureus*, *Candida* spp. and *Mycobacterium tuberculosis*. In contrast to abscesses that form during acute ascending pyelonephritis, hematogenously derived abscesses are usually cortical in location, are not prone to rupture into the perinephric space and are not associated with the characteristic clinical syndrome of pyelonephritis. Conversely, the typical pathogens of acute ascending pyelonephritis almost never cause renal abscesses in patients who have bacteremia arising from an extraurinary-tract focus.[1]

PREVENTION

Little is known about the prevention of pyelonephritis or renal abscess. Presumably, the same measures that can be recommended to non-compromised women who wish to reduce their risk of uncomplicated recurrent cystitis (e.g. avoiding spermicide-diaphragm contraception, use of chronic antimicrobial prophylaxis or early patient-initiated therapy for UTI symptoms) should decrease the risk of uncomplicated pyelonephritis.[18] Postmenopausal women can reduce their risk of bacteriuria with vaginal estrogen treatment; this might also prevent pyelonephritis. Complicated pyelonephritis may be prevented by removing the precipitating factor. Urinary catheters should be avoided whenever possible, used according to current guidelines when unavoidable, and removed as soon as no longer essential.[12]

Indwelling catheters coated with antimicrobial substances have been shown to prevent bacteriuria/funguria in select patients; however, their ability to prevent clinically apparent UTI or other end points of clinical relevance in a wider population is unproven.[19] Similarly, in a small study, an avirulent strain of *E. coli* was used successfully to prevent overgrowth with more pathogenic organisms in catheterized patients.[20] Further studies involving larger, more representative populations and clinically relevant end points would be useful.

Correction of urologic abnormalities (whether surgically or medically) may reduce the associated infection risk but treatment decisions must be carefully individualized and based on the expected risks and benefits of the planned intervention(s). It is not known whether improved glycemic control among patients who have diabetes reduces their increased risk of pyelonephritis but the other documented benefits of this therapy provide ample rationale for its use.

A recent Cochrane Review concluded that cranberry juice (or cranberry extract tablets) did reduce the incidence of symptomatic UTI. However, dropout rates in the reviewed studies were high, suggesting that although effective, these interventions may not be tolerated by all patients.[21] Patients desiring nonantimicrobial therapy can be advised that daily intake of cranberry juice is an option that may provide some benefit with regard to recurrent UTI, with minimal risk. Theoretically this may also decrease the risk of pyelonephritis, although this has not been studied.

Prophylactic antimicrobial therapy is useful in women who have recurrent uncomplicated cystitis[22] and in certain compromised hosts, for example renal transplant recipients in the early post-transplant period.[23] However, in many other compromised hosts antibiotic prophylaxis is without clear benefit and often selects for resistant organisms and causes drug-related adverse effects. Whether the experimental anti-UTI vaccines that are currently being evaluated will prevent cystitis or pyelonephritis is unknown.[24] At present there is no medically defined role for vaccines, receptor analogue therapy, *Lactobacillus* preparations or yoghurt in the prevention of UTI or pyelonephritis.[18]

CLINICAL FEATURES

The clinical manifestations of acute pyelonephritis vary considerably depending on the characteristics of the host and pathogen. A typical history for the classic pyelonephritis syndrome, which is most commonly observed with kidney infections in otherwise healthy young women, includes several days of progressive flank pain, malaise, fever and chills, prostration and possibly nausea and vomiting, often preceded and/or accompanied by symptoms of acute cystitis.[1]

The physical examination characteristically shows an ill-appearing, febrile, tachycardic patient, often with evidence of volume contraction. The pathognomonic physical finding of acute pyelonephritis is tenderness to palpation or percussion over one or both costovertebral angles. Mild to moderate abdominal and suprapubic tenderness are often also present.

Atypical presentations are common. Even otherwise healthy young women who have pyelonephritis may not have all of the classic symptoms or examination findings, and infants or young children, elderly or debilitated patients and patients who have underlying systemic illnesses or neurologic impairment often have an even less characteristic clinical picture.[1] Abdominal pain, headache, nonspecific constitutional symptoms, diffuse back pain, pelvic pain or respiratory complaints may predominate, obscuring the diagnosis and suggesting other processes. A deceptively benign presentation, including sometimes even the complete absence of suggestive symptoms, can mask the presence of severe renal infections in immunocompromised or sensory-impaired hosts.[1] On the other hand, even in patients who have a classic presentation for acute pyelonephritis, other entities must be considered in the differential diagnosis, including (in the appropriate setting) pelvic inflammatory disease, acute appendicitis, urolithiasis, basal pneumonia and acute pancreatitis or biliary tract disease. The decision whether to perform a pelvic examination in a woman suspected of having pyelonephritis must be individualized, taking into consideration the patient's demographic characteristics, the specifics of the history (including the sexual history) and the findings on general physical examination.

In addition to the varied combinations of symptoms and physical findings encountered in patients who have acute pyelonephritis, a wide range of severity of illness is seen. At one extreme, patients who seem healthy and have what otherwise appears clinically to be acute cystitis may demonstrate a slight elevation of body temperature or report mild malaise, suggesting early renal involvement. At the other extreme, patients may present in full-blown septic shock, with multisystem organ failure. The severity of illness has a significant influence on subsequent management, as described below.

Abscess

The initial history and physical examination usually provide few clues as to the presence of an intrarenal or perinephric abscess, although these entities should be kept in mind in high-risk patients. The presence of a palpable mass is suggestive of renal abscess but is neither a sensitive nor a specific finding. Failure of a patient who is thought to have ordinary pyelonephritis to improve substantially after treatment for 48 hours increases the likelihood of abscess sufficiently to warrant further diagnostic studies.[1]

DIAGNOSIS

Urinalysis and urine culture

Acute pyelonephritis is a clinical diagnosis based on a combination of characteristic symptoms and signs together with supporting laboratory tests.[1] The minimal laboratory evaluation needed to make this diagnosis in the appropriate clinical setting is microscopic examination (whether by urinalysis or Gram stain) of a voided urine specimen to evaluate for the presence of pyuria, followed by quantitative urine culture. The Gram stain is also helpful by confirming the presence of bacteria in the urine (which are seen in unconcentrated urine specimens when the urine bacterial concentration is >10⁵ cfu/ml) and by suggesting the likely bacterial type, although effective empiric treatment often can be selected without this information.[25]

In the absence of prior antimicrobial therapy, the urine culture almost always shows high concentrations (>10⁵ cfu/ml) of one or more bacterial species. Pure growth of a single uropathogenic organism is typical of infections in noncompromised hosts, whereas polymicrobial infections are more common in compromised hosts. Lesser bacterial concentrations are occasionally encountered and in the appropriate clinical context (e.g. a patient who has typical symptoms and examination findings, plus pyuria) do not exclude the diagnosis of pyelonephritis. Antimicrobial susceptibility testing of urine isolates is essential, both to confirm that the empirically selected treatment regimen is appropriate and for guiding selection of an effective oral agent for patients treated initially with a parenteral antimicrobial regimen.[25]

Ancillary tests

Other tests may be indicated depending on the severity of illness, the range of alternative diagnoses being considered and the presence of co-morbid conditions. Pre-therapy blood cultures are commonly collected although, interestingly, bacteremia (if present) predictably clears with appropriate therapy directed toward the urinary infection, and clinical outcomes are similar regardless of the presence or absence of bacteremia. A pregnancy test is useful if the patient might be pregnant and treatment is being considered with an agent (such as an aminoglycoside or a fluoroquinolone) that might be toxic to the fetus.[17]

Imaging studies

Imaging studies are not routinely indicated for the diagnosis or management of acute pyelonephritis.[1] For patients in whom the initial diagnosis is unclear, those who fail to respond appropriately to therapy and those in whom abscess or obstruction is suspected for other reasons, CT scan can be used to clarify the anatomy and guide a mechanical intervention, in addition to helping evaluate

for an alternative diagnosis.[1] Of all urinary tract imaging modalities, contrast-enhanced CT provides the best anatomic definition of inflammatory processes in the urinary tract, including sensitive detection of abscesses and differentiation of abscesses (water density) from simple inflamed tissue (tissue density; Figs 55.5–55.8). Inflamed regions of the pyelonephritic kidney appear on enhanced CT as streaky or wedge-shaped hypodense areas that fail to concentrate contrast material normally in comparison with surrounding renal tissue. Focal bulges or diffuse swelling of the entire kidney are common, as is inflammatory stranding in the perinephric fat. Terms coined by radiologists in the 1980s for these changes, such as 'focal' (or 'lobar') nephronia and 'focal' (or 'diffuse') bacterial nephritis, were often confusing to the clinician and were applied inconsistently by different radiologists. The Society of Uroradiology has defined a uniform terminology according to which all such changes are reported under the umbrella term 'acute pyelonephritis', with modifiers that describe the observed anatomic abnormalities. The extent and severity of such CT findings at the time of presentation are predictive of the clinical course, including the likelihood of bacteremia, progression to abscess formation and death.

Ultrasonography, although commonly used as an initial imaging test for patients who have a suspected focal infectious complication during pyelonephritis, is comparatively insensitive[1] and is often followed by a CT scan irrespective of the ultrasound results. Consequently, it may be best to omit this test and proceed directly to CT. (However, serial directed sonographic examinations can be used subsequently to follow the response of abscesses or hydronephrosis to therapy, without the higher cost and exposure to radiation and contrast material of repeated CT scans.) Single photon emission CT (SPECT) using technetium-99 dimercaptosuccinate (⁹⁹Tc-DMSA), the newest imaging modality for use in pyelonephritis, is slightly more sensitive than CT for identifying areas of inflammation within the kidney, which can be advantageous if the initial diagnosis is in question. However, it cannot distinguish between frank abscesses and inflamed but viable tissue, and so is of little help in evaluating the patient who fails to respond to therapy. Excretory urography and MRI have little role in the management even of complicated pyelonephritis.[1] Nonenhanced spiral CT is more sensitive than excretory urography in detecting urinary calculi and avoids exposing the patient to contrast material, and so may be the modality of choice (when available) if urolithiasis is a concern. Occasionally, antegrade or retrograde ureterography may be indicated, usually when stent placement or calculus removal is needed to relieve obstruction.

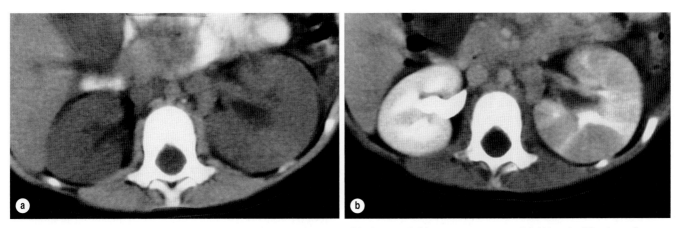

Fig. 55.5 Febrile urinary tract infection with white blood cell count of 36 000/ml (girl, 3 years). (a) Precontrast CT scan: left kidney is diffusely swollen; parenchymal attenuation is the same as that of the right kidney. (b) Postcontrast CT scan: wedge-shaped regions of hypoenhancing parenchyma in the left kidney are most pronounced in the posterior portion. Inflamed parenchyma enhances from 32 to 93 Hounsfield units (HU), whereas normal kidney enhances from 33 to 140 HU. The right kidney shows normal cortical enhancement and pronounced medullary blush. With permission from Talner et al.[24]

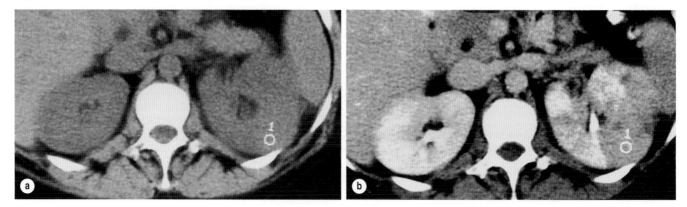

Fig. 55.6 Woman with clinical signs of acute pyelonephritis. (a) Precontrast CT scan: focal bulge present in anterolateral aspect of left kidney. Attenuation is the same as that of normal kidney parenchyma. (b) Postcontrast CT scan: rounded and streaky regions of hypoenhancing parenchyma in the left kidney are most pronounced anterolaterally. Attenuation in the region of interest (cursor) was 22 HU on precontrast scans and increased to 93 HU on postcontrast scans. Normal parenchyma increased from 25 to 130 HU. With permission from Talner *et al*.[24]

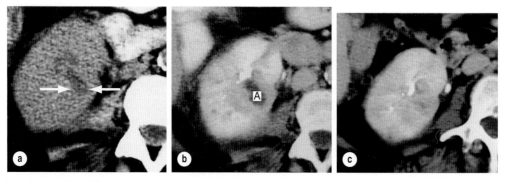

Fig. 55.7 Acute pyelonephritis with small intrarenal abscess. (a) Precontrast CT scan shows small region of low attenuation (arrows). (b) On the postcontrast CT scan, the abscess (A) fails to enhance at all. Surrounding inflamed parenchyma bulges and enhances less than adjacent normal parenchyma. (c) Follow-up CT scan obtained after prolonged antibiotic therapy. The abscess has resolved without drainage. The focal swelling is gone but the parenchyma still shows hypoenhancement. With permission from Talner *et al*.[24]

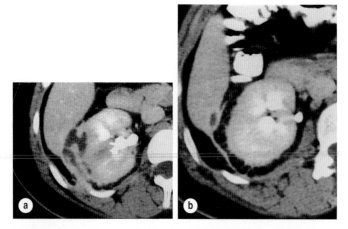

Fig. 55.8 Renal abscess perforating into subcapsular and perinephric spaces (woman, 29 years). (a) Postcontrast CT scan. Dumbbell-shaped nonenhancing region laterally in right kidney represents parenchymal abscess breaking through subcapsular and perinephric spaces. Note marked thickening of perinephric fascia posterolaterally. (b) CT section obtained caudal to (a). Note thickening of perinephric inflammation. At this level there is a small pararenal abscess pocket adjacent to the liver. With permission from Talner *et al*.[24]

MANAGEMENT

In comparison with the treatment of acute cystitis, which has been extensively studied, there have been relatively few large, high-quality treatment trials for acute pyelonephritis on which to base therapeutic recommendations.[25,26] Much of the prevailing wisdom regarding the treatment of pyelonephritis comes from tradition, anecdotal experience, extrapolation from animal models or pharmacokinetic studies, small clinical trials involving heterogeneous patient populations and *in-vitro* susceptibility test results. Nonetheless, some guidelines can be suggested for key management issues.

Inpatient versus outpatient and parenteral versus oral therapy

Traditionally, most patients who have pyelonephritis have been hospitalized and given intravenous antimicrobial therapy, at least initially. However, evidence is accumulating that oral therapy on an ambulatory basis (with or without initial parenteral treatment and observation in the emergency department or short-stay unit) is acceptable for the majority of patients who have acute pyelonephritis.[27] Outcomes with oral therapy for otherwise healthy ambulatory patients who are clinically stable and can take medications by mouth have been similar to those obtained with sicker patients given traditional in-hospital parenteral therapy, at a considerable cost saving. Oral therapy has even been used successfully with pediatric patients and with pregnant women in whom pyelonephritis has traditionally been considered to require in-hospital management.

Thus, there is no single right answer to the question of the optimal setting for treatment. The management plan must be individualized to the patient, taking into consideration the severity of illness (including the presence of nausea or vomiting), the patient's underlying host status and reliability level, and the availability of a support system at home and a mechanism for medical follow-up (Table 55.1). Women who have uncomplicated pyelonephritis and who are only mildly ill can sometimes be treated successfully from the outset with oral therapy alone (Table 55.2). Moderately ill patients can be can be rehydrated with intravenous fluids (if needed) in the clinic or emergency department, given an initial parenteral dose of antibiotic and observed. If after several hours their condition has failed to improve sufficiently they can be admitted to the hospital for continued parenteral therapy, whereas if they are feeling better and are able to take fluids by mouth they can be discharged to home with an appropriate oral antibiotic regimen (Table 55.2), with close follow-up arranged.

Men with pyelonephritis, or women who have complicating factors other than pregnancy, have previously been thought to require admission and treatment with parenteral antibiotics. However, even within these populations there may be a subset of patients (with mild symptoms, ability to take oral medications and otherwise without signs of severe disease) who may be treated as outpatients with oral medications. Little literature specifically addressing this issue exists; therefore, most such patients probably should be admitted to the hospital initially for parenteral therapy, particularly if they are more than minimally ill.

Table 55.1 Indications for hospital admission in patients with acute pyelonephritis

Indication	Rationale
Severly ill, unstable (1)	Needs close monitoring and aggressive resuscitation
Moderate or severe host compromise	At risk of poor response to therapy, progression to 1
Suspected abscess, obstruction, stone	Needs diagnostic evaluation and intervention; at risk of progression to 1
Pregnant women*	At risk of progression to 1
Children*, men*	At risk of poor response to therapy, progression to 1
Persistent vomiting (despite antipyretic therapy and intravenous hydration)	Needs iv or im therapy†
No suitable oral therapy available	Needs iv or im therapy†
Unsuitable home situation, unreliable follow-up, or unreliable/noncompliant patient	At risk of progression to 1

*Selected patients with mild illness and suitable home situations may be treated orally as outpatients, with or without a first iv dose in the emergency department or clinic.
†Home parental therapy acceptable (where available) for mildly or moderately ill patients.

Antimicrobial regimen

Because urine culture and susceptibility testing takes several days to complete, the initial antimicrobial regimen for acute pyelonephritis is usually selected empirically (from among those agents that have suitable pharmacokinetic characteristics and a good 'track record' in pyelonephritis treatment trials) on the basis of the predicted susceptibility patterns of the expected organism(s) (Table 55.2).[1,25,26] For all patients, activity against 'ordinary' Gram-negative bacilli is essential in the empiric regimen. For patients who have complicated UTI or recent antimicrobial therapy, Gram-positive organisms and drug-resistant Gram-negative organisms must also be anticipated.

Suitable initial regimens are shown in Table 55.2, which emphasizes aminoglycosides, fluoroquinolones, third-generation cephalosporins and β-lactam–β-lactamase inhibitor combination agents for parenteral use, and trimethoprim–sulfamethoxazole (TMP–SMX), fluoroquinolones and amoxicillin–clavulanate (co-amoxiclav) for oral use. Because of the high prevalence among uropathogens of resistance to ampicillin, other penicillins and first- or second-generation cephalosporins – as well as these agents' adverse pharmacokinetic properties and inconsistent performance in clinical trials[25,26] – these drugs should be avoided as empiric monotherapy for even mild or uncomplicated pyelonephritis. Emerging resistance to TMP–SMX among uropathogens has diminished this drug's utility in the USA for empiric oral therapy of UTIs, particularly pyelonephritis, since in-vitro resistance is associated with clinical failure rates of more than 50%.[28] Unfortunately, resistance to fluoroquinolones, which have traditionally been regarded as the 'fall-back' option for UTIs due to TMP–SMX-resistant Gram-negative uropathogens, is already quite prevalent in some places, and resistance to extended-spectrum cephalosporins among community-source E. coli also is emerging globally. How this will affect future recommendations for empiric therapy of pyelonephritis remains to be seen. Whether oral third-generation cephalosporins should have a role in the empiric therapy of pyelonephritis in outpatients has not been adequately studied.

Antimicrobial regimens can be simplified by using a single agent (there being little rationale for combination therapy except in patients who are thought to have both Gram-positive and Gram-negative pathogens)[29] and by using twice-daily dosing with ciprofloxacin, TMP–MX and co-amoxiclav, or once-daily dosing with ceftriaxone, levofloxacin, ertapenem and the aminoglycosides.

Conversion to oral therapy

Patients initially admitted to the hospital for intravenous therapy have traditionally been continued on parenteral therapy until susceptibility results are known. They are then placed on an oral agent selected on the basis of the susceptibility pattern of the urine organism, and are observed in the hospital for an additional 1–2 days to evaluate the success of oral therapy (Table 55.3). This approach leads to unnecessarily prolonged hospital stays in many patients. Conversion to oral therapy can be done safely as soon as the initial indications for parenteral therapy have resolved, as evidenced by the success of oral therapy for mildly ill ambulatory patients who have pyelonephritis. When the hospitalized patient is clinically ready for oral therapy before susceptibility results are available, an oral regimen can be selected empirically, much as is done in the emergency department for patients treated with an oral agent from the outset.[25,27] In most locales in the USA, the fluoroquinolones are predictably active against community-acquired E. coli. Thus, despite being slightly more expensive than TMP–SMX (which might be the preferred agent for a known susceptible organism), fluoroquinolones can yield a tremendous cost saving if they permit patients to be discharged sooner.

The practice of observing patients who have pyelonephritis in the hospital for 24 hours or longer on oral therapy before discharge is without empiric support. When examined retrospectively, this approach was found to detect relapse in only 1% of patients and intolerance of the new oral agent in only 4%.[30] Thus, patients can usually be safely

Table 55.2 Suggested empiric initial treatment regimens for acute pyelonephritis*

Modifying circumstances	Treatment setting	Empiric treatment options
Uncomplicated pyelonephritis		
Mild to moderate illness, no nausea or vomiting	Outpatient therapy acceptable	Oral[†] fluoroquinolone (not in children), TMP–SMX caution[§] or amoxicillin–clavulanate (co-amoxiclav) caution[§] for 7–14 days (co-amoxiclav preferred if Gram-positive cocci present)
Severe illness or possible urosepsis	Hospitalization required	Parenteral[‡] fluoroquinolone (not in children), third-generation cephalosporin, gentamicin (± ampicillin or piperacillin), piperacillin–tazobactam, aztreonam or carbapenem, TMP–SMX caution[§] until patient is better; then oral[†] agent (see above) to complete 14 days of therapy (Initial regimen should include ampicillin or piperacillin if Gram-positive cocci are present)
Complicated pyelonephritis		
Pregnancy, mild illness	Outpatient therapy acceptable	Oral[†] co-amoxiclav, cephalosporin or TMP–SMX caution[§] for 10–14 days (co-amoxiclav preferred if Gram-positive cocci present)
Pregnancy with moderate to severe illness	Hospitalization required	Parenteral[‡] third-generation cephalosporin, gentamicin (± ampicillin or piperacillin) caution,[§] piperacillin–tazobactam, carbapenem caution[§] or TMP–SMX caution[§] until patient is better; then oral[†] amoxicillin, co-amoxiclav, a cephalosporin or TMP–SMX caution[§] for 14 days (Initial regimen should include ampicillin or piperacillin if pre-therapy Gram stain shows Gram-positive cocci or no organisms, or is not done)
Not pregnant, mild illness, no nausea or vomiting	Outpatient therapy acceptable	Oral[†] fluoroquinolone (not in children) for 10–14 days
Not pregnant with moderate to severe illness or possible urosepsis	Hospitalization required; imaging studies and urologic consultation often needed	Parenteral[‡] gentamicin (± ampicillin or piperacillin), fluoroquinolone, third-generation cephalosporin, aztreonam, ticarcillin–clavulanate, piperacillin–tazobactam or carbapenem until patient is better; then oral[†] agent (see above) for 14–21 days (Initial regimen should include ampicillin, piperacillin or a carbapenem if pre-therapy Gram stain shows Gram-positive cocci or no organisms, or is not done)

*'Uncomplicated' is usually limited to noncompromised, nonpregnant adult women but can include carefully selected men and children who lack compromising conditions and are only mildly ill.
[†]**Oral regimens**: TMP–SMX, 160 mg + 800 mg q12h; norfloxacin, 400 mg q12h; ciprofloxacin, 500 mg q12h; ofloxacin 200–300 mg q12h; lomefloxacin, 400 mg q24h; levofloxacin, 500 mg q24h; amoxicillin, 500 mg q8h; amoxicillin–clavulanate (co-amoxiclav), 850 mg q12h or 500 mg q8h; cefpodoxime proxetil, 200 mg q12h.
[‡]**Parenteral regimens**: TMP–SMX, 160 mg + 800 mg q12h; ciprofloxacin, 200–400 mg q12h; ofloxacin, 200–400 mg q12h; levofloxacin, 500 mg q24h; gentamicin, 5 mg/kg q24h; ceftriaxone, 1–2 g q24h; ampicillin, mezlocillin or piperacillin, 1–2 g q6h; imipenem–cilastatin, 250–500 mg q8h–q6h; meropenem, 1 g q8h; ertapenem, 1 g q24h; doripenem, 500 mg q8h; ampicillin–sulbactam, 1.5–3 g q6h; ticarcillin–clavulanate, 3.2 g q8h–q6h; piperacillin–tazobactam, 3.375 g q8h–q6h; aztreonam, 1 g q12h–q8h.
[§]**Cautions**: fluoroquinolones (norfloxacin, ciprofloxacin, ofloxacin, levofloxacin and lomefloxacin) should not be used in pregnancy or in young children. TMP–SMX, although not approved for use in pregnancy, has been widely used (but should be avoided in the first trimester and near term). TMP–SMX and co-amoxiclav should be used only if susceptibility of urine organism is known or is highly (>95%) likely. Gentamicin should be used with caution in pregnancy because of its possible toxicity to eighth-nerve development in the fetus. The fluoroquinolones norfloxacin and lomefloxacin can only be administered po; ciprofloxacin, levofloxacin and ofloxacin can be administered iv or po. Imipenem/cilastatin is FDA class C in pregnancy, all other carbapenems (meropenem, ertapenem and doripenem) are FDA class B.
Adapted with permission from Stamm & Hooton.[26]

Table 55.3 Criteria for conversion to oral therapy

Patient no longer severely ill or unstable
Patient taking fluids by mouth; no vomiting; adequate gut function
Suitable oral agent available:
- documented or predicted activity against causative organism(s)
- highly bioavailable
- good 'track record' in UTI therapy
- no contraindication to use (i.e. no history of previous adverse reaction), no drug–drug interactions, no fetal toxicity (pregnant women), no age-related toxicities (e.g. fluoroquinolones in children)

discharged once they have demonstrated tolerance of the first dose of an appropriate oral agent, whether the drug is selected empirically or on the basis of known susceptibility results.

Expected clinical course

Nearly all patients who have pyelonephritis and who will ultimately be cured by antimicrobial therapy alone experience substantial clinical improvement within the first 2 days of therapy, sometimes even after the first liter of intravenous rehydration fluid and before receiving any antimicrobial agent. Patients commonly continue to have fever and flank pain for several days on effective therapy, but these manifestations should begin to wane and there should be improvement in the patient's energy level, appetite and sense of well-being.

If after 48 hours there is no improvement in any of these parameters, aggressive re-evaluation is required.[1] Possibilities to be considered include a mistaken diagnosis, a mismatch between the urine organism and the selected antimicrobial regimen and an anatomic complication such as obstruction or abscess. A directed history and physical examination are indicated, as is repeated laboratory testing (including blood cultures and chemistries, urinalysis and urine culture plus Gram stain) and urinary tract imaging studies, beginning with enhanced abdominal CT. In some patients this evaluation will reveal a focal process in need of an invasive procedure, such as drainage of an abscess (see Fig. 55.8) or an obstructed collecting system; in some patients, continued medical therapy (with or without adjustment) will suffice (see Fig. 55.7). Consultation with an infectious diseases specialist and/or a urologic surgeon or interventional radiologist can be extremely helpful in problematic cases to ensure that all relevant options are considered and the appropriate procedures performed.

Complications

Supportive care for patients who develop septic shock, ARDS and multisystem organ failure during pyelonephritis, which is not specific to pyelonephritis, is discussed in Chapter 44. When infection is present, obstruction to urine flow (e.g. by a stone or tumor) must be relieved, either by removal of the obstruction or by provision of alternative drainage. When possible, removal of urinary calculi from patients who have pyelonephritis is probably best delayed until the bacterial load can be reduced and the patient stabilized with medical therapy. Gas-forming UTIs have traditionally been managed surgically in most instances, often with nephrectomy in cases of emphysematous pyelonephritis (see Fig. 55.3). However, reports of successful medical therapy of gas abscesses[15] and emphysematous pyelonephritis indicate that even in these extreme situations therapy can be individualized.

Intrarenal (see Fig. 55.7) and perinephric (see Fig. 55.8) abscesses have also traditionally been managed with combined medical and surgical therapy. Recent experience with closed (catheter-assisted) drainage or medical therapy alone suggests the possibility of alternative approaches in this setting as well.[31] Small abscesses, especially those occurring in otherwise intact hosts, are most likely to respond to medical therapy, whereas large collections, particularly in compromised hosts or in patients who have severe illness, are likely to require drainage. The cost and morbidity of a drainage procedure must be weighed against the cost and morbidity of the protracted antibiotic therapy that is usually required when abscesses are treated with antibiotics alone. If an abscess is to be drained, the optimal method (open versus closed) depends in part on the anatomy, the host and local expertise. Perinephric abscesses (see Fig. 55.8) have been described as requiring a more aggressive interventional approach than intrarenal abscesses but published experience suggests that drainage is not always needed even here.

Duration of therapy

The optimal duration of therapy for acute pyelonephritis, unlike that for acute cystitis, is largely undefined and remains a source of controversy.[29] As with other aspects of the management of pyelonephritis, because of the highly variable nature of the illness and the host substrate, it is probably best to tailor duration of therapy to the individual patient.

Clinical trial data demonstrate that 14 days of a traditional sequential regimen that includes an intravenous aminoglycoside initially, followed by oral TMP–SMX or ampicillin, eliminates the initial infection in 100% of women who have moderate or severe uncomplicated pyelonephritis, with no relapses at the 6-week follow-up visit.[32] Thus, courses of therapy longer than 14 days should be unnecessary when similarly potent regimens are used in comparable hosts. In other trials, approximately 90% of patients who had uncomplicated

pyelonephritis and were treated for only 5 days with aminoglycosides, third-generation cephalosporins or fluoroquinolones were cured,[29] although some of the 10% failure rate was attributable to relapses with the initial pathogen.

Whether there is a real or clinically meaningful difference in success rates between 5–7 days and 10–14 days of therapy for uncomplicated pyelonephritis is unknown. Of note, a multicenter randomized clinical trial performed in the mid-1990s demonstrated that 7 days of oral ciprofloxacin (with or without an initial intravenous dose) was 96–99% effective for uncomplicated pyelonephritis of mild to moderate severity in ambulatory women. Similarly, 14 days of oral TMP–SMX (with or without an initial intravenous dose of ceftriaxone) was 92–96% effective if the urine organism was susceptible to TMP–SMX. However, these favorable findings are not necessarily applicable to women who have more severe uncomplicated infections or to patients who have complicating factors, for whom longer treatment duration may be preferable. Duration of therapy for abscesses must be individualized, taking into consideration underlying host status, the nature of the abscess, adequacy of drainage (if undertaken) and response to therapy (both clinical and as revealed by serial imaging studies).

Follow-up

Routine repeat urine cultures are commonly performed during therapy for pyelonephritis to confirm sterilization of the urine but may add little beyond what is apparent from clinical evaluation and possibly from inspection of the urine for pyuria.[33] It is prudent to confirm at least by telephone that patients who are sent out from the emergency department with oral therapy are improving as expected. Whether routine post-therapy clinic visits, urine cultures and urinalyses contribute to favorable outcomes has not been studied. However, as it has been argued that in the setting of uncomplicated acute cystitis these measures are unnecessary,[34] it is possible that the same may be true with pyelonephritis, at least for uncomplicated cases in seemingly reliable and responsible patients. Post-therapy evaluations still are advisable in children, pregnant women[17] and probably also in other compromised hosts.

Urologic evaluation for predisposing conditions

In addition to the management of the acute pyelonephritis episode, in selected patients it is worth searching for an underlying urologic abnormality, as the surgical correction of such an abnormality might prevent future infections. The cost and morbidity of such a search must be weighed against the likelihood of finding a correctable abnormality, the morbidity of the possible corrective procedure itself and the infectious morbidity that can be averted by a successful procedure. In the absence of firm data, opinions differ as to the indications for imaging studies and corrective surgery after pyelonephritis.[34] One approach is to investigate all children and men who develop pyelonephritis, as they are the most likely to have an important correctable abnormality. Women probably should be studied if they have a second (same-strain) relapse of pyelonephritis despite an extended course of appropriate antimicrobial therapy for a first relapse. Whether women who have multiple episodes of pyelonephritis caused by diverse organisms will benefit from urologic investigation is unknown.

SUMMARY

Acute pyelonephritis is a diverse entity that challenges the clinician to intervene sufficiently but not excessively, and for which the management approach must be tailored to the individual patient. New developments in the field – such as the use of at-home oral therapy, shorter treatment courses, single-daily-dose intravenous aminoglycoside, ertapenem or ceftriaxone therapy and early hospital discharge – provide opportunities for cost savings and enhanced patient convenience. Alertness is required to anticipate and detect complications in high-risk patients or in those who fail to respond to treatment as expected. Intrarenal and perinephric abscesses, gas-forming renal infections and infections superimposed on urinary obstruction are potentially lethal processes that require aggressive therapy, often including mechanical intervention.

REFERENCES

References for this chapter can be found online at http://www.expertconsult.com

Complicated urinary infection, including postsurgical and catheter-related infections

INTRODUCTION

This chapter discusses urinary tract infections (UTIs) occurring in individuals with abnormalities of the genitourinary tract, designated 'complicated UTI'. This includes UTIs following urologic surgery and infections associated with urinary catheterization, i.e. intermittent catheterization and both short-term (<30 days) and long-term (>30 days) indwelling catheters. Urinary infection in pregnant women is not addressed.

EPIDEMIOLOGY

Urinary tract infection is the most common bacterial infection in adults. In the setting of structural or functional abnormalities of the genitourinary tract or after urologic interventions, the frequency of UTI may be exceptionally high (Table 56.1).

Infection incidence on a population basis has not been reported. In a review of hospitalization for acute pyelonephritis in Manitoba for 1989–92,[7] the rate of admissions was 11 per 10 000 population for women and 3.3 per 10 000 for men. Of these, 34% of patients with pyelonephritis admitted to two tertiary care hospitals had complicating genitourinary factors. For patients admitted to hospital with a diagnosis of UTI other than pyelonephritis, 84% of subjects at one institution and 36% at a second had complicating factors.

Table 56.1 Infection rates after genitourinary surgery, extracorporeal shock wave lithotripsy or catheterization in the absence of antimicrobial prophylaxis

Procedure	Proportion infected postprocedure
Genitourinary surgery Transurethral prostatectomy[1] Transurethral procedure with instrumentation for stone extraction[2]	6–64% 25%
Extracorporeal shock wave lithotripsy (ESWL)[3] Negative urine culture before ESWL Positive urine culture before ESWL Sepsis	1.5% 21% 4.5%
Catheterization Urodynamic studies[4] Indwelling catheter[5] Intermittent catheterization[6]	1.5–36% 3–7%/day 4.06/100 patient days

The urinary tract is also the most common source of infection in elderly individuals presenting to the emergency department with bacteremia; it accounts for about one-third of all bacteremic episodes in this population.[8] Most of these bacteremic individuals have abnormalities of the urinary tract, primarily obstructing lesions and indwelling catheters.

Urinary tract infection is the most frequent hospital-acquired infection. Urinary infection accounts for 40% of all nosocomial infections, occurring at a rate of approximately 2 per 100 patient discharges.[9] Hospital-acquired UTI is associated with indwelling catheters in at least 80% of episodes, with acquisition of infection by 3–5% of exposed subjects per day of catheterization. Most catheter-associated infections are asymptomatic, but symptomatic infection, including bacteremia, sepsis syndrome and death, may occur. The catheterized urinary tract is the most frequent source of nosocomial Gram-negative rod bacteremia.[5] While bacteremia occurs in only 2–4% of patients who have catheter-acquired UTI, the high frequency of indwelling catheter use means that the absolute number of episodes of bacteremia secondary to catheter-acquired UTI is high.

Approximately 5% of individuals resident in long-term care facilities in North America have a chronic indwelling catheter. The prevalence of bacteriuria in these subjects is 100%. The urinary tract of residents with chronic indwelling catheters is the source of over half of all bacteremic episodes in these facilities. For individuals who have neurogenic bladders managed by intermittent catheterization, the reported rates of infection are 4.06 per 100 patient days[6] or 17.2 per patient year.[10]

PATHOGENESIS

The normal genitourinary tract, apart from the distal urethra, is sterile. The usual colonizing flora of the distal urethra – *Staphylococcus epidermidis*, diphtheroids, streptococci and certain anaerobes – are rarely uropathogens. The sterility of the urine and genitourinary tract is primarily maintained through the flushing action of normal urine voiding. Other variables that may contribute include the concentration and chemical composition of the urine, the bladder mucous layer, Tamm–Horsfall protein excreted from the kidneys, and the innate immune system. These additional factors are probably less important in the development of complicated UTI, where obstruction to normal urine flow overwhelms all other factors in promoting infection.

In complicated UTI, including postsurgical infection and catheter-related infections, the major factor contributing to the initiation and persistence of bacteriuria is an impaired ability to clear organisms from the urinary tract. This may be attributable to:

- obstruction of urine flow with a pool of urine remaining in the urinary tract after voiding;
- the presence of a protected environment, such as an infection stone or a bacterial biofilm on a catheter, from which organisms cannot be eradicated by usual antimicrobial therapy; or

- increased introduction of organisms into the bladder through interventions such as intermittent catheterization.

A wide variety of genitourinary abnormalities are associated with complicated UTI (Table 56.2). These are congenital or acquired functional, structural or metabolic abnormalities. The abnormality may be transient – for instance, the presence of a noninfected stone, a cystoscopy procedure or short-term catheterization. In this situation, once the abnormality is corrected there is no longer an increased risk of UTI. If the abnormality cannot be corrected, as in a patient who has an ileal conduit or with a neurogenic bladder maintained on intermittent catheterization, there is a continued risk of recurrent UTI.

Where UTI occurs in a patient who has an indwelling urethral catheter, the organisms may have gained access to the bladder by several routes:

- carried into the bladder from the periurethral flora or on contaminated equipment with initial introduction of the catheter;
- ascending the mucous sheath from the periurethral area on the outside of the catheter; or
- intraluminally by ascension up the catheter.

The intraluminal route appears to be more important in men than in women, in whom a shorter urethra probably facilitates extraluminal ascent.

When infection occurs in the presence of a foreign body in the genitourinary tract, such as a ureteral stent, nephrostomy tube or indwelling catheter, a bacterial biofilm forms on the inert material.[11] A biofilm is an adherent colony of organisms, with individual organisms encased in copious extracellular matrix which also incorporates urine constituents such as calcium, magnesium and Tamm–Horsfall protein. This biofilm provides a relatively protected environment for the bacteria by interfering with the diffusion of both antibiotics and host defenses, thus contributing to persistent and relapsing infection.

Urinary tract infection may also be acquired in urologic practice when organisms are transmitted between patients on inappropriately cleaned diagnostic or therapeutic equipment.[12] In particular, contamination is a risk where instruments are not appropriately changed or cleaned between patients and where fluid is left standing for prolonged periods at room temperature. Shared use of urinometers or urine collecting devices among patients with indwelling catheters has also been repeatedly identified as a cause of nosocomial outbreaks of infection.[13]

MICROBIOLOGY

The spectrum of micro-organisms isolated from individuals who have complicated UTI is more varied than observed in patients who have uncomplicated UTI.[14] Table 56.3 summarizes the organisms isolated in

Table 56.2 Genitourinary abnormalities associated with an increased frequency of urinary tract infection

Type of lesion	Examples
Obstructing lesion	Tumor, stricture, urolithiasis, prostatic hypertrophy, diverticulum, pelvicalyceal junction obstruction, congenital abnormality, renal cysts
Foreign body	Indwelling catheter, ureteric stent, nephrostomy tube
Functional abnormality	Neurogenic bladder, vesicoureteral reflux, cystocele
Metabolic illness	Diabetes mellitus, medullary sponge kidney, post renal transplantation
Urinary instrumentation and urologic surgery	Prostatectomy, cystoscopy
Urinary diversion	Ileal conduit

Table 56.3 Bacteria isolated in complicated urinary tract infection

Organism	Proportion of total organisms isolated* (%)
Gram-negative organisms	
Escherichia coli	21–54
Klebsiella pneumoniae	1.9–17
Citrobacter spp.	4.7–6.1
Enterobacter spp.	1.9–10
Proteus mirabilis	0.9–10
Providencia spp.	1.9
Pseudomonas aeruginosa	2.0–19
Other Gram-negative organisms	6.1–23
Gram-positive organisms	
Enterococci	6.1–23
Coagulase-negative staphylococci	1.3–3.7
Staphylococci aureus	0.9–2.0
Group B streptococci	1.2–3.5
Other Gram-positive organisms	1.9
Yeast	0–7

* Data on frequency of isolation of different bacterial species derived from references[15-18].

several studies of varied populations with complicated UTI. Although *Escherichia coli* remains an important infecting organism, the frequency with which it is isolated is substantially lower than that reported for acute uncomplicated UTI. *Escherichia coli* has unique virulence characteristics which promote symptomatic infection in the person with a normal genitourinary tract (see Chapter 53). Where complete urine voiding is impaired, organisms without unique urovirulence properties may also become important uropathogens. Therefore, there is a lower prevalence of genotypic or phenotypic expression of virulence factors by *E. coli* isolated from individuals who have complicated genitourinary infection than by *E. coli* isolated from acute uncomplicated UTI.[19]

The distribution of other infecting organisms is determined by factors such as:

- whether organisms are isolated from initial or recurrent infection;
- whether acquisition is nosocomial or community-acquired;
- whether there is an indwelling urinary device; and
- previous antimicrobial exposure.

Common organisms isolated include Enterobacteriaceae such as *Klebsiella*, *Citrobacter*, *Serratia*, *Proteus* and *Providencia* spp., other Gram-negative organisms such as *Pseudomonas aeruginosa* and other nonfermenters, and Gram-positive organisms such as *Enterococcus faecalis* and group B streptococci. Coagulase-negative staphylococci are frequently isolated, although rarely in symptomatic infection, and their pathogenicity is seldom clear. Yeasts, primarily *Candida* spp., may be isolated, usually in individuals who have prolonged or repeated courses of antimicrobial drugs.[20] Anaerobic organisms are isolated rarely, and then in the setting of highly complex urologic abnormalities and abscess formation in the urinary tract.

The urease-producing organisms, principally *Proteus mirabilis*, *Providencia stuartii* and *Morganella morganii*, are important pathogens. Rarely, more unusual urease-producing organisms such as *Ureaplasma urealyticum* or *Corynebacterium urealyticum* D2 may be isolated. These organisms maintain an alkaline environment leading to the formation of struvite stones or catheter encrustation, and promoting persistence of infection.

In addition to the much wider variety of infecting species in complicated UTI compared with uncomplicated UTI, there is also often increased antimicrobial resistance among the infecting bacteria. Increased resistance is promoted by:

- repeated antimicrobial courses for recurrent UTI; and
- the high frequency of nosocomial acquisition.

Some of the infecting organisms, such as *P. aeruginosa*, are intrinsically more resistant to antimicrobials, while others such as *E. coli* or *K. pneumoniae* have acquired genetic elements for resistance.

PREVENTION

General measures

Urinary tract infection in the abnormal genitourinary tract occurs because of the presence of an underlying abnormality or intervention that breaches normal defenses and allows the introduction and persistence of micro-organisms. Therefore, the most important interventions to prevent UTI are:

- to identify and, wherever possible, correct underlying abnormalities; and
- to avoid nonessential interventional procedures.

It is important to follow appropriate aseptic technique for interventional procedures such as cystoscopy or urodynamic studies, as well as for operative procedures. All fluids used in urologic procedures must be handled in a manner that ensures sterility. In particular, equipment must be disassembled after a procedure and reassembled using sterile components before the next procedure, and aseptic technique must be maintained.[12] Institutions should establish and maintain appropriate infection surveillance programs to ensure that endemic infection rates are known and to facilitate early identification of potential outbreaks.[5]

Catheter-acquired infection

The single most important practice in preventing catheter-acquired UTI is not to use an indwelling catheter unless clearly indicated and, if a catheter must be used, to limit the duration of catheterization to as short a period as possible.[5] When a catheter is necessary, a closed urinary drainage system must be maintained. In addition, practicing aseptic technique at insertion is important (Table 56.4).

Patients who have indwelling catheters and are receiving antimicrobial therapy have a decreased incidence of infection acquisition during the initial 4 days of catheterization compared with patients who do not receive antimicrobials. After the first 4 days, the infection rates are similar, but patients receiving antimicrobials develop infection with more resistant organisms. Therefore, antimicrobial therapy to prevent infection when an indwelling catheter is *in situ* is currently not recommended.

Table 56.4 Interventions to prevent catheter-acquired infection

Proven effective	Avoid use of catheter
	Limit duration of catheterization
	Maintain closed drainage system
	Antibiotics first 4 days (not recommended)
Possibly effective	Aseptic insertion
	Antibiotics last 48 h of catheterization
	Antimicrobial decontamination of gut
Proven not effective	Daily meatal care with soap or antiseptic
	Disinfectant (formaldehyde, chlorhexidine, hydrogen peroxide) in drainage bag
	Antimicrobial-coated catheters
	Continuous antibiotic or antiseptic irrigation

Data from Pratt *et al.*[5]

Repeated evaluations of interventions using topical or local anti-infectives to prevent infection associated with indwelling catheters have consistently documented no benefit.[5] For instance, daily perineal cleansing with either soap or disinfectant does not decrease and may increase the rate of infection. Other measures that do not decrease the frequency of infection are the addition of disinfectants such as povidone–iodine or chlorhexidine to the drainage bag and routine irrigation with normal saline or antiseptics. The use of catheters impregnated with antimicrobial agents such as silver has been controversial. Some of these devices may decrease the occurrence of bacteriuria, but they have not been shown to decrease symptomatic UTI or other morbidity.[21] It is, in fact, remarkable how consistently local anti-infective measures have failed to modify the occurrence of catheter-acquired infection.

The use of antimicrobials for preventing infection in patients who have spinal cord injury and who are maintained on intermittent catheterization has also been controversial. Clinical trials report antimicrobial prophylaxis may prevent infection in the early postinjury months, but at the cost of increased antimicrobial resistance when infection occurs. Therefore, prophylactic antimicrobials are currently not recommended for these patients.[22] For spinal cord injured patients, cranberry juice has not been shown to prevent infection.[23] However, an educational program which included written educational material, self-assessment, telephone follow-up, review of catheter technique by an experienced nurse, and physician access for urinary infection care was associated with a sustained decreased frequency of infection.[24]

Indications for long-term catheterization include chronic obstruction, to assist with healing of decubitus ulcers and, occasionally, patient preference. Individuals with chronic indwelling catheters are consistently bacteriuric, usually with between two and five organisms. The incidence rate of acquisition of infection with a new organism is similar to that of short-term indwelling catheters, i.e. 3–5% per day. While it is recommended that procedures for catheter management should be similar for both long-term and short-term catheters, there are no studies reported for long-term catheters which document any specific practices that are effective in decreasing the risk of infection. In particular, systemic antimicrobial therapy does not decrease the risk of symptomatic infection, but does increase the likelihood of infection with resistant organisms.[25] It is, however, likely that avoiding trauma to the catheter and early identification of catheter obstruction will decrease the incidence of symptomatic infection for patients with long-term catheters.

Postoperative infection

The perioperative use of antimicrobials encompasses two issues:

- treatment of pre-existing bacteriuria to prevent the complications of invasive infection; and
- prophylaxis to prevent postoperative infection in individuals without positive pre-intervention urine cultures

Treatment of bacteriuria preoperatively in individuals undergoing genitourinary interventions is indicated to prevent postoperative bacteremia and sepsis. Postoperative sepsis was reduced from 6.2% to zero when appropriate antimicrobials were given before operation to patients whose urine was infected preoperatively.[26] Antimicrobial therapy should be selected on the basis of the infecting organism and antimicrobial susceptibilities, and initiated at least 1 hour before surgery.

There are some indications for the use of true prophylactic therapy in urologic surgery[27] (Table 56.5) Most authorities now suggest that antimicrobial prophylaxis is appropriate for transurethral prostatectomy even if the pre-procedure urine culture is negative,[27,28] although this recommendation was controversial in the past.[30] Renal transplant patients receive 6 months' postoperative prophylaxis with trimethoprim–sulfamethoxazole to prevent pneumocystis pneumonia and other infections.[29] This regimen also effectively prevents both asymptomatic and symptomatic UTI.

There is no generally accepted 'standard' antimicrobial regimen for prophylaxis.[27] Many different antimicrobials have been used. Generally, an aminoglycoside, with or without a cephalosporin, or a fluoroquinolone is used. Studies have documented the efficacy

Table 56.5 Prophylactic antimicrobial therapy in genitourinary surgery to prevent postoperative urinary tract infection

Procedure	Regimen	Infection rate with prophylaxis (%)	Infection rate without prophylaxis (%)
Transurethral instrumentation			
UTI with stone extraction[2]	Cefotaxime 1 g iv, one dose	8.5	25
Sepsis[26]	Cefotaxime 1 g iv, one dose	0	6.2
Prostatectomy			
Sterile urine preoperatively[28]	Various	3–22	6–70
Preoperative bacteriuria[28]	Various	35–41	65–92
Transplantation			
Renal transplantation[29]	Trimethoprim–sulfamethoxazole 160–800 mg q24h for 4 months	8	35

of second- and third-generation cephalosporins, including cefotaxime, ceftriaxone, cefotetan, cefoxitin and ceftazidime, as well as fluoroquinolones. It is not clear, however, that these agents are superior to less costly alternatives such as aminoglycosides and trimethoprim–sulfamethoxazole.

The recommended regimen is one dose 1–2 hours preoperatively.[27] The appropriate duration of antimicrobial therapy has not been defined. If an indwelling catheter remains *in situ* postoperatively some authors recommend continuation of antibiotics until the catheter is removed. However, recent studies suggest that, at least for some agents, a single dose is as effective as multidose therapy.[31,32] The shortest effective duration of therapy is preferred to limit cost and adverse effects, and the emergence of antimicrobial-resistant organisms.

CLINICAL FEATURES

The clinical presentations of complicated UTI are diverse, and vary along a spectrum from asymptomatic bacteriuria without a measurable host response to septic shock and death. Infection may be localized to the bladder or may involve the kidney and, in men, the prostate. In many patients with persistent abnormalities and recurrent infection, asymptomatic bacteriuria is the most common presentation. When symptomatic infection occurs, the clinical features are usually consistent with lower UTI including frequency, suprapubic discomfort, dysuria and urgency.

With renal infection the characteristic presentation of pyelonephritis, including fever and costovertebral angle tenderness, may occur. Urinary obstruction or trauma to the genitourinary mucosa may predispose to bacteremia and more severe infection.

Presenting symptoms may not, however, be straightforward. In males, recurrent bladder infection may be secondary to chronic bacterial prostatitis. Infection may also manifest as lower UTI irritative symptoms alone despite the presence of upper tract or renal infection. In individuals with uncomplicated UTI, fever is a reliable localizing symptom for upper UTI. This is not the case for complicated and postsurgical infection, or infection in the presence of an indwelling catheter. In these cases trauma to the bladder mucosa may lead to invasive infection and fever associated with lower UTI alone. In most cases, however, treatment decisions will not depend upon knowledge of the site of infection within the urinary tract.

Presentations in unique patient groups

Certain patient groups may demonstrate some unique clinical presentations of infection. For patients who have a spinal cord injury with a neurogenic bladder, the usual irritative lower tract symptoms may be absent because of altered sensation associated with the neurologic injury.[22] Signs and symptoms suggestive of UTI, in addition to fever, kidney pain or tenderness and bladder discomfort, may include a new onset or increase in urinary incontinence, increased sweating, increased spasticity and a general sense of being unwell. Autonomic dysreflexia may occur in patients with spinal cord injury at high thoracic or cervical levels. Patients with multiple sclerosis may present with increased fatigue and deterioration in neurologic function.

Infection may occasionally present as fever without any localizing genitourinary findings, usually in individuals who have indwelling catheters or obstruction. For patients without indwelling catheters, a diagnosis of UTI in the febrile patient who has a positive urine culture and no localizing findings must be assessed critically. In populations with a high prevalence of asymptomatic bacteriuria, the large majority of such episodes are not attributable to UTI.[33]

In patients who have undergone renal transplantation, symptoms and signs may be absent or mild in the early post-transplant period, despite the presence of bacteremia. This lack of symptoms may be due to immunosuppressive therapy or uremia.

Occasionally, symptoms of the underlying genitourinary abnormality may be prominent. For instance, if a UTI occurs in the setting of a ureteral stone, symptoms of renal colic may predominate. The bacteriuric patient with diabetes mellitus who develops papillary necrosis may also present with symptoms of renal colic. Infections with Enterobacteriaceae (usually *E. coli* and *K. pneumoniae*) in patients with diabetes mellitus and hyperglycemia with glycosuria may present as emphysematous cystitis or pyelonephritis. Acute bacterial prostatitis usually presents with prominent symptoms of urethral obstruction including retention.

Presentations with unique infecting organisms

Infection by selected organisms may also produce a unique clinical presentation. Catheter obstruction is associated with urease-producing organisms, the most common of which is *P. mirabilis*. *Corynebacterium urealyticum* infection is associated with the clinical syndrome of encrusted cystitis. This is encrustation of the bladder wall by struvite crystals precipitated by the alkaline urine generated by the urease of the organism. If a persistent fungal infection is identified, there may be a fungus ball in the bladder or kidney associated with obstruction.

Recurrent infection after antimicrobial therapy

Early recurrent infection after antimicrobial therapy is characteristic of individuals with persistent genitourinary abnormalities. Infection may be symptomatic or asymptomatic and may represent:

- relapse with recurrence of the pre-therapy infecting organism after therapy; or
- re-infection with a new organism.

Selected reports that document this high frequency of recurrent infection are summarized in Table 56.6. Bacteriologic cure rates at 4–6 weeks (long-term follow-up) are consistently less than 50% (i.e. recurrent infection is the expected outcome) if the underlying abnormality persists. If the underlying abnormality is transient or reversible, such as a single obstructing stone that is passed, permanent or long-term cure may be achieved. When the underlying abnormality promoting infection cannot be corrected, recurrent infection with organisms of increasing antimicrobial resistance is a common outcome. Some patients may ultimately have infections for years with acquisition of highly resistant organisms.

DIAGNOSIS

Clinical symptoms alone are not sufficient for a diagnosis of complicated UTI. For definitive diagnosis an appropriately collected urine specimen must be obtained for bacterial culture. The large variety of potential infecting organisms, together with the increased likelihood of antimicrobial resistance, means that obtaining a pre-therapy urine culture is essential for appropriate antimicrobial management of patients who experience complicated UTI. Blood cultures should also be obtained from patients who have evidence of sepsis, including symptoms such as high fever, rigors, hypothermia or acute confusion.

Urine specimen

The urine specimen must be collected before initiating antimicrobial therapy, using a urine collection method that limits contamination. Urine specimens should be forwarded promptly to the laboratory for semiquantitative culture and appropriate susceptibility testing. A clean-catch voided specimen or, if a voided specimen cannot be obtained, a specimen obtained through in and out catheterization, is usually appropriate. For individuals who have indwelling catheters, urine is collected by aseptic aspiration from the catheter port. Patients with obstruction for whom a urologic procedure for decompression is undertaken may have specimens obtained by ureteric catheterization or percutaneous aspiration of the renal pelvis. There is no completely satisfactory way of collecting specimens for culture from people who have an ileal conduit. Specimens collected through the conduit will always be contaminated with organisms colonizing the conduit, and clinical judgment is necessary to evaluate the significance of the organisms isolated.

Foreign material in the urinary tract, including indwelling urethral catheters, ureteric stents and nephrostomy tubes, are rapidly coated with a bacterial biofilm after insertion. Organisms isolated from urine specimens obtained through such devices reflect the microbiology of the biofilm on the inner surface of the catheter rather than bladder urine. Therefore, it is suggested that indwelling catheters should be changed before specimen collection and initiation of antimicrobial therapy.[36] The urine specimen is collected through the newly inserted catheter which is free of biofilm and samples bladder urine, leading to a more reliable identification of the infecting bacterial species.

Quantitative bacteriology

Current recommendations for interpretation of quantitative bacteriology in the diagnosis of complicated UTI are provided in Table 56.7. In the symptomatic patient, UTI may be diagnosed if the quantitative count of organisms in urine culture is 10^4 cfu/ml or more and there are symptoms consistent with genitourinary infection. For individuals who are asymptomatic, two specimens with a quantitative count of 10^5 cfu/ml or more with the same organism(s) isolated on two consecutive occasions are recommended for diagnosis.[25,37] In practice, however, a single specimen achieving counts of 10^5 cfu/ml or more is usually interpreted as bacteriuria.

Infections usually involve a single infecting organism, but there may be more than one bacterial species in the urine of patients with frequent recurrent infections. The patient who has a long-term indwelling catheter or other chronic device will usually have two to five organisms isolated.[5]

Rarely, less common organisms, such as yeast species, may be isolated in lower quantitative counts. Unusual uropathogens such as *U. urealyticum* or *Haemophilus influenzae*, which are uncommon causes of infection, will not be isolated by routine laboratory methods for urine culture. If there is complete ureteric obstruction with infection localized proximal to the obstruction, the culture may also be negative. Of course, urine cultures will also be negative with symptomatic infection if the patient has received effective antimicrobial therapy prior to collecting the urine specimens.

Pyuria

Pyuria is evidence for inflammation within the urinary tract, and may be attributed to many causes other than infection. Underlying abnormalities associated with complicated UTI, inflammation following a surgical procedure or a chronic indwelling catheter may all be associated with pyuria in the absence of infection. Thus, pyuria is not sufficient to confirm a diagnosis of a UTI in the absence of a positive urine culture. In addition, both symptomatic and asymptomatic UTI are usually associated with pyuria, so pyuria does not discriminate between symptomatic and asymptomatic infection. Therefore, a dipstick test or urinalysis that shows evidence of pyuria is consistent with but not diagnostic of UTI. A negative test for pyuria is, however, helpful to exclude a diagnosis of urinary infection.

Table 56.6 Bacteriologic outcome after antimicrobial therapy of complicated urinary tract infection

Regimen	Follow-up after therapy	Cure (%)	Re-infection (%)
Complicated urinary infection			
Lomefloxacin[16]	5–9 days	59	5.9
	4–6 weeks	43	19
Trimethoprim–sulfamethoxazole[16]	5–9 days	33	1.5
	4–6 weeks	28	9.2
UTI secondary to spinal cord injury			
Norfloxacin 14 days[34]	5–7 days	53	14
	8–12 weeks	16	NS
Various antimicrobials: 7–14 days[35]	1 week	47	NS
Various antimicrobials: ≥28 days[35]	1 week	41	NS
NS, not stated.			

Table 56.7 Quantitative bacteriology in the diagnosis of complicated urinary tract infection

Clinical presentation	Bacteriologic count
Asymptomatic bacteriuria	$\geq 10^5$ cfu/ml in two consecutive urine specimens
Symptomatic urinary infection	$\geq 10^4$ cfu/ml in one specimen or $\geq 10^5$ if collected by external catheter
Percutaneous aspiration in hydronephrosis	Any quantitative count
Diuresis, diuretic therapy, renal failure, selected infecting organisms (e.g. *Candida albicans*)	Lower quantitative counts ($<10^5$/ml) may occur in these situations

MANAGEMENT

Essential elements in approaching the management of UTI in the setting of an abnormal genitourinary tract include:

- initial clinical evaluation;
- appropriate pre-therapy diagnostic specimen collection;
- selection of initial antimicrobial therapy;
- appropriate supportive care;
- an assessment of the need for genitourinary investigation or urologic interventions to correct any abnormality; and
- review of urine culture results, once available, to ensure the optimal antimicrobial regimen is being given.

Supportive therapy should be given as appropriate depending on the severity of the clinical presentation. This may include hemodynamic monitoring, parenteral fluids, measurement of urine output, or antiemetic medication. If a chronic indwelling catheter is present, catheter replacement prior to initiating antimicrobial therapy is associated with more rapid defervescence and a decreased frequency of symptomatic relapse, as well as providing a more accurate urine specimen for culture.[36]

Asymptomatic bacteriuria

Asymptomatic bacteriuria should only be treated in patient groups where clinical studies have demonstrated a benefit. Table 56.8 summarizes current recommendations for treatment of asymptomatic bacteriuria for different patient populations. These recommendations are developed based on results of published clinical trials.[25]

Where treatment of asymptomatic bacteriuria is not indicated, antimicrobial therapy does not decrease morbidity of infection but is associated with a greater frequency of negative outcomes, including the emergence of resistant organisms and adverse drug effects. Studies in children, in fact, suggest that the treatment of asymptomatic bacteriuria may increase the frequency of symptomatic infection. Screening for bacteriuria is also not indicated except in populations for whom treatment of asymptomatic bacteriuria is recommended.

Table 56.8 Indications for the treatment of asymptomatic bacteriuria

Definite	Before an invasive genitourinary procedure
	Pregnancy
Not indicated	In the elderly
	For schoolgirls or healthy women
	Intermittent catheterization
	Indwelling urinary catheter
	Diabetic women

Data from Nicolle *et al.*[25]

Antimicrobial therapy

Whenever possible, empiric therapy should be avoided and antimicrobial therapy specific for the infecting organism(s) isolated in urine culture should be prescribed. This is usually possible if the patient has mild symptoms. When the patient's symptoms are severe enough to warrant immediate empiric therapy, it is essential that a urine culture be obtained before initiating therapy. The empiric antimicrobial regimen should be re-evaluated once culture results are available, usually 48–72 hours after the specimen was collected.

Initial parenteral therapy is preferred for individuals who have:

- hemodynamic instability;
- nausea and vomiting;
- questionable absorption of oral antimicrobials; or
- an infection by suspected resistant organisms for which oral therapy is not available.

The majority of patients can be managed without hospitalization or with a limited (24–72 hours) admission to a short-stay unit for initial parenteral therapy. Oral therapy is then started as soon as the patient is stable, often when pre-therapy urine culture results are available to assist in selecting the appropriate medication.

The antimicrobial agents appropriate for therapy are similar to those recommended in the treatment of acute uncomplicated UTI or acute nonobstructive pyelonephritis (Tables 56.9, 56.10). The selection of a specific antimicrobial agent is based upon clinical presentation, the known or suspected infecting organism and its susceptibilities, patient tolerance, documented efficacy and, in some cases, cost.

There are many clinical trials addressing the treatment of complicated UTI, but few of these are helpful in identifying a preferred regimen in a specific clinical situation.[14] One problem is the lack of an accepted 'standard' antimicrobial therapy with respect to agent, dose or duration to serve as a comparator for new agents. In addition, studies have generally enrolled diverse patient populations for whom different outcomes with therapy would be anticipated on the basis of underlying abnormalities. The severity of illness also varies, and subjects may have clinical presentations ranging from an increase in incontinence or bladder spasms to a life-threatening illness with bacteremia.

In view of the very high frequency of relapse, therapeutic trials should provide both short-term (1 week post-therapy) and long-term (4–6 weeks post-therapy) outcomes.[37] Frequently, studies of therapy for complicated UTI have provided only short-term therapeutic

Table 56.9 Oral therapeutic regimens for the treatment of complicated urinary tract infection

Agent	Dose
Amoxicillin	500 mg q8h
Amoxicillin–clavulanate	500 mg q8h or 875 mg bid
Cephalexin	500 mg q6h
Cefuroxime axetil	500 mg q12h
Cefpodoxime proxetil	100 mg q12h
Ceftibuten	400 mg q24h
Cefixime	400 mg q24h
Nitrofurantoin	50–100 mg q6h
Nitrofurantoin monohydrate/macrocrystals	100 mg q12h
Norfloxacin	400 mg q12h
Ciprofloxacin	250–500 mg q12h
Ciprofloxacin extended release	1 g q24h
Ofloxacin	400 mg q24h or 200 mg q12h
Levofloxacin	200–500 mg q24h
Trimethoprim	100 mg q12h
Trimethoprim–sulfamethoxazole	160 mg trimethoprim–800 mg sulfamethoxazole q12h

Table 56.10 Parenteral regimens for the treatment of complicated urinary tract infection in patients with normal renal function

Agent	Dose
Ampicillin	1 g q6h
Piperacillin	3 g q6h
Ticarcillin–clavulanate	3.1 g q6h
Piperacillin–tazobactam	4 g piperacillin–500 mg tazobactam q8h
Cefazolin	1–2 g q8h
Cefotaxime	1 g q8h
Ceftriaxone	1 g q24h
Ceftazidime	1 g q8–12h
Cefepime	1–2 g q12h
Imipenem	500 mg q6h
Meropenem	500 mg q6h or q8h
Ertapenem	1 g q24h
Gentamicin	5 mg/kg q12h or q24h
Tobramycin	5 mg/kg q12h or q24h
Amikacin	15 mg/kg q12h or q24h
Trimethoprim–sulfamethoxazole	160 mg trimethoprim–800 mg sulfamethoxazole q12h
Ciprofloxacin	400 mg q12h
Levofloxacin	500 mg q24h
Ofloxacin	400 mg q12h

outcomes. The many published studies, therefore, provide limited insight into the comparative efficacy of different antimicrobials. These studies do, however, document the effectiveness of a wide variety of antimicrobial agents.

Oral therapy

For oral therapy, the fluoroquinolone antimicrobials as a class have been widely studied and promoted.[14,27] Benefits of fluoroquinolones include a wide antimicrobial spectrum and good patient tolerance. The main concern is increasing antimicrobial resistance with widespread use of this class of antimicrobials. The isolation of a fluoroquinolone-resistant extended-spectrum β-lactamase producing *E. coli* or *K. pneumoniae* is an increasing problem and may be a therapeutic challenge. Amoxicillin–clavulanic acid is effective for the treatment of some of these strains and nitrofurantoin may be effective for *E. coli* bladder infections. Many of these strains remain susceptible to fosfomycin or pivmecillinam, but the clinical efficacy of these agents for complicated UTI has not yet been determined.

In studies of oral therapy for pyelonephritis, cell-wall-active agents such as amoxicillin or first-generation cephalosporins appear less effective than non-cell-wall-active agents such as trimethoprim–sulfamethoxazole or quinolones.[38] Appropriate comparative clinical trials have not shown whether these cell-wall-active agents have a lower efficacy for complicated UTI. For Gram-positive organisms such as group B streptococci and *Enterococcus* spp., amoxicillin orally or ampicillin parenterally would be the treatment of choice.

Nitrofurantoin may be used for patients who have lower tract symptoms. This agent should be avoided in subjects with pyelonephritis or renal impairment, and is not effective for *P. mirabilis*, *K. pneumoniae* or *P. aeruginosa* infection. It is effective for most strains of vancomycin-resistant *Enterococcus*.

Parenteral therapy

For parenteral therapy, an aminoglycoside antimicrobial remains the treatment of choice because of the documented efficacy of this group of drugs over many years of use, and the continued susceptibility of most uropathogens. The nephrotoxicity and ototoxicity of aminoglycosides

are seldom a problem if the duration of therapy is limited, with an early switch to oral therapy following initial clinical improvement and review of the urine culture.

Many other antimicrobial agents are effective as parenteral therapy including penicillins (piperacillin and piperacillin–tazobactam), cephalosporins (cefazolin, cefuroxime, cefotaxime, ceftriaxone and ceftazidime), carbapenems (imipenem, ertapenem, meropenem) and fluoroquinolones (levofloxacin, ciprofloxacin). If *Enterococcus* spp. may be present, ampicillin should be added. The increasing prevalence of ampicillin resistance in *E. faecium* and *E. faecalis* in many institutions means that vancomycin may be necessary to treat nosocomial enterococcal infection.

Duration of therapy

Few reported studies have directly addressed the question of the appropriate duration of therapy. The usual recommended duration is 7–14 days.[14,37] A prospective, randomized, clinical trial of spinal cord injured patients showed that 14 days of ciprofloxacin therapy resulted in fewer symptomatic relapses post-therapy than a 3-day course.[39] However, whether an alternate treatment duration between 3 and 14 days would be as effective is not yet known. In another prospective randomized study, 2 weeks of ciprofloxacin therapy was as effective as 4 weeks for men presenting with febrile urinary infection.[40]

There are selected clinical situations where alternative durations of therapy are appropriate:
- where relapsing infection is due to a prostate source, 6 or 12 weeks of antimicrobial therapy is recommended;
- if symptomatic infection associated with an indwelling catheter is treated while the catheter remains *in situ*, it is recommended that the duration of therapy is as short as possible, usually 5–7 days, to limit the emergence of resistant organisms; and
- after successful extracorporeal shock wave lithotripsy for an infected struvite stone, continuation of antimicrobial therapy is recommended for at least 4 weeks to prevent relapse and sterilize residual stone fragments.[41]

Treatment of patients with renal failure

Patients who have abnormalities of the genitourinary tract are more likely to have impaired renal function. Renal function should be evaluated, if not already known, for patients who present with possible complicated UTI. If there is renal impairment appropriate modifications in antimicrobial dose are necessary. Nitrofurantoin and tetracyclines other than doxycycline should be avoided.

In patients with renal failure, renal perfusion is decreased and antimicrobials may not reach infected renal tissue or achieve high urine levels. The aminoglycosides, in particular, may be less effective.[14] The fluoroquinolone antimicrobials, trimethoprim–sulfamethoxazole, trimethoprim and extended-spectrum β-lactam antimicrobials appear to be effective in the treatment of UTI in the presence of significant renal failure. A more prolonged duration of antimicrobial therapy may be necessary to cure UTI in these patients.

An additional potential therapeutic problem is the patient who has normal measured renal function and satisfactory urinary antimicrobial levels but disparate kidney function. If the function of one kidney is severely impaired relative to the other, blood flow is preferentially increased in the functioning kidney and, despite adequate bladder urine antibiotic levels, little antibiotic will be filtered by the poorly functioning kidney. Antimicrobial treatment may then not eradicate infection localized to the poorly functioning kidney. This is one potential explanation for relapsing infection.

Treatment of fungal infection

Treatment of asymptomatic funguria is not beneficial and is not recommended.[42] The current treatment options and reported cure rates for symptomatic infection are shown in Table 56.11.

Table 56.11 Treatment regimens for fungal urinary tract infection

Agent	Dose	Cure rate (%)
Amphotericin B: parenteral	0.3–1 mg/kg single dose or 6 mg/kg total dose	75
Amphotericin B: bladder irrigation	Continuous, 50 mg/1 for 5 days	72–88
Fluconazole	50–400 mg q24h for 7 days	70–80
5-Flucytosine	50–150 mg/kg q6h	70

Data from Malani & Kauffman.[43]

The treatment of choice is fluconazole, which is the only azole antifungal excreted in the urine. The usual dose is 200 mg/day for 7–14 days.[43] Some non-*albicans Candida* spp., particularly *C. krusei* and *C. glabrata*, have decreased susceptibility or are resistant to fluconazole. The efficacy of voriconazole or posaconazole, which are not excreted in urine, is not known. Flucytosine may be effective for some resistant strains, but flucytosine resistance may emerge rapidly when this agent is used alone. Previously, bladder irrigation with amphotericin B was a recommended therapy. This approach, however, is costly and time-consuming and is no longer considered optimal therapy.

For many infections with *Candida*, a single dose of amphotericin B may be effective, given its prolonged excretion.[44] Echinocandin antifungals, including caspofungin, anidulafungin and micafungin, are not excreted into the urinary tract. However, preliminary case reports suggest caspofungin may be effective for treatment of some fluconazole-resistant *Candida* strains causing UTI.[45]

Suppressive therapy

Suppressive therapy is long-term antimicrobial therapy given to individuals with underlying abnormalities to prevent morbidity from urinary infection when the infection cannot be definitively cured (Fig. 56.1).

When a patient who has an underlying abnormality that cannot be corrected experiences recurrent morbidity, suppressive therapy may prevent symptomatic episodes.[46] Renal transplant patients with persistent infection of a native kidney leading to symptomatic recurrences is one example where this approach might be considered. Suppressive therapy may also be considered for men who have frequent recurrent episodes of symptomatic urinary infection from a prostate source and prolonged antimicrobial therapy has failed to cure the infection. Continuous suppressive therapy is recommended for the few individuals with a struvite (infection) stone that cannot be completely removed to prevent further stone enlargement and preserve renal function.

Long-term suppressive therapy is, however, infrequently indicated and should be used selectively because of cost and the potential for adverse effects including development of infection with resistant organisms.

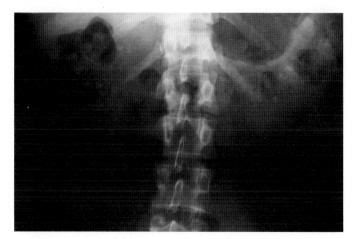

Figure 56.1 Nephrocalcinosis complicated by relapsing *Pseudomonas aeruginosa* infection. Plain film of the abdomen showing multiple bilateral renal stones. This woman has had recurrent stone formation since the age of 18 despite dietary manipulation and repeated lithotripsy. Urinary infection with *P. aeruginosa* was identified at 24 years of age with subsequent recurrent episodes of symptomatic upper tract infection. She has been maintained on suppressive ciprofloxacin therapy for over 10 years with control of symptomatic infection.

INDICATIONS FOR INVESTIGATION

An important aspect of the management of UTIs is determining when to undertake urologic or imaging investigations to characterize abnormalities in the genitourinary tract (see also Chapter 55). Single infections that respond promptly to antimicrobials are unlikely to be associated with significant underlying abnormalities. On other occasions the abnormality may be obvious, such as the presence of an indwelling catheter. In selected other patients, genitourinary investigation should be considered. These clinical scenarios include:

- delayed or incomplete response to appropriate antimicrobial therapy;
- early recurrence of infection after therapy; and
- symptomatic fungal infection, where a fungus ball in the bladder or kidneys should be excluded.

Some patients may have previously well-characterized abnormalities but present with a change in frequency or severity of infection. In these cases, repeat evaluation to identify any changes (e.g. development of new bladder or renal stones) should be considered. Patients presenting with sepsis and hemodynamic instability may require urgent evaluation to identify an abscess or obstruction requiring immediate source control.

REFERENCES

References for this chapter can be found online at http://www.expertconsult.com

Management of persistent symptoms of prostatitis

INTRODUCTION

'Prostatitis' is the diagnosis given to a large group of men presenting with varied complaints referable to the lower urogenital tract and perineum. By one estimate, 50% of adult men experience symptoms of prostatitis at some time in their lives. National Health Center for Health Statistics data indicate that there were 76 office visits per 1000 men per year for genitourinary problems, with prostatitis accounting for approximately 25% of these visits. Recent epidemiologic studies suggest that 2–10% of adult men in varied populations worldwide suffer from prostatitis symptoms at any time. Patients may experience symptoms for prolonged periods. Data also suggest that men with a history of prostatitis may prove substantially more likely to develop prostate cancer and lower urinary tract symptoms associated with benign prostate hyperplasia. Management of patients who experience persistent symptoms following repeated courses of treatment represents a clinical challenge.

PATHOGENESIS

Genitourinary tract infection and inflammation are important in the pathogenesis of prostatitis syndromes. However, the proportion of cases attributable to these causes remains subject to active debate. Most prostate infections occur by ascending through the urethra. Mechanical factors such as urethral length, micturition and ejaculation provide some protection, although the relative importance of such defenses is unclear. The oblique courses of the ejaculatory ducts and some prostatic ducts have also been proposed as mechanical defenses. Other host defenses include the antimicrobial activity in the prostatic secretions, particularly a zinc-containing polypeptide known as prostatic antibacterial factor. The prostate has higher concentrations of zinc than any other organ and prostatic secretions from normal men contain high zinc levels. Men with chronic bacterial prostatitis have low prostatic fluid zinc concentrations, but their serum zinc levels are normal and oral zinc supplements do not increase prostatic secretion zinc levels. Local immunoglobulin production by the prostate also appears to be an important host defense. Many patients with prostatitis have increased leukocyte numbers in their prostatic secretions or semen, but the role of cellular immunity in resolving chronic prostatitis remains uncertain.

Hematogenous dissemination of systemic infections may result in prostatic infection in patients with tuberculosis or other granulomatous infections. This route is especially common in patients who are immunosuppressed or who have HIV infection. Rare patients develop prostatic infection or abscesses due to involvement by infection of adjacent organs, for example with perforated appendicitis or diverticulitis.

MICROBIOLOGY

Uropathogenic bacteria

Bacteriuria is a hallmark of acute and chronic bacterial prostatitis. The agents are standard uropathogens associated with bacterial urinary tract infection (e.g. Enterobacteriaceae, pseudomonads, enterococci, etc.). Recurrent infections caused by the same organism are the sine qua non of chronic bacterial prostatitis. Between episodes of bacteriuria these organisms may be 'localized' to the prostate as described below. Unfortunately, patients with well-documented acute and chronic bacterial prostatitis constitute a minority of patients presenting with prostatitis (less than 10% in our clinic).

Other genitourinary pathogens

Other pathogens have been implicated as causes of prostatitis. The best evidence supports a role for sexually transmitted pathogens. In the pre-antibiotic era, *Neisseria gonorrhoeae* was a frequent cause of prostatitis and the most common cause of prostatic abscess. However, in current practice *N. gonorrhoeae* is seldom implicated. Some studies suggest a role for other sexually transmitted diseases (STDs), particularly *Chlamydia trachomatis*, *Ureaplasma urealyticum* and *Trichomonas vaginalis*. The proportion of cases attributable to these pathogens remains undefined.

Granulomatous infections

A few patients develop granulomatous prostatitis, an uncommon syndrome representing a characteristic histologic reaction of the prostate to a variety of insults. Granulomatous prostatitis is classified as 'specific' when associated with particular granulomatous infections, or as 'nonspecific' in other cases. Specific causes of granulomatous prostatitis include *Mycobacterium tuberculosis*, atypical mycobacteria, bacille Calmette–Guérin (BCG) (after topical therapy for transitional cell carcinoma) and the deep mycoses (especially blastomycosis, coccidioidomycosis and cryptococcosis). Causes of nonspecific granulomatous prostatitis include acute bacterial prostatitis, prostatic surgery and rheumatoid diseases.

The clinical point is that specific diagnostic studies are required to document STDs or granulomatous infections in patients with symptoms or signs of prostatitis. Accurate diagnosis is the prerequisite for successful treatment, which may require antimicrobials seldom prescribed for standard uropathogens.

CLINICAL FEATURES

Patients with prostatitis can be classified into four syndromes: acute bacterial prostatitis, chronic bacterial prostatitis, chronic prostatitis/chronic pelvic pain syndrome and asymptomatic prostatitis (Table PP26.1).

Acute bacterial prostatitis

The clinical features of acute bacterial prostatitis are readily apparent. Characteristic complaints include acute symptoms of urinary tract infection, such as urgency, frequency, dysuria and occasionally gross hematuria or acute urinary retention. Patients may also have systemic symptoms of a 'flu-like' syndrome, with fever, chills or other symptoms associated with bacteremia. Occasional patients experience bladder outflow obstruction due to acute edema of the prostate.

Physical examination may show a high temperature, lower abdominal or suprapubic discomfort due to bladder infection, or urinary retention. The rectal examination is often impressive, with an exquisitely tender, 'tense' prostate. Urinalysis reveals pyuria, and cultures will be positive for uropathogenic bacteria. Systemic leukocytosis is common, with increased numbers of segmented cells. Bacteremia may occur spontaneously or result from vigorous rectal examinations.

Chronic bacterial prostatitis

The characteristic clinical feature of chronic bacterial prostatitis is recurrent episodes of bacteriuria caused by the same organism. Between bouts of bacteriuria, the patient may be asymptomatic or have only minimal symptoms. The infected prostate remains a focus of organisms causing relapsing infection in such patients. The prostate is usually normal on either rectal or endoscopic evaluation.

On occasion, chronic bacterial prostatitis presents as a systemic illness. Small numbers of bacteria in the prostate do not cause systemic illness but represent the source of such systemic infection. With acute exacerbations, bladder bacteriuria and secondary sepsis may occur. This is especially true among older men, who may have the combination of prostatic obstruction and infection.

Chronic prostatitis

Chronic prostatitis/chronic pelvic pain syndrome is the National Institutes of Health consensus term for the largest group of patients with prostatitis symptoms. Chronic pelvic pain symptoms are the characteristic common presentation, especially perineal, lower abdominal,

testicular, penile and ejaculatory pain. Other genitourinary tract complaints include sexual dysfunction and voiding complaints. Some patients have inflammation in their prostatic secretions, post-prostate massage urine or semen (inflammatory subtype of chronic prostatitis/chronic pelvic pain syndrome, formerly termed 'nonbacterial prostatitis'), while others have no evidence of inflammation (noninflammatory subtype of chronic prostatitis/chronic pelvic pain syndrome, formerly termed 'prostatodynia').

Asymptomatic prostatitis

Asymptomatic prostatitis is the term used for men with inflammation diagnosed during evaluation for other genitourinary tract problems. For example, some patients undergoing evaluation for infertility have increased concentrations of leukocytes in their seminal fluid. Chronic prostatitis, characterized by inflammatory infiltrates in prostate specimens, represents the most common 'benign' diagnosis among men who undergo prostate biopsy for evaluation of elevated prostate-specific antigen levels or a digital rectal examination suggesting the possibility of prostate cancer.

INVESTIGATIONS

The critical practice point is to distinguish patients with lower urinary tract complaints associated with bacteriuria from the larger number of men without bacteriuria. Careful review of the history, physical examination and previous laboratory studies is helpful in making this distinction. Patients with bacteriuria may have acute or chronic bacterial prostatitis, while these conditions are rare in patients with no history of bacteriuria.

Document uropathogens

Urine culture and sensitivity testing is essential for men with acute lower urinary tract symptoms. Men with documented bacteriuria should have lower urinary tract localization studies, ideally the 'four glass' test described in Table PP26.2. A less sensitive alternative is to obtain pre- and post-prostate massage urine specimens. The purpose of these investigations is to document a prostatic focus of infection when the patient does not have bacteriuria. Documenting persistent prostatic infection supports the need for continued antimicrobial therapy.

Unequivocal diagnosis of bacterial prostatitis requires that the colony count of a recognized uropathogen in postmassage (VB_3) urine exceed the colony count in the first-void urine (VB_1) by at least

Table PP26.1 NIH consensus classification of prostatitis syndromes

Category	Characteristic clinical features	Bacteriuria	Inflammation*
Acute bacterial prostatitis	Acute urinary tract infection	+	+
Chronic bacterial prostatitis	Recurrent urinary tract infection caused by the same organism	+	+

Chronic prostatitis/chronic pelvic pain syndrome
    Inflammatory subtype[†]
    Noninflammatory subtype[‡]
	Primarily pain complaints, plus voiding complaints and sexual dysfunction	
		−
		−
			
			+
			−

Asymptomatic prostatitis	Diagnosed during evaluation of other genitourinary complaints	−	+

*Objective evidence of an inflammatory response in expressed prostatic secretions, post-prostate massage urine, semen, or by histology.
[†]Formerly termed 'nonbacterial prostatitis'.
[‡]Formerly termed 'prostatodynia'.

Table PP26.2 Lower urinary tract localization study

Specimen	Abbreviation	Procedure
Voided bladder 1	VB_1	Initial 5–10 ml of urinary stream
Voided bladder 2	VB_2	Midstream specimen
Expressed prostatic secretions	EPS	Secretions expressed from prostate by digital massage after midstream specimen
Voided bladder 3	VB_3	First 5–10 ml of urinary stream immediately after prostate massage

Unequivocal diagnosis of chronic bacterial prostatitis requires a 10-fold higher concentration of a uropathogen in the VB_3 of EPS specimen when compared to the VB_1 specimen. The organism is identical to organisms causing repeated episodes of bacteriuria.

10-fold. However, many men with chronic bacterial prostatitis harbor only small numbers of pathogenic bacteria in their prostates. Direct culture of the expressed prostatic secretions (EPS) is useful in this situation because colony counts in EPS are often 1 or 2 logs higher than comparable counts in the VB_3. The hallmark of chronic bacterial prostatitis is that the uropathogen present in VB_3 or EPS may be isolated on multiple occasions and is identical to the organism causing episodes of bacteriuria.

Document other infectious agents

Patients with risk factors for STD pathogens should have appropriate testing for *N. gonorrhoeae, C. trachomatis* and other agents. Serologic testing should be recommended for both syphilis and HIV infection. Patients who have clinical findings suggesting granulomatous prostatitis should have appropriate studies for specific agents associated with this condition (which often entails histologic studies and cultures of prostate tissue).

Document inflammation

Traditionally, microscopic evaluation has been recommended to identify EPS inflammation because this provides objective support for the diagnosis of chronic prostatitis. Although many authorities diagnose inflammation based on finding >10 or >20 leukocytes per high power field in the prostatic secretions, we prefer to define inflammation based on chamber counts with >1000 leukocytes/mm³ because this method is substantially more accurate than the traditional 'wet mount'. There appears to be little value in counting EPS leukocytes in patients with urethral inflammation, especially among men at risk for STDs. Therefore, we examine a urethral smear before proceeding with the lower urinary tract localization study. Diagnosis of urethral inflammation (or 'urethritis') by either VB_1 or urethral smear supports appropriate testing for STD pathogens. In contrast, the clinical utility of distinguishing between the inflammatory and noninflammatory subtypes of chronic prostatitis/chronic pelvic pain syndrome is subject to active debate because these two categories of chronic prostatitis have not been demonstrated to differ in their clinical presentation or response to therapy.

Other investigations

Our standard approach is to recommend a noninvasive uroflow study and postvoid residual testing (by ultrasound) to evaluate possible structural and functional obstructions that may contribute to the etiology or persistence of prostatitis symptoms. Patients with abnormal flow rates or significant postvoid residual urine have additional evaluation with a retrograde urethrogram to evaluate the possibility of urethral stricture. Video urodynamics is reserved for patients with abnormal uroflow findings and negative urethrograms.

Cystoscopy is not recommended for routine evaluation of men with prostatitis symptoms. We reserve cystoscopy for cases where bladder cancer or interstitial cystitis is considered likely (e.g. in older patients, those with hematuria or a history of chemical exposure, or patients in whom painful voiding complaints are prominent). Urinary cytology is obtained if transitional cell carcinoma *in situ* is considered prominently in the differential diagnosis. For patients undergoing cystoscopy, we prefer general or regional anesthesia and recommend hydrodistention with appropriate bladder biopsies. Prostate-specific antigen testing should be considered because occasional patients with carcinoma of the prostate present with persistent symptoms of prostatitis. However, such testing is not recommended for patients with more acute symptoms, since temporary elevation of prostate-specific antigen (and prostatic acid phosphatase) is common following acute episodes. Transrectal ultrasound evaluation may also be considered in selected patients to evaluate possible ejaculatory duct obstruction or complications such as prostatic abscess.

MANAGEMENT

Acute bacterial prostatitis

Appropriate therapy results in dramatic improvement. Many antimicrobials that do not penetrate the uninflamed prostate have proved effective. Thus, drugs appropriate for Enterobacteriaceae, pseudomonads or enterococci should be started once cultures are obtained. For men who require hospitalization, conventional therapy is the combination of an aminoglycoside plus a β-lactam. The fluoroquinolones or third-generation cephalosporins are attractive alternatives for monotherapy.

For less severe infections the conventional choice for outpatient therapy is the combination of trimethoprim and sulfamethoxazole. Because of increasing antimicrobial resistance, fluoroquinolones represent the preferred oral therapy for patients who do not require hospitalization. We usually prescribe one of the newer quinolones for outpatient management.

Patients with acute urinary retention require bladder drainage. In this situation we prefer a suprapubic cystostomy tube, placed using a percutaneous approach. Traditionally, it has been taught that an indwelling transurethral catheter would pass through and obstruct drainage of the acutely infected prostate, increasing the risk for bacteremia and prostatic abscess. However, this has never been evaluated in a controlled study. General measures are also indicated, including hydration, analgesics and bed rest.

Chronic bacterial prostatitis

Trimethoprim–sulfamethoxazole is the traditional 'gold standard'. Long-term therapy with trimethoprim (80 mg) plus sulfamethoxazole (400 mg) taken orally twice daily for 4–16 weeks was superior to shorter courses. Such therapy results in symptomatic and bacteriologic cure in approximately one-third of patients, symptomatic improvement during therapy in approximately one-third (who relapse after stopping treatment) and no improvement in the remaining patients. However, increasing rates of antimicrobial resistance in many areas have tarnished this gold standard.

During the last decade the fluoroquinolones have become the preferred treatment for chronic bacterial prostatitis in most settings. In contrast to the β-lactams, concentrations of many fluoroquinolones are relatively high in prostatic fluid, prostatic tissue and seminal fluid compared to plasma levels. Good results were reported for men with bacterial prostatitis, including patients who failed therapy with trimethoprim–sulfamethoxazole. Useful fluoroquinolones include ciprofloxacin, ofloxacin and levofloxacin. Currently our first choice for curative therapy for chronic bacterial prostatitis is usually an appropriate fluoroquinolone, at full-dose for at least 3 months.

Patients who are not cured benefit from long-term suppressive treatment using low-dosage antimicrobial agents. Since most patients are asymptomatic between episodes of bacteriuria, the goal of suppressive therapy is to prevent symptoms of bacteriuria. Very low doses of drugs are remarkably effective. Available agents include penicillin G, tetracycline, nitrofurantoin, nalidixic acid, cephalexin and trimethoprim–sulfamethoxazole. Although effective, we seldom recommend fluoroquinolones for chronic suppression, because of cost and the potential for development of antimicrobial-resistant organisms.

Chronic prostatitis/chronic pelvic pain syndrome

Therapy is often unsatisfactory because the etiology of chronic prostatitis/chronic pelvic pain syndrome remains unclear. As outlined above, an etiologic role has been suggested for many infectious agents. Prostaglandins, autoimmunity, psychologic abnormalities, neuromuscular dysfunction of the bladder neck or urogenital diaphragm, allergy to environmental agents, stress and other psychologic factors have all been suggested as causes.

Antimicrobial drugs are often considered the first-line treatment. Patients with recognized uropathogens may respond to such empiric therapy. For men without evidence of infection by recognized pathogens, antimicrobial treatment often results in temporary, if any, relief. Because long-term antimicrobial therapy offers limited benefit for patients with no evidence of urogenital infection, we recommend a thorough evaluation for infectious agents. We prescribe antimicrobials only for patients with documented infections rather than recommending repeated courses of empiric therapy.

Alpha-blocker therapy has been evaluated in case series and randomized clinical trials. These agents represent our second-line therapy, after antibiotics. A number of other medications have been supported by case series or nonrandomized studies, including anti-inflammatory drugs, anticholinergic drugs, allopurinol, muscle relaxants and chronic pain medications.

Other measures that have been reported to provide relief include acupuncture, prostate massage, sitz baths, diathermy, exercises, physiotherapy and psychotherapy. Anecdotal reports suggest that transurethral resection of the prostate, microwave or thermal therapy might provide relief for highly selected patients. Some clinicians recommend increased frequency of ejaculation to relieve 'congestion'. Others recommend abstinence from ejaculation, alcohol, coffee, tea, spicy foods, etc. There is little objective evidence that any of these measures changes the natural history of chronic prostatitis/chronic pelvic pain syndrome.

Asymptomatic inflammatory prostatitis

Some practitioners prescribe antimicrobial and/or anti-inflammatory treatment for patients with asymptomatic prostatitis. There are limited data that patients benefit from such treatment. Thus, most authorities do not recommend treatment of asymptomatic prostatitis because the risk of side-effects does not justify the theoretical benefit from such treatment.

CONCLUSION

Patients with documented bacteriuria may have acute or chronic bacterial prostatitis, while these conditions are rare in patients with no history of bacteriuria. Specific diagnostic studies are necessary to document uropathogens, STD agents or granulomatous infections. Other diagnoses are possible in certain patients. Accurate diagnosis is the prerequisite for successful treatment.

FURTHER READING

Further reading for this chapter can be found online at http://www.expertconsult.com

George J Alangaden
John David Hinze
Richard E Winn

Practice point | **27** |

Tuberculosis of the urogenital tract

DEFINITION OF THE PROBLEM

A 47-year-old man who was born in India and emigrated to the United States 5 years ago presents with painless swelling of the scrotum. He has no systemic symptoms. Examination reveals a nontender 3 cm firm mass involving the left epididymis. Urine examination demonstrates persistent pyuria with negative cultures.

INTRODUCTION

Genitourinary tuberculosis (TB) is a severe form of extrapulmonary TB that is uncommon in countries with a low prevalence of TB. In 2003 in the United States, genitourinary TB accounted for about 1% of the 14 874 cases of TB and 5% of the 3029 cases of extrapulmonary TB. However, genitourinary TB can account for up to 20% all TB cases in high TB-prevalence countries. It is uncommon in children and most cases present in adults older than 20 years, with a male:female predominance of 2:1.

PATHOGENESIS

Genitourinary TB is almost always caused by *Mycobacterium tuberculosis* (MTB) and results from hematogenous dissemination from the lungs to the kidneys during primary infection, with subsequent reactivation later in life. Infection initially involves the renal cortex, with granuloma formation and caseation necrosis. It progressively involves the medulla and papilla with development of macroscopic cavitary lesions. Subsequent MTB bacilluria results in infection of the ureters and bladder. Progressive disease can result in fibrosis affecting the ureters and bladder, and may lead to total destruction of the kidney, termed 'autonephrectomy'.

Descending infection from the kidneys in males can affect the epididymis, seminal vesicles, testes and prostate. TB of the penis is rare and can result from sexual contact. In women, hematogenous infection of the fallopian tubes occurs initially, followed by spread of infection to the endometrium, ovaries and cervix.

Rarely genitourinary TB can result from infection following intravesical immunotherapy with bacille Calmette–Guérin (BCG) for the treatment of transitional cell carcinoma of the bladder. Transmission of TB via donor kidney during renal transplantation has been reported.

CLINICAL FEATURES

Genitourinary TB is a slowly progressive infection that is clinically inapparent for decades. Many patients with pulmonary TB may have coexistent asymptomatic genitourinary TB. The symptoms of genitourinary TB are often localized to the organs involved and constitutional symptoms are uncommon. The commonest symptoms of genitourinary TB reported in large series of patients have included dysuria, frequency or urgency (31–65%), hematuria (30–43%) and flank pain (21–57%), with fever being infrequent (12–33%).

Genital TB in men generally presents with a scrotal mass due to infection of the epididymis and less frequently with prostatitis, orchitis or scrotal fistulas. In women with genital TB the most common presentation is infertility, followed by pelvic pain or dysmenorrhea.

DIAGNOSIS

The early diagnosis of genitourinary TB requires a high degree of clinical suspicion. A history of prior TB infection in the context of chronic urinary symptoms, scrotal mass in men or infertility in women should prompt consideration of genitourinary TB.

A tuberculin skin test should be performed in suspected cases, and will be positive in approximately 90% of patients with genitourinary TB.

Radiologic findings can help support the diagnosis of genitourinary TB. Chest radiographs to assess the presence of pulmonary TB may demonstrate abnormalities in about a third of cases. Simple abdominal radiography might show renal calcification. The most commonly used radiologic technique for evaluating genitourinary TB has been the intravenous pyelogram (IVP). Renal TB is suggested by the presence of abnormalities of both the upper and lower urinary tracts. An IVP may demonstrate calyceal distortion, delayed excretion, cavitation, 'moth-eaten' calyces or strictures with caliectasis. The characteristic 'phantom calyx' occurs when the IVP reveals an obstructed nonfunctioning calyx proximal to an infundibular stricture. A 'hiked-up' renal pelvis observed when the renal pelvis makes an acute angulation with the ureter is highly suggestive of renal TB. Another highly suggestive lesion is the 'putty kidney' consisting of a heavily calcified caseous mass surrounded by a thin parenchymal shell. Ureteral TB may manifest as strictures and obstructions, giving the appearance of 'beading', 'corkscrewing', straight 'pipe-stems', focal calcification or hydronephrosis. Commonly, the bladder appears thickened and fibrotic with small capacity.

Ultrasound, CT and MRI are increasingly being utilized in the evaluation of genitourinary TB and help to provide a guide for fine-needle aspiration biopsies.

- Ultrasound may demonstrate small focal kidney lesions in patients with renal TB. In women with TB of the fallopian tubes, ultrasonography demonstrates adnexal masses containing small scattered calcifications. Testicular and transrectal ultrasonography can be used to evaluate a scrotal mass and the prostate but the findings are nonspecific.
- The CT scan can provide details of the renal parenchyma and associated abnormalities in the genital tract, abdomen and pelvis. Typical CT findings are caliectasis and focal cortical scarring (>80%).
- On MRI scans tuberculous foci appear hypointense on T2-weighted images. In women with genital TB the hysterosalpingogram demonstrates characteristic abnormalities, displaying a contracted deformed uterine cavity with intrauterine adhesions. The fallopian tubes may have ragged outlines and appear beaded or rigid.

The finding of 'sterile' pyuria has been considered an important clue to the laboratory diagnosis of genitourinary TB. However, common bacterial uropathogens are often isolated from the urine of patients with genitourinary TB. This can obscure the diagnosis and result in unnecessary antibiotic therapy. The initial microbiologic testing should include at least three first-morning urine specimens for acid-fast bacillus (AFB) stain and culture. It is important to ensure that patients are not receiving antibiotics since commonly used agents such as fluoroquinolones can inhibit the growth of MTB. Mycobacterial cultures of the urine may be positive in about 77–92% cases of genitourinary TB. If urine, menstrual blood or seminal fluid cultures are negative, then ultrasound- or CT-guided fine-needle aspiration, uterine curettage or diagnostic laparoscopy should be used to obtain appropriate tissue for microbiologic and histopathologic testing.

The average time to isolation of MTB using liquid and solid media is about 2–4 weeks and susceptibility testing requires an additional 2–4 weeks. Polymerase chain reaction (PCR) assays targeting MTB DNA have been used for the rapid diagnosis of genitourinary TB on urine and tissue specimens. Reports suggest higher sensitivity and specificity compared to AFB smear and MTB cultures. However, cultures should be performed to obtain MTB isolates for susceptibility testing which is essential to guide therapy.

MANAGEMENT (SEE ALSO CHAPTERS 30 AND 143)

The primary management of genitourinary TB is medical. Short-course anti-TB therapy regimens have been shown to be effective for all forms of extrapulmonary therapy including genitourinary TB. The recommendations of the World Health Organization and the Centers for Disease Control and Prevention include initial intensive 2-month therapy with a three- or four-drug regimen using isoniazid, rifampin and pyrazinamide. Ethambutol may be utilized as the fourth agent in areas with a high prevalence of isoniazid resistance. The intensive phase is followed by 4 months of continuation therapy with isoniazid and rifampin (rifampicin). Therapy in the continuation phase should be guided by the results of susceptibility testing. The management of patients unresponsive to treatment or with drug-resistant TB should be carried out in close conjunction with an expert. Urine cultures should become negative after 2–3 months of therapy. Follow-up radiologic imaging to monitor for development of obstructive uropathy should be considered.

A common problem in the management of genitourinary TB is the progression of nephroureteric disease despite appropriate antimicrobial therapy. Fibrosis causing obstruction can occur anywhere along the urinary tract. Endoscopic balloon dilatation, ureteric stents and reconstructive urologic surgery have been utilized in the management of these sequelae. Nephrectomy is seldom necessary and may be indicated in cases of a nonfunctioning kidney, recalcitrant infection, life-threatening hematuria and uncontrollable hypertension secondary to renal TB.

FURTHER READING

Further reading for this chapter can be found online at http://www.expertconsult.com

Practice point | **28** | *George J Alangaden*

Urinary tract infections in kidney transplant recipients

DEFINITION OF THE PROBLEM

A 42-year-old woman with end-stage renal disease secondary to hypertension and diabetes mellitus underwent a cadaveric renal transplant. Five weeks after her transplant, while on antibiotic prophylaxis with trimethoprim–sulfamethoxazole she develops low-grade fever and dysuria. Urine examination reveals pyuria and bacteriuria, and *Escherichia coli* resistant to trimethoprim-sulfamethoxazole is isolated from urine culture.

INTRODUCTION

In the USA, 16 646 kidney transplants were performed in 2006. The 5-year patient and kidney graft survival rates are about 80%. Mortality related to infection in the first year following kidney transplant is less than 5%. Urinary tract infections (UTIs) are the most common infectious complication after kidney transplantation; they account for 47–61% of infections and a third of bacteremias. The cumulative incidence of UTI is about 17% for both men and women within 6 months and 60% for women and 47% for men at 3 years after transplantation.

The wide range of frequencies of UTI reported is the result of varying definitions of UTI, use of antibiotic prophylaxis and the duration of follow-up. If the presence of bacteriuria (10^5 organisms/ml) alone is used to define UTIs it overestimates the incidence. The inclusion of concomitant pyuria to bacteriuria may identify patients at risk for subsequent symptomatic UTI which occurs in about 25–47% of recipients. Use of trimethoprim–sulfamethoxazole prophylaxis results in slightly lower rates of UTIs. The incidence of UTI is greatest during the first 3 months following transplantation and may be related to surgical trauma, presence of urinary catheters and ureteric stents.

PATHOGENESIS AND RISK FACTORS FOR UTI

Host immune system deficiencies that predispose to infections including UTI among renal transplant recipients are termed as the 'net state of immune suppression' and include antirejection immune suppressive therapy, surgical trauma, presence of catheters and stents, metabolic factors such as hyperglycemia and immunomodulating viral infections such as cytomegalovirus. Women and diabetic transplant recipients are at greatest risk for UTIs and are more likely to develop bacteremias resulting from UTIs. Other specific risk factors include older age, prolonged pre-transplant dialysis, polycystic kidney disease, pre-transplant UTIs, allograft trauma, microbial contamination of cadaveric kidneys, complications related to ureteral anastomosis, presence of urinary catheters and ureteric stents, re-implantation and vesicoureteral reflux.

CLINICAL FEATURES OF UTI

Most UTIs in renal transplant recipients presents as cystitis with common symptoms such as frequency, urgency, dysuria and minimal fever. Pyelonephritis and bacteremias can occur and are more likely in the early period after transplantation. In the immediate post-transplant period, the time to development of UTIs in the presence of a urinary catheter is about 1 week. Recurrent UTIs occur in 5–27% of cases.

MICROBIOLOGY FOR UTI

The pathogens isolated from kidney transplant recipients with UTI are similar to those in the general population. Enterobacteriaceae account for 40–90% of UTIs, with *Escherichia coli* being the most common pathogen. Other Gram-negative uropathogens include *Klebsiella* spp., *Enterobacter* spp., *Pseudomonas aeruginosa*, *Serratia marcescens* and *Acinetobacter* spp. Gram-positive bacteria such as *Enterococcus* spp., coagulase-negative staphylococci and *Corynebacterium urealyticum* cause 7–22% of UTIs. *Candida* spp. are uncommon uropathogens in renal transplant recipients, accounting for 1–5% of UTIs.

Enterococcus spp. and antibiotic-resistant Enterobacteriaceae are being increasingly reported worldwide in association with UTIs in renal transplant recipients. Enterococcal UTIs appear to occur early after transplantation. Resistance to trimethoprim–sulfamethoxazole, ciprofloxacin and the production of extended-spectrum β-lactamases has been noted in *E. coli* and *E. cloacae*.

PREVENTION OF UTI

Good surgical technique and early removal of urinary catheters decrease the risk of UTI.

Trimethoprim–sulfamethoxazole has been shown to be cost-effective in preventing UTIs after renal transplantation. Moreover, trimethoprim–sulfamethoxazole prevents opportunistic infections caused by *Pneumocystis jirovecii*, *Listeria monocytogenes*, *Nocardia asteroides* and *Toxoplasma gondii*. Hence prophylaxis with trimethoprim–sulfamethoxazole has been recommended for 6–12 months after renal transplantation. The doses range from 80 mg/400 mg to 320 mg/1600 mg of trimethoprim–sulfamethoxazole administered daily. Ciprofloxacin in doses of 250–500 mg daily is as effective as trimethoprim–sulfamethoxazole. Antibiotic stewardship and infection control practices are necessary to forestall the emergence and spread of multidrug-resistant pathogens.

629

DIAGNOSIS AND THERAPY OF UTIs

The diagnosis of UTI should be based upon the presence of symptoms, pyuria and bacteriuria. Given the emergence of drug resistance among uropathogens, Gram stain, cultures and antimicrobial susceptibilities should be performed on clean-voided midstream urine specimens. Blood cultures should be obtained if systemic symptoms such as high fevers or clinical features of pyelonephritis are present.

Initial empiric therapy of symptomatic UTI should include antibiotics that are active against Enterobacteriaceae such as broad-spectrum penicillins, cephalosporins or fluoroquinolones. Nephrotoxic agents such as aminoglycosides should be avoided, especially since these patients are often receiving other potentially nephrotoxic agents (e.g. tacrolimus). Subsequent therapy should be adjusted based upon results of urine cultures and susceptibilities. A course of therapy of about 2 weeks is recommended except in cases of relapse or prostatitis when prolonged therapy for 4–6 weeks is appropriate. Hospitalization may be necessary based upon severity of illness.

Imaging studies such as renal ultrasound or CT are indicated if there is a poor response to appropriate antimicrobial therapy, or when a surgical complication such as a ureteral anastomosis leak or obstruction is suspected. Recurrent and relapsing UTIs or breakthrough UTI on prophylaxis may warrant further urologic investigations such as voiding cystourethrography to identify any correctable structural or functional defects of the urinary tract.

ASYMPTOMATIC BACTERIURIA AND CANDIDURIA

The natural history of asymptomatic bacteriuria in renal transplant recipients is poorly defined. In the absence of controlled studies to examine effectiveness of antibiotic treatment, the optimal management of asymptomatic bacteriuria remains controversial. Routine antibiotic treatment is not recommended as it appears to have no impact on renal function and does not appear to decrease the rate of symptomatic UTIs.

Likewise the management of asymptomatic candiduria is controversial. Routine treatment of candiduria has been recommended in the past. However, in a recent study of 1738 kidney transplant recipients, of whom 11% had candiduria, no difference in outcomes was noted among treated or untreated patients with asymptomatic candiduria.

UTI IN KIDNEY–PANCREAS TRANSPLANT RECIPIENTS

Transplantation of the pancreas is increasingly used in the management of patients with type 1 diabetes mellitus with end-stage renal disease. The main types of pancreas transplantation are simultaneous kidney–pancreas transplantation (the most common), pancreas after kidney transplantation, or pancreas alone. In pancreatic transplantation, the drainage from the pancreas is diverted into the duodenum (enteric drainage) or into the urinary bladder.

Advances in surgical techniques and antirejection therapies have resulted in patient survival rates of greater than 95% and kidney and pancreas graft survival rates of 92–94% and 78–84%, respectively. Infections (especially UTIs) are more common in these patients compared to renal transplantation alone, due to the complexity of surgery and the structural and metabolic changes resulting from pancreatic secretions draining into the urinary bladder. Hence UTIs and urologic complications are more frequent in recipients with bladder drainage compared to those with enteric drainage. In contrast, recipients with enteric drainage have a higher rate of intra-abdominal infections.

Common uropathogens isolated from UTI in these patients are *E. coli*, *Klebsiella* spp., *Proteus* spp., *Pseudomonas* spp., coagulase-negative staphylococci and *Enterococcus* spp. The principles of management of UTI in these patients are the same as described in renal transplant recipients. UTIs are often recurrent and may result in epididymitis, prostatitis and prostatic abscesses. Such complications may necessitate conversion of urinary bladder drainage to enteric drainage.

CONCLUSION

UTIs are the most common infectious complication after renal transplantation and can occur despite trimethoprim–sulfamethoxazole prophylaxis. The epidemiology of UTIs varies based upon the time after transplantation. *Enterococcus* spp. and antibiotic-resistant Enterobacteriaceae have emerged as important uropathogens. Hence the antibiotic treatment of symptomatic UTIs in these patients should be guided by culture and susceptibility data. Until the natural history and optimal management of asymptomatic bacteriuria and candiduria are better defined, routine therapy of asymptomatic bacteriuria and candiduria may be unnecessary.

FURTHER READING

Further reading for this chapter can be found online at http://www.expertconsult.com

Chapter | 57 |

Khalil G Ghanem
George R Kinghorn

Syphilis

Venereal syphilis (from now on, referred to as 'syphilis') is a disease caused by the spirochete *Treponema pallidum* subspecies *pallidum* and is transmitted during sexual intercourse and other intimate contact; it may also be vertically transmitted by a pregnant woman to her fetus in utero or during birth.

Two other subspecies of *T. pallidum* – *pertenue* and *endemicum* – are responsible for yaws and endemic syphilis, respectively. The name 'syphilis' was drawn from a poem, 'Syphilis sive morbus gallicus', written by Fracastoro of Verona in 1530, in which the mythical swineherd Syphilis refused to make sacrifices to Apollo and was smitten as a result. In 1905, the association between *T. pallidum* and syphilis was first described by Schaudinn and Hoffman.[1]

EPIDEMIOLOGY

An epidemic of sexually transmitted syphilis spread across Europe at the end of the 15th century. There are conflicting views about its origin. Recent phylogenetic studies show that strains of *T. pallidum* subspecies *pallidum* are most closely related to yaws-causing strains found in South America rather than Old World strains.[2] This finding suggests that syphilis was most likely introduced to the Old World by Christopher Columbus and his men upon their return from the New World. The impact of syphilis in 16th century Europe was similar to the global impact of AIDS in the late 20th century. Syphilis had certainly become endemic in Europe by the 17th century, since then there have been several epidemic waves, notably during the Napoleonic wars and the period of industrialization in the 19th century, and during and after the two world wars of the 20th century.[3]

In North America and northern Europe, by the 1970s, syphilis had become predominately a disease of homosexual men. During the late 1980s, there were renewed outbreaks of heterosexual and congenital syphilis in North America in the wake of the HIV epidemic.[4] Syphilis rates reached a nadir in 2000, but began increasing shortly thereafter despite the introduction of a National Plan to Eliminate Syphilis. In 2006, 9756 primary and secondary syphilis cases (3.3 cases/100 000 population) were reported to the US Centers for Disease Control and Prevention (CDC), a 14% increase from the previous year.[5] From 2000 to 2005, these increases were predominantly among men (5.7 cases/100 000 men in 2006), with 60% occurring among men who have sex with men. In 2006, increases in women (1 case/100 000 women in 2006) and in cases of congenital syphilis (8.5 cases/100 000 live births in 2006) were noted after a steady decline.

In the UK there has been a substantial increase in syphilis cases: from 301 cases in 1997 to 3702 in 2006. The majority of cases are among men (8.2 cases/100 000 men in 2006). Almost a quarter of those with syphilis in the UK in 2006 were also infected with HIV.

Early on, cases were predominantly reported from London and the North West of England,[6] but recent increases have been documented throughout the UK.

The annual incidence of congenital syphilis in infants aged less than 1 year in the US increased from 3.0 per 100 000 live births in 1980 to a peak of 107.3 per 100 000 live births in 1990. The very large increase in reported cases was artificially elevated by the introduction of a new reporting system. From 1996 to 2005, a steady 14% yearly decrease in the number of congenital syphilis cases was observed in the US. However, in 2006, a 3.7% increase from the previous year was noted in conjunction with the increased rates seen in women.

The World Health Organization (WHO) estimates that the annual global incidence of syphilis is approximately 12.2 million cases, most of which occur in developing countries, where the disease has remained a prominent cause of genital ulcer disease in heterosexual men and women, of stillbirth, and of neonatal morbidity and mortality. The prevalence of pregnant seropositive women is 0.1–0.6% in developed countries, but it may exceed 10% in many developing countries.

Transmission

The organism is transmitted from the early mucocutaneous lesions, primarily via sexual contact, and enters the body through small breaches in epithelial surfaces of genital, anorectal, oropharyngeal and other cutaneous sites (Fig. 57.1). The probability of sexual transmission to an uninfected partner in early syphilis has been estimated to be ~60% (range 9–80%).[7] Syphilis is rarely transmitted during transfusion of blood or blood products or through needle sharing by intravenous drug users.

Prenatal transmission is greatest in cases of maternal infection of short duration, but it may also occur during the latent stages of syphilis. Disease manifestations are unusual before 18 weeks in utero. Stillbirth caused by congenital syphilis has a maximum incidence at 6–8 months of gestation. Even when a previous pregnancy has resulted in an uninfected child, congenital syphilis may occur in subsequent offspring, and it may affect only one of twins. It is preventable with maternal treatment during pregnancy.[8]

PATHOGENESIS AND PATHOLOGY

Treponema pallidum subsp. *pallidum* is microaerophilic with a unique wave-like cell body that is 6–15 μm long and 0.15–0.20 μm wide. It contains a periplasmic flagellum and can be identified in darkfield microscopy by its characteristic morphology and movements, which typically include angling. The organism has evolved to become a highly invasive and persistent pathogen with little toxigenic activity and an

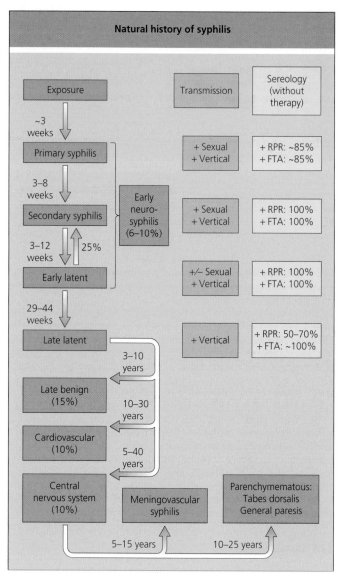

Fig. 57.1 The natural history of syphilis. FTA, fluorescent treponemal antibody absorbed test; RPR, rapid plasma reagin test.

inability to survive outside the mammalian host. It has extreme nutritional requirements, owing to deficiencies in biosynthetic pathways, and it has a narrow equilibrium between oxygen dependence and toxicity. It cannot be cultured on artificial media but it can be propagated in organ culture, such as rabbit testis. It has a slow growth rate, optimal at 91–95°F (33–35°C), with a doubling time of 30–36 hours.

Analysis of the genome, which is contained on a single circular chromosome with 1 138 006 base pairs, shows that the organism lacks lipopolysaccharide and lipid biosynthesis mechanisms, as well as many metabolic pathways, including pathways for the tricarboxylic acid cycle, for components of oxidative phosphorylation, and for most amino acids and vitamins. It requires D-glucose, maltose and mannose but cannot utilize other sugars. It is able to use exogenously supplied amino acids and is dependent on serum components such as fatty acids.

Treponema pallidum initiates an inflammatory response at the site of inoculation and is disseminated during the primary infection (reviewed by LaFond & Lukehart[9]). Animal studies have shown that treponemes appear within minutes in lymph nodes and blood,[10] and disseminate widely within hours. Eighteen hours following inoculation, treponemes are detectable in the cerebrospinal fluid (CSF) of

rabbits. Following inoculation, *T. pallidum* gains access to deeper tissues by inducing the production of matrix metalloproteinase-1 in dermal cells. The organism activates endothelial cells which then signal inflammatory and immune cells to migrate into infected tissues. Polymorphonuclear lymphocytes are the first cells that respond to pathogen invasion, but their presence is limited and transient. Toll-like receptor (TLR)-2 has been shown to recognize *T. pallidum* microbial patterns and is involved in mediating the innate response.[11] Dendritic cells are stimulated by the TLR-2 pathway. They phagocytize the organisms and migrate to lymph nodes where they activate T cells.

T. pallidum components also induce the production of tumor necrosis factor (TNF) by macrophages (and other proinflammatory cytokines), which further activates the immune response. Humoral responses consisting of IgM and IgG antibodies are detected within 6 days after infection and are specific for a broad range of *T. pallidum* surface molecules. These antibodies have been shown to have opsonizing activity as well as the ability (in the presence of complement) to immobilize the organisms and neutralize their ability to form lesions. These antibodies have not been shown to be treponemicidal. The number of organisms within a lesion begins to decline significantly 14–16 days following infection.

Evasion of the host immune response is thought to occur via several mechanisms:[9]

- the antigenic inertness of the *T. pallidum* surface;
- limited number of organisms causing disease below the 'critical antigenic mass' necessary to stimulate a robust immune response;
- the invasion of immune-privileged sites;
- the slow generation time of the organism; and
- the ability of the organism to bypass the host's iron-sequestration mechanisms.

Histologic appearances and pathology

Some manifestations of syphilis (e.g. neuropathy) are immune-complex mediated. In early lesions, perivascular infiltration by lymphocytes and plasma cells is accompanied by intimal proliferation in arteries and veins. This leads to ischemia and ulceration. Organisms are most numerous in the walls of capillaries and lymphatic vessels.

In late lesions, the characteristic lesion of mucocutaneous surfaces is the syphilitic gumma. Granulation tissue forms with histiocytes, fibroblasts and epithelioid cells. Endarteritis obliterans and necrotic areas are pronounced. Gummas most often originate in subcutaneous tissues and spread in all directions. Spirochetes are not readily demonstrable in these lesions.

Heubner's arteritis occurs in cardiovascular and meningovascular syphilis. It is characterized by lymphocytic and plasma cell infiltration of the vasa vasorum and adventitia of large and medium-sized vessels. Occlusion of the vasa vasorum results in medial necrosis and fibroblast proliferation. There is associated subintimal proliferation, which leads to luminal occlusion and thrombosis.

PREVENTION

The risk factors for acquisition of syphilis mirror those of other sexually transmitted diseases (STDs). Primary prevention depends on similar methods, such as reducing the number of sexual partners and consistent use of condoms. Single-dose intramuscular benzathine penicillin G and oral azithromycin have been used as treatment for incubating syphilis.[12] Administration of treponemicidal antibiotics to treat other STDs, such as gonorrhea and chancroid, may also abort incubating concurrent syphilis. The development of a vaccine against syphilis has long been inhibited by the inability to grow the organism on artificial media.

Secondary prevention by early diagnosis, treatment, partner notification, education and counseling remain the mainstay of prevention efforts. Access to prompt and appropriate services for infected persons is essential. In many developed countries, clinic-based specialist services have long been established. In developing countries, the WHO has recommended that STD management be integrated into basic health care and reproductive health services.

Serologic screening for syphilis remains a cost-effective measure for control. Congenital syphilis may be prevented by maternal screening and treatment during early pregnancy. In the US, screening is advocated at the first prenatal visit; among high risk women, it should be repeated twice during the third trimester (28–32 weeks' gestation and at delivery).[13] In developing countries, where congenital syphilis is more common, the disease occurs when there has been no maternal screening, when no treatment has been administered in response to positive tests, or when primary infection occurs later in pregnancy.

CLINICAL FEATURES

Studies conducted in the US and Europe in the early 20th century helped to define the natural history of syphilis,[14–16] summarized in Figure 57.1.

Incubation period

The time from transmission to the appearance of primary lesions averages 21 days (range 10–90 days); the incubation period varies inversely with the size of the spirochete inoculum.

Primary syphilis

The primary chancre appears at the site of initial treponemal invasion of the dermis. It may occur on any skin or mucous membrane surface and is usually situated on the external genitalia (Fig. 57.2). Initial lesions are papular but rapidly ulcerate. They are usually single, but 'kissing' lesions may occur on opposing mucocutaneous surfaces. Typically, the ulcers are nontender (unless there is coexisting infection) and indurated, and have a clean base and raised edges (Fig. 57.3). There is often surrounding edema, especially with vulval lesions. Chancres of the cervix, anorectum or oropharynx are commonly silent. Nontender, nonsuppurative, rubbery inguinal lymphadenopathy appears 1 week later and usually becomes bilateral after 2 weeks. The chancre usually heals spontaneously within 3–6 weeks but leaves a scar.

The differential diagnosis includes other sexually transmitted causes of genital ulcer disease (which may coexist) such as chancroid, lymphogranuloma venereum, donovanosis, genital herpes and HIV, as well as traumatic ulceration, pyogenic lesions, aphthous ulceration and malignancy.

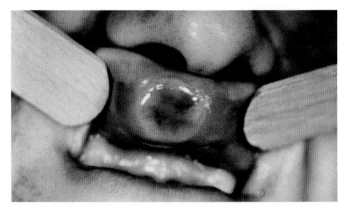

Fig. 57.3 Chancre of upper lip in primary syphilis. The chancre shows the characteristic features of a raised, rolled and everted edge, central ulceration and a granular base. From Kinghorn GR. Syphilis. Medicine 1995;24:64–8, with permission of The Medicine Group (Journals) Ltd.

Secondary syphilis

The manifestations of generalized treponemal dissemination first appear about 8 weeks after infection. Constitutional symptoms consist of fever, headache, and bone and joint pains. There is wide diversity in physical features.

Skin rashes are the most common feature. They are initially macular and become papular by 3 months. Lesions appear initially on the upper trunk (Fig. 57.4), the palms and soles (Fig. 57.5), and flexural surfaces of the extremities. The later papulosquamous eruptions typically have a coppery color and often follow skin cleavage lines, as in pityriasis rosea. Facial lesions follow the hairline of the temporal and frontal scalp (the so-called corona veneris) and cause split papules at the angles of the mouth (Fig. 57.6). There may be hypopigmented lesions on the lateral neck (collaris veneris). Lesions in hairy areas cause moth-eaten alopecia of the scalp, beard, eyebrows and eyelashes.

Condylomata lata are moist flat-topped papules that appear about 6 months after infection in the moist intertriginous areas around the genitalia, anus and axillae, and beneath the breasts. On mucous membranes, especially of the mouth, erythematous macules evolve into asymptomatic, slightly elevated, flat-topped lesions covered by a

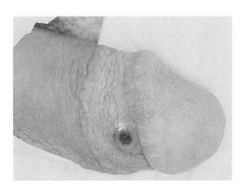

Fig. 57.2 Primary chancre in coronal sulcus in primary syphilis. A typical solitary lesion with raised everted edges, central ulceration and undermined base. From Kinghorn GR. Syphilis. Medicine 1995;24:64–8, with permission of The Medicine Group (Journals) Ltd.

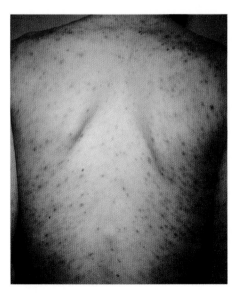

Fig. 57.4 Maculopapular rash on trunk in secondary syphilis. From Kinghorn GR. Syphilis. Medicine 1995;24:64–8, with permission of The Medicine Group (Journals) Ltd.

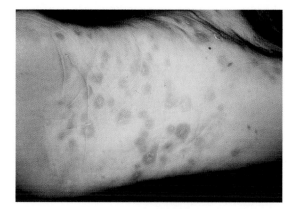

Fig. 57.5 Plantar syphilid in secondary syphilis. From Kinghorn GR. Syphilis. Medicine 1995;24:64–8, with permission of The Medicine Group (Journals) Ltd.

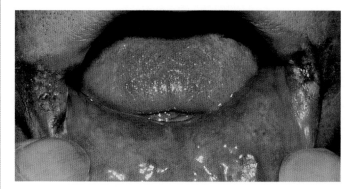

Fig. 57.6 Split papules at angle of mouth and mucous patch on lower lip in secondary syphilis. From Kinghorn GR. Syphilis. Medicine 1995;24:64–8, with permission of The Medicine Group (Journals) Ltd.

hyperkeratotic grayish membrane. These mucous patches may coalesce to form 'snail-track' ulcers.

Generalized lymphadenopathy occurs in 50% of cases of secondary syphilis. It has similar characteristics to the localized lymphadenopathy of primary infection. Other systemic features of secondary syphilis include panuveitis, periostitis and joint effusions, glomerulonephritis, hepatitis, gastritis, myocarditis and aseptic meningitis.

The lesions of secondary syphilis resolve spontaneously in a variable time period and most patients enter the latency stage within the first year of infection. In some, especially the immunocompromised, primary or secondary lesions may recur.

The differential diagnosis is broad and includes exanthema associated with many infectious diseases, including primary HIV infection, dermatoses (e.g. pityriasis rosea and guttate psoriasis) and connective tissue disorders such as systemic lupus erythematosus. Condylomata lata must be differentiated from viral warts, scabies and lichen planus.

Latent syphilis

In latent syphilis there are no clinical stigmata of active disease, although disease remains detectable by positive serologic tests. In early latency, within 1–2 years of infection, up to 25% of asymptomatic patients will experience secondary relapses, hence the distinction between early and late latency. Vertical transmission of infection may still occur, but sexual transmission is less likely in the absence of mucocutaneous lesions. The late manifestations of syphilis arise, often decades later, in about 30% of those who have latent syphilis.

Tertiary gummatous syphilis

The characteristic lesions of tertiary syphilis appear 3–10 years after infection and consist of granulomas or gummas. The granulomas appear as cutaneous plaques or nodules of irregular shape and outline (Fig. 57.7) and are often single lesions on the arms, back and face. Gummas are areas of granulomatous tissue, often arising from subcutaneous structures. They have a tendency for central necrosis and ulceration and for peripheral healing with tissue-paper scarring. Punched-out lesions appear most commonly on the scalp, face and sternoclavicular areas of the chest and on the lateral calf (Fig. 57.8). Gummas can also cause palatal perforation; destruction of nasal cartilage, producing saddle-nose deformity; painless testicular swelling, which may mimic a tumor; portal hypertension and portosystemic anastomoses; and diffuse interstitial glossitis and subsequent malignant neoplasms of the tongue.

Cardiovascular syphilis

The typical lesion of cardiovascular syphilis is aortitis affecting the ascending aorta and appearing 10–30 years after infection. The aortitis may be asymptomatic and detected as dilatation of the ascending aorta on chest radiography, often accompanied by linear calcification of the aortic wall, or it may lead to stretching and incompetence of the aortic valve, to left ventricular failure or to aneurysm formation.

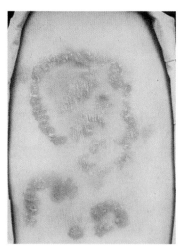

Fig. 57.7 Cutaneous nodular gummas of upper arm in tertiary gummatous syphilis. The lesions have a serpiginous outline. From Kinghorn GR. Syphilis. Medicine 1995;24:64–8, with permission of The Medicine Group (Journals) Ltd.

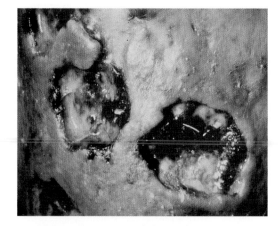

Fig. 57.8 Multiple gummatous ulcers of lower leg in tertiary gummatous syphilis. The lesions have a punched-out appearance with 'wash-leather' slough overlying a base of granulation tissue. They show a tendency for peripheral healing with thin tissue-paper scars. From Kinghorn GR. Syphilis. Medicine 1995;24:64–8, with permission of The Medicine Group (Journals) Ltd.

Aneurysms may be associated with a variety of syndromes caused by pressure on adjacent structures in the mediastinum, and they may cause sudden death from rupture. Other symptoms include angina pectoris from associated coronary ostial stenosis. Cardiovascular syphilis is more commonly associated with neurosyphilis than with gummatous disease.

The differential diagnosis of thoracic aortic aneurysm includes Behçet's disease, Takayasu's arteritis, ankylosing spondylitis and atheromatous disease. Similar histologic lesions may appear in other large arteries.

Neurosyphilis

Treponemes invade the central nervous system very early after infection[17,18] but the majority of patients are asymptomatic. Neurosyphilis is characterized by a number of heterogeneous syndromes. The onset can occur weeks or decades after treponemal dissemination.

Asymptomatic neurosyphilis precedes the development of clinically apparent disease and accounts for one-third of all neurosyphilis. It occurs in 10% of those with latent disease and has a peak incidence at 12–18 months after infection. It reverts spontaneously in 70% of patients.

Meningeal neurosyphilis usually has its onset during the early stages of disease and is characterized by symptoms of headache, confusion, nausea and vomiting, neck stiffness and photophobia. There may be focal seizures, aphasia, delirium and papilledema. Cranial nerve palsies cause unilateral or bilateral facial weakness and sensorineural deafness. Other manifestations include hydrocephalus, spinal pachymeningitis and spinal meningomyelitis.

Meningovascular syphilis occurs most frequently between 4 and 7 years after infection. Symptoms usually begin abruptly, and focal neurologic signs are most common in the territory of the middle cerebral artery. Less commonly, focal ischemia affects the basilar or spinal arteries. The clinical features of hemiparesis, seizures and aphasia reflect multiple areas of infarction from diffuse arteritis.

Gummatous neurosyphilis is the least common syndrome. Lesions arise from the pia mater and subsequently invade the brain or spinal cord, resulting in features typical of a space-occupying lesion of these structures.

Parenchymatous syphilis appears later and has become rare in its classic forms in the antibiotic era. The peak incidence of general paresis from parenchymatous disease of the brain used to be 10–20 years after infection. It was more common in males. The onset is insidious with subtle deterioration in cognitive function and psychiatric symptoms that mimic those of other mental disorders. As the disease progresses, neurologic signs develop, including pupillary abnormalities, hypotonia of the face and limbs, intention tremors and hyperreflexia. In late disease, there is progressive dementia, onset of seizures and increasing weakness leading to an incontinent bedfast state.

Tabes dorsalis, the second form of parenchymatous neurosyphilis, was the most common form of neurosyphilis before antibiotics were available. It has an onset 15–25 years after primary infection. The most characteristic symptom is of lightning pains – sudden paroxysms of lancinating pain affecting the lower limbs. Other early symptoms include paresthesia, progressive ataxia, and bowel and bladder dysfunction. The clinical signs result from leptomeningeal infiltration of the preganglionic portion of the dorsal root ganglia, with subsequent atrophic change in the posterior columns of the spinal cord. The signs are hypotonia, areflexia, and impaired joint-position and vibration sense. Pupillary abnormalities are usual, and 50% of patients have the classic Argyll Robertson pupil (small, irregular pupils that are unreactive to light but constrict normally to accommodation–convergence). Optic atrophy is also common. Later features of tabes dorsalis include visceral crises in 10–15% of patients, characterized by recurrent episodes of epigastric pain and vomiting, mimicking an acute abdomen; acute urinary retention; progressive ataxia with a wide-based slapping gait; the appearance of neuropathic joints and perforating ulcers; and coexisting palsies of the third, sixth and seventh cranial nerves.

The differential diagnosis of neurosyphilis covers the whole spectrum of neurologic and psychiatric conditions. Routine serologic screening tests for syphilis are indicated in patients who exhibit any of these features.

Congenital syphilis

Many infants with congenital syphilis are asymptomatic at birth. The placenta may show proliferative vascular changes and there may be acute inflammation of the umbilical cord (funisitis). Early congenital syphilis manifests itself as rhinitis with serosanguinous nasal discharge, vesiculobulbous eruptions of the skin and oral mucous patches. Skin lesions on the lips, nostrils and anus heal with radiating scars (rhagades). In addition, there are often bone abnormalities, characterized by diaphyseal periostitis, osteochondritis and a positive Wimberger's sign, which may present with limb pseudoparesis. Other features include chorioretinitis, visceral lesions causing pneumonia alba, hepatosplenomegaly associated with jaundice and the nephrotic syndrome.

In late congenital syphilis (presenting after 2 years of age) there may be a variety of skeletal developmental defects, including a high-arched palate, a protruding mandible, frontal bossing of the skull and saddle-nose deformity resulting in a characteristic facies (Fig. 57.9); additionally, there can be bilateral hydroarthoses of the knees (Clutton's joints), sabre tibiae from osteoperiostitis, perforation of the palate and nasal septum, and sternoclavicular thickening. Dental abnormalities occur with peg-shaped permanent incisors (Hutchinson's teeth) and mulberry multicusped molars; together with interstitial keratitis and eighth nerve deafness, these dental abnormalities form Hutchinson's triad. Other features include hydrocephalus and mental retardation, as well as other typical lesions of gummatous syphilis and neurosyphilis.

Syphilis and HIV infection

Some 16–25% of patients infected with syphilis in the US and the UK are estimated to be co-infected with HIV (reviewed by Zetola & Klausner[19]). The diagnosis of one condition requires immediate testing for the other. The presence of syphilitic ulcers increases the risk of HIV transmission and acquisition.[20] Several studies have reported differences in clinical manifestations among HIV-infected and uninfected patients.[21,22] The major finding consistently reported by these studies is the collapse of the usual timeline of the natural history of syphilis – it is not uncommon to find patients presenting with classic manifestations of primary and secondary syphilis concomitantly. In addition,

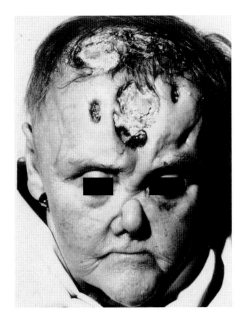

Fig. 57.9 Typical facies in late congenital syphilis. There is frontal bossing, an underdeveloped maxilla, a prominent jaw and a depressed nasal bridge, with multiple gummatous ulcers of scalp. From Kinghorn GR. Syphilis. Medicine 1995;24:64–8, with permission of The Medicine Group (Journals) Ltd.

several studies highlighted the increased frequency of early symptomatic (meningeal) neurosyphilis among dually infected patients.[23]

Diagnosis of syphilis in HIV-infected patients is similar to HIV-uninfected patients, but there is an increased frequency of false-positive reaginic tests[24] (see below). Very rarely, false-negative reaginic and treponemal tests have been reported.[25]

DIAGNOSIS

Microscopic identification

Treponema pallidum can be identified from genital lesions of primary syphilis and lesions from secondary or early congenital syphilis by darkfield microscopy. Darkfield microscopy is the gold-standard test to diagnose the genital chancres of primary syphilis as serologic tests may be negative in up to 30% of patients. The specificity of darkfield microscopy in diagnosing syphilis from oral or rectal mucosal lesions is much lower given the presence of nonpathogenic treponemes at those sites. Lesions are thoroughly cleansed with saline and scarified if necessary. Lymph node aspirates are also useful for microscopic examination in secondary syphilis.

The organism can also be identified by direct immunofluorescent antibody testing where no facilities for darkfield microscopy exist.

In biopsy specimens from late syphilis or in atypical early lesions, it may be possible to identify the organism by silver stains such as Warthin–Starry preparations or by direct immunofluorescent antibody testing.

Diagnosis using the polymerase chain reaction (PCR) has been based on primers and probes prepared from the 47 kDa gene. This technique is not routinely available.

Serologic testing

The serologic tests for syphilis can be subdivided into two types: standard nontreponemal (reaginic) tests and the specific treponemal antibody tests (Table 57.1). The former tests are sensitive but not specific and they provide titers that can be followed after therapy. The latter are sensitive and specific but do not provide titers to monitor therapeutic response (reviewed by Larsen *et al.*[26]). As the relationship between microbiologic status (i.e. presence of treponemes) and serologic status is not well defined, serologic failure may not reflect microbiologic failure; similarly, serologic response to therapy may not reflect microbiologic eradication of the organism.[27]

Standard nontreponemal tests

The nontreponemal tests detect IgM and IgG antibodies to lipoidal material released from damaged host cells and to lipoidal-like antigens of *T. pallidum*. There are several tests available that use the VDRL antigen (consisting of cardiolipin, cholesterol and lecithin) as the principal component. These tests are quantitative and are useful in assessing response to treatment. Reactivity to these tests does not develop until 1–4 weeks after the chancre appears in primary syphilis. Titers are highest in secondary syphilis. The prozone phenomenon occurs in 2% of sera; undiluted sera give negative results because of antibody excess or the presence of blocking antibodies, or both. The titer slowly declines after the 1- to 4-week period following the appearance of the chancre, and it may spontaneously become negative in some cases of late latent syphilis and neurosyphilis (see Fig. 57.1).

The VDRL slide test is widely used and requires the microscopic demonstration of antigen–antibody flocculations in heat-inactivated serum.

The rapid plasma reagin (RPR) test uses charcoal added to the VDRL reagent to enhance visualization of the antigen–antibody flocculations. The flocculations are visible macroscopically.

Biologic false-positive reactions to these tests occur in a wide variety of conditions. They can be subdivided into acute reactions, lasting for 6 months or less, and chronic reactions (Table 57.2).

Specific treponemal antibody tests

Specific treponemal antibody tests are used for confirmatory testing. They detect IgG antibodies to antigenic determinants of treponemes. They are qualitative procedures and are not helpful in assessing treatment responses; once positive, they tend to remain positive for life, irrespective of treatment. They are used to differentiate true-positives from false-positives in the standard nontreponemal antibody tests.

The fluorescent treponemal antibody absorption (FTA-ABS) test and the FTA-ABS double-staining (FTA-ABS DS) test are both indirect immunofluorescent tests. The double stain test employs a fluorochrome-labeled counterstain for *T. pallidum* and an antihuman IgG conjugate labeled with tetramethyl rhodamine isothiocyanate to detect antibody in patient serum. False-positive results may occur in about 1% of sera; possible causes include technical error, Lyme borreliosis, pregnancy, genital herpes, alcoholic cirrhosis and connective tissue diseases such as systemic lupus erythematosus and scleroderma.

The microhemagglutination assay for antibodies to *T. pallidum* (MHA-TP) detects passive hemagglutination of erythrocytes sensitized with ultrasonicated Nichol's strain *T. pallidum*. In many laboratories, the TPHA has been replaced by the similar *T. pallidum* particle

Table 57.1 Serologic tests for syphilis

	SENSITIVITY*				Specificity*
	Primary	Secondary	Latest	Late	
Nonspecific reaginic tests					
VDRL	80	100	95	70	98
RPR	86	100	98	75	98
USR	80	100	94		98
TRUST	85	100	97		97
Specific treponemal antibody tests					
MHA-TP	76	100	96	95	99
FTA-ABS	84	100	100	96	97
FTA-ABS double-staining	80	100	100		98

*The values for sensitivity are the mean values in CDC (Centers for Disease Control and Prevention) tests. The values for specificity are mean values in nonsyphilis populations in CDC tests.

Table 57.2 Causes of biologic false-positive cardiolipin tests

	Acute	**Chronic**
Physiologic	Pregnancy	Old age
Spirochete infections	Leptospirosis Relapsing fever Rat-bite fever Lyme disease	
Other infections	Varicella zoster Herpes simplex Infectious mononucleosis Cytomegalovirus Toxoplasmosis Viral hepatitis HIV seroconversion illness *Mycoplasma* infection Malaria Other acute viral or bacterial sepsis	Lepromatous leprosy Tuberculosis Lymphogranuloma venereum Malaria Kala-azar Trypanosomiasis Tropical spastic paraparesis HIV or AIDS
Vaccinations	Smallpox Typhoid Yellow fever	
Autoimmune diseases		Systemic lupus erythematosus Polyarteritis nodosa Rheumatoid arthritis Sjögren's syndrome Primary biliary cirrhosis Hashimoto's thyroiditis Autoimmune hemolytic anemia Idiopathic thrombocytopenic purpura
Other		Malignancy Malnutrition Injecting drug use

agglutination (TPPA) test but uses gelatin particles rather than erythrocytes as the carrier. It is more sensitive than the FTA-ABS.

Treponemal enzyme immunoassay (EIA) commercial tests were initially designed as confirmatory tests for syphilis. Serum is added to microwells coated with a treponemal antigen. After incubation, an enzyme-labeled antihuman immunoglobulin conjugate and enzyme substrate are added to detect antigen–antibody reaction. The test also has advantages of automated or semiautomated processing and objective reading of results, and it can be interfaced with laboratory computer systems to allow electronic laboratory report generation. The test can be modified to detect specific IgM antibody.

There are many commercial tests in any given format whose performance characteristics vary.

Indications for examination of cerebrospinal fluid

Examination of cerebrospinal fluid (CSF) in syphilis should be considered if:[28]

- neurologic, ophthalmic or auditory symptoms and signs are present;
- other clinical evidence of active infection (e.g. aortitis, gumma, iritis) is present;

- serologic failure occurs despite adequate therapy (and no evidence of re-infection);
- HIV infection is present (especially if RPR = 1:32 and CD4 <350 cells/ml);
- serum nontreponemal titer >1:32 if duration of syphilis is more than 1 year; and
- nonpenicillin-based treatment regimen is planned.

The typical CSF findings of neurosyphilis consist of:

- moderate mononuclear pleocytosis (10–400 cells/ml);
- elevated total protein (0.46–2.0 g/l); and
- positive CSF VDRL.

The CSF VDRL is highly specific, and false-positive results are rare in the absence of blood contamination.[29] A negative CSF VDRL does not exclude neurosyphilis. Treponemal-specific tests performed on CSF may have higher sensitivity than CSF VDRL, but false-positives have been reported.[30]

Typical neuroimaging findings have been described for neurosyphilis.[31]

Evaluation of neonates for congenital syphilis

The definitions of congenital syphilis are listed in Table 57.3. It is recommended that the following investigations be carried out in a child born to a seropositive mother if there has been no documented completion of treatment at least 4 weeks before delivery, if a nonpenicillin regimen was administered, or if relapse or re-infection is suspected:[28]

- physical examination for stigmata of congenital syphilis;
- radiography of long bones for evidence of periostitis;
- examination of the CSF; and
- darkfield microscopic examination (or DFA staining) of suspicious lesions or body fluids

Infection of the neonate is also suggested if the serum (not cord blood) nontreponemal antibody titer is four or more times greater than the mother's, or if specific IgM treponemal antibody tests are positive. Passively transferred maternal IgG antibody can persist in the infant's serum for up to 12 months.

MANAGEMENT

Current treatment regimens are based on over 50 years of clinical experience with penicillin,[32] expert opinion, and open clinical studies rather than on randomized clinical trials. Thus, significant differences

Table 57.3 Definitions of congenital syphilis

Confirmed diagnosis	An infant in whom *T. pallidum* is identified by darkfield microscopy, fluorescent antibody or other specific stains in specimens from lesions, placenta, umbilical cord or autopsy material
Presumptive diagnosis	1. Any infant whose mother had untreated or inadequately treated syphilis at delivery, regardless of symptoms or signs in the infant 2. Any infant or child who has a reactive specific treponemal test for syphilis and one of the following: evidence of congenital syphilis on physical examination evidence of congenital syphilis on long-bone X-ray reactive CSF VDRL elevated CSF cell count or protein (without other cause) reactive test for FTA-ABS-IgM using fractionated serum

Table 57.4 Treatment of acquired syphilis comparing the US and UK recommendations

Stage	US CDC-recommended regimens	US alternative regimens	UK recommended regimens
Early syphilis (primary, secondary, early latent of <1–2 years' duration)	Benzathine penicillin G 2.4 million units im single dose	Tetracycline 500 mg po q6h for 14 days Doxycycline 100 mg po q12h for 14 days Azithromycin 2 g po single dose Ceftriaxone 1 g im q24h for 10 days	Procaine penicillin G 600 000 units im q24h for 10 days Benzathine penicillin G 2.4 million units im once
Late syphilis (latent syphilis of >1–2 years' duration, cardiovascular, gummatous syphilis)	Benzathine penicillin G 2.4 million units weekly for 3 weeks	Tetracycline 500 mg po q6h for 28 days Doxycycline 100 mg po q12h for 28 days	Procaine penicillin 600 000 units im q48h for 17 days Benzathine penicillin G 2.4 million units weekly for 3 doses
Neurosyphilis	Aqueous crystalline penicillin G 3–4 million units iv q4h for 10–14 days	Ceftriaxone 2 g im or iv q24h for 10–14 days	Procaine penicillin 1.8–2.4 million units im q48h plus probenecid 500 mg po q6h for 17 days Benzyl penicillin 3–4 million units iv q4h for 17 days

exist when comparing treatment guidelines from different countries (Table 57.4). Many antibiotics, with the notable exceptions of the aminoglycosides and sulfonamides, have some treponemicidal activity, and their administration for other conditions may abort or modify the natural history of syphilis.[27]

Parenteral penicillin G is the preferred drug at all stages of syphilis.[33] The preparations used, the dosage and the duration of treatment depend on the clinical stage and disease manifestations (see Table 57.4).[28] Adequate treatment requires the maintenance of serum concentrations in excess of 0.03 units/ml for at least 10 days.[34] A single intramuscular dose of 600 000 units of aqueous procaine penicillin gives an effective serum concentration for at least 24 hours; in comparison, a single intramuscular dose of 2 400 000 units of long-acting benzathine penicillin G maintains effective levels for about 2 weeks. Of note, the latter dose does not provide consistent treponemicidal levels in the CSF.

In patients who are hypersensitive to penicillin, regimens based on tetracycline, doxycycline,[35] erythromycin, ceftriaxone[36] and chloramphenicol have all been successfully used to treat syphilis; however, success is less assured than with penicillin. Azithromycin has been shown to be effective at treating early syphilis,[37] but emerging resistance may limit widespread use.[38]

Ceftriaxone, a third-generation cephalosporin, may be used as an alternate agent for the treatment of neurosyphilis,[39] but efficacy data are limited.

Desensitization of penicillin-allergic patients is recommended for the treatment of pregnant women and (may be considered for) neurosyphilis because parenteral penicillin G is the only treatment with well-documented efficacy in these situations.

Jarisch–Herxheimer reaction

The Jarisch–Herxheimer reaction is an acute febrile reaction that occurs in many patients within 24 hours of commencing treatment. It is mediated by cytokines. The fever may be accompanied by headache, myalgia, bone pains and an exacerbation of skin lesions. It must be differentiated from penicillin allergy. Patients should be advised that it may occur. Symptoms may be controlled by antipyretics.

In pregnant women the reaction may induce early labor or cause fetal distress. In late neurosyphilis and cardiovascular syphilis, the Jarisch–Herxheimer reaction can be more serious and may be associated with life-threatening sequelae. Many clinicians advocate a short course of corticosteroids to lessen its effects in these patients.

Treatment of congenital syphilis

The optimal treatment of congenital syphilis is unknown. Regimens that have been recommended for early congenital syphilis are intravenous aqueous crystalline penicillin G 50 000 units/kg every 8–12 hours for 10–14 days, or intramuscular procaine penicillin G 50 000 units/kg once daily for 10–14 days.[28] For infants with normal CSF findings, intramuscular benzathine penicillin G 50 000 units/kg in a single dose has also been successful. In children with late congenital syphilis presenting after 2 years of age, regimens should be the same as those recommended for late acquired disease.

Follow-up

The nontreponemal serologic test titers are followed after therapy at bi-yearly intervals to document response. Response is defined as a fourfold decline in titers at a pre-specified time (depending on stage) following therapy.[40] Failure is defined as a lack of fourfold decline during that interval, a fourfold increase in titers after appropriate therapy, or any clinical signs or symptoms consistent with syphilis.

For early syphilis, a serologic response is expected 6–12 months after therapy. For late stage disease, a decline is expected 12–24 months after therapy. An inappropriate serologic response may reflect treatment failure or re-infection. If treatment failure cannot be reliably ruled out, patients should undergo a CSF examination prior to retreatment. For patients diagnosed with neurosyphilis who had abnormalities in their CSF, repeat CSF examinations should be conducted every 6 months until resolution of all abnormalities. If there is worsening of CSF parameters or persistent abnormalities after 2 years, retreatment should be considered.

Treatment of syphilis in HIV-seropositive patients

The current recommendations are to treat HIV-infected patients with the standard therapeutic regimens used in HIV-uninfected patients; enhanced therapy was not shown to be beneficial.[41] Response to standard therapy in HIV-infected patients is a controversial topic, with several studies documenting increased serologic and clinical failure rates compared to HIV-uninfected patients.[42,43] Whether this reflects microbiologic failure or merely a delay in the response of the reaginic serologic titers to standard therapy is unclear. Currently, the main recommendation is to obtain more frequent serologic follow-up testing to ensure appropriate response to therapy. Thus, dually infected patients should have follow-up reaginic tests performed at 3, 6, 9, 12 and 24 months after therapy. In HIV-infected patients treated for neurosyphilis, a follow-up lumbar puncture 6 months after therapy is recommended and at 6-month intervals until abnormalities have resolved. Several studies have suggested that CSF and neurologic abnormalities may persist for a prolonged period despite adequate therapy.[44,45] Decisions on retreatment should be individualized.

Recent data suggest that reversal of immunosuppression by the use of highly active antiretroviral therapy may decrease the risk for syphilis serologic failure among HIV-infected patients.[46,47]

Management of sexual contacts

It is recommended that attempts be made to identify, trace and offer further investigation to at-risk sexual contacts. In early syphilis, these are those contacts occurring within 3 months plus the duration of symptoms for primary syphilis, within 6 months plus the duration of symptoms for secondary syphilis and within 1 year for early latent disease. All long-term partners of patients with late syphilis should be offered investigation.

Many clinicians recommend presumptive treatment of all sexual contacts within the 90-day period preceding patient presentation of early syphilis if serologic test results are not immediately available and if follow-up cannot be assured.

Prognosis

In the pre-HIV era, cure rates with initial treatment of early syphilis were better than 95%. The long-term outcome of adequately treated cases is excellent. In late syphilis, infection can usually be arrested, although some treponemes may persist in less accessible sites (e.g. the eye and nervous system). As long as immune function is normal, this persistence of treponemes rarely has clinical sequelae. The outlook for HIV-positive and other immunocompromised patients appears to be less assured.

REFERENCES

References for this chapter can be found online at http://www.expertconsult.com

Genital herpes

Genital herpes is one of the most common sexually transmitted diseases. Of these, the agents of genital herpes – herpes simplex virus (HSV) type 2 and, less commonly, HSV type 1 – are among the most frequently encountered human pathogens.[1,2]

EPIDEMIOLOGY

Genital herpes infections are common, with estimates of 500 000–700 000 cases of symptomatic first episodes/year in the USA.[3–7] Humans are the natural reservoir for HSV and virtually all cases of genital herpes are sporadic, acquired via person-to-person transmission. There are no reported epidemics of genital herpes.[2]

Herpes simplex virus infections have a worldwide distribution, with seroprevalence to either HSV-1 or HSV-2 approaching 90% in some age and sex groups.[3–7] Herpes simplex virus-1 infection is common early in life, typically as orolabial 'cold sores' with antibodies appearing in childhood and prevalence increasing with age; HSV-2 antibodies increase in prevalence with increasing age after the onset of sexual activity. Approximately one in every four adults in the USA is seropositive for HSV-2.[3–7] Overall, however, HSV-2 seroprevalence decreased approximately 19% in the USA by 2004, compared to surveys done 10 years previously (overall seroprevalence to HSV-2 of 17.0%, compared a previous overall seroprevalence of 21.0%).[8] Herpes simplex virus-2 seroprevalence rates in the USA differ for some racial, sex and ethnic groups. Women acquire HSV-2 infections more readily than men and overall have a higher seroprevalence rate.[6,9] Other risk factors for genital herpes include lower socioeconomic status, increased number of sexual partners, African-Caribbean race and Hispanic ethnicity.[4–7] The highest prevalence of HSV-2 antibodies is among commercial sex workers and up to 70% of prostitutes in the USA have the infection. The lowest HSV-2 prevalence is in sexually abstinent groups, including nuns, where seroprevalence is 3% or lower.[4–7]

The incidence of seroconversion is approximately 5–10%/year when discordant couples are followed longitudinally. Among HSV-naive females with male partners who have the infection, seroconversion is as high as 15–30%/year. However, when the female partner has the infection first, less than 5% of male partners seroconvert/year.[9]

After infection with an HSV, antibodies to HSV-1 and HSV-2 type common antigens provide partial protection to infection with the counterpart virus. In prospective studies, women who have HSV-1 infection have a 5–20%/year lower rate of seroconversion to HSV-2 than women who do not have HSV infection.[9] Seroconversion to HSV-1 during childhood has decreased, particularly in upper and middle class socioeconomic groups in developed countries, whereas symptomatic infection with HSV-2 during adulthood has increased, and first visit for medical care of genital herpes remains on the rise.[4,5]

PATHOGENESIS

Herpes simplex viruses are large enveloped DNA viruses with a diameter of approximately 150 nm, a dsDNA core, an icosahedral capsid composed of 162 capsomers, an amorphous tegument layer and a lipid envelope. There are 11 different glycoproteins projecting from the envelope that are crucial for virion-cell surface attachment and cell-to-cell spread (Fig. 58.1; see also Chapter 155).[1,10]

Herpes simplex viruses are spread by direct contact, including contact with infected secretions:

- HSV-1 is typically spread through close contact with infected oral secretions, and genital herpes due to HSV-1 is usually due to oral–genital contact; and
- HSV-2 is primarily spread through intimate contact with infected genital secretions and tissues.

Intact skin is fairly resistant to virus infection, but abraded skin or mucous membranes are more susceptible.

The virus attaches to the cell surface and the viral envelope fuses with the cell membrane using a specific cellular receptor. Virion–cell surface attachment and virus intracellular penetration are mediated by viral surface glycoproteins. The viral nucleocapsid is released into the cytoplasm where it is transported to the nuclear pores of the cell. Following viral DNA replication and gene expression in the cell nucleus, the replicated nucleocapsid is assembled and buds through the nuclear membrane, acquiring an envelope. The enveloped nucleocapsid is translocated across the cytoplasm and cell membrane, acquiring surface glycoproteins at both the nuclear membrane and cell surface.[1,10]

Herpes simplex virus then infects and replicates in parabasal and intermediate skin cells. Replication results in lysis of the infected cell. Infection may spread locally by direct cell-to-cell invasion or to more distant sites via sensory nerve pathways. As virus replication spreads to involve the local autonomic and sensory nerve endings, retrograde transmission of virions (or possibly nucleocapsids) occurs with transport of virus particles to the regional sensory ganglia. Transient virus replication may occur in the ganglia at this point. From the sensory ganglia, antegrade virion migration along sensory nerves allows viral spread to other sites. By this method of spread, crops of herpetic lesions may arise at nonadjacent sites such as the thighs or buttocks. Virus replication is associated with cell lysis, cell destruction and local inflammation of all tissues except the sensory ganglia.[2,11,12]

Central nervous system disease may occur as an aseptic meningitis with primary HSV-2 or as a necrotic focal encephalitis with HSV-1 via spread through the cribriform plate to the temporal horns. Recurrent aseptic meningitis has been described, but is rare. Rarely, hematogenous dissemination may occur with visceral organ involvement, most commonly in immune compromised patients.[2]

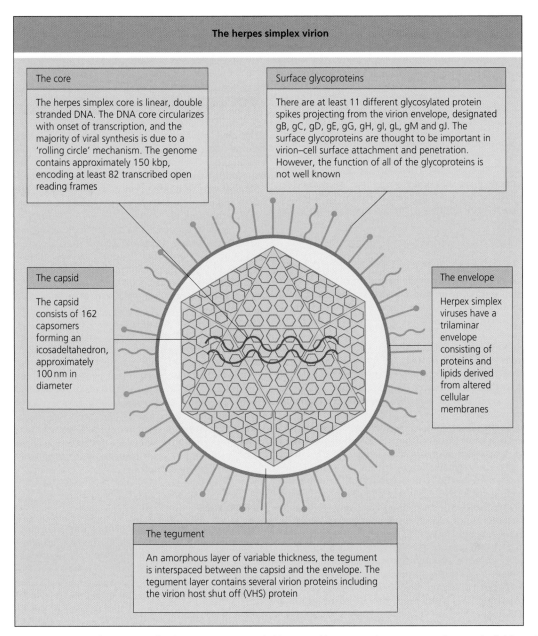

Fig. 58.1 The herpes simplex virion. This consists of a dsDNA core surrounded by a capsid, an amorphous tegument layer and a lipid envelope with numerous glycoprotein spikes. The overall diameter is 150–200 nm. Virus replication takes place within the nucleus of the infected cell. The envelope is gained as the virion passes through the nuclear membrane. Replication of virus within the host cell results in cell lysis and destruction. Latent virus does not cause neural cell lysis within ganglia.

Immune response

Both cellular and humoral host immune responses appear to be elicited by genital herpes infection.[10–17] The lysis of infected epithelial cells results in local inflammation, macrophage recruitment and T-cell activation. In a murine model, there is induction of natural killer lymphocytes. Lymphocyte activation results in the appearance of antibodies, including virus-neutralizing antibodies and antibodies that provide passive protection against infection when given to animals who are then challenged with virus.[1,10] T-cell responses, including cytotoxic T-cell responses, appear to be crucial in limiting and clearing disease.[14] Murine models also indicate that the degree of macrophage function at the site of local invasion may contribute to limiting the spread of infection.[1]

Cytokine induction is less well described. In cell culture models, HSV-infected cells express the cytokines interleukin-2, tumor necrosis factor and interferon-γ.[14] Peripheral blood mononuclear cells have been shown to produce interferon-α within hours of exposure to HSV virions.[12] Individuals with limited cellular immunity, including those at the extremes of life, patients with AIDS and bone marrow transplant recipients, tend to have prolonged severe disease with extensive tissue involvement and a higher rate of dissemination.[15]

Human humoral immune responses to HSV include the rapid generation of IgM antibodies following infection, with the appearance of detectable IgG and IgA antibodies approximately 10–14 days later. Antibodies appear first to certain structural proteins, and then sequentially to the various surface glycoproteins. Seroconversion to all virus antigenic determinants after infection may require months as measured by Western blot.[5,13,16] Lifelong virus neutralizing anti-bodies and antibody-dependent cellular cytotoxic antibodies are detectable approximately 1 month after infection. Lack of antibody-dependent cellular cytotoxic antibodies has been correlated with a poor clinical outcome and may be a factor in severe disease in the newborn.[1,17,18]

Histology

The characteristic lesion of HSV infection is an erythematous mac-ular or papular lesion, which progresses to a thin-walled vesicle on an erythematous base. Histologically, HSV infection is characterized by edema, multinucleate giant cells and Cowdry type A intranuclear inclusions. The inflammatory reaction present within HSV lesions consists of a mononuclear cell infiltrate of predominantly CD4+ T cells (Fig. 58.2).[19]

Latency

Lifelong latency is a unique property of the herpesviruses and is char-acterized by persistence of virus or viral DNA in aquiescent state in sensory and autonomic ganglia.[1] Viral transcription is limited to three latency-associated transcripts[1] and antiviral medications are unable to eradicate latent virus.[1,2,10]

Periodic recurrences of symptomatic disease are due to reactivation of latent virus. Latent virus begins to replicate and form active virus particles. The virus particles are transported by antegrade axonal flow from the ganglion to the epithelium in the genital tract. Following reactivation, fully infectious virus may be detected in cutaneous lesions at the site of recurrence.

Reactivation of latent virus tends to be site and virus specific. HSV-2 reactivates much more readily from the sacral ganglia than HSV-1 and HSV-1 reactivates more readily from the trigeminal ganglia.[2,10,20] How the virus remains latent within the ganglia and how reactivation occurs are not fully understood. In the epithelial cell, actively replicating virus DNA exists in a circular form. During latency the viral DNA assumes a linear configuration and latent viral DNA is episomal. Latency is not a wholly quiescent period, however, as some herpes simplex genes thought to be regulatory transcripts are expressed during this time.[1,2,10] Sequences within the herpes sim-plex genome specify 'latency-associated transcripts', which may be important in reactivation of virus replication. These sequences are highly divergent between HSV-1 and HSV-2 and may account for the preferential reactivation of virus type with its corresponding ganglion following latency.[2,10,20]

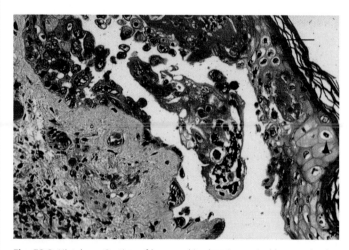

Fig. 58.2 Histology. Section of human skin showing typical herpes simplex virus effects: multinucleated giant cells (arrowhead) and intranuclear inclusion (arrow).

Virtually all recurrent genital herpes is due to reactivation of latent infection rather than to re-infection.[21] Several events may contribute to reactivation, including trauma to the ganglia, immunosuppression, UV light, fever and possibly sexual activity.[2,20]

PREVENTION

The only proven prevention strategy is avoidance of skin-to-skin contact when HSV is present in the genital tract. This includes avoidance of close physical contact during clinically symptom-atic outbreaks when virus is present in high concentrations. Most patients can recognize symptomatic clinical outbreaks even when their symptoms are 'atypical' or mild and can avoid intimate contact during this time.

Frequent, intermittent asymptomatic or subclinical shedding of low titers of virus from the genital tract occurs in both men and women,[22] and accounts for most cases of transmission of genital herpes.[22-24] There is no current method to predict when asymptom-atic virus shedding is occurring. It has been demonstrated that use of suppressive aciclovir, valaciclovir or famciclovir decreases both the number of days of virus shedding and the quantity of virus shed in an immunocompromised host.[25-27] In a landmark study, decreased shedding due to chronic suppressive antiviral therapy has been shown to lead to decreased transmission in a randomized, placebo-controlled trial among immunocompetent heterosexual couples where one person had genital HSV-2 and the sexual part-ner did not.[28] Valaciclovir was given at a dose of 500 mg daily in the treatment group, which resulted in 48% reduction in transmission in the susceptible partner. There are no data on risk of transmis-sion between homosexual couples; however, the safety of the anti-viral therapy and the data on decreased viral shedding regardless of sex would tend to favor routine use of suppressive therapy among HSV-2 discordant couples.

Vaccines

Protective vaccines may become important preventive options. The increasing incidence of genital herpes, the large number of HSV-2-seropositive individuals who are unaware of their infection status and the risk of disease transmission from asymptomatic shedding underscore the need for an effective vaccine.[23,24]

In vaccine studies, various animal models, including a guinea-pig vaginal HSV-2 model and a mouse footpad inoculation or scarifica-tion model, indicate that certain vaccine candidates provide protec-tion from acquiring infection or ameliorate disease.[29,30] When studied in humans, these vaccine candidates have not been as effective as in the animal models. In a previous controlled trial in discordant cou-ples, an inactivated HSV-2 glycoprotein vaccine failed to provide protection.[31] Recently, human trials have been completed or phase III trials are underway to evaluate recombinant surface glycoprotein vaccines.[32,33] No vaccine for HSV-2 is currently licensed and none has currently been shown to be effective.

Barrier contraception

Barrier contraception such as latex condoms can reduce the risk of dis-ease transmission by decreasing contact with the partner's infected skin or mucous membranes or infected secretions. Frequent condom use decreased the risk of HSV-2 acquisition in persons with high-risk behav-ior, such as four or more partners per year or those with a history of a sexually transmitted disease.[34] Because herpesvirus may be present out-side the portion of genital tract protected by barrier contraception, con-dom use is not infallible, and many couples may not place a condom until sexual activity is already underway. However, condom use should be encouraged as one arm of a multifactorial approach to decrease risk of transmission.

CLINICAL FEATURES

Genital herpes is a lifelong infection characterized by an initial infection followed by latency, and frequent recurrences. Infection may range from severe and symptomatic to asymptomatic. Herpes simplex virus disease is defined as:

- primary disease when a person lacking any antibodies to HSV acquires an infection with HSV-1 or HSV-2; and
- nonprimary first-episode disease when an individual with pre-existing antibodies to one serotype, typically HSV-1, acquires disease with the second type.

As the presence of pre-existing type common antibodies and cell-mediated immune responses modifies the course of disease, first-episode nonprimary disease is typically less severe than primary disease.[2,10]

Genital herpes may recur from none to six or more times/year. Recurrent disease tends to be milder than symptomatic first-episode disease, with fewer vesicles, less discomfort and a shortened duration of symptoms.[2,10]

Transmission of HSV-2 to a sexual partner or a neonate may be the first indication of the presence of genital herpes infection in an asymptomatic source partner.[24,35] The time and source of disease acquisition are often difficult to prove conclusively because:

- genital herpes can have a prolonged asymptomatic phase after acquisition and may be transmitted via asymptomatic shedding; and
- clinically silent or unrecognized disease is common.

Primary first-episode genital herpes

Primary genital herpes is most often seen as a disease of sexually active teenagers and young adults. Following exposure, a clinically silent incubation period lasts for 2–7 days. Onset of clinically apparent disease may be heralded by fever, headache and local genital pain and burning. Patients may appear to be systemically ill. In general, females tend to have more severe disease than males, with estimates of urinary retention occurring in approximately 10% of females. Up to 25% of females manifest symptoms of aseptic meningitis.[2,10]

The characteristic painful lesions in the genital area initially present as erythematous macules, which then progress to vesicles on an erythematous base, pustules, ulcers and finally to crusts (Fig. 58.3). Each crop of lesions takes an average of 8 days to heal completely, and successive crops of lesions may arise during the course of the disease. Untreated genital herpes may require weeks to resolve, averaging 3 weeks to cessation of lesions. Healing is usually complete, although particularly severe or large ulcers may result in scarring.[2]

In the male, lesions typically appear on the penis and glans penis (Fig. 58.3). In females, lesions may be present throughout the genital tract including the perineum, vulva, labia, perianal regions and buttocks. The vesicles are typically distributed bilaterally in primary disease. Cervical involvement is usually present and may escape detection if limited external disease is present and a complete pelvic examination is not performed. A vaginal discharge may accompany cervical and, less commonly, vaginal herpes. In either sex, the perianal and rectal mucosa may be involved, especially if exposure was due to rectal intercourse. Tender bilateral inguinal adenopathy is generally present. Vesicles may also be present on the thighs.

If herpetic involvement of the urethra occurs, severe dysuria may result. Sacral radiculopathy may occur during the course of primary genital herpes, with urinary retention, neuralgias, dysesthesia and diminished rectal tone. Tenesmus and rectal pain may be present with rectal herpes.[2,10]

In HSV-naive individuals, primary genital disease due to either HSV-1 or HSV-2 is clinically indistinguishable, making identification of infection by genital cultures and virus typing important for diagnosis. Atypical symptoms are quite common, with up to 30% of genital herpes presenting as paresthesias or urinary retention rather than the classically described vesicular genital lesions.[2,9,10,36]

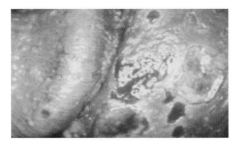

Fig. 58.3 Primary HSV. Multiple painful, erythematous, ulcerating lesions on shaft and head of penis. Exudative crust is visible over one lesion.

Nonprimary first-episode disease

Nonprimary first-episode genital HSV-2 infection is typically intermediate in severity when compared with that of primary and recurrent genital herpes.[2] Untreated disease lasts for approximately 10–14 days, with fewer lesions and fewer crops of lesions than are typical for primary disease. Systemic symptoms, including fever, are less common than in primary genital herpes, and virus can be cultured less frequently from the cervix and genital tract.[2,10]

Recurrent genital herpes

In approximately 50% of patients, a prodrome of symptoms heralds the onset of recurrent disease. Commonly reported prodromal symptoms include local burning and itching, tingling and dysesthesia. Patients may have their own recognizable cluster of symptoms. The prodromal symptoms may occur without the development of noticeable lesions or may be followed by the typical vesicular eruption lasting 6–10 days. In contrast to the widely distributed bilateral lesions of primary genital herpes, the crop of vesicular lesions in recurrent disease tends to be localized and unilateral. Lesions are typically present on the vulva in women and the glans penis and penile shaft in men, although lesions may also present on the thigh or buttocks, in the rectum and at other sites. Paresthesia, dysesthesia, local edema, pain, regional adenopathy and local swelling may accompany recurrent cutaneous herpes.[2,10]

Recurrence rates vary widely from none to six or more episodes/year, with some individuals having one or more recurrences each month. Recurrences may be triggered by sexual activity, with high rates of recurrent disease in commercial sex workers. Immunocompromised patients may experience frequent, prolonged and severe recurrences.[37] Genital herpes due to infection with HSV-2 reactivates much more readily than genital herpes due to HSV-1. Recurrent genital herpes has been reported in over 80% of individuals following primary genital HSV-2, whereas recurrence in patients who had HSV-1 primary genital herpes was less than 50%.[2] Recurrence of genital herpes averages 0.33/month with HSV-2 disease, but only 0.02/month for HSV-1 genital disease.[20]

Asymptomatic shedding

Landmark studies have demonstrated both by culture and by polymerase chain reaction (PCR) that herpesvirus is frequently present in the genital tract when lesions are absent and skin is intact, or when small or unrecognized lesions are present (Fig. 58.4).[38,39] During periods of asymptomatic virus shedding, virus titers are typically lower than during a symptomatic acute outbreak. When detected by virus culture, asymptomatic shedding occurs on an average of 4% of days, whereas women with primary genital herpes may shed virus on up to 17% of days in the first few months following their primary outbreak.[22,23]

Uncommon sites of infection

Although the majority of herpes virus infections occur in the genital and orolabial regions, cutaneous disease may occur in virtually any site, causing localized to widespread disease. Genital herpes may present as:

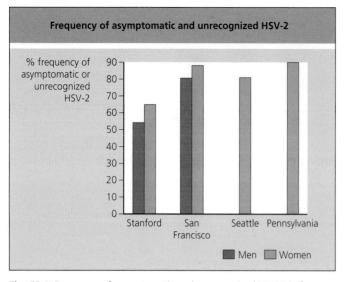

Fig. 58.4 Frequency of asymptomatic and unrecognized HSV-2 in four major US cities.[4,36,40–42]

Table 58.1 Differential diagnosis of genital herpes

Disease	Diagnostic clues
Syphilis	Lesions usually single and painless; positive darkfield microscopy
Chancroid	Nonindurated ulcers, positive bacterial cultures for *Haemophilus ducreyi*
Lymphogranuloma venereum	Constitutional symptoms follow onset of lesions; responds to doxycycline
Genital warts	Chronicity of lesions: no vesiculation; minimal pain
Fixed drug eruption	History; viral culture negative
Contact dermatitis	History; lack of systemic symptoms; no adenopathy
Trauma	History; lack of systemic symptoms; no adenopathy
Psoriasis	Chronicity of lesions; lesions elsewhere on body

- rectal herpes, with symptoms of proctitis, including rectal discharge, anal pain and pain on defecation;
- sacral paresthesia with urine retention; and
- painful anal fissures.

Males with rectal herpes may also present with impotence as a manifestation of neurologic involvement with HSV.[2,10]

Neonatal herpes is a rare complication of genital herpes resulting from exposure of a newborn to HSV-2 from the maternal genital tract (see Chapter 52). Acquisition may occur during maternal primary genital disease via exposure to infectious virus in the birth canal during labor and delivery. Less commonly, the fetus acquires the infection during gestation. The incidence of neonatal herpes is approximately 1/3500 live births. An increased incidence is noted in pre-term infants. Maternal acquisition of genital herpes during the third trimester of pregnancy increases the risk of neonatal transmission more than 10-fold compared with the risk of transmission from longstanding maternal HSV infection.[35,43]

Disease in the immunocompromised host

Herpes simplex viruses may be significant pathogens in immunocompromised hosts. Patients who have HIV disease may have both frequent and increased duration of recurrences of HSV mucocutaneous disease. Delayed healing and continued virus replication lead to local spread and large, painful ulcers extending through the cutaneous and subcutaneous layers. In patients with CD4+ lymphocyte counts <100 cells/mm³, treatment of genital herpes may be complicated by emergence of aciclovir-resistant HSV strains.[2,10,37,44]

DIAGNOSIS

Despite an overall increasing awareness of sexually transmitted diseases, recognition of genital herpes by both the patient and the health-care provider is often limited, and the majority of infections are undiagnosed or unrecognized (Table 58.1).[4,5,36] Diagnosis of herpes simplex disease is important:

- to establish presence or absence of infection;
- to guide treatment considerations; and
- to allow the health-care practitioner an opportunity to intervene in disease transmission.

Diagnosis may be accomplished by serologic and microbiologic methods.

Viral culture

Viral culture and typing is the preferred method for identifying infection, as it is the most accurate and most widely available diagnostic modality. It is recommended for all patients who have not had previous virologic confirmation of disease, including those with first-episode genital disease. Culture provides confirmation of the clinical diagnosis, and typing of virus predicts subsequent recurrence patterns. Culture of body fluids, vesicles and tissues from patients with symptomatic disease yields positive results in most cases when obtained early in the disease. Cervical cultures are positive in up to 90% of women with primary or first-episode genital herpes during the first week of symptoms, with decreasing rates of virus recovery during disease resolution. Virus may be recovered from mucocutaneous ulcers, cutaneous vesicles, cerebrospinal fluid (CSF), rectum, urethra, urine and elsewhere in the genital tract.[2,45]

In recurrent disease, virus may not be present in readily detectable quantities. Culture of multiple sites such as urethra, rectum and genital tract improves the chance of virus recovery. Growth and typing of virus requires less than 5 days, and modified culture techniques that detect herpes antigens (the shell-vial assays) yield preliminary results in 1–2 days.[38,45]

Serologic assays

Type-specific serologic diagnosis is important:

- for serosurveys to gauge prevalence rates;
- for identification of asymptomatic patients;
- in situations where culture is not feasible or available; and
- for patient counseling in scenarios of sexually transmitted disease and other public health clinics.

Herpes simplex antibodies are readily detectable following infection, but it may take several months for complete antibody development to all antigenic determinants. Differentiating HSV-1 from HSV-2 antibodies is more problematic due to the antigenic similarity of the viruses.[1,10,16] Antibody responses in general are broadly cross-reactive between HSV-1 and HSV-2.[45] Antibodies to glycoprotein G are type specific, as are antibodies to portions of glycoprotein B.[46] Recently developed tests using glycoprotein G-based serologic assays are now commercially available and include both ELISA and immunoblot formats. Sensitivities for HSV-2 using IgG antibody development range from 80% to 98%, and perform worst in low-risk groups where false-positives are more common. One recent study of a low-risk group comparing the Focus HSV-1 and -2 ELISA to type-specific Western blot showed a specificity of 94%, a sensitivity of close to 100%, but a positive predictive value of only 37.5%, indicating that commercially available tests must be interpreted with caution in low-risk populations.[47] Overall, serologic assays that rely on virus-specific antibodies to IgG have a specificity approaching 96%. Older assays do not discriminate between HSV type 1 and 2 and have little to no practical value.[46,48]

Other diagnostic techniques

The advent of the PCR allows amplification and detection of HSV gene segments even when present in virus copy numbers too low for detection by culture. Assays based on PCR are rapid and sensitive, but strict control measures are necessary to avoid false-positive results. Detection of HSV by PCR is most useful for herpes meningitis, encephalitis and other central nervous system infections that are not readily diagnosed by CSF culture or would otherwise require brain biopsy for diagnosis. The sensitivity of HSV PCR approaches that of biopsy for the diagnosis of herpes encephalitis. HSV-2 can be detected by PCR in a high proportion of people with recurrent aseptic meningitis.[1,10,49,50]

Use of PCR to detect and quantify virus sequences on the skin and in the genital tract in the absence of lesions has provided important information about the duration and amount of asymptomatic virus shedding as the virus copy number is often below the threshold of detection by culture.[22] Neonatal herpes infection may also be diagnosed by PCR amplification of HSV gene segments in the serum and CSF.

MANAGEMENT

Currently, the practitioner has a choice of effective, safe and well-tolerated medications (Table 58.2). Antiviral therapy is effective:

* in the treatment of primary and first-episode genital herpes;
* for episodic treatment of recurrences; and
* for suppression of frequent recurrences.

Continuous antiviral therapy has also been shown to decrease viral shedding. Antiviral therapy has not yet been shown to affect latency or 'cure' genital herpes. Recent data are encouraging that continuous antiviral therapy may decrease, but not eliminate, the risk of transmission. The combination of education, counseling, barrier contraception and antiviral therapy has the potential to greatly decrease the risk of partner-to-partner transmission and potentially the anxiety and decreased quality of interpersonal interactions that may accompany a diagnosis of genital herpes.

Pharmacologic agents (see also Chapter 146)

Aciclovir is the acyclic analogue of the nucleoside guanosine. In order to be active, it must first be phosphorylated by the virus-encoded enzyme, thymidine kinase, to aciclovir monophosphate. The monophosphorylated form is then further phosphorylated by cellular enzymes to the di- and triphosphate form. The active form, aciclovir triphosphate, inhibits the HSV-specific DNA polymerase and terminates the replicating DNA chain by competing with its analogue deoxyguanosine triphosphate. Aciclovir lacks the 3'-hydroxyl group necessary for subsequent phosphodiester linkages, so that extension of the replicating DNA chain is no longer possible.[39]

Aciclovir has proved to be a well-tolerated and effective medication with a wide margin of safety. Its safety and specificity result from the relative inability of cellular kinases to phosphorylate aciclovir to its active form and from the more potent inhibition of HSV DNA polymerase than human DNA polymerase by aciclovir triphosphate. Resistance to aciclovir occurs when HSV strains develop that lack thymidine kinase or, less commonly, by strains with an altered thymidine kinase or DNA polymerase.[39]

Aciclovir is currently available as an oral, topical and intravenous agent. Clearance is via the kidney, with approximately 90% of the drug excreted unchanged in the urine.[39] Side-effects for the oral and topical forms are minimal. Topical aciclovir may cause burning and is not approved for use on mucous membranes.[51] Oral aciclovir may

Table 58.2 Antiviral therapy

Medication	Indication	Dose, route	Side-effects
Aciclovir	Primary genital herpes	200 mg po five times daily or 400 mg po q8h for 7–10 days	Nausea
	Recurrent genital herpes	400 mg q8h for 5 days or 800 mg q12h for 5 days or 800 mg q8h for 2 days	Nausea
	Suppression of frequent recurrences	400 mg po q12h	Nausea
	Severe or disseminated disease	5 mg/kg slow iv q8h for 14 days	Reversible crystalline nephropathy, tremors
	Encephalitis	10 mg/kg slow iv q8h for 14–21 days	Reversible crystalline nephropathy, tremors
Valaciclovir	Primary genital herpes	1 g q12h for 7–10 days	Nausea
	Recurrent genital herpes	500 mg q12h for 3 days or 1 g q24h for 5 days or 1 g q12h for 1 day	
	Suppression of frequent recurrences	500 mg q24h or 1 g q24h	
Famciclovir	Primary genital herpes	250 mg po q8h for 7–10 days	Nausea
	Recurrent genital herpes	125 mg po q12h for 5 days or 1 g q12h for 1 day	
	Suppression of frequent recurrences	250 mg po q12h	
Foscarnet	Aciclovir-resistant herpes simplex virus	60 mg/kg q8h, infuse over 2h for 10 days	Azotemia, seizures, hypo- or hyperkalemia and hypo- or hyperphosphatemia

Note: The topical aciclovir 5% ointment available in the USA is of little value in the treatment of genital herpes and is not recommended as effective therapy. Valaciclovir 1 g q24h and 500 mg q24h are both approved for chronic suppressive therapy, but the authors recommend 500 mg q12h.

cause nausea, especially with high doses. These symptoms are generally mild and resolve over time with continued use of the drug.[52] Intravenous aciclovir may cause local pain and phlebitis if drug extravasates during administration.[39] The most common significant side-effect of intravenous aciclovir is a reversible nephropathy secondary to crystallization of aciclovir in the renal tubules. Administration of intravenous doses slowly over 1 hour decreases the incidence of nephropathy. Aciclovir nephropathy is rarely seen in normal adults, but is more common in the elderly and in those with underlying renal dysfunction. Intravenous aciclovir may rarely cause neurologic complications, including lethargy, delirium and tremors.[39]

Other therapeutic agents

Antiviral medications that have recently become available include valaciclovir, penciclovir and famciclovir.

Valaciclovir

Oral bioavailability of aciclovir is limited, with only 15–20% of the oral dose absorbed. Valaciclovir, a prodrug of aciclovir, was developed to increase the oral bioavailability and is absorbed at levels three to five times greater than those for aciclovir. Following absorption, valaciclovir is then hydrolyzed to aciclovir. Oral administration of valaciclovir can lead to serum levels of aciclovir approaching those following intravenous administration of aciclovir.[53]

Penciclovir

Penciclovir is also an acyclic nucleoside analogue and is available in oral and topical forms. Topical penciclovir is a treatment option for orolabial HSV-1 but has not been approved for use in genital herpes. Like aciclovir, the drug must first be phosphorylated by the HSV-encoded thymidine kinase to penciclovir monophosphate. Cellular kinases then phosphorylate the compound to the di- and triphosphate forms. Like aciclovir triphosphate, penciclovir triphosphate is an inhibitor of HSV DNA polymerase. Although penciclovir is phosphorylated by thymidine kinase much more readily than aciclovir, this benefit is offset by reduced activity against the viral polymerase compared with that of aciclovir. DNA chain termination is not a significant property of penciclovir triphosphate. The intracellular half-life of penciclovir triphosphate is much longer than that of aciclovir triphosphate. It is still unclear whether these differences have an effect on the effectiveness or safety of penciclovir compared with those of aciclovir.[54,55]

Famciclovir

Famciclovir is an oral prodrug of penciclovir. Similar to valaciclovir, famciclovir was developed in an effort to increase oral bioavailability. Following ingestion, famciclovir is rapidly converted by deacetylation to penciclovir. Approximately 60–70% of the dose is excreted in the urine as penciclovir.[56]

Foscarnet

Foscarnet is a pyrophosphate analogue that inhibits viral DNA polymerase.[57] Because it does not require phosphorylation to become active, its efficacy is not dependent on the presence of HSV-specific thymidine kinases. As such, foscarnet is one of the few drugs available for the treatment of aciclovir-resistant herpes simplex due to thymidine kinase or thymidine kinase-altered strains. Foscarnet is only available as an intravenous preparation. The most common side-effects include nephrotoxicity, electrolyte abnormalities, seizures and penile ulcers. Saline hydration decreases the renal toxicity and is recommended to diminish the risk of azotemia. Foscarnet-resistant HSV strains have occasionally developed in immunosuppressed hosts.[58]

Cidofovir or (S)-9-(3-hydroxy-2-phosphonylmethoxypropyl) cytosine

Cidofovir is an acyclic nucleoside phosphonate antiviral agent currently used in the treatment of cytomegalovirus retinitis. Cidofovir is active *in vitro* against HSV and has activity against thymidine kinase-negative and thymidine kinase-altered HSV strains. Trials of cidofovir in humans for the treatment of resistant genital herpes have not been completed. The primary toxicity of cidofovir at doses used to treat cytomegalovirus is nephrotoxicity. The doses of cidofovir necessary to treat aciclovir-resistant genital herpes have not been established.[59,60]

Ineffective therapies

Ineffective therapies include bacille Calmette–Guérin (BCG) vaccination, topical povidone–iodine (Betadine), topical vidarabine, topical idoxuridine and gammaglobulin. Topical therapy with foscarnet has been disappointing, with recent studies of treatment of recurrent genital herpes showing little to no benefit.[61] Lysine is a popular over-the-counter supplement purported to decrease the symptoms of genital herpes. Well-controlled clinical trials of lysine, including a double-blind cross-over study, have failed to demonstrate efficacy.[62,63]

General treatment guidelines

Antiviral therapy decreases both the duration of symptoms and viral shedding in genital herpes. Maximum benefit occurs when antiviral therapy is initiated promptly, ideally with the first prodromal symptoms with recurrent genital herpes. With the wide margin of safety of the oral antiviral medications and the need to initiate therapy promptly, it is appropriate to begin medication before receiving culture results or other confirmatory test results.

Aciclovir, famciclovir and valaciclovir are all appropriate agents for the treatment of genital herpes. For some indications, valaciclovir and famciclovir offer more convenient dosing regimens. However, for many health-care providers, generic aciclovir remains the drug of choice for the treatment of genital herpes due to the extensive clinical experience with the drug, its excellent safety and efficacy profiles, wide availability and lower cost (Table 58.3).

Treatment of primary genital herpes

Antiviral therapy is clearly of benefit in the treatment of primary genital herpes. When compared with placebo it has been shown to reduce median:

- duration of viral shedding by 7 days;
- duration of pain by 4 days; and
- time to healing by 7 days.[64]

Antiviral therapy does not prevent the establishment of latency or affect the likelihood and frequency of recurrences when compared with placebo.[71] Higher than recommended doses of antiviral medications are no more effective in the treatment of genital herpes and may be associated with an increased risk of nausea.[52] Treatment for longer than 10 days in the normal host does not improve outcome when compared with the standard regimen.

Primary or first-episode genital herpes may be adequately treated with a variety of oral regimens, including aciclovir at doses of 200 mg five times daily or 400 mg q8h for 10 days. Alternatively, valaciclovir 1 g q12h for 7 days or famciclovir 250 mg q8h for 7–10 days is also effective treatment for primary genital herpes.[63,65]

Individuals with severe disease or who are unable to take oral medications should be treated with intravenous aciclovir at doses of 5 mg/kg administered over 1 hour q8h. Topical aciclovir is of little value in the treatment of primary disease.[64] The combination of oral and topical aciclovir offers no therapeutic advantage.[63,72]

Oral famciclovir and oral valaciclovir have been compared with oral aciclovir for the treatment of first-episode genital herpes in recent clinical studies. Oral famciclovir in doses of 125, 250 or 500 mg q8h for 10 days has been shown to be as effective as aciclovir 200 mg five times daily for 10 days.[63,73] Valaciclovir 1 g q12h was also as effective as aciclovir 200 mg five times daily in the treatment of first-episode genital herpes.[63,74] Neither famciclovir nor valaciclovir appears any more effective than aciclovir.

Table 58.3 Drug comparison trials

Medications	Indication	Authors	Results	Conclusions
Aciclovir 200 mg po five times daily for 10 days versus placebo	First-episode genital herpes	Corey et al.[64]	With po or iv aciclovir, pain decreased by 4 days, viral shedding decreased by 7 days, time to healing reduced by 7 days, 60% fewer new lesions; topical aciclovir of limited value	Oral aciclovir significantly effective in treatment of first-episode genital herpes
Famciclovir various doses po q8h versus aciclovir 200 mg po five times daily	First-episode genital herpes	Loveless et al.[65]	Famciclovir 125, 250 or 500 mg q8h equal to aciclovir 200 mg five times daily, each given for 10 days; famciclovir 250, 500 or 750 mg q8h equal to aciclovir 200 mg five times daily, each given for 5 days	Famciclovir equal in efficacy to standard dose aciclovir and required less frequent dosing interval
Valaciclovir 1 g po q12h po versus aciclovir 200 mg po five times daily	First-episode genital herpes	Fife et al.[66]	Valaciclovir q12h doses as effective as aciclovir five times daily	Valaciclovir as effective as aciclovir, but required less frequent dosing interval
Valciclovir 1 g po q12h versus aciclovir 200 mg po five times daily versus placebo	Recurrent genital herpes	Smiley et al.[67]	Time to healing equivalent for valaciclovir and aciclovir (115–116 hours) and shorter than with placebo (144 hours); duration of viral shedding also decreased in treated group	Treatment with valaciclovir or aciclovir significantly more effective than with placebo, and no difference between the two drug treatments (valaciclovir 500 mg q12h now shown to be as effective as 1 g q12h in a separate study)
Famciclovir 125, 250 or 500 mg po q12h compared with placebo	Recurrent genital herpes	Sacks et al.[68]	Time to healing reduced by 1.1 days in treated group; significant reduction in shedding	Famciclovir effective in treatment of recurrent genital herpes
Aciclovir 400 mg po q12h versus placebo	Suppression of frequent recurrences	Mertz et al.[69]	Mean number of recurrences 11.4/year for placebo group, 1.8/year for treated group; number free from recurrences for 1 year: 2% for placebo group, 44% for treated group	Aciclovir highly effective at suppressing recurrences; minimal side-effects, frequent high patient compliance and satisfaction with treatment
Famciclovir various doses po versus placebo	Suppression of frequent recurrences	Mertz et al.[70]	Time to first recurrence 82 days for placebo, greater than 120 days for treatment; 250 mg q12h most effective and 78% of patients with no recurrences at 120 days versus 42% of those treated with placebo	Famciclovir 250 mg q12h effective for suppressing frequent recurrences
Aciclovir 400 mg po q12h versus placebo	Suppression of asymptomatic viral shedding	Wald et al.[25]	Five of 34 treated shed virus during therapy compared with 25 of 34 in placebo group; days shed were 6.9% with placebo, 0.3% with aciclovir	Aciclovir dramatically decreases asymptomatic viral shedding

Episodic treatment of recurrent genital herpes

Recurrent genital herpes is generally milder and of shorter duration than primary disease, so the expected benefits of treating individual episodes with antiviral therapy are not as profound as those seen in primary disease. Episodic treatment of recurrent genital herpes with antiviral therapy results in only a modest decrease in disease severity, with a mean decrease in the duration of symptoms of 1 day or less.[73]

Aciclovir at a dose of 200 mg five times daily or 400 mg q8h for 5 days remains the recommended therapy.[75] Patient-initiated therapy at the time of onset of prodromal symptoms has been shown to be of significantly greater benefit than therapy delayed to initial lesion onset.[73]

Both valaciclovir and famciclovir have been evaluated for effectiveness in the treatment of recurrent genital herpes. Recent clinical trials comparing valaciclovir (1 g q12h) with either aciclovir (200 mg five times daily) or placebo showed the following in both treatment arms when compared with placebo:

- decreased time to lesion healing;
- decreased duration of pain; and
- reduced duration of viral shedding.[67]

Oral famciclovir at doses of 125, 250 or 500 mg q12h reduced viral shedding and duration of symptoms and reduced time to healing when compared with placebo.[76] The lowest effective dose, 125 mg q12h for 5 days, is the currently approved treatment dose. Recently, a 1-day course of famciclovir 100 mg twice over 24 hours was found to be more effective than the standard 3-day course of valaciclovir.[77] A convenient 1-day course of valaciclovir at a dose of 2 g twice daily, for a total of 4 g over 24 hours, was found to be safe and effective, but has not been evaluated in comparison trials.[67] Neither famciclovir nor valaciclovir appears to offer any therapeutic advantage over aciclovir in the immunocompetent host.

The 5% topical aciclovir ointment available in the USA is not effective at reducing viral shedding, symptoms or time to healing, and is not licensed or recommended for treatment of recurrent genital herpes.[78] A different preparation available in Europe, a 5% topical aciclovir cream, has been shown to be effective and may be an appropriate alternative to oral therapy if available to the patient.[79]

Suppression of frequently recurring genital herpes

Chronic antiviral therapy has proven to be a safe and well-tolerated mechanism for suppressing symptomatic recurrences in patients with moderate to frequently (more than five episodes per year) recurring genital herpes.

Aciclovir

Aciclovir was the first antiviral agent evaluated for effectiveness in suppressing recurrent disease. In one study, patients with frequent recurrences had a reduction of recurrences from more than 12/year to an average of 1/year when treated with aciclovir 400 mg q12h.[69]

Suppressive therapy is safe and well tolerated, with no long-term effects on sperm motility, no noted laboratory abnormalities and minimal side-effects.[69,80]

Aciclovir has now been used for suppressive therapy for up to 10 years and has not been associated with development of tolerance or with any significant development of resistant strains in the normal host.[69,81,82] However, interruption of therapy at 1- or 2-year intervals is suggested to assess the frequency of episodes and the need for suppressive therapy. It has recently been shown that suppressive therapy with aciclovir decreases the frequency of asymptomatic viral shedding in women.[25] Aciclovir is now available as a generic prescription in most places, which may provide significant cost-saving considerations when deciding on pharmacotherapy.

Famciclovir

Famciclovir is now licensed in the USA for suppressive therapy at a dose of 250 mg q12h, the most effective dose tested in a dose-ranging study of famciclovir compared with placebo for suppression of frequently recurring genital herpes in women.[70] In this trial, once-daily dosing regimens were not as effective as the q12h dosing regimens at equal or higher cumulative daily doses. A subsequent 1-year trial in men and women also found that the 250 mg q12h dosage was effective and well tolerated. At present, there are no results available of trials comparing the efficacy of suppressive therapy with famciclovir to therapy with valaciclovir or aciclovir.

Valaciclovir

Valaciclovir has also been used for suppression of genital herpes and has recently been licensed in the USA at a dose of 500 mg or 1 g orally daily for suppression of genital herpes in the normal host. The 500 mg daily dose appears to be effective in persons with a history of 6–10 episodes/year. This regimen appears to be less effective than aciclovir 400 mg orally q12h or valaciclovir 1 g daily or 250 mg q12h in patients with very frequent recurrences (10 or more episodes/year). Once-daily dosing with valaciclovir 1 g appears to have acceptable efficacy in the normal host, but should not be used in the immunocompromised host because there is evidence of reduced efficacy in people who have HIV infection. Valaciclovir 1 g daily or 250 mg q12h and aciclovir 400 mg q12h appeared equivalent in efficacy, even among people with frequent recurrences. Valaciclovir was found to decrease viral shedding by 71% at a dose of 1 g daily in immunocompetent persons.[83] Valaciclovir 500 mg q12h was found to be safe and was also significantly more effective than valaciclovir 1 g daily in suppressing genital herpes in people who have HIV infection and a median CD4+ lymphocyte count of 320 cells/mm.[3,84]

Summary

In summary, there are no data at present suggesting that suppressive therapy with either famciclovir or valaciclovir at the licensed doses is more effective than suppressive therapy with aciclovir 400 mg q12h. In addition, cost comparisons favor the use of generic aciclovir rather than the newer agents.

CONCLUSION

Genital herpes is one of the most commonly encountered sexually transmitted diseases. Its management requires:

- recognition of disease;
- patient education about the unique features of the disease, including latency and virus shedding; and
- judicious use of antiviral medications.

REFERENCES

References for this chapter can be found online at http://www.expertconsult.com

Chapter | 59 |

Sten H Vermund
Madhav P Bhatta
Vikrant V Sahasrabuddhe

Papillomavirus infections

INTRODUCTION

Human papillomavirus (HPV) is the most common viral sexually transmitted infection (STI) in humans.[1] Mild disease includes genital warts (condyloma acuminata), verruga or cytologically evident dysplasia of the cervix or anus. Persistent anogenital infection with certain 'high-risk' HPV types is associated with advanced cervical neoplastic disease and invasive carcinoma of the anogenital region, most notably the cervix.[2] Oncogenic 'high-risk' HPV genotypes (notably types 16, 18, 31, 33, 35, 39, 45, 51, 52, 56, 58, 59, 66, 73 and 82) are likely to be responsible for a high proportion of carcinomas of the cervix, vagina, vulva, anus and penis worldwide.[3] Other HPV genotypes termed 'low-risk' and nongenital types of HPV cause benign epithelial warts, as well as a number of other dermatologic conditions[4] not reviewed in this chapter (see Chapter 156).

HPV-associated anogenital disease

Human papillomavirus represents a family of DNA viruses with more than 120 related genetic types, more than 40 of which infect the anogenital tract.[3] The genome consists of a circular double-stranded DNA about 8000 base pairs long within an icosahedral protein coat with no membrane envelope. Most HPV genotypes have three regions:
- a transcription and replication control region;
- an early region encoding proteins for replication, regulation and modification of the host cytoplasm and nucleus; and
- a late region encoding capsid proteins.[5]

HPV is a strictly epitheliotropic virus with various HPV genotypes targeting specific epithelial targets (e.g. soles of feet, nongenital skin, anogenital skin, anogenital/oropharyngeal mucosa).

Strong epidemiologic and molecular evidence identifies HPV as a necessary but insufficient cause of cervical cancer.[2,3] Cervical cancer is the second most common cancer among women worldwide. Globally, an estimated 500 000 new cases and 275 000 deaths occurred in 2002, with developing countries accounting for more than 80% of cases (Fig. 59.1). In the absence of screening programs, 85% of women with cervical cancer will die given the advanced stage of the disease at the time of diagnosis. Despite widespread screening, it is estimated that there are still more than 12 000 new cases of cervical cancer and 4000 deaths due to the disease annually in the USA. For every case of invasive cervical cancer found by Papanicolaou-type cervical cell examination testing (Pap smear), an estimated 50–100 cases of squamous intraepithelial lesions are detected. In the USA about 35% of invasive cervical cancers and 57% of deaths occur in women older than 55 years of age. The lifetime risk for acquiring invasive cervical cancer in the USA is 0.85% and the risk of dying from it is 0.30%. However, black women are 61% more likely to develop invasive disease and have about twice the risk (0.56% vs 0.27%) of dying from invasive cervical cancer than white women in the USA.[6] The racial disparity in the incidence of cervical cancer becomes more prominent among women older than 40 years.

Cervical cancer development involves four major steps: HPV infection, viral persistence, progression of persistently infected cells to pre-cancer cancer, and invasion. Therefore, HPV infection is the single most important and necessary risk factor for cervical squamous intraepithelial lesions (SILs) and cancer. Although most women with cervical cancer are well into their forties when diagnosed, HPV infection and disease pathogenesis are known to begin at the onset of sexual activity.[7] Early signs of cervical intraepithelial neoplasia (CIN) are detectable through cervical cytology screening programs that provide periodic Pap smear or other screening modalities. An overwhelming majority of cervical cancer cases occur in women receiving suboptimal cervical screening and treatment regimens. Older women, women from ethnic or racial minorities, and women from poor and disadvantaged backgrounds are more likely to be diagnosed with advanced-stage disease as a direct consequence of fewer or absent early detection opportunities.

EPIDEMIOLOGY, PATHOGENESIS AND PATHOLOGY

Epidemiology

Genital HPV is a common infection among sexually active adults and adolescents.[1] The estimates of HPV prevalence vary greatly depending on the methods used for HPV detection and the populations sampled. Diagnostic limitations, subclinical cases, repeated and multiple infections, and the phenomenon of inconsistent HPV types noted at separate clinical encounters make the incidence and prevalence estimates for HPV infection imprecise. In the latter circumstance, one cannot be sure whether a new viral type has been acquired or whether it was missed at a prior diagnosis.

Estimates based on visible warts grossly underreport prevalence, while estimates based on molecular evidence of infection (presence of HPV DNA in exfoliated genital tract cells) show the highest rates (20% in a general or 75% in a very high-risk population of women or adolescents). The estimates of HPV prevalence, based on the polymerase chain reaction (PCR) test for HPV DNA among asymptomatic women in the general population, have ranged from 2% to 44% in various populations.[8] A meta-analysis of studies from around the world estimates the global HPV prevale nce to be 10.4%, with an estimated 291 million HPV-infected women.[9] In the USA, approximately 20 million women are estimated to be infected with HPV at any one time. A 2007 survey using PCR for HPV DNA detection found an overall HPV

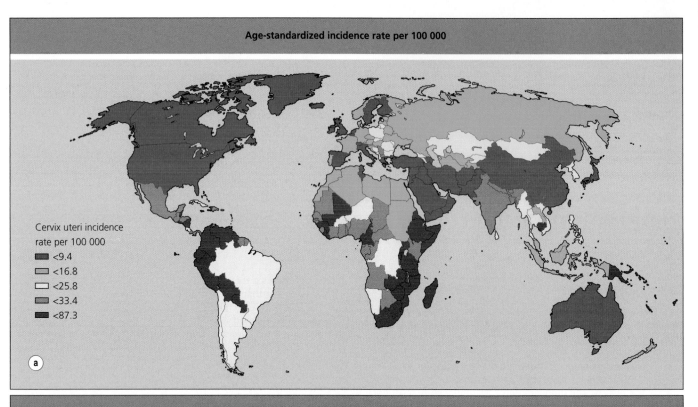

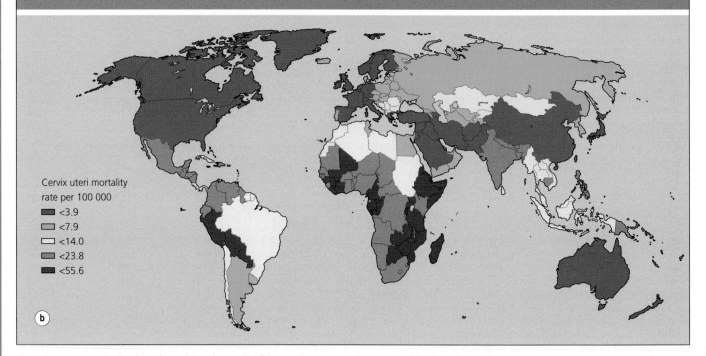

Fig. 59.1 Age-standardized incidence (a) and mortality (b) rates due to cervical cancer worldwide. Adapted from GLOBOCAN 2002, International Agency for Research on Cancer; Parkin DM, Bray F, Ferlay J, Pisani P. Global cancer statistics, 2002. CA Cancer J Clin 2002;55:74–108.

prevalence of 26.8% among US females aged 14–59 years.[10] The prevalence showed an increasing trend, starting at age 14 years and peaking at 44.8% among women aged 20–24 years. The prevalence gradually declined thereafter, through age 59. A longitudinal study of HPV infection in a cohort of college women in the USA found an average annual incidence of 14% and that about 60% of the women were infected with

HPV at some time during the 3-year follow-up period.[11] Similar results were also observed in a slightly older cohort (mean age 32 years) of women with a cumulative incidence of 54% after 3 years.[12]

There is considerable regional variation in both overall prevalence and type-specific distribution of HPV among women in the general population. For example, a study of worldwide distribution of HPV types based on the PCR test for HPV DNA found an age standard-ized HPV prevalence of 1.4% in Spain versus 25.6% in Nigeria.[13] HPV prevalence rates as high as 97% have been reported in some studies among specific populations, such as HIV-infected women. The rate of active HPV infection decreases with age; sexually active women under age 25 consistently show the highest rates. Both acquired genital tract immunity and diminishing behavioral risk with age may be responsi-ble for this strong inverse prevalence–age relationship. Other risk fac-tors associated with HPV infections include a higher number of recent and lifetime sexual partners, higher frequency of sexual intercourse, compromised immune status, high-risk characteristics of the sex part-ner including partner genital warts, and a high number of lifetime sex partners of the partner.

Genital HPV infections are primarily transmitted by skin-to-skin contact; penetrative sexual intercourse is not always necessary for transmission. The rate of HPV transmission per sexual contact is not known but is likely to be high, with similar transmission rates for vari-ous HPV types. A high proportion (20–30%) of concurrent infections with multiple HPV types has been observed when women in general populations are sampled. Most sexually active women are probably infected with at least one if not several HPV types during their life-time.[1] HPV infection in women is typically short lived, with a 70% clearance rate in 12 months and greater than 90% clearance rate in 2 years. Whether the virus is totally cleared or simply suppressed by cell-mediated immunity to a latent state without full viral expression is unclear.

The degree and duration of immunity conferred by a natural HPV infection is not known. It is estimated that only 50–60% of women develop serum antibodies to HPV after natural infection.[14] The tran-sient nature of HPV DNA detection, lack of all infections producing humoral response and inaccurate serology make it difficult to measure total exposure to HPV infection. Estimates based on HPV DNA detec-tion methods suggest that the prevalence of HPV and concurrent HPV infections in men may be similar to that found in women.

Persistence of type-specific HPV infection is an important risk fac-tor for cervical cancer development and progression. Though method-ologically challenging to assess, screening studies show that the median time of clearance of HPV infections ranges from 6 to 18 months.[15] The longer an HPV type persists, the less likely the virus will subse-quently clear up over a fixed interval, and the risk of precancer diagno-sis increases.[15] While both prevalence and incidence of HPV are higher among younger women, it is older women who seem to be at higher risk of persistent HPV infection. There is not yet an accepted defini-tion of persistence, particularly one that is clinically relevant. Of all the carcinogenic HPV infections, only a small portion (about 10%) is associated with a high absolute risk of precancer diagnosis. HPV type risk factors for persistence of infection and progression to precan-cer are not well understood. Other factors associated with persistence of infection may include older age, immunosuppression, higher HPV virus load and infection with multiple HPV types.

Human papillomavirus transmission can also occur intrapartum due to vaginal delivery.[16] Viral load in cervical and vaginal cells may be an important determinant for the risk of perinatal HPV transmission. Whether acquisition of HPV during the perinatal period predisposes to an increased risk of CIN among female infants in later life is unclear, as the evidence for high-risk HPV transmission and persistent infec-tion throughout childhood is uncertain. Juvenile laryngeal papillo-matosis may result from vertical transmission resulting in obstructive warts years later. Genital warts in children, in contrast, do not seem to occur from perinatal transmission and are typically the consequence of child sexual abuse when seen in immunocompetent children.

Oncogenesis and co-factors for oncogenesis

Molecular studies demonstrate that HPV has a direct mechanistic role in oncogenesis.[17] The integration of viral DNA is critical for malignant transformation, while continued expression of HPV proteins is neces-sary for maintenance of the transformed state. In benign warts and in preneoplastic lesions, the HPV genome is maintained in a circular non-integrated form, whereas in cervical cancer cells the previously circular viral DNA is often found integrated into the linear host cell genome. Proteins from both HPV and endogenous origins can deregu-late cell cycles and enable carcinogenesis to occur. The expression of some of the 'early' genes (E6/E7) of high-risk HPV types (16, 18 and others) seems to be an essential factor for malignant conversion of the cervical epithelium. The viral DNA will integrate into the host DNA within the E1/E2 open reading frame of the viral genome.[5] Because the E2 region of the viral DNA normally represses the transcription of the E6 and E7 early viral genes, HPV integration causes overexpression of the E6 and E7 proteins of high-risk HPV types. Transformation can occur when these expressed E6 and E7 proteins bind the products of tumor suppressor genes *p53* and retinoblastoma (*pRB*), respectively. This modifies or inactivates their normal cell-regulating functions, namely the transcription of genes involved in cell cycle control. The E6/*p53* and E7/*pRB* interactions cause genomic instability, resulting in the accumulation of chromosomal abnormalities followed by clonal expansion of malignant cells.

Human papillomavirus DNA from oncogenic viral types is found in nearly all cervical cancer cells. Infection with a high-risk HPV type is a necessary cause for both squamous cell carcinoma and adeno-carcinoma of the cervix. HPV-16 and HPV-18 are the two most com-mon high-risk types, accounting for 70% of cervical cancers and about 50% of CIN grade 3.[18] Since high-risk HPV type infection is common in women with normal cervical cytology and only a fraction of HPV-infected women develop cervical cancer, HPV infection is a necessary but not sufficient cause of cervical and many other anogenital cancers. However, carcinogenic risk may be enhanced by a number of addi-tional factors.

Women infected with more than one HPV type are at a higher risk of precancer than women with a single infection. Co-infections with *C. trachomatis* and herpes simplex virus type-2 may increase carcinoma risk in women with HPV infection. Local inflammation from infec-tious or other causes may stimulate cytokine responses that impact HPV expression. Retinoids such as β-carotene, antioxidants such as vitamin C and methylation agents such as folic acid have been impli-cated in cervical disease, but the role of nutritional factors is still unclear. There is evidence of higher folate levels in blood having a pro-tective effect against precancer. Smoking has been shown to increase the risk of squamous cell carcinoma twofold among HPV-infected women. Long-term use of oral contraceptive hormones is associated with an almost threefold increase in the risk of cervical cancer in HPV-infected women. Women with seven or more full-term pregnancies are four times more likely than nulliparous women, and two times more likely than women with one to two full-term pregnancies to develop squamous cell carcinoma.

A 'male factor' is apparent in increased cervical cancer risk to women. Women married to men whose first wives died of cervical cancer, monogamous women married to men who are frequently away from home, and female sexual partners of men with penile can-cer all have a higher than expected cervical cancer risk.[19] Lack of male circumcision is associated with higher penile HPV infection rates and increased risk of cervical cancer in their female sex partners. Unlike other STIs, condom use is neither strongly nor consistently associated with HPV prevention, perhaps indicating higher infectiousness per contact of HPV or the possibility of genital transmission from perineal or other noncoital sexual contact.[20] Sexual couples can be discordant in HPV infection status or type, demonstrating the transient nature of infection in many persons, its low level in at least one partner and/or resistance to HPV by the uninfected partner through local immune or genetic factors.[21] HPV-related genital cancers can cluster in families due, perhaps, to shared risk factors and/or host immunogenetics.

Host genetics and immunosuppression

A current research challenge is to investigate the role of host genetics in HPV acquisition, retention and disease pathogenesis. Theoretically,

HLA type or other host cell receptor genetic profiles may affect the degree of host cell susceptibility, efficiency of viral replication, nature of host immune responses and likelihood that infection will persist. Molecular techniques have improved the precision and affordability of immunogenetic assessments within epidemiologic and clinical studies. There may be a protective effect of HLA DRB1*1301 on HPV clearance and precancer development.[22]

Impaired immunity increases susceptibility to many infections and malignancies. Immunosuppressed persons, including those with low CD4[+] T-cell counts due to HIV infection, cancer chemotherapy, renal transplant or rheumatology on immunosuppressive drugs, may have an impaired ability to clear up HPV, permitting longer duration of infection and increased likelihood of oncogenic integration of HPV into the host genome. Immunosuppression can exacerbate the severity of epithelial warts and facilitate the persistence, pathogenicity and progression of HPV-induced neoplasia.[23,24] HIV-infected women have higher prevalence, incidence, regression and recurrence of HPV infection, cervical neoplasia and cervical cancer than HIV-uninfected women with comparable risks. Invasive cervical cancer was added to the list of acquired immunodeficiency syndrome (AIDS)-defining conditions by the US Centers for Disease Control and Prevention (CDC) in 1993. Women with lower CD4[+] T-cell level are more likely to manifest HPV infection and cervical neoplasia.

The magnitude of HPV prevalence is proportional to the severity of immunosuppression, although HPV-16 is more weakly associated with immune status than other high-risk HPV types. A meta-analysis of HPV types among HIV-infected women found an overall prevalence of 56.6% in African women compared to 31.4% in women in North America.[25] Additionally, studies from different populations suggest that HIV-infected women may also be infected with a broader range of HPV types than HIV-uninfected women. The proportion of HPV prevalence attributable to HPV-16 is lower in HIV-infected women, including those with high-grade SIL, than in women in the general population.[25]

Cervical cytology is now deemed an adequate screening tool for CIN in HIV-positive women, but the high recurrence rate and multifocal nature of this disease reinforces the need for annual screening. Highly active antiretroviral therapy (HAART) does not seem to impact the natural history of HPV infection or reduce the risk of cancer or precancer in HIV-infected women. However, prolonged exposure of the cervix to high-risk HPV in a relatively immunosuppressed state in HIV-infected women may confound this relationship.

Other genitourinary cancers

Anal cancers in women and men are strongly associated with HPV, with 80–95% reported HPV prevalence in anal carcinomas.[26] A high level of HPV infection may be important for the development of anal intraepithelial neoplasia. Men and women who practice receptive anal intercourse have higher anal cancer rates, but anal disease in women can occur even without anal intercourse, presumably through perineal HPV spread. Prior to the era of highly active antiretroviral combination chemotherapies, the HIV epidemic was associated with a huge rise in anal cancer rates affecting both men and women. Cytologic screening for anal disease with a Pap smear-type anal swab is advocated for high-risk persons, especially for sexually active homosexual men; the utility of HPV for anal disease screening is not established.

Invasive squamous carcinoma is not common in the vulva or vagina. Using PCR methods, the prevalence of HPV infection in vaginal cancer is about 60–65% and in vulvar cancers 20–50%. Both HPV types 16 and 18 are associated with vulvar squamous cell carcinoma, although the prevalence of HPV-16 is less than in cervical carcinoma. Primary squamous cell carcinoma of the ovary is rare; most cases represent malignant transformation of ovarian teratomas and are not HPV related.

Oncogenic HPV types can be detected in 40–50% of carcinoma of the penis and urethra. Other malignancies may be HPV related.[27] Other urologic malignancies (e.g. prostate and bladder) may not have

an HPV etiology, although this continues to be studied. It has been suggested, but not clearly demonstrated, that HPV can act as an oncogenic agent in persons who are already predisposed to bladder cancer for other reasons.

Additionally, infection with HPV is most likely a risk factor for a subset of squamous cell carcinoma of the head and neck.[28] However, further research is needed to elucidate the full role of HPV in the development of nongenital tract cancers. 'Low-risk types' such as HPV-11 can nonetheless cause severe non-neoplastic disease including juvenile laryngeal papillomatosis. The non-anogenital disease spectrum of HPV is discussed in Chapter 156.

PREVENTION

Primary HPV prevention is promoted through vaccination as well as through measures to prevent or reduce exposure. Measures for preventing exposure are not absolute, but reduce risk of transmission, nonetheless. These measures include encouraging sexual abstinence or delaying sexual debut among sexually inexperienced youth, mutual monogamy in couples, correct and consistent condom use, and other sexual risk reduction strategies. Measurable successes in reducing the incidence of cervical cancer have been achieved in industrialized nations through screening by cervical cytology, followed by clinical treatment when indicated. In countries where screening has been extensive, the mortality rate from cervical cancer has fallen markedly since the 1950s. However, lower-income women may have higher sexual risk profiles and the lowest rates of access to preventive health services, thus resulting in cervical cancer death rates greater than those seen among socioeconomically higher women.

As a medical screening procedure, Pap smears have numerous operational challenges in developing country settings.[29] A proper Pap smear requires a pelvic examination, an adequate sample of cells, including those from the transformation zone (the squamocolumnar junction), proper fixing of the cells, excellence in cytopathologic processing and assessment, adequacy of the clinical response to the results, and appropriate follow-up by patients. This operational complexity, combined with the Pap smear's only moderate sensitivity, has motivated a search for improved cervical cancer screening approaches.[29] In western industrialized settings, liquid-based cytology (Thin Prep™ Pap smear) is now the test of choice among many clinicians and laboratories for cervical cytology due to its relative ease of standardization and increased sensitivity (over conventional Pap smear); however, the high costs of infrastructure and maintenance, as well as the need for multiple visits, make it difficult to use in resource-limited settings.[30]

Visual inspection with acetic acid (VIA) stands out as one of the most promising low-cost alternatives to conventional Pap smears, especially for use in low-resource settings.[29] VIA involves the application of 3–5% dilute acetic acid (common household vinegar) to the cervix after examination through a vaginal speculum, and observing the color changes on the cervix after 1 minute. Due to reversible protein coagulation and increased reflectivity of precancerous cells having a high nuclear:cytoplasmic ratio, precancerous areas of the squamocolumnar junction appear white in color (Fig. 59.2). Trained nonphysician health-care workers can perform the screening. VIA gives immediate results, which can help in linking screening and treatment in the same visit, through the use of cryosurgery, an ablative treatment method for cervical precancerous lesions that has been proven to be safe, acceptable and feasible for large-scale implementation in developing countries. Other modifications to VIA have been proposed, including use of Lugol's iodine instead of acetic acid (visual inspection with Lugol's iodine, VILI) or visual inspection with magnification (VIAM). VILI seems to have comparable or better accuracy measures than VIA, while VIAM does not seem to offer any additional benefits. Digital camera imaging of the cervix has been proposed as another adaptation to enhance the accuracy of VIA. This method provides visual documentation for medical records, a measure of quality control, patient and nursing education, and also allows distance consultation (telecervicography).

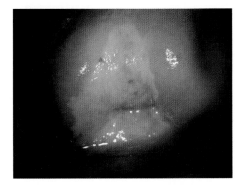

Fig. 59.2 Appearance of the cervix after application of 3–5% acetic acid. Note the well-defined, opaque acetowhite area, with regular margins, involving a large part of the visible squamocolumnar junction. Courtesy of Dr Mulindi Mwanahamuntu.

Current screening guidelines

Molecular HPV screening of cervicovaginal samples is most sensitive and objective. Many HPV DNA tests are used and others are being developed, but the only Food and Drug Administration (FDA)-approved, commercially available HPV detection kit as of 2008 is Digene/Qiagen Corporation's Hybrid Capture-2® (HC-2). This assay utilizes a non-radioactive chemiluminescence method that stratifies HPV genotypes into the following risk strata:

- high/intermediate-risk oncogenic HPV types (types 16, 18, 31, 33, 35, 39, 45, 51, 52, 56, 58, 59, and 68); and
- low-risk non-oncogenic HPV genotypes (types 6, 11, 42, 43, and 44).

Multiple studies across the world have used HPV HC-2 for categorizing patients into low- and high-risk groups. Whether HPV HC-2 has value as a stand-alone screening tool, can complement cytology screening or is too cost-ineffective for use has been the subject of intense investigation; it has been shown to be a useful triage tool for patients with minor cytologic abnormalities on Pap smears in clinical practice. Results from the Atypical Squamous Cells of Undetermined Significance (ASCUS) Low-grade Squamous Intraepithelial Lesion (LSIL) Triage Study (ALTS), a consensus report crafting revised guidelines for reporting cervical cytologies (2001 Bethesda System), another consensus report for management of women with abnormal cervical cytology, many meta-analyses, reports and cost-effectiveness/decision analysis models have now suggested logical roles for HPV testing in clinical practice and cervical cancer screening programs.[31–33] Based on the ALTS results, the 2001 Bethesda System subdivides the previous ASCUS cytopathologic category into two: 'atypical squamous cells of undermined significance' (ASCUS) and 'atypical squamous cells, cannot exclude high-grade SIL' (ASC-H).

Liquid-based cytologic assessment makes possible retention of the Pap test specimen for subsequent HPV screening. Thus, a valuable role for HPV testing is use of the Pap test using the liquid cytology method and testing the remaining sample should the cytology result demand further HPV testing analyses. Note that a second patient visit and examination are not needed with this approach. A large expert panel developed the 2006 consensus management guidelines, recommending HPV testing as the preferred method of follow-up evaluation for women aged 20–30 years with ASCUS cytology. HPV DNA testing as a primary screening test for women above age 30 is also approved and the test is being marketed in selected countries as a primary cervical cancer screen, with or without cytology. The sensitivity of a single lifetime HC-2 test for detection of high-grade SIL is around 80–90% (higher than for cytology) and specificity has ranged from 57% to 89%. Human papillomavirus testing holds promise as a cost-effective tool in resource-limited settings, especially since it needs much less quality control and assurance than cytology.

Cost-effectiveness of both primary and secondary prevention through cervical cancer screening has been used to evaluate public policy.[34,35] Analyses in countries with existing screening programs have focused on identifying the optimal screening interval, the ages for starting and stopping screening, and consideration of the various recommended roles for HPV testing. Analyses for resource-poor settings with infrequent or no screening have focused on strategies that enhance the linkage between screening and treatment, consider non-cytologic alternatives such as VIA, VILI and HPV DNA testing, and target women between the ages of 35 and 45 years for screening one, two or three times per lifetime. Cervical cancer screening strategies incorporating visual inspection of the cervix with acetic acid or HPV DNA testing for HPV in one or two clinical visits are cost-effective alternatives to conventional three-visit cytology-based screening programs in resource-poor settings.[35,36] Single lifetime screening is as cost-effective as hepatitis B vaccination, second-line treatment regimens for tuberculosis and malaria prevention with bed nets.[35,36]

Vaccination against HPV

Immunization with the L1 protein of the HPV virus induces a strong and long-lasting immune response and, as of 2008, two prophylactic vaccines are commercially available for public health application.[37–39] Both are composed of HPV type-specific L1 proteins that self-assemble into noninfectious, recombinant virus-like particles (VLPs).[39] Gardasil® (Merck) is a quadrivalent HPV-6/11/16/18 L1 VLP vaccine manufactured in a yeast system. Each injection includes 20 µg of HPV-6, 40 µg of HPV-11, 40 µg of HPV-16 and 20 µg of HPV-18 in an adjuvant of 255 µg of aluminum hydroxyphosphate sulfate.[39] Cervarix® (GlaxoSmithKline) is an HPV-16/18 L1 VLP vaccine manufactured in an insect-cell system and includes 20 µg of HPV-16 and 20 µg of HPV-18 VLP in an adjuvant of 500 µg of aluminum hydroxide with 50 µg of 3-deacylated monophosphoryl lipid A (ASO4).[39] For both vaccines, administration of three doses induces high levels of serum antibodies in virtually all vaccinated individuals.

In women who have no evidence of past or current infection with the HPV genotypes in the vaccine, both vaccines show >90% protection against persistent HPV infection for up to 5 years after vaccination, which is the longest reported follow-up so far.[39] The CDC Advisory Council for Immunization Practices (ACIP) recommends the use of Gardasil® to girls as young as 9 years old, before the initiation of sexual activity, and women up to 26 years of age (for 'catch-up' vaccination, in case they were not vaccinated when they were younger).[40]

As yet, the duration of antibody protection induced by vaccination is unknown, as is the need for future booster doses. Other biologic issues include unknown vaccine efficacy in pre-adolescents/adolescents, for whom the vaccine is recommended but no efficacy end points were assessed in the original trials. 'Bridging studies' have shown high immunogenicity and favorable safety profiles in this age group (9–15 years), but it is not known whether this higher immune response in younger children translates into detectable differences in clinical efficacy or duration of protection. The vaccine performance in immunocompromised individuals is unclear, an important issue for Africa and elsewhere given the frequency of immunosuppression due to HIV/AIDS. The 'cross-protection' against other, nonvaccine HPV types is now reported as only partial, and limits the initially projected claims of wider applicability of the vaccine.[41] In particular, the impact of HPV-16/18 eradication on the predominance of other HPV types in cervical cancer will be known only after decades, unless a broadly neutralizing antibody response against several high-risk types can be generated by second-generation prophylactic vaccines. Clinical trials are already ongoing to evaluate a nine-valent vaccine (types 6, 11, 16, 18, 31, 35, 45, 52, 58).

Finally, real-world implementation suggests that vaccine 'roll-out' will be difficult. Overcoming patient, parent and provider level attitudes that do not favor vaccination, especially against a sexually transmitted infection, is a formidable challenge. It is also critical to study optimal policies on male vaccination (assuming future approval of the vaccine for male patients) and determining whether HPV vaccines should be available for adolescents without requiring parental consent or if HPV vaccines should be mandated for school entry. Tiered pricing for HPV vaccines, innovative financing mechanisms and multi-disciplinary partnerships will be essential in order for the vaccines to reach populations in greatest need, especially in developing countries. Prices in 2008 are among the highest of any commonly used vaccine. Since HPV vaccines do not eliminate the risk of cervical cancer, cervical screening will still be required to minimize cancer incidence.

Prophylactic (VLP-based) antibody-generating vaccines do not eliminate pre-existing persistent infections.[42] Vaccines proposed as immunomodulators or therapeutic adjuncts to radiation therapy, termed therapeutic vaccines, are thus being investigated for impacting established HPV infection and its consequences. Based on successes in several animal models, phase I trials of the safety and immunogenicity of multiple therapeutic vaccine candidates have been undertaken. Various approaches are being investigated.[43]

CLINICAL FEATURES

Human papillomavirus infection may be asymptomatic or manifested in various benign or malignant lesions on cutaneous and mucosal surfaces. Genital warts can be flat (condyloma lata), as is common in the cervix, or more papillary (condyloma acuminata), as is typical in the vulva, vagina or anus. Human papillomavirus is present in a wide variety of clinical circumstances: subclinical latent infection, clinically apparent warts, neoplasia or carcinoma, with normal or abnormal genital cytology[44] (Fig. 59.3). Condyloma acuminata and condyloma lata are often caused by low-risk HPV types 6, 11 or related types. Most tend to regress naturally and are rarely associated with malignant progression. They are often multifocal, can be large and have a high rate of recurrence after treatment.

Cervical intraepithelial neoplasia that exhibits nuclear atypia possesses potential for progression to invasive carcinoma if not removed. The transformation zone of the cervix has neither the protective qualities of the keratinized squamous cells nor the vascular and immunologic milieu of the columnar epithelia and is particularly susceptible to HPV infection and subsequent neoplastic transformation. The usual cervical lesion is flat with warty colposcopic and cytopathic features and may be visualized when painted with 5% acetic acid to reveal acetowhite thickening. Both CIN I and II may precede CIN III and carcinoma in situ, and a small proportion progress to invasive carcinoma.[1] The majority of lower-grade CIN regresses to normal. The trend in cytopathology and gynecologic pathology is to use full descriptions of biopsy results, acknowledging the limitations of the CIN system that may not capture the complexity of a given cervical specimen. In addition, the 2001 Bethesda System for cytology results merges CIN II and III, as did the older system, since interobserver reliability in distinguishing these is poor.[45]

High-risk HPV types have been associated with all grades of CIN, whereas low-risk HPV types have segregated primarily in condylo-

Table 59.1 Human papillomavirus types and associated diseases	
HPV-associated diseases	**HPV types**
Skin warts	1, 2, 3, 4, 7, 10, 26, 27, 28, 29, 41, 48, 57, 60, 63, 65, 75, 76, 77, 78
Epidermodysplasia verruciformis benign lesions	3, 5, 8, 9, 12, 14, 15, 17, 19, 20, 21, 22, 23, 24, 25, 36, 47, 49, 50
Epidermodysplasia verruciformis squamous cell carcinoma	5, 8, 14, 17, 20, 47
Periungual squamous cell carcinoma	16, 34, 35
Laryngeal papillomas	6, 11
Oral focal epithelial hyperplasia	13, 32
Squamous cell carcinoma (tonsil)	16, 33
Anogenital warts	6, 11, 40, 42, 43, 44, 54, 55, 74
Low-grade anogenital intraepithelial neoplasia	6, 11, 16, 18, 30, 31, 33, 34, 35, 39, 40, 45, 51, 52, 56, 57, 58, 59, 61, 64, 66, 67, 68, 70, 71, 72, 73, 74
High-grade anogenital intraepithelial neoplasia	16, 18, 31, 33, 34, 35, 39, 45, 51, 52, 56, 58, 59, 68
Squamous cell carcinoma (cervix mostly)	16, 18, 31, 33, 35, 39, 45, 51, 52, 56, 58, 59, 68
Adenocarcinoma (cervix mostly)	16, 18

mata and CIN I (Table 59.1). However, discrepancies between HPV type and morphology do exist, and cytology and histology provide variable and, at times, conflicting, information. Cells with inflammatory changes but no neoplastic characteristics are termed abnormal squamous cells or atypical cells (Fig. 59.4) and their management was the topic of the clinical trial (ALTS) described earlier.[46,47]

HPV infections occasionally are clinically recognized by the characteristic raised appearance of the accompanying warts. Acetowhitening is helpful to clinicians examining the cervix, vagina, vulva, anus or penis, especially under magnification. This is done following an abnormal cytology result in order to identify lesions requiring biopsy. A valid reference standard for grading HPV-related anogenital pathology remains elusive, as clinical and pathologic results are prone to observer interpretation and misclassification (Figs 59.5–59.9).[3]

On microscopic examination of a Pap test or biopsy, the diagnosis of HPV infection can sometimes be made by finding neoplasia or dysplasia. The term koilocytotic dysplasia is still used widely if cells pathognomonic for HPV infection are seen. Koilocytes are large cells with a clear enlarged cytoplasmic space. The nucleus is hyperchromatic, often irregular and larger than normal. It may appear smaller than normal, though it is not, because the nucleus is within a larger-than-normal cell and cytoplasmic space.[3]

DIAGNOSIS

As HPV cannot be cultured *in vitro* in animal models, detection relies on molecular analyses of presence and sequencing of HPV DNA.[48] Early HPV tests used nucleic acid probes labeled with radioactive phosphorus (^{32}P) in a slot/dot-blot hybridization format and nucleic acid *in-situ* hybridization. On the other hand, newer target nucleic acid amplification techniques can detect individual HPV genotypes based on specific primer sequences.[49] Polymerase chain reaction is the

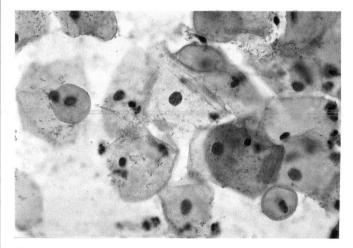

Fig. 59.3 Normal squamous cells and inflammatory cells. (Pap stain.) Courtesy of Dr William H Rogers.

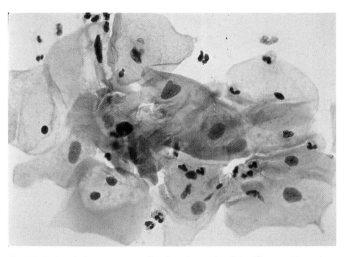

Fig. 59.4 Atypical squamous cells of undetermined significance. Here the cells are slightly enlarged and irregular relative to the cells in Figure 59.3 and contain perinuclear clear areas suggestive, but not diagnostic, of HPV infection. (Pap stain.) Courtesy of Dr William H Rogers.

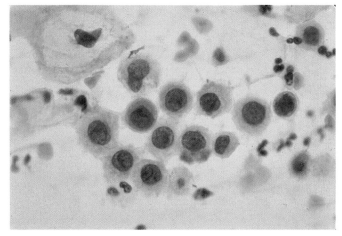

Fig. 59.6 High-grade squamous intraepithelial lesion. This contains small cells with an increased nuclear to cytoplasmic ratio and marked nuclear hyperchromasia; in the classic terminology, this would be considered a severe dysplasia or CIN III. (Pap stain.) Courtesy of Dr William H Rogers.

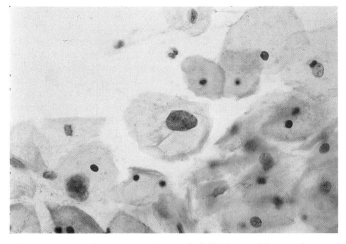

Fig. 59.5 Low-grade squamous intraepithelial lesion. In this case, the lesion would classically be called a mild dysplasia; the cell in the center of the photograph has a nucleus that is enlarged more than four times the size of the surrounding normal squamous cells; in addition, the nucleus has irregular nuclear outlines and hyperchromasia. (Pap stain.) Courtesy of Dr William H Rogers.

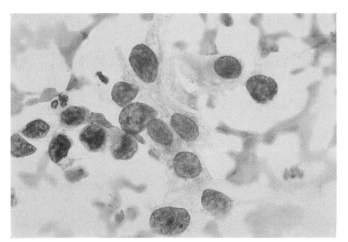

Fig. 59.7 Carcinoma in situ. The abnormal hyperchromatic cells have indistinct cell borders and form a pseudosyncytial arrangement. (Pap stain.) Courtesy of Dr William H Rogers.

'gateway technology' to all genotyping methods and can be harnessed for multiple applications, including HPV viral detection, quantitative measurement of HPV viral load, HPV DNA sequencing, analyzing mutations, etc.[49]

The L1 gene segment is used most often in genotyping assays based on PCR, wherein primers are selected from conserved or consensus sequences that flank polymorphic, type-specific sequences. Once PCR using consensus primers is performed, genotype determination can be accomplished by several methods, including restriction fragment length polymorphism (RFLP) reverse hybridization using a line-probe/dot-blot assay or cycle sequencing and assignment of genotypes by sequence comparison.[48] Polymerase chain reaction has been used as a diagnostic tool in epidemiologic investigations of HPV, but associated costs and technology requirements are often inappropriate for large screening programs. Although PCR-based methodology can detect very small amounts of HPV DNA, strict laboratory procedures and controls are critical in reducing contamination-related false-positive findings. Various PCR techniques can allow detection of more than 37 genotypes, including high-risk (HR) HPV types (16, 18, 31, 33, 35,

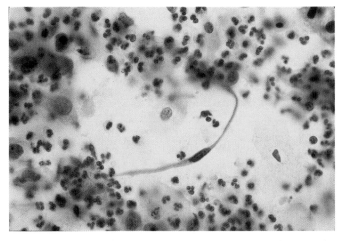

Fig. 59.8 Squamous cell carcinoma. This shows highly atypical, enlarged, abnormal keratinized cells. (Pap stain.) Courtesy of Dr William H Rogers.

Fig. 59.9 Genital HPV infection. (a) Vulvovaginal HPV infection. (b) Penile HPV infection.

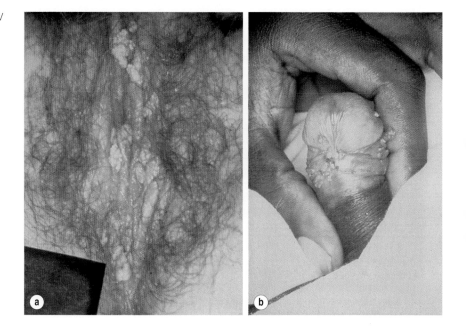

39, 45, 51, 52, 56, 58, 59, 66, 73, 82), probable high-risk (PHR) types (26, 53, 68), low risk (LR) types (6, 11, 40, 42, 54, 55, 61, 70, 72, 81, and CP6108) and HPV types with as yet undefined risk (UR) (62, 64, 67, 69, 71, 83, 84, and IS39).

The sensitivity of PCR can result in DNA detection in a very large proportion of sexually active women (often 20–60%). Although it is the most sensitive technique for identifying HPV, a loss of specificity for predicting cervical disease means that the appropriate use of PCR in clinical screening remains to be determined. Cell sampling strategies include scrape, swab, brush, cervicovaginal lavage, home lavage and even sampling from vaginal tampons. In many epidemiologic and clinical investigations, high sensitivity of HPV assessment is desired to avoid false-negative assessments. In such circumstances, use of the cervicovaginal lavage increases sensitivity method related directly to cellular yield. In routine cervical screening, the Pap test-style approach of cervical scrape and swab, using DNA-based diagnostics, seems sufficiently sensitive for clinical purposes.

Serology may become a tool to evaluate treatment successes, but it is not yet an adequate clinical diagnostic tool due to its suboptimal sensitivity and specificity. Seroepidemiologic studies have assessed antibody response to HPV-16 and HPV-18, and HPV-6 and HPV-11 for the most part. A variety of test formats have been employed, including ELISA, Western blot, radioimmunoprecipitation assays and IgG and IgA levels in serum and in cervical secretions. Standardization is in progress for antibody and DNA measurements to harmonize laboratory procedures; an international standard reference reagent could improve test performance and comparability.[50]

MANAGEMENT

An accurate diagnosis and appropriate treatment plan can help eliminate the long-term sequelae of HPV disease. Current forms of treatment attempt to ablate the pathologic lesions and eliminate HPV. The first goal is realistic in a large majority of patients, whereas the second is elusive given multifocal infection and the ease of re-infection with HPV. Ablation of frank warts or pathologic lesions identified visually or by biopsy can be achieved by topical application of chemicals, cold (cryosurgery), heat (loop electrosurgery, laser) or surgery (cone biopsy, hysterectomy). Topical treatments include salicylic acid, cantharidin, podophyllin liquid, podophilox gel, trichloroacetic acid and topical 5-fluorouracil.[51,52] Success in treating condylomata can be increased if the area is first soaked with 5% acetic acid to show the extent of the local infection.[53] Topical therapies work better against warts occurring on moist mucosal surfaces than on lesions found on heavily keratinized epithelia. Cryosurgery applies pressurized liquid nitrous oxide or liquid carbon dioxide with a swab, freezing superficial squamous epithelium and killing many of the HPV-inhabited cells. Loop electrosurgical excision procedure (LEEP), also called large loop excision of the transformation zone (LLETZ), has gained repute over the past few years as a treatment modality for high-grade CIN, since it is a safe and effective outpatient procedure carried out by removing broader areas than can be ablated and also providing tissue for histopathologic analysis. LEEP is much preferred over cold knife conization (removal of a large, cone-shaped part of the lower cervix), especially for cryotherapy-ineligible cervical lesions. Warts of the vagina, urethral meatus, anus and oral mucosa are often treated with cryotherapy initially, while topical agents may be used to treat warts of the vagina, vulva, anus, and urethral meatus and penis in men, when the evidence implicates low-risk HPV types.[52] Recurrence rates associated with all modalities are high because these methods often fail to eradicate the subclinical or latent reservoir of HPV remaining in adjacent epithelial cells and mucous membranes. Other methods such as laser vaporization have been studied and show adequate efficacy yet are limited in their widespread availability due to high costs. Surgery is reserved for patients with either extensive or refractory lesions.

During pregnancy, removal of visible warts is often advisable due to their propensity to proliferate and become friable.[54] Similarly, high-grade CIN may need intervention even during pregnancy. In contrast, treatment for subclinical genital HPV infection and lower-grade CIN during pregnancy is not recommended since spontaneous improvement postpartum is common.[54]

Immunologic therapy with interferons can be directed against all sites of infection, including clinical, subclinical and latent disease. Interferons have been used successfully as monotherapy or in combination with traditional modalities to treat anogenital condyloma acuminata. Persons with severe or recurrent disease are far more likely to receive interferon therapy in combination with other therapeutic modalities than monotherapy alone. Cost and side-effects inhibit the widespread use of interferon therapy.[55]

In the absence of HIV co-infection, currently available therapeutic methods (all modalities) are moderately successful in the treatment of frank genital warts, with recurrence rates of 25% within 3 months, and in clearing up HPV. Recrudescence is higher in HIV-infected and immunocompromised individuals. Fortunately, cytologic successes are higher than HPV clearance rates. Patient follow-up is based on colposcopy and cytology, while the best use of HPV diagnostics for post-therapeutic prognosis and management remains to be defined.

Chemoprevention

Chemoprevention is the use of agents to prevent or retard neoplastic progression. The desired effect for chemopreventive agents is complete regression or at least the prevention of progression. However, spontaneous high regression rates, the subjective nature of CIN diagnosis, the impact of biopsy on regression and the low threshold for ablative intervention complicate evaluation of such approaches.

Several processes in the HPV infection cycle are appropriate targets for the development of antiviral and/or antineoplastic agents.[56] The development of chemical compounds active against HPV could prevent the benign and malignant diseases associated with HPV infection. Use of retinoids such as dietary vitamin A (retinol) and carotenoids is being studied early in the neoplastic process (either systemically or locally) to maintain normal cervical cell function and inhibit disease progression. Retinoids do not seem to act to inhibit proliferation of HPV-immortalized cervical cells via effects on HPV E6 and E7, but they may act to inhibit cervical proliferation by suppressing the activity of epidermal growth factor and insulin-like growth factor signaling pathways. Combined interferon–retinoid therapy might provide an enhanced anticancer benefit due to the fact that each agent inhibits cervical cell proliferation.

SUMMARY

Human papillomavirus is a ubiquitous, often transient infection that can cause anogenital carcinoma under conditions favoring persistence of high-risk genotypes. Simpler screening approaches now enable expansion of programs to high-prevalence, resource-limited settings. Availability of preventive HPV vaccines gives additional hope for radical reductions in cervical and other anogenital cancers. However, control of HPV-related cancers is realistic only with a concerted global effort to expand screening, treatment and vaccination to all women.

REFERENCES

References for this chapter can be found online at http://www.expertconsult.com

Lymphogranuloma venereum, chancroid and granuloma inguinale

Cutaneous lesions are common on the external genitalia.[1] Such lesions may be restricted to the genital region, part of a generalized skin eruption or a local manifestation of a systemic disorder (see Table 60.1).

A thorough medical history and physical examination often provide the necessary keys to correctly diagnosing genital lesions. A history of multiple or new sexual partners or contact with commercial sex workers increases the likelihood of venereal disease. A history of recent drug intake or recurrence of a lesion at the same location upon re-introduction of the causative drug is characteristic of a fixed drug eruption or erythema multiforme. A history of trauma, such as from shaving, scratching or vigorous masturbation may suggest traumatic ulcers. A history of trauma also helps to distinguish the white lesions of postinflammatory hypopigmentation from those of vitiligo. Contact dermatitis is usually accompanied by a history of contact with an irritant or allergen. These can include soaps, lotions,

lubricants, condoms or spermicides or perhaps less obvious irritants if they have been inadvertently transferred to the genital region by the hands. A history of pruritus may be obtained with contact dermatitis, scabies, lichen planus or lichen sclerosis. Local tingling or paresthesia may precede the appearance of recurrent lesions due to herpes simplex virus (HSV). A history of systemic involvement will usually accompany the diagnosis of Behçet's syndrome and Crohn's disease.

On physical examination, genital lesions can be broadly categorized as raised, flat or ulcerative (see Table 60.1). Raised lesions such as condylomata lata, pearly penile papules or molluscum contagiosum may be mistaken for genital warts. Hyperpigmented lesions, though usually benign, should be biopsied to rule out squamous cell carcinoma, Kaposi's sarcoma or malignant melanoma. Flat hypopigmented lesions that are not morphologically characteristic of vitiligo or postinflammatory hypopigmentation also should undergo biopsy to seek a diagnosis of lichen sclerosis or lichen planus. Ulcerative

Table 60.1 Differential diagnosis of cutaneous genital lesions

Category		Lesion	Usual morphology	Comments
Flat lesions	Erythematous	Contact dermatitis	Red edematous patch, may be vesicular	Recent contact with an irritant or allergen
		Seborrheic dermatitis	Ill-defined, erythematous, scaly patches or plaques with crusting	Idiopathic inflammation of the sebaceous glands
		Tinea cruris (dermatophytosis)	Well-demarcated scaling plaques, with an erythematous border, over the inner thighs	See Chapter 179
		Psoriasis	Well-demarcated erythematous plaques with scales on keratinized skin, and without scales on nonkeratinized skin	Typically involves the scalp, elbows, knees, back and buttocks
		Candidal balanitis	Red papules or plaques on penile shaft	See Chapter 178
		Plasma cell (Zoon's) balanitis	Glistening, moist, erythematous patch over the glans penis or coronal sulcus	Benign, chronic balanitis
	Hyperpigmented	Pigmented nevi	Well-demarcated lesions with regular borders and homogeneous pigmentation	Biopsy to rule out malignant melanoma
	Hypopigmented	Lichen sclerosis	Hypopigmented plaques of atrophic skin with progressive scarring over the vulva or penis (balanitis xerotica obliterans)	Benign chronic dystrophic disease, more common in postmenopausal women
		Lichen planus	Reticulated, white branching striae on nonkeratinized skin	Presents as inflammatory papules on keratinized skin
		Vitiligo	Depigmented well-demarcated patches with no skin surface changes	Absence of melanocytes, possibly autoimmune
		Postinflammatory hypopigmentation	Flat ill-defined demarcated patches with partial or total loss of pigment	Follows healing of some inflammatory lesions

Table 60.1 Differential diagnosis of cutaneous genital lesions—cont'd

Category		Lesion	Usual morphology	Comments
Raised lesions	Normal pigmentation	Genital warts	Cauliflower-like (condylomata acuminata), flat-topped or rounded papules	See Chapter 59
		Secondary syphilis	Moist, hypertrophic, flat-topped papules (condylomata lata)	May also be ulcerative; see Chapter 57
		Molluscum contagiosum	Smooth, firm, shiny umbilicated nodules	See Chapter 159
		Pearly penile papules	Crownlike arrangement of dome-shaped papules around the corona of the penis	Benign angiofibromas usually appearing in adolescence
		Prominent sebaceous (Tyson's) glands	Clustered pale papules on the corona and inner surface of prepuce	Aberrant sebaceous glands, normal anatomic variant
		Cysts	Dome-shaped nodules or papules	Common, benign growths
		Fordyce spots	Purplish or reddish telangiectatic papules on scrotum, penis or vulva	Occurs in late puberty, normal anatomic variant
		Sclerosing lymphangitis	Firm translucent cord encircling the penis proximal to the corona	Result of trauma or friction
	Erythematous	Scabies	Elongated papules (female's burrow) with surrounding excoriation	Look for corresponding lesions on wrists or in fingerwebs; see Chapter 11
		Hidradenitis suppurativa	Tender inflamed nodules at base of hair follicles	Recurrent abscesses of apocrine glands
		Pyogenic granulomas	Pedunculated vascular masses usually on the scrotum	Benign tumors
	Hyperpigmented	Seborrheic keratosis	Brown, keratotic, verrucous lesions	Benign lesions usually occurring after age 40
		Lichen planus	Pruritic, flat-topped violaceous papules on keratinized skin	Idiopathic, inflammatory eruption, often associated with oral lesions
		Squamous cell carcinoma *in situ* (three forms)	Large, red-brown scaly or crusted verrucous lesion, usually solitary	Bowen's disease
			Smaller, flat verrucous lesions, usually multifocal	Bowenoid papulosis
			Erythematous, raised, irregular plaques	Erythroplasia of Queyrat
		Kaposi's sarcoma	Violaceous indurated plaques or nodules	See Chapter 95
Ulcerative lesions	Nonvenereal diseases	Aphthous ulcers	Painful irregular ulcers with erythematous borders and a white fibrin base	Commonly associated with oral ulcers
		Behçet's syndrome	Painful, shallow, irregular ulcers with erythematous borders and a white fibrin base on the glans penis or labia minora	Associated with oral ulcers, uveitis, arthritis, vasculitis or chronic meningoencephalitis
		Reiter's syndrome	Painless, serpiginous, shallow erosions of the penis with raised, erythematous borders (circinate balanitis)	Typically associated with urethritis, arthritis or conjunctivitis
		Erythema multiforme	Superficial vulvar, vaginal or penile erosions	Associated with stomatitis or bullous eruption over palms and soles
		Fixed drug eruption	Well-demarcated dusky red shallow erosion	History of drug intake
		Erosive lichen planus	Nonspecific shallow ulcerations	Commonly associated with oral lesions
		Trauma	Variable morphology	History of recent trauma
		Crohn's disease	Ulcerative perineal granulomas; may form scars, sinuses or fistulas	Inflammatory bowel disease; anal fissures may be present
		Squamous cell carcinoma	Irregular, friable ulceration	Elderly patients with an indolent nonhealing ulcer
	Venereal diseases	Primary syphilis	Single painless ulcer with indurated edges and clean base	See Chapter 57
		Secondary syphilis	Multiple painless shallow ulcers	See Chapter 57
		Herpes simplex virus	Painful shallow ulcers, may be crusted	See Chapter 76
		Chancroid	Painful irregular, nonindurated ulcer with necrotic base; may have multiple ulcers	Commonly associated with inguinal buboes
		Granuloma inguinale	Painless nonindurated, 'beefy-red' ulcer with a clean base; may have multiple ulcers	May develop groin abscesses (pseudobuboes)
		Lymphogranuloma venereum	Primary lesion usually unnoticed but may present as a small painless ulcer or papule	Usually presents with painful inguinal lymphadenopathy

lesions may be classified as painful or painless. Syphilis and granuloma inguinale are typically painless, unless secondarily infected by other bacteria. Painful ulcers include chancroid, HSV, aphthous ulcers and Behçet's syndrome. In addition to genital ulceration, Behçet's syndrome may manifest with oral ulcers, panuveitis, large joint arthritis, erythema nodosum or chronic meningoencephalitis.

HIV and genital ulcer disease have reciprocal and synergistic effects. By disrupting the epithelial barrier and drawing immune cells (including CD4+ cells) to the site of infection, genital ulcers facilitate the transmission of HIV.[2,3] Conversely, the immune suppression caused by HIV infection may alter the presentation and course of genital ulcer disease as well as the response to conventional therapy. Individuals with HIV may present with multiple, larger and more invasive genital ulcers which are slow to resolve. Ulcers due to HSV, for example, may become chronic and present as painless lesions due to destruction of local nerve endings.[4,5] Conventional therapies for genital ulcer disease in HIV-infected individuals may be complicated by slower healing and increased risk of treatment failure. While many advocate longer courses of therapy for HIV-positive individuals with genital ulcers, guidelines on appropriate durations are lacking. In most cases, therapy should be continued until complete resolution of the ulcer with close follow-up after discontinuing antibiotics.

The management of cutaneous genital lesions generally depends on making an accurate diagnosis. However, a syndromic approach to the management of genital ulcer disease has proved both feasible and useful in light of the cost and logistics required to make a definitive microbiologic diagnosis in resource-limited settings.[6] The management of syphilis and HSV is discussed elsewhere in this text. The remainder of this chapter will deal with lymphogranuloma venereum, chancroid and granuloma inguinale.

Lymphogranuloma Venereum

Lymphogranuloma venereum (LGV) is a sexually transmitted disease caused by three serovars of *Chlamydia trachomatis*: L1, L2 and L3.

EPIDEMIOLOGY

Lymphogranuloma venereum is endemic in West and East Africa, India, South East Asia, South America and some Caribbean islands. Until recently it occurred only sporadically in North America and Europe, usually in returning travelers. Beginning in 2003, outbreaks of LGV have been reported from across Western Europe[7,8] as well as from the United Kingdom, Canada, the United States and Australia. More than 98% of cases have been in men who have sex with men (MSM) and the majority of these appeared to be from high-risk sexual networks. In all jurisdictions, risk factors have included older age (median 40 years), white race and co-infection with HIV and other sexually transmitted infections, most notably gonorrhea. Most men infected with LGV have reported both receptive and insertive anal intercourse without condoms with multiple sexual partners. Whether the high prevalence of HIV among men diagnosed with LGV represents co-transmission, more symptomatic disease among those co-infected with HIV, or introduction of LGV into HIV-assortative sexual networks is not clear. Recent data from the UK suggest that LGV infection among MSM may have settled to a stable endemic rate.[9]

PATHOGENESIS AND PATHOLOGY

Lymphogranuloma venereum is acquired sexually by direct contact with infected lesions although transmission through contaminated fomites has been documented. Unlike other *Chlamydia trachomatis* infections of the urogenital system (due to serovars D through K) which are confined to the mucosal layer, the LGV serovars invade the submucosal connective tissue and lymphatic system. After exposure, epithelial abrasions allow the organism to penetrate into the submucosal tissues where they are taken up by macrophages and subsequently carried to the regional lymph nodes.

CLINICAL FEATURES

Lymphogranuloma venereum begins in the genital region and spreads through the regional lymphatics. Clinical disease classically occurs in three stages. The transient primary lesion is a small, painless genital papule which may ulcerate, and occurs at the site of inoculation. It appears 3–21 days after exposure and generally goes unnoticed. It usually occurs on the coronal sulcus in men and on the cervix, posterior vaginal wall or vulva in women. Urethral involvement may cause urethritis with discharge and dysuria.

The second stage generally occurs 2–6 weeks after the primary infection. It is characterized by painful regional lymphadenopathy and systemic symptoms. In men, the inguinal lymph nodes are affected and node enlargement on either side of the inguinal ligament produces the characteristic 'groove sign'. In women, lymph drainage from the rectum and vagina results in pelvic lymphadenopathy. Involvement of these deep nodes causes lower abdominal and back pain. Initially, the lymph nodes are mobile and discrete, but with progressive inflammation they become fixed and suppurative with bubo formation. Buboes, enlarged fluctuant nodes, may spontaneously rupture or form chronically draining sinuses. Hematogenous dissemination has been documented by the recovery of organisms from the blood and cerebrospinal fluid. Such patients experience nonspecific constitutional symptoms or, less commonly, present with meningoencephalitis, pneumonitis, arthritis or hepatitis.

The third stage is marked by subsequent scarring and fibrosis of affected tissue and results in lymphatic obstruction and genital edema (Fig. 60.1). This can lead to severely disfiguring conditions such as thickening and fibrosis of the labia in women (esthiomene) and distortion of the penis in men. Regional spread of LGV to the pelvis in women may cause salpingitis, pelvic adhesions and infertility.

Anorectal infection with LGV is predominantly seen in women and homosexual men and occurs by direct inoculation from either anal intercourse or contaminated fomites. Patients present with fever, rectal pain and mucopurulent or bloody anal discharge. Mucosal ulcerations and friable granulation tissue within the rectum are evident on sigmoidoscopy and resemble inflammatory bowel disease. The rectal ulcers are sharply demarcated with a mixed inflammatory infiltrate in the adjacent lamina propria and occasional crypt abscess formation. Crohn's disease, syphilis and herpetic proctitis should be considered in the differential diagnosis. Untreated LGV infection of the anorectum can result in perirectal abscesses, anal fissures, fistulae, and fibrosis causing rectal stricture.

Interestingly, the majority (70–96%) of LGV infections reported among MSM in western countries have presented exclusively with proctitis. The urogenital symptoms typically associated with LGV

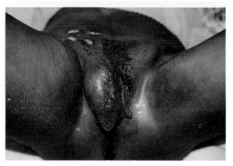

Fig. 60.1 Lymphogranuloma venereum causing unilateral vulvar lymphedema and inguinal buboes.

have been notably absent and testing of urethral swabs and urine by polymerase chain reaction (PCR) for serovars L1, L2 and L3 in the majority of cases has been negative. This absence of genital ulcers and enlarged inguinal lymph nodes may mislead the clinician from considering LGV as the cause of proctitis and thereby delay diagnosis and treatment. While the preponderance of rectal cases among men who report experiencing both receptive and insertive anal intercourse may suggest a failure to recognize penile lesions and inguinal adenopathy due to LGV, the propensity for LGV to remain asymptomatic or present as a typical 'non-gonococcal' urethritis may also be unappreciated. Notably, in one study from the Netherlands, 32 men were found to have LGV infection of the rectum on routine screening, yet 40% had no anoscopic abnormalities and 56% reported no anal discharge.[10]

Conjunctival or oropharyngeal infection occurs rarely and may be a result of autoinoculation or orogenital sex. The regional mandibular and cervical lymph nodes are involved and subsequent spread to supraclavicular and mediastinal nodes has been reported to cause pericarditis.

DIAGNOSIS

LGV is diagnosed clinically with the exclusion of other causes of genital ulcer disease. While detection of LGV serovars by nucleic acid amplification followed by DNA sequencing or restriction fragment length polymorphism (RFLP) analysis is highly sensitive and specific, the availability of these assays varies. Where these tests are available, swabs of the primary lesion as well as vaginal or urethral swabs should be stored dry at –20°C and sent immediately to the laboratory. Aspirates of inguinal nodes and urine should also be stored frozen. Although not currently approved for use with rectal or oropharyngeal swabs, some reference laboratories may offer nucleic acid testing from these sites for research purposes. Growth of the organism in cell culture is labor intensive, with a recovery rate of only 50%[11] and is generally not offered by most laboratories.

Serology is often the mainstay for the diagnosis of LGV. Complement fixation is currently the most sensitive and widely used test and a titer of 1:64 or greater in the appropriate clinical setting provides a probable diagnosis. Other *Chlamydia* infections may result in a positive complement fixation test, but a titer of less than 1:16 essentially excludes acute LGV. Microimmunofluorescence is more specific but less sensitive than complement fixation and titers of 1:256 or greater are required to provide a probable diagnosis.

MANAGEMENT

Although LGV infections resolve spontaneously, this occurs over several weeks and may be complicated by fibrosis, stricture formation or superinfection. Antimicrobial therapy decreases the incidence of complications, but has not been shown to affect the rate of healing. The recommended therapy irrespective of site of infection is oral doxycycline 100 mg twice daily for 3 weeks. Treatment recommendations for HIV-infected patients are the same. Oral erythromycin 500 mg four times daily is the treatment of choice during pregnancy. Successful treatment with oral azithromycin 1 g once weekly for 3 weeks has been reported but clinical studies are lacking. Trimethoprim–sulfamethoxazole (TMP-SMX; co-trimoxazole) is generally not recommended as it is not sterilizing and treatment failures have occurred. Patients should be followed to document clinical resolution. Anyone who had sexual contact with a patient with LGV within 60 days of the patient's onset of symptoms should be evaluated and, if asymptomatic, treated with doxycycline 100 mg twice daily for 7 days. Repeated aspiration of buboes may be necessary to relieve pain and prevent rupture. Surgical intervention may be required for fistula or stricture, or for management of chronic local edema.

Chancroid

Chancroid is an acute genital ulcer disease typically associated with regional lymphadenitis. The etiologic agent is *Haemophilus ducreyi*, a fastidious, pleomorphic, Gram-negative coccobacillus.

EPIDEMIOLOGY

Chancroid, endemic in Africa, Asia and the Caribbean, is the most common cause of genital ulcers in many developing countries and accounts for 23–56% of cases.[12] It is much less frequent in North America and Europe where it occurs in sporadic outbreaks associated with prostitution, illicit drug use, travel and returning military personnel.

Chancroid occurs predominantly in heterosexuals and outbreaks are related to frequent sexual partner change and the number of sexual partners of an infected person, as occurs in prostitution. Indeed, female sex workers appear to be the main reservoir of infection.[13] Women are often asymptomatic and commercial sexual activity may continue despite active infection and ulceration.[13] Also, PCR testing on cervical specimens from high-risk women without genital ulcers has confirmed that asymptomatic carriage of *H. ducreyi* does occur.[14] Likely the result of exposure to mucosal surfaces, uncircumcised men are more susceptible to infection.

PATHOGENESIS AND PATHOLOGY

Chancroid is transmitted from person to person by direct contact. A break or microabrasion in the skin or mucosa is necessary for the organism to penetrate the epidermis and establish infection. Virulence factors have not been well defined. Pili have been demonstrated, but their role in cellular adhesion is unknown. The production of superoxide dismutase and hemolysin may contribute to tissue damage and ulceration, while evasion of immune defenses and phagocytosis may be mediated in part through lipo-oligosaccharides and outer membrane proteins.

Once within the epidermis, *H. ducreyi* incites a cellular immune response with infiltrates consisting of CD4$^+$ and CD8$^+$ lymphocytes along with macrophages. The inflammatory lesion appears first as an erythematous papule which eventually pustulates and undergoes central necrosis, creating the pathognomonic painful, nonindurated ulcer. Three distinct histologic zones have been classically described on biopsy:

- the superficial zone, in which the organism is most readily seen, contains necrotic debris, fibrin and degenerated neutrophils;
- the middle zone is characterized by edematous inflammatory tissue with neovascularization; and
- the deep zone exhibits a dense cellular infiltrate.

CLINICAL FEATURES

Patients who have chancroid generally present with painful genital ulcers within 4–7 days of exposure. The initial tender, erythematous papule develops into a pustule and progresses to form a painful ulcer about 1–2 cm in size (Fig. 60.2). The ulcer margins, typically undermined and raised, are irregular and sharply demarcated. Because the ulcer edge is not indurated, it is known as a 'soft chancre'. The friable, granular base is often covered with a gray or yellow necrotic exudate. Approximately one-third of patients develop multiple lesions, which may coalesce to form giant ulcers. Autoinoculation may result in 'kissing lesions' on opposing surfaces.

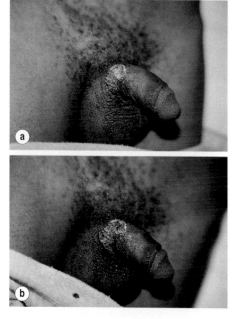

Fig. 60.2 Chancroid ulcer. (a) Before and (b) after the performance of a swab, demonstrating the friability of the ulcer base.

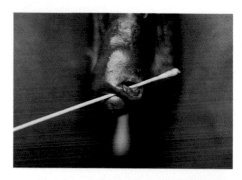

Fig. 60.4 Phagedenic chancroid with extensive tissue destruction.

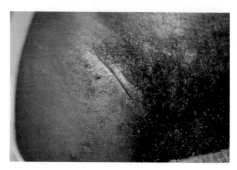

Fig. 60.5 Healed inguinal bubo with scar formation from previous chancroid infection.

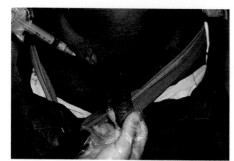

Fig. 60.3 Typical chancroid ulcer. Unilateral lymphadenitis and demonstration of the aspiration of a bubo.

The clinical picture varies with gender, and men tend to be more symptomatic than women. In men, the ulcer is visible and usually located on the prepuce, urethral meatus, glans, coronal sulcus or penile shaft (Fig. 60.3). The scrotum and perineum are less frequently involved. In women, the clinical presentation may be atypical, with symptoms of dyspareunia or dysuria. Ulcers in women may be found on the fourchette, labia, vaginal wall, perineum, perianal region and the medial aspect of the thigh. Involvement of the cervix is rare. The ulcers may resemble those of genital herpes or granuloma inguinale (GI).

Inguinal lymphadenitis is seen in about 50% of men and 35% of women and may be bilateral. Lymph nodes progressively enlarge to become necrotic and fluctuant (buboes), and may spontaneously rupture forming draining sinuses or inguinal ulcers. Systemic symptoms are characteristically absent. Extragenital ulcers are rare, but have been described in the mouth, and on the fingers and breasts. Patients co-infected with HIV are more likely to have multiple genital lesions and may experience a delayed response to treatment. Disseminated infection does not occur even in the immunocompromised. Although untreated ulcers usually heal spontaneously, they can be complicated by secondary bacterial infection, extensive tissue destruction and scarring (Figs 60.4, 60.5).

DIAGNOSIS

H. ducreyi is a fastidious, temperature-sensitive organism that survives for only a short time outside the human host. Growth *in vitro* requires specialized culture conditions and achieves a sensitivity of only 70–80%. In spite of this, culture remains the gold standard for diagnosis.

Specimens are obtained by first cleansing the ulcer by flushing with saline and then exudate is collected on a swab from the base of the ulcer. Ideally, specimens should be inoculated onto culture media at the bedside. If this is not possible, specimens should be transported to the laboratory promptly as *H. ducreyi* will survive on swabs for only 2–4 hours.[15] Bacterial contamination reduces the accuracy of the Gram stain and its overall sensitivity and specificity are less than 50%. Specific media are required to grow *H. ducreyi in vitro* and gonococcal agar supplemented with 2% bovine hemoglobin plus 5% fetal calf serum, or Mueller–Hinton agar supplemented with 5% chocolatized horse blood have been used.[15] Culture plates are incubated at 33°C in 5% CO_2. Growth is usually seen within 72 hours, but plates should be kept for 5 days before being reported negative. Colonies are raised, nonmucoid, yellow-gray in color and very self adherent. *H. ducreyi* is oxidase-positive and catalase-negative. A positive culture may be confirmed by demonstrating the presence of nitrate reductase, cytochrome oxidase, alkaline phosphatase and the requirement for heme.

PCR techniques have been developed to detect *H. ducreyi* with a sensitivity of 83–96% and a specificity of 100%.[16] A commercially available multiplex PCR assay for the simultaneous detection of *H. ducreyi*, *Treponema pallidum* and herpes simplex virus simplifies the diagnosis and management of genital ulcer disease.

MANAGEMENT

The treatment of chancroid has been complicated by antimicrobial resistance and HIV co-infection. There are wide regional variations in antimicrobial susceptibilities, but increasing global resistance to tetracycline, aminoglycosides, sulfonamides and amoxicillin–clavulanic acid has been documented.

Current recommendations for treatment include oral azithromycin 1 g in a single dose, intramuscular ceftriaxone 250 mg in a single dose, oral ciprofloxacin 500 mg twice daily for 3 days or oral erythromycin base 500 mg four times daily for 7 days.[6] Ease of administration and compliance make single-dose therapies preferable and there is good evidence that single-dose ciprofloxacin 500 mg orally is effective regardless of HIV serostatus.[17] Erythromycin and ceftriaxone may be used in pregnancy.

Response to treatment is characterized by a decrease in pain within 48 hours. Complete ulcer healing may take approximately 10 days, depending on the size of the ulcer. The development of fluctuant buboes may occur on treatment and these should be aspirated by needle or drained by incision.

Granuloma Inguinale

Granuloma inguinale (or donovanosis) presents as a painless genital ulcer that bleeds easily. It is caused by the Gram-negative pleomorphic bacterium *Klebsiella granulomatis.*

EPIDEMIOLOGY

Granuloma inguinale is endemic in tropical and subtropical regions such as Papua New Guinea and India. It is also found in South Africa, parts of Brazil, the Caribbean, and among aboriginals in central Australia. Granuloma inguinale is rare in North America and Europe.

The prevalence of granuloma inguinale is highest among adults aged 20–40 years. It is widely believed to be sexually transmitted because of its predominance in sexually active persons, especially those with multiple sexual partners or contact with prostitutes, its predilection for the genital region and the high incidence of co-infection with other STDs. The possibility of nonsexual transmissibility has been inferred from its occurrence in persons such as children and the elderly presumed sexually inactive.[18]

PATHOGENESIS AND PATHOLOGY

K. granulomatis invades epidermal and dermal tissues causing local inflammation but little is known about its virulence factors or the immune response to infection. On histopathology, large mononuclear cells containing inclusion bodies (Donovan bodies) are characteristic. The associated epithelial changes include ulceration, microabscesses, acanthosis, irregular elongation of the rete pegs and pseudoepitheliomatous hyperplasia. Untreated lesions may become hyperkeratotic. The dermal layer exhibits inflammatory changes, with a dense cellular infiltrate and varying degrees of fibrosis and edema.

CLINICAL FEATURES

The initial lesion of granuloma inguinale (GI) is a small firm papule at the site of infection which appears after an incubation period of 3–50 days. This typically erodes to form a painless ulcer (Fig. 60.6). The ulcer is granulomatous and 'beefy-red' with a nonpurulent base and bleeds readily when manipulated. Occasionally the ulcers may become necrotic and foul smelling with significant tissue destruction. Multiple lesions may develop on opposing surfaces or along skin folds. In men, ulcers are generally found at the coronal sulcus and are more common in uncircumcised men. In women, the labia minora and fourchette are most commonly affected but lesion may appear in the upper genital tract, including the cervix. Vaginal bleeding or discharge, pelvic inflammatory disease or a pelvic mass are not uncommon presentations. Less typically GI may present as a raised, hypertrophic ulcer with an irregular edge. The dry appearance of these lesions may be confused with genital warts.

Infection of extragenital sites accounts for 6% of cases and include the oropharynx, nose, larynx and neck. Abscess formation in the groin mimics lymphadenitis (pseudobuboes), but the lymph nodes themselves are rarely involved. The typical clinical picture may be altered if the genital lesions become secondarily infected, resulting in pain, purulent exudate and tender lymphadenopathy.

Without treatment, GI is slowly progressive, often resulting in soft tissue destruction and extensive scarring (Fig. 60.7). Possible sequelae include genital adhesions, stenosis of the urethral, vaginal or anal

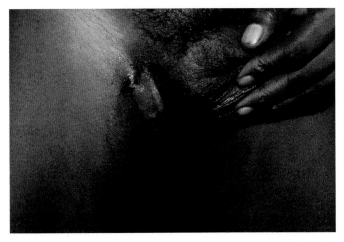

Fig. 60.6 Granuloma inguinale. The chronic, granulomatous, beefy-red ulcer without suppuration is typical. Photo kindly supplied by J K Maniar.

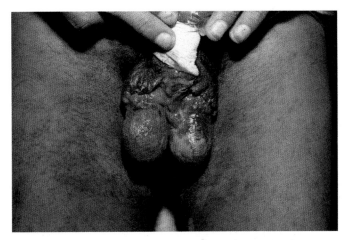

Fig. 60.7 Granuloma inguinale. Lack of treatment has permitted progressive destruction of the scrotum. Photo kindly supplied by J K Maniar.

orifices, and rectovaginal fistulas. Contiguous pelvic spread may result in a 'frozen pelvis' and hematogenous spread to the bones or liver may occur albeit rarely. During pregnancy, GI is often more aggressive, with a higher rate of dissemination and a slower response to treatment. Perinatal infection is rare, but prophylactic antibiotics should be administered to the infant.

DIAGNOSIS

The diagnosis of GI is made clinically and confirmed by the presence of intracellular Donovan bodies seen within large mononuclear cells on smear or biopsy. Reliable culture techniques and serologic tests are not available. To obtain a smear for diagnosis, debris should first be gently removed from the base of the ulcer with a cotton swab. A second swab is then used to scrape the surface of the ulcer without causing bleeding. The granulomatous tissue is spread directly onto a slide, air dried, and stained with Wright or Giemsa stain. Donovan bodies are identified as darkly staining, intracellular ovoid organisms, with or without a capsule. The smear is more likely to be negative if the lesion is early, sclerotic or secondarily infected. In such cases, a histologic diagnosis should be sought.

MANAGEMENT

Treatment regimens are empiric, as *in-vitro* susceptibility testing is not available. Currently recommended regimens include oral azithromycin 1 g followed by 500 mg daily, oral doxycycline 100 mg twice daily, a double-strength tablet of TMP-SMX twice daily, oral ciprofloxacin 750 mg twice daily or erythromycin 500 mg four times daily.[6,19] Erythromycin is the drug of choice in pregnancy. The rapid clinical response achieved with azithromycin and once daily administration has made this drug the treatment of choice.[6,20] Intravenous or intramuscular gentamicin may be added briefly in treatment of lesions that resolve slowly, and for HIV-infected persons. Duration of therapy has not been established but a minimum of 3 weeks or until all lesions have completely resolved is recommended.

Relapses are common and may occur up to 2 years after apparently successful treatment, requiring an additional course of antibiotics. Complications such as strictures, sinus formation, extensive superinfection or disfiguration may require surgical intervention.

REFERENCES

References for this chapter can be found online at http://www.expertconsult.com

Management of gonorrhea

INTRODUCTION

Gonorrhea is caused by *Neisseria gonorrhoeae*, a Gram-negative intracellular diplococcus which is an obligate human pathogen. It is the second most commonly reported bacterial sexually transmitted infection (STI). Those individuals most at risk of gonococcal infection are women younger than 25 years, a previous diagnosis of gonorrhea or other STI, new or multiple sex partners, inconsistent condom use, commercial sex work, drug use and overseas travel to countries of higher prevalence.

CLINICAL MANIFESTATIONS

There is a broad spectrum of clinical manifestations of gonorrhea: asymptomatic and symptomatic, local infection of the anogenital area and pharynx, and disseminated infection. The incubation period is short, ranging from 1 to 14 days, with males likely to present with symptoms within 5 days and females within 10 days in those who become symptomatic.

Urethral infection in males is usually symptomatic and presents with a mucopurulent discharge followed shortly by dysuria in 20% after a single sexual exposure. The severity of symptoms is determined by the infecting strain. Common complications of urethritis are epididymitis and acute or chronic prostatitis. In the pre-antibiotic era, gonococcal urethritis in the male resolved over several weeks, with 95% of cases becoming asymptomatic within 6 months. Subsequent episodes of gonorrhea in those not treated are more likely to result in urethral stricture. However, as males are more likely to be symptomatic and present for care, such complications are now rare.

In females the endocervical canal, urethra, periurethral and Bartholin's glands are the most common sites of infection. The transmission rate to females after a single encounter is high at 50%. If symptoms are present, the patient will present with vaginal discharge, dysuria, postcoital and intermenstrual bleeding. Females are more likely to be asymptomatic and therefore screening of those at high risk of infection is an important aspect of control. Local complications include pelvic inflammatory disease (PID) in 10–20% of infections. Long-term sequelae of PID are ectopic pregnancy, infertility and chronic pelvic pain. Pregnant women with gonorrhea have an increased risk of spontaneous abortion and premature delivery. Gonococcal ophthalmia neonatorum is the most common complication in the newborn. Although *Chlamydia trachomatis* is the most common cause of neonatal infectious conjunctivitis, there is an overlap in incubation period and symptoms and therefore both diagnoses should be considered.

Rectal infection may be the only site of infection in up to 40% of men who have sex with men and presents with pruritus, mucopurulent discharge and rectal pain. Symptomatic infection in females is uncommon.

Gonococcal infection of the pharynx is transmitted by orogenital contact and occurs in 10–25% of patients with gonorrhea at another site. Over 90% of pharyngeal infections are asymptomatic and its transmission to others is inefficient and rare.

The most common systemic complication is disseminated gonococcal infection (DGI) which occurs in 0.5–3% of untreated local infection. Clinical manifestation is a triad of migratory polyarthritis, tenosynovitis and dermatitis. As the bacteremia is not continuous, only 20–30% of patients have positive blood cultures; however, 80% will have evidence of local infection at one of the sites outlined above. Gonococcal endocarditis, meningitis and perihepatitis are all rare.

LABORATORY DIAGNOSIS

The diagnosis of gonorrhea is dependent on the identification of the organism by Gram stain, culture, nucleic acid hybridization tests and nucleic acid amplification techniques (NAAT).

Gram staining showing intracellular Gram-negative diplococci in urethral specimens of symptomatic males is highly sensitive and specific for *N. gonorrhoeae*; however, as staining of specimens from endocervical, rectal and pharyngeal swabs is less sensitive, other diagnostic methods are necessary.

Culture and nucleic acid hybridization testing can be used on male urethral and endocervical specimens. Culture is best for rectal and pharyngeal specimens and has the additional benefit of antimicrobial susceptibility data. In cases of persistent gonococcal infection, culture is essential. NAAT can be used in a wide variety of specimens; however, limitations are cost, contamination and cross-reaction with nongonococcal *Neisseria* leading to false-positive results.

The recommendation is that patients being tested for gonorrhea should be offered testing for all other STIs, particularly *C. trachomatis*, HIV and syphilis. Co-infection with *Chlamydia* can occur in 25–38% of patients with gonococcal infection and gonorrhea facilitates the transmission of HIV.

TREATMENT

Control of gonorrhea has depended on the use of effective single-dose therapy administered at the time of diagnosis to ensure maximal patient compliance. This is done in conjunction with the diagnosis of other STIs and treatment of sexual partners. The rates of dual infection with *C. trachomatis* in those infected with *N. gonorrhoeae* are high. If *Chlamydia* results are not available or if a non-NAAT is negative for *Chlamydia*, patients should be treated for both gonorrhea and *Chlamydia*.

The availability of antimicrobial agents for the treatment of gonorrhea in the late 1930s has been persistently followed by sequential development of drug resistance to antimicrobial classes commonly used for treatment. The ongoing problem of antimicrobial resistance was recognized and in 1986 the Centers for Disease Control and Prevention (CDC) set up the Gonococcal Isolate Surveillance Project (GISP) to monitor trends in antimicrobial susceptibility and to provide a rational basis on which to select gonococcal therapies. This project has been instrumental in determining key policy changes in treating and thus controlling this infection over the past two decades.

Before 1976 antimicrobial resistance was not usually checked as the isolates were invariably susceptible to penicillin which was the drug of choice for treatment of the infection. The types of penicillin resistance that subsequently emerged were chromosomally mediated penicillin- and tetracycline-resistant *N. gonorrhoeae* (CMRNG), plasmid-mediated penicillinase-producing *N. gonorrhoeae* (PPNG) and tetracycline-resistant *N. gonorrhoeae* (TRNG), leading to abandonment of these drugs for eradication of infection. Since the 1990s, chromosomally mediated high-level resistance to quinolones (QRNG) resulting from mutations in gyrA (DNA gyrase) and par C (topoisomerase IV) has increased dramatically. The quinolones, as a class of drugs, are no longer recommended for the treatment of gonorrhea. Based on susceptibility patterns, current CDC guidelines for the treatment of gonorrhea are confined to a single class of drugs, the cephalosporins.

Uncomplicated gonococcal infection

Gonococcal infection of the urethra, cervix and rectum

- Ceftriaxone 125 mg intramuscularly in a single dose *or* cefixime 400 mg orally in a single dose *or* spectinomycin 2 g intramuscularly in a single dose, *plus*
- treatment of chlamydial infection if not excluded as a diagnosis.

Gonococcal infection of the pharynx

Gonococcal infection of the pharynx is more difficult to eradicate than from the anogenital area and the treatment recommendations differ. The treatment of choice, which clears infection in over 90% of cases, is:

- ceftriaxone 125 mg intramuscularly in a single dose, *plus*
- treatment of chlamydial infection if not excluded as a diagnosis.

Patients treated for uncomplicated gonococcal infection with one of the above regimens who have symptomatic relief do not need a test of cure. Those who are persistently symptomatic despite appropriate treatment require re-evaluation by culture to determine antimicrobial susceptibility patterns as well as sex partner evaluation.

Complicated gonococcal infection

Disseminated gonococcal infection

A cephalosporin-based regimen is recommended for DGI for a minimum of 1 week with parenteral administration for the first 24–48 hours until there is clinical improvement, followed by a switch to an oral regimen as outlined below:

- Ceftriaxone 1 g intramuscularly or intravenously q24h *or* cefotaxime 1 g intravenously q8h *or* ceftizoxime 1 g intravenously q8h *or* spectinomycin 2 g intramuscularly q12h, *followed by a switch to*
- cefixime 400 mg orally twice daily *or* cefpodoxime 400 mg orally twice daily.

As epididymitis can be caused by *N. gonorrhoeae* or *Chlamydia*, particularly in those under 35 years of age, antimicrobial therapy should cover both infections. The recommended regimen for sexually acquired infection is:

- ceftriaxone 250 mg intramuscularly in a single dose, *plus*
- doxycycline 100 g orally twice daily for 10 days.

Gonococcal conjunctivitis

This is a rare complication often resulting from autoinoculation. The treatment recommendation is based on a consensus opinion as there is only one published study on its treatment:

- ceftriaxone 1 g intramuscularly in a single dose, *plus*
- saline solution lavage of the infected eye.

Pelvic inflammatory disease

The mode of antimicrobial administration in women with PID is determined by the severity of the infection. Parenteral and oral regimens appear to be equally efficacious and a switch to oral therapy is recommended after 24 hours of symptomatic improvement. Duration of therapy is 14 days.

Parenteral therapy

- Cefotetan 2 g intravenously q12h *or* cefoxitin 2 g intravenously q6h *plus*
- doxycycline 100 mg orally *or* intravenously q12h

or

- clindamycin 900 mg intravenously q8h *plus*
- a loading dose of gentamicin 2 mg/kg intravenously or intramuscularly, followed by a maintenance dose of 1.5 mg/kg q8h.

Oral therapy

- Ceftriaxone 250 mg intramuscularly in a single dose *or* cefoxitin 2 g intramuscularly and probenecid 1 g orally, *plus*
- doxycycline 100 mg orally twice daily for 14 days, *with or without*
- metronidazole 500 mg orally twice daily for 14 days.

There are few data to support the use of an alternative regimen to cephalosporins in the treatment of gonorrhea. In the uncommon event that an individual has a history of a serious adverse event to cephalosporin, desensitization is recommended. If this is not possible, azithromycin 2 g orally as a single dose can be used in uncomplicated infection; however, there are concerns over emerging macrolide resistance, it causes significant gastrointestinal symptoms and it is costly. Use of azithromycin should be strictly limited to rare situations. Fluoroquinolones should only be considered as an alternative treatment option if antimicrobial susceptibilities are available on specimens.

PREVENTION

Public health programs designed to control gonorrhea aim to reduce harm to the infected individual and their sex partners by early detection and treatment at the time of diagnosis with contact tracing. In addition, public health policy at a population level aims to educate on prevention, promote screening programs and facilitate easy access to treatment clinics. Correct and consistent use of male latex condoms markedly reduces the risk of transmission of discharging diseases including gonorrhea.

At an individual level, an important aspect of care is the treatment of patients' sex partners to prevent further transmission or re-infection. Any sex partners within 60 days of the onset of symptoms or diagnosis of gonorrhea should be screened and treated. If the sexual contact is greater than 60 days then the most recent sex partner should be treated. Patients and their sex partners should avoid sexual contact until they are treated and their symptoms have resolved. Treatment regimens are outlined in treatment of uncomplicated gonorrhea above.

FURTHER READING

Further reading for this chapter can be found online at http://www.expertconsult.com

Persistent/recurrent vaginal discharge

INTRODUCTION

Vaginal discharge is one of the cardinal symptoms of lower tract gynecologic exudative infections. These disorders are classified by anatomic site of origin. For example, gonorrhea and chlamydial infections are cervical infections; bacterial vaginosis (BV), trichomoniasis and vaginal yeast infections are vaginal disorders. Herpes simplex and human papillomavirus can cause epithelial lesions on the external genitalia, but they can also cause cervicitis with discharge (see Chapter 49).

Initial steps

The first step in assessing a complaint of recurrent vaginal discharge is to differentiate between a normal physiologic discharge, a vaginal discharge and cervical infections. Many women have a small amount of vaginal discharge (physiologic leukorrhea), which is clear or white, does not have an odor, and is composed predominantly of squamous epithelial cells; this may vary with the menstrual cycle.

Patients do not differentiate from cervical and vaginal disorders, but often report 'vaginal discharge', which may represent either cervical or vaginal pathology. Therefore, initial evaluation of a patient who has recurrent or persistent discharge should include assessment for cervical infection. 'Recurrent' chlamydial and gonococcal infection is most often due to patient noncompliance with treatment regimens, re-exposure to an untreated sexual partner or re-exposure (i.e. new-incident infection). New-incident chlamydial and gonococcal infection is particularly common among adolescents.

Assuming that gonococcal and chlamydial infection has been ruled out and that the problem has been localized to the vagina, the next step in managing recurrent vaginal discharge is to determine the specific etiology of the vaginitis. This involves taking a careful history, with attention to recent douching, antimicrobial use (including use of over-the-counter antifungal medications) and reproductive history, followed by a clinical examination, which should include microscopic evaluation of vaginal discharge and determination of vaginal pH. The differential algorithm proposed by Sobel (see Further reading) is the standard in clinical assessment. The clinical and microscopic evaluation of recurrent vaginitis is shown in Figure PP30.1.

RECURRENT VAGINITIS DUE TO INFECTION

Recurrent trichomoniasis

Recurrent infection with *Trichomonas* spp. is most commonly due to re-infection from an untreated male partner or to re-exposure. Trichomoniasis in men is usually asymptomatic, and it is therefore imperative that all male partners of women who have trichomoniasis be treated with metronidazole, 2 g orally, as a single dose.

Metronidazole-resistant trichomoniasis is rare (<1% of clinical isolates) and should be considered only after re-infection has been ruled out and the patient has failed two courses of therapy. In these patients, metronidazole resistance should be confirmed, and they will respond frequently to a prolonged course of metronidazole (2–4 g daily for 10–14 days). Alternatively, tinidazole has been used successfully to treat resistant *Trichomonas* infection, at 2–3 g orally for 7–10 days.

Recurrent candidal vaginitis

Candidal vaginitis is extremely common and recurrences are frequent, in up to 45–50% of cases in some studies. Recurrent candidiasis is found more frequently in women who are taking antimicrobial agents and in those who have uncontrolled diabetes mellitus. Immunosuppressed

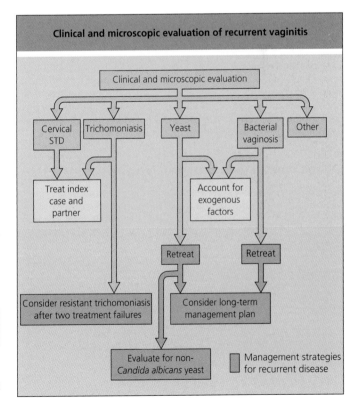

Fig. PP30.1 Clinical and microscopic evaluation of recurrent vaginitis.

patients, such as persons who have advanced HIV disease, are also at a modest risk of recurrent candidiasis as well as recurrent BV (see below).

After potential precipitating factors have been considered, there remains a subset of women who continue to get frequent recurrences. Careful microbiologic evaluation, with identification of the fungal species, may rarely reveal a yeast that is resistant to the commonly used imidazole and triazole therapies, such as *Candida glabrata* or *Candida tropicalis*. These investigations are expensive and should be reserved for use only after the clinical and epidemiologic risks have been identified. Persons who have chronic, recurrent candidiasis that is known to be caused by *Candida albicans* benefit from a course of long-term prophylaxis with fluconazole, 100–200 mg weekly (see also Chapter 49).

Recurrent bacterial vaginosis

Bacterial vaginosis is a disorder due to ecologic disturbances among the vaginal flora. Bacterial vaginosis is particularly prone to relapse. As above, the management of recurrent BV should account for the following:

- assurance that appropriate antimicrobial treatment was given initially – for example, many practitioners currently use a single-dose regimen of metronidazole (2 g orally) which has a treatment failure rate of up to 20%; persons who have suspected recurrence should be treated with a full multiday regimen of metronidazole 500 mg orally every 12 hours, or metronidazole vaginal gel (0.75%) 5 g every 12 hours for 5 days, or 2% clindamycin cream 5 g every 12 hours for 7 days;
- removal of exogenous factors that contribute to the pathogenesis of BV, including douching – douching is particularly associated with the development of BV because of the disruption of the local mucosal surfaces and flora, and women who use spermicides are at higher risk for BV and must balance the risk and benefits of their use;
- ruling out the presence of cervical infection – infections in the lower genital tract induce an inflammatory response, which in turn can cause BV; therefore, as above, ruling out cervical gonococcal and chlamydial infection is important early in the evaluation of persons who have recurrent BV.

The majority of women have primary BV (i.e. BV without an identifiable cause). Primary BV responds to treatment, but recurs frequently in these patients. Recurrence rates are as high as 20–30% 1 month after treatment. In these cases, long-term treatment with topical metronidazole should be considered. In nonpregnant women, treatment should take into account the impact of symptoms on the patient's lifestyle. In pregnant women, because of the potential for perinatal complications, periodic evaluation and treatment for recurrences is recommended.

Other causes of recurrent vaginitis

Bacterial vaginosis and yeast vaginitis are the most common types of recurrent vaginitis. Uncommon causes include hypersensitivity vaginitis, especially to latex, which is managed by avoiding latex exposure.

This is one situation in which natural membrane condoms may be appropriate. Desquamative inflammatory vaginitis is an uncommon disorder that is diagnosed by a high vaginal pH, a negative amine test, the absence of clue cells, and the presence of polymorphonuclear leukocytes and parabasal cells. These patients may respond to intravaginal 2% clindamycin cream, 5 g every 12 hours for 1 week; however, they are prone to frequent recurrence.

USE OF BIOLOGIC REMEDIES

Women who have frequently recurrent vaginitis occasionally turn to biologic remedies obtained from health food shops or over the Internet. These have included (among others) yoghurt douches, lactobacilli for vaginal instillation and prescriptions for eating large quantities of yoghurt. Controlled studies to date have failed to demonstrate any benefits of these remedies.

PATIENT COUNSELING

By the time they see a medical specialist, patients who have recurrent vaginal discharge have typically been seen by many medical care providers with limited results, and they are therefore often frustrated. Counseling on the etiology and pathogenesis of the disorder with frank explanation of the expected impact of therapy is a critical component of management. Issues of sexuality should also be explored, because patients may find intercourse either uncomfortable or embarrassing.

SUMMARY

Important points to remember are:

- take a complete history;
- account for exogenous factors;
- account for systemic diseases;
- rule out cervical sexually transmitted diseases;
- perform a complete evaluation including microscopy;
- consider episodic management and suppressive management; and
- counsel the patients intensively.

FURTHER READING

Further reading for this chapter can be found online at http://www.expertconsult.com

Persistent or recurrent nongonococcal urethritis in men and women

DEFINITION

There are an estimated 2 million cases of nongonococcal urethritis (NGU) in the USA per year, of which about 30–50% are caused by *Chlamydia trachomatis*; however, in the remaining *Chlamydia*-negative NGU cases, the microbiologic etiology is not well understood. It had been suspected that a proportion of *Chlamydia*-negative NGU cases may have been false-negative cases of *Chlamydia* urethritis; however, several lines of evidence have suggested that this is not the case, or is at least uncommon. Cervical cultures of female partners of men with *Chlamydia*-negative NGU have been repeatedly negative. In 25–30% of *Chlamydia*-negative NGU, no organisms have been recovered, although some additional etiologies have been proposed (Table PP31.1).

Chlamydia-negative NGU has been less well described in women. Women with persistent symptoms of a lower urinary tract infection yet with negative urine specimens from the bladder are all too often considered to have psychological problems, and thus are not adequately evaluated.

There are no widely accepted definitions for persistent or recurrent NGU. The 2006 Centers for Disease Control and Prevention (CDC) treatment guidelines for sexually transmitted diseases (STD) do not provide any definitions for these two clinical syndromes. In reviewing the literature, there are some 'loosely' applied defining terms for both entities:

- persistent urethritis refers to urethritis that fails to resolve or substantially improve within 2 weeks of initiating appropriate treatment regimens; and
- recurrent urethritis is defined as return of urethritis within 6 weeks following an initial response to appropriate treatment.

Most of the time these terms are used interchangeably since the duration of symptoms in relation to prior treatment may be unclear, although the median time for recurrence after completing treatment has been estimated at 2 weeks. Most men with recurrent NGU are culture negative for *Chlamydia* unless the interval following treatment is more than 2 weeks and they have had sexual intercourse with an untreated partner. The likelihood of resistant organisms playing a role in persistent or recurrent NGU is not known, with only infrequent cases reported over the past 10 years.

Table PP31.1 Etiologic agents for nongonococcal *Chlamydia*-negative urethritis (NGU) in men

Etiologic agent	Estimated prevalence	Preferred method of diagnosis	Comments
Mycoplasma genitalium	7–50%	Polymerase chain reaction (PCR)	In the 1990s, the advent of PCR-based assays for detecting *M. genitalium*, several studies reported the prevalence of *M. genitalium* being significantly higher in symptomatic men with acute *Chlamydia*-negative NGU than in asymptomatic men (13–42% versus 0–15%).
Trichomonas vaginalis	6–20%	PCR	*T. vaginalis* is not routinely diagnosed in men because of the apparent limited ability of culture to detect this organism in the male genital tract. One study found *T. vaginalis* in 17% of urethritis cases and 12% of those without evidence of disease. Another study reported a prevalence of *T. vaginalis* urethritis in men of 17%, but in men with *Chlamydia*-negative NGU, the prevalence reported was 19.9%.
Ureaplasma urealyticum	2–43%	PCR	The association between *U. urealyticum* and NGU remains controversial; it is suggested that serovar 2 is associated with NGU. The most convincing evidence linking *U. urealyticum* to NGU comes from human experimental studies. Results from a volunteer experiment showed that *U. urealyticum* may cause disease the first time it gains access to the urethra, but subsequent invasion results in colonization, without disease
Herpes simplex virus (HSV)	3–10%	PCR Serology	The possibility of HSV urethritis should be considered in persistent urethritis since symptoms from primary HSV urethritis last for about 2 weeks. Both HSV types 1 and 2 can be a cause of *Chlamydia*-negative NGU and urethral symptoms can occur without any obvious vulvar or penile lesions.

CLINICAL FEATURES

In contrast to the lack of definitions for the two clinical syndromes, the clinical presentations are much more specific, and similar to any acute inflammation of the urethra. Symptoms are prominent and detected earlier in men than in women, and include dysuria and urethral discharge, ranging from clear to mucopurulent. It is important to note that urethral discharge may not be present in all patients. In men, a spontaneous urethral discharge is frequently present prior to voiding.

DIFFERENTIAL DIAGNOSIS

Chronic bacterial prostatitis is a consideration; however, less than 5% of patients with persistent or recurrent *Chlamydia*-negative urethritis have microbial etiologies that can cause prostatitis. The clinical signs and symptoms of chronic prostatitis may resemble persistent or recurrent urethritis, and the prostate could possibly function as a sanctuary site for an indolent infectious process; however, the actual role of the prostate in persistent or recurrent urethritis is unknown. There is very little benefit in placing these patients on prolonged antibiotic therapy.

Acute bacterial cystourethritis may occur, mostly in patient with anatomic and functional lower urinary tract anomalies, but these patients tend to present with dysuria, urinary frequency and suprapubic pain, but without urethral discharge. Pyuria and positive urine cultures are common, although bacterial culture numbers may not reach 10^5 cfu/ml of urine. Treatment of this entity requires at least 7 days of antibiotics targeting uropathogens as well as attention to the urethral anomaly.

Rarer problems such as retained urethral foreign bodies, periurethral fistulas and periurethral abscesses should be excluded by palpation.

LABORATORY INVESTIGATIONS

Documenting laboratory evidence of urethritis is critical. The laboratory criteria for the diagnosis of urethritis are the presence of five or more polymorphonuclear cells (PMNs) per high power field in a urethral specimen and the absence of Gram-negative intracellular diplococci. If a urine sample is obtained, the presence of leukocyte esterase and of more than 10 white blood cells (WBC) per high power field on spun urine sediment are suggestive of urethral inflammation.

Testing for *N. gonorrhoeae* and *C. trachomatis* should be performed to exclude the possibility of re-infection with these organisms but not be repeatedly undertaken. In most clinical settings, testing for *Ureaplasma urealyticum* and *Mycoplasma genitalium* is not widely available. Routine testing for herpes simplex virus (HSV) is not recommended; however, polymerase chain reaction (PCR) testing or type-specific serology can be undertaken if there is a clear urethral discharge in the context of recent contact with a known HSV-positive sex partner, or if there is a urethral discharge at the same time as a genital HSV outbreak. The diagnostic tool of choice for suspected *Trichomonas vaginalis* urethritis is PCR testing either of a urethral specimen or urine.

MANAGEMENT OF PERSISTENT OR RECURRENT URETHRITIS

The management of persistent or recurrent urethritis is largely empiric and frustrating since often no organism is identified; however, it is important to confirm the presence of urethritis clinically

Table PP31.2 Recommended treatment regimens for persistent and recurrent urethritis

Persistent/ recurrent urethritis	Important steps	Recommended treatment regimens
First episode	Look for indicators for re-exposure and re-infection; if present, repeat testing for gonorrhea and chlamydia	Metronidazole 2 g or tinidazole 2 g po (one dose), plus either azithromycin 1 g po (one dose) or erythromycin 500 mg po q6h for 7 days
Second or any subsequent episodes	Look for indicators for re-exposure and re-infection; if present, repeat testing for gonorrhea and chlamydia	Erythromycin 500 mg po q6h for 3 weeks, or ofloxacin 300 mg po q12h for 3 weeks

and by laboratory criteria. This is a critical step to help exclude patients with functional complaints, who have urethral symptoms but no evidence of urethritis, who may benefit from reassurance. Revisiting the sexual exposure history and medication compliance may shed light into the possibilities of re-infection from an untreated partner and relapses secondary to inadequate treatment courses, as well as the presence of potentially resistant organisms.

Management of the initial persistent or recurrent episode of urethritis includes re-evaluating for the presence of gonococcal and/or chlamydial organisms, and empirically treating for *T. vaginalis*. The optimal regimen for covering potentially tetracycline-resistant organisms (i.e. mycoplasmas and ureaplasmas) has not been defined, and different regimens have not been compared. Table PP31.2 outlines the recommended regimens for first and subsequent persistent or recurrent urethritis episodes.

If symptoms persist after 3 weeks of empiric treatment with no infectious agents identified, continued antibiotic therapy is not beneficial. Moreover, there are no data to support retreating previously treated asymptomatic sex partners. Many cases resolve after 3 weeks of antibiotics.

Reassuring and encouraging patients that symptoms will resolve spontaneously over time, that most recurrences will arise independent of resumption of sexual activity, that the risk of transmission to a partner is low, and that the likelihood of long-term sequelae such as infertility or cancer appears to be exceedingly low, is important.

FURTHER READING

Further reading for this chapter can be found online at http://www.expertconsult.com

Section | 3 |

Jonathan Cohen & Steven M Opal

Special Problems in Infectious Disease Practice

Chapter | **61** | *Aric L Gregson*
Philip A Mackowiak

Pathogenesis of fever

HISTORICAL CONSIDERATIONS

Akkadian cuneiform inscriptions confirm that fever has been recognized as a sign of disease since at least the 6th century BC.[1] Although various theories to explain the source of fever were advanced over the centuries, it was not until the 1850s that Claude Bernard correctly attributed the source of fever to metabolic processes within the body itself.

Our ability to measure body temperature progressed more quickly than our understanding of its source and regulation. Early devices used the expansion property of air to measure temperature, probably first in the 2nd century BC. In 1592, Sanctoria Sanctoria, a colleague of Galileo's at Padua, employed such a device in clinical studies, leading him to hypothesize the existence of a 'normal' body temperature. These early devices were prone to changes in barometric pressure until a closed thermometer employing alcohol was invented by Cornelius Drebbel in 1608. Some of the earliest closed liquid thermometers used scales based upon the freezing point of water and the oral temperature of a healthy human.[2] It was not until the early 18th century that Gabriel Daniel Fahrenheit popularized a reliable mercury-based thermometer with a scale based on the freezing and boiling points of water.

Clinical thermometry was not fully integrated into medical practice until Carl Reinhold August Wunderlich published his sentinel work, *Das Verhalten der Eigenwärme in Krankenheiten* (The course of temperature in diseases), in 1868. In it he reportedly examined some 25 000 patients from whom he obtained nearly 1 million individual measurements. These observations led him to propose 98.6°F (37°C) as the 'normal' body temperature and temperatures of 100.4°F (38°C) or above as fever.[3,4] Despite the fact that these observations were made more than 130 years ago, were based on axillary temperatures and were obtained using thermometers calibrated 2.6–4.0°F (1.4–2.2°C) higher than contemporary thermometers, many continue to regard Wunderlich's observations as definitive.[5]

FEVER VERSUS HYPERTHERMIA

Fever is defined as 'a state of elevated core temperature, which is often, but not necessarily, part of the defensive responses of multicellular organisms (host) to the invasion of live (micro-organisms) or inanimate matter recognized as pathogenic or alien by the host'.[6] More simply, fever is a regulated rise in core temperature in response to a physiologic threat to the host. The febrile response, of which fever is a component, is characterized by a cytokine-mediated rise in core temperature, accompanied by increases in acute-phase reactants and a host of other immunologic, endocrinologic, neurologic and physiologic changes.

'Hyperthermia' is defined as a disturbance in temperature regulation when core temperature is above the range specified for the normal active state of the species.[6] It may be regulated (e.g. as in fever) or forced (as in heat stroke) when total heat production exceeds the capacity for heat loss. Forced hyperthermia is characterized by a sustained elevation of core temperature lacking the diurnal fluctuations characteristic of both fever and normal body temperature, and does not respond to antipyretic drug therapy.[7,8]

Heat stroke, a form of forced hyperthermia, often occurs in association with exertion and drugs, such as phenothiazines, anticholinergics or cocaine, which alter the body's ability to regulate heat. Classic heat stroke is most often seen in persons at the extremes of age with co-morbid conditions. It is associated with a lack of sweating, moderate rhabdomyolysis and lactic acidosis, and rarely causes renal failure. In the exertional form of heat stroke, sweating is profuse, making its detection more difficult. Rhabdomyolysis may be severe in exertional heat stroke and, along with marked lactic acidosis, leads to a significant risk of renal failure. Common to both types of heat stroke is extreme hyperthermia, in which core temperatures may exceed 106°F (41.1°C).

Malignant hyperthermia, induced by general anesthetics in predisposed persons, and the closely related neuroleptic malignant syndrome are other types of forced hyperthermia. Malignant hyperthermia is a rare autosomal dominant disorder, usually triggered by inhalational anesthetic agents and often fatal, which is the result of heat production in skeletal muscle which accumulates because of limitations of active heat dissipation during anesthesia. It manifests clinically as elevated core temperature, lactic acidosis, myoglobinemia and muscular rigidity. Because muscular rigidity follows the development of hyperthermia in a majority of cases, the increased core temperature is believed to be due initially to increased metabolism and disturbances of cellular permeability, not muscle contraction. Temperature increases rapidly, at approximately 1.8°F (1°C) each minute. Core temperatures reaching 114.8°F (46°C) have been reported.[9] Hyperthyroid storm can also lead to hyperthermia, although in such cases temperatures rarely exceed 104°F (40°C).

CLINICAL THERMOMETRY

In clinical practice, fever is defined as a core temperature above the normal range. Presently, no physical examination is considered complete without some measurement of body temperature. When interpreting the significance of such measurements, clinicians should consider important variables such as the anatomic site of measurement, the time of day and the type of instrument used to obtain the temperature recording. Thermometers must be tested periodically according to the manufacturer's recommendations to ensure proper calibration.[10,11] When measurements are taken, thermometers must be allowed adequate time to equilibrate with the test site. For mercury thermometers, rectal measurements require 1–5 minutes for optimal readings, whereas axillary and oral measurements require up to 11 minutes.[12,13] Newer thermistor-based electronic thermometers have shorter equilibration times than traditional mercury thermometers. Tympanic membrane thermometers equilibrate in seconds and are convenient to use. Unfortunately, their results are inconsistent and correlate poorly with concurrent rectal, axillary and oral measurements.[2,14–16]

Core temperature is an amalgam of temperatures derived from the various internal organs, all having different metabolic rates. Under normal physiologic conditions such differences are small. However, during shock or in the face of extreme thermal stress, regional and organ-specific differences in temperature can be marked.[17] Because core temperature readings are difficult to obtain, peripheral measurements are used to approximate core temperature. Mean rectal temperatures exceed oral by 0.8°F (0.4°C) and tympanic membrane temperatures by 1.6°F (0.8°C).[18,19] During shock, rectal temperature may underestimate an elevated core temperature because of poor rectal perfusion.[20] Moreover, rectal measurements are associated with a small but significant risk of infection due to cross-contamination.[21]

Oral temperature measurements have been standard practice because of accessibility and reasonable accuracy. Mastication and smoking both increase oral temperature. Ice-water ingestion decreases oral temperature, although only briefly.[19] Two studies of the effect of tachypnea and open-mouth breathing on oral temperature found that open mouth breathing, but not tachypnea per se, lowers oral temperature.[22,23] Because oral measurements require the subject's cooperation, they are difficult to obtain in critically ill and uncooperative patients.

NORMAL BODY TEMPERATURE

What constitutes normal body temperature remains the subject of debate. A temperature of 98.6°F (37°C) continues to be regarded as normal by many physicians and health care professionals, as a result of Wunderlich's original studies. 'Normal body temperature', however, is not a specific temperature but a range of temperatures, the parameters of which vary from one person to another.[24] One of the largest studies of oral temperature in healthy subjects yielded a mean temperature of 98.2°F (36.8°C).[24] Only 8% of the temperatures recorded were 98.6°F (37°C). The mean temperature varied diurnally with a nadir at 0600h and a peak at 1600–1800h, a mean amplitude of variability of 0.9°F (0.5°C), and a range of 0.1–2.4°F (0.05–1.3°C). Women had slightly higher mean temperatures than men [98.4°F (36.9°C) versus 98.1°F (36.7°C), p <0.001] but did not have greater diurnal variability. In this study population, 98.6°F (37°C) had no special significance with regard to normal body temperature (Fig. 61.1). The upper limit of normal temperature (i.e. greater than the 99th percentile) varied according to the time of day, from an early morning low of 99.0°F (37.2°C) to an evening peak of 100°F (37.8°C).

THERMOREGULATION

Mammals employ various thermogenic mechanisms to increase heat production during episodes of cold exposure and during the initiation of fever. Shivering is a principal thermogenic mechanism, except in neonates. Nonshivering thermogenesis is most closely linked to brown adipose tissue, so named because of its brown color, which is due to a profuse vascular supply and a high concentration of mitochondria. Brown adipose tissue is most prominent near the shoulder blades, neck, adrenal glands and deep blood vessels. Noradrenaline (norepinephrine) induces enzymatic hydrolysis of triglycerides to glycerol and free fatty acids in brown adipose tissue. These free fatty acids are the primary substrate oxidized by mitochondria to produce adenosine triphosphate (ATP) and heat. They also act as a signal to uncouple oxidative phosphorylation, thereby generating excess heat.

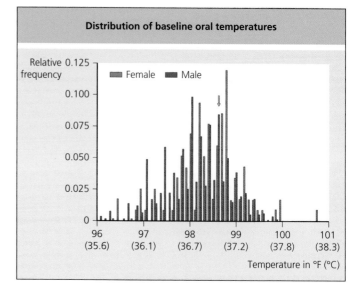

Fig. 61.1 Distribution of baseline oral temperatures in healthy men and women. Frequency distribution of 700 baseline oral temperatures obtained during two consecutive days of observation in 148 healthy young volunteers. Arrow indicates location of 98.6°F (37°C). With permission from Mackowiak et al.[24] Copyright 1992, American Medical Association.

In the resting state, approximately 72% of basal metabolic heat is produced by vital organs. Heat is distributed throughout the body via the circulatory system. Variations in cutaneous blood flow determine the amount of heat lost at the skin surface by radiation, evaporation, convection and conduction.[25] When environmental temperature exceeds body temperature, evaporation is the most effective means of heat dissipation. The balance between heat production and heat loss, largely under control of the autonomic nervous system, maintains body temperature near the hypothalamic set-point of 98.2°F (36.8°C). When it is necessary to decrease core temperature, blood flow is preferentially directed to the skin and sweating mechanisms are activated. In cold environments or at the onset of fever, blood flow is directed away from the surface towards the internal vital organs to minimize heat loss.

More than 60 years of investigation have suggested that no single, central location is responsible for temperature regulation. Rather, a series of hierarchical structures appear to control body temperature (Fig. 61.2). This hierarchical system includes a continuum of structures from the hypothalamus and limbic system extending through the brain stem, reticular formation, spinal cord and sympathetic ganglia. The rostral hypothalamus, referred to as the 'preoptic' region, is actually composed of the medial and lateral aspects of the preoptic area, the anterior hypothalamus and the septum. Many, although not all, thermophysiologists consider the preoptic region to be a central thermoregulation region, having greater thermosensitivity than other structures. The preoptic region orchestrates thermoregulatory responses in other effector areas via signals transmitted through the median forebrain bundle, a bidirectional pathway within the lateral hypothalamus.[26] Indeed, the median forebrain bundle has been shown to manage efferent signals controlling shivering and cutaneous blood flow.[27] Afferent signals ascend to the brain stem reticular formation via the lateral spinothalamic tract. The preoptic region of the hypothalamus, in turn, receives this information and integrates afferent and efferent signals to maintain the appropriate body temperature.

Thermoregulation is coordinated via a subset of temperature-sensitive preoptic neurons. There are three basic types of such neurons, which differ according to their responses to temperature changes. So called 'warm-sensitive neurons', accounting for approximately 30% of the preoptic neuronal population, increase their firing rates in response to increases in preoptic temperature. Their efferent output initiates heat

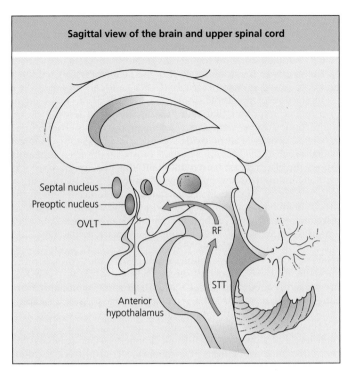

Fig. 61.2 Sagittal view of the brain and upper spinal cord. The figure shows the multisynaptic pathway of skin and spinal thermoreceptors through the spinothalamic tract (STT) and reticular formation (RF) to the anterior hypothalamus, the preoptic region and the septum. OVLT, organum vasculosum laminae terminalis. Redrawn with permission from Mackowiak.[1]

loss responses proportional to increases in body temperature over a certain threshold. A smaller number of 'cold-sensitive neurons' present in the preoptic region comprise less than 5% of total neurons. These neurons increase their firing rates as body temperature decreases. Cold-sensitive neurons are under synaptic inhibition from warm-sensitive neurons and, as the firing rates of warm-sensitive neurons decrease, so does the synaptic inhibition on cold-sensitive neurons. The net result is an increase in the firing rates of the cold-sensitive neurons[26,28] (Fig. 61.3). It may be that only the warm-sensitive neurons are truly thermosensitive and that thermoregulation is accomplished through their inhibitory and excitatory signals.[29–31] The majority of preoptic neurons do not demonstrate changes in firing rates in response to changes in preoptic temperature.

Pyrogens

Although peripheral neuronal input is of paramount importance during normal homeostatic thermoregulation, soluble 'endogenous pyrogens' (pyrogenic cytokines) exert a pronounced effect on temperature regulation during fever. These pyrogens have long been thought to mediate fever by elevating the hypothalamic set-point temperature (see also Chapter 2).

Traditionally, pyrogens have been classified as either 'endogenous' or 'exogenous'. Pyrogenic cytokines are endogenous immunoregulatory polypeptides, such as interleukin (IL)-1β, IL-6 and tumor necrosis factor (TNF). They are primarily derived from stimulated mononuclear cells and directly interact with the anterior hypothalamus to elevate the core temperature set-point. Exogenous pyrogens are the usual stimuli that induce mononuclear cells to produce and release pyrogenic cytokines. They include substances such as lipopolysaccharide (LPS), peptidoglycan, lipopeptides and numerous other microbial products. The distinction between endogenous and exogenous pyrogens and their ability to initiate fever is artificial, as some endogenous molecules can themselves induce the production of pyrogenic

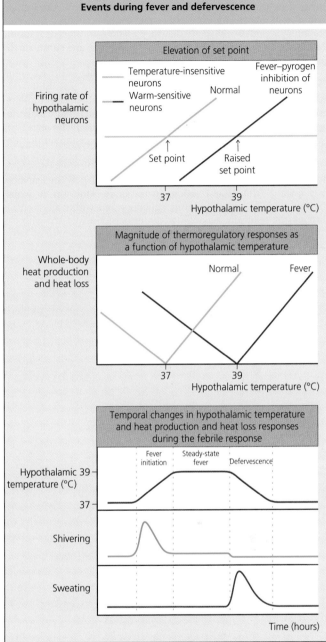

Fig. 61.3 Events during fever and defervescence. When pyrogens are present in the preoptic region the whole body and neuronal responses are as shown by the purple lines. Upper: Normally the firing rates of warm-sensitive and temperature-insensitive neurons functionally overlap at 98.6°F (37°C), the set-point of thermoregulatory neurons. During pyrogen inhibition of warm-sensitive neurons, this overlap occurs at the raised set-point of 102.2°F (39°C). Center: During fever, heat production is initially great but, as body temperature rises towards 102.2°F, heat production diminishes and should cease at 102.2°F. Lower: During fever initiation, shivering causes an increase in hypothalamic temperature and then ceases as the temperature reaches 102.2°F. During defervescence the hypothalamus activates heat loss responses such as sweating. Adapted with permission from Boulant.[28]

cytokines. Antigen–antibody complexes, complement, inflammatory bile acids and androgenic steroid metabolites are examples.

Pyrogenic cytokines have numerous activities other than pyrogenesis, including autocrine, paracrine and endocrine functions that determine the character of the febrile response. As such, they coordinate gene expression and cellular activities that drive the inflammatory response to infection (and other forms of injury). However, preliminary evidence suggests that they might also prevent immune destruction of certain pathogenic micro-organisms[32] and stimulate the growth of others.[33]

Although expression of Toll-like receptors (TLRs) in the organum vasculosum laminae terminalis (OVLT) raises the possibility that exogenous pyrogens induce fever directly, independent of proinflammatory cytokines, considerable data have suggested that exogenous pyrogens primarily exert their pyrogenic effect indirectly by increasing circulating pyrogenic cytokines, which in turn elevate the set-point of the thermoregulatory center (Fig. 61.4).

Because pyrogenic cytokines are large, hydrophilic molecules, they do not easily cross the blood–brain barrier, and it is unclear how they interact with central regions in the brain. One way in which they might gain access to thermoregulatory sites within the brain is through the relatively leaky blood–brain barrier associated with the OVLT. However, even in this region, and with the assistance of active

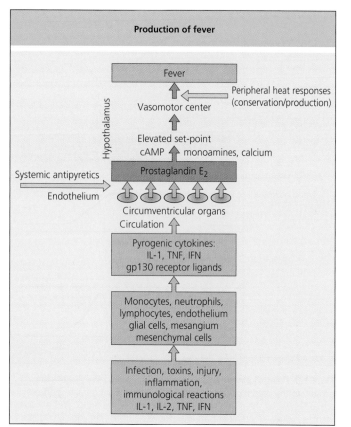

Fig. 61.4 Production of fever. Microbial agents, inflammatory agents and some cytokines induce the synthesis and release of pyrogenic cytokines from a variety of cells. These cytokines, in turn, trigger specialized endothelial cells of the hypothalamic vascular organs, which release prostaglandin E_2 (PGE$_2$). Elevated PGE$_2$ then brings about increases in cyclic adenosine monophosphate (cAMP) monoamines and calcium in the thermoregulatory center of the anterior hypothalamus, resulting in a resetting of the thermostatic temperature from normothermia to febrile levels. These neurotransmitters then activate the vasomotor center, which brings about vasoconstriction (heat conservation) and increased heat production, both resulting in an increase in blood temperature (fever). Regardless of the cause of fever, antipyretics inhibit this pathway by preventing the increase in cytokine-mediated PGE$_2$ production in the hypothalamus. IFN, interferon; IL, interleukin; TNF, tumor necrosis factor.

transport, passage of pyrogenic cytokines across the blood–brain barrier is too slow and modest to account for the initial rapid onset of fever seen following the intravenous administration of LPS, IL-1 or IL-6.[34] Endothelial and microglial cells at the blood–brain barrier have IL-1 receptors and, in response to IL-1 and LPS, synthesize TNF, IL-1β and IL-6, as well as cyclo-oxygenase (COX)-2 mRNA.[30,35]

Interaction of pyrogenic cytokines with cells at the OVLT might also induce responses that route the febrile signal inward toward the preoptic area via secondary cytokine production, phospholipase A$_2$/COX-2 activity, a nitric oxide secondary messenger, or via direct neural input to the preoptic region.[36] Prostaglandin (PG) E$_2$ readily crosses the blood–brain barrier and inhibiting PGE$_2$ synthesis blocks cytokine-induced fever, supporting its primary role in the pathogenesis of fever. Nitric oxide is generated by endothelial cells in the blood–brain barrier in response to IL-1 and IL-6. However, its role as a secondary messenger of the fever response is uncertain.[37]

Multiple pyrogenic mechanisms likely activate the OVLT. In certain experimental models, circulating levels of IL-1 do not correlate with the initial fever peak, although IL-6 may correspond to subsequent peaks.[30,38] Such observations suggest that IL-1 and TNF are paracrine modulators and IL-6 an endocrine modulator.[39] Yet other models suggest that bacterial superantigens, such as staphylococcal enterotoxin B, induce cell-associated cytokines that activate endothelial and microglial cells at the OVLT in the absence of high levels of circulating, cell-free cytokines.[40] Thus, it is possible that different combinations of mechanisms control fever in different situations.

In the case of endotoxin-induced fever, the febrile response seems to be initiated when Gram-negative bacteria and/or their products arrive in the liver, are taken up by Kupffer cells and activate the complement cascade to generate C5a.[34] This, in turn, rapidly stimulates Kupffer cells to release PGE$_2$. In such models, TNF and other pyrogenic cytokines are produced later and do not appear to be the immediate triggers of fever. One theory is that the Kupffer cell-generated PGE$_2$ is transported by the bloodstream to the ventromedial preoptic anterior hypothalamus (POA), and diffuses into the thermoregulatory regions to raise the thermal set-point. If this is so, PGE$_2$ would be the final, central fever mediator. However, it is also possible that PGE$_2$ activates hepatic vagal afferents projecting to the medulla oblongata, thence to the POA via the ventral noradrenergic bundle. Noradrenaline (norepinephrine) consequently secreted might then stimulate α_1-adrenoceptors on thermoregulatory neurons to evoke a rapid initial rise in core temperature not associated with any change in POA PGE$_2$.

Although these models address the mechanisms responsible for the induction phase of fever, the mechanisms responsible for the plateau or descending phases of fever remain obscure. The explanation for the tendency of fevers to oscillate in circadian fashion, even during infections such as bacterial endocarditis, remains unclear. In endocarditis the circulating levels of exogenous pyrogens (bacteria) remain remarkably constant throughout the day and night.

Acute-phase response

Fever is just one component of the febrile response, collectively referred to as the 'acute-phase response'. Often fever and the acute-phase response are linked, as in trauma or infection. However, they can also exist independently, suggesting that, although pyrogenic cytokines have the capacity to elicit both responses, fever and the acute-phase response are, nevertheless, independently regulated entities (see also Chapter 2).

A wide array of physiologic and endocrinologic alterations occurs during the febrile response. These include anorexia and sleepiness, and altered synthesis of glucagon, insulin, adrenocorticotropic hormone, cortisol, catecholamines, growth hormone, thyroid-stimulating hormone, thyroxine, aldosterone and arginine vasopressin. Inhibition of bone formation, negative nitrogen balance, gluconeogenesis and altered lipid metabolism also occur. Serum levels of zinc and iron fall,

Table 61.1 Acute phase proteins

Positive acute-phase proteins*	
CRP	Ferritin
Serum amyloid A	Phospholipase A$_2$
Haptoglobin	Plasminogen activator inhibitor-1
α_1-Acid glycoprotein	Fibronectin
α_1-Protease inhibitor	Hemopexin
Fibrinogen	Pancreatic secretory trypsin inhibitor
Ceruloplasmin	Inter-alpha protease inhibitor
Complement (C3 and C4)	Mannose binding protein
C-1 esterase inhibitor	LPS binding protein
C4b binding protein	
α_2-Macroglobulin	
Negative acute-phase proteins†	
Albumin	Transferrin
Transthyretin	α_2-HS glycoprotein

*Proteins exhibiting increased plasma concentrations during the acute-phase response.
†Proteins exhibiting decreased plasma concentrations during the acute-phase response.
Adapted from Kushner & Rzewnicki.[42]

whereas copper levels rise. Decreased erythropoiesis, in part responsible for 'anemia of chronic disease' (or, more appropriately 'anemia of chronic inflammation'), thrombocytosis and leukocytosis are additional features.[41]

Like fever, the acute-phase response is a tightly regulated response activated by a variety of stimuli (e.g. surgery, trauma, infection, cancer, burns). It is further characterized by production of an array of acute-phase proteins. These proteins are designated 'positive' or 'negative', depending on whether their levels rise or fall during the acute-phase response (Table 61.1). Those belonging to the former category are substantially more prominent than those belonging to the latter. The major positive acute-phase proteins are C-reactive protein (CRP) and serum amyloid A. Negative acute-phase proteins include albumin, pre-albumin (transthyretin) and transferrin. C-reactive protein and serum amyloid A normally exist in only minute concentrations but increase more than 1000-fold during the acute-phase response. C-reactive protein enhances phagocytosis by binding phosphocholine, present on foreign pathogens and damaged host cells, and activates complement. In certain situations, CRP stimulates thrombosis and promotes inflammatory cytokine production and the release of tissue factor by monocytes. Nevertheless, considerable evidence suggests that, *in vivo*, CRP functions primarily as an anti-inflammatory mediator.[43,44] Serum amyloid A enhances phagocyte adhesion and chemotaxis. Complement components, another group of acute-phase proteins, influence chemotaxis, opsonization and vascular permeability. The antioxidants and anti-inflammatory molecules, haptoglobin and ceruloplasmin, also appear to function as both positive acute-phase proteins and modulators of the inflammatory response. The thrombocytosis, decrease in iron and zinc levels and other features of the acute-phase response all appear to be important components of the defense against bacterial pathogens.[45]

Endogenous antipyretics

Core temperature rarely if ever reaches, far less exceeds, 106.0°F (41.1°C) during fever. This suggests that fever has a thermal ceiling, perhaps designed to protect the host against the deleterious effects of temperatures higher than 106.0°F (41.1°C).[38] Indeed, the warm-

sensitive neurons in the preoptic region reach their peak firing rates and the cold-sensitive neurons in the same region are maximally suppressed at 107.6°F (42°C), suggesting that the anterior hypothalamus is incapable of thermoregulation at temperatures higher than 107.6°F (42°C).[46] Various mechanisms, including pyrogen tolerance, circulating cryogens and modification of effector synthesis, appear to work to prevent core temperature from rising above 106°F (41.1°C). The pyrogenic effects of IL-1 and TNF are attenuated after repeated or prolonged exposures. Moreover, an important feature of tolerance to LPS is a decrease in pyrogenic cytokine production by macrophages.[38,47]

The best characterized endogenous antipyretics are α-melanocyte stimulating hormone (αMSH), arginine vasopressin (AVP), lipocortin-1, glucocorticoids and IL-10.[48–50] IL-10 has been shown to prevent LPS-induced fever by attenuating the production of TNF, IL-6 and IL-1 and increasing release of soluble IL-1-receptor antagonist, and through direct interaction with microglial cells in the central nervous system.[51] Arginine vasopressin appears to exert its antipyretic effects as a neurotransmitter of specialized neurons projecting into the ventroseptal area. Firing of such neurons increases during fever.[52] Moreover, neutralization of AVP during experimental fever is associated with increases in both the height and the duration of fever, all of which suggest an antipyretic role for AVP.[53] The melanocortin αMSH is a neurotransmitter of neurons with projections to the hypothalamic paraventricular nucleus, the integrative output nucleus for fever and numerous autonomic stress responses. Under experimental conditions, peripheral and intracerebral administration of αMSH blocks IL-1- and LPS-induced fever. Centrally administered αMSH-receptor blockers inhibit the antipyretic effect of αMSH.[53]

Arachidonic acid liberated from cell membranes by the action of phospholipase can be metabolized either by COX to pyrogenic PGE$_2$ or via an alternative cytochrome p450-mediated pathway to antipyretic eicosanoids (epoxyeicosanoids). Induction of cytochrome p450 shifts arachidonic acid metabolism away from COX and toward the cytochrome p450 pathway, thereby reducing core temperature through a combination of diminished PGE$_2$ production and an increase in production of antipyretic epoxyeicosanoids.[54]

ANTIPYRETICS

Aspirin and acetaminophen (paracetamol) have been a mainstay of antipyretic drug therapy since the turn of the 20th century. A host of nonsteroidal anti-inflammatory drugs (NSAIDs) also possess antipyretic properties. Despite the popularity of these drugs among both health-care workers and the general public, it is still not clear that reducing core body temperature benefits febrile patients. Although antipyretic therapy assumes that fever is, at least in part, noxious and that suppression of fever will eliminate or reduce its noxious effects, neither assumption has been validated experimentally. Consequently, rational guidelines for suppressing fever have been slow in coming.

Fever creates a number of potential metabolic challenges for the host. During the chill or ascending phase of fever, activation of the sympathetic nervous system causes peripheral vasoconstriction and an associated increase in mean arterial pressure.[55] Oxygen consumption increases, as does carbon dioxide production.[56] External cooling can attenuate these effects, but only if shivering is prevented.[57] If shivering is not prevented, external cooling reduces skin temperature faster than core temperature and initiates vasoconstriction and shivering, which can paradoxically increase core temperature, oxygen consumption and the respiratory quotient. Importantly, external cooling can also cause vasospasm of diseased coronary arteries.[58] Unfortunately, certain antipyretic drugs also cause coronary vasoconstriction in patients who have coronary artery disease. Friedman *et al.*[59] observed significant increases in mean arterial pressure, coronary vascular resistance and myocardial arteriovenous oxygen difference after administration of intravenous indometacin (0.5 mg/kg) in such patients. Mean coronary blood flow decreased simultaneously from 181 ± 29 to 111 ± 14 ml/min ($p < 0.05$). Thus, in this investigation, myocardial oxygen demand increased in the face of a fall in coronary blood flow following indometacin administration.

Aspirin, acetaminophen and the NSAIDs all inhibit COX-mediated synthesis of inflammatory thromboxanes and prostaglandins from arachidonic acid. Cyclo-oxygenase has at least two distinct isoforms, COX-1 and COX-2. Cyclo-oxygenase-1 was long regarded as a constitutively expressed cellular enzyme involved in various housekeeping functions, whereas COX-2 was touted as an inducible enzyme responsible for hypothalamus-mediated fever and produced as part of the inflammatory process by a variety of cell lines, including macrophages, synoviocytes and endothelial cells. However, this dichotomous concept of a constitutive COX-1 and an inducible proinflammatory COX-2 has proved to be oversimplified. Not only do some cells express COX-2 constitutively, but under certain conditions COX-2 has also been shown to promote healing of mucosal lesions and the resolution of inflammation.[60]

The distinctive affinities of the various categories of antipyretic drug for the different COX variants are thought to determine their relative antipyretic and analgesic potencies. Acetaminophen and aspirin, for example, are equally potent inhibitors of central COX but only 10% as potent in this regard as indometacin. Acetaminophen selectively inhibits a third COX variant, a close relative of COX-1 derived from the same gene and referred to as 'COX-3'.[61] The importance of the discovery of COX-3 is that it explained the pharmacologic actions of acetaminophen and other antipyretic analgesic drugs, which are weak inhibitors of COX-1 and COX-2 but penetrate easily into the central nervous system. NSAIDs, such as diclofenac or ibuprofen, are also potent inhibitors of COX-3 expressed in cultured cells, but being highly polar, are unlikely to reach brain COX-3 in effective concentrations.[62] Only aspirin irreversibly inhibits COX and does so via acetylation within the active site of the enzyme. Other NSAIDs and acetaminophen inhibit COX reversibly.[63]

Aspirin and the NSAIDs also have COX-independent antipyretic activity. Aspirin induces cytochrome p450, which might augment its antipyretic effect by shifting arachidonic acid metabolism toward cytochrome p450-mediated production of cryogenic epoxyeicosanoids. Additionally, acetylation of COX-2 by aspirin increases the production of 15R-hydroxyeicosatetraenoic acid, which neutrophils use to form aspirin-triggered lipoxins (ATL). These lipoxins have potent anti-inflammatory activity, independent of aspirin. Heat shock proteins have been shown to reduce transcription of IL-1β *in vitro*, and therapeutic doses of aspirin and certain NSAIDs increase heat shock factor-1 concentration *in vitro*. These same drugs also diminish the activity of transcriptional activator nuclear factor-κB.[63] The latter is involved in the transcription of pyrogenic cytokines, adhesion molecules, inducible nitric oxide synthase and COX-2 in certain cell lines. Production of adenosine, an anti-inflammatory mediator produced by leukocytes, is enhanced by aspirin and NSAIDs. The clinical implications of these alternative antipyretic pathways remain to be determined.

Antipyretic therapy is commonly administered to enhance patient comfort. General experience with antipyretic drugs, which are for the most part also analgesic agents, seems to support this rationale. However, carefully controlled efficacy studies have never quantified the degree to which antipyretic therapy enhances the comfort of patients who have fever. Moreover, the relative cost of such symptomatic relief, in terms of drug toxicity and adverse effects of the antipyretic agents on the course of the illness responsible for the fever, has never been determined. The importance of these negative drug effects is underscored by studies demonstrating prolonged time to crusting of varicella skin lesions in children,[64] and increased rhinovirus shedding and decreased neutralizing antibody formation following acetaminophen use in adults.[65,66] Paracetamol use has been reported to prolong parasite clearance time in children infected with *Plasmodium falciparum*, presumably by decreasing production of TNF and oxygen radicals.[67] The risks of antipyretic drug therapy, including direct and indirect drug toxicity, increased morbidity from infection and the masking of a possible underlying infection, must be weighed against any possible benefit.

Antipyretic therapy has never been shown to be effective in preventing febrile seizures, perhaps reflecting the fact that the etiology of such seizures has more to do with the disorders responsible for the fevers than fever per se.[68] Camfield *et al.*[69] conducted a randomized double-blind study comparing single daily-dose phenobarbital plus antipyretic instruction with placebo plus antipyretic instruction in preventing recurrent febrile seizures following an initial simple febrile seizure. In children treated with phenobarbital and antipyretics, the febrile seizure recurrence rate was 5%, whereas in those receiving placebo and antipyretics the rate was 25%, suggesting that a single daily dose of phenobarbital is more effective than counseling parents about antipyretic therapy in preventing recurrent febrile seizures. More recent studies in children have shown that, whether given in moderate doses or in relatively high doses, neither acetaminophen[70] nor ibuprofen[71] reduces the rate of recurrence of febrile seizures.

Antipyretic drugs to modulate the activity of pyrogenic cytokines have been studied in bacterial sepsis.[72] In certain animal models, COX inhibitors confer protection when given soon after bacterial challenge, presumably by blunting the adverse effects of TNF and IL-1. In a large clinical trial, Bernard *et al.*[73] found that 48 hours of intravenous therapy with the COX inhibitor, ibuprofen, lowered core temperature, heart rate, oxygen consumption and blood levels of lactic acid. However, ibuprofen did not decrease the incidence of organ failure or 30-day mortality rate in patients who have sepsis.

Several tentative conclusions regarding the benefits and relative risks of antipyretic therapy seem justified in light of the limited data available. Clearly short courses of approved doses of standard antipyretic drugs carry a low risk of toxicity. Most antipyretic drugs have analgesic as well as antipyretic properties. Therefore, if not otherwise contraindicated (as is, for instance, aspirin in young children because of the risk of Reye's syndrome), such drugs can be used to provide symptomatic relief in patients who have fever, to reduce the metabolic demands of fever in chronically debilitated patients and possibly to prevent or alleviate fever-associated mental dysfunction in the elderly. To minimize antipyretic-induced fluctuations in temperature and the risk of recurrent shivering and its increased metabolic demands, antipyretic agents should be administered to patients who have fever at regular intervals to preclude abrupt recurrences, rather than as needed for temperatures above some arbitrary level. When prescribing such medications, physicians must recognize that each carries its own risk of toxicity and may prolong the course of at least some infections. There is no compelling evidence that a response to antipyretic medications is useful diagnostically in distinguishing serious from self-limited illnesses, nor is there evidence that such medications are effective in suppressing febrile seizures, even if given prophylactically.

In view of the capacity of external cooling measures to induce a cold pressor response, it is questionable whether this form of antipyretic therapy should ever be administered to patients who have fever. If external cooling is used to treat fever, care must be taken to prevent shivering because of its associated increase in metabolic work. Intravascular cooling devices may reduce variation in body temperature as compared to external cooling devices, although their effect on shivering and oxygen consumption has not been evaluated.[74,75] Unfortunately, even if shivering is prevented, there is no guarantee that a cold pressor response will be averted. In view of indometacin's capacity to cause coronary vasoconstriction in patients who have coronary artery disease, NSAIDs should be used with caution, if at all, to suppress fever in such patients.

REFERENCES

References for this chapter can be found online at http://www.expertconsult.com

Clinical approach to acute fever

Fever is one of the most frequent symptoms leading to consultation with a health professional. Vast numbers of febrile illnesses are of short duration and benign outlook, and few of these are diagnosed. However, in the midst of this mass of minor illness are patients whose illness is serious or likely to become so. Some of these serious illnesses also present a danger to others, and thus have a significance beyond that of the individual patient. This is the challenge of acute fever: to distinguish the threatening from the trivial in acute illnesses in which fever is a main feature.

In some cases, of course, the fever becomes prolonged and this topic of more long-lasting fever (fever of unknown origin; FUO) is discussed in Chapter 63. The distinction between fevers of short and those of longer duration is important in considering diagnostic possibilities. Many acute and short-lived fevers are of viral origin, and conversely viral fevers without particular diagnostic features rarely last longer than 1 or 2 weeks; thus, prolonged fever without distinguishing features is rarely caused by a virus, at least in immunologically normal patients.

HISTORY

As with any other medical problem, the history is the most productive component of the initial encounter. Hypotheses are generated from the patient's account and the physician's observations, and are successively pursued or rejected in the light of emerging data. In the case of acute fever, however, a few special features of the history stand out. One of these is the common difficulty in reaching agreement on the meaning of words and phrases used in this context. It is rare for the phrase 'I have a fever' to mean that the body temperature has been measured by a reliable method. More often, the phrase means that the patient has a subjective sensation of warmth, or a feeling of chilliness or undue sweating. 'Flu' is another word in common use and usually describes aching muscles, chills and shivering, but sometimes is used to denote upper respiratory symptoms such as a runny nose or scratchy throat, and sometimes to indicate a fever. And, of course, different meanings are attached to these and other words in different cultures and languages.

A second distinctive point when taking the history of a patient with acute fever relates to the time-honored 'systems review'. This is usually employed, if at all, at the end of a history taking, but often has so little to contribute that it is discarded. In the case of acute fever, however, because the range of possibilities is so much wider than for many presenting symptoms, the systems enquiry is useful early in the history taking; it often reveals the only relevant localizing evidence, as patients may have forgotten or thought insignificant symptoms that provide valuable clues. Among the apparently minor clues that may emerge on direct enquiry are minor respiratory, abdominal or urinary symptoms, a transient rash or previous episodes of illness of a similar nature. Apparent localizing features that are actually symptoms of the raised temperature may, however, give false leads. Thus, dark urine in a febrile patient may simply denote dehydration, and some patients, especially women, experience burning and discomfort passing urine when they are febrile. Muscle and joint pains are also hard to interpret during fever: severe pains suggest viral infections such as influenza or dengue, but they are also a feature of some enteroviral infections (Bornholm disease) and of leptospirosis. Neurologic features are especially difficult. Some patients regularly experience headache when febrile, and many children and some older patients become delirious with a high fever; whether such clinical features indicate a specifically neurologic involvement obviously needs careful observation.

A history of medication may be important in acute febrile disease. A large number of drugs may themselves cause fever, often without a rash or other clear indicators. Among antimicrobial agents, penicillins, cephalosporins and sulfonamides are especially notable, but many others may be implicated. Anti-infective agents may suppress or modify infections, and so confound a diagnosis, and antipyretic agents may greatly modify the pattern of fever in an infection.

Travel history

As rapid movements of vast numbers of people throughout the world have been made possible in the era of air travel, so have the possibilities of an infection developing in one country when it was acquired in another. A travel history must never be omitted in a patient who has fever, and many tragic deaths from *Plasmodium falciparum* malaria testify to its importance. The history should be accurate as to time and place. The name of a country is not enough; a stay in a four-star hotel in a capital city presents different risks from those of a camping trek in rural areas of the same country.

Timing is especially helpful, even though many infections have a wide range of recorded incubation periods. For example, an illness beginning more than about 10 days after return is unlikely to be one of the common acute respiratory infections, with the exception of *Mycoplasma pneumoniae* and perhaps Q fever; dengue, too, and other arbovirus infections would have developed by this time. An incubation period of more than 3 weeks excludes the hemorrhagic virus infections, such as Lassa fever, and almost excludes typhoid. On the other hand, longer periods still leave open the possibility of viral hepatitis, Katayama fever (acute schistosomiasis) and primary HIV infection. As to malaria, the incubation period of *P. falciparum* infection may be as little as 1 week, but after 6 or 8 weeks a first presentation of this form of malaria becomes uncommon. *Plasmodium vivax* and *Plasmodium malariae* infections may develop months or years after travel to a malarial area.

Other important aspects of the travel history are the immunization record and an account of medications, with special emphasis on antimalarial prophylaxis.

It is sometimes necessary to begin treatment before a definite diagnosis has been made, or when the causal organism but not its antibiotic susceptibility is known. The travel history is important here too, as the pattern of antibiotic resistance in many pathogens varies greatly from country to country, and will determine an appropriate choice of therapy. Notable examples are the differences in drug resistance in malaria in different countries, the spread of multiresistant typhoid and shigellosis and the erratic distribution of pneumococcal resistance to penicillin. In each of these examples, the area in which infection was acquired may limit the options available for chemotherapy.

Every physician who sees a febrile traveler cannot be expected to have an up-to-date knowledge of the precise infective risks, let alone the antibiotic resistance patterns of possible pathogens, and therefore easy communication with a Tropical and Infectious Diseases Unit and with one of the specialized information services dealing with travel medicine, which are available in many countries, is essential. Nevertheless, it is wise to keep up to date with prevalent trends; witness the large epidemic of chikungunya affecting large areas of Asia.[1] Free online resources such as ProMED (www.promedmail.org) provide enormously valuable real-time information on current outbreaks and ongoing epidemics.

What are the actual causes of acute fever in returning travelers? (As this chapter focuses on illnesses with a large element of fever, primarily diarrheal diseases, or sexually transmitted diseases with mainly local symptoms and signs, and many other health risks of travel are not discussed here, see Section 6.) Contrary to popular myth, the 'classic' tropical diseases are rarely acquired by short-term travelers, with the vital exception of malaria. This ranks first among diagnoses of acute fever in returning travelers, followed by a large group of short-lived fevers for which no etiology is ever established. Other diagnoses obviously vary in their frequency with the pattern of travel to and from a particular country. As the traveler is exposed not only to exotic pathogens, but also to a changing ecologic background of widely distributed pathogens, it is not surprising that ordinary respiratory infections, ranging from colds to pneumonia, are common. So too are initially febrile presentations of diarrheal diseases and prodromes of hepatitis. Urinary infection, as one of the most common causes of fever in women not always accompanied by localizing symptoms, must also be remembered. Some diagnoses encountered with widely variable frequency in different units are listed in Table 62.1.

Contact history

Contact history may be relevant in travelers and in people staying at home. Information about local endemic or epidemic infections should be sought. Most frequent of all, especially in the winter months, is a history of contact with acute respiratory infection, which is possibly relevant because so many respiratory infections begin with 1 or 2 days of indeterminate fever, but the very frequency of such infections makes this aspect of the history difficult to interpret. Even in places with high uptakes of routine immunization, measles is encountered, and tends then to be missed because of its low prevalence and because it may occur in older subjects in highly immunized populations. Measles is especially important when the patient, or a contact, is immunosuppressed. Rubella, a more difficult and uncertain clinical diagnosis, is clearly of the greatest import if the patient or a contact is pregnant. Known contact with meningococcal disease obviously demands immediate attention, although, owing to the vagaries of meningococcal carriage and immunity, few patients who have this disease have a direct contact history. A story of 'food poisoning' or diarrheal disease in contacts may be relevant as shigellosis, salmonellosis and *Campylobacter jejuni* infections may all begin with a febrile phase, while ingestion of raw milk and some cheeses raises the possibilities of brucellosis and listerial infection. The long incubation periods of most forms of viral hepatitis should be remembered in exploring possible contact history. Of those most commonly associated with travel, the incubation period of hepatitis A is from 2 to 6 weeks, that of hepatitis B from 4 weeks to many months.

Occupational history

Many occupational exposures are not particularly relevant to acute febrile presentations, but many of the points about contact history just discussed are especially applicable to health workers and to those involved in child care. Other specific risks arising from occupation that may present as an acute fever include leptospirosis in sewage workers and fish farmers, and the many infective risks in veterinary and abattoir work, including brucellosis and *Streptococcus suis* infection. Fever may be the first clinical manifestation of tuberculosis relevant to health professionals, especially those involved with the care of patients who have HIV, and to carers of the homeless.

Some fevers associated with occupation are not infective. Fever and chills may be caused by inhalation of metal fumes or breakdown products of polymers. Many occupational lung diseases manifest with primarily respiratory features, but in extrinsic allergic alveolitis fever and influenza-like symptoms may dominate the picture. These conditions are characterized by recurrent episodes related to the particular exposure. Further detail is given in Chapter 67.

Bioterrorism and fever

Several agents that might be involved in bioterrorism are likely to cause nonspecific fever as their initial manifestation (Table 62.2). In smallpox, after the incubation period of 12 days, there is nearly

Table 62.1 Diagnoses made in travelers returning from tropical countries with fever as a principal symptom

Common
Malaria
No diagnosis made
Respiratory infection
Diarrheal disease (fever before or accompanying gut symptoms)
Urinary tract infection
Viral hepatitis; febrile prodrome

Uncommon
Dengue
Typhoid
Tuberculosis
Acute HIV infection
Acute schistosomiasis
Rickettsial infections
Amebiasis

Table 62.2 Bioterrorism and fever

Agent	Main early features
Smallpox	Nonspecific fever for 2–3 days followed by rash slowly progressing to vesicles or pustules OR hemorrhages, system failure and death within a few days
Pulmonary anthrax	Rapidly progressive systemic illness with fever, dyspnea, sometimes wide mediastinum and pleural effusions
Pneumonic plague	Rapidly progressive systemic illness with respiratory features prominent from the second day. Extensive, often bilateral, pneumonia

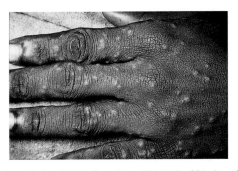

Fig. 62.1 The early focal rash of smallpox. This is the fifth day of the fever and the third day since the rash began to appear.

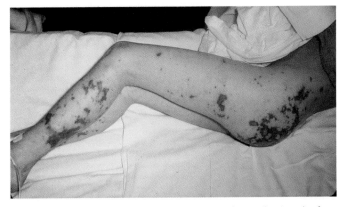

Fig. 62.2 Fully developed, almost pathognomonic hemorrhagic rash of meningococcal sepsis.

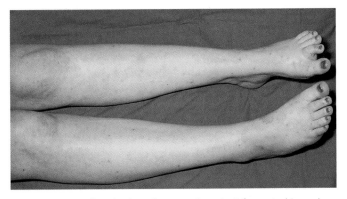

Fig. 62.3 Very early rash of meningococcal sepsis. A few petechiae only, but meningococcal sepsis nonetheless. It can progress to the appearance of Figure 62.2 within minutes or hours. This is the window of opportunity for early treatment.

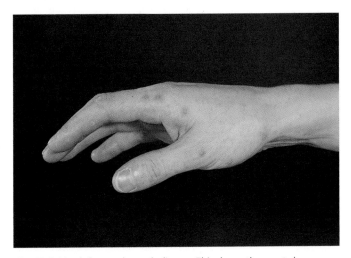

Fig. 62.4 Hand, foot and mouth disease. This shows the scanty lax vesicles found at these sites. There is often a maculopapular rash too, especially on the buttocks.

always a period of 2–3 days of fever and chills, perhaps rigors, headache and backache, before the focal rash begins to emerge. In the most severe forms, hemorrhagic manifestations appear and the patient dies without ever developing the focal rash. An early focal rash is illustrated in Figure 62.1. The onset of plague is also very acute, with chills, rigors, headache and generalized pains. Signs of system failure including generalized hemorrhages become apparent early in the septicemic form, but are also often seen together with enlarged nodes in bubonic plague. Pulmonary anthrax usually has a very acute onset, with early respiratory and systemic symptoms, but less acute presentations are now known to occur. Chest radiography may show mediastinal widening. (For a further discussion of bioterrorism, see Chapter 71.)

PHYSICAL EXAMINATION

Temperature

Depending on the duration of the illness, few temperature measurements may be available for evaluation. Recorded temperatures of higher than 102.2°F (39.0°C) are more likely to be caused by a significant infection than are lesser degrees of fever, but very high fever must raise suspicion of a noninfectious cause such as heat stroke or substance abuse. The pattern of fever is much less valuable than is commonly supposed. This aspect is discussed more fully in Chapter 63, but a few points relevant to short-term fevers may be mentioned. A dramatic fever with wild swings between readings is suggestive of pyogenic infection (especially abscess formation) and of acute pyelonephritis, but may also be seen in other conditions, including malaria and disseminated tuberculosis, as well as in Still's disease and occasionally in drug fever. Perhaps the most common reason for this kind of chart, however, is the use of antipyretics in a febrile patient, which often gives rise to this feature.

The most important caveats relate to malaria, and they cannot be emphasized enough. The temperature pattern in *P. falciparum* infections is often quite erratic, and this diagnosis must be considered in all febrile and some nonfebrile patients coming from a malarial area. Regular tertian or quartan fevers (meaning every other day and every third day, respectively) are not found in the early stages of malaria, and are a feature of relapse rather than initial infection. On the other hand, when present they are very characteristic of malaria.

Rashes

Many acute febrile illnesses are accompanied by a rash, which aids greatly in establishing a diagnosis. A few, notably those of meningococcal sepsis, are of vital importance in determining the need for urgent treatment or the protection of contacts (Figs 62.2, 62.3). Some are pathognomonic, others only indicative (Figs 62.4, 62.5), and the features of the rash must be placed in context with other features of the illness. In hand, foot and mouth disease the distribution is pathogno-

monic. Tables 62.3–62.5 provide information about rashes associated with acute fevers, including those encountered in returning travelers, but a few specific points are worth emphasizing.

In measles, easily forgotten in well-immunized populations but important to remember in older age groups, fever precedes the Koplik spots and the exanthem by 2 or 3 days but sometimes by as much as 1 week, although respiratory features are prominent for most of this time. In rubella and in enteroviral infections, general symptoms only rarely precede the rash, and then only by 1 day or so. In dengue, the

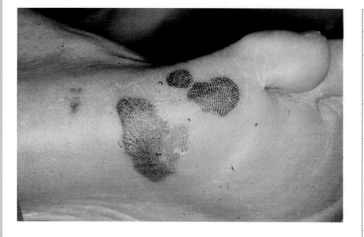

Fig. 62.5 Purpuric skin lesions in staphylococcal endocarditis.

Table 62.4 Rashes associated with acute bacterial infections

Agent	Rashes	Comment
Neisseria meningitidis	Petechial/purpuric	Also non-hemorrhagic early rashes
Neisseria gonorrhoeae	Hemorrhagic vesicles, pustules	
Staphylococcus aureus	Pyogenic skin lesions Scalded skin syndrome Peripheral purpura Erythema	In staphylococcal endocarditis In toxic shock syndrome
Streptococcus pyogenes	Erysipelas Erythema	Local erythema, bullae In toxic shock syndrome
Salmonella typhi	Rose spots	
Pseudomonas aeruginosa	Ecthyma gangrenosum Cellulitis ± blebs	Also in *Aeromonas* and other Gram-negative bacillary infections
Haemophilus aegyptius	Brazilian purpuric fever	

Table 62.3 Rashes associated with acute viral infections

Virus	Syndrome	Comment
Measles	Measles	Maculopapular followed by staining
Rubella	Rubella/German measles	Macular, often general facial flush
Herpesvirus 6	Roseola infantum	Macular or maculopapular after several days of fever
Erythrovirus B19*	Erythema infectiosum	Slapped cheeks, lacy on trunk and limbs, often rubelliform or hemorrhagic
Varicella-zoster	Chickenpox Shingles	Vesicular, rarely hemorrhagic Neurologic distribution, premonitory pain, erythema
Herpes simplex	Disseminated herpes Eczema herpeticum	
Epstein–Barr virus		Occasionally macular rash; severe rashes usually ampicillin-induced
Enteroviruses		Usually macular or maculopapular, sometimes hemorrhagic and/or vesicular (hand, foot and mouth disease; see Fig. 62.4)
Primary HIV	Mononucleosis-like illness	(Maculopapular rashes in chronic HIV infection; see Chapter 89)
Viral hemorrhagic fevers	(See Chapter 126)	Purpura, ecchymoses

*Also called Parvovirus B19 (Chapter 158).

rash characteristically appears in the second phase of the biphasic illness. Infections associated with pathognomonic or at least characteristic rashes may, however, also occur with nonspecific rashes; the early rash of meningococcal sepsis may be macular or maculopapular, and Lyme disease may exhibit nonspecific rashes in addition to erythema chronicum migrans.

Mouth

The mouth may show useful signs in a febrile patient (Table 62.6, Fig. 62.6). Especially in infancy and childhood, the tongue and mouth give some indication of dehydration, although mouth breathing and tachypnea often produce a similar appearance. The tongue is notably raw and red in scarlatina, in Kawasaki disease and in toxic shock syndrome. Vesicles are found, especially on the soft palate and anterior fauces, in some enteroviral infections (hand, foot and mouth disease). Palatal petechiae are fairly nonspecific, but are common in infectious mononucleosis and rubella. Many important signs in HIV infection are to be found in the mouth and these are discussed in Section 5.

Eyes

Some degree of conjunctival suffusion is common in people with a high temperature. This is often prominent in measles, rubella, some adenovirus infections and in leptospirosis. In infections with a hemorrhagic rash, conjunctival hemorrhages may be present in addition to skin petechiae or purpura; this is especially helpful in patients with dark skin, when petechiae are difficult to see. Other ocular signs that may be important in acute febrile illness are uveitis in acute sarcoid (although many patients with acute sarcoid do not show ocular involvement) and in Still's disease. Choroiditis occurs in histoplasmosis and in toxoplasmosis. Although choroidoretinitis in toxoplasmosis is most frequently a late marker of congenital infection, it is now clear that a few patients with acute acquired toxoplasmosis (and not HIV-infected) do have acute choroiditis. Miliary tuberculosis, with

Table 62.5 Rashes associated with acute spirochetal and rickettsial infections

Agent	Rashes	Comments
Leptospirosis	Hemorrhages Also other rashes	Weil's disease
Borrelia recurrentis (relapsing fever)	Petechiae	Often no rash; sometimes severe hemorrhages
Borrelia burgdorferi (Lyme disease)	Erythema migrans	Sometimes secondary annular or nonspecific rashes
Spirillum minus (rat-bite fever)	Blotchy macular, papular and urticarial rashes, beginning near the bite and spreading	Rashes also in the *Streptobacillus moniliformis* form of rat-bite fever
Rickettsial infections	Macular, papular petechial	Primary eschar (*tache noir*) in some syndromes

Table 62.6 Oral signs in acute fever

Sign	Diagnosis
Dehydration	Any fever
Herpes simplex	Common in meningococcal and pneumococcal infection
Raw tongue	Scarlatina Kawasaki's disease Toxic shock syndrome
Ulcers, vesicles	Varicella Herpes simplex Enteroviruses (herpangina, hand, foot and mouth disease) Aphthous stomatitis Secondary syphilis Erythema multiforme
Palatal petechiae	Nonspecific, but common in infectious mononucleosis and rubella

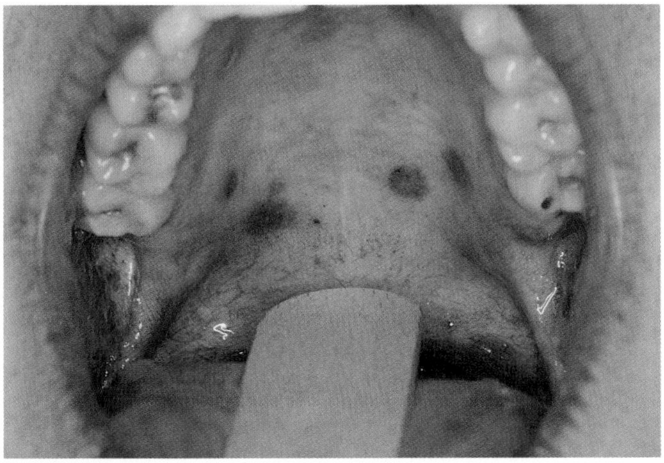

Fig. 62.6 Oral signs in hand, foot and mouth disease.

or without tuberculous meningitis, sometimes manifests as fever and general ill health; the diagnosis is immediately established if choroidal tubercles are seen. If, as often, they are scanty, they will be missed on perfunctory examination; a systematic search of both fundi with the pupils dilated is needed.

Lymph nodes

Generalized node enlargement is relatively uncommon in acute febrile illness. Among the common infections of children and young adults, rubella, Epstein–Barr virus mononucleosis and cytomegalovirus infection are notable causes, to which must be added cat-scratch disease and, in those at risk, secondary syphilis and primary HIV infection. These latter infections are especially important to remember in returning travelers. General node enlargement is also seen in some more specifically tropical diseases, of which dengue is the most likely to affect a short-term traveler. Acute histoplasmosis is another possibility after a first visit to an endemic area.

Focal nodes must direct a careful search of the relevant drainage area. For example, tender enlarged inguinal nodes may be more prominent than the source of infection, which may be insignificant-looking streptococcal lesions of the feet, perhaps superimposed on insect bites or fungal infection. Acquired toxoplasmosis in the immunocompetent host, although usually subclinical, manifests as a febrile illness with localized lymphadenopathy, most often in one or other cervical group but sometimes in nodes elsewhere. The persistent myth that toxoplasmosis is a cause of a 'glandular fever' syndrome must be firmly laid to rest. It is rare for the lymphadenopathy of acquired toxoplasmosis to be generalized, and atypical mononuclear leukocytes, if found at all on the blood film, are few in number.

Spleen

Acute and longer-term febrile illnesses make a contrast here. Splenomegaly is found in so many of the infections and other conditions causing FUO as to be of limited diagnostic value. By contrast, splenomegaly in a patient with fever of a few days' duration certainly merits further attention. It may indicate a particular infection, such as infectious mononucleosis, rubella, a hepatitis prodrome (in which splenomegaly is especially common in children) or, in a returning traveler, malaria. Splenomegaly may be attributable to an underlying hematologic condition, perhaps a hemolytic anemia or a lymphoma, itself the cause of the fever or a reason for increased susceptibility to infection.

MAKING A DECISION

Some specific factors in the history and examination suggest the need for a plan of management that goes beyond symptom relief. This may mean repeated observation, investigation or investigation combined with provisional treatment. The factors are:

- recent travel, especially to a malaria-risk country (see Chapter 111);
- chills and rigors;
- height of fever;
- fever and rash;
- extremes of age;
- any known or suspected immunosuppression;
- neurologic features;
- dehydration;
- parental or partner concern; and
- physician's impression.

Chills are common enough at the onset of respiratory infections, particularly at the onset of influenza. Nevertheless, the rapid rise in body temperature they denote is also common in some more serious infections, and this caution applies with greater force if the patient has rigors. A temperature of more than 102.2°F (39°C) is common enough in the early stage of an ultimately minor infection, but higher temperatures sustained for more than a short time are more likely to be associated with serious infections.

The combination of fever and any kind of hemorrhagic rash, be it only a few petechiae, is especially important.

Many patients on immunosuppressive therapy are living and working normally in the community but are at increased risk of infection. In some conditions, notably asplenia from any cause, infection may take a fulminant course and any fever demands very prompt attention (see Chapter 82). In addition, some forms of immunosuppression may initially manifest with a febrile illness, and the possibility of a first presentation of HIV infection has to be borne in mind.

Depression of consciousness, meningism or localizing neurologic signs are clearly important. Children with high fever may exhibit mild confusion and experience hallucinations; this is seen less commonly at older ages. Whether such clinical features denote specific neurologic involvement needs careful assessment.

Children and the elderly are at greater risk of dehydration, but patients of any age with fever, especially in warm conditions and if anorexic or vomiting, may become fluid deficient.

Whatever the level of anxiety in patient or carer, someone close to the patient may well have an accurate notion of whether the illness is out of the ordinary, and their opinions should be carefully considered.

The physician may form the impression that the illness is unusual, or serious, or likely to become serious. This is so common a problem as to merit more detailed discussion.

Is the patient ill?

Even after the most meticulous history taking, physical examination and attention to the issues just discussed, there are large numbers of patients with fever of short duration in whom no particular warning features are present. Fortunately, most patients who have fever of a few hours' or a few days' duration recover uneventfully without sequelae and without a diagnosis other than a meaningless attribution to 'viral infection'. How should one judge, in the home, in the health center or practice premises, or in the hospital Emergency Room, which of these patients should be further investigated, or investigated and given provisional empiric treatment? This must be one of the most frequent decisions that has to be made by clinicians all over the world and yet it is ignored in books about diagnosis. Decision theory is largely silent in this context because the elements of the decision involve multiple factors, usually heuristic in character, few of which can be assigned a numeric value.

It seems that the most common factor affecting the physician's decision is the impression that the patient has an infection with systemic and potentially hazardous features – for which the word 'toxic' is often used as shorthand – and this is the main determinant of further investigation and treatment in patients who have acute febrile illness. Indeed, algorithms on this problem often begin with the question: 'Is the patient toxic?'

Attempts to analyze what this means have been more often pursued in children than in adults. This work had its origin in the increased use of blood culture in infants and children, most of whom did not look ill, taken to 'walk-in' clinics or hospital Emergency Rooms in the USA. Positive blood cultures were found in 2.8–8% of these patients. In most places the main organisms were *Streptococcus pneumoniae, Neisseria meningitidis* and, before general immunization against this organism, *Haemophilus influenzae*. A few of these children, perhaps 4–7%, went on to develop meningitis or other focal infections.[1] These findings spawned a vast amount of work on the early detection of potentially serious illness in febrile infants and on developing management plans for their care. Observations which commonly raise concern in doctors and parents about the possibility of serious illness are the child's reaction to handling and to social overtures, the skin color and state of hydration,[2] while in one study the most sensitive predictors of serious illness were poor feeding and restlessness.[3]

A qualitative study of 83 cases of meningococcal disease seen in general practice in South Wales showed how, even in the absence of a rash, clinical and contextual features helped to differentiate these patients from the many with acute self-limiting febrile illnesses.[4] Many of the patients showed 'features not normally expected in children with acute self-limiting illnesses'; these included lethargy, poor eye contact, altered mental state and abnormal cry. Detecting early pointers of serious illness is especially important in meningococcal disease because an apparently mild illness may progress within hours to life-threatening sepsis. A large study of 448 children with meningococcal disease found that 72% had features of sepsis, leg pains, cold hands and feet, and abnormal skin color, preceding by many hours the classic signs of meningococcal disease.[5]

Attempts to analyze what experienced physicians do without conscious thought have tended to confirm the value of clinical judgment in predicting or excluding a high risk of serious disease in older infants and children, but more work of this kind is needed in adults. It seems impossible to dispense with the elusive but crucial clinical impression of illness, although even this may deceive in either direction. One reason for disasters associated with *P. falciparum* malaria and with meningococcal septicemia is the apparently good condition of the patient which may precede a rapid decline whereas, conversely, patients may look much more ill than they are after an exhausting long journey or a lively party. When, as so often, there is doubt about the assessment, a total leukocyte count of greater than 15×10^9/l has been valuable in some, but not all, studies in indicating an increased post-test probability of bacteremia.

Beyond the basic need for time and care in clinical assessment, a confident relationship between patient and physician, and easy access for further consultation are perhaps the most important factors in ensuring that major illness is not missed.

A decision tree for the management of acute febrile illness is given in Figure 62.7.

LABORATORY INVESTIGATIONS

With few exceptions, among them the classic infectious diseases such as measles and varicella, most acute and short-lived infections have no specific features that enable a clinical diagnosis to be made. Few of these illnesses are investigated. Facilities to do so are not available in most of the world and, when they are available, are unnecessary in patients who have mild and self-limiting illnesses. It follows that most of these infections remain undiagnosed, although a specific diagnosis can be assigned to a substantial number of them in research projects in which full virologic investigations are undertaken. This is the case especially in acute infections in children, who may experience a remarkably large number of infections, most of them viral, in the course of a year.

Investigations are certainly indicated when any of the 'danger points' just described are present, and in any febrile patient whose general condition gives concern. The precise range of investigations chosen will obviously vary depending on the facilities available and on the vagaries of the clinical situation, but even a small and frequently accessible range of investigations (Table 62.7) greatly increases the possibility of establishing a diagnosis. When the features of the illness give no specific direction, the most useful investigations are a routine blood count together with careful examination of a stained blood film, blood culture, urine examination, and posteroanterior and lateral radiographs of the chest. When blood is taken, a serum specimen should be saved for later study.

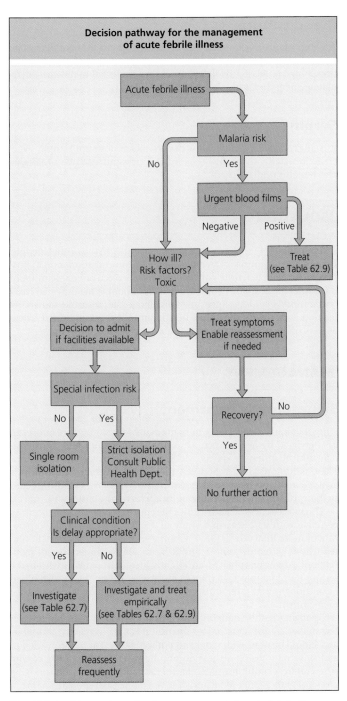

Decision pathway for the management of acute febrile illness

Acute febrile illness →
Malaria risk
— No
— Yes → Urgent blood films
— Negative
— Positive → Treat (see Table 62.9)

How ill? Risk factors? Toxic →

Decision to admit if facilities available

Treat symptoms Enable reassessment if needed → Recovery? — No / Yes → No further action

Special infection risk
— No → Single room isolation
— Yes → Strict isolation Consult Public Health Dept.

Clinical condition Is delay appropriate?
— Yes → Investigate (see Table 62.7)
— No → Investigate and treat empirically (see Tables 62.7 & 62.9)

→ Reassess frequently

Fig. 62.7 Decision pathway for the management of acute febrile illness.

Initial investigations are often, of course, much more extensive depending as they do on available resources and initial clinical clues. These will most commonly include liver function tests, stool microscopy and culture, antigen detection and serologic tests for particular

Table 62.7 Basic laboratory investigations in patients who have acute fever

- Routine blood count
- Stained blood film
- Urine microscopy and culture
- Chest radiograph
- Save serum

pathogens, and relevant imaging, especially abdominal ultrasound and CT scanning or MRI. The more extensive range of investigations is fully discussed in the context of FUO (see Chapter 63).

Total and differential leukocyte count

Modest degrees of neutrophilia, up to about $15 \times 10^9/l$, are of little help. More definite neutrophilia is principally found in pyogenic bacterial infections, but also in amebiasis, leptospirosis and in many noninfectious conditions such as thromboembolism, rheumatic fever, Still's disease, exacerbations of chronic liver damage and mechanical tissue damage (Table 62.8). Neutropenia is common in many viral infections, including rubella and influenza, and, among infections of travelers, is often found in malaria, typhoid, brucellosis, rickettsial diseases and visceral leishmaniasis. Leukopenia is also a feature of severe and overwhelming sepsis, but the serious condition of patients who show this feature is usually only too evident. Thrombocytopenia is a very frequent feature of the blood film in malaria and in sepsis. A substantial number of atypical mononuclear cells is found most commonly in acute Epstein–Barr virus and cytomegalovirus infections, whereas eosinophilia points to the tissue-invasive stage of many parasitic infections.

Specific diagnoses from the blood film

Malaria is by far the most important finding from examination of the blood in those at risk, but other diagnoses that can sometimes be made in this way are listed in Table 62.9. In addition to examination of the blood, a diagnosis may occasionally be aided by direct examination of material from a skin lesion, for example in meningococcal sepsis.

Urine examination

Small degrees of proteinuria are of no significance in febrile patients. Dipsticks can be used to detect Gram-negative infections and pyuria, but should not be used alone in the diagnosis of fever because of the high false-negative rate of the nitrate test for bacteriuria. Urinary infection is best diagnosed by direct microscopy of a drop of urine with the finding of heavy pyuria, often some hematuria and visible organisms. The presence of organisms in association with pyuria in a freshly obtained specimen indicates significant bacteriuria and a Gram stain can help in distinguishing positive

Table 62.8 Value of total and differential leukocyte count in acute fever*

Neutrophilia	Neutropenia
Sepsis	Severe sepsis
Abscess	Malaria
Amebiasis (usually)	Typhoid
Leptospirosis (usually)	Brucellosis
Still's disease	Visceral leishmaniasis
Lymphoma (uncommon)	Rickettsial infections
Atypical mononuclear cells	**Eosinophilia**
Epstein–Barr virus	Schistosomiasis (Katayama fever)
Cytomegalovirus	Visceral larva migrans (toxocariasis, etc.)

*This table concerns acute illnesses in which fever is a principal feature; it does not include conditions such as tropical eosinophilia in which respiratory features are dominant.

Table 62.9 Specific diagnoses from the blood film*

- Malaria
- Babesiosis
- Trypanosomiasis
- Filariasis
- Leptospirosis (darkfield)
- Relapsing fever (darkfield or staining)
- Bartonellosis
- Ehrlichiosis
- Meningococcemia
- Histoplasmosis, candidemia

*Etiologies of acute fever are sometimes established by examination of the blood film.

cocci from negative bacilli. Urinary infection is one of the most common infections that can manifest as a febrile illness with no localizing symptoms or signs.

Chest radiograph

The most important findings in a febrile but previously healthy patient are areas of consolidation, since general symptoms and fever may precede respiratory symptoms and signs by several days, and radiographic changes may be surprisingly prominent in patients with few or no respiratory symptoms. This is especially likely in 'atypical' pneumonia, such as that associated with Q fever or *Mycoplasma pneumoniae* infection (Fig. 62.8). The other crucial finding is that of pulmonary tuberculosis, in some communities to be suspected throughout the population, and in others more especially in the indigent and those infected with HIV. Other diagnoses may also be made, such as *Pneumocystis jirovecii* (formerly *P. carinii*) infection in HIV infection before respiratory features become evident, allergic pneumonias, visceral larva migrans and pulmonary emboli. Chest radiography is especially important in older patients, who may develop serious pneumonia in the absence of any indicative clinical features.

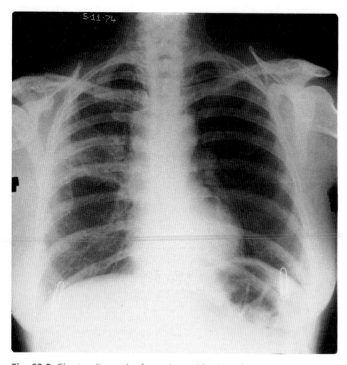

Fig. 62.8 Chest radiograph of a patient with *Mycoplasma* pneumonia. Respiratory symptoms are often scanty or absent in the first few days of the illness.

Blood culture

The importance of blood culture in febrile patients thought ill enough to need investigation is evident but, important as it is, the information gained is necessarily delayed and thus irrelevant to the immediate management decisions.

Serum

It is always sensible, if blood is drawn, to save a serum sample, especially for later comparative tests if the illness proves to be prolonged and remains undiagnosed.

ISOLATION

A few patients who have infections present a risk to other people. Because the diagnosis is often obscure at the time of admission to hospital of an acutely febrile patient, isolation is often advisable initially, if facilities are available. Sometimes, as for example in suspected Lassa fever, more elaborate measures involving the control-of-infection team in liaison with the public health authorities are indicated. These aspects of the management of infection are discussed in Chapter 6.

MANAGEMENT

Symptomatic treatment

Drug therapy is unnecessary in many acute fevers, but discomfort can be alleviated by agents such as aspirin, paracetamol and nonsteroidal anti-inflammatory agents, which act as cyclo-oxygenase inhibitors. There is little to choose between their effect on fever, but aspirin is avoided in infants because of its association with Reye's syndrome, and in many older patients because of its effects on the gastric mucosa.

The effectiveness of antipyretics in reducing fever does not seem to correlate with its cause. In a study of 1559 children with a temperature of more than 101 °F (38.4 °C) on arrival at the Emergency Room, reductions of temperature 1 and 2 hours after a single dose of paracetamol (acetaminophen) were slightly greater in patients who had a serious bacterial infection than in those who did not,[6] although it had been thought that fever with a serious cause might be less responsive to an antipyretic.

Sponging is still sometimes used as a method of reducing fever. A few studies confirm that it does this, but it is often very uncomfortable, and should be done with tepid and not iced water. The vasoconstriction and shivering causing distress do not, however, produce a rise of core temperature. Combining paracetamol (acetaminophen) with sponging gives a slightly greater reduction of temperature than sponging alone.[7]

It is useful to know the timing of antipyretic action, especially if the aim is to reduce the likelihood of febrile convulsions. Both antipyretic drugs and sponging show an appreciable effect within about 30 minutes and have their maximal effects in 2–3 hours.

Corticosteroids are effective antipyretics but should be used only for specific indications in conjunction with appropriate anti-infective therapy for the known or presumed cause of the fever.

Maintaining hydration is important and not always easy in a warm climate as patients who have fever are often anorexic and sometimes vomiting.

Empiric treatment

One of the most taxing and common decisions that has to be taken in acute febrile illness is whether to start empiric treatment based on one or more hypotheses about the diagnosis. On one side is the fear of rapid and perhaps irreversible deterioration, especially in *P. falciparum*

Table 62.10 Some dangerous features in patients who have acute fever

- Petechial/purpuric rash
- Travel involving risk of malaria
- Chills and rigors
- Extremes of age
- Neurologic signs
- Asplenia
- Hypogammaglobulinemia
- Post bone marrow transplant

Table 62.11 Suggested empiric regimens for use when urgent treatment is indicated in patients who have acute fever

Presumed diagnosis	Action
Meningococcal sepsis	1. Blood culture if possible 2. Penicillin G (benzylpenicillin)
Septic shock in asplenia	1. Blood culture if possible 2. Penicillin G (benzylpenicillin) or cephalosporin*
Streptococcal sepsis	1. Blood culture if possible 2. Local lesion, Gram stain and culture if possible 3. Penicillin G (benzylpenicillin) ± clindamycin
Staphylococcal sepsis	1. Blood culture if possible 2. Local lesion, Gram stain and culture if possible 3. Flucloxacillin or similar agent*
Severe malaria	1. Blood films 2. Quinine (or artemether or artesunate; see Chapter 111)
Lassa fever	1. Strict isolation 2. Tribavirin (ribavirin) 3. Inform public health authorities

*Knowledge of local resistance patterns and antibiotic policy needed.

malaria and in sepsis. On the other are the confounding effects of possibly inappropriate treatment, and the added problem of adverse drug reactions. If immediate treatment is given, it is nearly always possible to take blood before starting and this can be used for diagnostic tests.

Some indications for immediate treatment (Table 62.10) in acutely febrile patients can be firmly stated; others are contingent and depend on the precise details of the clinical and epidemiologic situation. The most urgent are the possibility of meningococcal sepsis and that of serious infection in asplenic subjects. Next in urgency are indications pointing toward streptococcal sepsis and, in returning travelers, the possibility of *P. falciparum* malaria. Immediate treatment should also be seriously considered if there is evidence of any immunologic disorder and, more generally, if other indicators of severe illness such as those already discussed are present. Table 62.11 gives some recommendations for action in these circumstances. The antibiotic choice, as always, must take account of local susceptibility patterns, and for this reason, more than one option is given. For example, penicillin is no longer the agent of first choice in many places for serious pneumococcal infection, and the spread of meningococcal resistance to penicillin would make future changes necessary in the national policy in the UK for the immediate treatment of suspected meningococcal sepsis.[8]

It has been written (by Garrison) that Wunderlich, the founder of clinical thermometry, 'found fever a disease and left it a symptom'. This chapter shows that fever remains an important and challenging symptom that demands meticulous analysis so as to achieve the best prospects for accurate diagnosis and treatment.

REFERENCES

References for this chapter can be found online at http://www.expertconsult.com

Chapter | **63** | Chinh Nguyen
Alan Cross

Fever of unknown origin

INTRODUCTION

Fever of unknown origin (FUO) is one of the most challenging tests of the diagnostic acumen of the physician. The workup can be long and arduous, leading to frustration on the part of both clinician and patient. There have been many reports spanning over 70 years (Table 63.1). The case mix of FUO patients has changed significantly over this period as technologic and radiographic advances have occurred.

The Petersdorf and Beeson criteria for FUO, which standardized its definition in 1961,[7] are:

- a body temperature of more than 101°F (38.3°C) for at least 3 weeks; and
- failure to establish a diagnosis after 1 week of investigation.

These criteria were designed to eliminate self-limited diseases that might have been represented in earlier series.[1-6] Because of changes in modern medicine, two modifications of the classic definition have been proposed:

- allowing 3 outpatient days to be the equivalent of 1 week's inpatient workup;[26] and
- shortening the 3-week febrile period to 2 weeks.[27]

These quantitative definitions are, by their nature, arbitrary. As such, recent literature has put an emphasis on changing the definition of FUO from a quantitative to a qualitative one, to specify a minimum negative diagnostic workup before the febrile illness can qualify as an FUO.[23] Patients who are neutropenic (see Chapter 73), who have HIV (see Chapter 92) or who acquired their fevers in a nosocomial setting (see Chapter 28) are now considered as separate categories, as the approach in these patient populations is different.

CLASSIC FEVER OF UNKNOWN ORIGIN

Disease categories

An etiology of FUO is identified in the majority of cases in each published series on FUO (average 73%, range 30–93% of cases). The principal disease categories include infection, neoplasms and collagen diseases, with the remaining diverse range of cases being grouped together as 'miscellaneous'. Table 63.1 summarizes the variations in select case studies on FUO which have been published over the years since its original description.

Figure 63.1 summarizes the relative contributions of the various disease categories to the final diagnosis. Trends are difficult to assess as they vary depending on the inclusion or exclusion of different series. The recommendation to change the definition of FUO to facilitate an ambulatory evaluation does not alter the relative contribution of various disease categories to the final diagnoses in one review.[23]

This same review emphasizes 14 clinical entities that comprise the majority of final diagnoses: endocarditis, tuberculosis, abdominal abscess, Epstein–Barr virus (EBV) and cytomegalovirus (CMV) infection, lymphoma, leukemia, adult-onset Still's disease, systemic lupus erythematosus (SLE), polymyalgia rheumatica and giant cell arteritis, sarcoidosis, Crohn's disease, subacute thyroiditis, habitual hyperthermia and drug fever.

Infections

The major infections represented in older papers – tuberculosis (TB), endocarditis and abdominal abscesses – continue to make up a significant proportion of FUO in recent series.[13,14] Tuberculosis is a leading infectious cause of FUO, particularly in developing countries.[16,17,19,21,22,25,28] The types of infection causing FUO have become more diverse,[11-25] including HIV infection, Lyme disease, and diseases such as typhoid fever and amebiasis in patients who have resided in or traveled to developing countries.

In one series in which TB represented 40% of all cases of FUO,[22] TB manifested in all its myriad forms, including Pott's disease, TB lymphadenitis, primary and postprimary pulmonary TB, with miliary TB predominating. Current BACTEC technology allows for easier isolation of the organism than in the past. Occasionally, the diagnosis was established via clinical improvement with antituberculous therapy.[17]

In the diagnosis of miliary tuberculosis, the probability of a positive smear for mycobacteria increases with the number of sites sampled. On histopathology, granulomas are present in liver biopsies from 90% to 100% of cases, whereas they are seen in 60–70% of transbronchial biopsies (though more transbronchial biopsies are performed than liver). Anemia is present in as many as 50% of patients and leukopenia is not infrequent. Occasionally marked leukocytosis has led to the misdiagnosis of leukemia. Granulomas are seen in roughly 50% of bone marrow biopsies, but the yield increases to greater than 80% when hematologic abnormalities are present. Serial chest imaging may reveal infiltrates not initially present.

In earlier series, the most common cause of native-valve endocarditis was viridans streptococci; however, with the decreased incidence of rheumatic valvular heart disease, this etiology has become less common. More recent studies have seen an increase in *Staphylococcus aureus*, driven, in part, by intravenous drug abuse and the changing epidemiology of *S. aureus* in the community setting.[16,17] The continued finding of streptococcal species in more recent series places a premium on withholding antibiotics in clinically stable patients so that multiple blood cultures can be drawn.

Other infectious etiologies of FUO in recent series include occult osteomyelitis, intra-abdominal and retroperitoneal abscesses, pyelonephritis, enteroviral infections, rickettsial infections (including scrub and murine typhus, Mediterranean spotted fever), CMV, EBV

Table 63.1 Diagnoses in selected series of FUO reported in the literature

	Country	Total	Infection	Neoplasm	Collagen	Miscellaneous	Undiagnosed
Alt & Barker 1930[1]	USA	57	14	6	0	1	36
Hamman & Wainwright 1936[2,3]	USA	54	32	12	0	0	10
Keefer 1939[4]	USA	80	51	19	0	10	0
Bottiger 1953[5]	Sweden	68	16	11	4	4	33
Geraci et al. 1959[6]	USA	70	15	21	0	20	14
Petersdorf & Beeson 1961[7]	USA	100	36	19	15	23	7
Petersson 1962[8]	Finland	81	15	5	5	0	56
Sheon & Van Ommen 1963[9]	USA	60	12	11	8	6	23
Fransen & Bottiger 1966[10]	Sweden	60	8	19	2	4	27
Jacoby & Swartz 1973[11]	USA	128	51	26	19	22	10
Larson et al. 1982[12]	USA	105	32	33	9	18	13
Knockaert et al. 1992[13]	Belgium	199	45	14	42	47	51
Kazanjian 1992[14]	USA	86	28	21	18	11	8
De Kleijn et al. 1997[15]	Netherlands	167	43	21	33	20	50
Zhiyong et al 2003[25]	China	208	66	35	46	11	50
Liu et al. 2003[19]	Taiwan	78	33	5	16	6	18
Tabak et al. 2003[22]	Turkey	117	40	22	27	12	16
Vanderschueren et al. 2003[23]	Belgium	290	57	29	68	38	98
Saltogu et al. 2004[21]	Turkey	87	51	12	16	2	6
Arce-Salinas et al. 2005[20]	Mexico	45	19	8	12	1	5
Ertern et al. 2005[17]	Turkey	57	24	10	17	0	6
Ammari 2006[28]	Jordan	52	26	8	6	12	0
Chin et al. 2006[16]	Taiwan	94	54	8	7	8	17
Bleekers-Rovers et al. 2007[29]	Netherlands	73	12	5	16	3	37
Total		2416	780	380	386	279	591

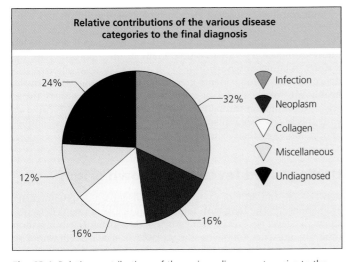

Fig. 63.1 Relative contributions of the various disease categories to the final diagnosis.

and parvovirus B19 infection, as well as fastidious bacteria, mainly brucellosis.[16–25,29] In many instances, the reliability of the microbiologic diagnosis is not always clearly defined.

Neoplasia

Lymphoma (both Hodgkin's and non-Hodgkin's) remains the most common malignant disease causing FUO.[12–15] Its insidious presentation and protean manifestations may explain why lymphoma continues to account for a sizable number of cases despite new diagnostic modalities. For example, fever in some cases persists for months before a lymph node becomes sufficiently large enough for detection. In addition, it may be difficult to locate an involved lymph node on physical examination and it is impossible when the retroperitoneal nodes or bone marrow are the only site of disease. A directed percutaneous needle biopsy of an involved lymph node or bone marrow may contain insufficient material to reveal diagnostic histopathology.[30] Thus, lymphoma may elude clinical detection for several weeks.

Other neoplasms and solid tumors are less common causes of FUO.[12–15] The peripheral blood smear of certain leukemias and myelodysplastic syndromes may reveal no definitive findings (e.g. aleukemic leukemia). Consequently, establishing the diagnosis requires bone marrow examination.[31]

Renal cell carcinoma is a primary malignancy of the renal cortex. The classic triad of flank pain, hematuria and a palpable renal mass is present only in a minority of cases.[32] Up to 20% of patients will experience fever.[33] Metastatic adenocarcinoma in the liver, regardless of the primary site, may also cause FUO.[31] In most situations, but not all, there is elevated hepatic alkaline phosphatase, hepatomegaly, or both. Other solid tumors that can cause FUO include leiomyosarcomas of the gastrointestinal tract, pheochromocytomas, hepatomas, sarcomas and atrial myxomas.

Other rare causes of FUO from this category include malignant histiocytosis, angioimmunoblastic lymphadenopathy with dysproteinemia and a variety of CNS tumors.

Rheumatologic disorders

Adult Still's disease, for which there is no definitive laboratory test, remains the most common rheumatologic cause of FUO.[17,19,22,23,34] As there is no single diagnostic test for adult Still's disease, the diagnosis is largely clinical, requiring the presence of major and minor criteria, or a combination of both, as well as certain exclusions.[35] Proposed major criteria include fever of at least 102°F (39°C) lasting 1 week or longer, arthralgias and arthritis lasting 2 weeks or longer, characteristic rash, and a leukocytosis with granulocyte predominance. Minor criteria include sore throat, recent lymph node swelling, hepatomegaly and/or splenomegaly, abnormal liver function tests and a negative antinuclear antibody and rheumatoid factor. Temperature changes can be dramatic, sometimes as much as 4°C in 4 hours. The characteristic rash of adult Still's disease is described as an evanescent salmon pink, macular or maculopapular eruption, classically appearing only during febrile episodes.

Temporal arteritis, with or without polymyalgia rheumatica (PMR), should be considered in febrile patients over 50 years of age; the erythrocyte sedimentation rate (ESR) is nearly always elevated. While the diagnosis of PMR is largely clinical, the gold standard for temporal arteritis is temporal artery biopsy. Cardinal features, which are not always present, include jaw and tongue claudication, and visual and temporal artery abnormalities. The diagnosis of PMR rests on several diagnostic criteria, including elevated ESR, elderly age, and bilateral pain and stiffness in the shoulders, neck and hips, though these are not universally accepted.[36] The classic presentation of headache, jaw claudication, visual loss or a palpable temporal artery may be absent in one-third of patients who have temporal arteritis.

Systemic lupus erythematosus (SLE) has been variably present in more recent series on FUO, occasionally surpassing adult Still's disease.[20,29] With the widespread availability of the antinuclear antibody test, however, it has become less frequent as a cause of FUO. Lupus is a chronic inflammatory disease of unknown origin which can affect multiple organs, including the skin, joints, nervous system, lungs and serous membranes; the diagnosis is based upon a combination of compatible clinical and serologic criteria.

Other less common rheumatologic causes of FUO include Wegener's granulomatosis and cryoglobulinemia. Polyarteritis nodosa should be considered if there is mononeuritis multiplex, myalgias, skin lesions, abdominal pain (which is due to small intestinal ischemia) and azotemia.[37] A variety of other autoimmune diseases such as mixed connective tissue disease, small vessel and median vessel vasculitis, and erythema nodosum present initially as prolonged fever.

Miscellaneous

A diverse array of conditions, including granulomatous diseases, inflammatory illnesses and drug-related fevers may cause FUO. Crohn's disease and sarcoidosis are examples of granulomatous diseases.[38] Previous studies occasionally list granulomatous hepatitis as a final diagnosis in FUO. However, it should be regarded as a histologic

finding, with its own broad differential diagnosis, including infections, like tuberculosis and brucellosis. It should not be regarded as a diagnosis unto itself.

Other conditions that must be considered include alcoholic hepatitis, pulmonary emboli, subacute thyroiditis, Sweet's syndrome and familial Mediterranean fever. Leukocytosis may occur with these conditions but it is often especially prominent in alcoholic hepatitis and familial Mediterranean fever. A number of hereditary periodic fever syndromes have become better elucidated within the past decade. Besides familial Mediterranean fever, other autoinflammatory diseases include TRAPS (tumor necrosis factor receptor-associated periodic fever syndrome, formerly known as familial Hibernian fever), HIDS (hyper-IgD syndrome), the cryopyrin diseases and all of their variants, including Muckle–Wells syndrome. These latter inflammatory disorders are a result of altered interleukin 1 production. Their clinical features are summarized in Table 63.2. Genetic testing for these conditions is now available to assist in the diagnosis, although it should be noted that these assays have not yet been validated.[39]

Subacute thyroiditis may be difficult to diagnose because there are usually no systemic features of thyrotoxicosis and the thyroid function tests are usually normal in its initial phase. The thyroid gland may be nontender; however, it is commonly diffusely enlarged. Schnitzler syndrome (hyperostosis, lymph node enlargement and monoclonal IgM gammopathy) is a rare cause of FUO.[40] In children, a new syndrome, PFAPA (periodic fever, aphthous stomatitis, pharyngitis and cervical adenitis), has been described.[41] This syndrome can be difficult to distinguish from familial Mediterranean fever but lacks serositis and episodes respond to steroids.

Hematomas and drug fever may cause FUO. Hematomas causing FUO may occur as a result of hemorrhages into the abdominal cavity or retroperitoneal space, but bleeding within the wall of an aneurysm or dissection of the thoracic or abdominal aorta has also been reported as being responsible. In these cases, persistent fever and anemia typically follow an episode of chest, back or abdominal pain that spontaneously resolves. Trauma may predispose to the formation of hematomas in extravascular spaces.

Kikuchi's necrotizing lymphadenitis is an infrequent cause of FUO. It is a benign, often self-limiting condition whose important clinical features include fevers and cervical lymphadenopathy. Fevers are typically low grade and can occasionally be accompanied by systemic symptoms. Diagnosis is usually established via lymph node biopsy.[42]

Drug fever can occur with virtually any medication, even those administered for long periods without previous problems (Table 63.3).[43] Despite common belief, eosinophilia, rash and/or relative bradycardia are not always present. There are no distinctive clinical features associated with drug fever that help to distinguish it from the other causes of fever mentioned above. The diagnosis often rests upon correction of fever upon discontinuation of the responsible drug.

Endocrinologic causes of FUO include hyperthyroidism and adrenocortical insufficiency.[40] Factitious fever comes in two forms: falsely elevated thermometer recordings without fever, and self-inflicted injury to induce fever or infection. Many of these patients have the features of Munchausen syndrome.[44] In order to provide objective evidence of fever, some patients may warm the thermometer when the health-care worker is not in attendance. Others may subject themselves to mutilation through such maneuvers as injecting themselves with specimens contaminated with micro-organisms. These entities appear almost exclusively in health-care workers.

Undiagnosed fever of unknown origin

Between 7% and 30% of cases remain undiagnosed despite intensive evaluations.[1–15] The long-term follow-up, available in two FUO series, shows that fever resolves in the majority of these patients within a short time.[45] In one series, follow-up was available for eight cases in whom no diagnosis was established.[14] Fever resolved within 3 weeks of the period of FUO in 87% of cases and within 4 months in all patients. The other series investigated the long-term follow-up of 49 cases of undiagnosed

Table 63.2 Familial autoinflammatory syndromes

	FAMILIAL MEDITERRANEAN FEVER (FMF)	MEVALONATE KINASE DEFICIENCIES			TUMOR NECROSIS FACTOR-RECEPTOR-ASSOCIATED PERIODIC SYNDROME	CRYOPYRIN DISEASES		
		Classic hyper-immunoglobulin D syndrome (HIDS)	Mevalonic aciduria	Variant HIDS		Familial cold autoinflammatory syndrome (FCAS)	Muckle–Wells syndrome (MWS)	Chronic infantile neurologic cutaneous and articular syndrome (CINCA)
Age at onset (yrs)	<20	<1	<1	<10	<20	<1	<20	<1
Cutaneous involvement	Erysipelas-like erythema	Maculopapular rash	Morbilliform rash	Maculopapular rash	Migratory rash, overlying area of myalgia	Cold-induced urticaria-like lesions	Urticaria-like rash	Urticaria-like lesions
Musculoskeletal involvement	Monoarthritis common	Arthralgia, occasional oligoarthritis	Arthralgia common	Arthralgia	Severe myalgia common; occasional frank monoarthritis	Arthralgia common; occasional mild myalgia	Lancing limb pain, arthralgia common; arthritis can occur	Epiphyseal bone formation
Abdominal involvement	Sterile peritonitis common	Splenomegaly, severe pain common	Splenomegaly, pain may occur	May occur	Severe pain very common	None	May occur	Hepatosplenomegaly
Eye involvement	Uncommon	Uncommon	Uncommon	Uncommon	Conjunctivitis and periorbital edema very common	Conjunctivitis	Conjunctivitis, sometimes optic nerve elevation	Papilledema with possible loss of vision, uveitis
Distinguishing clinical symptoms	Erysipelas-like erythema	Prominent cervical lymphadenopathy	Dysmorphic features, neurologic symptoms	Lymphadenopathy may occur	Migratory nature of myalgia and rash, periorbital edema	Cold-induced urticaria-like lesions	Sensorineural hearing loss	Chronic aseptic meningitis, sensorineural hearing loss, arthropathy
Gene involved	MEFV	MVK	MVK	?	TNFRSF1A	CIAS1	CIAS1	CIAS1
Protein involved	Pyrin (marenostrin)	Mevalonate kinase	Mevalonate kinase	?	Type 1 TNF-receptor	Cryopyrin	Cryopyrin	Cryopyrin

Reproduced and adapted from Simon et al.[39] with permission.

Table 63.3 Drugs associated with drug fever

Common	Less common
Atropine	Allopurinol
Amphotericin	Hydralazine
Penicillins	Isoniazid
Cephalosporins	Rifampin (rifampicin)
Phenytoin	Macrolides
Procainamide	Clindamycin
Quinidine	Vancomycin
Sulfonamides	Aminoglycosides
Interleukin-2, interferon	

FUOs taken from a larger cohort of 199 cases.[45] Fever resolved within a few weeks of discharge in 31 of the 49 cases (63%) and within 2 years of discharge in 83%. In the remaining 8 patients (17%), fever recurred and required repeated courses of nonsteroidal anti-inflammatory drugs (NSAIDs) and corticosteroids. Despite the lack of diagnosis in these patients, the mortality rate 5 years after discharge was small – only 3%. Thus, in most of these patients the fever abated without treatment, and rarely did a serious disorder emerge later.[14,45]

Despite advances in diagnostic techniques over the past decade, there continues to be a high proportion of undiagnosed cases in developed countries, sometimes exceeding 50%.[14,23,29,45] These same advances may allow for the diagnosis for a variety of conditions before they meet the definition of FUO. Moreover, the relatively good prognosis in patients with FUO may suggest the need for long-term clinical follow-up and diagnostic abstinence after life-threatening diseases have been reasonably ruled out.

FEVER OF UNKNOWN ORIGIN IN OTHER GEOGRAPHIC REGIONS

The clinician must consider diseases more common in specific geographic regions when evaluating patients from these areas. A compilation of all FUO series in Spain over 25 years, including 914 patients, demonstrated that brucellosis accounted for 16% of infectious diagnoses and that 8% were due to parasitic causes, including hydatid disease, leishmaniasis and fasciola infection.[46] Studies conducted in hospitalized patients who had fever in India and in Nigeria reported a *Brucella abortus* seroprevalence of 0.8–5.2%, leading the authors to speculate that brucellosis might account for a percentage of cases of undiagnosed FUO in these regions as well.[47,48] Studies of prolonged fever in Egypt note that 16% of cases were diagnosed with a parasitic infection.[49] In addition to typhoid fever and tuberculosis, melioidosis has been reported as a common cause of FUO in South East Asia.[50,51] HIV infection is an important consideration throughout the developing and developed world. Thus, patients from these parts of the world who present with FUO should be evaluated for infections caused by these organisms.

The literature on FUO in developing countries is limited. Several series have been published that characterize the specific diagnoses associated with prolonged fevers in other countries. Not all of the FUOs published from the developing world meet the revised Petersdorf and Beeson criteria requiring absence of a diagnosis despite an initial workup. Patients often present late in disease, and there is limited access to diagnostic tests, including accurate blood culture methods, limited treatment facilities, and variable patient follow-up. Endemic disease and inadequate immunizatons may complicate the workup of FUO in developing countries. For example, typhoid fever is often diagnosed by serologic methods (the Widal test). However, in endemic areas, 12–29% of patients may have a positive titer at baseline. Convalescent titers are difficult to obtain because of poor follow-up, and misinterpretations of these tests frequently occur.

In three series on FUO from Bangladesh, India and China, and in a pooled analysis of all the series from Turkey, infections were the leading cause.[25] In all of these, tuberculosis is the leading infectious diagnosis. Other diagnoses included typhoid fever, malaria, visceral leishmaniasis, amebiasis, syphilis, leprosy and filariasis. The finding that infectious diagnoses comprise a greater proportion of cases of FUO in developing countries is supported in other series as well.

GENERAL APPROACH TO DIAGNOSIS

There is no universally accepted approach to patients with FUO. Many series have proposed a variety of algorithms, and though many of them are prospective studies, no approach has been validated in randomized trials. The approach to the patient with FUO needs to be individualized on a case-by-case basis. Typical Bayesian theory may not apply, as there may be no high probability diagnosis, and thus one can expect a high false-positive rate.

It is necessary to perform a thorough history and physical examination with a baseline set of laboratory tests and imaging, with further testing being directed by potential diagnostic clues (PDCs) generated from this initial evaluation. The aggressiveness of the workup and the necessity of certain tests should be dictated by the clinical status of the patients, with the pacing accelerated to the use of more invasive studies in those individuals who are more ill.

In the elderly, an aggressive workup is often more warranted, as a diagnosis is possible in 80–90% of cases[52] (Table 63.4), though these data have not been updated recently and the case series in question were small. Similar to individuals with HIV, a separate definition for FUO in the elderly has been advocated based on several principles. The hypothalamus in the elderly is less responsive to pyrogens, and so the febrile response may be more blunted or delayed.[53] Further, the baseline temperature can be lower than in younger individuals, particularly in those who are more frail.[54]

History and physical findings

Thorough and repeated medical history and physical examinations are essential. Particular attention should be paid to travel, both recent and remote, exposure to animals and pets, occupation, sick contacts, family history of similar illnesses, as well as a thorough drug list looking for potential causes of drug fever. Many of these elements, besides providing valuable tools to guide laboratory testing, can also change and add to the differential diagnosis of potential illnesses. For example, melioidosis, a disease typically restricted to South East Asia, can be latent for up to 29 years. A family history of similar illness may point to one of the growing number of periodic fever syndromes.

The patient should be questioned regarding symptoms such as myalgias, arthralgias/arthritis, rash and oral ulcers, as such clinical features can assist in the diagnosis of many diseases, including PMR and SLE.

Table 63.4 Pooled data from three studies of FUO in the elderly (%)

Diagnosis	Knockaert	Barrier	Esposito
Infections	25	41	36
Neoplasms	12	13	23
Multisystem	31	30	25
Miscellaneous	10	2	7
No diagnosis	12	13	5

Adapted from Tal et al.[52]

A thorough physical examination follows. For instance, in series on miliary tuberculosis, choroid tubercles were present in as many as 50% of patients on autopsy.[55] Particular attention should be paid to the presence of any rashes and their appearance, which is an important diagnostic clue to many infectious and noninfectious entities, including adult Still's disease and SLE.

The thorough history and physical examination is used to generate PDCs and pursue abnormalities with directed testing, or, in the words of the bank robber Willie Sutton, to 'go where the money is'. If the diagnosis is not made immediately, a thorough history and physical examination should be repeated, as many abnormalities which were not present initially or missed altogether may declare themselves during subsequent examinations. History and observation of the evolution of a clinical identity led to the diagnosis in 44% of patients in one series.[23] This number should not be regarded as 'low yield' effort, which is an arbitrary designation, as a 40% yield in instances where it is difficult to establish a final diagnosis should not be ignored. Another study found that PDCs, however, are frequently misleading.[29]

Verification of fever

Verification that a fever exists seems intuitive, but its importance cannot be overlooked. Up to 35% of patients referred for evaluation of prolonged fevers were found not to have fevers at all or to have factitious fevers. Temperature recordings should be made with a healthcare worker in attendance. The lack of physiologic responses associated with fever (chills, diapheresis, tachycardia, tachypnea) should alert the clinician to the possibility of factitious fever. Patients undergoing evaluation for FUO should measure and record their temperatures daily in a log book.

While the fever pattern was once considered useful in the diagnosis of FUO, such characterizations are highly nonspecific and cannot be used to make a diagnosis.[56] The only exception to this statement is relapsing temperature elevations. This is characteristic of malaria, trypanosomiasis, relapsing fever, brucellosis, cyclic neutropenia or fever patterns in lymphoreticular malignancies. Characterization of fevers as either continuous or intermittent may allow the clinician to at least provide the patient with some prognostic counseling, as a diagnosis is much more likely to be reached in the former than in the latter.[23,29]

Laboratory and imaging evaluation

While there is no agreed upon 'standard' set of laboratory studies required for the evaluation of FUO, a number of determinations have been frequently recommended:

- complete blood count, including differential and platelets
- routine blood chemistries, including assessment of hepatic and renal function
- erythrocyte sedimentation rate (ESR) and C-reactive protein (CRP)
- protein electrophoresis
- antinuclear antibody (ANA) and rheumatoid factor (RhF)
- urinalysis
- at least three blood cultures separated in time by several hours
- chest X-ray
- abdominal ultrasound or CT imaging
- tuberculin skin test.

Additionally, all patients should be screened for HIV infection. In the following section select tests will be discussed in further detail. Table 63.5 summarizes the 'minimum' diagnostic workup as suggested by the authors of this chapter.

Erythrocyte sedimentation rate (ESR)

Several factors will elevate the ESR besides inflammation or infection,[57] including renal failure, hyperlipidemia, female gender, advanced age and even technical factors, such as tilting the test tube

Table 63.5 Suggested minimum workup

- Complete blood count, including differential and platelets
- Routine serum chemistries, including assessment of hepatic and renal function
- Erythrocyte sedimentation rate (ESR) and C-reactive protein (CRP)
- Antinuclear antibody (ANA) and rheumatoid factor (RhF)*
- Urinalysis with urine culture
- Three blood cultures separated in time by several hours
- Chest X-ray
- Abdominal ultrasound or CT imaging
- Tuberculin skin test*
- HIV ELISA with Western blotting for confirmation

*These tests can be ordered at the discretion of the consultant.

by an angle of 3° from the vertical, which may accelerate the ESR by as much as 30 mm/h. Conversely, factors that will lower the ESR include morphologically abnormal red cells and extremely elevated leukocyte counts. However, there are only a few infectious diseases that are known to drive the ESR to greater than 100 mm/h, and these include osteomyelitis and endocarditis.[58,59] Although a nonspecific test, many clinicians will use a low ESR to rule out a significant inflammatory disorder. Some individuals with giant cell arteritis can have a normal ESR.[60]

C-reactive protein

C-reactive protein (CRP) is an acute phase protein which plays a role in the recognition of foreign pathogens and phospholipid constituent of damaged cells. Advantages that CRP offers over ESR include less variation with changes in size, shape and number of red cells, more rapid changes with improvement in clinical condition, and less variation between gender.

The utility of ESR versus CRP in the diagnosis of FUO has never been systemically evaluated. This is likely to be more useful if there is a high pretest probability of a rheumatologic or hematologic disorder. It is probably also prudent to check these laboratory studies if the patient is older than 50 years, where the possibility of diseases such as PMR and temporal arteritis is higher.

Blood cultures

The earliest series on FUO emphasized endocarditis as one of the primary infectious etiologies of FUO, though it has become a less prominent entity in more recent studies, being absent from some altogether. Blood culture remains the primary method of detecting endocarditis. In the past, fastidious organisms such as the nutritional variant streptococci (e.g. now being renamed to the genus *Abiotrophia* and *Granulicatella*) and HACEK (*Haemophilus*, *Actinobacillus*, *Eikenella*, *Cardiobacterium*, *Kingella* spp.) organisms constituted a number of cases of culture-negative endocarditis. However, with modern technology, they are more easily grown and are isolated, on average, between 5 and 7 days.[61] This, along with the increased use of the Duke criteria and transesophageal echocardiography (TEE), and a decline in acute rheumatic fever and subsequent valvular heart disease, accounts for the decline in the overall cases of endocarditis which meet the definition of FUO.

Except for those individuals treated inappropriately with antibiotics, the most common causes of culture-negative endocarditis are *Bartonella*, *Brucella* and *Coxiella* spp., anaerobes and fungi. The primary method of diagnosis of Q fever is serologic, as isolating the organism in cell-free medium is difficult. However, it is still possible to attempt to grow *Bartonella* and *Brucella* species; hence communication with the laboratory in order to optimize collection and growth is still useful.

Filamentous fungi are also difficult to grow, though this entity is seen almost exclusively in intravenous drug abusers.

The overall yield of blood culture in the FUO patient population is low, often less than 5%, even in older series. Thus, unless there is a strong clinical suspicion of endocarditis, more than the requisite three blood cultures is probably not required.

CT imaging

Historically patients with FUO in whom no diagnosis was established were eventually referred for exploratory laparotomy. This practice has been almost entirely replaced in modern settings by CT scanning. CT scanning is effective for diagnosing many of the conditions which were etiologic in older series of FUO, including occult abscesses, hematomas and intra-abdominal lymphadenopathy. The diagnostic yield of abdominal imaging in a recent series on FUO was 20%,[29] comparable to older series that looked at the utility of this modality.

Some reviews use abdominal ultrasound in place of abdominal CT. In one such review, it was clinically helpful in 10% of cases where it was used.[62] Another study tabulated the number of abdominal imaging studies at more than three CT scans and/or ultrasound examinations per patient.[13]

Tuberculin skin test

It may be useful to place a tuberculin skin test (TST) in all patients with FUO. This should be done with the understanding that the presence or absence of a reactive skin test does not necessarily rule in or rule out the diagnosis of tuberculosis, which in the past was a leading infectious cause of FUO. In one series from Turkey, where there is a high incidence of tuberculosis, the TST was positive in 37% of patients overall, with 54% of these individuals having active tuberculosis and 24% without.[22] The TST is known to have a poor sensitivity in patients with miliary tuberculosis.

QuantiFERON-TB Gold test

This is an interferon gamma-based *in-vitro* T-cell assay, whose principle rests on the T cells of individuals previously sensitized to TB antigens producing interferon gamma on rechallenge. Thus far, it has only been studied for use in the diagnosis of latent TB, where it may have the advantage of being negative in those individuals with prior history of BCG vaccination[63,64] and less susceptible to false-positive results due to infection with nontuberculous mycobacteria. It also has the advantage of requiring only a single visit. What role it will play in algorithms for evaluating patients with FUO who are suspected of having TB is yet to be determined.

Additional investigations

Occasionally other forms of testing are warranted, including:
* serologies
* nuclear imaging
* biopsy.

Serologies

Antibody testing only indicates whether or not a patient has been exposed to a microbial agent, but does not indicate whether that agent is necessarily the cause of the FUO. In a study involving 73 patients, serologies were sent in 53, totaling 509 microbiologic serologic tests. With the exception of testing for *Yersinia enterocolitica*, serologic testing was never helpful in establishing the diagnosis.[29] This emphasizes that serologies should not be sent unless there is a high pretest probability that the patient has a given condition; even then, it is usually confirmatory of the diagnosis being made on some other basis. 'Blind' serologic testing may actually be misleading, resulting in further unnecessary diagnostic procedures. For example, serologic testing for zoonotic infections such as tularemia, Lyme disease or Rocky Mountain spotted fever should be performed only if the patient has been exposed to a relevant animal or tick. Brucellosis, bartonellosis, leptospirosis and some cases of hepatitis B or C, histoplasmosis or coccidioidomycosis can occasionally be detected by serologic diagnosis in FUO.

By contrast, antigen testing is usually more suggestive of active disease, as is the case with cryptococcal antigenemia. However, CMV antigenemia requires clinical correlation, as patients with HIV can be antigenemic without having CMV disease.

Radionuclide scans

The use of nuclear imaging in the diagnosis of patients with FUO has yielded variable results, in part because of low numbers, few randomized trials and differences in the timing of testing during evaluation.

Gallium scans are based on the principle that gallium is bound to transferrin, with increased blood flow and permeability at a given site of inflammation resulting in a subsequent increase in uptake of the radioisotope. Imaging is then obtained 18–72 hours after injection of the substance. In one study published before CT scanning came into widespread use, gallium 67 (^{67}Ga) scanning contributed to the final diagnosis in 14% of cases; however, false-positives led to unnecessary testing in 21% of patients.[12] In a more recent study of 145 patients with FUO, ^{67}Ga contributed to the diagnosis in 24–29% of cases.[65]

Leukocytes can be labeled with either indium 111 (^{111}In) or technetium 99m (^{99m}Tc). The process requires whole blood from the patient. The white cells are then isolated and incubated with radiolabel, washed and re-injected into the patient. Results over the years have been mixed, with sensitivity ranging anywhere from 45% to 82%, and specificity ranging from 69% to 86%.

Both CT and ultrasound can be done almost immediately, whereas radionuclide studies require anywhere between 24 and 48 hours between tracer injection and imaging.[66] Hence the delay implies a certain stability in the patient. Even in the event of an abnormal radionuclide scan, anatomic imaging such as CT is frequently required before intervention such as biopsy can be performed,[66] as was the case in many of the studies that examined the utility of nuclear imaging.[67]

The most promising nuclear study for the diagnosis of FUO is positron emission tomography using 2-(^{18}F)-fluoro-2-deoxy-D-glucose (FDG-PET). The application of FDG-PET is based on the observation of increased glucose metabolism in both malignant and inflammatory cells.[66] As part of a structured protocol, FDG-PET was deemed clinically helpful in 33% of cases.[62] Results in other studies have varied widely, with FDG-PET contributing to the diagnosis in 16–55% of cases.[62,67] Two prospective studies found FDG-PET to be superior to ^{67}Ga scanning, while another found it inferior to ^{111}In granulocyte scintigraphy, due to frequent false-positives.[68]

Some technical aspects may guide the selection of one form of nuclear scanning over another. Theoretically, ^{67}Ga scanning would be better able to detect both tumor and infection, whereas intuitively one would expect that leukocyte scanning would be more specific for infection. Malignancies have also been detected with white blood cell scans.[66] While the data are sparse as to whether one form of scintigraphy outperforms another, FDG-PET does offer the advantage that imaging can be completed within 2 hours of administration of the radioisotope.

Biopsy

Most PDCs are used to eventually point to biopsy of specific organs. The yield of such biopsies has varied depending on the series. Biopsy material can provide both culture and/or histologic evidence as a cause of FUO. Of note, in two clinical series of FUO published by the same investigator, tissue biopsy was required to make the diagnosis in the second series as often as in the first reported 20 years earlier.[12]

In a prospective study from the Netherlands, bone marrow biopsy established the diagnosis in 2 of 19 patients.[29] Other reports indicate a yield of anywhere from 0% to 18%.[69,70] In a pooled analysis of 857 published cases of FUO in Turkey, bone marrow biopsies were positive in roughly 30% of cases. In many instances in which biopsy was low yield, the biopsies were blinded and not guided necessarily by suspicion for a given condition. In areas with a low prevalence of tuberculosis, leishmaniasis, salmonella, brucellosis, etc., the yield of bone marrow biopsy for infectious etiologies of FUO would be expected to be low.

Liver biopsies in older series were stated to be useful without a number being given; more recent studies demonstrate a 14–17% yield.[71,72] Some reviews recommend liver biopsy in FUO investigations,[73] while others are against its routine use.[29,73] Physical or laboratory abnormalities have not been helpful in predicting which patients will have an abnormal liver biopsy.[71] The use of liver biopsy should again be dictated by the clinician and the entity to be diagnosed.

No study has evaluated the overall yield of temporal artery biopsy in those suspected of having temporal arteritis. Given that it is causative of up to 15% of cases of FUO in older patient populations, temporal artery biopsy should be considered in those older than 55 years with an elevated ESR.

Outside of the liver and bone marrow, biopsies of other sites should be guided by PDCs, i.e. if the patient has a rash or lymphadenopathy, then the site should be biopsied and sent for histopathology as well as appropriate cultures. The yield of such biopsies, even when there is palpable lymphadenopathy, has varied widely.

Other diagnostic studies in FUO

There are few data on the use of echocardiography or MRI in patients with FUO. In one study, echocardiography seemed to facilitate the diagnosis of endocarditis.[23] However, false-negatives have also been noted in other studies.[29]

No study has systemically looked at the overall yield of bilateral lower extremity ultrasound looking for deep venous thrombosis (DVT), even in the absence of symptoms. Given that DVT was etiologic of FUO in up to 6% of cases in some series, and the fact that the procedure is inexpensive and low risk, it could be given some consideration.[12,29] Pelvic CT is useful for the diagnosis of septic thrombophlebitis of pelvic veins when clinically indicated.

Drug-related fevers

When a drug-related fever is suspected, necessary drugs can be changed to alternatives of a different class. Upon initial presentation, a reasonable initial intervention is discontinuing as many drugs as possible. After stopping the agent that is responsible for the fever, the fever will usually resolve within 3 days, although it may take as long as 2 weeks. Persistence of fever beyond this time should direct the clinician to investigate an alternate source. If the fever remits, the clinician can definitively confirm the diagnosis by re-instituting the agent, which characteristically elicits fever again within a few hours. This procedure is safe unless drug-induced organ damage, such as interstitial nephritis or hepatitis, has occurred.

THERAPEUTIC INTERVENTIONS

The principle of a therapeutic trial is that the response to an intervention is both diagnostic and therapeutic. This requires that the intervention be as specific as possible. For instance, while isoniazid is fairly specific for mycobacteria, rifampin (rifampicin) has activity against a wide range of bacteria. The empiric use of agents such as these may be misleading for several reasons:

- medical intervention makes it difficult to determine whether a new finding has resulted from the treatment or from the underlying disease;

- fall of temperature may be fortuitous or it may result from the antipyretic effects of corticosteroids or NSAIDs; and
- improper use of antibiotics may lead to a false sense of therapeutic and diagnostic security and interfere with finding a diagnosis.

Thus, therapeutic trials should be discouraged in the early course of investigation in fevers of unknown origin.

The 'naproxen' test was used to differentiate fevers secondary to malignancies from those of infectious etiology.[74] This test has not been validated, and in a recent study of 77 patients with FUO,[75] though it caused a partial/complete response in 73% of patients with malignancies, this was also the case in 80% of patients with infections (including tuberculosis) and 55% of inflammatory states (including adult Still's disease). Overall, the sensitivity of the naproxen test was 55% for neoplastic fever with a specificity of 62%.

If patients are clinically suspected of having a pulmonary embolism or DVT as the cause of their fevers, defervescence should occur rapidly after the initiation of anticoagulation.

Prolonged empiric therapy may have multiple deleterious consequences beyond the unnecessary expense, inconvenience or iatrogenic complications for the patient. In addition, complications resulting from unnecessary interventions may confuse further diagnostic strategies based on abnormalities on physical examination or laboratory findings. For these reasons, therapeutic interventions should be discouraged in stable patients. If, however, a patient has a rapidly progressive, potentially fatal illness, empiric therapy becomes unavoidable.

PROGNOSIS

The prognosis of FUO is dependent on the patient population and the underlying diagnosis. In a disease process where a diagnosis may not be reached in up to 50% of cases, both clinicians and patients can easily get frustrated. Thus it is important to counsel patients about the relative positive outcome for those individuals in whom no diagnosis is reached after a reasonably thorough workup. In one study of 199 patients with FUO, 61 were eventually discharged with no diagnosis, of whom six died.[45] However, the deaths were thought to be related to the fever-causing process in only two of these cases. In a study of 34 patients discharged from hospital without a diagnosis and followed for up to 7 years, there was only one case of malignancy and two others had continuous illness. The diagnosis was found with certainty in only two cases, both within the first year.[76]

This is true in recent studies as well, though with shorter follow-up. In one prospective study of 73 patients with FUO, a diagnosis could not be reached in 37, of whom only one died at long-term follow-up.[29] The cause of death and whether or not it was related to the fever was not elucidated. In another study of 290 immunocompetent patients with FUO, follow-up information was available for 80 without a diagnosis.[23] Death occurred in three, but was presumably not linked to the initial febrile illness.

Prognosis is worse in those whose febrile illness is found secondary to a malignancy. In one of the above series, hematologic malignancies represented only 11.5% of the final diagnoses, but were responsbile for 58.3% of the fatalities.[23] Diagnostic delay has also been associated with adverse outcomes in such infections as miliary tuberculosis, disseminated fungi and intra-abdominal processes.

REFERENCES

References for this chapter can be found online at http://www.expertconsult.com

The potential role of infectious agents in diseases of unknown etiology

INTRODUCTION

Ultimately all human diseases are the result of a deleterious interaction between our genomes and the environment in which we exist. A critical component of that environment are the other living things that share the biosphere with us. We are exposed to a multitude of microbial pathogens over a lifetime and carry with us a remarkably complex and highly variable complement of endogenous micro-organisms (the microbiota) with the potential to do harm if our defenses falter. The microbiota of the average adult human is estimated to contain 10^{14} organisms and consists of at least 1000 different species, of which nearly half have yet to be successfully isolated and cultivated.[1,2]

When Pasteur, Koch and many other microbiologists of the latter half of 19th century first confirmed the 'germ theory' of disease, they revolutionized medicine and the way we think about disease. The fatalistic perception of human illness as a passive, inevitable consequence of life was replaced by the notion that at least some diseases were active, and possibly even preventable and reversible processes caused by invading micro-organisms. The search for the microbial etiology of all human maladies was on and continues to the present time.[3] The most recent, dramatic example of this search is the discovery of the infectious cause of peptic ulcer disease. Generations of physicians and surgeons considered it axiomatic that ulcers were the result of excess gastric acidity ('no acid, no ulcer'). When Marshall and Warren[4] finally convinced a skeptical scientific and medical community in the 1980s that most cases of chronic gastritis and peptic ulcer were actually caused by spiral bacterial organisms (*Helicobacter pylori*) inhabiting the gastric mucosa, they revolutionized the management of peptic ulcer disease.[5] Are there other common, or not so common, chronic idiopathic disease states waiting to be revealed as infectious diseases? Many elements of enigmatic clinical illnesses such as chronic fatigue syndrome (Chapter 70) suggest a microbial etiology, yet the nature of these illusive, potential pathogens and proof of their causation in disease pathogenesis remain ill-defined.

The genomic era in both human and microbial genetics has rekindled an interest in the discovery of micro-organisms as a cause of human disease. Many chronic inflammatory, neoplastic, and neurologic diseases carry tantalizing hallmarks suggestive of an underlying infectious cause.[6] This renewed discovery process may force us to re-examine the dynamic relationship that exists between human physiology and the myriad of exogenous and endogenous organisms surrounding all of us.

THE DEFINITION OF DISEASE CAUSATION AND ETIOLOGIC AGENTS IN THE PRE-GENOMIC ERA

In 1890, Koch first formally presented his famous postulates to define the requisite evidence needed to confirm the causative role of a microorganism in human disease.[3] This was the culmination of decades of seminal work by Koch and his mentor Friedrich Henle, along with many other scientists of the time, including Louis Pasteur and Edwin Klebs. Koch correctly surmised that such unambiguous guidelines were necessary to bring clarity and consistency into the newly emerging field of microbial pathogenesis. He initially proposed three essential elements to define a pathogen (or 'parasite' using his original terminology):

- Postulate 1: That the parasite is found in every case in which the disease occurs and accounts for the clinical and pathologic features of the disease;
- Postulate 2: That the parasite is not found in other diseases as a non-pathogen or fortuitous parasite; and
- Postulate 3: After being isolated from the body and repeatedly passed in pure culture, the parasite can induce the disease anew (in animal models or even in intrepid human volunteers).

A fourth postulate was subsequently added, apparently by others, necessitating the ability to re-isolate the same parasite from the diseased animal model. Koch's postulates have served us well and certainly helped solidify the germ theory of disease. The components are of particular value for obligate pathogens that are not highly species-specific, thereby allowing for animal models of human disease. Many microbiologists consider these postulates to be sacrosanct, even up to the present time. Yet it is worth noting that even Koch himself recognized from the beginning that these guidelines were not relevant for all pathogens. Koch famously observed that leprosy was likely caused by the mycobacterial-like bacillus (*Mycobacterium leprae*) that was readily identifiable on tissue stains of involved skin, yet he (or anyone else for the next century) was never able to grow the organism on artificial media. This violated his own third postulate; nonetheless, he was comfortable assigning a pathogenic role to these readily visible leprosy bacilli.

A myriad of well-known human pathogens, including many viruses, rickettsia, spirochetes and other pathogens, do not fulfill all of Koch's postulates and yet their etiologic identities are well established. The fact that many opportunistic potential pathogens colonize people for prolonged periods without causing disease (e.g. *Candida albicans*, *Staphylococcus aureus*, etc.) was not appreciated in the early days of clinical microbiology. This violates Koch's second postulate. Moreover, many human diseases caused by well-known microbial pathogens lack comparable animal models (e.g. rheumatic fever, progressive multifocal leukoencephalopathy) and therefore do not meet all of Koch's postulates.

ALTERNATIVE VIEWS OF MICROBIAL CAUSATION OF HUMAN DISEASE IN THE GENOMIC ERA

Many common infectious diseases result from a synergistic combination of variable numbers of different species of micro-organisms. Some examples include bacterial vaginosis, periodontitis or hepatitis D, a deficient virus requiring co-infection with a helper virus (hepatitis B virus) for replication. These infectious diseases violate the principle of serial passage in pure culture and then reproducing the disease in animal models. Periodontitis is a good example of the complexity that underlies the pathogenesis of some common infectious diseases.

Periodontitis is among the most prevalent infectious diseases afflicting 30–70% of adults worldwide.[7] This oral infection has been extensively studied by both culture-dependent and culture-independent methods.[8] A consistent pattern of microbial pathogens has now emerged as the cause of periodontitis. Despite the fact that Koch's postulates could not be applied to define the etiology of this common pathologic process, the genomic evidence strongly supports this 'communal' model of periodontal disease. Biofilms consisting of *Streptococcus mutans* and other oral streptococci residing in a mono- or disaccharide-rich environment in the oral cavity express exotoxins that gradually induce dental caries over time. A synergistic combination of bacterial pathogens living within the biofilm lining the gingival crevice then gives rise to periodontal disease. A combination of *Treponema denticola, Porphyromonas gingivalis, Tannerella forsythia,* and *Actinobacillus actinomycetemcomitans* gradually leads to gingivitis, bone resorption and the full expression of periodontitis. Later disease progression often involves additional noncultivable bacterial strains and a methanogenic Archaea organism (the first example of a member of the Archaea kingdom associated with a human disease).[1,2]

Important human illnesses are the result of long term-sequelae of remote infections (the 'hit and run' hypothesis) that occur months or even years after the infection has cleared. Examples include Guillain–Barré syndrome following enteric infection with specific serotypes of *Campylobacter* spp., Sydenham's chorea as a late manifestation of the non-suppurative complications of *S. pyogenes* pharyngitis, or post-infectious reactive arthritis (formerly known as Reiter's syndrome) following enteric infections. The pathogen is usually no longer cultivatable from these patients when the disease is manifest and yet their immunologic footprint clearly identifies the etiologic organism in each case.[1,6] A large number of immune-mediated, inflammatory and neoplastic diseases may have, as their proximate cause, a specific pathogen or group of micro-organisms as an inducer or essential propagator of human illness.

Exposure of the susceptible host with the appropriate genotype, and the fortuitous concurrence of the necessary set of environmental and epidemiologic circumstances conspire together to initiate and maintain an aberrant host response leading to overt clinical disease. Sarcoidosis might be an example of a disease induced by environmental and generally nonpathogenic bacterial organisms in some genetically susceptible individuals.[9–11] A specific genetic locus has been recently identified that appears to be linked with sarcoidosis.[12] Excessive and aberrant granulomatous reactions to common microorganisms such as *Propionibacterium acnes*[13–15] or tuberculous or environmental, non-tuberculous, mycobacterial antigens[16,17] might induce sarcoidosis in these susceptible patients. Similarly, genetic susceptibility to inflammatory bowel disease is well described in association with NOD2 polymorphisms and other mutations in pattern recognition receptors, resulting in defective clearance of enteric bacteria and microbial antigens and mediators along the mucosal epithelium of the small and large bowel.[18–20] This genetic predisposition to inflammatory bowel disease, in concert with alterations in the microenvironment and enteric microbial flora, is currently one of the favored hypotheses to explain the pathogenesis of Crohn's disease.[21–23]

Endemic Burkitt's lymphoma in children in sub-Saharan Africa provides another unfortunate example of a confluence of permissive environmental conditions and collaboration between two widely disparate pathogens to cause neoplasia. Burkitt's lymphoma is common in African children living in holoendemic regions where mosquito-borne falciparum malaria exists. Neoplastic transformation to lymphoma is generally attributed to an aberrant host response to Epstein–Barr virus (EBV) infection. Recent evidence indicates that *Plasmodium falciparum,* via its major erythrocyte protein PfEMP-1, induces general immunosuppression and profound B cell proliferation which activates productive infection with EBV. High level replication of EBV promotes the translocation and activation of the potent oncogene *c-myc,* resulting

Table 64.1 Microbial disease associations and possible causations – neoplastic diseases

Possible pathogen	Neoplasia	Level of evidence of causation*
Helicobacter pylori	Gastric adenocarcinoma	+++
	Gastric lymphoma	++
Epstein–Barr virus	Burkitt's lymphoma (with *Plasmodium falciparum*)	+++
	Hodgkin's disease	++
	Nasopharyngeal carcinoma	++
	Primary CNS lymphoma	+++
	Immunoblastic lymphoma	++
Hepatitis B	Hepatoma	+++
Hepatitis C	Hepatoma	+++
Schistosoma haematobium	Bladder carcinoma	++
Human papilloma virus 16/18	Cervical carcinoma	+++
	Colorectal cancer	+
Helicobacter bilis	Biliary tract cancer	+
Human T-cell leukemia/ lymphoma virus-1	Acute T-cell leukemia/ lymphoma	+++
	Invasive cervical carcinoma	+
	Small cell carcinoma of the lung	+
Human endogenous retrovirus-K10	Testicular cancer	+
Kaposi's sarcoma-associated herpes virus (human herpesvirus-8)	Kaposi's sarcoma	+++
	Primary effusion lymphoma	++

*Level of evidence: epidemiologic link only +; some evidence of causation ++; clear evidence of causation +++.

in malignant transformation to Burkitt's lymphoma.[24,25] The potential role of other viral, bacterial and parasitic infectious diseases in the pathogenesis of other neoplastic diseases is surveyed in Table 64.1.[26]

There are a large number of clinical settings in which a specific micro-organism or group of micro-organisms might be necessary and sufficient to cause a variety of human illnesses, yet go unnoticed when relying upon standard diagnostic techniques.[1–5] A number of epidemiologic features and histopathologic findings suggest a microbial cause for a variety of idiopathic diseases. Such diseases as sarcoidosis,[9–11] Kawasaki disease,[27] multiple sclerosis, Kikuchi–Fujimoto disease[28–30] and numerous other diseases suggest an underlying infectious cause.

Caution needs to be exercised before it can be unequivocally concluded that an implicated organism is in fact the true etiologic agent.[3,6] Chronic disease syndromes and neoplastic diseases are frequently associated with a myriad of infectious diseases, yet the link between association as a mere bystander and actual microbial causation is often difficult to define clearly. Certain organisms could be highly associated to a specific disease entity, yet simply occupy a unique ecologic niche created by the disease itself. *Streptococcus bovis* (recently renamed *S. gallolyticus*) is highly associated with neoplastic lesions in the colonic mucosa, yet there is little evidence to suggest that this organism causes colon tumors. The organism takes the opportunity

Table 64.2 Mechanisms by which causative microbial pathogens might escape detection

Mechanism	Examples	Comments
'Hit and run hypothesis'	*Streptococcus pyogenes* – chorea minor in rheumatic fever Measles – subacute sclerosing panencephalitis	Disease manifestations induced by infection but separated from body site and in time by months to years
Difficult to culture or noncultivable	*Tropheryma whipplei* –Whipple's disease *Bartonella henselae* – cat-scratch disease	Genomic studies indicate enormous numbers of microbial genomes that have yet to be successfully cultured
Commensal organisms that rarely cause disease in susceptible hosts	*Sacrocystis* spp. – enteritis or myositis Non-tuberculous mycobacteria – respiratory infections	Difficult or impossible to prove Koch's postulates
Disease occurs with microbial communities	Periodontitis Bacterial vaginosis	Synergistic combinations of microorganisms cause disease
Micro-organism induces immunologic or neoplastic alterations	Kaposi's sarcoma-associated herpes virus (human herpesvirus-8) *Helicobacter pylori* Gastric carcinoma	Microbial pathogen may serve as promoter or essential inducer
Human endogenous retrovirus (HERV)	HERV-E and systemic lupus erythematosus	Widely prevalent in human genome – possible inducer or propagator for chronic diseases
Different micro-organisms trigger illness only in genetically susceptible patients	Possibly sarcoidosis Kawasaki disease Multiple sclerosis, etc.	A variety of possible microbial pathogens may induce disease at critical time intervals in susceptible individuals

to colonize the unique microenvironment adjacent to the neoplastic tissue. A survey of potential mechanisms by which the microbial cause of disease could go unrecognized using conventional diagnostic methods is provided in Table 64.2.

THE HYGIENE HYPOTHESIS AND THE PATHOGENESIS OF INFLAMMATORY DISEASES

It should also be acknowledged that, paradoxically, heavy exposure to some elements of the microbiota, particularly at a young age, may actually protect against a number of inflammatory and allergic diseases later in life. The incidence of asthma, Crohn's disease, diabetes and multiple sclerosis has progressively increased over the last half century in developed nations as vaccine-preventable and food and waterborne enteric infections have dramatically decreased.[31] These inflammatory diseases are much less common in developing countries where the incidence of childhood infection remains high. The 'hygiene hypothesis' suggests that improved hygiene fails to prime innate immune responses to common microbial antigens in early life. This impairs mucosal immune maturation, promotes a Th2-type cytokine response and facilitates inappropriate cellular tolerance to many common microbial antigens. The end result is excessive and disordered inflammation to many of these environmental antigens later in childhood and adulthood, with resultant increased risk of inflammatory diseases. The hygiene hypothesis seems plausible yet still lacks extensive experimental evidence in support of this appealing notion.[31–34]

CULTURE-INDEPENDENT TECHNIQUES TO DETECT NOVEL PATHOGENS

In the genomic age in which we now live, Koch's postulates need to be modified or even discarded as an obsolete system to define the essential elements of what identifies a microbial pathogen. The evolving definition of what constitutes a human pathogen has moved from a formal requirement to fulfill all of Koch's postulates to a genomic expression of Descartes' assertion, 'I clone, therefore I am.' This is best evidenced by the remarkable discovery of hepatitis C as the most common cause of non-A, non-B post-transfusion hepatitis by Choo and colleagues in 1989.[35] After decades of concerted, yet futile, efforts to isolate the implicated virus using standard virologic techniques, Choo *et al.* decided to attempt to clone the genome of the unknown agent directly from the serum of a chimpanzee experimentally infected and known by serial serum dilution and animal challenge to contain high titers of infectious non-A, non-B hepatitis.

After treating the serum with reverse transcriptase, they generated a large number of sequences of amplified nucleic acids to create a comprehensive cDNA library. It was not known at the time if the presumed hepatitis-causing agent was an RNA or DNA virus or perhaps a noncultivable bacterium. The resulting battery of lambda phage cDNA clones were then tested against the serum of a patient with chronic severe non-A, non-B hepatitis. It was hoped that this human serum would provide a source of antibodies that would recognize at least some of the expressed viral peptides derived from the cloned sequences. After screening nearly one million clones, the reactive peptide sequence was identified. They then showed that this was an RNAse- but not DNAse-sensitive genome and, by overlapping hybridization experiments, they confirmed that this was a positive-stranded RNA virus of approximately 10 000 base pairs. This newly discovered virus shared unexpected homologies with a number of arthropod-borne viral pathogens. The viral agent was confirmed to be a previously unknown member of the flavivirus family. The mystery of post-transfusion, non-A, non-B hepatitis was finally solved by cloning, unencumbered by the need to fulfill Koch's postulates.[3,35]

A similar cloning strategy has now been adapted from work done with genome searches for comparative microbial ecology, environmental biology and molecular phylogeny studies.[2,3] Microbial DNA sequences are isolated and amplified by polymerase chain reaction (PCR) using broad range bacterial primers for essential target sequences such as ribosomal RNA genes. These amplified, novel bacterial sequences are then cloned in a DNA library where comparative sequence analysis is performed with highly conserved and well-characterized sequences from known classes of micro-organisms. The genes for 16S RNA, other essential ribosomal RNA sequences, or highly conserved enzymes are scanned for sequence homologies throughout the Bacteria and Archaea domains.

Sequence homologies and genomic groupings can now be exploited to identify shared genetic space and evolutionary distance between essentially any unknown pathogen and all identifiable, genome-characterized micro-organisms. These culture-independent methodologies are now employed to search for novel, difficult to culture or noncultivable microbial pathogens that might cause human disease. Such unbiased genome searches have been instrumental to the work of Relman, Fredricks and others[3] discovering the etiology of longstanding diseases of known microbial cause but with noncultivable organisms such as the Whipple's disease bacillus (*Tropheryma whipplei*)[36,37] or newly recognized, emerging pathogens such as the causative agents of bacillary angiomatosis (*Bartonella henselae*) and human monocytic ehrlichiosis (*Ehrlichia chaffeensis*).[3] The resulting genomic evidence about the predicted metabolic requirements of *T. whipplei* was then exploited to develop a cell-free medium to successfully culture the Whipple's disease bacillus for the first time.[38] The basic strategy employed in these genome searches is depicted in Figure 64.1. Current sequencing machinery now permits the simultaneous sequencing of over 200 000 short unique nucleotides from small samples of DNA without the need for preparatory cloning.[3] This facilitates rapid genome screens with known sequences of viruses, rickettsia and numerous other difficult to culture microbial genomes for potential pathogens.

Another genomic technique that can be used to detect and define novel microbial pathogens is DNA subtraction techniques.

This methodology was successfully employed to link a previously unknown herpes-like virus (HHV-8), now known as Kaposi's sarcoma-associated herpes virus (KSHV) as the cause of HIV-related Kaposi's sarcoma.[2,3] The DNA sequences derived from diseased tissues and a similar set of DNA sequences from normal tissues are subjected to subtractive hybridization and PCR amplification to enrich the DNA complement of DNA sequences found in the diseased sample only. Unique sequences are then analyzed to determine if any sequence homologies exist with known pathogens. As the known genomic universe of micro-organisms continues to expand, it is likely that this and related culture-independent methods will reveal new pathogens associated with human illness.

KOCH'S POSTULATES REDEFINED

A new set of more practical guidelines to assign causation of potential pathogens to diseases of unknown cause is needed in the genomic era of the 21st century. Numerous diagnostic schemes have been proposed to complement or replace Koch's postulates for defining pathogens. A modification of the Hill[39] and Evans[40] criteria to supplement Koch's postulates is a reasonable framework upon which to build a more logical and practical diagnostic system to define disease causation. This set of criteria can readily be modified to include genomic evidence for noncultivable pathogens (Table 64.3). Each criterion need not be met to determine disease causation of each suspect human pathogen. The more criteria that are satisfied, the more convincing the link becomes between the suspected pathogen as the etiologic agent responsible for the disease process. A more integrated system that takes into account variations in the host response along with the microbial agent responsible for disease causation may be needed in the future.[6]

THE ROLE OF HUMAN ENDOGENOUS RETROVIRUSES IN HEALTH AND DISEASE

The human genome is replete with endogenous retroviruses (HERVs, also known as retrotransposons) that have entered the human germline at various times in the evolutionary past and now occupy 8.3% of the genome.[41] They maintain the basic structure of retroviruses with long terminal repeats (LTR) flanking the open reading frames for polymerase (*pol*), including reverse transcriptase, envelope (*env*) and core matrix (*gag*) genes along with various regulatory genes. They have accumulated loss of function point mutations in structural and regulatory genes, rendering them incapable of exogenous viral production. It is possible to 'resurrect' some recently inherited HERVs from the human genome but this is unlikely to occur spontaneously.[42] However, these endogenous retroviruses are far from genetically or metabolically dormant. Some HERVs have physiologic roles including syncytiotrophoblast formation in placental development and intrinsic resistance to exogenous retrovirus infection.[43]

HERVs also have the potential to contribute to pathologic reactions in their hosts.[41] The LTR regions are transcriptionally active and serum antibodies are detectable to Env and Gag proteins from a number of HERVs, indicating that these structural genes are transcribed and expressed. Transposition of HERVs can inactivate cellular genes at other loci in the human genome. Moreover, the LTRs of HERVs can have polar effects in *cis* and promote transcriptional activation of adjacent cellular genes. Lastly, transcriptional activators are found within HERVs that might have the capacity to activate cellular genes in *trans*.

HERVs have been implicated in induction of malignant transformation by activating oncogenes or inactivating apoptosis-inducing genes. HERVs might contribute to immune-mediated diseases such as multiple sclerosis (MS), rheumatoid arthritis (RA) and systemic lupus erythematosus (SLE) by the generation of HERV antigens that cross-react with endogenous antigens and break tolerance to normal autoantigens. The *gag* p30 of class I HERVs bear striking homology

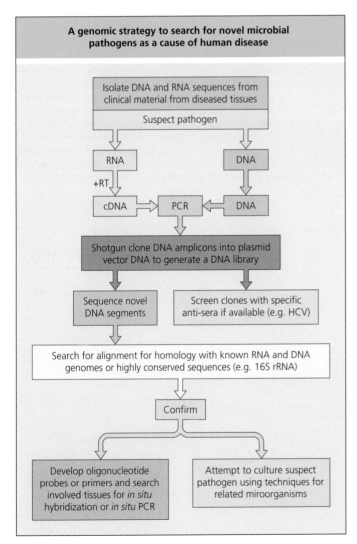

A genomic strategy to search for novel microbial pathogens as a cause of human disease

Isolate DNA and RNA sequences from clinical material from diseased tissues

Suspect pathogen

RNA → +RT → cDNA → PCR ← DNA ← DNA

Shotgun clone DNA amplicons into plasmid vector DNA to generate a DNA library

Sequence novel DNA segments

Screen clones with specific anti-sera if available (e.g. HCV)

Search for alignment for homology with known RNA and DNA genomes or highly conserved sequences (e.g. 16S rRNA)

Confirm

Develop oligonucleotide probes or primers and search involved tissues for *in situ* hybridization or *in situ* PCR

Attempt to culture suspect pathogen using techniques for related miroorganisms

Fig. 64.1 A genomic strategy to search for novel microbial pathogens as a cause of human disease. cDNA, complementary DNA; HCV, hepatitis C virus; PCR, polymerase chain reaction; RT, reverse transcriptase.

Table 64.3 Koch's postulates revisited: microbial causation in the genomic era

Modified Hill[39] and Evans[40] criteria	Genomic criteria[3]
Prevalence of disease higher in patients exposed to suspect pathogen(s) than those not exposed	Nucleic acid sequence of suspect pathogen should be present in diseased tissues
Incidence of disease should be higher in patients exposed to suspect pathogen(s) than controls in prospective studies	No or few copies of nucleic acid sequences of suspect pathogen should be found in the absence of disease and normal tissue
The disease should be temporally linked to exposure to suspect pathogen(s)	If suspect pathogen sequences predate onset of disease, the copy number of sequences should increase with onset of clinical illness (temporal relationship)
A spectrum of disease should be found after exposure from mild to severe disease (dose–response relationship)	Copy number of suspect pathogen sequences should correlate to disease severity (gene copy–host response relationship)
A measurable host response should occur following exposure to suspect pathogen(s)	The suspect pathogen sequences should localize by *in situ* hybridization to affected tissues
Experimental reproduction of disease should occur in models or human volunteers	Suspect pathogen sequences should be reproducibly found in patients with similar illnesses and in animal models (if available)
Prevention of transmission of suspect pathogen should decrease incidence of disease and eradication of pathogen should decrease the disease	Resolution of clinical illness should be accompanied by reduction or elimination of suspect pathogen sequences
The whole process should make biologic sense and fit the epidemiology of disease	The suspect pathogen determined by nucleic acid homology searches should fit the biology and pathology of genetically related micro-organisms

with the human 70K ribonucleoprotein (RNP) U1 snRNP, a frequently recognized autoantigen in SLE.[44] It is tempting to speculate that SLE is induced in some patients by molecular mimicry when expressed HERVs Gag proteins induce antibodies that cross-react with epitopes found on the 70K RNP. HERVs may facilitate epitope spreading and loss of Fas-mediated apoptosis of self-reacting T cells which might further contribute to the progression of autoimmune disease.

HERVs may collaborate with other viruses such as EBV to induce the synthesis of endogenous superantigen motifs encoded by HERVs.[45] This process is hypothesized to contribute to the immune-mediated CNS pathology in MS. HERV-K18 has superantigenic activity in its envelope peptide; expression of this Env protein is transactivated by B-cell clonal expansion by co-infection with EBV. This type of immune dysregulation in the CNS is implicated in the pathogenesis of plague formation within the white matter in MS.[41,45,46] Finally, recent evidence suggests that the Env protein of HERV-W can act as a ligand for the pattern recognition receptors CD14 and Toll-like receptor 4 (TLR-4).[47] Activation of effector cells of the innate immune system via TLR-4 with cytokine and chemokine generation might further contribute to injurious CNS inflammation in MS and other demyelinating disorders. A brief review of the known and possible infectious diseases that are associated with or cause inflammatory and vasculitic diseases is presented in Table 64.4[48] and Table 64.5.[49–52]

Table 64.4 Microbial disease associations and possible causation – inflammatory diseases

Possible pathogen	Disease	Level of evidence of causation*
Propionibacterium acnes	Sarcoidosis	+ (environmental mycobacteria also implicated)
Human herpesvirus-6 (HHV-6)	Multiple sclerosis (relapsing–remitting type)	+/++ (HERV-W also implicated in association with Epstein–Barr virus or HHV-6)
Mycobacterium paratuberculosis	Inflammatory bowel disease	+ (high concentrations of enteric bacteria also implicated)
Human endogenous retrovirus (HERV)-W	Psoriasis	+
HERV-K18	Type 1 diabetes	+ (enteroviruses also implicated)
Bacterial superantigens	Kawasaki disease	+
Yersinia enterocolitica	Kikuchi–Fujimoto disease	++ (KSHV also implicated)
Kaposi's sarcoma-associated herpes virus (KSHV)	Multicentric Castleman's disease	++
Mixed enteric aerobes and anaerobes	Necrotizing enterocolitis[48]	+

*Levels of evidence: epidemiologic link only +; some evidence of causation ++; clear evidence of causation +++.

Table 64.5 Microbial disease associations and possible causations – vasculitis

Microbial agent	Disease	Level of evidence of causation*
Hepatitis B	Polyarteritis nodosa	++/+++
Hepatitis C	Mixed cryoglobulinemia	++/+++
Staphylococcus aureus	Wegener's granulomatosis Churg–Strauss eosinophilic vasculitis	++ +
Epstein–Barr virus (EBV)	Rheumatoid arthritis	++ (HERV also implicated)
Cytomegalovirus[49]	Atherosclerosis	+ (*Chlamydia pneumoniae* also implicated[50])
Human endogenous retrovirus (HERV)-E	Systemic lupus erythematosus	+ (EBV also implicated)
Parainfluenza virus	Giant cell arteritis[51]	+ (parvovirus B19 also implicated)
Bacterial lipopolysaccharide	Anti-neutrophil cytoplasmic antibody – associated crescentic glomerulonephritis[52]	+

*Levels of evidence: epidemiologic link only +; some evidence of causation ++; clear evidence of causation +++.

CONCLUSIONS

The number of potential pathogens that might cause disease in some susceptible human populations has expanded by an order of magnitude with the recognition of a multitude of noncultivable micro-organisms in our environment and even among our endogenous microbiota. It seems likely that at least some human diseases of unknown cause that currently exist will eventually be attributable to one or more of these as yet noncultured organisms. Synergistic combinations of viral, bacterial and even parasitic infections are now known to cause specific clinical disease entities and hopefully additional conditions, currently regarded as 'idiopathic', will be found to be of microbial cause. Aberrant host responses to common micro-organisms might explain many inflammatory and perhaps even some neoplastic diseases. The role of human endogenous retroviruses in human disease alone or in combination with other potential pathogens remains a fertile area of research in the coming years.

The discovery of previously unrecognized infectious diseases as a cause of human illness is certainly worth the time and expense. Microbial causation holds out hope for specific and improved treatments and even prevention of illness. This discovery work will be more complicated than that of the microbe hunters of the past century, but the new tools of systems biology and genomics offer unique opportunities to decipher human disease as never before. The challenge of discovery of new agents in microbial pathogenesis has been rekindled and significant advances in this field are fully anticipated in the coming years.

REFERENCES

References for this chapter can be found online at http://www.expertconsult.com

Philip S Barie
Steven M Opal

Chapter | **65** |

Infectious complications following surgery and trauma

Significant tissue injury substantially increases the risk of infection for several reasons. The net host response to injury is predominantly immunosuppressive; transgression of natural epithelial barriers (e.g. skin, respiratory mucosa, gut mucosa) creates a portal of entry for invasion by potential pathogens; tissue injury, foreign bodies and ischemia provide optimal conditions for bacterial proliferation; well-intentioned therapies can have adverse consequences; and lapses of infection control often occur under emergency conditions. These risks can be apportioned as patient-derived risks, environment-derived risks or treatment-derived risks. The polytrauma patient is often subjected to multiple surgical procedures, creating additive risks for adverse outcome.

Some infective complications are unique to surgery (e.g. surgical site infections (SSIs), infection of traumatic wounds and burns, post-operative intra-abdominal infections), whereas others are common to all critically ill patient populations (e.g. health-care related infection, catheter-related infection, etc.). Management of the surgical patient presents some special challenges:

* it can be particularly difficult to distinguish sterile inflammation with or without bacterial colonization from invasive infection; and
* prevention of infection at the site of tissue injury is of utmost importance, especially after severe trauma and before high-risk elective surgery.

The incidence of infection following surgery or trauma is context-sensitive. The incidence of SSI following minor, clean, elective surgery is approximately 2% and that of other infectious complications is practically nil.[1] In contrast, the overall incidence of infection following major trauma is about 25%.[1,2] Infection is common and the leading cause of late death after trauma accompanied by multiple organ dysfunction syndrome (MODS).[3-5] It is generally stated that the development of postoperative nosocomial infection, especially with a multidrug-resistant pathogen, increases the risk of death three- to five-fold;[5] however, the attributable risk of mortality from infection remains controversial and not universally accepted.[6]

PATIENT-DERIVED RISK FACTORS

Risk factors that result from intrinsic attributes of the host are listed in Table 65.1. Among these factors are age, chronic medical conditions (especially diabetes mellitus) and hypocholesterolemia. The contribution of age to infection risk is increasingly being recognized.[7] In a multicenter, preoperative risk assessment for the development of postoperative pneumonia, age was found to be the most powerful independent predictor of risk.[7] Substantial evidence indicates that perioperative hyperglycemia increases the risk of infection, even if mild or transient. Failure to maintain euglycemia during open heart surgery triples the risk of sternal wound infection.[8] While some

Table 65.1 Host factors that contribute to the development of nosocomial infection

Nonmodifiable	Modifiable
Ascites	Chronic inflammation
Obesity	Corticosteroid therapy
Diabetes mellitus	(controversial)
Extremes of age	Hypocholesterolemia
Peripheral vascular disease	Hypoxemia
(especially for lower extremity	Postoperative anemia
surgery)	Prior site irradiation
Extent of tissue trauma or burns	Recent operation
	Remote infection
	Skin carriage of staphylococci
	Undernutrition
	Transfusions
	Antibiotics

controversy persists over the risk–benefit ratio in the maintenance of euglycemia in the critically ill surgical patient, avoidance of significant hyperglycemia (>150 mg/dl or 8.3 mmol/l) is advised. Hypocholesterolemia is rapid and dramatic after surgical stress, and has been associated with an increased risk of SSI and pneumonia[9] and independently with an increased risk of death in critically ill patients with systemic inflammatory response syndrome (SIRS). The possible mechanisms underlying this risk are several, including dysfunction of lipid-laden macrophages or decreased binding of endotoxin by apolipoproteins.

The surgical stress response

Surgical stress is associated with a stereotypical response.[10] The stress hormone response to surgical stress or tissue injury augments cardiovascular function through the sympathetic nervous system, enhances glycogenolysis, mobilizes peripheral lean tissue and fat for use as fuel, enhances coagulation to limit hemorrhage and stimulates a proinflammatory cytokine response to begin the process of tissue repair. Cellular immunity is depressed in large part by the actions of cortisol, catecholamines, a shift to Th2-type cytokines and the actions of regulatory T cells (T_{reg}). Three major events characterize the initial inflammatory response:

* activation of coagulation;
* increased microvascular endothelial permeability with tissue edema formation; and
* chemotaxis, margination and transvascular migration of neutrophils.

The first step in the process is recognition of a foreign antigen, either by elements of the adaptive immune system (e.g. T cells, preformed antibodies, classic complement pathway) or by innate immune elements (e.g. myeloid cells, Toll-like receptors, alternative complement and mannose-binding lectin pathways). The inflammatory response is then amplified in a complex process regulated by cytokines, plasma enzymes (e.g. complement, coagulation, kinin and fibrinolytic pathways), lipid mediators (e.g. prostaglandins, leukotrienes) and mediators derived from mast cells and platelets. Fast-acting mediators, such as vasoactive amines and bradykinin, modulate the immediate response. Several hours later, mediators such as leukotrienes, chemokines and platelet-activating factor are involved in the accumulation and activation of phagocytes. Once neutrophils have arrived at a site of inflammation, they release macrophage chemoattractants that, in turn, control the later accumulation and activation of monocytes and macrophages.

The acute-phase response is a dynamic homeostatic process that involves the immune, cardiovascular and central nervous systems. Normally, the acute-phase response lasts only a few days. Two physiologic responses are closely associated with acute inflammation: the first involves the alteration of the temperature set-point in the hypothalamus and the generation of fever; the second involves alterations in metabolism and gene expression in the liver. Interleukin (IL)-1, IL-6 and tumor necrosis factor regulate the febrile response through the induction of prostaglandin E2, possibly as a protective mechanism against bacterial infection (see Chapters 2 and 61). At the same time, IL-1 and IL-6 act on the hypothalamic–pituitary–adrenal axis to generate corticotropin and stimulate cortisol production. This provides a negative feedback loop, because corticosteroids inhibit cytokine gene expression.

The second important aspect of the acute-phase response is altered hepatic protein synthesis. Production of numerous proteins is upregulated, whereas synthesis of others is suppressed. Acute-phase reactants (APRs) thus may be 'positive' or 'negative'. Positive APRs include fibrinogen, clotting elements, proteases and some protease inhibitors, complement components, lipopolysaccharide-binding protein, serum amyloid A and C-reactive protein. Negative APRs (e.g. albumin, antithrombin, inter-α inhibitor, protein C) are decreased in synthetic rate to allow an increase in the capacity of the liver to synthesize the induced APRs. Although most APRs are synthesized by hepatocytes, some are produced by other cell types such as myeloid cells, endothelial cells, fibroblasts or adipocytes.

Acute-phase reactants contribute to host defense in several ways, including direct neutralization of inflammatory mediators, thereby minimizing tissue damage and facilitating tissue repair. For example, increased synthesis of complement proteins mobilizes neutrophils and macrophages. Fibrinogen plays an essential role in hemostasis and the promotion of wound healing. Protease inhibitors (e.g. α_1-antitrypsin) neutralize elastase and lysosomal proteases released following the infiltration of activated neutrophils and macrophages, thus mitigating the activity of the proinflammatory enzyme cascades. Increased plasma concentrations of metalloproteases help to prevent iron loss during infection and injury, minimize the amount of heme iron available for bacterial metabolism and scavenge reactive oxygen species.

PATHOGENESIS OF INFLAMMATION AND ORGAN DYSFUNCTION

The acute response to injury is characterized by a syndrome of:
- fever (≥100.4 °F (38° C)) or hypothermia (≤96.8 °F (36° C));
- leukocytosis (>12 000/mm³), leukopenia (<4000/ml) and excess bands (>10% immature neutrophils);
- increased heart rate (<90 beats/minute); and
- increased respiratory rate (>24/minute) or, if mechanically ventilated, P_{aCO_2} <32 mmHg.

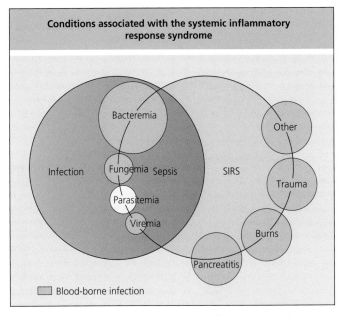

Fig. 65.1 The interactions between systemic inflammation, sepsis and multiple organ dysfunction syndrome. SIRS, systemic inflammatory response syndrome.

Systemic inflammatory response syndrome[11] is the name given to this constellation if at least two of the parameters are present. Among surgical patients, there are many causes of tissue injury-induced inflammation (e.g. trauma, burns, pancreatitis) (Fig. 65.1) that have no relation to infection on initial presentation. Recovery from general anesthesia can produce symptoms indistinguishable from true SIRS, but the effect is transitory. While the diagnostic value of SIRS is often criticized for being nonspecific, in the surgical setting the persistence of SIRS is important prognostically. The presence and magnitude of SIRS in the trauma bay has been associated with increased risk of nosocomial infection. Moreover, among critically ill surgical patients, persistent SIRS was associated with prolonged stay in intensive care units (ICU), worsening SIRS was associated with MODS and a higher mortality (see also Chapter 44).

The proinflammatory response can be incited by either tissue injury or infection. The same pattern recognition receptors of the innate immune system (the TLRs and receptor for advanced glycation end products) that detect infection-related, pathogen-associated molecular patterns (PAMPs) can also recognize numerous host-derived damage-associated molecular patterns (DAMPs) (see Chapter 44). Host-derived DAMPs include heat shock proteins, high-mobility group box 1 protein (HMGB1), heme, fibronectin extra domain A, calgranulins, heparan monomers, β-defensins and many other molecules released from damaged host cells and cells undergoing apoptosis.[12] Inflammation is modulated by a complex interrelationship of activation of the coagulation, kinin, complement and other systems, generating numerous already-known and probably yet-to-be-discovered mediators, including prostaglandins, leukotrienes, reactive oxygen and nitrogen species, lipid peroxides, coagulation factors, adhesion molecules and cytokines. Consequently, phagocytic cells, platelets and endothelial cells are activated, in part to contain the inflammatory response (e.g. to localize and eradicate a nascent infection). Containment is also the likely role of the counter-regulatory anti-inflammatory response, downregulating the potentially injurious, systemic, proinflammatory response. The anti-inflammatory response is mediated by cortisol, IL-4, IL-10, myeloid colony-stimulating factors, transforming growth factors and other mediators. The counter-regulatory response results in the activation of genetic programs ('suicide' genes) that cause phagocytic cells to undergo apoptosis (i.e. programmed cell death). Apoptosis causes inflammation to subside; several adverse clinical events such

Fig. 65.2 Hypothetical interactions of proinflammatory and anti-inflammatory responses. Pathogenesis of immunosuppression, nosocomial infection, organ dysfunction and outcome.

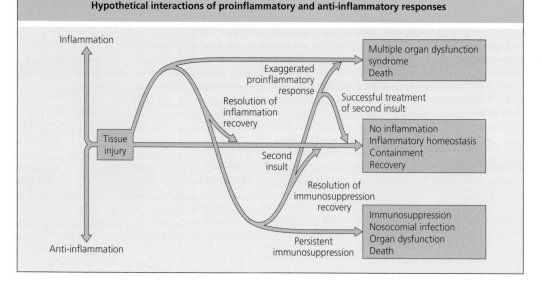

as hypoxemia or blood transfusions may delay apoptosis, promote inflammation and contribute to adverse outcomes.[13]

Details of the regulatory control of the anti-inflammatory response over the proinflammatory response and the promotion of subsequent tissue repair remain incomplete. Elements that likely contribute to the inflammatory ebb and flow are depicted in Figure 65.2. There is substantial experimental evidence that an accentuated neutrophil proinflammatory response occurs by neutrophils that are first 'primed' by an inflammatory stimulus and then respond in an exaggerated, deleterious manner in response to a second insult. Examples of a primary insult include a period of hypoxia or blood transfusion, or the initial injury (e.g. a femur fracture), whereas an example of a second insult would be a postoperative nosocomial pneumonia.[13] The dysfunctional inflammatory response results in release of mediators that, among other effects, induce adherence of neutrophils and platelets to microvascular endothelium; entrap microthrombi of fibrin, platelets, neutrophils and cellular debris; and cause tissue hypoperfusion, ischemia and edema as a result of loss of microvascular integrity.[14] Resuscitation and natural fibrinolysis may restore microvascular flow before tissue necrosis occurs, but re-introduction of molecular oxygen to the ischemic bed may result in the generation of reactive oxygen species. These highly toxic mediators have innumerable deleterious effects, including the ability to oxidize lipid components of cell membranes.

The splanchnic bed is especially susceptible to ischemia, and ischemia and reperfusion of the gut may be central to the pathogenesis of inflammation and organ dysfunction.[13] The intestine is an immunologically active organ that serves to protect the host from ingested bacteria as well as the potentially lethal bacterial inoculum contained in feces. Ischemic reperfused intestine becomes dysfunctional, with ileus and the ensuing putative release of mediators, bacterial toxins (e.g. endotoxin) or live bacteria ('bacterial translocation'). Although the existence of bacterial translocation is well documented in murine models it does not appear to occur in humans. Increased intestinal permeability of luminal products does occur in humans and may account for the gut-derived, persistent proinflammatory stimulus following severe injury or hypotension. Under catabolic conditions, the dysfunctional gut no longer provides trophic support of hepatic function, and maintenance of hepatic reticuloendothelial host defense function is impaired.

The clinical manifestations of MODS are protean (see Fig. 65.2) and the consequences are grave. No longer conceptualized as an 'all-or-nothing' phenomenon in which organ 'failure' is recognized after a threshold of dysfunction is reached, MODS can affect several organs to varying degrees and the effects are cumulative.[11] As many as 50%

of critically ill surgical patients and nearly 100% of critically ill non-survivors develop some degree of MODS. The development of MODS prolongs ICU stay even among patients who develop only minimal organ dysfunction, and mortality increases as it progresses.

ENVIRONMENT-DERIVED RISK FACTORS

The importance of colonization with bacteria or active remote infection as a risk factor for subsequent infection cannot be over-emphasized. Patients who are chronic carriers of staphylococci and streptococci are at increased risk of SSIs after elective surgery,[15] as are patients with active soft tissue infections at tissue sites remote from the surgical wound. In hospitalized patients, colonization of the skin, lower airway and gut with pathogenic bacteria and fungi is common and occurs rapidly even among immunocompetent hosts. Aided and abetted by breaks in infection control measures, these potential pathogens colonize and then invade vulnerable hosts. The risk of SSI and intra-abdominal infection is increased by prolonged pre-event hospitalization. Nosocomial pneumonia is promoted by pre-existing colonization of the lower airway by the same pathogen.[16] The same can be said for invasive fungal infections of surgical patients, which are often preceded by multiple-site colonization and invasive infection with vancomycin-resistant enterococci. There is little doubt that antibiotic selection pressure leads to nosocomial infections with multidrug-resistant bacteria, which are a threat to vulnerable patients.[17]

TREATMENT-DERIVED RISK FACTORS

Modern therapy is often invasive and disruptive of homeostasis even as treatment tries to restore it (Table 65.2). Clinicians must be cognizant of the adverse consequences of therapies that may impair host defenses or disrupt commensal flora, increasing the risk of nosocomial infection. Among several factors of importance are the control of serum glucose concentration, the avoidance of blood transfusion, maintenance of normoxia and normothermia, minimized duration of mechanical ventilation, and rational antibiotic prophylaxis and therapy. Also crucial are maintenance of the operating room environment and adherence to the principles of infection control and universal precautions. There are published guidelines for the prevention of SSI[17] and vascular catheter-related infection (see also Chapter 45).[18]

Table 65.2 American Society of Anesthesiologists (ASA) physical status score

Score	Description	Examples
ASA 1	A normal healthy patient	
ASA 2	A patient with a mild to moderate disturbance that results in no functional limitations	Hypertension, diabetes mellitus, chronic bronchitis, morbid obesity, extremes of age
ASA 3	A patient with a severe systemic disturbance that results in functional limitations	Poorly controlled hypertension, diabetes mellitus with vascular complications, agina pectoris, prior myocardial infaction, pulmonary disease that limits activity
ASA 4	A patient with a severe systemic disturbance that is life threatening with or without the planned procedure	Congestive heart failure, unstable angina pectoris, advanced pulmonary, renal or hepatic dysfunction
ASA 5	A moribund patient not expected to survive with or without the operative procedure	Ruptured abdominal aortic aneurysm, pulmonary embolism, head injury with increased intracranial pressure
E	Any patient in whom the procedure is an emergency	

Blood transfusion

Evidence is substantial and increasing that allogenic transfusion of red blood cell concentrates is immunosuppressive and increases the risk of nosocomial infection. Transfusion requirements are understandable in the trauma and surgery environment and alternatives are few. Nonetheless, transfusions should be avoided if possible, especially in hemodynamically stable patients who are not bleeding. Leukoreduced red blood cell transfusion has reduced but not eliminated the adverse immune consequences of transfusion and now is considered the standard of care in developed countries.[19]

Protection of the hypoxic wound

A fresh surgical incision is a hypoxic, ischemic environment. Blood vessels are divided at the wound margins and use of electrocautery leaves a surrounding margin of coagulation necrosis. Maneuvers to support the oxygenation and perfusion of the incision have demonstrated benefit. Hypothermia (body temperature under 94.1°F (34.5° C)) leads to MODS and increased mortality after major abdominal vascular surgery and to an increased incidence of SSI.[20] Intraoperative hypothermia should be avoided at all costs with use of fluid warmers, forced-air blankets and other maneuvers to avoid body cooling.

ANTIBIOTIC PROPHYLAXIS AND THE RISK OF SURGICAL SITE INFECTION

The administration of antibiotics before surgery is commonplace and of proven benefit to prevent postoperative SSI. However, it is only the surgical incision that is afforded protection, and antibiotics are not a panacea. If not administered properly, antibiotic prophylaxis will not be effective and may be harmful.

Most commonly, the risk of SSI, as categorized by the National Nosocomial Infections Surveillance program, is defined by three risk factors:[1]

- a contaminated or dirty wound;
- poor overall medical condition of the patient; and
- a prolonged operative time (longer than the 75th percentile for operations of the type).

Surgical incisions are classified as clean (class I), clean–contaminated (class II), contaminated (class III) or dirty (class IV). A poor overall medical condition of the patient is categorized by an American Society of Anesthesiologists (ASA) score of more than 2 (see Table 65.2). Prolonged surgery has implications for the degree of tissue injury, antibiotic pharmacokinetics and intraoperative repeat dosing, and it provides a prolonged opportunity for wound inoculation. An increased risk of SSI occurs with an increasing degree of wound contamination (e.g. clean wounds have less risk than contaminated wounds), regardless of other risk factors (Table 65.3),[21] and as the number of risk factors increases for a given type of operation (Table 65.4).

Antibiotic prophylaxis is indicated clearly for most clean–contaminated and contaminated (or potentially contaminated) operations. Dirty operations are those in which surgery and antibiotics represent treatment for an infection, not prophylaxis against it. An example of a potentially contaminated operation is lysis of adhesions for mechanical small bowel obstruction – intestinal ischemia cannot be predicted accurately before surgery, and the possibility exists of an enterotomy during adhesiolysis, which increases the risk of SSI twofold. An example of a clean–contaminated operation in which antibiotic prophylaxis is not always indicated is elective cholecystectomy. Antibiotic prophylaxis is indicated only for high-risk biliary surgery; patients at high risk include those over the age of 70 years, diabetic patients and patients whose biliary tract has recently been instrumented (e.g. during biliary stenting). The vast majority of patients who undergo laparoscopic cholecystectomy do not require antibiotic prophylaxis. Laparoscopic clean–contaminated operations are generally at decreased risk of infection.[1] The potential reasons are several, including a diminished surgical stress response, decreased tissue injury and smaller incisions.

Table 65.3 Incidence of surgical site infection as a function of wound classification

Traditional class	NNIS RISK INDEX				
	0	1	2	3	All
Clean	1.0%	2.3%	5.4%	NA	2.1%
Clean–contaminated	2.1%	4.0%	9.5%	NA	3.3%
Contaminated	NA	3.4%	6.6%	13.2%	6.4%
Dirty	NA	3.1%	8.1%	12.8%	7.1%
All	1.5%	2.9%	6.8%	13.0%	2.8%

NNIS, National Nosocomial Infections Surveillance Program; NA, not applicable (by definition, because the traditional wound classification is one of the risk factors, patients with clean wounds cannot have three risk factors, nor can those with dirty wounds have no risk factors).
From Martone & Nichols.[21]

Table 65.4 Surgical site infection percentage rates for selected procedures

Procedure	Time cutpoint (hours)	NUMBER OF RISK FACTORS			
		0	1	2	3
Coronary artery bypass graft (chest or leg)*	5	1.20	3.57	5.68	9.63
Laparotomy	2	1.71	3.29	5.16	7.77
Open reduction and internal fixation of fractures[†]	2	0.73	1.35	2.51	4.85

*Pooled incidence of surgical site infection for both incisions.
[†]Overall incidence.
From National Nosocomial Infections Surveillance System.[1]

Antibiotic prophylaxis of clean surgery is controversial. When bone is incised (e.g. in a craniotomy or sternotomy) or a prosthesis is inserted, antibiotic prophylaxis is generally indicated.

Choice of antibiotic

Most SSIs are caused by Gram-positive cocci. The most common pathogens are *Staphylococcus aureus*, followed by *Staph. epidermidis*, *Enterococcus faecalis* and *Escherichia coli*, the latter two of which are common pathogens after clean–contaminated surgery. The antibiotic chosen should be directed against staphylococci for clean cases and high-risk clean–contaminated elective surgery of the biliary and upper gastrointestinal tracts. A first-generation cephalosporin is the preferred agent for most patients, with clindamycin preferred for patients with a history of anaphylaxis to penicillin. Although methicillin-resistant *Staph. aureus* (MRSA) has been isolated in the community from never-hospitalized patients, vancomycin prophylaxis is appropriate only in institutions where the incidence of MRSA is high. In regions where community-acquired (CA-MRSA) is high, screening patients for MRSA carriage before selected, high-risk, elective surgical procedures (e.g. total hip arthroplasty, neurosurgery with ventriculoperitoneal shunt placement) may be appropriate so that attempts at decontamination of CA-MRSA prior to surgery can be initiated.

Elective colon surgery is a special circumstance and one in which practices are in evolution. Mechanical bowel preparation to reduce bulk feces made colon surgery safe for the first time. Antibiotic bowel preparation, standardized in the 1970s by the oral administration of nonabsorbable neomycin and erythromycin base, reduced the risk of SSI further to its present rate of approximately 4–8%, depending on the number of ASA risk factors. Although outpatient mechanical preparation is now the norm, three doses of oral antibiotics are still given to most patients at approximately 18, 17 and 10 hours preoperatively so that fecal bacterial counts are minimal at the time of surgery. A dose of parenteral second-generation cephalosporin (or a quinolone or monobactam plus metronidazole for the penicillin-allergic patient) is given before skin incision, and the benefit appears to be additive.[22] Moreover, there is less reticence to operate on the less-than-perfectly-prepared colon, extrapolating from good results from primary repair of penetrating colon injuries.

Timing and duration of parenteral antibiotics

It is firmly established that the optimal time to give cephalosporin prophylaxis is within 2 hours before the time the incision is made (Table 65.5).[23] Antibiotics given sooner (except possibly for longer half-life agents such as quinolones and metronidazole) are not effective, nor are agents that are given after the incision is closed. Antibiotics with short half-lives should be re-dosed during surgery if the operation is prolonged or bloody, and there is still some benefit if the initial antibiotic dose is given intraoperatively.

Considering the exigencies of surgical hemostasis and that the fresh surgical incision is ischemic, the postoperative administration of antibiotics is questionable owing to hypoperfusion that results from divided vessels. Single-dose prophylaxis should be standard. Other than in solid-organ transplant surgery, in which therapeutic immunosuppression has made 48-hour regimens standard, there is no indication for prolonged antibiotic prophylaxis.

Topical antiseptics and antibiotics may also help prevent SSI. A preoperative shower with an antiseptic soap (e.g. povidone–iodine) is a mainstay of perioperative preparation. Topical mupirocin ointment applied to the nares of patients who are chronic carriers of *Staph. aureus* reduces the increased incidence of SSI that is characteristic of chronic staphylococcal carriage.[15]

Prolongation of antibiotic prophylaxis beyond 24 hours not only provides no benefit, but can also be associated with a number of complications. *Clostridium difficile*-associated disease (CDAD) has been associated with disruption of the normal balance of gut flora and overgrowth of the enterotoxin-producing *C. difficile*. The incidence and severity of nosocomial CDAD is increasing.[24] The spectrum of disease is broad, ranging from asymptomatic to life-threatening pancolitis with infarction or perforation. Although virtually every antibiotic has been implicated in the pathogenesis of CDAD, even after administration of a single dose, prolonged antibiotic prophylaxis

Table 65.5 Risk of the development of surgical site infection relative to the timing of antibiotic prophylaxis

Timing	No. patients	No. (%) infections	RR (95% CI)	OR (95% CI)
Early	369	14 (3.8)*	6.7* (2.9–14.7)	4.3* (1.8–10.4)
Preoperative	1708	10 (0.59)	1.0	
Perioperative	282	4 (1.4)	2.4 (0.9–7.9)	2.1 (0.6–7.4)
Postoperative	488	16 (3.3)*	5.8* (2.6–12.3)	5.8* (2.4–13.8)
All	2847	44 (1.5)		

Early, administration more than 2 hours preoperatively; Preoperative, administration during the recommended interval (≤2 hours before skin incision); Perioperative, administration within 2 hours after the skin incision; Postoperative, administration more than 2 hours after the skin incision.
*$p <0.0001$ compared with preoperative group.
From Classen et al.[23]

clearly increases the risk. Prolonged prophylaxis also increases the risk of later nosocomial infections unrelated to the surgical site and the emergence of multidrug-resistant pathogens. Both pneumonia and catheter-related infections have been associated with prolonged antibiotic prophylaxis, as has the emergence of SSI caused by MRSA.[25]

ANTIBIOTIC PROPHYLAXIS OF TRAUMA-RELATED INFECTIONS

Traumatic injury is profoundly immunosuppressive and injured patients are at very high risk of infection. The overall incidence of infection after trauma is approximately 25%,[4,10,13] with infection of a wound (or an incision made as treatment) and nosocomial infection equally likely. Certain patterns of injury are independently associated with infectious morbidity in particular, including hemorrhagic shock, the need for blood transfusion, heavy wound contamination, central nervous system injury, colon injury, combined thoracoabdominal injuries, four or more organs injured, and increasing injury severity.[4] Co-morbid factors of importance include hyperglycemia, hypothermia and hypoxemia.

Certain characteristics of trauma make the situation more complex. Antibiotics are administered after injury, but there is a period when injured tissues may be vulnerable before antibiotics are administered. Trauma patients may be hypotensive and vasoconstricted owing to shock and tissue penetration may be decreased. Ongoing blood loss may result in ongoing antibiotic loss, especially if the agent is highly protein-bound and tissue redistribution is slow, or if the antibiotic is administered before major hemorrhage is controlled. Postinjury fluid shifts and hypoalbuminemia can cause major fluctuations in volume of distribution that can be difficult to estimate. As a result, it has been postulated that higher doses of antibiotics should be administered for the prophylaxis of post-traumatic infection, although controlled studies to support this contention are lacking.

Despite the high risk, the basic principles of antibiotic prophylaxis still apply – use a safe, narrow-spectrum agent for a defined brief period (no more than 24 hours), preferably one that has a limited role in the therapy of infection (e.g. a first- or second-generation cephalosporin).[4] Multiple studies indicate unequivocally that 24 hours of prophylaxis with a cephalosporin is all that is necessary following penetrating abdominal trauma, even in the presence of a colon injury and shock.[3,4] Other injuries in which appropriate antibiotic prophylaxis is beneficial include high-grade open fractures, animal bites and, possibly, chest injuries when an emergency tube thoracostomy is required.[3]

Following a human bite, the risk of infection is so high that 7–10 days of therapy with an agent effective against oral anaerobic flora is commonplace (see PP34). Injuries in which there is demonstrated to be no benefit of antibiotic prophylaxis include clean lacerations (even if primary repair is delayed) and skull fracture with or without leakage of cerebrospinal fluid.

Tetanus prophylaxis should be administered for high-risk wounds, such as soft tissue wounds with fecal contamination (e.g. injury caused by farm implements). If tetanus immune status is inadequate or unknown in high-risk wounds, administration of tetanus toxoid alone will be insufficient and tetanus immune globulin should be co-administered (see Chapter 21).

Prophylaxis of postsplenectomy sepsis is another special circumstance, albeit an increasingly rare one owing to the development of successful protocols for the nonoperative management of blunt splenic injuries. Postsplenectomy sepsis can be fulminating and lethal, and is most commonly caused by encapsulated organisms such as *Streptococcus pneumoniae* (see Chapter 82). The incidence is sufficiently low in adults (<1%) for long-term antibiotic prophylaxis not to be indicated. In infants and children where the incidence is higher, daily oral penicillin prophylaxis may be indicated (see Chapter 82 for details). Polyvalent pneumococcal vaccine is administered both to adults and to children, usually postoperatively, although the asplenic host has a blunted immune response to vaccination.

THE POSTOPERATIVE PERIOD

Several circumstances conspire to make fever the most common postoperative complication. A proinflammatory response follows tissue injury. Pulmonary defense mechanisms are impaired during anesthesia and recovery, and small-volume pulmonary aspiration of gastric contents unquestionably occurs. Wound hematoma is one of many known noninfectious causes of fever,[26] and other potential postoperative complications, including venous thromboembolic disease, pancreatitis, myocardial infarction, visceral ischemia and atelectasis, can also cause fever in the absence of infection. In this milieu it is challenging, but crucial, to distinguish inflammation from infection so as to treat patients appropriately. Confounding the evaluation of patients further is that hospitalized patients become colonized rapidly with potential pathogens.[27] Colonization is known to precede invasive infection. However, the high incidence of colonization, especially of the upper aerodigestive tract, makes it impossible to equate the mere isolation of a pathogen with the diagnosis of nosocomial infection, especially in critically ill patients.

Postoperative prophylaxis of infection

Surgical patients are at especially high risk of nosocomial infection. Judicious preoperative antibiotic prophylaxis decreases the risk of infection, but this prophylaxis in the absence of other techniques will not accomplish much. Proper infection control practice cannot be emphasized enough. The use of fast-drying alcohol gels for hand disinfection improves compliance, and can be used in the operating room and at the bedside.[26]

Surgery is invasive and surgical patients are often immunosuppressed owing to illness or injury;[10,13] the surgical stress response augments the immunosuppression. Many standard interventions impair host defenses (see Table 65.1). Surgical care must minimize the possibility of iatrogenic infection, while supporting the patient until host defenses can recover.

Catheters and drains should be removed as soon as possible. Each time a natural epithelial barrier to infection (e.g. skin, respiratory tract mucosa, gut mucosa) is breached, a portal is created for potential invasion of the host by pathogens. Subcutaneous drains increase the risk of SSI.[28] Prolonged central venous catheterization increases the risk of bacteremia; prolonged intubation and mechanical ventilation increase the risk of pneumonia. Moreover, prolonged urinary catheterization increases the risk of urinary tract infection. These devices should be removed as soon as feasible.[4] Improved catheter designs and endotracheal tubes (e.g. silver impregnated tubes and tubes that aspirate subglottic secretions via an extra lumen) might decrease the risk of nosocomial infection further.

Although cumbersome and therefore not popular, topical antiseptics and antibiotics appear to decrease the risk of nosocomial infection in seriously ill, high-risk patients. Data demonstrate that topical 0.12% chlorhexidine mouthwash (a bactericidal, viricidal and fungicidal antiseptic), applied to the oropharynx and the exposed surface of the endotracheal tube, decreases the incidence of postoperative pneumonia. Selective digestive decontamination, described in various forms nearly two decades ago, utilizes an oral paste of multiple antibiotics, enteral administration of the same antimicrobial agents by gavage and sometimes a short course of intravenous antibiotics. Infection rates are reduced unequivocally[27] and it may be appropriate in high-risk situations.

Prophylaxis of fungal infections is controversial. Although surgical patients are immunosuppressed and are frequently exposed to antibiotics, invasive fungal infections are unusual. Although *Candida* spp. are frequently isolated from the peritoneal fluid of patients with peritonitis, specific antifungal therapy is generally not indicated unless *Candida* spp. are isolated in pure culture from blood, from peritoneal fluid or from an abscess. Fungemia can be associated with indwelling central venous catheters, but on the rare occasions where fungemia complicates surgery (solid-organ transplant patients excepted), the patient is usually debilitated from a protracted serious illness and has already been exposed to multiple courses of antibiotics. Most surgical patients who are potential candidates for antifungal prophylaxis, apart from their routine use with organ transplant protocols, are those who become colonized with yeast at two or more sites (e.g. skin and urine). Empiric antifungal agents such as fluconazole are often used in this situation, despite convincing evidence of efficacy.[26] Fluconazole has numerous drug interactions (e.g. ciclosporin, macrolides, quinolones). Widespread use of fluconazole has been associated with the emergence of azole-resistant strains of *Candida*, especially *C. krusei*.[29]

Blood transfusion

In surgery and trauma, blood transfusions are given commonly and may be life-saving; alternatives to transfusions in the acute setting are few, but for hemodynamically stable postoperative patients hemoglobin concentrations >7 g/dl are well tolerated.[19] Erythropoietin administration may decrease transfusion requirements of the 'chronically critically ill' patient. An expanding body of evidence suggests that blood transfusion should be avoided, if possible. The immunosuppressive effects of allogeneic blood transfusions have been demonstrated in both solid-organ transplant recipients (in whom graft survival has been prolonged) and colon cancer surgery patients (in whom survival is decreased).

Observations that blood transfusions are associated with increased rates of nosocomial infection are numerous. Blood transfusions have been associated with an increased risk of infection following penetrating abdominal trauma independent of related factors such as shock or acute blood loss, and they have been related to increasing injury severity and increasing transfusion volume in unselected trauma patients. Data suggest that blood transfusion therapy of 6–20 units in the first 12 hours following multiple trauma is associated with an increased risk of nosocomial infection.[30] The risk of infection increased as the total transfusion volume increased, especially when units were transfused after more than 14 days of storage. The postulated 'storage lesion' is complex but includes changes in oxygen affinity, red blood cell deformability, shortened circulation time and the biologic consequences of cytokine generation and release. Recently, observational studies have suggested that transfusion of critically ill patients increases the risk of nosocomial infection,[31] and may worsen MODS and increase mortality.[32]

Hyperglycemia and control of blood sugar

Hyperglycemia has several deleterious effects on host immune function, most notably impaired function of neutrophils and mononuclear phagocytes. It is possible also that hyperglycemia is a marker of the catabolism and insulin resistance associated with the surgical stress response, and that exogenous insulin administration may ameliorate the catabolic state. Increasing evidence indicates that poor control of blood glucose during surgery and in the perioperative period increases the risk of infection and worsens outcome from sepsis. Diabetic patients have a higher risk of infection of both the sternal incision and the vein harvest incisions on the lower extremities.[8] Tight control of blood glucose by the anesthesiologist during surgery must be accomplished to decrease the risk, and that control must extend into the immediate postoperative period as well.

The need to manage carbohydrate metabolism carefully has important implications for the nutritional management of surgical patients. Gastrointestinal surgery may render the gastrointestinal tract unusable as a route for feeding, sometimes for prolonged periods. Ileus is common in surgical ICUs, whether from traumatic brain injury, narcotic analgesia, prolonged bed rest, inflammation in proximity to the peritoneal envelope (lower lobe pneumonia, retroperitoneal hematoma, fractures of the thoracolumbar spine, pelvis or hip) or other causes. Parenteral nutrition is relied on for feeding, despite evidence of a lack of efficacy[33] and the possibility of hepatic dysfunction; hyperglycemia

may be an important complication as well. Every effort should be made to provide enteral feeding, as substantial evidence indicates that enteral feeding reduces the risk of nosocomial infection by nearly one-half among critically ill and injured patients.[34]

The diagnosis of postoperative infection

The evaluation of a patient for possible infection usually begins with the report of a fever. The clinical response is too often the reflexive ordering of multiple cultures of various body fluids, even at times when the likelihood of infection and therefore the yield of the cultures is low. The only intervention mandated by new-onset fever is a history and physical examination.[26] All additional evaluations, whether radiologic or microbiologic, should be dictated by the findings of the evaluation at the bedside.[35] Fever related to infection in the immediate postoperative period (<48–72 hours after the operation) is rare unless the patient was operated upon for an active infection. The exception is necrotizing SSI caused by *Strep. pyogenes* or *Clostridium* spp., for which inspection of the incision is mandatory. The yield of blood cultures is known to be very low in the immediate postoperative period, and obtaining cultures to evaluate fever less than 72 hours postoperatively is not recommended.[26] After 72 hours, the possibility of nosocomial infection increases, but even then there is still the possibility that fever may be due to a noninfectious cause (e.g. venous thromboembolic disease, wound hematoma) and diagnostic rigor must be maintained. Overall, postoperative fever may be due to a noninfectious cause in as many as one-half of circumstances.[26]

Intra-abdominal infection

Intra-abdominal infection is a recognized complication following abdominal surgery. After an abdominal operation, an existing infection may persist or recur. Potential causes include severe illness, inadequate antibiotic dosing, resistant pathogens, inadequate source control, technical shortcomings, tissue ischemia and complete failure of intra-abdominal host defenses. Most patients with community-acquired intra-abdominal infections (e.g. secondary peritonitis from, for instance, appendicitis or diverticulitis) are infected by sensitive Enterobacteriaceae and anaerobic Gram-negative bacilli such as *Bacteroides fragilis*. Such patients rarely harbor multidrug-resistant pathogens; if surgery is required for a good-risk patient and is performed properly, the patient will usually recover regardless of which of several appropriate antibiotic regimens may be chosen.[36]

Source control is an emerging concept in the management of intra-abdominal infection.[35] Simply stated, adequate source control is the correct operation performed at the correct time in the correct manner. In practice, however, it is much more difficult to define. Whereas the surgical management of complicated appendicitis has relatively few permutations, this is not the case for complex entities such as perforated diverticulitis. Issues surrounding whether to resect, perform an anastomosis or a colostomy, or place drains make it impossible to declare that there is one 'correct' surgical approach, but it may be possible to describe management attributes that are clearly not appropriate. Studies suggest that source control is inadequate in approximately 10% of cases of complicated intra-abdominal infection; therefore, failure of source control is more likely as a cause of failure of treatment of intra-abdominal infection than any shortcoming of the antibiotic regimen.

In circumstances in which involvement of the peritoneal cavity is generalized and at least one source control procedure has failed to control a nosocomial intra-abdominal infection, the patient may be considered to have tertiary peritonitis.[37] Diffuse peritonitis, infected serosanguinous fluid rather than pus, poorly localized collections and isolation of enterococci, coagulase-negative staphylococci, yeast and *Pseudomonas aeruginosa* are characteristic. Local peritoneal host defenses are nonfunctional. The management of tertiary peritonitis is controversial. Some experts believe that the peritoneal cavity is colonized rather than infected, and that peritoneal toilet should be provided by daily saline lavage with the abdomen left open,[38] but randomized studies are nonexistent. What is clear, however, is that the typical mortality rate of about 30% is more than 10-fold higher than that usually reported for secondary peritonitis.

Ischemic enteropathies (e.g. acute pancreatitis, acalculous cholecystitis, ischemic colitis, ischemic hepatitis) can complicate the management of critical surgical illness. Patients have usually sustained a period of splanchnic hypoperfusion and the consequences can be devastating. Such patients usually manifest SIRS owing to tissue ischemia, and whether the patient is infected or becomes infected at some point can be very difficult to discern. Acute pancreatitis can complicate cardiopulmonary bypass or upper abdominal surgery (e.g. gastrectomy, splenectomy); most patients do not become infected and the administration of prophylactic antibiotics to patients with acute pancreatitis remains controversial.[26]

Outcomes of postoperative pancreatitis vary widely, depending on the severity of the attack. Acute acalculous cholecystitis has been reported as complicating virtually any operation but has a predilection for patients with trauma, burns, shock and emergency cardiac and peripheral vascular surgery.[39] The diagnosis is made most efficiently by bedside ultrasonography, and the treatment of choice is evolving to percutaneous cholecystostomy. The mortality rate of acute acalculous cholecystitis is approximately 30%.

Ischemic colitis is the most dangerous of these entities. The distribution and severity vary widely; sometimes the presentation can be as subtle as occult blood in the stool or an unexplained fever. When it does manifest itself, it usually does so within 72 hours of the insult that puts the patient at risk. The diagnosis is made most frequently by flexible lower gastrointestinal endoscopy but, because only the mucosa is inspected, endoscopy is not quantitative. Mild cases are probably noninfectious – there are no data to demonstrate that antibiotic therapy alters the course of mild ischemic colitis. Transmural colitis can lead to perforation; at worst, when severe ischemic colitis necessitates an emergency colectomy in the context of critical illness, the mortality rate may be as high as 80%.[40]

CT scan is probably the most useful modality for imaging the abdomen of seriously ill patients, particularly when there is substantial uncertainty as to the precise diagnosis. The benefits of imaging must be weighed against the formidable logistics and inherent risk of transporting a critically ill patient within the hospital for an imaging study. Moreover, it is possible to image the abdomen too soon (before about 7 days postoperatively) and thereby achieve a false-negative result. Fewer than one-half of abdominal-pelvic CT studies performed on critically ill patients yield meaningful information about diagnoses that are amenable to further intervention.[26]

Pneumonia

Although SSI is probably the nosocomial infection most closely associated with surgery, hospital-associated pneumonia (HAP) or specifically ventilator-associated pneumonia (VAP) is probably more common and certainly more dangerous. Long-term observational studies suggest that HAP is more common than SSI among surgical patients, and indicate clearly that the incidence of VAP is higher in surgical ICUs than in medical or pediatric ICUs.[1] In surgical subspecialty units (e.g. burns units, trauma units, neurosurgical units, cardiothoracic units), the incidence of VAP exceeds 15 cases/1000 days of mechanical ventilation (Table 65.6).[1] The increased incidence of VAP among surgical patients occurs despite comparable rates of mechanical ventilation in the ICU, which may reflect that intraoperative mechanical ventilation is not captured in ICU statistics if the patient is extubated early after surgery. However, surgical patients are at increased risk with respect to airway reflexes (because of anesthesia, analgesia and sedation), hypoventilation and atelectasis (because of the above factors plus painful chest or upper abdominal incisions), gastric intubation, ileus and numerous other factors. Trauma patients are at especially increased risk if they sustain a head or chest injury (e.g. pulmonary contusion, rib fractures) or are intoxicated with drugs or alcohol. The risk of VAP is increased

Table 65.6 Incidence of ventilator-associated pneumonia

Type of ICU	Ventilator utilization	Pooled mean	Median
Medical	0.49	7.3	6.0
Pediatric	0.45	4.9	3.9
Surgical	0.47	13.2	11.6
Cardiothoracic	0.47	10.5	9.5
Neurosurgical	0.38	14.9	11.9
Trauma	0.58	16.2	15.3
Burn	0.33	15.9	

Utilization, number of ventilator days per number of patient days; rates are per each 1000 days of indwelling artificial airway (e.g. endotracheal tube, tracheostomy tube).
From National Nosocomial Infections Surveillance System.[1]

by aspiration during endotracheal intubation, high severity of injury, blood transfusions, hyperglycemia, prolonged mechanical ventilation and the acute respiratory distress syndrome.

Meticulous infection control to minimize the spread of pathogens around the unit, minimized sedation, daily sedation 'holidays', keeping the head of the patient's bed at an angle of 30° at all times, antiseptic or antibiotic decontamination of the oropharynx, endotracheal extubation at the earliest possible opportunity, early tracheostomy if extubation cannot occur promptly, early enteral nutrition and meticulous pulmonary toilet, including continuous aspiration of subglottic secretions, can all be part of a comprehensive program for the prevention of pneumonia (see Chapter 28).[40]

Bloodstream infection

Bacteremia is an unusual complication of most surgical infections. Bacteremia accompanies only 8% of intra-abdominal infections overall, although less common infections such as ascending cholangitis are characterized by positive blood cultures in about 90% of cases. Clostridial bacteremia can complicate emphysematous cholecystitis or occult perforation or neoplasm of the gastrointestinal tract.[41] Surgical site infections have been described as potential sources of staphylococcal or enterococcal bacteremias,[42] and staphylococcal or pseudomonal bacteremia can complicate pneumonia caused by those organisms. Suppurative phlebitis, a bacteremic complication of infected vascular access sites, usually a peripheral intravenous site, is a rare but potentially serious form of postsurgical bacteremia.[43]

Catheter-related bloodstream infection is relatively uncommon in surgical units compared with medical or pediatric units, despite the high reliance on central venous access and monitoring (Table 65.7).[1] According to the US Centers for Disease Control and Prevention, the operator inserting a central catheter must wear a cap, mask and sterile gown and gloves for all insertion procedures and the operative field must be draped widely.[18] Central venous catheter insertion under emergency conditions (e.g. trauma resuscitation, cardiac arrest) almost always has lapses of infection control, and therefore catheters inserted under such conditions should be removed (and replaced at a different site, if needed) as soon as the patient has been stabilized.

PRINCIPLES OF ANTIBIOTIC THERAPY

The decision to start empiric antibiotic therapy in the surgical patient should be made with great care. An occasional patient will develop an early infection, but when it occurs it is usually the delayed

Table 65.7 Incidence of central line-associated bloodstream infections, National Nosocomial Infections Surveillance System, 1995–2001

Type of ICU	Central line utilization	Pooled mean	Median
Medical	0.51	5.9	5.2
Pediatric	0.46	7.6	6.8
Surgical	0.66	5.3	4.9
Cardiothoracic	0.79	2.9	2.4
Neurosurgical	0.44	4.7	4.5
Trauma	0.63	7.9	7.0
Burn	0.49	9.7	

Utilization, number of central venous catheter days per number of patient days; rates are per 1000 days of indwelling catheter.
From National Nosocomial Infections Surveillance System.[1]

manifestation of a community-acquired infection that was occult at the time of admission. In the case of pneumonia that develops within 3 days after surgery, the clinician must be alert to the possibility of a pneumococcal pneumonia. However, 'atypical' pneumonia is almost unheard of in surgical practice unless the patient is profoundly immunosuppressed, and so there is seldom a consideration to administer a macrolide antibiotic for that indication.

Early-onset HAP is more likely to be caused by antibiotic-susceptible strains of *Staph. aureus*, *Haemophilus influenzae*, *E. coli* and *Klebsiella pneumoniae*, whereas late-onset HAP and VAP are more likely to be caused by multidrug-resistant pathogens such as MRSA, *P. aeruginosa*, *Acinetobacter* spp. and others. Considering that *Staph. aureus* and *P. aeruginosa* are the two most common health-care-associated pneumonia pathogens, initial empiric antibiotic therapy must account for both pathogens, meaning two-drug anti-MRSA and anti-pseudomonal treatment in institutions with a high prevalence of MRSA, until targeted therapy is feasible based upon the microbiology laboratory findings.

Because the consequences of overtreatment (primarily later nosocomial infections with multidrug-resistant bacteria or opportunistic pathogens such as fungi) can be as severe as undertreatment, ongoing antimicrobial therapy should be reviewed every day in every patient with a bias to stopping treatment as soon as the patient improves. It may be possible to withhold or truncate antibiotic therapy by the use of a propensity score, such as the Clinical Pulmonary Infection Score.[44,45]

It has been hypothesized that 'antibiotic heterogeneity' – changing the pattern of antibiotic use either randomly by computerized decision support or by scheduled change of antibiotic class (e.g. antibiotic 'rotation' or 'cycling' programs) – may be a valid alternative to antibiotic control or restriction programs to prevent the emergence of multidrug-resistant bacteria. Initial data in surgical patients provide support for the 'cycling' hypothesis. Quarterly cycling of cefepime, ciprofloxacin, imipenem–cilastatin and piperacillin–tazobactam resulted in decreased use of aminoglycosides, vancomycin and antifungal agents.[46] Moreover, infections caused by resistant bacteria were reduced, as was mortality. It is not known which attribute or attributes (drug, order of administration, duration of cycle, omission of other drugs for potential empiric use) contribute to the effect. Further clinical studies will be needed to confirm the safety and effectiveness of such antibiotic usage strategies in the surgical patient.

REFERENCES

References for this chapter can be found online at http://www.expertconsult.com

Recreational infections

INTRODUCTION

At the end of the first decade of the 21st century we still eagerly await the arrival of the predicted age of leisure. However, even with major time pressures, people continue to spend their restricted leisure hours in more adventurous and imaginative ways. This chapter examines how these activities expose them to increased risks of infection and disease. Along with many other factors that predispose to clinical infection, recreational behavior may either expose the host to infective organisms or modify the immune response, thereby increasing susceptibility to infection and disease. Recreational infection can be classified by recreational activity or according to the particular infections (or systems infected – Table 66.1) Inevitably there is considerable overlap with other sections of this book, such as international medicine (see Chapters 101–128), sexually transmitted diseases (Chapters 57–60) and zoonotic infections (Chapter 164).

TRAVEL

Travel is a common recreational activity either as an end in itself or in order to participate in other recreations. Travelers may be exposed to infection either during the journey or at their destination. During travel there may be exposure to gastrointestinal pathogens in mass-produced

Table 66.1 Recreational activity associated with infection

Activity	Risk
Travel (especially 'adventure travel')	Infection during travel (gastrointestinal and respiratory pathogens) Geographic (tropical) infection
Animal contact: keeping pets, zoo/farm visits, etc.	Zoonotic infection
Outdoor activities: camping, trekking, barbeques, etc.	Zoonoses acquired by ingestion, inoculation, inhalation and arthropod transmission
Water contact: bathing, jacuzzi, canoeing, sailing, etc.	Ingestion, inoculation and inhalation
Contact sports: rugby, wrestling, football, etc.	Skin infection, blood-borne viruses
Vigorous exercise	Possibly respiratory infection

food or exposure to respiratory pathogens from air-conditioning units and fellow travelers. In addition, the general fatigue of long-distance travel may perhaps lower resistance to infection in a nonspecific manner.

Outbreaks of food poisoning from airline food occur frequently and are well described,[1] and even cholera has been transmitted in this way.[2] An estimated 4.5 million North Americans travel on cruise ships each year and a recent review has drawn attention to the incidence of respiratory and gastrointestinal infection associated with this activity. Outbreaks of gastrointestinal illness have been caused by contaminated food and water,[3] and in addition there have been descriptions of more prolonged outbreaks of infection associated with the possibility of person-to-person transmission and environmental contamination. This type of outbreak is usually thought to be due to viral infection with organisms such as astroviruses, caliciviruses (norovirus) and reoviruses (rotavirus). The classification of these gastrointestinal viral pathogens is complex and changes rapidly.[4-7] Historically, a number of bacterial infections including cholera and typhoid have been associated with ship-borne spread.

Respiratory infection, including multidrug-resistant pulmonary tuberculosis, has also been transmitted during aircraft flight,[8,9] and there is a well-recognized association between outbreaks of *Legionella* infection and air-conditioning systems in holiday hotels.[10]

Western travelers increasingly seek more exotic destinations where, as a result of poverty and poor infrastructure in the local population, they may be at risk of infection with common pathogens (particularly of the gastrointestinal and respiratory tracts). They may also be at risk of more exotic infections that do not exist in their own country (e.g. malaria). By the nature of the travel, the patient with infection often may not have access to the level of diagnostic and therapeutic interventions that would be regarded as standard in the developed world, so empiric treatment of presumed infections is often required. These risks are discussed in detail in Chapter 102.

ZOONOSES

Zoonoses are infections of animals which can be transmitted to humans, who may act either as a dead-end host or may propagate the infection further. The resulting infection may or may not be clinically apparent. This topic is addressed in Chapters 110, 119–128, 160 and 164 but issues specifically related to recreation are discussed here. Many leisure activities increase the opportunity for contact between humans and animals, with consequent increased risk of infection. Keeping pet animals is a common recreational pastime and increases risks of zoonotic infection.

Hiking and camping (particularly light-weight 'backpacking') increase the risk of zoonoses. People may hike in a temperate climate or, increasingly, may choose to trek in a tropical or developing country.

These activities increase the potential for contact with infected animals. Infection can then be transmitted by a number of possible routes, such as:

- inhalation (e.g. Q fever, anthrax);
- ingestion of contaminated food or water (e.g. *Salmonella*, *Brucella*, *Toxoplasma*);
- animal bites (e.g. rabies, skin infections);
- exposure of skin to contaminated water (e.g. leptospirosis, schistosomiasis, mycobacteria)
- exposure of skin to sand (e.g. strongyloides, cutaneous larva migrans and jigger flea); and
- via arthropod vectors (e.g. arboviruses, Lyme disease).

Zoonotic infection acquired by inhalation

Inhaled zoonoses that can be acquired by the intrepid outdoor explorer include Q fever (caused by *Coxiella burnetii*) and brucellosis (more commonly acquired by ingestion). Rarer problems include plague, anthrax, tularemia and psittacosis.[11]

Zoonotic infection acquired by ingestion

Many of the common 'food poisoning' organisms are zoonoses, and these are discussed in detail in Chapters 34 and 109. However, there are certain recreational activities that particularly expose participants to increased risks of ingesting pathogenic organisms (which are often zoonotic, although they may be exclusively human parasites). Backpackers drinking inadequately boiled or purified water may become infected with *Cryptosporidium* spp., *Giardia* spp., hepatitis A, *Aeromonas* spp. and *Salmonella* spp. Barbecues are particularly notorious for leading to inadequately cooked meat (or fish) and consequent infection with *Salmonella* spp.,[12] *Campylobacter* spp.[13] and other more exotic organisms such as *Trichinella* spp. There have been well-documented outbreaks of cryptosporidial infection in children enjoying recreational visits to farm open days.[14,15]

Arthropod-borne zoonoses

Viruses that must spend some of their life cycle in a blood-sucking arthropod are known as arboviruses (see Chapter 164). Over 200 such viruses have been identified and over 70 have been reported as affecting humans. In 1994, 100 cases of presumed or confirmed arboviral disease were reported from 20 states of the USA.[16] These were all encephalitis viruses (mainly Californian and St Louis encephalitis), principally spread by mosquitoes. In 2001 there was a large outbreak of West Nile virus in the Eastern USA with 48 human cases and numerous infections of birds (principally crows)[17] and West Nile virus is now seen throughout the USA and Southern Europe. Yellow fever is a life-threatening mosquito-borne, zoonotic viral infection and the illness remains a risk for travelers and residents during outdoor activities in endemic regions of Africa and South America. In Europe, tick-borne encephalitis is regularly reported from Austria and southern Germany.[18] A major risk factor is outdoor recreation (in particular, walking through long grass while wearing short trousers). An inactivated vaccine is available.

Tick-borne rickettsiae (see Chapters 122 and 176) are also potential pathogens among those who enjoy 'the great outdoors'.[19] They are mainly of the spotted fever group. In southern Europe, Africa and India, the disease is called tick typhus or boutonneuse fever and is caused by *Rickettsia conorii*. In the USA, it is Rocky Mountain spotted fever, caused by *Rickettsia rickettsii*. New rickettsioses identified during the past decade include Japanese spotted fever, Astrakhan fever, Flinders Island spotted fever, California flea typhus, African tick-site fever and *R. slovaca* infections in central France.

Scrub typhus may affect the trekker in eastern Asia. The infective organism is *Orientia tsutsugamushi*. The reservoir is rodents and the vector is the larva (chigger) of the trombiculid mite. Clinically the disease resembles other rickettsial infections, and prevention and treatment strategies are similar.

Lyme disease (see Chapter 43), caused by infection with *Borrelia burgdorferi*, is another condition that may be acquired by recreational exposure, especially in the northern hemisphere. The reservoir consists of mammals such as rodents and deer, with infection being spread by hard ticks (the *Ixodes ricinus* complex).

INFECTIONS CAUSED BY EXPOSURE TO WATER

A large number of infections can be caused by exposure to water (Table 66.2), and some of these have already been discussed in the section on zoonoses. Exposure to water can take place in a variety of recreational contexts. Trekkers and fishermen may wade through infected water, people may bathe in fresh water or sea water, and people may undertake other non-bathing recreational activities in water (e.g. water skiing, sailing, canoeing). There is also an increasing popularity of spa baths, whirlpool baths and jacuzzis.

As with arthropod-borne infections, infections related to water may be acquired by a number of routes, including ingestion, aspiration, inhalation of aerosols, and penetration of skin or mucous membranes by invasive organisms. A variety of clinical infections, including gastrointestinal infection, hepatitis, conjunctivitis, pneumonia, skin and soft tissue infection, may result, and numerous diverse organisms have been implicated.

Table 66.2 Infections spread via recreational contact with water

Mode of spread	Bacteria	Virus	Protozoa	Helminths
Fecal–oral spread (accidental ingestion)	*Escherichia coli* *Salmonella* spp. *Vibrio* spp. *Aeromonas* spp. *Shigella* spp.	Enteroviruses (including polio) Hepatitis A Norovirus	*Cryptosporidia* *Giardia* spp.	
Direct inoculation	*Leptospira* *Mycobacterium marinum* *Pseudomonas* spp. *Vibrio* spp. *Aeromonas* spp.		*Naegleria* *Acanthamoeba*	*Schistosoma*
Aerosol or aspiration	*Legionella* spp. *Pseudomonas*	Adenoviruses		

Pathogenic organisms may enter the water from exogenous sources such as human contamination (e.g. sewage), animal and bird contamination, and farm effluent. Organisms may also come directly from aquatic animals or protozoa or be free living in the water supply.

Infection associated with whirlpools

Jacuzzis, whirlpool baths and spa baths, which are increasingly found in leisure resorts, are all based on the principle of being bathed in warm water through which jets of water and bubbles of air are blown in order to produce feelings of relaxation and pleasure. They therefore share the potential for the transmission of cutaneous, mucosal and respiratory infection. The main pathogens implicated in these infections are *Pseudomonas aeruginosa* and *Legionella pneumophila*. *Pseudomonas* infections of the skin were initially described in the early 1980s.[20] The first reports were of folliculitis, but infection of wounds, eyes, ears and urinary tract have now been described.[21] Fatal *Pseudomonas* pneumonia in an immunocompetent male has been associated with jacuzzi exposure.[22]

Legionella spp. (mainly *L. pneumophila*, but other species are also implicated) cause two distinct syndromes:

- legionnaires' disease (or legionnaires' pneumonia), which is usually a severe pneumonic illness requiring appropriate antibiotic treatment; and
- Pontiac fever, which is generally a more benign self-limiting illness causing myalgia, fever and headache.

The latter syndrome has frequently been associated with whirlpool use, although a prolonged outbreak of legionnaires' pneumonia among cruise ship passengers associated with exposure to a contaminated whirlpool spa has been described.[23]

Infection from bathing

Numerous case reports and reviews have associated bathing in swimming pools, natural fresh water and the sea with gastrointestinal, respiratory and cutaneous infection. In swimming pools there have been reports of infection with *Shigella*, *Giardia* and *Cryptosporidium* spp., and various viruses including hepatitis A virus.[24]

The association of sea bathing and disease is a major political issue as millions of dollars are spent in the developed world in an effort to improve sewage disposal and enhance the quality of bathing water. Microbiologic standards now exist for bathing water in Europe and North America. There is certainly a risk of infection from swimming in heavily contaminated water but the risk of minor symptomatic infection from swimming in less heavily polluted water remains contentious.[25] In the 1950s the UK Public Health Laboratory Service used a case-controlled method and showed no link between polio and sea bathing.[26] Cabelli's classic work under the aegis of the US Environmental Protection Agency in the 1970s suggested a dose–response relationship between the microbiologic contamination of bathing water and self-reporting of gastrointestinal symptoms.[27] These studies have been criticized for looking at self-reported symptoms in self-selected groups, with no control for other risk factors for gastrointestinal symptoms.

More recently, a large UK study attempted to address these criticisms by randomizing holiday makers to be 'swimmers' or 'non-swimmers'.[28] This study showed a significantly higher rate of gastroenteritis in the swimmers and demonstrated a dose–response relationship between occurrence of symptoms and concentrations of fecal streptococci (although only with the concentration measured at chest height). Currently, coliform counts are used to assess water quality and the authors of the above study could not demonstrate a correlation between symptoms and the coliform count.

In addition to gastroenteritis, an Australian study showed increased reporting of respiratory, eye and ear symptoms amongst swimming beach-goers as opposed to non-swimming ones. The incidence of the reported symptoms increased with increasing levels of pollution.[29] The authors of the UK study have now published their results of non-enteric illness acquired during bathing and their results are in broad agreement with those of the Australian study.[30]

Infection in non-swimming recreational water activities

In addition to the hazards of bathing detailed above, many people are exposed to infection by recreational use of water where swimming is not the primary purpose. Such activities include angling, canoeing, water skiing, sailing and white water rafting.

Leptospirosis (see Chapters 124 and 171) is traditionally regarded as a significant risk. It is estimated that on average in the UK there are 5 million recreational water users each year exclusive of bathers, and yet among this at-risk population there are only 2.5 cases of leptospirosis a year.[31] The annual total incidence of leptospirosis in England and Wales is more than 10 times that figure; it occurs principally among agricultural workers. Leptospirosis is a zoonotic infection that is mainly carried by rodents. It is estimated that about 25% of the rats in UK are infected. The risk of contracting infection relates less to the overall water quality than to the density of the local rodent population. Triathlon and other forms of 'adventure racing' have also led to outbreaks of leptospirosis. Sejvar *et al.* described the outbreak that occurred during the 2000 'Eco-Challenge' event in Sabah, Borneo. Of 304 competing athletes, 42% met the case definition for leptospirosis.[32] The authors suggest that taking 200 mg of doxycycline weekly during exposure may limit infection and disease (a strategy previously demonstrated to be effective by the US military).

By the nature of the sport, canoeing involves high level exposure to water and, in addition to leptospirosis, other infections can be acquired. There is an increased incidence of gastrointestinal symptoms, and it has been shown that more than 50% of canoeists had experienced 'flu-like' symptoms shortly after canoeing.[33] An outbreak of blastomycosis has been reported amongst canoeists in Wisconsin rivers.[34]

Miscellaneous water-related infections

Naegleria and *Acanthamoeba* spp. are free-living amebae with no insect vector or human carrier state. They have been isolated on a worldwide basis from water and soil, and rarely can produce a severe amebic meningoencephalitis that is usually fatal (see Chapter 182). Schistosomiasis is dealt with in detail in Chapter 112. The cercariae of human schistosomes penetrate intact human skin and then migrate to their favored site to commence their maturation. Within 24 hours the penetration of the skin can produce a pruritic papular rash that is called 'swimmers' itch'. Avian schistosomes are found in temperate climates, including in the Great Lakes of North America, and although they are unable to mature past the cercarial stage in a human host and therefore cannot give rise to later stage schistosomiasis, they can be responsible for producing a significant 'swimmers' itch'.

Katayama fever occurs typically 4–8 weeks after infection and is associated with fever, chills, headache and cough. There is hepatosplenomegaly and lymphadenopathy, and usually a significant eosinophilia. It is caused both by *Schistosoma japonicum* and *S. mansoni*, the latter being particularly recognized in swimmers who have bathed in Lake Malawi and the other rivers and lakes of East Africa.

INFECTION SPREAD BY DIRECT CONTACT

Many sports require close physical contact on the sports field and may also involve close contact in the changing rooms with shared towels, shaving equipment, etc. Tetanus is caused by contamination of a wound by the spores of *Clostridium tetani*. After contamination, the organism then elaborates a toxin that produces the clinical syndrome of tetanus. Although immunization against tetanus is widely practiced, there is still a risk to those playing contact sports (especially rugby and football), as well as to those pursuing more leisurely activities such as gardening.

The close contact in the scrum of rugby football may transmit herpes simplex virus and cause a condition called scrumpox or herpes gladitorium. This is highly infectious and may spread rapidly between players. Aciclovir is effective treatment. Staphylococcal infection (including methicillin-resistant *Staphylococcus aureus*) may also be spread in similar circumstances.

The moist atmosphere of changing rooms may promote the transmission of respiratory infections as well as a number of cutaneous infections such as verrucas, athlete's foot (*Tinea pedis*) and dhobie itch (*Tinea cruris*). The spread of these tineal infections may be facilitated by sharing towels and washing equipment.

Gardening is usually considered a fairly safe pastime, but tetanus is a potential risk and sporotrichosis (see Chapter 179) can be acquired by scratches from rose thorns and similar injuries.

Blood-borne infection transmission in contact sport

The risk of transmission of blood-borne pathogens during contact sport is thought to be extremely low. There were large outbreaks of hepatitis amongst orienteers in Sweden from 1956 to 1966, and on the basis of the clinical and epidemiologic picture these were assumed to be due to hepatitis B virus (HBV), although a serologic test was not available.[35] As part of these outbreaks, 568 cases of hepatitis occurred between 1957 and 1963. Several modes of transmission were postulated, including twigs contaminated with infected blood inoculating subsequent competitors, contaminated water in stagnant pools and transmission during washing after competition. It was established that 95% of orienteers received scratches or wounds during the competition. The outbreak was curtailed by the introduction of regulations that banned competitors who had hepatitis from competing for 15 months and that specified compulsory protective clothing. More cases were reported when these regulations were relaxed. There has also been a report of an outbreak of HBV infection among sumo wrestlers in Japan.[36] There is one report from Italy of an HIV-positive football player transmitting infection to another player during a collision when both players were bleeding profusely,[37] but the risks are generally considered to be negligible.

Numerous guidelines exist to limit the risk still further.[36] In rugby football, for example, a player with an open or bleeding wound must leave the field until the wound is covered and the bleeding controlled.

EFFECT OF EXERCISE ON THE IMMUNE SYSTEM

Although it is clear from the above that recreational activity can expose participants to numerous infective agents that they might not otherwise encounter, it is by no means so obvious whether recreation (in particular, vigorous exercise) has any clinically significant effect on immune function.[38] There is increasing evidence that physical exercise may bring benefit in terms of cardiovascular health. However, the evidence from the immunologic perspective is less obvious.

There are numerous anecdotal reports of increased incidence of upper respiratory infection in athletes and there have been attempts to examine this systematically. However, despite numerous reviews there is no consistent association between physical activity and incidence of clinical upper respiratory infection. Nor has any consistent immunologic abnormality been demonstrated in high-level athletes. This inconsistency has many parallels with the situation in chronic fatigue syndrome, and many top athletes who have recurrent infections develop a clinical condition indistinguishable from chronic fatigue syndrome.

The overall message from anecdotal reports, from case-controlled studies of symptoms, from animal studies and from laboratory testing of immune function seems to be that moderate regular exercise enhances immunity whereas sudden unusual exertion or consistent, very high-grade training may have a deleterious effect. This is described as the 'J-shaped curve' correlating exercise and immunity.[38,39] Animal studies suggest that exercising before infection is beneficial, whereas exercising when infected is harmful. Some of the reported immunologic effects of exercise are listed in Table 66.3.

It is generally advised that people who are suffering from acute infections do not participate in vigorous exercise. This seems common

Table 66.3 Effects of exercise on the immune system

Symptoms/self-reported infections (anecdote and case-control)	Most studies suggest that moderate regular exercise reduces frequency and severity of upper respiratory tract infections but excessive training increases it Many studies are subjective and it may be that athletes are more aware of their symptoms than are controls Some increase in infection may be due to local factors such as mouth breathing rather than to any change in systemic immunity
Animal studies	Exhaustive exercise during experimental viral infection increases mortality and morbidity from that viral infection; the effect may be attenuated by exercise prior to infection Similar results have been shown in pneumococcal infection – exercise prior to infection protected against mortality but forced exercise after infection enhanced mortality
Immune function studies	Moderate exercise in HIV-positive people has been shown to produce some increase in CD4+ lymphocyte counts Excessive training in non-HIV-infected people has been shown to suppress CD4+ lymphocyte counts Heavy exercise decreases lymphocyte proliferation and levels of IgA; the decreased levels of IgA may correlate with increased incidence of upper respiratory tract infections Regular moderate exercise will increase levels of natural killer lymphocytes Exercise generally increases the release of proinflammatory cytokines and acute phase proteins

sense and most people would probably not feel like doing so, although definite evidence of harm remains contentious.

CONCLUSION

Recreational activities can expose participants to novel infectious agents that they are less likely to encounter in other contexts. In many of these the diagnosis may not be very obvious unless the condition is considered. Physicians need to add 'recreational history' to the already extensive list of travel, occupational and animal exposure details about which they need to enquire when evaluating a patient with a suspected infection. Whether recreational activity can alter immune function remains more controversial, although there seems to be increasing consensus that regular physical exercise may be of benefit but that excessive exercise may increase risks of infection.

REFERENCES

References for this chapter can be found online at http://www.expertconsult.com

Tar-Ching Aw
Iain Blair

Chapter | **67** |

Occupational infections

The traditional model of infectious disease causation is the epidemiologic triangle. It has three components: an external agent, a susceptible host and environmental factors that bring the host and the agent together to produce an infection.[1]

Occupational infections are defined by two of these components. Particular infectious agents or organisms may be associated with a workplace or occupational setting and specific work activities may predispose the worker to exposure, resulting in an occupational infection.

THE IMPORTANCE OF OCCUPATIONAL INFECTIONS

Although difficult to quantify, occupational infections are probably uncommon when compared to those that result from non-occupational activities or environments.

Infections can only be confidently attributed to occupational exposure as a result of careful epidemiologic investigation. Case reports, surveillance data and cross-sectional surveys may lead to a hypothesis that a particular infection is diagnosed more commonly in one or other group of workers. However, in order to accurately estimate an odds ratio or relative risk, a carefully designed, adequately powered, case-control or cohort study will be required. Assuming that bias and confounding factors can be adequately controlled, it may then be possible to satisfy the Bradford Hill criteria for causation. Few infections have been subject to this rigorous approach.

In the individual case where an occupational infection is suspected, it is important to take an adequate occupational history. A workplace visit to assess the system of work can help confirm the likelihood of the infection being acquired through workplace factors.[2] A high index of suspicion will ensure that occupational infections are not missed. If an occupational source is not recognized, there will be a continuing risk to other workers in the same work area, and the affected individual may be at risk of re-infection on return to work, especially if full immunity following the initial infection does not occur.

A number of occupational infections that are of historical interest in developed countries are still found in less developed parts of the world, and staff who are traveling to work in those areas may acquire these infections. As the working environment becomes ever more complex, there is the potential for new occupational infections to emerge.

Infections acquired occupationally may spread to other workers or the workers' families or social contacts. As with any infection, occupational infections are controlled by controlling the source of infection, its route of transmission and by protecting susceptible persons. Most occupational infections can be prevented if appropriate measures are implemented. Some occupational infections, especially those for which vaccines are available (e.g. hepatitis B), are more amenable to prevention than others (e.g. hepatitis C). Health education and preventive programs in the workplace provide a good system for minimizing the risk of occupational infections. The largest employer in the United Kingdom – i.e. the National Health Service – has a requirement for every health-care facility to have access to an occupational health service. This has helped in reducing the burden of occupationally acquired infections in the health-care community.[3] The system is not as well developed in other industries where there is a recognized risk of occupational infections (e.g. in farming).

This chapter is written from a United Kingdom perspective and describes the arrangements and structures for public health and occupational health practice that will be found in the UK. Similar arrangements can be expected in most industrialized countries. For example, the US Centers for Disease Control and Prevention (CDC) have published guidelines for preventing the transmission of infectious diseases in the health-care workplace. These are available at http://www.cdc.gov/ncidod/dhqp/worker.html.

The US National Institute for Occupational Safety and Health (NIOSH), which is part of CDC, has published research and recommendations on most aspects of work-related injury and illness including infections (see http://www.cdc.gov/niosh/topics/diseases.html).

The Australian Safety and Compensation Council (ASCC) provides policy advice on all aspects of occupational health and safety to allow local legislators to enact and enforce laws. A recent ASCC report focuses on the more common and important infections associated with occupations in Australia.[4]

CLASSIFICATION OF OCCUPATIONAL INFECTIONS

Mode of transmission, occupations and examples of infections are outlined in Table 67.1.

SURVEILLANCE OF OCCUPATIONAL INFECTIONS

Surveillance of occupationally acquired infection is problematic. A range of data sources are available. The examples described here are from the United Kingdom but similar systems may be found in other countries.

It is a legal requirement for clinicians to notify certain specified infectious diseases to local health authorities. The current list of notifiable infections for the UK covers common infections (including viral hepatitis and tuberculosis) that may be occupationally acquired, as well as rarities such as leptospirosis, rabies and anthrax. Microbiology laboratories also report micro-organisms of public health significance to local health authorities. Outputs from these surveillance schemes can be viewed at http://www.hpa.org.uk/infections/topics_az/noids/menu.htm.

Table 67.1 Occupational infections

Mode of transmission	Occupations	Examples of infections
Contact with animals and animal products (zoonoses)	*Source of infection and route of transmission:* Contact with material from infected animals, by inhalation, ingestion, bite or scratch Contact with contaminated animal product (carcasses, placental tissue, hair, wool or hides) from endemic area Contact with animal excreta by fecal–oral or percutaneous route or in water *Occupation types:* Farm worker[1] Poultry worker Veterinarian Butcher Slaughterman Wool and leather worker Zoo worker Animal handler Sewage worker	*Salmonella* Cryptosporidiosis *Escherichia coli* O157 *Campylobacter* *Yersinia* Brucellosis Leptospirosis Q fever Psittacosis Ovine chlamydia Cat-scratch fever Pasteurellosis *Capnocytophaga canimorsus* Anthrax Rabies *Echinococcus* Schistosomiasis Avian influenza Newcastle disease *Streptococcus suis* B-virus infection Monkeypox Glanders Hendra and Nipah viral diseases Rat bite fevers Rodents main reservoir, transmission by inhalation of excreta: • arenaviral hemorrhagic fevers • hantavirus infection • lymphocytic choriomeningitis • Lassa fever Exposure to sewage is not a risk factor for *Helicobacter pylori* or hepatitis A or E viruses in sewage workers who are properly trained and provided with personal protective equipment[2,3]
Exposure to vectors	*Source of infection and route of transmission:* Exposure to tick, flea, or mites through work in infested area or in rodent-infested building *Occupation types:* Farm worker Forestry worker Overseas worker Pest control worker	Borrelia infections (Lyme disease, relapsing fever) Babesiosis Ehrlichiosis Tularemia Plague Scrub typhus Typhus Tick-borne rickettsial infections Bartonella infection Arthropod-borne viral fevers (Over 100 arboviruses cause disease in humans, often as an incidental host in a zoonotic cycle. Infection can occur in those working in endemic areas and also through laboratory exposure) (see Chapter 164)
Care of patients	*Source of infection and route of transmission:* Contact with patients, respiratory or blood-borne Contact with human excreta Skin-to-skin contact with infected patient	HIV Hepatitis B Hepatitis C Staphylococcal infection, e.g. methicillin-resistant *Staphylococcus aureus* (MRSA), Panton–Valentine leukocidin (PVL)

Table 67.1 Occupational infections—cont'd

Mode of transmission	Occupations	Examples of infections
	Occupation types: Health-care worker[4,5] Dental worker Embalmer Teacher[6] Sewage worker Laboratory worker	Typhoid/paratyphoid Hepatitis A Cryptosporidiosis Norovirus Tuberculosis Mycoplasma infection Scabies West Nile virus infection[7] Influenza Measles Mumps Meningococcus Parvovirus[8] Cytomegalovirus[9] There is some evidence that working in a child day-care centre is associated with higher seroprevalence of antibodies to cytomegalovirus infection but not erythrovirus (formerly parvovirus) B19 infection, although both of these infections are common in the general population[10] Pertussis Varicella Rubella Adenovirus Diphtheria Ebola–Marburg viral infection Lassa fever Monkeypox Severe acute respiratory syndrome (SARS)
Environmental sources, exposure to soil	*Source of infection and route of transmission*: Ploughing, digging or excavating soil in endemic area Contact with dust containing rodent feces, bird roosts, chicken coops or bat-inhabited caves in endemic area *Occupation types*: Building cleaning worker Construction worker Archaeologist	Tetanus Listeria Histoplasmosis Coccidioidomycosis Paracoccidioidomycosis Blastomycosis Hookworm
Occupational skin infections	*Source of infection and route of transmission*: Cleaning pools or aquarium Dental work in patients' mouths Barefoot contact with contaminated soil in endemic area Working continuously with wet hands Touching infected farm animals, plants containing thorns, splinters or sphagnum moss, infected meat or poultry, infected fish or shellfish *Occupation types*: Dental worker Farm worker Veterinarian Florist Slaughterer Butcher Fisherman Aquarium worker	Orf Ringworm Herpetic whitlow Erysipeloid *Mycobacterium marinum* skin infection Viral warts *Candida paronychia* Chromomycosis Cutaneous larva migrans Sporotrichosis *Vibrio vulnificus* infection Cutaneous anthrax

In neither of these systems is the occupation of the case requested or recorded. Local and national health authorities may enhance the data that are collected as part of case investigation and management, and this may include occupation and other relevant risk factors. However, such additional data are not consistently collated, analyzed or disseminated and, when available, are susceptible to ascertainment and reporting bias.

To overcome these shortcomings, active surveillance of selected occupationally acquired infections is carried out by the Surveillance of Infectious Diseases at Work (SIDAW) Project at the University of Manchester. Data are contributed by local public health staff each month. Most reports relate to diarrheal disease and scabies in health-care workers but legionellosis, tuberculosis and cutaneous anthrax have been reported.

Other occupational surveillance schemes also occasionally report occupational infections. Outputs from these surveillance schemes can be viewed at http://www.hse.gov.uk/statistics/indexoftables.htm.

Acute illnesses due to biologic agents encountered during a specified work activity – for example Lyme disease, Q fever, rabies, *Streptococcus suis*, tetanus, tuberculosis, anthrax, brucellosis, avian chlamydiosis, ovine chlamydiosis, hepatitis, legionellosis and leptospirosis – are reportable to the Health and Safety Executive under Reporting of Injuries, Diseases and Dangerous Occurrences Regulations 1995 (RIDDOR 95).[5] This legal requirement to notify is intended to provide information on trends and to facilitate prevention. More information and links to outputs can be viewed at http://www.hse.gov.uk/statistics/sources.htm. Reports on infections are infrequent.

The Industrial Injuries Disablement Benefit (IIDB) Scheme provides benefits to employees if they develop a prescribed occupational disease. Diseases are prescribed when there is a recognized risk to workers in an occupation and where the risk is uncommon or absent in the general population. For some occupational diseases there is a strong association with occupation and the disease may rarely occur outside work (e.g. mesothelioma, coal miner's pneumoconiosis). However, most infections are common in the general population and it is difficult to establish a causal link with the occupation. In lay terms an infection will be attributed to an occupation if it is *more likely than not* to be caused by that occupation. In epidemiologic terms this means an attributable fraction (the proportion of the additional risk that can be attributed to the exposure in the exposed population) of 50% or more which equates to a relative risk of 2 (a doubling of the background risk caused by exposure).

Prescribed infections include:

* anthrax where work involves contact with animals infected with anthrax, or the handling of animal products or residues;
* glanders where work involves contact with equine animals or their carcasses;
* leptospirosis where work involves places liable to be infested by rodents or other small mammals, handling dogs, or contact with pigs or bovine animals or meat products;
* hepatitis A virus infection where work involves contact with raw sewage; and
* hepatitis B or C virus infection where work involves contact with human blood products or other sources.

Ancylostomiasis where work involves work in or about a mine is included in the list of UK prescribed diseases, although there is scant evidence that mining carries an increased risk of hookworm infestation. Earlier observations indicated a risk of anemia in Cornish tin miners, attributed to a lack of toilet facilities in the mines leading to spread of hookworm infestation.[6] Interestingly, this risk was not seen in coal mines. It has also not been reported as a risk in tin mines in other countries (e.g. Malaysia), even though hookworm infestation in the tropics is prevalent. The methods used for tin mining in different countries can, however, be different.[7] Most of the coal mines and tin mines in the UK are now closed, although ancylostomiasis remains on the prescribed diseases list. A complete list of prescribed infections can be viewed at http://www.dwp.gov.uk/advisers/db1/appendix/appendix1.asp.

The UK Labour Force Survey (LFS) is a national survey of 52 000 households on self-reported work-related illness. THOR-GP is a UK-wide surveillance scheme in which 270 participating general practitioners report cases of work-related ill health. Participants make a judgment as to whether a new case should be attributed to work on the balance of probabilities. Additional information and links to outputs can be viewed at http://www.hse.gov.uk/statistics/sources.htm. Again, reports on infections are infrequent.

PREVENTION AND CONTROL OF OCCUPATIONAL INFECTIONS

The control of any occupational infection requires a detailed knowledge of its epidemiology, clinical features, reservoir, mode of transmission, incubation period and communicable period. To prevent and control infection, measures are necessary to eliminate the source of infection and the route of transmission. Susceptible workers can be offered protection with antibiotics or immunization.

The Control of Substances Hazardous to Health (COSHH) Regulations 2002 require employers to assess the risks from exposure to all hazardous substances (including biologic agents) and to implement measures to protect workers and others from those risks as far as is reasonably practicable.[8] Following a workplace risk assessment, exposure to potential infection should be eliminated by changing working practices and removing hazardous products or waste. Residual risk is controlled by promoting good occupational hygiene and environmental hygiene, and by focusing on design and engineering controls. Staff training and provision and use of personal protective equipment (PPE) are key measures (Table 67.2).

Table 67.2 Control of occupational infection

Controlling the source of infection	In the case of zoonoses, best practice should be observed with respect to animal husbandry, biosecurity of animal houses, feed and water, hygiene of animal houses and equipment, inspection, testing and certification and quarantine. Codes of practice are available and some of these are backed by legal measures In the case of human sources, prompt action is needed to isolate the case while infectious and to treat if possible to render the case noninfectious.
Controlling the route of transmission	Guidelines are available which detail the measures that should be implemented to prevent transmission, including handwashing and use of appropriate personal protective equipment. In the health-care workplace, standard precautions are widely promoted in addition to enhanced measures for specific infections
Protecting susceptible workers	Antibiotic or antiviral chemoprophylaxis may be required. All staff should be up to date with their routine immunizations (tetanus; diphtheria; polio; measles, mumps and rubella). Immunization is cost-effective for some groups of workers, particularly health-care workers and laboratory workers. Health warning cards may be issued to at-risk workers

Immunization

All workers should be fully immunized according to the routine immunization schedule.[9] In UK this comprises diphtheria; tetanus; pertussis; polio; measles, mumps and rubella (MMR); *Haemophilus influenzae* b (Hib); meningitis C (MenC) and pneumococcal vaccines. See: http://www.immunisation.nhs.uk/Immunisation_Schedule for further details.

In addition, selective immunization may be recommended for groups of workers at increased risk[10] (Table 67.3).

Immunization for laboratory and pathology staff

Laboratory and pathology staff handle pathogens or potentially infected specimens, and mortuary staff are potentially exposed to infected cadavers.[11] Other laboratory personnel include cleaners, porters and administrative staff. Guidelines for morticians and embalmers can be viewed at http://www.hpa.org.uk/webw/HPAweb&HPAwebStandard/HPAweb_C/1200660060264?p=1200660029736.

All staff should have had all routinely recommended immunizations, which in the UK include tetanus, diphtheria, polio, MMR and MenC. Staff handling fecal specimens who may be exposed to polio viruses should have a reinforcing polio immunization every 10 years. Staff who may be exposed to diphtheria should have antibody levels tested 3 months after immunization. The recommended level is 0.01 IU/ml for those involved in routine diagnostic testing and 0.1 IU/ml for those exposed to toxigenic strains. A reinforcing dose is recommended every 10 years. Additional recommendations for laboratory and pathology staff are summarized in Table 67.4.

Table 67.4 Immunization of laboratory and pathology staff against specific occupational infections

Bacille Calmette–Guérin (BCG)	Recommended for microbiology and pathology staff, mortuary staff and others at high risk
Hepatitis B	Recommended for laboratory staff who have direct contact with patients' blood or tissues. Antibody levels should be checked after immunization
Hepatitis A, Japanese encephalitis, cholera, meningococcal serogroups A, C, Y, W135, smallpox, tick-borne encephalitis, typhoid, yellow fever, influenza, varicella, anthrax, rabies	Recommended for staff handling or carrying out research on specific organisms and those working in reference laboratories or infectious disease hospitals

Table 67.3 Immunization for groups of workers at increased risk

Immunization	Occupational groups
Anthrax	Those handling imported infected animal products or working with infected animals
Cholera	Relief or disaster aid workers
Diphtheria, polio, tetanus	Laboratory and health-care workers who may be exposed in the course of their work in laboratories and clinical infectious disease units
Hepatitis A	Laboratory workers who work with hepatitis A virus, staff of large residential institutions for those with learning difficulties, sewage workers, people who work with primates Consider for food packagers and handlers, staff in day-care facilities and some other categories of health-care workers based on risk assessment
Hepatitis B	Health-care workers in the UK and overseas, including students and trainees who have direct contact with patients' blood or tissues, laboratory staff who handle material that may contain the virus, staff of residential accommodation for those with learning difficulties, morticians and embalmers, prison service staff in contact with prisoners Consider for other staff groups such as the police and fire and rescue services based on risk of exposure
Influenza	Health and social care staff directly involved in patient care
Japanese encephalitis	Laboratory staff who may be exposed to the virus
Measles, mumps, rubella (MMR)	Health-care staff should be immune to measles, mumps and rubella for their own benefit and also to prevent them from spreading infection to patients
Rabies	Pre-exposure immunization should be offered to laboratory workers handling the virus, those who may handle imported animals, people who regularly handle bats in the UK, those working abroad whose work may bring them into contact with rabid animals and health-care workers who may be exposed to body fluids from a patient with rabies
Smallpox	Workers in laboratories where pox viruses (such as monkeypox or genetically modified vaccinia) are handled. Not recommended for people exhuming bodies in crypts
Tick-borne encephalitis (TBE)	In endemic areas recommended for those engaged in forestry, woodcutting, farming and the military. Recommended for laboratory workers who may be exposed to TBE
Tuberculosis	Bacille Calmette–Guérin (BCG) recommended for unvaccinated, tuberculin-negative persons aged under 35 with increased risk of exposure to persons with tuberculosis, including health-care workers, laboratory staff, veterinary and abattoir workers (who may handle infected animal species), prison staff, staff of care homes, staff of hostels for homeless people and refugees

Table 67.5 Selected infections with occupational significance

Infection	Description of infection in humans and public health importance	Risk factors, source and route of transmission	Surveillance/occurrence	Prevention and control
Brucellosis	Zoonosis. Acute febrile illness, fever or unknown origin or chronic bone or joint infection	Different species found in goats, sheep, cattle, pigs, dogs Contact with infected animals, animal tissues or consumption of unpasteurized milk Infectious aerosols occur in abattoirs No human-to-human spread	Approximately 20 cases reported annually in England and Wales (E&W) in recent years but still common worldwide Farmers and veterinarians at risk Prevalence of *Brucella* antibodies is elevated in Tanzanian abattoir workers[11]	Eliminate infection from domestic animals by testing, slaughter and immunization Pasteurize milk Precautions for those handling infected animals No immunization for humans
Varicella	Viral infection producing characteristic rash Occurs mainly in children; may have serious sequelae in adults, pregnancy and the immunocompromised	Direct and respiratory spread from human cases	Common; epidemics every 1–2 years 90% of adults are naturally immune as a result of childhood infection	Health-care staff with varicella and nonimmune health-care staff who have been exposed to varicella require active management to prevent spread to vulnerable patients Immunization is available and may be used universally or selectively In E&W varicella immunization is recommended for susceptible health-care workers who have direct contact with patients
Human seasonal influenza	Acute viral respiratory illness caused by influenza A or B viruses New strains may produce winter epidemics of varying size and severity Outbreaks can occur in hospitals, schools, prisons and other closed communities High attack rate with potential for staff absenteeism	Spread by respiratory secretions from human cases by large droplet or direct spread. Spread by airborne aerosol may also occur	Worldwide distribution In the UK in recent years primary care consultation rates for influenza-like illness have peaked at about 30/100 000 per week in January or February. In epidemic years rates may be 200/100 000 per week or higher	Affected staff should stay away from work during the infectious period (approximately 5 days in adults) Hygiene measures may reduce spread through coughing and contaminated hands and environmental surfaces. Guidelines on PPE should be followed Vaccines active against prevalent strains are manufactured each year and are used selectively Antivirals are available for treatment and prophylaxis and guidelines on their use have been published Annual immunization is recommended for health-care workers directly involved in patient care
Avian influenza	Zoonosis mainly affecting wild waterfowl and domestic poultry, caused by avian strains of influenza A virus Potential for transformation of avian strains into new human pandemic strain by genetic intermixing with seasonal human strains	Spread to humans occurs rarely through close contact with material from affected poultry or other birds Disease may be a severe respiratory illness (H5N1) or conjunctivitis (H7N2, H7N3)	Since 2003, H5N1 has been endemic in poultry worldwide The disease is rare in humans, albeit with a high case-fatality rate. To date 14 countries have reported 361 human cases of H5N1 with 221 deaths	Avian influenza is controlled in poultry by surveillance, testing and culling affected flocks Workers involved in culling activities should be provided with appropriate PPE; they should receive antiviral prophylaxis, seasonal influenza immunization and medical follow-up Detailed guidelines are available http://www.hpa.org.uk

Pandemic influenza	Global pandemics of influenza A occurred in 1918, 1957 and 1968 with high attack rates and significant morbidity and mortality, with effects on health services and other national infrastructure	Until a new pandemic strain emerges it is not possible to predict how it will behave in terms of attack rate, virulence and clinical features. The World Health Organization and most national governments have published planning assumptions based on experience from previous pandemics	In the UK, planning assumptions are for a 50% clinical attack rate, with an initial wave lasting about 15 weeks with the peak in weeks 6 and 7, when 22% of cases will occur each week	In the UK, services are planning for business as usual for as long as possible. Persons with influenza will be urged to stay at home, cough etiquette and enhanced hygiene will be encouraged, all affected persons will receive a course of antiviral treatment, business continuity plans will mitigate the effects of absenteeism, nonessential services will be suspended, social distancing measures may be introduced. National strategic plans and detailed guidance can be viewed at http://www.dh.gov.uk
Hepatitis B and C viruses[12]	Hepatitis B is an acute viral infection of the liver. The initial illness may be severe and a chronic carrier state may develop, leading after some years to cirrhosis and hepatocellular carcinoma. Hepatitis C is also a viral infection of the liver. The initial illness is often asymptomatic but 80% of those infected develop chronic infection that may result in cirrhosis and hepatocellular carcinoma	Human cases and carriers are the source of infection and transmission is by the blood-borne route. Hepatitis B is also transmitted by the sexual route and vertically from mother to infant. Health-care workers and laboratory staff who are exposed to blood and tissues from infected patients are at risk. Other groups of workers such as tattooists and body piercers may also be at risk. Nigerian butchers had an HBsAg seroprevalence rate of 9.4% compared with 3.3% in a control group[13]. In the UK there is a reporting system for occupational exposure to blood-borne viruses	The incidence of acute hepatitis B in Europe varies from 1 to 30 per 100 000 per year. The prevalence of chronic infection varies from <1–2%. Some seroprevalence studies have suggested a higher prevalence in health-care workers but this may be explained by confounding factors such as ethnicity and country of origin rather than risk of occupational exposure. Reliable estimates of hepatitis C incidence are not available. Prevalence of past infection in the UK is 0.1% in blood donors and 0.2% in health-care workers. In the UK there have been 11 cases of hepatitis C seroconversion in health-care workers following percutaneous exposure	Some groups of patients are screened for evidence of infection. Standard infection control precautions should be followed (including use of PPE and safe handling of needles and sharp instruments). Hepatitis B vaccination is recommended for health-care workers who may have direct contact with patients' blood or body fluids. It is also recommended for workers who are at risk of injury from blood-contaminated sharp instruments, or of being deliberately injured or bitten by patients. Guidelines are available. Guidelines are also available for the management of health-care workers who have had percutaneous exposures. Infection may spread from health-care workers to patients and for this reason pre-employment screening has been introduced in some countries

Continued

Table 67.5 Selected infections with occupational significance—cont'd

Infection	Description of infection in humans and public health importance	Risk factors, source and route of transmission	Surveillance/occurrence	Prevention and control
Human immunodeficiency virus[14]	A chronic viral infection which leads to depletion of CD4 lymphocytes and immunosuppression resulting in AIDS	Humans are the source of infection and spread is by the blood-borne, sexual or vertical route. Health-care workers and laboratory staff who are exposed to blood and tissues from infected patients are at risk	The incidence of HIV infection in the UK is not known. The cumulative incidence of HIV infection in mid-2007 was about 90 000 and there are about 7500 new diagnoses each year	Standard infection control precautions should be followed (including use of PPE and safe handling of needles and sharp instruments). Postexposure prophylaxis (PEP) with antivirals is recommended for health-care workers who may have contact with HIV-infected patients' blood or body fluids. Guidelines are available
			The prevalence of anti-HIV varies depending on the population subgroup that is tested. In pregnant women in the UK the prevalence is between 0.5% and 5%. In the UK there have been five reports of HIV seroconversion following percutaneous exposure in health-care workers	Spread of infection from an HIV-infected health-care worker to a patient has been reported and in some countries HIV-infected health-care workers are not permitted to carry out exposure-prone surgical procedures. Guidelines are available
Tuberculosis (TB)	Infection of lungs and other organs with Mycobacterium tuberculosis or rarely other species including Mycobacterium bovis. TB can cluster in health-care settings and other closed communities	Transmission is by inhalation of respiratory droplets from an infectious case. Bovine TB may be contracted by consumption of milk from or contact with an infected animal	In 2006 in E&W there were 8051 cases of TB. Regional rates vary from 5 to 45 per 100 000 per year. Health-care workers have twice the expected incidence of TB, allowing for age, sex and ethnic factors[15]	Infection control procedures should be followed. BCG vaccine is recommended for health-care workers who may have close contact with infectious patients but not for nonclinical staff. Guidelines are available
Leptospirosis	Zoonosis with wide clinical spectrum caused by one of many serovars of Leptospira	Many different animal reservoirs. Transmission is percutaneous from urine of affected animals	In 2006 there were 44 laboratory-confirmed cases in E&W. Most cases were recreational but seven were farmers, all of whom reported contact with livestock or rats. Other risks included clearing streams or drains	Those at risk should use appropriate PPE. Guidelines are available
Anthrax	Infection in humans affects skin, respiratory and gastrointestinal tract	Spread from infected animals by spores of Bacillus anthracis through contact with animals or animal products. Spores survive in the environment	Rare. Nineteen cases reported in the UK in 1975–96 in workers handling imported infected animal products or working with infected animals	Control anthrax in livestock and disinfect imported animal products. Processing of products reduces risk of infection; bone meal used as fertilizer should be sterilized; PPE should be used. Immunization is available for those at risk

Ovine and avian chlamydiosis (psittacosis)	Zoonosis. Potentially serious respiratory and systemic infection caused by *Chlamydophila psittaci*	Spread from psittacine birds (parrots etc.) and other mammals which may be asymptomatic by inhalation of aerosols of bird dropping and other material from infected species. Human-to-human spread is very rare	Worldwide distribution 100 cases reported in E&W each year	Affected birds should be quarantined, treated or culled. Caution is required when handling birds and cleaning cages
Avian and ovine chlamydiosis	Zoonosis. Respiratory infection and may lead to miscarriage in pregnancy, caused by *Chlamydophila abortus*	Spread by inhalation of aerosols from infected and aborting sheep. Cattle and goats may also be affected	Worldwide distribution, particularly in sheep-rearing countries. Commonest cause of infectious abortion in sheep in the UK but human infection is rare (1–2 cases per year in E&W)	Pregnant women should not help to lamb or milk ewes; they should avoid contact with aborted or newborn lambs (and placenta) and should not handle clothing that has been in contact with ewes or lambs. A live vaccine for use in sheep is available. This should not be handled by pregnant women or women of child-bearing age
Diarrheal disease	There are many causes of infectious intestinal disease. Some are zoonoses, others have only human reservoirs	Transmission is by the direct or indirect fecal–oral route.	Refer to surveillance data for specific infections. http://www.hpa.org.uk/infections/topics_az/gastro/menu.htm. Norovirus infection is a common occupational infection amongst health-care staff	Infection control procedures should be followed, including handwashing and use of PPE Guidelines are available
Methicillin-resistant *Staphylococcus aureus* (MRSA)	A spectrum of infection from minor skin infection to life-threatening bacteremia caused by methicillin-resistant *S. aureus*	The reservoir is colonized or infected humans. Spread is direct on hands, fomites, equipment or the environment. Acquisition of MRSA infection has been described as result of occupational contact with pigs[16]	MRSA is common in hospitals and in other care settings. In England in the most recent 12-month period there were 5366 cases of bacteremia, a rate of 1–2 per 10 000 hospital bed days. Health-care staff may become infected or colonized with MRSA and may act as source of infection for nosocomial transmission	Infection control procedures should be followed, including handwashing and use of PPE Guidelines are available
Hepatitis A	Infection of liver caused by hepatitis A virus. Asymptomatic disease is common in children; severity increases with age. Improved standards of hygiene have resulted in a decline in incidence in the UK in recent years	Transmitted by the fecal–oral route through person-to-person spread or contaminated food or drink	In 2004 there were 669 cases in E&W. A high proportion of adults and adolescents in developed countries are susceptible. Most cases are sporadic although clusters have been reported amongst men who have sex with men, intravenous drug users and hostel dwellers. Travel to endemic areas is also a risk factor. In some studies work with sewage has been shown to be a risk factor but this has been disputed[17]	Observing appropriate infection control precautions including use of PPE will minimize occupational spread of hepatitis A infection. Immunization is recommended for laboratory workers who may be exposed to hepatitis A, staff of large residential institutions for those with learning difficulties, sewage workers and people who work with primates. Immunization may be considered for food packagers and handlers, staff in day-care facilities and some other categories of health-care workers based on local risk assessment

Continued

Table 67.5 Selected infections with occupational significance—cont'd

Infection	Description of infection in humans and public health importance	Risk factors, source and route of transmission	Surveillance/occurrence	Prevention and control
Orf[18,19]	Caused by parapoxvirus Presents as a self-limiting subacute papulovesicular cutaneous lesion usually on the hands	Associated with lambs, sheep and goats	Groups affected include farmers, children visiting farms, meat industry workers	Proper hand hygiene; use of gloves Quarantine of affected animals.
Q fever[20,21]	Caused by highly infectious bacterium *Coxiella burnetii*. Incubation period 2–3 weeks Acute cases present as high fever with malaise, myalgia, sore throat, chills, vomiting, and diarrhea. Some develop pneumonia, liver function abnormalities or hepatitis, and endocarditis 50% of infected humans are asymptomatic. Chronic cases are rare	Transmitted by inhalation of organisms in dried placental material and birth fluids from infected sheep Cattle, sheep and goats are main reservoirs Consumption of raw unpasteurized milk has been a cause of a few cases Individuals with pre-existing heart valve disease are especially vulnerable if they develop chronic Q fever	Notifiable disease in the USA and the UK Occupational groups at risk are farmers, veterinarians and abattoir workers	Vaccine available for groups at risk, and also for animals Preventive measures include proper disposal of products of conception from sheep, and quarantine of imported livestock
Nipah[22] and Hendra virus	Closely related paramyxoviruses Nipah virus causes encephalitis and both Nipah and Hendra virus cause respiratory effects High case-fatality rate	Nipah virus transmitted from infected pigs. Abattoir workers also at risk. Hendra virus from horses Certain species of fruit bats are reservoirs 2004 Nipah virus outbreak in Bangladesh suggests possible person-to-person transmission, although no specific evidence for this	First major outbreak of Nipah virus in humans reported in Malaysian pig-farmers in 1998 Hendra virus first isolated in 1994 following outbreak in horses and three cases in humans in Australia	In an outbreak, PPE advised for workers dealing with infected animals, and as a precautionary measure for health-care staff dealing with infected patients
Lyme disease	Infection with spirochaete *Borrelia burgdorferi* causing rash which may progress to polyarthritis and nervous system involvement	Deer and sheep are reservoir Transmission is bite of *Ixodes* tick	Widespread in Europe and North America In E&W in 2006 there were 768 reports	In endemic areas avoid tick bites Guidelines are available
Japanese encephalitis (JE)	JE is a mosquito-borne viral encephalitis Very common cause of childhood encephalitis in Asia Can spread in laboratory workers	Reservoir is pigs and birds Spread is by mosquito vector	There have been reports of laboratory-acquired JE virus infection	Immunization is recommended for laboratory staff who may be exposed to the virus

Rabies	Acute viral encephalomyelitis caused by Lyssavirus (classic rabies virus) or bat-related Lyssavirus	Infection is via the bite or scratch of a rabid animal Person-to-person spread does not occur although rabies has spread through corneal grafts and other transplanted tissues from infected persons	Worldwide there are 40 000–70 000 cases of rabies each year In the UK, deaths occur in people infected abroad, with 24 reports since 1902 Very rarely deaths are reported following exposure to bat-related Lyssavirus	Pre-exposure immunization with rabies vaccine should be offered to laboratory workers handling the virus, those who may handle imported animals, people who regularly handle bats in the UK, those working abroad whose work may bring them into contact with rabid animals and health-care workers who may be exposed to body fluids from a patient with rabies
Tick-borne encephalitis (TBE)	Flavivirus infection of central nervous system ranging from mild febrile illnesses to meningoencephalitis	Reservoir is small mammals, domestic livestock and birds Spread is by bite of infected tick or by ingestion of unpasteurized milk from infected animals, especially goats	The virus is restricted to parts of Central Europe and Asia Those working or traveling in forested parts of endemic areas during spring and summer are at risk	Awareness of risk areas is essential Minimize tick bites by covering arms, legs and ankles, and using insect repellents on socks and outer clothes Attached ticks should be removed as soon as possible; seek local medical advice Immunization is recommended for those engaged in forestry, woodcutting, farming and the military in endemic areas Laboratory workers who may be exposed to TBE should also be immunized
Meningococcal infection[23]	Meningitis, septicemia and rarely pericarditis and arthritis caused by *Neisseria meningitidis* Serogroups B and C are most common in the UK, overseas A, Y, W135 occur Overall mortality remains around 10% in the UK	Meningococci colonize the nasopharynx Transmission is by respiratory droplets from a person carrying the organism, usually requiring prolonged close contact	In E&W notified cases of meningococcal infection have declined from a peak of nearly 3000 cases in 1999 to 1275 cases in 2006 Seasonal epidemics of group A infection are common in sub-Saharan Africa. Epidemics of group W135 infection have occurred in association with Hajj pilgrimages to Saudi Arabia Health-care workers exposed to infected cases are at increased risk but absolute risks are very low	Persons aged under 25 years and others of any age at increased risk should be immunized with a single dose of MenC conjugate vaccine. It is also recommended for long-stay visitors to high-incidence countries who will be working with local people. This group should also be offered ACWY quadrivalent polysaccharide vaccine Health-care workers should minimize exposure by use of PPE when carrying out procedures that may produce aerosols Chemoprophylaxis is recommended if the mouth or nose is directly exposed to respiratory secretions from a case

BCG, bacille Calmette–Guérin; PPE, personal protective equipment.

725

CONCLUSIONS

There are many infections that can be acquired through work activities or from workplaces (Table 67.5). The recognition of occupational factors as an important component in the transmission of these infections will aid in the management of affected cases, and in prevention. Continuing vigilance for new occupational infections, advances in preventive measures and an experienced occupational health team working with infection control specialists are key to the successful prevention of these infections.

REFERENCES

References for this chapter can be found online at http://www.expertconsult.com

Infections from pets

INTRODUCTION

Domestic pets, particularly dogs and cats, have dated back prior to Ancient Egypt. Currently, more than a third of US households keep some pet, including 53 million dogs, 57 million cats and a plethora of other animals from birds to fish to reptiles.[1] In Cheshire, England, 24% of households own a dog and 52% a pet of some type,[2] while in Australia, 66% of households have a domestic pet.[3] It is therefore not surprising that transmission of infection from animals to humans and humans to animals is common.

DOG-ASSOCIATED INFECTIOUS DISEASES

Dog bites

Table 68.1 lists some of the infectious organisms associated with dogs and canine contact. Of the over four million Americans bitten annually by a dog, only 15–20% will seek, or need, medical attention and 3–18% will become clinically infected. Dog bites account for 1% of all Emergency Department visits and result in ~10 000 hospitalizations and 1–10 deaths annually.[1] Most dog bites are inflicted by the victim's own pets or an animal known to them, often while separating the dog in a fight with another dog.[4] Half of dog bite wounds are to the hands and pose a special risk for penetration into the bones and joints and potential spaces of the hand. It is possible for nerves and/or blood vessels to be damaged. Approximately 15% of dog bites are to the head and neck, 20% to the leg or foot and 15% to the upper extremity.[1,3,4]

The incidence of dog bite wounds peaks in the summer months and on weekends. The median age of dog bite victims is 28 years old and more than 60% are male. Most dog bite wounds are punctures (~60%), lacerations (10%) or both (30%). Most patients attempt some form of self-therapy before presenting for medical attention, which include washing with soap and water, applying a topical iodophor or alcohol product. The median time for presentation for medical care is 35 hours post injury, usually after the onset of clinical signs of infection.

At presentation approximately 60% of wounds exhibit a purulent exudate, 30% have other signs of infection and 10% are abscesses. Approximately one-third of patients reporting to an Emergency Department will require hospitalization for intravenous antibiotics. When cultured, these wounds yield an average of five isolates, usually three aerobes and two anaerobes. Mixed aerobic/anaerobic infection occurs in 50% of dog bite wounds and 35% grow only aerobes. Common aerobic isolates include *Pasteurella* species, 50% (*P. canis* 26%; *P. multocida* subspecies *multocida* 12%; *P. stomatis* 12%; *P. multocida* subspecies *septica*, 10%), streptococci, 46%, staphylococci, 46% (half of which are *Staphylococcus aureus*) and *Neisseria* spp., 16%.[1,4] Methicillin-resistant *Staphylococcus aureus* (MRSA) carriage and infection in companion animals, including dogs and cats, is common and the isolates are indistinguishable from human isolates; transmission of MRSA from humans to animals and vice versa has been reported.[5,6] In addition, dog bite wounds with multidrug-resistant *Escherichia coli* and enterococci have also occurred. *Capnocytophaga canimorsus* from dog bites is able to escape from human immune surveillance[7] and has been associated with fatal sepsis, especially in asplenic patients and those with liver disease.

Common anaerobes isolated include *Fusobacterium* spp., 32%, *Bacteroides* spp., 30% (especially *B. tectum*), *Porphyromonas* spp., 28%, *Prevotella* spp., 28% (especially *P. heparinolytica*) and peptostreptococci, 16%.[1,3,4] Mycoplasmas (e.g. *Mycoplasma canis* and *Mycoplasma spumans*) and other atypical isolates may also be present in dog bite wounds.[8]

Table 68.2 outlines susceptibility patterns of common bite isolates. MRSA isolates are, at present, unusual. For those patients hospitalized,

Table 68.1 Infections transmissible from dogs

Bacteria	Fungi	Parasites	Viruses
Normal flora	*Blastomyces* spp.	*Giardia* spp.	Rabies
Pasteurella spp.	*Microsporum* spp.	*Babesia* spp.	Lymphocytic choriomeningitis
Capnocytophaga canimorsus	*Trichophyton* spp.	*Toxocara* spp.	Influenza
Tularemia		*Dipylidium canium*	Mumps
Ehrlichiosis		Echinococcosis	
Brucellosis		*Ancyclostoma* spp.	
Mycobacterium fortuitum		Scabies	
Campylobacter spp.		*Cheytelliella*	
Anaerobiospirillum thomasii			
Yersinia spp.			

Table 68.2 Activity of selected antimicrobials against animal bite isolates

	Pasteurella multocida	*Staphylococcus aureus*	Streptococci	*Capnocytophaga* spp.	Anaerobes
Penicillin	+	–	+	+	V
Ampicillin	+	–	+	+	V
Amoxicillin–clavulanate	+	+	+	+	+
Ampicillin–sulbactam	+	+	+	+	+
Dicloxacillin	–	+	+	–	–
Cephalexin	–	+	+	–	–
Cefuroxime	+	+	+	+	–
Cefoxitin	+	+	+	+	+
Tetracyclines	+	V	–	V	V
Moxifloxacin	+	+	+	+	+*
Erythromycin	–	+	+	+	–
Azithromycin	+	+	+	+	–
Clarithromycin	V	+	+	+	–
Trimethoprim–sulfamethoxazole	+	+	V	+	–
Clindamycin	–	+	+	–	+

+, active; –, poor or no activity; V, variable activity against listed pathogen.
* Except *Fusobacterium canefelinum*.

the mean length of stay is 3 days with ~30% requiring incision and drainage and 25% requiring debridement of the wound. Severely penicillin-allergic patients may need a combination of agents. Fluoroquinolones, tetracyclines and sulfa drugs are relatively contraindicated in pregnant patients; tetracyclines and fluoroquinolones should be avoided in patients younger than 18 years. Agents (monotherapy) associated with therapeutic failure include first-generation cephalosporins and macrolides.

The duration of therapy will depend upon the severity of the wound. For wounds that are seen less than 8 hours post-injury and require 'prophylaxis' (moderate to severe wounds), the duration of prophylaxis is usually 3–5 days. Therapy for a cellulitis is usually 7–10 days, while the therapy for septic arthritis and osteomyelitis is often 4–6 weeks. Cases of endocarditis and infection of prosthetic joints following bites have been reported, albeit rarely. The principles of wound care are noted in Table 68.3.

Rabies

Approximately 7000 animals per year test positive for rabies in the USA. Most are wild animals, such as raccoons, foxes and bats. Dog-associated rabies is uncommon in developed countries as a result of stray animal control programs and widespread rabies vaccine use by dog owners. Dog rabies has occurred in areas where endemic foci of infected raccoons and skunks are common. Canine transmission of rabies to humans infrequently occurs in the USA, but it is not uncommon in Latin American countries, Africa and particularly in the Indian subcontinent and other regions in Asia. The World Health Organization reported over 55 000 deaths/year due to endemic canine rabies worldwide (see Chapter 160).[9,10]

Enteric diseases from dogs

Giardiasis

Giardia lamblia is a flagellated protozoan parasite that is an important cause of diarrheal disease worldwide and can cause diarrhea in many mammalian species including dogs and humans. In many hospitals that have pet visitation programs, *G. lamblia* is the most frequent infectious agent identified on screening. The disease is transmitted by fecal–oral spread and causes flatulence, foul-smelling stools, abdominal discomfort and malaise in humans. Diagnosis is by stool examination. Therapy is with metronidazole; relapses are not infrequent.

Echinococcosis

Echinococcus granulosis is a dog tapeworm found in the small intestine, the ova of which are shed into the stool. The illness is associated with dogs found in sheep-raising areas, especially if the dogs are fed offal. These ova may remain viable for up to 1 year in appropriate climatic conditions. Humans can ingest the ova, which hatch in the small intestine into oncospheres that penetrate the bowel wall. Humans will act as an intermediate host. Usually these oncospheres reach the liver (60%) and occasionally the lung (25%) and other organs (15%).

Rupture of a hydatid cyst can cause catastrophic disease and anaphylaxis. A variety of serologic tests are available to assist in diagnosis. However, the presence of septation in a liver cyst (indicating daughter cysts) is considered diagnostic. Therapy for this disease includes surgery. Some suggest aspiration is acceptable, although there is a risk of spillage and complications. Scolicidal agents such as albendazole and mebendazole remain as adjunctive therapies.

Echinococcus multilocularis causes a severe form of alveolar hydatid disease, again often involving the human liver. This parasitic infection is found primarily in the artic regions of the northern hemisphere and often necessitates aggressive surgical resection for successful removal. *Echinococcus vogeli* is found in canines of Columbia, Ecuador, Panama and Venezuela, and can also cause human disease. The diagnosis and management of echinococcosis is further reviewed in detail in Chapter 114.

Miscellaneous enteric infections acquired from dogs

Isospora spp. infection of the gastrointestinal tract is common in dogs and while transmission to humans is not proven, it remains possible, especially in the immunocompromised patient. *Trichuris vulpis*, the whipworm of dogs, resembles the human whipworm *Trichuris trichuria*. However, the ova of the former are twice the size of the latter, and

Table 68.3 Components of care for animal bites

History	Situation, pet ownership/identity
Geographic location	
Examination	Nerve function
	Tendon function
	Blood supply (pulses)
	Presence of edema, crush injury
	Proximity to joint
	Bone penetration
Diagram (or photograph) of wound(s) for the record	
Wound care	Irrigation (important)
	Debridement (cautious)
	Elevation (important)
Antimicrobials	Prophylaxis, 3–5 days (po)
	Therapy for established infection (po vs im initial dose)
	Empiric vs specific (animal specific)
Management:	
Culture (if infected)	
Baseline radiograph	
Tetanus toxoid (0.5 ml im) if required	
Rabies prophylaxis (rabies immune globulin/human diploid cell vaccine) if needed	
Health Department report (if required)	
Decision regarding need of hospitalization	Fever >100.5°F (38°C)
	Sepsis
	Compromised host
	Advance of cellulitis
	Patient noncompliance
	Acute septic arthritis
	Acute osteomyelitis
	Severe crush injury
	Tendon/nerve injury or severance
	Tenosynovitis

have been reported in children, institutionalized patients, and rarely in immunocompetent adults associated with dog contact.

Toxocara canis is a ubiquitous roundworm in dogs that causes both cutaneous larva migrans and visceral larva migrans in humans, and affects many puppies (often less than 6 months old) and adult dogs (via ingestion of embryonated ova). Infection in humans is usually associated with children who have pica (1–6 years old) who acquire it from backyards and contaminated sandboxes. Most infection in humans is asymptomatic and eosinophilia (>30%) may be the only sign. However, the larvae may migrate anywhere in the human body and their final location determines the associated symptoms. Some patients develop an asthma-like illness; others present with pallor, weight loss, hepatomegaly or pruritic skin lesions. Diagnosis is based on a compatible history coupled with specific serology. Dogs may also transmit *Ancyclostoma canium* and *Ancyclostoma brazilense*, which also cause cutaneous larva migrans.

Infections from contact with dog urine

Leptospirosis

Leptospires are finely coiled, motile spirochetes that can be carried asymptomatically for many months by dogs, and the prevalence of leptospirosis increased significantly from 2002 to 2004, especially in suburban and rural areas.[11] Dogs may also become ill, manifested by fever, jaundice, conjunctivitis and hematuria. Dogs are often vaccinated for leptospirosis, but vaccine failures (>1 year postvaccination) have been reported. Humans may become infected through contact from the urine of an infected dog, from contact with infected tissues or indirectly from contaminated soil or water. Slightly alkaline or neutral pH, warm temperatures and moist soil favors survival of leptospires in the environment.

Most humans will have subclinical infection or an anicteric 'viral type' illness. Some may develop the classic biphasic illness and proceed onto Weil's disease. During the first phase, leptospires may be isolated from the blood, urine and spinal fluid. Later, antibodies may develop and recrudescent fever, arthralgia, hepatitis, skin rash and conjunctival suffusion may appear along with other complications (see Chapters 124 and 171). Some studies suggest that therapy with penicillin G or doxycycline may shorten the course of disease if started within the first 4 days of illness. Jarisch–Herxheimer reaction can occur after the first dose of therapy.

Brucellosis

Brucellosis is a disease of both wild and domestic animals that is transmitted to humans. Dogs may be infected with *Brucella canis*, a small Gram-negative coccobacillary organism that is found in kennel-raised dogs and is the least common cause of human brucellosis. Many infections with *B. canis* are laboratory animal acquired. Dogs may have persistent carriage of the organism and shed it in urine and gestational tissues. It can be transmitted between dogs during mating. Human disease occurs 2–4 weeks after exposure and has protean manifestations with both an acute and a chronic form (see Chapter 123).

Tick/flea-borne infectious diseases associated with dogs

Ehrlichiosis

Canine ehrlichiosis was first described in 1932 in Algeria. Since then it has been noted that dogs can be hosts to a variety of tick-borne, intraerythrocytic parasites including *Ehrlichia canis*, *Ehrlichia chaffeensis* (associated with human monocytic ehrlichiosis), *Anaplasma phagocytophilia* (associated with human granulocytic ehrlichiosis), *Ehrlichia ewingii* and *Ehrlichia platys* that cause canine pancytopenia and have a worldwide distribution. While dog to human transmission is unlikely, the disease has that potential. In humans, ehrlichiosis is contracted by a tick bite that inoculates the organism into the skin and which then spreads via the lymphatics. In humans it causes fever, headache, chills and malaise and has an associated leukopenia, thrombocytopenia and elevated liver enzymes. Therapy in humans is tetracycline or doxycycline.

Infections acquired from direct contact with dogs

Canine scabies due to *Sarcoptes scabiei* var. *canis* is also known as mange. The mites feed on the stratum granulosum of the skin and deposit the eggs in a burrow. After hatching, the larval forms migrate to the surface. Transmission to humans has been noted and is manifested as an erythematous, nonfollicular dermatitis, in part due to hypersensitivity. Skin scrapings will often not demonstrate the mite and diagnosis rests upon history and clinical response to scabicides. Dogs should also be treated with the application of a scabicidal agent. A similar condition known as 'walking dandruff' in dogs is due to *Cheyletiella* (mites). These mites do not burrow and disease is manifested in humans with erythematous macules, which may become pustular or vesicular or have other manifestations of allergic reaction such as urticaria and erythema multiforme (see Chapter 11).

CAT ASSOCIATED INFECTIOUS DISEASES

Cat bites

Cats can transmit a number of diseases to humans as listed in Table 68.4. Most physicians will encounter cat bites as the most common cat-related disease, with approximately 500 000 cat bites in the United States alone on an annual basis, usually when handling their own cat. Most wounds are trivial and do not need medical care. Cat bites affect more women (72%) than men, with an average age of 39 years for the victim.[1] At the time of presentation a nonpurulent wound with cellulitis (42%) is the most common condition encountered; however, the wounds may also develop into a purulent cellulitis (39%) and even have abscess formation (19%). An associated lymphangitis may be present in 28% of cases. An average of six bacterial species is isolated in the typical wound (range, 0–13). Approximately 85% of cat bite injuries involve puncture wounds, less than 5% are lacerations and ~10% are combinations of both.[3,4] Cats' teeth are small but sharp and easily penetrate the bones, tendons and joints of the hand and lead to osteomyelitis, tendonitis and septic arthritis, respectively.

The bacteriology of these wounds reflects the normal oral flora of the biting cat. Several recent studies[1,12,13] have shown *Pasteurella* species to be present in 75% of cases, with *P. multocida* subspecies *multocida* in 54% of wounds and *P. multocida* subspecies *septica* in 28%. These two subspecies are associated with more severe injury and have a propensity for bacteremia and central nervous system infections, respectively. Other common aerobic isolates include oral streptococci (46%), staphylococci (35%), *Neisseria* spp. (especially *N. weaverii*), *Moraxella* species (35%) and *Corynebacterium* spp. (28%). *Capnocytophaga canimorsus* is an unusual nonfermentative Gram-negative aerobic rod that is associated with bacteremia and significant mortality in compromised patients such as those with asplenia or liver disease.

Anaerobes are present in 63% of cases, usually in mixed culture, and when present were associated with more severe infection and abscess. Common anaerobic isolates include *Bacteroides tectum* (28%), *Fusobacterium* spp. (33%), especially *F. nucleatum* and *F. russii*, *Porphyromonas* spp. (30%) and *Prevotella* spp. (19%).[12–14] Most anaerobes isolated from cat bites are not producers of β-lactamase, but cat-associated *F. nucleatum* spp. are notably often resistant to fluoroquinolones and a new subspecies (*F. nucleatum* subspecies *canifelium*) has been proposed.[15]

In addition, *Erysipelothrix rhusiopathiae* has been isolated from cat bites. While usually a localized infection manifested by painful ulceration and a papular skin lesion, a disseminated form exists. Anthrax uncommonly infects cats and results from contact with infected soil, especially associated with herbivores. The differential diagnosis of the cutaneous papular lesion that starts as a vesicle and can progress to brawny edema and central necrosis also includes brown recluse spider bite, cat-scratch disease,[16] tularemia and plague. Tularemia has been associated with cat bites.

Antimicrobial selection is delineated in Table 68.2. Severely penicillin-allergic patients may need a combination of agents. The principles of wound care are noted in Table 68.3. Pain, out of proportion to the injury and in proximity to a bone or joint, suggests periosteal penetration.

Rabies

Rabies is a widespread zoonotic infection affecting numerous wild animals in many regions of the world. Domestic cats account for less than 5% of rabid animals and usually acquire it from a 'spillover effect' from exposure to infected wildlife. This disease is covered in Chapter 160.

Cat-scratch disease

Bartonella henselae is a fastidious Gram-negative rod that is the etiologic agent of cat-scratch disease (CSD) in the general population and bacillary angiomatosis in HIV-infected individuals. CSD is of worldwide distribution, has an autumn and winter prevalence in temperate climates and may be transmitted by direct inoculation (scratch or bite) and/or by fleas. Over 80% of cases are in people younger than 21 years old; children younger than 14 years old are typically infected after exposure to a newly acquired pet cat/kitten. Strays and cats from pounds have a higher frequency of infection and may be bacteremic (>40% in one San Francisco study) compared to household cats (6% in one New York City study). Most infections in cats are asymptomatic and can last for several months.[16] Domestic dogs, while accidental hosts, may also act as an important reservoir.

Approximately 1 week (range 3–10 days) after injury/exposure, 25–60% of patients may develop a primary inoculation papule at the site of injury, which may become vesicular or crust. In approximately 2 weeks (5–12 days) tender, regional lymphadenopathy may develop. These nodes may be the only manifestation in approximately half of the cases, often lasts more than 3 weeks (6–12 weeks) and usually resolves spontaneously but may suppurate in ~15% of cases. Accompanying symptoms include fatigue and malaise (28%), fever of 101–106°F (38.3–41.1°C) (12%), exanthem (4%), parotid swelling (2%) and seizures (<1%). Other manifestations may include ocular granuloma, erythema nodosum, thrombocytopenic purpura and osteomyelitis.[17] Endocarditis due to *Bartonella quintana*, a related organism, and rarely *B. henselae*, both associated with cat fleas, has been reported in homeless men (see Chapter 176).

Diagnosis is usually on clinical grounds coupled with a history of cat exposure. The organism is very difficult to isolate (chocolate media or CDC agar after 2–3 weeks) except in the research setting and serologies are of variable reliability. Biopsies are sometimes performed to exclude diseases such as Hodgkin's lymphoma, and show granuloma formation with stellate microabscesses. While the Warthin–Starry stain has been recommended, it is difficult to interpret, especially in the absence of a positive control specimen. Serology using EIA IgG antibodies may remain positive for over 1 year, while IgM antibodies usually resolve in less than 3 months.[18]

Table 68.4 Possible infections transmissible from cats

Inhalation	Vector-borne	Fecal–oral	Bites, scratches	Direct contact
Bordetellosis (*Bordetella bronchiseptica*) Plague Q fever	Ehrlichosis Cat-scratch disease Bacillary angiomatosis	Campylobacterosis *Helicobacter* spp. Cryptosporidiosis Toxoplasmosis Salmonellosis *Anaerobiospirillum* diarrhea Yersiniosis Toxocariasis Opisthorchiasis Dipylidiasis	Normal floral isolates (including *Pasteurella* spp.) Rabies *Erysipelothrix rhusiopathiae* Anthrax Tularemia	Plague Histoplasmosis Dermatophytosis Scabies *Cheyletiella* mites

Therapy is usually supportive. Antimicrobial therapy with azithromycin has been reported to diminish the size and duration of the adenopathy. Doxycycline and rifampin (rifampicin) have been used for CSD-associated retinitis. *In-vitro* resistance to first-generation cephalosporins has been correlated with clinical therapeutic failure. Prevention is by control of fleas in pets and sometimes treatment of the pet at the time of acquisition.

Bacillary angiomatosis is CSD in a severally immunocompromised (usually HIV-infected) host that manifests either as purplish skin lesions resembling Kaposi's sarcoma or as colorless subcutaneous nodules. Biopsy of the lesions yields a characteristic histopathologic picture of vascular proliferation. DNA probes have also been used to diagnose this disease. These patients may also be symptomatic from disease and have associated fever and even peliosis hepatitis. Antimicrobial therapy, although its efficacy is poorly defined, is usually employed in this situation and includes macrolides, quinolones or doxycycline (Chapter 176).

Cat-associated enteric infections

Cats may acquire salmonellosis from infected foods, especially offal, live prey (such as songbirds), uncooked meat or fishmeal, or contaminated water. Kennel transmission has also occurred. Cats may shed *Salmonella* species via the feces, the conjunctiva or the oral route. In addition, their fur may become contaminated and pass infection as can their water dishes. Newly acquired young cats are more likely to carry *Campylobacter jejuni* than older cats. *Helicobacter bizzozeronii* and *Helicobacter felis* are found in cat stomachs and association with human cases have been noted, albeit rarely. *Helicobacter pylori* has also been isolated from cats and is thought to have been transmitted to them by human caretakers. Cryptosporidiosis can affect cats that, along with other animals, are definitive hosts. Naturally infected cats exhibit watery diarrhea and some cats can be colonized. Transmission between cats and humans has been reported.[19]

Cats are definitive hosts for *Toxoplasma gondii* and millions of oocysts may be excreted daily in their feces. Approximately 1% of US cats are thought to be excreting oocysts on any given day. While ingestion of undercooked meat is the usual mode of transmission of toxoplasmosis, infection may develop from exposure to fecal oocysts when changing litter boxes or gardening in soil contaminated with oocysts by cat feces. The oocysts that pass from the feces are noninfectious and nonsporulated. However, 2–3 days after shedding, the oocysts may sporulate depending on temperature (>39.2 and <98.6°F; >4 and <37°C) and climactic factors. These may remain infective in soil for up to 1 year.

Less common isolates include *Anaerobiospirillum thomasii*, which causes diarrhea in cats and is associated with bacteremia in humans. Cats may be asymptomatic carriers or infected with *Yersinia pseudotuberculosis*, which can cause diffuse diarrhea and abdominal pain in humans. *Toxocara cati* is a helminthic parasite that affects cats with which humans may become incidentally infected when ingesting infected cat feces (usually children in the ages of pica). Most human infection is asymptomatic but can present as asthma, abdominal pain, hepatomegaly and/or eosinophilia. The disease is usually self-limiting. The cat liver fluke, *Opisthorchis felineus*, can be transmitted to humans from ingestion of rare or raw fish infected with the parasite. *Dipylidium caninum* is a cat tapeworm that can be transmitted to humans, usually children, when they ingest infected fleas. Patients develop mild abdominal discomfort and eosinophilia. Demonstrating proglottids upon parasitologic examination of the feces makes the diagnosis (see Chapter 184).

Infectious diseases associated with direct contact with cats

Dermatophytosis

Domestic cats can harbor a wide variety of dermatophytes on the hair of their coat and skin. They may also acquire human dermatophytosis from their owners and transmit it to others with an incubation period of 1–3 weeks. Asymptomatic, as well as symptomatic

carriage occurs. *Microsporum canis* has been found in up to 90% of longhaired show cats. Up to 50% of exposed humans will develop symptomatic infection, including ringworm and tinea capitis. Other organisms isolated include *Epidermophyton floccosum*, *Microsporum* spp. and *Trichophyton* spp. Infectious arthrospores can disseminate from the hair and skin to the local environment where they remain viable for months. Contaminated fomites may also act as vectors of transmission. In cats, dermatophyte infection can manifest as patchy alopecia or even a scaly dermatitis.

To break a cycle of transmission, cats may be treated with topical antifungals and on occasion oral antifungals. In addition, cleaning areas of cat hair and removal of dander from carpets and restriction of pet cats from the bedroom may facilitate control. Diagnosis is by skin scrapings and microscopic examination after potassium hydroxide addition or by use of a Wood's lamp. Human infection can be treated by topical or oral antifungals.

Cats may also directly transmit *Dermatophilus congolensis*, an actinomycete that can cause cutaneous exudative or pustular dermatitis. In cats, the hair around the lesion should be clipped and the lesion kept dry. The human dermatitis is usually self-limiting but on occasion antimicrobial therapy (penicillin) may be required if extensive skin involvement with cellulitis develops.

Cryptococcus neoformans can infect cats and cause feline disease that sheds viable organisms into the environment. However, human transmission from infected cats has not, as yet, been documented.[20]

Mites

Cats may become infected with *Sarcoptes scabiei* (scabies) and transmit this to humans. The mites cause a hypersensitivity reaction in humans, manifested by pruritic papular lesions and nocturnal itching. As cat scabies do not burrow into human skin, skin scrapings will not be diagnostic and diagnosis is by clinical presentation. Therapy is by removal of the mites from the cat and laundering the household bedding and clothing. *Cheyletiella* spp. are another type of animal mite that can be transmitted from cat to humans.

Cat infections acquired by inhalation

Bordetella bronchiseptica is a Gram-negative coccobacillus that can be found in the respiratory tracts of domestic cats and for which they should be vaccinated. In dogs it has been associated with 'kennel cough' but its clinical manifestations are often less prominent in cats. When cough appears in cats there may be an associated pneumonia. This organism can cause a pertussis-like (whooping cough) illness in humans, especially children or compromised hosts (HIV, etc.). Although cross-immunity may exist in humans from pertussis immunization during childhood, immunity wanes by adulthood. Human illness may range from a mild upper respiratory tract infection to frank pneumonia. The organism can be cultured but requires special media and can be misidentified in routine clinical laboratories.

Yersinia pestis is the Gram-negative coccobacillus that causes plague. Cat fleas are considered poor vectors for transmission but the cats themselves may contract the illness, especially in the summer months by exposure to rat fleas. Fatal cases in humans of inhalation plague and exposure to infected cats have been reported.

Humans directly exposed to infected material from parturient or aborted tissue from cats infected with Q fever (*Coxiella burnetii*) may also acquire disease. Cats may acquire infection from a tick bite or from infected material in the environment.

INFECTIOUS DISEASES ASSOCIATED WITH BIRD EXPOSURE

Contact with pet birds may vary from kissing or feeding the bird from the owner's mouth to cleaning cages or allowing the bird free range of a home or a yard. It is difficult to determine how often some of the organisms, such as *Campylobacter jejuni, P. multocida* or *Mycobacterium tuberculosis*, are passed to humans, but *Chlamydia psittaci* is regularly transmitted, as are *Salmonella* spp.

Inhalation infections from birds

Psittacosis

Chlamydia psittaci can be carried by any bird – pet or wild – not just psittacine birds such as parakeets or parrots, and all birds that carry the organism can pass it on to humans. The disease is better called ornithosis rather than psittacosis. Ducks and turkeys have been responsible for outbreaks of ornithosis in humans as well as birds kept in the home. Although respiratory symptoms are usually the result of transmission from birds to humans, there have been reports of human-to-human transmission, but apparently this is not common. Too little is known about the incidence of infection with *C. psittaci* because few studies have been done of different human populations using modern, accurate serologic techniques. If the respiratory symptoms are mild, the infection is often undiagnosed. Even in patients who have pneumonia, the diagnosis needs to be confirmed by showing a fourfold rise in acute and convalescent serum titers 2–4 weeks apart, but this is seldom pursued.

The diagnosis of acute disease is dependent on a high index of suspicion, and therapy must be empiric, because rapid diagnostic techniques are not available. A history of contact with a sick bird is highly suggestive, but well birds can carry the disease and a number of cases have been reported without a history of bird contact, presumably from inapparent environmental contact with bird excreta. Pigeon and other birds' feces abound in many urban environments, as do chicken and duck feces in rural environments.

The pneumonia in humans can be severe, and is often lobar accompanied by high fevers and chills. The sputum may be purulent with a lack of potential pathogens on smear, because *C. psittaci* does not take the Gram stain. Once empiric therapy is decided upon, tetracycline is preferred, although erythromycin has been reported to be effective. A safe duration of therapy is 2 weeks, although a shorter period may be adequate. Complications such as meningoencephalitis, arthritis or endocarditis may occur.

A specific diagnosis is important because epidemiologic factors may need to be investigated. A bird dealer may be importing carriers without appropriate quarantine and/or treatment and cases of human-to-human transmission may be uncovered, including possible nosocomial spread. Control measures for *C. psittaci* infection of birds and humans have been detailed by the US Public Health Service.

Histoplasmosis

Histoplasma capsulatum has been found in bird droppings, especially from chicken and blackbirds. *Histoplasma capsulatum* has been found throughout the world, but it is especially common in river valleys of central North America, parts of Mexico and in the Caribbean, and is thus considered a 'regional' fungus. Histoplasmosis is usually not due to exposures to pets, with the exception of exposure to chickens, which are sometimes kept and regarded as pets. The fungus grows in the feces of chickens, but does not infect them. Most human infections are asymptomatic but others may result in an influenza-like illness or rarely a progressive pneumonia (see Chapters 31 and 178). The majority of symptomatic infections are self-limiting; however, treatment when necessary (especially in the immunocompromised host) can begin with amphotericin B followed by itraconazole or fluconazole for acute, progressive infections or itraconazole or fluconazole alone for more indolent disease. Prevention strategies should include advising immunocompromised people to avoid bird feces, especially from chickens.

Cryptococcosis

Cryptococcus neoformans in found in soil throughout the world, but it appears to thrive in pigeon feces.[20] Pigeon fanciers who keep flocks of pigeons for sport are exposed to *C. neoformans* more than the general population, as demonstrated by serologic testing; however, an increased incidence of disease has not been documented in these people. Cryptococcosis initially begins as a self-limiting respiratory infection. The fungus may disseminate widely to multiple organs including the central nervous system. It has a predilection for people who have CD4+ T-helper-1 lymphocyte defects, and if untreated the meningitis it causes is associated with high mortality (up to 50%). There may be significant morbidity and sequelae (e.g. noncommunicating hydrocephalus, blindness) (see Chapter 91).

The diagnosis is aided by the presence of cryptococcal polysaccharide antigen in the blood or cerebrospinal fluid, and a decrease in antigen titer is usually associated with a response to therapy. Amphotericin B with or without flucytosine is the treatment of the acute episode, followed by fluconazole for more chronic therapy. Prevention should include advising immunocompromised people to avoid contact with pigeons.

Tuberculosis has been seen in patients in households where tuberculosis has been recognized in macaws.[21] It is difficult to determine whether spread is from birds to humans or vice versa. Other psittacine birds may become infected with *M. tuberculosis*.

Enteric diseases associated with bird exposure

All of the organisms listed in Table 68.5 have been isolated from birds; some, such as *Salmonella* spp. and *Giardia lamblia*, are clearly implicated in transmission to humans. Parasites that may spread to humans from birds include *G. lamblia* and *Cryptosporidium* spp., although direct spread from the latter is not as well documented as the former (see Chapters 180 and 181 for treatment guidelines). Mites may be spread by direct and indirect contact with infested birds.

Table 68.5 Organisms carried by small mammal pets

Bacteria	Fungi	Parasites	Viruses
Campylobacter spp.	*Sporothrix schenckii*	*Cryptosporidium* spp.	Lymphocytic choriomeningitis virus
Spirillum minus	*Penicillium marneffei*		Hantavirus
Streptobacillus moniliformis			
Salmonella spp.			
Leptospira interrogans			
Francisella tularensis			
Yersinia pestis			
Listeria monocytogenes			
Pasteurella multocida			
Burkholderia pseudomallei			

Viral diseases from pet birds

Identical strains of influenza virus have been found in both humans and domestic ducks and chickens where contact has been documented. The incidence of ducks or other birds serving as reservoirs for influenza is not certain. Since 1998, when a large outbreak of avian influenza A (H5N1) in Hong Kong was associated with several human deaths, millions of birds have been slaughtered in an attempt to control the infection.

SMALL MAMMAL PETS

Small mammal pets include mice, rats, hamsters, gerbils, guinea pigs and rabbits. People may also keep more exotic animals such as mink, ferrets and ocelots. These animals carry organisms similar to those carried by mice and rats; ocelots carry organisms similar to those carried by cats. Table 68.5 lists organisms carried by small mammal pets.

Most pets, regardless of type, can carry *Salmonella* spp. and *Campylobacter* spp. Many, including rabbits, carry *P. multocida* as part of their mouth flora. There are some that are more likely to carry certain organisms.

Rat-bite fever

Rats can carry *Spirillum minus* and *Streptobacillus moniliformis*. Rat-bite fever due to *S. minus* (also known as spirillary fever and sodoku) is seen worldwide but is most common in Asia.[22] A rash with reddish or purplish plaques accompanies the fever. The healed bite wound may reactivate when fever develops. The diagnosis requires highly specialized laboratories for confirmation. Treatment consists of penicillin or tetracycline.

Rat-bite fever due to *S. moniliformis* (also called Haverhill fever) is more common in the USA and may be due to a rat bite or to exposure to contaminated milk or water during an outbreak. The fever is usually accompanied by a maculopapular or petechial rash that is most pronounced on the extremities. Arthritis of large joints is common, as are relapses. Focal abscesses and endocarditis may occur. A specialized laboratory can confirm the diagnosis if a sterile site (i.e. joint fluid or blood) is positive on culture. Treatment is with penicillin or tetracycline.

Lymphocytic choriomeningitis virus (LCMV) is carried by mice and other rodents, including pet Syrian golden hamsters. It has been isolated from guinea pigs and dogs. Infection in humans results from exposure to the urine, feces or saliva of the rodent and may result in no symptoms, although a flu-like syndrome or meningitis may occur. The flu-like syndrome may be followed by recovery and then relapse with meningitis. Orchitis, parotitis and thrombocytopenia have also been observed. Diagnosis of LCMV is made by isolation of the virus from a sterile site such as the cerebrospinal fluid or acute and convalescent serum specimens showing a fourfold rise in titer. There is no treatment. If a case occurs in a pet hamster, the entire colony should be screened for LCMV.

MISCELLANEOUS PETS

Monkeys

The most insidious and disastrous viral infection that a pet monkey can pass to a human is cercopithecine herpesvirus type 1 (herpesvirus simiae; B virus). This latent infection of often-asymptomatic monkeys can be passed to humans by saliva or by a bite. It is almost always fatal in humans, in whom it causes progressive encephalitis which, if not fatal, will leave severe sequelae in most cases (see Chapter 155). If diagnosed early, treatment with aciclovir or other antiviral herpes agent, may result in improvement and even recovery. Although it is a legal requirement to screen imported pet monkeys, this does not always occur and may even miss carriers.

Nonhuman primates (and prairie dogs) can also transmit hepatitis A and B, and monkeypox, which is clinically indistinguishable from smallpox. Patients with bites or scratches are more likely to have a shorter incubation period (9 days vs 13 days) and more severe disease and require hospitalization than 'non-invasive' exposures from cleaning cages, etc.[23] Monkeys may also transmit salmonellosis, shigellosis, campylobacteriosis, amebiasis, strongyloides, giardiasis, yersiniosis, and dermatophyte infection.

Reptiles, amphibians and fish

Any reptile or amphibian may carry *Salmonella* spp., which are excreted in the feces and may infect humans caring for the pet. This has been best exemplified by outbreaks in humans who have pet turtles.

Fish may harbor *Salmonella* spp., including multidrug-resistant isolates, *Aeromonas hydrophila*, *Citrobacter diversus*, *Pseudomonas aeruginosa*, *Providencia stuartii* and *Vibrio* spp. including *Vibrio. vulnificus* (which can cause a rapidly fatal infection in patients with liver dysfunction) and other halophilic bacteria (salt water). In addition, *Mycobacterium marinum* has been found in fish tanks (both fresh and salt water) and can cause a purplish rash with granulomatous lesions, usually on the hands of those cleaning the tanks and handling the fish. The diagnosis is made when the skin lesion is biopsied and cultured. Treatment with rifampin (rifampicin) and ethambutol, minocycline or trimethoprim–sulfamethoxazole (co-trimoxazole) has been successful in eradicating this infection.

Erysipelothrix rhusiopathiae is an uncommon infection of food handlers, especially fishmongers. It causes erysipeloid, painful, indurated, irregular skin lesions, usually on the hands. It is very susceptible to penicillin. Penicillin-allergic patients can be treated with clindamycin.

REFERENCES

References for this chapter can be found online at http://www.expertconsult.com

Infections acquired from animals other than pets

Zoonotic infections may be acquired from farm animals, beasts of burden, fish and wild animals via a number of routes (Fig. 69.1). Many of the emerging infectious diseases are zoonotic in origin.

The approach to the patient with a potential zoonotic infection involves the generation of a reasonable differential diagnosis that includes those infectious agents that are potentially transmissible from the specific animal to which the patient was exposed. This may be a challenging task for the clinician when the exposure has been to a rarely encountered animal. Historical points worth considering are summarized in Table 69.1.

Although the number of infectious agents potentially transmissible from a specific animal to humans may be great, many of these

infections are limited geographically and need not be considered in the differential diagnosis. Examples include the lack of plague transmission outside endemic areas such as the Western USA, countries that are free of brucellosis and the limitation of tularemia to the northern hemisphere. In some cases a good history of animal exposure will be elicited but a review of the medical literature will not be able to identify a published reference on zoonotic transmission of any relevant diseases from that specific animal. One additional difficulty is that the lack of an effective veterinary or human public health system in a given country may result in a lack of knowledge of zoonotic infections transmitted from even commonly encountered animals. In such cases, it is worthwhile considering similar animals with known flora or from

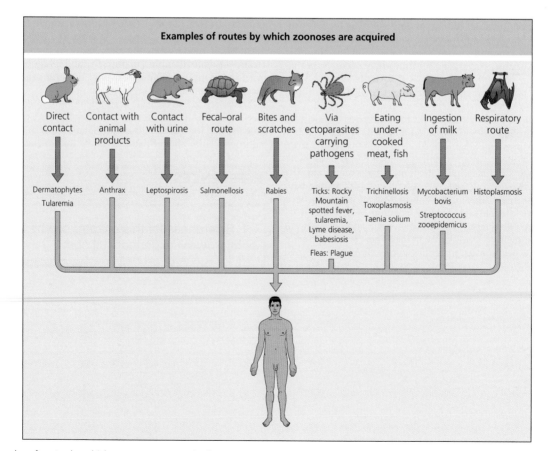

Fig. 69.1 Examples of routes by which zoonoses are acquired.

Table 69.1 Selected historical points in patient exposure history

Historical finding	Worth adding to differential diagnosis
Contact with any vertebrate, especially reptiles	Salmonellosis
Exposure to urine, either directly or via contaminated water	Leptospirosis, as essentially all mammals can become infected with *Leptospira interrogans* and shed infectious organisms in the urine
Bites from wild mammals, with the exception of those from rodents other than groundhogs (*Marmota monax*)	Evaluate risk of rabies and the potential need for rabies prophylaxis
Itching and a history of cutaneous contact with a mammal	Allergic reaction, dermatophyte infection or infestation with ectoparasites, such as species-specific varieties of *Sarcoptes scabiei*
Consumption of undercooked wild mammals	Trichinellosis and toxoplasmosis
Consumption of fermented fish or marine mammals	Botulism, most commonly due to the type E toxin
Consumption of uncooked fish	Any of more than 50 parasitic infections, depending upon the species of fish eaten and the geographic locale

which zoonoses have been acquired and infections of the animal with known zoonotic agents. Examples include the following.

- *Escherichia coli* O157:H7 infections have been most commonly transmitted to humans via the ingestion of undercooked ground beef. Deer, like cattle, are large grazing herbivores. They have transmitted this infection to humans via the consumption of venison.
- Camels have been noted to have serologic evidence of infection with *Coxiella burnetii*, but human cases of Q fever as a result of contact with camels have not been documented. It is possible that this is, in part, due to the lack of active case finding in those parts of the world in which camels are common.
- The environment of the animal, which may include exposure to fresh water or salt water, is important. For example, shark bite wounds may be infected with *Vibrio* spp., which are commonly found in salt water and as part of the normal oral flora of sharks, whereas fresh-water alligator bites are most commonly infected with *Aeromonas hydrophila*, an organism that is found in fresh water and as part of the normal alligator oral flora.
- Consider the diet of the animal. Cattle that have been fed material that includes nervous tissue are at increased risk of having bovine spongiform encephalopathy (BSE).
- Consider other species with which the animal has had contact, including contact with humans while in captivity. Tuberculosis, measles and shigellosis are not thought to normally be infectious agents of nonhuman primates. Rather, they are acquired from human contact. Similarly, the housing of camels indoors with cattle increases the risk that the camels will acquire bovine tuberculosis.

Good communication with the clinical microbiology laboratory is essential in the diagnosis of zoonotic infections. In some cases the

diagnosis is established serologically, whereas in others a particular pathogen, perhaps one that requires special culture media or handling, may be found. In addition to increasing the probability of correctly identifying the etiology of the patient's illness, good communication is essential for safety, especially when infections due to *Francisella tularensis*, *Brucella* spp., cercopithecine herpesvirus type 1 (herpesvirus simiae; B virus) and other highly biohazardous agents are under consideration.

The following discussion is organized by type of animal, as this is helpful for the clinician who is attempting to generate a reasonable differential diagnosis.

DOMESTICATED HERBIVORES (CATTLE, SHEEP, GOATS, PIGS, CAMELS, HORSES AND RELATED ANIMALS)

Bacterial infections

Brucella melitensis is most commonly acquired from goats but has been acquired from sheep and dromedary camels. *Brucella abortus* is associated with cattle and, although horses can occasionally become infected, transmission to humans from horses, if it occurs, is very rare. *Brucella suis* can be transmitted to humans from both domesticated and feral pigs. Of note, the specificity of the association between the species of *Brucella* and the animal host is far from absolute. Examples include the occurrence of *B. melitensis* in cattle in parts of southern Europe, Israel, Kuwait and Saudi Arabia and the establishment of *B. suis* biovar 1 in cattle in Brazil and Colombia.[1] Many other animals have contracted brucellosis. Infection of bison in Yellowstone Park has been of concern to cattle ranchers in Western USA who worry that their cattle will be infected from contact with the bison. There have not, however, been documented cases of transmission of brucellosis in the area of the park from bison to cattle nor from bison to humans. In other geographic locations, *Brucella* infections of caribou have been known to spread disease to humans.

Transmission of anthrax by large domesticated herbivores is the normal means by which the infection is acquired by humans. Cutaneous anthrax, inhalation anthrax (woolsorter's disease) and gastrointestinal anthrax all are most commonly associated with the domestication of sheep, goats and cattle. In parts of the world in which water buffalo are domesticated, these animals have served as the source of outbreaks of human anthrax, as have oxen. Animal products can transmit the disease. For example, during the early 1900s cutaneous anthrax was transmitted via contaminated shaving brushes made of animal hair.

Yersinia pestis has been (rarely) transmitted to humans from both camels and goats in Libya and from camels in endemic areas of the former Soviet Union via direct contact and in individuals who consumed the infected animals.[2]

Epizootics of tularemia, associated with heavy infestation by the wood tick, *Dermacentor andersoni*, occur in sheep. Human cases of tularemia have included cases in sheep shearers, owners and herders. In a review published in 1955, 189 human cases of tularemia were reported in association with the sheep industry.[3] Tularemia has rarely been transmitted from pigs to humans.[4]

Tuberculosis due to *Mycobacterium bovis* subsp. *bovis* was the impetus for pasteurization of cow's milk. *Mycobacterium tuberculosis* infection can occur in cattle, but does not typically result in systemic infection. Infection with *M. bovis* is also associated with occupational exposure, as with slaughterhouse workers. The related *M. bovis* subsp. *caprae* has caused human infections after contact with cattle.[5]

Infection with *Listeria monocytogenes* may result from the ingestion of contaminated meat and dairy products or via direct cutaneous exposure during parturition. In the latter case, cutaneous listeriosis has been reported among veterinarians and other individuals delivering animals.[6] Infections transmitted by ingestion of animal milk are listed in Table 69.2.

Table 69.2 Agents transmitted via milk products and cheese

Disease	Source
Clostridium botulinum toxin	Yogurt, cheese
Brucella spp.	Many animals' milk and cheese
Campylobacter fetus	Cow's milk
Campylobacter jejuni	Cow's milk, cheese from goats
Campylobacter laridis	Cow's milk, contaminated by birds
Central European tick-borne encephalitis	Goat's milk, cheese from goats and sheep
Corynebacterium diphtheriae	Cow's milk
Corynebacterium ulcerans	Cow's milk
Escherichia coli O157:H7 and other strains	Cow's and goat's milk, cream, cheese
Listeria monocytogenes	Cow's milk, cheese
Mycobacterium bovis subsp. *bovis*	Cow's milk
Salmonella spp.	Many animals' milk, cheese, ice cream
Staphylococcus aureus	Cow's milk
Streptobacillus moniliformis	Cow's milk (single outbreak in 1926)
Streptococcus zooepidemicus	Cow's milk, cheese
Toxoplasma gondii	Goat's milk
Yersinia enterocolitica	Cow's milk

Yersinia enterocolitica, normally found in the fecal flora of pigs, has been transmitted from pigs to humans via contact and by ingestion of chitterlings (pig intestines).[7]

Erysipelothrix rhusiopathiae has been transmitted to humans from many different animals and animal products. It typically is an occupational illness, often acquired via a hand wound while handling animal material. Alerting the clinical microbiology laboratory to its possibility is of great help, as the organism's identification is not difficult if it is suspected.[8]

Streptococcus suis, especially type 2, a pathogen of pigs, is a common cause of bacteremia and bacterial meningitis among individuals working with pigs in Asia. *Rhodococcus equi* is commonly found in the feces of horses and in the soil. Exposure to farm animals, including horses, has been reported in some cases of human infection. The association of leptospirosis with swine is well known and one name for the illness is swineherd's disease. Cattle, goats, camels, dogs and rats are also potential sources of human infection.

Exposure of pregnant women to the birth products of sheep and goats that are infected with *Chlamydophila abortus* (formerly named *Chlamydia psittaci*, serotype 1) has resulted in illness. Human infection with this organism has been reported in both Europe and the USA, and can be severe, resulting in abortion.[9]

Salmonellosis has been transmitted to humans by each of these animals, including camels. Pigs have been documented as a source of human cases of multidrug-resistant *Salmonella enterica* serotype *typhimurium* definitive phage type 104 (DT104) infection.[10]

Escherichia coli O157:H7 is often present in the gastrointestinal tract of cattle. The most common route of transmission is via ingestion of undercooked ground beef. Transmission due to fecal contamination of food products can occur, such as via unpasteurized apple

cider prepared from apples that were on the ground in a cattle pasture and used for cider production. Deer, like cattle, are large grazing herbivores and have been reported to transmit this infection to humans who have consumed venison. Outbreaks have been associated with visits to petting zoos. It has become increasingly understood that Shiga toxin-producing *E. coli* other than *E. coli* O157:H7 is responsible for approximately half of human Shiga toxin-producing *E. coli* infections.

Pasteurella aerogenes is the most commonly isolated organism from human infections following the bites of swine.[11] A number of other Gram-negative organisms have also been isolated from these infections. Camel bite injuries are typically infected and are particularly likely from male camels during the rutting season. Members of the genus *Actinobacillus* have been recovered from bites from horses and cattle and *Pasteurella caballi* has been isolated from wounds following horse bites. Rabies has been reported in all of these animals as well as in llamas.

Pig-bel, or enteritis necrotans, has been associated with the consumption of large quantities of pork in populations that have a low protein diet, such as in the highland Melanesians of Papua New Guinea and in Germany immediately following the Second World War. Evidence suggests that the major etiologic agent is *Clostridium perfringens* type C. Human cases of Q fever are acquired from sheep, goats and cattle, as well as from cats. Infection can be transmitted for significant distances via the wind. The data on human acquisition via contaminated milk are less compelling.

Glanders, due to *Burkholderia mallei*, has been transmitted to humans via equids. The disease is now quite limited geographically and the isolation of this agent from a patient in North America or Europe must be assumed to be due to bioterrorism until proven otherwise.

Viral infections

Localized cutaneous involvement can be due to infection with the parapoxviruses orf virus (which causes contagious ecthyma and is transmitted by sheep and goats either directly or via fomites), bovine papular stomatitis virus and pseudocowpox virus; and by the orthopoxviruses cowpox virus (which is more commonly transmitted to humans via cats than cattle) and buffalopox virus. The host range of influenza A virus includes many other mammals, including birds, swine and horses.

Variant Creutzfeldt–Jakob disease (variant CJD) has been reported from the UK, France, Japan and other countries and appears to be associated with the consumption of meat from cattle that were infected with BSE. Although cases of BSE have been identified in the USA, no cases of variant CJD have been found to be due to consumption of US cattle. Prion diseases of large herbivores in the USA, including chronic wasting disease of cervids, have raised the possibility of the introduction of prion diseases into the human food supply. A detailed discussion of the molecular aspects of prion-associated disease and the clinical manifestations of the spongiform encephalopathies are found in Chapter 22.

Rift Valley fever, which infects domestic ruminants, can be transmitted to humans both by mosquitoes and by contact with the tissues of slaughtered, infected animals such as sheep.[12] Similarly, Crimean-Congo hemorrhagic fever infects a variety of animals, including cattle and sheep, and is transmitted to humans via ticks (especially *Hyalomma* spp.), via contact with blood of infected animals and, if appropriate precautions are not taken, in the hospital setting.

Hendra virus, a paramyxovirus, caused an infection of horses and a few individuals in contact with these horses in Australia. The natural reservoir has been identified as a flying fox (bat). Nipah virus was the cause of an epidemic of encephalitis that affected more than 250 people in Malaysia and Singapore, killing 105 people. More recent outbreaks have occurred in India in West Bengal in 2001 when it killed three-fourths of the 66 infected people and in Bangladesh in 2004 when it killed 18 of 30 infected people. Subsequently, there have been additional outbreaks in West Bengal during 2007 and in Bangladesh in 2008. The vast majority of those infected had contact with pigs, which were culled in order to stop the epidemic. There has been concern about the possibility that some cases were due to person-to-person transmission. The natural reservoir of Nipah virus, a paramyxovirus that is related most closely to the Hendra virus, has been identified as a bat. Menangle virus, a recently described paramyxovirus, caused an infection of pigs and infection in humans in contact with the pigs in Australia. The natural reservoir has been identified as a flying fox (bat).

Recent concern has been generated over the possibility of certain endogenous porcine retrovirus infections causing disease in humans following xenotransplantation of organ tissues from pigs. Some of these retroviruses can propagate in human cell lines and they could potentially induce immunodeficiency in experimental systems.[13] This poses a potential risk of activation of porcine retroviruses in the setting of an unnatural host such as an immunosuppressed, solid organ, human transplant recipient. Fortunately, it appears that commonly utilized porcine heterografts for heart valve replacement surgery are unlikely to be complicated by inadvertent activation of porcine retroviruses. The currently employed glutaraldehyde fixation and sterilization method for porcine heart valves eliminates infectivity of endogenous retroviruses.[14]

Parasitic infection

An epidemic of cryptosporidiosis occurred in 1993 in Milwaukee, Wisconsin, in which the public water supply was contaminated and more than 400 000 people were infected. The epidemic was traced to untreated water from Lake Michigan, from which the causative organism was incompletely removed by the water filtration process. Possible sources included cattle along two rivers, slaughterhouses and human sewage.[15] In addition to water-borne epidemics, human infections occur via direct contact with cattle and sheep (the disease primarily occurs in lambs), including infection as a result of farm visits.

Echinococcal disease, although not transmitted to humans from sheep, occurs in areas of the world in which sheep serve as an intermediate host and in which dogs ingest sheep viscera, subsequently excreting infective eggs in their feces. A different echinococcal strain occurs in dromedary camels.

The demonstration of the eggs of *Dicrocoelium dendriticum*, the lancet liver fluke of cattle, sheep and goats, in human feces may be due to a true infection (dicrocoeliasis) but is more often due to a pseudo-infection. In pseudoinfections, eggs obtained via the consumption of liver (sometimes eaten raw) are passed per rectum without causing an actual infection in the human.

The pig ascarid *Ascaris suum* has been reported to cause human infection. Illness, including pulmonary infiltrates as a result of larval migration, resulted in intubation in students who ingested intestinal contents of pigs as a result of a fraternity 'prank'.[16]

Taenia solium, the pork tapeworm, is acquired via the ingestion of undercooked infected pork. *Trichinella spiralis* is most commonly acquired from eating undercooked pork, but has also been acquired following the ingestion of bear and horsemeat.[17] *Taenia saginata*, the beef tapeworm, is acquired via the ingestion of undercooked beef. Toxoplasmosis can be acquired via the ingestion of undercooked meat, especially lamb, as well as from contaminated goat's milk.

Dermatophyte infection

Infection with zoophilic dermatophytes commonly occurs in people in contact with these animals. These include, for example, *Trichophyton verrucosum* spread from cattle to humans, and *T. equinum* from horses,[18] among others.

BATS

Rabies virus is known to occur in many species of bat and transmission to humans via bite, scratch and inhalation of aerosolized saliva has been reported. Bats also account for many cases of rabies in livestock. Other Lyssaviruses that have been transmitted to humans from

bats include European bat Lyssavirus-1, European bat Lyssavirus-2 and, most recently, Australian bat Lyssavirus.[19] Most recent reports of human rabies from bat exposure find no clear evidence of a documented bat bite. Transmission apparently occurs from inadvertent bites or from unrecognized contact with the bat saliva. This is the rationale for the administration of rabies immune globulin and rabies vaccine when a bat is found in the room upon awaking from sleep, in the room of a small child or in the room of an intoxicated or mentally challenged person[20] (see Chapter 160). As noted above, bats have been found to be reservoirs of the zoonotic paramyxoviruses Nipah virus, Hendra virus and Menangle virus.[21]

Many outbreaks of histoplasmosis due to *Histoplasma capsulatum* have been associated with exposure to bat guano in caves. Other bat-associated outbreaks have been the result of disturbing piles of bat guano from old buildings[22] and clearing debris from a bridge.[23]

NONHUMAN PRIMATES

The numerous pathogens that have been isolated from nonhuman primates (NHPs) include many human pathogens. Documented transmission of human pathogens include bacterial (*Shigella* and *Salmonella* spp.), mycobacterial (*M. tuberculosis*), viral (hepatitis A virus), parasitic (*Entamoeba histolytica*) and fungal (dermatophyte) agents. In addition, there are infectious agents of human origin that infect NHPs and that have not been reported to be transmitted back to humans. These include measles virus and (human) herpes simplex virus type 1.

Of concern are those infectious agents that are not normally regarded as human pathogens. Many of these are particularly virulent. Historically, it is worth noting that molecular evidence suggests that HIV-1 was originally a pathogen of chimpanzees, *Pan troglodytes troglodytes*, and that HIV-2 was originally a pathogen of sooty mangabees. There are numerous simian immunodeficiency virus (SIV) strains and it is possible that one or more might be transmitted to humans via contact, ingestion or by growing the pathogen. Transmission of SIV to a human has occurred in a laboratory accident.[24]

The possibility of life-threatening infection with cercopithecine herpesvirus-1 must be considered in bites, scratches and contact with saliva from Asiatic macaques, especially from the rhesus monkey, *Macaca mulatta*. It is hypothesized that there are distinct genotypes of the virus and that the isolates from different species vary in their pathogenicity for humans. Institutions that work with macaques should have plans in place to prevent and treat infections with cercopithecine herpesvirus-1[25] and have access to testing by laboratories with special expertise in the isolation and serologic testing of this virus. The NIH B Virus Resource Laboratory at Georgia State University (phone (404) 413-6550, fax (404) 413-6556, website http://www2.gsu.edu/~wwwvir/Diagnostics/forms.html, e-mail bvirus@gsu.edu or jhilliard@gsu) is the reference laboratory for the USA.

Filovirus infections with both Ebola and the Reston strain of Ebola, which is less pathogenic for humans than other strains of Ebola, have been transmitted from NHPs to humans. Marburg virus, a filovirus causing hemorrhagic fever with high mortality, has been transmitted from vervet (or green) monkeys to humans. The reservoir in nature of Ebola and Marburg viruses appears to be bats.

Monkeypox, an orthopoxvirus, was initially identified in human cases of illness that were clinically consistent with smallpox. It is found in NHPs and in squirrels and other rodents in Africa and has been transmitted from human to human. Tanapox (benign epidermal monkeypox) has been transmitted to humans both via mosquitoes and by direct contact with monkeys in primate centers in the USA, but has not been transmitted from human to human. Yabapox virus has, rarely, caused subcutaneous growths at the site of inoculation.

Kyasanur forest disease virus, a member of the tick-borne encephalitis subgroup, is found in Karnataka State, India, and has a number of NHP reservoirs. The presence of dead monkeys in the endemic area may precede an epidemic.

737

Rabies has been reported in NHPs but, with the exception of a recent report in which the white-tufted-ear marmoset (*Callithrix jacchus*) was the source of eight human cases of rabies in Brazil,[26] there are only isolated case reports of transmission of rabies from NHPs to humans.

MUSTELIDS (FERRETS, SKUNK, OTTER, MINK, WEASEL, BADGER, MARTENS)

Influenza A virus has been transmitted in a laboratory setting in which a researcher was infected by a ferret that had been infected with a strain of influenza A virus and which 'sneezed violently at close range' while it was being examined.[27] Ferrets are susceptible to influenza A and B viruses. Mink on mink farms have been found to be infected with influenza A viruses.[28]

There is a report of *M. bovis* infection of the right palm more than 20 years following a ferret bite.[29] *Mycobacterium bovis* is known to infect wild ferrets and badgers. There is a case report of sporotrichosis complicating a badger bite. Rabies infection is known to occur in skunks, otters, badgers, weasels, mink and ferrets, including pet ferrets, in the USA. Transmission of rabies from skunks to humans has been documented.[30] A rabies vaccine has been licensed for use in ferrets and the National Association of State Public Health Veterinarians recommendations are for primary immunization at 3 months and booster immunizations annually.[31] The recommendations regarding a healthy ferret that bites a human are the same as those for dogs and cats with respect to confinement and observation for 10 days, with evaluation by a veterinarian at the first sign of illness.[31]

Rat-bite fever as a result of ferret and weasel bites was reported in the medical literature between 1910 and 1920. Only in a report of a weasel bite was there isolation of an organism from the patient's blood.[32] Trichinellosis has been reported in people who ate inadequately cooked or raw liver, spleen, blood and muscle of a badger.[33]

RODENTS

Yersinia pestis is transmitted in epidemics from rats to humans via the rat flea, *Xenopsylla cheopis*. Numerous rodents other than rats serve as reservoirs, some of which have been responsible for human plague. Similarly, tularemia is widely distributed in nature and has been transmitted to humans by many different rodents.

Leptospirosis is commonly associated with skin or mucous membrane exposure to water contaminated by the urine of rodents, including rats, mice and voles. It has rarely been reported to be transmitted via rodent bite.[34] Other uncommonly reported bacterial infections following rodent bites include *Pasteurella multocida*, the *Pasteurella* 'SP' group and sporotrichosis. Rat-bite fever can be due to either *Streptobacillus moniliformis* or *Spirillum minus*. The former has been transmitted to humans not only by wild rats but also by laboratory rats, mice and other rodents.

It is unclear how often rodents cause cases or outbreaks of human salmonellosis. However, given that *Salmonella* spp. are commonly recovered from rodent feces, the serotypes commonly recovered from rodents are similar to those recovered from cases of human disease, and rodents often infest human dwellings, restaurants and food production facilities, it is likely that they account for some fraction of human illness.

Many of the tick-borne relapsing fevers have wild rodents as reservoirs. This is also the case for *Babesia microti*, Lyme disease and human granulocytic ehrlichiosis. The reservoirs of Colorado tick fever include a number of squirrels, chipmunks and other rodents. Similarly, Powassan encephalitis, tick-borne encephalitis and Omsk hemorrhagic fever virus are transmitted via ticks and have small mammals as reservoirs. *Leishmania* spp. are transmitted by sandflies and often have rodents as reservoirs.

Those members of the Hantavirus genus that are known to cause hantavirus pulmonary syndrome (HPS) are carried by New World rats and mice, family Muridae, subfamily Sigmodontinae, and are transmitted via the inhalation of rodent excreta or saliva or, rarely, via rodent bite. In the USA and Canada, the viruses include Sin Nombre virus, the main cause of HPS, transmitted by the deer mouse (*Peromyscus maniculatus*); New York virus, transmitted by the white-footed mouse (*Peromyscus leucopus*); Black Creek Canal virus, transmitted by the cotton rat (*Sigmodon hispidus*); and Bayou virus, transmitted by the rice rat (*Oryzomys palustris*).[35] In South America, viruses include Andes virus in Argentina, Chile and Uruguay transmitted by the long-tailed pygmy rice rat (*Oligoryzomys longicaudatus*), a virus for which there is epidemiologic evidence of person-to-person transmission; Juquitiba virus in Brazil; Laguna Negra virus in Paraguay, transmitted by the vesper mouse (*Calomys laucha*); and Bermejo virus in Bolivia.[36] Hantaviruses that are associated with hemorrhagic fever with renal syndrome in Europe and Asia include Hantaan virus, transmitted by the murine field mouse (*Apodemus agrarius*); Dobrava virus transmitted by the murine field mouse (*Apodemus flavicollis*); Seoul virus, transmitted by the Norway rat (*Rattus norvegicus*) in Asia; and Puumala virus transmitted by the bank vole (*Clethrionomys glareolus*).[37]

Arenaviruses are transmitted from rodents via the excreta and urine. These include lymphocytic choriomeningitis virus, which is found worldwide and has been transmitted to humans by hamsters[38] as well as mice; Machupo virus, which causes Bolivian hemorrhagic fever and is transmitted by *Calomys callosus*; Junin virus, which causes Argentinian hemorrhagic fever and is transmitted by *Calomys* spp.; Guanarito virus, which is found in Venezuela; Lassa fever virus, which is found in Africa and is transmitted by the multimammate rat, *Mastomys natalensis*; and a recently described New World arenavirus that caused three fatal infections in California and shared 87% identity with the Whitewater Arroyo virus at the nucleotide level.[37]

Reservoirs of cowpox virus include several rodents. This is consistent with the epidemiology of cowpox in which cat contact is implicated. Cowpox, or a similar virus, has also been transmitted via rat bite.[39] A multi-state outbreak of more than 70 cases of monkeypox occurred in the United States following the importation of exotic rodents from Ghana and affected people who had contact with pet prairie dogs that had been in contact with the African rodents at an animal distributor.

Rickettsialpox has been associated with infestation of mice (*Mus musculus*) with mites which serve as the vector for human disease.[40] Rodents serve as reservoirs for many other rickettsial diseases, including murine typhus in which rats are the principal reservoir and the flea *X. cheopis* the principal vector; *Rickettsia prowazekii*, which has been associated with flying squirrels;[41] scrub typhus, in which rats are hosts of the trombiculid mite vectors; and members of the spotted fever group.

Although the issue of whether giardiasis is commonly zoonotic in origin is debated, beavers may have been the source of an outbreak of water-borne giardiasis.[42]

Ingestion of rodents has been associated with rare cases of trichinellosis, such as due to the ingestion of squirrel and bamboo rat.[43] There has been speculation on whether consumption of squirrel brains causes a spongiform encephalopathy, but data are limited.[44] Eating fermented beaver has resulted in botulism.[45]

Trichophyton mentagrophytes var. *mentagrophytes* is a common zoophilic dermatophyte, infecting humans and domestic animals. Rodents are regarded as the reservoir of infection.

LAGOMORPHS (RABBITS, HARES)

Tularemia, also known as rabbit fever, is acquired from rabbits and hares as a result of cutaneous contact and skinning of rabbits, presumably entering via microabrasions in the skin or conjunctiva, and via ingestion.[4,46] Transmission via infectious aerosol has also been reported as a result of mowing over a rabbit.[47] Tularemia transmission to humans has not been reported from domesticated rabbits. Although uncommon, eight cases of human bubonic plague from 1950 to 1974 were reported as a result of contact (e.g. skinning) with rabbits and hares[48] in plague-endemic areas of the USA. Q fever has been transmitted to humans following contact with wild rabbits.[49]

A patient with *Bordetella bronchiseptica* respiratory infection was shown to have a strain that was indistinguishable by pulsed-field gel electrophoresis from the strain isolated from a respiratory tract isolate from one of 20 farm rabbits that slept with a cat with which she had contact.[50]

RACCOONS

The raccoon ascarid, *Baylisascaris procyonis*, has caused cases, including fatal ones, of meningoencephalitis, usually in young children who accidentally ingest infectious ova.[51] Ocular involvement has also been reported. Leptospirosis has been reported from contact with raccoons.[52] Rabies is common in raccoons, although direct transmission to humans in the USA has not been reported.

MONGOOSES

Leptospirosis is common among mongooses in Hawaii[53] and a number of Caribbean islands.[54] Rabies is quite common among many species of mongoose and accounts for a significant number of cases of human exposure to rabies in the Caribbean. It is the principal rabies reservoir in South Africa and it may be an important source of wildlife rabies in India.[55]

INSECTIVORES

Hedgehog contact has transmitted salmonellosis[56] and dermatophyte infections due to *Trichophyton erinacei*.[53] In an outbreak of leptospirosis in Italy in which 32 of 33 confirmed cases were contracted by drinking water at the same water fountain, a dead hedgehog was found in a water reservoir connected to the system, although isolation of *Leptospira* spp. from the hedgehog was not attempted.[57]

The Asian house shrew, *Suncus murinus*, has been found to be infested with the oriental rat flea, *Xenopsylla cheopis*, and infected with *Yersinia pestis*. It may well be important in the maintenance of plague between epidemics. Insectivores also appear to be reservoirs of tick-borne encephalitis and tularemia.

MARINE MAMMALS (SEALS, SEA LIONS, WALRUS, WHALES, DOLPHINS, PORPOISES, MANATEES)

At the case report level, there are several infections that have been transmitted from marine mammals to humans. Leptospirosis, which is commonly encountered in seals and California sea lions, has been transmitted from an infected sea lion pup to a human. Two people developed leptospirosis after performing a necropsy on a sea lion that died of leptospirosis.[58] Human infection with *Erysipelothrix rhusiopathiae* has been reported on a few occasions among veterinarians and veterinary students caring for or performing autopsies on cetaceans.[59] In these reports, the isolation of the organism was not made from the human cases. Two of three people who cared for affected gray seals developed 'single milker's nodule-like lesions' on the fifth finger of the right hand. The lesions from the seal handlers demonstrated virus particles that were identical with the virus particles from the seals' pox lesions and were characteristic of the paravaccinia subgroup of poxviruses.[60]

Pulmonary tuberculosis due to a member of the *Mycobacterium tuberculosis* complex that is similar to *M. bovis* has been transmitted from seals in a marine park in Western Australia to a seal trainer who developed pulmonary tuberculosis 3 years after his last exposure to the animals with an isolate of the *Mycobacterium* that could not be distinguished from the seal isolates on the basis of DNA restriction endonuclease analysis.[61] Seal trainers are in very close contact with seals who, by barking and coughing, are potentially able to transmit infection via the aerosol route.

Four people involved in necropsies of harbor seals from which influenza A virus A/Seal/Mass/1/80 (H7N7) was isolated, developed purulent conjunctivitis but did not have detectable antibodies in single serum samples 3–6 months after the exposure to the influenza A virus isolated from the seals.[62] A seal that was known to be infected with the influenza A virus sneezed into the face and right eye of a person who subsequently developed conjunctivitis from which the virus was isolated.[63] Influenza A virus has also been isolated from cetaceans.

Numerous cases of 'seal finger' have been reported in people who have been bitten or scratched by seals and from skinning or handling seals. Seal finger often responds to tetracycline therapy. The etiologic agent has not been established. Other organisms that have been transmitted via the bite of marine mammals include a single case report of *Mycoplasma phocacerebrale*, which was isolated from the drainage material from a patient's fingers and swabs from the seal's front teeth.[64]

Consumption of whale, seal and walrus meat is not uncommon among the Inuit in Canada, Alaska, Greenland and Siberia. There have been large epidemics of salmonellosis resulting from consumption of whale meat from floating and beached whale carcasses that have been used as the source of food. Trichinellosis (trichinosis) has been acquired following the consumption of raw or undercooked walrus meat. The clinical presentation in arctic trichinellosis due to *Trichinella nativa* differs from that of classic trichinellosis caused by *Trichinella spiralis* in that the most prominent clinical symptoms in arctic trichinellosis are gastrointestinal, with prolonged diarrhea.[65] Food-borne botulism, typically due to *Clostridium botulinum* type E, has been acquired from the consumption of fermented foods included beluga whale meat, seal meat, seal flippers and walrus meat.

ARMADILLOS

Both experimental and naturally occurring leprosy in nine-banded armadillos has been noted and there has been a body of literature (reviewed by Blake *et al.*[66]) which suggests that contact with armadillos may have been the source of leprosy in some patients in the USA and Mexico. Sporotrichosis has been found to be highly associated with armadillo contact in Uruguay.[67]

BIRDS

Psittacosis is transmitted to humans not only via pet birds but also via turkeys, wild and domestic pigeons, ducks and other birds.[68]

Salmonellosis has been acquired from contact with birds and from consumption of birds (e.g. chicken, turkey) and eggs.[69] *Campylobacter jejuni* and *C. laridis* infections have been associated with both the consumption of birds and, interestingly, consumption of milk that has been pecked by magpies (*Pica pica*) and jackdaws (*Corvus monedula*).[70] *Erysipelothrix rhusiopathiae* has been acquired from bird contact. Newcastle disease virus of fowl, an occupational disease, causes an acute conjunctivitis which may be associated with pre-auricular adenitis.[71]

Histoplasmosis, often in large outbreaks, has been the result of inhalation of bird excreta.[72] Infection with *Cryptococcus neoformans*, which is known to be found in bird droppings, has at the case report level been linked to exposure to pet birds[73] and fancy pigeons.[74]

Q fever has been reported in five members of a family as a result of exposure to either aerosolized, contaminated pigeon excreta or infected ticks, or both.[75]

Avian strains of influenza A virus represent a global concern, as the host range of the viruses may include humans. There exists the potential for pandemic influenza as a result of the introduction of an avian virus with a hemagglutinin to which humans lack immunity.[76] In 1997 in Hong Kong, there were 18 human cases of influenza A H5N1 infection and six deaths. The outbreak ended after the institution of control measures that included the culling of poultry in Hong Kong. In 1999 an H9N2 strain, closely related to a quail virus which co-circulated with H5N1 viruses in live poultry markets in Hong Kong in late 1997 and shown to possess a set of internal genes similar to those of the H5N1 viruses, infected two children.[77] More recently, avian strains have caused infections not only in birds in multiple countries but also in people, continuing to raise the specter of pandemic influenza. As of this writing, there has not been efficient person-to-person spread of these strains.

The recent epidemic of West Nile virus infection in the USA is largely attributable to the introduction of this flavivirus into a new ecologic niche in wild birds in North America. Blackbirds, crows, other wild birds and domestic chickens are susceptible to this viral illness and this forms the reservoir for this mosquito-transmitted infection that is responsible for a potentially lethal form of viral encephalitis.[78]

Tularemia has been, at the several case report level, acquired from wild birds. A case of Crimean–Congo hemorrhagic fever in an ostrich farm worker who was involved in the slaughter of ostriches, *Struthio camelus*, and handled the fresh blood and tissues of the birds, has been reported. There were numerous adult *Hyalomma* ticks on the ostriches and he likely was infected either directly due to skinning the ostriches or as a result of the presence of the ticks on the ostriches.[79]

FISH

In addition to the normal flora of the fish, a wound can become infected with environmental bacteria. The species of bacteria that live in water are dependent on both salinity and temperature. Free-living estuarine and fresh-water bacteria include the genera *Vibrio*, *Aeromonas* and *Plesiomonas*. As a result, the etiologic agents isolated from an infected wound from a fish bite, spine or fin injury that occurs in salt water may well be different from one that occurs in fresh water. The normal flora of teeth in salt-water sharks includes, for example, *Vibrio* spp., including *V. harveyi* (formerly *V. carchariae*), an organism that was the cause of infection following the bite of a great white shark.[80] By contrast, *Edwardsiella tarda* is commonly isolated from catfish injuries occurring in fresh water. Other organisms that have caused wound injuries as a result of injuries from fish include *Aeromonas* spp., *Erysipelothrix rhusiopathiae*, *Mycobacterium marinum*, *Mycobacterium terrae*, *Streptococcus iniae*, *Vibrio vulnificus* and *Vibrio vulnificus* serovar E (biotype 2; indole-negative) from eels.[81] *Vibrio alginolyticus*, *Photobacterium damselae* subsp. *damselae* (formerly *Vibrio damsela*), *Shewanella putrefaciens*, *Pseudomonas aeruginosa* and *Halomonas venusta* have all been isolated from fish bites and injuries. It is not always clear whether the source of the organism is the fish or the water.

Ingestion of fish or fish products can pose a significant risk of acquiring both bacterial and parasitic infections unless the fish has been well cooked.

Vibrio spp., including *V. fluvialis*, *V. hollisae*, *V. parahaemolyticus* and *V. cholerae* O1,[82] have all been associated with fish consumption, as has *P. shigelloides*. Eel consumption has been associated with *Photobacterium damselae* subsp. *damselae* (formerly *Vibrio damsela*).[83] *Listeria monocytogenes* infections have been associated with the consumption of fish, including vacuum-packed salmon and cold-smoked rainbow trout.[84]

Fish-associated botulism is usually due to type E toxin and in the USA is most common among Alaskans. Fermented fish eggs, fish eggs, home-marinated fish and dry salted fish have all been implicated. Consumption of apparently fresh (unpreserved and unfermented) fish in Hawaii resulted in three adults with botulism due to type B toxin.[85] Numerous parasitic infections have been reported following

Table 69.3 Selected parasites transmitted via consumption of fish

Parasite	Type of parasite	Types of fish
Diphyllobothrium latum	Cestode	Salmon, pike, perch, burbot
Diphyllobothrium pacificum	Cestode	Marine fish
Diphyllobothrium ursi	Cestode	Salmon
Nanophyetus salminicola	Trematode	Usually salmonids
Heterophyes heterophyes	Trematode	Mullet, tilapia, mosquito fish
Haplorchis yokogawai	Trematode	Mullet
Haplorchis taichui	Trematode	Mullet
Clonorchis sinensis	Trematode	Fresh-water fish
Opisthorchis viverrini	Trematode	Fresh-water fish
Opisthorchis felineus	Trematode	Fresh-water fish
Metorchis conjunctus	Trematode	Fresh-water fish
Anisakis simplex	Nematode	Salmon, tuna, herring, mackerel, others
Pseudoterranova decipiens	Nematode	Cod, pollock, haddock, salmon, Pacific rockfish
Eustrongyloides spp.	Nematode	Killfish, estuarine fish, minnows
Dioctophyma renale	Nematode	Fresh-water, estuarine fish
Capillaria philippinensis	Nematode	Fresh-water, estuarine fish
Gnathostoma spinigerum	Nematode	Fresh-water fish

the consumption of raw, undercooked, pickled and lightly or cold-smoked fish. Selected cestodes, trematodes and nematodes acquired from the consumption of fish are listed in Table 69.3.

AMPHIBIANS

Contact with amphibians has transmitted sparganosis, due to *Diphyllobothrium* (*Spirometra*) *mansoni*, which has been transmitted by the use of contaminated frog flesh as a poultice (reviewed by Huang and Kirk[86]), and far less commonly with intraocular *Alaria* spp. in a woman with a long history of frog collection and food preparation.[87]

Ingestion of amphibians has transmitted sparganosis. Infection with the trematode *Fibricola seoulensis* has been reported from Korea, including a report in which 10 Korean soldiers who ate raw or undercooked flesh of snakes or frogs during survival training acquired the infection.[88] A single case of a fatal infection in a 24-year-old man due to *Alaria americana* has been attributed to the consumption of undercooked frogs' legs, although there was no documentation of consumption. Two cases of intraocular infection with an *Alaria* spp. were reported in Asian-Americans in California who consumed cooked frogs' legs in Chinese dishes.[89] Although frogs' legs have a very high rate of contamination with *Salmonella*, there are few published reports of salmonellosis attributed to their ingestion. *Salmonella* infections remain a potential risk when handling reptiles, such as turtles, lizards and snakes.

BEARS

There is a single published report of transmission of leptospirosis to two zoo employees in which the most likely source was an ill polar bear cub.[90] There is a notable lack of published reports on infections following the bites of bears. A case report in which a man shot and killed a grizzly bear in Alaska and scratched his left index finger on one of the bear's teeth while removing the bear's tongue resulted in an infection with *Mycobacterium chelonae* subsp. *abscessus*.[91]

Consumption of undercooked bear meat has been associated in multiple reports with trichinellosis. Bear steaks are often served rare, in part because they are somewhat 'tough' if they are fully cooked. Bears are known to have a high rate of toxoplasmosis and the possibility of a dual infection (trichinellosis and toxoplasmosis) in a person who ingested undercooked bear meat has been reported.[92] It is worth noting that acute hypervitaminosis A has been reported following the ingestion of polar bear liver.

LARGE HERBIVORES (ELEPHANTS, RHINOCEROSES)

Few infections have been transmitted from elephants and rhinoceroses to humans. These include documented transmission of *M. tuberculosis* from elephants,[93] *M. bovis* from rhinoceroses[94] and an orthopoxvirus (possibly cowpox). It is likely that cases of tuberculosis in elephants, which are almost all reportedly due to *M. tuberculosis*, are the result of human-to-elephant transmission. In the United States, approximately 3% percent of elephants are infected with *M. tuberculosis*.[95]

REFERENCES

References for this chapter can be found online at http://www.expertconsult.com

Chapter | **70** | *Jos WM van der Meer*
Gijs Bleijenberg

Chronic fatigue syndrome

INTRODUCTION

Fatigue is one of the most common complaints of patients with all kinds of underlying disease, but physicians often tend to ignore the complaint because they are unable to deal with it properly.

Chronic fatigue syndrome (CFS) is a syndrome characterized by persistent and unexplained fatigue associated with severe impairment in daily functioning.[1] Patient organizations tend to prefer the term ME (myalgic encephalomyelitis) or CFIDS (chronic fatigue and immune dysfunction syndrome) which are both misnomers, because they refer to pathological processes that have not been proven (inflammation of the central nervous system; immunodeficiency).

Because a substantial proportion of patients with CFS (around 75%) report a sudden onset starting with or following an infection, infectious disease specialists are often consulted by patients with CFS. This also justifies a chapter on CFS in a textbook like this. However, not all patients attribute the start of the symptoms to an infection and a more gradual onset is not uncommon.

The pathogenesis of CFS is still poorly understood (see below) and among physicians and lay people some considerable controversy surrounds the syndrome. Some doctors feel that it is a nonexistent illness, others consider it a mental illness, whereas still others (among them many patients) are convinced that it is a somatic disorder. Because older textbooks did not deal with CFS or coin it as a psychiatric illness ('neurasthenia'), a number of doctors are not diagnosing patients as suffering from CFS; patients may return with the self-diagnosis of CFS or ME, and this may lead to friction within the doctor–patient relationship. Because of the controversies mentioned, many patients with CFS will have had negative experiences with doctors that voiced their doubts regarding CFS. Such negative experiences will often enforce the patient's attributions to a somatic explanation for the illness.

The literature on CFS reinforces this controversy; however, it also struggles with a number of mediocre studies in which unsubstantiated claims regarding pathogenesis, diagnosis and therapy are made. These studies are often readily accepted as true by patients and their organizations as they desperately look for solutions to their illness. Physicians who take care of CFS patients should be aware of these issues, and – as is stressed in the guideline from the UK National Institute of Health and Clinical Excellence (NICE) – need good communication skills to enable patients to participate as partners in decisions about their health care.[2] In addition, this guideline recommends a timely and accurate diagnosis and early symptom management.

CASE DEFINITION AND DIAGNOSTIC APPROACH

Descriptions of CFS-like illness can be found in the older literature, some dating back centuries.[3] Although there are several case definitions used around the world, the most widely accepted and used is the consensus definition published by Fukuda *et al.*[4] (Table 70.1). This case definition, which was primarily meant for clinical and epidemiologic research on CFS, has not been validated for use in individual patients. An intrinsic problem with classifications like this is that the way the criteria are scored makes a substantial difference; by spontaneous reporting the average score is considerably lower than when systems are systematically asked for, either orally or by questionnaire.[5]

A second problem of which clinicians should be aware, is that the number of positive criteria does not reflect the severity of fatigue and impairment.[5] This means that to assess the severity of illness other

Table 70.1 Diagnostic criteria for chronic fatigue syndrome (CFS)

To diagnose CFS the following criteria should be fulfilled:
- Clinically evaluated, unexplained, persistent or relapsing fatigue that is of new or definite onset (not lifelong) lasting 6 or more consecutive months
- The fatigue is not the result of ongoing exertion
- The fatigue is not substantially alleviated by rest
- The fatigue results in substantial reductions in previous levels of occupational, educational, social or personal activities

Four or more of the following symptoms are concurrently presented for >6 months
- Impaired memory or concentration
- Sore throat
- Tender cervical or axillary lymph nodes
- Muscle pain
- Multi-joint pain
- 'New' headaches
- Unrefreshing sleep
- Postexertion malaise

After Fukuda *et al.*[4]

questions must be asked. A better alternative is to use the validated questionnaires that are available. We prefer the Checklist Individual Strength for fatigue and the Sickness Impact Profile (SIP-8) or Medical Outcomes Survey Short Form-36 (MOS SF-36) to assess functional impairment.[5,6]

The criteria of the case definition[4] cover most of the symptoms that occur within the context of CFS. Most prominent are incapacitating fatigue and postexertional malaise lasting more than 24 hours; patients may further suffer from myalgia, arthralgia, headache, sleep disturbances (such as unrefreshing sleep, insomnia), and problems with memory and concentration. In addition, CFS patients have abdominal complaints (as in irritable bowel syndrome), hyperhidrosis, frequent micturition and slightly elevated body temperature.[7] Sore throat and painful lymph nodes, although listed in the American literature and in the Fukuda case definition,[4] are rare and usually not found by physical examination. It is not uncommon for patients to report that they have become allergic, but this also is hard to substantiate.[8] Patients with primary fibromyalgia often suffer from fatigue and accompanying symptoms similar to those of CFS patients.[9] Many authorities consider CFS and fibromyalgia part of a spectrum in which either fatigue or pain is most prominent.

A major difficulty for the physician is that CFS is – to a large extent – a diagnosis of exclusion. Over the years there have been a series of claims in the literature on diagnostic markers (e.g. RNAse-1, microbial serology or polymerase chain reaction, immunologic tests), but so far none has proven useful. Likewise, testing the function of the pituitary–adrenal axis or imaging the CNS (see below) is not fruitful outside the research setting as the abnormalities that have been reported are too subtle to be of diagnostic significance. Thus, there is no gold standard for the diagnosis and the differential diagnosis is a long one. In Table 70.2, a systematic differential diagnosis of chronic

fatigue is presented. It is clear that most alternative diagnoses can be excluded by taking a thorough history from the patient and performing a meticulous physical examination and a limited set of diagnostic tests. If the duration of the illness is longer than a year, the number of additional investigations may be more limited, since a range of diagnoses (e.g. bacterial endocarditis, malignancy) are becoming highly unlikely in the absence of any specific accompanying signs and without overt deterioration of the somatic state. Extensive serology also becomes unnecessary since most infections do not remain symptomatic for such a prolonged period.

EPIDEMIOLOGY

Although CFS has received most attention in the western world, it seems to occur everywhere. In the older literature there are a number of small outbreaks of CFS, the causes of which have not been elucidated.[3] The recent literature deals merely with sporadic cases.

There is a clear female preponderance in CFS: at least 70% of the patients are female.[4] Most patients are in the third decade of life, but CFS occurs in the young (mainly adolescents) and also in people of older age.[4]

The prevalence of CFS has been found to vary between countries but this may be due to the different methodologies of the various studies, as well as ethnic and sociologic differences. With regard to the latter, perceptions of illness, attributions and the tendency of labeling a complex of symptoms CFS/ME greatly differ between countries. Through questionnaires sent to general practitioners, we found a prevalence of 1.95 per 1000 in the Netherlands.[10] From community-based studies in adults in the USA, prevalence rates of 2.3 and 4.2 per 1000 have been reported, whereas a prospective study in primary care in the UK found 26 per 1000.[11–13] After correction for co-morbid psychological disorders the prevalence in the latter study became 5.0 per 1000, which still is remarkably high.

ETIOLOGY AND PATHOGENESIS

There are many hypotheses regarding the etiology and pathogenesis of CFS, but few are supported by evidence. So far, the search for a unifying explanation (e.g. a chronic infection by persisting micro-organism) has not been successful. Some 15 years ago it occurred to us and others that – when investigating the etiology and pathogenesis of CFS – it is more fruitful to discern a series of factors:
- predisposing factors;
- precipitating factors; and
- perpetuating factors.

From a theoretical point of view, this does not preclude the possibility that ultimately the precipitating factors and perpetuating factors are the same, but in the research setting and for our current understanding this distinction is more appropriate.

Predisposing factors

Predisposing factors comprise genetic factors, some of which are emerging from studies using modern genetic techniques but still arouse considerable controversy.[14–17] So far these genetic factors have not led to greater insight into the molecular substrate of CFS. As mentioned, there is a strong gender predisposition for CFS: at least 70% of the patents with CFS are female. Personality characteristics such as neuroticism and introversion are considered to contribute to the risk of developing CFS.[1] Likewise, inactivity during childhood and infectious mononucleosis are contributing factors.[18,19] Childhood traumas are associated with an increased risk of CFS.[20]

Table 70.2 Systematic differential diagnosis of chronic fatigue

Localized organ dysfunction	Endocrine: • Pituitary: hypopituitarism • Adrenal: adrenal insufficiency, hypercorticism • Thyroid: hypo- and hyperthyroidism • Parathyroid: hypo- and hyperparathyroidism • Diabetes mellitus Heart: heart failure Lung: emphysema, chronic obstructive pulmonary disease, other causes of respiratory insufficiency Liver: chronic hepatitis, cirrhosis Kidneys: renal insufficiency
Generalized disorder	Infection Noninfectious inflammatory disease Intoxication Storage disease Neoplasm Anemia
Neurologic	Multiple sclerosis Narcolepsy Myasthenia gravis
Psychologic/psychiatric	Mood disorder Sleep disorder Somatoform disorder
Drug-induced	Side-effect of drug Psychotropic agents
Idiopathic	Chronic fatigue syndrome

Precipitating factors

Precipitating factors are the factors that start the illness. These precipitating factors, which are largely attributions of patients, seem to be heterogeneous: infection, physical trauma, intoxication (including medication), operation and/or anesthesia, and serious life events are all considered to be instigators of CFS. Although these attributions are often very plausible, there is only circumstantial evidence that they are the starting point of CFS. The typical history of the patient with CFS is that it all started with a flu-like illness that was accompanied by severe fatigue; when the flu resolved, the fatigue remained. Evidence for infection as a starting point comes from studies in infectious mononucleosis, caused by Epstein–Barr virus (EBV).[21,22] In the acute phase, this infection – when symptomatic – is often accompanied by fatigue that wanes over a period of weeks to months. A small minority of patients (approximately 10–15%) experience fatigue beyond 6 months and develop the characteristic chronic fatigue syndrome. How many of these patients spontaneously recover between 6 months and 1 year is not clear.

The severity of the acute infection but no other clinical, demographic or psychological factors have been found to be risk factors for developing CFS.[21] A more rapid IgG response to EBV-associated nuclear antigens and a slower development of the peak interferon gamma (IFN-γ) response to latent cycle EBV peptides seems to predispose to the development of CFS.[23] Recently, in a small study using microarrays, activation of mitochondrial function of a number of genes, fatty acid metabolism and cell cycle were found to predispose to CFS in EBV infection.[24]

Another relevant question is whether certain infections do lead more often to CFS than others. Although EBV infections are commonly incriminated as a starting point for CFS, other infections are also associated with CFS. In fact, fatigue after 6 months is as common in EBV infection as in Q fever and Ross River virus infection.[25]

Although a number of metabolic abnormalities (mitochondrial defects such as carnitine deficiency) have been claimed to underlie CFS, none of these has been supported by solid scientific evidence.[26]

Perpetuating factors

Perpetuating factors are responsible for the chronicity of CFS and can be divided into somatic and psychological perpetuating factors. With regard to the former, one may ask the question whether microbial pathogens, especially those that persist after acute infection, may act as perpetuating factors. For EBV there is no evidence in this respect: virologic studies[27] as well as interventions with antiviral drugs[28] do not point to EBV as a perpetuating factor. There is no evidence for a role of other micro-organisms (e.g. *Helicobacter pylori*, *Borrelia* spp., *Brucella* spp., *Coxiella burnetii*, *Candida* spp., *Mycoplasma* spp.) as a persisting cause. Nevertheless, the hypothesis could be entertained that an as yet unknown persistent microbe acts as the precipitating and perpetuating factor for CFS.

A number of claims have been made regarding immunologic factors in CFS but few have been independently reproduced. In well-controlled studies, only minor differences have been found.[29,30] One area of controversy is the sensitivity to dexamethasone and production of cytokines such as interleukin-10 and IFN-γ production; in these areas at least there are profound differences between adults and adolescents with chronic fatigue.[31,32]

In most studies the immunologic abnormalities are not great and such subtle changes do not automatically imply causality or a role as a perpetuating factor. It may well be that such findings are a consequence of change in activity and/or behavior.

There are more controversial findings regarding the pathophysiology of CFS. For instance, the finding of an abnormal RNAse-1 response has not been substantiated by independent investigations.[33,34]

There is a subtle derangement of the hypothalamic-pituitary-adrenal (HPA) axis, with a relatively low glucocorticoid response (albeit within the normal range) despite a relatively high adrenocorticotropic hormone (ACTH).[35,36] These changes are not present during the early stages of fatiguing illness and are reversed during successful cognitive behavioral therapy.[36] Intervention studies with low-dose steroids have not provided unequivocal answers[37,38] and are listed as strategies not to be used in the NICE guideline.[2]

There are controversial reports in the literature regarding the growth hormone pathway, but no abnormalities were found in well-controlled studies.[39–41] Abnormalities within the serotonin pathway have also been implicated in the pathogenesis of CFS. Evidence for enhanced serotonin metabolism has been reported,[42–44] but interference with a 5-HT$_3$ inhibitor failed to demonstrate an effect in a placebo-controlled trial in well-defined CFS patients, despite an earlier positive pilot study.[45,46]

From the preceding paragraphs it may be clear that so far few, if any, somatic factors have been found to play a role in the pathogenesis of CFS.

With regard to psychological factors, Vercoulen *et al.*[47] were able to provide a model of CFS on the basis of a Lisrel analysis of a large number of measurements in patients with CFS (Fig. 70.1). This model appears to be specific for CFS, as it is statistically rejected for fatigue secondary to other diseases. Factors that were found to contribute to chronicity are strong somatic attributions ('I know that it is a pure somatic disorder'), a low self-efficacy ('I cannot influence my complaints') and a strong focus on bodily sensations. The latter is one of the most prominent features of CFS, and the avoidance of physical activity is a consequence of perceptions and expectations rather than of the actual physical condition. The role of perception will be discussed in more detail below.

In the older literature, CFS was sometimes considered to be atypical depression, but the current view is that CFS and depression are different conditions.[48] At time of diagnosis, depression is present in 25% of patients, while 50–75% of CFS patients have a lifetime history of major depression.[49] In patients with CFS a number of typical symptoms of depression, such as anhedonia, guilt and lack of motivation are not found, and the changes in the HPA axis are opposite. Antidepressants such as fluoxetine are neither effective against the fatigue nor against the symptoms of depression.[50]

CENTRAL FATIGUE IN CFS

The fatigue in CFS is considered centrally located as the subjective sense of fatigue is perceived at the level of the central nervous system.[51,52] There are few if any arguments for peripheral fatigue, the

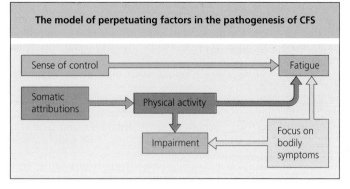

Fig. 70.1 The model of perpetuating factors in the pathogenesis of chronic fatigue syndrome. Using a Lisrel analysis of empiric data a model was established in which fatigue is a consequence of a lack of sense of control ('I don't have control over my symptoms'), decreased physical activity and a focus on bodily sensations (the patients are very tuned in to bodily symptoms and feel there is something wrong with their body). Strong somatic attributions ('I know this is a physical illness') leads to decrease in physical activity. The lack or avoidance of physical activity and the focus on bodily sensations also lead to the impairment. Reprinted with permission from Vercoulen *et al.*[47]

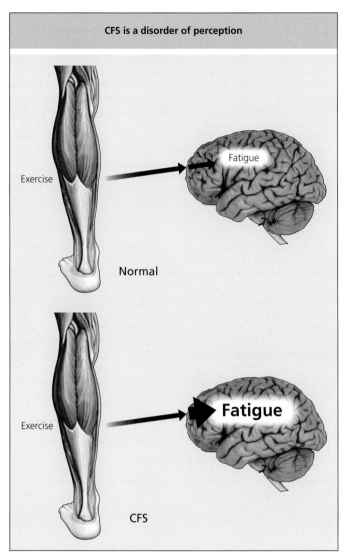

Fig. 70.2 Chronic fatigue syndrome (CFS) as a disorder of perception. The upper panel depicts the normal situation: muscle activity as in exercise is perceived as physiologic fatigue. In CFS the same signal from the muscle is perceived as severe fatigue; apparently the signal is amplified at the level of the brain. Similarly, other bodily signals are also perceived in an amplified fashion.

fatigability that occurs in disorders of muscle and neuromuscular junctions, as the motor power during voluntary muscle contraction is essentially normal.

The central localization of the fatigue is in agreement with the findings that point to a disturbed perception of fatigue (Fig. 70.2), as well as of other signals from the body (pain, sleep quality, memory). In well-controlled studies on exercise capacity, neuropsychological functioning, and sleep physiology, several investigators have found that CFS patients perceive the performance of their body as miserable or at least not to the level to be expected.[53–55] The finding of failing central activation of maximal voluntary contraction also fits into this concept.[56]

A key question in this respect is what the neurobiologic substrate is for this disturbance in perception. In the previous section we have already discussed a number of mediator systems (neurotransmitters, hormones) that could play a role, but it is clear that more research is needed here. A number of studies have addressed the question whether structural and functional abnormalities can be demonstrated in the brain of CFS patients, using modern high-resolution imaging techniques. Older studies reported white matter hyperintensities on MRI and cerebral blood flow abnormality using SPECT imaging, but

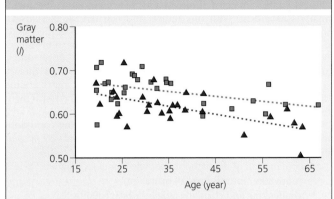

Fig. 70.3 The loss of gray matter during aging in patients with chronic fatigue syndrome (red symbols) compared to matched controls (green symbols). Adapted with permission from De Lange et al.[60]

well-controlled studies were not able to confirm these findings.[57,58] Recent MRI studies by two independent groups have detected diminished gray matter volumes in CFS patients compared to matched controls (Fig. 70.3).[59,60] These differences are, however, too small to be used for diagnosis in individual patients. The relevance of these findings for the pathophysiology of CFS is underscored by the observation that these changes are – at least to some extent – reversible with successful cognitive behavioral therapy (see below).[61]

On functional MRI it was found that in patients with CFS a motor imagery task evoked stronger responses in visually related structures than matched controls.[62] In addition, the ventral anterior cingulate cortex became active when healthy controls made an error, but remained inactive in CFS patients during erroneous performance.[62] These results point to dysfunctional motor planning and motivational disturbances in CFS.

In another functional MRI study, CFS patients were also shown to utilize more extensive areas of the brain to process auditory information than controls.[63] Likewise, greater activity in cortical and subcortical regions of the brain was found during a fatiguing cognitive task.[63] These imaging findings are corroborated by electrophysiologic data showing higher delta wave activity in the left uncus and parahippocampal gyrus and higher theta in the cingulate gyrus and right superior frontal gyrus.[64]

ABNORMALITIES OF THE AUTONOMIC NERVOUS SYSTEM

There have been speculations about abnormalities of the autonomic nervous system in CFS for many years as evidenced by some of the accompanying symptoms (hyperhidrosis, palpitations, dizziness and orthostatic intolerance). Research findings are somewhat controversial but it is probably safe to conclude that signs of postural tachycardia or (pre)syncope can be found in a minority of CFS patients.[65,66] The higher heart rate that may be encountered in many patients at baseline, together with a marked decrease in stroke volume in response to head-up tilt testing, may point to deconditioning.[65] Tests like the head-up tilt test should not be done routinely in the diagnostic process.[2]

PROGNOSIS AND TREATMENT

Without treatment, less than 10% of patients recover over time, even though some improvement is not rare.[67] A strong belief in a physical cause of illness and a long duration of illness are associated with a poor outcome.[68]

Although a great number of claims have been made regarding a variety of treatments for CFS, few are supported by results of solid clinical trials.[69] At least three systematic reviews and one meta-analysis have dealt with this subject and reached the conclusion that (only) cognitive behavioral therapy (CBT) and graded exercise therapy (GET) are of proven benefit.[69-72] There is no evidence-based drug treatment (hormones, immunomodulatory drugs, antimicrobials, psychotropic drugs, vitamins and other dietary supplements) for CFS.[2] The same holds for diets (e.g. the 'Candida diet') that are largely being advised by proponents of complementary medicine.

CBT is a form of psychotherapy directed at changing condition-related cognitions and behaviors. The key components of CBT according to Prins et al.[1] are:

- explanation of the pathophysiologic model (see Fig. 70.1);
- motivation for this form of treatment;
- challenging and changing fatigue-related cognitions;
- achievement and maintenance of a basic degree of physical activity, followed by
- gradual increase of physical activity; and
- planning work rehabilitation or rehabilitation in other personal goals.

With CBT patients should learn to gain control over their symptoms; graded increase of activity is an intrinsic part of the treatment. In that sense CBT for CFS always includes a graded activity component, which is the only therapeutic ingredient in GET while cognitions are not explicitly treated. The improvement rates for CBT are around 70%; in GET they are lower (around 50%). Indicators of failure are a strong focus on physical symptoms and a poor sense of control. Likewise, patients claiming disability-related benefits have a poor treatment outcome.[73]

An important issue with regard to efficacy is the aim of CBT. In many studies improvement and rehabilitation is the treatment goal. Our CBT studies[73-77] aimed to cure (i.e. disappearance of symptoms and functional impairment as its defined goal, ability to return to work and other activities and no longer considering oneself as a patient).[1] It should be realized that if cure is not the goal of treatment, it will never be attained. Of great interest is our recent observation that – as mentioned above – there is a regain of gray matter with successful CBT, underscoring that the loss of gray matter in CFS is neurobiologically important, that CBT induces morphologic changes that point to plasticity of the brain.[60]

Another important question is whether the effect of CBT is lasting; a number of follow-up studies have shown that there is a sustained effect.[78,79] However, there are a couple of problems with CBT. The first one is availability; although the term cognitive behavioral therapy is widely used, specific CBT, tailor-made for CFS is hard to get. A second major problem – fed by some patient organizations – is that many CFS patients have strong somatic attributions and reject the idea that a psychological intervention may help them.

CONCLUSION

Over recent years, although our insight into the pathogenesis of CFS increased and we have made progress with regard to our abilities to manage and treat the disorder, our knowledge of the syndrome is still too limited. Controversies about CFS between doctors, researchers and patients have not been particularly helpful in facilitating solid research and further solving the enigmas of the syndrome. In addition, such controversies are harmful to patients; health-care workers should do their utmost to facilitate effective management of the condition, as proposed in the NICE guidelines.[2]

REFERENCES

References for this chapter can be found online at http://www.expertconsult.com

Andrew W Artenstein

Chapter | **71** |

Bioterrorism and biodefense

INTRODUCTION

Bioterrorism can be broadly defined as the deliberate use of microbial agents or their toxins as weapons against noncombatants outside the setting of armed conflict. The concept is analogous to biologic warfare in a combat theater. The broad scope and mounting boldness of worldwide terrorism was impressively demonstrated by the massive attacks on New York City and Washington DC on September 11, 2001; the multifocal anthrax attacks that followed shortly thereafter, while not known to be directly related to 9/11, awakened civilized society to the threats posed by these 'weapons of mass terror'. This realization, in concert with recent revelations regarding the apparent willingness of terrorist organizations to acquire and deploy biologic weapons, constitutes ample evidence that the specter of bioterrorism poses a persistent global threat.

Biologic weapons have been used against both military and civilian targets throughout history. It has been variously speculated that at least some of the plagues visited upon ancient Egypt, as documented in the biblical book of Exodus, represented natural outbreaks of endemic infectious diseases that were recast as supreme forms of bioterrorism. In the 14th century Tatars attempted to use epidemic disease against the defenders of Kaffa by catapulting plague-infected corpses into the city.[1] British forces gave Native American tribespeople blankets from a smallpox hospital in an attempt to affect the balance of power in the 18th century Ohio River Valley.[1] In addition to their well-described use of chemical weapons, Axis forces purportedly infected livestock with anthrax and glanders to weaken Allied initiatives during the First World War. Perhaps the most egregious period in the history of biologic weaponry involved the Japanese program in Manchuria from 1932 to 1945. Based on survivor accounts and confessions of Japanese participants, thousands died as a result of experimental infection with a multitude of virulent pathogens at Unit 731, the code name for the biologic weapons facility there.[2]

The USA maintained an offensive biologic weapons program from 1942 until 1969, when the program was terminated by President Nixon. The Convention on the Prohibition of the Development, Production, and Stockpiling of Biological and Toxin Weapons and on Their Destruction (BWC) was ratified in 1972 and formally banned the development or use of biologic weapons, with enforcement the responsibility of the United Nations.[1] Unfortunately, the BWC has not been effective in its stated goals; multiple signatories, including the former Soviet Union and Iraq, have violated the terms and spirit of the agreement. The accidental release of aerosolized anthrax spores from a military plant in Sverdlovsk in 1979, resulting in at least 68 human deaths from inhalational anthrax, verifies the existence of an active Soviet offensive biologic weapons program.

THREAT ASSESSMENT

Biologic agents are considered weapons of mass destruction (WMD) because, as with certain conventional, chemical and nuclear weapons, their use may result in large-scale morbidity and mortality. In a World Health Organization (WHO) assessment model of the hypothetical casualty estimates from the intentional release of 50 g of aerosolized anthrax spores upwind from a population center of 500 000 (analogous to Providence, Rhode Island, USA), nearly 200 000 people might be killed or incapacitated by the event.[3] Biologic weapons possess unique properties among all WMD. Unlike other forms, biologic agents are associated with a clinical latency period of days to weeks in most cases, during which time exposed individuals are asymptomatic and early detection is quite difficult with currently available technology. Additionally, specific antimicrobial therapy and, in select circumstances, vaccines are available for the treatment and prevention of illness caused by biologic weapons; casualties from other forms of WMD can generally only be treated by decontamination, trauma mitigation and supportive care.

Nations adhering to democratic principles are vulnerable to bioterrorism because of the inherent freedoms that their citizens and visitors enjoy. This freedom of movement and access to public and private institutions can be exploited by rogue nations, terrorist organizations or malicious individuals intent on untoward acts. When coupled with worldwide cultural tensions, geopolitical conflicts and economic instability, open societies provide fertile ground for terrorism.

Recent events have established bioterrorism as a credible and ubiquitous threat and, in some quarters, as a potential tool for political coercion. The intentional contamination of restaurant salad bars with *Salmonella* by a religious cult trying to influence a local election in The Dalles, Oregon, in 1984;[4] the revelations that Aum Shinrikyo, the Japanese cult responsible for the sarin gas attack in the Tokyo subway system in 1995, experimented on multiple occasions with spraying anthrax from downtown Tokyo rooftops; and the findings of the United Nations weapons inspectors of massive quantities of weaponized biologic weapons in Iraq during the first Gulf War and its aftermath[5] served as sentinel warnings of a shift in terrorism trends. The anthrax attacks in the USA in October and November 2001, following the catastrophic events of September 11th, elevated bioterrorism to the fore of the international dialogue.

The aims of bioterrorism are those of terrorism in general: morbidity and mortality among civilian populations, disruption of societal fabric, and exhaustion or diversion of resources.[6] A 'successful' outcome, from a terrorist standpoint, may be achieved without furthering all of these aims and, in fact, may be accomplished simply by the credible threat of action or by a small-scale agent deployment. The anthrax attacks in 2001 evoked fear and anxiety and diverted public health and health-care resources away from other critical activities despite the limited number of casualties associated with the event.

Biologic weapons offer other, significant advantages to terrorists:

- they are relatively inexpensive to acquire as compared with conventional or nuclear weaponry;
- they can be deployed in a stealth fashion due to a variable clinical latency period, thus allowing the perpetrator opportunity to escape if desired; and
- they clearly evoke anxiety and panic in a population that is, in some instances, out of proportion to their physical effects.

From a rogue government's standpoint, the technology for bioterrorism is 'dual use', i.e. it can serve legitimate functions such as vaccine or pharmaceutical production as readily as biologic weapons production, thus making detection by inspectors all the more difficult.

To be employed in large-scale bioterrorism, biologic agents must undergo complex processes of production, cultivation, chemical modification and weaponization. For these reasons state sponsorship or direct support from governments or organizations with significant resources, contacts and infrastructure would predictably be required in large-scale events.[6] However, some agents may be acquired by terrorist groups on the black market and in other illicit settings.[7] Although an efficient mode of delivery has traditionally been felt to be necessary, the anthrax attacks in the USA in late 2001 illustrated the devastating results that can be achieved with relatively primitive delivery methods, e.g. high-speed mail sorting equipment and mailed letters.

Numerous attributes contribute to the effectiveness of a biologic weapon:

- availability or ease of large-scale production;
- ease of dissemination, especially by the aerosol route;
- stability in storage and delivery;
- cost; and
- clinical virulence.

The last refers to the reliability with which the pathogen causes high mortality, morbidity or social disruption. The Centers for Disease Control and Prevention (CDC) have prioritized biologic agent threats based upon the aforementioned characteristics,[8,9] and this has influenced current preparedness strategies (Table 71.1). Category A agents, considered the highest priority, are associated with high mortality and the greatest potential for major impact on public health. Category B agents are considered 'incapacitating' because of their potential for moderate morbidity but relatively low mortality. Most of the category A and B agents have been experimentally weaponized in the past. Category C agents include emerging threats and pathogens that may be available for development in the future.

Another factor that must be addressed in assessing future bioterrorism risk and predicted agents is the historical track record of experimentation with specific pathogens, an area that has been informed from the corroborated claims of various high-level Soviet defectors and data released from the former offensive weapons programs of the USA and the UK.[1,7,10] It is apparent from these sources, combined with the burgeoning fields of molecular biology and genomics, that future risk scenarios may have to contend with genetically altered and 'designer' pathogens that may be equipped with enhancements in virulence, such as antimicrobial resistance or augmented toxin production, or modifications that enhance dissemination, such as prolonged aerosol stability. To this end the author has added a miscellaneous grouping of potential threat agents to the extant CDC categories (see Table 71.1). The most cautious approach to assessing risk may be to remain open to additional, novel possibilities.

BIOTERRORISM RECOGNITION

By definition bioterrorism is insidious; absent advance warning or specific intelligence information, clinical illness will be manifest before the circumstances of a release event are known. For this reason health-care providers are likely to be the first responders to this form of terrorism. This is in contrast to the more familiar scenarios in which police, firefighters, paramedics and other emergency services personnel are deployed to the scene of an attack with conventional weaponry or a

natural disaster. Physicians and other health-care workers must therefore maintain a high index of suspicion of bioterrorism and recognize suggestive epidemiologic clues and clinical features to enhance early recognition, disseminate information rapidly and guide initial management of casualties. This remains the most effective way to minimize the deleterious effects of bioterrorism on individual patients and on the public health.

Early recognition is hampered for multiple reasons. Terrorists have an unlimited number of targets in most open, democratic societies; it is unrealistic to expect that without detailed intelligence data, all of these can be secured at all times. Certain sites, such as government institutions, historic landmarks or large events may be predictable targets, but there are other, less predictable possibilities. Metropolitan areas are considered vulnerable, but owing to the expansion of suburbs, commuters, and the clinical latency period between exposure and symptoms inherent with biologic agents, casualties of bioterrorism are likely to present for medical attention in diverse locations and at varying times following a common exposure. An event in New York City on a Wednesday morning may result in clinically ill individuals presenting over the ensuing weekend to a variety of emergency rooms within a 60-mile radius. Additionally, our mobile society ensures that affected individuals will likely present for medical care thousands of miles away from the original release point of the bioterrorist's weapon. This adds layers of complexity to managing a bioterrorism event and illustrates the critical importance of surveillance, cooperation and real-time communication in this setting.

Further hindering the early recognition of bioterrorism is that initial symptoms may be nondiagnostic. In the absence of a known exposure, many symptomatic individuals may not seek medical attention early on or may be misdiagnosed with a flu-like illness if they do. Once beyond the early stages many of these illnesses progress quite rapidly and treatment may be less successful. Most of the diseases caused by agents of bioterrorism are rarely, if ever, seen in clinical practice; physicians are, therefore, likely to be inexperienced with their clinical presentation. Additionally, these agents, by definition, will have been laboratory-manipulated and may not present with the classic clinical features of naturally occurring infection. This was dramatically illustrated by differences in the clinical presentations of some of the inhalational anthrax cases in the USA in October 2001 as compared with those described in earlier outbreaks.[11]

Early identification of bioterrorism is facilitated by the recognition of epidemiologic and clinical clues. Clustering of patients with common symptoms and signs, especially if these are unusual or known to be associated with bioterrorism agents, should prompt expeditious notification of local public health authorities. This approach may not only detect malicious events but will also lead to the recognition of outbreaks of naturally occurring disease or novel, emerging pathogens. The recognition of a single case of a rare or nonendemic infection, in the absence of a travel history or other potential natural exposure, should raise the specter of bioterrorism and should prompt notification of public health authorities. Finally, unusual patterns of disease, such as unusual age distributions, more severe clinical forms of infection or concurrent illness in human and animal populations, should raise suspicions for bioterrorism or another form of emerging infection. In fact for some category A, B or C agents of bioterrorism, available evidence supports the potential role of animals as early warning sentinels of an attack or as markers of persistent exposure risks to humans.[12]

Infectious diseases specialists are uniquely suited to play pivotal roles in the recognition, investigation and mitigation of bioterrorism, based on:

- an understanding of epidemiologic principles and risk assessment;
- expertise in specific threat agents, their clinical presentations and diagnostic approaches;
- knowledge of communicability and infection control principles; and
- an understanding of the tenets of treatment and prophylaxis of infectious diseases.

Table 71.1 Agents of concern for use in bioterrorism

Highest priority: category A (based upon potential mortality, morbidity, virulence, transmissibility, aerosol feasibility and psychosocial implications of an attack)

Microbe/toxin	Disease
Bacillus anthracis	Anthrax: inhalational, cutaneous
Variola virus	Smallpox and its variants
Yersinia pestis	Plague: pneumonic, bubonic, septicemic
Clostridium botulinum toxin	Botulism
Francisella tularensis	Tularemia: pneumonic, typhoidal
Viral hemorrhagic fevers	
Filoviruses	Ebola, Marburg
Arenaviruses	Lassa fever, South American hemorrhagic fevers
Bunyaviruses	Rift Valley fever, Congo–Crimean hemorrhagic fever
Flaviviruses	Dengue

Moderately high priority: category B (based upon potential morbidity, aerosol feasibility, dissemination characteristics, and diagnostic difficulty)

Microbe/toxin	Disease
Coxiella burnetti	Q fever
Brucella spp.	Brucellosis
Burkholderia mallei	Glanders
Burkholderia pseudomallei	Melioidosis
Alphaviruses (e.g. EEE, VEE)	Viral encephalitides
Ricinus communis toxin	Ricin intoxication
Staphylococcal enterotoxin B	Staphylococcal toxin illness
Salmonella spp., *Shigella dysenteriae*, *Escherichia coli* O157:H7, *Vibrio cholerae*, *Cryptosporidium parvum*, *Listeria monocytogenes*, *Campylobacter jejuni*, *Yersinia enterocolitica*	Food- and waterborne gastroenteritis
Rickettsia prowazekii	Epidemic typhus
Chlamydia psittaci	Psittacosis
Epsilon toxin of *Clostridium perfringens*	*C. perfringens* intoxication

Emerging threat agents: category C (based upon potential for production and dissemination, availability, morbidity/mortality)

Microbe/toxin	Disease
Hantaviruses	Viral hemorrhagic fevers
Flaviviruses	Yellow fever, West Nile virus
Mycobacterium tuberculosis	Multidrug-resistant tuberculosis
Nipah virus	Systemic flu-like illness

Miscellaneous (other examples of candidate threat agents that possess some elements of bioterrorism concern)

Genetically engineered vaccine- and/or antimicrobial-resistant category A or B agents
HIV-1
Adenoviruses
Influenza
Rotaviruses
Molecular hybrid pathogens (e.g. smallpox–plague, smallpox–ebola)
Severe acute respiratory syndrome coronavirus

EEE, eastern equine encephalomyelitis; VEE, Venezuelan equine encephalomyelitis.
Adapted from Patrozou & Artenstein.[26]

Nonetheless, an effective response to bioterrorism requires coordination of the medical system at all levels, from the community physician to the tertiary care center, with active engagement of public health, emergency management and law enforcement infrastructures.

THREAT AGENTS

This section will cover the biologic threat agents felt to be of major current concern, largely the CDC category A agents. Extensive coverage of specific pathogens can be found in related chapters in this text (cross-referenced in Table 71.2) and in other sources.[13,14] Data concerning clinical incubation periods, transmission characteristics and infection control procedures for agents of bioterrorism are provided in Table 71.2. Syndromic differential diagnoses for select clinical presentations are detailed in Table 71.3.

Anthrax

Anthrax results from infection with *Bacillus anthracis*, a Gram-positive, spore-forming, rod-shaped organism that exists in its host as a vegetative bacillus and in the environment as a spore. Details of the microbiology and pathogenesis of anthrax are found in Chapter 128 of this text. In nature anthrax is a zoonotic disease of herbivores that is prevalent in many geographic regions; sporadic human disease results from environmental or occupational contact with endospore-contaminated animal products.[15] Anthrax is uncommon in developed countries. In developing areas the cutaneous form of anthrax is the most common presentation; gastrointestinal and inhalational forms are exceedingly rare in naturally acquired disease. Cutaneous anthrax is rarely seen in current-day industrialized countries due to importation restrictions. The last known case of naturally occurring inhalational anthrax in the USA occurred in 1976.[16]

The recent attacks in the USA were on a relatively small scale, and nearly 40% of the confirmed cases were of the cutaneous variety.[17] The serious morbidity and mortality, however, were related to inhalational disease, as was noted in the Sverdlovsk outbreak in 1979. Therefore, planning for larger-scale events with aerosolized agent continues to be warranted.

The clinical presentations and differential diagnoses of cutaneous and inhalational anthrax are described in Table 71.3. The lesion of cutaneous anthrax may be similar in appearance to other lesions, including cutaneous forms of other agents of bioterrorism; however, it may be distinguished by epidemiologic as well as certain clinical features. Anthrax is traditionally a painless lesion, unless secondarily infected, and associated with significant local edema (Fig. 71.1). The bite of *Loxosceles reclusa*, the brown recluse spider, shares many of the local and systemic features of anthrax but is typically painful from the outset and lacks significant edema.[18] Cutaneous anthrax is associated with systemic disease and its attendant mortality in up to 20% of untreated cases, although with appropriate antimicrobial therapy, mortality is less than 1%.[16]

Once the inhaled endospores reach the terminal alveoli of the lungs, generally requiring particle sizes of 1–5 μm, they are phagocytosed by macrophages and transported to regional lymph nodes, where they germinate into vegetative bacteria and, subsequently, disseminate hematogenously.[15] The bacteria generate potent exotoxins, lethal toxin and edema toxin, which lead to hemorrhagic mediastinitis, systemic illness and death. Spores may remain latent for extended

Table 71.2 Epidemiologic characteristics for selected category A and B bioterrorism-associated diseases

Disease	Incubation period range (days)	Person-to-person transmission	Infection control precautions for patients	Case fatality rate
Inhalational anthrax (see Chapter 128)	2–43*	No	Standard	Untreated 100% Treated 45%
Cutaneous anthrax (see Chapter 128)	1–12	No	Standard	Untreated 20% Treated <1%
Botulism (see Chapter 21)	12–72 hours	No	Standard	6%
Primary pneumonic plague (see Chapter 120)	1–6	Yes	Droplet	Untreated 100% Treated ~50%
Bubonic plague (see Chapter 120)	2–8	No	Standard	Untreated 60% Treated <5%
Smallpox	7–19	Yes	Contact and airborne	Unvaccinated 30% Vaccinated 3%
Tularemia pneumonia (see Chapter 121)	1–21	No	Standard	Untreated 60% Treated <4%
Viral hemorrhagic fevers (see Chapter 126)	2–21	Yes	Contact and airborne	Marburg 25% Ebola 80% Other forms 2–30%
Viral encephalitides (see Chapter 19)	1–14	No	Standard	10–35%
Q fever (see Chapter 176)	2–41	No	Standard	3%
Brucellosis (see Chapter 123)	5–60	No	Standard	Untreated 5%
Glanders	1–21	Yes	Contact and droplet	Untreated – approaches 100% Treated – low

*Based on limited data from human outbreaks; experimental animal data support clinical latency periods of up to 100 days.
Adapted from Patrozou & Artenstein.[26]

Table 71.3 Syndromic differential diagnoses and clinical clues for category A agents of bioterrorism

Syndrome	Clinical presentation	Differential diagnosis	Bioterrorism-associated disease	Disease-specific clues
Influenza-like illness	Nonspecific constitutional and upper respiratory symptoms: malaise, myalgias, nausea, emesis, dyspnea, cough with or without chest discomfort, without coryza or rhinorrhea, leading to abrupt onset of respiratory distress, with or without shock, mental status changes, with chest radiograph abnormalities (wide mediastinum or infiltrates or pleural effusions)	Influenza, community-acquired bacterial pneumonia, viral pneumonia, *Legionella*, Q fever, psittacosis, *Mycoplasma*, *Pneumocystis* pneumonia, tularemia, dissecting aortic aneurysm, bacterial mediastinitis, SVC syndrome, histoplasmosis, coccidioidomycosis, sarcoidosis, ricin and staphylococcal enterotoxin B (pulmonary edema/ARDS), Nipah virus	Inhalational anthrax	• 3-day average symptom duration before presentation • Abdominal pain, headache, mental status abnormalities, hypoxemia common • Mediastinal adenopathy: ~90% (Fig. 71.2) • Hemorrhagic pleural effusions: ~70% • CT more sensitive than chest X-ray in early hemorrhagic mediastinal adenopathy • Meningoencephalitis: possibly ~50% • Blood cultures positive in untreated; pleural fluid cultures or antigen-specific immunohistochemical stain usually positive
Skin lesion(s)	Pruritic, painless papule on exposed areas leading to vesicle(s), ulcer, then edematous black eschar, with or without massive local edema and regional adenopathy and fever, evolving over 3–7 days	Recluse spider bite, staphylococcal lesion, atypical Lyme disease, orf, glanders, tularemia, plague, rat-bite fever, ecthyma gangrenosum, rickettsialpox, atypical *Mycobacteria*, cutaneous diphtheria, cutaneous leishmaniasis	Cutaneous anthrax	• Painless; spider bite is a painful lesion • Nonpitting local edema may be massive (Fig. 71.1) • If untreated, may progress to systemic involvement • Blood cultures, skin biopsy (from vesicular edge or erythema at edge of eschar)
Fulminant pneumonia	Abrupt onset of constitutional symptoms and rapidly progressive respiratory illness with cough, fever, rigors, headache, sore throat, myalgias, dyspnea, pleuritic chest pain, GI symptoms, lung consolidation, with or without hemoptysis, shock; variable progression to respiratory failure	Severe community-acquired bacterial or viral pneumonia, inhalational anthrax, pulmonary infarct, pulmonary hemorrhage, influenza, *Mycoplasma* pneumonia, *Legionella*, Q fever, bacterial pneumonia, SARS, tuberculosis, melioidosis	Pneumonic plague Pulmonary tularemia	• Lobar or multilobar involvement, with or without buboes • Hemoptysis common • Characteristic sputum Gram stain • Cough generally nonproductive • Pulse–temperature dissociation in 40%

(Continued)

Table 71.3 Syndromic differential diagnoses and clinical clues for category A agents of bioterrorism—cont'd

Syndrome	Clinical presentation	Differential diagnosis	Bioterrorism-associated disease	Disease-specific clues
Sepsis with bleeding diathesis and capillary leak	Sepsis syndrome, GI symptoms, mucosal hemorrhage, altered vascular permeability, DIC, purpura, acral gangrene, hepatitis, hypotension, with or without CNS findings, multiorgan system failure	Meningococcemia; Gram-negative sepsis; streptococcal, pneumococcal or staphylococcal bacteremia with shock; malaria; leptospirosis; typhoid fever; borreliosis; typhoidal tularemia; overwhelming postsplenectomy sepsis; acute leukemia; Rocky Mountain spotted fever; fulminant hepatitis; TTP; hemolytic uremic syndrome; SLE; hemorrhagic smallpox; hemorrhagic varicella (in immunocompromised); dengue.	Septicemic plague	• Occurs in minority of aerosol exposures • Cutaneous findings as late sequelae, with or without buboes • High-density bacteremia
			Viral hemorrhagic fever	• Maculopapular rash in Ebola, Marburg • Certain organ systems preferentially involved with specific VHF etiologies
Febrile prodrome with generalized exanthem	Fever, malaise, prostration, headache, myalgias and enanthema followed by development of synchronous, progressive, centrifugal papular, leading to vesicular/pustular rash on face, mucous membranes, extremities more than trunk, leading to generalization with or without hemorrhagic component, with systemic toxicity	Varicella, drug eruption, Stevens–Johnson syndrome, measles, secondary syphilis, erythema multiforme, severe acne, disseminated herpes zoster or simplex, meningococcemia, monkeypox, generalized vaccinia related to smallpox vaccination, insect bites, coxsackievirus, vaccine reaction	Smallpox	• Palms and soles involved • Rash is denser peripherally even after fully evolved • Lesions are well circumscribed, firm and almost nodular • Secondary bacterial infection common • Hemorrhagic variant in pregnant and immunocompromised patients associated with severe systemic toxicity, bleeding diathesis, and early mortality
Progressive weakness	Acute onset of afebrile, symmetric, descending flaccid paralysis that begins in bulbar muscles, dilated pupils, diplopia or blurred vision, dysphagia, dysarthria, ptosis, dry mucous membranes leading to airway obstruction and respiratory muscle paralysis. Clear sensorium and absence of sensory changes	Myasthenia gravis, brain stem CVA, polio, Guillain-Barré syndrome variant, tick paralysis, chemical intoxication	Botulism	• Expect dearth of GI symptoms in aerosol attack as opposed to food-borne botulism • Low-dose inhalation exposure may delay symptom onset • Prominent anticholinergic effects.

ARDS, acute respiratory distress syndrome; CVA, cerebrovascular accident; DIC, disseminated intravascular coagulation; GI, gastrointestinal; SLE, systemic lupus erythematosus; SVC syndrome, superior vena cava syndrome; TTP, thrombotic thrombocytopenic purpura; VHF, viral hemorrhagic fever.

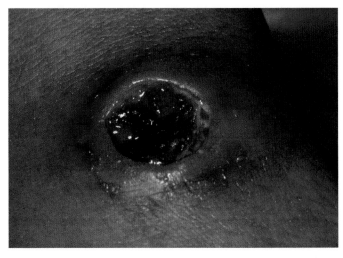

Fig. 71.1 Lesion of cutaneous anthrax. © Diepgen TL, Yihune G, *et al.* Dermatology Online Atlas (http://www.dermis.net). Reprinted with permission.

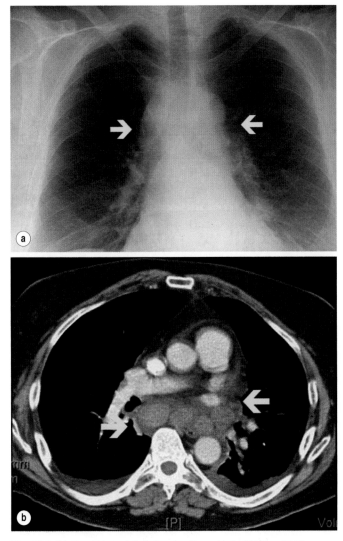

Fig. 71.2 (a) Chest X-ray, inhalational anthrax, United States, 2001 demonstrating mediastinal widening (arrows). (b) Chest CT scan demonstrating mediastinal widening (arrows) and bilateral pleural effusions. From Jernigan *et al.*[11]

periods of time in the host, up to 100 days in some experimental animal exposures[17] This has translated into prolonged clinical incubation periods following exposure to endospores; cases of inhalational anthrax occurred up to 43 days after exposure in the Sverdlovsk experience, although the average incubation period is 2–10 days, perhaps influenced by exposure inoculum.[15,17]

Prior to the anthrax attacks in the USA in October 2001, most of the clinical data concerning inhalational anthrax derived from Sverdlovsk, the largest outbreak recorded in humans. While the clinical experience derived from the US anthrax attacks in 2001 had much in common with the clinical manifestations of inhalational anthrax noted in the Sverdlovsk cases, more detailed data are available from the recent US experience and some novel findings were noted. There were 11 confirmed cases of inhalational anthrax, 5 (45%) of whom died. Although this contrasts with a case fatality rate of greater than 85% reported from Sverdlovsk, the reliability of reported data from the latter outbreak is questionable[17] and, perhaps more importantly, patients in the 2001 outbreak were more likely to receive appropriate treatment at an earlier stage. Patients with inhalational anthrax almost uniformly present for medical attention an average of 3.3 days after symptom onset with fevers, chills, malaise, myalgias, nonproductive cough, chest discomfort, dyspnea, nausea or vomiting, tachycardia, peripheral neutrophilia and liver enzyme elevations.[11,19]

Many of these findings are nondiagnostic and overlap considerably with those of influenza or other common viral respiratory tract infections. Data suggest that discrimination between inhalational anthrax and benign, influenza-like illnesses may be possible on the basis of presenting symptoms; shortness of breath, nausea, and vomiting are significantly more common in anthrax while rhinorrhea is uncommonly seen in anthrax but noted in the majority of community-acquired viral respiratory infections.[20]

Other common clinical manifestations of inhalational anthrax as informed by the recent attacks include abdominal pain, headache, mental status abnormalities and hypoxemia. Abnormalities on chest radiography appear to be universally present, although these may only be identified retrospectively in some cases. Pleural effusions are the most common abnormality; infiltrates, consolidation and/or mediastinal adenopathy/widening are noted in the majority (Fig. 71.2a). The latter is felt to be an early indicator of disease, but CT scan appears to provide greater sensitivity than chest radiographs for this finding (Fig. 71.2b). In the recent outbreak of inhalational anthrax, more than 80% of cases were noted to have mediastinal widening with or without pleural effusions or infiltrates.

The clinical manifestations of inhalational anthrax generally evolve to a fulminant septic picture with progressive respiratory failure. *B. anthracis* is routinely isolated in blood cultures if obtained

prior to the initiation of antimicrobials (Fig. 71.3). Pleural fluid is typically hemorrhagic; the bacteria can either be isolated in culture or documented by antigen-specific immunohistochemical stains of this material (Fig. 71.4) in the majority of patients.[11] The average time from hospitalization until death was 3 days (range 1–5 days) in the five recent US fatalities, consistent with other reports related to the clinical virulence of this infection. Autopsy data typically reveal hemorrhagic mediastinal lymphadenitis and disseminated metastatic infection. Pathology data from the Sverdlovsk outbreak confirm meningeal involvement, typically hemorrhagic meningitis, in 50%[21] and, in fact, meningoencephalitis was the presenting diagnosis (Fig. 71.5) in the index case of the 2001 attacks.[22]

The diagnosis of inhalational anthrax should be entertained in the setting of a consistent clinical presentation in the context of a known exposure, a possible exposure or epidemiologic factors suggesting bioterrorism, e.g. clustered cases of a rapidly progressive systemic illness. The diagnosis should also be considered in a single individual with a consistent or suggestive clinical illness in the absence of another etiology. Table 71.3 delineates a detailed differential diagnosis with specific discriminating features. It should be noted that multiple bioterrorism threat agents are included in the differential diagnosis of inhalational anthrax.

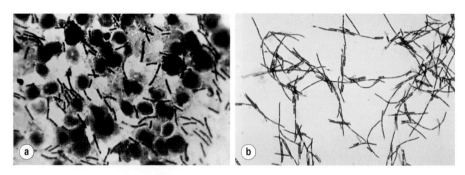

Fig. 71.3 *Bacillus anthracis*. (a) *Bacillus anthracis* appearing as Gram-positive bacilli. (b) The typical 'jointed bamboo-rod' appearance of the organism from blood cultures. Courtesy of CDC and Dr William A Clark.

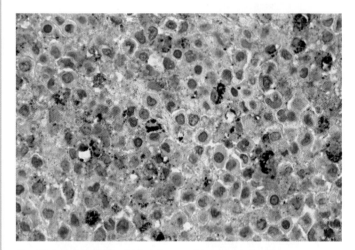

Fig. 71.4 Pleural fluid cell block immunohistochemical stain demonstrating *Bacillus anthracis* antigen (red) within a mononuclear inflammatory cell infiltrate. From Jernigan *et al*.[11]

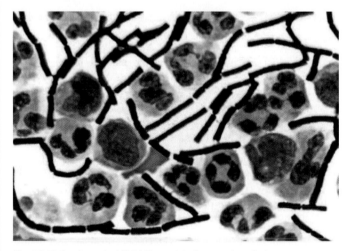

Fig. 71.5 Cerebrospinal fluid Gram stain from anthrax index case, United States, 2001, demonstrating numerous Gram-positive rods and neutrophils. From Jernigan *et al*.[11]

The early recognition and treatment of inhalational anthrax appear to be associated with a survival advantage;[11] in the US experience patients who received appropriate antimicrobials within 4.7 days of symptom onset had a mortality rate of 40% as compared with a mortality rate of 75% for those treated after that period.[23] Therefore, prompt empiric antimicrobial therapy should be initiated if infection is clinically suspected. Combination parenteral therapy is appropriate in the ill individual for a number of reasons:[11]

- to cover the possibility of antimicrobial resistance;
- to target specific bacterial virulence properties, e.g. the theoretical effect of clindamycin on toxin production;
- to ensure adequate drug penetration into the central nervous system; and
- to favorably impact survival.

In order to optimize the outcome in inhalational anthrax it is likely that novel therapies, such as toxin inhibitors or receptor antagonists, will need to be developed and deployed.[24] A variety of such strategies, guided by the pathogenesis of the organism and its disease-producing toxins, has shown promise in animal studies to date and will likely be components of effective therapeutic regimens in the future.[25]

Detailed therapeutic and postexposure prophylaxis recommendations for adults, children and special groups have been recently reviewed elsewhere.[17,26] Anthrax vaccine adsorbed (AVA), the current product in use for select indications, has been proven to be effective in preventing cutaneous anthrax in human clinical trials and in preventing inhalational disease after aerosol challenge in nonhuman primates.[27] The vaccine has generally been found to be safe but requires six doses over 18 months with the need for frequent boosting. Because of the aforementioned dosing issues and the limited availability of AVA, second-generation anthrax vaccines employing recombinant protective antigen and humanized antiprotective antigen monoclonal antibodies are in production.

Smallpox

The last known naturally acquired case of smallpox occurred in Somalia in 1977; in 1980, as the culmination of a 12-year, intensive campaign by the World Health Organization (WHO), the disease became the first in history to be officially certified as 'eradicated' as a scourge of humans.[28] However, because of concerns that variola virus stocks may have either been removed from or sequestered outside of their WHO-designated repositories, smallpox is considered to be a potential agent of bioterrorism. Smallpox is an attractive biologic weapon as its re-introduction into human populations would be a global public health catastrophe. It is stable in aerosol form with a low infective dose; case fatality rates approach 30%; secondary attack rates among unvaccinated close contacts are 37–88% and are amplified, especially in health-care settings; and much of the world's population is susceptible. Routine civilian vaccination was terminated more than two decades ago and vaccine-induced immunity appears to wane over time in vaccinees.[29] Vaccine supplies remain limited, and there are currently no antiviral therapies of proven clinical effectiveness against this pathogen.

Following an average incubation period of 10–12 days (range 7–19 days), patients experience the acute onset of a 2- to 3-day prostrating prodrome consisting of fever, rigors, malaise, vomiting, headache and backache. They subsequently develop a centrifugally distributed eruption that initially involves the face and extremities and then generalizes as it evolves through macular, papular, vesicular and pustular stages in synchronous (i.e. lesions progress concurrently and have similar appearances diffusely) fashion over approximately 8 days, with umbilication in the latter stages (Fig. 71.6). Enanthema in the oropharynx typically precede the exanthem by a day or two; this represents high titer viral replication in the upper respiratory tract and correlates with high infectivity. The rash generally remains denser peripherally and typically involves the palms and soles early on, a potentially useful clue in narrowing the differential diagnosis (Fig. 71.7). The umbilicated pustules begin crusting during the second week of the eruption; separation of scabs is usually complete by the end of the third week, but the course of the systemic illness may be attenuated and the appearance of the exanthem milder in those with partial, pre-existing immunity or more progressive and virulent in those with immunodeficient states.

The differential diagnosis of smallpox is extensive (see Table 71.3) but may be aided by a number of features of the disease: synchronous lesions, umbilicated appearance in the pustular stage, early involvement of palms and soles, and the centrifugal distribution of the eruption. Historically, varicella and drug reactions posed the most diagnostic dilemmas,[29] although the recent importation of monkeypox to the USA from its animal reservoir in Africa elevates this entity to a loftier position on the differential diagnosis list.[30] While the diagnosis of smallpox is suggested by clinical features, definitive diagnosis is accomplished by vaccinated clinicians acquiring samples of blood and lesional contents or scrapings from crusts for analysis by electron microscopy, viral antigen immunohistochemistry, polymerase chain

reaction and viral isolation. Because processing and evaluation of specimens from a suspected case of smallpox requires high-level biocontainment facilities, collaboration with public health authorities is necessary.

Smallpox is transmitted from person-to-person by respiratory droplet nuclei and, less commonly, by contact with lesions or contaminated fomites. Airborne transmission by fine-particle aerosols has, under certain conditions, been documented[31] and should be assumed as a potential mode of spread in a bioterrorism event. The virus is communicable from the onset of the enanthem, generally one or two days prior to the rash, until all of the scabs have separated, although patients are felt to be most contagious during the first week of the rash due to high titers of replicating virus in the oropharynx. Household members, other face-to-face contacts and health-care workers have traditionally been at highest risk for secondary transmission; the last group is obviously of greatest concern with regards to amplification of infection, especially among medically vulnerable populations. Thus, hospitalized cases of suspected smallpox must immediately be placed in negative-pressure rooms with contact and airborne precautions; those not requiring hospital-level care should remain isolated at home in order to avoid infecting others.

The suspicion of a single smallpox case should prompt immediate notification of local public health authorities and the hospital epidemiologist. Containment of the disease is predicated on the 'ring vaccination' strategy, which was successfully deployed in the WHO

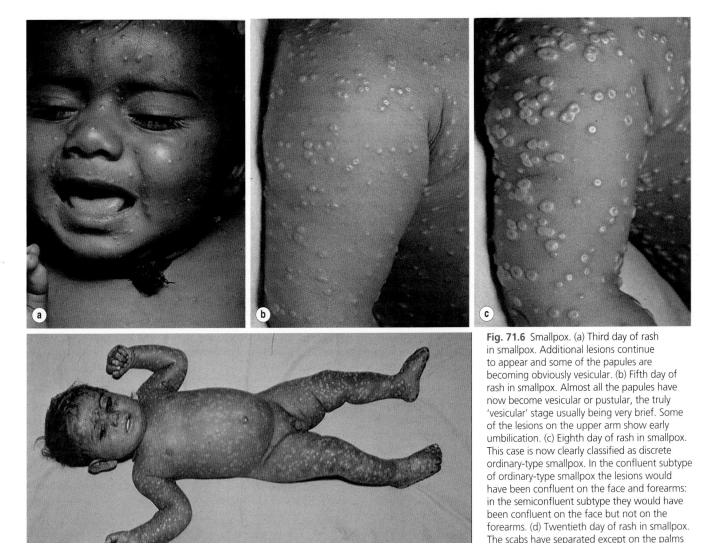

Fig. 71.6 Smallpox. (a) Third day of rash in smallpox. Additional lesions continue to appear and some of the papules are becoming obviously vesicular. (b) Fifth day of rash in smallpox. Almost all the papules have now become vesicular or pustular, the truly 'vesicular' stage usually being very brief. Some of the lesions on the upper arm show early umbilication. (c) Eighth day of rash in smallpox. This case is now clearly classified as discrete ordinary-type smallpox. In the confluent subtype of ordinary-type smallpox the lesions would have been confluent on the face and forearms: in the semiconfluent subtype they would have been confluent on the face but not on the forearms. (d) Twentieth day of rash in smallpox. The scabs have separated except on the palms of the hands and the soles of the feet, leaving depigmented areas. From Fenner et al.[28]

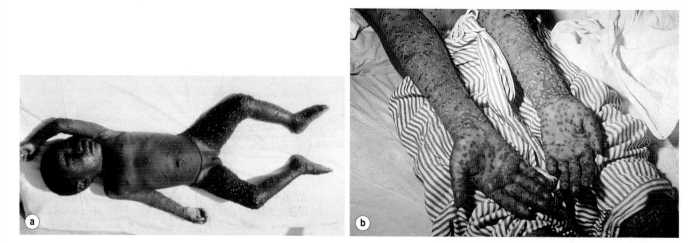

Fig. 71.7 (a) Typical centrifugal distribution of the rash in smallpox. (b) Patient with smallpox, Kosovo, Yugoslavia epidemic, March and April 1972. The scabs will eventually fall off leaving marks on the skin that will become pitted scars. The infection is transmissible until all scabs have fallen off. (a) Courtesy of CDC and Dr Paul B Dean; (b) Courtesy of CDC and Dr William Foege.

global eradication campaign and which mandates the identification and immunization of all directly exposed persons or those at high risk of exposure, including close contacts, health-care workers and laboratory personnel. Vaccination of infected individuals, if deployed within 4 days of infection during the early incubation period, can significantly attenuate or prevent disease and may favorably impact secondary transmission.[29] Because the disease does not exist in nature, the occurrence of even a single case of smallpox would be tantamount to bioterrorism and would warrant an epidemiologic investigation to ascertain the perimeter of the initial release, so that tracing of those initially exposed can be accomplished.[32]

Botulism

Botulism is an acute neurologic disease resulting from intoxication with *Clostridium botulinum* that occurs sporadically and in focal outbreaks throughout the world. Generally, the illness is associated with wound contamination by the bacterial form or ingestion of preformed, food-borne toxin. A detailed discussion of botulism is found in Chapter 21. Aerosol forms of the toxin, a rare mode of acquisition in nature, have been weaponized for use in bioterrorism although their actual use has never been documented.[5] Botulinum toxin is considered to be the most toxic molecule known; it is lethal to humans in minute quantities and acts by blocking the release of the neurotransmitter acetylcholine from presynaptic vesicles, thereby inhibiting muscle contraction.[33]

Botulism presents with the clinical features of an acute, afebrile, symmetric, descending, flaccid paralysis without mental status or sensory changes. The disease manifests initially in the bulbar musculature; fatigue, dizziness, dysphagia, dysarthria, diplopia, dry mouth, dyspnea, ptosis, ophthalmoparesis, tongue weakness and facial muscle paresis are early findings seen in more than 75% of cases. Progressive muscular involvement leads to respiratory failure in untreated cases. The clinical presentations of food-borne and inhalational botulism are indistinguishable in experimental animals.[33]

The diagnosis of botulism is based largely on epidemiologic and clinical features and the exclusion of other possible differential diagnoses (see Table 71.3); there is no commercial assay currently available to confirm intoxication. While sporadic or clustered cases occur regularly, albeit infrequently in developed countries, it must be recognized that any single case of botulism could be the result of bioterrorism or could herald a larger scale 'event'. Certainly, large numbers of epidemiologically unrelated, geographically dispersed or multifocal cases should raise the specter of an intentional release of the agent, either in food/water supplies or as an aerosol.

The mortality from food-borne botulism has declined from 60% to 6% over the last four decades, probably as a result of improvements in intensive and supportive care. Because the need for mechanical ventilation may be prolonged in these patients, the finite resource of ventilators would be rapidly overwhelmed in the event of a large-scale bioterrorism event using botulism toxin, even though these devices are part of the Strategic National Stockpile in the USA for such incidents. New developments in ventilator technology may mitigate some of the predicted shortfalls. Treatment with an equine antitoxin is available in limited supply from the CDC and may ameliorate disease if given early.

Plague

Plague, a systemic disease caused by the Gram-negative pathogen *Yersinia pestis*, presents in a variety of clinical forms in nature as detailed in Chapter 120. Plague is endemic in parts of South East Asia, Africa and the western USA. While naturally acquired disease results from a variety of exposure modes, bioterrorism carried out using aerosolized preparations of the agent would likely result in cases of primary pneumonic plague occurring outside of endemic areas. As was the case with the anthrax attacks in the USA in 2001, however, unexpected forms of the disease, such as bubonic and septicemic plague, might also occur in an event.

Primary pneumonic plague classically presents as an acute, febrile, pneumonic illness with prominent respiratory and systemic symptoms; gastrointestinal symptoms, purulent sputum production or hemoptysis occur variably.[34] Chest roentgenogram typically shows patchy, bilateral, multilobar infiltrates or consolidations (Fig. 71.8). Untreated or inappropriately treated patients progress rapidly to develop respiratory failure, vascular collapse, purpuric skin lesions, necrotic digits and death. The differential diagnosis is essentially one involving etiologies of rapidly progressive pneumonia and includes clinical syndromes caused by a number of other agents of bioterrorism (see Table 71.3). The diagnosis may be suggested by observing the characteristic small, Gram-negative, coccobacillary forms in sputum specimens with bipolar or 'safety pin' uptake of Giemsa or Wright stain (Fig. 71.9).[35] Culture confirmation is necessary to confirm the diagnosis; the microbiology laboratory should be notified in advance if plague is suspected, as special techniques and precautions must be employed to prevent inadvertent transmission to laboratory personnel.

Treatment recommendations for plague have been reviewed elsewhere.[26,35] Pneumonic plague can be transmitted from person-to-person by respiratory droplet nuclei, thus placing close contacts, such as patients and health-care workers in the health-care setting,

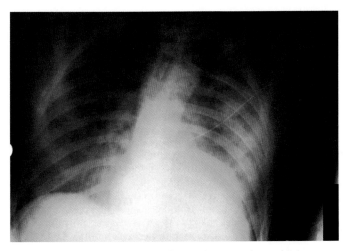

Fig. 71.8 Chest X-ray, pneumonic plague, demonstrating multilobar infiltrates. Courtesy of CDC and Dr Jack Poland.

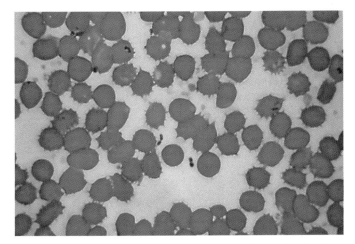

Fig. 71.9 Peripheral blood smear demonstrating bipolar uptake of stain, the so-called 'safety pin' appearance of *Yersinia pestis*. Courtesy of CDC and Dr Jack Poland.

at risk. Domestic cats may participate in maintaining a transmission chain during a bioterrorism event.[12] Prompt recognition and treatment of plague cases, appropriate deployment of postexposure prophylaxis, and early institution of droplet precautions for infected individuals will interrupt secondary transmission.

Tularemia

The causative agent of tularemia, *Francisella tularensis*, is another small Gram-negative coccobacillus that would be predicted to cause a primary pneumonic illness if delivered as an aerosol in a bioterrorism event. Once again, however, vigilance is necessary as naturally occurring disease can be acquired by a variety of routes and present in many clinical forms; therefore an intentional release of bacteria may also result in more than one form of tularemia. Pulmonic tularemia presents with the abrupt onset of a febrile systemic illness with prominent upper respiratory symptoms, pleuritic chest pain, and the variable development of pneumonia, hilar adenopathy and progression to respiratory failure and death in approximately 30% of inappropriately treated patients.[36] The diagnosis is generally established on clinical features, based on the differential diagnosis (see Table 71.3) and microbiologic data; laboratory personnel should be notified in advance if tularemia is suspected, as the organism can be very infectious when manipulated in laboratory conditions. This agent is discussed in depth in Chapter 121.

Viral hemorrhagic fevers

Pathogenic members of four distinct families of RNA viruses are potential agents of viral hemorrhagic fevers (VHF): the agents of Ebola, Marburg, Lassa fever, Rift Valley fever and Congo–Crimean hemorrhagic fever. These syndromes are discussed in detail in Chapter 126. VHF cause clinical syndromes with many common features: fever, malaise, headache, myalgias, prostration, mucosal hemorrhage and other signs of increased vascular permeability, leading to shock and multiorgan system failure in advanced cases.[37] Additionally, specific pathogens are associated with specific target organ effects.

Hemorrhagic fever viruses have generally been viewed as emerging infections in nature due to their sporadic occurrence in focal outbreaks throughout the world and environmental disruption by expanding human populations. These viruses are also potential weapons of bioterrorism for a number of reasons:[10]

* they are highly infectious in aerosol form;
* they are transmissible in health-care settings;
* they cause high morbidity and mortality; and
* they are purported to have been successfully weaponized.

Blood and other body fluids from infected patients are infectious. As such, person-to-person airborne transmission may occur and strict contact and airborne precautions should be instituted in these cases.[37] Transmission in health-care settings is a well-described risk with these agents. Treatment is largely supportive and includes the early use of vasopressors as needed. Ribavirin is effective against some forms of VHF but not those caused by Ebola and Marburg viruses. Nonetheless, this drug should be initiated empirically in patients presenting with a consistent clinical syndrome until an alternate etiology is confirmed.

ASSOCIATED ISSUES AND SEQUELAE OF BIOTERRORISM

Surveillance

Surveillance is perhaps the most critical element in the early recognition and identification of bioterrorism events. In the context of the individual clinician surveillance is analogous to clinical vigilance; in the broader context of communities and larger populations, it involves a public health system and infrastructure designed to detect perturbations in the baseline occurrence of either symptoms, as is the case with syndromic surveillance systems, or diseases, as is the case with a standard public health system of reportable diseases. Syndromic surveillance systems have been used recently for monitoring influenza activity and other emerging infectious diseases, and various real-time, electronic platforms are currently in use by a number of organizations to detect early, sensitive indicators of disease activity.

Quarantine

Quarantine, the physical separation and geographic restriction of groups of uninfected individuals potentially exposed to a communicable illness, has been variably considered to be one management strategy following bioterrorism. The potential effectiveness, feasibility, legality and consequences of quarantine have recently been reviewed.[38] The logistics of this approach are complex and impractical, and it can be associated with adverse consequences, such as increased risk of disease transmission among a quarantined group or riots. It seems clear that there are only limited scenarios in which the potential public health benefits of the imposition of quarantine may outweigh the potential problems engendered by this approach; these largely revolve around highly transmissible, lethal agents. In most situations a disease-specific containment strategy, based on transmission epidemiology and disease prevention approaches, is preferable.

Management of special patient populations

The approach to the management of diseases of bioterrorism must include provisions for children, pregnant women and immunocompromised individuals. Specific recommendations for treatment and prophylaxis of these special patient groups for selected bioterrorism agents have recently been reviewed.[16,26,35,36] A general approach requires an assessment of the risk of using certain drugs or products in select populations versus the potential risk of the infection in question, accounting for the extent of exposure and agent involved. Live virus immunizations such as the smallpox vaccine pose higher risk to these special groups than to others. This consideration will impact mass vaccination decisions and, like most other aspects of medicine, will require an assessment of risk versus benefit.

Psychosocial morbidity

An often overlooked but vitally important issue is that of psychosocial morbidity related to bioterrorism. These sequelae may take the form of acute anxiety reactions and exacerbations of chronic psychiatric illness during the stress of the event, or post-traumatic stress disorder (PTSD) in its aftermath, and may involve clinical victims of bioterrorism as well as health-care workers and other first responders. Nearly half of the emergency department visits during the Gulf War missile attacks in Israel in 1991 were related to acute psychological illness or exacerbations of underlying problems.[39] Data from recent acts of terrorism in the USA suggest that PTSD and/or depression may develop in more than 35% of those impacted by the events.[40,41] Although close proximity to an event and personal loss appear to be directly correlated with PTSD and depression, respectively, those indirectly involved also experience substantial morbidity.[41] The long-term psychosocial impact of these events and of the persistent threat of terrorism in general remains to be determined.

CONCLUSION

The response to bioterrorism is unique among weapons of mass destruction because it necessitates management strategies common to all disasters as well as the application of basic infectious diseases principles: disease surveillance, infection control, antimicrobial therapy and prophylaxis, and vaccine prevention. For these reasons, we, as physicians (and specifically infectious diseases specialists), are likely first responders to bioterrorism and must keep our diagnostic and clinical skills current and our clinical vigilance active regarding potential threat agents. We are expected to be reliable sources of information for our patients, colleagues and public health authorities.[42] As a group we must guard against the inexorable 'bioterrorism fatigue' that may otherwise result from a persistent state of heightened readiness without an actual event taking place.[6]

REFERENCES

References for this chapter can be found online at http://www.expertconsult.com

Management of candiduria in the ICU

INTRODUCTION

Candiduria can be defined as the presence of greater than 10^5 fungal cfu/ml urine, though as little as 10^3 cfu/ml can result in disease in certain 'at risk' groups. The prevalence of candiduria varies between 6.5% and 20% amongst hospitalized patients and presents a dilemma to clinicians, who must decide if the finding represents colonization alone, or is a feature of invasive fungal infection. Probably only 3–4% of cases of candiduria lead to candidemia, but 10% of all cases of candidemia are associated with a prior episode of candiduria. Indeed, studies based in the intensive care unit (ICU) have shown that candiduria can be associated with a rise in mortality from 19% to 50%.

PATHOGENESIS

Candiduria can arise in several ways. Contamination of specimens by perineal colonization is less common in the ICU, since most patients are catheterized, though this does not obviate the need for a confirmatory second specimen. Colonization of the urinary tract may occur in the catheterized patient and this is commoner in those who have had antimicrobial exposure. Local infection of both the lower urinary tract (cystitis, urethritis) and upper tract (pyelonephritis) with *Candida* spp. is encouraged by urologic instrumentation, including catheterization. Other factors predisposing to ascending infections include ongoing broad-spectrum antibiotic therapy, diabetes mellitus, renal insufficiency, and any obstructive anomaly of the urinary tract. Importantly, patients with disseminated candidiasis may seed the urinary tract from bloodstream spread; in up to one-tenth of patients, candiduria may herald candidemia (Table PP32.1).

MICROBIOLOGY

The majority (50–70%) of *Candida* isolates from urine in the ICU are *C. albicans*, which is sensitive to fluconazole. Indeed, provided that patients have not previously been exposed to fluconazole, it is reasonable to assume that any germ tube-positive yeast will be sensitive to fluconazole. However, increasing numbers of yeasts other than *C. albicans* occur in the ICU setting and the prevalence varies between units. In particular, *C. tropicalis* and *C. glabrata* account for 10–20% of such isolates, the latter species being notable for its resistance to azole drugs.

CLINICAL FEATURES

Candiduria alone does not cause symptoms; local infection can cause classic cystitis or urethritis and pyelonephritis may lead to flank pain. Patients who have candiduria as a feature of disseminated candidiasis may have evidence of systemic candidal disease, which should be assiduously checked for: clinical features include sepsis, fever, lesions of the optic fundi, skin lesions and hepatosplenomegaly.

INVESTIGATIONS

It is clear from Table PP32.1 that a repeat fresh urine sample must be sent to the microbiology laboratory to confirm candiduria. Microscopy for the presence of white blood cells may be useful in differentiating

Table PP32.1 Etiology of candiduria and laboratory investigation

Source of candiduria	Laboratory investigations
Inadvertent contamination	Repeat sample: clear
Colonization of lower tract	Repeat sample may be positive Patient well No WBCs in urine (catheterization will affect this) Check for *Candida* colonization at other sites
Infection of lower tract	Repeat sample will be positive WBCs in urine Ultrasound if not instrumented Screen for diabetes, renal disease Check for *Candida* colonization at other sites
Infection of upper tract	WBCs + casts in urine Ultrasound Screen for diabetes, renal disease Check for *Candida* colonization at other sites
Disseminated *Candida* infection	Check for *Candida* colonization at other sites Blood cultures/other sterile site: positive for *Candida* CXR, abdominal ultrasound High CRP

colonization from urinary tract infection, but the finding can be non-specific in a catheterized patient; the presence of hyphae-containing granular casts is a rare finding which would confirm true renal infection. If the patient has not been catheterized or had urologic instrumentation recently, it is prudent to screen for diabetes mellitus and renal insufficiency by biochemical testing, and anatomic anomalies using ultrasound. Ultrasound of the renal tract can also demonstrate the presence of fungal balls in patients who have persistent candiduria. Simple tests to screen for the possibility of disseminated candidiasis would include a chest X-ray, abdominal ultrasound, C-reactive protein, cultures of other potentially infected sites (e.g. tracheal aspirate or bronchial lavage, bile, surgical drains, intravascular line tips) and blood cultures.

The 'Candida colonization index' (ratio of the number of 'Candida-positive' samples to total number of surveillance samples sent to the laboratory) can be used to predict those that may benefit from pre-emptive systemic therapy; although the approach has not been extensively validated in all types of ICU, it provides a useful guide for borderline cases.

MANAGEMENT

Modern management of candiduria in the ICU setting is determined by the likely source of fungi (Table PP32.2). It is clear that colonization can be treated by simply replacing the urinary catheter or, better, permanent removal. In all cases, rational reduction in the spectrum of antibacterial agents administered to patients will help eliminate fungal colonization and infection. These simple measures allow up to 40% of patients with candiduria to clear fungi from the urine.

True infection of the urinary tract should be treated with a definitive 2-week course of an antifungal, usually fluconazole, in addition to catheter removal or exchange. Fluconazole can be administered intravenously in the ICU or via the nasogastric tube in the oral form, if the patient's gastrointestinal system is functioning. Isolation of a germ tube-negative Candida spp. raises the possibility of a fluconazole-resistant yeast, necessitating recourse to intravenous amphotericin B. Although of increasing favor in hospitals, neither voriconazole nor the echinocandin agents reach high concentrations in the urinary tract and therefore, at present, are not advised routinely. Despite anecdotal reports, there is no clear case for local intermittent or continuous bladder irrigation with amphotericin B; the procedure necessitates instrumentation of the urinary tract which might otherwise be unnecessary. Furthermore, although local irrigation with amphotericin B can achieve prompt clearance of funguria, the effect is short lived compared with clearance rates achieved by fluconazole.

Finally, the canduric patient who may have invasive fungal infection warrants more aggressive 'pre-emptive' antifungal therapy. This must be based on careful assessment of combined clinical and laboratory findings; a Candida colonization index of above 0.5 is used by some to guide therapy. If C. albicans is isolated and the patient is stable, it is reasonable to treat with high-dose fluconazole for 2–6 weeks (400–800 mg/day for a 70 kg adult). However, if the same patient is clinically unstable, or if the isolate is non-albicans, it would be prudent to treat with amphotericin B, as indicated in Table PP32.2. Although

Table PP32.2 Management of candiduria in the ICU

Suspected cause of candiduria	Action	Additional considerations
Contamination	None	–
Colonization	No antifungal Remove/replace catheter Stop antibacterials if possible	If patient is at risk of infection (e.g. neutropenia) or undergoing urologic procedure, low birth weight infant: fluconazole 200 mg q24h for 7–14 days
Lower UTI	Fluconazole 200 mg q24h for 7–14 days if C. albicans	–
Upper UTI	Fluconazole 6 mg/kg q24h for 2–6 weeks if C. albicans	Surgical drainage may be needed. Amphotericin B if patient unstable or if non-albicans
Disseminated infection likely	Fluconazole 6–12 mg/kg q24h (if C. albicans) or amphotericin B 0.7–1.0 mg/kg q24h, depending on severity, for at least 2–6 weeks	If dissemination confirmed: follow up for at least 3–6 months after discharge from ICU in case of distant seeding Use of lipid formulations of amphotericin B necessitates doses of 3–5 mg/kg q24h

newer agents such as voriconazole or the echinocandins provide alternative treatment options for non-albicans infection, urinary tract clearance may be more effective using systemic amphotericin. The appropriate duration of therapy in this setting is unclear, and must be determined according to the individual clinical situation and response to therapy.

FURTHER READING

Further reading for this chapter can be found online at http://www.expertconsult.com

Infections associated with near drowning

At least 100 million North Americans use the marine environment for recreation each year. Recreational use of water is probably responsible for the bulk of the 8000 deaths from drowning per annum in the USA (1500 in children) and for many of the estimated 150 000 deaths worldwide. The epidemiology of 'near drowning' is less well known but is thought to be up to 500 times as common. Drowning is death from suffocation as a result of submersion in liquid. In the majority of cases water is aspirated into pulmonary air spaces. This produces a variety of pathologies depending on whether fresh or sea water is inhaled, but the end result is alveolar dysfunction, causing venous blood to be shunted into the systemic circulation past under-ventilated alveoli to cause hypoxemia. In a minority of cases hypoxemia can result from apnea caused by several different mechanisms. Although 'near drowning' by definition means that the victim survives the initial hypoxic insult (for more than 24 hours), a number of complications may then ensue from the aspiration and hypoxia, including pulmonary edema, convulsions and infective problems such as pneumonia or sepsis. There may be additional problems from hypothermia although paradoxically this may have a protective benefit against cerebral hypoxia. Many of these complications may result in an ultimately fatal outcome.

PATHOGENESIS

Lung damage following aspiration of either sea water or fresh water produces inflammation and edema, which damage alveolar defense mechanisms and enhance the risk of infection. The relatively anaerobic conditions may also favor infection. Infecting organisms may include those already colonizing the lungs or upper airways, which have been carried distally with the aspiration and have then taken advantage of improved conditions for growth. Alternatively, organisms in the aspirated water may give rise to infective problems. Finally, an ill patient with lung damage may be admitted to hospital (and to an intensive care unit) and therefore be exposed to all the risks of nosocomial pneumonia.

MICROBIOLOGY

The literature on the microbiology of near drowning consists mainly of single case reports rather than large-scale reviews but common themes do emerge. Organisms that have been implicated are shown in Table PP33.1, and these can be divided into those that are characteristically associated with pneumonia (either community-acquired or nosocomial) and those that are more specifically associated with immersion incidents. Gram-negative organisms predominate in the aquatic environment (both sea water and fresh water) but anaerobic organisms and *Staphylococcus* spp. can also be found. Some organisms are more likely according to whether immersion took place in sea water or fresh water and depending on whether the water was clean or contaminated. Certain organisms may be more common in particular geographic areas. For example, one might anticipate exposure to *Burkholderia pseudomallei* following a near-drowning episode in the paddy fields of South East Asia (see Chapter 119).

Several cases of infection with *Aeromonas* spp. exist in the literature and these are associated with a high proportion of positive blood cultures and a high mortality. Fungal infections can also cause problems and there are reports of *Aspergillus* pneumonia and disseminated aspergillosis particularly affecting the central nervous system (CNS) after immersion incidents. *Pseudallescheria boydii* is also reported. This is the sexual form of *Scedosporium apiospermum* and is also associated with frequent CNS invasion and a high mortality.

Infection is commonly polymicrobial and this is particularly reflected in the multiple case reports that emerged after the tsunami hit South East Asia in December 2004.

CLINICAL FEATURES

The clinical features of infection after near drowning are similar to those seen when the particular infection arises from more conventional causes and depend on the site of infection. The main complication is pneumonia (as might be predicted from the portal of entry) but there is often an associated bacteremia, which may produce clinical features of sepsis. There have also been case reports of meningitis after near drowning. Skin and soft tissue infection may also result from immersion, especially when associated with trauma such as after the tsunami.

Noninfective pulmonary edema is a common complication of near drowning and can progress to full adult respiratory distress syndrome. Pulmonary edema can be difficult to distinguish clinically and radiographically from pneumonia. In one series of 125 near drowning episodes, the incidence of pulmonary edema was 43% whereas the incidence of pneumonia was 14.7%. These figures are sensitive to changes in case definition and clearly many patients who initially have pulmonary edema may subsequently go on to develop pneumonia, which tends to be a later complication.

Most patients who have pneumonia have fever (although recognition of this may be confounded if there is any residual hypothermia from the immersion). They may have clinical features of pulmonary consolidation or edema, or both.

Table PP33.1 Micro-organisms implicated in pneumonia or sepsis after near drowning

Conventional respiratory pathogens (including atypical organisms and those associated with nosocomial pneumonias)
Staphylococcus aureus *Haemophilus influenzae* *Streptococcus pneumoniae* *Escherichia coli* *Pseudomonas* spp. *Moraxella* spp. *Klebsiella* spp. *Legionella* spp.
Pathogens specifically related to immersion
Aeromonas spp. *Pseudomonas putrefaciens* *Francisella philomiragia* *Chromobacterium violaceum* *Burkholderia pseudomallei* *Vibrio* spp. *Pseudallescheria boydii* *Aspergillus* spp. *Acinetobacter baumanii*

Table PP33.2 Antibiotic regimens for pneumonia and sepsis associated with near drowning

	Dose for average adult patient
Clindamycin	900 mg q8h
Ciprofloxacin	400 mg q12h
Ticarcillin–clavulanate	3 g q6h
Gentamicin	5 mg/kg q24h
Ceftazidime	2 g q8h
Metronidazole	500 mg q8h
Meropenem	500 mg q8h

All these antibiotics are administered intravenously.

INVESTIGATIONS

Near-drowning victims should have a chest radiograph on admission and this may well be clear or show nonspecific shadowing. They should also have a full blood count and arterial blood gas analysis. Leukocytosis is usual in patients who have pneumonia but is not specific for infection.

Pulmonary secretions must be examined microbiologically; these may include expectorated sputum or tracheal aspirates in intubated patients. There may be pus cells in the samples and it is common to find infecting micro-organisms by stain and by subsequent culture. Blood cultures must always be taken because there is a high rate of bacteremia. CNS involvement is a common complication and therefore there should be a low threshold for CNS imaging and obtaining of appropriate specimens by lumbar puncture or neurosurgery.

MANAGEMENT

Patients who have survived a near drowning episode require emergency evaluation to determine whether they are at risk of subsequent delayed complications. If they are asymptomatic, with no abnormalities on physical examination and with a normal chest radiograph, arterial blood gases and full blood count, they can be safely discharged because they are at low risk of pulmonary problems. However, any abnormality on this initial evaluation should prompt hospital admission for observation.

If hypoxemia is present, supplemental oxygen should be given. If this does not correct the situation, it may be necessary to admit the patient to an intensive care unit for further respiratory support.

In common with many other intensive care situations, there used to be a widespread practice of administering glucocorticoids to patients who had undergone aspiration. There has never been evidence of benefit in near-drowning incidents and this practice is not recommended.

ANTIBIOTICS

Prophylactic antibiotics have been shown to be of no benefit and their use is not recommended. However, there should be a low threshold for instituting antimicrobial therapy if there is any suspicion of developing pneumonia or sepsis (Table PP33.2). Features giving rise to concern include deteriorating arterial blood gases, new infiltrates on chest radiograph, hemodynamic disturbance or the development of fever or leukocytosis. It is likely that antibiotics will have to commence before any microbiologic information is available from the laboratory (although initial Gram stains may be helpful). Therefore, broad-spectrum empiric cover with good pulmonary penetration is indicated. However, given the unusual microbiology with resistant organisms and the polymicrobial nature of the infections discussed above, it is essential that appropriate samples are taken prior to starting anti-infectives.

Numerous antibiotics have been used, including aminoglycosides, monobactams, carbapenems, cephalosporins and extended-spectrum penicillins (with and without β-lactamase inhibitors). There are no large-scale trials to guide rational therapy. I suggest the use of clindamycin, which has good penetration and will provide good Gram-positive cover as well as treating anaerobic infection. This should be combined with ciprofloxacin to cover the Gram-negative organisms and also provide some cover against *Legionella* spp. Other reasonable combinations would be ticarcillin–clavulanate with gentamicin, and ceftazidime with metronidazole, although neither of these two regimens offers cover against *Legionella* spp. Clearly, the initial regimen may need to be modified in the light of subsequent information from the microbiology laboratory, but it is important to remember that polymicrobial infection is common. If there is no adequate response or fungi are isolated, it may be necessary to consider the use of antifungal treatment and intravenous voriconazole can be valuable in this context.

FURTHER READING

Further reading for this chapter can be found online at http://www.expertconsult.com

Management of human bites

EPIDEMIOLOGY

As with animal bites, bites from humans are relatively common injuries that can lead to severe infection with significant morbidity. Furthermore, human bites have a higher complication and infection rate than animal bites. The epidemiology of patients with human bite infections presenting to emergency departments was outlined in a prospective multicenter study of 50 patients by Talan *et al.* (see Further reading). Seventy per cent of the patients were men and the median age was 27 years. The hands were involved in 86% of these bite-related injuries; 56% and 44% were due to clenched fist and occlusive bite injuries, respectively.

Hand bites are especially prone to infection because of the numerous compartments and the absence of significant soft tissue separating the skin from bones and joints. The reported rate of infectious complications in human bites of the hand is 25–50% and in bites of the face 2.5%. The majority of infections already exist when the patient first presents for care.

MECHANISMS OF INJURY

Human bites may occur from accidental injuries, purposeful biting or closed fist injuries. Wounds may be either occlusive injuries, in which the teeth actually bite the body part, or clenched fist injuries. The clenched fist injury is a ragged laceration most often found over the metacarpal joints of the middle and ring fingers. It results when an individual strikes another person's mouth with a closed fist. An apparently innocuous 3–5 mm laceration over a dorsal metacarpophalangeal joint may overlie a deep bacterial inoculum, tracked deep into the wound with extension. Penetration of the joint occurs in up to 62% of wounds; up to 58% involve injury to the bone.

MICROBIOLOGY

Infected wounds are polymicrobial, with an average of five organisms per wound (Table PP34.1). At least 42 different species of bacteria have been identified in human saliva, and 190 species have been found when gingivitis or periodontitis is present. Anaerobes include *Prevotella*, *Peptostreptococcus*, *Fusobacterium*, *Veillonella*, *Porphyromonas*, *Bacteroides fragilis* and *Clostridium* spp. Anaerobes are found in more than 50% of human bite wounds and frequently produce β-lactamase, unlike those from animal bites. Common pathogenic aerobes include β-hemolytic streptococci, *Staphylococcus aureus* and *Haemophilus* spp. *Eikenella corrodens*, a facultative anaerobic, slow-growing, Gram-negative rod, is

Table PP34.1 Bacteriology of human bite wounds: aerobic and anaerobic micro-organisms isolated from 50 patients with infected human bites

Micro-organism	No. of patients with pathogen (%)
Anaerobes	
Prevotella spp.	18
Fusobacterium spp.	17
Veillonella spp.	12
Peptostreptococcus spp.	11
Eubacterium spp.	8
Actinomyces spp.	4
Lactobacillus spp.	4
Bacteroides spp.	2
Microaerophilic bacteria	
Campylobacter spp.	8
Aerobes	
Streptococcal species	**42**
S. anginosus	26
S. oralis	7
S. pyogenes	7
S. intermedius	6
S. constellatus	4
Staphylococcal species	**27**
S. aureus	15
S. epidermidis	11
Other aerobic organisms	
Eikenella corrodens	15
Haemophilus spp.	11
Corynebacterium	6
Gemella morbiliform	6
Neisseria	4
Enterobacter cloacae	4
Candida spp.	4

Modified with permission from Talan *et al.*

frequently implicated in fight–bite injury infections and has been found in 10–29% of human bite wounds. It acts synergistically with aerobic organisms, most frequently streptococci, and is thought to account for greater morbidity in these wounds. *E. corrodens* is usually resistant to first-generation cephalosporins, macrolides, clindamycin and aminoglycosides, and these agents should be avoided as monotherapy.

MANAGEMENT

Human bites do not typically cause immediate symptoms besides the laceration injury. Infection can develop rapidly, however, because of direct inoculation of oral and skin flora into the wound. Signs and symptoms of infection, including redness, swelling and a clear or purulent discharge, may develop 24–72 hours after the bite. Lymph nodes adjacent to the wound may become enlarged and range of motion in the area may be reduced. Leukocytosis may occur.

The approach to the human bite depends on the location and the mechanism of injury. Important prognostic factors for the development of infection include the extent of tissue damage, the depth of the wound and which compartments are entered, and the pathogenicity of the inoculated oral bacteria.

Wound care

The mainstays of bite wound management are as follows:
* *Cleansing*: To reduce the high inoculum of oral flora, wounds should be vigorously cleansed with soap or a quaternary ammonium compound and water.
* *Exploration*: Under topical anesthesia, the wound should be explored in a bloodless field to look for foreign bodies, tendon laceration or joint penetration. It is essential that the wound be examined through the full range of motion, including the position at the moment of injury. Wounds that demonstrate tendon lacerations should be presumed to have joint involvement as well, and this finding should prompt consultation with a hand surgeon. Hand radiographs should be obtained, looking for fractures, dislocations, retained teeth or foreign bodies, or air in the joint.
* *Irrigation*: Wounds should be irrigated with 150 ml or more sterile normal saline or lactated Ringer's solution.
* *Debridement*: Devitalized tissue should be removed through debridement.
* *Delayed suturing* (*except for facial bites*): Although there are no controlled studies on suturing human bites, the high rate of infection and complications of human bites on the hand mandate that they be left open. The wound should be covered with a dry sterile dressing and the hand splinted in a position of function, either with a plaster splint or by packing the palm with bulky gauze and wrapping the hand in a mitten-type dressing. The wound can be closed later with sutures if needed after infection has cleared and granulation tissue is present.
* *Facial bites*: Facial wounds are at low risk for infection, and a large series of sutured facial human bites treated in a plastic surgery clinic had an infection rate of only 2.5%. Treatment should include aggressive debridement, irrigation and suturing. Cosmetic considerations are important.

Antiviral agents

Human bites have resulted in the transmission of herpes simplex, hepatitis C, hepatitis B and HIV. Victims of bites from persons potentially infected with HIV or hepatitis should receive rapid, vigorous and thorough wound cleansing with soap and water to remove saliva, and irrigation with virucidal agents such as 1% povidone–iodine. A baseline HIV blood test and hepatitis antibodies at the time of injury should be obtained or arranged, along with a follow-up test in 6 months.

If the bite involved blood, hepatitis B and HIV prophylaxis may be warranted. The potential risk of HIV transmission from the bite victim to the person inflicting the bite should also be considered.

Prophylaxis

Human bites are tetanus-prone wounds. A tetanus toxoid booster should be administered if the patient has been adequately immunized in the past, with last dosage given within the past 10 years. Adults aged 19–64 years who require a tetanus toxoid-containing vaccine should receive combined tetanus, diphtheria and acellular pertussis vaccine (Tdap) instead of tetanus, diphtheria vaccine (Td), if they have not previously received Tdap. Adults who have never received tetanus and diphtheria toxoid-containing vaccine should receive a series of three vaccinations (Table PP34.2). Tetanus immune globulin is required if tetanus immunization has not taken place or is inadequate.

The role of antibiotic prophylaxis in uncomplicated bite wounds is controversial. In general, when the patient is seen within 3 hours, the wound is clean and does not involve the hand, antibiotic prophylaxis can be avoided. However, antibiotic prophylaxis is recommended for all human bites of the hand. One randomized, placebo-controlled study of hospitalized patients with uninfected human bites on the hand found no infections in patients who received antibiotics, whereas those who received placebo had a 47% infection rate. Antibiotics are indicated for high-risk human bite wounds elsewhere on the body, including deep punctures, severe crush injuries, contaminated wounds, older wounds and wounds in patients with underlying illnesses. The antibiotic selected should provide coverage for Gram-positive organisms and *E. corrodens*, such as a second-generation cephalosporin or amoxicillin–clavulanate, and should be given for 5 days with close follow-up.

Antimicrobial therapy

Infected human bites of the hand require both aerobic and anaerobic cultures, and the patient should be treated with antibiotics that cover Gram-positive organisms, *E. corrodens* and anaerobes.

Table PP34.2 Antitetanus prophylaxis

	Previously received three or more doses of Td or DT	Incomplete or unknown vaccination history
Clean or minor wound, age of wound <6 h	Td* if last dose administered more than 10 years ago	Primary vaccination series†
All other wounds	Td* if last dose administered more than 5 years ago	Tetanus immune globulin (260 units im) *and* primary vaccination series

*Adults aged 19–64 years who require a tetanus toxoid-containing vaccine as part of wound management should receive combined tetanus, diphtheria and acellular pertussis vaccine (Tdap) instead of tetanus, diphtheria vaccine (Td) if they have not previously received Tdap.
†Adults who have never received tetanus and diphtheria toxoid-containing vaccine should receive a series of three vaccinations. The preferred schedule is a single dose of Tdap followed by Td >4 weeks later and a second dose of Td 6–12 months later. Tdap can substitute for Td for any one of the three doses in the series. Tdap is not licensed for use among adults aged >65 years. The safety and immunogenicity of Tdap among adults aged >65 years was not studied during US prelicensure trials.

Treatment options include oral amoxicillin–clavulanate, or intravenous ampicillin–sulbactam or ertapenem. β-lactam-allergic patients can receive fluoroquinolones plus clindamycin, or trimethoprim–sulfamethoxazole plus metronidazole.

The duration and route of antibiotic therapy should be individualized based on the site involved, the culture results and response to treatment. All patients with infected human bites of the hand should be hospitalized. High-risk patients, such as those with delayed presentation or deep structure involvement, require prophylactic parenteral antibiotics and close evaluation. Localized infections from human bites not involving the hand can usually be treated without hospitalization if the patient is reliable and has no evidence of lymphangitis, tendon, joint or bone damage or systemic symptoms. Discharge instructions should include immobilization, elevation and sterile dressing changes every 6 hours, and a follow-up visit in 1–2 days.

When cellulitis is already present, a therapeutic course of 10–14 days may be necessary, extended to 3 weeks for tenosynovitis, 4 weeks for septic arthritis and 6 weeks for osteomyelitis. In practice intravenous therapy until the C-reactive protein (CRP) falls to less than 50 mg/l is a pragmatic and objective indication to change to oral antibiotics. If CRP does not fall rapidly or remains static, clinical reappraisal and a second debridement are advisable.

HUMAN BITE FORENSICS

Although many human bites are a consequence of mutual aggression, the physician must keep in mind that the patient may be the victim or perpetrator of child, spousal or elder abuse. All countries require reporting of suspected child abuse; laws vary for spousal or elder abuse. Bite-mark evidence has become accepted as a powerful tool in the investigation of crime. The examining physician should document the appearance of the bite carefully, including its shape, color and size. The physician must determine if a criminal act may have occurred; if so, the wound should be photographed. Counseling or referral should be offered when appropriate.

FURTHER READING

Further reading for this chapter can be found online at http://www.expertconsult.com

Factitious fever

Obtaining an accurate clinical history is the essence of good practice in infectious diseases. When deception on the part of the patient is introduced into a consultation or an episode of care, there is a risk that the real needs of the patient are not addressed. The underlying psychopathology may go unrecognized and untreated. The costs to both the patient and the health-care provider can be substantial.

Factitious disorder is defined in the ICD-10 and the DSM-IV-TR (Table PP35.1) as the intentional production or feigning of symptoms, either physical or psychological, in order to assume the sick role. The patient is not conscious of the motive for the abnormal illness behavior. This is in contrast to malingering, where the production or simulation of illness produces an identifiable advantage to the patient, such as avoiding a criminal trial or an examination or discharge from hospital. In somatoform disorders, the symptoms themselves are produced unconsciously.

Factitious fever is either fraudulent or self-induced. In the former, there is manipulation of the processes of measuring the temperature and the latter is achieved by the injection or ingestion of an infectious agent or pyrogen (Table PP35.2). In the earliest case reports, the majority of cases were fraudulent fevers. With the routine use of electronic thermometers, there is a preponderance of self-induced infection.

EPIDEMIOLOGY

The true incidence of factitious fever is unknown. The collection of accurate scientific data on the condition is hindered by patients' secrecy and by the unwillingness or lack of confidence of physicians to document or report their suspicions. Much of the medical literature consists of retrospective case series and case reports. Prevalence data are derived from case series in highly selected patient groups, such as patients with 'fever of unknown origin' or patients seen by tertiary or quaternary psychiatric referral services. These provide estimates that factitious fever represents 2.2–9.3% of fevers of unknown origin, depending on the setting or level of care (Table PP35.3). In a national survey in Germany, physicians perceived that 1.3% of their annual case load consisted of factitious disease and that 11% of these cases had factitious fever (Fliege 2007).

Between 70% and 95% of factitious fevers reported in the literature are in females, usually in their third or fourth decade and with a high level of education. Male cases are usually older and are more likely to present with fraudulent fever than with self-induced infection.

Associations with other psychiatric conditions, such as borderline personality, depressive or anxiety disorders and eating disorders have been observed by some authors.

Factitious fever by proxy (see Table PP35.1) is usually induced by the female parent.

PATHOPHYSIOLOGY

The tendency to factitious disease often starts in early adulthood, sometimes following a period of hospitalization for a genuine medical condition.

The majority of cases are in individuals employed in health care, which may be an effect of the preoccupation with illness, rather than a risk factor in itself.

The unconscious need to assume the sick role may result from family disruption or emotional or physical abuse in early childhood.

Table PP35.1 DSM-IV-TR criteria for factitious disorders

Factitious disorder	Factitious disorder by proxy
• Intentional production or feigning of physical or psychologic signs or symptoms • The motivation for the behavior is to assume the sick role • External incentives for the behaviour are absent	The intentional production or feigning of physical or psychologic symptoms in another person who is under the individual's care for the purpose of indirectly assuming the sick role

Table PP35.2 Mechanisms of factitious fever

Fraudulent fever	Self-induced fever
Manipulation of thermometer Switching thermometers External heat source Shaking mercury column Friction at site of thermometer placement	**Injection of pyrogen** Contaminated body fluids Bacterial cultures Nonsterile substance, e.g. milk
Fraudulent documentation	**Ingestion of pyrogen**
Fever by proxy	Thyroxine Phenolphthalein Antibiotics Phenytoin Atropine

Adapted from Sarwari & Mackowiak (1997).

Table PP35.3 The prevalence of factitious fever (FF) in case series of fever of unknown origin

Author	Year of publication	Number of cases in series	Prevalence of FF (%)	Setting	Data collection
Petersdorf & Beeson	1961	100	3	University hospital	Retrospective
Rumans & Vosti	1978	506	2.2	University hospital	Retrospective
Aduan et al.	1979	343	9.3	University hospital	Prospective
Larson et al.	1982	105	2.9	University hospital	Retrospective
Knockaert et al.	1992	199	3.5	University hospital	Prospective
Zenone	2006	144	4.7	Nonuniversity hospital	Retrospective

PRESENTATION

Although fever may be the presenting complaint, often it develops over the course of an illness. The history is often elaborate but inconsistent and, upon direct questioning, vague. Some patients are conversant with medical terminology and may form an inappropriately strong bond with the physician. Factitious fever is a recognized presentation of an extreme form of factitious disease, Münchhausen's syndrome, a condition first described by Asher in 1951 and inspired by the exaggerated chronicles of the exploits of the German cavalry officer Baron Karl Friedrich Hieronymus von Münchhausen. Such patients exhibit pseudologia fantastica (pathologic lying), dramatic presentations and aggressive behavior. Often, they have a history of multiple hospital admissions and self-discharges against medical advice.

Physical examination may be surprisingly normal. There may be evidence of previous presentations (historical accounts refer to the 'grid iron abdomen' from multiple previous operations) or unusual scars from self-inflicted lesions.

Fraudulent fever has notable characteristics (Table PP35.4). Patients with self-induced fever may have a true bacteremia, but no identifiable source. There may be evidence of local infection at the site of injection (cutaneous abscess, nonhealing wounds).

INVESTIGATIONS

Standard blood tests and imaging may be unremarkable. The unusual and inconsistent history and examination can lead to extensive and risky investigations as the search for the underlying cause progresses. In the pursuit of the sick role, the patient undergoes these procedures willingly, despite their invasive nature.

DIAGNOSIS

The differential diagnosis is wide (Table PP35.5) and there may be some overlap between different syndromes. An expert psychiatric opinion should be sought.

Table PP35.4 Characteristics of fraudulent fever

- Lack of normal diurnal variation
- Absence of tachycardia during spikes of temperature
- Rapid defervescence, unaccompanied by diaphoresis
- Fever greater than 41°C

Table PP35.5 Differential diagnosis of factitious fever

- True fever
- Somatization
- Malingering
- Eating disorder
- Chemical dependency
- Personality disorder
- Psychosis

Prior to the advent of digital tympanic thermography, fraudulent fever was revealed by simultaneous readings of oral and rectal temperature, measuring the temperature of freshly voided urine or by close observation of the patient whilst the temperature is being taken. The diagnosis may be suspected early because of inconsistencies in the history and examination. Patients may be recognized from previous hospital admissions, but 'hospital hopping' is common and a history of multiple previous admissions can go unrecognized. A room search, if acceptable, may reveal injection paraphernalia and even bacterial culture media that the patient has used for auto-inoculation. Ultimately, if obtainable, a patient confession provides the diagnosis.

MANAGEMENT

Patients may present with genuine medical conditions (e.g. septic emboli or endocarditis), which coexist with or result from the abnormal illness behavior; their prompt management is the priority.

It is important to recognize that the patient's intention is to assume the sick role rather than to gain gratification from the deception of the caregivers. Therefore, management should be directed to address this need.

Opinions vary regarding the importance and risk of confronting the patient with the suspicion that their illness is factitious. There is consensus that early psychiatric consultation is advisable. However, outcome studies show that the uptake of long-term psychiatric treatment in this patient group is poor.

Intervention studies are hindered by the difficulty of case identification and the lack of a reliable control group.

PROGNOSIS/OUTCOME

There is a recognized mortality from factitious fever, particularly from direct intravenous injection of bacterial cultures or contaminated body fluids. Patients may be left with permanent disability resulting from self-induced disease or from invasive investigations and interventions. Health-care-associated illness becomes a risk in the event of prolonged hospital admission.

Although not easily quantifiable, repeated assessments, hospital admissions, unnecessary investigations and legal proceedings constitute a considerable cost to the health-care provider.

An awareness and early recognition of factitious disease is important to direct appropriate psychiatric referral and treatment.

MEDICOLEGAL ISSUES

It is advisable to consult a medicolegal organization if factitious fever is suspected. If the fraudulent nature of the illness could readily be inferred from the evidence in a patient's medical notes, the physician may be held responsible for unnecessary treatments or investigations. Ultimately, the patient may seek to sue their practitioner in order to legally sanction their pursuit of the sick role.

FURTHER READING

Further reading for this chapter can be found online at http://www.expertconsult.com

Methicillin-resistant *Staphylococcus aureus* (MRSA) colonization

Since its initial report in 1962, MRSA has been considered a hospital-related phenomenon for a few decades. Mostly sporadic cases and small outbreaks were reported. In the late 1980s MRSA rates started to increase and nowadays MRSA has become endemic in hospitals worldwide, with only a few exceptions. This is associated with high morbidity, mortality and additional costs to society. In addition, there are increasing reports of community-onset disease that primarily affects younger people and may sometimes be fatal.

Staphylococcus aureus is a commensal micro-organism that is found in healthy people. Carriage of *S. aureus* in healthy individuals is mainly located in the nose (Fig. PP36.1).[1] A recent survey in the USA in a random sample of the population found that 32.4% carried *S. aureus*

and 0.8% MRSA.[2] Carriage of *S. aureus* rarely causes disease in healthy people but is associated with an increased risk for the development of infections in various patient populations.[1] Carriage of MRSA is associated with an even higher risk than carriage of methicillin-susceptible *S. aureus* (MSSA). In patients colonized with MRSA at admission, 19% develop an infection with MRSA during the hospitalization period. In carriers of MSSA this is only 1.5% and in noncarriers 2.0%.[3]

Although the risk of carriage has been clearly established, there is an ongoing debate regarding the effects of eradication of carriage. There are two possible objectives to eradicating carriage:

1. *To control the spread of MRSA*: As most of the individuals that carry MRSA are asymptomatic, control of spread includes

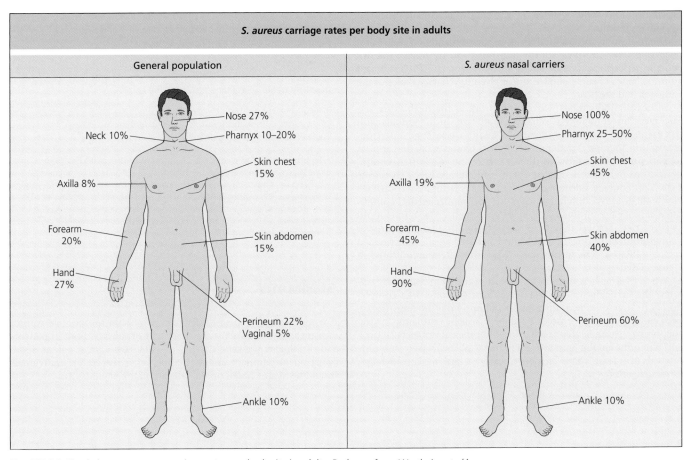

Fig. PP36.1 *Staphylococcus aureus* carriage rates per body site in adults. Redrawn from Wertheim *et al.*[1]

both infected and colonized individuals. This also includes health-care workers. Numerous reports have identified colonized health-care workers as the source of MRSA outbreaks.[4] Therefore, successful control of MRSA should include identification and treatment of colonized patients and health-care workers. Using this strategy, the MRSA rates in Scandinavia and The Netherlands have remained extremely low.

2. *To prevent the development of infection in patients who are at high risk* (e.g. patients in the intensive care unit or patients scheduled for high-risk surgery): Although this makes sense considering the proven risk of MRSA carriage, the strategy has not been studied sufficiently for its effectiveness.

The best studies in this field have included patients carrying *S. aureus* in general, mainly consisting of MSSA. A review integrating the results of these studies concluded that there is a significant reduction of the *S. aureus* infection rate in carriers treated before surgery or while on hemodialysis or peritoneal dialysis.[5] These studies used mupirocin nasal ointment. The study in surgical patients only showed a significant effect in carriers, although this was not the primary objective of the investigators. The protective effect of mupirocin in surgical patients is very likely; however, the final evidence should come from an intervention study treating carriers only. At present, the prophylactic use of mupirocin in patients is recommended in MRSA carriers undergoing high-risk surgery in several national guidelines. The studies in hemodialysis and peritoneal dialysis did show a significant reduction of the infection rate but the prolonged use of mupirocin carries a substantial risk for the development of resistance to this precious compound. To date, the optimal treatment schedule has not been defined and extremely careful monitoring for mupirocin resistance is mandatory when it is used in this setting.

Recently a guideline for the treatment of carriage has been developed, based on a systematic review of the literature and expert opinion.[6] This resulted in the following conclusions and recommendations.

The indication for eradication of carriage depends on the consequences of MRSA carriage for the individual and for others, the risk and the seriousness of side-effects of treatment and the estimated a-priori chance of successful treatment given the characteristics of the pathogen and the host.

In healthy individuals who do not work in the health-care setting, eradication therapy is usually not advised. In individuals with risk factors for the development of an MRSA-associated infection, eradication therapy is generally indicated. However, as this applies to patients with underlying diseases there are also often contraindications because the risk of treatment failure is high. Therefore, a division is made into uncomplicated versus complicated carriage (Table PP36.1). Treatment strategies for uncomplicated and complicated carriage are outlined in Tables PP36.2 and PP36.3. In complicated carriers, topical therapy is combined with a combination of two systemic antibiotics. Details of the preferred agents are provided in Table PP36.4. This results in a treatment strategy as outlined in Figure PP36.2.

When treatment is complete, its effectiveness is measured by cultures. The first cultures are obtained at least 48 hours after completion of treatment. At least three sets of cultures from the nose, throat, perineum, sputum (in case of productive cough, ventilation or tracheostomy), wounds, skin lesions, insertion sites of catheters (if present) and urine (in the presence of a urinary catheter), taken with time intervals of at least 7 days, are needed before a carrier is considered to be treated effectively.

Table PP36.1 Definitions of uncomplicated and complicated MRSA carriage[6]

Uncomplicated carriage

MRSA carrier who:

- has no active infection caused by MRSA and no active skin lesions and no invasive material with a connection between the interior and exterior environment (e.g. urinary catheter, external fixator); *and*
- MRSA carriage is located in the nose (apart from other sites); *and*
- MRSA strain is *in-vitro* susceptible for mupirocin

Complicated carriage

MRSA carrier who:

- has active skin lesions or invasive material with a connection between the interior and exterior environment; *or*
- failed earlier treatment according to the guideline for uncomplicated carriers; *or*
- MRSA carriage is not located in the nose; *or*
- MRSA strain is *in-vitro* resistant to mupirocin

Table PP36.2 Recommendations for treatment of uncomplicated carriage[6]

Recommendations	Level*
Mupirocin nasal ointment in both nostrils q8 h for 5 days	1
During treatment daily washing of skin and hair with a disinfecting soap (chlorhexidine soap solution 40 mg/ml or povidone–iodine shampoo 75 mg/ml)	3
Clean underwear, clothing, washcloths and towels daily, and a complete change of bedding on days 1, 2 and 5 during treatment	4
If therapy fails, explore the situation at home for reservoirs, i.e. humans and/or pets (a reservoir at home has to be treated simultaneously with the carrier)	3
If second treatment fails, the person becomes a complicated carrier and treatment as outlined in Table PP36.3 is recommended	4

*The strength of the recommendations given is according to the handbook of the Dutch Institute for Healthcare Improvement (CBO). Level 1: conclusion supported by at least two independent randomized clinical trials of good quality or by a meta-analysis; level 2: supported by at least two randomized clinical trials of mediocre quality or insufficient power or other comparative studies (cohort study, patient-control study); level 3: not supported by comparative studies mentioned in levels 1 and 2; level 4: expert panel opinion.

SUMMARY

To control the spread of MRSA, it is important to optimize control measures. One measure is the treatment of carriage, both in patients and health-care workers. Carriers of MRSA who are at risk of developing an infection or contaminating other susceptible individuals should be treated based on the relevant national guidelines.

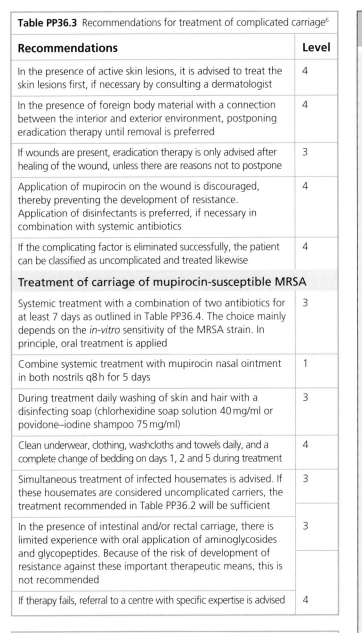

Table PP36.3 Recommendations for treatment of complicated carriage[6]

Recommendations	Level
In the presence of active skin lesions, it is advised to treat the skin lesions first, if necessary by consulting a dermatologist	4
In the presence of foreign body material with a connection between the interior and exterior environment, postponing eradication therapy until removal is preferred	4
If wounds are present, eradication therapy is only advised after healing of the wound, unless there are reasons not to postpone	3
Application of mupirocin on the wound is discouraged, thereby preventing the development of resistance. Application of disinfectants is preferred, if necessary in combination with systemic antibiotics	4
If the complicating factor is eliminated successfully, the patient can be classified as uncomplicated and treated likewise	4

Treatment of carriage of mupirocin-susceptible MRSA

Systemic treatment with a combination of two antibiotics for at least 7 days as outlined in Table PP36.4. The choice mainly depends on the *in-vitro* sensitivity of the MRSA strain. In principle, oral treatment is applied	3
Combine systemic treatment with mupirocin nasal ointment in both nostrils q8h for 5 days	1
During treatment daily washing of skin and hair with a disinfecting soap (chlorhexidine soap solution 40 mg/ml or povidone–iodine shampoo 75 mg/ml)	3
Clean underwear, clothing, washcloths and towels daily, and a complete change of bedding on days 1, 2 and 5 during treatment	4
Simultaneous treatment of infected housemates is advised. If these housemates are considered uncomplicated carriers, the treatment recommended in Table PP36.2 will be sufficient	3
In the presence of intestinal and/or rectal carriage, there is limited experience with oral application of aminoglycosides and glycopeptides. Because of the risk of development of resistance against these important therapeutic means, this is not recommended	3
If therapy fails, referral to a centre with specific expertise is advised	4

Table PP36.4 Oral combination therapy for eradication of MRSA carriage[6]

Antibiotic 1	Antibiotic 2	Recommendation
Trimethoprim 200 mg q12h Doxycycline 200 mg q24h Clindamycin 600 mg q8h Clarithromycin 500 mg q12h Ciprofloxacin 750 mg q12h	First choice: rifampin (rifampicin) 600 mg q12h In case of resistance: fusidic acid 500 mg q8h	Recommended
Fusidic acid 500 mg q8h	Rifampin (rifampicin) 600 mg q12h	Alternative

The dosages in this table are the recommended dosages for an adult patient of about 70 kg. Combination therapy is preferred because of better effectiveness and a decreased risk of resistance.

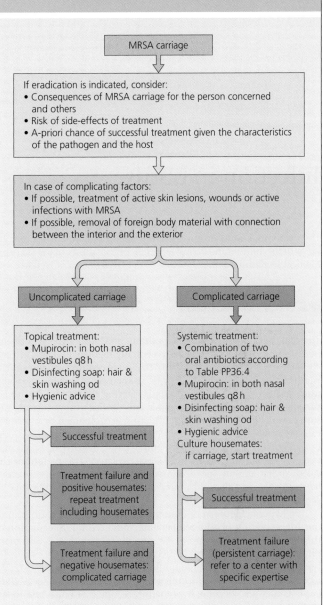

Fig. PP36.2 Antibiotic eradication of MRSA carriage.

REFERENCES

References for this chapter can be found online at http://www.expertconsult.com

David J Barillo
Kevin K Chung

Practice point **37**

Infection in burns

The opinions and assertions herein contained represent the private views of the authors and do not represent official policy of the US Army Medical Department, the US Army or the Department of Defense.

PATHOPHYSIOLOGY

Thermal injury results in a significant and sustained hypermetabolic response, possibly related to centrally mediated release of catecholamines, glucagon and cortisol.[1] The initial cardiovascular response is a decrease in cardiac output with an increase in systemic vascular resistance secondary to hypovolemia. During the second 24 hours, the patient becomes hypermetabolic and cardiac output increases to supernormal (2–2.5 times normal) levels, accompanied by a reciprocal drop in systemic vascular resistance to 40–80% of normal.[2] Cardiac output remains elevated until the burn wounds are closed, which may take weeks to months if the burn surface is large.[1] This pattern of elevated cardiac output and decreased systemic vascular resistance is a *normal response* to thermal injury, and is not, of itself, indicative of sepsis.

The hypermetabolism of burn injury results in increased heat production, elevation of core temperature and a central upregulation of the thermoregulatory set-point. Fever in the burn patient is thus often physiologic and not related to infection.[3] Burn centers do not consider burn patients as being febrile until core temperature exceeds 102.5°F (39.2°C) and do not perform 'fever workups' below this level. Burn patients may also become hypothermic secondary to heat loss to the environment as a consequence of lost skin integrity. Burn hypermetabolism causes increased clearance of many medications, including antibiotics and anticonvulsant, and dosing should be based upon serum measurements where available.

Thermal injury suppresses essentially all aspects of the immune system. The multiple immunologic consequences of burn injury are summarized in Table PP37.1 Leukocyte counts in the range of 14 000–18 000/mm³ or higher are typically seen in burn patients in the absence of infection; the white blood cell (WBC) trend, rather than the absolute WBC count, should be followed if infection is suspected. Moreover, bacterial colonization of the burn wound is an expected and unavoidable consequence, which may or may not lead to wound infection.

In summary, the pathophysiology of burn injury makes the timely diagnosis of infection difficult. Elevated temperature, WBC count, and cardiac output combined with a low systemic vascular resistance and presence of bacteria in the burn wound may indicate serious systemic infection, or may simply represent normal physiologic response. Acute infection is best suggested by a *change* in hemodynamic status, body temperature or clinical condition, increased need for ventilatory support, new onset of ileus, glycosuria or glucose intolerance.

DIAGNOSTIC WORKUP OF THE POTENTIALLY SEPTIC BURN PATIENT

A septic workup starts with a complete physical examination with specific attention directed at the burn wound (see below) and to any current or previous site of intravenous cannulation. Rectal examination should be performed to rule out prostatitis in males and perirectal disease in both sexes. Cultures of blood, sputum and urine are obtained, along with a chest radiograph. A timeframe of initial presentation of infection by site is presented in Figure PP37.1

In addition to acalculous cholecystitis and pancreatitis, burn patients occasionally develop short-segment small bowel necrosis by a mechanism which remains unclear. An adjunct to abdominal CT is diagnostic peritoneal lavage, which has a sensitivity of 0.86, a specificity of 1.00 and an overall accuracy of 94% in the diagnosis of intraperitoneal infection in burn patients.[4]

Drug resistance is a continuing problem, with emergence of extended-spectrum β-lactamase-producing, enteric Gram-negative organisms as well as multidrug-resistant *Pseudomonas*. Multidrug-resistant *Acinetobacter* species are also becoming common, although the presence of this organism does not independently affect mortality.[5] For empiric coverage, a burn center-specific antibiogram should be developed as drug susceptibilities will differ from the remainder of the hospital. Empiric *Acinetobacter* coverage may necessitate inhaled colistin (for pneumonia) combined with oral minocycline and intravenous colistin for severe infection.

Children may develop idiopathic fevers in the 103°F (39.5°C) range early in the course of burn injury, usually resolving without identifiable source. Persistent fever suggests otitis media, urinary tract infection or burn wound cellulitis. Oropharyngeal colonization with *Streptococcus pyogenes* is a theoretical concern, as spread of streptococci to the burn wound results in a rapidly spreading cellulitis. Routine penicillin prophylaxis of pediatric burn patients has been advocated but is probably unnecessary. Alternately, penicillin can be administered until admission throat cultures return as negative.

Electrical burn injury may result in muscle necrosis (under intact or uninjured skin) along the route of current passage. Sepsis workup should include prompt surgical exploration of body regions known or suspected to be in the path of current flow if another source is not immediately apparent.

Positive blood cultures in the absence of wound infection should prompt examination of intravenous cannulation sites and consideration of endocarditis. Gram-negative bacteremia, but not Gram-positive bacteremia in burn patients is significantly associated with increased mortality.[6] The association of fungemia with increased mortality is equivocal.[6]

Table PP37.1 Impact of thermal injury on immune function

Circulating	IL-1	Initial increase in serum levels followed by decreased production
		Increased local production at sites of inflammation
	IL-2	Suppressed production
	TNF	Increased serum levels in severely infected burn patients
	IL-6	Increased serum levels in severely infected burn patients
		Increased local production at sites of inflammation
	Neopterin	Serum levels increased (nonspecific marker of macrophage stimulation)
	Circulating immunoglobulins	Decreased serum levels
	Prostaglandin E_2	Increased serum levels of prostaglandin E_2
	Thromboxane B_2	Increased serum levels
	Activation/depletion of alternative complement pathway	
	Secondary elevation of fibronectin levels	
	Reduction in serum opsonic activity	
Cellular	Initial leukopenia (margination) followed by leukocytosis	
	Generalized activation of circulating granulocytes by multiple pathways	
	Depression of neutrophil chemotaxis, phagocytosis and bactericidal activity	
	Depression of helper T cells	
	Generation of suppressor inducer T cells	
	Increased production of suppressor effector T cells	
	Suppression of IL-2 production by lymphocytes	
	Activation of macrophages	
Other	Loss of cutaneous skin barrier to infection	
	Smoke inhalation	Increased risk of pneumonia (impaired mucociliary clearance mechanisms, defective alveolar macrophage function, distal airway obstruction, alveolar collapse, segmental atelectasis, increased requirements for airway intubation and mechanical ventilation)
	Requirement for long-term intubation of bladder and vascular system	
	Nutritional deficits	
	Impairment of reticuloendothelial system function	
	Multiple blood transfusions	

IL, interleukin; TNF, tumor necrosis factor.

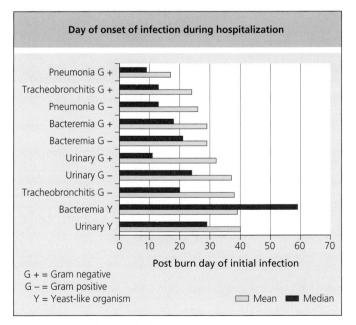

Fig. PP37.1 Day of onset of infection during hospitalization.

Radionucleotide studies such as indium or tagged leukocyte scans, in general, are not useful in burn patients. Burn wound or skin donor sites will frequently concentrate isotopes, making interpretation difficult.

EVALUATION OF THE BURN WOUND

The burn wound is the key to management of the burn patient. The physiologic, metabolic and immunologic changes seen in burn injury are proportional to the size of the wound, and do not return to normal until the burn wound is successfully closed. The burn wound is the first site to examine when sepsis is suspected.

The thick leathery nonviable coating of a burn, termed eschar, is warm, protein rich, moist and avascular, representing an excellent culture medium unaffected by parenterally administered antibiotics or by circulating elements of the immune system.[1] For this reason, the eschar of full thickness burns should be expeditiously excised. Eschar normally becomes colonized with the patient's own flora (Gram-positive bacteria) within 3–5 days of injury.[7] This initial colonization is subsequently replaced by Gram-negative flora over a variable interval. The principal concern is eventual colonization of the subeschar space. When bacterial densities at the interface of eschar and underlying viable tissue reach a level of >10^5 cfu/gram of tissue, wound infection with systemic microbial spread is likely.[1] The goals of burn wound management are to contain microbial colonization to a manageable level with topical agents pending surgical debridement and wound closure with skin autografts or other modalities.[1]

Because the presence of bacteria in the burn wound per se is not a pathologic finding, specialized procedures and terms have been developed to quantify the potential for wound infection:

- *burn wound colonization* is the term given to the presence of micro-organisms within the eschar and does not imply active local or systemic infection;
- *burn wound invasion* occurs when micro-organisms invade viable tissue adjacent to the burn eschar, an infrequent event in contemporary burn practice; and
- invasion accompanied by a positive blood culture or by distant spread of micro-organisms or toxic products is termed *burn wound septicemia*.

Cultures of the burn surface or of debrided tissue are useful for epidemiologic purposes to document resident flora in the event of true infection. Quantitative wound cultures (cfu/gram of tissue) have limited diagnostic utility in burn wound care. A negative quantitative culture (bacterial density $<10^5$ cfu) correlates well (96.1% negative predictive power) with absence of invasive infection on histopathologic tissue evaluation; however, the agreement between positive cultures and positive histologic examination is only 35.7% (positive predictive power).[7] Thus, only a negative quantitative culture has clinical significance.

The *sine qua non* of wound evaluation is histopathologic examination of a biopsy specimen to determine the presence of micro-organisms in viable tissue.[1] This is performed as a bedside procedure under local anesthesia. A 500 mg sample of eschar (ellipse measuring 1–2 cm) is excised to include the underlying viable tissue. Frozen section technique provides results in 30 minutes but has a 3.6% false-negative rate, and should be confirmed by permanent sections.[8] A rapid section technique that produces permanent sections in 4 hours has been described.[9] Results with either technique are communicated to the clinician using standardized nomenclature (Table PP37.2).

Cellulitis is diagnosed by the presence of expanding erythema at the margins of the burn wound. Erythema surrounding second- or third-degree burn injury that does not increase in size may also represent areas of first-degree burn. Burn wound cellulitis usually responds to β-lactams. Occasionally, cellulitis is poorly controlled until the adjacent burn is excised.

True burn wound infection is suggested by early eschar separation, conversion of partial thickness to full thickness injury, subeschar hemorrhage, degeneration of granulation tissue, dark red, brown or black discolorization of eschar (Fig. PP37.2), violaceous discoloration of the unburned skin at the wound margins or ecthyma gangrenosum. Diagnosis is confirmed by wound biopsy and histologic examination. When invasive bacterial infection (Stage 2A, 2B or 2C) is diagnosed, the wound should be immediately excised. Gram-negative organisms are most frequently implicated.

Fungal infection of the burn wound is most commonly caused by *Aspergillus*, *Candida*, *Mucor* or *Rhizopus* spp. Invasive fungal wound infection is an independent predictor of mortality.[10] Wound colonization involving *Candida* spp. is commonly treated with topical nystatin or clotrimazole with little supportive evidence. *Aspergillus* spp. characteristically produce superficial colonization or infection of necrotic tissue, which should be promptly excised. *Mucor* spp. may produce a rapidly spreading fascial infection with early microvascular involvement and its presence in a burn wound is an indication for immediate, radical and repeated surgical excision.

Table PP37.2 Histologic classification of burn wound infection

Class 1 – Colonization	1A Superficial	Superficial bacterial colonization of the wound Micro-organisms present on wound surface
	1B Penetration	Penetration of the eschar by bacteria in variable thickness of eschar
	1C Proliferation	Multiplication of micro-organisms present in the subeschar space
Class 2 – Invasion	2A Microinvasion	Micro-organisms present in viable tissue immediately subjacent to subeschar space
	2B Generalized	Multifocal or widespread penetration of micro-organisms deep into viable tissue
	2C Microvascular	Involvement of small vessels and lymphatics

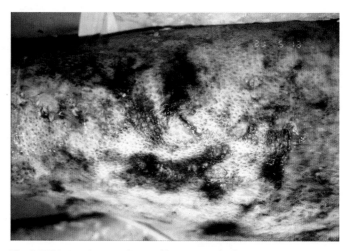

Fig. PP37.2 Invasive pseudomonal burn wound infection, stage 2C.

REFERENCES

References for this chapter can be found online at http://www.expertconsult.com

Transfusion-related infections

Disturbingly, transmission of HIV and the hepatitis viruses may occur from blood donors in an often asymptomatic phase after infection when neither the pathogen nor its antigens, nor host-specific immunologic markers are detectable by conventional screening tests. This is known as the window period (WP). The addition of nucleic acid testing (NAT) to screening tests has decreased the duration of the WP, resulting in less than one case of HIV transmitted per million units transfused in developed countries. Current risk estimates are based on mathematical models calculating the probability of donors presenting in the WP. Estimating infection risks by testing donor blood for all potential pathogens or observing the recipients for illness are impractical and prohibitively expensive because of the large sample sizes required (see Table PP38.1 and annotations).

Acellular 'manufactured' blood products, such as fresh frozen plasma (FFP), albumin, gamma globulins and clotting factor concentrates, are usually pooled from multiple donors. The risk of contamination of such large pools is offset by rigorous physicochemical sterilization procedures. In contrast, cellular products – packed red

Table PP38.1 Risk of transfusion-transmitted diseases in the United States

Pathogenic agent	Average estimated risk per unit
Hepatitis A virus (HAV)	Unknown, presumably <1:1 000 000
Hepatitis B virus (HBV)	1:205 000*
Hepatitis C virus (HCV)	1:1 935 000[†]
Human immunodeficiency virus-1 (HIV-1)	1:2 135 000[†]
Human T-cell lymphotrophic virus 1 and 2 (HTLV-1, HTLV-2)	1:2 993 000
Cytomegalovirus (CMV)	Infrequent[‡]
Parvovirus B19	Unknown, presumably <1:1 000 000
West Nile virus (WNV) and other arboviruses	Unknown, presumably <1:1 000 000[†]
Plasmodium spp. (agents of malaria)	1:4 000 000
Babesia	<1:1 000 000
Trypanosoma cruzi (agent of Chagas disease)	Unknown, presumably <1:1 000 000
Agent of Creutzfeldt–Jakob disease (CJD), variant CJD (vCJD)	Unknown, presumably <1 000 000
Bacteria associated with symptomatic sepsis	1:500 000 for red blood cell units 1:15 400 for apheresis platelet units[§]

Case of infection per unit of blood product transfused:
Calculated by the incidence rate/window period (IR/WP) model, which measures the residual risk of a given viral pathogen by multiplying the IR (new infections in the specific blood donor population per year) by the length of the WP in fractions of a year. These calculations assume that:
- timing of donation is independent of the time of infection;
- rate of transmission is nearly 100%;
- testing is flawless with no infections missed due to immunologically silent state or variant strains; and
- no infections are missed due to inherent decreased lifespan of transplant recipients because of co-morbidities.
*Estimates for HBV reflect risk projections before implementation of blood donor screening with nucleic acid testing (NAT) in 1999.
[†]Estimates for HIV and HCV indicate risk projections following implementation of NAT for these agents in 1999 and West Nile virus in 2003.
[‡]In association with CMV risk-reduced components.
[§]Risk estimate for symptomatic sepsis associated with transfusion of apheresis platelet units reflects the experience of a single US medical center (Johns Hopkins) before implementation of a bacterial detection system.
Data from Ness *et al.* (2001).

Table PP38.2 Methods for reducing risk of transmission

Method	Comment
Deferral of high-risk patients	Sole method available for CJD by exclusion of patients who have lived in the UK or Europe Important in prevention of malaria, babesiosis, HIV-2 and HIV serogroup O infection
Exclusion of patients with history of disease	Exclusion of patients with history of intravenous drug use or of jaundice prevents HIV-, HCV- and HBV-related illnesses
Screening of blood products with serologic tests	Selection of seronegative donors for the immunocompromised Effective in reducing transmission of viruses of the herpesvirus family (CMV, EBV, hepatitis viruses, HIV) Seronegative blood donors may harbor intracellular viruses such as CMV with undetectable antibody titers Transient viremia may bind circulating antibody, rendering it undetectable
Pathogen-reduction methods in the manufacturing process	
Heat (pasteurization) Nanofiltration Leukocyte reduction	Ineffective for prions and non-enveloped viruses Effective in viral illness Effective in reducing transmission of viruses of the herpesvirus family (CMV, EBV). Not as good as blood from seronegative donors Cells of granulocyte–macrophage lineage are a common source of CMV infection
Physicochemical processes	
Solvent/detergent treatment Photodynamic treatment Selective-affinity resin	Effective against lipid-enveloped viruses (HIV, HBV, HCV) Ineffective against non-enveloped viruses (HAV, parvovirus B19) Pooling of products with >2500 donors risks contamination of large batches Allows single-unit treatment Photosensitive compounds (S-303, inactine, riboflavin, psoralens) activated by ultraviolet light inactivate pathogens by oxidation (methylene blue) or binding to nucleic acids (riboflavin and psoralens) Adsorbs scrapie prion protein

CJD, Creutzfeldt–Jakob disease; CMV, cytomegalovirus; EBV, Epstein–Barr virus; HAV, hepatitis A virus; HBV, hepatitis B virus; HCV, hepatitis C virus.

blood cells (RBCs), platelets and granulocytes – are mostly single-donor derived and have limited sterilization options (Table PP38.2).

THE VIRAL PATHOGENS (TABLE PP38.3)

Hepatitis A virus (HAV)

Rare cases of HAV may occur in clotting factor concentrates treated with the solvent/detergent method (see Table PP38.2). The lack of a viral envelope enables this RNA virus to survive pasteurization and chemical inactivation by photodynamic treatment.

Hepatitis B (HBV)

In transcutaneous exposures, HBV is significantly more infective than HCV and HIV. In the USA, 5% of the population is seropositive and over a million people have chronic infection. Serum hepatitis B surface antigen (HbsAg) is detectable 30–60 days after transmission and persists up to 4 months following acute infection. IgM anti-HBc antibodies are present at symptom onset and signal high-level viremia. Anti-HBsAg antibodies (anti-HBs) become detectable after an often asymptomatic window period of 37–87 days. They protect against re-infection but cannot achieve tissue eradication. Anti-HBc is detectable in chronic carriers. It is possible for a donor to be HBsAg negative yet still be infective. Rare HBV mutants that do not produce HBsAg are undetectable by routine HBsAg and anti-HBc testing but are still pathogenic. Novel antibody and NAT-based assays detect these mutants.

Hepatitis C (HCV)

This RNA flavivirus has six genotypes. Genotype 1 responds less favorably to treatment and is predominant in North America. Overall,

3.9 million Americans are seropositive for HCV, resulting in chronic disease in 2.7 million and up to 40 000 new cases per year. Approximately two-thirds of HCV carriers have a history of intravenous drug use. Among blood donors, 0.07–0.09% have confirmed infection. Prior to seroconversion, fluctuating viral levels, often even below NAT thresholds, result in a residual risk of HCV transmission by blood transfusion.

Human retroviruses

HIV infections were first diagnosed in hemophiliacs and other transfusion recipients in 1982. Fortunately, timely policies of high-risk donor deferral by detailed history in 1983 and HIV antibody testing in 1985 decreased transmission dramatically, even before the disease became a part of the public consciousness. Improved screening methods with sensitive immunoassays, p24 antigen testing and RNA testing on pooled blood products have reduced transmission further since the 1990s (see Chapter 163).

While HIV-1 antibody tests may detect 60–91% of HIV-2 infections, these and HIV-1 group O (outlier group) are mainly prevented by donor deferral from high-risk areas.

Human T-cell lymphotrophic virus (HTLV)-1 and -2 infections

HTLV-1 and -2 have 60–70% sequence homology and a shared tropism for T lymphocytes. In contrast with HIV, HTLV is rarely present in cell-free plasma. Screening for HTLV-1 antibodies began in 1988. A sensitive HTLV-1/2 combination assay introduced in 1998 detects close to 100% of HTLV-2 infections, making these infections from blood transfusions very rare indeed. Prevalence of markers in screened blood has decreased recently.

Table PP38.3 The viral pathogens

Pathogen	Associated disease	Notes
Common hepatitis viruses		
HAV	Infectious hepatitis, 15- to 40-day incubation period Only 20–30% new infections are symptomatic Peak viremia occurs 2 weeks before jaundice Signs or symptoms may persist for 2 months	No chronic carrier state At risk: seronegative patients and travelers Infection prevented by donor deferral by history of acute disease, chemical evidence of hepatitis or serology
HBV	Incubation period ranges from 5 weeks to 6 months 30% of those infected are symptomatic Up to 10% of adults and 30–90% of infants develop chronic infection Acute hepatitis, vasculitis, glomerulonephritis Cirrhosis and hepatocellular carcinoma Chronic carrier state and chronic active hepatitis	Risk factors for the newly infected: • 40% infected partners • 15% MSM • 14% intravenous drug users • 1/3 no identifiable risk At risk are seronegative individuals by sexual, vertical, parenteral, transcutaneous routes Infection prevented by donor deferral by history of acute disease or chemical evidence of hepatitis
HCV	Chronic hepatitis develops in 75–85% of persons infected after 45 years of age and in 50–60% of those infected as children or young adults HCV causes hepatitis, vasculitis, rashes, cirrhosis and hepatocellular carcinoma	As HBV 3–7% of infants have vertically transmitted maternal infection from HCV Hepatocellular carcinoma yearly incidence rate 1–4% in cirrhotic patients with HBV
Other viral pathogens		
Deltavirus (HDV)	Acute on chronic (HBV) infection, fulminant disease	Parenteral, co-transmission with HBV, or superinfection of chronic carriers of HBV
CMV (HHV-5)	Mild viral illness with lymphadenopathy in the immunocompetent Pneumonitis, hepatitis, gastroenteritis, and retinitis in advanced HIV and immunosuppressed seronegative patients	Seronegative unit selection may prevent transmission Cell-depleted blood components (plasma, cryoprecipitate) do not transmit CMV; leukocyte reduction by filtration has a similar degree of protection Platelets also have a low risk of transmission
Neonatal CMV	Severe CMV disease including hemolytic anemia	Premature infants (<1200 g) born to CMV-seronegative mothers
Congenital CMV	Congenital malformation, jaundice, hepatosplenomegaly, microencephalopathy, thrombocytopenia Occasional severe malformation with high mortality rates	Fetuses of seronegative mothers
EBV (HHV-4)	Infectious mononucleosis associated with Burkitt's lymphoma, nasopharyngeal carcinoma and post-transplantation lymphoproliferative disease	Seronegative individuals
KSHV (HHV-8)	Kaposi's sarcoma, body cavity-based lymphoma and Castleman's disease	Seronegative individuals
HIV	These and other regionally limited variants such as HIV-2 and HIV-1 group O cause AIDS	Blood donors are deferred if they had risk exposures to HIV-1 group O in Central and West Africa Specific HIV-2 antibody test kits detect >99% of HIV-2
HTLV-1	Adult T-cell leukemia, lymphoma, tropical spastic paraparesis, chronic arthritis Mild immunosuppression opportunistic infections	Regional exposures (Southern Japan, Caribbean)
HTLV-2	As per HTLV-1 but no hematologic malignancy	HTLV-2 epidemic in intravenous drug users in the Americas and Europe in the past 50 years Parenteral exposures, and sexual and vertical transmission
Parvovirus B19	Fifth disease, a childhood exanthem Hypoplastic/aplastic crises and/or chronic severe anemia secondary to persistent infection	Patients with immunosuppression with HIV or hematologic malignancies or RBC abnormalities with shortened RBC lifespan; sickle cell anemia, thalassemia
Congenital	Fetal loss, malformation or congenital illness	Seronegative pregnant patients

CMV, cytomegalovirus; EBV, Epstein–Barr virus; HAV, hepatitis A virus; HBV, hepatitis B virus; HCV, hepatitis C virus; HDV, hepatitis D virus; HHV, human herpesvirus; HTLV, human T-cell lymphotrophic virus; KSHV, Kaposi's sarcoma-associated herpes virus; MSM, men who have sex with men.

Human herpesviruses (HHV)

These enveloped, double-stranded DNA viruses are associated with lifelong carrier states and reactivation. Herpes simplex and varicella-zoster viruses are rarely, if ever, transmitted by transfusion. Cytomegalovirus, Epstein–Barr virus (EBV) and HHV-8, widely prevalent in the adult population, may be transmitted in blood products and affect the seronegative young or immunocompromised.

Cytomegalovirus (CMV)

Anti-CMV antibodies are present in up to 50% of donors. Seronegative recipients of unscreened cellular blood components have an overall relative risk of approximately 1% of primary CMV infection. This ranges from zero to 50% of infants and 30% of bone marrow transplant recipients. In solid-organ transplant recipients, the risk of CMV by the transplanted seropositive organs overshadows the relatively smaller risk posed by transfusions. Second-strain infections remain theoretically possible even in seropositive recipients.

Other herpesviruses

About 90% of the adult population is EBV seropositive. Infection is deterred by host virus-specific cytotoxic T lymphocytes and transfusion-associated EBV infection is rare. HHV-8 infects B-lymphocytes and monocyte/macrophage cell types. Data about HH-8 infection risk from transfusion are sparse, but in a recent study of 991 transfusion recipients in Kampala, Uganda, 425 recipients received a blood product from a single seropositive donor. HHV-8 seroconversion occurred in 41 recipients.

Parvovirus B19

Parvovirus is present in 1/50 000 to 1/20 000 donors, with surges during epidemics. About 50% of the adult population has antibodies indicating exposure and immunity to this erythrotropic virus. Prospective studies have demonstrated a persistent 40% infection risk in untreated hemophiliacs who received virus-attenuated clotting factor concentrates. Either donor or recipient antibodies may prevent infection, however, as these antibodies are ineffective in large plasma pools and albumin preparations.

This virus is non-enveloped and hence resistant to most physico-chemical sterilization methods. Exclusion of high viral load source plasma by NAT, and subsequent novel heating methods and nano-filtration may make these transfusion products safer. Fortunately, infection in most recipients is of little consequence.

West Nile virus (see Chapter 19)

In the 2002 West Nile virus (WNV) US epidemic, 23 infections were transmitted by blood components. Predictably, outcomes were severe in the elderly and the immunocompromised. Meningoencephalitis developed in 12 patients, and several patients died. In acute infection, viremia often lasts up to 2 weeks, making transfusion-related transmission possible. Due to swift policies implemented for product quarantine and improved NAT screening, the outbreak was contained. Potential arboviral epidemics with pathogens such as dengue may be halted by similar policies.

BACTERIAL CONTAMINATION OF BLOOD PRODUCTS

This is the second most frequent cause of transfusion-related fatalities reported to the US Food and Drug Administration (FDA) (Table PP38.4). Bacterial proliferation is more efficient in platelet concentrates typically stored at room temperature for up to 5 days than in

Table PP38.4 Bacterial contaminants and associated blood products

Contaminating pathogens	Comments
Yersinia enterocolitica *Pseudomonas fluorescens* *Staphylococcus epidermidis* *Serratia liquefaciens*	Red blood cell transfusions: *Y. enterocolitica* accounts for about 75% of all reported cases of transfusion of contaminated red blood cells Siderophoric growth enhanced by storage >25 days in cold storage (4°C)
Coagulase-negative staphylococci *Salmonella choleraesuis* *Escherichia coli* *Serratia marcescens*, *S. liquefaciens* *Bacillus* spp. *Enterobacter cloacae* *Brucella*	Platelet transfusions (1 in 4200): storage at room temperature for 4–5 days enhances growth of these organisms, mostly skin saprophytes 85% of fatal reactions are caused by Gram-negative organisms; predominant mechanism is endotoxic shock Prevalence: most common bacteria are 25% coagulase-negative staphylococci, 13.5% *Salmonella* spp.
Yersinia spp.	Desferrioxamine: *Yersinia* spp. are siderophoric (iron-loving) organisms and iron uptake is essential for growth Iron overload conditions have an increased risk of invasive yersiniosis

RBCs stored for 42 days because they are refrigerated at lower temperatures. Bacteria enter blood products due to:
- inadequate disinfection during phlebotomy;
- transient bacteremia during donation;
- breaks in technique during pooling or sealing; or
- disruption of container integrity.

PARASITES

Malaria is not transmitted by RBC-free components. Interestingly, these tropical parasites remain viable both in platelet concentrates stored at room temperature and in RBCs stored at 4°C. They also survive cryopreservation and thawing. Post-transfusion incubation period is 7–50 days. Babesiosis is a malaria-like, tick-borne zoonosis (Table PP38.5). No screening test currently exists to detect asymptomatic carriers of these parasites. Donor deferral by history of residence in endemic areas prevents most transmission.

Approximately 20–25% of the US population is seropositive for *Toxoplasma gondii*, and screening for antibodies prevents transmission.

Visceral leishmaniasis is reported in 1990 Persian and 2003 Iraq war veterans. *Leishmania tropica* survives for at least 25 days in blood stored under standard conditions. Transfusion-transmitted *L. donovani* and *L. infantum* infection has been reported. Deferral policies from blood donation should prevent transmission from Gulf War veteran blood donation.

Chagas disease is widespread in Latin America. Low-level *Trypanosoma cruzi* parasitemia usually persists for life and may be transmitted by immigrants from endemic regions. Treatment is only effective during the acute stage. Of seven cases in immunocompromised patients reported in the US since 1989, five were due to platelet products. *T. cruzi* remains viable in refrigerated blood for 18 days

Table PP38.5 Parasitic diseases

Parasite	Causative organism and presenting symptoms	People at risk and risk reduction
Malaria	*Plasmodium falciparum*, *P. vivax*, *P. ovale* and *P. malariae* Chills, fever, splenomegaly, fatigue, nausea, vomiting, headache and diarrhea	Blood donation deferral of travelers, military personnel and immigrants from endemic countries
Babesiosis	*Babesia microti* in North America, *Babesia divergens* in Europe Usually asymptomatic or mild flu-like symptoms	Severe disease in the immunocompromised, asplenic patients and the elderly Risk reduced by preventive measures against tick bites during outdoor activity
Toxoplasmosis	*Toxoplasma gondii* causes transfusion-related infection, usually related to whole blood or WBC transfusion	May cause serious disease in the immunocompromised Risk reduced via serologic screening
Chagas disease	*Trypanosoma cruzi* infection causes an acute phase illness varying from no symptoms to fever, skin rash, conjunctivitis and hepatosplenomegaly A chronic phase occurs in up to 30–40% of infected patients and can be transmitted by blood donation	Screening donors by history of travel or residence, or antibody testing is not routine. Pathogen reduction with psoralens or other agents and blood filtration offer alternative approaches One-time serologic testing of donors with risk factors is a possible alternative to testing each donation

There are few reliable serologic tests for screening, and prevention is mainly based on donor deferral from endemic regions.

and for more than 8 months in citrated samples at room temperature, and survives freezing and thawing. In South America where up to 49% of recipients of parasitemic blood become infected, 3–4% of donors with risk factors (see Table PP38.5) had *T. cruzi* antibodies. A study in California reported that 1 of 340 donors had a risk factor for Chagas disease but transmission risks are unclear. The American Red Cross tested nearly 149 000 blood donations between August 2006 and January 2007, with a *T. cruzi* enzyme-linked immunosorbent assay (ELISA) system. Sixty-three specimens from 61 donors (roughly 1 in 2365 donations) were positive. Based on early study analysis, the FDA has licensed this assay in the USA for blood donor screening.

CREUTZFELDT–JAKOB DISEASE

All forms of Creutzfeldt–Jakob disease (CJD) are transmissible by transplanted organ tissues including sporadic CJD. While classic CJD may not be transmitted by transfusion, the variant from of CJD behaves differently. A bovine spongiform encephalopathy (BSE) epidemic affecting 250 000 cattle occurred in the UK between 1980 and 1996 and was passed on to 145 patients who developed vCJD by consumption of tainted beef (see Chapter 22). Fifteen of the patients had donated blood before the diagnosis; two of the 48 recipients of these blood components have developed vCJD. Conventional pathogen reduction methods do not affect the transmission of vCJD.

Following discovery of additional vCJD in continental Europe, a policy initially implemented in 1999 for deferring donors from the UK was recently revised to include donors who spent more than 5 years in Europe between 1980 and 1996.

CONCLUSIONS

The risk of transfusion-transmitted infection is at an all time low in developed nations. Newer pathogen reduction methods promise further protection at an escalating cost. Decision making regarding blood screening policies must be based on accurate estimates of the incremental safety benefit, balanced with a need for affordability. Finally, in the era of global migration, it is critical to ensure overall safety of blood products by directing resources to help developing nations establish sustainable blood collection, processing and transfusion systems.

FURTHER READING

Further reading for this chapter can be found online at http://www.expertconsult.com

Kawasaki disease

INTRODUCTION

Kawasaki disease is the most common cause of acquired heart disease in children living in the developed world. First described by Dr Tomisaku Kawasaki in Japan in 1967, the illness presents as an acute, self-limited, febrile vasculitis. It is not clear whether this entity newly emerged around the time of the initial report, or whether it was unrecognized as a distinct syndrome from common childhood febrile exanthems such as measles and scarlet fever prior to the era of vaccination and antibiotics. Although a host of potential bacterial and viral pathogens have been examined as the single causative agent for Kawasaki disease, the etiology of this important illness remains unknown.

EPIDEMIOLOGY

Kawasaki disease is a pediatric illness and over 80% of cases occur in patients under the age of 5 years, with nearly all cases occurring by the age of 8 years. The diagnosis is rare and may be delayed in older children and adults. A meta-analysis from 2005 described a total of 57 published reports of adult Kawasaki disease. Kawasaki disease has a male to female ratio of 1.5:1 and occurs in all racial and ethnic groups. Reported incidence rates vary widely from 3 per 100 000 in South America to 134 per 100 000 in Japan which reports the highest annual incidence.

After intensive search spanning four decades, a single etiology has not yet been identified as leading to Kawasaki disease, but many epidemiologic features suggest an infectious cause. The age distribution supports this hypothesis as Kawasaki disease is rare in infants under 3 months of age who might be protected by passively acquired maternal antibodies and rare in adults which suggests widespread immunity. Also, Kawasaki disease has a winter/spring seasonal predominance in temperate climates and has been associated with epidemics. The organisms listed in the differential diagnosis (Table PP39.1) are among those that have been studied as potential causative agents, but have not been found to be indisputably associated with the illness.

It is likely that a common exposure precipitates the syndrome only in genetically predisposed individuals. Whether that exposure is to a new, unidentified agent or is a response to bacterial toxins acting as superantigens continues to be widely debated. Some investigators have suggested that multiple causes may lead to the final common pathway of the clinical syndrome.

CLINICAL MANIFESTATIONS (FIG. PP39.1)

Kawasaki disease is a triphasic illness. The clinical signs and symptoms evolve over an acute febrile phase of 7–14 days then gradually spontaneously resolve even in the absence of directed therapy. Coronary artery aneurysms are the principal sequelae of the disease, and occur in 20–25% of untreated patients and in <5% of patients who receive appropriate therapy with intravenous immunoglobulin (IVIG).

There is no diagnostic test for Kawasaki disease, and diagnosis in the acute phase is based on the presence of fever for at least 5 days, and four of the five classic clinical findings. Other associated physical and laboratory characteristics may be supportive (Table PP39.2). The subacute phase occurs from about 10 to 25 days after the initial febrile period, and is marked by periungual desquamation, arthritis and thrombocytosis. The convalescent phase continues until all signs of illness have resolved and the erythrocyte sedimentation rate (ESR) has normalized, typically 6–8 weeks in total.

Adult patients with Kawasaki disease have been noted to present with similar findings, but arthralgia, lymphadenopathy and elevated liver enzymes occurred more commonly in adults, and cheilitis, meningitis and thrombocytosis were seen less often than in pediatric cases.

Not all patients present with four of the five classic features of Kawasaki disease, and these presentations are termed 'incomplete' Kawasaki disease. Incomplete presentations are most common in infants.

Table PP39.1 Differential diagnosis of Kawasaki disease	
Viruses	Measles Echovirus Adenovirus Epstein–Barr virus
Bacteria	*Staphylococcus aureus* *Streptococcus pyogenes* *Rickettsia rickettsii* *Leptospira interrogans*
Drug reactions	Serum sickness Stevens–Johnson syndrome
Rheumatologic disease	Systemic-onset juvenile idiopathic arthritis
Heavy metal toxicity	Mercury hypersensitivity (acrodynia)

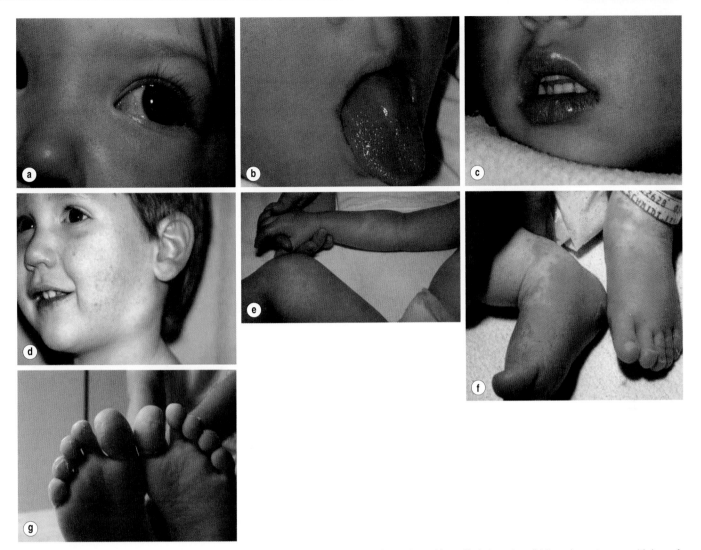

Fig. PP39.1 Features of Kawasaki syndrome. (a) Bilateral, nonexudative conjunctival injection with perilimbal sparing. (b) Strawberry tongue with loss of filiform papillae and persistence of fungiform papillae ('seeds' of strawberry). (c) Erythematous, fissured lips. (d) Unilateral enlarged left jugulodigastric nodes. (e) Erythematous rash. (f) Erythema of soles, swelling of dorsa of feet. (g) Periungual desquamation of toes in convalescent phase. Reproduced with permission from Burns & Glodé (2004). Reprinted from the Lancet. Copyright Elsevier 2004.

Although these patients do not fulfill the complete clinical criteria for the diagnosis of Kawasaki disease they do remain at risk for cardiovascular sequelae, and the syndrome must always remain a diagnostic consideration for children with prolonged, unexplained fever.

MANAGEMENT

IVIG is the mainstay of therapy, and is given as a single infusion of 2 g/kg. Aspirin is given adjunctively for its anti-inflammatory effects in the acute phase and antiplatelet effects in the subacute and convalescent phases of illness. The dosing for aspirin in the acute phase ranges from 30 to 100 mg/kg/day in four divided doses. The American Academy of Pediatrics/American Heart Association (AAP/AHA) guidelines suggest 80–100 mg/kg/day for 14 days or until the patient has been afebrile for 48–72 hours. This is followed by low-dose aspirin (3–5 mg/kg/d), typically for 6–8 weeks or until after convalescent echocardiography documents the absence of ongoing cardiac involvement and laboratory evidence of inflammation has resolved.

Despite their usefulness in other forms of vasculitis, corticosteroids have not been consistently shown to improve the outcomes of patients treated for Kawasaki disease and are not recommended as standard therapy.

There is clear evidence that delays in diagnosis and treatment contribute to the development of coronary artery aneurysms, and prompt treatment within the first 10 days of fever is recommended. In fact, United States and Japanese experts agree that treatment may commence after only 4 days of fever when the classic criteria are met. Importantly, treatment is still recommended for patients with evidence of coronary artery involvement or ongoing acute inflammation who present after 10 days of fever.

Most patients will respond with rapid clinical improvement and defervescence after IVIG infusion, but about 10% will have persistent or recrudescent fevers. These patients are at increased risk of coronary artery aneurysms. Although there is no clear evidence to establish the efficacy of further treatments, most experts recommend a second infusion of 2 g/kg IVIG for patients who remain febrile 36–48 hours after their initial infusion. Additional treatment approaches have been suggested for refractory cases including corticosteroids, plasma exchange,

Table PP39.2 Clinical and laboratory features of Kawasaki disease

Classic diagnostic criteria	Fever for at least 5 days *and* at least four of the following five physical findings: • polymorphous exanthem • conjunctival injection without exudate • oropharyngeal erythema, lips cracking, 'strawberry tongue' • extremity changes including erythema, edema and induration of hands and feet, periungual desquamation (subacute) • cervical lymphadenopathy >1.5 cm, typically unilateral
Other associated clinical findings	Cardiovascular: coronary artery ectasia or aneurysms, pericarditis, myocarditis, valvular regurgitation, aneurysms of noncoronary arteries CNS: aseptic meningitis, extreme irritability Gastrointestinal: hepatitis, diarrhea, gallbladder hydrops Genitourinary: urethritis, hydrocele Musculoskeletal: arthritis, arthralgia Dermatologic: erythema and induration at site of previous bacille Calmette–Guérin (BCG) vaccination, erythema with subsequent desquamation of groin Ocular: anterior uveitis
Associated laboratory findings	Blood findings: • elevated erythrocyte sedimentation rate, C-reactive protein • anemia (normocytic, normochromic) • leukocytosis with neutrophilia and band forms • thrombocytosis (subacute phase) • hypoalbuminemia • elevated serum transaminases Urine findings: sterile pyuria CSF findings: neutrophilic pleocytosis Synovial findings: neutrophilic leukocytosis

abciximab, infliximab, ulinastatin and cytotoxic agents, but their utility remains uncertain due to a paucity of controlled data.

LONG-TERM CARE

Cardiac follow-up for Kawasaki disease patients is individualized based on severity of coronary involvement. Coronary artery aneurysms will resolve in about 50% of patients, but functional and histologic changes in these affected segments remain. For patients with persistent aneurysms, progressive stenosis can lead to occlusion and myocardial infarction. Aneurysm rupture occurs rarely. Antithrombotic therapy is continued for patients with persistent coronary abnormalities.

It is necessary to defer any live-viral vaccines for 11 months after the infusion of IVIG, but other childhood immunizations need not be delayed.

FURTHER READING

Further reading for this chapter can be found online at http://www.expertconsult.com

Section | 4 |

Thierry Calandra & Kieren A Marr

Infections in the Immunocompromised Host

Steven M Holland
Sergio D Rosenzweig
Richard-Fabian
Schumacher
Luigi Notarangelo

Chapter | **72** |

Immunodeficiencies

INTRODUCTION

White blood cells (WBC) can be easily classified into lymphoid (T, B and natural killer (NK) cells) and myeloid (neutrophils, eosinophils, basophils and monocytes/macrophages) by virtue of their lineage-restricted progenitor's origin. Several recent, comprehensive reviews on the role of innate and adaptive immunity in host defense against microbial invasion are now available and interested readers are referred to these publications[1-3] and to Chapters 2 and 88 of this textbook. Defects in these cells lead to defects in their respective pathways of host defense, and specific and reproducible patterns of infection susceptibility. Therefore, the study of mechanisms of resistance to infection is best and most precisely approached through the study of monogenic immunodeficiencies.

MYELOID CELLS AND DEFECTS

Mature neutrophils develop in the bone marrow from a myeloid stem cell over about 14 days, but spend only 6–10 hours in the bloodstream before exiting by diapedesis to sites of inflammation. Myeloid disorders can be generally divided into those of number and those of function. Neutrophilia (>7500 neutrophils/μl in adults) is typically dependent on causes extrinsic to the neutrophils, such as acute or chronic infection, steroids and adrenaline (epinephrine). On the other hand, neutropenia (mild: <1500 neutrophils/μl, moderate: 1500–1000 neutrophils/μl, severe: <500 neutrophils/μl) can be intrinsic or extrinsic to neutrophils or their progenitors. Although neutropenia can accompany many immunodeficiencies, the most common causes are drug induced (e.g. chemotherapy, drug toxicity).

Myeloid disorders should be suspected in patients who have recurrent, severe, bacterial or fungal infections. Unusual organisms (e.g. *Burkholderia cepacia*, *Chromobacterium violaceum*) or uncommon locations (e.g. liver abscess) should always prompt questions about neutrophil integrity (Table 72.1). Severe viral and parasitic infections are not typically increased in these patients and should direct attention to disorders involving lymphocytes or monocytes. Laboratory evaluation should be guided by the clinical presentation and patterns of infection. Some assays, such as repeated WBC counts with differentials or microscopic evaluation of neutrophils, are relatively simple and can readily identify or exclude certain disorders. Assays such as oxidative burst testing, phagocytosis, chemotaxis or flow cytometry are more specialized, and few laboratories do them routinely.

SEVERE CONGENITAL NEUTROPENIA

Severe congenital neutropenia (SCN) (Online Mendelian Inheritance in Man (OMIM) #202700; see http://www.ncbi.nlm.nih.gov/omim) comprises a heterogeneous group of disorders with variable inheritance patterns that share bone marrow maturation arrest at the promyelocyte or myelocyte stage and severe chronic neutropenia (<200 neutrophils/μl). Some are associated with an increased susceptibility to acute myeloid leukemia. In 1956, Kostmann described a Swedish kindred with severe congenital neutropenia inherited in an autosomal recessive pattern.[4] However, the majority of cases of severe congenital neutropenia are sporadic or autosomal dominant due to heterozygous mutations in neutrophil elastase (*ELA2*, located at 19p13.3). Surprisingly, mutations in this same gene also cause cyclic neutropenia.[5]

The clinical manifestations of SCN appear promptly after birth: 50% are symptomatic in the first month and 90% within 6 months. Omphalitis, upper and lower respiratory tract infections, and skin and liver abscesses are common. Subcutaneous granulocyte colony-stimulating factor (G-CSF; 5μg/kg per day; range 1–120μg/kg depending on patient response) has dramatically reduced infections and hospitalizations and increased survival. Somatic mutations in the G-CSF receptor occur in some patients with elastase mutations and are associated with myeloid leukemias. The etiology of these mutations is unclear, but they are acquired and not germline. An elastase interacting protein, growth factor independent 1 (GFI-1, OMIM *600871), acts as a repressor of elastase production. Dominant GFI-1 mutations that block elastase repression are associated with neutropenia and abnormal lymphocyte function.[6]

An X-linked form of severe congenital neutropenia (XLN) due to discrete mutations in the Wiskott–Aldrich syndrome protein (WASP) has also been identified.[7]

CYCLIC NEUTROPENIA/CYCLIC HEMATOPOIESIS

Cyclic neutropenia (OMIM #162800) is an autosomal dominant disease characterized by regular cyclic fluctuations in all hematopoietic lineages, but symptoms are only due to reduced neutrophil counts. Neutrophil counts cycle about every 21 days (range 14–36 days); severe neutropenia (<200/μl) lasts 3–10 days.[5] Most patients become symptomatic in early childhood with aphthous oral ulcers, gingivitis, lymphadenopathy, pharyngitis, tonsillitis or skin lesions. Permanent teeth may be lost due to chronic gingivitis and periapical abscesses. Bone marrow aspirates during neutropenia show maturation arrest

Table 72.1 Infecting agents and myeloid defects

Disease or syndrome	Defect	Characteristic infections
Chediak–Higashi syndrome	CHS1/LYST	*Staphylococcus aureus* *Streptococcus pneumoniae* Other streptococcal infections *Haemophilus influenzae* Gram-negative rods (skin and lung)
Specific granule deficiency	cEBPe/others	*Staph. aureus* *Strep. pneumoniae* Other streptococcal infections *H. influenzae* Gram-negative rods (skin and lung)
Myeloperoxidase deficiency	MPO	*Candida* (when accompanied by diabetes mellitus)
Leukocyte adhesion deficiency 1	CD18	*Staph. aureus* *Pseudomonas aeruginosa* Gram-negative rods (skin and bowel)
Chronic granulomatous disease	NADPH oxidase	*Staph. aureus* (skin, liver, lymph nodes) *Serratia marcescens* (lung, skin, bone, sepsis) *Burkholderia cepacia* (lung, sepsis) *Chromobacterium violaceum* (skin, sepsis) *Nocardia* spp. (lung) *Aspergillus* spp. (other filamentous fungi; lung, bone)

Hyper-IgE syndrome (Job's)	STAT3	Primary pathogens:
		  S. aureus (lung and skin)
		  Strep. pneumoniae (lung)
		  H. influenzae (lung)
		  Pneumocystis jirovecii (lung)
		Secondary pathogens in lung cavities:
		  P. aeruginosa
		  Aspergillus spp.

Interferon-γ/IL-12 pathway	Multiple	Nontuberculous mycobacteria *Salmonella* spp. *Mycobacterium tuberculosis* Some DNA and RNA viruses

at the myelocyte stage or, less frequently, bone marrow hypoplasia. Granulocyte colony-stimulating factor lifts counts in cyclic neutropenia, dramatically improving quality of life and survival in these patients. Interestingly, infections and hospitalizations tend to lessen with age.

KOSTMANN SYNDROME

In 1956, Kostmann described a Swedish kindred with severe congenital neutropenia inherited in an autosomal recessive pattern.[4] Although the literature has been very confusing about whether Kostmann syndrome is caused by *ELA2*, and there has been a tendency in the past to use SCN and Kostmann syndrome interchangeably, the Kostmann gene has now been identified in the original family and in a large Kurdish cohort as being due to recessive mutations in *HAX-1* (1q21.3), the function of which is anti-apoptotic.[8]

IMMUNE-MEDIATED NEUTROPENIAS

Alloimmune neonatal neutropenia

Alloimmune neonatal neutropenia (ANN) is caused by the transplacental transfer of maternal antibodies against NA1 and NA2, two isotypes of the immunoglobulin receptor FcγRIIIb, leading to immune destruction of neonatal neutrophils.[9] This problem typically arises in otherwise normal children of apparently normal healthy mothers. The mothers do not express FcγRIIIb on their own neutrophils, leading to the elaboration of antibodies against FcγRIIIb expressed on fetal neutrophils to which the mother is sensitized during pregnancy. Antibody-coated neutrophils are phagocytosed and removed from the circulation, leading to neutropenia and infections. These antineutrophil antibodies can be detected in 1 in 500 live births and should be sought in all infants with neutropenia. Omphalitis, cellulitis and pneumonia within the first 2 weeks of life may be the presenting infections. Detection of neutrophil-specific alloantibodies in maternal serum is diagnostic. Parenteral antibiotics and G-CSF should be given; intravenous gamma globulin may not be effective in reversing ANN. With the normal waning of maternal antibody levels in the infant, ANN resolves spontaneously.

Primary autoimmune neutropenia

Primary autoimmune neutropenia (AIN) is the most common cause of chronic neutropenia (absolute neutrophil count <1500/μl lasting at least 6 months) in infancy and childhood.[10] It has a slight female preponderance and occurs in about 1:100 000 live births. Antibodies directed against different neutrophil antigens can be detected in almost all patients, almost 85% of which are IgG. Detection of granulocyte-specific antibodies may require repeated testing. Approximately one-third of these autoantibodies are directed against NA1 and NA2. Other antigens include CD11b/CD18 (Mac-1), CD32 (FcγRII) and CD35 (C3b complement receptor).

The average age at diagnosis is 8 months. The majority of patients present with skin or upper respiratory infections, but the diagnosis may be incidental, as patients may remain asymptomatic despite low neutrophil counts; severe infections are infrequent. Neutrophil counts are usually between 500 and 1500/μl at the time of diagnosis. The neutrophil count may transiently increase during severe infections and bone marrow may be normal or hypercellular. The prognosis of primary AIN is good, since it is usually self-limited. The neutropenia remits spontaneously within 7–24 months in 95% of patients, preceded by the disappearance of autoantibodies. Antibiotics for infections are usually sufficient. In severe infections or for emergency surgery G-CSF is used.

Secondary autoimmune neutropenia

Secondary AIN can be seen at any age but is more common in adults and has a more variable clinical course. Systemic lupus erythematosus, Hodgkin's disease, large granular lymphocyte proliferation or leukemia, Epstein–Barr virus (EBV) infection, cytomegalovirus (CMV) infection, HIV infection and parvovirus B19 infection have been associated with secondary AIN. Antineutrophil antibodies typically have pan-FcγRIII specificity, rather than to the FcγRIII subunits, making the resulting neutropenia more severe. Anti-CD18/11b antibodies have been detected in a subset of patients. Secondary AIN responds best to therapy directed at the underlying cause.

DEFECTS OF GRANULE FORMATION AND CONTENT

Chediak–Higashi syndrome

Neutrophil granules house critical enzymes for bacterial and fungal killing, and are mobilized to the phagosome immediately after ingestion of an invader (Fig. 72.1). This intracellular trafficking requires

molecular motors which move granules inside the cell. The Chediak–Higashi syndrome (CHS) is a rare and life-threatening autosomal recessive disease, clinically characterized by oculocutaneous albinism, frequent pyogenic infections, neurologic abnormalities and a relatively late onset lymphoma-like 'accelerated phase'.[11] Affected patients show hypopigmentation of the skin, iris and hair. The latter is light brown to blonde, with a characteristic metallic silver-gray sheen. Under light microscopy, CHS hair shafts show pathognomonic small aggregates of clumped pigment that are disorderly spaced, instead of the central shaft distribution in normals. Giant azurophilic granules form from the fusion of multiple primary granules in neutrophils, eosinophils and basophils, but enlarged cytoplasmic granules are found in all granule-containing cells. Mild neutropenia is common and due to intramedullary destruction of neutrophils.

Chediak–Higashi syndrome is due to mutations in the lysosomal trafficking regulator gene, *LYST* or *CHS1* (1q42.1–q42.2; OMIM #214500),[11] but the mechanism and pathophysiology of CHS are still elusive. Monocyte and neutrophil chemotaxis are diminished. Phagocytosis is normal or increased, but bacterial killing is delayed, probably due to low levels of primary granule enzymes. Natural killer (NK) cells show very low cytotoxicity, but neutrophil and monocyte antibody-dependent cellular cytotoxicity is intact. B-cell function is usually unaffected. Progressive degeneration of the peripheral and central nervous systems is common, with neuropathy of the legs, cranial nerve palsies, seizures, mental retardation and autonomic dysfunction.

The 'accelerated phase' is one of the main causes of death in CHS and is clinically indistinguishable from other hemophagocytic syndromes. It is characterized by fever, hepatosplenomegaly, lymphadenopathy, cytopenias, hypertriglyceridemia, hypofibrinogenemia, hemophagocytosis and tissue lymphohistiocytic infiltration. Etoposide (VP16), steroids and intrathecal methotrexate have been effective. However, without successful bone marrow transplantation, the accelerated phase usually recurs. Unfortunately, although bone marrow transplantation cures the immune defect and the accelerated phase in CHS, it does not prevent the central or peripheral neurologic problems.[12]

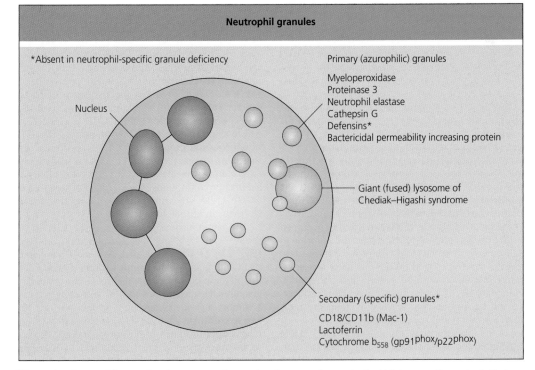

Fig. 72.1 Neutrophil granules. Neutrophils contain primary, secondary and tertiary granules, each of which has specific contents that are produced at different points in myeloid ontogeny. The larger, azurophilic primary granules contain a host of proteins, only several of which are listed here. Note that secondary granule deficiency affects both all secondary granule contents as well as the primary granule defensins. Primary granules fuse in Chediak–Higashi syndrome, along with a smaller number of secondary granules to give the characteristic cell inclusions.

Neutrophil-specific granule deficiency

The CCAAT/enhancer binding proteins (C/EBPs) are transcription factors that guide myelopoiesis and cellular differentiation. Neutrophil-specific granule deficiency (OMIM #245480) is a rare, heterogeneous, autosomal recessive disease characterized by the profound reduction or absence of neutrophil-specific granules and their contents, as well as the primary granule product, defensins. In several cases a homozygous recessive mutation was found in C/EBPε (14q11.2).[13] However, other cases do not have mutations in C/EBPε, suggesting genetic heterogeneity. These patients have markedly increased susceptibility to pyogenic infections of the skin, ears, lungs and lymph nodes. Neutrophils show bilobed nuclei (pseudo-Pelger–Huët anomaly). Electron microscopy shows absent peroxidase-negative granules in some patients and empty peroxidase-negative granules in others. Staphylococcidal activity may be reduced due to poor phagocytosis, but candidacidal activity and superoxide production are normal. Hemostatic abnormalities due to reduced levels of platelet-associated high molecular-weight von Willebrand factor and platelet fibrinogen and fibronectin, may occur.[13]

The diagnosis of specific granule deficiency is suggested by recurrent infections with Gram-positive cocci and Gram-negative rods particularly involving the skin. The peripheral smear shows large hypogranulated neutrophils and is confirmed by electron microscopy and specific granule enzyme detection by ELISA (e.g. lactoferrin or specific defensins). Eosinophils may not be detectable on routine smears because of the lack of specific granules. Management is complicated by poor inflammatory responses. Aggressive diagnosis of infections, prolonged therapy and early use of surgical excision are necessary. Bone marrow transplantation is appropriate to consider early.

DEFECTS OF OXIDATIVE METABOLISM

Chronic granulomatous disease

Nicotinamide-adenine dinucleotide diphosphate (NADPH) oxidation is the main process by which superoxide and its metabolites hydrogen peroxide and bleach are generated (Fig. 72.2). The nascent NADPH oxidase enzyme complex exists as two groups of components: a heterodimeric membrane-bound complex (cytochrome b_{558}) embedded in the walls of secondary granules and four distinct cytosolic proteins.[14] The structural components are referred to as *phox* proteins for phagocyte oxidase. Cytochrome b_{558} is composed of a 91 kDa glycosylated β chain (gp91^{phox}) and a 22 kDa nonglycosylated α chain (p22^{phox}). When bound together, these two proteins span the membrane and bind heme and flavin on the cytosolic side. The cytosol contains the structural components p47^{phox}, p67^{phox} and the regulatory components p40^{phox} and rac. On cellular activation the cytosolic components p47^{phox} and p67^{phox} are phosphorylated and bind tightly together. In association with p40^{phox} and rac, these proteins combine with the cytochrome complex (gp91^{phox} and p22^{phox}) to form the intact NADPH oxidase. Following assembly, an electron is taken from NADPH and donated to molecular oxygen, leading to the formation of superoxide. In the presence of superoxide dismutase, this is converted to hydrogen peroxide, which, in the presence of myeloperoxidase and chlorine in the neutrophil phagosome, is converted to hypochlorous acid (bleach). Phagocyte production of reactive oxygen species facilitates activation of the primary granule proteins neutrophil elastase and cathepsin G inside the phagocytic vacuole. This paradigm for NADPH oxidase-mediated microbial killing suggests that reactive oxidants are most critical as intracellular activation and signaling molecules.

Mutations in any of the four structural components of the NADPH oxidase cause chronic granulomatous disease (CGD), a disease characterized by recurrent life-threatening infections due to catalase-positive bacteria and fungi, and exuberant granuloma formation (OMIM #306400, 233690, 233700, 233710). Mutations in the X-linked gp91^{phox} account for about two-thirds of cases.[15] The rest of the cases are autosomal recessive; there are no autosomal dominant cases of

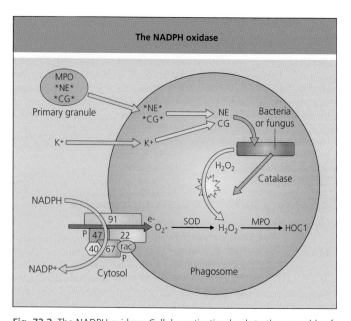

Fig. 72.2 The NADPH oxidase. Cellular activation leads to the assembly of the nascent NADPH oxidase, by joining of secondary granule membrane and cytosolic components. The generation of an intravacuolar charge is rectified by potassium influx, which in turn liberates neutrophil elastase (NE) and cathepsin G (CG) from their associated matrix (**). As classically conceived, an ingested organism is shown degrading its own hydrogen peroxide, thereby eliminating a supplement to the defective metabolic pathway in chronic granulomatous disease. However, the pathologic relevance of the role of catalase in bacterial or fungal virulence is unclear.

CGD. The frequency of CGD in the United States may be as high as 1:100 000. Clinically, CGD is quite variable with the majority of patients presenting in early childhood, but later presentations are increasingly common.[15]

The lung, skin, lymph nodes and liver are the most frequent sites of infection (see Table 72.1). In North America, the overwhelming majority of infections in CGD are due to only five organisms: *Staphylococcus aureus*, *Burkholderia cepacia*, *Serratia marcescens*, *Nocardia* and *Aspergillus* spp. In other countries *Salmonella* and bacille Calmette–Guérin (BCG) infections are also common.[16] Trimethoprim–sulfamethoxazole (TMP–SMX) prophylaxis reduces the frequency of bacterial infections in general and staphylococcal infections in particular. Staphylococcal liver abscesses encountered in CGD are dense, caseous and difficult to drain, requiring surgery in almost all cases. With the success of antibacterial prophylaxis and therapy, fungal infections, typically those due to *Aspergillus* spp., became the leading cause of mortality in CGD.[15] Itraconazole prophylaxis and other highly active oral antifungal triazole compounds have significantly reduced fungal mortality in CGD.[17] CGD is the only primary disease in which invasive aspergillosis occurs in normal lung tissue.

The granulomatous manifestations of CGD are particularly troublesome, often involving the gastrointestinal and genitourinary tracts (Fig. 72.3). Esophageal, jejunal, ileal, cecal, rectal and perirectal involvement with granulomata mimic Crohn's disease. Gastric outlet obstruction is common and can be the initial presentations of CGD.[18] Bladder granulomata, ureteral obstruction and urinary tract infection are also common. Steroid therapy (e.g. prednisone 1 mg/kg/day then tapered to a low dose on alternate days) is quite effective and surprisingly well tolerated for treatment of obstructive lesions. The frequency of relapse/recurrence of gastrointestinal granulomatous disease is high, so prolonged low-dose maintenance is often necessary. Other therapies for severe granulomatous complications include cyclosporin A and colostomy for refractory rectal disease. Several cases have been treated with infliximab. The latter therapy must be used with great caution, as infliximab increases the rates of severe fungal and bacterial infections in CGD.

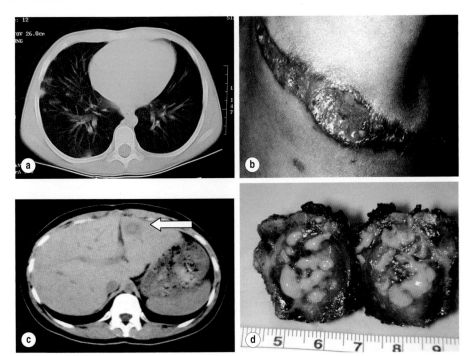

Fig. 72.3 Manifestations of chronic granulomatous disease (CGD). (a) Pneumonia due to *Aspergillus* can present subtly, both clinically and radiographically. This patient was asymptomatic but had multifocal pneumonia due to *A. fumigatus*. (b) Wound dehiscence typically presents 5–10 days postoperatively. It is an exuberant granulation tissue on biopsy and is best treated with short courses of corticosteroids. (c) Liver abscesses due to staphylococci are quite common in CGD (arrow) and typically require en bloc resection due to their dense, granulomatous nature (d).

X-linked carriers of gp91^phox have two populations of phagocytes: one that produces superoxide and one that does not, yielding a characteristic mosaic pattern on oxidative burst testing. Discoid lupus erythematosus-like lesions, aphthous ulcers and photosensitive rashes have been seen in gp91^phox carriers. Infections are not usually seen in these female carriers unless the normal neutrophils are below 5–10%, at which stage these carriers are at risk for CGD-type infections.[15]

The diagnosis of CGD is made by a measure of superoxide production. Currently, we prefer the dihydrorhodamine (DHR) assay because of its relative ease of use, its ability to distinguish X-linked from autosomal patterns of CGD on flow cytometry, and its sensitivity with low numbers of functional neutrophils.[19] Immunoblot and mutation analysis are required to identify the specific affected protein and genetic lesion, respectively. Male sex, earlier age at presentation and relatively severe disease suggest X-linked disease. Autosomal recessive forms of CGD (mostly p47^phox deficient) have a significantly better prognosis than X-linked disease. Mortality for X-linked CGD is about 5% per year, compared to 2% per year for the autosomal recessive varieties.[15] The precise gene defect should be determined in all cases, as it is critical for genetic counseling and is prognostically significant. Complete myeloperoxidase deficiency gives a DHR assay that looks like CGD, but has normal superoxide production.[20]

Prophylactic TMP–SMX (5 mg/kg per day based on TMX) reduces the frequency of major bacterial infections from about once every year to once every 3.5 years without increasing serious fungal infections in CGD. The greatest cause of mortality in CGD in developed countries remains *Aspergillus* pneumonia, but oral triazoles as prophylaxis can prevent fungal infection in CGD. A large, multicenter, placebo-controlled study showed that interferon gamma (IFN-γ) reduced the number and severity of infections in CGD by 70% compared to placebo regardless of inheritance pattern of CGD or use of prophylactic antibiotics, level of superoxide generation, bactericidal activity or cytochrome b levels.[21] Therefore, our current recommendation is to use prophylaxis with TMP–SMX, itraconazole and IFN-γ (50 μg/m²) in CGD.[22] Azole antifungals (itraconazole, voriconazole, posaconazole) are preferred to amphotericin B for the treatment of active fungal infections.

A microbiologic or histopathologic diagnosis is critical in managing complications in CGD. In severe infections, leukocyte transfusions are often used, although their efficacy is anecdotal. Bone marrow transplantation leading to stable chimerism has been successfully performed in patients with CGD.[23] Bone marrow transplantation can be successful for refractory infection, predominantly from *Aspergillus*.[24] Gene therapy for p47^phox and gp91^phox deficiencies have been successful, but not durable.[25]

Myeloperoxidase deficiency

Myeloperoxidase (MPO; 17q23) is synthesized in neutrophils and monocytes, packaged into primary granules and released either into the phagosome or the extracellular space where it catalyzes the conversion of H_2O_2 to hypochlorous acid. Myeloperoxidase deficiency (OMIM #254600) is the most common primary phagocyte disorder: 1/4000 individuals have complete MPO deficiency and 1/2000 have a partial defect.[26] It is an autosomal recessive trait with variable expressivity. Despite *in vitro* studies showing that MPO-deficient neutrophils are markedly less efficient than normal neutrophils in killing *Candida albicans* and hyphal forms of *Aspergillus fumigatus*, clinical infection in MPO deficiency is rare. Of the MPO-deficient patients who have had clinical findings, candidiasis is the most common problem, and diabetes mellitus appears to be a critical co-factor.[26] Definitive diagnosis is established by neutrophil or monocyte peroxidase histochemical staining or specific protein detection. There is no specific treatment for MPO deficiency. Dihydrorhodamine gives an abnormal signal in complete MPO deficiency.[20]

THE LEUKOCYTE ADHESION DEFICIENCIES

For over a century, leukocyte movement from the bloodstream toward inflamed sites has been recognized as critical in preventing and fighting infections. Leukocyte adhesion to the endothelium, to other leukocytes

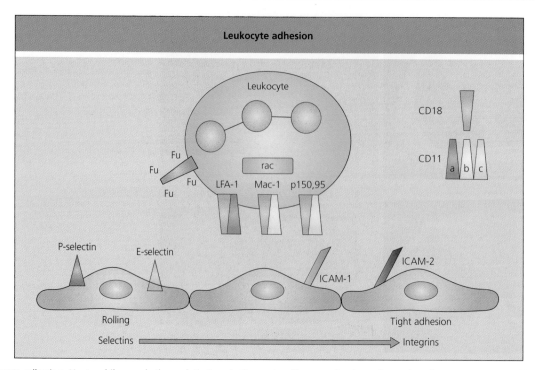

Fig. 72.4 Leukocyte adhesion. Neutrophils sample the endothelium in the postcapillary venules through a series of receptors. Depicted here are the selectin and integrin pathways, which are critical for neutrophil adhesion (monocytes and eosinophils have other ligand and receptor options). CD15s binds to selectins on the endothelium with loose adhesion, allowing closer sampling of the endothelium for tight adhesion in the setting of endothelial activation, mediated through the integrins. Neutrophil integrins bind to intercellular adhesion molecules (ICAMs).

and to bacteria is critical in the ability of leukocytes to travel, communicate, inflame and fight infection. Different families of adhesion molecules mediate these processes, critical among which are the integrins and selectins (Fig. 72.4).

Leukocyte adhesion deficiency type 1

The leukocyte β2 integrins are heterodimeric molecules on the surface of neutrophils, monocytes and lymphocytes that bind to intercellular adhesion molecules (ICAMs) on the endothelial surface in order to attach and exit the circulation.[27] ICAMs can also be expressed on other leukocytes, allowing for cell–cell adhesion. In addition, certain β2 integrins can bind directly to pathogens or to complement. Leukocyte integrins are composed of an α chain (CD11a, CD11b or CD11c), noncovalently linked to a common β2 subunit, CD18, encoded by ITGB2 on 21q22.3. The αβ heterodimers of the β2 integrin family include CD11a/CD18 (lymphocyte function associated antigen 1 (LFA-1)), CD11b/CD18 (macrophage antigen 1 (Mac-1) or complement receptor 3 (CR3)) and CD11c/CD18 (p150,95 or complement receptor 4 (CR4)). Since CD18 is required for normal expression of the αβ heterodimers, recessive mutations in CD18 lead to either very low or no expression of CD11a, CD11b and/or CD11c, with resulting inability to bind to endothelium, each other, certain pathogens or complement opsonized particles. This disease is known as leukocyte adhesion deficiency type 1 (LAD1; OMIM #116920).[27]

LAD1 has severe (less than 1% of normal expression of CD18 on neutrophils) and moderate (up to 30% of normal expression of CD18 on neutrophils) phenotypes. In addition, patients with normal cell surface expression of a nonfunctional CD18 have been described, indicating that functional assays must be performed if the clinical suspicion of LAD1 is high.

Patients with the severe phenotype of LAD1 characteristically have delayed umbilical stump separation and omphalitis, persistent leukocytosis (>15 000/μl), destructive gingivitis and periodontitis with associated loss of dentition and alveolar bone. Recurrent infections

of the skin, lung, bowel and perirectal area are common from *Staph. aureus* or Gram-negative bacilli. Necrosis and ulceration without pus accumulation or neutrophil invasion of the infected site are common (Fig. 72.5). Impaired wound healing is characteristic of LAD1: scars tend to be dystrophic and have a 'cigarette-paper' appearance. In contrast to the severe phenotype, patients with the moderate phenotype tend to be diagnosed later in life, have normal umbilical stump separation, have fewer life-threatening infections and live longer. However, leukocytosis, periodontal disease and delayed wound healing are still common. Aggressive medical management with antibiotics, and surgery when indicated, are requisite. Neutrophil transfusions may be helpful in severe cases.

Complement-mediated phagocytosis is severely impaired due to absence of CD18/CD11b (CR3/Mac-1) and antibody-dependent cell-mediated cytotoxicity (ADCC) is diminished. However, IgG-mediated phagocytosis is unaffected as is superoxide production and primary and secondary granule release. At present, bone marrow transplantation is the only definitive corrective treatment. Gene therapy of LAD1 is not yet of clinical benefit.

Other defects in leukocyte adhesion

Selectins are the molecules that mediate the loose, rolling adhesion of neutrophils along postcapillary venules.[27] Leukocyte adhesion deficiency type 2 (LAD2) is a metabolic defect now referred to as congenital disorder of glycosylation type IIc (CDG-IIc) due to recessive mutations in the GDP-fucose transporter (FUCT-1; 11p11q11; OMIM #266265).[28] This fucosylation defect is apparent on several molecules, most notably the neutrophil ligand sialyl-Lewis[x]. Patients have infections of the skin, lung and gums, leukocytosis and poor pus formation, as well as mental retardation, short stature, distinctive facies, and the Bombay (hh) blood phenotype. *In vitro*, LAD2 cells show impaired neutrophil migration, aggregation and adherence to endothelial cells. Fucose supplementation may be helpful. Infections appear to moderate with age.

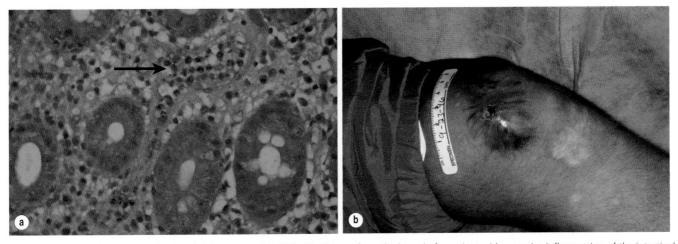

Fig. 72.5 Examples of leukocyte adhesion deficiency type 1 (LAD1). (a) A biopsy from the bowel of a patient with extensive inflammation of the intestinal ulceration. Note the abundance of neutrophils intravascularly (arrow), but the paucity of neutrophils in the parenchyma. (b) Charactristic dystrophic or 'cigarette paper' scarring following skin ulceration in a boy with LAD1.

Defects in endothelial expression of E-selectin[29] and in the Rho GTPase RAC2 (RAC2, 22q12.13–q13.2; OMIM #602049)[30,31] also lead to abnormalities in adhesion and increased infections.

INTERFERON-γ/IL-12 PATHWAY DEFECTS

The mononuclear phagocyte is critical for protection against intracellular infections. It mediates antigen presentation, lymphocyte stimulation and proliferation, and cytokine production and response. Mycobacteria infect macrophages leading to production of interleukin (IL)-12, which in turn stimulates T cells and NK cells to produce interferon gamma (IFN-γ). IFN-γ increases production of tumor necrosis factor (TNF), IL-12 and other cytokines as well as mediating mycobacterial killing, through unknown mechanisms. IFN-γ signaling depends on the signal transducer and activator of transcription 1 (STAT1), while TNF signaling depends on the nuclear factor kappa B (NF-κB) essential modulator (NEMO) (Fig. 72.6). Defects in several critical members of the pathway involving IFN-γ, IL-12, TNF and their respective receptors and signaling molecules have been clearly identified at the functional and genetic levels as being responsible for infections with mycobacteria, salmonellae and certain viruses.[32]

The IFN-γ receptor is composed of ligand binding (IFN-γR1) and signal transducing (IFN-γR2) chains. Autosomal recessive mutations in either chain that lead to abolition of IFN-γ signaling have severe infection phenotypes, predominantly with mycobacteria. Patients with complete defects present early in life, often after BCG vaccination. They have poor or absent granuloma formation (but normal tuberculin skin tests) and typically develop repeated, disseminated, life-threatening infections due to mycobacteria, salmonellae and some viruses. Mortality is overwhelmingly due to mycobacterial disease. Treatment relies upon antimicrobial agents and bone marrow transplantation if possible. Rare recessive mutations with partial function have intermediate phenotypes and more curable infections.[33]

The most common mutation in IFN-γR1 is due to a four-base deletion at or around base 818 (818del4), located just inside the intracellular domain of the molecule. This mutation allows the nonfunctional protein to remain stuck on the cell surface where it binds with the normal protein and impedes signaling[34] (Fig. 72.7). Patients with this autosomal dominant mutation in IFN-γR1 usually present in childhood with pulmonary nontuberculous mycobacterial infection and recurrent multifocal nontuberculous osteomyelitis. IFN-γ signaling persists, but at a greatly reduced level compared to normal.

IFN-γ therapy, sometimes at high dose, can be effective.[33] Long-term prophylaxis against environmental mycobacteria with a macrolide seems prudent.

Recessive mutations in IL-12p40 and IL-12 receptor β1 and dominant mutations in STAT1 are typically not as severe as complete IFN-γ receptor defects. Mutations affecting IL-12 signaling may present with more *Salmonella* infections.[35] Because these defects have preserved IFN-γR function, IFN-γ can be used therapeutically.

NUCLEAR FACTOR KAPPA B PATHWAY DEFECTS

Immune signaling through the receptors for IL-1, IL-18, TNF, CD40 and the Toll-like receptors (TLRs), as well as signaling for ectodermal (teeth, hair, sweat gland) formation converge at the activation of NF-κB, a process dependent on the proper phosphorylation and degradation of its inhibitor, IκB. The X-linked gene for the NF-κB essential modulator (NEMO) is necessary for this process. Defects in NEMO may cause ectodermal dysplasia along with a complex and overlapping set of immunodeficiencies with dysfunction in the innate TLRs, tumor necrosis factor receptor (TNFR), IL-1R and acquired (CD40, IL-18) immune systems, due to disruption of their common signaling pathway.[36] These patients typically require intravenous immune globulin, due to ineffective immunoglobulin class switching, as well as antibiotics.[37] Macrolide prophylaxis to prevent the acquisition of environmental mycobacterial infection appears prudent.

While defects in NF-κB, which is at the convergence of TLRs, lymphocyte activation and ectodermal signaling, give a complex phenotype of immune and somatic abnormalities, defects in TLR signaling give phenotypes that are exclusively immunologic. Recessive mutations in interleukin receptor 1 associated kinase 4 (IRAK-4) lead to profound susceptibility to sepsis and meningitis with encapsulated bacteria (*Streptococcus pneumoniae, Neisseria meningitidis, Haemophilus influenzae*) early in life.[38] Clinically, these patients are remarkable for a paucity of inflammatory responses despite severe infection, due to inability to transduce IL-1 and TNF signals.[39] Recessive mutations in the more proximal signaling molecule MyD88 lead to a similar phenotype.[40] While IRAK-4 and MyD88 are required for bacterial defense, recessive mutations in TLR3 and Unc-93B predispose to cases of familial herpes simplex encephalitis.[41,42]

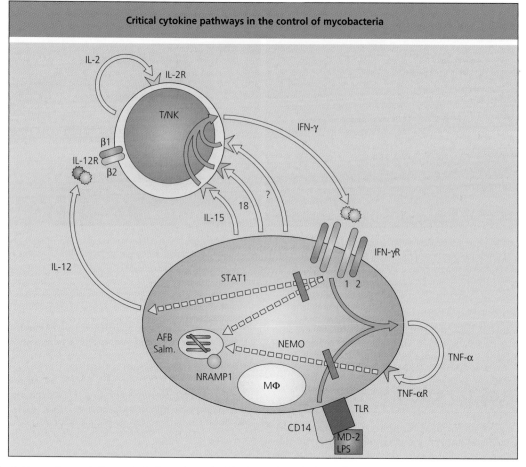

Critical cytokine pathways in the control of mycobacteria

Fig. 72.6 Critical cytokine pathways in the control of mycobacteria. Mycobacteria and salmonellae stimulate the elaboration of IL-12 by infected macrophages, leading to the production of IFN-γ by T cells and NK cells. IFN-γ in turn stimulates macrophages to produce TNF and IL-12. The critical signaling molecules STAT1 and NEMO are also indicated. IL-12 independent pathways for IFN-γ production are also indicated (IL-15, IL-18), which work in concert with IL-12 for lymphocyte stimulation. Other, as yet undefined pathways are also suggested.

HYPER-IgE RECURRENT INFECTION SYNDROME

Immune signaling for activation of the inflammatory response is highly dependent on IL-6 for its upregulation and IL-10 for its down-regulation. The shared signal molecule STAT3 mediates not only signaling for IL-6 and IL-10, but also the key mediators of inflammation IL-17, IL-21 and IL-22. Therefore, mutations in STAT3 affect a large number of pathways that both increase and diminish inflammation, as well as control the expression of epithelial defenses, and cause the hyper-IgE recurrent infection syndrome (HIES; Job's syndrome).[43] It is an autosomal dominant disorder characterized by recurrent infections, typically of the lower respiratory system and skin, eczema, extremely elevated levels of IgE, eosinophilia, and abnormalities of the connective tissue, skeleton and dentition[44] (Fig. 72.8). The majority of patients have characteristic facial abnormalities including a broad, somewhat bulbous nose. Failure of primary dental deciduation, leading either to failure of secondary dentition eruption or retention of both sets of teeth is common. Many patients also have abnormalities of bone formation and metabolism, which may result in fractures, scoliosis, kyphosis and osteoporosis. HIES occurs spontaneously in all racial and ethnic groups.

IgE is greatly elevated at some point in the life of all patients with HIES, but about 20% have been observed to drop their IgE levels below 2000 IU/ml as they get older while retaining their susceptibility to infection.[44] The clinical manifestations of HIES are quite distinct (Table 72.2). Eczema usually presents within the first days to months of life. Other early signs include mucocutaneous candidiasis and severe diaper rash. Sinus or pulmonary infections, predominantly with *Staph. aureus* or *H. influenzae*, are common, as are postinflammatory pneumatoceles. Otitis media and externa are common. Other pathogens that have been recovered include *Aspergillus* spp., *Pseudomonas aeruginosa*, *Strep. pneumoniae*, group A streptococci, *Cryptococcus neoformans*, *Pneumocystis jirovecii* and *C. albicans*. Mucocutaneous candidiasis involving the mouth, vagina, intertriginous areas, fingernails and toenails affects about 50% of HIES patients. Bony abnormalities are frequent, as are pathologic fractures. IL-17, a critical proinflammatory cytokine made by CD4 T cells is STAT3 dependent, so is not produced in HIES.[45]

High-dose intravenous antibiotics for a prolonged course are required for eradication of infection and to prevent bronchopleural fistula formation and bronchiectasis. Empiric coverage should consider *Staph. aureus*, *H. influenzae* and *Strep. pneumoniae*. Infection of pneumatoceles and bronchiectatic lung with *P. aeruginosa* and *Aspergillus* spp. is especially problematic. Most experts use prophylactic antibiotics (e.g. TMP–SMX) to cover *Staph. aureus*.

LYMPHOCYTE IMMUNE DEFICIENCIES

Lymphocyte immune deficiencies have provided the paradigms for understanding immunology, tolerance and transplantation for decades. The nomenclature is dense and confusing because diseases originally

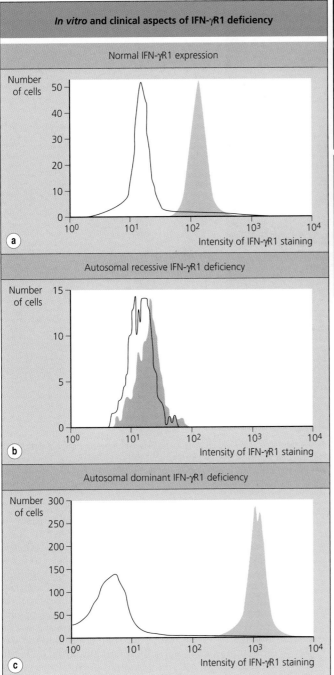

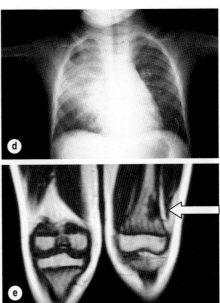

Fig. 72.7 *In vitro* and clinical aspects of IFN-γR1 deficiency. (a–c) Flow cytometry for the IFN-γR1 on peripheral blood monocytes. Dotted lines indicate the background fluorescence of the sample with an irrelevant antibody. (a) Normal IFN-γR1 fluorescence intensity. (b) Monocytes from a child with complete IFN-γR1 deficiency. Note the lack of specific staining for IFN-γR1. (c) Increased intensity of IFN-γR1 staining on monocytes from a patient who has MAC osteomyelitis. (d) Chest radiograph from the same patient showing extensive right lung infection with MAC. (e) The corresponding MRI of his distal femur (arrow indicates the infected lesion).

described phenotypically have turned out to be due to numerous separate genetic defects (e.g. interleukin 2 receptor common gamma chain, JAK3, interleukin 7 receptor alpha chain).[46] The confused terminology is unavoidable as the clinical syndrome is described first, followed by detailed genetics. The application of DNA diagnostics has demonstrated that defects in one gene may result in several different phenotypes (phenotypic heterogeneity) and that the same phenotype can be caused by different gene defects (genetic heterogeneity). Therefore, both syndromic and molecular diagnoses should be pursued in all cases.

DNA cleavage, polymerization and repair resulting in recombination are critical for lymphocyte diversity and antigen specificity.[47] Therefore, defects that affect lymphoid ligand binding, signaling or any of the steps of successful DNA recombination may present as defects in acquired immunity.

When considering the diagnosis of severe combined immunodeficiency (SCID), it is important to keep several things in mind:

- SCID is a medical emergency. If the patient with SCID is to survive transplantation, it is important to avoid community viral infections, which can be devastating.

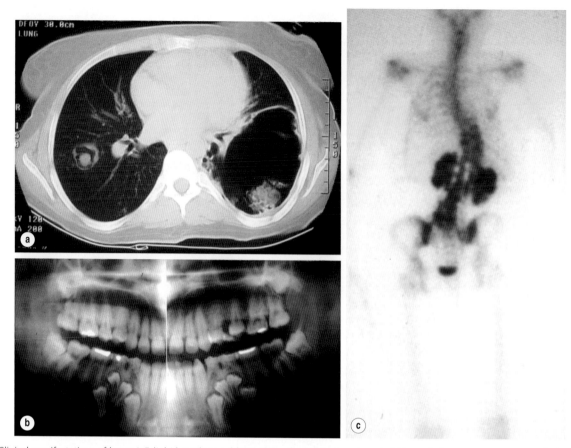

Fig. 72.8 Clinical manifestations of hyper-IgE (Job's) syndrome. (a) CT of the chest showing characteristic postinflammatory pneumatocele formation. Note the development of bilateral aspergillomata with inflammation of the cavity walls. (b) Panoramic radiograph of the dentition of a 33-year-old woman with HIES shows the characteristic retention of primary teeth due to failure of deciduation of the retained primary teeth. (c) Extensive scoliosis is demonstrated in this radionuclide bone scan in a 25-year-old woman with HIES. A list of some of the characteristic features of the syndrome is included in Table 72.2.

Table 72.2 Features of hyper-IgE syndrome	
Feature	**%**
Eczema	100
Characteristic facies (>16 years)	100
Skin boils	87
Pneumonias	87
Mucocutaneous candidiasis	83
Lung cysts	77
Scoliosis (>16 years)	76
Delayed dental deciduation	72
Pathologic fractures	57

- Persistent maternal engraftment is both a sign of SCID and a cause of many of the symptoms, such as failure to thrive and rash.
- The phenotype of infections and clinical illness are the presentation of the patient; laboratory tests are efforts to confirm the genetics.
- Missense mutations may produce proteins that are still present in normal amount but nonfunctional.

Therefore, the clinical scenario, typically developed out of the infection profile and laboratory studies, must be used to guide decisions about which genes to sequence.[48]

T lymphocytes are not only crucial for resistance to intracellular pathogens, but also interact with B lymphocytes and antigen-presenting cells. Consequently, defects in T-cell development or function result in combined immune deficiencies. The forms with the most severe T-cell depletion are medical emergencies that lead to increased susceptibility to severe infections from birth. Failure to thrive, chronic diarrhea and interstitial pneumonia (due to opportunistic infections, such as *Pneumocystis jirovecii* or viruses) are typical (Fig. 72.9). The overall frequency of SCID is estimated to be about 1 in 50 000 live births. Lymphopenia in the setting of severe infection in an infant should raise suspicion. Quantification of the absolute CD3+ cell count, analysis of HLA-DR expression and T-cell activation allow identification of almost 98% of all SCID babies (Fig. 72.10).

Vaccination with live attenuated viruses or BCG may lead to fatal disseminated infection (Fig. 72.11). Graft-versus-host disease (GvHD), due to transplacental passage of alloreactive maternal T lymphocytes or transfusion of unirradiated blood products, can cause skin rash, diarrhea, hepatitis or bone marrow failure. Untreated, patients with SCID die within the first years of life. Prophylactic TMP–SMX (to prevent *Pneumocystis jirovecii* pneumonia) and aciclovir (for herpes viruses), immunoglobulin replacement therapy and aggressive treatment of all infections prolongs survival, but only early allogeneic bone marrow transplantation or (in selected cases) gene therapy or enzyme replacement therapy offers a chance for cure.

In recent years molecular diagnosis has been achieved for most immune deficiencies (Fig. 72.12) and mutation databases have been established that are constantly updated and accessible via the world wide web.

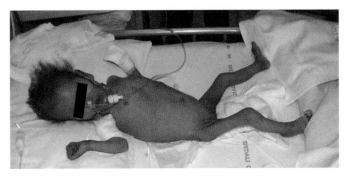

Fig. 72.9 Typical severe combined immunodeficiency baby. Note the wasting and malnutrition.

Severe combined immunodeficiency

In typical SCID, severe intestinal infections with malabsorption and failure to thrive are prominent. The intestinal mucosa shows variable degrees of villous atrophy. The most frequently isolated pathogens include *Campylobacter*, *Salmonella*, *Shigella*, *Cryptosporidium parvum* and *Giardia lamblia*. The liver is often involved, ranging from hepatomegaly with elevated transaminases, to sclerosing cholangitis due to *Cryptosporidium parvum*. CNS involvement can also occur, mostly due to viral infections (herpes simplex virus, enteroviruses and adenoviruses). SCID has been classically defined by the numbers of T cells, B cells and NK cells. The advantage to this system is that with one simple flow cytometric study one can determine which pathways are most likely to be affected. The nomenclature for SCID is complex at a cellular, genetic and molecular level but has important implications for prenatal and carrier testing, transplant success and genetic correction.

X-linked SCID, γc deficiency (T⁻B⁺NK⁻)

The most common SCID phenotype is absence of mature T and NK lymphocytes in the blood and peripheral lymphoid organs, with a normal to increased number of B cells (T⁻B⁺ SCID).[48] Most com-

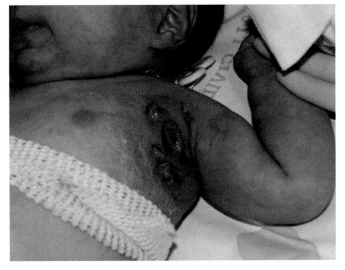

Fig. 72.11 Axillary BCGitis in a T⁻B⁺ severe combined immunodeficiency baby with generalized BCG infection. Note the extensive cutaneous ulceration.

monly, this disease is inherited as an X-linked trait (SCID-X1, OMIM #300400). SCID-X1 has an estimated incidence between 1:150 000 and 1:200 000 live births and accounts for 35–40% of all cases of SCID. It is caused by mutations in the *IL2RG* gene which encodes the chain of the IL-2 receptor that is common to multiple other cytokine receptors as well, hence its designation as the common gamma chain (γc). Located at Xq13, this cytokine receptor subunit is shared by the receptors for IL-2, IL-4, IL-7, IL-9, IL-15 and IL-21 and is therefore involved in the growth and maturation of T, B and NK cells[49] (Fig. 72.13). Since these cytokine receptors lack intrinsic catalytic activity, they partner with an intracellular signal transducer, JAK3, a member of the Janus associated kinase (JAK) family of protein tyrosine kinases. Therefore, absence of γc leads to marked impairment of signaling for multiple cytokines.

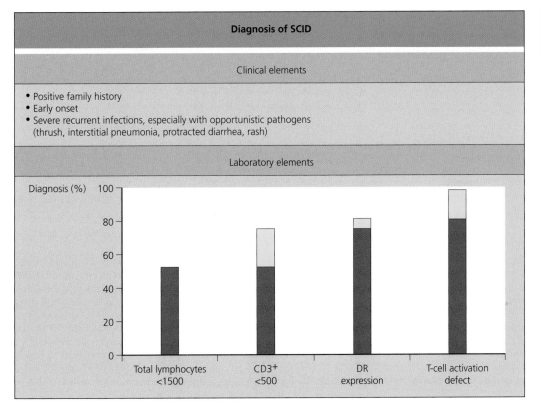

Diagnosis of SCID
Clinical elements
• Positive family history • Early onset • Severe recurrent infections, especially with opportunistic pathogens (thrush, interstitial pneumonia, protracted diarrhea, rash)
Laboratory elements

Diagnosis (%) — bar chart with categories: Total lymphocytes <1500; CD3⁺ <500; DR expression; T-cell activation defect

Fig. 72.10 Clinical and laboratory elements useful in the diagnosis of severe combined immunodeficiency.

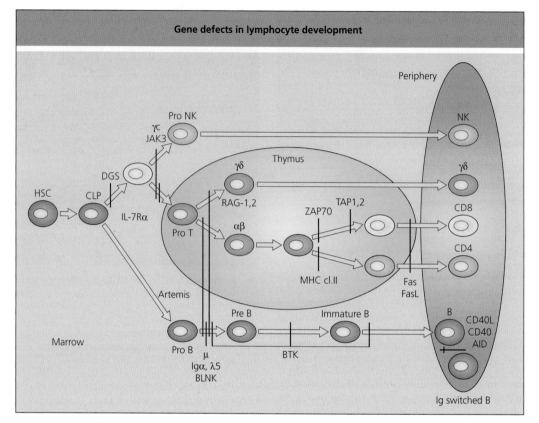

Fig. 72.12 Model of lymphocyte development with the relative gene defects that may lead to immune deficiencies shown in red (for details see text).

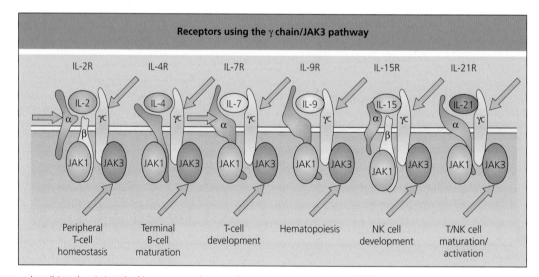

Fig. 72.13 Diagram describing the six interleukin receptors that use the common gamma-chain/JAK3 pathway for signaling.

As in all forms of SCID, clinical onset of SCID-X1 is usually within the first few months of life with persistent diarrhea, pneumonia, failure to thrive and severe or persistent candidiasis. The diagnosis is usually suspected because of lymphopenia, with low to absent T and NK cells and normal to elevated B cells. Mitogen-induced proliferation is virtually absent and serum immunoglobulin levels are low to undetectable. Serum IgG may initially be normal due to persistence of transplacentally passed maternal antibodies. The thymus lacks a clear cortical–medullary demarcation, Hassall's corpuscles are absent, and in general there is a severe depletion of lymphoid tissues with absent lymph nodes.

The diagnosis can be made by flow cytometry for γc expression on the surface of lymphocytes or monocytes. However, some *IL2RG* gene mutations allow expression of nonfunctional γc on the cell surface. Therefore, normal γc expression does not rule out a diagnosis of SCID-X1. Further complicating matters, engraftment of maternal T cells (observed in as many as 50% of cases of SCID) may lead to an atypical immunologic phenotype, representing a diagnostic challenge. HLA typing and molecular analysis at highly polymorphic DNA loci can identify the presence of maternal T cells. Other forms of SCID may present with the same cellular phenotype (T⁻B⁺ SCID) and should be considered if γc expression is normal. Detection of a mutation in *IL2RG*, most often inherited from the mother, confirms the diagnosis. Mutations found in different families are listed at http://www.nhgri.nih.gov/DIR/GMBB/SCID/IL2RGbase.html.

The standard treatment for SCID-X1 is allogeneic human stem cell (usually bone marrow) transplantation (BMT), with success rates near 100% when an HLA-identical sibling is used as donor.[50] Excellent results are also achieved with BMT from matched unrelated donors, but since early treatment is crucial and the search for a compatible donor often takes several months without a guarantee of finding one, haploidentical family donors have been increasingly used.[50] GvHD prevention by elimination of T-cells from the donor marrow or the use of positively selected peripheral blood stem cells after mobilization is crucial to successful HLA-mismatched transplantation and is now successful in as many as 70–80% of patients. Even in the absence of myeloablation, engraftment of donor T (and often NK) cells is easily achieved. In contrast, engraftment of donor-derived B cells is facilitated by chemotherapy or irradiation conditioning of the recipient. When functional B-cell deficiency persists in patients without donor B-cell engraftment, regular intraveous immunoglobulin substitution is required. In utero stem cell transplantation has been successfully performed in affected fetuses with good clinical and laboratory T-cell reconstitution.[51]

Because functional γc expression provides a strong proliferative advantage to lymphocyte precursors, SCID-X1 is an ideal model for gene therapy. A number of patients have been successfully treated and have achieved normal T- and NK-cell counts and function after retroviral-mediated γc gene transfer into autologous CD34+ bone marrow cells.[52] However, the development of leukemias due to gene insertion in some of the recipients has raised concern about the safety of gene therapy.[53]

JAK3 deficiency (T⁻B⁺NK⁻)

Similar to the case with other transmembrane receptors, γc signals through an intracellular cascade including JAK3 and STAT5 molecules (Fig. 72.14). After the X-linked form, autosomal recessive *JAK3* mutations are the second most common form of T⁻B⁺ SCID (JAK3 deficiency, 19p12–13.1, OMIM #600173).[54] Because γc and JAK3 are linked components in the same signaling pathway, JAK3 deficiency is clinically and immunologically similar to SCID-X1. Diagnosis of JAK3 deficiency is established by immunoblot for JAK3 in patient lymphocytes or cell lines and/or demonstration of *JAK3* gene mutations. Since JAK3 deficiency is compatible with the presence of significant numbers of circulating, although poorly functioning, T lymphocytes, JAK3 deficiency should be considered in all undefined cases of combined immune deficiency, especially those presenting with a high proportion of peripheral B lymphocytes. Prenatal diagnosis based on DNA analysis of chorionic villus biopsies has been performed. As is the case for SCID-X1, definitive treatment of JAK3-deficient SCID is allogeneic BMT. *JAK3* gene transfer into hematopoietic stem cells in *jak3* knockout mice has been successful, indicating the possibility for *JAK3* gene therapy in humans. The mutations in JAK3 are listed at http://bioinf.uta.fi/JAK3base.

IL-7Rα (CD127) deficiency (T⁻B⁺NK⁺)

Interleukin-7 is produced by stromal cells in the bone marrow and the thymus and provides survival and proliferative signals to IL-7 receptor bearing (IL-7R⁺) cells. The IL-7 receptor consists of two subunits, the γc chain and the IL-7Rα chain, which maps to chromosome 5p13. IL-7Rα is specific for the IL-7R, is expressed by lymphoid precursor cells and is essential for differentiation of early thymocytes. Consequently, mutations that impair expression of IL-7Rα result in an early block in T-cell development, leading to SCID with absent T cells but normal to elevated B cells.[55] NK cells are preserved due to

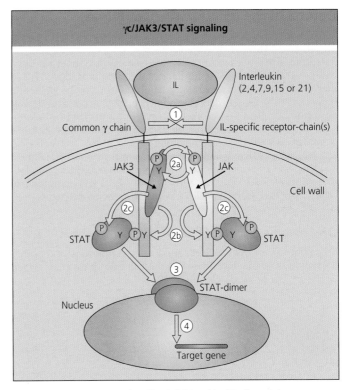

Fig. 72.14 γc/JAK3/STAT signaling is initiated by binding of the cytokine to its receptor. Heterodimerization (1) of the receptor chains (one interleukin-specific chain and the γc) allows for reciprocal tyrosine phosphorylation (2a) of JAK3 and other JAK molecules leading to their activation. Activated JAKs then phosphorylate (2b) tyrosine residues on both receptor subunits creating docking sites for the STATs. These signaling elements are themselves tyrosine phosphorylated by the JAKs (2c) in order to dimerize and translocate to the nucleus (3), where they bind to consensus sequences within regulatory regions of cytokine-inducible genes, and act as transcription factors driving transcription of the target genes.

retained IL-15 signaling. The diagnosis is suggested by flow cytometry for CD127 on T, B, NK cells or macrophages, and confirmed by mutation detection. The clinical picture is similar to other forms of SCID. Allogeneic stem cell transplantation is the only curative treatment.

IL-2Rα (CD25) deficiency (T⁻B⁺NK⁺)

IL-2Rα (CD25) is a low affinity IL-2 receptor and another member of the complete IL-2 receptor complex required for IL-2-mediated signaling and peripheral T-cell homeostasis. Therefore, the defect caused by loss of IL-2α is relatively limited to T lymphocytes, leaving a normal number of B and NK cells[56] (OMIM *147730). This also makes for persistent lymphadenopathy and abnormal apoptosis. Unlike the case for γc and JAK3 defects, CD25 deficiency has significant autoimmunity. These patients can have a progressive lymphoproliferative syndrome reflecting disturbed peripheral immune homeostasis.

CD45 deficiency (T⁻B⁺NK⁻)

CD45 is a protein tyrosine phosphatase, also known as the leukocyte common antigen since it is expressed on all nucleated hematopoietic cells, and makes up to 10% of the cell surface area of T and B cells. Not only does it govern T-cell receptor (TCR) signaling through regulation of the Src family kinases p56lck and p59fyn, it also downregulates integrin-mediated adhesion and dephosphorylates JAK kinase complexes. The immunologic phenotype is one of complete lack of T cells, with normal to increased B-cell counts.[57]

Defects of the p56lck/ZAP-70 pathway

Stimulation of T cells through the CD3/T-cell receptor (CD3/TCR) complex (Fig. 72.15) results in a complex series of activations focusing on p56lck, an Src tyrosine kinase, immunoreceptor tyrosine-based activation motifs (ITAMs) and ZAP-70, an intracellular tyrosine kinase.[58] ZAP-70 itself becomes phosphorylated by Src family protein tyrosine kinases. In humans, ZAP-70 is required for development of CD8+ T cells in the thymus and peripheral blood T-cell proliferation in response to mitogens and antigens. Defective expression of p56lck leads to hypogammaglobulinemia, lymphopenia with a reduced proportion of CD4+ T cells, and reduced *in vitro* proliferation. Defects in ZAP-70 result in impaired T-cell development and function.[58,59] Infants with ZAP-70 deficiency present with typical clinical features of SCID, virtual absence of CD8+ T cells, and nonfunctional CD4+ T lymphocytes. Both p56lck and ZAP-70 are autosomal recessive.

DNA repair defects (T⁻B⁻ SCID)

Recombination of DNA in T cells and B cells is required for the generation of the immune diversity that is the hallmark of the mammalian immune system.[60] This process requires specific gene products that cut and recombine DNA as well as specific sites to be acted upon. The genes that control these processes are responsible for phenotypes of SCID causing complete absence of both T and B lymphocytes in the periphery. The majority of these patients have a defect in the recombination process.[61] To recognize foreign antigens, B and T cells use specialized receptors: the immunoglobulin (Ig) and the TCR, respectively. These are characterized by highly polymorphic antigen-recognition sites, which are the coding products of variable (V), diversity (D) and joining (J) gene segments that undergo somatic rearrangement due to a mechanism known as V(D)J recombination.[60] V(D)J recombination is crucial for the differentiation of T and B lymphocytes and is triggered by the lymphocyte-specific proteins recombinase activating genes (RAG)1 and RAG2. These gene products act together to recognize specific recombination signal sequences (RSS) that flank each of the V, D and J gene elements in the Ig and TCR genes and break the DNA double strand there. Several ubiquitously expressed DNA repair proteins (including Ku70, Ku80, DNA-PKcs, XRCC4, DNA ligase I and IV, and Artemis – the last involved in another form of SCID) then mediate the final steps of the V(D)J recombination process.

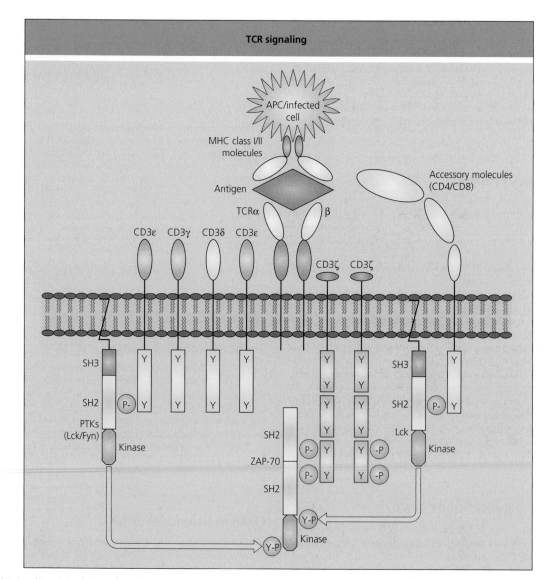

Fig. 72.15 TCR signaling. Stimulation of T cells through the CD3/T-cell receptor (CD3/TCR) complex results in activation of p56lck, an Src tyrosine kinase, that mediates tyrosine phosphorylation of immunoreceptor tyrosine-based activation motifs (ITAMs) in the CD3-γ, -δ, -ε and -ζ chains. ZAP-70, an intracellular tyrosine kinase, is then recruited into the CD3/TCR complex through binding of its SH2 domains to phosphorylated ITAMs of the ζ chain. ZAP-70 itself becomes phosphorylated by Src family protein tyrosine kinases. Phosphorylation triggers ZAP-70 activation, allowing phosphorylation of downstream signaling molecules such as linker for activation of T cells (LAT) and SLP-76.

Complete RAG1/RAG2 deficiency (T⁻B⁻NK⁺)

The clinical presentation of complete RAG-deficient SCID (11p13, OMIM #601457) is very similar to the other autosomal recessive forms of SCID with early onset severe respiratory infections, chronic diarrhea leading to failure to thrive, and persistent candidiasis.[61] Frequent transplacental passage of maternal T lymphocytes leads to cutaneous manifestations suggestive of GvHD. The immunologic phenotype is characterized by severe lymphopenia, with virtual absence of T and B lymphocytes. Almost all autologous circulating lymphocytes are NK cells, since they do not require any DNA rearrangement. No specific immunoglobulins can be produced. Curative treatment is bone marrow transplantation.

Omenn syndrome (T⁺B⁻NK⁺)

Omenn syndrome (OS, OMIM #603554) affects infants of both sexes who present with a prominent, generalized papular skin eruption or scaling exudative erythroderma, alopecia, enlarged lymph nodes, hepatosplenomegaly, hypoproteinemia with edema, and eosinophilia, associated with severe respiratory infections, chronic diarrhea and failure to thrive[62] (Fig. 72.16). It is an important example of genotype–phenotype correlation in immune function, since this syndrome is clinically distinct from complete RAG1/2 deficiency, but is due to 'leaky' mutations in *RAG1/RAG2*. This clinical phenotype may mimic histiocytosis X of the Letterer–Siwe type, or GvHD, and may occasionally be seen in SCID infants with transplacental passage of alloreactive maternal T cells (referred to as Omenn-like syndrome).

The molecular pathogenesis of OS long remained a mystery. However, the demonstration of a variable number of autologous, oligoclonal, autoreactive, activated T cells in OS infants, and the simultaneous occurrence of OS and T⁻B⁻ SCID in two siblings suggested a genetic relationship. This hypothesis was proven when mutations in *RAG1* and *RAG2* were demonstrated in OS patients.[63] In contrast to T⁻B⁻ SCID, each patient carried at least one mutant allele that allowed expression of a partially functioning RAG protein resulting in a leaky V(D)J rearrangement defect, with reduced, but not abolished, intrathymic T-cell differentiation.

In contrast to other forms of SCID, OS may have leukocytosis with marked eosinophilia and variable (up to normal) T-cell counts. A characteristic finding in OS is the coexpression of activation/memory markers (HLA-DR, CD45RO, CD25, CD95, CD30) on the surface of T lymphocytes, which predominantly secrete T helper (Th)2-type cytokines, such as IL-4 and IL-5. B lymphocytes are typically absent

from peripheral blood and lymphoid tissues and immunoglobulin levels are markedly diminished, but IgE is usually elevated. Lymph nodes show lymphoid depletion and an increased proportion of interdigitating reticulum cells, eosinophils and histiocytes. Thymus shows lymphoid depletion, lack of corticomedullary demarcation and lack of AIRE staining, a critical protein for the induction of self-tolerance.[64]

OS is diagnosed by its characteristic features after engraftment of allogeneic T cells has been excluded. Mutation analysis of *RAG1* and *RAG2* confirms the diagnosis and can be used for prenatal diagnosis in affected families. Interferon gamma may reduce the Th2-type T-cell activity and ameliorate the clinical status, but unless treated by BMT, OS is usually fatal within the first year of life. Steroids and cyclosporin A may be used for treatment of the GvHD-like skin reaction.

Radiation-sensitive SCID (Artemis deficiency; T⁻B⁻NK⁺)

Mutations in the RAG genes do not account for all V(D)J recombination defects in T⁻B⁻ SCID patients. A subgroup of patients also show increased cellular radiosensitivity (even in nonlymphoid lineages) due to mutations in *Artemis* (10p, OMIM #602450) that participates in the later phases of V(D)J recombination.[65] This latter form of T⁻B⁻ SCID is relatively common among Athabascan-speaking Native Americans (e.g. Navajo), among whom the incidence is estimated to be approximately 1 in 2000 live births. The encoded protein seems to be involved in the opening of the hairpin necessary to join the selected V(D)J regions. To date, *Artemis* mutations have been severe, resulting in a complete T⁻B⁻ SCID phenotype. However, hypomorphic mutations have been associated with an Omenn-like phenotype and others with lymphomas.[66]

DNA ligase IV deficiency (OMIM #606593) also leads to defects in DNA recombination and radiation sensitivity, known as the LIG4 syndrome.[67] Patients also have developmental delay and chromosomal instability.

Purine metabolic defects

Adenosine deaminase (ADA) and purine nucleotide phosphorylase (PNP) work in series to handle the products of purine metabolism. ADA is ubiquitously expressed and transforms adenosine into inosine and deoxyadenosine to deoxyinosine. PNP then converts inosine and deoxyinosine to hypoxanthine, which can either enter the purine salvage pathway or be excreted as uric acid.

Adenosine deaminase deficiency (T⁻B⁻NK⁻)

Adenosine deaminase (ADA) deficiency (20q13, OMIM *102700) is autosomal recessive and has a highly variable disease presentation depending on the degree of residual ADA activity.[68] Complete ADA deficiency presents early in life, with low enzyme activity, high accumulated adenosine levels, marked panlymphopenia without significant lymphoid tissues, and only maternally transferred IgG. SCID-type infections are common. Partial ADA defects may result in less severe clinical presentations with delayed (in infancy) or late (during adolescence or even adulthood) onset. Since the enzyme is ubiquitously expressed, nonhematopoietic organs such as kidney, bone, cartilage and the central nervous system may also be involved. Half of cases have characteristic bony abnormalities including flared, cupped costochondral junctions, best seen on lateral films, leading to a 'rachitic rosary' (bony prominences at the costochondral junctions, reminiscent of the beads of a rosary), similar to that seen in rickets.

Optimal treatment is BMT from an HLA-identical family donor. When this is not available, enzyme substitution treatment with pegylated bovine ADA (PEG-ADA) results in effective and sustained reduction of toxic metabolite levels and immune reconstitution.[69] *ADA* was the first SCID-causing gene to be cloned and ADA deficiency was the

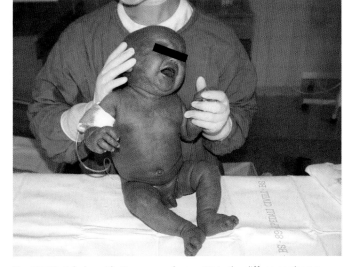

Fig. 72.16 A baby with Omenn syndrome. Note the diffuse erythema.

first human disease to be treated with gene therapy, although it was not curative.[70] Significant improvements in vector design, cell targeting and recipient preparation have resulted in improved outcome of gene therapy for ADA deficiency.[71]

Purine nucleoside phosphorylase deficiency

Purine nucleoside phosphorylase (PNP) works downstream of ADA to convert guanosine to guanine and deoxyguanosine to deoxyguanine. PNP deficiency (14q13, OMIM +164050) is an autosomal recessive disease characterized by the accumulation of deoxyguanosine and guanosine (dGTP in particular) that are directly toxic to lymphocytes. The accumulation of these metabolites inhibits ribonucleotide reductase, whose activity is essential to DNA synthesis. Although PNP is widely expressed, its deficiency is particularly deleterious to lymphoid development, especially T cells. Consequently, patients with PNP deficiency experience a dramatic and progressive T-cell lymphopenia during the first years of life, leading to a SCID phenotype.[72] Toxicities of the metabolites also involve the CNS, with symptoms ranging from behavioral problems, low cognitive function, to ataxia or tetraparesis. BMT is the only therapeutic option, since enzyme replacement therapy is not yet available.

DEFECTS IN ANTIGEN PRESENTATION

Major histocompatibility complex class II deficiency

T cells recognize foreign antigens in the context of self-MHC class II molecules expressed by antigen-presenting cells. MHC class II molecules are critical for numerous aspects of immune function, including antibody production, T-cell-mediated immunity, induction of tolerance and inflammatory responses. Therefore, MHC class II deficiency leads to an inability of T cells to recognize foreign antigens that would normally be presented by MHC class II molecules and a combined humoral and cellular immune deficiency. This autosomal recessive immunodeficiency (OMIM #209920), also referred to as the bare lymphocyte syndrome type II (BLS II), is genetically heterogeneous and may be due to mutations in any of four components of transcription factors that control MHC class II gene expression: class II transactivator (CIITA), RFXANK/RFX-B, RFX5 and RFXAP.[73] The hallmark of MHC class II deficiency is the absence of HLA-DR, -DQ and -DP molecules on B cells, monocytes and dendritic cells (which constitutively express HLA class II), and IFN-γ activated cells. CD4$^+$ T-cell counts are low, whereas CD8$^+$ T-cell counts are normal to increased. *In vitro* response to mitogens is often reduced and immunoglobulin levels are low. In the absence of allogeneic BMT, patients generally die between 5 and 18 years. A moderate phenotype has also been described with survival into adulthood.[74]

TAP deficiency

HLA class I molecules are polymorphic cell surface glycoproteins that play an essential role in presenting antigenic peptides to cytotoxic T lymphocytes and in modulating the activity of NK cells that bear HLA class I-binding receptors. HLA class I molecules are composed of a polymorphic heavy chain, encoded by *HLA-A*, *HLA-B* and *HLA-C* genes, associated with the invariant β_2-microglobulin (β_2M). The assembly of HLA class I molecules occurs in the lumen of the endoplasmic reticulum (ER), where they are loaded with peptides derived from the degradation of intracellular organisms or proteins. These peptides are transported into the ER via transporter-associated-with-antigen presentation (TAP) proteins.[75] The TAP complex consists of two structurally related subunits (TAP1 and TAP2), which interact to form a functional peptide transporter system. Defects in either TAP1 or TAP2 result in impaired peptide-HLA class I/β_2M complex formation and cause reduced surface expression of HLA class I molecules.

Patients with defective HLA class I molecule expression due to defects in either TAP1[75] or TAP2[76] have a far less severe clinical phenotype than observed in MHC class II expression. They often have nasal polyposis and bronchiectasis with recurrent sinopulmonary infections caused by *H. influenzae*, *Strep. pneumoniae*, *Staph. aureus*, *Klebsiella* and *P. aeruginosa*. Deep skin ulcers may also occur. The diagnosis is made by demonstration of profoundly low expression of HLA class I molecules on mononuclear cells.

IMMUNE DEFECTS WITH PREDOMINANT IMMUNOGLOBULIN DEFICIENCY

B-cell differentiation is a multistage process regulated by transcription factors which orchestrate a complex scheme of gene activation resulting in specific intracytoplasmic and membrane-bound proteins. While B-cell differentiation in the bone marrow is antigen independent, later stages of B-cell development in the periphery depend upon contact between the B cell and its cognate antigen (Fig. 72.17).

X-linked agammaglobulinemia (T$^+$B$^-$NK$^+$)

X-linked agammaglobulinemia (XLA), the prototype humoral immunodeficiency, was first described in 1952 by Bruton (OMIM *300300).[77] The most important clinical features are shown in Table 72.3. A block in B-cell differentiation at the pre-B-cell stage due to a mutated tyrosine kinase of the Src family (named Bruton tyrosine kinase, BTK) leads to a complete lack of circulating B lymphocytes and virtually no immunoglobulin production.[78] XLA should be considered in males with recurrent bacterial infections, low immunoglobulin levels and absent B cells. A positive family history on the maternal side is suggestive. T-cell count and function are usually normal. Diagnosis can be confirmed by analysis of BTK protein expression (immunoblotting or flow cytometry) and DNA mutation analysis. No genotype–phenotype correlation has yet emerged, and this diagnosis can be made later in life. Therapy consists of lifelong immunoglobulin replacement, usually 400–500 mg/kg every 3 weeks. Despite this, patients remain at risk for certain enteroviral infections of the CNS that can be especially devastating. The mutations are listed at http://www.uta.fi/laitokset/imt/bioinfo/BTKbase.

Autosomal recessive agammaglobulinemia

The recognition of females with agammaglobulinemia and the fact that in some kindreds boys and girls are equally affected, led to the search for autosomal recessive causes of agammaglobulinemia, which account for 5–10% of all patients with complete B-cell deficiency.

The clinical picture is similar to XLA, with a somewhat earlier onset and perhaps a more severe progression. The disease is genetically heterogeneous, with defects identified in the genes that encode for the µ heavy chain, the λ5-chain (part of the surrogate light chain), the Igα chain of the membrane expressed pre-B-cell receptor (BCR; involved in signal transduction) and in BLNK, an intracytoplasmic adapter that is phosphorylated by the tyrosine kinase Syk upon BCR signaling.[78]

Common variable immune deficiency

Common variable immune deficiency (CVID) has an incidence of 1:10 000 to 1:100 000 live births and is characterized by low IgG and IgA levels associated with defective specific antibody production in the setting of a normal to low B-cell count. In about 30% of patients, IgM levels are also low. The inability to produce specific antibodies puts patients at risk for frequent bacterial infections, predominantly in the respiratory and gastrointestinal tracts. The clinical picture is often complicated by autoimmune disorders

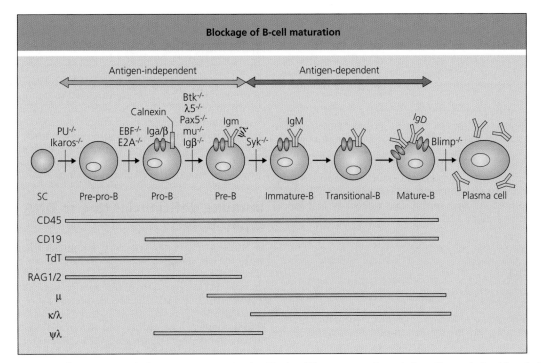

Fig. 72.17 Model of B-cell differentiation with the various proteins involved in the different stages shown below. The vertical red lines indicate a maturation block caused by the molecules indicated above.

Table 72.3 Characteristics of X-linked agammaglobulinemia
• Onset after 6 months of life (when maternal antibodies wane)   • Lack of tonsils and B lymphocytes (<2%)   • Recurrent bacterial infections of the upper and lower respiratory tract   • Risk of development of bronchiectasis   • Gastrointestinal *Giardia lamblia*   • Susceptibility to enteroviral encephalitis (echovirus, poliovirus)   • Susceptibility to arthritis caused by enteroviruses and mycoplasmas

like hemolytic anemia, thrombocytopenia, inflammatory bowel disease and others. There are early-onset (usually between 1 and 5 years) and late-onset (during adolescence) clinical phenotypes, suggesting that there may be different molecular mechanisms underlying CVID.[79] Recent work has identified causative mutations in the *CD19* and *ICOS* genes in a small number of cases. Sequence changes in *TACI* are widely recognized, but their role in CVID is still debated.[80]

Selective IgA deficiency

Selective IgA deficiency (IgAD) occurs in 1:700 live births and is characterized by low IgA levels in the serum (<5 mg/dl) and absent secretory IgA. IgG and IgM levels are normal, but defects in IgG_2 and IgG_4 have been described in a subgroup of patients. Circulating B cells are normal in number. In general, IgA deficiency is a benign disorder, with only 30% of affected patients being susceptible to bacterial infections, usually confined to the respiratory and gastrointestinal tract, or to autoimmune manifestations. A minor defect in IgA production (with levels ≤2 SD), partial IgA deficiency, is characterized by a good prognosis, with a tendency of IgA levels to normalize with age.[81] Little is known about the molecular basis of IgAD or CVID. However, given

the fact that both may occur in the same family and that some cases of selective IgA deficiency have developed CVID, a common pathogenic mechanism for both forms of humoral immune defect has been hypothesized. Environmental factors, such as anti-inflammatory and antirheumatic drugs or perhaps viral infections may accelerate the development of IgAD and CVID.

The hyper-IgM syndromes

B cells start out producing IgD and IgM and then switch their antibody production to IgG, IgA or IgE depending on interactions with T cells and other mononuclear cells. Failure to adequately undergo class switch recombination leads to overaccumulation of B cells making IgM and hence the hyper-IgM (HIGM) syndromes.[82] However, IgM elevation is an inconsistent and unnecessary part of the syndrome; what is central is the interaction of B cells with mononuclear cells for the generation of mature antibody and the killing of intracellular pathogens. The four distinct genetic defects identified as HIGM are typically characterized by low IgG and IgA levels, normal to increased IgM and a normal number of circulating B cells. Both X-linked and autosomal forms of the disease are known. The clinical picture is variable but most patients suffer from recurrent bacterial infections of the respiratory and gastrointestinal tracts.[82] Some forms of HIGM convey susceptibility to opportunistic pathogens including *Pneumocystis jirovecii*, *Cryptosporidium parvum* and CMV.

HIGM1, XHIM, CD40L and CD154 deficiency

CD40 ligand (CD40L), encoded by the X-linked *TNFSF5* (OMIM #308230), is predominantly expressed by activated CD4+ T cells. Interaction of CD40L with CD40 on B cells, dendritic cells, monocytes and some activated epithelial cells is necessary for immunoglobulin isotype switching, high affinity immunoglobulin production, somatic hypermutation and the formation of germinal centers in secondary lymphoid organs.[82] In addition, CD40L plays a crucial role in efficient interaction between T cells and

801

antigen-presenting cells, guiding the adaptive immune response to intracellular pathogens. HIGM1 is one of the two X-linked variants of HIGM. CD40L deficiency usually presents within the first year of life, and neutropenia is common. By the end of the first decade sclerosing cholangitis due to *Cryptosporidium parvum* infection is common. Later in life, the incidence of gastrointestinal tumors is elevated.[83]

The diagnosis is made by demonstration of absent CD40L on activated T lymphocytes and confirmed by mutation analysis of the *TNFSF5* gene. Mutations are catalogued at http://www.uta.fi/imt/bioinfo/CD40Lbase. Despite regular administration of immunoglobulins, mortality is as high as 40% by age 25. BMT should be pursued in appropriate cases. In murine models, unregulated CD40L expression has led to an increased incidence of autoimmune and lymphoproliferative diseases, making optimism for human gene therapy without the authentic regulatory elements premature. Trials with soluble trimeric CD40L are underway.

CD40 deficiency

CD40 is the cognate receptor for CD40L. Consequently, lack of CD40 expression (20q12, OMIM #606843) results in clinical and immunologic features very similar to those seen with CD40L deficiency.[84] Lack of isotype switching, impaired somatic hypermutation, defective memory B-cell generation and lack of germinal center formation are typical features. The diagnosis is made by analysis of CD40 expression and is confirmed by mutation analysis. Similar to X-linked HIGM1, treatment requires regular administration of intravenous immunoglobulin (IVIG), prophylactic antibiotics and use of sterile/filtered water to prevent *Cryptosporidium* spp. infection. Bone marrow transplantation should be considered in view of the poor long-term prognosis. Since CD40 is also expressed on some nonhematopoietic cells, unlike CD40L, patients with defective expression of CD40 are not fully corrected by BMT.[85] The clinical implications of this remain to be determined.

Ectodermal dysplasia with immunodeficiency

Nuclear factor kappa B essential modulator (NEMO, Xq28, OMIM #300291) sits at the juncture of innate immunity, acquired immunity and somatic development.[37] Affected boys have defects in the sweat glands, relatively thin hair, dental abnormalities (conical or peg teeth) and suffer from a wide range of infections such as pneumonia, osteomyelitis and meningitis. Since complete functional absence of NEMO in males leads to intrauterine death, those boys with the NEMO form of HIGM must have some degree of NEMO function due to hypomorphic mutations. In contrast, females heterozygous for nonfunctional mutations have incontinentia pigmenti, a syndrome that may include inflammatory lesions involving the skin, eyes and brain.[86] Skewed X-inactivation in hematopoietic cells in females usually, but not always, avoids manifestation of the immune defect.

Activation-induced cytidine deaminase deficiency

This autosomal recessive form of HIGM is characterized by a pure B-cell defect, with lack of immunoglobulin isotype switching, impaired somatic hypermutation and absence of high affinity antibodies (12p13, OMIM #606258). Activation-induced cytidine deaminase deficiency (AICD) encodes an mRNA editing protein that co-localizes with DNA repair enzymes and is selectively expressed in activated B cells in germinal centers.[87] Clinical symptoms include recurrent respiratory and gastrointestinal infections, but systemic bacterial infections such as meningitis and sepsis are also common. In contrast to the HIGM syndromes involving CD40–CD40L interactions, germinal centers are large, leading to hyperplasia of secondary lymphoid organs (tonsils).

SYNDROME-ASSOCIATED IMMUNE DEFICIENCIES

Immune deficiency may also be part of a broader clinical syndrome. In some of these disorders, signs related to immune deficiency predominate and direct the clinical evolution of the disease; in other cases, immune deficiency is variable and does not represent the most important clinical problem. In spite of their complexity, most of these diseases are monogenic, with the affected gene encoding a protein with pleiotropic functions. Alternatively, as in DiGeorge syndrome, the disease may result from a chromosomal microdeletion.

Immune deficiencies due to DNA repair defects

In addition to Artemis deficiency, immunodeficiencies due to DNA repair include ataxia telangiectasia (AT) and several related disorders.[88] Ataxia telangiectasia is due to mutations in the ataxia-telangiectasia-mutated (*ATM*) gene (11q22–23, OMIM #208900; mutations catalogued at http://ccr.coriell.org/Sections/BrowseCatalog/GeneDetail.aspx?PgId=414&gene=ATM). AT is typically associated with increased chromosome radiosensitivity and defective DNA repair, leading to somatic translocations that involve the T-cell receptor and immunoglobulin loci. Translocation between chromosomes 7 and 14 is particularly common. IgA, IgG$_2$, IgG$_4$ and IgE levels are low, and a progressive decline in T-cell number and function is typically observed. Most patients do not survive beyond young adulthood due to lymphomas and leukemia. Neurologic problems are a predominant sign of the disease.

The same clinical phenotype can be caused by mutations in the nearby gene *hMRE11*, which accounts for the so-called AT-like syndrome (OMIM #600814).[89] *hMRE11* encodes a protein involved in the earmarking of DNA double strand breaks. Mutations in *Nbs* (or nibrin) are the cause for the Nijmegen breakage syndrome (OMIM #251260), another immunodeficiency characterized by growth failure, microcephaly and a characteristic bird-like facies. The DNA ligases are also involved in DNA repair, and mutations can cause immunodeficiency.[90]

DiGeorge syndrome; velocardiofacial syndrome

This syndrome (22q11.21–23, OMIM #188400) has a wide range of clinical presentations, including thymus and parathyroid defects (hypocalcemia), overt facial abnormalities, growth failure, neurologic and neuropsychiatric manifestations, and heart defects, such as tetralogy of Fallot.[91] The predominant immunologic feature is a variably low T-cell count predisposing to *Candida* and other infections. The molecular defect lies in a heterozygous microdeletion on chromosome 22 that contains many genes (in 90% of the patients this occurs de novo). A critical gene in this cluster is TBX-1. However, this is a very common syndrome with quite variable expressivity. The frequency in the general population is thought to be 1:3000 live births and it can be transmitted as an autosomal dominant trait.

Wiskott–Aldrich syndrome

The Wiskott–Aldrich syndrome (WAS) protein is expressed selectively by hematopoietic cells. It is involved in the activation-induced reorganization of the cytoskeleton, particularly actin polymerization. Eczema, thrombocytopenia and immunodeficiency are the main features of WAS (Xp11.2;, OMIM #301000).[92] Microthrombocytes (low mean platelet volume) in a male with thrombocytopenia and eczema are highly suspicious, even before the immune deficiency characterized by recurrent bacterial airway infections is manifest. Immunoglobulin responses to polysaccharides are typically impaired and immune globulin replacement is often needed. Later in life there is an elevated incidence of leukemia, lymphoma and autoimmune diseases.

A relatively benign variant of WAS, X-linked thrombocytopenia (XLT), occurs without eczema or immunodeficiency. Most patients with this variant show missense mutations in *WASP* exons 1 or 2 that permit some gene expression. In some less severe cases, thrombocytopenia is intermittent,; however, mean platelet volume is consistently low.

X-linked lymphoproliferative syndrome (Duncan's syndrome)

Patients with X-linked lymphoproliferative syndrome (Xp25, OMIM *308240) show an increased susceptibility to severe manifestations after EBV infections.[93] Hepatitis, lymphomas and/or hemophagocytic lymphohistiocytosis (HLH) kill about 70% of affected males in their first decade. Those who survive, mostly affected by a milder variant, may present with hypogammaglobulinemia. The defective gene, *SH2D1A*, encodes the SLAM-associated protein (SAP), an SH2 domain containing protein expressed selectively in lymphocytes. The mutations are cumulated at http://www.uta.fi/imt/bioinfo/SH2D1Abase. SAP has a regulatory effect on cytokine production and is essential for the cytotoxic activity of NK cells.[93] Herpes viruses other than EBV have also been shown to trigger XLP. Several mutational hot-spots have been identified, but so far no genotype–phenotype correlation has been recognized. BMT should be considered before EBV infection if an HLA-compatible donor is available.

Familial hemophagocytic lymphohistiocytosis

Similar to X-linked lymphoproliferative syndrome, familial hemophagocytic lymphohistiocytosis is an autosomal recessive disease characterized by hepatosplenomegaly, acute bone marrow failure with histiocytic activation, coagulopathy and hypertriglyceridemia, often in response to viral infection. Onset is during the first few months of life; accelerated phases occur repeatedly, often with life-threatening hemorrhagic episodes.[94] The clinical presentation can be very difficult to differentiate from acute infection, as it is often accompanied by fever and hematologic signs of inflammation. The immunologic defect consists in virtually absent NK cytotoxicity due to a functionally deficient perforin (encoded by *PRF1* at 10q21–22), a protein normally released from the intracytoplasmic granules after the membranes of effector NK or T cells have fused to target cells. The resulting prolonged contact between infected and 'intended' cytotoxic cells leads to increased cytokine production that is thought to activate macrophages and histiocytes. Forms of this disease that do not have clear genetic predispositions may be triggered by various infections or by drugs. Accelerated phases of hemophagocytic lymphohistiocytosis (HLH) are true medical emergencies that may be brought into remission by chemotherapy and maintained with immunosuppression; however, they generally require BMT.[95]

Autoimmune lymphoproliferative syndrome (Canale Smith syndrome)

At the core of normal development is the proper coordination of cell death. When cell death occurs in a programmed way (i.e. not due to lysis by infecting agents or necrosis due to toxic events), it is referred to as apoptosis. Proper Fas/Fas ligand (FasL) interaction is critical for normal apoptosis (Fig. 72.18). The correct interaction Fas/FasL leads to the formation of the death inducing signaling complex (DISC), which acts through different caspases to induce mitochondrial damage and finally proteolytic cell death. Fas (CD95), encoded by *APT1* (*TNFRSF6*), is a transmembrane protein with an intracellular death domain. Death signaling requires assembly of homotrimers.

The autoimmune lymphoproliferative syndrome type I (ALPS I) is caused by heterozygous mutations in the receptor Fas that lead to disruption of normal homo-oligomerization resulting in deranged lymphoid homeostasis due to defective apoptosis.[96] In this autosomal

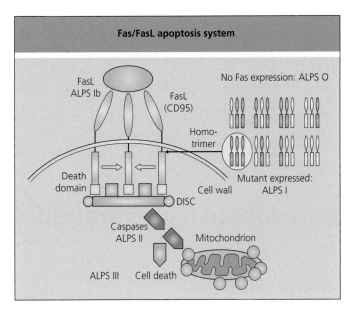

Fig. 72.18 The Fas/FasL apoptosis system and the various forms of ALPS caused by defects in it.

dominant disorder, only one in eight homotrimers will have three normal Fas molecules. However, the story remains quite complex, as the mutations in Fas have variable penetrance and expressivity. ALPS usually presents with lymphadenopathy, hepatosplenomegaly and hematologic autoimmunity such as hemolytic anemia, autoimmune neutropenia and immune thrombocytopenia. There is a markedly increased risk (up to 50 times) of lymphoma and leukemia.[97] Diagnostic findings include increased numbers of T cells that lack both CD4 and CD8 molecules, referred to as double negative T cells.

ALPS Ib is caused by mutations in the ligand for Fas, FasL (*TNFSF6*). Defects in certain caspases lead to a similar failure of lymphocyte apoptosis denominated ALPS II. ALPS III is the name currently used for the ALPS phenotype for which genetic defects have not been identified. ALPS-causing mutations have been found to have occurred outside of the germline, indicating somatic mutation leading to ALPS.[98]

IPEX

The clinical entity characterized by *i*mmunodysregulation (anemia, lymphadenopathy), autoimmune *p*olyendocrinopathy (diabetes, thyroiditis), *e*nteropathy and *X*-linked transmission is named IPEX and is due to defects in *FOXP3*, which encodes scurfin, a protein expressed predominantly in the thymus and spleen (OMIM: #304930, #304790).[99] It appears to have a key role in the generation of T regulatory cells, which repress T-cell activation and cytokine expression. Severely affected boys usually die in childhood. There is a somewhat milder phenotype associated with mutations sparing the coding sequence but affecting the polyadenylation signal. Opportunistic infections are not a typical part of IPEX, indicating that this is less a defect in protective immunity than a defect in regulation of immune response and cytokine production. Immunosuppression has proved beneficial in some patients with IPEX, underlining the importance of *FOXP3* in the control of autoreactive cell clones.

REFERENCES

References for this chapter can be found online at http://www.expertconsult.com

Chapter | **73** | *Oscar Marchetti*
Thierry Calandra

Infections in the neutropenic cancer patient

INTRODUCTION

Cancer occurs in one of every four people and is one of the leading causes of death in developed countries. Cancer can be subdivided in two main categories: solid tumors and hematologic malignancies, which include leukemias, lymphomas and multiple myeloma. Solid tumors account for more than 90% of all new cancer cases and hematologic malignancies for the remaining 5–10%.[1] Over the past decades, joint efforts of basic science and clinical research have resulted in substantial improvements of prevention, early detection and treatment of cancer. Indeed, overall 5-year survival rates in cancer patients improved from 39% in the 1960s to 60% in the 1990s.[1] Solid tumors are frequently treated with combined treatment modalities including surgery, radiation therapy and chemotherapy. In contrast, chemotherapy is the cornerstone of the management of patients with hematologic malignancies. New therapeutic options, such as immunotherapy and gene therapy, are being developed.

Infections frequently occur during treatment of cancer. Many factors contribute to increase the risk of infection: poor clinical and nutritional status, mechanical obstruction of natural passages, damage to anatomic barriers (surgery, use of prosthetic and intravascular devices), and defects of humoral and cell-mediated immunity, that are either disease associated or secondary to radiotherapy or chemotherapy. Cytotoxic agents exert their effects on both malignant cells and normally replicating progenitor cells and thus also cause major toxicity to normal tissues with high turnover (i.e. bone marrow and mucous membranes) resulting in myelosuppression and alteration of physiologic barriers. Historically, hemorrhage and infections have been major complications and leading causes of chemotherapy-related mortality (10–20% and 50–80%, respectively).[2] In the 1960s, both the severity and duration of granulocytopenia were identified as major determinants of infectious complications.[3] In the early 1970s, prompt empiric antibiotic treatment became the cornerstone of management of febrile neutropenic patients, resulting in drastic reduction of the mortality of bacterial infections.[4] Since then, major progress has been made in the understanding of the pathogenesis, prevention and treatment of infectious complications of cancer patients. Development of novel diagnostic and treatment strategies continues to improve the outcome of febrile neutropenic cancer patients.[5,6] However, new developments in anticancer therapy, especially new immunomodulating agents, increase the risk of opportunistic infections and represent new challenges for the prevention, diagnosis and management of infectious complications in neutropenic cancer patients.

EPIDEMIOLOGY

The majority of infections in granulocytopenic cancer patients are caused by micro-organisms of the patient's endogenous flora.[5] However, exogenous air-borne and food-borne pathogens, acquired either in the community or in the health-care system, can also cause infection.

Bacterial infections

Gram-positive and Gram-negative bacteria are the predominant pathogens in this clinical setting (Table 73.1).[5] Polymicrobial bloodstream infections, often consisting of mixed aerobic and anaerobic infections,

Table 73.1 Most common pathogens in neutropenic cancer patients

Gram-positive aerobic bacteria

Coagulase-negative staphylococci
Staphylococcus aureus
Viridans streptococci
Other streptococci (*S. pneumoniae*, *S. pyogenes*)
Enterococcus species
Corynebacterium spp. (*C. jeikeium*)
Bacillus spp.
Listeria monocytogenes

Gram-negative aerobic bacteria

Escherichia coli
Klebsiella spp.
Pseudomonas spp.
Other Enterobacteriaceae (*Proteus*, *Enterobacter*, *Serratia*, *Citrobacter* spp.)

Anaerobic bacteria

Bacteroides spp.
Clostridium spp.
Fusobacterium spp.
Propionibacterium spp.

Fungi

Candida spp.
Aspergillus spp.
Other molds (*Fusarium*, *Pseudallescheria boydii*, *Scedosporium*, *Rhizopus*, *Mucor* spp.)
Pneumocystis jirovecii

Viruses

Herpes simplex virus
Varicella-zoster virus
Respiratory viruses (influenza, respiratory syncytial virus)

Parasites

Strongyloides stercoralis
Other parasites in endemic areas (e.g. *Leishmania*)

occur in 5–20% of cases.[7] In past decades, most cancer centers have experienced major changes in the etiology of bacterial infections in the neutropenic host.[5–8] While Gram-negative bacteria were predominant in the 1970s and early 1980s, the frequency of Gram-positive bacteria markedly increased in the late 1980s and early 1990s, when they became the prevalent pathogens in many institutions. This trend has been recently confirmed by the results of a North American survey.[9] However, this trend reversed in the late 1990s in Europe, where Gram-negative and Gram-positive pathogens now account for an equal proportion of infections (Fig. 73.1).[8]

Many factors are involved in these epidemiologic shifts. The increasing incidence of infections due to coagulase-negative staphylococci and other Gram-positive skin colonizers has been associated with the increased use of intravascular access devices. The emergence of viridans streptococcal infections, sometimes associated with acute respiratory distress syndrome (ARDS) and septic shock, has been attributed to several factors, including the toxicity of high-dose chemotherapy with cytosine arabinoside on oral mucous membranes, the reactivation of oral herpes simplex virus (HSV) infection, and the use of fluoroquinolone prophylaxis.[10] Among Gram-negative bacteria, *Escherichia coli, Klebsiella* species and *Pseudomonas aeruginosa* are the most common bloodstream isolates. However, the incidence of *Pseudomonas aeruginosa* infections, a predominant cause of bacteremia in the 1960s and 1970s, has substantially declined over the last 30 years. The use of fluoroquinolone prophylaxis has undoubtedly played a major role in the decreasing incidence of Gram-negative infections observed in the late 1980s and early 1990s.[11]

The recent re-emergence of Gram-negative infections is probably due to the reduced use of fluoroquinolone prophylaxis in many centers out of concern for increased resistance.[12] Some centers have reported the emergence of infections due to multiresistant extended-spectrum β-lactamase (ESBL)-producing Gram-negative bacteria.[13] Superinfections due to *Stenotrophomonas maltophilia*, a nonfermentative Gram-negative microorganism likely to develop *in-vitro* resistance after extensive exposure to broad-spectrum antibiotics including β-lactams, have been associated with poor outcome in neutropenic cancer patients.[14]

Fungal infections

Fungal infections are a major threat to neutropenic cancer patients. Disseminated mycoses have been demonstrated in 10–40% of autopsies in patients with hematologic malignancies, especially in patients who have been treated with broad-spectrum antibiotics and corticosteroids.[2] Classically occurring as secondary infections in patients with prolonged and profound neutropenia, fungal infections also account for approximately 5% of initial infectious episodes.[15] Mixed fungal and bacterial infections may occur and the fungal infection may manifest as persistent fever after eradication of the bacterial pathogen.

Over 90% of all invasive mycoses are caused by *Candida* species (mainly *C. albicans, C. tropicalis, C. glabrata, C. krusei, C. parapsilosis* and *C. pseudotropicalis*) and *Aspergillus* species (mainly *A. fumigatus* and *A. flavus*), which account for 30–80% and 10–60% of cases of fungal infections, respectively. Azole-resistant non-*albicans Candida* species (*C. krusei, C. glabrata*) have emerged in some cancer centers, usually in conjunction with several predisposing factors including fluconazole prophylaxis.[16] Infections due to *A. terreus*, a species with reduced susceptibility to amphotericin B, have been recently reported in some centers.[17] *Fusarium, Pseudallescheria boydii, Scedosporium* and zygomycetes (e.g. *Rhizopus* and *Mucor*) are emerging fungal infections.[2] The occurrence of zygomycosis has been associated with the use of voriconazole prophylaxis.[18]

Other pathogens

Reactivation of latent herpes simplex virus (HSV) and varicella-zoster virus (VZV) infections are common in patients with hematologic malignancies, especially after chemotherapy or treatment with corticosteroids.[5] In contrast to other immunocompromised patients, especially transplant recipients, cytomegalovirus (CMV) infections play a minor role in neutropenic cancer patients, as acquired immunity is less severely suppressed than innate immunity. Other viral infections such as respiratory viruses (Influenza, Respiratory syncytial virus) and Erythrovirus (formerly Parvovirus) B19 occur occasionally. Primary parasitic infections as well as reactivation of latent infections, in particular those due to *Strongyloides* or *Leishmania* spp., only occur in patients who have lived in or visited endemic areas.

PATHOGENESIS

Underlying conditions

Microbial invasion and development of infection are facilitated by the presence of co-morbidities, immunosuppression and damage to anatomic barriers caused by the cancer itself or induced by chemotherapy

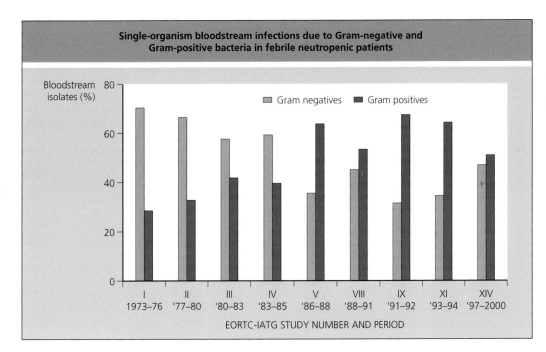

Fig. 73.1 Proportion of single-organism bloodstream infections due to Gram-negative and Gram-positive bacteria in febrile neutropenic patients: EORTC-IATG studies (1973–2000). Adapted from reference[8].

or invasive procedures.[5] Obstruction of the lumen of natural body passages (i.e. urinary, biliary, respiratory or digestive tract) by cancer impairs the flow of body fluids and secretions, creating conditions that promote microbial growth. Cytotoxic chemotherapy damages the epithelial tissue lining, resulting in loss of the integrity of the mucous membrane barrier. Development of mucositis therefore predisposes to infection by the patient's endogenous commensal flora and colonizing pathogens. Injury to the skin by venous puncture, presence of indwelling vascular access devices, bone marrow aspiration, lumbar puncture and other surgical interventions can also promote skin and soft tissue infections.

Defects of innate and acquired immunity

Neutropenia

Phagocytes (neutrophils, monocytes, macrophages and dendritic cells) are a critical component of the host innate immune defenses against infections. Thus, any alteration in function or number of these cells, especially neutrophils, will result in an increased risk of infection.[5] Neutropenia is defined as a neutrophil count <500 cells/mm³ or <1000 cells/mm³ with expected decrease to <500 cells/mm³ within 48 hours. Studies performed in the 1960s have shown that there is an inverse relationship between the number of circulating neutrophils and the incidence of infections.[3] As the neutrophil count decreases to <1000 cells/mm³, the incidence of infections increases markedly (Fig. 73.2). The risk of severe infectious complications such as bloodstream infections is greatest during agranulocytosis, i.e. when the neutrophil count drops below 100 cells/mm³.

The duration of neutropenia is also a major determinant of the risk of infection.[3] As shown in Figure 73.2, the longer the duration of neutropenia, the greater the risk of infection. Profound and prolonged neutropenia (i.e. <500 cells/mm³ for more than 10 days) is considered to be a major risk factor for both primary and secondary bacterial or fungal infections. Patients with neutropenia lasting less than 7–10 days are at low risk of complications.[5] Indeed, 95% of patients with neutropenia lasting less than 1 week respond to the initial empiric antibiotic therapy, while two-thirds of those with neutropenia for more than 2 weeks may require treatment modifications.[5,19] Moreover, the risk of recurrence of fever and infection is also substantially lower (<1%) in patients with a neutropenia of short duration than in those

with neutropenia lasting more than 2 weeks (38%).[19] In addition, the risk of death associated with superinfections is five times higher than that of primary infections.[15]

Yet factors other than the severity and duration of neutropenia also help to identify those patients at low or high risk of infectious complications (see Risk assessment pp.12–13).

Other immune defects

Neutropenia is the main immune defect of cancer patients. In general, defects of the humoral or cell-mediated components of acquired immunity are not predominant in these patients. However, specific immune defects directly associated with the underlying malignancy (e.g. hypogammaglobulinemia in chronic lymphocytic leukemia or multiple myeloma) or its management (e.g. therapy with high-dose corticosteroids) may occur and further increase the risk of infections in conjunction with neutropenia.[5]

New immunomodulating anticancer agents such as rituximab, fludarabine, imatinib, alemtuzumab and temozolomide have become available in recent years and are associated with cell-mediated immune defects, increasing the risk of infection. Temozolomide, a prodrug of dacarbazine, fludarabine, a purine analog and 2-chlorodeoxyadenosine induce selective CD4+ T-cell dysfunction, resulting in an increased risk of opportunistic infections.[20,21] VZV reactivation, *Nocardia* infection and tuberculosis have been reported in patients receiving imatinib, a potent inhibitor of tyrosine kinase. Immunotherapy with alemtuzumab, an anti-CD52 monoclonal antibody, has been associated with increased incidence of viral, bacterial and fungal infections.[22] Combining rituximab with cytotoxic chemotherapy for non-Hodgkin's lymphoma has been associated with an increased risk of bacterial infections.[23]

Genetic immune defects also predispose cancer patients to infectious complications. Deficits in mannose-binding lectin, a critical component of the lectin pathway of complement, have been associated with severe infections during prolonged neutropenia.[24] Polymorphisms of Toll-like receptor 4 have been associated with an increased risk of invasive aspergillosis in allogeneic hematopoietic stem cell transplant recipients.[25] These observations highlight the impact that genetic screening may have in the prevention and management of infections in cancer patients.

CLINICAL FEATURES

Fever

During neutropenia, fever develops in virtually all patients with hematologic malignancies and in about half of those with solid tumors.[5] Although any temperature distinctly above baseline is indicative of fever, fever has been arbitrarily defined as a single temperature >101.3°F (38.5°C) or >100.4°F (38°C) on two or more occasions during a 12-hour period by the Consensus Expert Panel of the Immunocompromised Host Society, or as a single temperature reading >100.9°F (38.3°C) or >100.4°F (38.0°C) during at least 1 hour by the Fever and Neutropenia Guidelines Panel of the Infectious Diseases Society of America.[5] Temperature should be measured orally or by auditory canal probe. More than two-thirds of the febrile episodes are likely to be caused by infection, which may occur with or without focal symptoms or signs. Because of the impaired host response, the classic signs of inflammation (i.e. pain, heat, redness, swelling, and purulent discharge) are often reduced or may even be absent. Therefore, fever is generally the first and frequently the only sign of infection.

Fever occurring in the context of neutropenia is considered to reflect ongoing infection unless proven otherwise. However, there are noninfectious causes of pyrexia, of which the most frequent are the underlying malignancy itself, cytotoxic chemotherapy, transfusion of blood products, antifungal and occasionally other antimicrobial agents,

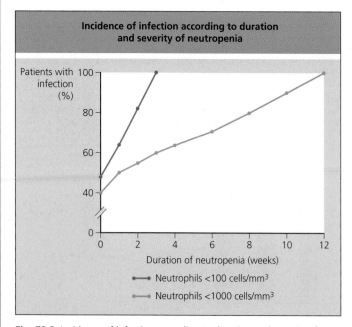

Fig. 73.2 Incidence of infection according to duration and severity of neutropenia. Adapted from reference[3].

colony-stimulating factors or allergic drug reactions. Uncommonly, infection may develop in the absence of fever because of the lack of inflammatory response such as during therapy with high-dose corticosteroids or when caused by certain micro-organisms (e.g. *Clostridium septicum*).

Types of infection

Classically, infections have been subdivided into three main categories:[5]

- *Microbiologically documented infections* (MDI), subdivided into those with and without bloodstream infection. Bloodstream infections, caused predominantly by bacteria (bacteremia) and occasionally by fungi (fungemia), may be either primary (in the absence of a nonhematogenous focus of infection) or secondary to a proven focus of infection (e.g. pneumonia, cellulitis, catheter-related infection, urinary tract infection).
- *Clinically documented infections* (CDI) defined by the presence of a site of infection (e.g. pneumonia, cellulitis, oropharyngeal mucositis, enterocolitis, catheter-exit site infection) without microbiologic proof of the nature of infection.
- *Fever of unknown origin* (FUO), also designated as fever of undetermined origin, unexplained fever or pyrexia of unknown origin, and defined as a febrile episode that is not accompanied by clinical or microbiologic evidence of infection.

Figure 73.3 shows the proportions of MDI, CDI and FUO in febrile neutropenic patients with hematologic malignancies (mainly acute

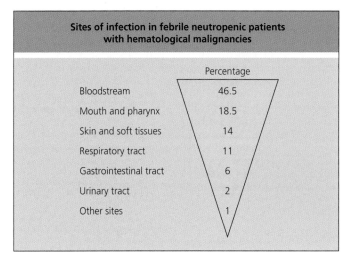

Fig. 73.4 Sites of infection in febrile neutropenic patients with hematologic malignancies (n=889). Data are derived from three consecutive studies of the EORTC-IATG conducted between 1991 and 2000.[26–28]

leukemia) or solid tumors in four consecutive multicenter studies conducted in the 1990s in Europe, the Middle East and North America.[26–30] Generally, MDI account for approximately 25–35% and 10–20%, CDI for 20–30% and 10–20% and FUO for 40–60% and 50–70% of the episodes of fever occurring in neutropenic patients with hematologic malignancies or solid tumors, respectively.[26–30] Most episodes of MDI consist of bloodstream infections (Fig. 73.4) that occur almost exclusively in patients with profound neutropenia (<100 cells/mm³).[3,26–28] Although the etiology of fever remains by definition unclear in FUO, the fever was probably of infectious origin if it resolved with antimicrobial therapy.

Sites of infection

In studies conducted in the 1990s the most frequent sites of infection in neutropenic cancer patients with hematologic malignancies or solid tumors with a first episode of fever were, by decreasing order of frequency, the bloodstream, the oral cavity and nasopharynx, the skin and soft tissues, the respiratory tract, the gastrointestinal tract and the urinary tract (Fig. 73.4).[26–28] Although similar data have been reported in recent randomized therapeutic trials, these may not reflect the whole spectrum of the clinical manifestations of infections during neutropenia. Different proportions of the site of origin of infection are expected in selected patient populations and in patients with secondary infections.

Bloodstream

Bloodstream infections account for 80–90% of microbiologically documented infections (Fig. 73.3) and for half of the febrile episodes for which a site of infection can be identified (Fig. 73.4). In primary bloodstream infections, the source remains unknown, but disrupted physiologic barriers (i.e. mucous membranes of the gastrointestinal tract and skin) are the most likely portals of entry. Bacteria are the most frequent blood isolates, accounting for over 90% of bloodstream infections. A single micro-organism is implicated in the majority of bloodstream infections, but polymicrobial infections occur in approximately 5–10% of cases.

As previously mentioned, the epidemiology of single-organism bacteremia in neutropenic cancer patients has changed over the last 30 years and may vary from center to center (see Fig. 73.1). Today, Gram-positive and Gram-negative bacteria cause an equal proportion of infections in many European centers. The most common Gram-positive bacteria are coagulase-negative staphylococci, viridans

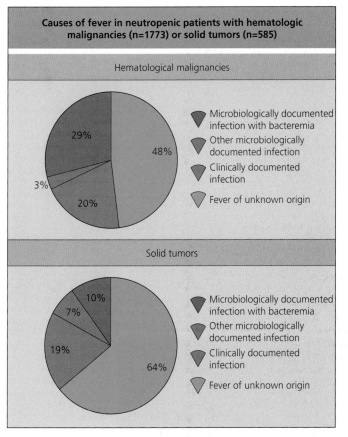

Fig. 73.3 Causes of fever in neutropenic patients with hematologic malignancies (n=1773) or solid tumors (n=585). Data are derived from four consecutive studies of the EORTC-IATG conducted between 1991 and 2000 and from a North American study conducted between 1992 and 1997.[26–30]

streptococci and *Staphylococcus aureus*. Among Gram-negative pathogens, *E. coli, Klebsiella* species and other Enterobacteriaceae are predominant, while *P. aeruginosa* has declined progressively (Table 73.1). Resistant bacteria (such as ESBL-producing enteric Gram-negative bacilli or *Stenotrophomonas maltophilia*) or fungi are classically isolated from blood in secondary febrile episodes occurring during antibiotic treatment.[14] In some countries, multiresistant ESBL-producing Gram-negative bacilli have emerged as a frequent cause of infection in neutropenic patients.[13]

Bloodstream infections are potentially life-threatening, but with prompt administration of empiric antibiotics at fever onset, severe complications such as severe sepsis and septic shock rarely occur today. Mortality rates between 1% and 3% have been reported in recent studies in febrile neutropenic cancer patients.

Mouth and pharynx

Maintenance of good oral hygiene and proper dental care are essential for the prevention of oral and systemic infections. Dental septic foci, such as braces and periodontitis, which may promote or facilitate the development of local and systemic infections, should be removed or treated prior to the initiation of chemotherapy. Indeed, infections of the oral cavity (e.g. mucositis, gingivitis, periodontitis) and pharynx occur in 15–25% of neutropenic cancer patients (Fig. 73.4).

The frequency and severity of these infections is correlated with the degree of mucosal damage induced by cytotoxic chemotherapy and with the severity of neutropenia. Mucous membranes of the mouth and pharynx are heavily colonized with viridans streptococci, Gram-positive rods, and aerobic and anaerobic Gram-negative bacilli. Loss of integrity of the mucosal barrier is therefore a major portal of entry for infection. Neutropenic patients with no or minimal mucosal damage are at much lower risk of infection than patients with severe chemotherapy-induced mucositis. *Candida* spp. also play an important role in infections of the oropharynx, especially under the selective pressure of broad-spectrum antibiotics. Oral lesions caused by reactivation of HSV infection may mimic chemotherapy-induced mucositis and also serve as a portal of entry for bacterial infection.

Skin and soft tissues

Cutaneous infections are common in neutropenic cancer patients, causing about 10–20% of all septic episodes for which a source of infection is identified (Fig. 73.4). Primary skin and soft tissue infections often result from a disruption of the integrity of the cutaneous barrier caused by needle punctures (venous or lumbar puncture, bone marrow biopsy) or by the presence of intravascular access devices. The anal and axillary areas are frequent foci of cutaneous infections as moisture, high bacterial colonization, relative skin frailty and microtrauma all facilitate the development of infection. Anal fissures are often complicated by perirectal cellulitis, classically caused by the fecal flora, including Gram-negative bacilli (Enterobacteriaceae, *P. aeruginosa*), enterococci and anaerobic Gram-negative bacilli. Axillary hidradenitis is a classic infection of neutropenic hosts caused by skin commensals and Gram-negative bacteria, including *P. aeruginosa* (Fig. 73.5a).

Disseminated cutaneous infections may reflect the development of septic skin foci in patients with bacterial, fungal or viral bloodstream infections. Clinically, these skin lesions appear as papules or nodules (Fig. 73.6), which are usually associated with classic symptoms and signs of sepsis (i.e. fever, chills, headache, backache, myalgia and muscle tenderness). Ulcers, vesicles, hemorrhagic or crusted lesions that are either isolated (with or without dermatome distribution) or disseminated are typically associated with herpetic skin infections, but may occasionally occur with staphylococcal or streptococcal infections.

A bacterial (e.g. *Pseudomonas* and *Aeromonas* spp.) or fungal etiology (*Fusarium, Aspergillus, Mucor* and *Rhizopus* spp.) should be suspected in cases of disseminated necrotic skin lesions. For example, ecthyma gangrenosum is a classic cutaneous complication in patients with *Pseudomonas* sepsis (Fig. 73.5b). Necrotizing fasciitis and metastatic musculoskeletal infections complicating bacteremia or fungemia have also been reported, albeit infrequently (Fig. 73.7a).

Intravascular access devices

Indwelling intravenous catheters, especially those inserted for prolonged periods of time (e.g. Broviac, Hickman, Port-a-cath) are a major source of infections, which most commonly arise at the exit site, but may also occasionally affect the tunneled section of the catheter. Clinical manifestations include pain, erythema and tenderness with no or minimal swelling during marrow aplasia. Microbes of the skin flora (i.e. coagulase-negative staphylococci, *Propionibacterium, Corynebacterium* and *Bacillus* spp., and viridans streptococci), *S. aureus*, Gram-negative bacteria and *Candida* species are the most frequent pathogens. When skin necrosis occurs, infections due to *P. aeruginosa*, mycobacteria (especially *M. chelonae* and *M. fortuitum*) or to molds (*Aspergillus, Fusarium* or *Mucor* spp.) should be suspected. Infection of intravascular access devices may be complicated by septic thrombophlebitis.

Respiratory tract

Respiratory infections account for 10–15% of the identified sites of infection in febrile neutropenic cancer patients (Fig. 73.4). Infections of the upper respiratory tract (sinusitis, otitis, epiglottitis, laryngitis and tracheitis) are uncommon, occurring in only 1% of episodes. Sinusitis and otitis are mainly due to common community-acquired

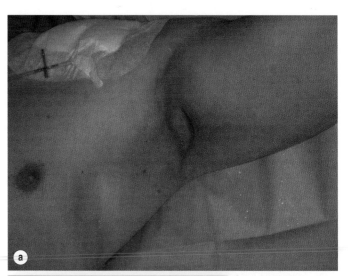
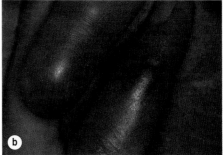

Fig. 73.5 Cutaneous bacterial infections in neutropenic patients with acute leukemia. (a) Axillary *Pseudomonas aeruginosa* hidradenitis. (b) Ecthyma gangrenosum of fingers in a patient with *Pseudomonas aeruginosa* sepsis.

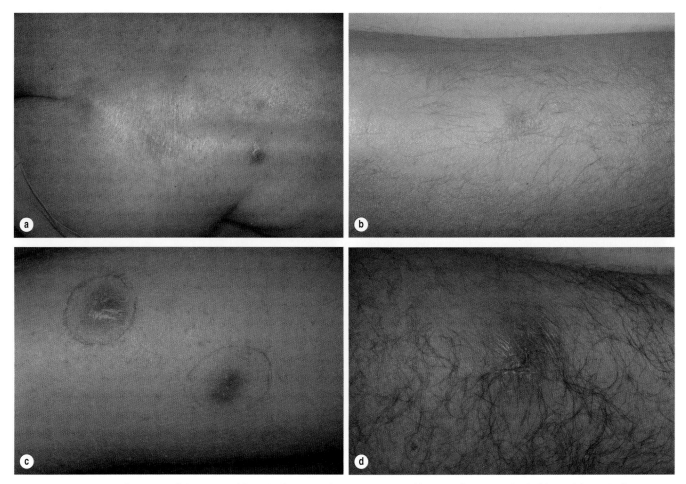

Fig. 73.6 Cutaneous manifestations of disseminated fungal infections in leukemic patients. (a) *Aspergillus terreus*, back. (b) *Candida tropicalis*, arm. (c) *Fusarium*, leg. (d) *Pseudallescheria boydii*, leg.

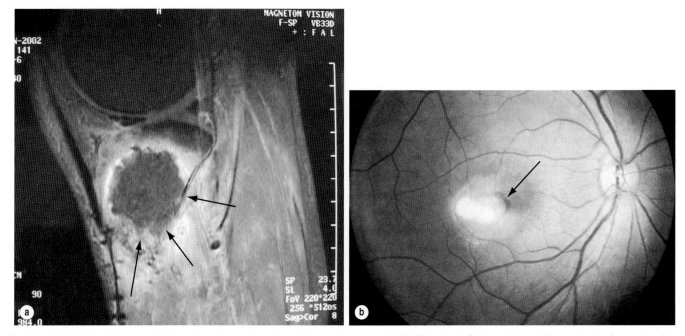

Fig. 73.7 Disseminated *S. aureus* infection in a leukemic patient. (a) Muscular abscess, MRI. (b) Retinal infectious lesion with macular involvement and secondary bleeding (arrow), fundoscopy.

bacteria, but infections due to *Pseudomonas* species and anaerobes can occur. Fungal (*Aspergillus, Mucor, Rhizopus* spp.) sinusitis is a severe and potentially life-threatening infection of patients with profound and prolonged neutropenia. It is often invasive and can infiltrate the nearby bone and skin and soft tissue structures of the orbit and extend into the central nervous system (Fig. 73.8).

Most frequently, lower respiratory tract infections (bronchopneumonia and pneumonia) are primary infections and account for about 10% of documented infections. However, they may occasionally be secondary to bloodstream infections. Due to the impaired inflammatory response, the classic symptoms and signs of pneumonia (such as fever, cough, dyspnea, chest pain, sputum and radiologic infiltrates) are often attenuated or delayed, and present in only half to two-thirds of the patients. Patients with profound neutropenia (<100 cells/mm³) rarely produce sputum. The proportion of infections due to pneumonia tends to be lower in the first febrile episodes than in subsequent ones. Moreover, early-onset pneumonia is more likely to be of bacterial origin, while late-onset pneumonia is more likely to be due to fungi or other opportunistic pathogens (Figs 73.9, 73.10a). Respiratory viruses (respiratory syncytial virus, influenza virus, parainfluenza virus, adenovirus) are rare, but may be associated with severe morbidity and mortality (Fig. 73.11a).

Another classic pulmonary complication in febrile neutropenic cancer patients is the development of adult respiratory distress syndrome after viridans streptococcal bacteremia (Fig. 73.11b). This syndrome occurs despite appropriate antibiotic therapy and is associated with important morbidity (i.e. respiratory failure requiring mechanical ventilation) and high mortality.[10]

Gastrointestinal tract and intra-abdominal organs

The gastrointestinal tract is the largest reservoir of micro-organisms of the human body and the endogenous gastrointestinal flora plays an important role in the pathogenesis of infection in the neutropenic cancer patient. Extended chemotherapy-induced mucosal damage is therefore a major portal of entry of systemic infections.

The gastrointestinal tract itself accounts for 4–8% of documented infections (Fig. 73.4). Esophagitis and enterocolitis are the two most frequent gastrointestinal infections in the neutropenic host. Esophagitis presents with severe retrosternal pain and dysphagia and is usually caused by the commensal bacterial flora, *Candida* species

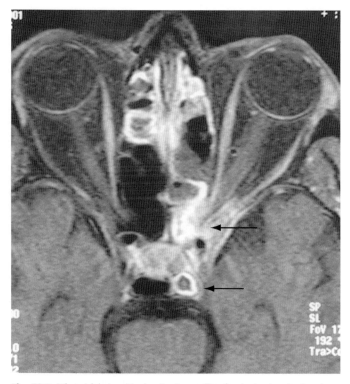

Fig. 73.8 Ethmoidal sinusitis due to *Aspergillus fumigatus* in a leukemic patient. The MRI shows bone destruction with invasion of the orbit, optical nerve (upper arrow) and central nervous system (lower arrow).

or reactivation of HSV. Symptoms and signs of enterocolitis include nausea, vomiting, bloating, abdominal discomfort, cramps, pain, constipation or diarrhea (often severe in the case of antibiotic-associated colitis). Typhlitis, a life-threatening necrotizing enterocolitis affecting the cecum or other bowel segments, typically occurs in patients with severe and prolonged neutropenia postchemotherapy for acute leukemia (Fig. 73.12).[31] The clinical manifestations are fever, abdominal pain (initially localized to the lower right abdominal quadrant, but becoming diffuse as the infection progresses) and diarrhea, which are often associated with a profound alteration of the patient's

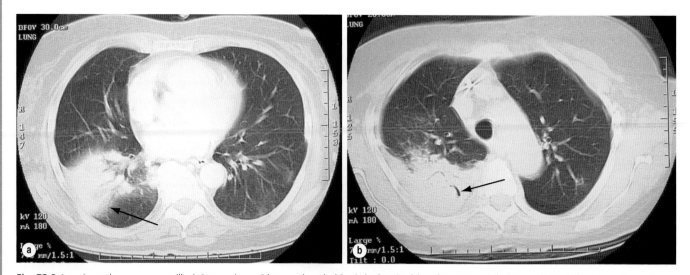

Fig. 73.9 Invasive pulmonary aspergillosis in a patient with acute lymphoblastic leukemia. (a) Early stage with halo sign (arrow) during neutropenia, CT scan. (b) Late stage with air crescent sign (arrow) after bone marrow recovery, CT-scan.

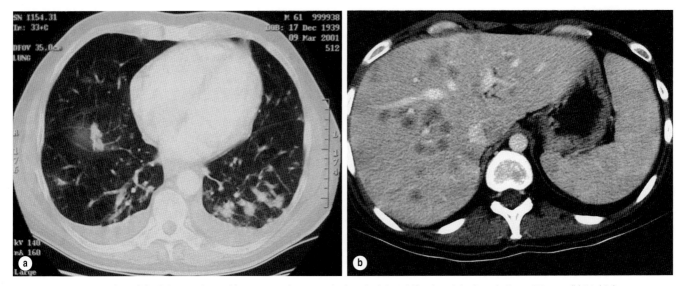

Fig. 73.10 Disseminated candidiasis in a patient with acute myelogenous leukemia. (a) Multifocal nodular lung lesions, CT scan. (b) Multiple hepatosplenic abscesses, CT-scan.

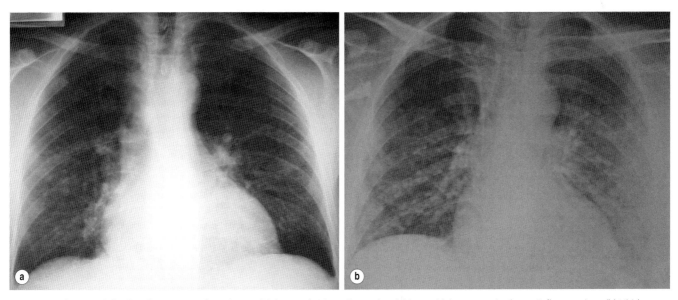

Fig. 73.11 Pulmonary infections in neutropenic patients with hematologic malignancies. (a) Interstitial pneumonia due to Influenza virus. (b) Viridans streptococcal bacteremia with acute respiratory distress syndrome.

clinical condition. Typhlitis is caused by the endogenous gut aerobic and anaerobic bacterial flora, but yeasts and molds may also be implicated.

In patients with neutropenic enterocolitis, the thickness of the intestinal wall as assessed by radiologic imaging has been correlated with morbidity and mortality.[32] Bleeding and perforation are the two major complications. Necrotizing fasciitis and septic shock can also occur, especially with clostridial infection, notably with *C. septicum*. Antibiotic-associated colitis due to *C. difficile* is a frequent cause of profuse diarrhea in neutropenic cancer patients exposed to multiple and prolonged antibiotic treatments. Severe complications

such as bleeding, perforation or toxic megacolon occur in 5–10% of cases.[33]

Bacterial liver abscesses and viral hepatitis are rare in neutropenic cancer patients. Hepatosplenic candidiasis, a disseminated fungal infection mainly observed in patients with acute leukemia, classically becomes manifest at the time of marrow recovery after a prolonged period of neutropenia. Diagnosis should be suspected in patients with persistent fever, lack of appetite, abdominal discomfort or frank pain, hepatosplenomegaly and elevated alkaline phosphatase.[34] Imaging techniques – ultrasonography, CT or MRI – show typical multiple target-like or bull's-eye lesions of the liver and spleen (Fig. 73.10b).

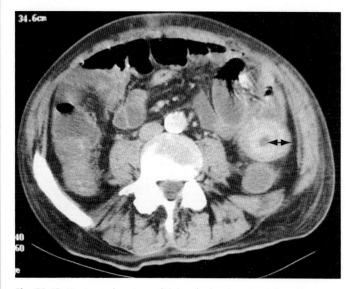

Fig. 73.12 Neutropenic enterocolitis in a leukemic patient. Prominent thickening of a segment of ileum (arrow), CT-scan.

Urinary tract

Urinary tract infections are rare (1–3%) in neutropenic patients (Fig. 73.4) and are mainly due to common uropathogens, such as Enterobacteriaceae. They occur with minimal symptoms, and dysuria is frequently absent as is pyuria because of neutropenia. Thus, diagnosis often relies on a positive urine culture in a febrile patient without evidence of another site of infection.

Other sites

Infections of the central nervous system, eye, heart, vasculature and bone are uncommon causes of sepsis in neutropenic patients with hematologic malignancies and solid tumors (1% of all episodes, Fig. 73.4). Infections of the central nervous system comprise bacterial meningitis and fungal or parasitic focal brain lesions. Acute primary bacterial meningitis occurs at a frequency similar to that of the general population. Bacterial meningitis also may occur in the context of bloodstream infections or as a complication of intrathecal chemotherapy. Infectious foci in the retina are observed in patients with disseminated bacterial and fungal infections (Fig. 73.7b). Endocarditis may occur even in the absence of risk factors, but is notably uncommon despite the frequency of bacteremia with organisms known to cause endocarditis. Clavicular osteomyelitis may be seen in patients with tunnel infections of subclavian intravascular access devices.

PREVENTION

Environmental measures

Preventive measures aimed at reducing the acquisition or transmission of nosocomial pathogens play an important role in reducing the risk of infection in neutropenic patients.[5] Special emphasis should be placed on careful hand washing by personnel, which can substantially diminish the risk of transmission of pathogens. Education of patients, family members, medical and nursing staff is essential. Contact with persons with overt respiratory or cutaneous infections must be avoided.

Patients should receive a well-cooked and low-microbial food diet and have access to safe water and ice supply. For patients with severe and prolonged neutropenia, air ultrafiltration may be desirable in settings where Aspergillus infections are frequently observed. When an optimal protective environment is required, clean air is provided by means of constant positive-pressure air flow and/or high-efficiency particulate air filtration. In addition, intensive disinfection measures are generally employed in high-risk patients. These include the use of antimicrobial mouth wash solutions, disinfectant soaps, creams and sprays. Proper oral and dental hygiene and careful nursing of the anal region are essential. Insertion and manipulations of intravascular access devices and bone marrow aspiration should be performed with great care and under strict aseptic conditions. Whenever possible, the use of nasogastric tubing and urinary catheters should be avoided.

Surveillance cultures of oropharynx, stools, urine and skin are of limited utility for the management of individual neutropenic patients, as they lack sensitivity and specificity for predicting and identifying the etiologic agent of infection and are costly and time-consuming. However, these cultures might be useful for epidemiologic studies and infection control purposes.

Antimicrobial prophylaxis

Prophylactic antimicrobial therapy has been used to suppress colonization by potential pathogens in high-risk neutropenic patients. Different strategies have been employed to prevent bacterial and fungal infections and reactivation of latent viral infections with mixed results. Thus, considerable controversy still surrounds the topic of antimicrobial prophylaxis for the prevention of infection in the neutropenic host.

Antibiotic prophylaxis

Oral nonabsorbable antibiotics have been used to achieve gut decontamination, since the bowel is the main reservoir of endogenous flora and an important source of infection in granulocytopenic cancer patients. However, the use of antibiotics such as vancomycin, gentamicin, polymyxin B, nystatin or colistin is associated with several problems. These antibiotics are nonpalatable and poorly tolerated, so that compliance is poor. Clinical efficacy has not been clearly demonstrated. Furthermore, administration of prophylactic oral antibiotics may induce resistance among endogenous bacteria, such as resistance to vancomycin among enterococci. Thus, prophylaxis with nonabsorbable antimicrobial agents has been abandoned in most institutions.

Alternatively, attempts have been made to 'selectively' decontaminate the alimentary tract using antibiotics such as trimethoprim–sulfamethoxazole (TMP-SMX; co-trimoxazole) to maintain the anaerobic flora, thereby preserving the 'colonization resistance' against aerobic bacteria and fungi. Results of initial studies suggested that TMP-SMX could decrease the incidence of infections, but this was not confirmed in subsequent studies. Furthermore, TMP-SMX is ineffective against P. aeruginosa, may prolong the duration of the bone marrow aplasia, and promote the emergence of resistant organisms. Current guidelines recommend the use of TMP-SMX only in patients at high risk of Pneumocystis jirovecii (formerly P. carinii) infection.[5]

In contrast to all other antibiotics used for prophylaxis of bacterial infections, fluoroquinolones have been unequivocally shown to reduce the incidence of Gram-negative infections, but the impact on the occurrence of fever, microbiologically or clinically documented infections, or infection-related mortality is less clear. The results of four meta-analyses are summarized in Figure 73.13.[35] Moreover, the use of fluoroquinolone prophylaxis was associated with an increased incidence of viridans streptococcal infections and emergence of resistance.[10,12] Levofloxacin, a fluoroquinolone with extended anti-Gram-positive activity, was recently found to reduce the incidence of febrile neutropenia when used as prophylaxis in patients with hematologic malignancies or solid tumors. The number needed to treat to prevent one febrile episode was 5 and 23, respectively.[36,37] However, the impact of levofloxacin prophylaxis on the morbidity and mortality associated with febrile neutropenia is limited, may vary from center to center and is in fact marginal in solid tumor patients.[38] Based on these data and on a recent meta-analysis, fluoroquinolone prophylaxis has been recommended for prevention of infection in patients with

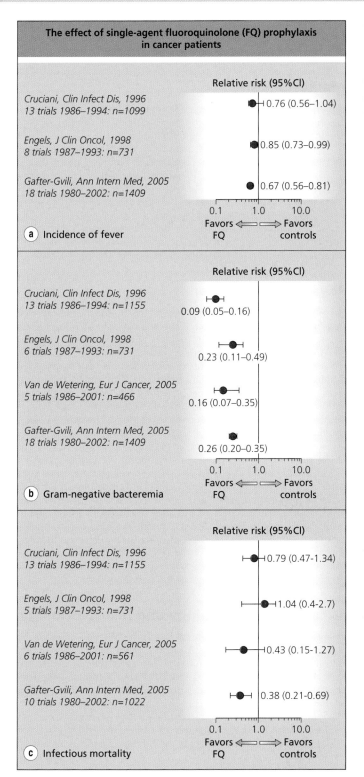

The effect of single-agent fluoroquinolone (FQ) prophylaxis in cancer patients

Relative risk (95%CI)

Cruciani, Clin Infect Dis, 1996
13 trials 1986–1994: n=1099 — 0.76 (0.56–1.04)

Engels, J Clin Oncol, 1998
8 trials 1987–1993: n=731 — 0.85 (0.73–0.99)

Gafter-Gvili, Ann Intern Med, 2005
18 trials 1980–2002: n=1409 — 0.67 (0.56–0.81)

0.1   1.0   10.0
Favors ⟸ ⟹ Favors
FQ   controls

(a) Incidence of fever

Relative risk (95%CI)

Cruciani, Clin Infect Dis, 1996
13 trials 1986–1994: n=1155
0.09 (0.05–0.16)

Engels, J Clin Oncol, 1998
6 trials 1987–1993: n=731
0.23 (0.11–0.49)

Van de Wetering, Eur J Cancer, 2005
5 trials 1986–2001: n=466
0.16 (0.07–0.35)

Gafter-Gvili, Ann Intern Med, 2005
18 trials 1980–2002: n=1409
0.26 (0.20–0.35)

0.1   1.0   10.0
Favors ⟸ ⟹ Favors
FQ   controls

(b) Gram-negative bacteremia

Relative risk (95%CI)

Cruciani, Clin Infect Dis, 1996
13 trials 1986–1994: n=1155 — 0.79 (0.47-1.34)

Engels, J Clin Oncol, 1998
5 trials 1987–1993: n=731 — 1.04 (0.4-2.7)

Van de Wetering, Eur J Cancer, 2005
6 trials 1986–2001: n=561 — 0.43 (0.15-1.27)

Gafter-Gvili, Ann Intern Med, 2005
10 trials 1980–2002: n=1022 — 0.38 (0.21-0.69)

0.1   1.0   10.0
Favors ⟸ ⟹ Favors
FQ   controls

(c) Infectious mortality

Fig. 73.13 Meta-analyses of the effect of single-agent fluoroquinolone (FQ) prophylaxis compared with that of placebo or no prophylaxis on the incidence of fever (a), Gram-negative bacteremia (b) and infectious mortality (c) in neutropenic cancer patients with hematologic malignancies. Red circles and black bars show relative risks with 95% confidence intervals in patients receiving fluoroquinolone prophylaxis compared to patients receiving placebo or other regimens. Adapted from references[11,35,40,81].

Table 73.2 Arguments in favor and against the use of fluoroquinolones and azoles for prophylaxis of infections in neutropenic patients

In favor	Against
Prevention of documented bacterial and fungal infections	Severe morbidity and mortality of bacterial and fungal infections infrequent in many centers
Prevention of febrile neutropenia	Exposure of large number of patients to routine antibacterial or antifungal prophylaxis: toxicity, resistance, costs
Reduced use of empirical antibacterial and antifungal therapy	Prophylaxis precludes use of the same class of agents for empirical therapy
Prevention of severe complications and mortality	New management strategies allow a targeted use of anti-infective agents

acute leukemia and haemopoietic stem cell transplantation (HSCT) recipients by experts of the first European Conference on Infections in Leukemia (ECIL-1).[39,40]

Clinicians remain divided on the utility and safety of antibiotic prophylaxis. While some consider that it should be strongly discouraged for the reasons mentioned above, others favor the use of fluoroquinolones, especially in high-risk patients with hematologic malignancies. Of note, once used as prophylaxis, fluoroquinolone antibiotics can no longer be used for empiric therapy of febrile neutropenia. This is a significant drawback for solid tumor patients in whom these agents are a key component of oral empiric regimens for outpatient therapy. The decision to use prophylaxis in a single center should therefore be based on a comprehensive evaluation of multiple factors including the frequency of severe complications. While this strategy may be efficacious in some settings, it may be of marginal utility in others. Arguments in favor and against the use of antibacterial prophylaxis are summarized in Table 73.2.

Antifungal prophylaxis

There is a lack of evidence suggesting a benefit of oral nonabsorbable antifungal agents and this practice has been abandoned in many institutions. In allogeneic hematopoietic transplant recipients, systemic antifungal prophylaxis with fluconazole (400 mg/d) has been shown to prevent infection with *C. albicans* and *C. tropicalis*, but not with *C. krusei*.[41] The activity of fluconazole against *C. glabrata* is unpredictable.

The utility of antifungal prophylaxis in patients with hematologic malignancies not undergoing bone marrow transplantation is less clear. Prophylaxis with ketoconazole, intravenous amphotericin B, fluconazole or itraconazole was found to reduce the incidence of superficial infections, but no consistent effects were observed on the incidence of invasive fungal infections, empiric use of amphotericin B or mortality of invasive fungal infections.[42] In some centers, the use of fluconazole prophylaxis was linked to a shift towards non-*albicans* *Candida* strains with either reduced *in-vitro* susceptibility (*C. glabrata*) or intrinsic resistance (*C. krusei*) to azoles, which may be associated with increased mortality.[16,43] Micafungin, a member of the echinocandin class of antifungal agents with activity against *Candida* and *Aspergillus* spp., was found to be superior to fluconazole for a composite end point (i.e. absence of suspected invasive fungal infection requiring empiric antifungal therapy and absence of documented breakthrough invasive mycoses) in hematopoietic stem cell transplant recipients.[44] However, this study failed to demonstrate a significant difference in the incidence of invasive mycoses or in mortality.

Few data are available on the use of other echinocandins (e.g. caspofungin, anidulafungin) as prophylaxis. Posaconazole, a new triazole with activity against *Candida* and *Aspergillus* spp. and emerging molds such as zygomycetes, was superior to fluconazole or itraconazole for the prevention of invasive fungal infections and reduced fungal-related deaths in allogeneic hematopoietic transplant recipients with graft-versus-host disease and in patients with acute leukemia and neutropenia.[45a, 45b]

Despite these overall encouraging results, antifungal prophylaxis remains a matter of great debate among experts. The arguments in favor and against antifungal prophylaxis are summarized in Table 73.2.[18,46] Antifungal prophylaxis is reasonable in selected high-risk conditions such as allogeneic hematopoietic stem cell transplantation or induction chemotherapy for acute leukemia. The choice of the antifungal agent (coverage of *Candida* or of both *Candida* and *Aspergillus*) should be guided by local epidemiologic data and by the patient's condition.[5]

Antiviral prophylaxis

Viral serology tests should be performed at the onset of chemotherapy to determine whether patients with hematologic malignancies have been previously infected with HSV, VZV or CMV as these may reactivate during therapy. Reactivation of HSV infection occurs in 70–80% of patients with acute leukemia receiving chemotherapy. Aciclovir prophylaxis is therefore recommended for HSV-seropositive individuals.[47] Oral valaciclovir is an alternative to oral aciclovir. Patients unable to take oral medications should be switched to intravenous aciclovir. CMV-seronegative patients with leukemia who may benefit from allogeneic hematopoietic stem cell transplantation should receive leukocyte-depleted blood products to prevent CMV transmission. Those interested in further reading on antiviral prophylaxis should refer to Chapter 146.

Immunoglobulins

Replacement therapy with intravenous immunoglobulins may be indicated for patients with low serum concentrations of immunoglobulins (e.g. IgG <50% of the lower normal limit or <4 g/l) or a history of severe bacterial infections in the context of chronic lymphocytic leukemia, multiple myeloma or bone marrow transplant patients in the post-engraftment period. This topic, along with vaccine strategies in the immunocompromised host, is discussed in detail in Chapter 83.

Vaccinations

The routine vaccination of oncohematologic patients with the 23-valent pneumococcal vaccine is generally recommended; similar recommendations exist for patients following HSCT after immune reconstitution (i.e. within 12–24 months after engraftment). During the influenza season, the vaccination of cancer patients – and especially of family members, health-care workers and other close contacts – may reduce transmission and infection-related morbidity and mortality[48] (see Chapter 83).

Prevention of mucositis

Palifermin, a recombinant epithelial growth factor, has been shown recently to protect hematopoietic stem cell recipients undergoing total body irradiation against severe oropharyngeal mucositis and to reduce the incidence of associated febrile neutropenic episodes.[49] Whether this observation applies to other populations of neutropenic patients remains to be investigated.

DIAGNOSIS

Evaluation of the febrile neutropenic cancer patient follows the universal principles guiding medical practice, including a prompt and thorough medical history and physical examination and use of rigorous diagnostic measures. However, in contrast to the non-neutropenic patient, empiric broad-spectrum antibiotic therapy should be administered without delay after the onset of fever and before the results of the microbiologic investigations become available.

Medical history

It is critical that cancer patients are thoroughly investigated at presentation with a special emphasis on the assessment of risk of infection. Medical history should include information on:
- travels to, or residence in, areas where infectious diseases (such as tuberculosis, fungal or parasitic infections, e.g. leishmaniasis or strongyloidiasis) are endemic, as these may reactivate during neutropenia;
- immunization history; and
- presence of vascular access devices.

Upon development of fever, the physician must obtain a meticulous history, and be aware of the fact that symptoms may be modified because of the impaired inflammatory response.[5]

Physical examination

Physical examination should be particularly thorough and must be performed keeping in mind that the classic signs of infection are markedly attenuated (e.g. pain, redness and induration) or absent (pus) because of neutropenia.[5] The physician should look for subtle inflammatory signs at common sites of infection (e.g. oropharynx, esophagus, respiratory tract, skin, insertion site of intravascular catheters, gastrointestinal tract, perianal region). The mouth and pharynx should be examined for erythema, mucositis, gingivitis, white patches and pseudomembranes, vesicles and ulcerations. The anterior nares should be inspected for signs of congestion, rhinorrhea, crusts, bleeding and ulcers. The skin may present features of a localized (i.e. primary) infection or multiple lesions in distant areas suggestive of a disseminated infection (Figs 73.5b, 73.6). Special attention should be paid to the presence of erythema, swelling and tenderness in the anal, perineal, axillary and periungual regions (Fig. 73.5a). Insertion sites of intravascular access devices and sites of cutaneous injury due to needle punctures or bone marrow aspiration should be thoroughly examined. Fundoscopy should be performed as it may reveal the presence of signs of systemic infection (Fig. 73.7b). Physical examination should be repeated frequently as clinical signs of infection may become manifest only a few days after the onset of fever.

Microbiology, radiology and histopathology

At least two sets of blood cultures should be obtained prior to the administration of antibiotics in the febrile neutropenic patient. Blood cultures are recommended even in the absence of fever in any patient with suspected infection. Blood should be drawn from a peripheral vein and also from intravascular catheters, if present.[5] It is prudent to draw blood from every port of multilumen intravascular devices. Qualitative cultures are performed routinely, but quantitative cultures might be helpful for the diagnosis of catheter-related bloodstream infections.[50] However, the yield of blood cultures in patients already on broad-spectrum antibiotics is notoriously poor. New molecular diagnostic methods such as polymerase chain reaction (PCR) may improve our ability to document the etiology of infection in these patients or in patients infected with micro-organisms that are difficult to grow.

Specimens (aspirate or biopsy) should be obtained from any site suspected of infection. The physician should carefully evaluate the benefits and risks (mainly bleeding in the thrombocytopenic patient) of initial (i.e. at the onset of fever) versus delayed (i.e. in those patients who are not responding to empiric therapy) invasive procedures to diagnose infections in poorly accessible sites. Exit sites of catheters should be cultured for bacterial, fungal and nontuberculous mycobacterial pathogens. Skin lesions should be aspirated or, whenever possible, biopsied for culture and/or histopathologic examination. Lesions of the oral cavity, pharynx and paranasal sinuses can be brushed or biopsied. In the presence of severe dysphagia, endoscopy with brushing and biopsy for cultures and histopathology should be considered. Stools from patients with diarrhea should be tested for *Clostridium difficile* toxins and cultured for bacteria (*Clostridia, Salmonella, Shigella, Campylobacter, Aeromonas* and *Yersinia* spp.) and protozoa (*Cryptosporidium*). Urinalysis and urine cultures should be performed routinely, even in the absence of urinary symptoms or of pyuria, a rare finding in neutropenic patients even when infection is present.

A chest radiograph is part of the standard workup of febrile neutropenic patients. Whether or not, and when, to obtain additional radiologic imaging is guided by the patient's clinical condition and response to empiric broad-spectrum antibiotics. For example, severe abdominal complaints in neutropenic patients will prompt thorough investigations with standard radiography, ultrasonography, CT or MRI scans. Patients with lesions of the liver and spleen suggestive of hepatosplenic candidiasis should undergo CT-guided or laparoscopic liver biopsy. The presence of lung infiltrates has important implications for the management of neutropenic patients. Several studies have shown that CT scanning is superior to conventional radiography for revealing the presence of lesions indicative of invasive aspergillosis that should prompt further investigations (bronchoalveolar lavage, transbronchial, transthoracic or open lung biopsy) to obtain samples for diagnosis.[51] Persistent or complicated sinusitis, otitis and suspected osteomyelitis or myositis are other indications for additional radiologic imaging and tissue sampling. Once again, it should be remembered that radiologic signs are attenuated and delayed in neutropenic patients, and may become apparent only after bone marrow recovery. Classic examples are hepatosplenic candidiasis and invasive pulmonary aspergillosis.[34]

Baseline viral (HSV, VZV, CMV, EBV) and parasitic (*Toxoplasma gondii*) serology should be obtained in patients with hematologic malignancies, especially when allogeneic hematopoietic transplant is contemplated, but not in those with solid tumors as they are not at high risk of developing severe viral or parasitic infections.

Novel nonculture diagnostic tests including molecular and serologic techniques have been described recently. These include the use of PCR for the diagnosis of bacterial and fungal infections and the serologic detection of circulating antigens (e.g. mannan for *Candida* species, galactomannan for *Aspergillus* species, and β-1,3-D-glucan for *Candida, Aspergillus* and other fungal species), metabolites (e.g. D-arabinitol for *Candida* species), and antibodies directed against fungal antigens (e.g. antimannan antibodies).[52–56] Variable diagnostic performances of these new tools have been reported. False-negative results have been associated with the use of antifungal prophylaxis, prompt initiation of antifungal therapy, localized infections and with infections caused by fungal species lacking or expressing low amounts of these markers. Conversely, false-positive results have been described in patients colonized by fungi at nonsterile sites or treated with semisynthetic penicillins. Whereas galactomannan is now routinely used in many institutions, additional studies are needed before the use of the other noninvasive tools can be recommended.

Circulating biologic markers of inflammation, such as C-reactive protein and proinflammatory cytokines (such as tumor necrosis factor, interleukin-1, 6 and 8) are not helpful for differentiating infectious from non-infectious causes of fever because of a lack of sensitivity and specificity. Procalcitonin, a circulating calcitonin precursor whose blood concentrations are markedly increased during sepsis and much less so during the course of inflammatory diseases, looks promising. Yet, at the time of onset of fever in neutropenic patients (i.e. when start of empiric antibiotic therapy is recommended), procalcitonin levels are not elevated in the majority of patients with bacterial infections. Moreover, procalcitonin remains low in infections due to coagulase-negative staphylococci. Clinical studies have suggested that procalcitonin might be useful when reassessing the etiology of persistent fever after the first 48 hours of empiric antibacterial therapy. However, further investigations on procalcitonin-guided management strategies in febrile neutropenic cancer patients are needed.

Other investigations

Hematology (complete blood count and differential) and chemistry tests (including electrolytes, tests of liver and kidney function) are an integral part of the monitoring of toxic reactions to cytotoxic and antimicrobial agents and should therefore be repeated at regular intervals. Moreover, measurement of blood levels of antimicrobial agents should be undertaken, especially in patients with renal or hepatic dysfunction. This recommendation is particularly important for agents with narrow therapeutic windows, such as aminoglycosides, glycopeptides, some β-lactams and some triazole antifungals, and when the patient does not respond to therapy despite demonstration of *in-vitro* susceptibility.[5]

MANAGEMENT

Neutropenic patients with suspected infection, whether febrile or not, must receive prompt empiric antibiotic therapy with broad-spectrum antibiotics. The concept of treating these patients with empiric antibiotics as soon they develop fever has radically changed the otherwise fulminant and almost uniformly fatal course of Gram-negative sepsis.[2,4] This is the single most significant advance made over the last 30 years in the area of supportive care for cancer patients.

Risk assessment

Serious and potentially life-threatening complications may occur during the course of bone marrow aplasia, including hemorrhage, disseminated intravascular coagulation, thrombosis, pulmonary embolism, organ dysfunction (such as congestive heart failure, renal insufficiency, respiratory failure) and septic complications (such as severe sepsis, septic shock, adult respiratory distress syndrome), that may require admission to the intensive care unit.[57–59] Until recently, all febrile neutropenic cancer patients have been treated in a uniform fashion. Today, risk assessment is an important aspect of the evaluation of the febrile neutropenic patient. It is important to determine whether the patient is at low or high risk of serious infections or other medical complications because this will influence the treatment modalities and will have an impact on the patient's hospital course and length of stay. Several factors have been identified that can be used to classify a given patient into a low- or high-risk category.

Factors associated with a *low risk* of complications are shown in Table 73.3.[5,57,58] Typically, a low-risk profile is defined by the following characteristics: cancer in remission, absence of severe co-morbidities, outpatient status at onset of fever and neutropenia not likely to last for more than 7 days. Conversely, uncontrolled cancer, the presence of concomitant medical conditions (severe mucositis, hemorrhage, dehydration, renal, hepatic, respiratory, cardiac or circulatory failure, altered mental status), inpatient status and neutropenia expected to last for more than 7 days are factors likely to be associated with a *high risk* of complications.

Different scoring systems have been proposed for risk stratification.[57,58] The Multinational Association for Supportive Care in Cancer (MASCC) score is based on seven clinical factors derived and validated from prospective analyses of 756 and 383 episodes of febrile neutropenia, respectively.[58] A MASCC score greater than or equal to 21, on a maximum score of 26, was used to identify patients at low risk (<5%) of severe complications (sensitivity: 71%, specificity: 68%, positive predictive value: 91%, negative predictive value: 36%) and who might be candidates for outpatient empiric antimicrobial therapy. However, the experience with this and other scoring systems is still limited.[57,58] According to a recent single-center study, about 50% of low risk febrile cancer patients, as assessed by the MASCC score, can be treated orally and 25% can be safely managed on an outpatient basis.[60]

Additional prospective studies are needed to more fully evaluate and finely tune the use of these risk assessment systems. It will be

Table 73.3 Factors associated with a low risk of severe complications in febrile neutropenic cancer patients

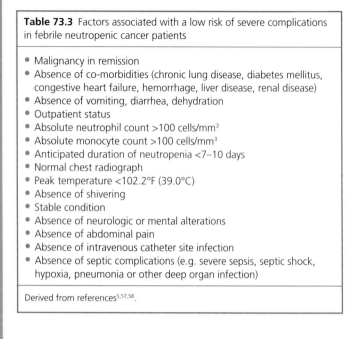

- Malignancy in remission
- Absence of co-morbidities (chronic lung disease, diabetes mellitus, congestive heart failure, hemorrhage, liver disease, renal disease)
- Absence of vomiting, diarrhea, dehydration
- Outpatient status
- Absolute neutrophil count >100 cells/mm³
- Absolute monocyte count >100 cells/mm³
- Anticipated duration of neutropenia <7–10 days
- Normal chest radiograph
- Peak temperature <102.2°F (39.0°C)
- Absence of shivering
- Stable condition
- Absence of neurologic or mental alterations
- Absence of abdominal pain
- Absence of intravenous catheter site infection
- Absence of septic complications (e.g. severe sepsis, septic shock, hypoxia, pneumonia or other deep organ infection)

Derived from references[5,57,58].

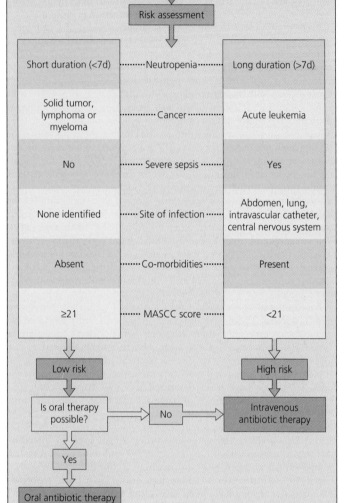

Fig. 73.14 Selection of intravenous or oral empiric antibiotic therapy based on risk assessment in febrile neutropenic patients. Severe sepsis and septic shock are defined according to reference[59]. Adapted from reference[6].

important to make sure that low-risk patients may be safely treated with oral antibiotics on an outpatient basis (see Oral antibiotic therapy, below). An algorithm for risk assessment may be used for guiding the choice of oral versus parenteral empiric antibiotic therapy (Fig. 73.14).

Empiric antibiotic therapy

Intravenous antibiotics

Over 90% of the first episodes of infection in neutropenic cancer patients are caused by Gram-positive and Gram-negative bacteria (Table 73.1 and Fig. 73.1). Empiric antibiotic regimens must be broad-spectrum and bactericidal, achieve high circulating and tissue levels and be nontoxic. For more than two decades, combinations of two or more intravenous antibiotics have been the 'gold standard' of empiric antibiotic therapy. Numerous combinations of antipseudomonal penicillins (e.g. mezlocillin, ticarcillin with or without clavulanic acid, azlocillin or piperacillin with or without tazobactam) or third- or fourth-generation cephalosporins (ceftazidime, ceftriaxone, cefpirome, cefepime) plus an aminoglycoside (gentamicin, tobramycin, netilmicin or amikacin) have been frequently utilized.[4,26,61] No regimen was shown to be superior to the others. For example, ceftazidime and amikacin was a popular antibiotic combination in the late 1980s and 1990s. However, aminoglycoside-containing regimens are associated with renal and auditory toxicity, especially in patients concomitantly receiving other toxic agents and often require monitoring of drug levels.

Thus, new treatment approaches have been explored to avoid these complications, such as once-daily dosing of aminoglycoside or β-lactam monotherapy. An international, multicenter trial of the EORTC-IATG showed that once-daily ceftriaxone and amikacin was as effective as, and at least no more toxic than, a combination of ceftazidime and amikacin given thrice daily.[62] Monotherapy with broad-spectrum and highly bactericidal agents, such as third- or fourth-generation cephalosporins (ceftazidime, cefepime, cefpirome), carbapenems (imipenem and meropenem) or antipseudomonal penicillins combined with a β-lactamase inhibitor (piperacillin–tazobactam) were found to be as effective as and less toxic than combinations of β-lactam and aminoglycoside.[28,63] The third-generation cephalosporin ceftazidime displays a limited activity against Gram-positive bacteria and no anti-anaerobic activity. Recent studies have suggested that ceftazidime may be less efficacious than carbapenems.[63,64]

Choices of intravenous empiric antibiotic therapy for high-risk patients, typically those with hematologic malignancies and long-duration neutropenia, are shown in Figure 73.15. Choices should be guided by the patient's clinical condition and local epidemiologic data. Consider using an aminoglycoside-containing regimen in critically ill patients, such as those with severe sepsis or septic shock, when a *P. aeruginosa* infection is suspected or when resistant Gram-negative bacteria prevail, including ESBL-producing strains. Consider using a glycopeptide antibiotic (vancomycin or teicoplanin) in patients with catheter-related infections, when penicillin-resistant streptococcal or methicillin-resistant staphylococcal infections are suspected or in critically ill patients with severe sepsis or septic shock. However, outside of these well-defined clinical circumstances encountered in a minority of patients, routine use of glycopeptide antibiotics is strongly discouraged. Empiric use of vancomycin has not been shown to improve patient outcome and is associated with increased costs, toxicity and

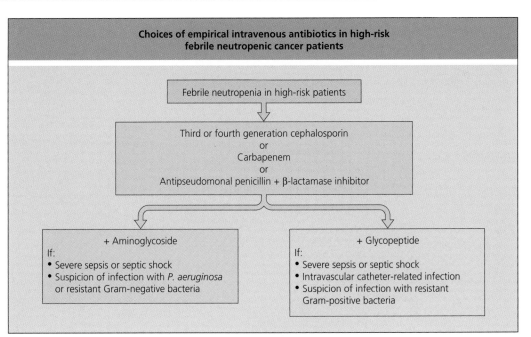

emergence of resistance. Whether new anti-Gram-positive agents (linezolid, quinupristin–dalfopristin, daptomycin, telavancin or dalbavancin) will provide new treatment options in neutropenic patients needs to be investigated.

After proper investigations and microbiologic cultures, it is reasonable to empirically use:

- an antifungal and/or antiviral agent in patients with esophagitis;
- a macrolide or 'respiratory' fluoroquinolone and/or TMP-SMX and/or an antifungal agent for coverage of opportunistic respiratory pathogens in patients with lung infiltrates;
- metronidazole in patients with an abdominal or perianal focus of infection and/or severe diarrhea; and
- TMP-SMX in severely ill patients with relapsing fever who are at risk of superinfection due to multiresistant *Stenotrophomonas maltophilia*.

The role of new parenteral broad-spectrum antibacterial agents such as ertapenem, doripenem, tigecycline, ceftobiprole, and telithromycin in febrile neutropenic patients remains to be determined.

Oral antibiotic therapy

Several studies have examined the role of oral absorbable antibiotics as empiric therapy of fever and suspected infections in low-risk adult patients with solid tumors and neutropenia expected to be of short duration (less than 7 days). Oral antibiotic therapy is possible when the patient is compliant, can swallow tablets, has normal gastrointestinal motility and function, and can be monitored for response to therapy, development of secondary infections and adverse reactions. Ofloxacin or ciprofloxacin given either alone or combined with amoxicillin–clavulanic acid have been studied in adult patients.[65,66] However, ofloxacin and ciprofloxacin have suboptimal activities against Gram-positive bacteria and should not be used as monotherapy. In contrast, oral ciprofloxacin plus amoxicillin–clavulanic acid was found to be as efficacious and safe as standard parenteral treatment in two large studies of low-risk patients in an inpatient setting.[29,30] New 'extended-spectrum' fluoroquinolones (i.e. moxifloxacin and gatifloxacin) with improved activity against Gram-positive bacteria are being investigated as monotherapy in febrile neutropenic patients. Of note, fluoroquinolone-containing oral regimens cannot be considered in neutropenic patients in whom fever develops during fluoroquinolone prophylaxis.

Despite preliminary favorable clinical observations, it has not yet been unequivocally demonstrated that management of low-risk febrile patients on a fully outpatient basis is safe.[60] At the present time, it is reasonable to discharge compliant patients who have responded to therapy, despite persistence of neutropenia, provided that the patient is not alone at home, is under careful medical supervision and lives within a short distance of a hospital.

There are no data on upfront oral antibiotic therapy of fever in children with neutropenia. Limited information is available on early discharge of selected children on oral cefixime 48 hours after intravenous antibiotic therapy in a hospital setting.[67]

Reassessment of therapy

The appropriateness of the empiric antibiotic regimen should be reassessed within 24–72 hours based on the results of microbiologic cultures and the patient's response to antibiotic therapy.

Therapeutic modifications based on culture results

If a pathogen has been isolated, antibiotic therapy is adapted based on *in-vitro* susceptibility tests and clinical response (Fig. 73.16). Vancomycin (or teicoplanin, a glycopeptide antibiotic not approved by the US Food and Drug Administration, which has been studied and used in some European countries) should be added if cultures grew methicillin-resistant staphylococci, penicillin-resistant streptococci or enterococci not covered by the empiric regimen. Recently introduced antibiotics such as quinupristin–dalfopristin (a streptogramin), linezolid (an oxazolidinone), daptomycin (a lipopeptide antibiotic), tigecycline (a tetracycline derivative) and other anti-Gram-positive drugs under development (e.g. telavancin, dalbavancin, ceftobiprole) exhibit excellent *in-vitro* activities against penicillin-resistant streptococci, methicillin-resistant staphylococci and vancomycin-resistant enterococci and might offer new therapeutic options for febrile neutropenic cancer patients. However, there is limited clinical experience with these antibiotics in these patients. Moreover, linezolid may cause thrombocytopenia and anemia when used for more than 2 weeks.

Three studies have now clearly shown that there is no indication for empiric use of vancomycin in centers where resistance of Gram-positive bacteria to β-lactam antibiotics is rare.[27,68,69] However, as

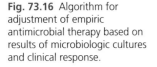

Fig. 73.16 Algorithm for adjustment of empiric antimicrobial therapy based on results of microbiologic cultures and clinical response.

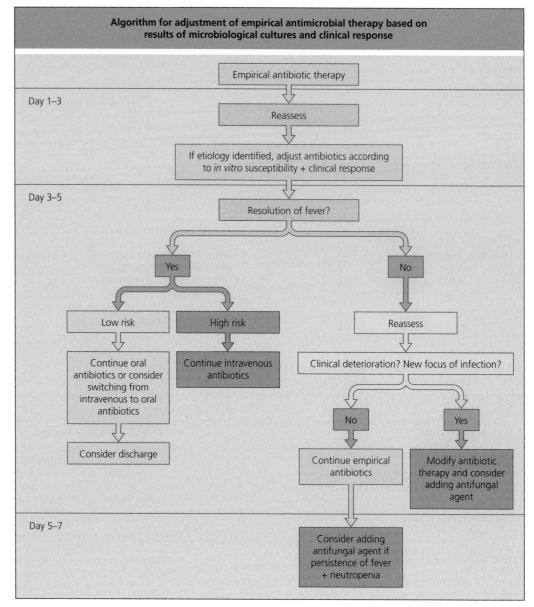

mentioned previously, the empiric use of vancomycin is justified in critically ill patients with severe sepsis or septic shock, in the presence of a catheter-related infection and in centers with high levels of β-lactam resistance among Gram-positive bacteria other than common skin colonizers such as coagulase-negative staphylococci. If suspicion of resistant Gram-positive infection is disproved by culture results, empiric vancomycin should be rapidly discontinued. Likewise, empiric use of an aminoglycoside should be stopped as soon as β-lactam-resistant Gram-negative bacteria are ruled out.

Therapeutic modifications based on initial response to empiric antibiotic therapy

It is necessary to treat patients for 3–5 days before one can begin to evaluate the response to therapy with some degree of confidence. However, earlier treatment adjustments may be required if the patient's condition deteriorates. Treatment recommendations for patients who have become afebrile and for those who remained febrile within 3–5 days after initiation of empiric therapy are presented in Figure 73.16.

Resolution of fever

Intravenous (high risk) or oral (low risk) antibiotics should be continued in patients who have responded to therapy (Fig. 73.16). In low-risk patients receiving intravenous antibiotics, switching to oral antibiotics, such as ciprofloxacin and amoxicillin–clavulanic acid or monotherapy with new-generation fluoroquinolones with extended anti-Gram-positive activity (e.g. moxifloxacin, levofloxacin, gatifloxacin), should be considered. In the absence of microbiologic proof and identified site of infection (i.e. FUO), it is usually not necessary to continue broad-spectrum antibiotics for longer than 7 days, if fever resolved quickly and the neutrophil count has returned to normal levels. Antibiotics can be stopped when the patient is afebrile for more than 48 hours and the neutrophil count is >500/mm³ for two consecutive days.[5]

Opinions differ regarding the optimal duration of therapy in patients with persistent neutropenia. Some physicians discontinue therapy in afebrile and clinically stable patients, while others prefer to continue broad-spectrum intravenous or oral antibiotics until recovery of neutrophils. Yet, the evidence supporting continuation of broad-spectrum antibiotics is not strong and is based on data obtained 20 years ago in a limited number of patients with FUO. In that study, nearly half of the patients with persistent neutropenia became febrile again within 3 days of stopping treatment and breakthrough infections and severe septic complications occurred.[70] Patients with microbiologically or clinically documented infections are usually treated for a total of 10–14 days (i.e. until cultures become sterile and clinical response is complete). However, prolonged antibiotic courses are costly and may be associated with toxicity and emergence of resistant bacterial or opportunistic fungal infections.

Persistence of fever

It is important to keep in mind that the median time to defervescence is 5 days in high-risk patients with hematologic malignancies. Therefore, persistence of fever may not necessarily indicate that treatment is failing. If a specific causal organism or an infection site has been identified, treatment should be continued or modified, as appropriate.[5]

Considerable controversy surrounds the optimal management of a stable patient with unexplained fever after 3 days of empiric therapy. Persistence of fever may be due to a slow response, suboptimal levels of antibiotics, resistant pathogens, nonbacterial infection, development of a secondary infection or a noninfectious etiology (such as cancer, transfusion reaction or drug fever). A thorough clinical examination, follow-up microbiologic cultures, extensive radiologic imaging (including a CT scan of the chest and abdomen) and invasive investigations, whenever possible, are an integral part of the workup of the persistently febrile neutropenic patient.

If the patient's clinical condition is deteriorating, management depends on whether or not the patient has developed a clinically obvious focus of infection. If a focus of infection has been found, attempts should be made to identify the causative pathogen by culture or biopsy. The antimicrobial treatment should then be modified accordingly. Moreover, withdrawal of an infected intravascular catheter is indicated, when the local signs of infection are extending, when the patient is clinically unstable, when a septic thrombophlebitis is documented or when infection is due to pathogens other than common skin colonizers.[5] In contrast, the utility of antibiotic lock solutions or rotation of antibiotic delivery via the different ports of multilumen catheters is controversial.

If there is no obvious site of infection, the patient is not deteriorating and reassessment does not reveal a new focus of infection, the physician has the choice between several treatment options:

- *continue* the initial empiric antibiotics for 2 more days;
- *change the antibiotics* (change of broad-spectrum β-lactam, addition of a glycopeptide or of an aminoglycoside);
- *add empirically an antifungal agent* (intravenous amphotericin B deoxycholate, lipid formulations of amphotericin B, itraconazole, voriconazole or caspofungin).

In this situation, our approach is to continue the initial antibiotic regimen and initiate early (i.e. within 48–96 hours after the onset of fever) empiric antifungal treatment, especially in the following circumstances:

- expected long-lasting neutropenia (>10 days);
- recurrent episodes of fever during the same episode of neutropenia;
- prolonged therapy with broad-spectrum antibiotics;
- *Candida* colonization of the oropharynx or gastrointestinal tract and severe mucositis or neutropenic enterocolitis;
- presence of one or multiple lung infiltrates;
- positive circulating fungal markers such as galactomannan, β-1,3-D-glucan, mannan/antimannan; or
- epidemiologic data indicating a high incidence of mold infections.

Fungal infections due to *Candida* or *Aspergillus* species are a frequent cause of persistent fever in this setting. Unfortunately, early diagnosis is difficult and infections are *often diagnosed at autopsy*.[2]

Studies conducted in persistently febrile neutropenic patients in the 1980s have suggested that empiric intravenous amphotericin B may reduce the morbidity and mortality due to invasive fungal infections.[71] Yet, the patient population has changed (e.g. due to evolving myeloablative

regimens, frequent use of antifungal prophylaxis and availability of new diagnostic tools) and no contemporary randomized controlled studies have definitively shown improved outcomes compared to placebo. Treatment guidelines recommend starting empiric amphotericin B after 4–7 days of unexplained fever, but this is purely arbitrary as the optimal timing for starting therapy is unknown.[5] The potential advantage of an early start must be balanced against the risk of unnecessary toxicity, emergence of resistant fungi and the not insignificant costs of a broad use of antifungal agents. Once started, it is recommended to continue empiric antifungal therapy until bone marrow recovery, at which time investigations (i.e. thoracic and abdominal CT scan) should be repeated to confirm or rule out the presence of an until then occult fungal infection. No further therapy is needed if an invasive fungal infection can be reasonably excluded. Conversely, any lesion suggestive of invasive mycosis after neutrophil recovery, such as cavitating pulmonary lesions or multiple hepatosplenic lesions, should, whenever possible, undergo extensive workup such as bronchoalveolar lavage and tissue biopsies for culture and histopathology. Treatment should be then reassessed if a fungal pathogen is isolated. Prolonged antifungal therapy is often necessary when an invasive mycosis has been diagnosed, as the patient is likely to undergo multiple cycles of chemotherapy. On the other hand, surgical resection should be considered in between two cycles of chemotherapy in the case of invasive pulmonary aspergillosis, especially in patients with a single lesion, with lesions at high risk of bleeding due to close contact with hilar blood vessels or in presence of hemoptysis.[51]

For decades, amphotericin B deoxycholate, a fungicidal agent active against most species of *Candida* and *Aspergillus*, has been the standard treatment for fungal infections. However, renal and infusion-related toxicity often lead to suboptimal dosing or discontinuation of therapy and emergence of resistant fungi has been reported. Lipid formulations of amphotericin B (lipid-complex, colloidal dispersion and liposomal form) are better tolerated, but costly.[72] Factors limiting the use of fluconazole as empiric antifungal treatment in persistently febrile neutropenic patients are its fungistatic activity for *Candida* species, lack of activity on *Aspergillus* and an increasing incidence of azole-resistant *Candida* species. Recent studies have shown that itraconazole and voriconazole are treatment alternatives to amphotericin B in this indication.[73,74] Voriconazole has been shown to prevent breakthrough fungal infections during neutropenia, to be efficacious for candidemia in non-neutropenic patients and to be a first choice therapy for invasive aspergillosis in immunocompromised hosts.[75] However, azole prophylaxis precludes the use of any agent of this class as empiric therapy for persistent febrile neutropenia. One should also keep in mind that azoles are fungistatic against *Candida*, which might reduce their efficacy in the context of neutropenia. Echinocandins, a new class of antifungal agents that inhibit fungal cell wall synthesis, show promising efficacy and toxicity profiles. Caspofungin has recently been licensed for salvage therapy of refractory invasive aspergillosis. A recent trial also showed that caspofungin was as effective as and less toxic than amphotericin B for the treatment of invasive candidiasis.[76] Finally, caspofungin has been shown to be as efficacious as and better tolerated than liposomal amphotericin B for empiric therapy of persistently febrile neutropenic patients.[77]

Evidence-based guidelines from the European Consensus Conference on Infections in Leukemia have proposed the following grading of recommendations for empiric antifungal therapy according to the grading system of the Centers for Disease Control:

- AI (strongly recommended) for liposomal amphotericin B and caspofungin;
- BI (generally recommended) for amphotericin B deoxycholate, lipid complex or colloidal dispersion, voriconazole and itraconazole;
- CI (optional) for fluconazole; and
- DI (generally not recommended) for amphotericin B deoxycholate in the presence of renal impairment or risk factors for increased nephrotoxicity.

Other new compounds, including posaconazole, anidulafungin and micafungin are approved for clinical use, but no data are so far available on their empiric use in persistently febrile neutropenic patients. Moreover, the efficacy and safety of combinations of antifungal agents of different classes are being intensively investigated. Although there is no indication for their use in empiric therapy, combinations of liposomal amphotericin B or voriconazole with caspofungin have yielded promising results in case-control studies of salvage therapy of invasive aspergillosis.[78] These observations need to be confirmed in prospective, randomized studies in documented infections as the use of these costly strategies will have major economical implications.

Supportive care

Hematopoietic growth factors

The main goal pursued with the use of hematopoietic colony-stimulating factors (CSFs) is the acceleration of hematopoietic recovery to reduce the severity and duration of neutropenia and thus the risk of infections. Several studies have examined the role of granulocyte colony-stimulating factor (G-CSF, filgrastim) and granulocyte–monocyte colony-stimulating factor (GM-CSF, sargramostim) in the treatment of cancer patients not receiving bone marrow transplantation. Treatment with G-CSF or GM-CSF was found to moderately shorten the duration of neutropenia when given to patients with acute leukemia. Results were less striking in patients with solid tumors and other hematologic malignancies. In some, but not all, of these studies, a shorter duration of neutropenia was associated with a reduction of infections, use of antibiotics and length of stay, but without clear-cut benefit on the incidence of severe infections and infectious mortality. Moreover, no consistent effects on the duration of fever or antibiotic therapy, infectious morbidity or mortality, and costs have been demonstrated using CSFs in febrile neutropenic patients.

Recommendations for the use of CSFs have been published by the American Society for Clinical Oncology, the European Society of Medical Oncology and the European Organization for Research and Treatment of Cancer.[79-80] At the present time, the evidence supporting the use of CSFs in neutropenic patients not undergoing bone marrow transplantation is limited and opinions of experts remain divided.[5] Yet, high-risk patients with profound, long-lasting neutropenia and severe deep organ infections (e.g. pneumonia, typhlitis, invasive mycosis) not responding to appropriate antimicrobial therapy may benefit from an accelerated recovery of neutrophils. Although we occasionally use CSFs under such circumstances in our own institution, we acknowledge the fact that there is no definitive evidence to support the administration of CSFs in these clinical conditions. Intermittent administration of CSFs may be considered in patients with a myelodysplastic syndrome and recurrent infections due to chronic neutropenia.

Granulocyte transfusions

Some experts consider the transfusion of granulocytes in patients with profound neutropenia and life-threatening bacterial or fungal infections not responding to an adequate antimicrobial treatment. However, evidence of efficacy is lacking, and several problems are associated with this procedure, including transmission of CMV, alloimmunization, graft-versus-host reaction, and damage of lung capillaries with risk of acute respiratory distress syndrome.

Acknowledgments

We are thankful to Drs Frank Bally, Alain Cometta, Giorgio Merlani, Fabio Nessi and Owen Robinson, who kindly provided clinical and radiologic illustrations.

REFERENCES

References for this chapter can be found online at http://www.expertconsult.com

Kieren A Marr

Chapter | **74** |

Infections in hematopoietic stem cell transplant recipients

HEMATOPOIETIC STEM CELL TRANSPLANTATION: BACKGROUND AND CURRENT PRACTICES

Hematopoietic stem cell transplantation (HSCT) has been increasingly used to treat hematologic and nonhematologic malignancies and inherited immunodeficiencies. Multiple practices, including conditioning regimens, stem cell sources and supportive care strategies have changed since the first successful bone marrow transplantations, owed principally to an evolving understanding of how overall success is achieved and to the development of new technologies. As these factors impact on the severity and duration of infectious risks, and sometimes even the clinical presentations and outcomes, clinicians involved in the care of HSCT patients benefit greatly from a baseline understanding of transplant practices.

In order to allow for donor hematopoiesis to establish in the recipient, a conditioning regimen must be applied before infusion of stem cells. The primary aim of the conditioning regimen is to suppress recipient T cells that could ultimately mediate rejection of the graft. It was also hypothesized that myeloablative conditioning regimens could effectively eliminate residual malignant disease. To accomplish these goals, conventional regimens have been highly myeloablative, employing total body irradiation (TBI) and high-dose chemotherapy (e.g. busulphan, cyclophosphamide). In this setting, severe and protracted neutropenia, and regimen-related organ toxicities can contribute to early infectious complications.

The type of conditioning therapy has been shown to impact on overall risks and timing of infectious complications. Recently, nonmyeloablative or reduced-toxicity conditioning regimens have been used, especially for patients who are not eligible for conventional myeloablative HSCT. Success of this strategy relies on the therapeutic potential of graft-versus-host (GVH) effects, which are produced when donor-derived immune cells recognize and eventually destroy host tumor cells and tissues.[1] Although graft-versus-host disease (GVHD) negatively impacts on overall survival by causing organ injury, necessitating the need for increasingly immunosuppressive therapies, GVH effects also induce the beneficial effects of 'graft versus tumor', sometimes to a degree that can result in complete remission.[2] A number of alternative conditioning regimens have been developed which typically are associated with fewer organ toxicities (e.g. gastrointestinal tract mucositis) and shorter (if any) duration of neutropenia.[3–7]

The most common causes of death in allogeneic HSCT recipients are infection (frequently in the setting of GVHD) and relapsed malignancy. One method transplantation groups use to minimize the risks for relapse and GVHD is manipulation of the cells that compose the infused graft. Cellular composition is dependent on stem cell source

and treatment of the stem cell product before infusion. Peripheral blood stem cells (PBSCs) can be used instead of bone marrow; these are harvested from peripheral blood of granulocyte colony-stimulating factor (G-CSF or filgastrim)-mobilized donors. Peripheral blood stem cell products often undergo *ex-vivo* manipulation in order to decrease donor T cells (T-cell depletion), thereby decreasing the risk of GVHD, or to select for specific stem cell precursors, such as CD34+ cells. The latter has been shown to reduce the incidence of relapse of malignancy by decreasing the number of contaminating tumor cells.[8,9] However, as expected, T-cell depletion through either method impacts on overall immune reconstitution and increases the risk for infections.

New technologies have allowed for the performance of more high-risk HSCTs, enabling transplantation from unrelated, human leukocyte antigen (HLA)-mismatched or even haploidentical donors. As these patients have relatively high rates of severe GVHD, the overall infectious risks and duration of susceptibility are expanded. Supportive care practices and the general approach to patients must then consider the primary risk periods, with consideration of the pace of immune reconstitution and how that impacts on the risk of infections.

RISK FOR INFECTIONS: IMPACT OF THE GRAFT, THE HOST AND TRANSPLANT COMPLICATIONS

The risk of infections post-HSCT is associated with a number of factors, defined largely by the type of graft received, the host and transplant complications – determinants of the 'net state of immunosuppression'. These risk factors vary according to the time after transplanation. Overall risks are dictated by the net state of immunosuppression, along with exposure to both exogenous and endogenous organisms.

The graft and type of transplant

Donor and HLA-matching of the graft impact on overall risks for infection, primarily by dictating the likelihood and severity of GVHD and the need for and intensity of immunosuppressive therapy. The cellular composition of the graft (stem cell source and *ex-vivo* manipulation) dictates the risks for infection through effects on immune reconstitution and the pace and severity of GVHD.

Transplantation with PBSCs may yield faster reconstitution of platelets, CD4+ T cells, neutrophils and monocytes.[10–14] A large study compared immune reconstitution and coincident infection after myeloablation followed by either peripheral blood stem cell transplant (PBSCT) or bone marrow transplant. During the first year after transplantation, most lymphocyte subsets, especially CD4+ T cells, were higher in PBSCT recipients. This was accompanied by fewer bacterial and fungal infections in patients who received PBSCT than in recipients of bone marrow transplants.[14] However, there is concern that the success of PBSCT, especially from unrelated or HLA-mismatched donors, may be limited by a more rapid onset of severe GVHD.[10,11]

Cord blood transplantation, which is increasingly performed in patients who lack suitable related donors, is associated with delayed hematopoietic recovery. With this, slow engraftment and impaired neutrophil function may work together to increase the risk of infection, particularly early after transplantation.[15–18] Studies have reported high risk for aspergillosis, candidiasis and infections due to adenovirus and human herpesvirus (HHV)-6 in cord blood transplant recipients.[15,19,20] Patients who receive cord blood after nonmyeloablative conditioning regimens that incorporate antithymocyte globulin (ATG) appear to be at particularly high risk for Epstein–Barr virus (EBV)-related complications.[21] On the other hand, the low rates of GVHD may confer a relative protection from infection late after transplantation.[22]

Although T-cell depletion (TCD) decreases the pace and severity of GVHD, T-cell depletion itself is associated with delayed immune reconstitution and an increased risk for infections.[23–26] A recent large study comparing infectious complications in patients treated with TCD bone marrow from unrelated donors to those of patients treated with GVHD suppressive therapies found that TCD was associated with a particularly high risk for both cytomegalovirus (CMV) infection and aspergillosis.[27] Because CD34$^+$ selection results in removal of T cells, natural killer (NK) cells and monocytes, this practice may increase the risk for infections after allogeneic and autologous transplantation.[28,29]

It appears that immune reconstitution is similar after nonmyeloablative and myeloablative HSCT, although few large comparative studies have been performed, and reconstitution depends on multiple host and therapeutic variables.[30,31] Results of at least one study suggested that nonmyeloablative HSCT may be associated with more rapid reconstitution of immune responses assessed *in vitro*.[31] Results of another study suggested that although the total numbers of lymphocytes and antibodies was not different during the first 180 days after nonmyeloablative and myeloablative HLA-identical HSCT, recipients of nonmyeloablative regimens had relatively higher numbers of CMV T-helper cells during the early time period, raising the possibility of a protective effect of donor T cells that survive the less ablative conditioning regimen.[32] Of course, the short duration of neutropenia and differences in organ toxicities are important determinants of infectious risks. One case-control study suggested fewer early bacterial and candidal infections after nonmyeloablative conditioning.[4,33] Late-onset GVHD after nonmyeloablative HSCT poses increased risks for late CMV disease and aspergillosis.[4,33,34] Infections (e.g. CMV) may occur at increased frequency early after nonmyeloablative transplant in patients who receive certain conditioning regimens (e.g. the antibodies anti-CD52 or Campath-1H).[35]

Host factors that impact on infection risks

Underlying disease is one of the most important factors impacting on risks for infection post-HSCT by virtue of the immunologic defects associated with the hematologic condition itself and previous cytotoxic therapies. Patients who receive HSCT for a hematologic malignancy beyond first remission, for aplastic anemia and for myelodysplastic syndromes have higher risks for aspergillosis.[19,36–40] Patients who have protracted courses of primary immunodeficiencies may also have increased risks, although few large studies have been performed.

Multiple studies have reported that older people have increased risks for infections after HSCT.[19,36,39] Although it is not clear why older age predicts higher risks, factors that have been suggested include

cumulative exposure to previous cytotoxic therapy, underlying disease, severity of GVHD, baseline organ dysfunction, previous microbial exposure and waning cellular immunity. On the other hand, youth may present increased risks for other infections; for example, adenoviral complications occur at increased frequency in young transplant recipients.[41,42] This may be explained by an increased likelihood of primary infection in the young, or even the eventual elimination of adenovirus infection with age.[41,43]

Other genetic factors may play a role in modulating risks for infectious complications. Factors that control innate immune responses in the host and donor may impact the risk for infection and for GVHD. This has become an active area of research. Polymorphisms in specific genes in stem cell transplant recipients, and in donor genes, have been associated with post-transplant risks for infection. For instance, risks for infectious complications after chemotherapy and stem cell transplantation have been reported to be associated with polymorphisms in the Fc gamma receptor, myeloperoxidase gene promoter, CXCL10, interleukin-10, DC-SIGN and multiple Toll-like receptors (TLR).[44–47] Studies to determine how host and donor defense polymorphisms impact on the risk for infection post-HSCT should provide novel therapeutic targets and allow for more personalized approaches to infection prevention in the future.

Transplant complications that impact on infection risks

Multiple complications that occur after HSCT alter the risk for infections. These complications may cause organ dysfunction and immune modulation and the need for potentially toxic and immunosuppressive therapies.

The most obvious organ dysfunction that occurs immediately following conditioning therapy is mucositis involving the gastrointestinal (GI) tract. Breakdown of the mucosa of the gut is a primary mode of entry for bacteria and *Candida* spp. that colonize the GI tract. Other, subtle manifestations of organ toxicities may also lead to subsequent infection risks. Patients with renal or hepatic dysfunction may not tolerate typical doses of prophylactic or empiric antibiotics or antifungals. Other biologic variables such as iron overload or metal chelating therapy may have an effect, especially on bacterial and filamentous fungal infections.[48]

Graft-versus-host disease and corticosteroid-based therapies are perhaps the most important post-HSCT complications leading to infections. Risk for all infections – bacterial, fungal and viral – are increased in patients with severe GVHD. These risks increase yet further in patients who receive high doses of corticosteroids. Most likely, this represents the combined impact of the direct immunosuppressive effects of GHVD, as well as the corticosteroid-induced impairment in neutrophil and monocyte/macrophage immunity and cell-mediated immunity. Corticosteroids administered for other post-HSCT complications, such as bronchiolitis obliterans, and 'idiopathic' pulmonary syndromes may also lead to equivalent, high risks for infections. The negative impact of corticosteroid exposure is not limited to the above risks; cumulative exposure to high-dose corticosteroids is an important variable predicting persistent infection and poor prognosis of treatment for viral or fungal disease.[49–51]

It has been hypothesized that infection with herpesviruses, especially CMV, may directly impact on the risk for other infections by modulating immune responses. Historically, the association between CMV disease and subsequent infections was largely attributed to the myelosuppressive effects of antiviral drugs administered for prophylaxis or therapy. However, high risk for subsequent bacterial and fungal infections have been noted in patients with active CMV or latent CMV disease, even after controlling for secondary neutropenia in multivariable models.[19,40,52] Cytomegalovirus-seronegative recipients of stem cells from seropositive donors (D+/R−) have increased risk for both bacterial and fungal infec-

Table 74.1 Approximate incidence of selected infectious complications in hematopoietic stem cell transplant (HSCT) recipients

Infection	Autologous HSCT	Allogeneic HSCT
Bacterial*		
Gram-positive	5–10	10–20
Gram-negative	5–10	5–10
Mycobacterial		
Mycobacterium tuberculosis	<2	<2
Nontuberculous	<2	<5
Fungal*		
Candida spp.	<2	<5
Aspergillus spp.	<10	5–15
Pneumocystis jirovecii	<2	<3
Viral		
Cytomegalovirus infection*		
R+ (auto)/R+/D+ or D– (allo)	25–40	70
R– (auto)/R–/D+ (allo)	3–5	15–25
R–/D– (allo)	NA	3–5
Cytomegalovirus disease*		
R+ (auto)/R+/D+ or D– (allo)	5–7	35–40
R– (auto)/R–/D+ (allo)	1–3	10
R–/D– (allo)	NA	1–3
Herpes simplex virus (HSV)*		
Without prophylaxis, HSV+	60–80	60–80
Varicella-zoster virus (VZV)*		
Without prophylaxis, VZV+	20–40	17–60
Influenza virus†	<5	<5
Respiratory syncitial virus†	<5	5–15
Parainfluenza virus†	<5	5–10
Adenovirus	<5	5–20
BK virus	<5	5–40
Epstein–Barr virus	<5	5–25
Human herpesvirus 6		
Infection	35–60	35–60
Disease	<3	<3 – 12
Parasitic		
*Toxoplasma gondii*ial*	<2	<2

Shown are estimates of disease incidence (%), unless indicated otherwise.[55–68]
*Dependent on prophylaxis;
†Episodic incidence during the year; NA, not applicable.

Table 74.2, and a more detailed discussion pertaining to diagnostic and therapeutic approaches for infectious complications are presented in other chapters.

BACTERIAL INFECTIONS IN HSCT PATIENTS: EPIDEMIOLOGY, MANIFESTATIONS AND MANAGEMENT

Patients are at highest risk for bacterial infections early after HSCT, with GI tract mucositis and neutropenia leading to translocation of endogenous pathogens, and during the later periods of GVHD, when risks for encapsulated organisms are particularly high. Bacteria most frequently become blood-borne through the GI tract and/or intravenous catheter, or through the respiratory tract. Risks are related to antibacterial prophylaxis patterns, degree of GI tract mucositis and presence of indwelling intravenous catheters. Late after HSCT, the epidemiology of infection largely depends on the severity of GVHD, application of prolonged prophylaxis and efficacy of immunization. There are numerous aerobic and anaerobic bacteria that cause infection in these patients, as outlined in more depth in Chapter 73. Overall risks are dependent on the type of transplant, degree of immunosuppression and post-transplant complications, and exposure; general estimates are provided in Table 74.1.

In patients with cancer and HSCT, the epidemiology of bacterial infections has changed over two decades, with large European and North American studies suggesting an increase in the incidence of infections caused by Gram-positive bacteria concurrent with a decrease in infections caused by Gram-negative bacteria.[72,73] Recent studies are demonstrating a potential reversal in trends, with more infections caused by Gram-negative bacteria.[74] Unfortunately, much of this increase appears to be associated with high rates of infection caused by multidrug-resistant (MDR) bacteria. A large multicenter Brazilian study showed that 37% of Gram-negative bacteria recovered from HSCT recipients were MDR; risks for these infections were increased with use of third-generation cephalosporins.[75] The outcomes of these infections can be particularly poor, especially in the setting of severe GVHD; for instance, *Pseudomonas aeruginosa* infections (lung and bloodstream) recur in 16% of patients who are treated with 14-day courses of appropriate antibiotics, with associated mortality estimated at 36%.[76]

Bacterial infections involving the GI tract are relatively common in these patients, as occurs in the setting of neutropenia after cytotoxic therapy; neutropenic enterocolitis occurs after conditioning therapy, with similar infectious causes. Diarrhea is also common after conditioning therapy for HSCT; recent reports suggest that 47–100% of autologous or allogeneic HSCT recipients develop diarrhea at some point during therapy.[77–81] Conventional bacterial pathogens, parasitic pathogens and viruses cause diarrhea in these patients; however, in allogeneic HSCT recipients, GVHD impacts the duration and magnitude of risks for infectious colitis and the differential diagnosis of diarrhea. For instance, GVHD has been reported to be an important risk factor for *Clostridium difficile*-associated disease (CDAD) in allogeneic HSCT recipients; in this population, complications such as CDAD-associated enteric bacteremia and mortality appear particularly high.[78,80] The contemporary burden of this infection is unknown in this population, as few large studies have been performed since recognition of highly toxigenic *C. difficile* strains.

Finally, management of allogeneic HSCT patients with acute diarrhea is more complex, as the differential diagnosis includes GVHD involving the GI tract; in a study of 169 HSCT recipients, an infectious cause of diarrhea was documented in only 45 (29%).[82] GVHD can be indistinguishable from infectious diarrhea using signs and symptoms alone; empiric immunosuppressive therapies often exacerbate and 'uncover' infectious causes (e.g. CMV, discussed below).

tions, even in the absence of CMV-specific therapy.[53] Donor or recipient seropositivity may have the most impact on survival in patients who receive HSCT from unrelated donors.[54]

Thus, multiple factors related to both host and transplant contribute to the 'net state of immunosuppression'. This net state, which changes according to the timing of the transplant and to exposures, dictates overall infectious risk, as summarized in Table 74.1 and Figure 74.1.

The remainder of this chapter will discuss major issues regarding the epidemiology, manifestations and management of specific infections after HSCT. As many concepts that apply to neutropenic cancer patients (as outlined in Chapter 73 by Marchetti and Calandra) also apply in this setting, this discussion will focus primarily on issues that are specific to stem cell transplant recipients. Commonly employed prevention strategies for different types of infection are outlined in

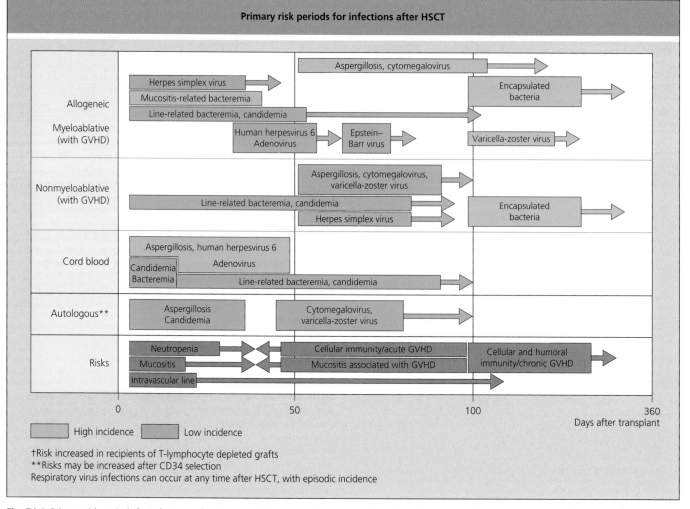

Primary risk periods for infections after HSCT

Fig. 74.1 Primary risk periods for infections after hematopoietic stem cell transplantation. Typical risk periods for the most common infections after each type of HSCT are shown. Risks are based on typical prophylaxis strategies, which include trimethoprim–sulfamethoxazole for *Pneumocystis jirovecii*, screened or filtered blood products and ganciclovir for cytomegalovirus, aciclovir for herpes simplex virus, and fluconazole for candidemia. Courtesy of R Bowden.[69]

VIRAL INFECTIONS IN HSCT PATIENTS: EPIDEMIOLOGY, MANIFESTATIONS AND MANAGEMENT

Infections caused by endogenous viruses (e.g. herpesviruses) and exogenous viruses (e.g. those acquired through the GI and respiratory tracts) are common in the HSCT population (see Table 74.1). The incidence of disease thus depends on mode of infection, recipient and donor CMV seropositivities, and immunosuppression. These host–pathogen interactions dictate the risk, timing and incidence of infection caused by latent herpes viruses, while exposure factors impact the epidemiology of exogenously acquired viruses. In the latter group, degree of immunosuppression more often impacts the severity of infection (i.e. whether a virus is contained within the upper respiratory tract or invades lung tissue).

Herpes virus infections

Herpesviruses are exceedingly important in HSCT recipients, with clinically significant infections caused by CMV, herpes simplex virus (HSV), varicella-zoster virus (VZV), EBV and HHV-6, -7 and -8.

Perhaps the most important infectious complication is caused by CMV; historically, mortality caused by CMV disease was approximated at roughly 25%. The risk for primary infection by blood products has been significantly reduced by screening and leukocyte depletion. Currently, the risk of CMV disease is primarily related to reactivation of infected recipient or donor cells during periods of low CMV-specific T-lymphocyte function during immune reconstitution or to exogenous immunosuppressive therapies. Allogeneic HSCT recipients, who have the highest risk during GVHD, most commonly develop interstitial pneumonitis and gastroenteritis, and less commonly, other manifestations such as retinitis, isolated fever, pancytopenia, hepatitis and encephalitis. However, retinitis appears to be increasingly recognized, especially late after allogeneic HSCT in the setting of severe GVHD and recurrent CMV reactivation.[83]

Infection caused by CMV has also been associated with 'indirect effects', which include higher mortality related to other infections.[53] For these reasons, prevention strategies have been an active area of research, especially in recipients of allogeneic HSCT (see Table 74.2). Antiviral drug strategies, which include both universal prophylaxis and pre-emptive therapy, are effective and have lowered CMV-related mortality; however, both prophylaxis and pre-emptive therapies have specific limitations, including emergence of drug resistance and toxicities associated with antiviral drugs. Unfortunately, no strategy is 100%

Table 74.2 Prevention strategies commonly employed in HSCT recipients

Indication	Strategy
Decreased duration of neutropenia	Colony-stimulating factors WBC transfusions
Bacterial infections	Antibiotic prophylaxis during neutropenia Empiric therapy (fever during neutropenia) Antibiotic prophylaxis during GVHD IVIG Vaccination
Cytomegalovirus disease	Screening (or filtering) of blood products in seronegative recipients Antiviral prophylaxis PCR or antigen-based screening for reactivation with pre-emptive therapy IVIG Safe sex practices Vaccination (experimental)
Herpes simplex virus (HSV)-1 and HSV-2	Antiviral prophylaxis Safe sex practices
Varicella-zoster virus	Antiviral prophylaxis Postexposure prophylaxis IVIG Immunization
Epstein–Barr virus (EBV)/post-transplant lymphoproliferative disorders	PCR screening for reactivation, reduce immunosuppression if possible, consider rituximab and therapy with EBV-specific cytotoxic T lymphocytes (experimental)
Adenovirus infections	PCR screening for reactivation with pre-emptive therapy
BK infection	PCR screening for reactivation, reduce immunosuppression if possible, pre-emptive strategies
Respiratory virus infections	Enhanced infection control measures Prophylaxis, pre-emptive therapy for influenza Vaccination
Fungal infections	Antifungal prophylaxis Prophylaxis to prevent *Pneumocystis jirovecii* pneumonia
Toxoplasmosis	Prophylaxis with seropositivity and GVHD
Other	Infection control measures to prevent food-borne illness and respiratory acquisition of infection

Listed are strategies that are in common use or have suggested potential in recent clinical studies.
GVHD, graft-versus-host disease; IVIG, intravenous immunoglobulin; PCR, polymerase chain reaction; WBC, white blood cell.

during prophylaxis or pre-emptive therapy has been reported, but appears to be less common than in other populations, such as in organ transplant recipients. The kinetics of viral reactivation, dictated by pathogen-specific cellular immunity and antiviral exposure, impacts the likelihood of viral resistance, especially in the settting in which resistance mutations impact viral 'fitness'.[85]

As control of CMV infection and risk for development of disease are primarily associated with both CD8+ and CD4+ T-cell immune responses, efforts are underway to develop strategies to enhance immunity, both as an effort to augment therapy of disease and to develop preventive strategies. Live-attenuated CMV vaccines, canarypox-vectored vaccines, recombinant gB vaccines and, more recently, DNA vaccines have been or are currently in development,[86,87] and may have efficacy in preventing both CMV disease and other 'secondary' manifestations associated with CMV immune modulation.

Both HSV and VZV infections occur and cause localized disease in seropositive hosts; reactivation and primary infection can also cause disseminated disease (e.g. hepatitis, pneumonitis, encephalitis). Prolonged antiviral prophylaxis is usually employed in seropositive patients; one randomized trial documented a decrease in VZV disease with 1 year of prophylaxis after allogeneic HSCT.[88] Rebound disease, and HSV and VZV antiviral resistance appear to be infrequent in this population.[89,90] An inactivated varicella vaccine given before receipt of autologous stem cells and 90 days thereafter has been shown to reduce the risk of VZV disease.[91]

Human herpes virus 6 (HHV-6), the cause of exanthem subitum, infects nearly everyone by 3 years of age and becomes latent in the brain. This virus (especially variant B) has been increasingly implicated in disease in adult and pediatric HSCT recipients. Although early reports associated HHV-6 with pneumonitis, rash, bone marrow suppression (especially involving megakaryotic lineage) and fever, most recent studies have shown more definitive associations with neurologic manifestations, including seizures, multifocal encephalitis and 'post-transplant acute limbic encephalitis'. The latter, 'PALE', is a recently described syndrome characterized by anterograde amnesia, syndrome of inappropriate production of antidiuretic hormone (SIADH), mild cerebrospinal fluid (CSF) pleocytosis and temporal EEG abnormalities.[92] Multiple issues surrounding HHV-6 including pathogenesis of disease, epidemiology and prevention, and the role of antiviral therapies remain under current investigation. One interesting observation is that this virus can be transmitted from a donor to an HSCT recipient by means of chromosomally integrated virus, also confounding the interpretation of HHV-6 viremia.[55]

Community-acquired respiratory viruses

Respiratory viruses, acquired within the community or nosocomially in association with institutional outbreaks, impose a significant burden of morbidity and mortality in this population. Biology of the viruses, pathogenesis of disease, diagnosis and therapies are discussed elsewhere in this text (Chapters 161 and 162). There are a few concepts specific to this population that are worthy of discussion.

Approximated incidence of respiratory tract 'infection' is listed in Table 74.1. However, incidence of pneumonia and related mortality is variable for specific viruses and is largely impacted by underlying immunity. Respiratory syncitial virus (RSV), influenza and parainfluenza (especially parainfluenza 3) have been reported to have the highest rates of pneumonia and related mortality in HSCT patients. These three viruses account for the bulk of infections in this patient population, progressing to pneumonia in 35% of patients.[93] Progression from upper to lower respiratory tract infection with RSV is dependent on lymphopenia, older age, allogeneic HSCT and degree of GVHD, but outcomes are also particularly poor when infection is established early after HSCT. In recent studies,[56,93,94] attributable mortality was estimated to be about 18%. Definitive recommendations of how to prevent progression of pneumonia are elusive in the absence of large randomized trials. Methods that have been explored and reported to

effective, largely because the duration of time at risk for CMV disease is progressively extended in patients who receive suppressive therapies without effective immune reconstitution. CMV disease has largely become a 'late' complication of allogeneic HSCT, occurring most commonly during the period of GVHD.[84] CMV resistance to ganciclovir

be safe include systemic and aerosolized administration of ribavirin, administration of intravenous immunoglobulin and use of neutralizing antibody, palivizumab.[56,95] Similarly, although no randomized trials have been performed to establish efficacy, oseltamivir is tolerated by HSCT recipients and used frequently to prevent disease caused by influenza viruses in outbreak settings.[96]

Human metapneumovirus has been recognized as a cause of previously undiagnosed 'idiopathic pneumonia' in HSCT recipients;[94,97] this virus, as well as parainfluenza 3, can persist in respiratory secretions for extended periods of time in asymptomatic HSCT recipients,[98,99] presenting challenges to both diagnostics and effective infection control. One caveat complicating the care of these patients is that diagnostic parsimony does not always apply in patients with diagnosed upper respiratory tract infections and pulmonary abnormalities. Both parainfluenza and influenza lower respiratory tract infections are frequently associated with 'co-pathogens', including bacteria and fungi, which require different therapies. In one study, parainfluenza 3 pneumonia was associated with other pathogens in 53% of cases.[100] Diagnostic bronchoscopy is wise, when feasible.

Adenovirus can cause disease after primary infection (gastroenteritis, interstitial pneumonitis) and after reactivation, with propensity to cause disease in the kidneys and liver. Incidence is variable and dependent on age, with higher rates in the young and older age groups, and degree of T-cell dysfunction related to cellular depletion or GVHD.[57]

Lower respiratory tract disease caused by respiratory viruses can present differently with different diagnostic imaging techniques. Disease may be inapparent on chest radiograph (Fig. 74.2a), with early pneumonia better shown on CT scan (Fig. 74.2b); CT scan can also show both nodular and 'ground glass' infiltrates, representative of bronchiolitis and pneumonia (Fig. 74.2c,d).

BK virus

Reactivation of polyoma BK virus (BKV) has been associated with post-engraftment hemorrhagic cystitis in allogeneic HSCT recipients.[101] Frequency of disease is dependent on the type of transplant and HLA match, type of conditioning agent, GVHD and pretransplant serologies.[58,102] Disease may be preceded by viral reactivation in urine and serum, presenting options for monitoring and 'pre-emptive' therapy.[103] Unlike renal transplant recipients, interstitial nephritis appears rarely (for a detailed discussion about BK virus, see Practice Point 43).

Hepatitis viruses

Hepatitis virus infections can be acquired from infected stem cell donors, although rates of transmission are variable and dependent on donor viral reactivation at time of stem cell recovery; effective prevention by treating donors with antiviral drugs and recipient vaccination has been reported.[104] Hepatitis C virus has recently been recognized as one of the two most common viral infections (with VZV) late after

HSCT, in one series occuring in 10% of long-term survivors of allogeneic HSCT recipients from matched related donors.[105]

FUNGAL INFECTIONS IN HSCT PATIENTS: EPIDEMIOLOGY, MANIFESTATIONS AND MANAGEMENT

Overall risks for fungal infections are contingent upon variables that modulate the pace of immune reconstitution, organ toxicities and microbial exposures.

Infections caused by *Candida* species

Although the yeasts that cause infection in HSCT patients include multiple other organisms, such as *Cryptococcus neoformans*, the vast majority of superficial and invasive yeast infections are caused by *Candida* spp. Invasive *Candida* infections can be separated into two primary syndromes: acute candidiasis (bloodstream infection) and chronic candidiasis (hepatosplenic infection). The pathogenesis and clinical characteristics of candidiasis are discussed in Chapter 178. In this population, bloodstream infections occur either through an indwelling intravascular catheter or through a damaged GI tract. Acute infection usually manifests as fever and signs of sepsis. Adequate antifungal therapy is essential, not only to cure the acute episode, but also to decrease the likelihood of late embolic manifestations (e.g. chorioretinitis, endocarditis).[106]

The widespread use of fluconazole, which is supported by numerous randomized trials carried out in the early 1990s,[107,108] has decreased the incidence and mortality rate attributable to both acute and chronic infections caused by *Candida albicans*.[40,109,110] This practice has resulted in improved overall survival in allogeneic HSCT patients.[107] However, the decreased incidence of early candidiasis due to azole-susceptible species (*C. albicans* and *C. tropicalis*) and improved survival late after HSCT with GVHD has allowed for an increase in infections due to fluconazole-resistant *Candida* spp., such as *C. glabrata* and *C. krusei*.[40,110–113] There has also been a shift from *Candida* spp. to molds as the primary fungal pathogens. Thus, the appearance of azole-resistant organisms is not a failure of prophylaxis but reflects the success of supportive care strategies. In patients who underwent allogeneic HSCT from unrelated donors for chronic myelogenous leukemia (CML), two of the most important variables predicting HSCT survival in the 1990s were use of ganciclovir-based strategies and fluconazole.[114]

Infections caused by filamentous fungi

Infections with filamentous fungi are usually acquired through the respiratory route, although filamentous fungi can also invade through a damaged GI tract.[115,116] The most common cause of fungal infection in HSCT patients is currently *Aspergillus fumigatus*.[36,117] The day of onset

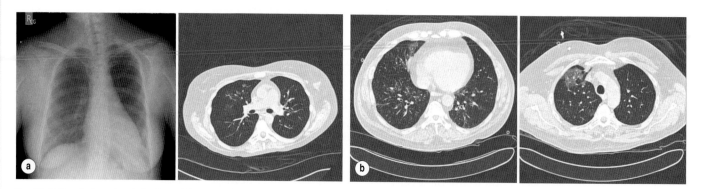

Fig. 74.2 Respiratory virus infections. (a) CXR and CT scan of documented human metapneumovirus infection in a patient with acute myelogenous leukemia. (b) CT scans of adenoviral infection complicating severe GVHD in a recipient of an HLA-matched unrelated donor transplant. In these scans, taken on the same day, both centrilobular nodules (left) and ground glass infiltrates (right) were apparent.

of aspergillosis has changed, from primarily the early neutropenic period to later after allogeneic transplant.[5,19,36] The risk factors for early and late disease are different; risks for early disease are primarily those that impact on the pace of engraftment, such as the specific stem cell product. There is also some indication that a portion of patients who present with aspergillosis early after HSCT may have been exposed to the organism before conditioning therapy. This may explain some of the impact of 'host' variables, such as age and underlying diseases on the risk of aspergillosis. Risks during the late period are largely those associated with GVHD and its therapies. Other infections, such as CMV disease, may pose both direct and indirect risks for subsequent disease. There has been an increase in invasive infections caused by zygomycetes and *Fusarium* spp.[117] Patients who receive transplants from an unrelated or an HLA-mismatched donor and patients with severe GVHD have particularly high risk for zygomycete infections.[117]

Most recent efforts have been directed towards preventing mold infections by using universal or targeted prophylaxis with different mold-active drugs (e.g. azoles, echinocandins or polyenes) or 'pre-emptive therapy' driven by screening for fungal antigens or nucleic acids. Success has been reported in large randomized trials applying azole antifungals, although there is concern of breakthrough infection with organisms that demonstrate innate or acquired drug resistance.[118,119] Specific concerns that have been reported in this context include infections with azole-resistant *Candida* species, zygomycetes with resistance to voriconazole, and *Trichosporon* and *Candida* spp. that have resistance to echinocandins. Currently, there are many issues of debate concerning preventative therapies, including which antifungal drug is best, which patients benefit and the optimal duration of therapy.

Fungal infections present with the typical appearance of nodular infiltrates on radiographs. In neutropenic patients, who have been studied most extensively, resolution of neutropenia may result in increased size of lesions and cavitation. Fungal pneumonia that occurs in non-neutropenic hosts can present with multiple radiographic abnormalities, including focal or multifocal consolidation. Nodular lesions and consolidations have multiple infectious and noninfectious etiologies (Fig. 74.3); bronchoscopic examination is necessary in order to optimize therapy. Recently, immune reconstitution syndrome has been recognized as a cause of progressive infiltrates in HSCT recipients with pulmonary aspergillosis.[120]

Pneumocystis infections

In the absence of prophylaxis, *Pneumocystis jirovecii* pneumonia (PCP) is a common cause of infection after allogeneic HSCT, particularly during lymphopenia and GVHD. Infections may manifest with multiple typical and atypical abnormalities, including ground glass infiltrates, pneumothorax, pleural effusions and nodular infiltrates.[121] Death attributable to PCP is particularly high after HSCT, emphasizing the importance of effective prevention. Trimethoprim–sulfamethoxazole is most frequently administered using a twice weekly algorithm, although the drug is only moderately tolerated due to allergic manifestations and bone marrow toxicity. Alternatives explored included pentamidine (aerosolized and intravenous), dapsone and atovaquone, although the latter strategies may not be as effective.[122] Importantly, patients who do not receive the trimethoprim–sulfamethoxazole formulation also do not have the added benefits of prevention of other pathogens, such as *Nocardia* spp. and *Toxoplasma gondii* infection; these patients can present with combined pulmonary and CNS lesions (Fig. 74.4).

SUMMARY

Infections remain a leading cause of death in HSCT patients, but the timing of onset and the spectrum of pathogens have evolved over the past two decades. Changes in transplantation practices, different hosts and the development of effective strategies to prevent early CMV disease and candidiasis have increased survival rates. Late after transplantation, severe

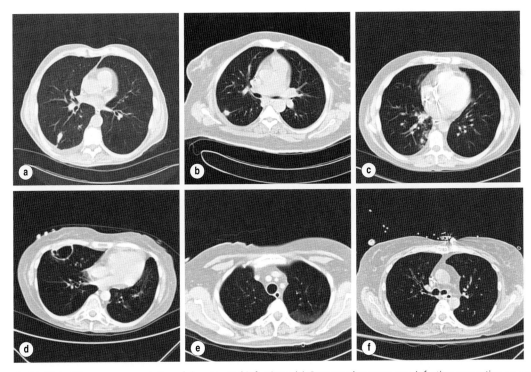

Fig. 74.3 Pneumonia. Multiple CT scans representative of documented infections. (a) *Stenotrophomonas* spp. infection presenting as a nodular lesion in patient with acute myelogenous leukemia (AML) and neutropenic fever. (b) Nodular lesion in a patient with AML and documented aspergillosis. (c) Cytomegalovirus pneumonitis presenting with focal, 'patchy', nodular infiltrate in a patient with graft-versus-host disease (GVHD). (d) Necrotic lesion diagnosed as *Aspergillus fumigatus* in a patient with Hodgkin's lymphoma. (e and f) Progression of scattered patchy peripheral ground glass infiltrate (e), followed by diffuse airway thickening and mild bronchiectasis (f) in a patient with GVHD after nonmyeloablative HSCT, who presented with obstructive symptoms and had *A. fumigatus* tracheobronchitis.

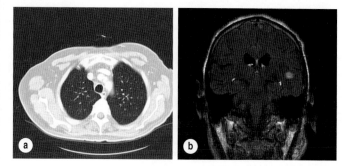

Fig. 74.4 (a, b) Toxoplasmosis. Nodular lung lesions and multiple foci of enhancement with associated edema in a patient treated with rituximab for mantle cell lymphoma who developed fevers and confusion as presenting symptoms of toxoplasmosis.

GVHD dominates the clinical presentation and is often accompanied by the emergence of other organisms, such as molds and other opportunistic pathogens. The approach to this patient population requires not only an understanding of the pathogens, but also a complete appreciation for the host and associated immunosuppression, which defines risk periods, differential diagnosis and appropriate therapies.

REFERENCES

References for this chapter can be found online at http://www.expertconsult.com

Chapter | **75** |

Nina E Tolkoff-Rubin
Robert H Rubin

Infection in solid organ transplantation

INTRODUCTION

The remarkable success of organ transplantation today (~90% 1-year allograft survival for kidney, heart and liver grafts, with long-term survival approaching 20 years) is changing the approach to an increasing number of illnesses that produce end-organ failure – the best chance for many of these patients is now transplantation.[1]

Three major barriers to success in organ transplantation are closely linked: *availability of organs* for transplantation, *allograft rejection* and *life-threatening infection*. The worldwide shortage of organs results in attempts to extend eligibility and use of organs, despite possible injury and/or infection, which in the past would have disqualified a particular donor (or allograft). The use of non-heart-beating donors, older donors and those with pre-existing cardiovascular disease is becoming more common, which places even greater emphasis on the evaluation of potential donors. Successful organ transplantation is predicated on a number of factors, particularly surgical excellence, creation of a protected environment and careful use of both antirejection and antimicrobial agents (Table 75.1).[2–4]

The great irony in transplantation is that transplant patients are not so much at risk from their primary illness but rather have a new concern – microbial invasion. Immunosuppressive and anti-inflammatory therapy, the cornerstones of post-transplant therapy,

amplify the extent and effects of invasive infection, while at the same time decreasing the signs and symptoms that could lead to early diagnosis (Fig. 75.1).

The current immunomodulating/anti-inflammatory agents are discussed in Practice Point 40.

PRINCIPLES OF ANTIMICROBIAL THERAPY IN TRANSPLANTATION

Antimicrobial agents play a critical role in the therapeutic prescription for the transplant recipient. This prescription has two components: an immunosuppressive strategy to prevent and treat rejection, and an antimicrobial strategy to make it safe. Flexibility is built into this prescription: any increase in immunosuppression should be linked to an increase in the antimicrobial regimen, particularly in determining the duration of therapy.[2–4]

Table 75.1 Advances in clinical transplantation

- Optimal tissue typing and matching of donor and recipient, with particular attention to presensitization issues
- Careful donor evaluation, technically impeccable procurement and preservation of the donor organ
- Precise attention to the surgical challenges, resulting in a minimum of tissue injury, secure vascular, bladder, ureteral, biliary or bronchial anastomoses, and the prevention and/or aggressive drainage of fluid collections
- Precise, individualized management of the immunosuppressive regimen: on the one hand, preventing and treating rejection; on the other hand, minimizing the adverse effects on host defenses and establishing the therapeutic prescription
- Prevention of infection whenever possible by instituting a program of environmental protection and preventive antimicrobial strategies, and early diagnosis/aggressive therapy of microbial invasion when prevention fails

Modified from Rubin.[2]

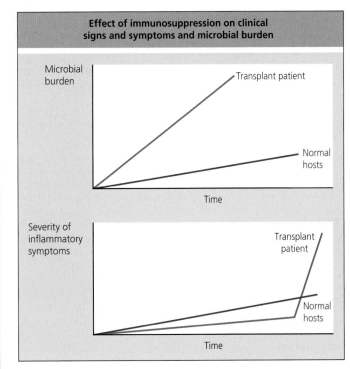

Fig. 75.1 Effect of immunosuppression on clinical signs and symptoms and microbial burden.

Antimicrobial agents can be prescribed in three different modes:[2,4]

- therapeutic mode, in which antimicrobial agents are administered as curative treatment for active infection;
- prophylactic mode, in which antimicrobial agents are administered to an entire population because of perceived risk. For such a strategy to be successful three criteria must be met: (1) the infection to be prevented must be common enough and important enough to justify the intervention; (2) the antimicrobial agent is nontoxic enough to make it safe; and (3) the use of this drug can be shown to be cost-effective; and
- pre-emptive mode, in which antimicrobial agents are administered to patients at risk for life-threatening infection, as determined by a clinical–epidemiologic assessment or a laboratory marker.

The most effective prophylactic program that has been tested is the use of low-dose trimethoprim–sulfamethoxazole post-transplant, which effectively eliminates *Pneumocystis jirovecii* from the differential diagnosis (as opposed to an incidence of 15% in the first 6 months post-transplant without prophylaxis). Significant protection against listeriosis, nocardiosis, toxoplasmosis and urinary tract infection is also provided at the same time.[2–4]

Pre-emptive therapy takes advantage of two separate approaches to the prevention of cytomegalovirus (CMV) disease. Clinical–epidemiologic studies have demonstrated that administration of OKT3 or ATG to CMV-seropositive patients results in reactivation of latent CMV infection and a significant rate of clinically important CMV disease. Initiation of ganciclovir therapy pre-emptively effectively limits CMV invasion. Alternatively, because viremia is usually demonstrable by polymerase chain reaction (PCR) assay 2–7 days before clinical disease is apparent, initiation of pre-emptive ganciclovir therapy on the basis of PCR results can be a useful way to manage antiviral therapy for those patients most in need of such an intervention.[2,4]

A similar situation exists when the active viral infection, such as that due to CMV, is present. Duration of therapy is determined by initial microbial burden, level of immunosuppression already present, and evolution of rejection while antiviral treatment is being administered. When immunosuppression is maintained at too high a level, resistance to antiviral therapy is particularly likely to develop; when antiviral therapy is administered for too short a period of time or at too low a dose, infection relapse occurs.[2,4]

RISK OF INFECTION

Factors have been defined that contribute to the occurrence and extent of infection in the organ transplant recipient (Table 75.2).[2]

Technical/anatomic problems

The occurrence of technical/anatomic problems can lead to devitalized tissue, formation of fluid collections, the need for invasive drainage catheters, indwelling vascular access devices and other foreign bodies that compromise the normal mucocutaneous barriers to infection. The incidence of such infections is determined by the complexity of the surgery being done, the wound healing capability of the patient and the technical skill of the surgeon. Antimicrobial prophylaxis provides some degree of protection for these patients, but nothing takes the place of technically impeccable surgery.

Environmental exposure

Environmental exposures, both in the community and in the hospital, can play an important role in the occurrence of clinically important infection in the transplant patient. In the community, inhalation of infection-laden air can be an important cause of morbidity and mortality. Thus, the geographically restricted, systemic mycoses (e.g. coccidioidomycosis and histoplasmosis) and acute infection with such

Table 75.2 Classification of infections occurring in organ transplant recipients

Infections related to technical complications	Transplantation of a contaminated allograft Anastomotic leak or stenosis Wound hematoma Vascular access device infection Iatrogenic damage to the skin Mismanagement of endotracheal tube leading to aspiration Infection related to biliary, urinary and drainage catheters
Infection related to excessive nosocomial hazard	*Aspergillus* spp. *Legionella* spp. *Pseudomonas aeruginosa* (and other Gram-negative bacilli, particularly extended β-lactamase producing Gram-negatives) *Nocardia asteroides* *Pneumocystis jirovecii* Methicillin-resistant *Staphylococcus aureus*
Newly emerging pathogens	*Fusarium* *Scedosporium* *Zygomycetes*

Infection related to exposures within the community	Dimorphic, geographically restricted, endemic mycoses:
	  Histoplasma capsulatum
	  Coccidioides immitis
	  Blastomyces dermatitidis
	  Strongyloides stercoralis

Community-acquired opportunistic infection resulting from ubiquitous saprophytes in the environment	*Cryptococcus neoformans* *Aspergillus* spp. *Nocardia asteroides* *Pneumocystis jirovecii*
Newly emerging infections	West Nile virus Avian influenza
Respiratory infections circulating in the community	*Mycobacterium tuberculosis* Influenza Parainfluenza Respiratory syncytial virus Adenovirus
Infections acquired by the ingestion of contaminated food/water	*Salmonella* spp. *Listeria monocytogenes*
Viral infections of particular importance in transplant patients	Herpes group viruses Hepatitis B and C Papillomaviruses and papovaviruses Human immunodeficiency virus

The incidence and severity of these infections and, to a lesser extent, the other infections listed are related to the net state of immunosuppression present in a particular patient.
Modified from Rubin.[2]

respiratory viruses as influenza and respiratory syncytial virus (RSV) will have a greater impact on transplant patients than on the rest of the community. The incidence of disseminated infection, the occurrence of progressive lung disease and the importance of secondary infection with *Staphylococcus aureus*, *Pseudomonas aeruginosa* and other Gram-negative bacteria are all increased in transplant patients.[2,4]

Other exposures of importance within the community include the enteric pathogens, particularly *Salmonella* spp. and *Listeria monocytogenes*, and such opportunistic pathogens as *Aspergillus* and *Nocardia*, which can be acquired from aerosols created in gardening and other recreational activities.[2]

As important as community exposures are in the acquisition of infection, nosocomial exposures are both more common and more dangerous. Such infections tend to be opportunistic and relatively resistant to antimicrobial infection. Two patterns of environmental exposure have been identified: domiciliary and nondomiciliary.[2,4,5]

Domiciliary exposure

Domiciliary exposures occur in the room or on the ward where the patient is housed, and are usually caused by contamination of the air supply or the potable water by such opportunistic organisms as *Aspergillus* spp., *Scedosporium*, *Fusarium* and zygomycetes. Such contamination can occur because of construction; because of the presence of plants and flowers contaminated with Gram-negative bacteria within the patient's room; because of shower and toilet facilities that create aerosols of Gram-negative bacilli or *Legionella* spp.; and because of contaminated water systems or air handling systems. The net result is that these immunosuppressed patients inhale aerosols contaminated by excessive numbers of potential pathogens.[2,4,5] Outbreaks of this type are characterized by clustering of cases in time and space.

Nondomiciliary exposure

Nondomiciliary exposures occur when patients are taken from their rooms to such central facilities as the operating room, radiology suite, cardiac catheterization laboratory and other locations. Excessive exposures of this type are more common than domiciliary exposures and more difficult to identify because of lack of clustering of cases in time and space.

Both domiciliary and nondomiciliary exposures can expose patients to potential pathogens.

Net state of immunosuppression

The net state of immunosuppression is a complex function that integrates a number of factors frequently present in transplant patients that can influence the ability to fight infection. The prime determinant is the immunosuppressive regimen employed – the dose, duration and temporal sequence of the drugs prescribed. Table 75.3 delineates the various factors that can contribute to the net state of immunosuppression.

Table 75.3 The net state of immunosuppression

Immunomodulatory effects of the underlying condition	Effects of the anti-rejection regimen
	Neutropenia
	Metabolic factors
	Protein–calorie malnutrition
	Uremia
	Iron overload
	Hyperglycemia
Immunomodulating infection	Cytomegalovirus
	Epstein–Barr virus
	Human herpesvirus 6
	Other herpes group viruses
	Hepatitis viruses
Other factors	Age (at the two extremes of life)
	Ethnic background (immune response gene effect)

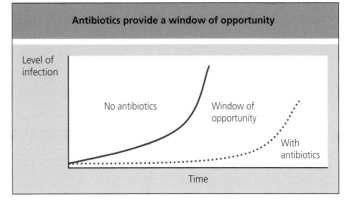

Fig. 75.2 Antibiotics provide a window of opportunity.

Particularly noteworthy in these patients are nutritional/metabolic factors and active infection with immunomodulating viruses such as CMV, Epstein–Barr virus (EBV), hepatitis viruses and human immunodeficiency virus (HIV). Thus, patients with protein–calorie malnutrition (as defined by a serum albumin <2.5 g/dl) have a 10-fold greater incidence of life-threatening infection; 90% of transplant patients with opportunistic infection do so in the context of systemic viral infection. Indeed, the exceptions are usually found to have been exposed to a previously unrecognized excessive environmental hazard.[2–4]

Darwinian factors

Bacteria and fungi compete with each other for nutrients and growth factors. These factors include glucose, iron and the products of red cell lysis. For example, the availability of iron will greatly increase the incidence of infection with such organisms as the zygomycetes, *Aspergillus* and *Listeria*, and other micro-organisms.[6] Similarly, hyperglycemia will greatly increase the level of *Candida* on the skin, in the gut, the pharynx and the female genital tract. A relatively minor break in the integrity of these tissues will lead to significant clinical infection because of the high microbial burden[2,4–6] (Fig. 75.2)

CHOOSING ANTIBIOTIC THERAPY

Choosing the best antibiotic regimen before the results of initial culturing are available can be a daunting process. The first consideration is whether the patient presents a 'therapeutic emergency' or a 'diagnostic dilemma'. If an emergent situation is present, then broad-spectrum therapy is indicated, and issues of cost and toxicity are of little concern. Such therapy is operative for the first 3–4 days, at which time culture information is usually available, the patient is clinically improved and a switch to narrower spectrum therapy, usually via the oral route, is appropriate.[2–4]

TIMETABLE OF INFECTION AFTER ORGAN TRANSPLANTATION

Based on the program of immunosuppression utilized, a 'timetable' (Fig. 75.3) can be constructed that delineates when in the post-transplant course different infections are likely to occur; that is, although pneumonia can occur at any point in the post-transplant course, the etiology will be very different at different times. Unexplained exceptions to the timetable should be regarded as clues to the presence of an unexpected environmental hazard that requires attention.[2–4]

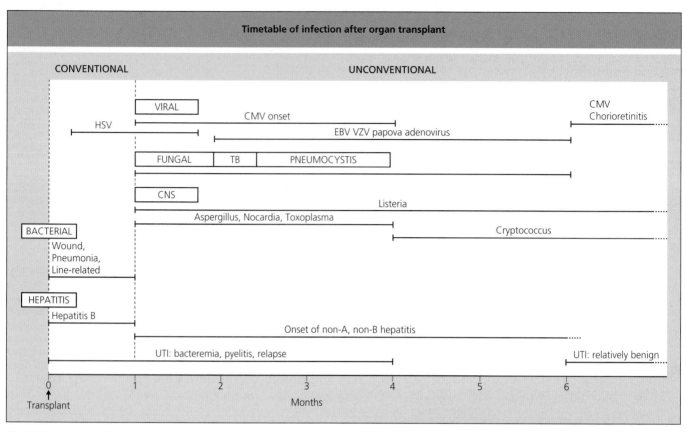

Timetable of infection after organ transplant

CONVENTIONAL — UNCONVENTIONAL

VIRAL
HSV
CMV onset
EBV VZV papova adenovirus
CMV Chorioretinitis

FUNGAL | TB | PNEUMOCYSTIS

CNS
Listeria
Aspergillus, Nocardia, Toxoplasma
Cryptococcus

BACTERIAL
Wound, Pneumonia, Line-related

HEPATITIS
Hepatitis B
Onset of non-A, non-B hepatitis

UTI: bacteremia, pyelitis, relapse
UTI: relatively benign

0 — 1 — 2 — 3 — 4 — 5 — 6
↑ Transplant
Months

Fig. 75.3 Timetable of infection after organ transplant. Exceptions to this timetable should initiate a search for an unusual hazard. CMV, cytomegalovirus; CNS, central nervous system; EBV, Epstein–Barr virus; TB, tuberculosis; HSV, herpes simplex virus; UTI, urinary tract infection; VZV, varicella-zoster virus. From Rubin.[2]

Infection in the first month post-transplant

In the first month post-transplant, the three major causes of infection in the organ transplant recipient are:

- infection in the recipient present before transplant;
- active infection conveyed with the allograft; and
- the same wound-, catheter-, vascular access-related infection and pneumonia encountered in nonimmunosuppressed patients subjected to comparable amounts of surgery.[2,4]

Donor-derived infection

Donor-derived infection is a major concern. On the one hand, there is a severe shortage of organs; on the other, objective assessment of the risk of infection from a particular donor in a timely fashion remains a challenge. At present, a detailed epidemiologic history is probably the best tool available, with the following categories of infection requiring consideration:

- Bloodstream infection from the donor is usually related to intensive care support during the donor's terminal illness. Vascular access devices are particularly vulnerable to this form of infection, with such organisms as *Candida* spp., *Staph. aureus* and *Staph. epidermidis*, and Gram-negative organisms such as *P. aeruginosa* being particularly important. In addition to the expected consequences of bacteremia, infection of the vascular suture line, with the development of mycotic aneurysms at risk for catastrophic rupture, is a major concern.[2,4]
- Allograft infection, although less common, can have similar adverse effects. The organs commonly transplanted (kidneys, liver, heart, lung and pancreas) receive a significant portion of the cardiac output. This is reflected in the frequency with which

disseminated infection seeds the allograft. Such micro-organisms as the endemic mycoses, the opportunistic fungi, mycobacteria and *Nocardia* can remain dormant for prolonged periods, only to become clinically important at a later time.[2,4]

- Viral infection has become the most important class of infection affecting organ transplant patients. The herpes group viruses, particularly CMV and EBV, hepatitis viruses B and C (HBV and HCV), HIV and community-acquired respiratory viruses are major pathogens for the transplant patient. Assessing the potential role of these viruses for both donor and recipient has become an important aspect of donor evaluation.[2,3]
- Newly emerging pathogens are playing an increasing role in transplant recipients. First, such pathogens as influenza (including avian flu and H1N1) and RSV have an increased incidence and severity in the transplant patient (see Fig. 75.1). What is new is the occurrence of clusters of fatal cases of rabies, lymphochoriomeningitis virus and the recognition of hitherto unrecognized viruses in the lungs. In addition, unrecognized lymphoma in the donor has been transferred via transplantation.[7–11]

Although we have entered an era of molecular diagnostics, which can provide the timely information required, the number of assays needed constitutes a formidable challenge. For the present, detailed clinical and epidemiologic evaluations remain the best tools available to prevent catastrophic donor-derived infection, with the available diagnostic assays serving as supplementary information.

Infection 1–6 months post-transplant

This is a period of great vulnerability to infection, a reflection of the fact that the net state of immunosuppression is markedly increased.

Table 75.4 Direct and indirect effects of cytomegalovirus infection in the organ transplant recipient

Direct effects	Mononucleosis/fever of unknown origin
	Pneumonia
	Enterocolitis
	CNS effects
	  Aseptic meningitis
	  Cerebritis
	  Transverse myelitis
	  Guillain–Barré syndrome

Indirect effects	Contributes to the net state of immunosuppression and the risk of opportunistic infection Contributes to allograft injury, with a particular emphasis on a vasculopathy Oncogenesis

There are two reasons for this: the sustained effects of exogenous immunosuppressive therapy now render the recipient particularly susceptible, and this is the time period when the immunomodulating viruses are most active. These include CMV, human herpesvirus (HHV)-6, EBV, HBV, HCV and HIV. The clinical syndromes that are important fit into two general categories:

- the direct and indirect effects of one or more of these viruses (Table 75.4); and
- opportunistic infection that is related to the increased level of immunosuppression, not to unusual environmental exposures.[2,4]

Infection more than 6 months post-transplant

Three categories of patients in this late period need to be considered:

- ~75% of patients will have had a satisfactory result from their transplant;
- 10–15% of patients have chronic liver disease; and
- ~10% of patients will have had a poor outcome from transplantation.

These patients are at particular risk for both opportunistic infections and community-acquired respiratory viruses.[2,4]

VIRAL INFECTIONS OF PARTICULAR IMPORTANCE FOR ORGAN TRANSPLANT RECIPIENTS

Herpes group viruses

The eight human herpes group viruses (CMV, EBV, herpes simplex virus (HSV)-1, HSV-2, varicella-zoster virus (VZV) and HHV-6, HHV-7 and HHV-8) share a number of properties, as follows.[2,4,5,12–16]

Latency

This describes the behavior of viruses when active replication is replaced by a nonreplicating state in a variety of cells within the patient. The viral genome is present in latently infected cells, but gene expression is limited, infectious virus is not produced and the virus is unavailable for immune attack. All patients with latent infection are seropositive for the particular virus. Latent virus is capable of being reactivated, producing fully functional virus. The stability of latency is an important consideration. Cytomegalovirus is stable in latency, requiring exposure to tumor necrosis factor (TNF) and other proinflammatory influences to begin full replication. Any cause of TNF release (e.g. rejection,

ATG, sepsis) can be involved in this process. Other viruses, particularly EBV and HSV, can reactivate in response to minimal exposures or even spontaneously. Once viral reactivation occurs, the extent of the viral replication, and the subsequent clinical effects, are determined by the patient's net state of immunosuppression.[2,3,17–19]

Cell association

The term 'cell association' emphasizes that these viruses are spread between individuals by intimate contact, transfusion or transplantation. Spread within an individual is accomplished by the direct contact of infected cells with other susceptible cells.[2,4]

Oncogenicity

All herpes group viruses should be considered potentially oncogenic. In the case of post-transplant lymphoproliferative disease (PTLD) and Kaposi's sarcoma (KS), EBV and HHV-8 play a major role in the pathogenesis of these malignancies. In addition, CMV disease has been shown to increase the incidence of EBV-associated PTLD as much as 10-fold.[2,4,5,15–26]

Clinical significance

Both direct and indirect effects of these viruses on the transplant patient must be considered (see Table 75.4). Direct effects include viral pneumonia, mononucleosis, hepatitis, enterocolitis and meningoencephalitis. These are thought to be due to lytic viral infection, tissue invasion and the host response to these events. The term 'indirect effects' refers to those caused by the cytokines, chemokines and growth factors produced as a consequence of viral replication and invasion. These effects include immunomodulation, allograft injury and oncogenesis. In many patients, the indirect effects are at least as important as the direct effects.[2,4,12–16]

Indirect effects of particular importance are those that affect the allograft: rejection and vascular injury due to the consequences of endothelial cell infection. In lung transplants, bronchiolitis obliterans is also associated with CMV and can be limited by an effective antimicrobial strategy.[2,4]

Cytomegalovirus

Epidemiology

Cytomegalovirus (CMV) can be transmitted in three ways:

- transfusion (of viable, latently infected leukocytes);
- transplantation (of an organ from a seropositive donor); and
- reactivation of virus from a seropositive (and hence latently infected) individual.

Uncommonly, the virus can be acquired through intimate contact between an actively infected individual and a CMV-naive transplant recipient. Three epidemiologic patterns of CMV infection are recognized in transplant patients: primary infection, reactivation CMV disease and superinfection.[2,4]

- Primary infection involves the transfer of viable cells from a seropositive donor into a seronegative recipient; 90% of the time, the allograft is the source of the latently infected cells. In addition, viable leukocyte-containing blood products can be the source of the virus. This latter form of transmission should be avoided by using 'pedigreed' blood products that come from CMV-seronegative donors or those that are administered though highly efficient leukocyte filters. Overall, ~50% of patients at risk of primary infection as a result of transplantation become clinically ill.
- Reactivation CMV infection occurs when the transplant recipient is seropositive prior to transplant and the virus that is activated is of endogenous origin. The great majority of patients in this category will have some evidence of viral replication, but only 10–20% will have evidence of clinical disease.[2,4,16]
- Superinfection occurs when an allograft from a CMV-seropositive donor is transplanted into a seropositive recipient and the virus

that is activated is of donor origin. Superinfection appears to cause more symptoms than reactivation disease. In any case, if intensive immunosuppression is required, both reactivation and superinfection will have greater effects.[2,4,]

Another important clinical problem that is currently appearing is the late onset of CMV after prophylaxis.[27,28]

Pathogenesis of CMV infection

The pathogenesis of CMV infection has two key steps: reactivation from latency, and amplification and dissemination of actively replicating virus. The key mediator in initiating this process is TNF, which binds to the TNF receptor of latently infected cells, resulting in a downstream signaling process that includes the activation of protein kinase C and nuclear factor kappa B (NF-κB). Activated p65/p50 NF-κB heterodimer translocates into the nucleus and binds to the CMV immediate early enhancer region, which initiates viral replication. Such conditions as sepsis, fulminant hepatic failure, allograft rejection and the 'cytokine storm' associated with OKT3 and ATG administration are associated with the elaboration of large amounts of TNF (and other proinflammatory mediators, such as catecholamines and prostaglandins).[2,4]

Once replicating virus is present, the degree of amplification that occurs is determined by the net state of immunosuppression and the subsequent immunosuppressive program. The critical host defense is the major histocompatibility complex (MHC)-restricted, CMV-specific cytotoxic T-cell response. A rapid viral replication rate prior to antiviral intervention, a high viral load and a slow rate of viral clearance on therapy are all associated with a relatively poor outcome to conventional courses of therapy and a high rate of relapse. It has been suggested that the production of interferon gamma (IFN-γ) by CD8+ T cells is reduced in patients with viremia, and that this deficit (termed 'specific interferon gamma impairment', SIGI) has predictive value prior to the initiation of antiviral therapy.[2,4,5,25–27]

Clinical effects of CMV infection

Direct effects Clinical CMV disease typically begins 1–4 months post-transplant, and is similar in all forms of organ transplantation, with one notable exception: the organ transplanted is more affected than the native organ (see Table 75.4).

The most common clinical syndromes include mononucleosis, interstitial pneumonia, bone marrow dysfunction, and both functional (poor motility) and structural damage to the gut (enterocolitis and poor gastric and small bowel motility). Perhaps most interesting is the possible bidirectional relationship between CMV and hepatitis C virus: infection with one results in an upregulation of the viral burden of the other.[2,4] However, a recent study argues against an association between HCV and CMV infections after transplantation.[29]

Indirect effects The indirect effects of CMV are of three types: allograft injury, promotion of opportunistic infection and oncogenesis. There is now a consensus that allograft injury can occur as a consequence of CMV infection. The most convincing data on this subject come from studies of heart transplant patients in whom both acute rejection and accelerated coronary atherosclerosis are linked to both symptomatic and asymptomatic CMV infection. CMV-infected endothelial cells are thought to play an important role in the vascular injury that can occur. Similar associations are found in liver and lung transplantation.[30–32]

Perhaps the most compelling information on this subject comes from human studies in which anti-CMV prophylaxis clearly decreased both acute and chronic rejection among kidney allograft recipients, and that ganciclovir therapy in cardiac transplant recipients decreased the incidence and severity of coronary artery atherosclerosis post-transplant. In summary, an ever-expanding body of evidence has linked CMV infection to allograft injury. There is a bidirectional relationship between these two processes, with a similar array of mediators being elaborated and a similar pathologic picture being produced by both; that is, although the initial stimuli may be different, the ultimate signaling pathway that causes injury is the same. A question that has long been debated has finally been answered – 'Which comes first,

CMV or rejection?' The answer is either or both. What also becomes a reasonable hypothesis is that other infections (e.g. HHV-6) could have similar effects and that ultimately the extent of allograft injury is the integration of a number of different processes that include ischemia, infection and classic rejection, with room in this model for other as yet to be defined processes.[2–4,33–42]

The potential effects of herpesviruses on oncogenesis

Cytomegalovirus and several other herpesviruses have been thought of as potentially oncogenic for many years. Epstein–Barr virus and HHV-8, in particular, have been linked to post-transplant lymphoproliferative disease (EBV) and KS (HHV-8), respectively. In addition, the incidence of PTLD is increased 7–10-fold in individuals with symptomatic CMV disease. An uncommon form of malignancy linked to EBV is smooth muscle neoplasia of the gut.[20–23,25]

Clinical management of CMV: diagnosis and treatment

Diagnosis The three general approaches to the diagnosis of CMV are serologic, virologic and pathologic. Serologic approaches are useful in assessing the past experience with the virus and the possibility of latent infection (all patients with circulating antibody against CMV should be considered as harboring latent virus that is capable of being reactivated). There is little need for serologic testing post-transplant.[2,3]

The CMV antigenemia assay and a quantitative PCR assay both offer same-day diagnosis, with a sensitivity and specificity of >95%, as well as a useful measurement of microbial burden. There are, however, some drawbacks to these assays: lung and gastrointestinal infection do not yield reliable results (and hence colonoscopic and/or lung biopsy for both immunofluorescent and standard pathologic assessment is still needed for evaluation of the patient with signs and symptoms of inflammation at these sites).[2,3]

Whether it is determined by PCR or antigenemia, the key measurement is viral load. Viral load determinations are useful in several ways:

- as a stratification device in determining the dose and duration of therapy;
- serial viral load measurements can be used to monitor the response to therapy, to guide pre-emptive therapy; and
- to predict the chance of relapsing disease and the need for more therapy.[2,3]

In occasional cases renal dysfunction occurs with a biopsy picture revealing cells laden with CMV inclusions, typically in the tubular epithelium and interstitium. Renal biopsies without CMV at the time of acute functional deterioration of the kidney revealed classic tubulointerstitial findings of acute cellular rejection; however, a patient with viremic CMV had a distinctive glomerular lesion on biopsy. CMV-infected recipients who are viremic have about twice the frequency of glomerulopathy versus those who are nonviremic. Renal dysfunction associated with glomerular lesions is less likely to respond to antirejection therapy. In liver transplantation, this issue is even more complicated as the direct and possible indirect effects of CMV on the liver may be obscured by allograft rejection and hepatitis C infection.

Treatment Strategies for controlling CMV include both preventive and therapeutic approaches (Table 75.5). In the preventive category such interventions as 'protective matching', 'pedigreed blood products', hyperimmune gamma globulin and antiviral therapy have been shown to offer some degree of protection. The term protective matching applies to the allocation of organs so that the transplantation of an allograft from a CMV-seropositive donor into a seronegative recipient is avoided. This strategy is effective, but limits the pool of potential donors at a time when there is already a shortage of organs. At present this approach is largely reserved for children.[2–5,42–51]

There are three groups of antiviral compounds that can be used to prevent or treat the consequences of CMV infection: aciclovir and valaciclovir; ganciclovir and valganciclovir; and foscarnet.[2,3]

Table 75.5 Prevention and treatment of cytomegalovirus infectious dose in the organ transplant recipient

Intervention	Effectiveness
Prevention	
Hyperimmune anti-CMV globulin	2+ (attenuated by anti-thymocyte globulin)
High-dose oral aciclovir or valaciclovir	1+
Valganciclovir	4+
Therapy	
Hyperimmune anti-CMV globulin	1+
Valaciclovir	1+
Valganciclovir	3+
Number of + = degree of effectiveness.	

Table 75.6 Clinical syndromes due to Epstein–Barr virus in organ transplant recipients

Benign viral diseases	Mononucleosis Interstitial pneumonia Syndromes of fever and adenopathy Meningitis and meningoencephalitis Leukopenia/thrombocytopenia Hepatitis Gastrointestinal bleeding Guillain–Barré syndrome
Post-transplant lymphoproliferative disease	Continuum from benign polyclonal process to malignant disease with monoclonal cells Leukopenia/thrombocytopenia Adenopathy Gastrointestinal bleeding due to tumor mass in the wall of the gut with perforation and/or intussusception Pneumonia Focal and diffuse central nervous system disease

Ganciclovir is the most useful anti-CMV drug currently available. Oral formulations of ganciclovir have the same bioavailability issues as oral aciclovir (<15% bioavailability, which rises to 50–60% when the valine ester is employed). Valganciclovir is the drug of choice for both the prevention and treatment of CMV disease. It is effective both pre-emptively and prophylactically.[2,3]

Primary resistance to ganciclovir is most unusual. However, when too low a dose and/or too short a duration of therapy are utilized, particularly when a high viral burden is present, secondary resistance can develop. In this circumstance, foscarnet becomes the treatment of choice, either alone or in combination with oral valganciclovir. Foscarnet is highly nephrotoxic, hence the hesitation for prescribing it unless resistance to the other antivirals is present.[2–4,43–52]

Epstein–Barr virus

The epithelial cells of the upper respiratory tract are the site of EBV replication and likely the natural reservoir for EBV infection. Transmission of the virus is effected by the exchange of virus-laden saliva. This infection is lytic in character, resulting in the release of replicating virus. These events result in continuing replication of the virus in the upper respiratory tract epithelium, with long-lived B lymphocytes becoming infected during their travel through the lymphoid tissues of the pharynx.[2,3,21–24]

In the nonimmunosuppressed host, clinical disease is initiated by infection of the epithelial cells and B lymphocytes, which then incites an intense, cytotoxic T-cell response to the latently infected B lymphocytes, which are widely distributed throughout the body. This immune response is responsible for most of the manifestations of infectious mononucleosis, as well as providing an explanation for the lack of efficacy of antiviral chemotherapy in dealing with the mononucleosis clinical syndrome.[2,3,21]

Although most adults who are EBV seropositive harbor latently infected, transformed B lymphocytes that have the potential for unlimited growth, lymphoproliferation is blocked by the activity of an active surveillance mechanism based primarily on an MHC-restricted, EBV-specific, cytotoxic T-cell response. High-dose immunosuppression, particularly with calcineurin inhibitors and with ATG, effectively blocks this mechanism, increasing the risk of PTLD. Similarly, primary EBV carries an increased risk of PTLD because the viral burden is greater and the immunologic response to the primary infection is still immature. There is increasing evidence that proinflammatory cytokines generated by such common events as CMV infection, allograft rejection and HCV infection increase PTLD risk considerably.

For example, CMV disease is associated with a 7–10-fold increase in the occurrence of PTLD and HCV increases the risk more than fivefold in liver transplant recipients.[20–25]

There are, then, two interacting factors that determine the incidence of PTLD in the transplant patient: viral load, and the ability of the EBV-specific, cytotoxic T-cell surveillance system to eliminate the transformed cells.

The clinical presentation of PTLD can be quite variable (Table 75.6). Management requires a marked decrease (including cessation) in immunosuppression, particularly of the calcineurin inhibitors and ATG. If further therapy is needed, anti-B cell monoclonal antibody has proven to be the treatment of choice for the more severe cases of PTLD.[2,20–25]

Herpes simplex virus

Virtually all the instances of HSV infection post-transplant are due to reactivation of latent infection in seropositive individuals, occurring 2–4 weeks post-transplant. Not only do the lesions persist longer than comparable lesions in the normal host, but also the severity is increased, with large, painful crusted ulcerations that may bleed or cause difficulties with aspiration. The typical vesicles on an erythematous base may be absent in the transplant patient, with ulcerations being the more common lesion recognized (both with anogenital and orolabial disease). Intraoral and esophageal infections occur predominantly in patients whose mucosa has been traumatized by endotracheal and/or nasogastric tubes. Lesions that are thought to be responding poorly to aciclovir should be considered for biopsy to rule out the presence of squamous cell carcinoma.[2–4]

Anogenital HSV-2 infection is less common than orolabial infection due to HSV-1. Unusually severe anogenital infection with large, coalescing, ulcerative lesions may be present in patients who are undergoing intensive immunosuppression. An unusual form of cutaneous dissemination (termed eczema herpeticum or Kaposi's varicelliform eruption) may be observed due to HSV, in which the skin lesions occur at sites of previous skin trauma – burns, eczema or atopic dermatitis. Rarely primary infection can occur due to allograft infection.[2,4,5]

Varicella-zoster virus

The most important information that relates to VZV infection in the transplant patient is whether the patient is seropositive for this virus.

Reactivation infection due to VZV (as with herpes zoster) or super-infection due to VZV are relatively mild illnesses; in contrast, primary VZV infection is a devastating illness characterized by hemorrhagic pneumonia and skin lesions, encephalitis, pancreatitis and hepatitis. The traditional approach to a seronegative patient with a significant exposure history to chickenpox is to administer zoster immune globulin, which has an efficacy of >80%. Delays in administering this agent can lead to attenuation of the preventive effects (e.g. the lack of the characteristic skin rash while dissemination and visceral invasion are occurring). Valaciclovir therapy is effective and can be combined with the vaccine in seronegative individuals.[2,3,12–14]

Human herpesviruses 6, 7 and 8

Human herpesvirus (HHV)-6 is a beta-herpesvirus closely related to CMV (66% DNA homology) that infects a variety of cell types, most notably CD4$^+$ cells. Replicating HHV-6 provides a strong stimulus for the release of an array of proinflammatory cytokines, most notably TNF, interleukin (IL)-1 and IFN-γ. The range of clinical effects includes febrile syndromes similar to those produced by CMV (e.g. fever and mononucleosis, hepatitis, bone marrow dysfunction, encephalitis and pneumonia). In addition, HHV-6 is thought to produce a series of indirect effects, particularly the potentiation of opportunistic infections due to an increase in the net state of immunosuppression, and allograft injury.[34,40–42]

HHV-6 primary infection is usually acquired in the first year of life, when it causes roseola (exanthem subitum); reactivation of latent HHV-6 is thought to be the major form of infection encountered thereafter. Possible central nervous system (CNS) effects of HHV-6 have received particular attention, and include mental status changes, seizures and headache. An association between multiple sclerosis and other demyelinating conditions has also been reported. Uncommonly, low attenuation white matter changes similar to those seen with immunosuppression-associated leukoencephalopathy can be identified.[34,40–42]

HHV-7 is another beta-herpesvirus that resembles CMV and HHV-6. Primary infection occurs under the age of 5 due to infection of CD4 molecules. In some ways, HHV-7 might be best thought of as an 'orphan virus' of unclear clinical importance.[15,40,41]

HHV-8 is a gamma-herpesvirus, which is the causative agent of KS. Both primary and reactivation infection with this virus have been linked with KS, particularly in those receiving corticosteroids and/or OKT3 antirejection therapy. Clinical manifestations of KS in transplant patients are similar to those seen in other immunosuppressed patients: violaceous/black nodules are common, often accompanied by visceral lesions, which include bleeding, perforation, obstruction and protein-losing enteropathy. Antiviral therapy with one or more of the following drugs may be useful in the management of transplant-related KS: ganciclovir, foscarnet, adefovir, cidofovir and HPMA [(S)-1-(3)-hydroxy-2-phosphonylmethoxypropyadenine].[20]

Papovaviruses

The papovaviruses are DNA viruses that can be divided into two genera: the polyomaviruses and the papillomaviruses. The polyomaviruses include BK virus, JC virus and simian virus 40 (SV40), which appear to cause asymptomatic infection during childhood; later in life, immunosuppression results in replication of these viruses, which are closely related antigenically and structurally.[53–57]

BK virus

BK virus (BKV) replication has been associated with a variety of renal and urinary tract disorders, including ureteral strictures, renal cell carcinoma and, increasingly, tubulointerstitial nephritis of the renal allograft. With present forms of immunosuppression, the incidence of BKV nephritis approaches 10% (see Practice Point 43).

JC virus

JC virus (JCV) has been shown to be the cause of progressive multifocal leukoencephalopathy (PML), a demyelinating disease of brain white matter. JCV causes progressive motor and sensory deficits, dementia and, usually, death in 3–6 months. As with BKV, a decrease in immunosuppression is usually advocated.[2,58]

Papillomaviruses

Papillomavirus infection is responsible for the development of warts, which can be so numerous in immunosuppressed transplant patients as to be disfiguring. Malignant transformation, particularly in sun-exposed areas, has been well documented. Human papillomavirus DNA has been linked to the skin cancers of these patients, and it is likely that such cancers arise as a result of the combined effects of the virus, immunosuppression and ultraviolet irradiation.[2,4,58]

Hepatitis viruses

Hepatitis B virus

Hepatitis B virus (HBV) is a DNA virus of the Hepadna group that has long been recognized as a significant problem in transplantation: HBV is efficiently transmitted by transfusion and transplantation, a reflection of its ability to sustain viremia for a prolonged period. Person-to-person transmission can also occur through intimate mucosal contact between virus carriers and susceptible individuals. Biomarkers for susceptibility to HBV infection are now in standard use – HBsAg in the blood is a marker for the presence of infectious virus, while anti-HBs is a marker for immunity. However, it should be emphasized that anti-HBs positivity can revert to HBsAg positivity and full transmissibility in the face of intensive immunosuppression. The presence of HBcAb in the serum of liver allograft donors (but not other types of organ transplantation) carries the risk of infecting the recipient. With the exception of this uncommon event, the rate of HBV transmission is estimated to be ~0.002% per transfusion or transplant. Therapeutic intervention with anti-HBS antibody for a prolonged period, beginning at the time of transplant, has had a favorable effect on the course of these patients. Even more promising is the emergence of lamivudine as an effective therapy (until resistance develops).[59–64]

Clinical impact of HBV infection

The major challenge with HBV infection in transplantation is the management of those who are already infected with the virus at the time of transplant. Corticosteroid therapy stimulates the level of virus replication, with a rapid increase in HBV DNA polymerase activity, HBeAg levels, HBV DNA and HBsAg being observed.[2]

Liver transplantation in patients with HBV infection has been particularly problematic. Recurrence of HBV infection was essentially universal, with a number of reports of excessive mortality in the first year post-transplant, as well as the occurrence of hepatocellular carcinoma within 4 years of successful transplantation. There was also an increased rate of sepsis during these first years post-transplant, with a particularly poor result (>80% mortality in the first year) in patients with both hepatocellular carcinoma and chronic HBV infection.[2]

Two major advances have changed this dismal picture. The first was prolonged immunoprophylaxis with anti-HBs hyperimmune globulin, beginning during the anhepatic phase of the transplant operation. One-year survival rates greater than 80% could now be achieved. In the face of these successes, two major problems emerged: cost (as high as $25 000/year with some administration schedules) and, more important, the selection of viral mutants that are still pathogenic but have changes in HBsAg such that the hyperimmune globulin and/or the hepatitis B vaccine is rendered inactive.[2,56–61]

The biggest advance, however, is the advent of effective antiviral chemotherapy with lamivudine. This nucleotide analogue is a potent inhibitor of the viral polymerase/reverse transcriptase, is well tolerated, and is effective not only in lowering viral levels, but also in improving hepatic function and histology. Resistant virus begins to emerge after 1 year of therapy (these mutants are usually in a highly conserved region of the reverse transcriptase known as the YMDD motif). The higher the viral load, the more likely and more quickly resistance mutants will emerge. After 1 year of therapy, resistance rates of 14–31% are noted, and at 2 years this rises to 38%. Clearly, multidrug regimens will be necessary for complete control of HBV.[2–4,62–64]

Hepatitis C virus

Hepatitis C virus (HCV) is an RNA virus that is the cause of post-transfusion hepatitis, post-transplant liver disease and most of the cases of non-A, non-B hepatitis. HCV is a common cause of end-stage liver disease necessitating liver transplantation, may cause progressive liver disease following transplantation and is an important contributor to the net state of immunosuppression. The most effective therapy at present is the combination of pegylated interferon and ribavirin, which appears to favorably influence the course of ~50% of patients with chronic HCV infection.[65,66]

Clinical impact of HCV infection

Hepatitis C virus is the major cause of non-A, non-B hepatitis, as well as more than 80% of post-transplant liver disease. HCV is spread via parenteral contact with blood or by transplantation of an organ from an HCV-viremic donor. HCV appears to differ from hepatitis A virus (HAV) and HBV in rarely producing fulminant hepatitis. HCV infection carries a greater than 50% risk of chronicity, with end-stage liver disease or hepatocellular carcinoma developing as a consequence of this in ~20% of these patients.[2–4,65,66]

Risk factors that are correlated with increased morbidity and mortality include viral load; intensity of immunosuppression; allograft rejection; HCV genotype (genotype 1b having been associated with higher viral loads, a more accelerated course, and a poorer response to interferon-based therapy); the presence of quasispecies (the greater the heterogeneity in the HCV population, the greater the difficulty in containing the infection); CMV viremia; iron overload; and details of cytokine responses that are beginning to emerge from ongoing studies.[2–4]

Two uncommon complications of HCV infection can be devastating. The first – fibrosing cholestatic hepatitis – manifests as high levels of circulating HCV, rapidly progressive hepatic failure, mildly elevated serum aminotransferase level, extensive periportal fibrosis, intense cholestasis, minimal inflammatory infiltrate and no cirrhosis. The hepatocytes are choked with exceedingly high levels of HCV, which results in direct hepatocyte injury. This diagnosis requires immediate decrease in immunosuppression and the initiation of the best available antiviral therapy.[2–4]

The second of these complications is glomerulonephritis. The most common form of this is membranoproliferative glomerulonephritis, with or without mixed cryogobulinemia. Uncommon forms of renal injury associated with HCV infection include membranous glomerulonephritis, acute and chronic transplant glomerulonephritis and thrombotic microangiopathy with anticardiolipin antibody.[2–4]

Human immunodeficiency virus

Transplantation of an organ from an HIV-infected donor into an uninfected recipient is a highly efficient mechanism for transmitting the virus. Rarely, a false-negative HIV test can be obtained from a donor who transmits the virus with the allograft. A bigger issue is the donor who has received large numbers of transfusions in a desperate attempt to save the individual's life. By this time, blood bank blood will obscure the results of laboratory studies: false-negative results can be obtained in this situation since the blood actually tested does not reflect clinical events; that is, the allograft in this situation, despite negative serologies, is quite able to transmit both HIV and hepatitis B and/or C.

When primary HIV infection is acquired post-transplant, it not uncommonly produces a mononucleosis syndrome ~6 weeks post-transplant. The mean time for the development of overt AIDS in persons who acquire primary HIV infection at the time of transplant has been ~3 years. A far bigger issue is the optimal management of patients with asymptomatic HIV infection who present with end-stage renal, hepatic, pulmonary and/or heart disease. Thus far, the results of transplantation in these individuals have been remarkably good. Increasingly, transplant groups are establishing guidelines for transplanting the HIV-positive individual:[67–70]

- Transplantation of HIV-infected individuals should be carried out at centers with great expertise in both transplantation and HIV therapy, and where these skills can be brought to bear in the day-to-day care of these patients.
- HIV-infected patients accepted for transplantation should be on a stable highly active antiretroviral therapy (HAART) regimen, are known to be compliant and to have acceptable blood levels of virus.
- Careful ongoing assessment for opportunistic infection should be undertaken. Appropriate prophylaxis should be initiated (e.g. trimethoprim-sulfamethoxazole, fluconazole) as well as perioperative antibacterial prophylaxis.

FUNGAL INFECTIONS OF PARTICULAR IMPORTANCE FOR THE ORGAN TRANSPLANT RECIPIENT

Invasive fungal infection (Table 75.7) has become increasingly important to the transplant patient in recent years:[1]

- A wide variety of fungal species capable of invading the transplant patient are present in the environment, both in the community and in the hospital. Person-to-person spread of *Candida* spp. by medical personnel has increased the difficulty of patient management.[2]
- The net state of immunosuppression can be quite high in these patients, facilitating both transmission and amplification of infection.
- The anti-inflammatory (as well as immunosuppressive) effects of antirejection therapy tend to obscure the signs and symptoms of infection. Along with the bland nature of patient–fungal interactions, early diagnosis and treatment can be a major challenge.
- Several new therapies have been developed; however, guidelines for the treatment and prevention of invasive disease are still being established. Particularly important in formulating these guidelines is the therapeutic prescription – an antirejection program and an antimicrobial program to make it safe. Such an approach needs flexibility, in which changes in one of these will trigger changes in the other.
- Initial host defenses against these fungi are mediated by polymorphonuclear leukocytes and macrophages: definitive immune response mediated by MHC-restricted, fungus-specific, cytotoxic T cells – just the form of host defense most susceptible to antirejection therapy.

Environmental exposures play a major role in the occurrence of fungal infections, with the inhalation of infectious aerosols being the most effective means of acquiring invasive infection due to a wide range of fungi (the endemic mycoses, the opportunistic molds like *Aspergillus*, and newly emerging organisms such as *Fusarium* and *Scedosporium*).[2]

The other major route by which transplant patients acquire clinically important fungal infection is via candidal overgrowth on mucocutaneous surfaces. From that point, it is a relatively small step to penetration of the mucocutaneous barrier, with invasion followed by the possibility of disseminated infection.

837

Table 75.7 Clinical fungal infection in the organ transplant recipient

Challenges	Recognition of signs and symptoms of early fungal invasion
	Blandness of the host response to fungal invasion
	Anti-inflammatory effects of the anti-rejection therapy
	Mucocutaneous overgrowth with increased potential for invasion, dissemination and development of metastatic sites of infection
	Host responses:
	• Nonspecific ('innate immunity')
	  – Polymorphonuclear leukocyte response
	  – Macrophage and monocyte response
	• Specific (specific immunity)
	  – Key host defense: major histocompatibility complex (MHC) restricted, microbial restricted cytotoxic T-cell response
	  – Specific humoral response (B cell response)

Key prognostic sign	Microbial burden
Important clinical infections	Candidiasis (key species: *Candida albicans, C. tropicalis, C. krusei, C. glabrata*)
Mucocutaneous overgrowth with the potential for dissemination	Bloodstream invasion 5% rate of metastatic spread in nonimmunosuppressed host 20–50% rate of metastatic spread in transplant recipients Metastatic spread should be assumed in the presence of vascular access catheters and as a consequence of surgical manipulation of colonized sites Fluconazole susceptible (*C. albicans* and *C. tropicalis*) Fluconazole resistant (acquired resistance with prolonged exposure; person-to-person spread on hands of medical personnel; intrinsic resistance of *C. krusei* and *C. glabrata*)
Invasive opportunistic fungi (saprophytes from the environment)	Invasive aspergillosis (the model for molds, including the endemic mycoses and newly emerging fungi) Primary portals of entry: inhalation, damaged skin Vascular invasion Infarction, hemorrhage and metastatic spread Primary therapy: voriconazole ± echinocandin ± amphotericin
Endemic mycoses	Histoplasmosis, coccidioidomycosis and blastomycosis Inhalation of infectious particles Consequences: hypersensitivity syndromes, lung disease (primary disease, progressive disease, metastatic disease) Particular impact on transplant patients Therapy: induce remission with amphotericin (particularly a lipid formulation) followed by an azole for prolonged therapy
Newly emerging fungal pathogens	Similar events to invasive aspergillosis Examples: *Fusarium* spp., *Scedosporium* spp., zygomycetes Therapy: tend to be amphotericin resistant; therapy with either voriconazole or posaconazole

'Darwinian factors' are now recognized as contributing significantly to microbial pathogenesis. The most common example of this phenomenon is when broad-spectrum antibacterial therapy has been given in the setting of an anatomic problem that has not been corrected. Candidal superinfection is a common result, requiring surgical correction as well as systemic antifungal therapy. Another version of Darwinian influences is when excessive amounts of iron, an important growth factor, can potentiate mucormycosis, listeriosis and candidiasis. Elevated glucose levels will increase the microbial burden in diabetics, particularly on mucocutaneous surfaces, where candidal overgrowth can play an important role in the pathogenesis of invasive infection.[2,3]

Candidiasis

Candida albicans and *C. tropicalis* are the most common candidal species to cause human disease. Secondary infection due to azole-resistant species such as *C. glabrata* and *C. krusei* is common, particularly in circumstances where the underlying defect in mucocutaneous structures remains uncorrected. Typical sites of infection include a catheterized urinary tract, vascular access catheters, peritoneal dialysis catheters and drainage catheters, particularly in the setting of hyperglycemia. Removal of these foreign bodies in association with antifungal therapy has been strongly advocated. Normally present on mucocutaneous surfaces, the vagina and the gut, invasive candidal disease is associated with overgrowth and tissue damage. Bloodstream invasion is a not uncommon event, with an incidence of 5–60% of metastatic infection of the eyes, bone and other sites. Manipulation of sites colonized by these organisms is particularly associated with bloodstream entry and dissemination. For this reason, pre-emptive therapy in association with surgery is advocated. Fluconazole has long been the treatment of choice, but with the increasing incidence of resistance, the possible need for broader spectrum therapy should be considered.[2,3,5,71–73]

Cryptococcosis

Cryptococcosis is an important cause of opportunistic infection, being ubiquitous in the environment and easily inhaled when an aerosol is created. The portal of entry is the lungs, with infection causing minimal symptoms and most infections escaping medical attention. In the transplant patient, a variety of clinical syndromes may occur: in the lungs, asymptomatic nodules are most common, although progressive pneumonia can occur. Systemic infection with metastatic seeding is common, with a particular impact on the CNS (with both meningitis and cerebritis being seen). Diagnosis is greatly facilitated by the ability to measure the presence of the polysaccharide capsule in the blood and/or cerebrospinal fluid. This is useful for both primary diagnosis and as a measure of the microbial burden. Initial therapy is usually with the combination of flucytosine and an amphotericin for 1–2 weeks to 'gain control', followed by a prolonged course of fluconazole.[2,4]

Invasive aspergillosis

Although a variety of hypersensitivity and colonization syndromes have been associated with *Aspergillus* infection, in transplant patients the concern is primarily with invasive disease following inhalation of aerosolized organisms that are ubiquitous in the environment. Three species account for 95% of the cases of invasive aspergillosis: *A. fumigatus*, *A. flavus* and *A. niger*. More than 80% of the patients with invasive disease have a pulmonary portal of entry, ~10% have a nasal sinus portal of entry, with cutaneous sites accounting for most of the rest.[2,3,74–76]

Both neutropenia and corticosteroid administration predispose to invasive aspergillosis. Environmental hazards leading to excessive exposure are the rule: within the hospital (usually representing construction) or in the community where such activities as gardening can lead to invasive disease. The clinical behavior of this entity is determined by its ability to invade blood vessels, so that the results of this infection include infarction, hemorrhage and metastatic spread.[2,3]

In more than 50% of patients with invasive aspergillosis, metastatic spread is already present at the time of first diagnosis; in addition, a site of metastasis may be the first sign of disseminated disease. The typical radiologic finding in these patients is focal lung disease, with either a nodule or a consolidation being present, often with cavitation. Unlike the leukemia or bone marrow transplant patient with invasive aspergillosis, halo signs and air crescent signs are uncommon. At present, biopsy is required for diagnosis. Preliminary evaluation suggests that the galactomannan assay may be a reliable biomarker for this condition.[2,3]

Therapy is continuing to evolve: voriconazole (or posaconazole; very few data on posaconazole for therapy) is the single drug of choice at present. Combination therapy is being further evaluated, with an echinocandin and/or an amphotericin B preparation being added to the azole. If the clinical state of the patient is appropriate and the anatomy is favorable, surgical resection in combination with the antifungal drugs will yield improved results.[77,78]

Invasive aspergillosis is potentiated by steroids and/or neutropenia, and occurs only in patients who are significantly immunocompromised and/or exposed to a major environmental hazard. Other associations include the presence of *Aspergillus* in marijuana, which can lead to invasive disease. Direct inoculation of damaged skin (e.g. vascular access sites, burns and sites of inoculation) can likewise require treatment. In lung transplant recipients two additional forms of *Aspergillus* infection have been noted: infection of the suture line, with subsequent necrosis and disruption, and tracheobronchial disease.[2]

Invasive aspergillosis, then, primarily occurs in situations of poor leukocyte function or a sustained exposure to steroids. However, even patients whose net state of immunosuppression is minimal can develop invasive aspergillosis if the environmental exposure is great enough. An important corollary to this observation is that a single case of invasive aspergillosis occurring in the first month post-transplant (a 'golden period' during which opportunistic infection only occurs under conditions of unusually intense environmental exposure) should trigger a search for environmental hazards before more cases occur.[2,3,74]

Clinically, invasive aspergillosis of the lungs, the most common presentation of invasive disease, can occur as the primary event or as a superinfection after pulmonary injury due to virus or bacteria, or pulmonary infarction. In as many as 50% of cases metastatic spread has already occurred by the time of diagnosis, and a site of metastasis may be the first presentation of invasive disease. The typical radiologic finding of invasive aspergillosis of the lungs is focal lung disease, with either a nodule or a consolidation being present, often with cavitation. Unlike the patient with leukemia and aspergillosis, halo signs and air crescent signs are uncommon in organ transplant patients. Specific diagnosis requires a biopsy procedure. Other diagnostic approaches such as the galactomannan assay appear to be quite promising. If the early promise is confirmed, then early pre-emptive therapy will become an important part of patient management.[2,3,73–76]

The traditional view of *Aspergillus* syndromes is that a colonization syndrome or allergic bronchopulmonary disease does not turn invasive. It is now clear, however, that on occasion this 'overlap' or 'crossover' occurs. Voriconazole now makes it possible to treat any evidence of invasive disease and, in many patients, avoid surgery. Combining voriconazole with surgery is also a useful strategy, preventing complications of surgical manipulation.[78]

The standard of care for invasive disease due to aspergillosis has long been a prolonged course of intravenous amphotericin B. Sustained therapy of this sort was rendered difficult by the toxicities of this regimen: an acute infusion toxicity, with cytokine release, fever, rigors and malaise; and chronic, progressive renal toxicity. Fortunately, there has been a major advance in the availability of alternative antifungal drugs. Antifungal agents, such as lipid-associated amphotericin B products, therapeutic azoles and echinocandins are discussed in Chapter 149.[71]

Pneumocystis jirovecii

Pneumocystis jirovecii (Table 75.8), previously known as *P. carinii*, was found to be the cause of interstitial pneumonia in Central and Eastern Europe in the mid-1940s among severely malnourished and premature infants. Long recognized as an important pathogen in transplant patients and other immunocompromised patients, the HIV epidemic amplified the importance of this pathogen. It is only in the past few

---

Table 75.8 *Pneumocystis jirovecii*

- Long recognized as an important pathogen, responsible for pneumonia (PCP) in immunocompromised hosts
- Exists in three forms: trophozoite, sporozoite (which is a precystic form) and cystic. For many years, mistakenly called a protozoan
- Although officially classified as a fungus, *Pneumocystis* does not respond to antifungal therapy
- Asymptomatic infection acquired before age 5.
- With immunocompromise, either reactivated or re-infection can occur.
- Patients with immunocompromise should be protected from person-to-person spread.
- Setting for *Pneumocystis* pneumonia
  - Children with malnutrition and hypoglobulinemia
  - HIV infection and/or AIDS
  - Organ transplant recipients
- In organ transplant patients not receiving prophylaxis, the incidence of pulmonary infection is 10–15% in the first year post transplant
- Prophylaxis indicated for ≥6 months
- *Pneumocystis* pneumonia clinically and radiologically very similar to CMV
- Clusters of patients with the exact same organism can easily be identified. Immunocompromised patients should be protected from nonimmunized patients
- Antimicrobial therapy for *Pneumocystis*
  - Trimethoprim–sulfamethoxazole
  - IV pentamidine (aerosolized form less effective)
  - Clindamycin
  - Dapsone ± pyrimethamine + leucovorin
  - Solid organ transplant
  - Atovaquone
  - Caspofungin ±

years that the taxonomy of this organism has been firmly established: it is not a trypanosome or a protozoan, as previously thought, rather it is a unicellular fungus that is usually acquired in the first decade of life and exists in three distinct forms: trophozoite (often found in clusters), sporozoite and a cystic form that often contains spores. Asymptomatic colonization is well recognized, with clinical disease occurring in patients with deficits in cell-mediated and humoral immunity. For example ~15% of organ transplant patients not receiving *Pneumocystis* prophylaxis will develop *Pneumocystis* pneumonia in the first 6 months post-transplant, particularly those patients with active CMV infection.

After long debate, it is now accepted that both person-to-person and hospital-based epidemics can occur due to *Pneumocystis*, although sporadic cases due to activation of longstanding lung colonization are even more common. Infection control activities to prevent outbreaks among immunosuppressed patients are appropriate. *Pneumocystis* clinically has a subacute presentation over several weeks, with fever, increased dyspnea, a nonproductive cough, tachypnea and pulmonary infiltrates. Rarely in transplant patients, but not uncommonly in HIV patients, extrapulmonary findings may be present, especially if aerosolized pentamidine is used. Other than tachypnea, abnormalities on physical examination are subtle or not present. The typical laboratory findings include an elevated lactate dehydrogenase level, diffuse bilateral infiltrates on X-ray and the presence of the organisms on microscopic examination of induced sputum. If this is negative, then bronchoalveolar lavage is indicated.

Therapeutic decision making is an important issue. Prevention is usually accomplished with trimethoprim–sulfamethoxazole; systemic treatment with the same drug for symptomatic *Pneumocystis* disease is the regimen of choice. Prednisone as adjunctive therapy should be considered for patients with significant hypoxemia. A wide variety of drugs (including pentamidine, atovaquone, trimetrexate, dapsone and pyrimethamine) are available for patients not tolerating trimethoprim–sulfamethoxazole. Drugs such as caspofungin, which act by inhibiting fungal cell wall synthesis in a fashion analogous to the effects of penicillin on bacterial cell wall synthesis, may add considerably to the efficacy of standard treatment. Clinical studies of the utility of this approach are currently in progress.[79–81]

Endemic mycoses

The three endemic mycoses (blastomycosis, coccidioidomycosis and histoplasmosis) share a number of characteristics in common: the organisms are dimorphic, growing as a mold in the soil of a particular geographic area, and the infectious particles, the conidia, are liberated from the mold into an aerosol that is inhaled. The host defense response to this challenge is nonspecific, consisting of polymorphonuclear leukocytes and alveolar macrophages. The more potent specific responses of cytotoxic T cells and specific antibodies then appear. The attenuation of the specific immune response caused by immunosuppression will lead to an increased incidence and severity of progressive pulmonary and disseminated infection, as well as metastatic spread to the skin, the CNS, bones and joints. Appropriate amphotericin B therapy followed by a prolonged oral course of an azole is the treatment of choice.[82]

Blastomycosis

Blastomyces dermatitidis, the causative agent of blastomycosis, has a geographic distribution similar to histoplasmosis (midwest and the south-eastern USA). Physical manifestations of this infection include radiologic findings of invasive pulmonary disease, hilar adenopathy and skin abnormalities. Disseminated infection can cause large nodular skin lesions that undergo necrosis and fibrosis. Therapy is with amphotericin B, followed by itraconazole.[83,84]

Coccidioidomycosis

Coccidioides immitis is dimorphic, growing as a mesh of septate hyphae that bear the arthoconidia that are inhaled and that mature into spherules, the definitive tissue pathogen. These events take place in the desert soil of the Lower Sonoran life zone, which encompasses the San Joaquin Valley of California, the south-western USA, northern Mexico and various sites of Latin America. The range of infectivity can be greatly extended by wind and dust storms, as well as on dust-laden packages sent from the endemic area. Risk factors for clinical disease include immunosuppression, pregnancy and non-Caucasian racial status. Following inhalation by a transplant patient the primary forms of disease encountered are progressive pneumonia, bloodstream invasion and meningitis.

A diffuse granulomatous meningitis encasing the base of the brain, causing hydrocephalus, cranial nerve palsies and a cerebral vasculitis with focal neurologic findings is the most important consequence of this infection, although other sites of metastatic infection can occur. The skin, the skeleton and the genitourinary tract are the most common other sites of involvement. During the first year of residence in the endemic area, an estimated 5% rate of infection is noted, with an additional 2–3% per year thereafter. Dissemination, often with CNS involvement, is found in as many as 75% of these individuals. Although hypersensitivity syndromes are common with this organism, these are rare in transplant patients because of the immunosuppression.

High-dose and prolonged amphotericin B therapy has long been the standard of care for this infection, with relapse being expected. This situation has been improved by the availability of fluconazole. The present approach is to gain control with amphotericin B and then switch to an extended course of oral fluconazole. Prophylaxis of transplant patients with fluconazole is usually recommended.[85,86]

Histoplasmosis

Histoplasma capsulatum is a dimorphic fungus that can be found in soil enriched with bird, bat and starling droppings in the Ohio and Mississippi river valleys, with extension into Maryland and Virginia. The inhalation of aerosolized organisms is the first step in the evolution of this infection, producing in the transplant patient both progressive pulmonary disease and systemic dissemination. Infected mononuclear cells are efficient carriers of the organisms, particularly to sites where large numbers of reticuloendothelial cells are normally found: liver, spleen, lymph nodes, bone marrow, gut and adrenal glands. In addition, mucocutaneous and CNS infections are not uncommon.

Studies carried out in Indianapolis during an epidemic resulting from urban renewal projects have shown a rate of infection of 5–15% among renal transplant patients. Disseminated infection is common in this situation, with CNS infection being particularly common. The treatment of choice is initial therapy with amphotericin (particularly with a lipid formulation that can target reticuloendothelial infection), followed by a prolonged course of itraconazole.[87,88]

Newly emerging mycoses

Unusual fungal species like the zygomycetes (the causative agents of mucormycosis), *Fusarium* and *Scedosporium* are becoming more common in transplant patients.[89] These are predominantly molds that produce a clinical picture similar to that seen with *Aspergillus*: invasive disease with vascular invasion and metastatic infection. Unless there is evidence to the contrary, these organisms should be considered amphotericin B resistant. The therapy of choice is voriconazole or posaconazole. Posaconazole is particularly effective against mucormycosis (an important point if voriconazole therapy selects for zygomycetes).

Zygomycosis (also termed mucormycosis) is a rapidly progressive fungal infection that causes tissue infarction. This necrotizing infection is observed in the following situations:

- primary infection of the skin at a site traumatized by extravasation of intravenous fluids, water immersion injury or pressure dressings contaminated by *Rhizopus* sporangiospores;
- primary pulmonary infections following inhalation of fungal sporangiospores; and
- rhinocerebral zygomycoses in which the fungal aerosol establishes disease in the nasal sinuses, with progressive extension into intracranial structures.

The clinical hallmark of zygomycosis is rapidly progressive, necrotizing infection, often with eschar formation in the skin and mucosa overlying involved tissues. Risk factors include acidosis (particularly diabetic ketoacidosis), steroids, over-immunosuppression and devitalized tissues that can be secondarily infected. Therapy is with posaconazole, with or without ablative surgery.

CONCLUSIONS AND SUMMARY

Invasive fungal infections remain a major problem for transplant recipients, causing pneumonia and bloodstream infection at a considerable cost and with greater consequences if not diagnosed early and treated aggressively. A major improvement in the treatment of fungal infection is the three separate classes of drugs (lipid-associated amphotericin B, antifungal azoles and echinocandins) that can be utilized. Particularly appealing is the possibility that combination therapy, bringing together different mechanisms of action, will result in even better and more effective therapy. For example, the combination

of an echinocandin with trimethoprim–sulfamethoxazole appears to be more effective than either drug by itself. Similar observations are being seen with the treatment of *Aspergillus* spp. Early diagnosis, as with the galactomannan assay or a PCR-based technique, will improve the therapeutic results. Better diagnostics will help as well. High-definition chest CT scanning is proving to have a role in early diagnosis and is an example of utilizing existing technology in an innovative fashion. One word of caution: false-positive galactomannan assays are seen with piperacillin–tazobactam and amoxicillin–clavulanate up to a week after discontinuing the antibiotics.

REFERENCES

References for this chapter can be found online at http://www.expertconsult.com

Chapter | 76 |

Patricia Muñoz
Maddalena Giannella
Marian G Michaels
Emilio Bouza

Heart, lung and heart–lung transplantation

INTRODUCTION

According to the 2008 Registry of the International Society for Heart (HT) and Lung Transplantation (LT), >80 000 heart, 3342 heart–lung and 25 950 lung transplantation procedures have been performed worldwide. Approximately 5000 HT are performed each year. The slow decline in reporting of HT over the last 15 years appears to have finally stopped, with significant increases in the last 2 years.

The most common indication for adult *heart transplantation* is now noncoronary cardiomyopathy (50% vs 34% for January to June 2007) and the proportion of recipients aged more than 60 years has steadily increased, now accounting for almost 25% of all recipients. Congenital heart disease is the most common cause of HT in children. Patients arrive to the transplant procedure in a more critical situation: 41% were receiving intravenous inotropic support and 29% were on some type of mechanical circulatory support modality (22% on a left ventricular assist device, LVAD). These patients commonly receive perioperative antilymphocyte antibodies (51%), tacrolimus (57%), mycophenolate mofetil (77%) and prednisone (63%) at 1 year post-transplant.

The main indications for *lung transplantation* are chronic obstructive pulmonary disease (COPD, 36%), idiopathic pulmonary fibrosis (IPF, 20%), cystic fibrosis (CF, 16%) and α_1-antitrypsin deficiency emphysema (AAT, 8%). Bilateral transplantation accounted for 67% of transplant procedures in 2006 and its proportion has risen for each of the four major indications since 1994 (for CF, bilateral transplantation is the norm). The age of donors and recipients has shifted toward a larger portion of older recipients (in 2007 24% of recipients were >60 years of age). Induction therapy, usually with interleukin-2 receptor (IL-2R) antagonists and alemtuzumab (Campath) has risen (39–54%). Calcineurin inhibitor plus purine synthesis antagonist comprised the maintenance regimen for approximately 77% of recipients at 1 year. However, regardless of the maintenance drug regimen, acute rejection in the first year is common.

Overall, 1-year survival is 80% for both types of transplantation; after the second year, 3.5% of the patients die annually. Graft failure is the main cause of death in the first 30 days post-transplant (42% of deaths after HT and 28% after LT), followed by non-cytomegalovirus (CMV) infection (13% of deaths after HT and 20% after LT). From 31 to 365 days, non-CMV infection is the most important cause of mortality (33% of deaths after HT and 36.4% after LT), followed by graft failure (18% in both populations) and acute rejection (12% after HT and 1.8% after LT). Median duration of patient survival after HT is 10 years and 5.2 years after LT (13 years and 7 years for those surviving the first year, respectively).

Infection is a very important cause of morbidity and mortality in patients undergoing these procedures, and this is of special interest as infection is amenable to prevention and intervention. When one considers the cumulative incidences of individual causes of death, non-CMV infection represented the leading single cause of death from 6 months post-transplant through 10 years of follow-up. We will now briefly review some specific characteristics of infectious complications in these populations.

EPIDEMIOLOGY AND SPECIFIC RISK FACTORS FOR INFECTION

The incidence of infection after HT ranges from 30–60%, with a related mortality of 3–15%.[1] Patients undergoing lung or heart–lung transplantation are at a higher risk for developing infectious complications. These account for approximately 40–50% of all deaths in these patients.

The chronology of the infections after solid-organ transplantation (SOT) has been described in detail in other chapters (see also Chapter 75). In summary, early infections (≤1 month) are similar to those of other patients who have undergone cardiothoracic surgery (pneumonia, empyema, wound infection, mediastinitis, catheter-related infections, urinary tract infections, etc.). Intermediate infections (2–6 months) are usually caused by opportunistic micro-organisms (CMV, fungi, etc.). Finally, late infections (≥6 months) may be caused either by common community pathogens in healthy patients or by opportunistic micro-organisms in patients with chronic rejection (Table 76.1).

Risk factors for infection after thoracic transplantation are described in Table 76.2. They may be classified into factors related to the patient and those due to technical complications during the operative and perioperative periods. We also recommend ruling out hypogamma-globulinemia in these patients.[13–15] The need for ventricular assist devices is an important risk factor for infection in HT recipients. In some series, up to one-third of patients on biventricular assist devices died of sepsis; bacteremia (59%), driveline infection (28%) and pump infection (11%) are also common.

A unique feature of cystic fibrosis patients who are undergoing lung/heart–lung transplantation is that they may develop bacteremia with organisms that normally inhabit their airway (*Pseudomonas aeruginosa*, *Burkholderia cepacia*, *Alcaligenes xylosoxidans*, *Stenotrophomonas maltophilia*). Moreover, the pattern of infections of the late period is unique in lung/heart–lung transplantation compared to other organ recipients. The lung is the most important site of late infection in these patients and the presence of chronic rejection or bronchiolitis obliterans is a major risk factor. Pathogens found in these late pulmonary infections can be the same as those recovered from cystic fibrosis patients, regardless of their underlying disease (*P. aeruginosa*, *A. xylosoxidans*, *S. maltophilia* and *Aspergillus fumigatus*). The presence of one or more of these potential pathogens may be associated with asymptomatic colonization or fatal disease. Opportunistic infection with *Nocardia* or *Cryptococcus* spp. can also occur late after transplantation.

Table 76.1 Etiology, incidence and timing of infections in heart transplant patients

Etiology	Incidence (%)
Bacteria	44–60
Virus	40–45
Fungus	2–15
Pneumocystis jirovecii	0.5–8
Parasites	0.5–2

Chronology of infection	Most common syndromes
Early infection (first month)	Pneumonia Surgical wound infection Mediastinitis Urinary tract infection Catheter-related infection Bloodstream infection Antibiotic-associated diarrhea Herpes simplex stomatitis Infections transmitted with the allograft
Intermediate infections (2–6 months)	Opportunistic infections* (similar to other SOT)
Late infections (after 6 months)	Common community-acquired infections Respiratory tract infections Urinary tract infections Varicella-zoster infections Opportunistic micro-organisms

*See also Chapter 75. SOT, solid-organ transplant.

Regardless of the time period, differentiation between rejection and infection can often be difficult in thoracic transplant recipients. Accordingly, biopsy and cultures are essential for appropriate management.

SPECIFIC CLINICAL SYNDROMES

For the remainder of this chapter we will address only a few infectious problems of special interest in the thoracic transplant recipient.

Pneumonia

In recipients of thoracic transplantation, infections frequently involve the lung.[2,3] The patient's underlying lung disease impacts on the presentation and the type of infection that occur after these procedures. This is illustrated by the increased risk of early and severe pneumonia with multiple antibiotic-resistant bacteria seen in cystic fibrosis patients undergoing heart–lung or lung transplantation.

Unique among heart–lung and lung transplant recipients is the relationship between the presence of chronic rejection and bronchiolitis obliterans with chronic infection of the airway. This relationship may be explained in part by the fact that lung transplant recipients have altered lung immunity due to impaired ciliary clearance, poor cough reflex and abnormal lymphatic drainage that predispose these patients to lower respiratory tract infections. Clinical manifestations may be indistinguishable from rejection of the lung and may strongly resemble a classic 'pulmonary exacerbation' of cystic fibrosis: increased cough and sputum production with a measurable decline of pulmonary function.

Table 76.2 Risk factors for infection after thoracic transplantation

Recipient

Age

Diabetes, malnutrition, obesity

Hypogammaglobulinemia

Renal failure

Critically ill status and ventilation at transplantation

Pulmonary hypertension not responsive to vasodilators (heart transplant)

No immunity against CMV, *Toxoplasma*, EBV, VZV

Latent infection (TB, CMV, HSV, VZV, EBV, endemic mycosis)

Donor CMV-positive serology

Previous admissions and colonization with multi-resistant pathogens

Previous antimicrobial or immunosuppressive therapy

Transplantation

Allograft injury (ischemia, preservation)

Complexity and length of surgery

Bacterial or fungal allograft colonization

Allograft latent infection (*Toxoplasma*, CMV, other viruses)

Native lung colonization (unilateral transplantation)

Postsurgical care (mechanical ventilation, iv catheters, ventricular assist devices, drainages, indwelling bladder catheter)

Transfusions

Intensive care unit stay

Postsurgical technical complications

Re-intervention

Postsurgical renal failure

Immunosuppression

After transplantation

Immunosuppression

Immunomodulatory infections (CMV)

Rejection

CMV, cytomegalovirus; EBV, Epstein–Barr virus; HSV, herpes simplex virus; TB, tuberculosis; VZV, varicella-zoster virus.

In isolated heart transplants, the etiologic agents of pneumonia are similar to those of other SOT patients: 60% are caused by opportunistic micro-organisms (mainly CMV), 25% by nosocomial pathogens and 15% by community-acquired bacteria and mycobacteria.[2] Pneumonia is one of the leading causes of death after HT. Mechanical ventilation is required in 37% of these patients and death occurs in 23–31%. This rate varies widely depending on the etiology, *Aspergillus* pneumonia having the worse prognosis (50–62%), followed by nosocomial pneumonia (26%, even 50% for those patients receiving ventilatory support) and CMV pneumonia (13%).

Nodular lesions are detected in 10% of HT patients and are mainly caused by *Aspergillus*, *Nocardia* and CMV. The time of appearance and some clinical manifestations may suggest the etiology and may help determine empiric treatment in selected cases.[4] Other pathogens such as *Nocardia*, *Rhodococcus equi* and tuberculosis (incidence in HT 1% in Spain) should also be considered.[5]

Postsurgical mediastinitis and sternum osteomyelitis

HT patients have a higher risk of postsurgical mediastinitis and sternal osteomyelitis than other heart surgical patients.[6,7] This complication may manifest as early bacteremia, sternum instability or dehiscence. The main causes are bacterial pathogens (staphylococci, Gram-negative rods), but *Mycoplasma*, mycobacteria, *Candida* and other less common pathogens should be suspected in 'culture-negative' wound infections. A bacteremia of unknown origin during the first month after HT should always suggest the possibility of mediastinitis. Risk factors include prolonged hospitalization before surgery, early chest re-exploration, low output syndrome in adults and the immature state of the immune system in infants. In a recent study, antibiotic prophylaxis with ciprofloxacin alone (OR 15.8; 95% CI 1.2–216.9) was independently associated with the development of incisional surgical infection.[8] Therapy consists of surgical debridement and repair, and antimicrobial therapy given for 3–6 weeks.

Cardiovascular infections

Infective endocarditis is a relatively rare complication of HT (1.5–6%).[9] Most of the cases are associated with previous nosocomial infections, mainly venous access devices and wound infections. *Staphylococcus aureus* and *Aspergillus* are the most common pathogens involved.[9] Interestingly, 80% of SOT recipients who developed endocarditis in one series had no previous history of valvular disease. CMV, *Toxoplasma* and parvovirus B19 may cause myocarditis in this population.

CONSIDERATIONS RELATED TO MICRO-ORGANISMS

Viral infections

Cytomegalovirus

Cytomegalovirus is the second most common cause of infection in thoracic transplant recipients, after bacterial infection. When no prophylaxis is given, 30–90% of patients will have laboratory data of infection and 10–90% will develop associated clinical manifestations (CMV disease). It can cause primary infection in a previously sero-negative patient or secondary infection in a previously seropositive person. Primary infection is usually transmitted via the donor graft or blood products. For ethical aspects, seronegative donor/receptor selection is not indicated. However, if transfusions are needed, the use of leukoreduced blood products is recommended.

CMV infection typically occurs between 1 and 6 months after transplantation. Clinical presentation includes asymptomatic infection, CMV syndrome, with malaise, fever and bone marrow suppression, and focal organ disease, most frequently pneumonia (27%) or gastrointestinal disease (19%). CMV pneumonitis usually presents as fever, tachypnea and hypoxia, and should be differentiated from rejection in LT patients. Chorioretinitis due to CMV is infrequent in these patients. CMV disease is particularly severe in high-risk patients such as recipient negative/donor positive (R–/D+) individuals or those receiving OKT3, anti-thymocyte globulins or monoclonal antibodies for a rejection episode.

Symptomatic CMV infection may occasionally be associated with superinfection with bacteria or fungi, possibly as a consequence of viral modulation of immunity. Interestingly, CMV infection has also been associated with an increased frequency of acute and chronic allograft rejection (diffuse arteriosclerosis in HT and bronchiolitis obliterans in LT),[10,11] although there is still controversy around this point.[12]

Treatment and CMV prevention

Therapy and prevention of CMV disease in this population does not differ from other SOT patients; a full discussion is presented in Chapters 72 and 155. Some authors, including ourselves, recommend administering gammaglobulins to patients with pneumonitis, gastrointestinal disease and frequent relapses.

Prevention of CMV disease in thoracic transplantation is based on two types of strategy: universal prophylaxis and pre-emptive therapy. In *lung and heart–lung transplantation* most authors recommend initial universal prophylaxis followed by pre-emptive therapy. In the first 3–6 months, all patients should receive initial intravenous ganciclovir (5 mg/kg/q12h) followed by oral valganciclovir (900 mg/q12h). In high-risk patients (D+/R–), administration of intravenous gamma-globulins is recommended. Pre-emptive therapy based on follow-up with polymerase chain reaction (PCR) or antigenemia should then be performed. Weekly antigenemia assay is recommended until the sixth month. Late-onset CMV disease (>1 year) has been observed in lung recipients after long-term prophylaxis (6 months) and some authors recommend indefinite prophylaxis.[12]

After *heart transplantation*, mismatched recipients (D+/R–) should receive universal prophylaxis. Ganciclovir followed by valganciclovir (1–3 months), with or without gammaglobulins, seems to be the most effective combination. Pre-emptive therapy is recommended in seropositive patients. After corticosteroid-resistant rejection, a course of antiviral therapy is usually administered.

Epstein–Barr virus

The incidence of post-transplantation lymphoproliferative disease (PTLD) related to Epstein–Barr virus (EBV) in lung recipients varies between 1.6% and 20%, and is two to six times more frequent than in other SOT recipients. More than half of patients are symptomatic, presenting with a mononucleosis-like picture with lymph node swelling, isolated PTLD lesions in the lung or gastrointestinal tract, disseminated disease or lymphoma. Risk factors for PTLD are primary infection and therapy with OKT3 or anti-thymocyte globulins. When PTLD is suspected, CT of the neck, chest, abdomen and pelvis should be considered to identify occult lesions. Biopsies should be obtained from suspicious lesions. Patients with active EBV disease typically have an elevated EBV viral load, which may be detected before clinical onset and may remain persistently high even after resolution of PTLD.

The high rates of morbidity and mortality attributed to PTLD have prompted efforts aimed at the prevention or pre-emptive treatment of EBV. Serial monitoring of the EBV viral load using quantitative PCR assays has been shown to predict occurrence of PTLD in transplant populations and is increasingly being used to guide initiation of pre-emptive therapy. However, specific target levels of load and specific sites to sample (blood versus bronchoalveolar lavage), as well as therapeutic pre-emptive treatment regimens, need to be clarified in prospective, comparative studies. The management of patients with PTLD is controversial. Reduction of immune suppression is uniformly recommended in order to enhance a cytotoxic T-lymphocyte response. Concerns over the development of rejection can limit this approach. While frequently used, antiviral therapies (primarily nucleoside analogues – e.g. ganciclovir – and immunoglobulins) are probably of limited benefit for the treatment of EBV PTLD. The use of the new anti-CD20 monoclonal antibody (rituximab) appears very promising for these patients. The use of chemotherapy may be necessary for patients who fail to respond to reduction of immunosuppression or in whom the PTLD lesions are judged to be malignant.

Other viruses

Viruses other than CMV and EBV cause disease in up to one-third of all lung/heart–lung transplant recipients. An important feature of these infections is that they can mimic rejection.

Herpes simplex virus can reactivate or cause primary pneumonitis, which can be fatal. Aciclovir prophylaxis is effective in preventing this

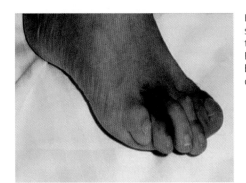

Fig. 76.1 Kaposi's sarcoma in a heart transplant recipient. Primary infection by HHV-8 was demonstrated.

problem. The incidence of Kaposi's sarcoma (KS) is 0.75% after HT, higher than after kidney transplantation (0.28%). KS was diagnosed a median of 24 months after SOT and mortality was 28.5% (Fig. 76.1). Primary infection with human herpesvirus 8 (HHV-8) was found to be an important risk factor.[16]

The community respiratory viruses such as respiratory syncytial virus (RSV), parainfluenza virus, influenza virus and adenovirus are also important causes of disease after thoracic transplantation. They often involve the lower respiratory tract and may be associated with significant morbidity and mortality. In addition, the insult from these viruses (particularly adenovirus) can lead to chronic sequelae such as bronchiolitis obliterans in lung recipients. The mainstay of treatment for community-acquired viruses is decreasing the immunosuppression and providing supportive care. Antiviral treatments are controversial and, while licensed therapies are available for RSV (ribavirin) and influenza (e.g. amantadine, rimantadine, oseltamivir, zanamivir), no well-proven therapies are available for parainfluenza or adenovirus.

Annual immunization with influenza vaccine or prophylaxis with amantadine is recommended in thoracic transplant patients. Varicella-zoster virus (VZV) infection should be prevented in seronegative patients who have contact with individuals with varicella or herpes zoster by the administration of hyperimmune globulin. VZV vaccine should be given to seronegative patients before transplantation.

Thoracic organ transplantation in serum hepatitis B surface antigen (HBsAg)-positive and hepatitis B virus (HBV) DNA-negative recipients is followed by HBV reactivation in a high percentage of cases. However, the clinical outcome and the availability of lamivudine and other anti-HBV agents suggest that infection is not an absolute contraindication (see Chapter 148).

Bacterial infections

Bacterial infections are the more frequent infectious complications after thoracic surgery, accounting for more than 40–50% of all infections. They occur early after transplant and are related to:

- pre-transplant donor and/or recipient colonization;
- invasive procedures (surgery, intubation, intravascular devices, etc.); and
- prolonged hospitalization.

Late bacterial infections in lung recipients are related to the severity of the obliterans bronchiolitis. Nosocomial pathogens, principally *P. aeruginosa* and methicillin-resistant *Staph. aureus* (MRSA), may be implicated. Cystic fibrosis patients represent an important cohort of LT recipients. These patients, as well as those with a prolonged intensive care stay before transplantation, are at high risk of being colonized with resistant pathogens (*Burkholderia cepacia*, *S. maltophilia*, *Alcaligenes xylosoxidans*). It is therefore important to obtain baseline cultures prior to transplant. A 2-week course of appropriate antimicrobial therapy is recommended for all patients with cystic fibrosis based upon these culture results. In LT recipients, it is very important to check for ischemic lesions of the anastomoses, since they increase the risk of infection and dehiscence. Nebulized antibiotics are recommended in these cases.

Some 'opportunistic' bacteria such as *Listeria monocytogenes*, *Rhodococcus equi* or *Nocardia* should also be considered in this population. In a recent review of nocardiosis, SOT (117, 26.1%) was the most common underlying condition (36 heart, 35 lung).[17] The disease is less common nowadays due to the widespread use of trimethoprim–sulfamethoxazole (TMP–SMX) in this population. However, it is important to remember that transplant patients may develop late nocardiosis, when TMP–SMX prophylaxis has been withdrawn. On the other hand, TMP–SMX prophylaxis is not uniformly protective against *Nocardia* spp. Nocardiosis may appear in patients with chronic rejection and intensive immunosuppressive treatment.

Finally, there is a group of bacteria that cause late infection, such as encapsulated micro-organisms including *Streptococcus pneumoniae* and *Haemophilus influenzae* (group b). Preventive vaccines should be offered to this population. Pneumococcal vaccination may be repeated 5 years after the first immunization.

Tuberculosis

Mycobacterium tuberculosis deserves a special mention. Lung transplant recipients have a high risk of tuberculosis (TB): 2072 (565–5306) cases per 10^5 inhabitants compared to 512 (317–783) for all SOT.[18] The incidence of tuberculosis in HT patients in Spain is 1.35 cases/100 heart transplant-years, more than 20-fold the national average.[19]

On average, TB developed 76 days after transplantation and extrapulmonary disease was common. Fever, dyspnea and alveolar infiltrates were the most common findings in a series of LT recipients with TB.[20] Reactivation may be triggered by antirejection therapy, although it may be acquired in the hospital environment or even from the allograft in heart–lung transplantation. TB should be considered in HT patients with prolonged and culture-negative febrile episodes. If the patient's condition deteriorates, prompt specific therapy should be initiated after obtaining samples for culture.

Besides the potential difficulty in establishing a diagnosis, due to its atypical presentation, the major problem of management of TB in this population is multiple drug interactions.[20,21] The benefit of rifampin (rifampicin) must be balanced against the problem it causes by interfering with the metabolism of immunosuppressive drugs, especially ciclosporin and tacrolimus. When the use of rifampin is mandatory, immunosuppressant levels should be monitored daily until they are stable.[18]

Fungal infections

Invasive fungal infections (IFI) after SOT used to be a major cause of morbidity and mortality after thoracic transplantation, although the incidence now appears to be decreasing.

Aspergillus species

The incidence of invasive aspergillosis (IA) in lung and heart transplant recipients varies, estimated to range between 3.9% and 26%. *Aspergillus* and other filamentous fungi have also been identified as causing colonization and disease in patients who develop bronchiolitis obliterans. The presence of fungi preoperatively is not a contraindication to transplantation; however, in double lung transplantation, the exclusion of the presence of mycetomas with a thoracic CT is mandatory. A characteristic clinical presentation in LT recipients is tracheobronchitis which can present in a simple, ulcerative, pseudomembranous or nodular form. In most cases it affects the anastomoses and may cause dehiscence, mediastinitis, hemorrhage and disseminated disease. IA of the residual native lung in recipients of single lung transplantation is difficult to detect and manage. In HT patients, the isolation of *Aspergillus* from any respiratory sample has a 60–70% positive predictive value for invasive aspergillosis.[22] Although other species may be involved, in our series *A. fumigatus* was recovered from 74% of the samples, but caused all episodes of invasive aspergillosis. In the first 6–9 months after LT, the recovery of *Aspergillus* spp. from respiratory secretions is an indication to perform an endoscopic study of the airways.

Risk factors for invasive lung aspergillosis after LT are *Aspergillus* spp. colonization, CMV pneumonia, airway ischemia and single lung transplantation. Risk factors after HT are reoperation, CMV disease, post-transplant hemodialysis and high environmental load reflected by the existence of an episode of IA in the HT program 2 months before or after the transplantation date. Itraconazole prophylaxis showed an independent protective value against developing IA (RR 0.2; 95% CI 0.07–0.9, *p*=0.03) and also determined a significantly prolonged 1-year survival (RR 0.5; 95% CI 0.3–0.8, *p*=0.01).[23]

Prompt recognition of this fungal infection is essential for achieving a successful outcome. However, both clinical symptoms and radiologic manifestations may be nonspecific at early stages of the disease. The isolation of *Aspergillus* spp. from nonsterile respiratory samples may indicate invasive infection, colonization or laboratory contamination, thus making treatment of symptomatic transplant recipients difficult. However, as mentioned, the isolation of *A. fumigatus* is highly predictive of invasive disease and should always be considered very seriously in this population. In our experience, all respiratory samples other than sputum proved to have the same predictive value, as has already been suggested by other authors. The choice of one or other technique should be based on the availability and expertise in each hospital, on the extent and location of the infiltrate and on patient characteristics. In previous studies we have demonstrated that in HT recipients with pneumonia, the sensitivity of bronchoalveolar lavage ranged from 58% to 89% and transthoracic aspiration reached 100% sensitivity. Clinical and microbiologic information should been combined with early CT scan, which provides more specific information than conventional chest X-ray (Fig. 76.2).

Although detection of galactomannan in serum has poor sensitivity for the diagnosis of invasive aspergillosis in LT recipients, detection of galactomannan in the bronchoalveolar lavage with a compatible clinical illness is highly suggestive of invasive disease.[24] Treatment of IA is discussed in depth in Chapters 72, 73 and 178. Voriconazole is the recommended first-line therapy in most patients. Parenteral liposomal amphotericin B (AMB), inhaled AMB or combination therapy may be considered as alternative or co-adjuvant therapies.[25,26] Duration of therapy depends on the extent of disease, the clinical response and the immunologic status of the patient. Most authors recommend prolonging the intravenous treatment until clinical response and radiologic normalization have been obtained and then continue with oral voriconazole or itraconazole for another 3–18 months. Regular monitoring of liver enzymes and serum concentrations of calcineurin inhibitors is required to avoid hepatotoxicity and nephrotoxicity. Inhaled AMB, with or without itraconazole, is employed in LT recipients with evidence of *Aspergillus* colonization, until the normalization

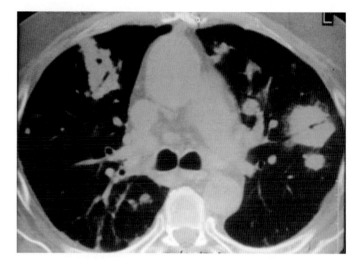

Fig. 76.2 Bilateral invasive aspergillosis in a heart transplant recipient.

of respiratory cultures.[27,28] For tracheobronchitis, treatment includes inhaled AMB combined with systemic voriconazole or itraconazole until bronchoscopic evidence of disease resolution.

Very few data on prophylaxis against *Aspergillus* in HT recipients are available. We have used oral itraconazole with good results and inhaled AMB is used at other institutions.[23,29] Inhaled AMB, with or without an oral antifungal, is predominantly used after LT.[27] A recent study has shown that universal prophylaxis with voriconazole was better than standard prophylaxis with itraconazole ± inhaled AMB (IA at 1 year 1.5% vs 23%, *p*=0.001) in patients at high risk (pre- or post-transplant *Aspergillus* colonization).[30]

Pneumocystis jirovecii

Pneumocystis jirovecii pneumonia is a severe pulmonary infection in immunocompromised hosts. Before the introduction of universal prophylaxis with trimethoprim–sulfamethoxazole, the incidence of *P. jirovecii* pneumonia in thoracic transplantation was 3–12% in heart recipients, and up of 80% in lung recipients. *P. jirovecii* pneumonia tends to occur within the first year after transplantation, but has occasionally been seen later, generally after rejection episodes. Symptoms range from isolated fever to serious respiratory distress leading to death. A summary of prophylactic strategies is presented in Table 76.3.

Table 76.3 Summary of the most commonly used prophylactic strategies in thoracic transplantation patients

Indication	Standard therapy	Dose and duration	Comments
Streptococcus pneumoniae, *Haemophilus influenzae*, influenza	Pre-transplant vaccination	As in other patients	*S. pneumoniae* vaccination should be repeated every 5 years Annual influenza vaccine
Perioperative prophylaxis	Cefazolin	1–2 g q8h iv for 48–72 h	LT recipients: active against *Staphylococcus aureus* and *Pseudomonas aeruginosa* (some centers recommend amoxicillin–clavulanate + ceftazidime) In cystic fibrosis patients, prophylaxis should include inhaled antibiotics (e.g. tobramycin) combined with systemic therapy selected with pre-transplant from donor and recipient cultures If cultures are negative, prophylaxis can be ended after 3–5 days; if positive, should be prolonged for 2 weeks

Table 76.3 Summary of the most commonly used prophylactic strategies in thoracic transplantation patients—cont'd

Indication	Standard therapy	Dose and duration	Comments
Pneumocystis jirovecii	Trimethoprim–sulfamethoxazole (TSX)	Double-strength TSX q24h or q12h on week-end days, or three times a week	May protect against *Nocardia* spp., *Listeria* spp., *Toxoplasma* and other bacteria Some groups recommend life-long prophylaxis for LT recipients For allergic or intolerant patients, see Chapter 75
Cytomegalovirus	Ganciclovir/valganciclovir	5 mg/kg/q12h iv for 15 days, followed by valganciclovir (900 mg/q12h) in D+/R– for the first 3–6 months	D+/R–: universal prophylaxis for 3 months; consider iv gammaglobulins R+: pre-emptive therapy in HT and universal prophylaxis in LT
Aspergillus spp. (Lung and heart–lung transplant)	Amphotericin B alone or with an oral antifungal	25 mg/q24h inhaled for 2–6 months, then once/15 days	Voriconazole, alone or combined with inhaled amphotericin, is also effective Patients who receive prophylaxis with voriconazole should be monitored for hepatoxicity
Mycobacterium tuberculosis	Isoniazid	300 mg/q24h po for 6–12 months	Low risk of toxicity
Toxoplasmosis (R–/D+)	Pyrimethamine plus folinic acid*	25 mg/q24h for 6 weeks	With folinic acid

D+, seropositive donor; HT, heart transplant; LT, liver transplant; R+, seropositive recipient; R–, seronegative recipient.
*Trimethoprim–sulfamethoxazole, three times a week, is effective protection for both *P. jirovecii* pneumonia and toxoplasmosis; high-risk HT patients should receive anti-*Aspergillus* prophylaxis.

REFERENCES

References for this chapter can be found online at http://www.expertconsult.com

Chapter | **77** |

Raymund R Razonable
Carlos V Paya

Liver transplantation

INTRODUCTION

Up to 70% of liver transplant recipients develop bacterial, viral, fungal and protozoal infections during the first year after transplantation.[1,2] The occurrence of these infections in liver recipients is influenced by two major factors: (1) the net state of immunosuppression, and (2) the epidemiologic exposures of the recipient and the donor. The complexities of liver transplantation surgery with the potential break in areas of high microbial load (i.e. gastrointestinal tract) and the common infectious indications for liver transplantation (e.g. chronic viral hepatitis) predispose to unique complications that may not be commonly observed among other solid-organ transplant (SOT) recipients.

PRETRANSPLANT INFECTIOUS DISEASE EVALUATION

Liver transplant candidates and their potential donors should undergo extensive infectious disease evaluation prior to transplantation (Table 77.1).[3] Among the many infections screened for are cytomegalovirus (CMV), herpes simplex virus (HSV) 1 and HSV2, Epstein–Barr virus (EBV), human immunodeficiency virus (HIV), human T-lymphotropic virus, hepatitis A–D viruses (HAV, HBV, HCV, HDV), *Treponema pallidum* and *Mycobacterium tuberculosis*. Individuals with identifiable risk factors such as residence in endemic areas undergo additional screening for *Coccidioides immitis*, *Trypanosoma cruzi* and *Strongyloides stercoralis*.

A unique characteristic of liver transplant candidates is the common occurrence of active infection during the pretransplant period. Cholangitis, peritonitis and abscesses are a few examples. In general, an underlying infection does not absolutely contraindicate liver transplantation, unless it is uncontrolled. However, all active infections should be controlled prior to, and if necessary, after transplantation. To illustrate, chronic HBV and HIV, which were once considered absolute contraindications to liver transplantation, are now adequately controlled after liver transplantation with the use of hepatitis B immunoglobulin (HBIg) and antiviral nucleosides (for HBV)[4] and highly active antiretroviral therapy (for HIV).[5]

RISK FACTORS

Epidemiologic exposures, underlying diseases and patient characteristics

Unlike other SOT patients, infection-related indications for liver transplantation are common. Indeed, the single most common indication for liver transplantation is HCV-induced cirrhosis.[6,7]

Table 77.1 Suggested measures to determine risks and exposures of liver transplant candidates and the suggested preventive measures prior to liver transplantation

Screening	Control measures, if susceptible
Standard screening tests	
HIV 1/2 ELISA	Highly active antiretroviral therapy
Hepatitis A serology	Hepatitis A vaccine
Hepatitis B serology	Hepatitis B vaccine
Hepatitis C serology	Assess for need of interferon alpha with or without ribavirin
Cytomegalovirus IgG	Advise the patient of risk of transmission and reactivation after transplantation. If susceptible to primary infection, use antiviral prophylaxis after transplantation
Epstein–Barr virus (EBV) serology	Advise the patient of risk of transmission and reactivation after transplantation. If susceptible to primary EBV infection, closely monitor for virus replication after transplantation; others use antiviral and immunoglobulin prophylaxis after liver transplantation
Varicella serology	Varicella vaccine; role of booster in immune individuals is not established
Purified protein derivative (PPD) skin test	Treat for latent tuberculosis infection prior to or after liver transplantation
Rapid plasma reagin	Treat syphilis if detected
Targeted screening tests	
Strongyloides stercoralis antibody	
Coccidioides immitis serology	
Human herpesvirus-8 serology	
Human T-cell lymphotropic virus	

Liver failure from HBV with or without superimposed HDV infection or from acute fulminant HAV or HBV or disseminated HSV hepatitis are other infection-related indications for liver transplantation. In the absence of effective therapy, the majority of patients with HBV develop recurrent infection after transplantation. Likewise, almost all HCV-infected recipients develop recurrence after transplantation. Fulminant hepatitis, regardless of etiology, is particularly associated with an increased risk for post-transplant viral and fungal super-infections.[8] Active or latent infection involving the donor or recipient liver (e.g. *Histoplasma capsulatum*, *C. immitis*, *Cryptococcus neoformans*, *Toxoplasma gondii*, *M. tuberculosis*) may be unrecognized prior to, and manifest with severe atypical disease after, liver transplantation. Interestingly, the risk of opportunistic infections is not significantly increased among HIV-infected liver recipients,[5] and the risk of infection is similar between recipients of liver allografts from deceased or living donors.[9]

Surgical factors and the hospital environment

A prolonged and complicated surgical procedure and the volume of blood loss directly correlate with infection risk after liver transplantation (Table 77.2).[2,8,10,11] The urgent nature of the procedure, such as during transplantation for fulminant hepatitis, could lessen the time to optimally prepare patients for liver transplantation. Abdominal re-exploration surgery (for re-transplantation, abdominal bleeding and other complications) and the type of biliary anastomosis (e.g. choledochojejunostomy) increases the risk of bacterial and fungal infections.[2,8,10,11] The length of hospital stay, the presence of indwelling vascular, genitourinary and percutaneous catheters, and nosocomial infections further contribute to infections after liver transplantation.

Net state of immunosuppression

The net state of immunosuppression is influenced by host factors, viral factors and pharmacologic immunosuppression. Muromonab-CD3 (OKT3), antithymocyte globulin (ATG), mycophenolate mofetil (MMF) and alemtuzumab increase the risk of CMV disease[12,13] and other opportunistic infections such as human herpesvirus (HHV)-6, *C. neoformans*, *Aspergillus* spp., and *Pneumocystis jirovecii*. The combination of OKT3 and MMF may accelerate the course of recurrent HCV.[7,14]

Contributing to the net state of immunosuppression are patient age, underlying diseases such as diabetes and HIV, and inherent immunologic deficiencies.[6,15,16] Drug-induced myelosuppression (i.e. leukopenia from trimethoprim–sulfamethoxazole, valganciclovir and MMF) and infections with immunomodulating viruses further increase the risk of infection.[17–19] Infections with HHV-6 and CMV, whose levels of replication are enhanced by immunosuppressive drugs, paradoxically increase immunosuppression and the risk of opportunistic superinfections.[17–21] Unique to liver transplantation is the interaction among CMV, HHV-6 and HCV, leading to the accelerated course of recurrent HCV.[7,14,22,23]

CLINICAL PRESENTATION

Characteristically, infections follow a temporal pattern that is predicted based on the time to onset after liver transplantation (Fig. 77.1). The post-transplant period is generally divided into three characteristic periods when certain types of infection typically occur. This period reflects the net state of immunosuppression, although the clinical course of many infections has been modified by antimicrobial prophylaxis.

First month

Liver transplantation is unique because the surgical procedure is performed in close proximity to areas of high microbial content. Spillage of gastrointestinal contents may cause intra-abdominal infections. Infected bilomas, intra-abdominal abscesses and surgical site infections caused by drug-susceptible and -resistant bacteria (e.g. *Staphylococcus aureus*, coagulase-negative staphylococci, enterococci, Gram-negative bacilli, anaerobic organisms) and fungi (e.g. *Candida albicans*, *Candida glabrata*) may occur. Clinical manifestations include fever and sepsis, although in many instances, atypical presentation may be observed such as isolated leukocytosis. Erythema, purulence and dehiscence of surgical wounds may occur. The risk of infection is particularly increased in patients who require abdominal re-exploration (i.e. hepatic artery or portal vein thromboses, biliary leak, re-transplantation). Prolonged hospitalization increases the risk of nosocomial pneumonia, catheter-associated urinary and bloodstream infections, and antibiotic-related *Clostridium difficile*-induced diarrhea.

HSV reactivation disease is the most common viral infection during this period, although antiviral prophylaxis has markedly reduced its incidence. Recurrence of HCV viremia is manifested during this period, and the degree of HCV replication has been correlated with the severity of recurrent HCV hepatitis and cirrhosis.

Second to the sixth month

This is the period when opportunistic infections, with CMV as the most common pathogen, typically occur.[24] CMV and other β-herpesviruses (HHV-6 and HHV-7) reactivate within 2–6 weeks after liver transplantation, although antiviral prophylaxis has delayed the onset of clinical disease.[24] HHV-6 and HHV-7 reactivations are mostly asymptomatic, although fever, myelosuppression and tissue-invasive diseases have been observed.[18] In contrast, CMV commonly presents with symptomatic illness characterized by fever and myelosuppression (CMV syndrome); in roughly 50% of cases, tissue invasion, particularly of the gastrointestinal tract and liver allograft, is a major manifestation.[12,24] If CMV hepatitis occurs, it can be confused with allograft rejection or drug toxicity.

Table 77.2 Risk factors for infections after liver transplantation

Preoperative period	Intraoperative period	Postoperative period
Lack of pathogen-specific immunity Severity of underlying clinical illness Fulminant hepatic failure Dialysis and renal insufficiency Anemia Previous or ongoing fungal infection (e.g. endemic mycoses) Chronic active infections (e.g. hepatitis B and C viruses) Latent infections (e.g. cytomegalovirus, herpes simplex virus, varicella zoster virus) Immune deficiencies (e.g. cytokine and chemokine deficiencies, immune receptor defects)	Presence of pathogens in the allograft (e.g. herpesviruses, fungal pathogens) Prolonged operative time Complicated surgical procedure Profound blood loss Choledochojejunostomy Infusion of large volume of blood products Prolonged ischemia time	Prolonged hospitalization Prolonged stay in intensive care unit Prolonged antibiotic use (e.g. resistant pathogens and fungi) Dialysis and renal insufficiency Gastrointestinal and biliary complications Vascular complications Allograft rejection Immunosuppressive drugs (e.g. muromonab-CD3, antithymocyte globulin, high-dose steroids, mycophenolate mofetil, alemtuzumab) CMV and HHV-6 reactivation Re-operation within 1 month after transplantation Re-transplantation

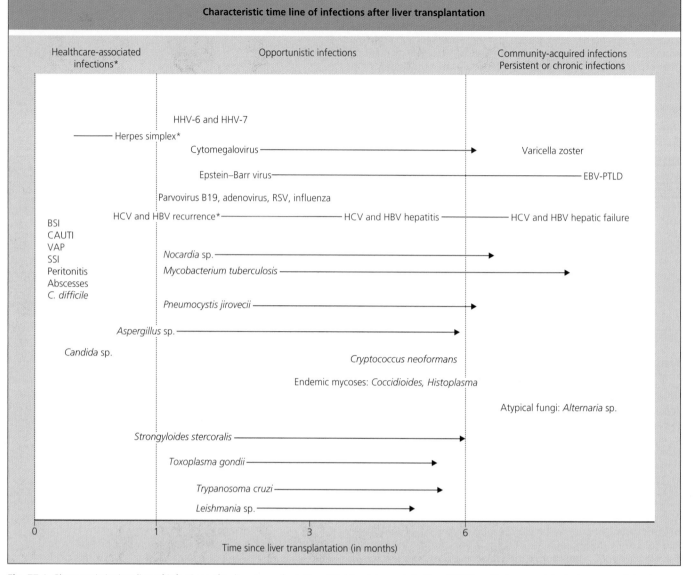

Fig. 77.1 Characteristic time line of infections after liver transplantation. BSI, bloodstream infection; CAUTI, catheter-associated urinary tract infection; EBV, Epstein–Barr virus; HBV, hepatitis B virus; HCV, hepatitis C virus; HHV, human herpesvirus; PTLD, post-transplant lymphoproliferative disorder; RSV, respiratory syncitial virus; SSI, surgical site infection. VAP, ventilator-associated pneumonia. *Healthcare-associated infections predominate during this period, with the exception of herpes simplex, HBV and HCV recurrence.

Hepatic dysfunction, from rejection, infection or drug toxicity, complicates the use of antimicrobial prophylaxis. In many instances, trimethoprim–sulfamethoxazole is withheld because of elevated serum transaminase levels, thereby predisposing the patients to *P. jirovecii*, *Nocardia* spp. and other bacterial infections. Other drugs that are often withheld because of hepatic dysfunction include isoniazid (for the prevention of tuberculosis) and antifungal medications (for prevention and treatment of fungal disease).

Invasive aspergillosis, most commonly due to *Aspergillus fumigatus*, is one of the most dreaded infections after liver transplantation. It is observed more commonly among liver recipients who were transplanted for fulminant hepatitis, those with profound immunosuppression, and those with epidemiologic exposures (such as close proximity to construction sites). Infection with endemic fungi (e.g. *H. capsulatum*, *C. immitis*) and *C. neoformans*, which have been transmitted occasionally through the transplanted allograft, may occur during this period. Cryptococcosis often presents as meningoencephalitis but can occur as an isolated pulmonary cryptococcoma or nonhealing cellulitis.

Virus-to-virus interactions are more commonly observed in liver compared to other SOT recipients.[7,17,19-23] The predisposition to a more severe form of CMV disease in patients with HHV-6 and HHV-7 co-infections is a classic example.[17,20,21] Also unique among the liver transplant population is the interaction between HCV, CMV and other herpes viruses, leading to rapid progression of recurrent HCV.[7,22,23]

Beyond the sixth month

Beyond the sixth month, the majority of liver recipients have good allograft function and their levels of immunosuppression have been reduced to the minimum. As a result, patients are no longer at high risk of opportunistic infections. In the minority of liver recipients, such as those with poor allograft function, those with recurrent chronic viral hepatitis, those with recurrent acute or chronic rejection, and those who remain on an intense immunosuppressive regimen, opportunistic infections similar to those observed during months 1–6 may occur.

Almost all HCV-infected liver recipients develop recurrent HCV viremia, and in many cases the severity of immunosuppression influences the progression of HCV replication to clinical hepatitis, fibrosis and allograft failure. In the HCV-infected population, recurrent HCV-associated allograft failure is the most common cause of death during the first 5 years after liver transplantation. Likewise, in the absence of anti-HBV therapy, recurrence of chronic HBV is characterized by a rapidly progressive course that results in allograft failure.

VZV reactivation, which manifests as mono- or multidermatomal zoster, typically occurs during the period between 6 and 12 months after liver transplantation. EBV-related post-transplant lymphoproliferative disorder may occur at any time, although it often peaks between 6 and 12 months and between 2 and 4 years after liver transplantation. In some cases, as exemplified by CMV, the onset of the typical infections has been delayed (i.e. late-onset CMV disease) by antimicrobial prophylaxis.[24,25]

DIAGNOSIS AND SURVEILLANCE

Surveillance

Surveillance cultures or other methods such as polymerase chain reaction (PCR) to identify infection before its clinical manifestation are utilized. Surveillance using rectal swab and stool specimen can identify colonization with drug-resistant bacteria, such as vancomycin-resistant enterococci, in an effort to interrupt nosocomial transmission.[26] Surveillance culture of biliary fluid is not recommended.[26]

Screening for CMV

CMV screening, either with PCR or pp65 antigenemia, is usually performed based on the risk of disease.[27] Because of poor sensitivity, viral culture should not be used to guide pre-emptive therapy.[27]

Hepatitis virus surveillance

HBV surveillance should be performed on all HBV-infected patients before and after transplantation to document HBV replication and to monitor effectiveness of therapy. Surveillance for HCV recurrence is performed using molecular methods that measure HCV replication.

Diagnostic methodologies

The etiology of an infectious syndrome is identified using culture, serology, histopathology, antigenemia testing (such as pp65 for CMV and galactomannan for aspergillosis) and molecular methods (such as PCR to detect CMV, HCV, HBV, HSV, VZV and bacterial pathogens). Generally, the utility of serology is limited by the inability of some transplant recipients to mount a humoral immune response. In contrast, molecular techniques provide a rapid, sensitive method for diagnosis.

MANAGEMENT

Prevention: vaccination, prophylaxis and pre-emptive therapy

Vaccination

All susceptible liver transplant candidates should receive necessary vaccinations prior to transplantation (Tables 77.1, 77.3). Susceptible patients should receive hepatitis A and B vaccines, varicella-zoster vaccine and tetanus vaccine prior to transplantation. Live attenuated vaccines are generally contraindicated after liver transplantation.

Table 77.3 Suggested measures for the prevention of infections after liver transplantation

Prophylaxis	Indications	Dose and duration	Comments
Cefotaxime	Perioperative antibacterial prophylaxis	1 g q8h iv for 48 h	Should be adjusted based on resistance patterns
Trimethoprim–sulfamethoxazole	*Pneumocystis jirovecii*	80 or 160 mg of trimethoprim component po q24h for 6 months	May protect against *Nocardia* spp., *Listeria* spp. and other bacteria; alternatives are inhaled or iv pentamidine or oral dapsone
Aciclovir	Herpes simplex virus	200–400 mg po q8h for 4 weeks	Should be withheld when ganciclovir is used; alternative is valaciclovir
Ganciclovir	Cytomegalovirus	1 g po q8h for 3 months	Used as prophylaxis or pre-emptive therapy; may protect against HHV-6 and herpes simplex virus
Valganciclovir	Cytomegalovirus	900 mg po q24h for 3 months	Not approved for this indication in the United States; may be used as prophylaxis or pre-emptive therapy; may protect against HHV-6 and herpes simplex virus
Fluconazole	*Candida* spp.	400 mg po q24h for 4 weeks	Targeted to patients with complicated and prolonged surgery with profound blood loss
Amphotericin B	Fungal pathogens including the filamentous *Aspergillus* spp.	0.2 mg/kg iv q24h	Administered to patients with fulminant hepatic failure; risk of nephrotoxicity; role of triazole such as voriconazole or echinocandins such as caspofungin not established
Oral selective bowel decontamination	Gram-negative bacilli and fungi	Variable; may be given prior to liver transplantation and for up to 4 weeks thereafter	Provides selective pressure favoring an anaerobic environment, with the goal of reducing the risk of bacterial and fungal superinfection
Hepatitis B immunoglobulin	Hepatitis B virus	10 000 IU q24h for first week then every 4 weeks	Maintain serum hepatitis B immunoglobulin level >100 IU; used in conjunction with antiviral nucleosides such as lamivudine and adefovir

Influenza virus vaccination should be given annually, although the live influenza virus vaccine should be avoided.

Oral selective bowel decontamination

A controversial practice after liver transplantation is the use of oral selective bowel decontamination (OSBD), a solution containing a combination of antimicrobials such as colistin, gentamicin and nystatin.[28,29] OSBD is administered to apply selective pressure to intestinal microflora (i.e. to decrease colonization with Gram-negative bacilli and fungi), thereby decreasing bacterial and fungal superinfections after liver transplantation.

Cytomegalovirus and herpes prevention

The two major approaches for preventing CMV disease after liver transplantation are antiviral prophylaxis and pre-emptive therapy.[30] Generally, CMV D+/R– liver recipients receive prophylaxis with a ganciclovir-based regimen for 3 months after transplantation. In the United States, valganciclovir is not approved for this indication, although most centers use the drug for prophylaxis. Newer agents such as maribavir are currently under investigation. In patients at lower risk of CMV disease, a pre-emptive approach is recommended wherein patients are monitored for CMV by PCR or pp65 antigenemia; if CMV is detected, antiviral therapy is provided. CMV prophylaxis is administered to patients receiving OKT3 for acute rejection. When ganciclovir is not used for prophylaxis, aciclovir should be given to prevent HSV disease.

Antifungal prophylaxis

In some centers, prophylaxis with fluconazole or low-dose amphotericin B is given to patients with fulminant hepatitis. Because of the risk of invasive fungal disease, particularly with candidiasis, fluconazole may be administered to liver recipients who require re-transplantation or re-operation, and those with prolonged surgical time or profound blood loss. This approach is supported by a meta-analysis demonstrating that fluconazole reduced invasive fungal (mainly due to *C. albicans*) infections by 75%.[10] Nonetheless, antifungal prophylaxis is not a widely accepted practice after liver transplantation. The utility of newer antifungal drugs such as the echinocandins have not yet been established.

Hepatitis B virus prevention

Prevention of recurrent HBV after liver transplantation is essential since it recurs with a progressive and fatal course. This can be accomplished with HBIg, which acts by neutralization of circulating HBV antigens. HBIg is usually administered with or without antiviral nucleosides such as lamivudine and adefovir which decreases HBV replication. The dose of HBIg is usually 10 000 IU/day for the first week after transplantation and, because it provides temporary protection, it is given at 4-week intervals with the goal of achieving serum HBIg levels above 500 IU for the first year and over 100 IU thereafter. Reinfection with HBV is estimated to occur in less than 10% of patients who were receiving HBIg and lamivudine therapy.[31] Prolonged use of HBIg and antiviral drugs before liver transplantation is discouraged because of the risk of selecting resistant mutants, such as the surface antigen and YMDD mutants, respectively.

Hepatitis C virus prevention

HCV recurrence is almost universal and its course is accelerated after liver transplantation. Progression to cirrhosis and allograft failure occurs in 30% of patients within 5 years after liver transplantation. There is currently no widely accepted measure to prevent HCV recurrence.[32] Pre-emptive treatment of early HCV infection with interferon alpha (IFN-α) may be a reasonable option; however, the risk of interferon-mediated acute rejection, contraindications to IFN-α and ribavirin use during the early transplant period, and the poor tolerance to IFN-α and ribavirin therapy are major limitations.

Therapy of established infection

Early administration of effective therapy is key to the management of infections after liver transplantation. Common bacterial infections such as catheter-related bloodstream and urinary infections should be treated aggressively with antimicrobial therapy tailored to the offending micro-organism and guided by susceptibility tests.

CMV disease, which is one of the most common infections in liver recipients,[24,30] is currently treated with intravenous ganciclovir for a duration dictated by clinical and virologic responses.[24,30] Valganciclovir has now been demonstrated to be as effective as intravenous ganciclovir for the treatment of non-severe forms of CMV disease in SOT recipients.[33]

Treatment of recurrent HCV is often initiated during acute or chronic phases of recurrent hepatitis. Combination therapy with IFN-α and ribavirin has yielded better results when compared to IFN-α monotherapy.[32] Studies on the efficacy of pegylated IFN-α, which provides more sustained levels of circulating interferon, possibly with fewer side-effects, are anticipated.

Reduction in the degree of pharmacologic immunosuppression should complement antimicrobial therapy. Drainage of infected fluid collections (e.g. infected hematoma and abscesses), debridement of surgical infections and removal of infected catheters are essential components of therapy.

CONCLUSION

Liver transplant recipients have characteristics that differentiate them from other SOT groups. The complexity of the surgical procedure places the liver recipient at higher risk of bacterial and fungal infections. The higher prevalence of infection-related indications for transplantation, such as HCV and HBV infection, among liver transplant recipients presents as a challenge that is not seen in other SOT groups. Recently, liver transplantation among HIV-infected patients with end-stage chronic HCV cirrhosis has become a reality. These characteristics and the diversity of the clinical indications for liver transplantation require a tailored and individualized approach to prophylaxis, surveillance and management of infections after liver transplantation.

REFERENCES

References for this chapter can be found online at http://www.expertconsult.com

Pancreatic transplantation

INTRODUCTION

Pancreas (more accurately pancreaticoduodenal allograft) transplantation is currently a widely accepted modality for the treatment of insulin-dependent diabetes mellitus.[1] While most patients undergo pancreas transplantation in combination with renal transplantation, selected nonuremic patients may also be candidates for pancreas transplantation alone. Although rejection rates have decreased with better immunosuppressive therapy, infections remain a source of major morbidity and are one of the leading causes of death in this population. In contrast to infections after kidney transplantation, much

of the infection-related morbidity in the pancreas allograft recipient is related to postsurgical intra-abdominal infections. Common postsurgical infectious complications include urine leak, abscess, infected pseudocyst, infected pancreatocutaneous fistula, infected pancreatic or lymphatic ascites, leakage of pancreatic exocrine secretions or enteric contents, and, rarely, infected pseudoaneurysms.

To handle pancreatic exocrine secretions, drainage into the bladder (bladder drainage, BD) or the small intestine (enteric drainage, ED) are the two most commonly used techniques (Fig. 78.1). Bladder drainage is associated with metabolic acidosis, intravascular volume depletion, reflux pancreatitis and urinary tract complications, including hematuria, urethritis, urethral strictures and urethral disruption,

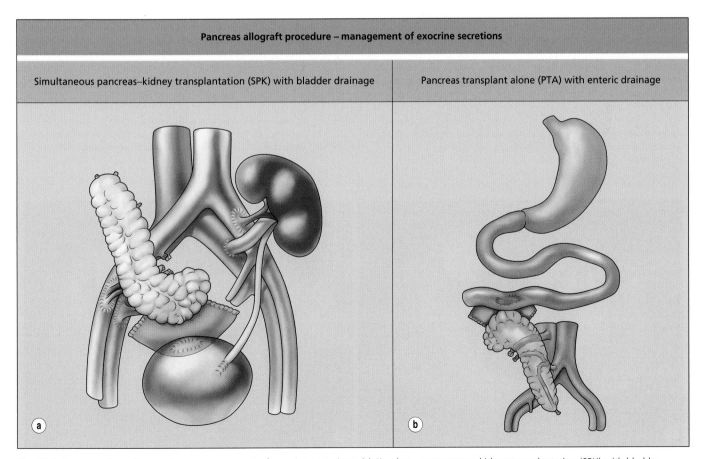

Pancreas allograft procedure – management of exocrine secretions

Simultaneous pancreas–kidney transplantation (SPK) with bladder drainage	Pancreas transplant alone (PTA) with enteric drainage
(a)	(b)

Fig. 78.1 Pancreas allograft procedure – management of exocrine secretions. (a) Simultaneous pancreas–kidney transplantation (SPK) with bladder drainage. (b) Pancreas transplant alone (PTA) with enteric drainage.

all of which may be compounded by infected urine and recurrent urinary tract infections (UTIs). On the other hand, ED is associated with significantly fewer urologic and metabolic complications than BD, and has therefore become the preferred technique.

Several factors contribute to the development of intra-abdominal infections after pancreas transplantation, including:

- intense immunosuppressive regimens;
- compromised defenses associated with diabetes;
- postreperfusion pancreatitis with local release of cytokines and digestive enzymes providing a favorable environment for micro-organisms;
- contamination of the operative field by micro-organisms present in the donor duodenum; and
- microbial translocation from the duodenum facilitated by postreperfusion edema, ischemia or rejection.

Infectious complications associated with pancreas transplantation include UTI, anastomotic leaks of the duodenal segment, intra-abdominal abscesses, mycotic aneurysms, infected pancreatic pseudocysts, infected pancreatocutaneous fistulae and infected abdominal ascites. In addition, cytomegalovirus may affect the pancreas allograft.

These infections typically present with nonspecific symptoms such as pain over the pancreas graft, dysuria, hematuria, fever, malaise, vomiting, etc., and signs such as elevated serum amylase, lipase and creatinine. Postoperative sepsis can be accompanied by mild hyperglycemia.

URINARY TRACT INFECTIONS

Urinary tract infections are a common problem in patients with primary BD of the duodenum segment in pancreas transplantation. Bladder-drainage pancreas transplants lead to significantly more UTIs than ED transplants do (63% vs 20% in the first postoperative year).[2] Urinary tract infections can occur either in the early or late post-transplant period, and they are frequently recurrent. The underlying pathophysiology includes impaired integrity of the bladder mucosa, alteration in urinary pH, urinary retention or stasis due to residual diabetic autonomic neuropathy, prolonged catheter drainage, microbial contamination by the contents of the donor duodenum, retained intravesical sutures and bladder stones. Activation of pancreatic enzymes in the bladder together with urinary alkalosis resulting from bicarbonate secretion appears to cause significant impairment of the mucosal defenses.[3]

The presentation of UTI in pancreas transplant recipients does not differ from the presentation in any other immunosuppressed patient. Symptoms of fever, urinary frequency, dysuria and urgency are common, although patients can be asymptomatic. Enterovesical fistula involving the duodenal segment of the pancreas allograft is a rare cause of recurrent UTI following ED pancreas transplant and can present with pneumaturia. The majority of UTIs are bacterial but fungal infections are also common. The most common bacteria encountered are *Escherichia coli* (27%) and other Gram-negative organisms, such as *Klebsiella*, *Proteus* and *Pseudomonas* spp.[4] Gram-positive organisms are present in approximately 20% of cases, primarily in males, and are probably related to the long-term use of indwelling catheters.[4] In BD pancreas transplants, 50–71% of patients developing a first UTI had a recurrence within the first 90 days. However, less than one-third of these recurrent infections were from the same pathogen as that responsible for the previous infection.[4] Occasionally, a simple lower UTI progresses to an upper UTI or pyelonephritis in the renal allograft, a process that may be accelerated by a diabetic neurogenic bladder and vesicoureteral reflux. Frequently, the donor duodenal segment is colonized with *Candida* spp., explaining the prevalence of fungal UTIs.

Most UTIs following pancreas transplantation can be treated successfully with appropriate antibiotics. Non-nephrotoxic antibiotics that concentrate in the urine, such as the fluoroquinolones, are first-line agents. Fungal UTIs can occasionally be successfully treated with fluconazole or amphotericin bladder irrigations; however, recurrence is common and systemic amphotericin B has been the mainstay of therapy. The role of newer triazole antifungals is undefined. Recurrent UTIs merit further investigation, including cystoscopy to exclude lower urinary tract pathologies such as bladder calculi, foreign bodies or suture granulomata at the duodenum–bladder anastomosis, or a fungus ball (see also Chapter 55). The diagnosis of enterovesical fistula involving the duodenal segment of the pancreas allograft can be made by cystoscopy (presence of bladder mucosal erythema), CT scan (Fig. 78.2) and a high urinary amylase level. In the absence of lower tract abnormalities, the upper tracts are examined by retrograde pyelography and CT scans of the transplanted and native urinary systems. Recurrent, problematic, resistant infections in BD pancreas transplant recipients or those causing renal allograft dysfunction are generally considered indications for conversion to ED.[5]

Multiple recurrent UTIs are associated with poorer long-term renal transplant outcomes.[6,7] Patients with chronic rejection have more UTIs per year, and an earlier onset of chronic rejection correlated with a higher incidence of UTI.[6] However, the pathophysiology uniting UTI

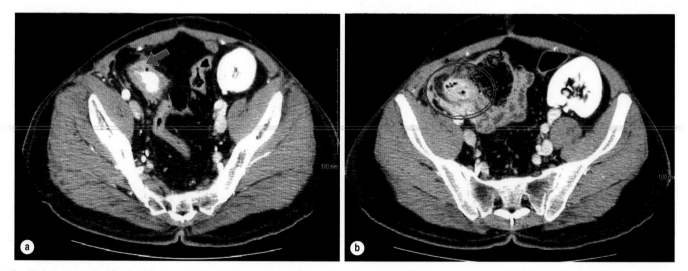

Fig. 78.2 Enterovesical fistula. (a) CT scan shows inflammation and air in wall of bladder. (b) CT scan shows a focus of air and fluid in a cavity adjacent to the bladder and neighboring duodenal segment of the pancreas allograft.

with chronic rejection remains unclear. Potential mechanisms include direct injury, mediated by inflammatory cytokines and chemokines, or enhanced alloreactivity, stimulated by inflammation.

Anastomotic duodenal segment leak: enteric drainage versus bladder drainage

Leakage of pancreatic exocrine secretions from the transplant results in severe life-threatening intra-abdominal infection requiring prompt surgical intervention. With greater experience and better immuno-suppression, this surgical complication has fortunately become less common. A retrospective study at our center compared the incidence of pancreatic enzyme leaks with BD with the incidence with ED. In patients with ED of the duodenum segment the leak rate was 6.3% whereas in BD patients it was 18.8% (p=0.0001; Table 78.1). Most ED leaks occur early post transplant (<4 weeks). In contrast, many leaks in BD transplants occur late (>4 weeks), usually months to years after transplantation, suggesting different etiologies between the two groups. In both groups, early post-transplant leaks are largely techni-cal, either related to ischemia of the duodenal segment or dehiscence of the anastomotic suture line. On the other hand, the precise etiology of late leaks in BD transplants is rarely identified and is probably mul-tifactorial. Whereas early leaks are more common at the anastomotic suture lines, late leaks may occur anywhere in the duodenal segment and are possibly related to immunologic rejection, chronic distention, cytomegalovirus (CMV) disease or chronic urine irritation.

In addition to differing in their time of presentation, anastomotic duodenal segment leaks in ED and BD pancreas allografts differ in presenting signs and symptoms. Leaks in BD pancreatic transplants present with rapid onset lower abdominal pain, fever and occasion-ally hematuria, reflecting sudden spillage of urine into the perito-neal cavity. A sentinel episode of gross hematuria is not uncommon. Concomitant elevation of serum creatinine and serum amylase are classic laboratory findings. In contrast, leaks in ED pancreatic trans-plants generally cause abdominal pain, fever and hyperamylasemia. An elevated serum creatinine is not part of the usual symptom com-plex, unless sepsis is severe.

In patients with BD transplants, the diagnosis is made by either a ^{99m}technetium (^{99m}Tc) voiding cystourethrogram (VCUG) or a CT cystogram. A ^{99m}Tc VCUG is performed by administering labeled diethylene-triamine-penta-acetic acid through an indwelling urinary catheter. Persistent radioisotope in the peritoneal cavity on delayed images indicates a bladder leak (Fig. 78.3). In ED transplants the CT scan detects a fluid collection surrounding the pancreas allograft, frequently in proximity to the duodenal segment (see Fig. 78.3). The presence of air or contrast material in the fluid collection is the sine qua non for enteric leak. However, the absence of these findings does not exclude a leak and an infected fluid collection. Determination of sterility depends on sampling the fluid, usually by percutane-ous aspiration or laparoscopy. The presence of fluid that is rich in amylase and bilirubin confirms the diagnosis of enteric content leak. Polymicrobial infections with enteric organisms are common and indicate an enteric leak until proven otherwise. On the other hand, if

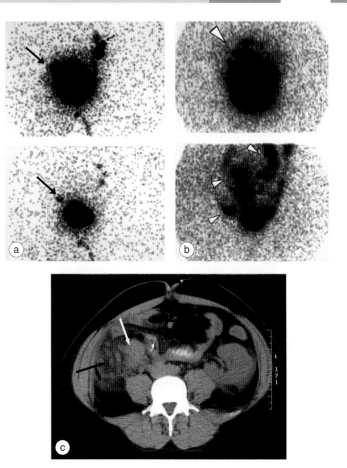

Fig. 78.3 ^{99m}Technetium voiding cystourethrograms. (a) Filling and voiding phases of normal ^{99m}Tc DTPA VCUG. The large arrow represents the duodenal segment of the bladder-drained pancreas transplant. The small arrow represents retrograde flow of radioisotope into the pelvis of the transplanted kidney. (b) Abnormal ^{99m}Tc VCUG. Persistence of radioisotope in the peritoneal cavity is consistent with bladder leak (multiple white arrow heads). Although sensitive for diagnosing urine leak, a radioisotope VCUG does not localize the site of leak. A follow-up contrast VCUG may provide localization, if necessary. (c) Abdominal CT scan demonstrating an enteric leak. The pancreas (white arrow) and a peripancreatic fluid collection (black arrow) are seen. Air and contrast material in the fluid collection are diagnostic of an enteric leak. The absence of these findings, however, does not rule out the possibility of a leak.

amylase content is high and bilirubin content is low, then pancreatic parenchymal injury causing leak of exocrine secretions is likely. This diagnosis is further supported if the fluid is sterile or contains only Gram-positive organisms.

Small leaks in BD transplants can occasionally be treated by Foley catheterization alone for 4–6 weeks. However, if symptoms do not

Table 78.1 Leaks in 747 consecutive simultaneous pancreas and kidney transplants at the University of Wisconsin from October 1983 to July 2000

	Bladder drainage (n=446)	Enteric drainage (n=301)	p value
Patients with leak (n)	84 (18.8%)	19 (6.3%)	0.0001
Patients with leak by 60 days	5.30%	5.50%	
Patients with leak by 1 year	16.1%	6.6%	
Patients with leak by 5 years	20.5%	6.6%	
Patients with leak by 10 years	22.9%	6.6%	
Graft salvage rate after leak	83/84 (98.8%)	6/19 (31.6%)	0.001
Candida-associated infection	15/84 (17.8%)	7/19 (38%)	0.01

resolve completely or if they recur after removal of the Foley catheter, patients may require surgical conversion to enteric drainage.[5] Leaks in ED transplants usually require urgent surgical intervention. In our experience, the most common organisms associated with leaks in ED transplants are *Candida* spp., including *C. glabrata* or *C. albicans* (38%), and vancomycin-resistant enterococci (14%). The mainstays of surgical treatment are debridement of devitalized tissue, tension-free re-closure of the duodenal segment, placement of continuous suction drains in conjunction with the use of appropriate antibiotics and construction of a Roux-en-Y intestinal diversion if this was not performed at the time of transplantation. However, despite these measures, the rate of re-leakage or failure to control sepsis is rather high, even in experienced centers. These complications may ultimately necessitate pancreatectomy in a significant number of patients.

The impact of duodenal segment leaks and associated intra-abdominal infections on renal and pancreas allograft survival is significant. These infections and their antimicrobial treatment commonly contribute to renal allograft dysfunction. Furthermore, in the current immunosuppressive era, leak is a major cause of graft loss since ED transplants that develop a leak may require graft pancreatectomy.

INFECTED FALSE ANEURYSM OF THE ARTERIAL GRAFT

Mycotic aneurysms that occur in immunocompetent patients are often thought to be from septic emboli of cardiac origin. In contrast, the origin of mycotic aneurysms after pancreas transplantation is thought to be due to local infection around the iliac Y graft interacting with tissue digestion by activated pancreatic enzymes. A locally invasive infection promoted by enzymatic tissue digestion leads to disruption of the arterial anastomosis culminating in massive bleeding. Candidiasis is commonly seen in these patients; however, other organisms, such as *Staphylococcus aureus*, *E. coli*, *Enterococcus faecalis*, *Pseudomonas aeruginosa* and *Enterobacter* spp., can also be present individually or in mixed infections. Reduced cell-mediated immunity in transplant recipients, enzymatic digestion of tissues, and adhesiveness and invasion of *C. albicans*[8] may contribute to this infectious complication.

Patients with infected false aneurysms usually present in the immediate postoperative period with hypotension associated with intra-abdominal bleeding and hemorrhagic shock. In some cases, gastrointestinal bleeding may also be present. A sentinel episode of mild intra-abdominal or gastrointestinal bleeding frequently presages a more life-threatening event. It is also occasionally preceded by a significant peripancreatic infection. Patients may also present with generalized sepsis, unilateral iliac vein thrombosis and rarely a tender or pulsatile mass.

An infected false aneurysm of the transplanted pancreas is difficult to diagnose. In stable patients with peripancreatic infection

and a sentinel bleeding episode, urgent iliac arteriography should be performed (Fig. 78.4). If unstable, an emergency laparotomy can be life saving. Ultrasound, CT and MRI are useful adjunctive tools to evaluate peripancreatic infection or bleeding, but only in the stable patient. Although they may show a dilated vessel in the region of the pancreatic arterial supply, CT angiography or conventional angiography is usually necessary to confirm the diagnosis (see Fig. 78.4). Samples of the aneurysm wall and contents should be cultured for aerobic and anaerobic bacteria and fungi.

The extent of active infection in the iliac artery or Y graft artery wall is difficult to determine at the time of surgery, and minimal intervention at the initial surgery is usually doomed to failure. Aggressive management is necessary in order to prevent death. Five general principles apply to the operative management of infected aneurysms:[9]

- control of hemorrhage;
- confirmation of the diagnosis by obtaining tissue specimens for culture;
- operative control of sepsis, including resection of the aneurysm and wide debridement of the infected tissue;
- prolonged antibiotic or antifungal therapy; and
- arterial reconstruction through uninfected tissue planes.

The recommended procedure for an infected Y graft associated with intra-abdominal bleeding or gastrointestinal bleeding is complete excision of the involved donor or recipient iliac arteries, and transplant pancreatectomy. Rarely, infected false aneurysms may present only as a pulsatile mass without peritoneal or gastrointestinal bleeding and this requires only aneurysmectomy without a pancreatectomy. In any case, limb blood flow is restored by surgical bypass of the recipient common iliac artery.[10] The conduit of choice is a blood-type compatible cadaver iliac graft from another donor or autogenous vein. Alternatively, an extra-anatomic femoral–femoral or axillary–femoral bypass with polytetrafluoroethylene can be used. The identification of *Candida* spp. in the peripheral blood or blood clot removed from the Y graft indicates systemic fungal involvement. Broad-spectrum antibiotic and antifungal therapy should be initiated immediately until organism-specific antibiotic therapy can be instituted.

INFECTED PANCREATIC PSEUDOCYST

Pancreatic pseudocyst is rare after pancreas transplantation. It is defined as a peripancreatic inflammatory fluid collection rich in pancreatic enzymes but devoid of enteric contents that is localized by a nonepithelial fibrous wall. Patients typically present with nonspecific abdominal complaints including generalized malaise and weakness, nausea, abdominal pain, fevers and weight loss; associated elevations of serum amylase and lipase are common. In cases of BD, malodor of the urine and a UTI may coexist. A CT scan should be obtained. Pseudocyst formation in the pancreas

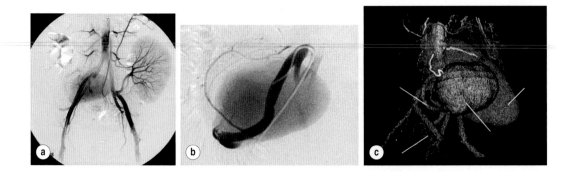

Fig. 78.4 Infected false aneurysm of a pancreas transplant. (a), (b) Arteriogram of an infected false aneurysm originating from the ligated superior mesenteric artery stump of the pancreas transplant. (c) Triphasic CT reconstruction (90° rotation) demonstrating the feeding vessels of the false aneurysm in relation to the pancreas transplant.

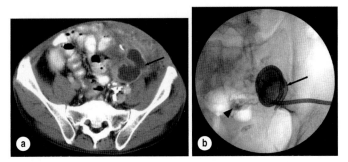

Fig. 78.5 Pancreatic pseudocyst. (a) CT scan demonstrating a pseudocyst of a pancreas transplant in the left pelvis (arrow). (b) Percutaneous drainage of a pancreas transplant pseudocyst. Injection of radiographic contrast material (arrow) demonstrates the pancreatic duct (arrowhead) in communication with the pancreatic pseudocyst.

transplant is thought to be similar in origin to that of the native pancreas – namely, inflammatory pancreatitis. Pancreatitis of the pancreas transplant is most commonly related to reflux and neurogenic bladder, alcohol or duct strictures. Biliary stone disease, while commonly contributing to native pancreatitis, is almost nonexistent in the transplant setting.

Loculated fluid encompassing the transplanted pancreas on CT scan suggests pancreatic pseudocyst (Fig. 78.5). A well-developed capsule of the pancreatic pseudocyst can sometimes be observed, as can a dilated pancreatic duct. Aspiration of the fluid collection is necessary to evaluate the presence of organisms as well as to determine the nature of the fluid (Fig. 78.6). The absence of bilirubin and the presence of amylase in the aspirate is the sine qua non in the diagnosis of pancreatic pseudocyst.

Management mimics that for pseudocyst of the native pancreas. If the pancreatic pseudocyst is infected, external drainage and antibiotic therapy are key. Sterile pseudocysts that are smaller than 6 cm in diameter in relatively asymptomatic patients can be managed expectantly. Persistent infection of the pancreatic pseudocyst can require prolonged antibiotic therapy (up to 6–8 weeks) and percutaneous drainage (Figs 78.5 and 78.6). Persistent high amylase drainage despite conservative measures suggests a possible communication with the pancreatic duct. To confirm this, a fistulogram through the percutaneous drainage catheter is indicated. If a communication with the pancreatic duct is identified and the infection has been treated, a definitive internal drainage procedure is indicated. Internal drainage of a pancreas transplant pseudocyst is optimally achieved via a Roux-en-Y cysto-enterostomy.[11] In BD cases, the pancreatic pseudocyst may alternatively be drained into the bladder by performing a pseudocyst–vesicostomy through a combined transurethral and trans-abdominal approach.[12] Enteric conversion may also be indicated. The long-term outcome from these procedures should be excellent.

INFECTED PANCREATICOCUTANEOUS FISTULA

Pancreaticocutaneous fistula (Fig. 78.7) is a rare complication that can occur after pancreas transplantation due to a pancreatic abscess, concomitant downstream flow obstruction of the pancreatic duct or to direct percutaneous drainage of a pancreatic pseudocyst in communication with duct of Wirsung. Treatment involves a switch to enteric drainage if the pancreas is bladder drained or, if enterically drained primarily, takedown of fistula tract and Roux-en-Y pancreaticojejunostomy. Endoscopic retrograde pancreatography (ERP) and a stent insertion may be effective therapy if a duct stricture exists in association with the enzyme leak. Octreotide may also help with closure of the fistula by diminishing the fistula output. If the pancreas is

nonfunctional, pancreatectomy is the best option. Treatment of the underlying or concomitant surrounding infection is usually required for definitive treatment and closure of the fistula tract.

INFECTED ABDOMINAL ASCITES

Lymphatic ascites after pancreas and kidney transplantation in uremic patients occurs in up to 15–20% of cases. This complication is attributed to the extensive lymphatic dissection necessary for surgical exposure during the operative procedure. It is exacerbated by a poorly absorptive peritoneal membrane if there has been prior peritoneal dialysis complicated by peritonitis. In addition, impaired peritoneal macrophage function and accumulation of peritoneal effluent following peritoneal dialysis may explain the high incidence of deep wound infections in this population.[13] In a comparison study at our institution, the rate of postoperative fluid collections in patients previously on peritoneal dialysis was significantly greater than the rate in patients who had not previously received peritoneal dialysis (24% vs 13%, $p<0.01$; personal communication, Y. Becker). In many instances, fluid collections were associated with Gram-positive or Gram-negative bacterial or fungal contamination and required antibiotic or antifungal therapy. Peritoneal dialysis patients have a greater incidence of intra-abdominal fluid collections infected with micro-organisms that colonize human skin.[14]

The initial diagnosis of ascites is based on physical examination. Abdominal radiographs will demonstrate a paucity of air or a ground-glass appearance. CT scanning or ultrasound confirms the diagnosis. The ascites fluid should be sampled for bacteria and fungi and evaluated for cell count, amylase, total protein and chylomicrons. Elevated pancreatic enzymes and total protein are characteristic of pancreatic ascites, whereas amylase-poor ascitic fluid is characteristic of lymphatic ascites.

Treatment of ascites is based on the use of therapeutic paracentesis, placement of a soft, small-caliber intraperitoneal, indwelling drainage catheter or judicious use of diuretic therapy, or both (see Fig. 78.6). For pancreatic ascites, cessation of oral feedings with the use of hyperalimentation and parenteral octreotide is usual. For infected ascites, percutaneous drainage and appropriate antibiotics usually result in complete resolution and excellent long-term outcomes. Polymicrobial or fungal infection suggests possible leak of enteric contents. Investigation for this entity should include injection of the percutaneous drain with contrast, a CT scan with oral contrast, or enteroclysis.

CYTOMEGALOVIRUS INFECTION OF THE PANCREAS ALLOGRAFT

Cytomegalovirus continues to be the most common viral pathogen affecting organ transplant recipients. The 1-year rate of CMV disease is 13–17% in prophylaxis-treated simultaneous pancreas–kidney transplant recipients.[15,16] As in bone marrow and other solid organ transplants, the relative risk of CMV infection in pancreas transplantation varies according to the CMV antibody status of donor and recipient. Nearly 80% of cases of CMV occur in recipients in the high-risk donor-positive–recipient-negative cohort.[15] Symptomatic CMV infection and CMV disease increases the risk for subsequent renal graft rejection (relative risk, 2.11; $p=0.0032$) and non-CMV infections (relative risk, 2.22; $p=0.0011$).[16] Despite the high frequency of systemic CMV infection, CMV infection of the pancreas allograft is uncommon.[17]

The clinical presentation of CMV infection of the pancreas allograft is characterized by abdominal pain and fever, associated with elevation of serum amylase and lipase, and leukopenia. Distinguishing CMV allograft pancreatitis from acute rejection on clinical grounds alone is difficult.[17] Evaluation of allograft histology is essential in this setting. Cytomegalovirus pancreatitis demonstrates multifocal, predominantly acinar mononuclear inflammatory infiltrates associated with characteristic cytopathic changes. Marked cellular enlargement, intranuclear acidophilic inclusions with surrounding halos, and

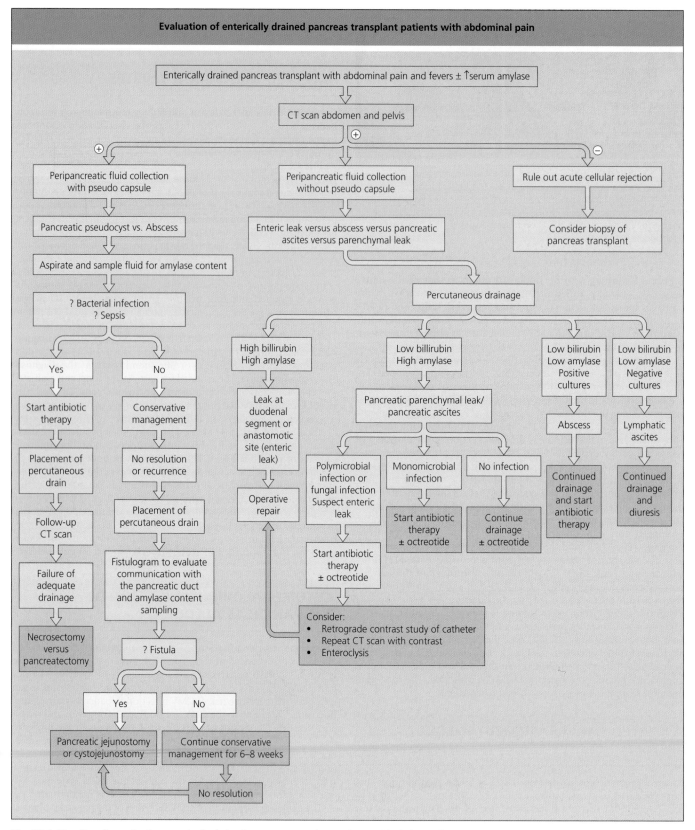

Fig. 78.6 Algorithm for evaluating enterically drained pancreas transplant patients with abdominal pain.

granular basophilic cytoplasmic inclusions are characteristic findings. Immunohistochemistry may be a useful adjunctive test in equivocal cases.[17]

Current CMV prophylaxis is based on the use of oral valganciclovir or intravenous ganciclovir for the first 10 days or while being treated with polyclonal antibody therapy. Doses are adjusted according to creatinine clearance. Long-term post-transplant prophylaxis (for 12 weeks) may be tailored to CMV antibody donor–recipient status, using valganciclovir or ganciclovir for high-risk patients, and aciclovir for those patients who have a low risk of CMV infection.

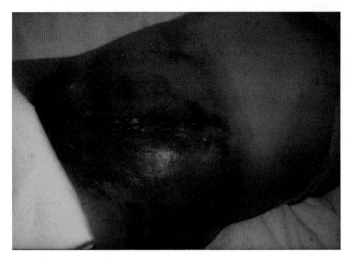

Fig. 78.7 Leakage of irritating pancreatic juices from the pancreas allograft into the surgical wound. Courtesy of Dr H Sollinger.

Treatment of tissue-invasive CMV disease, including allograft pancreatitis, includes lowering immunosuppression and using maximum antiviral treatment with either intravenous ganciclovir or oral valganciclovir. Persistent or recurrent cases may merit the addition of CMV immune globulin (starting dose of 100 mg/kg intravenously every other day for 3 days, then 100 mg/kg intravenously weekly as indicated).

In spite of adequate prophylaxis, CMV remains a problem following pancreas transplantation. Newer, more effective anti-CMV medications may help clinicians to achieve further reduction in symptomatic CMV infection and disease.

REFERENCES

References for this chapter can be found online at http://www.expertconsult.com

Klara M Posfay-Barbe
Marian G Michaels
Michael D Green

Chapter | **79** |

Intestinal transplantation

INTRODUCTION

Experimental models of intestinal transplantation (IT) in dogs were pioneered in the late 1950s; however, clinical trials in humans met with initial failure because of graft rejection, sepsis and/or technical problems.[1] The availability of tacrolimus in 1989 facilitated better control of rejection and allowed IT to become clinically feasible.[2,3] With more than 15 years of clinical experience, IT is being performed by a growing number of transplant centers.[4] However, both the procedure and postoperative care remain complex which likely accounts for the fact that more than 80% of patients undergoing these procedures have done so at only one of 10 major centers worldwide.[4,5]

EPIDEMIOLOGY

Intestinal transplantation is performed as treatment for intestinal failure, defined as a loss of its function manifest by an inability to maintain a normal state of fluid and electrolyte balance, nutrition, growth and development. Intestinal failure may be present on the basis of congenital (e.g. intestinal atresia) or mechanical (e.g. pseudo-obstruction syndrome) problems or as the consequence of an intestinal calamity (e.g. short gut syndrome following necrotizing enterocolitis or volvulus). While total parenteral nutrition (TPN) is available for patients experiencing intestinal failure, its use is associated with significant risks, including venous access complications, recurrent episodes of catheter-associated bloodstream infections and TPN-induced cholestatic liver disease.[6,7]

Intestinal transplantation can be performed as an isolated procedure, concomitant with a liver allograft or as a multivisceral (usually including stomach, duodenum, pancreas, liver and the small intestine) transplant procedure. The choice of procedure is individualized based on the underlying diagnosis associated with intestinal failure and the status of liver function in the presence of chronic TPN. Patient and graft survival vary according to which transplant procedure a patient receives; the best outcomes are in isolated IT and the worst are observed in recipients of multivisceral transplantation. Historically, 5-year survival for isolated IT, liver–intestine and multivisceral transplantation was around 50%. Improvements in surgical techniques along with innovations with immunosuppressive strategies have led to improved outcomes, with 5-year survival rates now more than 70% at some institutions.[5,8] The outcome of IT must be compared to the survival of potential candidates for this procedure without IT, which estimates 40% at 2 years,[9] depending on age and the presence or absence of liver disease. Given the poor outcomes without IT and the improving outcomes of IT itself, it is not surprising that the number of IT recipients in 2001–2005 rose fourfold compared to earlier time periods.[4]

Recipients of IT are, on average, younger than recipients of other types of organ transplantation; 66% of IT recipients are less than 18 years old[4] and 50% are less than 5 years.[1] The young age of these patients reflects the relatively high prevalence of intestinal failure in children due to congenital malformations or intestinal calamity during infancy. It also has important implications on the risk for infection. Patients may undergo IT prior to completion of standard vaccination regimens, putting them at increased risk for vaccine-preventable infections. Transplantation at a younger age also increases the likelihood that IT recipients will be immunologically naive against a variety of pathogens including cytomegalovirus (CMV) and Epstein–Barr virus (EBV). In addition, published experience suggests that younger children are at increased risk for the development of respiratory infections after IT.[10] The importance of this latter observation is further emphasized by the fact that respiratory infection accounted for 40% of infection-related deaths in one recent series of IT in children.[10] As a counterpoint to the potential risks associated with IT in children, undergoing this procedure at a younger age is associated with higher life expectancy and quality of life.[6]

PATHOGENESIS AND PATHOLOGY

Patients undergoing IT are at high risk for developing infectious complications. Unique among IT recipients is the relationship that has been observed between the presence of rejection of the intestinal allograft and the development of bloodstream infection.[11] This relationship may be explained in part by the development of breaks in the protective barrier of the intestinal mucosa that can be associated with rejection of the intestinal allograft. Historically, the overall incidence of rejection of the intestinal allograft has been extremely high (90%); an average patient experiences between one and five episodes per graft.[12] Accordingly, the high rejection rate is one of the major factors accounting for the high frequency of bloodstream infections seen in IT recipients. Recent modifications in immunosuppression, including the use of induction therapy, appear to have resulted in a decreased frequency of rejection[5,8] and a lower rate of bloodstream infections.[8]

Patients with rejection of the allograft can present with clinical signs and symptoms (including fever, abdominal pain or distention, nausea, vomiting and an increase in stomal output) that may be suggestive of infection. Because the presentation of intestinal rejection can mimic infection, it is critical to obtain endoscopic biopsy specimens to confirm the diagnosis. Empiric antibiotics should be considered in patients with severe rejection of the intestinal allograft until blood cultures are found to be negative. Bloodstream infections are also associated with the presence of EBV-associated post-transplant lymphoproliferative disease (PTLD) of the intestine in this patient population.[11] This association is likely also due to breaks in the protective barrier of the intestinal mucosa. Infections in IT recipients can also be attributed to technical complications such as anastomotic leaks resulting in bacterial peritonitis.

The intense immunosuppression required by IT recipients puts these patients at high risk for opportunistic pathogens that are typical after solid-organ transplant, including CMV, EBV and *Pneumocystis jirovecii*, as well as more unusual pathogens such as *Cryptosporidium*.[13] Finally, IT patients frequently require prolonged use of central venous catheters, increasing the risk for catheter-associated bloodstream infections. As in other settings, strategies to reduce these catheter-related bloodstream infections, such as antibiotic locks, have been studied[14] but have yet to demonstrate significant reduction in catheter-associated bloodstream infections in IT recipients.

TIMING AND PATTERN OF INFECTIOUS COMPLICATIONS

In general, the timing of infectious complications after IT follows the typical pattern described for any solid-organ transplant recipient (Table 79.1).[15] However, some differences in the typical timeline of infection are seen following IT, related in part to prolonged and intense immunosuppression. The most important difference is that bloodstream infections occur at a higher rate and continue to occur for a prolonged (if not indefinite) period compared to other organ transplant recipients. A second difference is that IT recipients are at higher risk for morbidity and mortality from CMV and EBV disease

Table 79.1 Timing of infection in intestinal transplant recipients	
	Frequency of infection (%)
Early (0–30 days after transplantation)	
Surgical site:	
• Intra-abdominal	10
• Superficial and deep wound	20–30
Catheter-associated infection	
• Bloodstream*	25
• Urinary tract	10
Ventilator-associated pneumonia	10
Rejection-associated bacteremia	5–10
Intermediate (1–6 months)	
Catheter-associated infection:	
• Bloodstream*	10–20
Rejection associated bacteremia	10–15
CMV*	20–50[†]
EBV/PTLD*	10–33[‡]
• Associated with bacteremia*	5
Late (> 6 months)	
Catheter-associated infection:	
• Bloodstream*	5–10
Rejection associated bacteremia	10–15
CMV*	<10
EBV/PTLD*	<5
• Associated with bacteremia*	<5
Community-acquired infection	Varies[§]

CMV, cytomegalovirus; EBV/PTLD, Epstein–Barr virus/post-transplant lymphoproliferative disease.
*Indicates difference from solid-organ transplant recipients.
[†]Incidence higher in adult intestinal transplant recipients.
[‡]Incidence higher in pediatric intestinal transplant recipients.
[§]Varies with age and community exposure.
Adapted from Fishman & Rubin.[15]

than other transplant recipients.[16–19] CMV may present much later after IT compared to other organ recipients and these patients can develop chronic or recurrent CMV disease (particularly of their graft). These differences between IT recipients and other solid-organ transplant patients is largely attributable to the young age and increased likelihood that IT recipients will be seronegative for CMV and EBV at the time of transplant. Thus, they are at risk for developing graft-related primary infection, which tends to be more severe. The differences may also be explained by the large amount of lymphoid tissue in the intestinal allograft and the generally higher levels of immunosuppression needed to prevent rejection in these patients.

INFECTIOUS SYNDROMES

More than 90% of children with IT present with a bacterial infection following transplantation, with an average of approximately three per patient.[20] However, fungal and viral infections also contribute to the infectious burden after IT.[10]

Bacteremia

Clinical presentation

Bacteremia has been reported to be the most frequent infectious complication following IT.[10] In one series, 277 episodes of bacteremia were identified in 123 children undergoing IT.[10] The rate of bacteremia in IT patients is much higher (about two episodes per patient)[21,22] than that reported for patients undergoing other types of organ transplantation.[23] Bacteremia, typically presenting as fever alone or in combination with signs of sepsis, occurs most frequently during the first 4 months after transplantation. However, episodes can occur even years after IT. Sepsis has been identified as the major cause of death in nearly 50% of cases reported to the International Intestinal Transplant Registry.[4]

The high incidence of bacteremia may be linked to the prolonged presence of central venous catheters as well as translocation of microbiologic flora from within the lumen of the intestinal allograft. In most studies, an obvious source of bacteremia is not identified but abnormal histologic findings in the allograft (rejection, PTLD or both) are frequently present at the time of bloodstream infection.[12] Enteric organisms are the most frequently recovered pathogens and are commonly resistant to multiple antibiotic classes. Some centers have observed a correlation between bacteria identified in the stool and those recovered from the blood. Bacterial overgrowth (defined as a bacterial count >10⁹ colony-forming units (CFU)/ml of stool) has been postulated to facilitate the development of translocation and has been recognized in nearly 90% of bacteremic episodes in these patients.[24] Bacterial overgrowth may be attributed to surgical manipulation of the transplanted bowel, absence of the protective ileocecal valve, abnormal gastrointestinal motility, lymphatic disruption, prolonged TPN and the use of antacid medication. In more than half the cases, the overgrowth includes both Gram-positive and Gram-negative bacteria.

Diagnosis

Blood cultures should be obtained from IT recipients presenting with fever or other clinical signs suggestive of systemic infection. If enteric pathogens are recovered, endoscopy should be performed to look for underlying causes such as rejection or PTLD.

Treatment

The initial empiric therapy for suspected bacteremia should take into account previous isolates obtained from that patient and their antimicrobial resistance patterns. Final treatment should reflect cultures and antimicrobial susceptibility testing performed at the time of clinical presentation. Attention should be paid to high rates of antimicrobial resistance present in bacterial isolates recovered from recipients of IT.

Abdominal infections

Due to mechanisms mentioned above (translocation, anastomotic leaks, increased rejection and mucosal damage), intra-abdominal infections (e.g. peritonitis, intra-abdominal abscesses or fluid collections) are more common in IT recipients than in other solid-organ transplant recipients. Staphylococci, enterococci, *Pseudomonas* spp. and a variety of different Enterobacteriaceae are the most frequent causative agents.[20] Imaging studies support microbiologic cultures obtained by targeted biopsies or other cultures to identify the infection. Again, attention should be paid to multidrug-resistant micro-organisms when starting antimicrobial therapy.

Cytomegalovirus

Epidemiology and clinical presentation

Experience in the 1990s identified that disease from CMV occurred in almost 25% of IT recipients and accounted for significant morbidity and mortality despite treatment with ganciclovir. However, rates of CMV disease have declined with aggressive use of CMV preventive strategies. One recent series reported that only one of 36 children undergoing IT developed symptomatic CMV disease.[8] When CMV disease occurs, up to 90% of patients may have involvement of their allograft as well as their native gastrointestinal tract.[16] Similar to other transplant recipients, CMV-negative recipients of organs from CMV-positive donors present with disease that is more likely to be invasive and more difficult to treat. Historically, primary CMV disease initially presents in the second month after IT, while reactivation episodes present later in the first post-transplant year.[16] However, the timing of both primary and secondary CMV disease may be delayed in patients who have been managed with CMV preventive strategies. Of importance, recurrent CMV disease has been observed frequently in IT recipients[16] and should be treated promptly with antiviral agents.

Diagnosis

Laboratory tests to diagnose viral infections are outlined in Table 79.2. Diagnosis of CMV disease is definitively made on histopathology but can be inferred with the finding of a positive pp65 antigenemia assay or detection of CMV DNA in the blood of a patient with a compatible clinical syndrome. Clinicians must be aware that results of viral cultures of the urine and even bronchoalveolar lavage specimens are difficult to interpret in previously infected patients since CMV is frequently shed asymptomatically in these secretions. Similarly, the presence of pp65 antigen and CMV DNA in the blood can be misleading, as these assays are often positive in asymptomatic patients. The specificity of these assays can be improved by quantitative determination of the pp65 antigen or CMV DNA. Because of the lack of specificity of these assays, histologic examination of involved organs to confirm the presence of CMV is critical when the diagnosis of invasive CMV is being entertained. The importance of histologic evaluation of the gastrointestinal tract should be further emphasized since antigenemia and/or CMV DNAemia may be absent from up to 50% of proven cases of CMV enteritis.[17]

Prevention

Strategies for the prevention of CMV disease vary amongst the various transplant centers. Current recommendations for the prevention of CMV in IT recipients at the Children's Hospital of Pittsburgh are shown in Table 79.3. CMV prevention is typically accomplished through the use of chemoprophylaxis with intravenous ganciclovir and/or valganciclovir, alone or in combination with CMV intravenous immunoglobulin (IVIG), or as pre-emptive therapy where antiviral therapy is initiated in response to a rising viral load, as measured by CMV antigenemia assay or nucleic acid amplification test. More intensive prophylaxis is recommended for patients at high risk for CMV (CMV-seronegative recipients of organs from CMV-seropositive donors).

At the present time, the use of oral valganciclovir is an alternative to prophylaxis with intravenous ganciclovir for adolescents and adult IT recipients. Pharmacokinetic studies for dosing oral valganciclovir suspension in children after transplantation are ongoing. Upon completion of these studies, use of valganciclovir suspension will likely be of merit as an alternative to intravenous treatment for younger children. Upon completion of ganciclovir chemoprophylaxis, some centers will continue to follow these patients using CMV viral load monitoring to inform pre-emptive antiviral therapy with ganciclovir (or valganciclovir). Finally, patients at risk for CMV (all patients except CMV-negative donor/CMV-negative recipient) treated for rejection with intravenous steroids or antilymphocyte antibodies should also receive a pre-emptive course of ganciclovir or valganciclovir.

Table 79.2 Laboratory evaluation of viral infections following intestinal transplantation

Organism	Frequency (%)	Diagnostic test	Follow-up
HBV	<1	HBV serologies, HBV PCR, histology	HBV PCR, liver function tests
HCV	<1	HCV serologies, HCV PCR	HCV viral load, liver function tests
RSV	Adults: <1 Children: 1–5	NP aspirate for antigen detection, culture, PCR	None
Parainfluenza	Adults: <1	NP aspirate for antigen, PCR	None
Adenovirus	30–50	Viral culture, histology, PCR	None
Enterovirus	Adults: <1 Children: 1–5	Viral culture, PCR	None
Influenza	1–5	NP aspirate for antigen detection, culture, PCR	None
HSV	1–5	Culture, antigen testing	Chronic aciclovir prophylaxis
CMV	>5	Culture, pp65 antigen, quantitative PCR, histology	Monitor pp65 antigen or quantitative CMV-PCR
EBV	>5	Quantitative PCR, histology, serology	Monitor EBV PCR, Imaging studies

CMV, cytomegalovirus; EBV, Epstein–Barr virus; HBV, hepatitis B virus; HCV, hepatitis C virus; HSV, herpes simplex virus; IS, immunosuppression; NP, nasopharyngeal; PCR, polymerase chain reaction; RSV, respiratory syncytial virus.

Table 79.3 Prophylactic strategies* in intestinal transplantation

Indication	Prophylaxis	Dose and duration	Comments
Cytomegalovirus			
Donor +, recipient −	Ganciclovir	5 mg/kg iv q12h for 14 days. Then 5 mg/kg iv q24h for 7–14 days if patient remains in hospital; start valganciclovir to complete 90–120 days of therapy once there is evidence of good gut function and absorption (adults: valganciclovir 900 mg po q24h; children: contact pediatric infectious disease specialist)	Adjust dose for renal function. Monitor CMV viral load after completion of prophylaxis until out 6 months from intestinal transplantation. Initiate pre-emptive ganciclovir if viral load becomes positive
	CMV-IVIG	150 mg/kg within 72 h of transplant and at 2, 4, 6 and 8 weeks post-transplant. 100 mg/kg at 12 and 16 weeks post-transplant	
Donor +, recipient +	Ganciclovir	5 mg/kg iv q12h for 14 days	Monitor CMV viral load after completion of prophylaxis until out 6 months from intestinal transplantation. Initiate pre-emptive ganciclovir if viral load becomes positive
Donor −, recipient −	No treatment		

*These are the strategies used at the Children's Hospital of Pittsburgh.

Treatment

Strategies for the treatment of CMV in IT recipients used at the Children's Hospital of Pittsburgh are shown in Table 79.4. CMV disease following IT should be managed using intravenous ganciclovir. Serial measurement of the CMV viral load using the pp65 antigenemia assay or a quantitative CMV PCR, along with follow-up endoscopic evaluation, should guide the duration of therapy. Use of CMV-IVIG in combination with ganciclovir should be considered for patients with involvement of the gastrointestinal tract (native or allograft) or of the lungs. Children have experienced a better outcome than adults after appropriate anti-CMV treatment, with successful outcomes approaching 90%.[25] The median time to resolution (defined as the absence of inclusions on biopsy) on ganciclovir treatment is approximately 20 days.[16] Immunosuppression should be maintained at baseline levels to avoid rebound rejection after treatment of CMV disease. Recurrence of disease is common, especially in CMV-positive donor/CMV-negative recipient patients. Long-term suppression with oral ganciclovir or valganciclovir may be helpful in patients who experience recurrent CMV disease, although few data are available to support this practice. Persistence of disease or of elevated CMV viral load despite treatment suggests the potential presence of ganciclovir resistance. The use of foscarnet or cidofovir should be considered in these cases.

Epstein–Barr virus

Epidemiology and clinical presentation

IT recipients are at high risk of developing EBV disease compared to other organ transplant recipients. EBV disease and PTLD are seen more commonly in children than adults and occur more frequently in recipients of multivisceral transplants > liver and intestinal transplant > isolated intestinal transplant. The International IT Registry identifies incidence rates of PTLD of 5.0% in adult compared to 15.3% in pediatric IT recipients.[4] However, the spectrum of EBV-related disease includes other clinical presentations in addition to PTLD (e.g. EBV enteritis, EBV hepatitis). Recent experience from our center found the current overall incidence of EBV disease to be approximately 20% although only half of these children met the histopathologic criteria for PTLD. These results represent an improvement from our earlier experience with EBV in IT recipients and likely reflect improved immunosuppression regimens and the use of an EB viral load monitoring protocol. Similar improvements in the incidence of EBV/PTLD have also been reported in the International IT Registry.[4]

EBV disease may present clinically as a febrile syndrome, mononucleosis, PTLD or malignant lymphoma. Diarrhea, which often contains occult blood, is a frequent finding in this patient population and may be associated with ulcerated nodular tumors of the intestinal tract. Nonspecific symptoms including fever, weight loss and malaise are common. Lymphadenopathy may also be present. Although the most frequent site of involvement is the intestinal tract, including the allograft, disseminated disease can also occur. Accordingly, it is important to note that EBV enteritis can be misdiagnosed as rejection. For this reason, it is recommended that Epstein–Barr encoded RNA (EBER) staining be considered on bowel biopsies with presumed rejection to rule out the possibility of EBV infection before treating for rejection.[26] This is particularly important in patients with a current or recent history of an elevated EB viral load in the peripheral blood.

There are three major differences between EBV/PTLD in IT recipients and other solid-organ recipients:

- EBV disease and PTLD are seen frequently in EBV-seropositive children undergoing IT. With other organ transplants EBV/PTLD is rarely seen in patients who are EBV-seropositive prior to transplant;
- EBV-associated disease including PTLD can occur concurrently with rejection after IT, whereas in other organ transplant recipients rejection tends to occur only after evidence of regression of the EBV disease; and
- as many as 30% of surviving IT patients will experience chronic and/or recurrent episodes of EBV disease in contrast to a recurrence rate of about 5–10% after other organ transplants.[27]

The last difference may be explained by the difficulty in reducing immunosuppressive treatment in the presence of concomitant rejection, limiting the body's ability to generate a cytotoxic T-lymphocyte response against EBV.

Diagnosis of Epstein–Barr virus post-transplant lymphoproliferative disease

When EBV disease (including PTLD) is suspected, CT scan of the neck, chest, abdomen and pelvis should be performed to identify occult lesions. Endoscopy should also be performed in IT recipients, especially

Table 79.4 Treatment strategies* in intestinal transplantation

Treatment	Dose and duration	Comments
Cytomegalovirus		
First-line therapy		
Ganciclovir	5 mg/kg iv q12h for minimum of 14–21 days	Maintenance therapy 5 mg/kg iv q24h or consider valganciclovir. Treat until pp65 or CMV PCR reverts to negative. Adjust dose for renal function
CMV-IVIG (for CMV pneumonitis, enteritis or retinitis)	100 mg/kg iv q48h for three doses	May repeat every 2 weeks depending on results
Alternative therapy		
Foscarnet	180 mg/kg iv q8h for 14–21 days	Maintenance therapy: 90–120 mg/kg iv q24h
Cidofovir	5 mg/kg iv once weekly for 2 weeks	Continuing therapy: 5 mg/kg iv once every 2 weeks as clinically needed
Epstein–Barr virus		
Initial treatment		
Reduction or elimination of immune suppression		Immune suppression reduced and maintained at low levels until resolution of disease unless rejection develops
Ganciclovir	5 mg/kg iv q12h for 14–21 days	Adjust for renal function. Treatment typically maintained until resolution of disease. Clinical efficacy unproven
Aciclovir	500 mg/m² iv q8h for 14–21 days	Adjust for renal function. Treatment typically maintained until resolution of disease. Clinical efficacy unproven
IVIG	300 mg/kg iv	May repeat every 2 weeks depending on results. Clinical efficacy unproven
Secondary treatment		
Rituximab	375 mg/m² iv once weekly for 4 weeks	The use of rituximab should be considered when patients fail to respond to initial treatment, or for those who develop concurrent rejection at the time of diagnosis or treatment for EBV/PTLD. Consultation with a subspecialist with experience in the management of EBV/PTLD (e.g. infectious disease, hematology/oncology) is recommended

*These are the strategies used at the Children's Hospital of Pittsburgh.

if the patient has diarrhea or other symptoms of gastrointestinal disease. Biopsies should be obtained from suspicious lesions and sent for histologic evaluation. The use of immunohistopathologic stains for the presence of EBV (e.g. EBER staining) is necessary to distinguish EBV-infected cells from nonspecific lymphocytic infiltrates. Patients with active EBV disease typically have an elevated peripheral blood EB viral load. However, results of these assays lack specificity as elevated EB viral loads also may be present in otherwise asymptomatic individuals.

Prevention of Epstein–Barr virus post-transplant lymphoproliferative disease

The high rates of morbidity and mortality attributed to EBV/PTLD have prompted efforts to prevent or pre-emptively treat EBV in IT recipients. Serial monitoring of the EB viral load using quantitative PCR assays has been shown to predict occurrence of PTLD. EB viral load surveillance is currently used to guide initiation of pre-emptive therapy at many centers.[19] However, specific target levels of viral load as well as therapeutic pre-emptive treatment regimens vary from center to center and remain to be evaluated in prospective, comparative studies. Pre-emptive therapy typically consists of reduction of immune suppression whenever possible. Ganciclovir and IVIG are also used by some

centers although definitive data demonstrating efficacy of these latter two agents are lacking.

Treatment of Epstein–Barr virus post-transplant lymphoproliferative disease

Strategies for the treatment of EBV/PTLD used at the Children's Hospital of Pittsburgh are shown in Table 79.4. Reduction of immune suppression is the major therapeutic manipulation for transplant recipients with EBV/PTLD and allows the body to develop EBV-specific cytotoxic T-cell lymphocytes to control the infectious process. Unfortunately, the high rates of rejection observed during attempts at immunomodulation of EBV may limit this approach in IT recipients. While frequently used, ganciclovir or aciclovir as well as IVIG are of unproven benefit for the treatment of EBV/PTLD. The use of anti-CD20 monoclonal antibody (rituximab) has been increasingly used in this population. Although rituximab appears quite promising, evidence of efficacy is limited to registry and anecdotal reports.[28–31] Historically, the mortality rate for IT patients with PTLD has been reported to be as high as 50%. However, the use of EB viral load monitoring to facilitate earlier diagnosis in association with evolving treatment strategies have led to improving rates of patient and graft survival, with rates approximating 75%.[10]

Adenovirus

Epidemiology and clinical presentation

Adenovirus infection has been observed frequently in pediatric recipients of IT. Rates of adenovirus infection in this population have ranged from 20.8%[32] to 100%.[33] However, the latter rate may have been attributable to the fact that viral cultures were obtained as part of routine screening of graft biopsies and not all of the patients were symptomatic. The presence of adenovirus has been identified much less commonly in adult IT recipients. The interpretation of a positive culture or histologic finding for adenovirus is made difficult by the frequent absence of any associated symptoms in IT recipients from whom evidence of adenovirus infection is demonstrated. When symptoms are found they most often include high stool output, alone or in the presence of fever.

Adenovirus can also present as an invasive disease.[34] Risk factors for invasive disease include failure to clear virus, isolating virus from more than one site and intensified immunosuppression.[33]

Diagnosis

It is very difficult to presumptively diagnose infection due to adenovirus in IT recipients, as fever, hepatitis and pneumonia may be caused by a variety of other pathogens. In addition, high stool output after IT is nonspecific and can also occur with rejection. The presence of high-grade fevers and symptoms suggestive of adenovirus infection should prompt serial cultures for viruses (including adenovirus) or PCR investigation and evaluation of graft biopsies. Unexplained hepatitis should warrant consideration of a liver biopsy. Similarly, an increase in stool output, with or without fever, should prompt endoscopic evaluation of the intestinal allograft. Histologic examination for the presence of adenoviral inclusions as well as the use of immunohistochemical stains of biopsy specimens from either site should be undertaken to help confirm this diagnosis.

Treatment

Unfortunately, there is no definitive treatment for adenoviral infection at this time. The most important component of therapy is supportive care along with a decrease in immunosuppression. The role of antiviral agents is unproven. A small number of case reports describe the use of ribavirin, ganciclovir and cidofovir in the treatment of single patients with adenoviral infection after solid-organ or bone marrow transplantation.[35,36]

Other pathogens

Similar to other organ transplant recipients, recipients of IT are at risk for infection from a wide variety of pathogens. Infection may develop from nosocomial exposures or once the patient has returned to the ambulatory setting. Infectious pathogens of the intestinal tract that can mimic intestinal rejection include adenovirus, rotavirus, *Clostridium difficile*, herpes simplex virus and nontuberculous mycobacteria.[21] An effort should be made to search for these pathogens by culture, histology and/or immunoassay before treating the patient for rejection.

Respiratory viruses (parainfluenza, respiratory syncytial virus, influenza) can be fatal in IT recipients.[22] While the relative frequency of acquisition is greater in the intermediate to late time periods after transplantation (after exposure to community-acquired pathogens), occurrence of disease in the early post-transplant period is most dangerous. Additional risks for severe disease with respiratory viruses include age less than 1 year, pre-existing lung disease and exposure to augmented immunosuppression.

REFERENCES

References for this chapter can be found online at http://www.expertconsult.com

Kidney transplant patients

INTRODUCTION

Kidney transplantation is the preferred strategy to treat end-stage renal disease. Improvement in surgical techniques, more efficacious immunosuppressive protocols, and a more accurate selection process of donors and recipients, have led to a remarkable improvement in both patient and graft survival, as well as in quality of life.[1] In parallel, a progressive reduction of morbidity and mortality caused by infectious diseases after transplantation has occurred, mainly as a consequence of improved prophylactic regimens. Nevertheless, infectious diseases are still a major cause of hospitalization after transplantation.[2] New infections have emerged and clinical and epidemiologic patterns of old infections have changed. BK virus has become an important viral pathogen after kidney transplantation, mostly due to the higher net state of immunosuppression associated with modern antirejection regimens and the lack of effective antiviral therapy.[3,4] Recent reports have appeared of donor to recipient transmission of rabies, lymphocytic choriomeningitis virus and West Nile virus infection.[5] Although cytomegalovirus (CMV)-associated morbidity and mortality have decreased due to the introduction of better diagnostic methods and new antiviral strategies, late-onset CMV disease remains a significant problem after kidney transplantation, particularly in high-risk recipients.[6]

While many infections following kidney transplantation are similar in nature to other organ transplant recipients, there are also specific problems found in patients with kidney disease.

- The majority of transplant candidates are undergoing dialysis before transplantation (except in cases of pre-emptive kidney transplantation). Patients on dialysis have frequent hospitalizations and are exposed to multiple medical procedures. They are more frequently colonized with methicillin-resistant *Staphylococcus aureus* and other resistant organisms and are at an increased risk for developing urinary tract infections and invasive fungal infections after transplantation.[7]
- Compared to native kidneys, the kidney allograft is more susceptible to nephrotoxic drugs and antimicrobial drugs can potentiate the nephrotoxicity of calcineurin inhibitors (ciclosporin and tacrolimus). For example, as shown in Table 80.1, drugs such as aminoglycosides, amphotericin B, foscarnet and cidofovir increase the risk of nephrotoxicity from calcineurin inhibitors. In addition, antimicrobials that inhibit the CYP3A4 enzyme (e.g. some macrolides or azoles) increase calcineurin inhibitor plasma levels, with a subsequent higher risk of nephrotoxicity. Conversely, drug inducers of the CYP3A4 system (e.g. rifampicin) may decrease levels of calcineurin inhibitors, resulting in allograft rejection. Clinicians must be aware of these and other drug interactions before starting antibiotic therapy in kidney transplant recipients.

- There are some infections seen predominantly in kidney transplantation. Recurrent urinary tract infections are frequently seen after kidney transplantation and may be due to the recipient's specific diseases (e.g. reflux nephropathy) or to anatomic changes produced during surgery. Although BK virus has been detected in the urine of other organ transplant recipients, it has rarely been associated with clinical nephropathy.

URINARY TRACT INFECTION

Urinary tract infection (UTI) is the most common bacterial infection after kidney transplantation.[8] Asymptomatic bacteriuria, acute cystitis and acute pyelonephritis are usually included in the definition of UTI. The incidence of UTI in kidney transplant recipients may vary between 20% and 75%. Although the major impact of UTI is seen in the early post-transplant period, it can appear months after transplant and has been associated with varying degrees of allograft dysfunction and a higher mortality.[9] Risk factors associated with UTI are female gender, diabetes mellitus, vesicoureteral reflux, duration of vesical catheterization and use of ureteral stenting.[10] As post-transplant urologic complications such as urinary leak or ureteral stricture are significantly reduced by ureteral stenting, this procedure is now in common use. The higher risk of UTI due to ureteral stenting can be reduced by antimicrobial prophylaxis.[11]

The microbial etiology of UTI after kidney transplantation is similar to that observed in the general population. *Escherichia coli* remains the most common pathogen of UTI, followed by other Enterobacteriaceae, such as *Klebsiella* or *Proteus* spp.[8,10] Other series have also identified *Enterococcus* and *Pseudomonas* spp. as common pathogens involved in UTI. *Corynebacterium urealyticum* is the cause of a rare entity reported as encrusted pyelitis and cystitis, where mucosal inflammation with encrustation of the mucosa by struvite crystals can be seen. Although candiduria is common after kidney transplantation, symptomatic infection is seen less frequently.

Clinical manifestations of UTI after transplantation may be attenuated due to the anatomic particularities of the kidney allograft and the immunosuppression-associated impaired inflammatory reactions. In kidney graft recipients with fever but without an evident clinical source, the urinary tract should be initially suspected as the potential cause of the infection.

The first step for preventing UTI after transplantation is an appropriate and timely removal of the urinary catheter. In addition, antibiotic prophylaxis is used in the majority of kidney transplant programs during the first 4–6 months after transplant (Table 80.2). Because co-trimoxazole is effective against common uropathogens and as prophylaxis for *Pneumocystis jirovecii* pneumonia and other pathogens such as *Nocardia*, *Toxoplasma* and *Listeria* spp., this drug is widely used

Table 80.1 Interaction between antimicrobial agents and immunosuppressive drugs

Antimicrobial drug	Interaction with immunosuppressive drugs	Comments
Aminoglycosides		
Aminoglycosides	Increase nephrotoxicity of calcineurin inhibitors	Aminoglycosides should be avoided in patients receiving calcineurin inhibitors. No published data available on interaction between aminoglycosides and sirolimus
Quinolones		
Ciprofloxacin	May increase ciclosporin levels	Mild interaction. Quinolones may potentiate the tubular toxicity of calcineurin inhibitors
Macrolides		
Clarithromycin	Increases calcineurin inhibitor and sirolimus levels	Important interaction. Azithromycin may be a better option
Azithromycin	May increase ciclosporin levels	Mild interaction
Antifungal agents		
Fluconazole	Increases calcineurin inhibitor and sirolimus levels	Moderate interaction
Voriconazole	Increases calcineurin inhibitor and sirolimus levels	Important interaction. Calcineurin inhibitors and sirolimus dose should be decreased 50–80% after starting voriconazole
Caspofungin, anidulafungin	Calcineurin inhibitors may increase echinocandin levels	Clinical relevance of this interaction is unknown
Amphotericin B	Increases nephrotoxicity of calcineurin inhibitors	Possibly lower toxicity with liposomal formulation
Antiviral agents		
Foscarnet	Increases nephrotoxicity of calcineurin inhibitors	Incomplete clinical data
Cidofovir	Increases nephrotoxicity of calcineurin inhibitors	Incomplete clinical data
Other antimicrobials		
Rifampicin	Decreases calcineurin inhibitor levels	If possible, rifampicin use should be avoided, due to high risk of rejection. Rifabutin may be a better option
Co-trimoxazole	May increase nephrotoxicity of calcineurin inhibitors	The risk of nephrotoxicity is higher with therapeutic than prophylactic doses

Calcineurin inhibitors: ciclosporin, tacrolimus and co-trimoxazole (trimethoprim–sulfamethoxazole, TMP–SMX).

Table 80.2 Preventive strategies after kidney transplantation

Prophylactic strategy	Recommendation	Comments
Antimicrobial prophylaxis	Co-trimoxazole 400/80 mg q24h or 800/160 mg three times a week for initial 3–6 months after transplant [In case of allergy to co-trimoxazole, a quinolone (ciprofloxacin, levofloxacin or moxifloxacin) can be used, along with a drug effective for *Pneumocystis jirovecii* pneumonia prophylaxis (dapsone 50–100 mg q24h, atovaquone 1500 mg q24h or inhaled pentamidine 300 mg every 3–4 weeks)]	Efficacy in preventing urinary tract infection, *Pneumocystis jirovecii* pneumonia, toxoplasmosis, *Listeria*, *Salmonella* spp.
Antiviral prophylaxis	Valganciclovir 450–900 mg* q24h for initial 3–6 months after transplant in D+/R– and/or after antilymphocyte therapy for rejection Valganciclovir 450–900 mg* q24h for initial 3–6 months after transplant in D+/R+ and D–/R+ Aciclovir 200 mg* q8h, valaciclovir 250 mg* q12h, or famciclovir 250 mg* q12h for initial 3 months after transplant for herpes prophylaxis in CMV D–/R– or in patients followed by pre-emptive approach	Usually recommended Optional. Some authors prefer using a pre-emptive approach in this setting Usually recommended
Antifungal prophylaxis	Fluconazole 200–400 mg* q24h in case of high risk for *Candida* infection, i.e. surgical complications (e.g. urinary leak), long intensive care unit stay, *Candida* colonization, use of parenteral nutrition, use of broad-spectrum antibiotic	Systemic antifungal prophylaxis generally not recommended

*Dose to be adapted for kidney function. D, donor; R, recipient.

after kidney transplantation.[12] In case of drug allergy or a high rate of co-trimoxazole-resistant organisms, a quinolone can be useful for prophylaxis. The management of asymptomatic bacteriuria after kidney transplantation remains controversial. Studies have failed to show a higher rate of symptomatic UTI in patients with untreated asymptomatic bacteriuria. Therefore, screening for or treatment of asymptomatic bacteriuria in renal transplant recipients is not recommended.[13]

Management of UTI should integrate a medical and a surgical approach. In general, prompt empiric antibiotic therapy is necessary in order to avoid progression to a more severe infection. Usually, broad-spectrum β-lactams (e.g. piperacillin) or a carbapenem is the antibiotic of choice to treat Enterobacteriaceae, *Pseudomonas* and *Enterococcus* spp. This antibiotic therapy should subsequently be adjusted when the etiologic pathogen is identified. The duration of therapy may vary from 7 to 10 days for uncomplicated UTIs to 4–6 weeks in cases of septic shock, presence of anatomic abnormalities or infections with resistant micro-organisms. An ultrasound of the allograft is also recommended to check for urologic complications such as obstruction or urinary leak, especially in cases of recurrent UTI or breakthrough infection during antibiotic prophylaxis. In patients with polycystic kidney disease, the native kidneys may be the cause of the UTI. If anatomic abnormalities are suspected or identified, a surgical or urologic consultation is indicated.

POLYOMAVIRUS INFECTION

BK virus, JC virus and the simian virus SV40 belong to the Papovaviridae family.[3] The main pathogen implicated in polyomavirus-associated nephropathy is BK virus, although some cases of JC-associated nephropathy have also been reported. Primary infection with either BK or JC virus usually occurs during childhood, and serologic studies have shown a prevalence of BK virus infection in 60–80% of adults. The prevalence of BK virus active infection in kidney transplant recipients measured by polymerase chain reaction (PCR) in plasma has been estimated to be approximately 10–15%. The prevalence of BK virus-associated nephropathy varies depending on the series and the immunosuppressive regimen, but is estimated to be between 1% and 10%.[4]

Clinical manifestations of BK virus infection in kidney transplant recipients include tubulointerstitial nephropathy and ureteral stenosis. A rising creatinine level is usually the only manifestation of BK virus-associated nephropathy; if unrecognized, this may lead to graft loss in 10–80% of cases.[4] In centers where universal screening for BK

virus is performed, current rates of graft loss due to BK virus-associated nephropathy are low because of appropriate management.

Identifiable risk factors are associated with BK virus-associated nephropathy. Although this nephropathy has occurred with all immunosuppressive regimens, it is more frequently associated with more intensive regimens such as those including tacrolimus, steroids and mycophenolate mofetil (MMF) at normal dosages. The use of antilymphocyte preparations as induction therapy and for treatment of acute rejection has also been suggested as a risk factor, but not in all series.[3]

The diagnostic certainty for BK virus-associated disease is classified at three levels – possible, presumptive and definitive BK virus-associated nephropathy.[4]

Possible Possible BK virus-associated nephropathy refers to a positive screening test, usually the presence of intranuclear viral inclusions in urogenital tract epithelial cells (decoy cells) in the urine. This test has an excellent negative predictive value, but lacks specificity.

Presumptive The term presumptive BK virus-associated nephropathy is used when an adjunct test is also positive (e.g. a quantitative BK viral load measured in urine or plasma by PCR). Plasma viral load appears to best correlate with an eventual diagnosis of BK virus-associated nephropathy.

Definitive The definitive diagnosis of BK virus-associated nephropathy requires a kidney biopsy to identify characteristic viral inclusions, as well as inflammatory infiltrates and cytopathic changes (Fig. 80.1). Histology of BK virus-associated nephropathy ranges from pattern A (minimal to mild viral cytopathic changes and inflammatory infiltrates) to pattern C (moderate to severe tubular atrophy and interstitial fibrosis, with variable inflammatory infiltrates).[4] Concurrent acute rejection can be present and is difficult to differentiate from the histologic changes due to BK virus.

The management of BK virus infection in kidney transplant recipients is discussed in more detail in Practical Point 43. Most programs recommend screening for BK virus, with or without urine cytology, every 3 months during the first 1–3 years after transplant, or when renal dysfunction occurs. If decoy cells are identified in urine, BK virus DNA should be quantified by PCR. Generally accepted thresholds predictive for BK virus-associated nephropathy are >10^7 DNA copies/ml in urine or >10^4 DNA copies/ml in plasma. Subsequently, a renal biopsy should be performed to confirm the diagnosis of BK virus-associated nephropathy.

There is no current etiologic treatment for BK virus-associated nephropathy. The most effective approach is to decrease immunosuppression, with close follow-up because of the risk of inducing acute

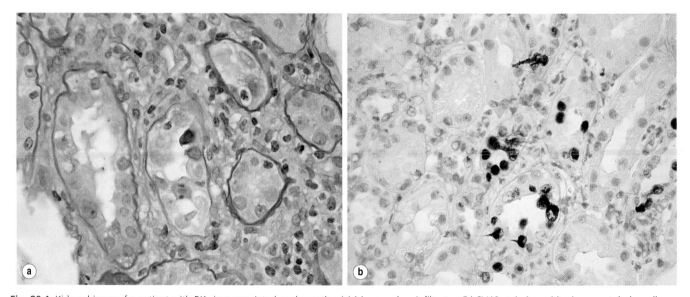

Fig. 80.1 Kidney biopsy of a patient with BK virus-associated nephropathy. (a) Mononuclear infiltrates. (b) SV40 stain is positive in some tubular cells (brown dots).

rejection. Some treatment options include switching from tacrolimus to ciclosporin, decreasing the dose of MMF (or replacing it by azathioprine) or discontinuing one of the drugs to maintain a two-drug regimen. Cidofovir at low doses (0.25–0.33 mg/kg given intravenously every 2–3 weeks) and leflunomide (a drug used for treatment of rheumatoid arthritis) have antipolyomavirus activity *in vitro* and some apparent benefit in small clinical series, but currently there is no consensus on their use.

HERPESVIRUS INFECTION

Cytomegalovirus infection remains a major problem in kidney transplantation.[14] In the absence of prophylaxis, around 50% of kidney transplant recipients may develop CMV active infection during the first 3 months after transplantation; this rate is as high as 80% in donor-positive, recipient-negative primary infections. Manifestations of CMV infection range from asymptomatic viral replication to symptomatic disease, including local tissue-invasive disease or generalized CMV syndrome. CMV syndrome is manifested by fever, malaise, leukopenia, thrombocytopenia and elevated liver enzymes. CMV tissue-invasive disease often presents as colitis or hepatitis. In kidney transplant recipients, CMV may produce allograft nephritis, although this is rare.

The major risk factor for developing CMV disease is the donor/recipient serostatus, the seronegative recipient with a seropositive donor being at the highest risk.[6] Other risk factors include the type of immunosuppressive regimen (e.g. the use of MMF), and the use of antilymphocyte agents as induction or antirejection therapy.[6]

Currently, there are two main strategies to prevent CMV disease: universal antiviral prophylaxis and pre-emptive therapy: universal prophylaxis (see Table 80.2) consists of administering an antiviral drug after transplantation to all at-risk patients, usually during the initial 3- to 6-month period; pre-emptive therapy consists of monitoring for CMV appearance in blood (e.g. with either CMV DNA PCR or antigenemia) and administering antiviral therapy only when significant CMV viremia is detected. Both strategies have not been compared in large-scale prospective randomized clinical trials. Drugs which have been used for the prevention of CMV infection in kidney transplantation are oral aciclovir or valaciclovir, and intravenous and oral ganciclovir. Recently, oral valganciclovir, a valyl-ester prodrug of ganciclovir with an improved bioavailability compared to oral ganciclovir, has been approved for CMV prophylaxis.[14,15] While intravenous ganciclovir (5 mg/kg twice a day) has been the preferred drug for the treatment of established CMV disease, recent reports show the equivalence of oral valganciclovir (900 mg twice a day, adapted for kidney function) for this indication.[16,17] However, caution is needed in cases of life-threatening infection and when oral absorption may be compromised. Monitoring of CMV viral load during treatment is a valuable tool to decide the duration of the antiviral therapy (usually 6–8 weeks), since the incidence of relapse is reduced if antiviral therapy is stopped when CMV viral load is undetectable.

Herpes simplex virus (HSV)-1 and -2 reactivation is common after kidney transplantation and its incidence is estimated to be approximately 50% in seropositive recipients. HSV may reactivate shortly after transplantation, and the lesions may be clinically atypical or more severe and may last longer, when compared to those seen in immunocompetent patients. HSV infection is seen less frequently in the era of CMV prophylaxis.

Several studies have described the epidemiology and clinical manifestations of varicella-zoster virus (VZV) infection after kidney transplantation. Incidence of VZV infection may vary between 3% and 10%, but primary infection (i.e. chickenpox) should be differentiated from secondary reactivation (i.e. herpes zoster). Since the majority of adult recipients are VZV seropositive, the most common manifestation of VZV infection after transplant is herpes zoster. Usually, zoster in kidney transplant recipients does not differ from that seen in the general population, although some series have highlighted a higher incidence of disseminated cutaneous reactivation (or visceral involvement) and

relapse can occur in up to 15% of patients. Postherpetic neuralgia also seems to be more frequent in this population. Diagnosis is often clinical; however, microbiologic confirmation by immunofluorescence or PCR may be useful to help distinguish it from HSV infection.

A more difficult problem is VZV primary infection in pediatric kidney transplantation, characterized by a high rate of visceral complications and mortality. Recent studies, however, have shown a reduction of VZV-associated complications, likely due to universal VZV screening and vaccination prior to transplantation.

The potential clinical significance of human herpes virus (HHV)-6 and -7 infection has not been convincingly established after kidney transplantation. A number of case reports of HHV-6-associated encephalopathy in solid-organ transplant recipients have been described.[18] Some reports have suggested an association between HHV-6 and -7 infections and CMV infection and disease in kidney transplant recipients.[19] The appropriate approach for screening and management of HHV-6 and -7 infections is currently unknown.

HEPATITIS B AND C VIRUS INFECTIONS

Infections with hepatitis B and C viruses (HBV and HCV) have been recognized as important health problems in end-stage renal failure and, consequently, in the kidney transplant population.[20] Transplant recipients develop HBV- or HCV-associated liver disease after transplantation as a result of progression of pre-existing infection or by transmission through blood products or organs from infected donors.

The introduction of blood donor screening, the increased use of erythropoietin and the adoption of strict infection control practices have significantly reduced the prevalence of HBV and HCV in most dialysis units. The availability and routine use of HBV vaccination has dramatically decreased the prevalence of HBV in dialysis units to <2%.[21] Owing to the lack of effective vaccination, HCV is still found in 5–40% of kidney transplant recipients.[22]

Liver disease associated with HBV and HCV infections (now mostly with HCV) is an important cause of morbidity and mortality after transplantation.[22,23] Chronic hepatitis and its sequelae are the main forms of liver involvement in these patients. In addition, an unusual form of liver disease called fibrosing cholestatic hepatitis, characterized by severe cholestasis and rapidly progressive liver failure, has been reported with both viruses after kidney transplantation.[24,25] These viruses have also been implicated in the pathogenesis of de novo or recurrent glomerular disease in the allograft, which may impair graft survival.[26] More recently, various reports have suggested an association between HCV infection and new onset diabetes mellitus after renal transplantation.[27] In spite of the detrimental effects of HBV and HCV on patient and graft survival, kidney transplantation still remains the best long-term option for HBV- and HCV-infected dialysis patients on the waiting list. Combined liver and kidney transplantation should be considered in the presence of liver cirrhosis.[23]

The diagnosis of chronic HBV infection is made or excluded on the basis of serologic markers such as HBsAg, HBsAb, HBeAg and anti-HBc-IgM/G. Measurement of hepatitis B viral load by PCR is an important guiding tool for the administration and monitoring of antiviral therapy. The diagnosis and screening of HCV infection is based on serologic testing with third-generation anti-HCV assays. As false-negative results may occur in immunocompromised patients, HCV RNA testing by PCR should be strongly considered. Genotyping and determination of hepatitis C viral load are helpful to evaluate potential efficacy and monitoring of antiviral treatment. Serum transaminase levels and viral load are poor markers of the severity of liver disease in HBV- and HCV-infected patients. Therefore, liver biopsy remains the gold standard for accurate grading and staging in these patients. CT scanning or duplex ultrasonography of the abdomen should be performed at regular intervals for early identification of portal hypertension, ascites and hepatocellular carcinoma.

The recommended antiviral treatment strategies in the nontransplant setting cannot be simply applied to kidney recipients. Interferon alpha (IFN-α, standard or pegylated) has been associated with triggering severe acute allograft rejection, often irreversible.[28] Therefore, antiviral treatment of HCV-infected transplant candidates while on dialysis remains the best option. It may be beneficial not only to prevent post-transplant liver disease, but also to possibly prevent post-transplant HCV-related glomerular disease and new onset diabetes. Currently, judicious use of combination therapy with pegylated IFN-α and low-dose ribavirin (adjusted according to hemoglobin levels and ribavirin plasma concentrations) is indicated when treating HCV-infected dialysis patients and is more effective than IFN-α monotherapy.[22,29]

Unlike interferon, lamivudine (100 mg/day) is safe and effective treatment for HBV after kidney transplantation.[23] However, the optimal timing to start or stop treatment remains obscure. Lamivudine use before transplantation has been shown to be associated with lower rates of reactivation than its use post-transplant in response to evidence of hepatitis. Survival post-transplant was also improved in patients who were treated with lamivudine in a pre-emptive strategy based on serial HBV DNA level measurements after transplantation.[30] The exact duration of antiviral therapy is not defined and long-term treatment is required in most of the patients. Unfortunately, the duration of antiviral therapy is related to both the likelihood of response and the development of resistance. Recently, adefovir (10 mg/day), tenofovir (300 mg/day) and entecavir (1 mg/day) have been used successfully for lamivudine-resistant HBV infection.[30,31] Adefovir therapy carries some risk of nephrotoxicity.

The doses of all antiviral agents need to be adjusted according to renal function.[30] Newer antivirals for both HBV and HCV are currently under study. These include antiproteases, immunomodulatory agents such as new interferons or therapeutic vaccines, alternatives to ribavirin for HCV and several new polymerase inhibitors including nucleosidic/nucleotidic inhibitors (e.g. clevudine, telbivudine, emtricitabine and valtorcitabine and their combinations) and peptide nucleic acids for HBV.[31,32]

Vaccination against HBV in nonimmune renal transplant candidates is essential and should be performed in all patients. Efficacious vaccines or specific immunoglobulin preparations are not yet available for HCV. However, hepatitis A and B vaccination should be recommended in HCV-infected patients before transplantation, since co-infection of HCV with other hepatotropic viruses results in worse clinical outcomes.[23]

OTHER INFECTIONS

The rate of tuberculosis in solid-organ transplant recipients has been estimated to be 50-fold higher than in the general population.[33] Management of tuberculosis is challenging in kidney transplant recipients. First, clinical manifestations can be atypical in immunocompromised patients and, therefore, delays in diagnosis are common. Second, therapy against *Mycobacterium tuberculosis* infection may be associated with significant toxicity and potential drug interactions with immunosuppressive agents. Thus, the diagnosis and treatment of latent tuberculosis infection in transplant candidates is of major importance.

In contrast with other organ transplants, invasive fungal infections are less common after kidney transplantation. The frequency of invasive aspergillosis has been estimated to be 0.7–4%, with the majority of cases occurring in patients with known risk factors, such as high-dose corticosteroids and graft failure requiring hemodialysis.[34] On the other hand, candidiasis is relatively more common, especially during the first month after transplant, in patients with surgical complications and long intensive care unit stay. Recommendations regarding antifungal prophylaxis are shown in Table 80.2. Arterial infection of the allograft by *Candida* spp. has rarely been reported and is associated with high morbidity and mortality due to hemorrhagic complications.[35] Asymptomatic candiduria is a common problem in kidney transplant recipients. A thorough search for invasive candidiasis and pre-emptive antifungal therapy is warranted in this setting. *Pneumocystis jirovecii* pneumonia has been practically eradicated since the introduction of universal prophylaxis with co-trimoxazole during the first months after transplantation. However, outbreaks of late-onset *Pneumocystis jirovecii* pneumonia have recently been described in patients without any new identifiable risk factor.[36]

Table 80.3 Vaccines in kidney transplantation

Timing of vaccination	Vaccine	Comments
Exclusively before transplant	Mumps, rubella, measles Varicella (chickenpox) Varicella-zoster (shingles)*	Live attenuated vaccines are contraindicated after transplant
Can be administered after transplant	Seasonal influenza vaccine, yearly Pneumococcal polysaccharide vaccine, every 3–5 years Hepatitis B Hepatitis A Polio (inactivated), tetanus, diphtheria, pertussis Human papillomavirus (HPV) vaccine*	Administer vaccines before transplant whenever possible to assure immunogenicity

*No data are currently available for this vaccine on immunogenicity and safety in transplant candidates.

PREVENTIVE STRATEGIES AND VACCINATION IN TRANSPLANTATION

Along with an integrated prescription of an immunosuppressive regimen to avoid rejection, prevention of infection is a cornerstone of the management of organ transplant recipients (see Tables 80.2 and 80.3). Vaccination in kidney transplant recipients should take into consideration two main aspects – namely safety and immunogenicity.[37] Live attenuated vaccines, like inhaled influenza vaccine or varicella vaccine, are generally contraindicated after organ transplantation. Inactivated vaccines can be safely administered after transplantation and studies have failed to show any possible relationship between vaccination and allograft rejection.

However, as immunogenicity may be reduced after organ transplant, a major effort should be undertaken in order to administer vaccines in transplant candidates before kidney transplantation, during the early course of their underlying renal disease, whenever possible. Household members should also be offered vaccination if there is no contraindication. The human papillomavirus virus vaccine deserves further evaluation in transplant candidates.[38]

Acknowledgments

The authors wish to thank Professor Atul Humar (Transplant Infectious Diseases, University of Alberta, Edmonton, Canada) and Professor Thierry Calandra (Infectious Diseases Service, Department of Medicine, University Hospital of Lausanne, Lausanne, Switzerland) for their critical review of the manuscript and helpful discussions, and Dr Samuel Rotman (Department of Pathology, University Hospital of Lausanne, Lausanne, Switzerland) for providing the BK nephropathy illustrations.

The Transplantation Center in Lausanne is supported by the 2004–2007 Strategic Plan of the Hospices-CHUV, Lausanne, Switzerland.

REFERENCES

References for this chapter can be found online at http://www.expertconsult.com

Vasculitis and other immunologically mediated diseases

INTRODUCTION

This chapter is concerned with a diverse group of conditions that have in common the fact that their cause is thought to be related to disordered immune processes, and that their treatment involves immunosuppressive therapy. In the past these diseases have been called 'autoimmune', 'collagen-vascular' or more frequently 'vasculitis', although as a group I think they are better referred to simply as immunologically mediated diseases (IMDs; Table 81.1). In addition, there is a large group of common disorders (e.g. asthma, eczema or inflammatory bowel disease) in which immunosuppressive therapy may be used, sometimes at high dose. Although not discussed in detail here, they are at risk from the same type of opportunistic infections as other immunosuppressed patients.

EPIDEMIOLOGY

The importance of IMDs to the infectious diseases practitioner lies in the fact that these patients frequently have severe multisystem disease and require high-dose immunosuppressive therapy, so the risk of opportunistic infection is high. Furthermore, they differ from other types of immunosuppressed patients in that they often receive several different modalities of immunosuppression (Table 81.2), and the duration of their treatment is much longer than that for a patient who has leukemia or cancer, in whom the neutropenic period is currently often not much more than 4 weeks (and sometimes much less). Infection is a major cause of morbidity and mortality in patients who have IMD but the incidence of infection in these patients varies considerably depending on the stage of the disease and the intensity of the immunosuppression.

In a study of 75 heavily immunosuppressed patients who had a variety of IMDs, we found a rate of 0.74 infections/patient/week,[1] and in the so-called catastrophic antiphospholipid syndrome, intercurrent infection is one of the major causes of death.[2] In contrast, a study of 200 outpatients with systemic lupus erythematosus (SLE) followed for 2 years found that infections only occurred in a third of cases. Most were single, minor and associated with disease activity.[3] In rheumatoid arthritis, the increased risk of infection is directly associated with the type of anti-inflammatory therapy that is used. Not surprisingly, the greatest risk is associated with glucocorticoids and cyclophosphamide.[4] The recent introduction of infliximab and adalimumab (monoclonal anti-tumor necrosis factor antibodies) into clinical practice for the management of moderate-to-severe

---

Table 81.1 Immunologically mediated diseases (IMDs)

Systemic lupus erythematosus	Mixed connective tissue disease
Polyarteritis nodosa	Progressive systemic sclerosis/scleroderma

Wegener's granulomatosis
  Lymphomatoid granulomatosis
  Bronchocentric granulomatosis
	Polymyositis/dermatomyositis

	Relapsing polychondritis
Antiglomerular basement membrane disease (Goodpasture's syndrome)	Behçet's syndrome
	Sjögren's syndrome
Mixed essential cryoglobulinemia	Inflammatory bowel disease

Rheumatoid arthritis
  Still's disease
  Felty's syndrome
	Churg–Strauss syndrome

	Henoch–Schönlein purpura
	Hemolytic–uremic syndrome/thrombotic thrombocytopenic purpura

High-dose immunosuppression is often used in the above IMDs and major opportunistic infection is a common problem. The list excludes generally less severe diseases such as asthma; although such patients may occasionally need high-dose immunosuppression, it is much less common.

Table 81.2 Immunosuppressive agents and procedures

Corticosteroids	Ciclosporin and related drugs
	  FK506 (tacrolimus)
	  Sirolimus

Thiopurines
  6-Mercaptopurine
  Azathioprine
	Total lymphoid irradiation

Alkylating agents	Antilymphocyte globulin
Mycophenolate mofetil	Intravenous immunoglobulin
Cyclophosphamide	Plasma exchange

Monoclonal antibodies
  Basiliximab
  Daclizumab
  Rituximab
  Infliximab
  Etanercept
  Adalimumab
  Natalizumab	

This list comprises types of immunosuppression typically used in patients who have IMD. It is common for several of these agents to be used in combination.

rheumatoid arthritis has led to the recognition that this confers an increased risk of infection, in particular due to tuberculosis.[5] Extensions of this approach, either by using different therapeutic targets (e.g. anti-interleukin-6 receptor) or different clinical applications (e.g. Crohn's disease) are in early phase development and will need to be monitored closely for other potential infective complications.

A wide range of opportunistic infections may occur in patients with IMD; indeed, one of the characteristics of this group is that there is a much wider differential diagnosis than typically occurs in bone marrow transplant recipients or other types of immunocompromised host. There are some associations of note: for instance, salmonellosis is a recognized complication of SLE and some other immunocompromised patients, although the mechanism is not at all clear.[6]

PATHOGENESIS AND PATHOLOGY

It is difficult to be certain whether the increased incidence of infection in patients with IMD is attributable to the abnormal immune function of the underlying disease or simply a consequence of the immunosuppressive therapy. Probably both are implicated.[7,8] Interestingly, there is a suggestion that part of the susceptibility to infection seen in patients with SLE is attributable to polymorphisms in the gene for mannose-binding lectin.[7]

In some cases, there may be an etiologic association between an infection and the disease itself. A good example of this is the role of the hepatitis viruses in the pathogenesis of cryoglobulinemia, polyarteritis nodosa and other types of systemic vasculitis,[9] and both Epstein–Barr virus and parvovirus B19 have been associated with various vasculitic illnesses.[10] There have also been intriguing reports suggesting that Wegener's granulomatosis may be caused by an abnormal response to an unknown infection, and that relapses of Wegener's granulomatosis can be prevented by chronic administration of trimethoprim–sulfamethoxazole (TMP–SMX).[11]

Although certain types of treatment are associated with particular defects in immune function, patients who have IMD commonly receive combinations of drugs, and this makes predictions very difficult. Certainly, high-dose corticosteroid therapy is complicated by infections such as *Listeria*, herpesviruses and fungi, whereas patients who develop neutropenia as a consequence of cyclophosphamide, for instance, are susceptible to the same kinds of infection as neutropenic patients. Plasma exchange (plasmapheresis) is a form of immunosuppression used particularly in these patients, and this has its own complications, in particular Gram-positive infections associated with intravenous access.[12,13]

It is not just the longer list of possible infections that makes assessment more difficult in these patients. It is frequently very hard to be sure whether the patient has infection or simply a relapse of the underlying disease. An acute flare-up of SLE involving the central nervous system can be indistinguishable from infective meningitis or encephalitis as a consequence of the immunosuppressive therapy. This leaves the clinician on the horns of an unpleasant dilemma; should the immunosuppression be reduced in order to allow antimicrobial therapy to be more effective, or should it be increased to bring the underlying disease back under control? It is helpful to ask whether the clinical features at this presentation are the same as on previous occasions when it was known to be disease activity. Individual patients tend to be consistent in the form of disease they get when it is active. No single investigation can be relied upon to distinguish infection from relapse. In SLE it is often said that an elevated C-reactive protein (CRP) is only seen in patients with intercurrent infection, but this is not an absolute distinction.[8]

A further complication is the phenomenon of 'infection provoked relapse' whereby in patients who have IMD an intercurrent infection can precipitate a relapse of the underlying disease;[14] conversely, flare-ups of SLE can be associated with dysregulated immune defenses,

thereby increasing the risk of infection. The infection and the vasculitis need to be treated simultaneously.

PREVENTION

Patients who have IMD, as with all immunosuppressed patients, are constantly at risk of a very wide range of infections but it is neither practicable nor desirable to try to prevent all of them. Tuberculosis is a particular problem because its presentation may be atypical and extrapulmonary disease is common. Patients who are receiving more than 15 mg/day of prednisolone for prolonged periods and who have a clinical history or radiologic evidence of past tuberculosis should be given prophylaxis with isoniazid 300 mg/day plus pyridoxine 10 mg/day.[15] If the risk is less clear, the complications of isoniazid need to be considered, although my practice is to err on the side of advising prophylaxis.[16] In the case of anti-tumor necrosis factor (TNF) therapy for rheumatoid arthritis, guidelines have been published that identify high-risk groups.[17]

In my opinion, the routine use of TMP–SMX as primary prophylaxis to prevent *Pneumocystis* pneumonia is not warranted in this population, even if they are receiving corticosteroids, because of the low incidence of the infection. Furthermore, in contrast to patients who have AIDS, relapse of *Pneumocystis* pneumonia is most uncommon in this population and secondary prophylaxis is not indicated.

CLINICAL FEATURES AND MANAGEMENT

Immunologically mediated diseases can represent a very complex challenge to the infectious diseases physician. Factors that need to be taken into account in assessing the patient include the nature of the underlying disease and the particular type of immunosuppression used, its duration and its dose (see Practice Point 40). Certain clinical syndromes merit particular attention.

Fever and pulmonary infiltrates

The development of fever and new pulmonary infiltrates is one of the most common and most difficult clinical syndromes that occur in patients who have IMD. The differential diagnosis is extraordinarily wide (Table 81.3), and includes infective and noninfective conditions. Details of specific infections may be found elsewhere in this book; here I consider some general principles that apply to the initial assessment and management of patients who have IMD who develop fever and pneumonia.

- There may be very rapid deterioration, from low-grade fever and cough to severe hypoxia needing mechanical ventilation within 12 hours, particularly if the patient is liable to develop pulmonary hemorrhage.
- Radiologic appearances are very nonspecific. It is rare to be able to 'guess' the diagnosis just on the basis of the chest radiograph, with the possible exception of *Pneumocystis* pneumonia.
- Multiple infections are common. Even if the physician correctly recognizes the clinical and radiologic features of *Pneumocystis* pneumonia, the patient may be co-infected with an additional, equally treatable pathogen such as cytomegalovirus (CMV).
- Sputum microbiology can be confusing. The presence of *Candida* spp., for instance, may indicate nothing more than colonization of the nasopharynx, whereas important pathogens such as *Aspergillus* or *Pneumocystis* often do not appear in the sputum.

Consideration of the nature of the underlying disease, the type of immunosuppression and epidemiologic features in the history are

Table 81.3 Causes of fever and pulmonary infiltrates in patients who have immunologically mediated disease*

Infective	Bacteria	Conventional respiratory pathogens[†] Mycobacteria *Nocardia*[18] 'Atypical' bacteria (*Mycoplasma* spp., *Coxiella* spp.) *Legionella* spp.
	Fungi	*Aspergillus* spp.[19†] *Candida* spp. *Cryptococcus neoformans* Zygomycetes Primary systemic fungi (*Histoplasma* spp., *Blastomyces* spp., etc.) Other systemic fungi (rarely; e.g. *Sporothrix schenckii*) *Pneumocystis*[†]
	Parasites	*Strongyloides stercoralis* *Toxoplasma*
	Viruses	Cytomegalovirus* Herpes simplex virus Varicella-zoster virus Respiratory syncytial virus Adenovirus Influenza and parainfluenza virus
Noninfective		Edema[†] Hemorrhage[20†] Infarction Emboli Tumor Radiation Chemotherapy Vasculitis Leukoagglutinin reaction

*The list is long but incomplete and, in practice, any organism isolated in pure or predominant culture from a bronchoalveolar lavage or open lung biopsy should be regarded as a pathogen until proved otherwise. Further details about some of the conditions are provided in the references, where indicated.
[†]Most common causes.

all helpful in guiding therapy. The single most important factor is gauging the speed of progression of the condition. It cannot be over-emphasized that in IMD patients a seemingly trivial community-acquired chest infection can proceed to life-threatening pneumonia and/or pulmonary hemorrhage within a frighteningly short period. Urgent evaluation and investigation is essential. All patients should have simple, basic laboratory investigations performed, including a full blood count, sputum and blood cultures, measurement of arterial oxygen saturation or formal blood gas concentrations and a chest radiograph.

Much has been written about the radiologic features of certain infections. It is perfectly true, for instance, that *Pneumocystis* pneumonia classically produces a bilateral 'ground glass' appearance, but so too does CMV infection and acute pulmonary hemorrhage in a patient who has pulmonary vasculitis. Combining the clinical and radiologic data results in a 'short list' of likely diagnoses, but too great a reliance on this is very hazardous. The main value of the chest radiograph is in indicating the extent and rate of progression of the process, not in guessing the pathogen.

Empiric antibacterial therapy is usually indicated if the clinical and epidemiologic evidence point to a simple community-acquired

pneumonia, and when the risk of a major opportunistic pathogen (e.g. invasive fungal infection or *Pneumocystis*) is judged to be low. *Pneumocystis* pneumonia is said to often have a very characteristic presentation, and some advocate empiric therapy. However, this strategy may be unwise in patients who have IMD because of the wide differential diagnosis and the possibility of co-infection with other pathogens.

In the majority of patients further specific investigations should be performed. Bronchoscopy with a bronchoalveolar lavage is valuable; close liaison with the laboratory is essential to ensure a rapid response and the maximum diagnostic yield.[21] High-resolution CT scans will undoubtedly give additional and sometimes useful information but in my experience are rarely diagnostic.[22] Pulmonary function tests can be very valuable in this group of patients, in particular measurement of carbon monoxide uptake (the KCO) to detect intrapulmonary hemorrhage.[23]

When a specific organism is identified the treatment follows conventional guidelines. 'Blind' empiric therapy is rarely advisable because of the wide differential diagnosis.

Acute neurologic problems

A wide differential diagnosis also exists for neurologic problems, and prompt evaluation, investigation and treatment are essential.[24] Knowledge of the nature of the immune deficit can narrow down the list of possibilities. This information can be linked to the clinical presentation to provide useful clues; thus, a patient who has a defect in cellular immunity as a result of high-dose steroid therapy who develops a subacute meningitis is likely to have *Listeria*, cryptococcal or tuberculous meningitis, whereas in a neutropenic patient *Aspergillus* or a pyogenic bacterial infection are more common.[25] These mental exercises are intellectually challenging, but in reality the clinician is faced with a patient in whom even the 'short list' of likely causes all demand quite different treatment. Clearly, it is most important to make the diagnosis as quickly as possible.

The initial assessment should include a detailed clinical and epidemiologic history and a careful neurologic examination. Key areas are:

- exposure to family members or others as a potential source;
- relevant foreign travel (not forgetting malaria);
- previous episodes of neurologic manifestations associated with relapse of underlying disease; and
- speed of progression of the disease.

Immediate investigations include a blood film and full blood count, blood and urine cultures and a chest radiograph. If there are new skin lesions they should be biopsied for immediate smear and culture. If a CT scan is available it is invaluable, and a lumbar puncture should be performed provided there are no contraindications.

Meningitis

Meningitis can be caused by common bacteria (*Streptococcus pneumoniae*, *Neisseria meningitidis*), but in immunosuppressed patients *Listeria monocytogenes* is particularly important. Despite the name, the cerebrospinal fluid (CSF) usually contains neutrophils, not mononuclear cells.

Polymicrobial meningitis (particularly with enteric Gram-negative bacteria) can be a clue to the presence of hyperinfection with strongyloidiasis, a complication of both corticosteroid therapy and also of infection with human T-cell leukemia/lymphoma virus. Enteroviruses are common causes of meningitis in normal hosts; rather curiously, they also occur in patients who have hypogammaglobulinemia.[26] Tuberculosis, cryptococcosis (and much more rarely, *Nocardia*) all manifest with a subacute picture and are recognized causes of meningitis in patients who have IMD.

Meningitis is rarely caused by relapse of the underlying disease, but it can occasionally be caused by drugs used in its treatment, notably nonsteroidal anti-inflammatory drugs (NSAIDs).[27]

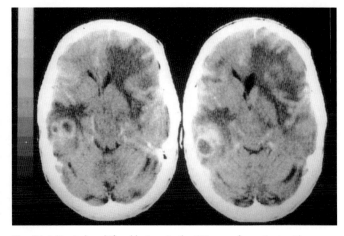

Fig. 81.1 Typical multifocal lesions in the CT scan of a patient with toxoplasmosis.

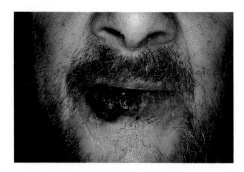

Fig. 81.2 A large necrotizing lesion caused by herpes simplex type 1 in a patient who has a teratoma. Herpetic stomatitis is common in immunosuppressed patients and is often atypical; any ulcerating lesion in the perioral region should be considered to be herpetic until proved otherwise.

Abscesses

In IMD patients, abscesses are usually nonbacterial. The commonest causes of focal neurologic lesions are fungi (especially *Aspergillus* spp.) and *Toxoplasma* (Fig. 81.1). *Nocardia* infections classically cause multiple focal abnormalities but occur less often. Tuberculoma and cryptococcoma are more common in textbooks than in patients. The diagnosis of single or multiple space-occupying lesions in IMD patients is particularly difficult. Neither the radiologic features nor the CSF findings are pathognomonic; it is rare for the causative organism to be identified from the CSF and, with the exception of the cryptococcal latex agglutination test, serologic tests are unhelpful. Particular care is needed in making a presumptive diagnosis of toxoplasmosis. Whereas in other groups of immunosuppressed patients the appearance of multiple enhancing lesions on the CT scan will often be sufficient grounds to commence empiric therapy, in patients who have IMD the differential diagnosis is much wider and if at all possible a tissue diagnosis should be obtained. Furthermore, *Toxoplasma* infection in SLE can mimic lupus cerebritis.[28]

Encephalitis

Encephalitis can be caused by infective and noninfective processes. Listeriosis and toxoplasmosis can manifest with an encephalitic picture, as can measles. Cerebral vasculitis (typically in SLE) is a particularly important consideration. It can cause a florid and life-threatening illness that can be extremely difficult to distinguish from an opportunist infection. Evaluation is complicated by the fact that high-dose corticosteroid therapy can itself cause neuropsychiatric manifestations. It is helpful if the patient is known to have a past history of cerebral vasculitis, but sometimes the only course of action is to treat with immunosuppression and antimicrobial agents until the picture becomes clearer. The use of monoclonal antibodies (particularly natalizumab to treat multiple sclerosis) has been associated with cases of progressive multifocal leukoencephalopathy (PML) due to JC virus[29] (see Chapter 157).

Two infections merit comment because of their rarity: herpes simplex encephalitis seems to be uncommon, despite the fact that local cutaneous reactivation often occurs, and likewise CMV encephalitis is very unusual in this population.

Gastrointestinal problems

Although immunosuppressed patients are susceptible to a wide range of bacterial, fungal, viral and protozoal infections of the gut,[30] it is largely those that are a feature of high-dose corticosteroid therapy that occur in patients who have IMD. The clinical features of common infections are often modified: herpetic stomatitis can be very severe, for instance (Fig. 81.2).

Extrapulmonary tuberculosis is more common in immunosuppressed patients and even if suspected (e.g. because a patient comes from the Indian subcontinent) can sometimes be hard to prove. The use of polymerase chain reaction to detect mycobacterial DNA in ascitic fluid is invaluable where it is available; meanwhile peritoneal biopsy is often the only diagnostic procedure of use. Not infrequently the only option is empiric therapy. Cytomegalovirus enteritis is perhaps underdiagnosed. It can affect any part of the gut, but particularly the colon.[31] Ganciclovir has been very effective.[32]

Strongyloides stercoralis can be present for many years without causing symptoms, but after corticosteroid therapy can cause subacute obstruction, pulmonary infiltrates and polymicrobial bacteremia or meningitis[33] (Fig. 81.3). Ivermectin is the drug of choice. Vasculitis (especially in SLE) can cause symptoms and signs indistinguishable from acute infection, including diarrhea, obstruction and perforation. Again, there are no diagnostic tests and management must depend on clinical evaluation and, if necessary, a therapeutic trial.

Skin, soft tissue and joints

Many organisms cause skin disease in immunosuppressed patients and the clinical manifestations are protean (Figs 81.4 and 81.5).[34] Many noninfective causes of skin rash need to be remembered, including cutaneous vasculitis and drug eruptions. Soft tissue infections are unusual except that patients who have hypogammaglobulinemia are susceptible to enterovirus polymyositis, although myositis is much more likely to be caused by the underlying disease (dermatomyositis, polymyositis or polyarteritis nodosa).

Acute arthritis is always an indication for aspiration to exclude infection: *Staphylococcus aureus* is the most common isolate. Once again, relapse of the underlying disease is an important part of the differential diagnosis.

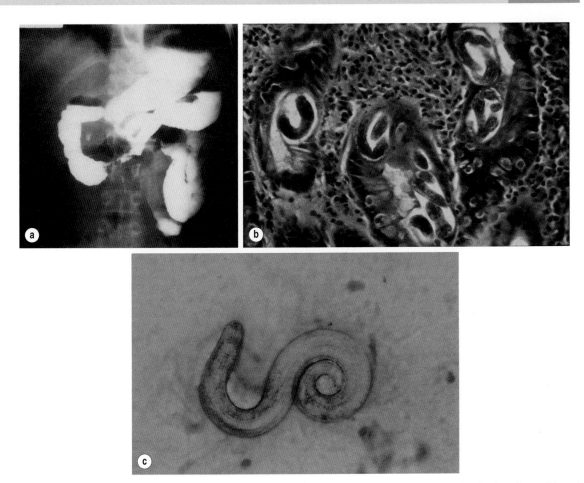

Fig. 81.3 *Strongyloides stercoralis.* (a) Barium meal examination of a patient with impaired cell-mediated immunity who developed a small bowel obstruction due to locally invasive *Strongyloides* infection. (b) Small bowel biopsy showing invasion by *Strongyloides.* (c) In some patients, the worms disseminate widely, leading to so-called hyperinfection syndrome. In this patient, who had an HTLV-1 lymphoma, worms were seen in sputum preparations.

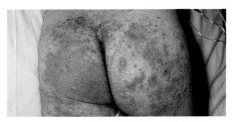

Fig. 81.4 Extensive dermatophyte infection in a bone marrow transplant recipient. Many other infections (and graft-versus-host disease) can give a similar appearance but the diagnosis is quickly established by biopsy and microscopy. This condition is limited to the skin but nevertheless requires systemic antifungal therapy.

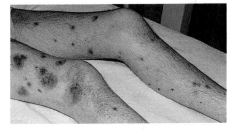

Fig. 81.5 Extensive skin lesions caused by *Mycobacterium chelonae* in a patient who had polyarteritis nodosa. The lesions were palpable but not especially painful.

REFERENCES

🖱 References for this chapter can be found online at http://www.expertconsult.com

Splenectomy and splenic dysfunction

INTRODUCTION

The spleen in postnatal life functions primarily as a specialized lymphatic organ. It clears particulate elements from the circulation and promotes a coordinated immune response to systemic antigens. The rapidly progressive and highly lethal syndrome of overwhelming postsplenectomy infection (OPSI) attests the critical importance of the spleen to host defense against disseminated infections in the systemic circulation.

EPIDEMIOLOGY

The incidence of fatal postsplenectomy sepsis has been estimated at approximately 1 per 300 patient-years in children and 1 per 800 patient-years in adults.[1] Serious infectious complications may also occur in patients who have splenic hypofunction found in a broad array of systemic disorders (Table 82.1).[2–7]

Functional asplenia is suggested by the presence of Howell–Jolly bodies (nuclear remnants within red blood cells) and target cells in the peripheral blood smear, and decreased uptake of radioactivity by spleen scan. Splenic hypofunction is more frequent than is commonly appreciated. A recent laboratory-based survey[8] analyzed over 100 000 blood smears per year and revealed that 0.5% of patient samples had Howell–Jolly bodies indicative of hyposplenism. This information was unknown to the majority of these patients and their physicians. The most common cause of functional asplenia is sickle-cell disease which leads to repeated infarction of splenic tissue over the first few years of life. Infants born with congenital asplenia are at particularly high risk of death from systemic infection within the first year of life.[7,9]

PATHOGENESIS AND PATHOLOGY

Structure–function relationships in the spleen

The spleen is organized to provide an optimal environment for particulate antigen clearance and immunologic surveillance within the systemic circulation. Although the spleen is a small structure that accounts for only 0.25% of body weight, it receives 5% of cardiac output and contains up to 25% of the total lymphocyte population within the body.[10] Blood enters the spleen through central arteries, which branch into penicillary arterioles (Fig. 82.1). These vessels are cuffed with T lymphocytes, forming a periarterial lymphocytic sheath. The white pulp of the spleen surrounds arterioles and consists of large populations of T cells with lesser numbers of B cells and natural killer (NK) cells. The marginal zone surrounds the white pulp and principally

Table 82.1 Conditions associated with functional asplenia

Atrophic spleen	Normal-sized or enlarged spleen
Ulcerative colitis	Hemoglobinopathies*
Celiac disease	Sarcoidosis
Graft-versus-host disease following bone marrow transplantation	Amyloidosis
Splenic irradiation	Systemic lupus erythematosus, rheumatoid arthritis
Thyrotoxicosis	Epstein–Barr virus infection
Dermatitis herpetiformis	Vasculitis with antineutrophil cytoplasmic antibodies
Idiopathic thrombocythemia	Liver disease – portal hypertension
Sickle-cell disease	AIDS, immunosuppressive agents

*Other than sickle-cell disease.

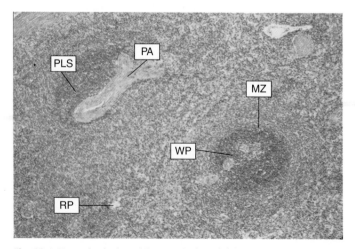

Fig. 82.1 Normal splenic architecture in the adult human. PLS, periarterial lymphatic sheath; PA, penicillary arteriole; MZ, marginal zone (B lymphocytes predominate); WP, white pulp (T cells predominate); RP, red pulp (vascular cords and venous sinuses). Hematoxylin and eosin stain.

consists of large concentrations of B cells with lesser numbers of T cells and antigen-presenting cells. Memory cells of the B-cell lineage are found primarily within the marginal zones of the spleen. The white pulp and marginal zone bring antigen-presenting cells, particulate antigens, T cells and B cells in close proximity. This microenvironment promotes a coordinated immune response to systemic antigens.[1,2,9]

The majority of the spleen consists of red pulp and venous sinuses. Before formed elements within the blood can reach the venous sinuses of the spleen, they must negotiate the red pulp with its tightly compact network of endothelial cells and macrophages (the cords of Billroth). This slow filtration process allows for careful immunologic surveillance and removal of damaged cellular elements and foreign particulate matter. The normal architecture of the spleen is depicted in Figure 82.1.

Immunologic defects and factors predisposing for postsplenectomy sepsis

A number of immunologic defects have been described in the postsplenectomy state (Table 82.2).[1-14] Hosea *et al.*[15] have demonstrated that the principal immunologic defect associated with the postsplenectomy state is an impairment in clearance of poorly opsonized particulate antigens. Invasive, encapsulated, bacterial pathogens possess an outer surface, polysaccharide capsule that impedes opsonization by immunoglobulin or complement upon entry to the systemic circulation. The spleen is much more efficient than the liver in removing poorly opsonized bacterial pathogens. Following splenectomy, decreased clearance of these encapsulated organisms results in disseminated intravascular infection and the OPSI syndrome.

Predisposing factors to postsplenectomy infection

Multiple host factors determine the cumulative risk of OPSI. A number of the most important host determinants of infection following surgical or functional asplenia are listed in Table 82.3. The principal determinant of risk of postsplenectomy sepsis is the age and immunologic experience of the patient before splenectomy.[7,15,16] In a recent review[17] of 19 680 patients followed for an average of 6.9 years after splenectomy, the overall risk of serious infections was found to be

Table 82.3 Risk factors for postsplenectomy sepsis

Risk factors	Comment
Patient age: the very young	Lack of immunologic experience (vaccines and naturally acquired infections) prior to splenectomy increases the risk
Patient age: the very old	Poor response to vaccines, immunosenescence, underlying diseases increase the risk in elderly
Absence of spleen at birth	Congenital asplenia results in serious bacterial infections in over 50% of patients in the first year of life if not managed with penicillin prophylaxis
Time interval following splenectomy	Greatest risk of infection is within the first 2–3 years following splenectomy
Traumatic versus other indications for splenectomy	Splenosis (splenic implants within the peritoneum) following trauma offers some protection against infection
Immunocompromised states	Patients with hematologic malignancies and continuing need for immunosuppressive medications increase the risk of postsplenectomy sepsis
Lack of presplenectomy vaccine	Immune responses to polysaccharide antigens better if administered before splenectomy

3.2% with a mortality risk of 1.4%. The highest fatality risk was in children with thalassemia major (5.1%) and sickle-cell disease (4.8%). A similar 12-year survey in Scotland calculated the overall incidence of severe postsplenectomy infection to be 7.0 per 100 person-years with an incidence of OPSI at 0.89 per 100 person-years.[18] The report emphasized a previously underappreciated observation that elderly patients are at significantly increased risk of severe infection when compared to young adults following splenectomy.

The spleen is particularly important in the primary immunologic response to polysaccharide antigens. These IgM and IgG$_2$ antibody responses are largely T-cell-independent B-cell responses that require the spleen for an optimal immune response.[19] This occurs in the marginal zone of the spleen where B cells are abundant for immunologic surveillance in the systemic circulation. This immune response is attenuated after splenectomy. T-cell-dependent B-cell responses to protein antigens and cellular immune responses are reasonably well preserved after splenectomy.[19,20] The end result is that carbohydrate neoantigens are not recognized and processed efficiently in the postsplenectomy state. This results in delayed clearance of virulent microbial pathogens and their toxins[14,15] as they first enter the systemic circulation.

If the growth rate of the pathogen exceeds the clearance rate of the host, overwhelming intravascular infection occurs with potentially lethal consequences. In experimental studies, macrophage synthesis of tumor necrosis factor (TNF) is upregulated after splenectomy. Enhanced TNF synthesis may increase the risk of systemic activation of the proinflammatory cytokines, and this may contribute to postsplenectomy sepsis.[21] Splenic macrophages are hard-wired via the vagal nerve where alpha-7 nicotinic receptors of the parasympathetic nervous system attenuate TNF and high mobility group box 1 (HMGB-1) synthesis. These early-acting (TNF) and late-acting (HMGB-1) cytokines are implicated in the pathogenesis of septic shock.[22,23] Splenectomy removes this cholinergic anti-inflammatory pathway and it is tempting to speculate that the loss of this inhibitory pathway could contribute to the exaggerated inflammatory response seen in OPSI.

Table 82.2 Immunologic defects found after splenectomy

Defect	Comment
Decreased clearance of particulate antigens	Hepatic Kupffer cells will partially correct this defect
Diminished clearance of poorly opsonized bacterial antigens	The spleen is the most efficient organ for this purpose
Diminished primary humoral immune response to neoantigens	IgM levels and T-cell-independent antibody responses decrease
Diminished antibody response to polysaccharide antigens	Increased risk from encapsulated bacterial organisms
Decreased tuftsin levels and fibronectin levels	Diminished levels of this tetrapeptide and serum protein reduces nonspecific attachment and phagocytosis
Quantitative and qualitative defects in the alternative complement pathway	Functional defects in the alternative complement pathway interferes with opsonization
Loss of vagally mediated cholinergic anti-inflammatory reflex	Neural control of inflammatory cytokine synthesis in the viscera is primarily mediated by the spleen

PREVENTION OF BABESIOSIS AND MALARIA

Individuals living in areas where *Babesia* spp. is endemic should be advised to avoid areas where ticks are common or, if unavoidable, to check daily for the presence of attached ticks. If the tick is removed within 24–48 hours it appears to protect against transmission of *Babesia* spp. Babesiosis can cause recalcitrant infections in splenectomized adults as well as children and in some cases has required exchange transfusion and prolonged treatment with antiprotozoan therapy (azithromycin–atovaquone or clindamycin and quinine). This infection needs to be prevented in splenectomized people. Chills, fever, anemia, leukopenia and thrombocytopenia can all accompany babesiosis. The diagnosis is usually evident if suspected and sought for on the blood smear. Babesiosis can be confused with *Plasmodium falciparum* malaria. Splenic function is important in clearing malaria parasites. Asplenic patients living or traveling to malaria-endemic areas should be meticulous in following malaria avoidance efforts (mosquito repellent, bed nets, screened windows, antimalarial chemoprophylaxis, etc.).

PREVENTION OF POSTSPLENECTOMY INFECTIONS

Splenic salvage method

The well-recognized risk of OPSI indicates a need to prevent these infections if at all possible. The most direct approach is to minimize the frequency with which splenectomy is performed.[24,25] Recent evidence suggests that the frequency with which splenectomy is undertaken has leveled off or decreased in North America,[8] perhaps with the recognition of the infectious risks associated with splenectomy. Elective splenectomy for congenital hemolytic disorders should be delayed until after the first 5 years of life if possible (Table 82.4). Surgical repair of splenic hematomas, conservative management of splenic trauma without splenectomy, percutaneous drainage of splenic abscesses and a decreased use of splenic irradiation have led to fewer patients at risk for postsplenectomy infectious syndromes.[26,27]

Partial splenectomy and surgical repair of splenic injury have been utilized along with autotransplantation of splenic tissue in an attempt to limit the risk of OPSI.[28,29] Enthusiasm for these splenic salvage maneuvers is tempered by the finding that these methods do not uniformly protect against sepsis in animal models[30] of splenectomy and case reports exist of overwhelming infections despite these maneuvers.[28–30] Preservation of residual splenic tissue, if possible, may still be preferable to total splenectomy in selected patients at high risk for infection.[31] The overall clinical applicability and practical value of splenic salvage techniques remain to be demonstrated in a large patient series.

Immunizations to prevent postsplenectomy sepsis

Immunization with the 23-valent pneumococcal polysaccharide (PPS) vaccine is safe and offers significant protection in children with sickle-cell disease.[32] The efficacy of the pneumococcal vaccine is reduced following splenectomy, yet protective antibody levels are achievable in the majority of patients following splenectomy for a variety of indications.[33–35] To optimize antibody response against T-cell-independent immunogens, it is recommended that the pneumococcal vaccine be administered at least 2 weeks before an elective splenectomy.[33] Postimmunization antibody levels should be measured to assess vaccine response. Nonresponders who do not develop antipneumococcal antibodies with repeated immunizations with PPS should consider other preventive measures against pneumococci (e.g. wear a medical alert bracelet, trial of the pneumococcal conjugate vaccine, carry a preemptive dose of a β-lactam antibiotic to presumptively treat if symptoms develop, seek early medical care for symptoms, etc.).[33,34] Current recommendations of the Task Force on Adult Immunization include repeat pneumococcal immunization every 5–6 years from the initial immunization.[35]

The role of polysaccharide–protein conjugate pneumococcal vaccine (PCV) in asplenic patients has yet to be fully evaluated in large clinical trials but preliminary results appear promising.[19,36] The conjugate protein linker allows for the development of T-cell-dependent B cell responses, with T-helper function amplifying the antibody response. Recent experimental studies[19] have verified that the conjugate vaccine produces peak antibody titers comparable to nonsplenectomized animals, albeit at a slower rate of increase. The secondary antibody response to subsequent doses of the vaccine is well preserved with the PCV formulation. Attempts to mix unconjugated pneumococcal antigens with the protein conjugated antigens were unsuccessful in boosting antibody titers to nonconjugated pneumococcal antigens. The current PCV has only seven serotypes while the standard PPS vaccine contains 23 serotypes. Further studies are warranted to determine if pneumococcal conjugate vaccines will be more efficacious than PPS vaccine in asplenic patients.[36] Current recommendations include the use of both PCV and PPS immunizations (separated by 2–3 months) in children and unimmunized adults with splenic hypofunction.[34]

Haemophilus influenzae type b conjugate vaccine is indicated in all children, including those who have functional or surgical asplenia. Immune responses to the conjugate vaccine are well preserved in the absence of splenic tissue or function.[37] It is unclear whether the *H. influenzae* type b vaccine is useful in adults who have not been vaccinated before splenectomy. The risk–benefit ratio would argue that it is reasonable to immunize children and adults who undergo splenectomy if they have not been previously immunized.[34,37] The same rationale is used to recommend meningococcal vaccine in children and young adults who undergo splenectomy,[38,39] particularly in those patients living or traveling in regions where meningococcal disease is prevalent.[40] The protein conjugate polysaccharide meningococcal vaccine may be a better option in high-risk asplenic patients but clinical data are limited at present.[39]

The duration of protection and vaccine efficacy against *Haemophilus*, pneumococci and meningococci in the asplenic patient have not been fully evaluated as yet. Vaccination is limited by variable antibody responses of uncertain duration and incomplete coverage of important serogroups within *Streptococcus pneumoniae* and *Neisseria meningitidis* (i.e. serogroup B). Vaccine failures are well known in

Table 82.4 Preventive measures in postsplenectomy patients	
Method	**Comment**
Salvage splenic tissue (splenorrhaphy, autotransplants)	Reasonable but unproven benefit
Delay elective splenectomy past early childhood	Greatest risk of OPSI is in early childhood; provide immunizations prior to splenectomy
Immunizations	Pneumococcal, meningococcal and *Haemophilus influenzae* vaccines provide partial protection
Antimicrobial prophylaxis	Indicated for asplenic young children (0–5 years); consider in high-risk adults for 1–3 years postsplenectomy
Early empiric therapy	Rational approach to rapidly progressive syndrome
Medical alert bracelet	Reminder for patient and health-care workers

splenectomized patients and therefore these preventive measures should not be entirely relied upon solely to fully protect asplenic patients. Annual influenza vaccines are now recommended for adults and children after splenectomy to avoid postinfluenza bacterial pneumonia.[39]

The efficacy of bacterial vaccines in the prevention of OPSI has not been adequately tested in large scale, randomized, controlled, clinical trials. The recommendations for these immunizations are largely based upon consensus opinion from expert committees and medical societies. Despite these recommendations, it is clear that the provision of adequate vaccine coverage for the asplenic host is less than perfect. A recent survey in the UK found that only 31% of splenectomized patients had received the pneumococcal vaccine.[41] A more concerted effort will be necessary to provide adequate immunizations to these susceptible patients.

Antimicrobial prophylaxis

The efficacy of long-term penicillin prophylaxis to prevent pneumococcal infections has been studied in detail in the pediatric age group. Sufficient clinical evidence now exists to support the recommendation of penicillin prophylaxis in the first 5 years of life in asplenic children.[34,42] Some authors suggest that prophylaxis be continued indefinitely in immunocompromised patients.[3,15,39,41] Amoxicillin may be preferable to penicillin as it is better tolerated and has activity against most strains of H. influenzae.[34] Co-trimoxazole or macrolide antimicrobials are suitable alternatives for patients allergic to β-lactams.

The value of penicillin prophylaxis in adults is more controversial. The uncertain benefits of penicillin prophylaxis in the adult must be weighed against the potential risk of acquisition of penicillin-resistant strains of S. pneumoniae and infections by other organisms not susceptible to penicillin.[1,34,39,41,42] This author recommends penicillin prophylaxis for 2 years following splenectomy in adult patients at high risk for OPSI (e.g. hematologic malignancies, severe liver disease, immunocompromised states). If inadequate antipneumococcal antibodies are found following immunizations, indefinite penicillin prophylaxis should be considered.[33,34]

Expectant management with early empiric therapy for symptoms suggestive of OPSI is a logical alternative for non-immunocompromised, asplenic adults. It is essential to educate and motivate patients and their families to administer an initial dose of oral amoxicillin or amoxicillin–clavulanate at the onset of symptoms compatible with systemic infection. Ideally, patients should have blood cultures taken before empiric antimicrobial therapy; however, this may not be feasible in all patients and treatment should not be delayed if symptoms compatible with OPSI exist.

A medical alert bracelet should be provided to patients following splenectomy. This bracelet serves to remind the patient as well as health-care workers that the patient is at risk for OPSI and that urgent management for this potentially devastating syndrome may be life saving. While most postsplenectomy infections occur 1–2 years after splenic excision, and severe infections related to asplenia are uncommon after 10 years, patients have developed severe infections up to six decades after splenectomy.[42] The alert bracelet should provide continued awareness of the risk of infection long after surgical removal of the spleen. A summary of preventative measures in the patient with functional or surgical asplenia is provided in Table 82.4.

CLINICAL FEATURES OF OVERWHELMING POSTSPLENECTOMY INFECTION

A large variety of bacterial, fungal and parasitic pathogens have been reported to cause serious infection in patients who have splenic hypofunction or asplenia (Table 82.5).[1,3,8,34] Streptococcus pneumoniae continues to account for the majority of bacterial infection associated with OPSI. Haemophilus influenzae and N. meningitidis contribute approximately 25% of bacterial infections in the postsplenectomy

Table 82.5 Microbial pathogens associated with postsplenectomy infections

Micro-organism	Comment
Streptococcus pneumoniae	Most common, highly lethal, characteristic presentation
Haemophilus influenzae	Increased risk – especially in childhood
Neisseria meningitidis	Possible increased risk – typical features of primary meningococcemia
Salmonella spp.	Increased risk – especially sickle cell disease
Other streptococci, enterococci	Possible increased risk of infection
Capnocytophaga canimorsus	Gram-negative rod may cause infection following dog bites
Babesia microti	Tick-associated or blood transfusion-associated protozoan parasite; may cause severe infection in asplenic patients
Plasmodium spp.	Sporadic reports of activation of latent malaria and fulminant course in non-falciparum malaria species
Anaerobes, Gram-negative enteric organisms, Pseudomonas, Burkholderia, Plesiomonas, Campylobacter spp., fungal, parasitic and viral pathogens	Case reports; true association is unclear

state. A large number of pathogens are particularly problematic for asplenic patients including babesiosis, salmonellosis and Capnocytophaga canimorsus infections.

The syndrome of overwhelming pneumococcal sepsis after splenectomy is one of the most dramatic and rapidly fatal infections in clinical medicine. Symptoms often begin with a vague sense of general malaise, sore throat, myalgia and gastrointestinal symptoms. Fever and true shaking chills are often seen during the prodromal phase of OPSI. While some patients note lower respiratory tract symptoms or symptoms of meningitis, the primary source of origin of the bacteremic infection is not localized in the majority of patients with OPSI.

Within 24–48 hours of onset of symptoms patients rapidly deteriorate with progressive hypotension, diffuse intravascular coagulation, purpuric lesions in the extremities, acute respiratory insufficiency, metabolic acidosis and coma. The rapidly progressive nature of the illness is suggestive of primary meningococcemia. The patient may develop refractory hypotension and die within hours of the onset of symptoms.[1,13,15] Long-term sequelae in survivors include gangrene of the extremities, bilateral adrenal hemorrhage, osteomyelitis from vascular insufficiency, endocarditis, meningitis and neurosensory hearing loss. The pneumococcal polysaccharide capsular serotypes 12, 22 and 23 account for the majority of cases of OPSI from S. pneumoniae.[15] All three serotypes are found in the current 23-valent pneumococcal polysaccharide vaccine but not the PCV-7 conjugate vaccine.

DIAGNOSIS OF OVERWHELMING POSTSPLENECTOMY INFECTION

The diagnosis of OPSI is often readily apparent upon clinical examination. Even a remote history of previous splenectomy should raise suspicion of possible OPSI. Supporting laboratory evidence includes consumptive coagulopathy, lactic acidosis, hypoxemia and acute renal

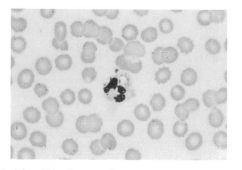

Fig. 82.2 Peripheral blood smear of a patient who has pneumococcal sepsis and meningitis. Note polymorphonuclear leukocyte with several bacterial diplococci in the cytoplasm. Wright stain.

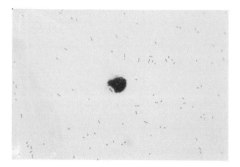

Fig. 82.3 Gram stain of cerebrospinal fluid from a patient who has pneumococcal meningitis. Note the numerous Gram-positive cocci in pairs and a single lymphocyte.

failure. Children are more likely to have concomitant bacterial pneumonia or meningitis than adults.[1,34] As a consequence of high-grade bacteremia, micro-organisms can often be identified in the peripheral blood smear (Fig. 82.2). The blood smear should be reviewed for evidence of parasitemia from *Plasmodium* or *Babesia* spp. A Gram stain of the buffy coat may readily reveal pneumococci as the level of bacteremia may exceed 1 million cfu/ml.

Patients who have concomitant bacterial meningitis may have large numbers of organisms in the cerebrospinal fluid (CSF) with minimal pleocytosis (Fig. 82.3). Blood cultures, bacterial cultures and results of antigen detection measures in the spinal fluid, sputum and urine will confirm the diagnosis.

MANAGEMENT OF OVERWHELMING POSTSPLENECTOMY INFECTION

This syndrome is a true medical emergency requiring immediate therapeutic administration of antimicrobial agents and intensive care support. High-dose intravenous penicillin has been the standard treatment for postsplenectomy pneumococcal sepsis. Vancomycin and ceftriaxone should be used empirically in areas where penicillin-resistant *S. pneumoniae* is prevalent or in patients who have received prolonged penicillin prophylaxis. Moreover, broad-spectrum bactericidal antimicrobial agents such as an extended-spectrum cephalosporin or a carbapenem should be considered in those cases where the suspected micro-organism cannot be identified on Gram strain of the buffy coat or CSF.

Passive immunotherapy with intravenous immunoglobulin has been shown to be of benefit in experimental models of postsplenectomy sepsis as has granulocyte–macrophage-colony stimulating factor (GM-CSF).[8,9] The therapeutic efficacy of passive immunotherapy, GM-CSF or other immunomodulators for human OPSI is worthy of further clinical investigation. Interleukin 18 (IL-18) protects animals from postsplenectomy pneumococcal sepsis by increasing IgM levels.[43] There is no clinical experience with IL-18 in asplenic patients as yet. Fluid resuscitation, vasopressor agents, hematologic support, ventilatory support and expert acid–base and electrolyte management are essential to survival in these critically ill patients.

The mortality rate for OPSI caused by *S. pneumoniae* has been reported to be between 50% and 70%.[1,2,11–15] With early recognition and treatment, combined with skilled supportive care, the mortality rate has decreased to as low as 10% in recent series.[42,44]

During the convalescent period, it may be necessary to surgically excise necrotic tissues that have been irreparably damaged by the prolonged hypotension and intravascular coagulation that often accompanies this syndrome. Late complications such as adrenal insufficiency, osteomyelitis and endocarditis should be sought in patients with persistent fever after an episode of OPSI. Patient education, vaccination and a medical alert bracelet should be offered to survivors to prevent recurrences.

REFERENCES

References for this chapter can be found online at http://www.expertconsult.com

Vaccination of the immunocompromised patient

INTRODUCTION

Immunosuppression is expected to downmodulate or to suppress responses to vaccination; consequently, immunizing the immuno-compromised host is a challenge. Unfortunately, experience with the immunocompromised host is often based on small and composite groups of patients with heterogeneous clinical conditions, differ-ent immunosuppressive regimens and diverse immunization back-grounds. This is in contrast to standard vaccinology data generated from large cohorts of healthy young subjects. The available informa-tion pertains mostly to immunogenicity, reactogenicity and safety of vaccinations. Data on protection are essentially missing, leaving the clinician wondering if the immunologic surrogates of protection derived from healthy vaccine recipients will apply to the immunocom-promised host as well.

The main focus of this chapter is to review the experience with vac-cinating patients suffering from different chronic conditions associ-ated with disease- or drug-induced immune depression. These include kidney and liver chronic diseases, long-term inflammatory and auto-immune diseases, malignancies and solid-organ grafts. The intent is to give a glimpse of what can reasonably be expected from immuniza-tion in such patients. Revaccination of hematopoietic stem cell trans-plant recipients and routine vaccination of children with congenital immune deficiency syndromes or HIV infection are also addressed.

BASIC RULES FOR VACCINATING THE IMMUNOCOMPROMISED HOST

1. Live vaccines are contraindicated for fear of uncontrolled disease caused by vaccine strain. Few conditions are sufficiently investigated to allow live vaccines under stringent criteria.
2. Inactivated vaccines can be used with no restrictions at all but the likelihood for them to be of any effectiveness is dependent on the degree of immunosuppression.
3. Immune responses to vaccination should be assessed at completion of vaccination. The common method of assessment is the determination of vaccine-induced antibody levels. Tests for diphtheria, tetanus, influenza and hepatitis B antibodies are available through routine laboratories, whereas tests for pneumococcal serotypes, *Haemophilus influenzae* type b and varicella are only performed in few specialized laboratories. Routine serology tests for measles, rubella, varicella and hepatitis A are commonly available but may be not sensitive enough for detecting vaccine-induced immunity. The ideal time for checking the antibody response to vaccination is 6–8 weeks after the last dose of vaccine.

4. Depending on the underlying disease, the therapeutic regimen and the vaccine's properties, re-establishment of vaccine-induced immunity to preimmunosuppression level may not be achieved by a single recall dose of vaccine and not immediately after cessation of therapy.
5. Hematopoietic stem cell transplant recipients require that the vaccination process be started all over again for all vaccines after engraftment.

IMPACT OF IMMUNOSUPPRESSIVE DRUGS ON THE RESPONSE TO VACCINATION

Corticosteroid therapy

On condition that no other immunosuppressive drug is given concom-itantly, the immune response to inactivated vaccines is insignificantly reduced in patients on systemic corticosteroid therapy, irrespective of the daily dose. Adequate antibody responses are reported after recall immunization (tetanus) as well as primary vaccinations (*H. influenzae* type b, influenza, pneumococcus) in both children and adults.

Immune response to live vaccines is less a concern than safety as the control of live antigens may be depressed to the extent that the tran-sient vaccine infection turns into a persistent infection. Live antigens are contraindicated if the daily dose of steroid is equivalent to ≥20 mg of prednisone (or ≥2 mg/kg in children weighing <10 kg) and therapy is applied (or planned) for 2 weeks or longer. Under such circum-stances, live vaccine administration should be delayed until 1 month after cessation of treatment. Patients receiving ≥20 mg (or ≥2 mg/kg in children weighing <10 kg) of prednisone for <2 weeks should not be immunized with a live vaccine while on treatment but may be vacci-nated at cessation of therapy or preferably 2 weeks later.[1]

Live vaccines are allowed regardless of treatment duration when low-dose steroids (<20 mg of prednisone, or <2 mg/kg in children weighing <10 kg) are applied. Topical treatments (including inhala-tion and intra-articular injection) and physiologic replacement are not contraindications to live vaccines.[1]

Other immunosuppressive drugs

Most investigations report that the reduction of the immune response is related to the number of immunosuppressive drugs at the time of immunization. Available data pertain mostly to adults with auto-immune diseases or solid-organ transplants receiving a primary pro-tein antigen (inactivated influenza vaccine), a polysaccharide antigen (pneumococcal polysaccharide vaccine) or a recall protein antigen (tetanus vaccine). Table 83.1 lists different immunosuppressive drugs (or drug combinations) and indicates the degree of impairment of

Table 83.1 Comparative impact of immunosuppressive drugs and drug combinations on response to vaccination in patients with organ transplants or autoimmune diseases

Immunosuppressive drugs	'PRIMARY' PROTEIN ANTIGEN Influenza		'RECALL' PROTEIN ANTIGEN Tetanus		POLYSACCHARIDE ANTIGEN Pneumococcus (23-V)	
	Impact	Context	Impact	Context	Impact	Context
Inhibition of T-cell signaling + prednisone						
Sirolimus + prednisone	Significant	Transplantation			Minimal	Transplantation
Ciclosporin A + prednisone	Significant	Transplantation	Minimal	Transplantation	Minimal	Transplantation
Inhibition of DNA synthesis ± prednisone	Impact	Context			Impairment	Context
Methotrexate	Minimal	Autoimmunity			Significant	Autoimmunity
Methotrexate + prednisone	Minimal	Autoimmunity			Significant	Autoimmunity
Azathioprine + prednisone	Minimal	Transplantation			Minimal	Transplantation
Mycophenolate + prednisone	Significant	Transplantation				
Inhibition of TNF activity ± prednisone	Impact	Context			Impact	Context
Adalimumab	Minimal	Autoimmunity				
Infliximab	Minimal	Autoimmunity				
Etanercept	Minimal	Autoimmunity				
Adalimumab + prednisone	Modest	Autoimmunity			Minimal	Autoimmunity
Infliximab + prednisone	Modest	Autoimmunity			Minimal	Autoimmunity
Etanercept + prednisone	Modest	Autoimmunity			Minimal	Autoimmunity
Inhibition of T-cell signaling and of DNA synthesis	Impact	Context	Impact	Context	Impact	Context
Ciclosporin A + prednisone + azathioprine	Significant	Transplantation			Significant	Transplantation
Ciclosporin A + prednisone + mycophenolate	Significant	Transplantation	Significant	Transplantation	Significant	Transplantation
Tacrolimus + prednisone + mycophenolate					Significant	Transplantation
Inhibition of DNA synthesis and of TNF activity	Impact	Context			Impact	Context
Methotrexate + infliximab	Significant	Autoimmunity			Significant	Autoimmunity
Methotrexate + prednisone + infliximab	Significant	Autoimmunity			Significant	Autoimmunity
Methotrexate + etanercept					Significant	Autoimmunity
Methotrexate + prednisone + etanercept	Significant	Autoimmunity			Significant	Autoimmunity
Methotrexate + prednisone + adalimumab	Significant	Autoimmunity			Significant	Autoimmunity
Inhibition of DNA synthesis and depletion of B-cells	Impact	Context				
Methotrexate + rituximab	Significant	Autoimmunity				

the antibody response to be expected from therapy. Not all double (respectively triple) regimens have an identical impact and some individual drugs exert different immunosuppressive effects depending on the combination.

ACUTE LYMPHOBLASTIC LEUKEMIA

Decline of previously induced vaccine immunity

The main determinant of antibody loss for diphtheria, tetanus and *H. influenzae* type b antibodies is thought to be dependent upon treatment intensity,[2-5] explaining why some investigators report no substantial negative effect,[2,6,7] while others report marginally protective or nonprotective antibody titers.[3,8] Another determinant is likely to be antibody levels at onset of chemotherapy. These are directly influenced by the patient's age and the number of vaccine doses previously received.

An accelerated decline of measles and rubella antibodies is observed in children immunized with a single dose of vaccine prior to the onset of treatment.[9,10] The true clinical significance of the loss of measles antibody is not clear. Indeed, immunoassays used for antibody measurements can be negative in the presence of positive neutralization tests that clearly correlate with protection.

Vaccination during therapy

Diphtheria and tetanus recall vaccination

A single recall dose of either toxoid induces a protective antibody level in all patients.

Haemophilus influenzae *type b vaccination*

Primary vaccination with the conjugate vaccine is associated with a low rate of response ranging from 50% to 60%. The likelihood of an adequate response is inversely related to the duration of therapy and its intensity.

Hepatitis B vaccination

The capacity to respond to hepatitis B vaccination is dependent on the intensity of therapy. Minimal requirements for these patients are double amounts of antigen for age and schedules comprising four to five doses. When these are met, only 35% of patients on intense therapy achieve a protective antibody level compared to 90% of patients with less intense regimens. The vaccination is protective in responders and, interestingly enough, in nonresponders to some extent as well, suggesting an undetected positive effect of cell-mediated immunity. The vaccination is totally ineffective in children receiving induction or consolidation therapy.

Influenza vaccination

The inactivated vaccine is no less immunogenic than in healthy controls but modestly so due to the vaccinees' young age.

Varicella vaccination

The live varicella vaccine was developed specifically for patients with acute lymphoblastic leukemia in remission. Minimal conditions for this vaccine to be used in leukemic children include all of the following:

* disease in remission;
* chemotherapy stopped for 1 week before and 1 week after vaccination;
* corticosteroid treatment stopped for 1 week before and 2 weeks after vaccination.

Overall, 85% of patients develop an immune response after a single dose and the proportion is higher among patients off chemotherapy at the time of vaccination. An additional 10% of children respond to a second dose of vaccine. An interval of 3 months is recommended between doses. The antibody response is accompanied by specific cell-mediated immunity. A sizeable proportion of patients (75%) retain detectable antibody levels for several years. Eighty-five percent of vaccine recipients escape chickenpox despite household exposure and if varicella does occur, symptoms are often mild or moderate. A mild vesicular rash can break out 1–6 weeks after the first vaccine dose. No relapses of leukemia are associated with the vaccination and the incidence of zoster is lower in vaccine recipients than in children experiencing natural infection.

Vaccination after cessation of therapy

A substantial immunologic rebound is usually observed shortly after cessation of therapy. Rarely, the immune depression persists for months affecting antibody or cell-mediated responses.

Diphtheria and tetanus recall vaccination

A single recall dose of either toxoid administered 3–6 months after cessation of therapy elicits protective antibody levels in most children. The immune response is excellent in patients who were at standard or intermediate risk but definitely weaker in high-risk patients. The capacity to respond is clearly correlated with the number of memory B cells left in the bone marrow at the end of treatment. Children who are able to develop a quantitatively adequate response produce fully functional antibodies. The timing of vaccination after cessation of therapy is not a critical factor as no differences are seen whether patients are vaccinated 1 or 6 months after treatment. The strategy for recall diphtheria and tetanus vaccination should be a single dose in standard and intermediate risk patients and a two-dose schedule and antibody measurement in high-risk children.

Haemophilus influenzae *type b recall vaccination*

The same observations and recommendations exist for *H. influenzae* b vaccination as described with diphtheria–tetanus vaccines.

Measles recall vaccination

A single recall dose of live vaccine given at least 3 months after the end of therapy induces a response rate as high as in healthy controls.

Influenza vaccination

Depending on the viral strain considered, between 45% and 88% of patients achieve protective antibody levels after a single dose of inactivated influenza vaccine. Contrary to observations with recall vaccinations, the timing of vaccination appears to be critical and responses rates are far higher and more homogeneous when vaccination is administered at least 6 months after treatment.

MULTIPLE MYELOMA

Vaccination during therapy

Haemophilus influenzae *type b vaccination*

Geometric mean concentrations of antibodies are comparable in multiple myeloma patients and healthy adults following a single dose of conjugate vaccine.

Influenza vaccination

Antibody concentrations are lower in multiple myeloma patients than in healthy controls. Immunization is totally ineffective if given within 7 days from chemotherapy. A delay of 2 weeks between the vaccine injection and the start of the next course of therapy is desirable.

Pneumococcal vaccination

Geometric mean concentrations of pneumococcal antibodies are lower in multiple myeloma patients than in healthy adults and the polysaccharide vaccine is essentially ineffective. A single dose of vaccine induces a serologic response in 50% of patients and despite vaccination serotype-specific antibody concentrations remain lower than in the unvaccinated age-matched healthy population.

SOLID TUMORS IN CHILDREN

Decline of previously induced vaccine immunity

An accelerated loss of antibody to tetanus, poliomyelitis, hepatitis B, measles, mumps and rubella is observed during therapy of various solid pediatric cancers.[11-13]

Vaccination during therapy

Diphtheria and tetanus vaccination

Primary vaccination of infants on therapy for a neuroblastoma induces protective immunity comparable to historic controls. No special immunization schedule is needed for these children.

Haemophilus influenzae type b vaccination

Primary immunization of preschool children with a single dose of conjugate vaccine is significantly less effective than in historic controls. An additional dose of vaccine is indicated in low responders.

Hepatitis B vaccination

Regular schedules are inadequate for primary immunization. The four-dose schedule (0, 1, 2 and 12 months) with 40 μg per dose (regardless of age) induces a protective level in over 70% of patients. The antibody response should be assessed 4 weeks after the third dose in order to detect low responders who will require an extra 40 μg dose (administered at 4 months).

Influenza vaccination

A single dose of inactivated vaccine is clearly insufficient. Two doses are needed and induce significantly lower responses than in healthy children.

Varicella vaccination

The vaccine is as immunogenic, well tolerated and safe in these children as in their healthy siblings on condition that the following criteria be fulfilled (blood lymphocyte count greater than $0.5 \times 10^9/l$; no chemotherapy for 2 weeks before and 2 weeks after vaccine administration).

Vaccination after cessation of therapy

Diphtheria, tetanus, poliomyelitis, hepatitis B, measles and rubella recall vaccination

A single dose of vaccine is sufficient to reactivate protective responses to diphtheria, tetanus, poliomyelitis and rubella in vaccine recipients who have lost vaccine-induced immunity during therapy. The impact of a single dose of hepatitis B and measles vaccine is less predictable so a follow up antibody measurement is indicated.

Hepatitis B vaccination

The primary immunization is effective with three or four doses (0, 1 and 6 months/0, 1, 2 and 6 months) on condition that 20 μg of antigen per dose be used regardless of age.

Influenza vaccination

Two doses of inactivated influenza vaccine induce similar responses in patients and age-matched controls.

Varicella vaccination

On condition that minimal conditions be met (at least 3 months after cessation of therapy, lymphocyte count greater than $0.7 \times 10^9/l$ and

normal age-adjusted serum IgG concentration), two doses of live vaccine administered 3 months apart are effective, well tolerated and safe in susceptible children recovering from therapy for a solid tumor.

SOLID TUMORS IN ADULTS

Lymphomas

Vaccination during therapy

Influenza vaccination

Regular immunization with the inactivated vaccine is unreliable in these patients. A single dose induces only a modest response and two doses are suggested to assure significant protective vaccine-induced immunity. It is prudent to maintain a 2-week delay between the vaccine injection and the start of the next course of chemotherapy.

Pneumococcal vaccination

Responses to a single dose of polysaccharide vaccine are clearly reduced and a second dose 1 month later does not increase the rate of response. A minimal interval of 2 weeks, and preferably 4 weeks, should be kept between the vaccine administration and the start of the next chemotherapy course.

Vaccination after cessation of therapy

Haemophilus influenzae type b vaccination

Patients recovering from a lymphoma are less likely to have a protective immunity than age-matched healthy controls, indicating a need for them to be immunized after therapy. Overall, a single dose of conjugate vaccine administered 2 years after treatment induces a protective antibody level in 90% of patients. A second dose to nonresponders is ineffective and likely related to the destruction of specific memory T cells during therapy.

Pneumococcal vaccination

The antibody response to a single dose of pneumococcal polysaccharide vaccine administered 2 years after therapy is similar in patients and in healthy age-matched controls. In contrast, the response to the 7-valent conjugate vaccine, in addition to being restricted to seven serotypes, is significantly inferior to that following the plain polysaccharide vaccine, possibly because of the lower antigen content in the former. However, the conjugate vaccine is able to exert a priming effect when administered prior to the polysaccharide vaccine.

OTHER SOLID MALIGNANCIES

Vaccination during therapy

Influenza vaccination

A single dose of inactivated vaccine is less efficient than in healthy controls. Rates of seroconversion are particularly low when vaccination is administered during a course of therapy. A delay of 2 weeks between the vaccine injection and the start of the next course of therapy is sufficient to ensure vaccine responsiveness. Rates of response are inversely correlated to the intensity of the immunosuppressive regimen. Yearly administration of a single dose of vaccine to elderly patients with intestinal cancer is associated with a significant reduction in the incidence of acute influenza pneumonia, a slight decrease in mortality and fewer interruptions of chemotherapy due to febrile episodes.

Pneumococcal vaccination

The effectiveness of a single dose of polysaccharide vaccine is clearly decreased in cancer patients compared to healthy controls but modestly so in comparison to individuals with various medical conditions not associated with immunosuppression. A minimal interval of 2 weeks, and preferably 4 weeks, should be kept between vaccine administration and chemotherapy courses in order to maintain vaccine efficacy.

SOLID ORGAN TRANSPLANTS IN CHILDREN

Decline of previously induced vaccine immunity

At comparable ages and time points in relation to the latest vaccine dose, the proportion of renal transplant recipients with protective levels of diphtheria, tetanus and poliomyelitis antibodies is lower than in healthy controls.[14–16] In contrast, the immunosuppressive therapy associated with liver transplantation has little impact on immunity to diphtheria and none on tetanus or poliomyelitis.[15]

Vaccination during therapy

Diphtheria and tetanus recall vaccination

Rates of protective response to a single recall dose of diphtheria toxoid range from 65% to 95% and rates to a single dose of tetanus vaccine range between 85% and 100%. In kidney transplant patients, the response to diphtheria, but not tetanus toxoid, is positively correlated to creatinine clearance. It is recommended that antibody levels be checked after recall vaccination in transplant patients and followed up in low responders. Both vaccinations are well tolerated and safe, triggering no episodes of acute rejection and no change in organ function.

Measles and rubella recall vaccination

In children successfully immunized prior to transplantation who become seronegative during treatment, a single dose of live vaccine administered 3 years after engraftment induces seroprotective responses in 85% of patients against measles and in all against rubella. The recall vaccination is safe.

Varicella recall vaccination

A single recall dose of live vaccine given 3 years after engraftment is fully effective and safe in children who were successfully immunized prior to transplantation and turn seronegative during therapy.

Hepatitis B vaccination

The regular three-dose schedule (0, 1 and 6 months) with the regular amount of antigen for age is not as immunogenic in liver transplant recipients as in historic controls. One extra dose of vaccine at 12 months with a double amount of antigen for age is required in nonresponders and brings protection to half of them. Response rates are significantly different in patients on single (100%), double (84%) or triple immunosuppressive therapy (66%).

Influenza vaccination

The influenza vaccination is effective in renal transplant patients but less so in liver transplant recipients, possibly because the latter are much younger. Not only is the antibody response modest in liver recipients but the cell-mediated response is significantly depressed, suggesting that additional measures such as vaccination of household contacts and postexposure chemoprophylaxis are needed to protect liver recipients. The vaccination is safe with no increase in acute graft rejections.

Measles vaccination

Two doses of live vaccine administered 4 years after engraftment induce seroconversion in 65% of susceptible children on single drug therapy and in 40% of patients on a two- or three-drug regimen.

Reactogenicity is comparable in transplant recipients and historic controls, and is characterized by minor adverse effects.

Pneumococcal vaccination

The sequential schedule consisting of two doses of 7-valent conjugate vaccine followed with one dose of 23-valent polysaccharide vaccine (all three doses every other month) results in a significant rise in antibody levels to all serotypes in all vaccine recipients. The need for the second dose of conjugate vaccine is questionable.

Varicella vaccination

Two doses of live vaccine administered 3 years after engraftment induce seroconversion in 73% of susceptible children on one-drug immunosuppressive therapy. The reactogenicity is comparable in transplant patients and controls with only minor local adverse effects. Seronegative children with an adequate lymphocyte count (at least 1500 cells/mm^3) can be immunized as early as 6 months after engraftment without modifying the immunosuppressive regimens. The antibody response rate is more modest (66%) in patients on double or triple immunosuppressive therapy but there is evidence of induced cell-mediated immunity. Interestingly, an additional 20% of patients seroconvert in a delayed fashion (6 months after completion of vaccination). Adverse reactions occur at increased frequency (vesicular rashes 55% and febrile episodes 25%) but are self-limited and benign.

SOLID ORGAN TRANSPLANTS IN ADULTS

Vaccination during therapy

Diphtheria, tetanus and poliomyelitis recall vaccination

A single recall dose of diphtheria–tetanus–poliomyelitis vaccine induces a protective response in 90% of patients to diphtheria and in all to tetanus and poliomyelitis. The diphtheria response is short lived compared to the other two. All vaccinations are well tolerated. Considering the possibility that a recall dose might induce a borderline response, it is imperative that the diphtheria antibody level be checked in all vaccine recipients and followed up in low responders.

Haemophilus influenzae type b vaccination

A single dose of conjugate vaccine is equally effective in inducing seroconversion among renal transplant recipients and controls but generates a protective level in only 35% of patients (on double or triple immunosuppressive therapy).

Hepatitis A vaccination

Two doses of inactivated vaccine administered 6 months apart are fully immunogenic in liver transplant recipients but less effective in renal transplant patients. In addition, and in contrast to immunocompetent individuals, only a minority of kidney recipients (24–40%) achieve a protective response following the first dose. The full two-dose schedule should then ideally be completed before exposure starts. The immune response is short lived in all patients. Between 60% and 75% of patients with a protective response at completion of vaccination do not maintain a protective antibody level 2 years later, suggesting that the immune memory has not been induced by vaccination.

Hepatitis B vaccination in liver transplant recipients with pre-existent hepatitis B-induced disease

These patients are presumed to receive life-long antiviral chemotherapy or immunotherapy. Hepatitis B vaccination targeting discontinuation of the antiviral therapy is a controversial issue and a complex process. First, the antiviral therapy has to be continued throughout the entire immunization process. Second, vaccines and vaccination schedules under investigation differ in many ways (number of doses

Table 83.2 Hepatitis B vaccination schedules in liver transplant adult recipients with pre-existent hepatitis B infection

Schedule	Concomitant therapy	Results at completion of vaccination (% of patients achieving a given level of anti-HBs antibody)
Conventional antigen and conventional adjuvant		
3 doses of 40 µg	Lamivudine	4–12% achieve level >10 IU/l. Several additional doses do not substantially increase rate of response
6 doses of 40 µg	Lamivudine	8% achieve level >10 IU/l
6 doses of 40 µg	Immunoglobulin	No increase above baseline value
9 doses of 40 µg	Immunoglobulin	8% achieve level >10 IU/l
Novel antigens and conventional adjuvant		
3 doses of 20 µg	Lamivudine	25% achieve level >10 IU/l
6 doses of 20 µg	Lamivudine	50% achieve level >10 IU/l
Conventional antigen and novel adjuvants		
6 doses of 20 µg	Lamivudine	12% achieve level >10 IU/l
5 doses of 40 µg	Immunoglobulin	40% achieve level >500 IU/l
>8 doses of 20 µg	Immunoglobulin	80% achieve level >500 IU/l. One dose of conventional vaccine given 2 years later induces anamnestic response

and/or amount of antigen per dose and/or novel antigen formulation and/or novel adjuvant formulation). The most pertinent features are commented below and summarized in Table 83.2.

- *Schedules based on the conventional HBs antigen*: an antibody level ≥10 IU/l is obtained in a small proportion of patients (<25%), irrespective of the number of doses and the amount of antigen, and there is no evidence that the antibody elevation is associated with a specific T-cell mediated response and correlated with long-term protection.
- *Schedules based on combinations of novel antigen and conventional adjuvant*: an antibody level ≥10 IU/l is induced in a somewhat higher but unpredictable proportion of patients and there is no evidence that the increase in antibody is a T-cell driven response.
- *Schedules based on combinations of novel adjuvant and conventional antigen*: these are likely to trigger a significantly higher antibody response on condition that they include a large number of doses (≥9) or a large amount of antigen per dose (≥40 µg). The priming effect of such schedules is suggested by the observation that a single dose of standard vaccine administered 2 years later is able to induce an anamnestic response.

The vaccination is well tolerated and safe regardless of antigen or adjuvant nature and quantity. Local reactions are occasional with the conventional vaccine and somewhat more frequent with novel adjuvants. No systemic adverse effects, no rejection episodes or alterations in liver enzyme profiles are reported following any of the above schedules.

Influenza vaccination

A single dose of inactivated vaccine has a two- to sixfold lower probability of inducing seroconversion in renal, heart and lung transplant recipients than in healthy controls. In renal patients, the magnitude of the immune response is directly related to the degree of graft function (a creatinine clearance >70 ml/min/1.73 m^2 correlates with high probability of protective response) and may be essentially unaltered

in patients with a well-functioning graft. Cell-mediated immunity is commonly maintained in renal graft recipients but severely depressed in lung transplant recipients. Most investigators report no improvement in seroconversion with an additional dose of vaccine. In heart transplant recipients, a three-dose schedule at monthly intervals increases somewhat the probability of achieving seroprotection. The MF59 adjuvanted vaccine formulation is no more immunogenic in transplant patients than the conventional vaccine.

Time elapsed after engraftment is an important determinant of efficacy. In lung transplant recipients, the overall rate of seroconversion is 45% when vaccination is given within 12 months of surgery and 75% after 1 year. Another determinant of efficacy is the intensity of the immunosuppressive therapy and the drug combination. Protection is demonstrated in heart transplant recipients and is similar with the conventional or the MF59 adjuvanted formulation. A single study in heart transplant recipients mentions a temporal association between vaccination and low-level histologic rejection episodes but these are strictly asymptomatic and respond to a single course of therapy. The rejection process appears to be unrelated to the time elapsed from engraftment, to the magnitude of the antibody response and to the number of vaccine doses administered.

Pneumococcal vaccination

Responses to a single dose of polysaccharide vaccine are heterogeneous and modulated by the intensity of the immunosuppressive therapy. Differences involve the proportion of patients responding to vaccination as well as the number and magnitude of serotype-specific responses. Even when nearly as effective as in healthy controls, responses are short-lived (2–3 years) and justify antibody monitoring. The presently available 7-valent conjugate vaccine does not significantly enhance the functional activity, duration or level of the antibody response in transplant recipients.

HEMATOPOIETIC STEM CELL TRANSPLANTS

Decline of previously induced vaccine immunity

The loss of vaccine-induced antibodies is rapid and relentless during the first 2 years after engraftment in both children [17,18] and adults [19-22] and affects all vaccine-induced antibodies that have been investigated (diphtheria, tetanus, poliomyelitis, H. influenzae type b, measles, mumps and rubella). Naturally acquired antibodies to pneumococcal serotypes wane in the same fashion. [23,24] Antibody waning may be accelerated by graft-versus-host reactions, depending on the vaccine considered: for instance, graft-versus-host disease (GVHD) has no impact on the decline of diphtheria and tetanus antibodies, but an enhancing effect on the loss of pneumococcal antibodies and poliomyelitis antibodies.

Revaccination

Declining vaccine-induced immunity is a clear indication for revaccinating all patients. Single doses of inactivated vaccines are insufficient to re-establish immunity to preimmunosuppression levels and complete revaccination schedules are needed. It is recommended that immunization be started 12 months after engraftment with inactivated vaccines, and no sooner than 24 months with live vaccines if the patient is deemed immunocompetent and free of GVHD. [25] Influenza immunization with the inactivated vaccine may be administered as early as 6 months after transplantation. A summary of recommendations is given in Table 83.3.

Usual revaccination schedules for inactivated vaccines (diphtheria, tetanus, pertussis in children younger than 7 years, poliomyelitis and hepatitis B) include three doses of vaccine with a '0, 2 and 10 months' timing. Revaccination schedules for live vaccines such as measles, mumps, rubella and varicella include two doses 6 months apart. [25] Interestingly a single dose of measles vaccine to previously unimmunized children induces seroconversion in 70% of patients. In contrast, a single dose to previously vaccinated children induces an antibody response in only 16%. However, protection is likely to be much better in the latter group than it appears because these patients have a strong

Table 83.3 Vaccination of children and adults after stem cell transplants

Vaccine	Age	Number of doses	Post-transplant schedule (months after engraftment)
Diphtheria vaccine	Any age	3 doses	12, 14 and 24 months
Tetanus vaccine	Any age	3 doses	12, 14 and 24 months
Pertussis vaccine	Any age <7 years	3 doses	12, 14 and 24 months
Poliomyelitis inactivated vaccine	Any age	3 doses	12, 14 and 24 months
Haemophilus influenzae type b conjugate vaccine	Any age	3 doses	12, 14 and 24 months
Hepatitis B vaccine	Any age	3 doses	12, 14 and 24 months
Influenza inactivated vaccine	Any age	1 dose (yearly)	6 months (or greater depending on epidemiologic circumstances)
Measles live vaccine	Any age >1 year	2 doses	24 and 30 months
Rubella live vaccine	Any age >1 year	2 dose	24 and 30 months
Varicella live vaccine	Any age >1 year	2 doses	24 and 30 months
Pneumococcus (polysaccharide vaccine schedule)	>5 years	2 doses	12 and 24 months
Pneumococcus (sequential conjugate/polysaccharide vaccine schedule)	<5 years	3 doses	12, 14 (conjugate vaccine) and 24 months (polysaccharide vaccine)

preferential T-helper 1 (Th1)-mediated activity which depresses antibody response but is capable of controlling wild-type viruses.

For some antigens (diphtheria, *H. influenzae* type b), priming the donor with a single dose of vaccine prior to harvest significantly accelerates the immune response in the recipient. Inactivated vaccines may be started sooner than 12 months following engraftment but, depending on the antigen and the timing of the first dose, the above mentioned three-dose schedule may be suboptimal and one additional dose may be required. Vaccination with the live measles vaccine sooner than 2 years post-transplant has been attempted only once (i.e. as early as 9 months after engraftment) in the setting of a measles outbreak in the community. A single dose was found to induce seroconversion in all seronegative patients and was well tolerated and safe.

Varicella vaccination sooner than 24 months after engraftment would be desirable in children since many cases of chickenpox and zoster occur within that period. If all the following prerequisites are met (no immunosuppressive therapy for past 3 months; lymphocyte count >1000 cells/mm³; T-cell count >700 cells/mm³; positive skin test with a recall antigen; total serum IgG level >5 g/l; no administration of gammaglobulin within past 6 weeks) a single dose of varicella vaccine administered 12–23 months after transplantation induces seroconversion in 77% of vaccine recipients and a second dose of vaccine augments it to 88%. The vaccine is well tolerated and appears safe.

CONGENITAL IMMUNE DEFICIENCY SYNDROMES

Principles

Sound theoretic considerations indicate that live vaccines may be insufficiently attenuated for these patients and unfortunate experiences with live products – bacille Calmette–Guérin (BCG), oral poliomyelitis, measles and smallpox vaccines – have confirmed this fear.[26,27] Consequently, patients with a T-cell function defect should not receive any live vaccines at all and patients with granulocyte or macrophage dysfunctions should not be given live-bacterial vaccines but may receive live-virus vaccines. In contrast, inactivated vaccines are never contraindicated in these patients, irrespective of the underlying immune deficiency, but their immunogenic effectiveness is likely to be attenuated or suppressed depending on the degree of B- and T-cell functional capacity.

Avoidance of live vaccines

Avoidance should be strictly abided by, particularly when substitution with inactivated vaccines is possible as is the case for influenza, poliomyelitis and typhoid vaccinations. However, recognition of the potential severity of wild-type virus infections like measles and chickenpox in these patients has led to investigating measles and varicella vaccines in individuals with partial T-cell functional defects such as DiGeorge anomaly. On condition that minimal criteria be met (>400 CD4 cells/mm³ and 15 months of age or older), these patients can be efficiently and safely immunized with live measles and varicella vaccines.[28] Furthermore, we have learned from inadvertent vaccinations that the immunogenic efficacy, the incidence and the severity of adverse effects are not significantly different in these patients and age-matched healthy controls.[28,29]

By analogy with measles and varicella vaccination in patients with partial T-cell defects, live measles and varicella vaccines are deemed acceptable in patients with a B-cell functional deficiency whose T-cell activity is normal. Two doses of each vaccine may be administered 3 months apart, starting at the age of 15 months.[30] In the setting of an outbreak, the first dose of measles vaccine may be given from 6 months of age and the first dose of varicella vaccine from 12 months.[30] There are no data suggesting that the two vaccines remain effective and safe when administered simultaneously. The measles–mumps–rubella formulation may be used instead of the monovalent measles vaccine.

Interference of concomitant immunoglobulin therapy

Live attenuated antigens, and particularly the further attenuated strain of measles virus, are at risk of neutralization by the immunoglobulin given as replacement therapy to some of these patients. Ideally, an interval of 8 months should be kept between immunoglobulin perfusion and live vaccine administration in order to prevent interference of the former with the latter.[30] When such an extended interval cannot be safely achieved owing to the child's clinical condition, measles or varicella vaccines should still be offered, in spite of probable reduced efficacy, with a minimal interval of 2 weeks between vaccination and the next dose of immunoglobulin.[30] Table 83.4 lists vaccines that are indicated in patients with congenital immune defects.

Table 83.4 Vaccination of infants and children with congenital immune defects

Legend:
1. No restriction
2. No restriction (immune response possibly reduced)
3. No restriction (immune response likely to be insufficient or absent)
4. Strict contraindication and no inactivated substitute vaccine available
5. Strict contraindication but inactivated substitute vaccine available
6. No strict contraindication (immune response possibly reduced)
7. No strict contraindication (immune response doubtful in case of concomitant immunoglobulin therapy)
8. No strict contraindication but inactivated substitute vaccine prefered

Vaccine	Granulocyte defects*	Partial antibody deficiency†	Complete antibody deficiency‡	Partial T lymphocyte deficiency§	Complete T lymphocyte deficiency¶
Diphtheria inactivated	1	2	3	2	3
H. influenzae b inactivated	1	2	3	2	3
Hepatitis A inactivated	1	1	3	3	3
Hepatitis B inactivated	1	2	3	2	3
Human papillomavirus inactivated	1	2	3	2	3
Influenza inactivated	1	2	3	2	3
Influenza live	1	8	5	5	5
Measles live	1	6	7	6	4
Meningococcal inactivated	1	2	3	2	3
Mumps live	1	6	7	6	4
Pertussis inactivated	1	2	3	2	3
Pneumococcus inactivated	1	2	3	2	3
Poliomyelitis inactivated (IPV)	1	2	3	2	3
Poliomyelitis live (OPV)	1	5	5	5	5
Rabies inactivated	1	2	3	2	3
Rotavirus live	1	6	4	4	4
Rubella live	1	6	7	6	4
Tetanus inactivated	1	2	3	2	3
Tick-borne encephalitis inactivated	1	2	3	2	3
Tuberculosis live (BCG)	4	4	4	4	4
Typhoid inactivated	1	2	3	2	3
Typhoid live	5	5	5	5	5
Varicella live	1	6	7	6	4
Yellow fever live	1	6	4	4	4

* e.g. Chronic granulomatous disease, leukocyte adhesion defects
† e.g. Immunoglobulin subclass deficiency, hypogammaglobulinemia, dysgammaglobulinemia
‡ e.g. Agammaglobulinemia
§ e.g. DiGeorge anomaly (without complete T cell absence), Wiskott–Aldrich syndrome
¶ e.g. Severe combined immunodeficiency

Congenital HIV infection

Routine vaccination of HIV-infected infants and toddlers with inactivated vaccines is recommended as per national schedules. Their immunogenic efficacy is proportionate to the patient's immune competence.[31] Asymptomatic and mildly symptomatic patients have normal antibody responses but the capacity to respond to vaccines decreases as the HIV infection advances. Live vaccines are to be avoided because of disastrous experiences in patients with severe immunodepression.[32–35] However, as wild-type measles and varicella infections are particularly dangerous and potentially lethal in patients who have become immunocompromised, routine vaccination with corresponding live vaccines is recommended as long as they have no evidence of severe immunosuppression (age-specific CD4 cell percentage greater than 15%).[30,36] When such criteria are met, vaccination is immunogenic, well tolerated and safe.[30,36] Consequently, both measles and varicella vaccines should be offered to children who are not severely symptomatic and not severely immunosuppressed (i.e. to those fitting into clinical categories N, A or B and immunologic categories 1 or 2) and have a sufficient number of CD4 cells (>750 CD4 cells/mm^3 before 1 year of age; >500 CD4 cells/mm^3 between 1 and 5 years; >200 CD4 cells/mm^3 from 6 years onwards). Two doses of each vaccine should be administered 3 months apart, starting at the age of 15 months.[30]

All above-mentioned precautions for the use of live vaccines in patients with inherited immune deficiencies (earlier vaccination in case of community outbreak and possible negative impact of immunoglobulin therapy) also apply to patients with a congenital HIV infection. Table 83.5 summarizes vaccines allowed or contraindicated in HIV-infected children.

CHRONIC KIDNEY DISEASES IN CHILDREN

Nephrotic syndrome

Pneumococcal vaccination

A single dose of polysaccharide vaccine is immunogenic in children with a steroid-sensitive disease and confers protection against peritonitis despite concomitant administration of low-dose prednisone. However, the decline of antibody is rapid and over half of the patients have antibody levels back to prevaccination values 3 years after vaccination. Responses obtained in children on high-dose prednisone are comparable to those obtained with lower corticosteroid dosage. Vaccination early in the disease process has no deleterious effect on disease activity. The antibody response is significantly lower in patients with a steroid-resistant disease.

Varicella vaccination

A single dose of live vaccine is immunogenic in children in remission (no corticosteroids for at least 6 weeks prior to vaccination), well tolerated and safe (no change in the relapse rate). In patients on uninterrupted low-dose prednisone, two doses of vaccine 4 weeks apart induce a protective response for at least 2 years in all vaccine recipients. Tolerance and safety (rate of relapse) are excellent in spite of the continued steroid treatment.

Chronic peritoneal dialysis

Diphtheria and tetanus vaccination

It is hypothesized that the earlier routine vaccination is started in infancy the better the immune response because of better renal function at the time of vaccination. Response rates to toxoids are slightly lower in infants and toddlers on peritoneal dialysis but modifications of routine schedules are deemed unnecessary.

Haemophilus influenzae type b vaccination

The conjugate vaccine induces protection in 90% of patients. However, considering the potential severity of invasive infections in children

under 5 years, it is recommended that the antibody titer be checked at completion of vaccination and at regular intervals thereafter. A single extra dose of vaccine is sufficient to reactivate a strong response.

Measles, mumps and rubella vaccination

Responses are clearly suboptimal. A single dose of triple vaccine induces seroconversion to measles, mumps and rubella in 80%, 50% and 80% of patients, respectively, with one-third seroconverting to all three viruses. It is recommended that levels of vaccine-induced antibodies be checked to assure protection.

Chronic hemodialysis

Impact of disease on vaccine-induced immunity

Chronic hemodialysis has little impact on immunity induced by routine vaccinations and booster immunizations. At comparable ages and time points after the last vaccine dose, the same proportion of patients and healthy controls have protective levels of diphtheria and tetanus antibodies. Similarly, pneumococcal vaccine responses are well preserved, yet antibody responses are very short lived and half of patients have inadequate levels 1 year later.

Varicella vaccination

Vaccination is indicated in anticipation of transplantation in view of the potential severity of chickenpox in transplant recipients. Nearly all patients develop a protective antibody level after two doses of vaccine administered 3 months apart. The few children who fail to respond to the initial two doses respond to a third. All patients vaccinated in anticipation of transplantation have a protective antibody level at the time of surgery. Vaccination prior to immunosuppression is protective. The incidence of chickenpox is significantly lower in vaccine recipients and the few breakthrough cases are significantly less severe. In addition, vaccination is clearly correlated with a reduced risk of zoster occurring during immunosuppressive therapy. The vaccination is well tolerated and causes only minor local reactions. Between 60% (patients on triple immunosuppressive therapy) and 100% of transplant recipients vaccinated prior to engraftment retain protective antibody levels 2–3 years after engraftment.

CHRONIC KIDNEY DISEASES IN ADULTS

Predialysis renal failure

Hepatitis B vaccination

Patients in renal failure are low responders to hepatitis B vaccination. At this stage responses are not correlated with the degree of functional insufficiency. The regular schedule (three doses at 0, 1 and 6 months with 20 μg of antigen/dose by the intramuscular route) is inadequate (57% protective responses) so that alternative schedules have been investigated.

- *Alternative 1*: Increasing the amount of antigen to 40 μg per dose provides an insignificant increase in rates of protective responses (67%).
- *Alternative 2*: Increasing the amount of antigen to 40 μg per dose and inserting an extra dose of vaccine at the time point '2 months' within the regular schedule results in a significantly higher rate of protective responses (80%).
- *Alternative 3*: The four-dose schedule (0, 1, 2 and 6 months) based on intradermal injections of a smaller amount of antigen per dose (10 μg) is as effective as the above-mentioned intramuscular schedule, with the advantage of requiring much less antigen altogether, but with the inconvenience of necessitating five concomitant injections of 2 μg each to provide the required amount of antigen intradermally.

Table 83.5 Vaccination of HIV infected infants and children

Vaccine	No immunosuppression*	Moderate immunosuppression†	Severe immunosuppression‡
Diphtheria inactivated	1	2	3
H. influenzae b inactivated	1	2	3
Hepatitis A inactivated	1	2	3
Hepatitis B inactivated	1	2	3
Human papillomavirus inactivated	1	2	3
Influenza inactivated	1	2	3
Influenza live	5	5	5
Measles live	1	6	4
Meningococcal inactivated	1	2	3
Mumps live	1	6	4
Pertussis inactivated	1	2	3
Pneumococcus inactivated	1	2	3
Poliomyelitis inactivated (IPV)	1	2	3
Poliomyelitis live (OPV)	5	5	5
Rabies inactivated	1	2	3
Rotavirus live	1	2	4
Rubella live	1	6	4
Tetanus inactivated	1	2	3
Tick-borne encephalitis inactivated	1	2	3
Tuberculosis live (BCG)	4	4	4
Typhoid inactivated	1	2	3
Typhoid live	5	5	5
Varicella live	1	6	4
Yellow fever live	4	4	4

1 No restriction
2 No retriction (immune response possibly reduced)
3 No restriction (immune response likely to be insufficient or absent)
4 Strict contraindication and no inactivated substitute vaccine available
5 Strict contraindication but inactivated substitute vaccine available
6 No strict contraindication (immune response doubtful in case of concomitant immunoglobulin therapy)

Age <12 months	
≥1500	
750–1499	
<750	

Age 1–5 years	
≥1000	
500–999	
<500	

Age 6–12 years	
≥500	
200–499	
<200	

* Number of CD4 cells/μl
† Number of CD4 cells/μl
‡ Number of CD4 cells/μl

Influenza vaccination

A single dose of inactivated vaccine is effective and induces a significant increase in antibody levels to all strains. The proportion of patients attaining the protective threshold is slightly lower than in healthy controls but the clinical significance of this finding is undetermined.

Long-term dialysis

Diphtheria and tetanus recall vaccination

Recall immunizations are imperative in these patients. Single recall doses of vaccine have a suboptimal efficacy. Patients do achieve protective antibody levels but responses are of primary type and short lived. One year later, the majority of patients are below the protection threshold for diphtheria and one-third for tetanus. Complete revaccination schedules are no more efficient than single doses, suggesting a failure to induce the immune memory. The suggested approach is to monitor antibody levels and to administer single recall doses of toxoid whenever needed.

Hepatitis B vaccination

Overall, the effectiveness of vaccination is inversely related to the patient's age. When adequate schedules (such as those mentioned below) are used, the probability of obtaining a protective response is close to 100% in patients aged less than 50 years, compared to 75% in those aged 60–74 years and 50% in those over 75 years of age. A functionally efficient hemodialysis is associated with a stronger response. A concomitant asymptomatic hepatitis C infection does not modify the response. Protective response rates are similar in hemodialysis and peritoneal dialysis patients provided that adequate schedules are used.

The regular vaccination schedule (three doses at 0, 1 and 6 months by the intramuscular route with 20 μg of antigen per dose) is grossly inadequate (55–65% protective responses). Repeating an unsuccessful regular schedule is of no benefit in these patients. Consequently, a number of alternative schedules were developed. In peritoneal dialysis patients, increasing the amount of antigen to 40 μg or 80 μg per dose is associated with a significant increase in adequate responses (80%). In hemodialysis patients it is necessary to increase both the number of doses (to four or five) and the amount of antigen per dose (to at least 40 μg) to augment the rate of protective responses to 70–80%. Based on historic comparisons, the five-dose schedule is not significantly more effective than the other.

The intradermal route of vaccination (5 μg of antigen per dose injected on a weekly or bi-weekly basis for several weeks) is as effective as intramuscular schedules on condition that the minimal amount of antigen administered over the entire immunization process is 50 μg in peritoneal dialysis patients and 80 μg in hemodialysis patients. The minimal number of injections required is 10 in peritoneal dialysis patients and may vary from 15 to 25 in hemodialysis patients.

Yet another approach is to give a 5 μg dose of vaccine intradermally on a weekly basis until attainment of the protective level. Intradermal schedules induce significantly earlier responses than intramuscular injections and should be considered when a rapid response is deemed essential. However, peak antibody levels are lower and the longevity of responses is shorter. Protection obtained from intradermal schedules should not be considered as definitive as that obtained after a successful intramuscular schedule. An additional intramuscular dose of 40–80 μg should be given 4–6 months after successful completion of the intradermal injection program and the antibody level should be checked in order to demonstrate that protection relies on the immune memory.

Influenza vaccination

A single dose of inactivated vaccine is associated with seroconversion rates and geometric mean antibody titers significantly lower for all strains than in healthy controls. However, protection is still achieved in a sizeable proportion of patients, varying between 45% and 90%

depending on the strain considered. One study suggests that patients on calcitriol therapy at the time of vaccination might have a stronger antibody response.

Pneumococcal vaccination

A single dose of polysaccharide vaccine induces immune responses of lower magnitude and shorter duration than in healthy individuals. These short-lived responses are clinically correlated with frequent breakthrough infections occurring approximately 2 years after vaccination. Vaccination is suspected to induce a phenomenon of immune tolerance to some of the pneumococcal serotypes.

Varicella vaccination

Vaccination of susceptible adults in anticipation of engraftment is indicated in view of the potential severity of chickenpox in these patients. The varicella vaccine is overall less immunogenic in adults than in children but still has a favorable impact. Between 65% and 75% of patients achieve a protective response after two doses administered 6 weeks apart.

CHRONIC LIVER DISEASES IN CHILDREN

End-stage hepatic failure

Diphtheria, tetanus, poliomyelitis, measles, mumps, rubella and varicella vaccination

Antibody responses to inactivated vaccines are not altered in infants and toddlers with chronic liver failure. Live vaccines (measles, mumps, rubella, varicella) are as effective and as safe as in healthy controls. Since geometric mean antibody concentrations generated by live vaccines are inversely related to the severity of liver dysfunction at the time of injection, immunization should be initiated as soon as possible following the first birthday.

Chronic hepatitis B (HBV) or hepatitis C (HCV) disease

Hepatitis A (HAV) vaccination

Immunization is indicated in children with a pre-existent chronic liver disease on the analogy of adults with identical conditions. The regular two-dose schedule (0 and 6 months) of inactivated vaccine is as effective as in healthy controls. Rates of response are independent of the hepatitis serologic status.

CHRONIC LIVER DISEASES IN ADULTS

Chronic hepatitis B (HBV) disease

Hepatitis A (HAV) vaccination

Immunization is indicated in patients with chronic HBV disease. The regular two-dose schedule (0 and 6 months) of inactivated vaccine is equally effective in patients and healthy adults. At 5 years, 88% of vaccine recipients maintain an antibody level above the protection threshold, indicating that the response is based on the stimulation of memory cells.

Chronic hepatitis C (HCV) disease

Hepatitis A (HAV) vaccination

It is recommended that adults with pre-existent HCV disease be vaccinated against HAV because of the increased probability of exposure and severe clinical course. Consequently, hepatitis A vaccination is considered complementary to hepatitis B immunization, and the combined vaccine is handy. The regular three-dose schedule (0, 1 and 6 months) of Twinrix®720/20 is much less effective in these patients than in healthy controls. At completion of vaccination, 88% of patients have a protective antibody level against HAV and 82% against HBV. Administration of a fourth dose does not significantly enhance the rate of response to either antigen. When exposure to either virus is deemed imminent, the accelerated three-dose schedule (0, 7 and 21 days) of Twinrix®720/20 is effective in providing short-term protection. Nearly 90% of patients develop a protective response against HAV and 80% against HBV. An additional dose administered shortly after the third one is of no benefit. Accelerated schedules are not protective in the long term and should be completed when long-term protection is sought.

Hepatitis B vaccination

Responses to the hepatitis B vaccine are less adequate in these patients than healthy adults so that specific schedules are required. Three intramuscular doses of 40 μg each (at monthly intervals) induce a protective antibody level in 72% of patients. Adding a fourth dose of 80 μg 1 month later enhances the probability of protection to 88%. However, as monthly injections over a rather short period of time do not set suitable conditions for induction of the immune memory, the protection obtained by such schedules is not reliable in the long run and an additional dose of vaccine should be offered 4–6 months later. Patients with a cirrhotic disease respond significantly less adequately to the above four-dose schedule (74% seroprotection). Patients who do not respond to the above four-dose schedule are still reasonably likely (72%) to develop a protective response when they receive monthly doses of 80 μg of antigen up to a maximum of 10 months. Concomitant treatment with pegylated interferon and ribavirin does not affect the immunogenic effectiveness of hepatitis B vaccination.

Chronic alcohol-induced cirrhosis

Hepatitis B vaccination

These patients have a severely impaired response to the hepatitis B vaccine. Three monthly doses of 40 μg administered intramuscularly induce a protective level of antibody in a mere 12% of individuals. Patients who do not respond to the above schedule may achieve a protective response with a monthly dose of 80 μg for a maximum of 10 months. Protection generated by monthly injections over a short period of time is not reliable in the long run and an additional dose of vaccine is required 4–5 months later to obtain a response based on memory cells. Neither of the above schedules is associated with significant adverse effects.

Influenza vaccination

No immunogenicity data are available in these patients. Immunization with the inactivated vaccine is modestly effective in reducing the incidence of influenza-like illness and that of culture-proven influenza infection.

CHRONIC INFLAMMATORY AND AUTOIMMUNE DISEASES IN CHILDREN

Inflammatory bowel diseases

Influenza vaccination

The immune response to a single dose of inactivated vaccine is significantly reduced in patients on immunosuppressive therapy compared to healthy controls. Inadequate responses are particularly likely with drug combinations associating an anti-tumor necrosis factor (TNF) agent and a drug interfering with DNA synthesis. When used as monotherapy (or in combination with prednisone), anti-TNF agents have a minimal impact on the antibody response.

Juvenile idiopathic arthritis

Hepatitis B vaccination

The regular three-dose schedule (0, 1 and 6 months) induces an antibody level ≥10 IU/l in virtually all patients but geometric mean antibody concentrations are significantly lower than in healthy individuals. Consequently, it is essential to check that the antibody level is greater than 100 IU/l at completion of vaccination in order to ensure that long-term protection can indeed be relied upon. The vaccination is very safe with no deterioration of disease activity indices and no flare ups observed during the entire immunization process and beyond.

Influenza vaccination

Yearly immunization is recommended in children on continuous salicylate treatment or on immunosuppressive therapy for a rheumatologic condition. After a single dose of inactivated vaccine, 95% of patients achieve a protective level to all strains, similar to age-matched healthy controls. Safety has been particularly investigated on the suspicion that wild-type influenza viruses might be rheumatogenic and found to be excellent with no increase in disease activity indices following vaccination.

Measles–mumps–rubella (MMR) vaccination

No data are available on the immunogenicity of the MMR vaccine in these patients. However, safety has been particularly investigated in order to relieve the fear that live attenuated viruses might aggravate disease activity. A retrospective study scrutinizing children during a period of 6 months before and after injection of the second dose of vaccine reveals no increase in disease activity or medication use, and no measles-like illness.

Meningococcal conjugate vaccination

A single dose of conjugate vaccine is as effective in these patients as in healthy controls. Furthermore, it is safe with no change in disease activity and no increase in the frequency of relapses over a 6-month observation period.

CHRONIC INFLAMMATORY AND AUTOIMMUNE DISEASES IN ADULTS

Rheumatoid arthritis

Hepatitis B vaccination

The regular three-dose schedule (0, 1 and 6 months) is modestly effective (68% seroconversion) and safe. It is necessary to check the antibody response after completion of immunization and to continue the vaccination process in low responders. A second vaccine cycle or a high-dose vaccine schedule can be used (such as for renal failure patients).

Influenza vaccination

A single dose of inactivated vaccine induces a lower geometric mean concentration of antibodies than in healthy controls. Antibody responses are minimally altered by concomitant treatment of prednisone and methotrexate but significantly depressed by a combination of methotrexate and rituximab. Reactogenicity is similar in patients and healthy controls, and safety is clearly established with no change in disease activity and no increase in autoantibodies or peripheral blood lymphocyte subpopulations.

Pneumococcal vaccination

The polysaccharide vaccine is unreliable in these patients (65% response) but perfectly safe with no deterioration of either clinical or laboratory disease activity indices.

Systemic lupus erythematosus

Tetanus recall vaccination

A single recall dose of toxoid induces a protective antibody level in over 90% of patients. The recall vaccination is no more reactogenic than in historic age-matched controls and has no impact on disease activity.

Hepatitis B vaccination

The regular three-dose schedule is effective and safe in these patients. No change in disease activity indices, or a need to resort to more aggressive therapies, has been reported following any dose of vaccine.

Influenza vaccination

Protection against influenza is desirable in systemic lupus erythematosus (SLE) patients because natural immunity to wild-type viruses is suspected of being weaker than in healthy individuals. A single dose of inactivated vaccine induces a similar response in patients and controls, and reactogenicity is similarly low in both groups. Numerous clinical studies have confirmed the vaccine's safety profile in SLE patients. The number of flares and mean disease activity indices were not modified over observation periods of up to 5 months. Autoantibodies are produced following vaccination (without clinical manifestations) yet antinuclear antibodies are not. It can be concluded that influenza vaccination is immunogenic and sufficiently safe to be recommended to SLE patients.

Pneumococcal vaccination

Recent studies with the 23-valent vaccine indicate that the immune response to pneumococcal vaccine is unreliable in relation to the number of serotype-specific responses. After a single dose, 80% of patients develop an adequate response while others develop a response to just one serotype or to none. The vaccination is well tolerated and safe. No deterioration of either clinical or laboratory disease activity indices and no production of autoantibodies are evidenced.

REFERENCES

References for this chapter can be found online at http://www.expertconsult.com

Immunodeficiencies associated with immunosuppressive agents

INTRODUCTION

This practice point reviews the immunologic effects (i.e. the degree of immunodeficiency) associated with therapeutic interventions of immunosuppressive agents commonly used in transplantation and in the treatment of rheumatic and autoimmune diseases (Fig. PP40.1). Differing mechanisms of action of specific immunosuppressive agents and of their immunologic target(s) reveal qualitative and quantitative differences in the type of immunodeficiency caused by these therapeutic interventions. Many immunosuppressive agents target multiple components of the immune system. Furthermore, the intensity of the immunodeficiency is substantially influenced by the number of agents administered since immunosuppressive agents are mostly used in combination.

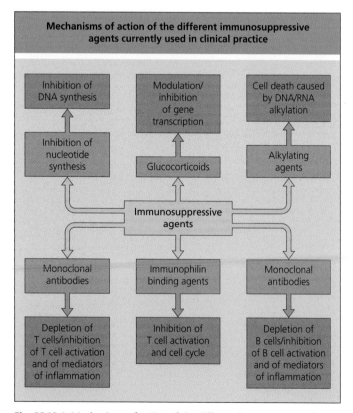

Fig. PP40.1 Mechanisms of action of the different immunosuppressive agents currently used in clinical practice.

HOST DEFENSES – GENERAL CONCEPTS

The immune system represents the primary mechanism of defense against a variety of pathogens (see Chapters 2 and 72). To understand the potential interference of immunosuppressive agents on the immune system, it is important to examine the different components of the immune system and the site of action of these agents. Immunologic dysfunctions can be anticipated depending upon the molecular target of each immunosuppressive treatment.

Anatomic barriers

The natural mechanisms of defense are mediated by anatomic barriers, primarily by the skin and mucosal (respiratory, gastrointestinal and urinary tract) barriers. The ability of these barriers to protect against invading pathogens is dependent upon their intrinsic physical structure as well as a series of factors, including the physical–chemical features of the environment (e.g. the pH and temperature), the local bacterial microflora and soluble local mediators such as secretory IgA and a variety of antimicrobial proteins.

Immunosuppressive treatment may severely compromise the integrity of the mucosal barrier because the particularly high turnover of cell division of the mucosal epithelium is very sensitive to the antiproliferative activity of immunosuppressive agents. This in turn may cause lesions of the epithelium, and the clinical picture may be complicated by the emergence of mucositis of variable severity. This type of complication is relatively frequent in cancer immunosuppressive regimens but is rare in the field of transplantation or immunologic diseases.

Innate immunity

This is an ancient system of defense that acts rapidly and does not require immunologic memory.[1] It is noteworthy that the innate immune system is not entirely nonspecific: the human (and vertebrate) innate immune system is able to recognize micro-organisms through pattern-recognition receptors (PRRs), and then is able to differentiate between self and pathogens. Pattern-recognition receptors recognize components of micro-organisms (known as pathogen-associated molecular patterns, PAMPs),[2] such as viral nucleic acids, components of bacterial or fungal cell walls, flagellar proteins. The first family of PRRs was the Toll-like receptor family. Toll-like receptors are transmembrane proteins that can recognize either extracellular or membrane-encased pathogens. Recently, two other families of PRRs have been described: the NOD-like receptors (NLRs) and the RIG-like helicases (RLHs) are soluble proteins that survey the cytoplasm in order to detect pathogens.

The effector components of innate immunity include soluble and cellular mediators. Amongst the former, the complement (C') proteins play a critical role in the recruitment and activation of neutrophils (C3a and C5a), in the opsonization of bacteria (C3bi) and in the destruction of certain micro-organisms through the membrane attack complex C5–C9. C-reactive protein (CRP) and lipopolysaccharide (LPS)-binding protein are additional soluble mediators of the innate immunity involved in the opsonization of bacteria or activation of C'.

The cellular effector components of innate immunity include neutrophils, monocytes/macrophages, dendritic cells, natural killer (NK) cells and gamma-delta T cells. These different types of cell, recruited at the site of infection and/or inflammation by the soluble mediators mentioned above, mediate either direct (e.g. phagocytosis and killing of bacteria) or indirect defense mechanisms (e.g. recruitment of other types of immune cell through the secretion of cytokines and chemokines).

Adaptive immunity

Adaptive immunity is very specific; it requires a certain time to become fully functional (the time is necessary for the generation, maturation and expansion of antigen-specific T and/or B cells) and is associated with the generation of immunologic memory following clearance of the pathogen.[3]

T lymphocytes are a critical component of adaptive immunity. The mechanisms of antigen (Ag) recognition by T lymphocytes are extremely specific. Following appropriate processing and presentation by professional antigen-presenting cells (APC), T lymphocytes recognize a complex formed by major histocompatibility complex (MHC) products and the Ag peptide on the surface of APC. Two major types of T lymphocyte (i.e. CD4 and CD8) are involved in the immune response against pathogens.

Based on their ability to produce different cytokines, CD4 T lymphocytes can generally be distinguished into three populations:
* T helper 1 (Th1), which are mostly characterized by the production of interferon gamma (IFN-γ) and interleukin (IL)-2;
* Th2, which produce mostly IL-4, IL-5 and IL-10; and
* Th17, which produce IL-17.

Th1 CD4 T cells are necessary for the maturation, expansion and maintenance of the CD8 T-lymphocyte response, of NK cells and for the activation of macrophages. Th2 CD4 T cells mediate the maturation and activation of pathogen-specific B lymphocytes. Th17 CD4+ T cells – a new T-cell subset secreting IL-17 – activate neutrophils and stimulate release of cytokines and chemokines by different cell types (e.g. macrophages, endothelial and epithelial cells) and probably play a pivotal role in inflammatory processes. CD8 T lymphocytes are the primary effector component of adaptive cell-mediated immunity. They are able to lyse virus-infected cells and tumor cells directly.

B lymphocytes mediate the immune response against pathogens through the production of immunoglobulins (Ig). Immunoglobulins may inhibit the entry of pathogens into target cells by binding to certain regions of the pathogen that are critical for the interaction with specific receptors on the surface of the target cells, a phenomenon known as neutralization. Furthermore, the primary role of Ig is the opsonization of bacteria and the activation of C' and the different components of innate immunity that may lead to the elimination of the pathogen.

It is therefore clear that immunosuppressive therapy, which is one of the primary causes of secondary immunodeficiency, may significantly impair B-cell or T-cell-mediated immunity and determine increased susceptibility to a variety of pathogens.

IMMUNOLOGIC EFFECTS AND CLINICAL ISSUES ASSOCIATED WITH IMMUNOSUPPRESSIVE THERAPY

In order to evaluate correctly the risk of infectious diseases associated with impairment of immune function(s), it is essential to know the degree of the defect and the component(s) of the immune system targeted by the immunosuppressive agents.

Glucocorticoids

Glucocorticoids (GC) are the cornerstone in the treatment of the majority of inflammatory diseases. Glucocorticoids are highly lipid soluble and thus penetrate easily through the cell membrane. They bind in the cytoplasm to a specific receptor (glucocorticoid receptor, GR) that is present in all nucleated cells.[4] The latter is the reason why it is not possible to dissociate the anti-inflammatory from the metabolic effects of GC.

The clinical picture of patients receiving treatment with GC may be complicated by a variety of infections caused by bacteria, fungi and viruses. The severity of these infectious complications depends upon the degree of immunosuppression resulting from GC treatment (Table PP40.1). Retrospective studies on large cohorts of patients treated with GC have clearly demonstrated that the risk of infection (including lethal infections) in these patients is significantly increased compared to patients not receiving GC.[5] Furthermore, it is important to emphasize that the dosage of GC is strictly linked to the risk of infection. A dosage of prednisone >20 mg/day is associated with a risk of infection twofold greater than that of a control group, while patients receiving a daily dosage of <10 mg/day do not show an increased risk of infection.

Alkylating agents

The alkylation of DNA is responsible for the cytotoxic, mutagenic and chemotherapeutic properties of this class of immunosuppressive agents. Cyclophosphamide (CYC) is effective on both 'resting' and dividing (i.e. activated) lymphocytes. Both T-cell (particularly T-helper) and B-cell functions are severely suppressed by CYC treatment.

The infectious complications associated with CYC treatment (see Table PP40.1) include bacterial, fungal and viral infections. The pathogens responsible for these infections are mostly typical opportunistic pathogens. It is important to emphasize that CYC is generally used in association with GC and therefore the risk for infectious complications is substantially increased, particularly if GC dosage is >0.5 mg/kg/day in patients aged more than 60 years and with a leukocyte nadir <3 × 10^9 cells/l. In order to prevent infectious complications, patients treated with CYC require close hematologic and immunologic monitoring and antimicrobial prophylaxis in certain conditions. Anti-*Pneumocystis* prophylaxis with trimethoprim–sulfamethoxazole is recommended in patients:
* undergoing continuous oral administration of CYC; and
* with a CD4 T-cell count of <200 cells/mm^3.

Although no definitive demonstration is available, the general perception is that continuous oral administration of CYC carries an increased risk of infection compared with intravenous pulses.

Immunophilin binding agents

Immunophilins are a large family of broadly expressed proteins that bind to certain immunosuppressive agents, such as ciclosporin A (CsA), tacrolimus and rapamycin. Due to their potent immunosuppressive effects that predominantly target T lymphocytes, these agents are fundamental components of immunosuppressive regimens in both solid organ and bone marrow transplantation.

Physiologically, T-cell receptor (TCR) signaling induces an elevation in the concentration of Ca^{2+} in the cytoplasm and activates the transcription factor AP-1. Ca^{2+} binds to calcineurin that in turn dephosphorylates the cytoplasmic form of the nuclear factor of activated T cells (NFAT). Once NFAT migrates into the nucleus, it forms a complex with AP-1, thus inducing the transcription of genes required for T-cell activation, including IL-2. When CsA is present in the cytoplasm, it forms a complex with cyclophilin (Cyp). The CsA–Cyp complex can bind to calcineurin, blocking its ability to activate NFAT and therefore inhibiting T-cell activation (Fig. PP40.2).

Table PP40.1 Type of infection related to immunosuppressive agents

Type of immunodeficiency	Type of immunosuppressive agent or chemotherapy	Type of infectious risk

Anatomic barriers (mucositis)	High-dose chemotherapy	Bacterial
		    Gram-positive – staphylococci (coagulase ±), streptococci
		    Gram-negative – Enterobacteriaceae, *Pseudomonas* spp.
		Fungal
		    Candida spp.
		Viral
		    Herpes simplex virus

Innate immunity (quantitative and qualitative defects)	High-dose chemotherapy/ radiotherapy	Bacterial
		    Gram-positive – staphylococci (coagulase ±), streptococci
		    Gram-negative – *Escherichia coli, Klebsiella, Pseudomonas* spp.
		Fungal
		    Candida
		    Aspergillus spp.

Adaptive immunity
  Cellular
	High-dose chemotherapy/ radiotherapy
	Immunosuppressive therapies (GC, CYC, CsA, FK-506, MTX, AZA, rapamycin, antilymphocyte serum, monoclonal antibodies)
		Bacterial
		    Legionella spp.
		    Mycobacterium tuberculosis
		    Atypical mycobacteria
		    Listeria monocytogenes
		    Salmonella spp.
		Fungal
		    Candida spp.
		    Cryptococcus neoformans
		    Histoplasma capsulatum
		    Coccidioides immitis
		Viral
		    Cytomegalovirus
		    Varicella zoster virus
		    Herpes simplex virus
		    Epstein-Barr virus
		    Live viral vaccines (measles, mumps, rubella, poliovirus)

Humoral	High-dose GC, CYC, MMF	Bacterial
		    Gram-positive – streptococci (*S. pneumoniae* and other streptococci)
		    Gram-negative – *Haemophilus influenzae, Neisseria meningitidis, Capnocytophaga canimorsus*
		Viral
		    Enterovirus
		Parasites
		    Giardia lamblia

AZA, azathioprine; CsA, ciclosporin A; CYC, cyclophosphamide; GC, glucocorticoids; MMF, mycophenolate mofetil; MTX, methotrexate; FK-506, tacrolimus.

Inhibitors of nucleotide synthesis

Azathioprine

Activated T lymphocytes are the primary target of azathioprine (AZA), which does not exert any cytotoxic effect on T lymphocytes prior to an antigen challenge, whereas the most potent immunosuppressive activities occur following antigen stimulation (Table PP40.2). On the basis of this mechanism of action, AZA has no effect on memory T lymphocytes. In addition to activated T lymphocytes, AZA exerts potent immunosuppression on B lymphocytes. Due to its selective effect on dividing cells, AZA rarely causes severe lymphopenia and only prolonged treatment may be associated with a substantial reduction in circulating lymphocytes.

Mycophenolate mofetil

Mycophenolate mofetil (MMF) is the prodrug of mycophenolic acid. Mycophenolate mofetil is a highly selective, noncompetitive inhibitor

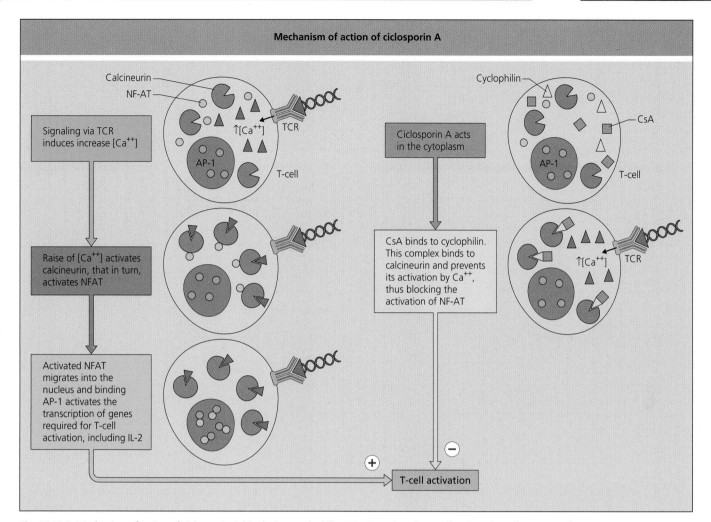

Fig. PP40.2 Mechanism of action of ciclosporin A (CsA). Cyp, cyclophilin; NF-AT, nuclear factor of activated T cells; TCR, T-cell receptor.

of the inosine monophosphate dehydrogenase involved in the de-novo synthesis of guanosine nucleotides (Table PP40.2, Fig. PP40.3). Purine synthesis may occur through two different pathways: de novo and salvage. Blood cells originating from the erythrocyte, megakaryocyte and myeloid lineages may use the salvage pathway if the de-novo pathway is inhibited. In contrast, the salvage pathway is not functional in B and T lymphocytes. From an immunologic standpoint, MMF has no effect on resting B and T lymphocytes but strongly suppresses proliferation of activated T lymphocytes by inducing apoptosis. It is a potent suppressor of primary and secondary T-cell responses. It also mediates potent inhibition of the primary humoral immune response but seems to be less effective in the inhibition of secondary humoral responses. Furthermore, due to the potent suppression of primary humoral immune responses, vaccination generally fails to induce humoral immune responses in patients undergoing MMF treatment.

Methotrexate

Originally developed as an anticancer agent, methotrexate (MTX) is an antifolate with a potent immunosuppressive action. MTX has a structure similar to the folates and uses the same mechanisms of transport to cross the membrane. In particular, two mechanisms have been identified:
- via a low affinity transporter; and
- via a folate-binding-protein (FBP) associated with the cell membrane.

In addition, MTX can also passively cross the membrane.

MTX has numerous enzymatic targets. The inhibition of dihydro-folate reductase (DHFR) is the primary mechanism of suppression of

pyrimidine synthesis. Inhibition of pyrimidine synthesis by MTX also occurs through the suppression of another enzyme, thymidylate synthase. Furthermore, MTX inhibits the de-novo synthesis of purines. Therefore, the immunosuppressive effect of MTX is mostly the result of suppression of pyrimidine and purine synthesis. With regard to the anti-inflammatory effect, it has been shown that MTX reduces the chemotaxis of neutrophils, inhibits the synthesis of leukotriene B4 and reduces the synthesis of IL-1. Finally, it has been shown that MTX induces apoptosis of activated but not resting CD4 and CD8 T lymphocytes (see Table PP40.2).

Monoclonal antibodies

Antilymphocyte antibodies are important therapeutic tools in the field of immunosuppression and transplantation. A major limitation of these agents is their lack of specificity and their partial efficacy. Another issue of serious concern is the toxicity profile with an increased risk for opportunistic infections and malignancies. On the basis of these limitations, polyclonal antibodies have been progressively replaced by the development of a series of monoclonal antibodies.

Numerous 'biologicals' are in development or in use in the field of oncology and rheumatology, such as abatacept (cytotoxic T-lymphocyte antigen-4 immunoglobulin) or tocilizumab (anti-IL-6 receptor). It is probably too early to establish the clinical safety of very new agents.[6] Currently, only a few are clinically relevant in transplantation and inflammatory diseases: anti-IL2 antibodies, inhibitors of tumor necrosis factor (TNF), rituximab and alemtuzumab.

Table PP40.2 Immunosuppressive drugs: mechanisms of action, indications and related adverse events

Immunosuppressive agents	Mechanisms of action	Indications for treatment	Infectious adverse events	Other significant adverse events
Glucocorticoids (GC)	Changes in circulating leukocyte populations (lymphocytopenia, monocytopenia, neutrophilia, eosinophilopenia, basophilopenia), Inhibition of synthesis of cytokines and proinflammatory molecules Inhibition of synthesis of the IL-2 receptor Suppression of Ag presentation by causing a reduction of expression of MHC molecules on the surface of APC Inhibition of lymphocyte proliferation by suppression of IL-2 production	Severe allergic reaction, inflammatory diseases, autoimmune diseases (connectivitis and vasculitis)	Gram-positive bacteria (*Staphylococcus aureus*, *Nocardia* spp., *Listeria monocytogenes*) Gram-negative bacteria (*Legionella pneumophila*, *Klebsiella pneumoniae*, *Pseudomonas* spp. or *Salmonella* spp.) Mycobacterial, fungal (*Pneumocystis jirovecii*, *Aspergillus fumigatus* and different types of *Candida* spp.) and viral infections	Metabolic diseases (osteoporosis, steroid-induced diabetes) Hormonal dysfunction Increase of cardiovascular risk factors (hypertension, dyslipidemia, diabetes) Changes in behavior Cataract Skin atrophy and striae rubrae distensae Gastrointestinal bleeding
Alkylating agents				
Cyclophosphamide (CYC)	Alkylation of purines within the DNA and RNA (the ultimate result is cell death due to a loss of the ability to divide)	Cyclophosphamide is largely used in the treatment of autoimmune and rheumatic diseases (severe manifestations of connectivitis or vasculitis)	Bacterial (*Staph. aureus*, *K. pneumoniae*), fungal (*Candida albicans*) and viral infections (herpes zoster)	Hematologic toxicity (myelodysplastic syndrome) and oncogenicity (bladder carcinoma) due to its antiproliferative and mutagenic properties Toxicity of CYC is dependent on dosage and duration of treatment (cumulative dose)
Immunophilin binding agents				
Calcineurin inhibitors				
Ciclosporin (CsA)	Lipophilic undecapeptide reversible inhibitor of T-cell activation that acts by interfering with calcineurin and thus IL-2 synthesis and release	Solid organ transplantation	Due to the selective immunosuppressive effects on T lymphocytes, infectious complications associated with immunophilin binding agents are predominantly caused by viral and fungal infections (see Table PP40.1)	Increased risk for cancer (lymphomas) directly related to EBV The incidence of post-transplant lymphoproliferative disease (PTLD) is caused by an EBV primary infection and depends on the intensity of immunosuppressive treatment (spontaneous regression of PTLD following the decrease of the intensity of immunosuppression) Renal toxicity and hypertension (CsA) can be explained on the basis of increased activity of the endothelin-converting enzyme that causes increased production of endothelin-1 (ET-1), a vasopressive and proinflammatory peptide. Neurotoxicity (tacrolimus)
Tacrolimus (FK-506)	Binds to immunophilins and in particular to the FK-506 binding proteins (FKBP) Although CsA and tacrolimus bind to different proteins, their mechanism of action is very similar since tacrolimus also inhibits calcineurin; however, it is 10- to 100-fold more potent than CsA	Occasionally used in the treatment of autoimmune and rheumatic diseases		

mTOR inhibitors

Agent	Mechanism	Indication	Infectious complications	Toxicity
Rapamycin (sirolimus) Everolimus	Sirolimus binds to the FKBP. However, the sirolimus/FKBP complex does not bind calcineurin but binds to a protein called the mammalian target of sirolimus (mTOR) that regulates the translation of mRNA necessary for cell division. A derivative of sirolimus (everolimus) has recently been developed	Solid organ transplantation	Since these agents are often used in combination with other classes of immunosuppressive agent, it is difficult to identify infectious complications specific for a particular class of immunosuppressors. Two viral infections, CMV and BK virus, are thought to be strictly related to immunosuppressive treatment with CsA or tacrolimus. Some studies have shown a lower incidence of CMV infection using sirolimus compared to other immunosuppressive regimens. Sirolimus has *in-vitro* antifungal activity (especially against *Cryptococcus neoformans*)	Although the immunosuppressive potency of sirolimus is very similar to that of CsA and FK-506, the toxicity profile is different. Sirolimus and everolimus toxicity includes hyperlipidemia, thrombocytopenia, delayed wound healing, mouth ulcers and pulmonary toxicity (interstitial pneumonitis). Sirolimus and everolimus may have antineoplastic effects

Inhibitors of nucleotide synthesis

Agent	Mechanism	Indication	Infectious complications	Toxicity
Azathioprine (AZA)	AZA and its metabolite, 6 mercaptopurine (6-MP), belong to the class of thiopurines. The targets of these drugs are the enzymes involved in the *de novo* synthesis of purines. In this way, AZA inhibits DNA replication in dividing cells including lymphocytes	Originally used in the field of transplantation, AZA has been progressively replaced by more potent purine inhibitors such as mycophenolate mofetil (MMF, see below). AZA is particularly effective against the hematologic, pulmonary and skin manifestations of autoimmune and rheumatic diseases	Infectious complications associated with AZA are predominantly caused by viruses (particularly Herpesviridae) and to a lesser extent by fungi and parasites, mostly observed in the field of renal transplantation. The most common infectious complication is CMV infection. Patients >60 years old represent an important risk factor for infectious complications during immunosuppressive therapy	Major side-effects are bone marrow suppression, hepatitis and infections. *Note:* Moderate severity of the toxicity profile of AZA, which rarely requires interruption of treatment, is rapidly reversed by the cessation of treatment. Severe bone marrow suppression has been reported in patients with concomitant treatment with allopurinol. Safely administered during pregnancy. No evidence for increased risk of malignancies
Mycophenolate mofetil (MMF)	Highly selective noncompetitive inhibitor of inosine monophosphate dehydrogenase, an enzyme involved in the *de novo* synthesis of guanosine nucleotides. The dual effect on T and B lymphocytes is responsible for the infectious complications associated with MMF therapy	Predominantly used in the field of solid organ transplantation. Occasionally used in the treatment of autoimmune and rheumatic diseases (lupus nephritis)	Frequency of CMV infection has been reported to be greater in patients receiving high (>3g/day) doses of MMF. In patients treated with MMF, but receiving aciclovir or ganciclovir anti-CMV prophylaxis, the incidence of CMV infection was not increased. MMF has potent *in-vitro* activity against *P. jirovecii*	Hematologic adverse events (thrombocytopenia) and gastrointestinal intolerance have been described

(Continued)

Table PP40.2 Immunosuppressive drugs: mechanisms of action, indications and related adverse events—cont'd

Immunosuppressive agents	Mechanisms of action	Indications for treatment	Infectious adverse events	Other significant adverse events
Methotrexate (MTX)	Antifolate agent with a potent immunosuppressive action MTX inhibits the *de novo* synthesis of purines by blocking the enzymatic activity of the 5-amino-imidazole-4-carboxamide-ribonucleotide transformylase (AICAR) The immunosuppressive effect of MTX is mostly the result of suppression of pyrimidine and purine synthesis The anti-inflammatory properties of MTX reduce the chemotaxis of neutrophils, inhibit the synthesis of leukotriene B4 and reduce the synthesis of IL-1	MTX at higher dosage (100–1000 mg/m^2 per cycle) has been extensively used in the field of oncology At lower doses (5–25 mg/week) it is essentially used as an anti-inflammatory agent and as an immunomodulator in the treatment of autoimmune diseases (rheumatoid arthritis) MTX together with CsA or FK-506 is used in the treatment of graft-versus-host disease	Infectious complications: upper respiratory tract infections, urinary tract infections	Severe liver and lung (interstitial pneumonitis) toxicity has been described in patients treated with MTX In addition, the defect in folate concentrations caused by MTX may be responsible for severe toxic effects such as myelosuppression, hepatotoxicity and diarrhea. These latter toxic effects can in part be prevented or controlled by the administration of folic or folinic acid which competes with the activity of MTX
Leflunomide	Inhibitor of the *de novo* pyrimidine synthesis	Used in the treatment of rheumatoid arthritis Efficacy and toxicity are comparable to those of MTX	Infectious complications affecting the upper respiratory tract; they are generally more frequent during the first year of treatment but only exceptionally cause interruption of therapy Leflunomide has *in-vitro* activity against CMV and BK virus, although its clinical use for CMV infection and BK virus-associated nephropathy has not yet been established	The most commonly reported adverse events are diarrhea, nausea, alopecia, headaches and elevation of LFTs
Monoclonal antibodies				
Anti-IL-2 receptor antibodies				
Basiliximab (BSL) Daclizumab (DCZ)	Antibodies directed against the α chain of IL-2R (anti-CD25 antibodies) BSL is a chimeric antibody that contains less than 10% murine sequences while DCZ is a humanized antibody	The primary goal of using anti-IL-2R antibody in the field of transplantation is to reduce the incidence of acute graft rejection and the dose of the other immunosuppressive agents	No increased risk for viral and bacterial infections has been reported	Therapy with IL-2R antibody is extremely safe and well tolerated

Inhibitors of tumor necrosis factor (TNF)			
Infliximab Etanercept Adalimumab	Infliximab is a chimeric (human/mouse) monoclonal antibody directed against TNF Etanercept is the human recombinant form of the soluble TNF receptor Adalimumab is a recombinant human IgG1 anti-TNF monoclonal antibody	Particularly used in rheumatoid arthritis (all), and in Crohn's disease (infliximab) Very effective in vasculitis like Behçet's syndrome and uveitis (infliximab)	Mycobacterial infections are commonly associated with the blocking of TNF activity especially with infliximab (re-activation of latent tuberculosis) Other infections associated with TNF inhibitor include those caused by *P. jirovecii herpes*, *Legionella* and *Listeria monocytogenes* There is an increased risk of fungal infections, such as invasive aspergillosis, especially in patients treated with anti-TNF monoclonal antibodies	Systemic (infliximab) or urticarial (etanercept) reactions rarely require interruption of treatment
Rituximab (anti-CD20)	Human/mouse chimeric monoclonal antibody that targets the B-cell CD20 antigen and causes rapid, long-term (2–9 months) specific B-cell depletion	Several reports of efficacy in rheumatoid arthritis, lupus nephritis, cryoglobulinemic vasculitis, pemphigus and Sjögren's syndrome	Uncommon. Bacterial (including sepsis, rarely), fungal and viral infections	Cytokine release syndrome (first administration), hypersensitivity syndrome B-cell depletion Occasionally, serum sickness (arthralgia, malaise, fever)
Alemtuzumab (Campath-1H)	Humanized CD52-specific complement fixing IgG1 monoclonal antibody The human CD52 antigen is found in variable concentrations on peripheral blood mononuclear cells Alemtuzumab especially depletes T cells, but also has a major effect on B cells, natural killer cells, monocytes and dendritic cells In summary, it has a very profound immunosuppressive effect	Initially used in oncology, alemtuzumab is actually not indicated for transplantation. However, it has been assessed as induction therapy in clinical trials in order to prevent acute rejection, and to avoid infectious complications by decreasing dosages of other immunosuppressive therapies (e.g. calcineurin inhibitors and steroids)	In very recently published studies, the most frequent infection was BK virus nephropathy, followed by fungal and CMV infections; mycobacterial infections were also observed. However, these rates were similar to rates reported with other regimens	Reported side-effects include profound thrombocytopenia and lymphopenia

APC, antigen-presenting cells; CMV, cytomegalovirus; EBV, Epstein–Barr virus; MHC, major histocompatibility complex.

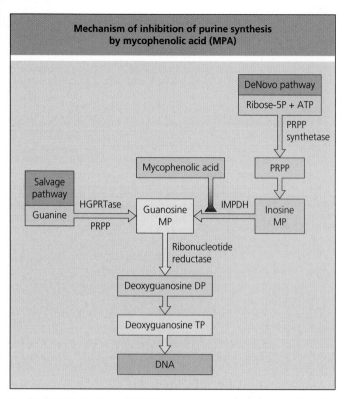

Fig. PP40.3 Mechanism of inhibition of purine synthesis by mycophenolic acid. HGPRTase, hypoxanthine–guanine phosphoribosyltransferase; IMPDH, inosine monophosphate dehydrogenase; PRPP, 5-phosphoribosyl-1(a)-pyrophosphate; ribose-5P, D-ribose-5'-phosphate.

Anti-interleukin-2 receptor antibodies

Interleukin (IL)-2 is a major T-cell growth factor necessary for the expansion of T lymphocytes following antigen-specific stimulation that represents a fundamental step in the generation of the T-cell-mediated immune response. Monoclonal antibodies have been raised against the α chain of the IL-2 receptor (IL-2R) (anti-CD25 antibody) to interfere with the initial expansion of T lymphocytes (see Table PP40.2). Anti-IL-2R monoclonal antibody formulations for clinical use have been developed in order to interfere with the initial expansion of T lymphocytes. These antibodies are directed against the α chain of the IL-2R.

Inhibitors of tumor necrosis factor

Tumor necrosis factor is a potent cytokine and a primary mediator of inflammatory reactions. Tumor necrosis factor plays a central role in many inflammatory diseases including inflammatory bowel and rheumatic diseases.[6] Several studies have demonstrated the fundamental role of TNF in the pathogenesis of rheumatoid arthritis (RA). Transgenic mice with a deregulation of the TNF gene develop a destructive arthritis similar to RA. In addition to RA, TNF is clearly implicated in the pathogenesis of juvenile rheumatoid and psoriatic arthritis and Crohn's disease.

Two specific classes of inhibitors of TNF function have been developed: infliximab and adalimumab, and etanercept. Infliximab is a chimeric (human/mouse) monoclonal antibody directed against TNF. The F_c portion of infliximab is a human IgG_1 while the antigen-binding variable domain that has a high affinity for human TNF is of murine origin. Adalimumab is a recombinant human IgG_1 anti-TNF monoclonal antibody. Etanercept is the human recombinant form of the soluble TNF receptor. It is a dimerized fusion protein formed by an extracellular domain of the TNF type II receptor (p75) and by the F_c portion of a human IgG_1. The mechanism of action of etanercept is the blocking of soluble and membrane-bound TNF and of lymphotoxin α.

Mycobacterial infections are commonly associated with the blocking of TNF activity, especially with infliximab administration. In the majority of cases, re-activation of latent tuberculosis has been observed. On the basis of these complications, the current guidelines for the therapeutic use of TNF inhibitors indicate that a purified protein derivative test or QuantiFERON-TB test should be performed before the initiation of treatment. The QuantiFERON-TB test (which measures the production of IFN-γ after incubation of whole blood with mycobacterial peptides) has recently been approved by the US Food and Drug Administration (FDA). In the case of a positive test without other signs of re-activation of the disease, treatment with isoniazid is advised before and during administration of infliximab. The number of cases of re-activation of tuberculosis seems to be less important following treatment with etanercept.[7]

Rituximab

Initially used in the treatment of non-Hodgkin's lymphoma (NHL), administration of anti-CD20 monoclonal antibodies is currently indicated in numerous rheumatologic (e.g. rheumatoid arthritis) and autoimmune diseases with predominant B-lymphocyte pathogenesis (systemic lupus erythematosus, Sjögren's disease, cryoglobulinemia, pemphigus, etc.). This antibody can cause prolonged depletion of B-cell responses, putting patients at risk for a variety of systemic bacterial and viral infections.[8]

CONCLUSIONS

Major advances have been made in the last two decades in the understanding of fundamental immunoregulatory mechanisms, in the development of novel immunosuppressive agents and in the prevention of infectious complications associated with immunosuppressive therapy. The future goals in the field of immunosuppression should include improvement in the management of infectious complications and the development of novel and more selective agents. The generation of highly selective agents is the only valid strategy to maximize immunosuppressive effects and minimize immunodeficiency.

REFERENCES

References for this chapter can be found online at http://www.expertconsult.com

Preventing tuberculosis and other serious infections in patients starting anti-tumor necrosis factor therapy

Therapies that inhibit tumor necrosis factor (TNF) have shown remarkable clinical efficacy against rheumatoid arthritis (RA), Crohn's disease, psoriasis, ankylosing spondylitis and other autoimmune diseases. Three anti-TNF compounds in current clinical use are infliximab, etanercept and adalimumab. Their use is now widespread, particularly in RA where over 40% of patients have been treated with such drugs. As a group, these drugs inhibit TNF, a proinflammatory cytokine involved in the pathogenesis of RA and other autoimmune diseases, but also integral to the host's innate immune system.[1–3]

TUMOR NECROSIS FACTOR AND ITS IMMUNE FUNCTION

Tumor necrosis factor is a proinflammatory cytokine expressed by activated immune cells in response to a variety of pathogens. It mediates systemic inflammatory responses via two cellular receptors (p55 and p75). TNF plays a crucial role in the host response against a variety of infections, in particular *Mycobacterium tuberculosis* (TB) and other intracellular pathogens,[1] as it stimulates inflammatory cell recruitment to areas of infection and the formation of granulomas that contain infection. In addition, TNF directly activates macrophages to phagocytose and kill mycobacteria and numerous other pathogens. In animal models, mice deficient in TNF or its p55 signaling pathway are highly susceptible to *Listeria monocytogenes*, *Histoplasma capsulatum* and numerous other pathogens including extracellular bacterial organisms like *Klebsiella pneumoniae* and *Streptococcus pneumoniae*.[1–3]

CURRENT ANTI-TNF DRUGS AND THEIR DIFFERENTIAL PROPERTIES

Infliximab and adalimumab are monoclonal antibodies, while etanercept is a soluble immunofusion construct of the p75 receptor. Infliximab is delivered as an infusion every 4–8 weeks. Adalimumab (given every 2 weeks) and etanercept (given weekly) are delivered by subcutaneous injection.[4] All three agents bind TNF, but important differences exist between these drug types with regard to their modulation of TNF activity. Compared with etanercept, infliximab binds TNF with greater avidity and for a longer duration. The half-life of infliximab is approximately 10.5 days and its biologic effect can persist for up to 2 months. Etanercept's half-life is 3 days and it binds TNF in a reversible manner, with disassociation of nearly 50% after only 10 minutes. These differences, coupled with differences in dosing, suggest that infliximab has greater, more sustained inhibition of TNF activity. Pharmacokinetically, adalimumab behaves similarly to infliximab. Further, infliximab and adalimumab appear to downregulate interferon gamma (IFN-γ) responses more than etanercept. In addition, it is anticipated that two new anti-TNF compounds, golimumab and certolizumab, will receive FDA approval prior to this chapter's publication.

Serious infections associated with anti-TNF agents

Infections from a variety of organisms have been reported in patients using these agents: *Coccidioides*, *Listeria*, *Histoplasma*, *Aspergillus*, *Nocardia* spp., nontuberculous mycobacteria (Fig. PP41.1), streptococci, *Staphylococcal aureus* and others.[2,3] Of serious concern is the development of active tuberculosis (TB) in some patients receiving these drugs. Similar to HIV-infected patients who develop TB, patients using anti-TNF compounds frequently present 'atypically' with extrapulmonary or disseminated disease. Accordingly, TNF antagonists should be used with caution in any person with risk factors for TB, and screening for latent TB infection (LTBI) should be undertaken before starting anti-TNF therapy.[3]

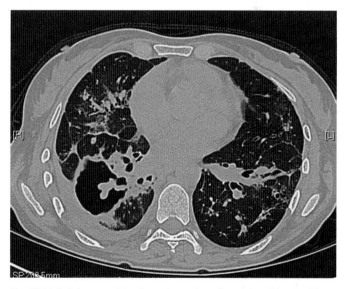

Fig. PP41.1 Pulmonary *Mycobacterium avium* disease in a 57-year-old female with rheumatoid arthritis treated with anti-TNF agents (courtesy of Dr. Michael Iseman). Chest CT shows extensive pulmonary parenchymal destruction and cavitation due to *M. avium* disease, first diagnosed while the patient was receiving infliximab. She subsequently initiated antimycobacterial therapy, briefly received adalimumab without good clinical response, and then continued to use etanercept for 1 year. Despite antimycobacterial therapy, her pulmonary disease continued to progress.

PREVENTION OF TUBERCULOSIS DURING ANTI-TNF THERAPY

Patients with latent TB are at risk for reactivation and progression to disease when exposed to anti-TNF therapy.[4] The risk depends upon the population studied and is greater in patient groups with higher background TB prevalence rates. This complication can be prevented by screening patients for LTBI and initiating preventive TB therapy prior to anti-TNF initiation. The usefulness of this screening, and the methodologies employed, vary by regional differences in TB prevalence and the usage of bacille Calmette–Guérin (BCG) vaccination, which can interfere with the interpretation of the tuberculin skin test (TST). BCG is known to cause false-positive skin tests, and in regions of low TB prevalence is likely responsible for a majority of positive TSTs where BCG is used. This is particularly true when interpreting TST positivity using a lower cut-off (i.e. 5 mm in the setting of immunosuppression).

Recently, new blood-based assays have been developed to detect latent TB infection. These tests, IFN-γ release assays (IGRAs), have a distinct advantage over the TST as they utilize proteins from the RD-1 genome of *M. tuberculosis*, a region that is not contained in BCG. Accordingly, this test is highly specific for *M. tuberculosis* and does not appear to be influenced by BCG vaccination.[5] In areas of high BCG usage, the IGRA reduces the false-positive TST results due to BCG. Some countries have adopted the IGRA as a preferred strategy in screening patients for LTBI in this setting. In other regions positive TST results are further evaluated with an IGRA if the patient has a history of BCG.

The relative sensitivities of TSTs and IGRAs for the diagnosis of LTBI in the anti-TNF setting have yet to be adequately studied. In patients with active TB disease, IGRAs have greater sensitivity, but relative performance is unknown in LTBI where there is no gold standard. Immunocompromised patients are more likely to have false-negative TST results, and similarly might also have false-negative or indeterminate IGRA results. Several small case series of patients receiving anti-TNF therapy suggest that the two methodologies might have at least similar sensitivities, and emerging evidence from other immunocompromised patients suggest that the IGRA might be more sensitive. Presently the US Public Health service recommends using IGRAs in any situation where the TST is employed.

SCREENING FOR LATENT TUBERCULOSIS BEFORE ADMINISTRATING ANTI-TNF THERAPY

Given the regional and national differences in TB prevalence, BCG usage and the potential usefulness of IGRAs in this setting, it is not surprising that screening guidance differs by region. Several points are worth emphasizing in screening[4] (Table PP41.1). The importance of taking a detailed history for TB risk factors cannot be understated. Patients born in or with a history of living in countries of high TB prevalence are at much higher risk for TB in this setting, and the positive predictive value of a TST or IGRA result is accordingly increased. Second, a 5 mm cut-off point should be used to define a positive TST result in these patients, as in other immunosuppressed hosts. Screening patients using both IGRAs and TSTs may be reasonable, with the knowledge that both tests have certain caveats and potential flaws. Chest radiography should be used to screen for active TB in any patient suspected to have LTBI.[5,6]

TREATMENT OF LATENT TUBERCULOSIS INFECTION

For patients with suspected LTBI, the presence of active TB disease should be excluded with appropriate diagnostic studies (i.e. sputum culture or other respiratory sampling). A 9-month course of daily therapy with isoniazid (INH) is the preferred treatment. One approach to treating patients with LTBI is to administer INH for at least 1 month prior to initiating anti-TNF therapy. This is to ensure that patients are taking and tolerating INH. Given the low bacillary load of LTBI, this recommendation seems reasonable and is based on the observational experience of Spanish investigators who adopted such a protocol and

---

Table PP41.1 Recommendations for screening, diagnosis and treatment of latent tuberculosis infection and tuberculosis in patients administered or scheduled to receive tumor necrosis factor (TNF) antagonists

- Screen patients for risk factors for *Mycobacterium tuberculosis* and test them for infection before initiating immunosuppressive therapies, including TNF antagonists. Risk factors include birth or extended living in a country where TB is prevalent, or history of any of the following:
  – residence in a congregate setting (e.g. jail or prison, homeless shelter or chronic-care facility)
  – a positive tuberculin skin test (TST) result
  – substance abuse (injection or noninjection)
  – health-care employment in settings with TB patients
  – chest radiographic findings consistent with previous TB.
- Utilize diagnostic aids in LTBI screening including the TST and/or interferon gamma release assays (IGRAs).
- Diagnosis and treatment of latent TB infection (LTBI) and TB disease should be in accordance with published guidelines.
- In patients who are immunocompromised (e.g. because of therapy or other medical conditions), interpret a TST induration of ≥5 mm as a positive result and evidence of *M. tuberculosis* infection.
- Interpret a TST induration of <5 mm as a negative result but not an exclusion for *M. tuberculosis* infection.
- Anergy panel testing is not recommended. Results from control-antigen skin testing (e.g. *Candida*) should not alter the interpretation of a negative TST result.
- Test to exclude TB disease before starting treatment for LTBI.
- Start treatment for LTBI before commencing TNF-blocking agents, preferably with 9 months of daily isoniazid.
- Consider treatment for LTBI in patients who have negative TST results but whose epidemiologic and clinical circumstances suggest a probability of LTBI.
- Pursue TB disease as a potential cause of febrile or respiratory illness in all patients receiving TNF-blocking agents.
- Consider postponement of TNF-antagonist therapy until the conclusion of treatment for LTBI or TB disease if possible. If not clinically possible, withhold TNF-antagonist therapy until the patient has demonstrated LTBI treatment adherence and tolerance, or in the case of TB disease, until the patient has shown adherence to appropriate anti-TB drugs to which their organism is known to be sensitive.

From Winthrop KL *et al.*, Arthritis Rheum 2005;52:2968–74.

subsequently saw an 85% reduction in TB cases associated with inflix- imab. A 4-month course of rifampin (rifampicin)-based therapy could be considered an alternative in patients who cannot tolerate 9 months of INH. While INH-related hepatotoxicity is not common, it should be monitored closely in those patients receiving methotrexate or other hepatotoxic drugs. Liver function testing should be performed at base- line and then periodically (e.g. monthly) in all such patients.

ANTI-TNF THERAPY AND OTHER SERIOUS INFECTIONS

Dimorphic fungal infections

Histoplasma capsulatum is an endemic fungus in many areas of the world, and is the second most commonly reported pathogen in association with TNF blockade.[2] Like TB, it can exist in a latent or slowly progressive state, and can progress to active disease, particularly during immuno- suppression. The role of routine serologic monitoring for prior evidence of histoplasmosis before starting an anti-TNF inhibitor is unclear and the value of empiric antifungal therapy is unknown. Currently, rou- tine serologic testing for histoplasmosis is not recommended in HIV- infected persons and recommendations about such screening or use of preventive therapy for histoplasmosis await further clinical study.

Coccidioides immitis is endemic to the southwestern US, Central and South America. Like *Histoplasma* spp., it too can exist in a latent or sub- clinical infectious state after exposure, and can later progress to disease during immunosuppression. Patients in endemic areas could poten- tially be screened with serology prior to initiation of TNF blockade. However, given that most of the coccidioidomycosis cases reported in association with TNF blockade are cases of acute infection, and not reactivation, the usefulness of pre-treatment serologic screening is unclear.

Bacterial pathogens

Listeria monocytogenes is an opportunistic, intracellular pathogen and fatal cases of listeriosis have occurred in persons taking TNF-blocking agents. Patients under TNF blockade should be advised to avoid raw meat, delicatessen meat and unpasteurized milk products.

Serious infections and death due to extracellular pathogens such as *Staph. aureus* and *Strep. pneumoniae* have also been reported in the anti-TNF setting. There are murine models suggesting that anti- TNF therapy could worsen such infections, and observational stud- ies suggest that serious bacterial infections (e.g. community-acquired pneumonia, skin/soft tissue infection, osteomyelitis) are elevated in patients receiving these therapies. Anti-TNF-treated patients are at increased risk of chronic furunculosis caused by *Staph. aureus*. Screening these patients for colonization and attempting to decol- onize them before anti-TNF therapy seems reasonable, yet no con- trolled studies have as yet clarified the value of this approach. With

regard to *Strep. pneumoniae*, it is widely recommended that patients receive 23-valent pneumococcal polysaccharide vaccine prior to ini- tiating these therapies. Vaccine immunogenicity can be diminished by methotrexate; if possible, therefore, patients should be vaccinated while not receiving this drug.

Other pathogens and perioperative infections

Anti-TNF products can reactivate or worsen hepatitis B. Prior to therapy, patients should be screened for hepatitis B and anti-TNF therapy should generally be avoided in infected patients. In contrast, for patients with chronic hepatitis C infection, it is thought that anti-TNF therapy might be used safely, albeit with caution and careful attention to hepatic enzymes. The development of herpes zoster might be slightly more common in patients using anti-TNF therapies, although there are conflicting data in this regard and any elevation in risk is likely small. Several small, retrospec- tive case series reported no increase in perioperative infection risk. Recently, however, two larger retrospective studies suggest a small increase in wound infections after orthopedic procedures and a delay in wound healing in patients who continued anti-TNF drugs. It seems prudent to discontinue anti-TNF therapy several weeks before surgery (depending on the drug's half-life), if possible, until the patient's surgical wounds are healed.[7,8]

Immune reconstitution inflammatory syndrome

The risk of immune reconstitution inflammatory syndrome (IRIS) upon discontinuation of anti-TNF therapy in patients with tuberculo- sis deserves mention. While it seems prudent to discontinue anti-TNF therapy when a patient is diagnosed with TB, it is unclear whether this is necessary or even beneficial to the patient, presuming the patient is receiving an appropriate multidrug anti-TB therapeutic regimen. There are case reports of IRIS occurring in TB patients in whom anti-TNF therapy was stopped,[7] and there is very limited evidence that concur- rent therapy of TB with anti-TNF compounds might be safe. Further, if anti-TNF therapy is stopped, there are no data to suggest when it is safe to resume such therapy. Generally it is appropriate to stop anti-TNF therapy when TB is diagnosed and remain vigilant for IRIS. Anti-TNF therapy can be resumed after the patient has demonstrable clinical improvement during an effective anti-TB regimen.

REFERENCES

References for this chapter can be found online at http://www.expertconsult.com

Lora D Thomas
J Stephen Dummer

Practice point | **42** |

Infectious diseases transmitted by grafts

INTRODUCTION

Recipients of transplants face two threats for infection not experienced by other surgical patients. One threat arises from the immunosuppression related to antirejection medications and the patient's underlying organ disease. The other threat arises from the multitude of pathogens that may be transmitted by the donor graft. Table PP42.1 presents a list of organisms that have been transmitted during transplantation.

BACTERIAL PATHOGENS

Donors may have bacterial infections at the time of organ procurement, either latent or symptomatic. Urinary infections in donors can cause graft infections in kidney recipients, particularly if the donor is infected with more virulent organisms such as *Staphylococcus aureus* and Gram-negative rods. Cadaveric donors are intubated and, as a result, nearly half will have evidence of airway or lung colonization. This issue is most pertinent in regards to lung transplant recipients,

Table PP42.1 Donor-transmitted pathogens

Bacteria	Urinary and pulmonary pathogens (*Staphylococcus aureus* and Gram-negative rods) *Mycobacterium tuberculosis* *Treponema pallidum* (syphilis)
Viruses	Herpesviruses (cytomegalovirus, herpes simplex virus, Epstein–Barr virus, human herpesvirus 6, 8) Hepatitis viruses (hepatitis B, C) Retroviruses (HIV-1, -2, human T-cell lymphotropic virus 1) Rhabdoviruses (rabies virus) Flaviviruses (West Nile virus) Arenaviruses (lymphocytic choriomeningitis virus)
Fungi	*Candida* spp. *Aspergillus* spp. *Histoplasma capsulatum* *Coccidioides immitis*
Parasites	*Toxoplasma gondii* *Trypanosoma cruzi* *Plasmodium* spp. *Strongyloides stercoralis*
Prions	Creutzfeldt–Jakob disease

and tailored antimicrobial therapy should be administered to the lung recipient in the setting of a positive donor sputum or bronchoalveolar lavage (BAL) culture. Most systemic bacterial infections in donors, such as bacteremia or meningitis, are not a contraindication for organ transplantation provided that the donor infection has been brought under control by appropriate antibiotics prior to organ procurement and the recipient is also treated after transplantation.

Transmission of *Mycobacterium tuberculosis* from a donor does occur; in one large series it accounted for 4% of post-transplant *M. tuberculosis* infections. Screening with tuberculin skin testing (TST) is recommended for living donors. As performing TST in cadaveric donors is not feasible, obtaining a history from the donor's relatives regarding previous active infection or exposure to tuberculosis is crucial. Prophylaxis in the recipient is generally recommended if the donor has a positive skin test or had a history of untreated active or latent tuberculosis.

VIRAL PATHOGENS

Herpesviruses are the most common and significant infectious agents encountered after transplantation. Herpesviruses cause persistent latent infections in their host and are efficiently transmitted during transplantation. Donor-transmitted infections of herpesviruses are most problematic if the recipient is seronegative, because a lack of immunity confers an opportunity for more severe or invasive disease. This phenomenon is true for many of the herpesviruses including cytomegalovirus (CMV), herpes simplex virus (HSV) and Epstein–Barr virus (EBV). Prophylaxis with antivirals in these individuals can dramatically reduce the risk of disease associated with these viruses. Transmission of other herpesviruses such as HHV-6 and -8 has also been described.

The risk of transmission of hepatitis B virus is greatest in donors with clear evidence of active infection, usually identified by either a positive surface antigen (HBsAg) or core IgM antibody (HBcIgM). The risk associated with receiving a graft from a donor who is positive for IgG antibody to core antigen (HBcIgG), but negative for HBsAg and HBcIgM is less clear, but can partially be predicted by the organ that is transplanted and the immune status of the recipient. Roughly half of all liver recipients will acquire hepatitis B infection from an HBcIgG-positive donor, while the transmission rate is low (<3%) for other solid-organ recipients. Pre-existing immunity in the recipient, either by vaccination or previous infection, reduces the risk of transmission. Donors who only have a positive surface antibody (HBsAb) are considered low risk for transmission. Donors are screened for hepatitis C virus (HCV) and organs from seropositive donors are usually rejected because the risk of transmission is high (roughly 50%), even in non-liver recipients. Organs from HCV-positive donors, however, are sometimes utilized in recipients who are severely ill or already seropositive for HCV.

Several cases of transmission of retroviruses, including human T-cell lymphotropic virus 1 (HTLV-1) and HIV, have been documented in transplant recipients. HTLV-1 can cause adult T-cell lymphoma/leukemia and tropical spastic paraparesis and myelopathy. Both diseases have been described in transplant recipients, who may have acquired their infection during transplantation, or from blood transfusions or hemodialysis. HTLV-1 infections are most prevalent in the Caribbean isles and in Southern Japan; there are also pockets of infection in parts of Africa, Asia and South America. Most reported cases of HIV transmission from organ donation occurred before 1985 when donor screening was first implemented. The transmission of HIV from an HIV-seronegative donor is rare. In reported cases, the donors were likely recently infected and in the early window of infection, usually in the first 2–8 weeks, when HIV antibodies are still undetectable. Most recently in 2007, four organ transplant recipients in Chicago acquired both HIV and hepatitis C from a seronegative donor. Cases like these have sparked increased interest in utilizing molecular methods, such as nucleic acid testing (NAT), to identify donors during the early window of infection when viremia is present, but antibodies have not yet developed. Such methods can potentially reduce the window period in detecting acute donor infections to 1–2 weeks.

In the past few years, cases of donor-transmitted rabies virus and West Nile virus have received attention. In 2004, four organ and tissue recipients with a common donor developed encephalitis within 30 days of transplantation. The donor died from a subarachnoid hemorrhage. All four recipients expired and had Negri bodies seen in brain tissue; three of the four had detectable antibodies against rabies virus. An investigation disclosed that the donor had told acquaintances of a bat bite. A similar episode of rabies transmission from an organ donor occurred in Germany. Rabies transmission has also been described after corneal transplantation. Four transplant recipients acquired West Nile virus infection from their common donor and three subsequently developed encephalitis within weeks of transplantation. The donor had been infected from a blood transfusion. Blood banks now screen for West Nile virus using a nucleic acid test. Routine testing of donors for West Nile virus or rabies virus is not recommended, but organ or tissue transplantation from a donor with an unexplained viral illness and encephalopathy should be avoided.

Lymphocytic choriomeningitis virus (LCMV) is an arenavirus usually acquired from exposure to rodents. Graft-transmitted infection with LCMV was described in two clusters of solid-organ recipients in 2003 and 2005. In all the recipients, symptoms began within 3 weeks of transplantation and included abdominal pain, mental status changes and fever. Peri-incisional erythema and pulmonary infiltrates were also encountered. Interestingly, neither of the two donors involved had laboratory evidence of infection, but prior to her death one donor had recent exposure to a pet hamster, which was infected with a LCMV genetically identical to the recipients' virus. Seven of the eight organ recipients died. One kidney recipient survived with immunosuppression reduction and ribavirin therapy. In 2008, a report from Australia described three organ recipients sharing a common donor, all of whom succumbed to a febrile, encephalopathic illness within 6 weeks of transplantation. The likely causative agent, identified using a high-throughput sequencing method, was an arenavirus closely related to LCMV.

FUNGAL PATHOGENS

Transmission of fungal infections during transplantation is rare. Donor infection with *Candida* spp., including *Candida albicans*, can be transmitted during transplantation, and has been associated with anastomotic and graft infections. Also, anastomotic infections from donor-derived *Aspergillus* colonization have been reported in lung transplantation; isolated cases of suspected *Aspergillus* acquisition from other organs (e.g. kidney) are in the literature, although risks are likely low. Transmission of endemic fungi from donor organs is also uncommon but isolated cases involving transmission of *Histoplasma capsulatum* and *Coccidioides immitis* have been documented. Since there is a high mortality rate associated with donor-transmitted coccidioidomycosis, donors from areas endemic for *C. immitis* should undergo serologic testing, and if positive, antifungal prophylaxis should be given to their organ recipients. Donor screening for *H. capsulatum* is not routinely recommended.

PARASITIC PATHOGENS

Toxoplasma gondii can be transmitted from transplanted organs, especially in heart grafts where cysts can lie dormant in myocardial tissue. Serologic screening is performed on heart and heart–lung donors prior to transplantation and prophylaxis is recommended in seronegative heart recipients who receive their graft from a seropositive donor.

Cases of donor-transmitted malaria infections, from *Plasmodium falciparum* and *Plasmodium vivax*, have been reported in solid-organ and bone marrow transplantation. Infections with *P. falciparum* usually cause earlier symptoms and parasitemia after transplantation (days) than *P. vivax* (weeks to months).

Trypanosoma cruzi is endemic in Latin America and causes Chagas disease. Five cases of donor-transmitted Chagas disease have been described in the United States (two heart, two kidney and one liver recipient). Similar to the cases involving malaria, the donors had either lived in or traveled to an endemic region. All five infected recipients were treated with nifurtimox, but one patient still succumbed to chagasic myocarditis.

PRION DISEASE

Multiple cases of Creutzfeldt–Jakob disease have been associated with cornea- and dura mater-related transplants. Transmission has not been described in solid-organ transplantation.

DONOR SCREENING

Table PP42.2 lists the current laboratory studies performed on all prospective donors, either living or cadaveric, and recommended individual measures to take in the case of a positive test. In addition to the

Table PP42.2 Donor screening

Mandatory tests of all donors	Appropriate actions in event of positive result
Rapid plasma reagin (RPR)	Prophylaxis in recipient
Cytomegalovirus serology	Depending on recipient's serology, consider prophylaxis
Epstein–Barr virus serology	Consider virologic monitoring in seronegative recipient
Hepatitis Bs Ag, core IgM	Consider use in critically ill recipient with prophylaxis
Hepatitis B, core IgG	Consider use in non-liver or immune recipient ± prophylaxis
Hepatitis Bs AB	Considered low risk
Hepatitis C serology	Consider use in critically ill recipient or seropositive recipient
HIV-1/2 serology	Avoid transplant
Human T-cell lymphotropic virus 1 and 2 serology	Avoid transplant
Toxoplasma serology	Prophylaxis in seronegative heart or heart–lung recipient
Blood cultures / Urine cultures / Bronchial alveolar lavage cultures (lung donor)	Directed antimicrobial therapy against isolated pathogen

laboratory evaluation for infection, a thorough behavioral and social questionnaire plays a crucial part in determining a donor's risk for certain transmissible pathogens. The recommendations, at present, reflect minimal requirements, with laboratory emphasis on serologic screening; currently efforts are underway to define optimal laboratory screening methodology, potentially employing sensitive platforms for nucleic acid testing, with the goal of optimizing and standardizing donor screening.

FURTHER READING

Further reading for this chapter can be found online at http://www.expertconsult.com

BK virus replication and disease in transplant patients

INTRODUCTION

The human polyomavirus type I, commonly known as BK virus (BKV), is a nonenveloped icosahedral particle of 40 nm diameter and fairly resistant to environmental inactivation.[1] Serologic studies indicate that BKV infects 60–90% of human populations worldwide during childhood without known symptoms or signs. The mode of natural transmission is unknown, but likely occurs via the oral or respiratory route. Subsequently, BKV establishes latent infection in cells of the urinary tract where the viral genome persists as a double-stranded circular DNA episome of 5 kb.

Reactivation of BKV replication is mediated by the viral noncoding control region which drives expression of the early genes consisting of the large and small T-antigen and the late genes consisting of the capsid proteins VP1, 2, 3 and the agnoprotein. Low-level asymptomatic urinary shedding is found in 5–10% of healthy non-immunosuppressed individuals ($<10^5$ genome equivalents (geq)/ml). In patients with impaired immune function, urinary shedding is more prevalent, ranging from 20% to >60%, and BKV loads are frequently $>10^7$ geq/ml.[1]

High-level BK viruria remains asymptomatic in most patients. However, BKV is linked to two major diseases, namely polyomavirus BK-associated nephropathy[2,3] and polyomavirus BK-associated hemorrhagic cystitis.[4,5] Both entities have been encountered sporadically in various types of immunodeficiency, but are consistently found after kidney and hematopoietic stem cell transplantation, respectively, suggesting the presence of specific risk factors linked to either procedure. BKV has been associated with rare cases of hemophagocytic syndrome, ureteric stenosis, pneumonitis, encephalitis, retinitis, multiorgan failure and a presentation reminiscent of progressive multifocal leukoencephalopathy.[1]

POLYOMAVIRUS-BK ASSOCIATED NEPHROPATHY

Polyomavirus-BK associated nephropathy (PVAN) has been diagnosed in 1–10% of kidney transplant recipients with a median time interval of 9 months post-transplantation.[6] Intense immunosuppression is the key risk factor synergizing with determinants of the patient (e.g. age >50 years, male gender, BKV-seronegative recipient), the graft (e.g. BKV-seropositive donor, human leukocyte antigen mismatches, ischemic or immune injury) and the virus (e.g. latent viral load, capsid serotype, rearrangement of control region, replicative fitness). The definitive diagnosis is made by demonstrating BKV replication in renal tubular epithelial cells in allograft tissues.[6] Most commonly,

the viral large T-antigen is identified by immunohistochemistry using antibodies cross-reacting with the homologous SV40 protein, but some centers use *in-situ* hybridization to detect the viral genome.

Three different histopathologic presentations have been distinguished:[6,7]

- PVAN A is defined by focal, frequently medullary BKV replication, with tubular epithelial cells with enlarged nuclei, rounding and occasionally sloughing from the basal membrane, and without significant inflammatory infiltrates. At this early stage, allograft function remains unaffected and progression to irreversible graft loss is <10%.
- PVAN B is characterized by extensive BKV replication with widespread cell necrosis, denudation of basal membranes and significant inflammatory cell infiltrates. This presentation is typically associated with impaired graft function and a 50% chance of graft loss.
- PVAN C is characterized by predominance of tubular atrophy, fibrosis and paucity of BKV replication which are associated with poor graft function and return to dialysis in >80% of cases.[6,8]

The histologic diagnosis is viewed as the gold standard for PVAN, but is challenged by:[9]

- false-negative results in 10–30% of cases of PVAN A due to the focality of BKV replication;
- confounding PVAN B and acute interstitial allograft rejection which significantly impacts on treatment and outcome;
- BKV-specific T-cell immune reconstitution after reduced immunosuppression mimicking acute rejection;
- the resemblance of PVAN C with chronic allograft nephropathy; and
- PVAN due to the closely related JC virus which appears to run a more benign course.

These limitations, together with the diverse risk factor profile and variable time of disease onset, have made the quantitative detection of BKV replication in urine and blood the pivotal tests for the management of kidney transplant patients.

As BK viruria and viremia have been demonstrated to precede the histologic PVAN diagnosis in kidney transplants by 12 weeks and 8 weeks, respectively,[2,6,9] it is recommended to screen for BKV replication in urine and plasma at least every 3 months during the first 2 years after transplantation, or if allograft dysfunction occurs prompting an allograft biopsy for a workup of BKV-associated kidney injury. The absence of BK viruria has a high negative predictive value to exclude PVAN. Confirmed BK viruria should trigger testing for BK viremia. Increasing plasma BKV loads persisting at levels greater than 4 log geq/ml for 4 weeks or longer has been used to define presumptive PVAN for which intervention should be considered, even in the absence of positive histologic findings.[6,9–12] Indeed, in patients with persisting high plasma BKV loads, BKV genomic variants emerge which are associated with higher replicative capacity and more extensive cytopathic damage.[13] Because of earlier manifestations, some centers prefer to screen bi-weekly or monthly during the first 6 months for a pre-emptive intervention strategy.

Intervention is currently based on the timely reduction of immunosuppression which needs to be tailored to the individual's transplant history and risk of rejection. Standard protocol reduction post-transplant probably clears high-level BKV replication in about a third of affected patients. Conversely, more extensive reductions are warranted in patients with persisting high-level viremia (i.e. >10^4 geq/ml) and histologically documented PVAN.[11,14] No validated protocols are available, but experts in the field recommend reducing the calcineurin inhibitor and the antiproliferative agent in documented PVAN (e.g. trough levels of tacrolimus <6 ng/ml or ciclosporin <125 μg/ml; daily dose of mycophenolate mofetil <1 g or azathioprine <75 mg).[6,15] Decline of plasma BKV loads can be expected to occur 4–12 weeks after tapering of immunosuppression and coincides with emerging BKV-specific T-cell responses to epitopes of the large T- and VP1 capsid antigens.[11,16] Thus, monitoring plasma BKV load every 2–4 weeks is generally predictive of the course of disease. Urine BKV loads usually follow plasma BKV load decline, with a variable delay of 8–16 weeks.

In cases of coexisting acute rejection, some centers have combined steroid pulse treatment with reducing maintenance immunosuppression in a second step. This presentation is associated with a more protracted course and poor outcome. The adjunct use of low-dose cidofovir[17] or switching from mycophenolate mofetil to leflunomide has been advocated.[18] However, given the long half-life and the risk of nephro-, hepato- and myelotoxicity of these drugs, randomized controlled trials are needed to demonstrate a benefit over timely reduction of maintenance immunosuppression.[19]

Re-transplantation after graft loss due to PVAN has been performed successfully, but recurrence of PVAN should be anticipated by screening for BKV replication. Allograft nephrectomy is required unless pre-emptive re-transplantation is considered. A period of reduced immunosuppression of 8–12 weeks is recommended to allow recovery of BKV-specific immune effectors prior to re-transplantation and can be correlated with clearance of BK viremia.[20]

POLYOMAVIRUS-BK ASSOCIATED HEMORRHAGIC CYSTITIS

Hemorrhagic cystitis causes significant morbidity after hematopoietic stem cell transplantation (HSCT) due to diffuse mucosal bleeding, inflammation, bladder wall thickening, immobilizing pain and progression to outright anemia and obstructive postrenal failure. The incidence of hemorrhagic cystitis ranges from <10% to >50% depending on the case definition, the conditioning regimen and the underlying etiology.[21] To distinguish hemorrhagic cystitis from mere hematuria, the symptoms of cystitis with pain and urge are required together with hematuria. Four grades of hematuria have been proposed:[4] grade I is defined as microscopic hematuria (>100 erythrocytes per high-power field), grade II as macrohematuria, grade III as macrohematuria with clots, and grade IV as macrohematuria with urinary obstruction and postrenal failure. In HSCT patients, early-onset hemorrhagic cystitis occurs pre-engraftment and has been linked to urotoxic conditioning regimens which include cyclophosphamide, ifosfamide, busulfan and/or total body irradiation.[4,5] By contrast, late-onset hemorrhagic cystitis occurs postengraftment and is associated with high-level local replication of viruses such as adenovirus, cytomegalovirus and BKV.[4]

The diagnosis of polyomavirus BK-associated hemorrhagic cystitis (PVHC) is typically made in HSCT patients with postengraftment cystitis, hematuria of grade II or higher, high-level BKV replication (i.e. >10^7 geq/ml) and exclusion of other pathogens. Histologic studies may show BKV replication in the uroepithelium, but are rarely performed during the acute stage, since urologic interventions are mostly aimed at hemostasis, clot removal and symptom management. BK viruria is not sufficient to define PVHC, since approximately 50% of HSCT recipients with BKV viruria are asymptomatic.[5] In patients with PVHC, urine BKV loads may be higher (e.g. >10^9 geq/ml) than in asymptomatic patients, but the levels frequently overlap.[22–25] Unlike in PVAN, genomic BKV variants seem to have no role in PVHC.[13,26] Recently, urine BKV loads peaking by more than 3 log increase over baseline within 2–3 weeks after onset have been proposed to correlate better with PVHC.[27] BK viremia has been detected in the plasma of one-third of HSCT recipients in the first 100 days after HSCT and sustained plasma BKV loads of 10^4 geq/ml or greater were associated with an increased risk of PVHC.[28–30] Clearly, both of the latter parameters require validation in independent prospective studies, as well as their potential to trigger pre-emptive interventions.

Risk factors for PVHC include allogeneic HSCT, acute graft-versus-host disease (GVHD), unrelated donor, myeloablative conditioning and a higher BKV recipient antibody titer pre-HSCT.[25,27,30] However, statistical significance was not reached for any of these factors in all studies. The pathogenesis of PVHC is not well understood. Late-onset PVHC postengraftment suggests a role of reconstituting immunity where BKV replication might play an important pathogenic role in the sequence of events:[1,5,31]

- damage of the uroepithelial lining by urotoxic conditioning;
- high-level BKV replication in the regenerating uroepithelial cell layer during the immunodeficient period; and
- extensive inflammation upon recovery of immunity postengraftment yielding the characteristics of PVHC.

Local uroepithelial damage and inflammation may also facilitate the leakage of BKV into the circulation, thereby explaining the diagnostic potential of plasma BKV loads.[1,28,29] This model of PVHC as an immune reconstitution syndrome has received widespread attention,[32] but clearly requires further corroborating evidence.

Current treatment of PVHC consists of analgesia, rehydration, forced diuresis and continuous bladder irrigation to prevent clot formation and urinary tract obstruction. Platelets and erythrocytes are administered as needed. PVHC with hematuria grade III–IV may require cystoscopy for cauterization and/or clot evacuation. In case of life-threatening intractable bleeding, selective arterial embolization or cystectomy must be considered. Treatment with steroids may alleviate the inflammatory component of PVHC, but will delay the immune control of BKV replication. Reducing immunosuppression may enhance the risk of acute GVHD. Local treatment with alum, formalin or hyperbaric oxygen has been reported, but these case reports are difficult to distinguish from spontaneous recovery. Intravenous cidofovir as bi-weekly dosing of 5 mg/kg together with probenecid or as a lower dose of 0.25 mg, 0.5 mg or 1 mg/kg given one to three times per week has been reported, but randomized controlled trials demonstrating efficacy are lacking.[19,33] However, in many cases, cidofovir was only applied some weeks after the start of PVHC. Moreover, clearance of clinical symptoms and BKV load decline appeared somewhat delayed and difficult to distinguish from a spontaneous course.

Although most centers would consider the off-label use of cidofovir for this indication, evidence from randomized controlled trials is lacking. Intravesical cidofovir instillation (5 mg/kg in 60–100 ml saline) has been described as a successful therapy option, but was neither well tolerated nor effective in our experience. Ciprofloxacin or levofloxacin may inhibit BKV replication in tissue culture and reduce the peaking of BKV loads in HSCT patients, but significant clinical benefit remains to be demonstrated.[19] In addition, ciprofloxacin is already widely used as antibacterial prophylaxis during neutropenia and seemingly resistant BKV isolates have been reported.[19,34]

CONCLUSION

Significant progress has been made in the diagnosis and timely management of PVAN after kidney transplantation, reducing the impact of this emerging complication. Similar progress seems to be underway for PVHC after HSCT, but diagnostic markers and treatment modalities require validation in randomized clinical studies. Both diseases are characterized by high-level BKV replication in different pathophysiologic settings, but their negative impact is likely to be significantly reduced once more efficacious and better tolerated antiviral therapies become available.

REFERENCES

References for this chapter can be found online at http://www.expertconsult.com

Index

Index

Index